	hydroxyzine	meperidine	metoclopramide	midazolam	morphine	nalbuphine	pentazocine	pentobarbital	prochlorperazine	promethazine	ranitidine	secobarbital	thiopental
	Y	Y	M	Y	M	Y	M	M	M	M	Y	—	—
	Y	M	—	Y	Y	—	Y	N	Y	Y	—	—	—
	M	M	M	Y	M	—	M	N	M	M	Y	—	N
	Y	Y	—	Y	Y	Y	Y	N	Y	Y	—	N	—
	N	M	M	N	M	—	M	N	N	N	Y	—	N
	M	M	Y	Y	M	—	M	N	M	M	Y	—	N
	Y	M	M	Y	M	—	M	N	M	M	Y	—	—
	Y	Y	—	Y	Y	—	N	N	Y	Y	Y	N	N
	—	N	M	—	N	—	N	—	—	N	—	—	—
	Y	M	M	Y	Y	Y	Y	N	M	M	N	—	—
	M	Y	M	Y	N	—	M	N	M	M	Y	—	N
	M	M	Y	Y	M	—	M	—	M	M	Y	—	—
	Y	Y	Y	Y	Y	Y	—	N	N	Y	N	—	—
	Y	N	M	Y	Y	—	M	N	M	M	Y	—	N
	Y	—	—	Y	—	Y	—	N	Y	N	Y	—	—
	Y	M	M	—	M	—	Y	N	M	Y	Y	—	—
	N	N	N	N	N	N	N	Y	N	N	N	—	Y
	M	M	M	N	M	Y	M	N	Y	M	Y	—	N
	M	M	M	Y	M	N	Y	N	M	Y	Y	—	N
	N	Y	Y	N	Y	Y	Y	—	Y	Y	Y	—	—
	—	—	—	—	—	—	—	—	—	—	—	Y	—
	—	N	—	—	N	—	—	Y	N	N	—	—	Y

N = Incompatible; do not mix in syringe   — = Information about compatibility is not currently available

2004
Lippincott's
Nursing
Drug Guide

2004
Lippincott's Nursing Drug Guide

Amy M. Karch, RN, MS

Assistant Professor of Clinical Nursing
University of Rochester School of Nursing
Rochester, New York

LIPPINCOTT WILLIAMS & WILKINS
A **Wolters Kluwer** Company

Philadelphia • Baltimore • New York • London
Buenos Aires • Hong Kong • Sydney • Tokyo

Staff

Publisher
Judith A. Schilling McCann, RN, MSN

Editorial Director
William J. Kelly

Senior Art Director
Arlene Putterman

Art Director
Elaine Kasmer

Clinical Manager
Eileen Cassin Gallen, RN, BSN

Drug Information Editor
Melissa M. Devlin, PharmD

Senior Associate Editor
Elizabeth P. Lowe

Clinical Editors
Lisa M. Bonsall, RN, MSN, CRNP;
Shari A. Cammon, RN, MSN, CCRN;
Christine M. Damico, RN, MSN, CPNP

Copy Editors
Amy G. Dinkel, Leslie Dworkin,
Thomas A. Groff, Patricia D. Nale,
Louise E. Quinn, Jane R. Smith,
Patricia Turkington

Manufacturing
Patricia K. Dorshaw (manager),
Beth Janae Orr (book prodution manager)

Digital Composition Services
Diane Paluba (manager),
Donald G. Knauss (project manager),
Joyce Rossi Biletz (senior desktop
assistant)

Editorial Assistants
Arlene P. Claffee (senior editorial coordinator)
Carol A. Caputo

The clinical procedures described and recommended in this publication are based on research and consultation with nursing, medical, pharmaceutical, and legal authorities. To the best of our knowledge, these procedures reflect currently accepted practice; nevertheless, they can't be considered absolute and universal recommendations. For individual application, all recommendations must be considered in light of the patient's clinical condition and, before the administration of new or infrequently used drugs, in light of the latest package-insert information. The authors and publisher disclaim responsibility for adverse effects resulting directly or indirectly from the suggested procedures, from undetected errors, or from the reader's misunderstanding of the text.

Visit our Web site at NursingDrugGuide.com

ISSN: 1081-857X
ISBN: 1-58255-260-6 (USA)
ISBN: 1-58255-295-9 (Canada)
LNDG—D N O S A J J
06 05 04 03 10 9 8 7 6 5 4 3 2 1

Contents

A quick-access full-color photoguide to pills and capsules is found between pages 716 and 717.

Consultants

Steven R. Abel, PharmD, FASHP
Professor and Head
Department of Pharmacy Practice
School of Pharmacy and Pharmacal
    Sciences
Purdue University
Indianapolis, Ind.

Tricia M. Berry, PharmD, BCPS
Associate Professor
St. Louis College of Pharmacy
St. Louis, Mo.

Lawrence Carey, PharmD
Assistant Professor
Physician Assistant Program
Philadelphia University
Philadelphia, Pa.

Elizabeth Chester, PharmD, BCPS
Clinical Pharmacy Specialist in Primary
    Care
Kaiser Permanente
Aurora, Colo.

Victor Cohen, PharmD
Assistant Professor of Pharmacy,
    Arnold & Marie Schwartz College of
    Pharmacy
Clinical Pharmacy Manager,
    Maimonides Medical Center
Brooklyn, N.Y.

Michele A. Danish, RPh, BS, PharmD,
BCPS
Pharmacy Clinical Manager
St. Joseph Health Services
North Providence, R.I.

Brenda Denson, PharmD
Clinical Coordinator, Pharmacy
Children's Hospital
Birmingham, Ala.

Ronald L. Greenberg, PharmD, BCPS,
RPh
Clinical Pharmacy Specialist
Fairview Ridges Hospital
Burnsville, Minn.

Tatyana Gurvich, PharmD
Clinical Pharmacologist
Glendale Adventist FPRP
Glendale, Calif.

AnhThu Hoang, PharmD
Pharmaceutical Consultant
Toronto, Ontario, Canada

Lisa M. Kutney, PharmD, RPh
Medical Writer
Robbinsville, N.J.

Kristi L. Lenz, PharmD
Oncology Clinical Pharmacy Specialist
Medical University of South Carolina
Charleston, S.C.

Marie Maloney, PharmD
Clinical Pharmacist
University Medical Center
Tucson, Ariz.

William O'Hara, RPh, BS, PharmD
Clinical Coordinator
Thomas Jefferson Hospital
Philadelphia, Pa.

Steven G. Ottariano, BS Pharm, RPh
Clinical Staff Pharmacist
Veterans Administration Medical Center
Manchester, N.H.

Jeffrey B. Purcell, PharmD
Clinical Lead Pharmacist, Harborview
  Medical Center
Clinical Associate Professor, University of
  Washington School of Pharmacy
Seattle, Wash.

Gary Smith, RPh, PharmD
Director of Pharmaceutical Manufacturer
  Relations
Medica
Minnetonka, Minn.

Preface

The number of clinically important drugs increases every year, as does the nurse's responsibility for drug therapy. No nurse can memorize all the drug information needed to provide safe and efficacious drug therapy. The *2004 Lippincott's Nursing Drug Guide* provides the drug information nurses need in a concise, ready-access format. This edition was completely updated and then it was reviewed by independent clinical reviewers, including pharmacists and nurses, to ensure that nurses will have the most up-to-date and accurate information possible.

This book presents nursing considerations related to drug therapy in the format of the nursing process, a framework for applying basic pharmacologic information to patient care. It is intended for the student nurse who is just learning how to apply pharmacologic data in the clinical situation, as well as for the busy practicing professional nurse who needs a quick, easy-to-use guide to the clinical use of drugs.

This book provides broad coverage of the drugs commonly encountered by nurses and of drugs whose use commonly involves significant nursing intervention. *Anatomy of a Monograph,* found at the end of this preface, explains how the information in each monograph can be used to implement the nursing process. Commonly used medical abbreviations are used throughout the book and are defined in the *Guide to Abbreviations* located after *Anatomy of a Monograph.* A handy guide to drug compatibility in syringes is found inside the front cover for ready access.

The first two chapters of this book provide a concise review of the nursing process and its application to pharmacologic situations, including guidelines for avoiding medication errors and concise examples of how to use the drug guide to apply the nursing process and to make a patient teaching guide. Next is a review of selected drug classifications, which provides a convenient, complete summary of the drug information pertinent to drugs in each class.

Complete Drug Monographs

Drug information is presented in monograph form, with the monographs arranged alphabetically by generic name. Each page of the book contains guide words at the top, much like a dictionary, to facilitate easy access to any drug. The right-hand edge of the book contains letter guides, again to facilitate finding a drug as quickly as possible.

Each drug monograph is complete in itself—that is, it includes all of the clinically important information that a nurse needs to know to give the drug safely and effectively. Every monograph begins with the drug's generic (nonproprietary) name; any alternate names follow in parentheses; an alphabetical list of the most common brand names, including common brand names found only in Canada (noted by the designation CAN); a notation indicating if the drug is available as an OTC drug; the drug's pregnancy category classification, and its schedule if it is a controlled substance. The names of drugs that are described in Appendix L, *Less Commonly Used Drugs,* appear alphabetically in the text and are cross referenced to the appropriate page.

Each monograph provides a commonly accepted pronunciation (after *USAN* and the *USP Dictionary of Drug Names, 2001*) to help the nurse feel more comfortable discussing the drug with other members of the health care team. After the pronunciation, each monograph gives you these features:
- The clinically important drug classes of each drug are indicated to put the drug in appropriate context.

- The therapeutically useful actions of the drug are described, including, where known, the mechanism(s) by which these therapeutic effects are produced; no attempt is made to list *all* of the drug's known actions here.
- Clinical indications for the drug are listed, including important unlabeled indications not approved by the FDA, as well as orphan drug uses where appropriate.
- Contraindications to drug use and cautions that should be considered when using the drug are listed.
- The pharmacokinetic profile of the drug is given in table form to allow easy access to such information as half-life, peak levels, distribution, and so on, offering a quick reference on how the drug is handled by the body.
- Dosage information is listed next, including dosages for adults, pediatric patients, and geriatric patients, and dosages for indications when these differ. A listing of the available forms of each drug serves as a guide for prescribing or suggesting alternate routes of administration. Details of drug administration that must not be overlooked for the safe administration of the drug (eg, "Dilute before infusing" or "Infuse slowly over 30 minutes") are included in the dosage section, but other aspects of drug administration (eg, directions for reconstituting a powder for injection) are presented under *Interventions* in the next section of the monograph. If there is a treatment for the overdose of this drug, that information is indicated in *Interventions*.
- The *IV Facts* sections give concise, important information that is needed for drugs given IV—dilution, flow rate, compatibilities—making it unnecessary to have a separate IV handbook.
- Commonly encountered adverse effects are listed by body system, with the most commonly encountered adverse effects appearing in *italics* to make it easier to assess the patient for adverse effects and to teach the patient about what to expect. Potentially life-threatening adverse effects are in **bold** for easy access. Adverse effects that have been reported, but appear less commonly or rarely, are also listed to make the drug information as complete as possible.
- Clinically important interactions are listed separately for easy access: drug-drug, drug-food, drug-lab test, drug-alternative therapy—for interferences to consider when using the drug and any nursing action that is necessary because of this interaction.

Clinically Focused Nursing Considerations

The remainder of each monograph is concerned with nursing considerations, which are presented, as stated above, in the format of the nursing process. The steps of the nursing process are given slightly different names by different authorities; this handbook includes: assessment (history and physical exam), interventions, and teaching points for each of the drugs presented.

CLINICAL ALERT provides important information about reported name confusions that have occurred with a given drug. This will alert the nurse to prevent potential medication errors.

- **Assessment:** Outlines the information that should be collected before administering the drug. This section is further divided into two subsections:

—**History:** Includes a list of those underlying conditions that constitute contraindications and cautions for use of the drug.

—**Assessment:** Provides data, by organ system, that should be collected before beginning drug therapy, both to allow detection of conditions that are contraindications or cautions to the use of the drug and to provide baseline data for detecting adverse reactions to the drug and monitoring for therapeutic response.

- **Interventions:** Lists, in chronological order, those nursing activities that should be undertaken in the course of caring for a patient who is receiving the drug. This includes interventions related to drug preparation and administration, the provision of comfort and safety measures, and drug levels to monitor, as appropriate.

- **Teaching points:** Includes specific information that is needed for teaching the patient who is receiving this drug. Proven "what to say" advice can be transferred directly to patient teaching printouts and used as a written reminder.

Evaluation

Evaluation is usually the last step of the nursing process. In all drug therapy, the patient should be evaluated for the desired effect of the drug as listed in the *Indications* section; the occurrence of adverse effects, as listed in the *Adverse Effects* section; and learning following patient teaching, as described in the *Teaching Points* section. These points are essential. In some cases, evaluation includes monitoring specific therapeutic serum drug levels; these cases are specifically mentioned in the *Interventions* section. The *Nursing Process Guidelines* chapter gives an example of how the drug monograph can be used to establish a nursing care plan, to develop a patient teaching printout, and to incorporate the nursing process into drug therapy.

Appendices

The appendices contain information that is useful to nursing practice but may not lend itself to the monograph format— alternative and complementary therapies; commonly used biologicals; guides to adult and pediatric immunizations; information about hormonal contraceptives; a detailed combination drug reference; topical agents; topical corticosteroids; laxatives; ophthalmic preparations; less commonly used drugs—as well as pregnancy categories (for U.S. drugs); schedules of controlled substances (for U.S. and Canadian drugs); formulas for pediatric dosage calculations; list of NANDA nursing diagnoses; recommended immunization schedules for adults and children; important drug-related dietary guidelines for patient teaching; a compendium of adverse drug effects with guidelines for nursing interventions; a new table of drugs that interact with grapefruit juice; and a listing of tablets and capsules that cannot be cut, crushed, or chewed. A suggested bibliography follows the appendices.

Index

An extensive index provides a ready reference to drug information. The **generic** name of each drug is highlighted in bold. If the generic name of a drug is not known, the drug may be found quickly by using whatever name is known. *Brand names* are listed in italics, commonly used chemical names and any commonly used "jargon" name (such as IDU for idoxuridine) are in parentheses after the generic name. In addition, the index lists drugs by clinically important classes—pharmacologic and therapeutic. If you know a patient is taking an antianginal drug and don't remember the name, reviewing the list of drugs under *Antianginals* may well help you recall the name. Chlorpromazine, for example, is listed by its generic name, by all of its brand names, and by classes as an Antipsychotic (a therapeutic classification), as a Phenothiazine (the pharmacologic class), and as a Dopaminergic Blocking Drug (a classification by postulated mechanism of action). The comprehensive index helps to avoid cross-referencing from within the text, which is time consuming and often confusing.

2004 Quick-Access Photoguide

The full-color photoguide presents nearly 400 pills and capsules, representing the most commonly prescribed generic and brand drugs.

What's New

The new features in the book include
- 35 new drugs
- Over 1,200 additions, changes, and updates on indications, dosage, and administration
- Updated and expanded nursing process section
- Expanded section on preventing medication errors
- All-new appendix of drugs that interact with grapefruit juice
- Expanded alternative and complementary therapies section
- Expanded *Less Commonly Used Drugs* appendix, which includes fertility drugs
- Updated list of drugs that cannot be cut, crushed, or chewed, including brand names
- Even more *Clinical Alert*s to point out possible name confusion to prevent medication errors
- Updated color insert section of commonly used drugs to facilitate recognition of drugs being used
- Three completely new continuing education tests on NursingDrugGuide.com Web site

Bonus Mini-CD-ROM

The free mini-CD-ROM contains the 200 most commonly prescribed drugs and 200 customizable patient-teaching printouts. This mini-CD-ROM is compatible with virtually all computer systems and can be used to prepare your own study aids, to develop nursing care plans, to prepare your own patient-teaching printouts, and to customize patient and staff teaching tools.

Added Benefit

With this guide comes access to free monthly drug updates delivered to you throughout the year via the NursingDrugGuide.com Web site. Get the hottest drug information available, including the latest FDA drug approvals and advances in clinical pharmacology.

This year you'll be able to take up to three new continuing education tests via the Web site and earn contact hours.

This ninth edition incorporates many of the suggestions and requests that have been made by the users of earlier editions of this book. It is hoped that the overall organization and concise, straightforward presentation of the material in the *2004 Lippincott's Nursing Drug Guide* will make it a readily used and clinically useful reference for the nurse who needs easily accessible information to facilitate the provision of drug therapy within the framework of the nursing process. It is further hoped that the thoroughness of the additional sections of the book will make it an invaluable resource that will replace the need for several additional references.

Amy M. Karch, RN, MS

Anatomy of a Monograph

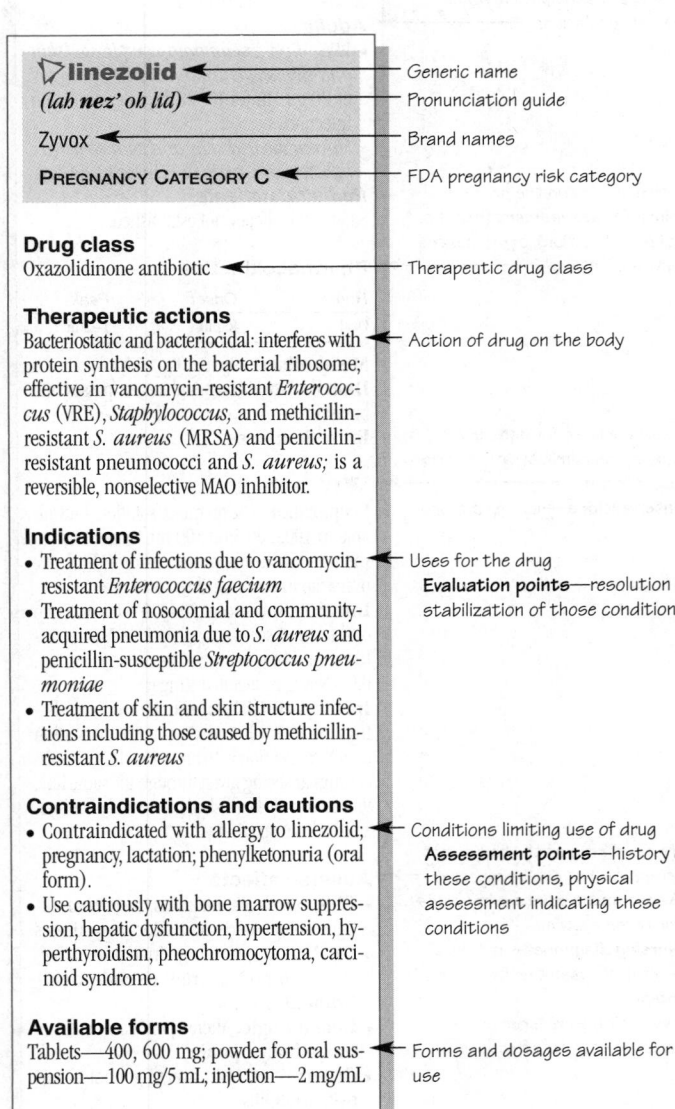

▽ **linezolid** ← Generic name
*(lah **nez**' oh lid)* ← Pronunciation guide
Zyvox ← Brand names
PREGNANCY CATEGORY C ← FDA pregnancy risk category

Drug class
Oxazolidinone antibiotic ← Therapeutic drug class

Therapeutic actions
Bacteriostatic and bacteriocidal: interferes with protein synthesis on the bacterial ribosome; effective in vancomycin-resistant *Enterococcus* (VRE), *Staphylococcus,* and methicillin-resistant *S. aureus* (MRSA) and penicillin-resistant pneumococci and *S. aureus;* is a reversible, nonselective MAO inhibitor. ← Action of drug on the body

Indications
- Treatment of infections due to vancomycin-resistant *Enterococcus faecium*
- Treatment of nosocomial and community-acquired pneumonia due to *S. aureus* and penicillin-susceptible *Streptococcus pneumoniae*
- Treatment of skin and skin structure infections including those caused by methicillin-resistant *S. aureus*

← Uses for the drug
Evaluation points—resolution or stabilization of those conditions

Contraindications and cautions
- Contraindicated with allergy to linezolid; pregnancy, lactation; phenylketonuria (oral form).
- Use cautiously with bone marrow suppression, hepatic dysfunction, hypertension, hyperthyroidism, pheochromocytoma, carcinoid syndrome.

← Conditions limiting use of drug
Assessment points—history of these conditions, physical assessment indicating these conditions

Available forms
Tablets—400, 600 mg; powder for oral suspension—100 mg/5 mL; injection—2 mg/mL ← Forms and dosages available for use

Recommended dose of drug for adults, pediatric patients, and special populations ⟶

Action of body on the drug—**points for assessment** (hepatic and renal function), cautions, and contraindications ⟶

Nursing actions for safe and appropriate administration of the drug in IV form ⟶
Interventions—nursing actions

Effects of drug on the body—not therapeutic but can be expected ⟶
Assessment points—baselines for these systems
Nursing diagnoses—potential alterations resulting from these effects
Evaluation—presence or absence of these effects

Dosages
No dosage adjustment is needed if switching between oral and IV forms.
Adults
- *VRE, MRSA, pneumonia, complicated skin and skin structure infections:* 600 mg IV or PO q 12 hr for 10–28 days, depending on infection.
- *Uncomplicated skin and skin structure infections:* 400 mg PO q 12 hr for 10–14 days.
Pediatric patients
Safety and efficacy not established.

Pharmacokinetics

Route	Onset	Peak
Oral	Rapid	1–2 hr

Metabolism: Hepatic; $T_{1/2}$: 5 hr
Distribution: Crosses placenta; passes into breast milk
Excretion: Urine

▼ IV facts
Preparation: Use premixed solution—available in 100, 200, and 300 mL forms; store at room temperature, protect from light, leave overwrap in place until ready to use.
Infusion: Infuse over 30–120 min, switch to oral form as soon as appropriate. May be infused into line using 5% dextrose injection, 0.9% NaCL, or lactated Ringer's.
Incompatibilities: Do not introduce additives into this solution; do not mix in solution or at Y-connection with any other drugs. If other drugs are being given through the same line, the line should be flushed before and after linezolid administration.

Adverse effects
- **CNS:** *Headache,* dizziness, *insomnia,* fatigue, somnolence, depression, nervousness
- **GI:** *Nausea,* vomiting, dry mouth, *diarrhea,* anorexia, gastritis, **pseudomembranous colitis**
- **Hematologic:** Altered prothrombin time, **thrombocytopenia**
- **Other:** Fever, rash, sweating, photosensitivity, tendinitis

Interactions ◄——

✳ Drug-drug • Risk of hypertension and related adverse effects if combined with drugs containing pseudoephedrine, SSRIs, MAOIs; use caution and monitor patient carefully if any of these combinations are used • Increased risk of bleeding and thrombocytopenia if combined with antiplatelet drugs (aspirin, dipyridamole, NSAIDs); monitor platelet counts carefully

✳ Drug-food • Risk of severe hypertension if combined with large amounts of food containing tyramine (see *Appendix O* for tyramine food lists); patient should be cautioned to avoid large amounts of these foods

Anticipated clinically important interactions
  Assessment points—history of use of these agents, physical response
  Evaluation—changes from anticipated therapeutic response related to drug interactions

■ Nursing considerations

 CLINICAL ALERT!
Name confusion has occurred between Zyvox (linezolid) and Vioxx (rofecoxib); use caution.

Directs nursing action to ensure safe and effective administration of this drug
  Interventions—nursing actions

Assessment ◄——

- **History:** Allergy to linezolid; hepatic dysfunction, bone marrow depression, hypertension, phenylketonuria, hyperthyroidism, carcinoid syndrome, pheochromocytoma, pregnancy, lactation
- **Physical:** Culture site; skin—color, lesions; body temperature; orientation, reflexes, affect; P, BP; mucous membranes, bowel sounds; liver function tests, CBC, and differential

Points to establish baselines, determine factors contraindicating drug use or requiring caution

Interventions ◄——

- Arrange for culture and sensitivity tests before beginning therapy.
- Reserve use of this drug for cases of well-documented bacteria-sensitive infections.
- Continue therapy as indicated for condition being treated.
- Monitor platelet counts regularly if drug is used for ≥ 2 weeks.
- Monitor blood pressure before and periodically during therapy if patient is on antidepressants or drugs containing sympathomimetics.

Nursing actions, in chronological order, for safe and effective drug therapy
  Evaluation—monitoring of these tests; effectiveness of comfort and safety measures

Drug-specific teaching points to include in patient teaching program

Nursing diagnosis—knowledge deficit regarding drug therapy
Evaluation—points patient should be able to repeat

- Advise patient to avoid foods high in tyramine to avoid risk of severe hypertension.
- Advise patient of high cost of drug and refer for financial support as needed.
- Monitor clinical response—if no improvement is seen or a relapse occurs, repeat culture and sensitivity.

Teaching points

- Take drug q 12 hr as prescribed; take the full course of the drug; drug may be taken with or without food.
- Avoid foods high in tyramine (a list will be provided) while you are on this drug.
- These side effects may occur: nausea, vomiting, abdominal pain (small, frequent meals may help, taking the drug with food may also help); diarrhea (consult nurse or physician if this occurs).
- Report rash, severe GI problems, weakness, tremors, anxiety, increased bleeding.

Guide to abbreviations

ACT	activated clotting time	DEA	Drug Enforcement Administration
ACTH	adrenocorticotropic hormone		
ADH	antidiuretic hormone	DIC	disseminated intravascular coagulation
ADLs	activities of daily living		
AIDS	acquired immunodeficiency syndrome	dL	deciliter (100 mL)
		DNA	deoxyribonucleic acid
ALA	delta-aminolevulinic acid	DR	delayed release
ALL	acute lymphocytic leukemia	DTP	diphtheria–tetanus–pertussis (vaccine)
ALT	alanine transaminase (formerly called SGPT)		
		DVT	deep venous thrombosis
AML	acute myelogenous leukemia	ECG	electrocardiogram
ANA	anti-nuclear antibodies	ECT	electroconvulsive therapy
APTT	activated partial thromboplastin time	ED	erectile dysfunction
		EEG	electroencephalogram
ARC	AIDS-related complex	EENT	eye, ear, nose, and throat
ARV	AIDS-related virus	EKG	electrocardiogram
AST	aspartate transaminase (formerly called SGOT)	ER	extended release
		EST	electroshock therapy
AV	atrioventricular	F	Fahrenheit
bid	twice a day	FDA	Food and Drug Administration
BP	blood pressure	FSH	follicle-stimulating hormone
BPH	benign prostatic hypertrophy	GABA	gamma-aminobutyric acid
BSP	bromsulphalein	GFR	glomerular filtration rate
BUN	blood urea nitrogen	GGTP	gamma-glutamyl transpeptidase
C	centigrade, Celsius	GI	gastrointestinal
CAD	coronary artery disease	g	gram
c-AMP	cyclic adenosine monophosphate	G-6-PD	glucose-6-phosphate dehydrogenase
CBC	complete blood count		
CDC	Centers for Disease Control and Prevention	gtt	drop
		GU	genitourinary
CGH	chorionic gonadotropic hormone	hr	hour
CHD	coronary heart disease	HBIG	hepatitis B immune globulin
CHF	congestive heart failure	Hct	hematocrit
CML	chronic myelogenous leukemia	HDL	high-density lipoproteins
CNS	central nervous system	Hg	mercury
COPD	chronic obstructive pulmonary disease	Hgb	hemoglobin
		Hib	*Haemophilus influenzae* type b
CPK	creatine phosphokinase	HIV	human immunodeficiency virus
CPR	cardiopulmonary resuscitation	HPA	hypothalamic–pituitary–adrenal (axis)
CR	controlled release		
CSF	cerebrospinal fluid	hs	at bedtime, at the hour of sleep (*hora somni*)
CTZ	chemoreceptor trigger zone		
CV	cardiovascular	HSV	herpes simplex virus
CVA	cerebrovascular accident	HTLVIII	human T-cell lymphotropic virus type III
CVP	central venous pressure		
CVS	cardiovascular system		

IHSS	idiopathic hypertrophic subaortic stenosis	PO	orally, by mouth *(per os)*
I & O	intake and output	PRN	when required *(pro re nata)*
IM	intramuscular	PT	prothrombin time
IOP	intraocular pressure	PTT	partial thromboplastin time
IPPB	intermittent (or inspiratory) positive pressure breathing	PVCs	premature ventricular contractions
IV	intravenous	q	each, every *(quaque)*
JVP	jugular venous pressure	qid	four times a day *(quarter in die)*
kg	kilogram	R	rate
L	liter	RAS	reticular-activating system
lb	pound	RBC	red blood cell
LDH	lactic dehydrogenase	RDA	recommended dietary allowance
LDL	low-density lipoproteins	RDS	respiratory distress syndrome
LH	luteinizing hormone	REM	rapid eye movement
LH-RH	luteinizing hormone–releasing hormone	RNA	ribonucleic acid
		RSV	respiratory syncytial virus
LRI	lower respiratory tract infection	SBE	subacute bacterial endocarditis
m	meter	SA	sinoatrial
MAO	monoamine oxidase	SC	subcutaneous
MAOI	monoamine oxidase inhibitor	SIADH	syndrome of inappropriate anti-diuretic hormone secretion
mcg	microgram		
mg	milligram	SLE	systemic lupus erythematosus
MI	myocardial infarction	SMA-12	sequential multiple analysis-12
min	minute	SR	sustained release
mL	milliliter	SRS-A	slow-reacting substance of anaphylaxis
mo	month		
MS	musculoskeletal	SSRI	selective serotonin reuptake inhibitor
ng	nanogram		
NMS	neuroleptic malignant syndrome	STD	sexually transmitted disease
NPO	nothing by mouth *(nihil per os)*	T	temperature
NSAID	nonsteroidal anti-inflammatory drug	$T_{1/2}$	half-life
		T_3	triiodothyronine
OC	oral contraceptive	T_4	thyroxine (tetraiodothyronine)
OTC	over the counter	TB	tuberculosis
P	pulse	TCA	tricyclic antidepressant
PABA	para-aminobenzoic acid	TIA	transient ischemic attack
PAT	paroxysmal atrial tachycardia	tid	three times a day *(ter in die)*
PBG	porphobilinogen	UPG	uroporphyrinogen
PBI	protein-bound iodine	URI	upper respiratory (tract) infection
PCWP	pulmonary capillary wedge pressure	UTI	urinary tract infection
		UT	ultraviolet
PDA	patent ductus arteriosus	VMA	vanillylmandelic acid
PE	pulmonary embolus	VLDL	very-low-density lipoproteins
PG	prostaglandin	WBC	white blood cell
pH	hydrogen ion concentration	WBCT	whole blood clotting time
PID	pelvic inflammatory disease	wk	week
PMS	premenstrual syndrome	yr	year

Acknowledgments

I would like to thank the many people who have worked so hard to make this book possible. Students and colleagues, past and present, who have helped me learn how to make pharmacology clinically useful; the many users of past editions of the book who have taken the time to offer suggestions and provide valuable comments; Arlene Claffee, the master organizer who keeps all the details in line and who always provides a ray of sunshine; Judy McCann, my new editor at the Springhouse office of Lippincott Williams & Wilkins; Eileen Gallen, Betsy Lowe, and Bill Kelly, who have helped me learn the ropes at Springhouse and have been patient and most helpful; Melissa Devlin, the pharmacy guru who keeps me on my toes and is always so quick to respond; Elaine Kasmer, Don Knauss, and Joe Clark, who provided their design expertise to this new edition; Joy Biletz and Diane Paluba, who applied their production skills to this book; Carol Caputo, who rounded up all of the permissions; copyeditors Amy Dinkel, Leslie Dworkin, and Trish Turkington; my best friend and husband, Dr. Fred Karch, who offers the needed sympathetic ear and the encouraging word when it is needed most; Pat Palmer and Connie Shimelonis, who managed to keep me real, grounded, and always laughing; Tim, Jyoti, Mark, Cortney, and Kathryn, who have grown up with deadlines, piles of paper, page proofs, and computer searches and think that is normal; and Duncan, whose endless energy and constantly wagging tail keep everything in perspective.

Nursing Process Guide

The delivery of medical care is in a constant state of change and sometimes in crisis. The population is aging, resulting in more chronic disease and more complex care issues. The population is transient, resulting in unstable support systems and fewer at-home care providers and helpers. At the same time, medicine is undergoing a technological boom (eg, CT scans, MRIs, experimental drugs). Patients are being discharged earlier from the acute-care facility or not being admitted at all for procedures that used to be done in the hospital with follow-up support and monitoring. Patients are becoming more responsible for their own care and for following complicated medical regimens at home.

Nursing is a unique and complex science and a nurturing and caring art. Traditionally, nurses minister to and soothe the sick; currently, nursing also requires using more technical and scientific skills. Nurses have had to assume increasing responsibilities involved not only with nurturing and caring, but with assessing, diagnosing, and intervening with patients to treat, prevent, and educate to help people cope with various health states.

The nurse deals with the whole person—the physical, emotional, intellectual, and spiritual aspects—considering the ways that a person responds to treatment, disease, and the change in lifestyle that may be required by both. The nurse is the key health care provider in a position to assess the patient—physical, social, and emotional aspects—to administer therapy and medications, teach the patient how best to cope with the therapy to ensure the most effectiveness, and evaluate the effectiveness of therapy. This requires a broad base of knowledge in the basic sciences (anatomy, physiology, nutrition, chemistry, pharmacology), the social sciences (sociology, psychology) and education (learning approaches, evaluation).

Although a [...] completely agree [...] the practice of nursin[...] key elements in the nu[...] elements are the basic c[...] decision-making or problem[...] assessment (gathering of infor[...] agnosis (defining that information[...] at some conclusions), intervention ([...] ministration, education, comfort measu[...] and evaluation (determining the effects [...] the interventions that were performed). The use of this process each time a situation arises ensures a method of coping with the overwhelming scientific and technical information confounding the situation and the unique emotional, social, and physical aspects that each patient brings to the situation. Using the nursing process format in each instance of drug therapy will ensure that the patient receives the best, most efficient, scientifically based holistic care.

Assessment

The first step of the nursing process is the systematic, organized collection of data about the patient. Because the nurse is responsible for holistic care, these data must include information about physical, intellectual, emotional, social, and environmental factors. They will provide the nurse with information needed to plan discharge, plan educational programs, arrange for appropriate consultations, and monitor physical response to treatment or to disease. In actual clinical practice, this process never ends. The patient is not in a steady state but is dynamic, adjusting to physical, emotional, and environmental influences. Each nurse develops a unique approach to the organization of the assessment, an approach that is functional and useful in the clinical setting and that makes sense to that nurse and that clinical situation.

Drug therapy is a complex, integral, and important part of health care today, and the

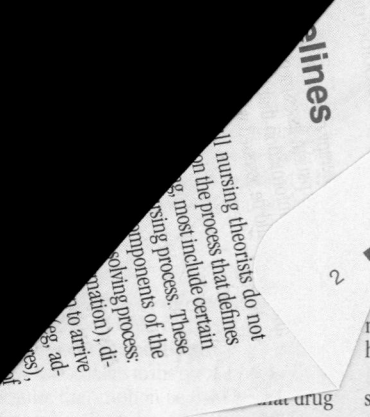

nursing theorists do not
...on the process that defines
...g, most include certain
...sing process. These
...sing components of the
...olving process:
...mation), di-
...g to arrive
...es), ad-

...n of health care: The way that
...eks health care will give the nurse
...formation to include in educa-
...rmation. Does this patient rou-
...k follow-up care or wait for emer-
...tuations?

...ical assessment

◆ **Weight:** Weight is an important factor
...en determining if the recommended
...sage of a drug is appropriate. The recom-
...nended dosage is based on the 150-lb adult
...male. Patients who are much lighter or much
heavier will need a dosage adjustment.

Age: Patients at the extremes of the age
spectrum—pediatric and geriatric—often
require dosage adjustments based on the
functional level of the liver and kidneys and
the responsiveness of other organs.

**Physical parameters related to
the disease state or known drug effects:** Assessment of these factors before beginning drug therapy will give a baseline level with which future assessments can be
compared to determine the effects of drug
therapy. The specific parameters that need
to be assessed will depend on the disease
process being treated and on the expected
therapeutic and adverse effects of the drug
therapy. Because the nurse has the greatest
direct and continual contact with the patient,
the nurse has the best opportunity to detect
the minute changes that will determine the
course of drug therapy and therapeutic success or discontinuation because of adverse
or unacceptable responses.

The monographs in this book include the
specific parameters that need to be assessed
in relation to the particular drug being discussed (see the sample monograph in the
preface). This assessment provides not only
the baseline information needed before giving that drug but the data needed to evaluate the effects of that drug on the patient.
The information given in this area should
supplement the overall nursing assessment
of the patient, which will include social, intellectual, financial, environmental, and other physical data.

Drug use: Prescription drugs, OTC
drugs, street drugs, alcohol, nicotine, and
caffeine all may have an impact on the effect of a drug. Patients often neglect to
mention OTC drugs, herbal and alternative
therapy, and contraceptives, not considering
them actual drugs, and should be asked
specifically about use of OTC drugs, herbals,
contraceptives, or any drug that might be
taken on a long-term basis and not mentioned.

Allergies: Past exposure to a drug or
other allergen can predict a future reaction
or note a caution for the use of a drug, food,
or animal product.

Level of education: This information will help to provide a basis for patient
education programs and level of explanation.

**Level of understanding of dis-
ease and therapy:** This information also
will direct the development of educational
information.

Social supports: Patients are being
discharged earlier than ever before and often need assistance at home to provide care
and institute and monitor drug therapy.

Financial supports: The financial
impact of health care and the high cost of
medications need to be considered when prescribing drugs and depending on the patient
to follow through with drug therapy.

Nursing diagnosis

Once data have been collected, the nurse must organize and analyze that information to arrive at a nursing diagnosis. A nursing diagnosis is simply a statement of the patient's status from a nursing perspective. This statement directs appropriate nursing interventions. A nursing diagnosis will show actual or potential alteration in patient function based on the assessment of the clinical situation. Because drug therapy is only a small part of the overall patient situation, the nursing diagnoses that are related to drug therapy must be incorporated into a total picture of the patient. In many cases the drug therapy will not present a new nursing diagnosis, but the desired effects and adverse effects related to each drug given should be considered in the nursing diagnoses for each patient. The North American Nursing Diagnosis Association (NANDA) produces a list of accepted nursing diagnoses (see Appendix O).

Interventions

The assessment and diagnosis of the patient's situation will direct specific nursing interventions. Three types of interventions are frequently involved in drug therapy: drug administration, provision of comfort measures, and patient and family teaching.

Drug administration

Drug: Ensuring that the drug being administered is the correct dose of the correct drug at the correct time, and is being given to the correct patient, is standard nursing practice.

Storage: Some drugs require specific storage environments (eg, refrigeration, protection from light).

Route: Determining the best route of administration is often determined by the prescription of the drug. Nurses can often have an impact on modifying the prescribed route to determine the most efficient route and the most comfortable one for the patient based on his or her specific situation. When establishing the prescribed route, it is im-

portant to check the proper method of administering a drug by that route.

Dosage: Drug dosage may need to be calculated based on available drug form, patient body weight or surface area, or kidney function.

Preparation: Some drugs require specific preparation before administration. Oral drugs may need to be shaken or crushed; parenteral drugs may need to be reconstituted or diluted with specific solutions; topical drugs may require specific handling before administration.

Timing: Actual administration of a drug may require coordination with the administration of other drugs, foods, or physical parameters. The nurse, as the caregiver most frequently involved in administering a drug, must be aware of and juggle all of these factors and educate the patient to do this on his or her own.

Recording: Once the nurse has assessed the patient, made the appropriate nursing diagnoses, and delivered the correct drug by the correct route, in the correct dose, and at the correct time, that information needs to be recorded in accordance with the local requirements for recording medication administration.

Each monograph in this book contains pertinent guidelines for storage, dosage, preparation, and administration of the drug being discussed.

Comfort measures

Nurses are in the unique position to help the patient cope with the effects of drug therapy.

Placebo effect: The anticipation that a drug will be helpful (placebo effect) has been proved to have tremendous impact on the actual success of drug therapy, so the nurse's attitude and support can be a critical part of drug therapy. A back rub, a kind word, and a positive approach may be as beneficial as the drug itself.

Side effects: These interventions can be directed at decreasing the impact of the anticipated side effects of the drug and promoting patient safety. Such interventions include environmental control (eg, temperature, lighting), safety measures (eg, avoiding driving, avoiding the sun, using side rails), physical comfort (eg, skin care, laxatives, frequent meals).

Lifestyle adjustment: Some drug effects will require that a patient change his or her lifestyle to cope effectively. Diuretic users may have to rearrange the day to be near toilet facilities when the drug works. MAOI users have to adjust their diet to prevent serious drug effects.

Each monograph in this book will include a list of pertinent comfort measures appropriate to that particular drug.

Education

With patients becoming more responsible for their own care, it is essential that they have all of the information necessary to ensure safe and effective drug therapy at home. Many states now require that the patient be given written information. Key elements that need to be included in any drug education include the following:

- Name, dose, and action of drug: With many people seeing more than one health care provider, this information is important for ensuring safe and effective drug therapy.
- Timing of administration: Patients need to know specifically when to take the drug with regard to frequency, other drugs, and meals.
- Special storage and preparation instructions: Some drugs require particular handling that the patient will need to have spelled out.
- Specific OTC drugs or alternative therapies to avoid: Many people do not consider these to be actual drugs and may inadvertently take them and cause unwanted or even dangerous drug interactions. Explaining problems will help the patient avoid these potential situations.
- Special comfort or safety measures that need to be considered: Alerting the patient to ways to cope with anticipated side effects will prevent a great deal of anxiety

and noncompliance with drug therapy. The patient also may need to be alerted to the need to return for follow-up tests or evaluation.

- Safety measures: All patients need to be alerted to keep drugs out of the reach of children. They also need to be reminded to tell any health care provider whom they see that they are taking this drug. This can prevent drug-drug interactions and misdiagnosing based on drug effects.
- Specific points about drug toxicity: Warning signs of drug toxicity that the patient should be aware of should be listed. He or she can be advised to notify the health care provider if any of these effects occur.
- Specific warnings about drug discontinuation: Some drugs with a small margin of safety and drugs with particular systemic effects cannot be stopped abruptly without dangerous effects. Patients taking these drugs need to be alerted to the problem and encouraged to call immediately if they cannot take their medication for any reason (eg, illness, financial).

Each drug monograph in this book lists specific teaching points that relate to that particular drug. An example of a compact, written drug card developed from the information in the monograph is shown on the next page.

Evaluation

Evaluation is part of the continual process of patient care that leads to changes in assessment, diagnosis, and intervention. The patient is continually evaluated for therapeutic response, the occurrence of drug side effects, and the occurrence of drug-drug, drug-food, drug–laboratory test or drug–alternative therapy interactions.

The efficacy of the nursing interventions and the education program must be evaluated. In some situations, the nurse will evaluate the patient simply by reapplying the beginning steps of the nursing process and analyzing for change. In some cases of drug therapy, particular therapeutic drug levels need to be evaluated as well.

Patient Drug Sheet: Oral Linezolid

Patient's Name: Mr. Kors
Prescriber's Name: J. Smith, ANP
Phone Number: 555-555-5555

Instructions:

1. The name of your drug is *linezolid*; the brand name is *Zyvox*. This drug is an antibiotic that is being used to treat your *pneumonia*. This drug is very specific in its action and is only indicated for your particular infection. Take the full course of your drug. Do not share this drug with other people or save tablets for future use.
2. The dose of the drug that has been prescribed for you is: *600 mg (1 tablet)*.
3. The drug should be taken *once every 12 hours*. The best time for you to take this drug will be *8:00 in the morning and 8:00 in the evening*. Do not skip any doses. Do not take two doses at once if you forget a dose. If you miss a dose, take the dose as soon as you remember and then again in 12 hours.
4. The drug can be taken with food if GI upset is a problem. Avoid foods that are rich in tyramine (list is below) while you are taking this drug.
5. The following side effects may occur:
    Nausea, vomiting, abdominal pain (taking the drug with food and eating small, frequent meals may help).
    Diarrhea (ensure ready access to bathroom facilities). Notify your health care provider if this becomes severe.
6. Do not take this drug with over-the-counter drugs or herbal remedies without first checking with your health care provider. Many of these agents can cause problems with your drug.
7. Tell any nurse, physician, or dentist who is taking care of you that you are on this drug.
8. Keep this and all medications out of the reach of children.

Notify your health care provider if any of the following occur:
    Rash, severe GI problems, bloody or excessive diarrhea, weakness, tremors, increased bleeding or bruising, anxiety

> Foods high in tyramine to avoid: aged cheeses, avocados, bananas, beer, bologna, caffeine beverages, chocolate, liver, over-ripe fruit, pepperoni, pickled fish, red wine, salami, smoked fish, yeast, yogurt.

Monographs in this book list only specific evaluation criteria, such as therapeutic serum levels, as they apply to each drug. Regular evaluation of drug effects, side effects, and the efficacy of comfort measures and education programs will not be specifically listed but can be deduced from information in the monograph regarding therapeutic effects and adverse effects. See *Nursing care plan: Patient receiving oral linezolid,* page 6. *Anatomy of a monograph,* in the preface, provides additional guidelines for using each section of a monograph as it applies to the nursing process.

Nursing care plan: Patient receiving oral linezolid

Assessment	Nursing diagnoses	Interventions	Evaluation
History (contraindications and cautions) Hypertension Hyperthyroidism Blood dyscrasias Hepatic dysfunction Pheochromocytoma Phenylketonuria Carcinoid syndrome Pregnancy Lactation Known allergy to linezolid	Imbalanced nutrition, less than body requirements, related to GI effects	Safe and appropriate administration of drug: Culture infection site to ensure appropriate use of drug	Monitor patient for therapeutic effects of drug: resolution of infection.
	Acute pain related to GI effects, headache	Provision of safety and comfort measures:	If resolution does not occur, reculture site.
	Ineffective tissue perfusion related to bone marrow effects	• Monitor BP periodically	Monitor patient for adverse effects of drug:
	Deficient knowledge related to drug therapy	• Monitor platelet counts before and periodically during therapy	• GI upset—nausea, vomiting, diarrhea
Medication History (possible drug-drug interactions) Pseudoephedrine SSRIs MAOIs Antiplatelet drugs		• Alleviation of GI upset • Ready access to bathroom facilities • Nutritional consult • Safety provisions if dizziness and CNS effects occur • Avoidance of tyramine-rich foods	• Liver function changes • Pseudomembranous colitis • Blood dyscrasias—changes in platelet counts • Fever • Rash • Sweating • Photosensitivity • Acute hypersensitivity reactions
Diet History (possible drug-food interactions) Foods high in tyramine		Patient teaching regarding: Drug Side effects to anticipate Warnings Reactions to report	Evaluate effectiveness of patient teaching program: patient can name drug, dose of drug, use of drug, adverse effects to expect, reactions to report.
Physical Assessment (screen for contraindications and to establish a baseline for evaluating effects and adverse effects) **CNS:** Affect, reflexes, orientation **CV:** P, BP, peripheral perfusion **GI:** Bowel sounds, liver evaluation **Hematologic:** CBC with differential, liver function tests **Local:** Culture site of infection **Skin:** Color, lesions		Support and encouragement to cope with disease, high cost of therapy, and side effects Provision of emergency and life-support measures in cases of acute hypersensitivity	Monitor patient for drug-drug, drug-food interactions as appropriate. Evaluate effectiveness of life-support measures if needed.

Preventing Medication Errors

A growing number of patients—and drugs—brings with it an increased risk of medication errors. Compounding this risk is the tremendous upsurge in the use of over-the-counter (OTC) drugs and herbal remedies. Physicians, pharmacists, and nurses serve as checkpoints for ensuring medication safety. A nurse is commonly the final check because nurses usually administer drugs and have responsibility for discharging patients to home to manage a potentially complicated drug regimen.

The monumental task of ensuring medication safety can be managed by consistently using the five rights of drug administration: the right drug, right route, right dose, right time, and right patient.

Right drug

- Always review a drug order before administering the drug.
- Do not assume that a computer system is always right and will protect the patient. Always double check.
- Make sure the drug name is correct. Ask for a brand name and a generic name. Because many drug names look and sound alike (note the Clinical Alerts throughout the monographs), the chance of reading the name incorrectly is greatly reduced if both generic and brand names are used.
- Avoid taking verbal orders whenever possible. If you must, have a second person listen in to verify and clarify the order.
- Abbreviations can be confusing between and even within health care facilities. Do not be afraid or embarrassed to ask the meaning of an abbreviation, even a common one. For instance, many errors have been reported with U and IU, which typically mean units and international units, respectively, but may be interpreted in many different ways. Many people use hs to mean hour of sleep, others may read it as every hour. As much as possible, spell out abbreviations for clarification.

- Also, consider whether the drug makes sense for the patient's diagnosis. If you do not know or you have questions, look the drug up and ask the patient what it is being used for.

Right route

- Review the available forms of a drug to make sure the drug can be given according to the order.
- Check the routes available and the appropriateness of the route.
- Make sure the patient is able to take the drug by the route indicated. If you know that the patient has trouble swallowing, for example, you also know that a liquid form of the drug may be better than a tablet or capsule.
- Do not use abbreviations for routes because the danger of confusion is too great. For example, SC is used to mean subcutaneous, but it has been misinterpreted to mean sublingual among other misinterpretations. Also, IV can be misinterpreted to mean IU, or international units.

Right dose

- Always place a 0 to the left of a decimal point, and never place a 0 to the right of a decimal point. For example, 0.5 is correct (not .5, which can be easily mistaken for 5) and 5 is correct (not 5.0, which can be easily mistaken for 50). If you see an ordered dose that starts with a decimal point, question it. And if a dose seems much too big, question that.
- Double check drug calculations. If a dose has to be calculated for pediatric or other use, always have someone double check the math, even if a computer did the calculations. This is especially important with drugs that have small margins of safety, such as digoxin.
- Check the measuring devices used for liquid drugs. Advise patients not to use kitchen teaspoons or tablespoons to measure drug doses.

- Do not cut tablets in half to get the correct dose without checking the warnings that come with the drug. Many drugs cannot be cut, crushed, or chewed because of the matrix systems that have been developed to prepare the drugs.

Right time

- Increased workloads, decreased nursing staffs, and constant interruptions can interfere with the delivery of medications at the right times. Even at home, patients are busy, have tight schedules, and may fail to follow a precise schedule. Ensure the timely delivery of the patient's drugs by scheduling dosage with other drugs, meals, or other consistent events to maintain the serum level.
- Teach patients the importance of timing critical drugs. Keep in mind that patients tend to take all of their daily drugs at once, in the morning, to reduce the risk of forgetting them. But with critical drugs, such as those with a small margin of safety, those that interact, and those that need meticulous spacing, you will need to stress the importance of accurate timing. As needed, make detailed medication schedules and prepare pill boxes.

Right patient

- Check the patient's identification even if you think you know who the patient is. Ask for the patient's full name, and check the patient's identification band if available.
- Review the patient's diagnosis, and verify that the drug matches the diagnosis. If a drug doesn't make sense for the patient's diagnosis, look it up and, if necessary, consult with the prescriber.
- Make sure all allergies have been checked before giving a drug. Serious adverse reactions can be avoided if allergies are known.
- Ask patients specifically about OTC drugs, herbal remedies, and routine drugs that they may not think to mention, such as oral contraceptives, thyroid hormones, and insulin. Serious overdoses, adverse reactions, and drug interactions can be avoided if this information is acquired early.

- Review the patient's drug regimen to prevent potential interactions between the drug you are about to give and drugs the patient already takes. If you are not sure about potential interactions, consult a drug reference.

The bottom line in avoiding medication errors is simple: "If in doubt, check it out." A strange abbreviation, a drug or dosage that is new to you, and a confusing name are all examples that signal a need for follow-up. Look up the drug in your drug guide or call the prescriber to double check. Never give a drug until you have satisfied yourself that it is the right drug, given by the right route, at the right dose, at the right time, and to the right patient.

Error reporting

In recent years, the incidence of medication errors has become a frequent media headline. As the population ages and more people are taking multiple medications—and as more drugs become available—the possibilities for medication errors seem to be increasing. Institutions have adopted policies for reporting errors, which protect patients and staff and identify the need for educational programs within the institution, but it is also important to submit information about errors to national programs. These national programs, coordinated by the U.S. Pharmacopeia (USP), help to gather and disseminate information about errors, to prevent their recurrence at other sites and by other providers. These reports might prompt the issuing of prescriber warnings to alert health care providers about potential or actual medication errors and to prevent these same errors from recurring. The reporting of actual or potential errors results in alerts and publicity about sound-alike drug names, problems with abbreviations, the need for clear writing of dosages and times, incorrect calculations, and transcribing issues.

If you witness or participate in an actual or potential medication error, it is important to report that error to the national clearinghouse to ultimately help other professionals avoid similar errors. To help streamline the process of reporting and make it as easy as possible for professionals to participate, the USP maintains one central reporting center, from which is disseminates information to the FDA, drug manufacturers, and the Institute for Safe Medication Practices (ISMP). You can report an actual error or potential error by calling 1-800-23-ERROR, the USP Medication Errors Reporting Program. Their office will send you a pre-addressed mailer to fill out and return to them. Or, you can log on to: www.usp.org to report an error on-line or to print out the form to mail or fax back to the USP. You may request to remain anonymous to all institutions to which to the report is subsequently disseminated if you feel uncomfortable sharing this information. If you aren't sure about what you want to report, you may report errors to the USP through the ISMP web site at www.ismp.org, which also offers a discussion forum on medication errors.

What kind of errors should be reported? Errors (or potential errors) such as administration of the wrong drug, strength, or dose of a drug; incorrect routes of administration; miscalculations; misuse of medical equipment; mistakes in prescribing or transcribing (misunderstanding of verbal orders); and errors resulting from sound-alike or look-alike names. In your report, you will be asked to include the following:

1. A description of the error or preventable adverse drug reaction. What went wrong?
2. Was this an actual medication accident (reached the patient) or are you expressing concern about a potential error or writing about an error that was discovered before it reached the patient?
3. Patient outcome. Did the patient suffer any adverse effects?
4. Type of practice site (hospital, private office, retail pharmacy, drug company, long-term care facility, etc)
5. Generic name (INN or official name) of all products involved
6. Brand name of all products involved
7. Dosage form, concentration or strength, etc
8. Where error was based on communication problem, is a sample of the order avail-

able? Are package label samples or pictures available if requested?
9. Your recommendations for error prevention.

You will also be asked to provide your name, title, facility address and email, fax, or phone location if someone wants to contact you about details. You can remain anonymous and no one will contact your employer to discuss the report. The ISMP publishes case studies and publicizes warnings and alerts based on clinician reports of medication errors. Their efforts have helped to increase recognition of the many types of errors, such as those involving sound-alike names, look-alike names and packaging, instructions on equipment and delivery devices, and others.

Report an actual or potential medication error: 1-800-23-ERROR or www.usp.org

For more information regarding warnings, error alerts, and case reports: www.ismp.org or www.fda.gov

Pharmacologic drug classification

Alkylating Agents

PREGNANCY CATEGORY D

Therapeutic actions
Alkylating agents are cytotoxic: they alkylate cellular DNA, interfering with the replication of susceptible cells and causing cell death. Their action is most evident in rapidly dividing cells.

Indications
- Palliative treatment of chronic lymphocytic leukemia; malignant lymphomas, including lymphosarcoma, giant follicular lymphoma; brain tumors; Hodgkin's disease; multiple myelomas; testicular cancers; pancreatic cancer; ovarian and breast cancers
- Used as part of multiple-agent regimens

Contraindications and cautions
- Contraindications: hypersensitivity to the drugs, concurrent radiation therapy, hematopoietic depression, pregnancy, lactation.

Adverse effects
- **CNS:** *Tremors, muscular twitching, confusion*, agitation, ataxia, flaccid paresis, hallucinations, seizures
- **Dermatologic:** *Skin rash, urticaria, alopecia*, keratitis
- **GI:** Nausea, vomiting, anorexia, **hepatotoxicity**
- **GU:** Sterility
- **Hematologic:** *Bone marrow depression,* hyperuricemia
- **Respiratory:** Bronchopulmonary dysplasia, **pulmonary fibrosis**
- **Other:** *Cancer, acute leukemia*

■ Nursing considerations
Assessment
- **History**: Hypersensitivity to drug, radiation therapy, hematopoietic depression, pregnancy, lactation

- **Physical:** T; weight; skin color, lesions; R, adventitious sounds; liver evaluation; CBC, differential, hemoglobin, uric acid, renal and liver function tests

Interventions
- Arrange for blood tests to evaluate hematopoietic function prior to and weekly during therapy.
- Restrict dosage within 4 wk after a full course of radiation therapy or chemotherapy due to risk of severe bone marrow depression.
- Ensure that patient is well hydrated before treatment.
- Arrange for small, frequent meals and dietary consultation to maintain nutrition if GI upset occurs.
- Arrange for skin care for rashes.

Teaching points
- Possible side effects: nausea, vomiting, loss of appetite (dividing dose may help; small, frequent meals may help; maintain fluid intake and nutrition; drink at least 10–12 glasses of fluid each day); infertility (potentially irreversible and irregular menses to amenorrhea and aspermia; discuss feelings with health care provider); this drug can cause severe birth defects; use birth control methods while on this drug.
- Report unusual bleeding or bruising; fever, chills, sore throat; cough, shortness of breath; yellowing of the skin or eyes; flank or stomach pain.

Representative drugs
altretamine
busulfan
carmustine
chlorambucil
cyclophosphamide
ifosfamide
lomustine
mechlorethamine
melphalan

Adverse effects in *Italics* are most common; those in **Bold** are life-threatening.

streptozocin
thiotepa

Alpha₁-Adrenergic Blockers

PREGNANCY CATEGORY C

Therapeutic actions

Alpha-adrenergic blockers selectively block postsynaptic alpha₁-adrenergic receptors, decreasing sympathetic tone on the vasculature, dilating arterioles and veins, and lowering both supine and standing blood pressure; unlike conventional alpha-adrenergic blocking agents (phentolamine), they do not also block alpha₂ presynaptic receptors, so they do not cause reflex tachycardia. They also relax smooth muscle of bladder and prostate.

Indications

- Treatment of hypertension (alone or with other agents)
- Treatment of BHP (doxazocin, terazosin, tamsulosin)
- Unlabeled uses: management of refractory CHF and Raynaud's vasospasm; treatment of prostatic outflow obstruction

Contraindications and cautions

- Contraindications: hypersensitivity to any alpha₁-adrenergic blocker, lactation. Use with caution in the presence of CHF, renal failure, pregnancy.

Adverse effects

- **CNS:** *Dizziness, headache, drowsiness, lack of energy, weakness,* nervousness, vertigo, depression, paresthesias
- **CV:** *Palpitations,* sodium and water retention, increased plasma volume, edema, dyspnea, syncope, tachycardia, orthostatic hypotension
- **Dermatologic:** Rash, pruritus, lichen planus
- **EENT:** Blurred vision, reddened sclera, epistaxis, tinnitus, dry mouth, nasal congestion
- **GI:** *Nausea,* vomiting, diarrhea, constipation, abdominal discomfort or pain
- **GU:** Urinary frequency, incontinence, impotence
- **Other:** Diaphoresis

Interactions

* **Drug-drug** • Severity and duration of hypotension following first dose of drug may be greater in patients receiving beta-adrenergic blocking drugs (propranolol), verapamil

■ Nursing considerations
Assessment

- **History:** Hypersensitivity to alpha₁-adrenergic blocker, CHF, renal failure, lactation
- **Physical:** Weight; skin color, lesions; orientation, affect, reflexes; ophthalmologic exam; P, BP, orthostatic BP, supine BP, perfusion, edema, auscultation; R, adventitious sounds, status of nasal mucous membranes; bowel sounds, normal output; voiding pattern, normal output; kidney function tests, urinalysis

Interventions

- Administer, or have patient take, first dose hs to lessen likelihood of first-dose syncope believed due to excessive postural hypotension.
- Have patient lie down, and treat supportively if syncope occurs; condition is self-limiting.
- Monitor patient for orthostatic hypotension: most marked in the morning, accentuated by hot weather, alcohol, exercise.
- Monitor edema, weight in patients with incipient cardiac decompensation, arrange to add a thiazide diuretic to the drug regimen if sodium and fluid retention, signs of impending CHF occur.
- Provide small, frequent meals, frequent mouth care if GI effects occur.
- Establish safety precautions if CNS, hypotensive changes occur (side rails, accompany patient).
- Arrange for analgesic for patients experiencing headache.
- Provide consultations to help patient cope with sexual dysfunction and priapism.

Teaching points

- Take drug exactly as prescribed. Take the first dose at bedtime. Do not drive a car or operate machinery for 4 hr after the first dose.
- Avoid OTC drugs (nose drops, cold remedies) while taking this drug. If you feel you need

one of these preparations, consult health care provider.

- Possible side effects: dizziness, weakness may occur when changing position, in the early morning, after exercise, in hot weather, and after consuming alcohol; tolerance may occur after taking the drug for a while, but avoid driving or engaging in tasks that require alertness while experiencing these symptoms; change position slowly, and use caution in climbing stairs; lie down for a while if dizziness persists; GI upset (frequent, small meals may help); impotence (discuss this with health care provider); dry mouth (sucking on sugarless lozenges, ice chips may help); stuffy nose. Most of these effects will gradually disappear with continued therapy.
- Report frequent dizziness or faintness.

Representative drugs
doxazosin
prazosin
tamsulosin
terazosin

Aminoglycosides

PREGNANCY CATEGORY D

Therapeutic actions

Aminoglycosides are antibiotics that are bactericidal. They inhibit protein synthesis in susceptible strains of gram-negative bacteria, appear to disrupt the functional integrity of bacterial cell membrane, causing cell death. Oral aminoglycosides are very poorly absorbed and are used for the suppression of GI bacterial flora.

Indications

- Short-term treatment of serious infections caused by susceptible strains of *Pseudomonas* species, *Escherichia coli,* indole-positive *Proteus* species, *Providencia* species, *Klebsiella-Enterobacter-Serratia* species, *Acinetobacter* species
- Suspected gram-negative infections before results of susceptibility studies are known

- Initial treatment of staphylococcal infections when penicillin is contraindicated or when infection may be caused by mixed organisms
- Neonatal sepsis when other antibiotics cannot be used (used in combination with penicillin-type drug)
- Unlabeled uses: as part of a multidrug regimen for treatment of *Mycobacterium avium* complex (a common infection in AIDS patients) and orally for the treatment of intestinal amebiasis; adjunctive treatment of hepatic coma and for suppression of intestinal bacteria for surgery

Contraindications and cautions

- Contraindications: allergy to any aminoglycosides, renal disease, hepatic disease, preexisting hearing loss, myasthenia gravis, parkinsonism, infant botulism, lactation. Use caution with elderly patients, patients with diminished hearing, decreased renal function, dehydration, neuromuscular disorders, pregnancy.

Adverse effects

- **CNS:** *Ototoxicity;* confusion, disorientation, depression, lethargy, nystagmus, visual disturbances, headache, fever, numbness, tingling, tremor, paresthesias, muscle twitching, convulsions, muscular weakness, neuromuscular blockade, apnea
- **CV:** Palpitations, hypotension, hypertension
- **GI:** Nausea, vomiting, anorexia, diarrhea, weight loss, stomatitis, increased salivation, splenomegaly
- **GU:** *Nephrotoxicity*
- **Hematologic:** Leukemoid reaction, agranulocytosis, granulocytosis, leukopenia, leukocytosis, thrombocytopenia, eosinophilia, pancytopenia, anemia, hemolytic anemia, increased or decreased reticulocyte count, electrolyte disturbances
- **Hepatic:** Hepatic toxicity; hepatomegaly
- **Hypersensitivity:** Purpura, rash, urticaria, exfoliative dermatitis, itching
- **Other:** *Superinfections, pain and irritation at IM injection sites*

Adverse effects in *Italics* are most common; those in **Bold** are life-threatening.

Interactions

✳ Drug-drug • Increased ototoxic and nephrotoxic effects if taken with potent diuretics and similarly toxic drugs (cephalosporins)

• Increased likelihood of neuromuscular blockade if given shortly after general anesthetics, depolarizing and nondepolarizing neuromuscular junction blockers

■ Nursing considerations
Assessment

• **History:** Allergy to any aminoglycosides, renal disease, hepatic disease, preexisting hearing loss, myasthenia gravis, parkinsonism, infant botulism, lactation, diminished hearing, decreased renal function, dehydration, neuromuscular disorders
• **Physical:** Arrange culture and sensitivity tests of infection prior to therapy; check renal function before, during, and after therapy, eighth cranial nerve function, and state of hydration, during and after therapy; hepatic function tests, CBC; skin color, lesions; orientation, affect; reflexes, bilateral grip strength; body weight; bowel sounds

Interventions

• Arrange for culture and sensitivity testing of infected area prior to treatment.
• Monitor duration of treatment: usual duration is 7–10 days. If no clinical response within 3–5 days, stop therapy. Prolonged treatment leads to increased risk of toxicity. If drug is used longer than 10 days, monitor auditory and renal function daily.
• Give IM dosage by deep injection.
• Ensure that patient is well hydrated before and during therapy.
• Establish safety measures if CNS, vestibular nerve effects occur (use of side rails, assistance with ambulation).
• Provide small, frequent meals if nausea, anorexia occur.
• Provide comfort measures and medication for superinfections.

Teaching points

• Take full course of oral drug; drink plenty of fluids.
• Possible side effects: ringing in the ears, headache, dizziness (reversible; safety measures need to be taken if severe); nausea, vomiting, loss of appetite (small, frequent meals, frequent mouth care may help).
• Report pain at injection site, severe headache, dizziness, loss of hearing, changes in urine pattern, difficulty breathing, rash or skin lesions.

Representative drugs

amikacin sulfate
gentamicin
kanamycin
neomycin (oral)
netilmicin
streptomycin
tobramycin (parenteral)

Angiotensin-Converting Enzyme (ACE) Inhibitors

PREGNANCY CATEGORY C (FIRST TRIMESTER)

PREGNANCY CATEGORY D (SECOND AND THIRD TRIMESTERS)

Therapeutic actions

ACE inhibitors block ACE in the lungs from converting angiotensin I, activated when renin is released from the kidneys, to angiotensin II, a powerful vasoconstrictor. Blocking this conversion leads to decreased BP, decreased aldosterone secretion, a small increase in serum potassium levels, and sodium and fluid loss; increased prostaglandin synthesis also may be involved in the antihypertensive action.

Indications

• Treatment of hypertension (alone or with thiazide-type diuretics)
• Treatment of CHF (used with diuretics and digitalis)
• Treatment of stable patients within 24 hr of acute MI to improve survival (lisinopril)
• Unlabeled uses: management of hypertensive crises; treatment of rheumatoid arthritis; diabetic nephropathy, diagnosis of anatomic renal artery stenosis, hypertension related to scleroderma renal crisis; diagnosis of primary aldosteronism, idiopathic edema; Bartter's syndrome; Raynaud's syndrome; hypertension of Takayasu's disease

Contraindications and cautions

- Contraindications: allergy to the drug, impaired renal function, CHF, salt or volume depletion, lactation, pregnancy, history of angioedema, bilateral stenosis.

Adverse effects

- **CV:** Tachycardia, angina pectoris, **myocardial infarction,** Raynaud's syndrome, CHF, hypotension in salt/volume-depleted patients
- **Dermatologic:** *Rash,* pruritus, pemphigoid-like reaction, scalded mouth sensation, exfoliative dermatitis, photosensitivity, alopecia
- **GI:** *Gastric irritation, aphthous ulcers,* peptic ulcers, dysgeusia, cholestatic jaundice, hepatocellular injury, anorexia, constipation
- **GU:** Proteinuria, renal insufficiency, renal failure, polyuria, oliguria, urinary frequency
- **Hematologic:** Neutropenia, agranulocytosis, thrombocytopenia, hemolytic anemia, **pancytopenia**
- **Other:** *Cough,* malaise, dry mouth, lymphadenopathy

Interactions

✳ **Drug-drug** • Increased risk of hypersensitivity reactions with allopurinal • Decreased antihypertensive effects with indomethacin
✳ **Drug-food** • Decreased absorption of selected agents if taken with food
✳ **Drug-lab test** • False-positive test for urine acetone

■ Nursing considerations
Assessment

- **History:** Allergy to ACE inhibitors, impaired renal function, CHF, salt or volume depletion, pregnancy, lactation
- **Physical:** Skin color, lesions, turgor; T, P, BP, peripheral perfusion; mucous membranes; bowel sounds; liver evaluation; urinalysis, renal and liver function tests, CBC and differential

Interventions

- Administer 1 hr before or 2 hr after meals; is affected by food in GI tract.

- Alert surgeon and mark patient's chart that ACE inhibitor is being taken; angiotensin II formation subsequent to compensatory renin release during surgery will be blocked; hypotension may be reversed with volume expansion.
- Monitor patient closely in situations that may lead to a fall in BP due to reduction in fluid volume (excessive perspiration and dehydration, vomiting, diarrhea) because excessive hypotension may occur.
- Arrange for reduced dosage in patients with impaired renal function.
- Arrange for bowel program if constipation occurs.
- Provide small, frequent meals if GI upset is severe.
- Provide for frequent mouth care and oral hygiene if mouth sores, alteration in taste occur.
- Caution patient to change position slowly if orthostatic changes occur.
- Provide skin care as needed.

Teaching points

- Take drug 1 hr before or 2 hr after meals; do not take with food.
- Do not stop taking the medication without consulting health care provider.
- Possible side effects: GI upset, loss of appetite, change in taste perception (limited effects; if they persist or become a problem, consult health care provider); mouth sores (frequent mouth care may help); skin rash; fast heart rate; dizziness, light-headedness (passes after a few days of therapy; if it occurs, change position slowly and limit activities requiring alertness and precision).
- Be careful in any situation that may lead to a drop in BP (diarrhea, sweating, vomiting, dehydration); if light-headedness or dizziness occurs, consult health care provider.
- Avoid OTC medications, especially cough, cold, allergy medications. If you need one of these, consult health care provider.
- Report mouth sores; sore throat, fever, chills; swelling of the hands, feet; irregular heartbeat, chest pains; swelling of the face, eyes, lips, tongue; difficulty breathing.

Adverse effects in *Italics* are most common; those in **Bold** are life-threatening.

Representative drugs
benazepril
captopril
enalapril
enalaprilat
fosinopril
lisinopril
moexipril
perindopril
quinapril
ramipril
trandolapril

Angiotensin II Receptor Blockers (ARBs)

PREGNANCY CATEGORY C (FIRST TRIMESTER)

PREGNANCY CATEGORY D (SECOND AND THIRD TRIMESTERS)

Therapeutic actions
ARBs selectively block the binding of angiotensin II to specific tissue receptors found in the vascular smooth muscle and adrenal gland. This action blocks the vasoconstriction effect of the renin-angiotensin system as well as the release of aldosterone leading to decreased blood pressure; may block vessel remodeling that occurs in hypertension and contributes to the development of atherosclerosis.

Indications
- Treatment of hypertension, alone or in combination with other antihypertensive agents

Contraindications and cautions
- Contraindications: hypersensitivity to any ARB, pregnancy (use during the second or third trimester can cause injury or even death to the fetus), lactation.
- Cautions: renal dysfunction, hypovolemia.

Adverse effects
- **CNS:** Headache, dizziness, syncope, muscle weakness, *fatigue, depression*
- **CV:** Hypotension
- **Dermatologic:** Rash, inflammation, urticaria, pruritus, alopecia, dry skin

- **GI:** Diarrhea, *abdominal pain,* nausea, constipation
- **Respiratory:** *URI symptoms,* cough, sinus disorders
- **Other:** Cancer in preclinical studies, urinary tract infections

Interactions
✳ **Drug-drug** • Decreased effectiveness if combined with phenobarbital

■ Nursing considerations
Assessment
- **History:** Hypersensitivity to any ARB, pregnancy, lactation, renal dysfunction, hypovolemia
- **Physical:** Skin lesions, turgor; body temperature; reflexes, affect; BP; R, respiratory auscultation; renal function tests

Interventions
- Administer without regard to meals.
- Ensure that patient is not pregnant before beginning therapy; suggest the use of barrier birth control; fetal injury and deaths have been reported.
- Find an alternative method of feeding infant if ARBs are given to a nursing mother. Depression of the renin-angiotensin system in infants is potentially very dangerous.
- Alert surgeon and mark patient's chart with notice that an ARB is being taken. The blockage of the renin-angiotensin system following surgery can produce problems. Hypotension may be reversed with volume expansion.
- If blood pressure control does reach desired levels, diuretics or other antihypertensives may be added to the drug regimen. Monitor patient's blood pressure carefully.
- Monitor patient closely in any situation that may lead to a decrease in blood pressure secondary to reduction in fluid volume—excessive perspiration, dehydration, vomiting, diarrhea—excessive hypotension can occur.

Teaching points
- Take drug without regard to meals. Do not stop taking this drug without consulting your health care provider.
- Use a barrier method of birth control while on this drug; if you become pregnant or de-

sire to become pregnant, consult with your physician.
- Know that the following side effects may occur: dizziness (avoid driving a car or performing hazardous tasks); nausea, abdominal pain (proper nutrition is important, consult with your dietitian to maintain nutrition); symptoms of upper respiratory tract or urinary tract infection, cough (do not self-medicate, consult with your nurse or physician if this becomes uncomfortable).
- Report: fever, chills, dizziness, pregnancy.

Representative drugs
candesartan
eprosartan
irbesartan
losartan
olmesartan
telmisartan
valsartan

Antiarrhythmics

PREGNANCY CATEGORY C

Therapeutic actions
Antiarrhythmics act at specific sites to alter the action potential of cardiac cells and interfere with the electrical excitability of the heart. Most of these drugs may cause new or worsened arrhythmias (proarrhythmic effect) and must be used with caution and with continual cardiac monitoring and patient evaluation.

Indications
- Treatment of tachycardia when rapid but short-term control of ventricular rate is desirable (patients with atrial fibrillation, flutter, in perioperative or postoperative situations)
- Treatment of noncompensatory tachycardia when heart rate requires specific intervention
- Treatment of atrial arrhythmias

Contraindications and cautions
- Reserve for emergency situations; there are no contraindications. Use caution during pregnancy or lactation.

Adverse effects
- **CNS:** *Light-headedness, speech disorder, midscapular pain, weakness, rigors*, somnolence, confusion
- **CV:** *Hypotension,* pallor, arrhythmias
- **GI:** *Taste perversion*
- **GU:** *Urinary retention*
- **Local:** *Inflammation,* induration, edema, erythema, burning at the site of infusion
- **Other:** Fever, rhonchi, flushing

Interactions
✳ **Drug-drug** • Monitor patients receiving antiarrhythmics for drug interactions; see specific drug for Interactions.

■ Nursing considerations
Assessment
- **History:** Cardiac disease, cerebrovascular disease
- **Physical:** P, BP, ECG; orientation, reflexes; R, adventitious sounds; urinary output

Interventions
- Ensure that more toxic drug is not used in chronic settings when transfer to another agent is anticipated.
- Monitor BP, heart rate, and rhythm closely.
- Provide comfort measures for pain, rigors, fever, flushing, if patient is awake.
- Provide supportive measures appropriate to condition being treated.
- Provide support and encouragement to deal with drug effects and discomfort of IV lines.

Teaching points
- Reserved for emergency use. Incorporate any information about drug into the overall teaching program for patient. Patients maintained on oral drug will need specific teaching. See individual monograph for details.

Representative drugs
Type I
moricizine
Type IA
disopyramide
procainamide
quinidine
Type IB
lidocaine

Adverse effects in *Italics* are most common; those in **Bold** are life-threatening.

mexiletine
phenytoin
tocainide
Type IC
flecainide
propafenone
Type II
acebutolol
esmolol
propranolol
Type III
amiodarone
bretylium
dofetilide
ibutilide
sotalol
Type IV
verapamil
Other
adenosine
digoxin

Anticoagulants

PREGNANCY CATEGORY C

Therapeutic actions

Oral anticoagulants interfere with the hepatic synthesis of vitamin K–dependent clotting factors (factors II, prothrombin, VII, IX, and X), resulting in their eventual depletion and prolongation of clotting times; parenteral anticoagulants interfere with the conversion of prothrombin to thrombin, blocking the final step in clot formation but leaving the circulating levels of clotting factors unaffected.

Indications

- Treatment and prevention of pulmonary embolism and venous thrombosis and its extension
- Treatment of atrial fibrillation with embolization
- Prevention of deep vein thrombosis
- Prophylaxis of systemic embolization after acute MI
- Prevention of thrombi following specific surgical procedures and prolonged bedrest (low-molecular-weight heparins)
- Unlabeled uses: prevention of recurrent transient ischemic attacks, and MI; adjunct to therapy in small-cell carcinoma of the lung.

Contraindications and cautions

- Contraindications: allergy to the drug; SBE; hemorrhagic disorders; tuberculosis; hepatic diseases; GI ulcers; renal disease; indwelling catheters, spinal puncture; aneurysm; diabetes; visceral carcinoma; uncontrolled hypertension; severe trauma (including recent or contemplated CNS, eye surgery, recent placement of IUD); threatened abortion, menometrorrhagia; pregnancy (oral agents cause fetal damage and death); or lactation (heparin if anticoagulation is required). Use caution in the presence of CHF, diarrhea, fever; thyrotoxicosis; senile, psychotic, or depressed patients.

Adverse effects

- **Bleeding:** *Hemorrhage;* GI or urinary tract bleeding (hematuria, dark stools; paralytic ileus; intestinal obstruction from hemorrhage into GI tract); petechiae and purpura, bleeding from mucous membranes; hemorrhagic infarction, vasculitis, skin necrosis of female breast; adrenal hemorrhage and resultant adrenal insufficiency; compressive neuropathy secondary to hemorrhage near a nerve
- **Dermatologic:** *Alopecia, urticaria, dermatitis*
- **GI:** *Nausea,* vomiting, anorexia, abdominal cramping, diarrhea, retroperitoneal hematoma, hepatitis, jaundice, mouth ulcers
- **GU:** Priapism, nephropathy, red-orange urine
- **Hematologic:** Granulocytosis, leukopenia, eosinophilia
- **Other:** Fever, "purple toes" syndrome

Interactions

✳ **Drug-drug** ● Increased bleeding tendencies with salicylates, chloral hydrate, phenylbutazone, clofibrate, disulfiram, chloramphenicol, metronidazole, cimetidine, ranitidine, cotrimoxazole, sulfinpyrazone, quinidine, quinine, thyroid drugs, glucagon, danazol, erythromycin, androgens, amiodarone, cefamandole, cefoperazone, cefotetan, moxalactam, cefazolin, cefoxitin, ceftriaxone, meclofenamate, mefenamic acid, famotidine, nizatidine, nalidixic acid ● Possible decreased anticoagulation effect with barbiturates, griseofulvin, rifampin, phenytoin, glutethimide, carbamazepine, vitamin K, vitamin E, cholestyramine, aminoglutethimide, ethchlorvynol ● Altered effects of warfarin with methimazole, propylthiouracil ● Increased activity and toxicity of phenytoin with oral anticoagulants

✳ **Drug-alternative therapy** ● Increased risk of bleeding with chamomile, garlic, ginger, gingko, ginseng therapy, turmeric, horse chestnut, green tea leaf, grape seed extract, feverfew, don guai

✳ **Drug-lab test** ● Red-orange discoloration of alkaline urine may interfere with some lab tests.

■ Nursing considerations
Assessment

- **History:** Allergy to the drug; SBE; hemorrhagic disorders; tuberculosis; hepatic diseases; GI ulcers; renal disease; indwelling catheters, spinal puncture; aneurysm; diabetes; visceral carcinoma; uncontrolled hypertension; severe trauma; threatened abortion, menometrorrhagia; pregnancy; lactation; CHF, diarrhea, fever; thyrotoxicosis; senile, psychotic, or depressed patients
- **Physical:** Skin lesions, color, T, orientation, reflexes, affect; P, BP, peripheral perfusion, baseline ECG; R, adventitious sounds; liver evaluation, bowel sounds, normal output; CBC, urinalysis, guaiac stools, prothrombin time, renal and hepatic function tests, WBCT, APTT

Interventions

- Monitor INR or APTT to adjust dosage.
- Do not change brand names once stabilized; bioavailability problems have been documented.
- Evaluate patient for signs of blood loss (petechiae, bleeding gums, bruises, dark stools, dark urine).
- Establish safety measures to protect patient from injury.
- Do not give patient IM injections. Monitor sites of invasive procedures; ensure prolonged compression of bleeding vessels.
- Double-check other drugs that are ordered for potential interaction: dosage of both drugs may need to be adjusted.

- Use caution when discontinuing other medications; dosage of warfarin may need to be adjusted; carefully monitor PT values.
- Maintain vitamin K on standby in case of overdose of oral agents; maintain protamine sulfate on standby for parenteral drug.
- Arrange for frequent follow-up, including blood tests to evaluate drug effects.
- Evaluate for therapeutic effects: PT, 1.5–2.5 times the control value; WBCT, 2.5–3 times control; INR, 2–3 times normal; APTT, 1.5–2 times normal.

Teaching points

- Many factors may change the body's response to this drug—fever, change of diet, change of environment, other medications. The dosage of the drug may have to be changed. Be sure to write down all changes prescribed.
- Do not change any medication that you are taking (adding or stopping another drug) without consulting health care provider. Other drugs affect the way anticoagulants work; starting or stopping another drug can cause excessive bleeding or interfere with the desired effects of the drug.
- Carry or wear a medical alert tag stating that you are on this drug. This will alert medical personnel in an emergency that you are taking this drug.
- Avoid situations in which you could be easily injured—contact sports, shaving with a straight razor.
- Possible side effects: stomach bloating, cramps (passes with time; if it becomes too uncomfortable, contact health care provider); loss of hair, skin rash (this is a frustrating and upsetting effect; if it becomes a problem, discuss it with health care provider); orange-red discoloration to the urine (this may be mistaken for blood; add vinegar to urine, the color should disappear).
- Arrange periodic blood tests to check on the action of the drug. It is very important that you have these tests.
- Use contraceptive measures while taking this drug; it is important that you do not become pregnant.
- Report unusual bleeding (when brushing your teeth, excessive bleeding from injuries, excessive bruising), black or bloody stools,

---

Adverse effects in *Italics* are most common; those in **Bold** are life-threatening.

cloudy or dark urine, sore throat, fever, chills, severe headaches, dizziness, suspected pregnancy.

Representative drugs
Oral
  warfarin sodium
Parenteral
  argatroban
  bivalirudin
  heparin
  lepirudin
Low-molecular-weight heparins
  dalteparin
  danaparoid
  enoxaparin
  tinzaparin

Antidiabetic Agents

PREGNANCY CATEGORY C

Therapeutic actions
Oral antidiabetic agents are called sulfonylureas. They stimulate insulin release from functioning beta cells in the pancreas; may improve binding between insulin and insulin receptors or increase the number of insulin receptors; second-generation sulfonylureas (glipizide and glyburide) are thought to be more potent than first-generation sulfonylureas. Other agents include: drugs that increase insulin receptor sensitivity (thiazolidinediones); drugs that delay or alter glucose absorption (acarbose, miglitol); and insulin, which is used for replacement therapy.

Indications
- Adjuncts to diet and exercise to lower blood glucose in patients with non–insulin-dependent diabetes mellitus (type 2)
- Adjuncts to insulin therapy in the stabilization of certain cases of insulin-dependent maturity-onset diabetes, reducing the insulin requirement and decreasing the chance of hypoglycemic reactions
- Replacement therapy in type 1 diabetes mellitus and when oral agents cannot control glucose levels in type 2 diabetes

Contraindications and cautions
- Contraindications: allergy to sulfonylureas; diabetes complicated by fever, severe infections, severe trauma, major surgery, ketosis, acidosis, coma (insulin is indicated); type 1 or juvenile diabetes, serious hepatic impairment, serious renal impairment, uremia, thyroid or endocrine impairment, glycosuria, hyperglycemia associated with primary renal disease; labor and delivery (if glipizide is used during pregnancy, discontinue drug at least 1 mo before delivery); lactation, safety not established.

Adverse effects
- **CV:** Increased risk of CV mortality
- **Endocrine:** *Hypoglycemia*
- **GI:** *Anorexia, nausea,* vomiting, *epigastric discomfort, heartburn, diarrhea*
- **Hematologic:** Leukopenia, thrombocytopenia, anemia
- **Hypersensitivity:** *Allergic skin reactions,* eczema, pruritus, erythema, urticaria, photosensitivity, fever, eosinophilia, jaundice

Interactions
✳ **Drug-drug** • Increased risk of hypoglycemia with sulfonamides, chloramphenicol, salicylates, clofibrate • Decreased effectiveness of both sulfonylurea and diazoxide if taken concurrently • Increased risk of hyperglycemia with rifampin, thiazides • Risk of hypoglycemia and hyperglycemia with ethanol; "disulfiram reaction" also has been reported.

✳ **Drug-alternative therapy** • Increased risk of hypoglycemia with juniper berries, ginseng, garlic, fenugreek, coriander, dandelion root, celery

■ Nursing considerations
Assessment
- **History:** Allergy to sulfonylureas; diabetes complicated by fever, severe infections, severe trauma, major surgery, ketosis, acidosis, coma (insulin is indicated); type 1 or juvenile diabetes, serious hepatic impairment, serious renal impairment, uremia, thyroid or endocrine impairment, glycosuria, hyperglycemia associated with primary renal disease
- **Physical:** Skin color, lesions; T; orientation, reflexes, peripheral sensation; R, ad-

ventitious sounds; liver evaluation, bowel sounds; urinalysis, BUN, serum creatinine, liver function tests, blood glucose, CBC

Interventions

- Administer drug before breakfast; if severe GI upset occurs may be divided and given before meals.
- Monitor urine and serum glucose levels to determine effectiveness of drug and dosage.
- Arrange for transfer to insulin therapy during periods of high stress (infections, surgery, trauma).
- Arrange for use of IV glucose if severe hypoglycemia occurs as a result of overdose.
- Arrange consultation with dietitian to establish weight loss program and dietary control as appropriate.
- Arrange thorough diabetic teaching program to include disease, dietary control, exercise, signs and symptoms of hypoglycemia and hyperglycemia, avoidance of infection, hygiene.
- Provide skin care to prevent breakdown.
- Ensure access to bathroom facilities if diarrhea occurs.
- Establish safety precautions if CNS effects occur.

Teaching points

- Do not stop this medication without consulting health care provider.
- Monitor urine or blood for glucose and ketones.
- Do not use this drug during pregnancy (except insulin).
- Avoid alcohol while on this drug.
- Report fever, sore throat, unusual bleeding or bruising, skin rash, dark urine, light-colored stools, hypoglycemia or hyperglycemic reactions.

Representative drugs

acarbose
acetohexamide
chlorpropamide
glimepiride
glipizide
glyburide
insulin
metformin
miglitol
nateglinide
pioglitazone
repaglinide
rosiglitazone
tolazamide
tolbutamide

Antifungals

PREGNANCY CATEGORY C

Therapeutic actions

Antifungals bind to or impair sterols of fungal cell membranes, allowing increased permeability and leakage of cellular components and causing the death of the fungal cell.

Indications

- Systemic fungal infections: candidiasis, chronic mucocutaneous candidiasis, oral thrush, candiduria, blastomycosis, coccidioidomycosis, histoplasmosis, chromomycosis, paracoccidioidomycosis, dermatophytosis, ringworm infections of the skin
- Treatment of onychomycosis, pityriasis versicolor, vaginal candidiasis; topical treatment of tinea corporis and tinea cruris caused by *Trichophyton rubrum*, *Trichophyton mentagrophytes*, and *Epidermophyton floccosum*; treatment of tinea versicolor caused by *Malassezia furfur* (topical); and reduction of scaling due to dandruff (shampoo)

Contraindications and cautions

- Contraindications: allergy to any antifungal, fungal meningitis, pregnancy, or lactation. Use with caution in the presence of hepatocellular failure (increased risk of hepatocellular necrosis).

Adverse effects

- **CNS:** Headache, dizziness, somnolence, photophobia
- **GI:** Hepatotoxicity, *nausea, vomiting*, abdominal pain
- **GU:** Impotence, oligospermia (with very high doses)

Adverse effects in *Italics* are most common; those in **Bold** are life-threatening.

- **Hematologic:** Thrombocytopenia, leukopenia, hemolytic anemia
- **Hypersensitivity:** Urticaria to anaphylaxis
- **Local:** *Severe irritation, pruritus, stinging* with topical application
- **Other:** *Pruritus,* fever, chills, gynecomastia

Interactions

✳ **Drug-drug** • Decreased blood levels with rifampin • Increased blood levels of cyclosporine and risk of toxicity with antifungals • Increased duration of adrenal suppression when methylprednisolone, corticosteroids are taken with antifungals

■ Nursing considerations

Assessment

- **History:** Allergy to antifungals, fungal meningitis, hepatocellular failure, pregnancy, lactation
- **Physical:** Skin color, lesions; orientation, reflexes, affect; bowel sounds, liver evaluation; liver function tests; CBC and differential; culture of area involved

Interventions

- Arrange for culture before beginning therapy; treatment should begin prior to lab results.
- Maintain epinephrine on standby in case of severe anaphylaxis after first dose.
- Administer oral drug with food to decrease GI upset.
- Administer until infection is eradicated: candidiasis, 1–2 wk; other systemic mycoses, 6 mo; chronic mucocutaneous candidiasis often requires maintenance therapy; tinea veriscolor, 2 wk of topical application.
- Discontinue treatment and consult physician about diagnosis if no improvement within 2 wk of topical application.
- Discontinue topical applications if sensitivity or chemical reaction occurs.
- Administer shampoo as follows: moisten hair and scalp thoroughly with water; apply sufficient shampoo to produce a lather; gently massage for 1 min; rinse hair with warm water; repeat, leaving on hair for 3 min.
- Provide hygiene measures to control sources of infection or reinfection.

- Provide small, frequent meals if GI upset occurs.
- Provide comfort measures appropriate to site of fungal infection.
- Arrange hepatic function tests prior to therapy and at least monthly during treatment.
- Establish safety precautions if CNS effects occur (side rails, assistance with ambulation).

Teaching points

- Take the full course of therapy. Long-term use of the drug will be needed; beneficial effects may not be seen for several weeks. Take oral drug with meals to decrease GI upset. Apply topical drug to affected area and surrounding area. Shampoo—moisten hair and scalp thoroughly with water; apply to produce a lather; gently massage for 1 min; rinse with warm water; repeat, leaving on for 3 min. Shampoo twice a week for 4 wk with at least 3 days between shampooing.
- Use hygiene measures to prevent reinfection or spread of infection.
- Possible side effects: nausea, vomiting, diarrhea (take drug with food); sedation, dizziness, confusion (avoid driving or performing tasks that require alertness); stinging, irritation (local application).
- Report skin rash, severe nausea, vomiting, diarrhea, fever, sore throat, unusual bleeding or bruising, yellowing of skin or eyes, dark urine or pale stools, severe irritation (local application).

Representative drugs

amphotericin B
butenafine
butoconazole
caspofungin
ciclopirox
clotrimazole
econazole
fluconazole
flucytosine
griseofulvin
itraconazole
ketoconazole
miconazole
naftifine
nystatin

oxiconazole
terbinafine
tolnaftate
voriconazole

Antihistamines

PREGNANCY CATEGORY C

Therapeutic actions
Antihistamines competitively block the effects of histamine at peripheral H_1 receptor sites, have anticholinergic (atropine-like) and antipruritic effects.

Indications
- Relief of symptoms associated with perennial and seasonal allergic rhinitis, vasomotor rhinitis, allergic conjunctivitis, mild, uncomplicated urticaria and angioedema
- Amelioration of allergic reactions to blood or plasma
- Treatment of dermatographism
- Control of nausea, vomiting, and dizziness from motion sickness (buclizine, cyclizine, diphenhydramine, meclizine)
- Adjunctive therapy in anaphylactic reactions
- Unlabeled uses: relief of lower respiratory conditions, such as histamine-induced bronchoconstriction in asthmatics and exercise- and hyperventilation-induced bronchospasm

Contraindications and cautions
- Contraindications: allergy to antihistamines, pregnancy, or lactation. Use cautiously with narrow-angle glaucoma, stenosing peptic ulcer, symptomatic prostatic hypertrophy, asthmatic attack, bladder neck obstruction, pyloroduodenal obstruction.

Adverse effects
- **CNS:** *Depression,* nightmares, sedation
- **CV:** Arrhythmia, increase in QTc intervals
- **Dermatologic:** Alopecia, angioedema, skin eruption and itching
- **GI:** *Dry mouth, GI upset,* anorexia, increased appetite, nausea, vomiting, diarrhea
- **GU:** Galactorrhea, menstrual disorders, dysuria, hesitancy

- **Respiratory:** *Bronchospasm, cough, thickening of secretions*
- **Other:** Musculoskeletal pain, mild to moderate transaminase elevations

Interactions
✳ **Drug-drug** ● Altered antihistamine metabolism with ketoconazole, troleandomycin ● Increased antihistaminic anticholinergic effects with MAO inhibitors ● Additive CNS depressant effects with alcohol, CNS depressants

■ Nursing considerations
Assessment
- **History:** Allergy to any antihistamines, narrow-angle glaucoma, stenosing peptic ulcer, symptomatic prostatic hypertrophy, asthmatic attack, bladder neck obstruction, pyloroduodenal obstruction, pregnancy, lactation
- **Physical:** Skin color, lesions, texture; orientation, reflexes, affect; vision exam; R, adventitious sounds; prostate palpation; serum transaminase levels

Interventions
- Administer with food if GI upset occurs.
- Provide mouth care, sugarless lozenges for dry mouth.
- Arrange for humidifier if thickening of secretions, nasal dryness become bothersome; encourage intake of fluids.
- Provide skin care for dermatologic effects.

Teaching points
- Avoid excessive dosage.
- Take with food if GI upset occurs.
- Possible side effects: dizziness, sedation, drowsiness (use caution driving or performing tasks that require alertness); dry mouth (mouth care, sucking sugarless lozenges may help); thickening of bronchial secretions, dryness of nasal mucosa (use a humidifier); menstrual irregularities.
- Avoid alcohol; serious sedation could occur.
- Report difficulty breathing, hallucinations, tremors, loss of coordination, unusual bleeding or bruising, visual disturbances, irregular heartbeat.

Adverse effects in *Italics* are most common; those in **Bold** are life-threatening.

Representative drugs

azatadine
azelastine
brompheniramine
buclizine
cetirizine
chlorpheniramine
clemastine
cyclizine
cyproheptadine
desloratadine
dimenhydrinate
diphenhydramine
fexofenadine
hydroxyzine
loratadine
meclizine
promethazine
tripelennamine

Antimetabolites

PREGNANCY CATEGORY D

Therapeutic actions

Antimetabolites are antineoplastic drugs that inhibit DNA polymerase. They are cell cycle phase specific to S phase (stage of DNA synthesis), causing cell death for cells in the S phase; they also block progression of cells from G_1 to S in the cell cycle.

Indications

- Induction and maintenance of remission in acute myelocytic leukemia (higher response rate in children than in adults), chronic lymphocytic leukemia
- Treatment of acute lymphocytic leukemia, chronic myelocytic leukemia and erythroleukemia, meningeal leukemia, psoriasis and rheumatoid arthritis (methotrexate)
- Palliative treatment of GI adenocarcinoma, carcinoma of the colon, rectum, breast, stomach, pancreas
- Part of combination therapy for the treatment of non-Hodgkin's lymphoma in children

Contraindications and cautions

- Contraindications: allergy to the drug, pregnancy, lactation, premature infants. Use cautiously with hematopoietic depression secondary to radiation or chemotherapy; impaired liver function.

Adverse effects

- **CNS:** Neuritis, neural toxicity
- **Dermatologic:** Fever, rash, urticaria, freckling, skin ulceration, pruritus, conjunctivitis, alopecia
- **GI:** *Anorexia, nausea, vomiting, diarrhea, oral and anal inflammation or ulceration;* esophageal ulcerations, esophagitis, abdominal pain, *hepatic dysfunction* (jaundice), acute pancreatitis
- **GU:** Renal dysfunction, urinary retention
- **Hematologic:** Bone marrow depression, hyperuricemia
- **Local:** Thrombophlebitis, cellulitis at injection site
- **Other:** *Fever, rash*

Interactions

✳ **Drug-drug** ● Decreased therapeutic action of digoxin with cytarabine ● Enhanced toxicity of fluorouracil with leucovorin ● Potentially fatal reactions if methotrexate is taken with various NSAIDs

■ Nursing considerations
Assessment

- **History:** Allergy to drug, hematopoietic depression, impaired liver function, lactation
- **Physical:** Weight; T; skin lesions, color; hair; orientation, reflexes; R, adventitious sounds; mucous membranes, liver evaluation, abdominal exam; CBC, differential; renal and liver function tests; urinalysis

Interventions

- Arrange for tests to evaluate hematopoietic status prior to and during therapy.
- Arrange for discontinuation of drug therapy if platelet count < 50,000/mm^3, polymorphonuclear granulocyte count < 1,000/mm^3; consult physician for dosage adjustment.
- Monitor injection site for signs of thrombophlebitis, inflammation.
- Provide mouth care for mouth sores.
- Arrange for small, frequent meals and dietary consultation to maintain nutrition when GI effects are severe.

- Establish safety measures if dizziness, CNS effects occur.
- Arrange for patient to obtain a wig or some other suitable head covering if alopecia occurs; ensure that head is covered in extremes of temperature.
- Protect patient from exposure to infections.
- Provide skin care.
- Arrange for comfort measures if anal inflammation, headache, or other pain associated with cytarabine syndrome occurs.
- Arrange for treatment of fever if it occurs.

Teaching points

- Prepare a calendar of treatment days for the patient.
- Possible side effects: nausea, vomiting, loss of appetite (medication may be ordered; small frequent meals may help; it is important to maintain nutrition); malaise, weakness, lethargy (these are all effects of the drug; consult your health care provider and avoid driving or operating dangerous machinery); mouth sores (frequent mouth care will be needed); diarrhea; loss of hair (you may wish to obtain a wig or other suitable head covering; keep the head covered in extremes of temperature); anal inflammation (consult with health care provider; comfort measures can be ordered).
- Use birth control; this drug may cause birth defects or miscarriages.
- Arrange to have frequent, regular medical follow-up, including frequent blood tests.
- Report black, tarry stools; fever, chills; sore throat; unusual bleeding or bruising; shortness of breath; chest pain; difficulty swallowing.

Representative drugs

capecitabine
cladribine
cytarabine
floxuridine
fludarabine
fluorouracil
gemcitabine
mercaptopurine
methotrexate

pentostatin
thioguanine

Antimigraine Agents (Triptans)

PREGNANCY CATEGORY C

Therapeutic actions

Triptans bind to serotonin receptors to cause vascular constrictive effects on cranial blood vessels, causing the relief of migraine in selective patients.

Indications

- Treatment of acute migraine attacks with or without aura
- Unlabeled use: treatment of cluster headaches

Contraindications and cautions

- Contraindications: allergy to any triptan, active coronary artery disease, uncontrolled hypertension, hemiplegic migraine, pregnancy.
- Cautions: the elderly, lactation.

Adverse effects

- **CNS:** *Dizziness, vertigo,* headache, anxiety, malaise or fatigue, *weakness, myalgia*
- **CV:** *Blood pressure alterations, tightness or pressure in chest*
- **GI:** Abdominal discomfort, dysphagia
- **Local:** *Injection site discomfort*
- **Other:** *Tingling, warm or hot sensations, burning sensation, feeling of heaviness, pressure sensation, numbness, feeling of tightness,* feeling strange, cold sensation

Interactions

✳ **Drug-drug** • Prolonged vasoactive reactions when taken concurrently with ergot-containing drugs, MAOIs, other triptans • Risk of increased blood levels and prolonged effects with hormonal contraceptives; monitor patient very closely if this combination must be used

✳ **Drug-alternative therapy** • Increased risk of severe reaction if combined with St. John's wort

Adverse effects in *Italics* are most common; those in **Bold** are life-threatening.

■ Nursing considerations
Assessment
- **History:** Allergy to any triptan, active coronary artery disease, uncontrolled hypertension, hemiplegic migraine, pregnancy, lactation
- **Physical:** Skin color and lesions; orientation, reflexes, peripheral sensation; P, BP; renal and liver function tests

Interventions
- Administer to relieve acute migraine, not as a prophylactic measure.
- Administer as prescribed—inhalation, injection, or orally.
- Establish safety measures if CNS, visual disturbances occur.
- Provide appropriate analgesics as needed for pains related to therapy.
- Monitor injection sites—pain and redness are common—for signs of infection or irritation.
- Provide environmental control as appropriate to help relieve migraine (lighting, temperature, etc).
- Monitor BP of patients with possible coronary artery disease; discontinue triptan at any sign of angina, prolonged high blood pressure, etc.

Teaching points
- Learn to use the autoinjector; injection may be repeated in not less than 1 hr if relief is not obtained; do not administer more than two injections in 24 hr (if appropriate).
- Be aware that this drug should not be taken during pregnancy; if you suspect that you are pregnant, contact physician and refrain from using drug.
- Be aware that the following side effects may occur: dizziness, drowsiness can occur (avoid driving or the use of dangerous machinery while on this drug); numbness, tingling, feelings of tightness or pressure.
- Maintain any procedures you usually use for a migraine—controlled lighting, etc.
- Report to physician immediately if you experience chest pain or pressure which is severe or does not go away.
- feelings of heat, flushing, tiredness, sickness, swelling of lips or eye-

Representative drugs
almotriptan
frovatriptan
naratriptan
rizatriptan
sumatriptan
zolmitriptan

Antivirals

PREGNANCY CATEGORY C

Therapeutic actions
Antiviral drugs inhibit viral DNA or RNA replication in the virus, preventing replication and leading to viral death.

Indications
- Initial and recurrent mucosal and cutaneous HSV 1 and 2 infections in immunocompromised patients, encephalitis, herpes zoster
- HIV infections (part of combination therapy)
- CMV retinitis in patients with AIDS
- Severe initial and recurrent genital herpes infections
- Treatment and prevention of influenza A respiratory tract illness
- Treatment of initial HSV genital infections and limited mucocutaneous HSV infections in immunocompromised patients (ointment)
- Unlabeled uses: treatment of herpes zoster, CMV and HSV infection following transplant, herpes simplex infections, infectious mononucleosis, varicella pneumonia, and varicella zoster in immunocompromised patients.

Contraindications and cautions
- Contraindications: allergy to the drug, seizures, CHF, renal disease, or lactation.

Adverse effects
Systemic administration
- **CNS:** Headache, vertigo, depression, tremors, encephalopathic changes
- **Dermatologic:** *Inflammation or phlebitis at injection sites,* rash, hair loss
- **GI:** *Nausea, vomiting,* diarrhea, anorexia
- **GU:** Crystalluria with rapid IV administration, hematuria

Topical administration
- **Skin:** *Transient burning at the site of application*

Interactions
✳ **Drug-drug** • Increased drug effects with probenecid • Increased nephrotoxicity with other nephrotoxic drugs
✳ **Drug-alternative therapy** • Decreased effectiveness if combined with St. John's wort

■ Nursing considerations
Assessment
- **History:** Allergy to drug, seizures, CHF, renal disease, lactation
- **Physical:** Skin color, lesions; orientation; BP, P, auscultation, perfusion, edema; R, adventitious sounds; urinary output; BUN, creatinine clearance

Interventions
Systemic administration
- Ensure that the patient is well hydrated with IV or PO fluids.
- Provide support and encouragement to deal with disease.
- Provide small, frequent meals if systemic therapy causes GI upset.
- Provide skin care, analgesics if necessary for rash.

Topical administration
- Start treatment as soon as possible after onset of signs and symptoms.
- Wear a rubber glove or finger cot when applying drug.

Teaching points
- Complete the full course of oral therapy, and do not exceed the prescribed dose.
- This drug is not a cure for your disease but should make you feel better.
- Possible side effects: nausea, vomiting, loss of appetite, diarrhea, headache, dizziness.
- Avoid sexual intercourse while visible lesions are present.
- Report difficulty urinating, skin rash, increased severity or frequency of recurrences.

Topical administration
- Wear rubber gloves or finger cots when applying the drug to prevent autoinoculation

of other sites and transmission of the disease.
- This drug does not cure the disease; application of the drug during symptom-free periods will not prevent recurrences.
- Avoid sexual intercourse while visible lesions are present.
- This drug may cause burning, stinging, itching, rash; notify health care provider if these are pronounced.

Representative drugs
abacavir
acyclovir
acyclovir sodium
adefovir
amantadine
amprenavir
cidofovir
delavirdine
didanosine
docosanol
efavirenz
famciclovir
fomivirsen
foscarnet
ganciclovir
imiquimod
indinavir
lamivudine
lopinavir
nelfinavir
nevirapine
oseltamivir
penciclovir
ribavirin
rimantadine
ritonavir
saquinavir
stavudine
tenofovir
valacyclovir
valganciclovir
vidarabine
zalcitabine
zanamivir
zidovudine

Barbiturates

Pregnancy Category D

C-II controlled substances

Therapeutic actions

Barbiturates act as sedatives, hypnotics, and anticonvulsants. They are general CNS depressants. Barbiturates inhibit impulse conduction in the ascending reticular activating system, depress the cerebral cortex, alter cerebellar function, depress motor output, and can produce excitation, sedation, hypnosis, anesthesia, and deep coma; at anesthetic doses, they have anticonvulsant activity.

Indications

- Sedatives or hypnotics for short-term treatment of insomnia
- Preanesthetic medications
- Anticonvulsants, in anesthetic doses, for emergency control of certain acute convulsive episodes (eg, status epilepticus, eclampsia, meningitis, tetanus, toxic reactions to strychnine or local anesthetics)

Contraindications and cautions

- Contraindications: hypersensitivity to barbiturates, manifest or latent porphyria, marked liver impairment, nephritis, severe respiratory distress, respiratory disease with dyspnea, obstruction, or cor pulmonale, previous addiction to sedative-hypnotic drugs, pregnancy (causes fetal damage, neonatal withdrawal syndrome), or lactation. Use cautiously with acute or chronic pain (paradoxical excitement or masking of important symptoms could result), seizure disorders (abrupt discontinuation of daily doses of drug can result in status epilepticus), fever, hyperthyroidism, diabetes mellitus, severe anemia, pulmonary or cardiac disease, status asthmaticus, shock, uremia.

Adverse effects

- **CNS:** *Somnolence, agitation, confusion, hyperkinesia, ataxia, vertigo, CNS depression, nightmares, lethargy, residual sedation (hangover), paradoxical excitement, nervousness, psychiatric distur-*bance, hallucinations, insomnia, anxiety, dizziness, abnormal thinking
- **CV:** *Bradycardia, hypotension, syncope*
- **GI:** *Nausea, vomiting, constipation, diarrhea, epigastric pain*
- **Hypersensitivity:** Skin rashes, angioneurotic edema, serum sickness, morbilliform rash, urticaria; rarely, exfoliative dermatitis, **Stevens-Johnson syndrome**
- **Local:** *Pain, tissue necrosis at injection site,* gangrene; arterial spasm with inadvertent intra-arterial injection; thrombophlebitis; permanent neurologic deficit if injected near a nerve
- **Respiratory:** *Hypoventilation, apnea, respiratory depression,* laryngospasm, bronchospasm, circulatory collapse
- **Other:** Tolerance, psychological and physical dependence; **withdrawal syndrome**

Interactions

✻ **Drug-drug** • Increased CNS depression with alcohol • Increased nephrotoxicity with methoxyflurane • Decreased effects of the following drugs given with barbiturates: oral anticoagulants, corticosteroids, oral contraceptives and estrogens, beta-adrenergic blockers (especially propranolol, metoprolol), theophylline, metronidazole, doxycycline, griseofulvin, phenylbutazones, quinidine

■ Nursing considerations
Assessment

- **History:** Hypersensitivity to barbiturates, manifest or latent porphyria; marked liver impairment; nephritis; severe respiratory distress; respiratory disease with dyspnea, obstruction, or cor pulmonale; previous addiction to sedative-hypnotic drugs; acute or chronic pain; seizure disorders; pregnancy; lactation; fever, hyperthyroidism; diabetes mellitus; severe anemia; pulmonary or cardiac disease; status asthmaticus; shock; uremia
- **Physical:** Weight; T; skin color, lesions, injection site; orientation, affect, reflexes; P, BP, orthostatic BP; R, adventitious sounds; bowel sounds, normal output, liver evaluation; liver and kidney function tests, blood and urine glucose, BUN

Interventions

- *Do not administer intra-arterially; may pro-* duce arteriospasm, thrombosis, gangrene.
- Administer IV doses slowly.
- Administer IM doses deep in a muscle mass.
- *Do not use parenteral dosage forms if solu-* tion is discolored or contains a precipitate.
- Monitor injection sites carefully for irritation, extravasation (IV); solutions are alkaline and very irritating to the tissues.
- Monitor P, BP, R carefully during IV administration.
- Provide resuscitative facilities on standby in case of respiratory depression, hypersensitivity reaction.
- Provide small, frequent meals, frequent mouth care if GI effects occur.
- Use safety precautions if CNS changes occur (side rails, accompany patient).
- Provide skin care if dermatologic effects occur.
- Provide comfort measures, reassurance for patients receiving pentobarbital for tetanus, toxic convulsions.
- Offer support and encouragement to patients receiving this drug for preanesthetic medication.
- Taper dosage gradually after repeated use, especially in epileptic patients.

Teaching points

When giving this drug as preanesthetic, incorporate teaching about the drug into general teaching about the procedure. Include:

- This drug will make you drowsy and less anxious.
- Do not try to get up after you have received this drug (request assistance if you must sit up or move about for any reason).

Outpatients

- Take this drug exactly as prescribed. This drug is habit forming; its effectiveness in facilitating sleep disappears after a short time. Do not take this drug longer than 2 wk (for insomnia), and do not increase the dosage without consulting health care provider. If the drug appears to be ineffective, consult health care provider.
- Avoid becoming pregnant while taking this drug. The use of oral contraceptives is not recommended as they lose their effectiveness while you are taking this drug.
- Possible side effects: drowsiness, dizziness, hangover, impaired thinking (these effects may become less pronounced after a few days; avoid driving a car or engaging in activities that require alertness); GI upset (taking the drug with food may help); dreams, nightmares, difficulty concentrating, fatigue, nervousness (these are effects of the drug that will go away when the drug is discontinued; consult your health care provider if these become bothersome).
- Report severe dizziness, weakness, drowsiness that persists, rash or skin lesions, pregnancy.

Representative drugs

amobarbital
butabarbital
mephobarbital
pentobarbital
pentobarbital sodium
phenobarbital
secobarbital

Benzodiazepines

PREGNANCY CATEGORY D

C-IV CONTROLLED SUBSTANCE

Therapeutic actions

Benzodiazepines are antianxiety agents, anticonvulsants, muscle relaxants, and sedative-hypnotics. Their exact mechanisms of action are not understood, but it is known that benzodiazepines potentiate the effects of gamma-aminobutyrate, an inhibitory neurotransmitter.

Indications

- Management of anxiety disorders, short-term relief of symptoms of anxiety
- Short-term treatment of insomnia
- Alone or as adjunct in treatment of Lennox-Gastaut syndrome (petit mal variant), akinetic and myoclonic seizures
- May be useful in patients with absence (petit mal) seizures who have not responded to succinimides; up to 30% of patients show

loss of effectiveness of drug within 3 mo of therapy (may respond to dosage adjustment)
- Unlabeled use: treatment of panic attacks, periodic leg movements during sleep, hypokinetic dysarthria, acute manic episodes, multifocal tic disorders; adjunct treatment of schizophrenia, neuralgias; treatment of irritable bowel syndrome

Contraindications and cautions
- Contraindications: hypersensitivity to benzodiazepines, psychoses, acute narrow-angle glaucoma, shock, coma, acute alcoholic intoxication with depression of vital signs, pregnancy (risk of congenital malformations, neonatal withdrawal syndrome), labor and delivery ("floppy infant" syndrome reported), or lactation (infants become lethargic and lose weight). Use cautiously with impaired liver or kidney function, debilitation.

Adverse effects
- **CNS:** *Transient, mild drowsiness initially; sedation, depression, lethargy, apathy, fatigue, light-headedness, disorientation, anger, hostility,* episodes of mania and hypomania, *restlessness, confusion, crying,* delirium, *headache,* slurred speech, dysarthria, stupor, rigidity, tremor, dystonia, vertigo, euphoria, nervousness, difficulty in concentration, vivid dreams, psychomotor retardation, extrapyramidal symptoms; mild paradoxical excitatory reactions during first 2 wk of treatment
- **CV:** Bradycardia, tachycardia, CV collapse, hypertension and hypotension, palpitations, edema
- **Dermatologic:** Urticaria, pruritus, skin rash, dermatitis
- **EENT:** Visual and auditory disturbances, diplopia, nystagmus, depressed hearing, nasal congestion
- **GI:** *Constipation, diarrhea, dry mouth,* salivation, *nausea,* anorexia, vomiting, difficulty in swallowing, gastric disorders, hepatic dysfunction, encopresis
- **GU:** Incontinence, urinary retention, changes in libido, menstrual irregularities
- **Hematologic:** Elevations of blood enzymes—LDH, alkaline phosphatase, AST, ALT; blood dyscrasias—agranulocytosis, leukopenia
- **Other:** Hiccups, fever, diaphoresis, paresthesias, muscular disturbances, gynecomastia; *drug dependence with withdrawal syndrome when drug is discontinued; more common with abrupt discontinuation of higher dosage used for longer than 4 mo*

Interactions
✳ **Drug-drug** ● Increased CNS depression with alcohol ● Increased effect with cimetidine, disulfiram, omeprazole, oral contraceptives ● Decreased effect with theophylline

■ Nursing considerations
Assessment
- **History:** Hypersensitivity to benzodiazepines, psychoses, acute narrow-angle glaucoma, shock, coma, acute alcoholic intoxication with depression of vital signs, pregnancy, lactation, impaired liver or kidney function, debilitation
- **Physical:** Skin color, lesions; T; orientation, reflexes, affect, ophthalmologic exam; P, BP; R, adventitious sounds; liver evaluation, abdominal exam, bowel sounds, normal output; CBC, liver and renal function tests

Interventions
- Keep addiction-prone patients under careful surveillance.
- Monitor liver function, blood counts in patients on long-term therapy.
- Ensure ready access to bathroom if GI effects occur; establish bowel program if constipation occurs.
- Provide small, frequent meals, frequent mouth care if GI effects occur.
- Provide measures appropriate to care of urinary problems (protective clothing, bed changing).
- Establish safety precautions if CNS changes occur (eg, side rails, accompany patient).
- Taper dosage gradually after long-term therapy, especially in epileptic patients; arrange substitution of another antiepileptic drug.
- Monitor patient for therapeutic drug levels; levels vary with drug being used.
- Arrange for patient to wear medical alert identification indicating epilepsy and drug therapy.

Teaching points

- Take drug exactly as prescribed; do not stop taking drug (long-term therapy) without consulting health care provider.
- Avoid alcohol, sleep-inducing, or OTC drugs.
- Possible side effects: drowsiness, dizziness (may become less pronounced after a few days; avoid driving or engaging in other dangerous activities); GI upset (take drug with food); fatigue; depression; dreams; crying; nervousness; depression, emotional changes; bed wetting, urinary incontinence.
- Report severe dizziness, weakness, drowsiness that persists, rash or skin lesions, difficulty voiding, palpitations, swelling in the extremities.

Representative drugs

alprazolam
chlordiazepoxide
clonazepam
clorazepate
diazepam
estazolam
flurazepam
lorazepam
oxazepam
quazepam
temazepam
triazolam

Beta-Adrenergic Blockers (β-Blockers)

PREGNANCY CATEGORY C (MOST), D (ATENOLOL), B (ACEBUTOLOL, PINDOLOL, SOTALOL)

Therapeutic actions

Beta-adrenergic blockers are antianginals, antiarrhythmics, and antihypertensives. Beta-blockers competitively block beta-adrenergic receptors in the heart and juxtaglomerular apparatus. They decrease the influence of the sympathetic nervous system on these tissues, the excitability of the heart, cardiac workload, oxygen consumption, and the release of renin; they lower BP. They have membrane-stabilizing (local anesthetic) effects that contribute to their antiarrhythmic action. They also act in the CNS to reduce sympathetic outflow and vasoconstrictor tone.

Indications

- Hypertension (alone or with other drugs, especially diuretics)
- Angina pectoris caused by coronary atherosclerosis
- Hypertrophic subaortic stenosis, to manage associated stress-induced angina, palpitations, and syncope; cardiac arrhythmias, especially supraventricular tachycardia, and ventricular tachycardias induced by digitalis or catecholamines; essential tremor, familial or hereditary
- Prevention of reinfarction in clinically stable patients when started 1–4 wk after MI
- Adjunctive therapy for pheochromocytoma after treatment with an alpha-adrenergic blocker, to manage tachycardia before or during surgery or if the pheochromocytoma is inoperable
- Prophylaxis for migraine headache (propranolol)
- Management of acute situational stress reaction (stage fright); essential tremor (propranolol)
- Unlabeled uses: treatment of recurrent GI bleeding in cirrhotic patients, schizophrenia, tardive dyskinesia, acute panic symptoms, vaginal contraceptive

Contraindications and cautions

- Contraindications: allergy to beta-blocking agents, sinus bradycardia, second- or third-degree heart block, cardiogenic shock, CHF, bronchial asthma, bronchospasm, COPD, pregnancy (neonatal bradycardia, hypoglycemia, and apnea have occurred in infants whose mothers received propranolol; low birth weight occurs with chronic maternal use during pregnancy), or lactation. Use cautiously with hypoglycemia and diabetes, thyrotoxicosis, hepatic dysfunction.

Adverse effects

- **Allergic reactions:** Pharyngitis, erythematous rash, fever, sore throat, laryngospasm, respiratory distress
- **CV:** *Bradycardia, CHF, cardiac arrhythmias, sinoatrial or AV nodal block, tachy-*

cardia, peripheral vascular insufficiency, claudication, **CVA,** pulmonary edema, hypotension
- **Dermatologic:** Rash, pruritus, sweating, dry skin
- **EENT:** Eye irritation, dry eyes, conjunctivitis, blurred vision
- **GI:** *Gastric pain, flatulence, constipation, diarrhea, nausea, vomiting,* anorexia, ischemic colitis, renal and mesenteric arterial thrombosis, retroperitoneal fibrosis, hepatomegaly, acute pancreatitis
- **GU:** *Impotence, decreased libido,* Peyronie's disease, dysuria, nocturia, frequency
- **Musculoskeletal:** Joint pain, arthralgia, muscle cramps
- **Neurologic:** Dizziness, vertigo, tinnitus, *fatigue,* emotional depression, paresthesias, sleep disturbances, hallucinations, disorientation, memory loss, slurred speech
- **Respiratory:** Bronchospasm, dyspnea, cough, bronchial obstruction, nasal stuffiness, rhinitis, pharyngitis
- **Other:** *Decreased exercise tolerance, development of antinuclear antibodies,* hyperglycemia or hypoglycemia, elevated serum transaminase, alkaline phosphatase, and LDH

Interactions
✳ **Drug-drug** • Increased effects with verapamil • Decreased effects with indomethacin, ibuprofen, piroxicam, sulindac, barbiturates • Prolonged hypoglycemic effects of insulin with beta-blockers • Peripheral ischemia possible if combined with ergot alkaloids • Initial hypertensive episode followed by bradycardia with epinephrine • Increased "first-dose response" to prazosin with beta-blockers • Increased serum levels and toxic effects with lidocaine, cimetidine • Increased serum levels of beta-blockers and phenothiazines, hydralazine if the two drugs are taken concurrently • Paradoxical hypertension when clonidine is given with beta-blockers; increased rebound hypertension when clonidine is discontinued • Decreased serum levels and therapeutic effects if taken with methimazole, propylthiouracil • Decreased bronchodilator effects of theophyllines • Decreased antihypertensive effects with NSAIDs (eg, ibuprofen, indomethacin, piroxicam, sulindac), rifampin

✳ **Drug-lab test** • Interference with glucose or insulin tolerance tests, glaucoma screening tests

■ Nursing considerations
Assessment
- **History:** Allergy to beta-blocking agents, sinus bradycardia, second- or third-degree heart block, cardiogenic shock, CHF, bronchial asthma, bronchospasm, COPD, hypoglycemia and diabetes, thyrotoxicosis, hepatic dysfunction, pregnancy, lactation
- **Physical:** Weight, skin color, lesions, edema, T; reflexes, affect, vision, hearing, orientation; BP, P, ECG, peripheral perfusion; R, auscultation; bowel sounds, normal output, liver evaluation; bladder palpation; liver and thyroid function tests, blood and urine glucose

Interventions
- Do not stop drug abruptly after long-term therapy (hypersensitivity to catecholamines may have developed, causing exacerbation of angina, MI, and ventricular arrhythmias). Taper drug gradually over 2 wk with monitoring.
- Consult with physician about withdrawing drug if patient is to undergo surgery (controversial).
- Give oral drug with food to facilitate absorption.
- Provide side rails and assistance with walking if CNS, vision changes occur.
- Position patient to decrease effects of edema, respiratory obstruction.
- Space activities, and provide periodic rest periods for patient.
- Provide frequent, small meals if GI effects occur.
- Provide comfort measures to help patient cope with eye, GI, joint, CNS, dermatologic effects.

Teaching points
- Take this drug with meals. Do not stop abruptly; abrupt discontinuation can worsen the disorder for which you are taking the drug.
- Possible side effects: dizziness, drowsiness, light-headedness, blurred vision (avoid driving or performing hazardous tasks); nausea, loss of appetite (frequent, small meals

may help); nightmares, depression (notify your health care provider, who may be able to change your medication); sexual impotence (you may want to discuss this with the health care provider).

• Report difficulty breathing, night cough, swelling of extremities, slow pulse, confusion, depression, rash, fever, sore throat.

• For diabetic patients, be aware that the normal signs of hypoglycemia (sweating, tachycardia) may be blocked by this drug; monitor your blood or urine glucose carefully; be sure to eat regular meals, and take your diabetic medication regularly.

Representative drugs
acebutolol
atenolol
betaxolol
bisoprolol
carteolol
esmolol
labetalol
metoprolol
nadolol
penbutolol
pindolol
propranolol
sotalol
timolol

Bisphosphonates

PREGNANCY CATEGORY C
(PARENTERAL), B (ORAL)

Therapeutic actions
Bisphosphonates inhibit bone resorption, possibly by inhibiting osteoclast activity and promoting osteoclast cell apoptosis; this action leads to decreased release of calcium from bone and decreased serum calcium level.

Indications
• Treatment of Paget's disease of bone (oral)
• Treatment of osteoporosis (oral) (postmenopausal and in males)
• Treatment of heterotopic ossification (oral)

• Treatment of hypercalcemia of malignancy in patients inadequately managed by diet or oral hydration (parenteral)
• Treatment of hypercalcemia of malignancy, which persists after adequate hydration has been restored (parenteral)

Contraindications and cautions
• Contraindications: allergy to bisphosphonates, hypocalcemia, pregnancy, lactation, severe renal impairment.
• Use cautiously in the presence of renal dysfunction, upper GI disease.

Adverse effects
• **CNS:** *headache,* dizziness
• **CV:** hypertension, chest pain
• **GI:** *nausea, diarrhea,* altered taste, metallic taste, *abdominal pain,* anorexia, esophageal erosion
• **Hematologic:** elevated BUN, serum creatinine, hypophosphatemia, hypokalemia, hypomagnesemia, hypocalcemia
• **Respiratory:** dyspnea, coughing, pleural effusion
• **Skeletal:** *increased or recurrent bone pain* (Paget's disease), focal osteomalacia, *arthralgia*
• **Other:** *infections* (UTI, candidiasis), *fever,* progression of cancer

Interactions
✳ **Drug-drug** • Increased risk of GI distress if taken with aspirin • Decreased absorption if oral form is taken with antacids, calcium, iron, multivalent cations; separate dosing by at least 30 min • Possible increased risk of hypocalcemia if parenteral form is given with aminoglycosides, loop diuretics; if this combination is used, monitor serum calcium levels closely

✳ **Drug-food** • Significantly decreased absorption and serum levels if oral form is taken with any food; administer on an empty stomach, 2 hr before meals

■ Nursing considerations
Assessment
• **History:** Allergy to bisphosphonates, renal failure, upper GI disease, lactation, pregnancy

- **Physical:** Muscle tone, bone pain, bowel sounds, urinalysis, serum calcium, renal function tests

Interventions

- Administer oral drug with a full glass of water, 2 hr before meals or any other medication; make sure that patient stays upright for at least 30 min after administration.
- Make sure that patient is well hydrated before and during therapy with parenteral agents.
- Monitor serum calcium levels before, during, and after therapy.
- Assure a 3-mo rest period after treatment for Paget's disease if retreatment is required; allow 7 days between treatments for hypercalcemia of malignancy.
- Ensure adequate vitamin D and calcium intake.
- Provide comfort measures if bone pain returns.

Teaching points

- Take drug with a full glass of water 2 hr before meals or any other medication; stay upright for at least 30 min after taking the drug.
- Periodic blood tests may be required to monitor your calcium levels.
- The following side effects may occur: nausea, diarrhea, bone pain, headache (analgesics may be available to help).
- Report twitching, muscle spasms, dark-colored urine, severe diarrhea, GI distress, epigastric pain.

Representative drugs

alendronate
etidronate
pamidronate
risedronate
tiludronate
zoledronic acid

Calcium Channel-Blockers

PREGNANCY CATEGORY C

Therapeutic actions

Calcium channel-blockers are antianginal and antihypertensive. They inhibit the movement of calcium ions across the membranes of cardiac and arterial muscle cells; this inhibition of transmembrane calcium flow results in the depression of impulse formation in specialized cardiac pacemaker cells, slowing of the velocity of conduction of the cardiac impulse, depression of myocardial contractility, and dilation of coronary arteries and arterioles and peripheral arterioles; these effects lead to decreased cardiac work, decreased cardiac energy consumption, and increased delivery of oxygen to myocardial cells.

Indications

- Treatment of angina pectoris due to coronary artery spasm (Prinzmetal's variant angina), chronic stable angina (effort-associated angina), hypertension, arrhythmias (supraventricular, those related to digoxin [verapamil]), subarachnoid hemorrhage (nimodipine)
- Orphan drug use in the treatment of interstitial cystitis, hypertensive emergencies, migraines, Raynaud's syndrome

Contraindications and cautions

- Contraindications: allergy to calcium channel-blockers, sick sinus syndrome, heart block, ventricular dysfunction, or pregnancy. Use cautiously during lactation.

Adverse effects

- **CNS:** *Dizziness, light-headedness, headache, asthenia,* fatigue, *nervousness,* sleep disturbances, blurred vision
- **CV:** *Peripheral edema, angina,* hypotension, arrhythmias, *bradycardia, AV block,* asystole
- **Dermatologic:** *Flushing, rash,* dermatitis, pruritus, urticaria
- **GI:** *Nausea, diarrhea, constipation,* cramps, flatulence, hepatic injury
- **Other:** *Nasal congestion, cough,* fever, chills, shortness of breath, muscle cramps, joint stiffness, sexual difficulties

Interactions

* **Drug-drug** • Increased effects with cimetidine, ranitidine • Increased toxicity of cyclosporine

■ Nursing considerations

Assessment

- **History:** Allergy to calcium channel-blockers, sick sinus syndrome, heart block, ventricular dysfunction; pregnancy; lactation
- **Physical:** Skin lesions, color, edema; orientation, reflexes; P, BP, baseline ECG, peripheral perfusion, auscultation; R, adventitious sounds; liver evaluation, normal GI output; liver function tests

Interventions

- Monitor patient carefully (BP, cardiac rhythm, and output) while drug is being titrated to therapeutic dose; the dosage may be increased more rapidly in hospitalized patients under close supervision.
- Ensure that patients do not chew or divide sustained-release tablets.
- Taper dosage of beta-blockers before beginning calcium channel-blocker therapy.
- Protect drug from light and moisture.
- Ensure ready access to bathroom.
- Provide comfort measures for skin rash, headache, nervousness.
- Establish safety precautions if CNS changes occur.
- Position patient to alleviate peripheral edema.
- Provide small, frequent meals if GI upset occurs.

Teaching points

- Do not chew or divide sustained-release tablets. Swallow whole.
- Possible side effects: nausea, vomiting (small, frequent meals may help); dizziness, lightheadedness, vertigo (avoid driving, operating hazardous machinery; avoid falling); muscle cramps, joint stiffness, sweating, sexual difficulties (should disappear when the drug therapy is stopped; discuss with health care provider if these become too uncomfortable).
- Report irregular heartbeat, shortness of breath, swelling of the hands or feet, pronounced dizziness, constipation.

Representative drugs

amlodipine
bepridil
diltiazem
felodipine
isradipine
nicardipine
nifedipine
nimodipine
nisoldipine
verapamil

Cephalosporins

PREGNANCY CATEGORY B

Therapeutic actions

Cephalosporins are antibiotics. They are bactericidal, inhibiting synthesis of bacterial cell wall, causing cell death in susceptible bacteria.

Indications

- Treatment of pharyngitis, tonsillitis caused by *Streptococcus pyogenes;* otitis media caused by *Streptococcus pneumoniae, Haemophilus influenzae, Moraxella catarrhalis, S. pyogenes;* respiratory infections caused by *S. pneumoniae, Haemophilus parainfluenzae, Staphylococcus aureus, Escherichia coli, Klebsiella, H. influenzae, S. pyogenes;* UTIs caused by *E. coli, Klebsiella pneumoniae;* dermatologic infections caused by *S. aureus, S. pyogenes, E. coli, Klebsiella, Enterobacter;* uncomplicated and disseminated gonorrhea caused by *Neisseria gonorrhoea;* septicemia caused by *S. pneumoniae, S. aureus, E. coli, Klebsiella, H. influenzae;* meningitis caused by *S. pneumoniae, H. influenzae, S. aureus, Neisseria meningitidis;* bone and joint infections caused by *S. aureus*
- Perioperative prophylaxis

Contraindications and cautions

- Contraindications: allergy to cephalosporins or penicillins, renal failure, or lactation.

Adverse effects

- **CNS:** Headache, dizziness, lethargy, paresthesias, seizures
- **GI:** *Nausea, vomiting, diarrhea, anorexia, abdominal pain, flatulence,* pseudomembranous colitis, liver toxicity

Adverse effects in *Italics* are most common; those in **Bold** are life-threatening.

- **GU:** Nephrotoxicity
- **Hematologic:** Bone marrow depression; decreased WBC, platelets, Hct
- **Hypersensitivity:** Ranging from *rash, fever* to **anaphylaxis;** serum sickness reaction
- **Local:** *Pain,* abscess at injection site, *phlebitis,* inflammation at IV site
- **Other:** *Superinfections, disulfiram-like reaction with alcohol*

Interactions

✳ **Drug-drug** • Increased nephrotoxicity with aminoglycosides • Increased bleeding effects with oral anticoagulants • Disulfiram-like reaction may occur if alcohol is taken within 72 hr after cephalosporin administration

✳ **Drug-lab test** • Possibility of false results on tests of urine glucose using Benedict's solution, Fehling's solution, *Clinitest* tablets; urinary 17-ketosteroids; direct Coombs' test

■ Nursing considerations
Assessment

- **History:** Allergy to any cephalosporin, liver and kidney dysfunction, lactation, pregnancy
- **Physical:** Skin status, liver and kidney function test, culture of affected area, sensitivity tests

Interventions

- Culture infected area and arrange for sensitivity tests before beginning drug therapy and during therapy if expected response is not seen.
- Administer oral drug with food to decrease GI upset and enhance absorption.
- Administer liquid drug to children who cannot swallow tablets; crushing the drug results in a bitter, unpleasant taste.
- Have vitamin K available in case hypoprothrombinemia occurs.
- Discontinue drug if hypersensitivity reaction occurs.
- Ensure ready access to bathroom and provide small, frequent meals if GI complications occur.
- Arrange for treatment of superinfections.

Teaching points
Oral drug

- Take full course of therapy.
- This drug is specific to an infection and should not be used to self-treat other problems.
- Swallow tablets whole; do not crush.
- Take the drug with food.
- Avoid drinking alcoholic beverages while taking and for 3 days after stopping this drug because severe reactions often occur (even with parenteral forms).
- Possible side effects: stomach upset or diarrhea.
- Report severe diarrhea with blood, pus, or mucus; rash; difficulty breathing; unusual tiredness, fatigue; unusual bleeding or bruising; unusual itching or irritation, pain at injection site.

Representative drugs
First generation
cefadroxil
cefazolin
cephalexin
cephapirin
cephradine

Second generation
cefaclor
cefmetazole
cefonicid
cefotetan
cefoxitin
cefpodoxime
cefprozil
cefuroxime
loracarbef

Third generation
cefdinir
cefditoren
cefepime
cefoperazone
cefotaxime
ceftazidime
ceftibuten
ceftizoxime
ceftriaxone

Corticosteroids

PREGNANCY CATEGORY C

Therapeutic actions
Corticosteroids enter target cells and bind to cytoplasmic receptors, initiating many complex reactions that are responsible for anti-

inflammatory, immunosuppressive (gluco-corticoid), and salt-retaining (mineralocorti-coid) actions. Some of these actions are con-sidered undesirable, depending on the indication for which the drug is being used.

Indications
Systemic administration

- Replacement therapy in adrenal cortical in-sufficiency
- Treatment of hypercalcemia associated with cancer
- Short-term management of various in-flammatory and allergic disorders such as rheumatoid arthritis, collagen diseases (SLE, etc.), dermatologic diseases (pemphigus, etc.), status asthmaticus, and autoimmune disorders
- Management of hematologic disorders—thrombocytopenic purpura, erythroblasto-penia
- Treatment of trichinosis with neurologic or myocardial involvement
- Treatment of ulcerative colitis, acute exac-erbations of multiple sclerosis, and pallia-tion in some leukemias and lymphomas

 Intra-articular or soft tissue adminis-tration: Treatment of arthritis, psoriatic plaques

 Retention enema: For ulcerative colitis, proctitis

 Dermatologic preparations: Relief of in-flammatory and pruritic manifestations of dermatoses that are steroid-responsive

 Anorectal cream, suppositories: Relief of discomfort from hemorrhoids and peri-anal itching or irritation

Contraindications and cautions

- *Systemic administration:* Infections, espe-cially tuberculosis, fungal infections, ame-biasis, hepatitis B, vaccinia, or varicella, and antibiotic-resistant infections; kidney dis-ease (predisposes to edema); liver disease, cirrhosis, hypothyroidism; ulcerative colitis with impending perforation; diverticulitis; recent GI surgery; active or latent peptic ul-cer; inflammatory bowel disease (drug may cause exacerbations or bowel perforation); hypertension, CHF; thromboembolitic ten-dencies, thrombophlebitis, osteoporosis, con-vulsive disorders, metastatic carcinoma, di-abetes mellitus; lactation.
- *Retention enemas, intrarectal foam:* Sys-temic fungal infections; recent intestinal sur-gery; extensive fistulas.
- *Topical dermatologic administration:* Fun-gal, tubercular, herpes simplex skin infec-tions; vaccinia, varicella; ear application when eardrum is perforated; lactation.

Adverse effects
Systemic administration

- **CNS:** *Vertigo, headache,* paresthesias, in-somnia, convulsions, psychosis
- **CV:** *Hypotension, shock,* hypertension and CHF secondary to fluid retention, thrombo-embolism, thrombophlebitis, fat embolism, cardiac arrhythmias secondary to electrolyte disturbances
- **Dermatologic:** *Thin, fragile skin; pe-techiae, ecchymoses,* purpura, striae, sub-cutaneous fat atrophy
- **Endocrine:** *Amenorrhea, irregular menses,* growth retardation, decreased car-bohydrate tolerance and diabetes mellitus, cushingoid state (long-term therapy), hypothalamic-pituitary-adrenal (HPA) sup-pression systemic with therapy longer than 5 days
- **Eye:** Cataracts, glaucoma (long-term ther-apy), increased intraocular pressure
- **GI:** *Peptic or esophageal ulcer, pancreati-tis,* abdominal distention, nausea, vomit-ing, increased appetite and weight gain (long-term therapy)
- **Hematologic:** *Na+ and fluid retention, hypokalemia,* hypocalcemia, increased blood sugar, increased serum cholesterol, decreased serum T_3 and T_4 levels
- **Hypersensitivity:** Anaphylactoid or hy-persensitivity reactions
- **Musculoskeletal:** *Muscle weakness,* steroid myopathy and loss of muscle mass, osteoporosis, spontaneous fractures (long-term therapy)
- **Other:** *Immunosuppression, aggrava-tion or masking of infections, impaired wound healing*

The following effects are related to specific routes of administration:

IM repository injections: Atrophy at injection site

Retention enema: Local pain, burning; rectal bleeding; systemic absorption and adverse effects (see above)

Intra-articular: Osteonecrosis, tendon rupture, infection

Intraspinal: Meningitis, adhesive arachnoiditis, conus medullaris syndrome

Intralesional therapy—head and neck: Blindness (rare)

Intrathecal administration: Arachnoiditis

Topical dermatologic ointments, creams, sprays, and so on: Local burning, irritation, acneiform lesions, striae, skin atrophy Systemic absorption can lead to HPA suppression (see above), growth retardation in children, and other systemic adverse effects. Children may be at special risk of systemic absorption because of their larger skin surface area–to–body weight ratio.

Interactions

✳ **Drug-drug** ● Increased steroid blood levels if taken concurrently with oral contraceptives, troleandomycin ● Decreased steroid blood levels if taken concurrently with phenytoin, phenobarbital, rifampin, cholestyramine ● Decreased serum level of salicylates if taken concurrently with corticosteroids ● Decreased effectiveness of anticholinesterases (ambenonium, edrophonium, neostigmine, pyridostigmine) if taken concurrently with corticosteroids

✳ **Drug-lab test** ● False-negative nitrobluetetrazolium test for bacterial infection (with systemic absorption) ● Suppression of skin test reactions

■ Nursing considerations
Assessment

● **History:** Infections, especially tuberculosis, fungal infections, amebiasis, hepatitis B, vaccinia, varicella, and antibiotic-resistant infections; kidney disease; liver disease, cirrhosis, hypothyroidism; ulcerative colitis with impending perforation; diverticulitis; recent GI surgery; active or latent peptic ulcer; inflammatory bowel disease; hypertension, CHF; thromboembolitic tendencies, thrombophlebitis, osteoporosis, convulsive disorders, metastatic carcinoma, diabetes mellitus; lactation

Retention enemas, intrarectal foam: Systemic fungal infections; recent intestinal surgery, extensive fistulas

Topical dermatologic administration: Fungal, tubercular, herpes simplex skin infections; vaccinia, varicella; ear application when eardrum is perforated

● **Physical:** *Systemic administration:* body weight, temperature; reflexes, affect, bilateral grip strength, ophthalmologic exam; BP, P, auscultation, peripheral perfusion, discoloration, pain or prominence of superficial vessels; R, adventitious sounds, chest x-ray; upper GI x-ray (history or symptoms of peptic ulcer), liver palpation; CBC, serum electrolytes, 2-hr postprandial blood glucose, urinalysis, thyroid function tests, serum cholesterol

Topical, dermatologic preparations: Affected area, integrity of skin

Interventions
Systemic administration

● Administer once a day before 9 AM to mimic normal peak diurnal corticosteroid levels and minimize HPA suppression.
● Space multiple doses evenly throughout the day.
● Do not give IM injections if patient has thrombocytopenia purpura.
● Rotate sites of IM repository injections to avoid local atrophy.
● Use minimal doses for shortest duration of time to minimize adverse effects.
● Arrange to taper doses when discontinuing high-dose or long-term therapy.
● Arrange for increased dosage when patient is subject to unusual stress.
● Use alternate-day maintenance therapy with short-acting corticosteroids whenever possible.
● Do not give live virus vaccines with immunosuppressive doses of glucocorticoids.
● Provide skin care if patient is bedridden.
● Provide small, frequent meals to minimize GI distress.
● Provide antacids between meals to help avoid peptic ulcer.
● Arrange for bed rails, other safety precautions if CNS, musculoskeletal effects occur.
● Avoid exposing patient to infection.

Topical dermatologic administration

- Use caution with occlusive dressings, tight or plastic diapers over affected area; these can increase systemic absorption.
- Avoid prolonged use, especially near eyes, in genital and rectal areas, on face and in skin creases.
- Provide careful wound care if lesions are present.
- Provide measures to deal with pain, discomfort on administration.

Teaching points
Systemic administration

- Take this drug exactly as prescribed. Do not stop taking this drug without notifying your health care provider; drug dosage must be slowly tapered to avoid problems.
- Take with meals or snacks if GI upset occurs.
- Take single daily or alternate-day doses before 9 AM; mark calendar or use other measures as reminder of treatment days.
- Do not overuse joint after intra-articular injections, even though pain may be gone.
- Arrange for frequent follow-up visits to your health care provider so that your response to the drug may be determined and the dosage adjusted if necessary.
- Know that the following side effects may occur: increase in appetite, weight gain (some of the weight gain may be from fluid retention, watching calories may be helpful); heartburn, indigestion (small, frequent meals, use of antacids between meals may help); increased susceptibility to infection (avoid crowded areas during peak cold or flu seasons and avoid contact with anyone with a known infection); poor wound healing (if you have an injury or wound, consult your health care provider); muscle weakness, fatigue (frequent rest periods may help).
- Wear a medical identification tag (applies to patients on long-term therapy) so that any emergency medical personnel will know that you are taking this drug.
- Report: unusual weight gain, swelling of lower extremities, muscle weakness, black or tarry stools, vomiting of blood, epigastric burning, puffing of face, menstrual irregularities, fever, prolonged sore throat, cold or other infection, worsening of symptoms.

- Know that with dosage reductions you may experience signs of adrenal insufficiency; report any of the following: fatigue, muscle and joint pains, anorexia, nausea, vomiting, diarrhea, weight loss, weakness, dizziness, low blood sugar (if patient monitors blood sugar).

Intra-articular, intralesional administration

- Do not overuse the injected joint even if the pain is gone. Follow directions you have been given for proper rest and exercise.

Topical dermatologic administration

- Apply sparingly and rub in lightly.
- Avoid eye contact.
- Report burning, irritation, or infection of the site, worsening of the condition.
- Avoid prolonged use.

Anorectal preparations

- Maintain normal bowel function by proper diet, adequate fluid intake, and regular exercise.
- Use stool softeners or bulk laxatives if needed.
- Notify your health care provider if symptoms do not improve in 7 days, or if bleeding, protrusion, or seepage occurs.

Representative drugs

alclometasone
amcinonide
beclomethasone
betamethasone
budesonide
clobetasol
clocortolone
cortisone
desonide
desoximetasone
dexamethasone
diflorasone
fludrocortisone
flunisolide
fluocinolone
fluocinonide
flurandrenolide
fluticasone
halcinonide
halobetasol
hydrocortisone
methylprednisolone
prednicarbate

prednisolone
prednisone
triamcinolone

Diuretics

PREGNANCY CATEGORY C

Therapeutic actions

Diuretics are divided into several subgroups. Thiazide and thiazide-related diuretics inhibit reabsorption of sodium and chloride in the distal renal tubule, increasing the excretion of sodium, chloride, and water by the kidney. Loop diuretics inhibit the reabsorption of sodium and chloride in the loop of Henle and in the distal renal tubule; because of this added effect, loop diuretics are more potent. Potassium-sparing diuretics block the effect of aldosterone on the renal tubule, leading to a loss of sodium and water and the retention of potassium; their overall effect is much weaker. Osmotic diuretics pull fluid out of the tissues with a hypertonic effect. Overall effect of diuretics is a loss of water and electrolytes from the body.

Indications

- Adjunctive therapy in edema associated with CHF, cirrhosis, corticosteroid and estrogen therapy, renal dysfunction
- Treatment of hypertension, alone or in combination with other antihypertensives
- Unlabeled uses: treatment of diabetes insipidus, especially nephrogenic diabetes insipidus, reduction of incidence of osteoporosis in postmenopausal women

Contraindications and cautions

- Contraindications: fluid or electrolyte imbalances, renal or liver disease, gout, SLE, glucose tolerance abnormalities, hyperparathyroidism, manic-depressive disorders, or lactation.

Adverse effects

- **CNS:** *Dizziness, vertigo,* paresthesias, weakness, headache, drowsiness, fatigue
- **CV:** Orthostatic hypotension, venous thrombosis, volume depletion, cardiac arrhythmias, chest pain
- **Dermatologic:** Photosensitivity, rash, purpura, exfoliative dermatitis
- **GI:** *Nausea, anorexia, vomiting, dry mouth, diarrhea, constipation,* jaundice, hepatitis, pancreatitis
- **GU:** *Polyuria, nocturia, impotence,* loss of libido
- **Hematologic:** Leukopenia, thrombocytopenia, agranulocytosis, aplastic anemia, neutropenia, fluid and electrolyte imbalances
- **Other:** Muscle cramps and muscle spasms, fever, hives, gouty attacks, flushing, weight loss, rhinorrhea, electrolyte imbalance

Interactions

✳ **Drug-drug** ● Increased thiazide effects and possible acute hyperglycemia with diazoxide ● Decreased absorption with cholestyramine, colestipol ● Increased risk of cardiac glycoside toxicity if hypokalemia occurs ● Increased risk of lithium toxicity ● Increased dosage of antidiabetic agents may be needed ● Risk of hyperkalemia if potassium-sparing diuretics are given with potassium preparations or ACE inhibitors ● Increased risk of ototoxicity if loop diuretics are taken with aminoglycosides or cisplatin

✳ **Drug-lab test** ● Monitor for decreased PBI levels without clinical signs of thyroid disturbances

■ Nursing considerations
Assessment

- **History:** Fluid or electrolyte imbalances, renal or liver disease, gout, SLE, glucose tolerance abnormalities, hyperparathyroidism, manic-depressive disorders, lactation
- **Physical:** Orientation, reflexes, muscle strength; pulses, BP, orthostatic BP, perfusion, edema, baseline ECG; respiratory rate, adventitious sounds; liver evaluation, bowel sounds; CBC, serum electrolytes, blood glucose; liver and renal function tests; serum uric acid, urinalysis

Interventions

- Administer with food or milk if GI upset occurs.
- Administer early in the day so increased urination will not disturb sleep.
- Ensure ready access to bathroom.
- Establish safety precautions if CNS effects, orthostatic hypotension occur.

- Measure and record regular body weights to monitor fluid changes.
- Provide mouth care, small frequent meals as needed.
- Monitor IV sites for any sign of extravasation.
- Monitor electrolytes frequently with parenteral use, periodically with chronic use.

Teaching points
- Take drug early in the day so sleep will not be disturbed by increased urination.
- Weigh yourself daily, and record weights.
- Protect skin from exposure to the sun or bright lights.
- Avoid foods high in potassium and the use of salt substitutes if taking a potassium-sparing diuretic.
- Take prescribed potassium replacement, and use foods high in potassium if taking a thiazide or loop diuretic.
- Increased urination will occur (stay close to bathroom facilities).
- Use caution if dizziness, drowsiness, feeling faint occur.
- Report rapid weight gain or loss, swelling in ankles or fingers, unusual bleeding or bruising, muscle cramps.

Representative drugs
Thiazide and related diuretics
bendroflumethiazide
benzthiazide
chlorothiazide
chlorthalidone
hydrochlorothiazide
hydroflumethiazide
indapamide
methyclothiazide
metolazone
polythiazide
Loop diuretics
bumetanide
ethacrynic acid
furosemide
torsemide
Potassium-sparing diuretics
amiloride
spironolactone
triamterene

Osmotic diuretic
mannitol

Fluoroquinolones

PREGNANCY CATEGORY C

Therapeutic actions
Fluoroquinolones are antibacterial. They are bactericidal, interfering with DNA replication in susceptible gram-negative bacteria, preventing cell reproduction and leading to death of bacteria.

Indications
- Treatment of infections caused by susceptible gram-negative bacteria, including *E. coli, Proteus mirabilis, K. pneumoniae, Enterobacter cloacae, Proteus vulgaris, Providencia rettgeri, Morganella morganii, Pseudomonas aeruginosa, Citrobacter freundii, S. aureus, S. epidermidis,* group D streptococci
- Unlabeled use: treatment of patients with cystic fibrosis who have pulmonary exacerbations

Contraindications and cautions
- Contraindications: allergy to any fluoroquinolone, pregnancy, or lactation. Use cautiously with renal dysfunction, seizures.

Adverse effects
- **CNS:** *Headache,* dizziness, insomnia, fatigue, somnolence, depression, blurred vision
- **GI:** *Nausea,* vomiting, dry mouth, *diarrhea,* abdominal pain
- **Hematologic:** Elevated BUN, AST, ALT, serum creatinine and alkaline phosphatase; decreased WBC, neutrophil count, hematocrit
- **Other:** Fever, rash, **photosensitivity**

Interactions
✳ **Drug-drug** • Decreased therapetic effect with iron salts, sucralfate • Decreased absorption with antacids • Increased serum levels and toxic effects of theophyllines with fluoroquinolones

Adverse effects in *Italics* are most common; those in **Bold** are life-threatening.

✻ Drug-alternative therapy • Increased risk of severe photosensitivity reactions with St. John's wort therapy

■ Nursing considerations
Assessment
- **History:** Allergy to fluoroquinolones, renal dysfunction, seizures, lactation
- **Physical:** Skin color, lesions; T; orientation, reflexes, affect; mucous membranes, bowel sounds; renal and liver function tests

Interventions
- Arrange for culture and sensitivity tests before beginning therapy.
- Continue therapy for 2 days after the signs and symptoms of infection have disappeared.
- Administer oral drug 1 hr before or 2 hr after meals with a glass of water.
- Ensure that patient is well hydrated during course of drug therapy.
- Administer antacids, if needed, at least 2 hr after dosing.
- Monitor clinical response; if no improvement is seen or a relapse occurs, repeat culture and sensitivity.
- Ensure ready access to bathroom if diarrhea occurs.
- Arrange for appropriate bowel training program if constipation occurs.
- Provide small, frequent meals if GI upset occurs.
- Arrange for monitoring of environment (noise, temperature) and analgesics, for headache.
- Establish safety precautions if CNS, visual changes occur.
- Encourage patient to complete full course of therapy.

Teaching points
- Take oral drug on an empty stomach, 1 hr before or 2 hr after meals. If an antacid is needed, do not take it within 2 hr of ciprofloxacin dose.
- Drink plenty of fluids.
- Possible side effects: nausea, vomiting, abdominal pain (small, frequent meals may help); diarrhea or constipation (consult health care provider); drowsiness, blurring of vision, dizziness (observe caution if driving or using hazardous equipment).

- Report rash, visual changes, severe GI problems, weakness, tremors.

Representative drugs
ciprofloxacin
gatifloxacin
levofloxacin
lomefloxacin
moxifloxacin
norfloxacin
ofloxacin
sparfloxacin
trovafloxacin

Histamine₂ (H₂) Antagonists

PREGNANCY CATEGORY B

Therapeutic actions
Histamine₂ antagonists inhibit the action of histamine at the histamine₂ receptors of the stomach, inhibiting gastric acid secretion and reducing total pepsin output; the resultant decrease in acid allows healing of ulcerated areas.

Indications
- Short-term treatment of active duodenal ulcer and benign gastric ulcer
- Treatment of pathologic hypersecretory conditions (Zollinger-Ellison syndrome) and erosive gastroesophageal reflux disease
- Prophylaxis of stress-induced ulcers and acute upper GI bleed in critically ill patients

Contraindications and cautions
- Contraindications: allergy to H₂ blockers, impaired renal or hepatic function, or lactation.

Adverse effects
- **CNS:** Dizziness, somnolence, headache, confusion, hallucinations, peripheral neuropathy, symptoms of brain stem dysfunction (dysarthria, ataxia, diplopia)
- **CV:** Cardiac arrhythmias, arrest; hypotension (IV use)
- **GI:** *Diarrhea*
- **Hematologic:** Increases in plasma creatinine, serum transaminase
- **Other:** Impotence (reversible with drug withdrawal), gynecomastia (long-term treat-

ment), rash, vasculitis, pain at IM injection site

Interactions

✳ **Drug-drug** • Increased risk of decreased white blood cell counts with antimetabolites, alkylating agents, other drugs known to cause neutropenia • Increased serum levels and risk of toxicity of warfarin-type anticoagulants, phenytoin, beta-adrenergic blocking agents, alcohol, quinidine, lidocaine, theophylline, chloroquine, certain benzodiazepines (alprazolam, chlordiazepoxide, diazepam, flurazepam, triazolam), nifedipine, pentoxifylline, tricyclic antidepressants, procainamide, carbamazepine when taken with H_2 blockers

■ Nursing considerations

Assessment
- **History:** Allergy to H_2 blockers, impaired renal or hepatic function, lactation
- **Physical:** Skin lesions; orientation, affect; pulse, baseline ECG (continuous with IV use); liver evaluation, abdominal exam, normal output; CBC, liver, and renal function tests

Interventions
- Administer drug with meals and hs.
- Decrease doses in renal dysfunction and liver dysfunction.
- Administer IM dose undiluted, deep into large muscle group.
- Ensure ready access to bathroom.
- Provide comfort measures for skin rash, headache.
- Establish safety measures if CNS changes occur (side rails, accompany patient).
- Arrange for regular follow-up, including blood tests to evaluate effects.

Teaching points
- Take drug with meals and at bedtime; therapy may continue for 4–6 wk or longer.
- Take prescribed antacids exactly as prescribed, be careful of the time.
- Inform health care provider about your cigarette smoking habits. Cigarette smoking decreases the effectiveness of this drug.
- Have regular medical follow-up while on this drug to evaluate your response.

- Report sore throat, fever, unusual bruising or bleeding, tarry stools, confusion, hallucinations, dizziness, muscle or joint pain.

Representative drugs
cimetidine
famotidine
nizatidine
ranitidine

HMG CoA Inhibitors

PREGNANCY CATEGORY X

Therapeutic actions
HMG CoA inhibitors are antihyperlipidemic. They are a fungal metabolite that inhibits the enzyme that catalyzes the first step in the cholesterol synthesis pathway in humans, resulting in a decrease in serum cholesterol, serum LDLs (associated with increased risk of coronary artery disease), and either an increase or no change in serum HDLs (associated with decreased risk of coronary artery disease).

Indications
- Adjunct to diet in the treatment of elevated total and LDL cholesterol in patients with primary hypercholesterolemia (types IIa and IIb) whose response to dietary restriction of saturated fat and cholesterol and other nonpharmacologic measures has not been adequate.

Contraindications and cautions
- Contraindications: allergy to HMG CoA inhibitors, fungal byproducts, pregnancy, or lactation. Use cautiously with impaired hepatic function, cataracts.

Adverse effects
- **CNS:** *Headache, blurred vision,* dizziness, insomnia, fatigue, muscle cramps, cataracts
- **GI:** *Flatulence, abdominal pain, cramps, constipation, nausea, vomiting,* heartburn
- **Hematologic:** Elevations of CPK, alkaline phosphatase, and transaminases
- **Musculoskeletal:** Rhabdomyolysis with possible renal failure

Adverse effects in *Italics* are most common; those in **Bold** are life-threatening.

Interactions

✳ **Drug-drug** • Monitor patients receiving HMG CoA inhibitors for possible severe myopathy or rhabdomyolysis if taken with cyclosporine, erythromycin, gemfibrozil, niacin

■ Nursing considerations

Assessment

- **History:** Allergy to HMG CoA inhibitors, fungal byproducts; impaired hepatic function; cataracts; pregnancy; lactation
- **Physical:** Orientation, affect, ophthalmologic exam; liver evaluation; lipid studies, liver function tests

Interventions

- Administer drug hs; highest rates of cholesterol synthesis are between midnight and 5 AM.
- Consult with dietitian about low-cholesterol diets.
- Arrange for diet and exercise consultation.
- Arrange for regular follow-up during long-term therapy.
- Provide comfort measures to deal with headache, muscle cramps, nausea.
- Arrange for periodic ophthalmologic exam to check for cataract development.
- Offer support and encouragement to deal with disease, diet, drug therapy, and follow-up.

Teaching points

- Take drug at bedtime.
- Institute appropriate diet changes.
- Possible side effects: nausea (small, frequent meals may help); headache, muscle and joint aches and pains (may lessen with time).
- Have periodic ophthalmic exams while you are on this drug.
- Report severe GI upset, changes in vision, unusual bleeding or bruising, dark urine or light-colored stools; muscle pain, weakness.

Representative drugs

atorvastatin
fluvastatin
lovastatin
pravastatin
simvastatin

Macrolide Antibiotics

PREGNANCY CATEGORY B, C
(DIRITHROMYCIN)

Therapeutic actions

Macrolides are antibiotics. They are bacteriostatic or bactericidal in susceptible bacteria; they bind to cell membranes and cause changes in protein function, leading to bacterial cell death.

Indications

- Treatment of acute infections caused by sensitive strains of *S. pneumoniae, Mycoplasma pneumoniae, Listeria monocytogenes, Legionella pneumophila;* URIs, LRIs, skin and soft-tissue infections caused by group A beta-hemolytic streptococci when oral treatment is preferred to injectable benzathine penicillin; PID caused by *N. gonorrhoeae* in patients allergic to penicillin; intestinal amebiasis caused by *Entamoeba histolytica;* infections in the newborn and in pregnancy that are caused by *Chlamydia trachomatis* and in adult chlamydial infections when tetracycline cannot be used; primary syphilis (*Treponema pallidum*) in penicillin-allergic patients; eliminating *Bordetella pertussis* organisms from the nasopharynx of infected individuals and as prophylaxis in exposed and susceptible individuals; superficial ocular infections caused by susceptible strains of microorganisms; prophylaxis of ophthalmia neonatorum caused by *N. gonorrhoeae* or *C. trachomatis*
- Treatment of acne vulgaris and skin infections caused by sensitive microorganisms
- In conjunction with sulfonamides to treat URIs caused by *H. influenzae*
- Adjunct to antitoxin in infections caused by *Corynebacterium diphtheriae* and *Corynebacterium minutissimum*
- Prophylaxis against alpha-hemolytic streptococcal endocarditis before dental or other procedures in patients allergic to penicillin who have valvular heart disease and against infection in minor skin abrasions
- Unlabeled uses: erythromycin base is used with neomycin before colorectal surgery to

reduce wound infection; treatment of severe diarrhea associated with *Campylobacter* enteritis or enterocolitis; treatment of genital, inguinal, or anorectal lymphogranuloma venereum infection; treatment of *Haemophilus ducreyi* (chancroid).

Contraindications and cautions

- Contraindications: allergy to any macrolide antibiotic. Use cautiously with hepatic dysfunction or lactation (secreted and may be concentrated in breast milk; may modify bowel flora of nursing infant and interfere with fever workups).

Adverse effects

- **CNS:** Reversible hearing loss, confusion, uncontrollable emotions, abnormal thinking
- **Dermatologic:** Edema, urticaria, dermatitis, angioneurotic edema
- **GI:** *Abdominal cramping, anorexia, diarrhea, vomiting,* pseudomembranous colitis, hepatotoxicity
- **Hypersensitivity:** Allergic reactions ranging from rash to **anaphylaxis**
- **Local:** *Irritation, burning, itching* at site of application
- **Other:** *Superinfections*

Interactions

✳ **Drug-drug** • Increased serum levels of digoxin • Increased effects of oral anticoagulants, theophyllines, carbamazepine • Increased therapeutic and toxic effects of corticosteroids • Increased levels of cyclosporine and risk of renal toxicity • Increased irritant effects with peeling, desquamating, or abrasive agents used with dermatologic preparations

✳ **Drug-lab test** • Interferes with fluorometric determination of urinary catecholamines • Decreased urinary estriol levels due to inhibition of hydrolysis of steroids in the gut

■ Nursing considerations
Assessment

- **History:** Allergy to macrolides, hepatic dysfunction, lactation, viral, fungal, mycobacterial infections of the eye (ophthalmologic)
- **Physical:** Site of infection, skin color, lesions; orientation, affect, hearing tests; R, adventitious sounds; GI output, bowel sounds, liver evaluation; culture and sensitivity tests of infection, urinalysis, liver function tests

Interventions

- Culture site of infection prior to therapy.
- Administer oral erythromycin base or stearate on an empty stomach, 1 hr before or 2–3 hr after meals, with a full glass of water (oral erythromycin estolate, ethylsuccinate, and certain enteric-coated tablets; see manufacturer's instructions; may be given without regard to meals).
- Administer drug around the clock to maximize therapeutic effect; scheduling may have to be adjusted to minimize sleep disruption.
- Monitor liver function in patients on prolonged therapy.
- Institute hygiene measures and treatment if superinfections occur.
- If GI upset occurs with oral therapy, some preparations (see previous) may be given with meals, or it may be possible to substitute one of these preparations.
- Provide small, frequent meals if GI problems occur.
- Establish safety measures (accompany patient, side rails) if CNS changes occur.
- Give patient support and encouragement to continue with therapy.
- Wash affected area, rinse well, and dry before topical application.

Teaching points

- Take oral drug on an empty stomach, 1 hour before or 2–3 hr after meals, with a full glass of water, or, as appropriate, drug may be taken without regard to meals. The drug should be taken around the clock; schedule to minimize sleep disruption. It is important that you finish the *full course* of the drug therapy.
- Possible side effects: stomach cramping, discomfort (taking the drug with meals, if appropriate, may alleviate this problem); uncontrollable emotions, crying, laughing, abnormal thinking (will end when the drug is stopped).
- Report severe or watery diarrhea, severe nausea or vomiting, dark urine, yellowing of the

---

Adverse effects in Italics are most common; those in Bold are life-threatening.

skin or eyes, loss of hearing, skin rash or itching.

- Wash and rinse area and pat it dry before applying topical solution; use fingertips or an applicator; wash hands thoroughly after application.

Representative drugs
azithromycin
clarithromycin
dirithromycin
erythromycin

Narcotics

PREGNANCY CATEGORY C

C-II CONTROLLED SUBSTANCE

Therapeutic actions
Narcotics act as agonists at specific opioid receptors in the CNS to produce analgesia, euphoria, sedation; the receptors mediating these effects are thought to be the same as those mediating the effects of endogenous opioids (enkephalins, endorphins).

Indications
- Relief of moderate to severe acute and chronic pain
- Preoperative medication to sedate and allay apprehension, facilitate induction of anesthesia, and reduce anesthetic dosage
- Analgesic adjunct during anesthesia
- A component of most preparations referred to as Brompton's cocktail or mixture, an oral alcoholic solution used for chronic severe pain, especially in terminal cancer patients
- Intraspinal use with microinfusion devices for the relief of intractable pain
- Unlabeled use: relief of dyspnea associated with acute left ventricular failure and pulmonary edema

Contraindications and cautions
- Contraindications: hypersensitivity to narcotics, diarrhea caused by poisoning until toxins are eliminated, during labor or delivery of a premature infant (may cross immature blood–brain barrier more readily), after biliary tract surgery or following surgical anastomosis, pregnancy, or labor (can cause respiratory depression of neonate; may prolong labor). Use cautiously with head injury and increased intracranial pressure; acute asthma, COPD, cor pulmonale, preexisting respiratory depression, hypoxia, hypercapnia (may decrease respiratory drive and increase airway resistance); lactation (may be safer to wait 4–6 hr after administration to nurse the baby); acute abdominal conditions; cardiovascular disease, supraventricular tachycardias; myxedema; convulsive disorders; acute alcoholism, delirium tremens; cerebral arteriosclerosis; ulcerative colitis; fever; kyphoscoliosis; Addison's disease; prostatic hypertrophy, urethral stricture; recent GI or GU surgery; toxic psychosis; renal or hepatic dysfunction.

Adverse effects
- **CNS:** *Light-headedness, dizziness, sedation,* euphoria, dysphoria, delirium, insomnia, agitation, anxiety, fear, hallucinations, disorientation, drowsiness, lethargy, impaired mental and physical performance, coma, mood changes, weakness, headache, tremor, convulsions, miosis, visual disturbances, suppression of cough reflex
- **CV:** Facial flushing, peripheral circulatory collapse, tachycardia, *bradycardia,* arrhythmia, palpitations, chest wall rigidity, hypertension, hypotension, orthostatic hypotension, syncope
- **Dermatologic:** Pruritus, urticaria, laryngospasm, bronchospasm, edema
- **GI:** *Nausea, vomiting,* dry mouth, anorexia, constipation, biliary tract spasm; increased colonic motility in patients with chronic ulcerative colitis
- **GU:** Ureteral spasm, spasm of vesical sphincters, urinary retention or hesitancy, oliguria, antidiuretic effect, reduced libido or potency
- **Local:** Tissue irritation and induration (SC injection)
- **Major hazards: Respiratory depression, apnea, circulatory depression, respiratory arrest, shock, cardiac arrest**
- **Other:** *Sweating,* physical tolerance and dependence, psychological dependence

Interactions

✳ Drug-drug • Increased likelihood of respiratory depression, hypotension, profound sedation, or coma in patients receiving barbiturate general anesthetics.

✳ Drug-lab test • Elevated biliary tract pressure (an effect of narcotics) may cause increases in plasma amylase, lipase; determinations of these levels may be unreliable for 24 hr

■ Nursing considerations
Assessment

• **History:** Hypersensitivity to narcotics; diarrhea caused by poisoning; labor or delivery of a premature infant; biliary tract surgery or surgical anastomosis; head injury and increased intracranial pressure; acute asthma, COPD, cor pulmonale, preexisting respiratory depression, hypoxia, hypercapnia; acute abdominal conditions; CV disease, supraventricular tachycardias; myxedema; convulsive disorders; acute alcoholism, delirium tremens; cerebral arteriosclerosis; ulcerative colitis; fever; kyphoscoliosis; Addison's disease; prostatic hypertrophy; urethral stricture; recent GI or GU surgery; toxic psychosis; renal or hepatic dysfunction; pregnancy; lactation

• **Physical:** T; skin color, texture, lesions; orientation, reflexes, bilateral grip strength, affect; P, auscultation, BP, orthostatic BP, perfusion; R, adventitious sounds; bowel sounds, normal output; urinary frequency, voiding pattern, normal output; ECG; EEG; thyroid, liver, kidney function tests

Interventions

• Caution patient not to chew or crush controlled-release preparations.
• Dilute and administer IV slowly to minimize likelihood of adverse effects.
• Direct patient to lie down during IV administration.
• Provide narcotic antagonist, facilities for assisted or controlled respiration on standby during IV administration.
• Use caution when injecting SC or IM into chilled areas or in patients with hypotension or in shock; impaired perfusion may delay absorption; with repeated doses, an excessive amount may be absorbed when circulation is restored.
• Monitor injection sites for irritation, extravasation.
• Instruct postoperative patients in pulmonary toilet; drug suppresses cough reflex.
• Monitor bowel function and arrange for anthraquinone laxatives for severe constipation.
• Institute safety precautions (side rails, assist walking) if CNS, vision effects occur.
• Provide frequent, small meals if GI upset occurs.
• Provide environmental control if sweating, visual difficulties occur.
• Provide back rubs, positioning, and other nondrug measures to alleviate pain.
• Reassure patient about addiction liability; most patients who receive opiates for medical reasons do not develop dependence syndromes.

Teaching points

When the drug is used as a preoperative medication, teach the patient about it when explaining the procedure.

• Take this drug exactly as prescribed. Avoid alcohol, antihistamines, sedatives, tranquilizers, OTC drugs.
• Possible side effects: nausea, loss of appetite (take the drug with food and lie quietly); constipation (notify health care provider if this is severe; a laxative may help); dizziness, sedation, drowsiness, impaired visual acuity (avoid driving or performing other tasks requiring alertness, visual acuity).
• Do not take any leftover medication for other disorders, and do not let anyone else take your prescription.
• Report severe nausea, vomiting, constipation, shortness of breath or difficulty breathing, skin rash.

Representative drugs

codeine
fentanyl
hydrocodone
hydromorphone
levomethadyl
levorphanol
meperidine
methadone

morphine sulfate
opium
oxycodone
oxymorphone
propoxyphene
remifentanil
sufentanil

Nitrates

PREGNANCY CATEGORY C

Therapeutic actions

Nitrates are antianginals. They relax vascular smooth muscle with a resultant decrease in venous return and decrease in arterial blood pressure, which reduces left ventricular workload and decreases myocardial oxygen consumption, relieving the pain of angina.

Indications

- Treatment of acute angina (sublingual, translingual, inhalant preparations)
- Prophylaxis of angina (oral sustained release, sublingual, topical, transdermal, translingual, transmucosal preparations)
- Treatment of angina unresponsive to recommended doses of organic nitrates or beta-blockers (IV preparations)
- Management of perioperative hypertension, CHF associated with acute myocardial infarction (IV preparations)
- Produce controlled hypotension during surgery (IV preparations)
- Unlabeled uses: reduction of cardiac workload in acute MI and in CHF (sublingual, topical) and adjunctive treatment of Raynaud's disease (topical)

Contraindications and cautions

- Contraindications: allergy to nitrates, angle-closure glaucoma, severe anemia, early MI, head trauma, cerebral hemorrhage, cardiomyopathy, pregnancy, or lactation. Use cautiously with hepatic or renal disease, hypotension or hypovolemia, increased intracranial pressure, constrictive pericarditis, pericardial tamponade, low ventricular filling pressure or low pulmonary capillary wedge pressure (PCWP).

Adverse effects

- **CNS:** *Headache,* apprehension, restlessness, weakness, vertigo, dizziness, faintness
- **CV:** Tachycardia, retrosternal discomfort, palpitations, **hypotension,** syncope, collapse, postural hypotension, angina
- **Dermatologic:** Rash, exfoliative dermatitis, cutaneous vasodilation with flushing, pallor, perspiration, cold sweat, contact dermatitis (transdermal preparations), topical allergic reactions (topical nitroglycerin ointment)
- **GI:** Nausea, vomiting, incontinence of urine and feces, abdominal pain
- **Local:** Local burning sensation at the point of dissolution (sublingual)
- **Other:** Ethanol intoxication with high dose IV use (alcohol in diluent)

Interactions

✴ **Drug-drug** • Increased risk of hypertension and decreased antianginal effect with ergot alkaloids • Decreased pharmacologic effects of heparin • Risk of orthostatic hypotension with calcium channel-blockers

✴ **Drug-lab test** • False report of decreased serum cholesterol if done by the Zlatkis-Zak color reaction

■ Nursing considerations
Assessment

- **History:** Allergy to nitrates, severe anemia, early MI, head trauma, cerebral hemorrhage, hypertrophic cardiomyopathy, hepatic or renal disease, hypotension or hypovolemia, increased intracranial pressure, constrictive pericarditis, pericardial tamponade, low ventricular filling pressure or low PCWP, pregnancy, lactation
- **Physical:** Skin color, T, lesions; orientation, reflexes, affect; P, BP, orthostatic BP, baseline ECG, peripheral perfusion; R, adventitious sounds; liver evaluation, normal output; liver function tests (IV); renal function tests (IV); CBC, Hgb

Interventions

- Administer sublingual preparations under the tongue or in the buccal pouch. Encourage the patient not to swallow. Ask patient if the tablet "fizzles" or burns. Check the expiration date on the bottle; store at room temperature, protected from light.

Discard unused drug 6 mo after bottle is opened (conventional tablets); stabilized tablets (*Nitrostat*) are less subject to loss of potency.

- Administer sustained-release preparations with water; tell the patient not to chew the tablets or capsules; do not crush these preparations.
- Administer topical ointment by applying the ointment over a 6 × 6-in area in a thin, uniform layer using the applicator. Cover area with plastic wrap held in place by adhesive tape. Rotate sites of application to decrease the chance of inflammation and sensitization; close tube tightly when finished.
- Administer transdermal systems to skin site free of hair and not subject to much movement. Shave areas that have a lot of hair. Do not apply to distal extremities. Change sites slightly to decrease the chance of local irritation and sensitization. Remove transdermal system before attempting defibrillation or cardioversion.
- Administer transmucosal tablets by placing them between the lip and gum above the incisors or between the cheek and gum. Encourage patient not to swallow and not to chew the tablet.
- Administer the translingual spray directly onto the oral mucosa; preparation is not to be inhaled.
- Withdraw drug gradually, 4–6 wk recommended period for the transdermal preparations.
- Establish safety measures if CNS effects, hypotension occur.
- Keep environment cool, dim, and quiet.
- Provide periodic rest periods for patient.
- Provide comfort measures and arrange for analgesics if headache occurs.
- Maintain life support equipment on standby if overdose occurs or cardiac condition worsens.
- Provide support and encouragement to deal with disease, therapy, and needed lifestyle changes.

Teaching points

- Place sublingual tablets under your tongue or in your cheek; do not chew or swallow

the tablet; the tablet should burn or "fizzle" under the tongue. Take the nitroglycerin before chest pain begins, when you anticipate that your activities or situation may precipitate an attack. Do not buy large quantities; this drug does not store well. Keep the drug in a dark, dry place, in a dark-colored glass bottle with a tight lid; do not combine with other drugs. You may repeat your dose every 5 min for a total of 3 tablets; if the pain is still not relieved, go to an emergency room.

- Do not chew or crush the timed-release preparations; take on an empty stomach.
- Spread a thin layer of topical ointment on the skin using the applicator. Do not rub or massage the area. Cover with plastic wrap held in place with adhesive tape. Wash your hands after application. Keep the tube tightly closed. Rotate the sites frequently to prevent local irritation.
- To use transdermal systems, you may need to shave an area for application. Apply to a slightly different area each day. Use care if changing brands; each system has a different concentration.
- Place transmucosal tablets between the lip and gum or between the gum and cheek. Do not chew; try not to swallow.
- Spray translingual spray directly onto oral mucous membranes; do not inhale. Use 5–10 min before activities that you anticipate will precipitate an attack.
- Take drug exactly as directed; do not exceed recommended dosage.
- Possible side effects: dizziness, lightheadedness (this may pass as you adjust to the drug; use care to change positions slowly); headache (lying down in a cool environment and resting may help; OTC preparations may not help); flushing of the neck or face (this usually passes as the drug's effects pass).
- Report blurred vision, persistent or severe headache, skin rash, more frequent or more severe angina attacks, fainting.

Representative drugs
amyl nitrite
isosorbide dinitrate

isosorbide mononitrate
nitroglycerin

Nondepolarizing Neuromuscular Junction Blockers (NMJ Blockers)

PREGNANCY CATEGORY C

Therapeutic actions

NMJ blockers interfere with neuromuscular transmission and cause flaccid paralysis by blocking acetylcholine receptors at the skeletal neuromuscular junction.

Indications

- Adjuncts to general anesthetics to facilitate endotracheal intubation and relax skeletal muscle; to relax skeletal muscle to facilitate mechanical ventilation.

Contraindications and cautions

- Contraindications: hypersensitivity to NMJ blockers and the bromide ion. Use cautiously with myasthenia gravis; pregnancy (teratogenic in preclinical studies; may be used in cesarean section, but reversal may be difficult if patient has received magnesium sulfate to manage preeclampsia); renal or hepatic disease, respiratory depression, altered fluid or electrolyte balance; patients in whom an increase in heart rate may be dangerous.

Adverse effects

- **CV:** *Increased heart rate*
- **Hypersensitivity:** Hypersensitivity reactions, especially rash
- **MS:** Profound and prolonged muscle paralysis
- **Respiratory:** *Depressed respiration, apnea,* bronchospasm

Interactions

✴ **Drug-drug** • Increased intensity and duration of neuromuscular block with some anesthetics (isoflurane, enflurane, halothane, diethyl ether, methoxyflurane), some parenteral antibiotics (aminoglycosides, clindamycin, lincomycin, bacitracin, polymyxin B, and sodium colistimethate), ketamine, quinine, quinidine, trimethaphan, calcium channel-blocking drugs (eg, verapamil), Mg^{2+} salts, and in hypokalemia (produced by K^+ depleting diuretics) • Decreased intensity of neuromuscular block with acetylcholine, cholinesterase inhibitors, K^+ salts, theophyllines, phenytoins, azathioprine, mercaptopurine, carbamazepine

■ Nursing considerations

Assessment

- **History:** Hypersensitivity to NMJ blockers and the bromide ion, myasthenia gravis, pregnancy, renal or hepatic disease, respiratory depression, altered fluid or electrolyte balance
- **Physical:** Weight, T, skin condition, hydration, reflexes, bilateral grip strength, pulse, BP, respiratory rate and adventitious sounds, liver and kidney function, serum electrolytes

Interventions

- Drug should be given only by trained personnel (anesthesiologists).
- Arrange to have facilities on standby to maintain airway and provide mechanical ventilation.
- Provide neostigmine, pyridostigmine, or edrophonium (cholinesterase inhibitors) on standby to overcome excessive neuromuscular block.
- Provide atropine or glycopyrrolate on standby to prevent parasympathomimetic effects of cholinesterase inhibitors.
- Provide a peripheral nerve stimulator on standby to assess degree of neuromuscular block, as needed.
- Change patient's position frequently, and provide skin care to prevent decubitus ulcer formation when drug is used for other than brief periods.
- Monitor conscious patient for pain, distress that patient may not be able to communicate.
- Reassure conscious patients frequently.

Teaching points

- Teaching points about what the drug does and how the patient will feel should be incorporated into overall teaching program about the procedure.

Representative drugs

atracurium

cisatracurium
doxacurium
mivacurium
pancuronium
rocuronium
tubocurarine
vecuronium

Nonsteroidal Anti-inflammatory Drugs (NSAIDs)

PREGNANCY CATEGORY B OR C

Therapeutic actions
NSAIDs have anti-inflammatory, analgesic, and antipyretic activities largely related to inhibition of prostaglandin synthesis; exact mechanisms of action are not known.

Indications
- Relief of signs and symptoms of rheumatoid arthritis and osteoarthritis
- Relief of mild to moderate pain
- Treatment of primary dysmenorrhea
- Fever reduction
- Unlabeled use: treatment of juvenile rheumatoid arthritis

Contraindications and cautions
- Contraindications: allergy to salicylates or other NSAIDs (more common in patients with rhinitis, asthma, chronic urticaria, nasal polyps); CV dysfunction, hypertension; peptic ulceration, GI bleeding; pregnancy or lactation. Use cautiously with impaired hepatic function, impaired renal function.

Adverse effects
- **CNS:** *Headache, dizziness, somnolence, insomnia,* fatigue, tiredness, dizziness, tinnitus, ophthalmologic effects
- **Dermatologic:** *Rash,* pruritus, sweating, dry mucous membranes, stomatitis
- **GI:** *Nausea, dyspepsia, GI pain,* diarrhea, vomiting, *constipation,* flatulence
- **GU:** Dysuria, renal impairment
- **Hematologic:** Bleeding, platelet inhibition with higher doses, neutropenia, eosinophilia, leukopenia, pancytopenia, thrombocytopenia, agranulocytosis, granulocytopenia, aplastic anemia, decreased hemoglobin or hematocrit, bone marrow depression, menorrhagia
- **Respiratory:** Dyspnea, hemoptysis, pharyngitis, bronchospasm, rhinitis
- **Other:** Peripheral edema, anaphylactoid reactions to **anaphylactic shock**

Interactions
✳ **Drug-drug** ● Increased toxic effects of lithium with NSAIDs ● Decreased diuretic effect with loop diuretics: bumetanide, furosemide, ethacrynic acid ● Potential decrease in antihypertensive effect of beta-adrenergic blocking agents

■ Nursing considerations
Assessment
- **History:** Allergy to salicylates or other NSAIDs; CV dysfunction, hypertension; peptic ulceration, GI bleeding; impaired hepatic function; impaired renal function; pregnancy; lactation
- **Physical:** Skin color, lesions; T; orientation, reflexes, ophthalmologic evaluation, audiometric evaluation, peripheral sensation; P, BP, edema; R, adventitious sounds; liver evaluation, bowel sounds; CBC, clotting times, urinalysis, renal and liver function tests, serum electrolytes, stool guaiac

Interventions
- Administer drug with food or after meals if GI upset occurs.
- Establish safety measures if CNS, visual disturbances occur.
- Arrange for periodic ophthalmologic examination during long-term therapy.
- Arrange for discontinuation of drug if eye changes, symptoms of liver dysfunction, renal impairment occur.
- Institute emergency procedures if overdose occurs (gastric lavage, induction of emesis, supportive therapy).
- Provide comfort measures to reduce pain (positioning, environmental control) and to reduce inflammation (warmth, positioning, rest).
- Provide small, frequent meals if GI upset is severe.

Adverse effects in *Italics* are most common; those in **Bold** are life-threatening.

Teaching points

- Use the drug only as suggested. Do not exceed the prescribed dosage. Take the drug with food or after meals if GI upset occurs.
- Possible side effects: nausea, GI upset, dyspepsia (take with food); diarrhea or constipation; drowsiness, dizziness, vertigo, insomnia (use caution when driving or operating dangerous machinery).
- Avoid OTC drugs while taking this drug. Many of these drugs contain similar medications, and serious overdosage can occur. If you feel that you need one of these preparations, consult with health care provider.
- Avoid alcohol while taking this drug.
- Report sore throat, fever, rash, itching, weight gain, swelling in ankles or fingers, changes in vision, black or tarry stools.

Representative drugs

celecoxib
diclofenac
diflunisal
etodolac
fenoprofen
flurbiprofen
ibuprofen
indomethacin
ketoprofen
ketorolac
meclofenamate
mefenamic acid
meloxicam
nabumetone
naproxen
oxaprozin
piroxicam
rofecoxib
sulindac
tolmetin
valdecoxib

Penicillins

PREGNANCY CATEGORY B

Therapeutic actions

Penicillins are antibiotics. They are bactericidal, inhibiting the synthesis of cell wall of sensitive organisms, causing cell death in susceptible organisms.

Indications

- Treatment of moderate to severe infections caused by sensitive organisms: streptococci, pneumococci, staphylococci, *N. gonorrhoeae, T. pallidum,* meningococci, *Actinomyces israelii, Clostridium perfringens, Clostridium tetani, Leptotrichia buccalis* (Vincent's disease), *Spirillium minus* or *Streptobacillus moniliformis, L. monocytogenes, Pasteurella multocida, Erysipelothrix insidiosa, E. coli, Enterobacter aerogenes, Alcaligenes faecalis, Salmonella, Shigella, P. mirabilis, C. diphtheriae, Bacillus anthracis*
- Treatment of syphilis, gonococcal infections
- Unlabeled use: treatment of Lyme disease

Contraindications and cautions

- Contraindications: allergy to penicillins, cephalosporins, other allergens. Use cautiously with renal disease, pregnancy, lactation (may cause diarrhea or candidiasis in the infant).

Adverse effects

- **CNS:** Lethargy, hallucinations, seizures
- **GI:** *Glossitis, stomatitis, gastritis, sore mouth,* furry tongue, black "hairy" tongue, *nausea, vomiting, diarrhea,* abdominal pain, bloody diarrhea, enterocolitis, pseudomembranous colitis, nonspecific hepatitis
- **GU:** Nephritis-oliguria, proteinuria, hematuria, casts, azotemia, pyuria
- **Hematologic:** Anemia, thrombocytopenia, leukopenia, neutropenia, prolonged bleeding time
- **Hypersensitivity:** *Rash, fever, wheezing,* **anaphylaxis**
- **Local:** *Pain, phlebitis,* thrombosis at injection site, Jarisch-Herxheimer reaction when used to treat syphilis
- **Other:** *Superinfections,* sodium overload, leading to CHF

Interactions

✳ **Drug-drug** • Decreased effectiveness with tetracyclines • Inactivation of parenteral aminoglycosides (amikacin, gentamicin, kanamycin, neomycin, netilmicin, streptomycin, tobramycin) if mixed in the same solution • Risk of increased serum levels if combined with aspirin, indomethacin, diuretics, sulfonamides

✳ **Drug-lab test** • False-positive Coombs' test (IV)

■ Nursing considerations
Assessment
- **History:** Allergy to penicillins, cephalosporins, other allergens, renal disease, lactation
- **Physical:** Culture infected area; skin rashes, lesions; R, adventitious sounds; bowel sounds, normal output; CBC, liver function tests, renal function tests, serum electrolytes, hematocrit, urinalysis; skin test with benzylpenicylloyl-polylysine if hypersensitivity reactions have occurred

Interventions
- Culture infected area before beginning treatment; reculture area if response is not as expected.
- Use the smallest dose possible for IM injection to avoid pain and discomfort.
- Arrange to continue treatment for 48–72 hr beyond the time that the patient becomes asymptomatic.
- Monitor serum electrolytes and cardiac status if penicillin G is given by IV infusion. Na or K preparations have been associated with severe electrolyte imbalances.
- Check IV site carefully for signs of thrombosis or local drug reaction.
- Do not give IM injections repeatedly in the same site; atrophy can occur. Monitor injection sites.
- Explain the reason for parenteral routes of administration; offer support and encouragement to deal with therapy.
- Provide small, frequent meals if GI upset occurs.
- Arrange for comfort and treatment measures for superinfections.
- Provide for frequent mouth care if GI effects occur.
- Ensure that bathroom facilities are readily available if diarrhea occurs.
- Maintain epinephrine, IV fluids, vasopressors, bronchodilators, oxygen, and emergency equipment on standby in case of serious hypersensitivity reaction.
- Arrange for the use of corticosteroids, antihistamines for skin reactions.

Teaching points
- Possible side effects: upset stomach, nausea, vomiting (small, frequent meals may help); sore mouth (frequent mouth care may help); diarrhea; pain or discomfort at the injection site (report this if it becomes too uncomfortable).
- Report unusual bleeding, sore throat, rash, hives, fever, severe diarrhea, difficulty breathing.

Representative drugs
amoxicillin
ampicillin
carbenicillin
cloxacillin
dicloxacillin
mezlocillin
nafcillin
oxacillin
penicillin G benzathine
penicillin G potassium
penicillin G procaine
penicillin V
piperacillin
ticarcillin

Phenothiazines

PREGNANCY CATEGORY C

Therapeutic actions
Mechanism of action of phenothiazines is not fully understood. Antipsychotic drugs block postsynaptic dopamine receptors in the brain, but this may not be necessary and sufficient for antipsychotic activity; depresses the RAS, including the parts of the brain involved with wakefulness and emesis; anticholinergic, antihistaminic (H_1), and alpha-adrenergic blocking activity also may contribute to some of its therapeutic (and adverse) actions.

Indications
- Management of manifestations of psychotic disorders
- Control of severe nausea and vomiting, intractable hiccups

Adverse effects in *Italics* are most common; those in **Bold** are life-threatening.

Contraindications and cautions

- Contraindications: coma or severe CNS depression, bone marrow depression, blood dyscrasia, circulatory collapse, subcortical brain damage, Parkinson's disease, liver damage, cerebral arteriosclerosis, coronary disease, severe hypotension or hypertension, prolonged QTc interval. Use cautiously with respiratory disorders ("silent pneumonia" may develop); glaucoma, prostatic hypertrophy; epilepsy or history of epilepsy; breast cancer; thyrotoxicosis; peptic ulcer, decreased renal function; myelography within previous 24 hr or scheduled within 48 hr; exposure to heat or phosphorous insecticides; pregnancy; lactation; children younger than 12 yr, especially those with chickenpox, CNS infections (children are especially susceptible to dystonias that may confound the diagnosis of Reye's syndrome).

Adverse effects
Antipsychotic drugs

- **Autonomic:** Dry mouth, salivation, nasal congestion, nausea, vomiting, anorexia, fever, pallor, flushed facies, sweating, constipation, paralytic ileus, urinary retention, incontinence, polyuria, enuresis, priapism, ejaculation inhibition, male impotence
- **CNS:** *Drowsiness,* insomnia, vertigo, headache, weakness, tremor, ataxia, slurring, cerebral edema, seizures, exacerbation of psychotic symptoms, extrapyramidal syndromes—*pseudoparkinsonism; dystonias; akathisia,* tardive dyskinesias, potentially irreversible (no known treatment) **neuroleptic malignant syndrome**
- **CV:** Hypotension, orthostatic hypotension, hypertension, tachycardia, bradycardia, cardiac arrest, CHF, cardiomegaly, **refractory arrhythmias,** pulmonary edema, prolonged QTc interval
- **EENT:** Glaucoma, *photophobia, blurred vision,* miosis, mydriasis, deposits in the cornea and lens (opacities), pigmentary retinopathy
- **Endocrine:** Lactation, breast engorgement in females, galactorrhea; syndrome of inappropriate ADH secretion; amenorrhea, menstrual irregularities; gynecomastia in males; changes in libido; hyperglycemia or hypoglycemia; glycosuria; hyponatremia; pituitary tumor with hyperprolactinemia;

inhibition of ovulation, infertility, pseudopregnancy; reduced urinary levels of gonadotropins, estrogens, progestins
- **Hematologic:** Eosinophilia, leukopenia, leukocytosis, anemia; aplastic anemia; hemolytic anemia; thrombocytopenic or nonthrombocytopenic purpura; pancytopenia
- **Hypersensitivity:** Jaundice, urticaria, angioneurotic edema, laryngeal edema, photosensitivity, eczema, asthma, anaphylactoid reactions, exfoliative dermatitis
- **Respiratory:** Bronchospasm, laryngospasm, dyspnea; suppression of cough reflex and potential for aspiration (**sudden death related to asphyxia** or cardiac arrest has been reported)
- **Other:** *Urine discolored pink to red-brown*

Interactions

✳ Drug-drug ● Additive CNS depression with alcohol ● Additive anticholinergic effects and possibly decreased antipsychotic efficacy with anticholinergic drugs ● Increased likelihood of seizures with metrizamide (contrast agent used in myelography) ● Increased chance of severe neuromuscular excitation and hypotension if given to patients receiving barbiturate anesthetics (methohexital, thiamylal, phenobarbital, thiopental) ● Decreased antihypertensive effect of guanethidine when taken with antipsychotics ● Increased risk of cardiac arrhythmias and serious adverse effects if combined with drugs that prolong the QTc interval.

✳ Drug-lab test ● False-positive pregnancy tests (less likely if serum test is used) ● Increase in protein-bound iodine, not attributable to an increase in thyroxine

■ Nursing considerations
Assessment

- **History:** Coma or severe CNS depression; bone marrow depression; blood dyscrasia; circulatory collapse; subcortical brain damage; Parkinson's disease; liver damage; cerebral arteriosclerosis; coronary disease; severe hypotension or hypertension; respiratory disorders; glaucoma, prostatic hypertrophy; epilepsy or history of epilepsy; breast cancer; thyrotoxicosis; peptic ulcer, decreased renal function; myelography within previous 24 hr or myelography scheduled within 48 hr; exposure to heat or phosphorous insecticides;

pregnancy; children younger than 12 yr, especially those with chickenpox, CNS infections

- **Physical:** Weight, T; reflexes, orientation, intraocular pressure; P, BP, orthostatic BP; R, adventitious sounds; bowel sounds and normal output, liver evaluation; urinary output, prostate size; CBC, urinalysis, thyroid, liver and kidney function tests, ECG analysis

Interventions

- Obtain baseline ECG with QTc interval noted.
- Dilute oral concentrate *only* with water, saline, 7-Up, homogenized milk, carbonated orange drink, and pineapple, apricot, prune, orange, V-8, tomato, and grapefruit juices; use 60 ml of diluent for each 16 mg (5 ml) of concentrate.
- Do *not* mix with beverages that contain caffeine (coffee, cola), tannics (tea), or pectinates (apple juice); physical incompatibility may result.
- Give IM injections only to seated or recumbent patients, and observe for adverse effects for a brief period afterward.
- Monitor pulse and BP continuously during IV administration.
- Do not change dosage in long-term therapy more often than weekly; drug requires 4–7 days to achieve steady-state plasma levels.
- Avoid skin contact with oral solution; contact dermatitis has occurred.
- Arrange for discontinuation of drug if serum creatinine, BUN become abnormal or if WBC count is depressed.
- Monitor bowel function, arrange therapy for severe constipation; adynamic ileus with fatal complications has occurred.
- Monitor elderly patients for dehydration and institute remedial measures promptly; sedation and decreased sensation of thirst related to CNS effects of drug can lead to severe dehydration.
- Consult physician regarding warning of patient or patient's guardian about tardive dyskinesias.
- Consult physician about dosage reduction, use of anticholinergic antiparkinsonian

drugs (controversial) if extrapyramidal effects occur.

- Provide safety measures (side rails, assist) if sedation, ataxia, vertigo, orthostatic hypotension, vision changes occur.
- Provide positioning to relieve discomfort of dystonias.
- Provide reassurance to deal with extrapyramidal effect, sexual dysfunction.

Teaching points

- Take drug exactly as prescribed. The full effect may require 6 wk–6 mo of therapy.
- Avoid skin contact with drug solutions.
- Avoid driving or engaging in activities requiring alertness if CNS, vision changes occur.
- Avoid prolonged exposure to sun or use a sunscreen or covering garments if exposure is necessary.
- Maintain fluid intake, and use precautions against heatstroke in hot weather.
- Report sore throat, fever, unusual bleeding or bruising, rash, weakness, tremors, impaired vision, dark urine (pink or reddish brown urine is to be expected), pale stools, yellowing of the skin or eyes.

Representative drugs

chlorpromazine
fluphenazine
mesoridazine
methotrimeprazine
perphenazine
prochlorperazine
promethazine
thioridazine
trifluoperazine
triflupromazine

Selective Serotonin Reuptake Inhibitors (SSRIs)

PREGNANCY CATEGORY C

Therapeutic actions

The selective serotonin reuptake inhibitors act as antidepressants by inhibiting CNS neuronal uptake of serotonin and blocking uptake of serotonin with little effect on norepinephrine; they are also thought to antagonize muscarinic, histaminergic, and alpha$_1$-adrenergic receptors. The increase in serotonin levels at neuroreceptors is thought to act as a stimulant, counteracting depression and increasing motivation.

Indications

- Treatment of depression; most effective in patients with major depressive disorder
- Treatment of obsessive-compulsive disorders, post-traumatic stress disorder, social anxiety, generalized anxiety disorder, panic disorder, PMDD
- Unlabeled uses: treatment of obesity, bulimia

Contraindications and cautions

- Contraindications: hypersensitivity to any SSRI; pregnancy. Use cautiously with impaired hepatic or renal function, diabetes mellitus, lactation

Adverse effects

- **CNS:** *Headache, nervousness, insomnia, drowsiness, anxiety, tremor, dizziness, light-headedness,* agitation, sedation, abnormal gait, convulsions
- **CV:** Hot flashes, palpitations
- **Dermatologic:** *Sweating, rash, pruritus,* acne, alopecia, contact dermatitis
- **GI:** *Nausea, vomiting, diarrhea, dry mouth, anorexia, dyspepsia, constipation, taste changes,* flatulence, gastroenteritis, dysphagia, gingivitis
- **GU:** *Painful menstruation, sexual dysfunction, frequency,* cystitis, impotence, urgency, vaginitis
- **Respiratory:** *URIs, pharyngitis,* cough, dyspnea, bronchitis, rhinitis
- **Other:** *Weight loss, asthenia, fever*

Interactions

✷ **Drug-drug** • Increased therapeutic and toxic effects of tricyclic antidepressants with SSRIs • Decreased therapeutic effects with cyproheptadine • Risk for severe to fatal hypertensive crisis with MAOIs; avoid this combination

✷ **Drug-alternative therapy** • Increased risk of severe reaction with St. John's wort therapy

■ Nursing considerations
Assessment

- **History:** Hypersensitivity to any SSRI; impaired hepatic or renal function; diabetes mellitus; lactation; pregnancy
- **Physical:** Weight; T; skin rash, lesions; reflexes, affect; bowel sounds, liver evaluation; P, peripheral perfusion; urinary output, renal function; renal and liver function tests, CBC

Interventions

- Arrange for lower dose or less frequent administration in elderly patients and patients with hepatic or renal impairment.
- Establish suicide precautions for severely depressed patients. Dispense only a small number of capsules at a time to these patients.
- Administer drug in the morning. If dose of > 20 mg/day is needed, administer in divided doses.
- Monitor patient response for up to 4 wk before increasing dose because of lack of therapeutic effect. It frequently takes several weeks to see the desired effect.
- Provide small, frequent meals if GI upset or anorexia occurs. Monitor weight loss; a nutritional consultation may be necessary.
- Provide sugarless lozenges, frequent mouth care if dry mouth is a problem.
- Ensure ready access to bathroom facilities if diarrhea occurs. Establish bowel program if constipation is a problem.
- Establish safety precautions (side rails, appropriate lighting, accompanying patient, etc.) if CNS effects occur.
- Provide appropriate comfort measures if CNS effects, insomnia, rash, sweating occur.
- Encourage patient to maintain therapy for treatment of underlying cause of depression.

Teaching points

- It may take up to 4 wk to get a full antidepressant effect from this drug. The drug should be taken in the morning (or in divided doses if necessary).
- The following side effects may occur: dizziness, drowsiness, nervousness, insomnia (avoid driving or performing hazardous tasks); nausea, vomiting, weight loss (small, frequent meals may help; monitor your weight loss—if it becomes marked, consult with your health care provider); sexual dys-

function (drug effect); flulike symptoms (if severe, check with your health care provider for appropriate treatment); photosensitivity (avoid exposure to sunlight).

- Do not take this drug during pregnancy. If you think that you are pregnant or you wish to become pregnant, consult with your physician.
- Report rash, mania, seizures, severe weight loss.

Representative drugs
citalopram
escitalopram
fluoxetine
fluvoxamine
paroxetine
sertraline

Sulfonamides

PREGNANCY CATEGORY C

PREGNANCY CATEGORY D (AT TERM)

Therapeutic actions
Sulfonamides are antibiotics. They are bacteriostatic; competitively antagonize paraaminobenzoic acid, an essential component of folic acid synthesis, in susceptible gram-negative and gram-positive bacteria, causing cell death.

Indications
- Treatment of ulcerative colitis, otitis media, inclusion conjunctivitis, meningitis, nocardiosis, toxoplasmosis, trachoma, UTIs
- Management of rheumatoid arthritis, collagenous colitis, Crohn's disease

Contraindications and cautions
- Contraindications: allergy to sulfonamides, sulfonylureas, thiazides; pregnancy (teratogenic in preclinical studies; at term, may bump fetal bilirubin from plasma protein binding sites and cause kernicterus); or lactation (risk of kernicterus, diarrhea, rash). Use cautiously with impaired renal or hepatic function, G-6-PD deficiency, porphyria.

Adverse effects
- **CNS:** Headache, peripheral neuropathy, mental depression, convulsions, ataxia, hallucinations, tinnitus, vertigo, insomnia, hearing loss, drowsiness, transient lesions of posterior spinal column, transverse myelitis
- **Dermatologic:** Photosensitivity, cyanosis, petechiae, alopecia
- **GI:** Nausea, emesis, abdominal pains, diarrhea, bloody diarrhea, anorexia, pancreatitis, stomatitis, impaired folic acid absorption, hepatitis, hepatocellular necrosis
- **GU:** Crystalluria, hematuria, proteinuria, nephrotic syndrome, toxic nephrosis with oliguria and anuria, oligospermia, infertility
- **Hematologic: Agranulocytosis, aplastic anemia,** thrombocytopenia, leukopenia, hemolytic anemia, hypoprothrombinemia, methemoglobinemia, megaloblastic anemia
- **Hypersensitivity: Stevens-Johnson syndrome,** generalized skin eruptions, epidermal necrolysis, urticaria, serum sickness, pruritus, **exfoliative dermatitis, anaphylactoid reactions,** periorbital edema, conjunctival and scleral redness, photosensitization, arthralgia, allergic myocarditis, transient pulmonary changes with eosinophilia, decreased pulmonary function
- **Other:** Drug fever, chills, periarteritis nodosum

Interactions
✴ **Drug-drug** • Increased risk of hypoglycemia when tolbutamide, tolazamide, glyburide, glipizide, acetohexamide, chlorpropamide are taken concurrently • Increased risk of folate deficiency if taking sulfonamides; monitor patients receiving folic acid carefully for signs of folate deficiency

✴ **Drug-lab test** • Possible false-positive urinary glucose tests using Benedict's method

■ Nursing considerations
Assessment
- **History:** Allergy to sulfonamides, sulfonylureas, thiazides; pregnancy; lactation; impaired renal or hepatic function; G-6-PD deficiency; porphyria
- **Physical:** T; skin color, lesions; culture of infected site; orientation, reflexes, affect, pe-

ripheral sensation; R, adventitious sounds; mucous membranes, bowel sounds, liver evaluation; liver and renal function tests, CBC and differential, urinalysis

Interventions
- Arrange for culture and sensitivity tests of infected area prior to therapy; repeat cultures if response is not as expected.
- Administer drug after meals or with food to prevent GI upset. Administer the drug around the clock.
- Ensure adequate fluid intake.
- Discontinue drug immediately if hypersensitivity reaction occurs.
- Establish safety precautions if CNS effects occur (side rails, assistance, environmental control).
- Protect patient from exposure to light (use of sunscreen, protective clothing) if photosensitivity occurs.
- Provide small, frequent meals if GI upset occurs.
- Provide mouth care for stomatitis.
- Offer support and encouragement to deal with side effects of drug therapy, including changes in sexual function.

Teaching points
- Complete full course of therapy.
- Take the drug with food or meals to decrease GI upset.
- Drink eight glasses of water per day.
- This drug is specific to this disease; do not use to self-treat any other infection.
- Possible side effects: sensitivity to sunlight (use sunscreens; wear protective clothing); dizziness, drowsiness, difficulty walking, loss of sensation (avoid driving or performing tasks that require alertness); nausea, vomiting, diarrhea (ensure ready access to bathroom); loss of fertility; yellow-orange urine.
- Report blood in the urine, rash, ringing in the ears, difficulty breathing, fever, sore throat, chills.

Representative drugs
balsalazide
sulfadiazine
sulfasalazine
sulfisoxazole

Tetracyclines

Pregnancy Category D

Therapeutic actions
Tetracyclines are antibiotics. They are bacteriostatic; inhibit protein synthesis of susceptible bacteria, preventing cell replication.

Indications
- Treatment of infections caused by rickettsiae; *M. pneumoniae;* agents of psittacosis, ornithosis, lymphogranuloma venereum, and granuloma inguinale; *Borrelia recurrentis, H. ducreyi, Pasteurella pestis, Pasteurella tularensis, Bartonella bacilliformis, Bacteroides, Vibrio comma, Vibrio fetus, Brucella, E. coli, E. aerogenes, Shigella, Acinetobacter calcoaceticus, H. influenzae, Klebsiella, Diplococcus pneumoniae, S. aureus;* when penicillin is contraindicated, infections caused by *N. gonorrhoeae, T. pallidum, Treponema pertenue, L. monocytogenes, Clostridium, B. anthracis, Fusobacterium fusiforme, Actinomyces, N. meningitidis*
- Adjunct to amebicides in acute intestinal amebiasis
- Treatment of acne
- Treatment of complicated urethral, endocervical, or rectal infections in adults caused by *C. trachomatis*
- Treatment of superficial ocular infections due to susceptible strains of microorganisms
- Prophylaxis of ophthalmia neonatorum due to *N. gonorrhoeae* or *C. trachomatis*

Contraindications and cautions
- Contraindications: allergy to any of the tetracyclines, allergy to tartrazine (in 250-mg tetracycline capsules marketed under brand names Panmycin, Sumycin, Tetracyn, and Tetracap), pregnancy (toxic to the fetus), lactation (causes damage to the teeth of infant). Use cautiously with hepatic or renal dysfunction, presence of ocular viral, mycobacterial, or fungal infections.

Adverse effects
- **Dermatologic:** *Phototoxic reactions, rash,* **exfoliative dermatitis**

- **GI:** *Discoloring and inadequate calcification of primary teeth of fetus if used by pregnant women, discoloring and inadequate calcification of permanent teeth if used during period of dental development,* fatty liver, liver failure, *anorexia, nausea, vomiting, diarrhea, glossitis, dysphagia,* enterocolitis, esophageal ulcers
- **Hematologic:** Hemolytic anemia, thrombocytopenia, neutropenia, eosinophilia, leukocytosis, leukopenia
- **Hypersensitivity:** Reactions from urticaria to **anaphylaxis**, including intracranial hypertension
- **Local:** *Transient irritation, stinging, itching,* angioneurotic edema, urticaria, dermatitis, superinfections with ophthalmic or dermatologic use
- **Other:** *Superinfections,* local irritation at parenteral injection sites

Interactions
✷ **Drug-drug** ● Decreased absorption with calcium salts, magnesium salts, zinc salts, aluminum salts, bismuth salts, iron, urinary alkalinizers, food, dairy products, charcoal ● Increased digoxin toxicity ● Increased nephrotoxicity if taken with methoxyflurane ● Decreased effectiveness of oral contraceptives (rare) with a risk of breakthrough bleeding or pregnancy ● Decreased activity of penicillins

■ Nursing considerations
Assessment
- **History:** Allergy to any of the tetracyclines; allergy to tartrazine; hepatic or renal dysfunction; pregnancy, lactation; ocular viral, mycobacterial, or fungal infections
- **Physical:** Site of infection, skin color, lesions; R, adventitious sounds; bowel sounds, output, liver evaluation; urinalysis, BUN, liver function tests, renal function tests

Interventions
- Administer oral medication on an empty stomach, 1 hr before or 2–3 hr after meals. Do not give with antacids. If antacids must be used, give them 3 hr after the dose of tetracycline.
- Culture infected area prior to drug therapy.

- Do not use outdated drugs; degraded drug is highly nephrotoxic and should not be used.
- Do not give oral drug with meals, antacids, or food.
- Provide frequent hygiene measures if superinfections occur.
- Protect patient from sunlight and bright lights if photosensitivity occurs.
- Arrange for regular renal function tests if long-term therapy is used.
- Use topical preparations of this drug only when clearly indicated. Sensitization from the topical use of this drug may preclude its later use in serious infections. Topical preparations containing antibiotics that are not ordinarily given systemically are preferable.

Teaching points
- Take the drug throughout the day for best results. The drug should be taken on an empty stomach, 1 hr before or 2–3 hr after meals, with a full glass of water. Do not take the drug with food, dairy products, iron preparations, or antacids.
- Finish your complete prescription; if any is left, discard it immediately. Never take an outdated product.
- There have been reports of pregnancy occurring when taking tetracycline with oral contraceptives. To be absolutely confident of avoiding pregnancy, use an additional type of contraceptive while on this drug.
- Possible side effects: stomach upset, nausea; superinfections in the mouth, vagina (frequent washing may help this problem; if it becomes severe, medication may help); sensitivity of the skin to sunlight (use protective clothing and a sunscreen).
- Report severe cramps, watery diarrhea, rash or itching, difficulty breathing, dark urine or light-colored stools, yellowing of the skin or eyes.
- To give eye drops: lie down or tilt head backward and look at the ceiling. Drop suspension inside lower eyelid while looking up. Close eye, and apply gentle pressure to inner corner of the eye for 1 min.
- Apply ointment inside lower eyelid; close eyes, and roll eyeball in all directions.
- This drug may cause temporary blurring of vision or stinging after application.

- Notify health care provider if stinging or itching becomes severe.
- Take the full course of therapy prescribed; discard any leftover medication.
- Apply dermatologic solution until skin is wet. Avoid eyes, nose, and mouth.
- You may experience transient stinging or burning; this will subside quickly; skin in the treated area may become yellow; this will wash off.
- Use cosmetics as you usually do.
- Wash area before applying (unless contraindicated); this drug may stain clothing.
- Report worsening of condition, rash, irritation.

Representative drugs
demeclocycline
doxycycline
minocycline
oxytetracycline
tetracycline

Tricyclic Antidepressants (TCAs)

PREGNANCY CATEGORY C, D
(AMITRIPTYLINE, IMIPRAMINE, NORTRIPTYLINE)

Therapeutic actions
Mechanism of action is unknown. The TCAs are structurally related to the phenothiazine antipsychotic drugs (eg, chlorpromazine), but in contrast to them, TCAs inhibit the presynaptic reuptake of the neurotransmitters norepinephrine and serotonin; anticholinergic at CNS and peripheral receptors; the relation of these effects to clinical efficacy is unknown.

Indications
- Relief of symptoms of depression (endogenous depression most responsive; unlike other TCAs, protriptyline is "activating" and may be useful in withdrawn and anergic patients)
- Unlabeled use: treatment of obstructive sleep apnea, panic disorder

Contraindications and cautions
- Contraindications: hypersensitivity to any tricyclic drug, concomitant therapy with an MAO inhibitor, recent MI, myelography within previous 24 hr or scheduled within 48 hr, pregnancy (limb reduction abnormalities reported), or lactation. Use cautiously with EST; preexisting CV disorders (severe CHD, progressive heart failure, angina pectoris, paroxysmal tachycardia); angle-closure glaucoma, increased intraocular pressure, urinary retention, ureteral or urethral spasm; seizure disorders (lower seizure threshold); hyperthyroidism (predisposes to CVS toxicity, including cardiac arrhythmias); impaired hepatic, renal function; psychiatric patients; schizophrenic or paranoid may exhibit a worsening of psychosis; manic-depressive disorder may shift to hypomanic or manic phase; elective surgery (discontinue as long as possible before surgery).

Adverse effects
- **CNS:** *Sedation and anticholinergic (atropine-like) effects* (dry mouth, blurred vision, disturbance of accommodation for near vision, mydriasis, increased intraocular pressure), *confusion* (especially in elderly), *disturbed concentration,* hallucinations, disorientation, decreased memory, feelings of unreality, delusions, anxiety, nervousness, restlessness, agitation, panic, insomnia, nightmares, hypomania, mania, exacerbation of psychosis, drowsiness, weakness, fatigue, headache, numbness, tingling, paresthesias of extremities, incoordination, motor hyperactivity, akathisia, ataxia, tremors, peripheral neuropathy, extrapyramidal symptoms, *seizures,* speech blockage, dysarthria, tinnitus, altered EEG
- **CV:** *Orthostatic hypotension,* hypertension, syncope, tachycardia, palpitations, MI, arrhythmias, heart block, precipitation of CHF, stroke
- **Endocrine:** Elevated or depressed blood sugar; elevated prolactin levels; inappropriate ADH secretion
- **GI:** *Dry mouth, constipation,* paralytic ileus, *nausea,* vomiting, anorexia, epigastric distress, diarrhea, flatulence, dysphagia, peculiar taste, increased salivation, stomatitis, glossitis, parotid swelling, abdominal cramps, black "hairy" tongue

- **GU:** Urinary retention, delayed micturition, dilation of the urinary tract, gynecomastia, testicular swelling; breast enlargement, menstrual irregularity, and galactorrhea; change in libido; impotence
- **Hematologic:** Bone marrow depression, including agranulocytosis; eosinophilia; purpura; thrombocytopenia; leukopenia
- **Hypersensitivity:** Skin rash, pruritus, vasculitis, petechiae, photosensitization, edema (generalized, face and tongue), drug fever
- **Withdrawal:** Symptoms with abrupt discontinuation of prolonged therapy; nausea, headache, vertigo, nightmares, malaise
- **Other:** Nasal congestion, excessive appetite, weight change; sweating, alopecia, lacrimation, hyperthermia, flushing, chills

Interactions

✱ Drug-drug • Increased TCA levels and pharmacologic effects with cimetidine, fluoxetine, ranitidine • Increased half-life and therefore increased bleeding with dicumarol • Altered response, including arrhythmias and hypertension, with sympathomimetics • Risk of severe hypertension with clonidine • Hyperpyretic crises, severe convulsions, hypertensive episodes, and death with MAO inhibitors • Decreased hypotensive activity of guanethidine

■ Nursing considerations
Assessment

- **History:** Hypersensitivity to any tricyclic drug; concomitant therapy with an MAO inhibitor; recent MI; myelography within previous 24 hr or scheduled within 48 hr; pregnancy; lactation; preexisting disorders; angle-closure glaucoma, increased intraocular pressure; urinary retention, ureteral or urethral spasm; seizure disorders; hyperthyroidism; impaired hepatic, renal function; psychiatric, manic-depressive disorder; elective surgery
- **Physical:** Weight; T; skin color, lesions; orientation, affect, reflexes, vision and hearing; P, BP, orthostatic BP, perfusion; bowel sounds, normal output, liver evaluation; urine flow, normal output; usual sexual function, frequency of menses, breast and scrotal examination; liver function tests, urinalysis, CBC, ECG

Interventions

- Ensure that depressed and potentially suicidal patients have limited access to drug.
- Reduce dosage if minor side effects develop; discontinue drug if serious side effects occur.
- Arrange for CBC if patient develops fever, sore throat, or other sign of infection.
- Ensure ready access to bathroom if GI effects occur; establish bowel program for constipation.
- Provide small, frequent meals, frequent mouth care if GI effects occur; provide sugarless lozenges for dry mouth.
- Establish safety precautions if CNS changes occur (side rails, assist walking).

Teaching points

- Take drug exactly as prescribed; do not stop taking this drug abruptly or without consulting the health care provider.
- Avoid alcohol, sleep-inducing drugs, OTC drugs.
- Avoid prolonged exposure to sunlight or sunlamps; use a sunscreen or protective garments if unavoidable.
- Possible side effects: headache, dizziness, drowsiness, weakness, blurred vision (reversible; safety measures may be needed if severe; avoid driving or performing tasks requiring alertness); nausea, vomiting, loss of appetite, dry mouth (small, frequent meals, mouth care, and sucking sugarless candies may help); nightmares, inability to concentrate, confusion; changes in sexual function.
- Report dry mouth, difficulty in urination, excessive sedation.

Representative drugs

amitriptyline
amoxapine
clomipramine
desipramine
doxepin
imipramine
nortriptyline
protriptyline
trimipramine

Adverse effects in *Italics* are most common; those in **Bold** are life-threatening.

▷abacavir sulfate
(ah **back'** a veer)

Ziagen

PREGNANCY CATEGORY C

Drug class
Antiviral drug

Therapeutic actions
Reverse transcriptase inhibitor; obstructs RNA and DNA synthesis and inhibits viral reproduction. Used in combination with other anti-HIV drugs to reduce the viral load as low as possible and decrease the chance of further viral mutation. Thought to cross the blood–brain barrier and be effective in the treatment of HIV-related dementia. There are no long-term studies on the effectiveness of this drug.

Indications
• Treatment of HIV infection in combination with other antiretroviral drugs

Contraindications and cautions
• Contraindicated with life-threatening allergy to any component.
• Use cautiously with renal and hepatic impairment, lactic acidosis, pregnancy, lactation.

Available forms
Tablets—300 mg; oral solution—20 mg/mL

Dosages
Adults
300 mg PO bid.
Pediatric patients
< 3 mo: Not recommended
> 3 mo– < 16 yr: 8 mg/kg PO bid; do not exceed 300 mg/dose.

Pharmacokinetics

Route	Onset	Peak
Oral	Slow	2–4 hr

Metabolism: Hepatic; $T_{1/2}$: 1–2 hr
Distribution: May cross placenta; may pass into breast milk
Excretion: Urine, feces

Adverse effects
• **CNS:** Headache, weakness
• **Dermatologic:** Rash
• **GI:** Diarrhea, nausea, GI pain, anorexia, vomiting, dyspepsia, liver enzyme elevations, liver enlargement, **risk of severe to fatal hepatomegaly**
• **Respiratory:** Dyspnea, pharyngitis, rhinitis, sinusitis
• **Other:** Severe hypersensitivity reactions—fever, malaise, nausea, vomiting, rash; **severe to fatal lactic acidosis**

Interactions
✱ **Drug-drug** • Risk of severe toxic effects if combined with alcohol

■ Nursing considerations
Assessment
• **History:** Life-threatening allergy to any component, impaired hepatic or renal function, pregnancy, lactation
• **Physical:** T; affect, reflexes, peripheral sensation; R, adventitious sounds; bowel sounds, liver evaluation; liver and renal function tests

Interventions
• Administer with meals or a light snack if GI upset occurs.
• Monitor patient for signs of hypersensitivity reaction; provide patient with hypersensitivity reaction card provided by manufacturer. Advise patient to stop drug at first sign of reaction. Do not attempt to try the drug again if a hypersensitivity reaction has occurred.
• Administer the drug concurrently with other anti-HIV drugs.
• Recommend the use of barrier contraceptives while on this drug.

Teaching points
• Take drug exactly as prescribed; take missed doses as soon as possible and return to normal schedule; do not double-up skipped doses; take with meals or a light snack if GI upset occurs.
• Be aware that these drugs are not a cure for AIDS or ARC; opportunistic infections may occur and regular medical care should be sought to deal with the disease.
• Be aware that the long-term effects of this drug are not yet known.

- Know that these side effects may occur as a result of drug therapy: nausea, loss of appetite, diarrhea (small, frequent meals may help; medication is available to control the diarrhea); dizziness, loss of feeling (take appropriate precautions).
- Be aware that this drug combination does not reduce the risk of transmission of HIV to others by sexual contact or blood contamination—use appropriate precautions.
- Consider the use of barrier contraceptives; this drug may block the effectiveness of oral contraceptives.
- This drug has been connected with severe hypersensitivity reactions, which usually occur early in the use of the drug. Keep your hypersensitivity list readily available, and stop the drug if any of these effects occur.
- Report extreme fatigue, lethargy, severe headache, severe nausea, vomiting, difficulty breathing, rash, fever.

▽ **abciximab**
(ab six' ah mab)

ReoPro

PREGNANCY CATEGORY C

Drug class
Antiplatelet drug

Therapeutic actions
Interferes with platelet membrane function by inhibiting fibrinogen binding and platelet–platelet interactions; inhibits platelet aggregation and prolongs bleeding time; effect is irreversible for life of the platelet.

Indications
- Adjunct to percutaneous transluminal coronary angioplasty or atherectomy for the prevention of acute cardiac ischemic complications in patients at high risk for abrupt closure of the treated coronary vessel; intended to be used with heparin and aspirin therapy
- Early treatment of unstable angina and non–Q-wave MI

Contraindications and cautions
- Contraindicated with allergy to abciximab; neutropenia; thrombocytopenia; hemostatic disorders; bleeding ulcer; intracranial bleeding; major trauma; vasculitis; pregnancy; severe, uncontrolled hypertension; administration of oral anticoagulants within 7 days (unless prothrombin time is ≤ 1.2 times control).
- Use cautiously with lactation.

Available forms
Injection—2 mg/mL

Dosages
Adults
0.25 mg/kg by IV bolus 10–60 min prior to procedure, followed by continuous infusion of 0.125 mcg/kg/min for 12 hr.
Pediatric patients
Safety and efficacy not established.

Pharmacokinetics

Route	Onset	Peak
IV	Rapid	30 min

Metabolism: Cellular; $T_{1/2}$: < 10 min, then 30 min
Distribution: Crosses placenta; may enter breast milk
Excretion: Unknown

▽ IV facts
Preparation: Withdraw the necessary amount through a 0.2- or 0.22-micron filter for bolus injection. Prepare infusion by withdrawing 4.5 mL through filter into syringe; inject into 250 mL 0.9% sterile saline or 5% dextrose. Do not use any solution that contains visibly opaque particles; discard solution after 12 hr. Do not shake; refrigerate solution.
Infusion: 10–60 min before procedure give bolus over at least 1 min; give continuous infusion at rate of 0.125 mcg/kg/min for 12 hr.
Incompatibilities: Do not mix in solution with any other medication; give through a separate IV line.

Adverse effects
- **CNS:** Dizziness, confusion

Adverse effects in *Italics* are most common; those in **Bold** are life-threatening.

- **CV:** bradycardia, hypotension, arrhythmias, edema
- **GI:** *Nausea, vomiting*
- **Hematologic:** Thrombocytopenia, **bleeding**
- **Local:** *Pain, edema*
- **Respiratory:** Pneumonia, pleural effusion

■ **Nursing considerations**

Assessment

- **History:** Allergy to abciximab, neutropenia, thrombocytopenia, hemostatic disorders, bleeding ulcer, intracranial bleeding, severe liver disease, lactation, renal disorders, pregnancy, recent trauma
- **Physical:** Skin color, lesions; orientation; bowel sounds, normal output; CBC, liver and renal function tests

Interventions

- Monitor CBC count before use and frequently while initiating therapy.
- Arrange for concomitant aspirin and heparin therapy.
- Establish safety precautions to prevent injury and bleeding (electric razor, no contact sports, etc.).
- Provide increased precautions against bleeding during invasive procedures—bleeding will be prolonged.
- Mark chart of any patient receiving abciximab to alert medical personnel to potential for increased bleeding in surgery or dental surgery.

Teaching points

- It may take longer than normal to stop bleeding while on this drug; avoid contact sports, use electrical razors, etc. Apply pressure for extended periods to bleeding sites.
- These side effects may occur: upset stomach, nausea.
- Report fever, chills, sore throat, rash, bruising, bleeding, dark stools or urine.

▽ **acarbose**

(a kar' boz)

Precose, Prandase (CAN)

PREGNANCY CATEGORY B

Drug class

Antidiabetic agent

Therapeutic actions

Alpha-glucosidase inhibitor obtained from the fermentation process of a microorganism; delays the digestion of ingested carbohydrates, leading to a smaller rise in blood glucose following meals and a decrease in glycosylated Hgb; does not enhance insulin secretion, so its effects are additive to those of the sulfonylureas in controlling blood glucose.

Indications

- Adjunct to diet to lower blood glucose in patients with non–insulin-dependent diabetes mellitus (type 2) whose hyperglycemia cannot be managed by diet alone
- Combination therapy with a sulfonylurea, metformin, or insulin to enhance glycemic control in patients who do not receive adequate control with diet and either drug alone

Contraindications and cautions

- Contraindicated with hypersensitivity to drug; diabetic ketoacidosis; cirrhosis; inflammatory bowel disease; existence of or predisposition to intestinal obstruction; type 1 diabetes; conditions that would deteriorate with increased gas in the bowel.
- Use cautiously with renal impairment, pregnancy, lactation.

Available forms

Tablets—50, 100 mg

Dosages

Adults

Give tid at the start of each meal; maximum dosage 100 mg PO tid. Initial dose of 25 mg PO tid at the start of each meal, increase as needed every 4–8 wk as indicated by 1 hr postprandial glucose levels and tolerance. For patient ≤ 60 kg, maximum dose is 50 mg tid; for patient > 60 kg, maximum dose is 100 mg tid.

- *Combination with sulfonylurea:* Blood glucose may be much lower; monitor closely and adjust dosages of each drug accordingly.

Pediatric patients

Safety and efficacy not established.

Pharmacokinetics

Route	Onset	Peak
Oral	Rapid	1 hr

Metabolism: Intestinal; $T_{1/2}$: 2 hr
Distribution: Very little
Excretion: Feces, small amount in urine

Adverse effects

- **Endocrine:** *Hypoglycemia*
- **GI:** *Abdominal pain, flatulence, diarrhea,* anorexia, nausea, vomiting
- **Hematologic:** *Leukopenia, thrombocytopenia,* anemia

Interactions

✷ **Drug-drug** • Possible decrease in digoxin levels if combined; monitor patients closely if this combination is used • Decreased effects of acarbose if taken with digestive enzymes or charcoal; avoid these combinations.

✷ **Drug-alternative therapy** • Increased risk of hypoglycemia if taken with juniper berries, ginseng, garlic, fenugreek, coriander, dandelion root, celery.

■ Nursing considerations
Assessment

- **History:** Hypersensitivity to drug; diabetic ketoacidosis; cirrhosis; inflammatory bowel disease; existence of or predisposition to intestinal obstruction; type 1 diabetes; conditions that would deteriorate with increased gas in bowel; renal impairment; pregnancy; lactation
- **Physical:** Skin color, lesions; T; orientation, reflexes, peripheral sensation; R, adventitious sounds; liver evaluation, bowel sounds; urinalysis, BUN, blood glucose, CBC

Interventions

- Give drug tid with the first bite of each meal.
- Monitor urine and serum glucose levels frequently to determine drug effectiveness and dosage; monitor liver function tests q 3 mo for 1 year, then periodically.
- Inform patient of likelihood of abdominal pain and flatulence.
- Consult with dietitian to establish weight loss program and dietary control.

- Arrange for thorough diabetic teaching program, including disease, dietary control, exercise, signs and symptoms of hypoglycemia and hyperglycemia, avoidance of infection, hygiene.

Teaching points

- Do not discontinue this drug without consulting health care provider.
- Take drug three times a day with first bite of each meal.
- Monitor urine or blood for glucose and ketones as prescribed.
- Continue diet and exercise program established for control of diabetes.
- These side effects may occur: abdominal pain, flatulence, bloating.
- Report fever, sore throat, unusual bleeding or bruising, severe abdominal pain.

▽acebutolol hydrochloride
(a se byoo' toe lole)

Monitan (CAN), Rhotral (CAN), Sectral

PREGNANCY CATEGORY B

Drug classes
Beta$_1$-selective adrenergic blocking agent
Antiarrhythmic drug
Antihypertensive drug

Therapeutic actions
Blocks beta-adrenergic receptors of the sympathetic nervous system in the heart and juxtaglomerular apparatus (kidney); decreases excitability of the heart, cardiac output and oxygen consumption, and release of renin from the kidney; and lowers BP.

Indications
- Hypertension, alone or with other drugs, especially diuretics
- Management of ventricular premature beats

Contraindications and cautions
- Contraindicated with bradycardia (HR < 45 beats per minute), second- or third-

---

degree heart block (PR interval > 0.24 sec), cardiogenic shock, CHF, asthma, COPD, lactation.

- Use cautiously with diabetes or thyrotoxicosis, hepatic impairment, renal failure, pregnancy.

Available forms
Capsules—200, 400 mg

Dosages
Adults
- *Hypertension:* Initially 400 mg/day in one or two doses PO; usual maintenance dosage range is 200–1,200 mg/day given in two divided doses.
- *Ventricular arrhythmias:* 200 mg bid PO; increase dosage gradually until optimum response is achieved (usually at 600–1,200 mg/day); discontinue gradually over 2 wk.

Geriatric patients
Because bioavailability doubles, lower doses may be required; maintain at ≤ 800 mg/day.

Patients with impaired renal or hepatic function
Reduce daily dose by 50% when creatinine clearance is < 50 mL/min; reduce by 75% when creatinine clearance is < 25 mL/min; use caution with hepatic impairment.

Pediatric patients
Safety and efficacy not established.

Pharmacokinetics

Route	Onset	Peak	Duration
Oral	Varies	3–4 hr	6–8 hr

Metabolism: Hepatic; $T_{1/2}$: 3–4 hr
Distribution: Crosses placenta; passes into breast milk
Excretion: Urine, bile, feces

Adverse effects
- **Allergic reactions:** Pharyngitis, erythematous rash, fever, sore throat, *laryngospasm, respiratory distress*
- **CNS:** Dizziness, vertigo, tinnitus, fatigue, emotional depression, paresthesias, sleep disturbances, hallucinations, disorientation, memory loss, slurred speech (Because acebutolol is less lipid soluble than propranolol, it is less likely to penetrate the blood–brain barrier and cause CNS effects.)
- **CV:** *Bradycardia, CHF, cardiac arrhythmias, sinoatrial or AV nodal block, tachycardia,* peripheral vascular insufficiency, claudication, CVA, pulmonary edema, hypotension
- **Dermatologic:** Rash, pruritus, sweating, dry skin
- **EENT:** Eye irritation, dry eyes, conjunctivitis, blurred vision
- **GI:** *Gastric pain, flatulence, constipation, diarrhea, nausea, vomiting,* anorexia
- **GU:** *Impotence, decreased libido,* Peyronie's disease, dysuria, nocturia, frequent urination
- **Musculoskeletal:** Joint pain, arthralgia, muscle cramp
- **Respiratory:** *Bronchospasm,* dyspnea, cough, bronchial obstruction, nasal stuffiness, rhinitis
- **Other:** *Decreased exercise tolerance, development of antinuclear antibodies,* hyperglycemia or hypoglycemia, elevated serum transaminase

Interactions
✳ **Drug-drug** • Increased effects of both drugs if combined with calcium channel blockers • Increased risk of orthostatic hypotension with prazosin • Possible increased BP-lowering effects with aspirin, bismuth subsalicylate, magnesium salicylate • Decreased antihypertensive effects with NSAIDs, clonidine • Possible increased hypoglycemic effect of insulin
✳ **Drug-lab test** • Possible false results with glucose or insulin tolerance tests (oral)

■ Nursing considerations
Assessment
- **History:** Sinus bradycardia, second- or third-degree heart block, cardiogenic shock, CHF, asthma, COPD, pregnancy, lactation, diabetes, or thyrotoxicosis
- **Physical:** Weight, skin condition, neurologic status, P, BP, ECG, respiratory status, kidney and thyroid function, blood and urine glucose

Interventions
- Give with meals if needed.
- Do not discontinue drug abruptly after long-term therapy. Taper drug gradually over 2 wk with monitoring (abrupt withdrawal may

cause serious beta-adrenergic rebound effects).

- Monitor apical pulse; do not administer if P < 50.
- Consult with physician about withdrawing drug if patient is to undergo surgery (withdrawal is controversial).
- Provide comfort measures for coping with drug effects.
- Provide safety precautions if CNS effects occur.

Teaching points

- Take drug with meals.
- Do not stop taking unless so instructed by health care provider.
- Avoid driving or dangerous activities if dizziness, weakness occur.
- These side effects may occur: dizziness, lightheadedness, loss of appetite, nightmares, depression, sexual impotence.
- Report difficulty breathing, night cough, swelling of extremities, slow pulse, confusion, depression, rash, fever, sore throat.

▽ acetaminophen (N-acetyl-p-aminophenol)

*(a seet a **min'** a fen)*

Suppositories: Abenol (CAN), Acephen, Children's Feverall

Oral: Aceta, Apacet, Atasol (CAN), Genapap, Genebs, Liquiprin, Mapap, Panadol, Tapanol, Tempra, Tylenol

PREGNANCY CATEGORY B

Drug classes
Antipyretic
Analgesic (non-narcotic)

Therapeutic actions
Antipyretic: reduces fever by acting directly on the hypothalamic heat-regulating center to cause vasodilation and sweating, which helps dissipate heat
Analgesic: site and mechanism of action unclear

Indications

- Analgesic-antipyretic in patients with aspirin allergy, hemostatic disturbances, bleeding diatheses, upper GI disease, gouty arthritis
- Arthritis and rheumatic disorders involving musculoskeletal pain (but lacks clinically significant antirheumatic and anti-inflammatory effects)
- Common cold, flu, other viral and bacterial infections with pain and fever
- Unlabeled use: prophylactic for children receiving DPT vaccination to reduce incidence of fever and pain

Contraindications and cautions

- Contraindicated with allergy to acetaminophen.
- Use cautiously with impaired hepatic function, chronic alcoholism, pregnancy, lactation.

Available forms
Suppositories—80, 120, 125, 300, 325, 650 mg; chewable tablets—80 mg; tablets—160, 325, 500, 650 mg; caplets—160, 500, 650 mg; gelcaps—650 mg; capsules—325, 500 mg; elixir—80 mg/2.5 mL, 80 mg/5 mL, 120 mg/5 mL, 160 mg/5 mL; liquid—160 mg/5 mL, 500 mg/15 mL; solution—80 mg/1.66 mL, 100 mg/mL; drops—80 mg/0.8 mL; sprinkle capsules—80, 160 mg

Dosages
Adults
By suppository, 325–650 mg q 4–6 hr or PO, 1,000 mg tid to qid. Do not exceed 4 g/day.
Pediatric patients
Doses may be repeated 4–5 times/day; do not exceed five doses in 24 hr; give PO or by suppository.

Age	Dosage (mg)
0–3 mo	40
4–11 mo	80
1–2 yr	120
2–3 yr	160
4–5 yr	240
6–8 yr	320
9–10 yr	400
11 yr	480

Adverse effects in *Italics* are most common; those in **Bold** are life-threatening.

Pharmacokinetics

Route	Onset	Peak	Duration
Oral	Varies	0.5–2 hr	3–4 hr

Metabolism: Hepatic; $T_{1/2}$: 1–3 hr
Distribution: Crosses placenta; passes into breast milk
Excretion: Urine

Adverse effects

- **CNS:** Headache
- **CV:** Chest pain, dyspnea, **myocardial damage** when doses of 5–8 g/day are ingested daily for several weeks or when doses of 4 g/day are ingested for 1 year
- **GI: Hepatic toxicity and failure,** jaundice
- **GU:** Acute kidney failure, renal tubular necrosis
- **Hematologic:** Methemoglobinemia—cyanosis; hemolytic anemia—hematuria, anuria; neutropenia, leukopenia, pancytopenia, thrombocytopenia, hypoglycemia
- **Hypersensitivity:** Rash, fever

Interactions

✱ **Drug-drug** ● Increased toxicity with long-term, excessive ethanol ingestion ● Increased hypoprothrombinemic effect of oral anticoagulants ● Increased risk of hepatotoxicity and possible decreased therapeutic effects with barbiturates, carbamazepine, hydantoins, rifampin, sulfinpyrazone ● Possible delayed or decreased effectiveness with anticholinergics ● Possible reduced absorption of acetaminophen with activated charcoal ● Possible decreased effectiveness of zidovudine

✱ **Drug-lab test** ● Interference with *Chemstrip* G, *Dextrostix*, and *Visidex II* home blood glucose measurement systems; effects vary

■ Nursing considerations
Assessment

- **History:** Allergy to acetaminophen, impaired hepatic function, chronic alcoholism, pregnancy, lactation
- **Physical:** Skin color, lesions; T; liver evaluation; CBC, liver and renal function tests

Interventions

- Do not exceed the recommended dosage.
- Consult physician if needed for children < 3 yr; if needed for longer than 10 days; if continued fever, severe or recurrent pain occurs (possible serious illness).
- Avoid using multiple preparations containing acetaminophen. Carefully check all OTC products.
- Give drug with food if GI upset is noted.
- Discontinue drug if hypersensitivity reactions occur.
- Treatment of overdose: Monitor serum levels regularly, N-acetylcysteine should be available as a specific antidote; basic life support measures may be necessary.

Teaching points

- Do not exceed recommended dose; do not take for longer than 10 days.
- Take the drug only for complaints indicated; not an anti-inflammatory agent.
- Avoid the use of other OTC preparations. They may contain acetaminophen, and serious overdosage can occur. If you need an OTC preparation, consult your health care provider.
- Report rash, unusual bleeding or bruising, yellowing of skin or eyes, changes in voiding patterns.

▽ acetazolamide
*(a set a **zole'** a mide)*

Apo-Acetazolamide (CAN), Dazamide, Diamox Sequels

PREGNANCY CATEGORY C

Drug classes

Carbonic anhydrase inhibitor
Antiglaucoma agent
Diuretic
Antiepileptic drug
Sulfonamide (nonbacteriostatic)

Therapeutic actions

Inhibits the enzyme carbonic anhydrase. This action decreases aqueous humor formation in the eye, intraocular pressure, and hydrogen ion secretion by renal tubule cells, and increases sodium, potassium, bicarbonate, and water excretion by the kidney, causing a diuretic effect.

Indications

- Adjunctive treatment of chronic open-angle glaucoma, secondary glaucoma
- Preoperative use in acute angle-closure glaucoma when delay of surgery is desired to lower intraocular pressure
- Edema caused by CHF, drug-induced edema
- Centrencephalic epilepsy
- Prophylaxis and treatment of acute altitude sickness

Contraindications and cautions

- Contraindicated with allergy to acetazolamide, antibacterial sulfonamides, or thiazides; chronic noncongestive angle-closure glaucoma.
- Use cautiously with fluid or electrolyte imbalance (specifically decreased Na+, decreased K+, hyperchloremic acidosis), renal disease, hepatic disease (risk of hepatic coma if acetazolamide is given), adrenocortical insufficiency, respiratory acidosis, COPD, lactation.

Available forms

Tablets—125, 250 mg; SR capsules—500 mg; powder for injection—500 mg/vial

Dosages
Adults

- *Open-angle glaucoma:* 250 mg–1 g/day PO, usually in divided doses. Do not exceed 1 g/day.
- *Secondary glaucoma and preoperatively:* 250 mg q 4 hr or 250 mg bid PO, or 500 mg followed by 125–250 mg q 4 hr. May be given IV for rapid relief of increased intraocular pressure—500 mg IV repeated in 2–4 hr then 125–250 mg PO q 4–6 hr.
- *Diuresis in CHF:* 250–375 mg (5 mg/kg) daily in the morning. Most effective if given on alternate days or for 2 days alternating with a day of rest.
- *Drug-induced edema:* 250–375 mg every day or once daily on alternate days or for 2 days alternating with a day of rest.
- *Epilepsy:* 8–30 mg/kg/day in divided doses. When given in combination with other antiepileptics, starting dose is 250 mg daily. Sustained-release preparation is not recommended for this use.

- *Acute altitude sickness:* 500 mg–1 g/day PO in divided doses of tablets or sustained-release capsules. For rapid ascent, the 1-g dose is recommended. When possible, begin dosing 24–48 hr before ascent and continue for 48 hr or longer as needed while at high altitude.

Pediatric patients

- *Secondary glaucoma and preoperatively:* 5–10 mg/kg IM or IV q 6 hr, or 10–15 mg/kg/day PO in divided doses q 6–8 hr.
- *Acute glaucoma:* 5–10 mg/kg IV q 6 hr or 8–30 mg/kg/day PO or 300–900 mg/m2/day PO in 3 divided doses.
- *Epilepsy:* 8–30 mg/kg/day in divided doses. When given with other antiepileptics, starting dose is 250 mg/day.
- *Drug-induced edema:* 5 mg/kg/dose PO or IV once daily in AM.

Pharmacokinetics

Route	Onset	Peak	Duration
Oral	1 hr	2–4 hr	6–12 hr
Sustained release	2 hr	8–12 hr	18–24 hr
IV	1–2 min	15–18 min	4–5 hr

Metabolism: $T_{1/2}$: 5–6 hr
Distribution: Crosses placenta; passes into breast milk
Excretion: Unchanged in the urine

▼IV facts

Preparation: Reconstitute 500-mg vial with 5 mL of sterile water for injection; stable for 1 week if refrigerated, but use within 24 hr is recommended.
Infusion: Give over 1 min for single injection, over 4–8 hr in solution.
Incompatibility: Do not mix with diltiazem or in multivitamin infusion.

Adverse effects

- **CNS:** Weakness, fatigue, nervousness, sedation, drowsiness, dizziness, depression, tremor, ataxia, headache, paresthesias, convulsions, flaccid paralysis, transient myopia
- **Dermatologic:** Urticaria, pruritus, rash, photosensitivity, erythema multiforme (Stevens-Johnson syndrome)

Adverse effects in *Italics* are most common; those in **Bold** are life-threatening.

- **GI:** Anorexia, nausea, vomiting, constipation, melena, hepatic insufficiency
- **GU:** Hematuria, glycosuria, *urinary frequency*, renal colic, renal calculi, crystalluria, polyuria
- **Hematologic:** Bone marrow depression
- **Other:** Weight loss, fever, acidosis

Interactions

✳ **Drug–drug** • Decreased renal excretion of quinidine, amphetamine, procainamide, TCAs • Increased excretion of salicylates, lithium • Increased risk of salicylate toxicity due to metabolic acidosis with acetazolamide

✳ **Drug–lab test** • False-positive results of tests for urinary protein

■ Nursing considerations

> **CLINICAL ALERT!**
> Name confusion has occurred between acetazolamide and acetohexamide; and between Diamox (acetazolamide) and Dymelor (acetohexamide); use caution.

Assessment

- **History:** Allergy to acetazolamide, antibacterial sulfonamides, or thiazides; chronic noncongestive angle-closure glaucoma; fluid or electrolyte imbalance; renal or hepatic disease; adrenocortical insufficiency; respiratory acidosis; COPD; lactation
- **Physical:** Skin color, lesions; edema, weight, orientation, reflexes, muscle strength, intraocular pressure; respiratory rate, pattern, adventitious sounds; liver evaluation, bowel sounds, urinary output patterns; CBC, serum electrolytes, liver and renal function tests, urinalysis

Interventions

- Administer by direct IV if parenteral use is necessary; IM use is painful.
- Give with food or milk if GI upset occurs.
- Use caution if giving with other drugs with excretion inhibited by urine alkalinization.
- Make oral liquid form by crushing tablets and suspending in cherry, chocolate, raspberry, or other sweet syrup, or one tablet may be submerged in 10 mL of hot water with 1 mL of honey or syrup; *do not use alcohol or glycerin* as a vehicle.

- Establish safety precautions if CNS effects occur; protect patient from sun or bright lights if photophobia occurs.
- Obtain regular weight to monitor fluid changes.
- Monitor serum electrolytes and acid–base balance during course of drug therapy.

Teaching points

- Take drug with meals if GI upset occurs.
- Arrange to have intraocular pressure checked periodically.
- Weigh yourself on a regular basis, at the same time of the day and in the same clothing. Record weight on calendar.
- These side effects may occur: increased volume and frequency of urination; dizziness, feeling faint on arising, drowsiness, fatigue (do not engage in hazardous activities like driving a car); sensitivity to sunlight (use sunglasses, wear protective clothing, or use a sunscreen when outdoors); GI upset (taking the drug with meals, having small frequent meals may help).
- Report weight change of more than 3 lb in 1 day, unusual bleeding or bruising, sore throat, dizziness, trembling, numbness, fatigue, muscle weakness or cramps, flank or loin pain, rash.

▽**acetohexamide**
(a set oh hex' a mide)

Dimelor (CAN), Dymelor

PREGNANCY CATEGORY C

Drug classes

Antidiabetic agent
Sulfonylurea—first generation

Therapeutic actions

Stimulates insulin release from functioning beta cells in the pancreas; may improve binding between insulin and insulin receptors or increase number of insulin receptors and lower blood glucose; has significant uricosuric activity.

Indications

- Adjunct to diet to lower blood glucose in non–insulin-dependent diabetes mellitus (type 2)

- Adjunct to insulin therapy in the stabilization of certain cases of insulin-dependent, maturity-onset diabetes, reducing the insulin requirement and decreasing the chance of hypoglycemic reactions

Contraindications and cautions

- Contraindicated with allergy to sulfonylureas; conditions in which insulin is indicated to control blood sugar—diabetes complicated by fever, severe infections, severe trauma, major surgery, ketosis, acidosis, coma; type 1 or juvenile diabetes; serious hepatic or serious renal impairment; uremia, thyroid, or endocrine impairment; glycosuria; hyperglycemia associated with primary renal disease; pregnancy or lactation.

Available forms

Tablets—250, 500 mg

Dosages

Adults

250 mg–1.5 g/day PO. Patients on < 1 g/day can be controlled with once-daily dosage; if patients are on 1.5 g/day, twice daily dosage, before morning and evening meals is appropriate; do not exceed 1.5 g/day.

- *Transfer from other oral antidiabetic agents:* initial dose of acetohexamide—one-half tolbutamide dose; 2 times chlorpropamide dose, then adjust dosage based on clinical response.
- *Transfer of type 2 patients on insulin to acetohexamide monotherapy:* insulin dose < 20 units—250 mg/day; insulin dose > 20 units—reduce dose by 25%–30%, start 250 mg/day; further reduce insulin based on response.

Pediatric patients

Safety and efficacy not established.

Geriatric patients

Geriatric patients tend to be more sensitive to the drug; start with a lower initial dose, monitor for 24 hr, and gradually increase dose as needed.

Pharmacokinetics

Route	Onset	Peak	Duration
Oral	1 hr	2–4 hr	12–24 hr

Metabolism: Hepatic; $T_{1/2}$: 6–8 hr
Distribution: Enters breast milk
Excretion: Renal

Adverse effects

- **Dermatologic:** Allergic skin reactions, eczema, pruritus, erythema, urticaria, photosensitivity
- **GI:** *Anorexia, nausea, vomiting, epigastric discomfort, heartburn*
- **Hematologic:** *Hypoglycemia,* leukopenia, thrombocytopenia, anemia
- **Hypersensitivity:** Fever, eosinophilia, jaundice
- **Other:** Possible increased risk of CV mortality, SIADH

Interactions

✳ **Drug-drug** • Increased risk of hypoglycemia with insulin, sulfonamides, chloramphenicol, oxyphenbutazone, phenylbutazone, salicylates, probenecid, MAOIs, clofibrate • Decreased effect with beta-adrenergic blocking agents (signs of hypoglycemia also may be blocked), rifampin • Decreased effectiveness of acetohexamide and diazoxide if taken concurrently • Increased risk of hyperglycemia with thiazides, other diuretics, phenytoin, nicotinic acid, sympathomimetics • Risk of hypoglycemia and hyperglycemia with alcohol; "disulfiram reaction" also has been reported ✳ **Drug-alternative therapy** • Increased risk of hypoglycemia if taken with juniper berries, ginseng, garlic, fenugreek, coriander, dandelion root, celery

■ Nursing considerations

 CLINICAL ALERT!
Name confusion has occurred between acetohexamide and acetazolamide; and between Dymelor (acetohexamide) and Diamox (acetazolamide); use caution.

Assessment

- **History:** Renal, hepatic, endocrine disorders
- **Physical:** Skin color, lesions; T; orientation, reflexes, peripheral sensation; R, adventitious sounds; liver evaluation, bowel

sounds; urinalysis, BUN, serum creatinine, liver function tests, blood glucose, CBC

Interventions

- Give drug before breakfast. If severe GI upset occurs or if dosage is 1.5 g/day, dose may be divided with one dose before breakfast and one before the evening meal.
- Monitor serum glucose levels frequently to determine effectiveness of drug.
- Transfer to insulin therapy during periods of high stress—infections, surgery, trauma, etc.
- Use IV glucose if severe hypoglycemia occurs as a result of overdose.

Teaching points

- Take this drug early in the morning before breakfast. If the drug is to be taken two times a day, take it before breakfast and before the evening meal.
- Do not discontinue this medication without consulting health care provider.
- Do not take this drug during pregnancy; if you think you are pregnant, consult health care provider.
- Monitor urine or blood for glucose and ketones as prescribed.
- Avoid alcohol while on this drug; serious reactions could occur.
- Report fever, sore throat, unusual bleeding or bruising, rash, dark urine, light-colored stools, hypoglycemic or hyperglycemic reactions.

▽acetohydroxamic acid (AHA)

(a see' toe hye drox am ik)

Lithostat

PREGNANCY CATEGORY X

Drug classes

Urinary tract agent
Urease inhibitor

Therapeutic actions

Inhibits the bacterial enzyme urease, inhibiting the production of ammonia in the urine and lowering the pH of urine infected with urea-splitting organisms. This enhances the effectiveness of antibiotics and increases the cure rate of these infections, which are often accompanied by kidney stone formation.

Indications

- Adjunctive therapy in chronic urea-splitting urinary tract infections

Contraindications and cautions

- Allergy to acetohydroxamic acid, physical conditions that are amenable to surgery or antimicrobial treatment, poor renal function, pregnancy (teratogenic—recommend the use of birth control methods while on this drug), lactation.

Available forms

Tablets—250 mg

Dosages

Adults

250 mg PO tid to qid for a total dose of 10–15 mg/kg/day; recommended starting dose is 12 mg/kg/day given q 6–8 hr; do not exceed 1.5 g/day.

Pediatric patients

Initial dose of 10 mg/kg/day PO; dose adjustment may be required by hematologic response.

Patients with renal impairment

Serum creatinine > 1.8 mg/dL: do not exceed 1 g/day with doses at 12-hr intervals; do not administer to patients with serum creatinine > 2.5 mg/dL.

Pharmacokinetics

Route	Onset	Peak
Oral	1 hr	15–60 min

Metabolism: Hepatic; $T_{1/2}$: 5–10 hr
Distribution: Crosses placenta, may enter breast milk
Excretion: Unchanged in the urine

Adverse effects

- **CNS:** *Headache, depression, anxiety, nervousness, malaise, tremulousness*
- **CV:** Superficial phlebitis of lower extremities
- **Dermatologic:** Nonpruritic, macular rash in the upper extremities and face (most common after ingestion of alcohol during long-term use), alopecia
- **GI:** *Nausea, vomiting, anorexia*

- **Hematologic:** Coombs' negative hemolytic anemia

Interactions
✳ Drug-drug ● Rash with alcohol ● Absorption of acetohydroxamic acid and iron decreased if both are taken; if needed, space doses at least 2 hr apart

■ Nursing considerations
Assessment
- **History:** Allergy to acetohydroxamic acid, physical conditions that are amenable to surgery or antimicrobial treatment, poor renal function, pregnancy, lactation
- **Physical:** Skin color, lesions; orientation, affect, reflexes; peripheral perfusion, veins in lower extremities; liver evaluation; CBC, liver and renal function tests

Interventions
- Arrange for culture and sensitivity tests of urine before beginning therapy; do not administer if urine is infected with non–urease-producing organisms.
- Ensure that patient is not pregnant or planning to become pregnant. Advise the patient to use birth control.
- Administer on an empty stomach—1 hr before or 2 hr after meals.
- Arrange for analgesics to relieve headache.

Teaching points
- Take the drug on an empty stomach—1 hr before or 2 hr after meals.
- These side effects may occur: headache (analgesics may help); nausea, vomiting, loss of appetite (small, frequent meals may help); rash (more common when alcohol is taken with this drug).
- This drug causes birth defects and should not be taken if you are, or are trying to become, pregnant; use of birth control methods is highly recommended; if you think you are pregnant, consult your physician immediately.
- Report unusual bleeding or bruising; malaise, lethargy; leg pain or swelling of the lower leg; severe nausea and vomiting.

▷acetylcysteine (*N*-acetylcysteine)
(*a se teel **sis'** tay een*)

Mucomyst, Mucomyst 10 IV, Mucosil-10, Mucosil-20, Parvolex (CAN)

PREGNANCY CATEGORY B

Drug classes
Mucolytic agent
Antidote

Therapeutic actions
Mucolytic activity: splits links in the mucoproteins contained in respiratory mucus secretions, decreasing the viscosity of the mucus
Antidote to acetaminophen hepatotoxicity: protects liver cells by maintaining cell function and detoxifying acetaminophen metabolites

Indications
- Mucolytic adjuvant therapy for abnormal, viscid, or inspissated mucus secretions in acute and chronic bronchopulmonary disease (emphysema with bronchitis, asthmatic bronchitis, tuberculosis, pneumonia), in pulmonary complications of cystic fibrosis, and in tracheostomy care; pulmonary complications associated with surgery, anesthesia, posttraumatic chest conditions; diagnostic bronchial studies
- To prevent or lessen hepatic injury that may occur after ingestion of a potentially hepatotoxic dose of acetaminophen; treatment must start as soon as possible, at least within 24 hr of ingestion. IV use approved as orphan drug for this indication.
- Unlabeled uses: as ophthalmic solution to treat keratoconjunctivitis sicca (dry eye); as an enema to treat bowel obstruction due to meconium ileus or its equivalent

Contraindications and cautions
- *Mucolytic use:* contraindicated with hypersensitivity to acetylcysteine; use caution and discontinue immediately if bronchospasm occurs.

- *Antidotal use:* no contraindications; use caution with esophageal varices, peptic ulcer.

Available forms

Solution—10%, 20%; injection—orphan drug availability

Dosages
Mucolytic use

- *Nebulization with face mask, mouthpiece, tracheostomy:* 1–10 mL of 20% solution or 2–20 mL of 10% solution q 2–6 hr; the dose for most patients is 3–5 mL of the 20% solution or 6–10 mL of the 10% solution tid–qid.
- *Nebulization with tent, croupette:* Very large volumes are required, occasionally up to 300 mL, during a treatment period. The dose is the volume or solution that will maintain a very heavy mist in the tent or croupette for the desired period. Administration for intermittent or continuous prolonged periods, including overnight, may be desirable.

Instillation

- *Direct or by tracheostomy:* 1–2 mL of a 10%–20% solution q 1–4 hr; may be introduced into a particular segment of the bronchopulmonary tree by way of a plastic catheter (inserted under local anesthesia and with direct visualization). Instill 2–5 mL of the 20% solution by a syringe connected to the catheter.
- *Percutaneous intratracheal catheter:* 1–2 mL of the 20% solution or 2–4 mL of the 10% solution q 1–4 hr by a syringe connected to the catheter.
- *Diagnostic bronchogram:* Before the procedure, give two to three administrations of 1–2 mL of the 20% solution or 2–4 mL of the 10% solution by nebulization or intratracheal instillation.

Antidotal use

- *For acetaminophen overdose:* administer acetylcysteine immediately if 24 hr or less have elapsed since acetaminophen ingestion, using the following protocol: • Empty the stomach by lavage or by inducing emesis with syrup of ipecac; repeat dose of ipecac if emesis does not occur in 20 min • If activated charcoal has been administered by lavage, charcoal may adsorb acetylcysteine and reduce its effectiveness • Draw blood for

acetaminophen plasma assay and for baseline AST, ALT, bilirubin, prothrombin time, creatinine, BUN, blood sugar, and electrolytes; if acetaminophen assay cannot be obtained or dose is clearly in the toxic range, give full course of acetylcysteine therapy; monitor hepatic and renal function, fluid and electrolyte balance • Administer acetylcysteine PO 140 mg/kg loading dose • See manufacturer's directions for preparation of oral dose using 20% solution and cola or other soft drink as diluent • Administer 17 maintenance doses of 70 mg/kg q 4 hr, starting 4 hr after loading dose; administer full course of doses unless acetaminophen assay reveals a nontoxic level • If patient vomits loading or maintenance dose within 1 hr of administration, repeat that dose. An IV form is being studied as an orphan drug • If patient persistently vomits the oral dose, administer by duodenal intubation • Repeat blood chemistry assays as described above daily if acetaminophen plasma level is in toxic range

Pharmacokinetics

Route	Onset	Peak	Duration
Oral	30–60 min	1–2 hr	
Instillation, Inhalation	1 min	5–10 min	2–3 hr

Metabolism: Hepatic; $T_{1/2}$: 6.25 hr
Excretion: Urine (30%)

Adverse effects
Mucolytic use

- **GI:** *Nausea*, stomatitis
- **Hypersensitivity:** Urticaria
- **Respiratory:** Bronchospasm, especially in asthmatics
- **Other:** *Rhinorrhea*

Antidotal use

- **Dermatologic:** Rash
- **GI:** *Nausea, vomiting, other GI symptoms*

■ Nursing considerations
Assessment

- **History:** Mucolytic use: Hypersensitivity to acetylcysteine, asthma Antidotal use: Esophageal varices, peptic ulcer
- **Physical:** Weight, T, skin color, lesions; BP; P; R, adventitious sounds, bowel sounds, liver palpation

Interventions
Mucolytic use
- Dilute the 20% acetylcysteine solution with either normal saline or sterile water for injection; use the 10% solution undiluted. Refrigerate unused, undiluted solution, and use within 96 hr. Drug solution in the opened bottle may change color, but this does not alter safety or efficacy.
- Administer the following drugs separately, because they are incompatible with acetylcysteine solutions: tetracyclines, erythromycin lactobionate, amphotericin B, iodized oil chymotrypsin, trypsin, hydrogen peroxide.
- Use water to remove residual drug solution on the patient's face after administration by face mask.
- Inform patient that nebulization may produce an initial disagreeable odor, but it will soon disappear.
- Monitor nebulizer for buildup of drug from evaporation; dilute with sterile water for injection to prevent concentrate from impeding nebulization and drug delivery.
- Establish routine for pulmonary toilet; have suction equipment on standby.

Antidotal use
- Dilute the 20% acetylcysteine solution with cola drinks or other soft drinks to a final concentration of 5%; if administered by gastric tube or Miller–Abbott tube, water may be used as diluent. Dilution minimizes the risk of vomiting.
- Prepare fresh solutions, and use within 1 hr; undiluted solution in opened vials may be kept for 96 hr.
- Treat fluid and electrolyte imbalance, hypoglycemia.
- Give vitamin K_1 if prothrombin ratio exceeds 1.5; give fresh-frozen plasma if PT ratio exceeds 3.
- Do not administer diuretics.

Teaching points
- These side effects may occur: increased productive cough, nausea, GI upset.
- Report difficulty breathing or nausea.

▷acitretin
See *Less Commonly Used Drugs,* p. 1336.

▷acyclovir (acycloguanosine)
(ay sye' kloe ver)

Alti-Acyclovir (CAN), Avirax (CAN), Zovirax

PREGNANCY CATEGORY B

Drug class
Antiviral

Therapeutic actions
Antiviral activity; inhibits viral DNA replication

Indications
- Initial and recurrent mucosal and cutaneous herpes simplex virus (HSV) 1 and 2 and varicella zoster infections in immunocompromised patients
- Severe initial and recurrent genital herpes infections in selected patients
- Herpes simplex encephalitis in patients > 6 mo
- Acute treatment of herpes zoster (shingles) and chickenpox
- Ointment: initial HSV genital infections; limited mucocutaneous HSV infections in immunocompromised patients
- Unlabeled uses: cytomegalovirus and HSV infection following transplant, herpes simplex infections, varicella pneumonia, disseminated primary eczema herpeticum

Contraindications and cautions
- Contraindicated with allergy to acyclovir, seizures, CHF, renal disease, lactation; use caution with pregnancy.

Available forms
Tablets—400, 800 mg; capsules—200 mg; suspension—200 mg/5 mL; powder for injection—500 mg/vial, 1,000 mg/vial; injection—50 mg/mL; ointment—50 mg/g

Dosages
Adults
Parenteral
5–10 mg/kg infused IV over 1 hr, q 8 hr (15 mg/kg/day) for 7 days.
Oral
- *Initial genital herpes:* 200 mg q 4 hr while awake (1,000 mg/day) for 10 days.
- *Long-term suppressive therapy:* 400 mg bid for up to 12 mo.
- *Acute herpes zoster:* 800 mg q 4 hr for 7–10 days.
- *Chickenpox:* 800 mg qid for 5 days.

Pediatric patients
Parenteral
< *12 yr:* 250–500 mg/m² infused IV over 1 hr, q 8 hr (750 mg/m²/day) for 7 days.
≥ *12 yr:* adult dosage.
Oral
Safety not established in children < 2 yr. ≥ 2 yr: 20 mg/kg per dose qid (80 mg/kg/day) for 5 days. Children > 40 kg should receive adult dose.

Geriatric patients or patients with renal impairment
Oral
Creatinine clearance < 10 mL/min: 200 mg q 12 hr.
IV

Creatinine Clearance (mL/min)	Dosage (IV)
> 50	5 mg/kg q 8 hr
25–50	5 mg/kg q 12 hr
10–25	5 mg/kg daily
0–10	2.5 mg/kg daily

Topical
Ointment (all ages): Apply sufficient quantity to cover all lesions 6 times/day (q 3 hr) for 7 days; 1.25-cm (0.5-in) ribbon of ointment covers 2.5 cm² (4 in²) surface area.

Pharmacokinetics

Route	Onset	Peak	Duration
Oral	Varies	1.5–2 hr	
IV	Immediate	1 hr	8 hr

Metabolism: $T_{1/2}$: 2.5–5 hr
Distribution: Crosses placenta; enters breast milk
Excretion: Unchanged in urine

▽ IV facts
Preparation: Reconstitute 500 mg vial in 10 mL sterile water for injection or bacteriostatic water for injection containing benzyl alcohol, 1,000 mg vial in 20 mL; concentration will be 50 mg/mL. Do not dilute drug with bacteriostatic water containing parabens. Use reconstituted solution within 12 hr; dilute IV solution to concentration of 7 mg/mL or less. Do not use biologic or colloidal fluids such as blood products or protein solutions. Warm drug to room temperature to dissolve precipitates formed during refrigeration.

Infusion: Administer by slow IV infusion of parenteral solutions; avoid bolus or rapid injection. Infuse over at least 1 hr to avoid renal damage.

Incompatibilities: Do not mix with diltiazem, dobutamine, dopamine, fludarabine, foscarnet, idarubicin, meperidine, morphine, ondansetron, piperacillin, sargramostim, vinorelbine.

Adverse effects
Systemic administration
- **CNS:** Headache, vertigo, depression, tremors, encephalopathic changes
- **Dermatologic:** *Inflammation or phlebitis at injection sites,* rash, hair loss
- **GI:** *Nausea, vomiting,* diarrhea, anorexia
- **GU:** Crystalluria with rapid IV administration, hematuria

Topical administration
- **Dermatologic:** *Transient burning at site of application*

Interactions
Systemic administration
✳ **Drug-drug** • Increased effects with probenecid • Increased nephrotoxicity with other nephrotoxic drugs • Extreme drowsiness with zidovudine

■ Nursing considerations
Assessment
- **History:** Allergy to acyclovir, seizures, CHF, renal disease, lactation, pregnancy
- **Physical:** Skin color, lesions; orientation; BP, P, auscultation, perfusion, edema; R, adventitious sounds; urinary output; BUN, creatinine clearance

Interventions
Systemic administration
- Ensure that the patient is well hydrated.
Topical administration
- Start treatment as soon as possible after onset of signs and symptoms.
- Wear a rubber glove or finger cot when applying drug.

Teaching points
Systemic administration
- Complete the full course of oral therapy, and do *not* exceed the prescribed dose.
- Oral acyclovir is *not* a cure for your disease but should make you feel better.
- These side effects may occur: nausea, vomiting, loss of appetite, diarrhea; headache, dizziness.
- Avoid sexual intercourse while visible lesions are present.
- Report difficulty urinating, rash, increased severity or frequency of recurrences.
Topical administration
- Wear rubber gloves or finger cots when applying the drug to prevent autoinoculation of other sites and transmission to others.
- This drug does not cure the disease; application during symptom-free periods will not prevent recurrences.
- Avoid sexual intercourse while visible lesions are present.
- This drug may cause burning, stinging, itching, rash; notify your physician if these are pronounced.

▷ adalimumab
(ad ah lim' you mab)

Humira

PREGNANCY CATEGORY B

Drug classes
Monoclonal antibody
Antiarthritis agent

Therapeutic actions
Monoclonal antibody specific for human tumor necrosis factor (TNF), it keeps the inflammatory response in check by reacting with and deactivating free-floating TNF released by active leukocytes. TNF is especially high in the synovial fluid of patients with rheumatoid arthritis.

Indications
- Reduction of the signs and symptoms and inhibition of the progression of structural damage in adult patients with moderately to severely active rheumatoid arthritis who have not responded adequately to disease-modifying anti-rheumatic drugs or methotrexate

Contraindications and cautions
- Contraindicated with allergy to any component of the preparation; presence of active infection including chronic or localized infections; lactation.
- Use cautiously with pregnancy, immune suppression, living in an area endemic with TB or histoplasmosis, pre-existing or recent-onset central nervous system demyelinating disorders.

Available forms
Preservative-free solution for injection—40 mg/mL; pre-filled syringes—40 mg/mL

Dosages
Adults
40 mg by SC injection every other week; patients who are not also receiving methotrexate may benefit from a dosage increase to 40 mg every week.
Pediatric patients
Safety and efficacy not established.

Pharmacokinetics

Route	Onset	Peak
SC	Slow	75–187 hr

Metabolism: Tissue; $T_{1/2}$: 10–20 days
Distribution: May cross placenta; may pass into breast milk
Excretion: Tissue

Adverse effects
- **CNS: CNS demyelinating disease,** *headache*
- **CV:** hypertension, arrhythmias

- **GI:** nausea, vomiting, abdominal pain
- **GU:** hematuria, UTI
- **Local:** *pain and swelling at the injection site, rash*
- **Metabolic:** hypercholesterolemia, hyperlipidemia
- **Respiratory:** *URI, sinusitis*
- **Other: serious to fatal infections including tuberculosis and fungal infections, malignancies,** flu-like syndrome, back pain, **allergic reactions,** increased alkaline phosphatase, autoantibodies, accidental injury

Interactions

* **Drug-drug** ● Risk of serious infection if combined with immune-suppressant drugs, including corticosteroids; if this combination must be used, follow patient very closely and discontinue drug at first sign of serious infection ● Do not use with live vaccines, possibility of serious illness

■ Nursing considerations
Assessment

- **History:** allergy to any component of the preparation; presence of active infection, lactation, pregnancy, immune suppression, living in an area endemic with TB or histoplasmosis; pre-existing or recent-onset CNS demyelinating disorders.
- **Physical:** temperature; skin—color, lesions; orientation, reflexes; BP; R; urinary output; lipid levels. CBC with differential

Implementation

- Arrange for pretreatment and periodic CBC levels to monitor for potential infection.
- Arrange for pretreatment tuberculin skin test; instruct patient to seek medical advice at any sign of tuberculin infection.
- Refrigerate drug; inspect solution for any particulate matter or discoloration prior to use, discard if any is found; discard vial after entry, the solution contains no preservatives.
- Administer by SC injection only; keep a map of injection sites and rotate sites between abdomen and upper thigh; do not use any area that is tender, bruised, red, or hard.
- Continue the use of other anti-arthritis drugs as appropriate.
- Protect patient from exposure to infection and ensure routine physical examination

and monitoring for potential cancers, infections, or autoimmune disorders.
- Discontinue drug and arrange for appropriate therapy at first sign of severe infection, lupus-like syndrome.
- Do not administer drug with any live vaccines; allow at least 2–3 wk between last vaccination and starting this drug.
- Suggest the use of barrier contraceptives to women of child-bearing age as the effects of this drug on a fetus are not known.
- Suggest another method of feeding the baby if the drug is needed in a lactating woman.

Teaching points

- Take this drug exactly as prescribed. This drug does not cure rheumatoid arthritis but may slow the damage caused by the disease; you will continue other therapies as appropriate. You and a significant other should learn how to prepare the drug and administer it by subcutaneous injection. The drug should be injected into the abdomen or upper thigh. Prepare a chart of injection sites and rotate the sites—do not use a site that is tender, bruised, red, or hard. Keep a calendar to remind you to inject the drug every other week.
- Refrigerate the drug; if you notice any particulate matter in the solution or if the solution is discolored, do not use it. Discard that solution. Use an appropriate disposal unit for the needles and syringes.
- Know that the following side effects may occur: headache (analgesics may be available to help); infections (you should avoid crowded areas or other people with known infections and use strict hand-washing techniques, you will be more susceptible to diseases); redness and swelling at injection site (rotating sites will help, warm soaks may be necessary if site is very uncomfortable).
- This drug may interact with other medications. Alert any health care provider caring for you that you taking this drug.
- Be aware that this drug should not be taken during pregnancy or when nursing a baby; use of barrier contraceptives is suggested, the effects of the drug on the human fetus or nursing baby are not known.
- You will need periodic blood tests to evaluate the effect of this drug on your system and to monitor for any infections, including TB.

- Report weight loss or wasting, persistent cough, low-grade fever, rash, infection, or swelling at injection sites.

▽adefovir dipivoxil
*(ah **def**′ o veer)*

Hepsera

PREGNANCY CATEGORY C

Drug class
Antiviral drug

Therapeutic actions
Antiviral activity; nucleotide analog which inhibits hepatitis B virus reverse transcriptase and causes DNA chain termination and blocked viral replication

Indications
- Treatment of chronic hepatitis B in adults with evidence of active viral replication and either evidence of persistent elevations in ALT or AST or histologically active disease

Contraindications and cautions
- Contraindicated in the presence of allergy to adefovir or any components of the product, lactation
- Use cautiously with pregnancy, renal impairment, signs of lactic acidosis, risk factors for severe liver disease

Available forms
Tablets—10 mg

Dosages
Adults
10 mg/day PO.
Pediatric patients
Safety and efficacy not established.
Patients with renal impairment
For creatinine clearance > 50 mL/min, 10 mg q 24 hr; creatinine clearance 20–49 mL/min, 10 mg q 48 hr; creatinine clearance 10–19 mL/min, 10 mg q 72 hr. For hemodialysis patients, 10 mg q 7 days following dialysis.

Pharmacokinetics

Route	Onset	Peak
Oral	Rapid	0.6–4 hr

Metabolism: Hepatic; $T_{1/2}$: 6.38–9.13 hr
Distribution: May cross placenta; may pass into breast milk
Excretion: Urine

Adverse effects
- **CNS:** headache, *asthenia*
- **GI:** nausea, diarrhea, abdominal pain, flatulence, dyspepsia, **severe hepatomegaly with steatosis, sometimes fatal; exacerbation of hepatitis if therapy is discontinued,** *elevated liver enzymes*
- **GU: nephrotoxicity,** hematuria, glycosuria
- **Metabolic: lactic acidosis, sometimes severe,** elevated creatine kinase, elevated amylase levels
- **Other:** HIV resistance if used to treat patients with unrecognized HIV infection

Interactions
✳ **Drug-drug** • Increased risk of nephrotoxicity if combined with other drugs that cause nephrotoxicity; if this combination is used, monitor renal function closely and evaluate risks vs. benefits of continuing the combination

■ Nursing considerations
Assessment
- **History:** allergy to adefovir or any component of the drug, renal or hepatic dysfunction, lactic acidosis, pregnancy, lactation.
- **Physical:** T; orientation, reflexes; abdominal exam, liver and renal function tests

Interventions
- Ensure that HIV antibody testing has been done before initiating therapy to reduce risk of emergence of HIV resistance.
- Caution patient not to run out of this drug; patients who stop taking it may develop worsened or severe hepatitis.
- Monitor patients regularly to evaluate renal function and liver enzymes.
- Withdraw drug and monitor patient if patient develops signs of lactic acidosis or hepatotoxicity, including hepatomegaly and steatosis.

Adverse effects in *Italics* are most common; those in **Bold** are life-threatening.

- Encourage women of child bearing age to use barrier contraceptives while on this drug as the effects of the drug on the fetus are not known.
- Advise women who are breast feeding to find another method of feeding the baby.
- Advise patient that this drug does not cure the disease and there is still a risk of transmitting the disease to others; advise the use of barrier contraceptives.

Teaching points

- Take this drug once a day.
- Take the full course of therapy as prescribed; if you miss a dose, take it as soon as you remember and then take the next dose at the usual time the next day. Do not double any doses.
- You will be asked to have an HIV antibody test if your HIV status is not known; some people with HIV who are treated with this drug develop resistant strains of HIV.
- This drug does not cure chronic hepatitis B infection; long-term effects are not yet known; continue to take precautions as the risk of transmission is not reduced by this drug.
- Do not stop taking this drug; you may experience very serious or worsening hepatitis B if the drug is stopped after you have been taking it. Consult your health care provider if your prescription is getting low and make sure that you do not skip any doses.
- These side effects may occur: nausea, diarrhea, abdominal pain, headache; try to maintain nutrition and fluid intake as much as possible—small, frequent meals may help.
- Report severe weakness, muscle pain, trouble breathing, dizziness, cold feelings in your arms or legs, palpitations.

▽adenosine
(a den' oh seen)

Adenocard, Adenoscan

PREGNANCY CATEGORY C

Drug classes
Antiarrhythmic
Diagnostic agent

Therapeutic actions
Slows conduction through the AV node; can interrupt the reentry pathways through the AV node and restore sinus rhythm in patients with paroxysmal supraventricular tachycardias; potent vasodilator that facilitates thallium uptake

Indications
- Conversion to sinus rhythm of paroxysmal supraventricular tachycardia, including that associated with accessory bypass tracts (Wolff–Parkinson–White syndrome), after attempting vagal maneuvers when appropriate (Adenocard)
- Assessment of patients with suspected CAD in conjuction with thallium tomography (Adenoscan)
- Orphan drug use: treatment of brain tumors in conjunction with BCNU

Contraindications and cautions
- Contraindicated with hypersensitivity to adenosine; second- or third-degree AV heart block, sick sinus syndrome (unless artificial pacemaker in place); atrial flutter, atrial fibrillation, ventricular tachycardia.
- Use cautiously with asthma (could produce bronchospasm in asthma patients).

Available forms
Injection—3 mg/mL

Dosages
For rapid bolus IV use only.
Adults
- *Conversion of arrhythmia:* Initial dose: 6 mg as a rapid IV bolus administered over 1–2 sec. Repeat administration: 12 mg as a rapid IV bolus if initial dose does not produce elimination of the supraventricular tachycardia within 1–2 min. 12-mg bolus may be repeated a second time if needed. Doses > 12 mg are not recommended.
- *Assessment of suspected CAD:* 140 mcg/kg/min IV infused over 6 min. Inject thallium at 3 min.
Pediatric patients
Not recommended.

Pharmacokinetics

Route	Onset	Peak	Duration
IV	Immediate	10 sec	20–30 sec

Metabolism: Hepatic; $T_{1/2}$: > 10 sec
Distribution: Rapidly picked up by red blood cells

▽ IV facts
Preparation: Store drug at room temperature; do not refrigerate. Solution must be clear at time of use; discard any unused portion of vial.
Infusion: By rapid IV bolus only, given over 1–2 sec; administer directly into a vein or as proximal as possible; follow with a rapid saline flush.

Adverse effects
- **CNS:** *Headache, light-headedness,* dizziness, tingling in arms, numbness, apprehension, blurred vision, burning sensation, heaviness in arms, neck and back pain
- **CV:** *Facial flushing, arrhythmias,* sweating, palpitations, chest pain, hypotension
- **GI:** *Nausea,* metallic taste, tightness in throat, pressure in groin
- **Respiratory:** Shortness of breath or dyspnea, chest pressure, hyperventilation

Interactions
✳ Drug-drug • Increased degree of heart block with carbamazepine • Increased effects of adenosine with dipyridamole • Decreased effects with methylxanthines (caffeine, theophylline), which antagonize adenosine's activity

■ Nursing considerations
Assessment
- **History:** Hypersensitivity to adenosine, second- or third-degree AV heart block, sick sinus syndrome, atrial flutter, atrial fibrillation, ventricular tachycardia, asthma (use caution)
- **Physical:** Orientation; BP, P, auscultation, ECG; R, adventitious sounds

Interventions
- Assess asthma patients carefully for signs of exacerbation of asthma.
- Monitor patient's ECG continually during administration. Be alert for the possibility of arrhythmias. These usually last only a few seconds.

- Maintain emergency equipment on stand-by at time of administration.
- Have methylxanthines available as antagonists if problems occur.

Teaching points
- These side effects may occur: rapid or irregular heartbeat (usually passes quickly), facial flushing, headache, light-headedness, dizziness, nausea, shortness of breath.
- Report chest pain, difficulty breathing, numbness, tingling so appropriate measures can be taken.

▽ albendazole
See *Less Commonly Used Drugs,* p. 1336.

▽ albumin, human (normal serum albumin)
(al byoo' min)

5%: Albuminar-5, Albunex, Albutein 5%, Buminate 5%, Normal Serum Albumin 5% Solution, Plasbumin-5
25%: Albuminar-25, Albutein 25%, Buminate 25%, Normal Serum Albumin 25% Solution, Plasbumin-25

PREGNANCY CATEGORY C

Drug classes
Blood product
Plasma protein

Therapeutic actions
Normal blood protein; maintains plasma osmotic pressure and is important in maintaining normal blood volume

Indications
- Supportive treatment of shock due to burns, trauma, surgery, and infections
- Burns: albumin 5% used to prevent hemoconcentration and water and protein losses in conjunction with adequate infusions of crystalloid
- Hypoproteinemia in nephrotic syndrome, hepatic cirrhosis, toxemia of pregnancy, post-

---

operative patients, tuberculous patients, pre-mature infants
- Adult respiratory distress syndrome: albu-min 25% with a diuretic may be helpful
- Cardiopulmonary bypass: preoperative blood dilution with 25% albumin
- Acute liver failure
- Sequestration of protein-rich fluids
- Erythrocyte resuspension: albumin 25% may be added to the isotonic suspension of washed red cells immediately before transfusion
- Acute nephrosis: albumin 25% and loop di-uretic may help to control edema
- Renal dialysis: albumin 25% may be useful in treatment of shock and hypotension
- Hyperbilirubinemia and erythroblastosis fe-talis: adjunct in exchange transfusions

Contraindications and cautions
- Contraindicated with allergy to albumin; se-vere anemia, cardiac failure, normal or in-creased intravascular volume, current use of cardiopulmonary bypass.
- Use cautiously with hepatic or renal failure.

Available forms
Injection—5%, 25%

Dosages
Administer by IV infusion only; contains 130–160 mEq sodium/L.
Adults
- *Hypovolemic shock:* 5% albumin: Initial dose of 500 mL given as rapidly as possible; additional 500 mL may be given in 30 min. Base therapy on clinical response if more than 1,000 mL is required; consider the need for whole blood. In patients with low blood volume, administer at rate of 2–4 mL/min. 25% albumin: Base therapy on clinical re-sponse. Administer as rapidly as tolerated; 1 mL/min may be given to patients with low blood volume.
- *Hypoproteinemia:* 5% albumin may be giv-en for acute replacement of protein; if ede-ma is present, use 25% albumin 50–75 g/day. Do not exceed 2 mL/min. Adjust the rate of infusion based on patient response.
- *Burns:* 5% or 25% albumin can be helpful in maintaining colloid osmotic pressure; suggested regimen has not been established.

- *Hepatic cirrhosis:* 25% may be effective in temporary restoration of plasma protein levels.
- *Nephrosis:* Initial dose of 100–200 mL of 25% albumin may be repeated at intervals of 1–2 days; effects are not sustained because of the underlying problem.
Pediatric patients
- *Hypovolemic shock:* 50 mL of 5% albumin; base dosage on clinical response.
- *Hypoproteinemia:* 25 g/day of 25% albu-min.
- *Hyperbilirubinemia and erythroblastosis fetalis:* 1 g/kg 1–2 hr before transfusion, or 50 mL of albumin may be substituted for 50 mL of plasma in the blood to be trans-fused.

Pharmacokinetics

Route	Onset	Peak
IV	Immediate	End of infusion

Metabolism: Tissue; $T_{1/2}$: unknown
Distribution: Crosses placenta; passes into breast milk
Excretion: Urine

▼ IV facts
Preparation: Swab stopper top with anti-septic immediately before removing seal and entering the vial. Inspect for particulate mat-ter and discoloration. Store at room tempera-ture; do not freeze. Do not dilute 5% albumin; 25% albumin may be undiluted or diluted in normal saline.
Infusion: Give by IV infusion slowly enough to prevent rapid plasma volume expansion 1–2 mL/min for adults, 0.25–1 mL/min for children. Give in combination with or through the same administration set as solutions of saline or carbohydrates. Do not use with alco-hol or protein hydrolysates—precipitates may form.

Adverse effects
- **CV:** Hypotension, CHF, **pulmonary ede-ma after rapid infusion**
- **Hypersensitivity:** Fever, chills, *changes in blood pressure*, flushing, nausea, vom-iting, changes in respiration, rashes

■ Nursing considerations

Assessment

- **History:** Allergy to albumin, severe anemia, CHF, current use of cardiopulmonary bypass, hepatic failure, renal failure
- **Physical:** Skin color, lesions; T; P, BP, peripheral perfusion; R, adventitious sounds; liver and renal function tests, Hct, serum electrolytes

Interventions

- Give to all blood groups or types.
- Consider using whole blood; infusion provides only symptomatic relief of hypoproteinemia.
- Monitor BP; discontinue infusion if hypotension occurs.
- Stop infusion if headache, flushing, fever, changes in BP occur; treat reaction with antihistamines. If a plasma protein is still needed, try material from a different lot number.
- Monitor patient's clinical response, and adjust infusion rate accordingly.

Teaching points

- Report headache; nausea, vomiting; difficulty breathing; back pain.

▽albuterol sulfate
(al byoo' ter ole)

AccuNeb, Novo-Salmol (CAN), Proventil, Proventil HFA, Proventil Repetabs, Salbutamol (CAN), Ventodisk (CAN), Ventolin, Ventolin HFA, Volmax

PREGNANCY CATEGORY C

Drug classes

Sympathomimetic drug
Beta$_2$-selective adrenergic agonist
Bronchodilator
Antiasthmatic drug

Therapeutic actions

In low doses, acts relatively selectively at beta$_2$-adrenergic receptors to cause bronchodilation and vasodilation; at higher doses, beta$_2$ selec-

tivity is lost, and the drug acts at beta$_2$ receptors to cause typical sympathomimetic cardiac effects.

Indications

- Relief and prevention of bronchospasm in patients with reversible obstructive airway disease
- Treatment of acute attacks of bronchospasm (inhalation)
- Prevention of exercise-induced bronchospasm
- Unlabeled use: adjunct in treating serious hyperkalemia in dialysis patients; seems to lower potassium concentrations when inhaled by patients on hemodialysis

Contraindications and cautions

- Contraindicated with hypersensitivity to albuterol; tachyarrhythmias, tachycardia caused by digitalis intoxication; general anesthesia with halogenated hydrocarbons or cyclopropane (these sensitize the myocardium to catecholamines); unstable vasomotor system disorders; hypertension; coronary insufficiency, CAD; history of stroke; COPD patients with degenerative heart disease.
- Use cautiously with diabetes mellitus (large IV doses can aggravate diabetes and ketoacidosis); hyperthyroidism; history of seizure disorders; psychoneurotic individuals; labor and delivery (oral use has delayed second stage of labor; parenteral use of beta$_2$-adrenergic agonists can accelerate fetal heart beat and cause hypoglycemia, hypokalemia, pulmonary edema in the mother and hypoglycemia in the neonate); lactation.

Available forms

Tablets—2, 4 mg; SR tablets—4, 8 mg; syrup—2 mg/5 mL; aerosol—90 mcg/actuation; solution for inhalation—0.083%, 0.5%, 1.25 mg/3 mL, 0.63 mg/3 mL; capsules for inhalation—200 mcg

Dosages

Adults

Oral

Initially, 2 or 4 mg (1–2 tsp syrup) tid–qid PO; may cautiously increase dosage if necessary to

4 or 8 mg qid, not to exceed 32 mg/day. Extended release tablets: 8 mg q 12 hr (*Volmax*); 4–8 mg q 12 hr (*Proventil*)

Inhalation

Each actuation of aerosol dispenser delivers 90 mcg albuterol; 2 inhalations q 4–6 hr; some patients may require only 1 inhalation q 4 hr; more frequent administration or larger number of inhalations not recommended.

- *Prevention of exercise-induced bronchospasm:* 2 inhalations 15 min prior to exercise.
- *Solution for inhalation:* 2.5 mg tid to qid by nebulization.
- *Inhalation capsules:* One 200 mcg capsule q 4–6 hr up to two 200 mcg capsules q 4–6 hr.
- *Prevention of exercise-induced asthma:* One 200 mcg capsule inhaled 15 min before exercise.

Pediatric patients

Oral, tablets

12 yr or older: Same as adult.
6–12 yr: 2 mg tid–qid. Do not exceed 24 mg/day.

Extended-release tablets

6–12 yr: 4 mg q 12 hr (*Volmax*).
6–11 yr: 4 mg q 12 hr (*Proventil*).

Oral, syrup

> 14 yr: Same as adult.
6–14 yr: 2 mg (1 tsp) tid–qid; if necessary, cautiously increase dosage. Do not exceed 24 mg/day in divided doses.
2–6 yr: Initially, 0.1 mg/kg tid, not to exceed 2 mg (1 tsp) tid; if necessary, cautiously increase stepwise to 0.2 mg/kg tid. Do not exceed 4 mg (2 tsp) tid.
< 2 yr: Safety and efficacy not established.

Inhalation

≥ 12 yr: Same as adult.
2–12 yr: 10–15 kg—1.25 mg; > 15 kg—2.5 mg

Solution for inhalation

10–15 kg: 1.25 mg bid–tid by nebulization.
> 15 kg: 2.5 mg bid–tid by nebulization.

Inhalation capsules

≥ 4 yr: One 200 mcg capsule inhaled q 4–6 hr.
- *Prevention of exercise-induced asthma:* One 200 mcg capsule inhaled 15 min before exercise.

Geriatric patients or patients sensitive to beta-adrenergic stimulation

Restrict initial dose to 2 mg tid–qid; individualize dosage thereafter. Patients > 60 yr are more likely to develop adverse effects.

Pharmacokinetics

Route	Onset	Peak	Duration
Oral	30 min	2–2.5 hr	4–8 hr
Inhalation	5 min	1.5–2 hr	3–8 hr

Metabolism: Hepatic; $T_{1/2}$: 2–4 hr
Distribution: Crosses placenta; passes into breast milk
Excretion: Urine

Adverse effects

- **CNS:** *Restlessness, apprehension, anxiety, fear, CNS stimulation,* hyperkinesia, insomnia, tremor, drowsiness, irritability, weakness, vertigo, headache
- **CV:** *Cardiac arrhythmias,* tachycardia, palpitations, PVCs (rare), anginal pain
- **Dermatologic:** *Sweating, pallor, flushing*
- **GI:** *Nausea,* vomiting, heartburn, unusual or bad taste
- **GU:** Increased incidence of leiomyomas of uterus when given in higher than human doses in preclinical studies
- **Respiratory:** Respiratory difficulties, pulmonary edema, coughing, bronchospasm, paradoxical airway resistance with repeated, excessive use of inhalation preparations

Interactions

❋ **Drug-drug** ● Increased sympathomimetic effects with other sympathomimetic drugs ● Increased risk of toxicity, especially cardiac, when used with theophylline, aminophylline, oxtriphylline ● Decreased bronchodilating effects with beta-adrenergic blockers (eg, propranolol) ● Decreased effectiveness of insulin, oral hypoglycemic drugs ● Decreased serum levels and therapeutic effects of digoxin

■ Nursing considerations
Assessment

- **History:** Hypersensitivity to albuterol; tachyarrhythmias, tachycardia caused by digitalis intoxication; general anesthesia with halogenated hydrocarbons or cyclopropane;

unstable vasomotor system disorders; hypertension; coronary insufficiency, CAD; history of stroke; COPD patients who have developed degenerative heart disease; diabetes ·mellitus; hyperthyroidism; history of seizure disorders; psychoneurotic individuals; lactation.

- **Physical:** Weight; skin color, temperature, turgor; orientation, reflexes, affect; P, BP; R, adventitious sounds; blood and urine glucose, serum electrolytes, thyroid function tests, ECG

Interventions

- Use minimal doses for minimal periods; drug tolerance can occur with prolonged use.
- Maintain a beta-adrenergic blocker (cardioselective beta-blocker, such as atenolol, should be used with respiratory distress) on standby in case cardiac arrhythmias occur.
- Prepare solution for inhalation by diluting 0.5 mL 0.5% solution with 2.5 mL normal saline; deliver over 5–15 min by nebulization.
- Do not exceed recommended dosage; administer pressurized inhalation drug forms during second half of inspiration, because the airways are open wider and the aerosol distribution is more extensive.

Teaching points

- Do not exceed recommended dosage; adverse effects or loss of effectiveness may result. Read the instructions that come with respiratory inhalant.
- These may occur: dizziness, drowsiness, fatigue, headache (use caution if driving or performing tasks that require alertness); nausea, vomiting, change in taste (small, frequent meals may help); rapid heart rate, anxiety, sweating, flushing.
- Report chest pain, dizziness, insomnia, weakness, tremors or irregular heart beat, difficulty breathing, productive cough, failure to respond to usual dosage.

▷ **aldesleukin (interleukin-2, IL-2)**
(al des loo' ken)

Proleukin

PREGNANCY CATEGORY C

Drug class
Antineoplastic

Therapeutic actions
Human interleukin produced by *Escherichia coli* bacteria; activates human cellular immunity and inhibits tumor growth through increases in lymphocytes, platelets, and cytokines (tumor necrosis factor and interferon)

Indications
- Metastatic renal cell carcinoma in adults
- Orphan drug use: treatment of adult patients with metastatic melanoma
- Unlabeled uses: treatment of Kaposi's sarcoma with zidovudine; treatment of metastatic melanoma with cyclophosphamide; treatment of non-Hodgkin's lymphoma with lymphokine-activated killer cells; treatment of phase I AIDS, advanced ARC with zidovudine

Contraindications and cautions
- Contraindicated with hypersensitivity to aldesleukin; abnormal thallium stress test; abnormal pulmonary function test; organ allografts; lactation.
- Use cautiously with renal, liver, or CNS impairment, pregnancy.

Available forms
Powder for injection—22 × 10^6 IU/vial

Dosages
Adults
Administer by 15 min IV infusion q 8 hr.
- *Metastatic renal cell carcinoma:* Each course of treatment consists of two 5-day cycles of 600,000 IU/kg q 8 hr IV over 15 min, separated by a rest, for a total of 14 doses, then 9 days of rest followed by 14 more doses. Treatment may be stopped because of toxicity. Retreatment may be considered after

all doses completed. Evaluate patient 4 wk after completion; if tumor shrinkage occurred, repeat treatments. Allow 7 wk from date of previous hospitalization.

Pediatric patients
Safety not established.

Pharmacokinetics

Route	Onset	Peak	Duration
IV	5 min	13 min	3–4 hr

Metabolism: Renal; $T_{1/2}$: 85 min
Distribution: Crosses placenta; passes into breast milk
Excretion: Urine

▼ IV facts

Preparation: Reconstitute each vial (22 million IU) with 1.2 mL sterile water for injection, USP; direct the sterile water at the side of the vial and swirl gently to avoid excess foaming; do not shake. Resultant liquid should be clear, colorless to yellow, containing 18 million IU/mL. Use plastic, not glass, containers and avoid in-line filters. Dilute in 50 mL of 5% dextrose injection, USP. Avoid dilution in bacteriostatic water or 0.9% sodium chloride injection; aggregation can occur. Do not dilute with albumin; do not mix with other drugs. Store vials in refrigerator before and after reconstitution; do not freeze. Administer within 48 hr of reconstitution; discard unused portions.
Infusion: Bring solution to room temperature before use; infuse over 15 min.
Incompatibility: Do not mix with other drugs.

Adverse effects

- **CNS:** *Mental status changes, dizziness,* sensory dysfunction, syncope, headache, conjunctivitis
- **CV: Capillary leak syndrome**—third spacing of fluids and severe hypotension, which may proceed to shock and death; *hypotension, sinus tachycardia, arrhythmias*
- **Dermatologic:** *Pruritus, erythema, rash,* dry skin, exudative dermatitis
- **GI:** *Nausea, vomiting, diarrhea, stomatitis, anorexia,* **GI bleed**
- **GU:** *Oliguria or anuria,* proteinuria, hematuria
- **Hematologic:** *Anemia, thrombocytopenia, leukopenia,* coagulation disorders
- **Respiratory:** *Respiratory difficulties, dyspnea,* pulmonary edema, coughing, bronchospasm
- **Other:** *Fever, chills, pain, fatigue, weakness, malaise, edema, infection*

Interactions

✳ Drug-drug • Increased hypotensive effects with antihypertensives • Decreased effectiveness with corticosteroids • Increased toxicity of cardiotoxic, hepatotoxic, myelotoxic, and nephrotoxic agents: doxorubicin, methotrexate, asparaginase, aminoglycosides, indomethacin

■ Nursing considerations
Assessment

- **History:** Hypersensitivity to aldesleukin; abnormal thallium stress test, pulmonary function test; organ allografts; lactation; renal, liver, or CNS impairment
- **Physical:** Weight; skin color, temperature, turgor; orientation, reflexes, affect; P, BP; R, adventitious sounds; bowel sounds; CBC, serum electrolytes, thyroid, liver and renal function tests; ECG, stress test, pulmonary function tests

Interventions

- Give only in intensive care settings with emergency life support available.
- Ensure that patient has normal thallium stress test and normal pulmonary function tests, including baseline blood gases, before giving drug.
- Monitor patient's vital signs, weight, cardiac monitoring (if BP falls), respiratory sounds, and pulse oximetry; cardiac sounds and perfusion evaluation; orientation.
- Tell patient to use birth control during drug use; women should not breast-feed.
- Monitor patient for signs of infection; advise patient to avoid exposure to crowds and to those with contagious diseases.
- Stop drug if patient becomes disoriented, somnolent, or very lethargic; continued use could result in a coma.
- Stop drug if severe side effects occur (arrhythmias, hypotension, chest pain, oliguria, liver failure, bullous dermatitis); drug may be restarted if a period of rest returns affected systems to normal.

Teaching points

- This drug is given in 5-day cycles with a 9-day rest period to allow the body to recover. This drug can only be given IV, and you will need to be closely monitored while it is given.
- You will need to have many tests to evaluate the effects of this drug and the advisability of continuing treatment.
- Avoid exposure to any infections or contagious diseases (eg, crowds); you will be more susceptible to infection.
- These side effects may occur: fever, chills, rash, fluid retention, difficulty breathing, nausea, vomiting, diarrhea.
- Report chest pain, dizziness, weakness, irregular heart beat, difficulty breathing, swelling, fever, malaise, fatigue, changes in stool or urine color.

▽alefacept

See *Less Commonly Used Drugs*, p. 1336.

▽alemtuzumab

See *Less Commonly Used Drugs*, p. 1336.

▽alendronate sodium
*(ah **len'** dro nate)*

Fosamax

PREGNANCY CATEGORY C

Drug classes
Bisphosphonate
Calcium regulator

Therapeutic actions
Slows normal and abnormal bone resorption without inhibiting bone formation and mineralization.

Indications

- Treatment and prevention of osteoporosis in postmenopausal women
- Treatment of men with osteoporosis
- Treatment of glucocorticoid-induced osteoporosis

- Treatment of Paget's disease of bone in patients with alkaline phosphatase at least two times upper limit of normal, those who are symptomatic, those at risk for future complications

Contraindications and cautions

- Contraindicated with allergy to biphosphonates; hypocalcemia, pregnancy, lactation.
- Use cautiously with renal dysfunction, upper GI disease.

Available forms
Tablets—5, 10, 35, 40, 70 mg

Dosages
Adults

- *Postmenopausal osteoporosis:* 10 mg/day PO in AM with full glass of water, at least 30 min before the first beverage, food, or medication of the day, or 70 mg PO once a week.
- *Males with osteoporosis:* 10 mg/day PO.
- *Prevention of osteoporosis:* 5 mg/day PO or 35 mg PO once a week.
- *Paget's disease:* 40 mg/day PO in AM with full glass of water, at least 30 min before the first beverage, food, or medication of the day for 6 mo; may retreat after 6-mo treatment-free period.
- *Glucocorticoid-induced osteoporosis:* 5 mg/day PO with calcium and vitamin D.

Pediatric patients
Safety and efficacy not established.

Patients with renal impairment
Dosage adjustment not necessary for creatinine clearance 35–60 mL/min; not recommended if creatinine clearance < 35 mL/min.

Pharmacokinetics

Route	Onset	Duration
Oral	Slow	Days

Metabolism: Not metabolized
Distribution: Crosses placenta; may enter breast milk
Excretion: Urine

Adverse effects

- **CNS:** *Headache*
- **GI:** *Nausea, diarrhea*

Adverse effects in *Italics* are most common; those in **Bold** are life-threatening.

- **Skeletal:** *Increased or recurrent bone pain,* focal osteomalacia

Interactions
✴ **Drug-drug** • Increased risk of GI distress with aspirin • Decreased absorption if taken with antacids, calcium, iron, multivalent cations; separate dosing by at least 30 min
✴ **Drug-food** • Significantly decreased absorption and serum levels if taken with food; separate dosing from food and beverage by at least 30 min

■ Nursing considerations
CLINICAL ALERT!
Name confusion has occurred between Fosamax (alendronate) and Flomax (tamsulosin); use caution.

Assessment
- **History:** Allergy to bisphosphonates, renal failure, upper GI disease, lactation, pregnancy
- **Physical:** Muscle tone, bone pain; bowel sounds; urinalysis, serum calcium

Interventions
- Give in AM with full glass of water at least 30 min before the first beverage, food, or medication of the day. Patient must stay upright for 30 min.
- Monitor serum calcium levels before, during, and after therapy.
- Recommend concomitant hormone replacement therapy in treatment of osteoporosis.
- Ensure 6-mo rest period after treatment for Paget's disease if retreatment is required.
- Ensure adequate vitamin D and calcium intake.
- Provide comfort measures if bone pain returns.

Teaching points
- Take drug in morning with a full glass of plain water (not mineral water), at least 30 min before any beverage, food, or medication, and stay upright for 30 min.
- These side effects may occur: nausea, diarrhea; bone pain, headache (analgesic may help).

- Report twitching, muscle spasms, dark-colored urine, severe diarrhea.

▽ alglucerase
See *Less Commonly Used Drugs,* p. 1336.

▽ allopurinol
*(al oh **pure'** i nole)*

Apo-Allopurinol (CAN), Purinol (CAN), Zyloprim

PREGNANCY CATEGORY C

Drug class
Antigout drug

Therapeutic actions
Inhibits the enzyme responsible for the conversion of purines to uric acid, thus reducing the production of uric acid with a decrease in serum and sometimes in urinary uric acid levels, relieving the signs and symptoms of gout

Indications
- Management of the signs and symptoms of primary and secondary gout
- Management of patients with malignancies that result in elevations of serum and urinary uric acid
- Management of patients with recurrent calcium oxalate calculi whose daily uric acid excretion exceeds 800 mg/day (males) or 750 mg/day (females)
- Orphan drug use: treatment of Chagas' disease; cutaneous and visceral leishmaniasis
- Unlabeled uses: amelioration of granulocyte suppression with fluorouracil; as a mouthwash to prevent fluorouracil-induced stomatitis

Contraindications and cautions
- Contraindicated with allergy to allopurinol, blood dyscrasias.
- Use cautiously with liver disease, renal failure, lactation, pregnancy.

Available forms
Tablets—100, 300 mg

Dosages
Adults
- *Gout and hyperuricemia:* 100–800 mg/day PO in divided doses, depending on the severity of the disease (200–300 mg/day is usual dose).
- *Maintenance:* Establish dose that maintains serum uric acid levels within normal limits.
- *Prevention of acute gouty attacks:* 100 mg/day PO; increase the dose by 100 mg at weekly intervals until uric acid levels are within normal limits.
- *Prevention of uric acid nephropathy in certain malignancies:* 600–800 mg/day PO for 2–3 days; maintenance dose should then be established as above.
- *Recurrent calcium oxalate stones:* 200–300 mg/day PO; adjust dose up or down based on 24-hr urinary urate determinations.

Pediatric patients
- *Secondary hyperuricemia associated with various malignancies:*
6–10 yr: 300 mg/day PO.
< 6 yr: 150 mg/day; adjust dosage after 48 hr of treatment based on serum uric acid levels.

Geriatric patients or patients with renal impairment
For geriatric patient or creatinine clearance 10–20 mL/min, 200 mg/day; for creatinine clearance < 10 mL/min, 100 mg/day; for creatinine clearance < 3 mL/min, intervals between doses will need to be extended, based on patient's serum uric acid levels.

Adverse effects
- **CNS:** *Headache, drowsiness,* peripheral neuropathy, neuritis, paresthesias
- **Dermatologic: Rashes—maculopapular, scaly or exfoliative—sometimes fatal**
- **GI:** *Nausea, vomiting, diarrhea,* abdominal pain, gastritis, hepatomegaly, hyperbilirubinemia, cholestatic jaundice
- **GU:** Exacerbation of gout and renal calculi, renal failure
- **Hematologic:** Anemia, leukopenia, agranulocytosis, thrombocytopenia, aplastic anemia, bone marrow depression

Interactions
* **Drug-drug** • Increased risk of hypersensitivity reaction with ACE inhibitors • Increased toxicity with thiazide diuretics • Increased risk of rash with ampicillin • Increased risk of bone marrow suppression with cyclophosphamide, other cytotoxic agents • Increased half-life of oral anticoagulants • Increased serum levels of theophylline • Increased risk of toxic effects with thiopurines, 6-MP (azathioprine dose and dose of 6-MP should be reduced to one-third to one-fourth the usual dose)

■ Nursing considerations
Assessment
- **History:** Allergy to allopurinol, blood dyscrasias, liver disease, renal failure, lactation
- **Physical:** Skin lesions, color; orientation, reflexes; liver evaluation, normal urinary output; normal output; CBC, renal and liver function tests, urinalysis

Interventions
- Administer drug following meals.
- Force fluids—2.5 to 3 L/day to decrease the risk of renal stone development.
- Check urine alkalinity—urates crystallize in acid urine; sodium bicarbonate or potassium citrate may be ordered to alkalinize urine.
- Arrange for regular medical follow-up and blood tests.

Teaching points
- Take the drug following meals.
- These side effects may occur: exacerbation of gouty attack or renal stones (drink plenty of fluids while on this drug, 2.5–3 L/day); nausea, vomiting, loss of appetite (take after meals or eat small, frequent meals); drowsiness (use caution while driving or performing hazardous tasks).
- Avoid OTC medications. Many of these preparations contain vitamin C or other agents that might increase the likelihood of kidney stone formation. If you need an OTC preparation, check with your health care provider.
- Report rash; unusual bleeding or bruising; fever, chills; gout attack; numbness or tingling; flank pain.

Adverse effects in *Italics* are most common; those in **Bold** are life-threatening.

▷ almotriptan
*(al moh **trip**' tan)*

Axert

PREGNANCY CATEGORY C

Drug classes
Antimigraine agent
Serotonin selective agonist
Triptan

Therapeutic actions
Binds to serotonin receptors to cause vascular constrictive effects on cranial blood vessels, causing the relief of migraine in selective patients.

Indications
• Treatment of acute migraines with or without aura

Contraindications and cautions
• Contraindicated in the presence of allergy to almotriptan, active coronary artery disease, Printzmetal's angina, peripheral vascular syndromes, uncontrolled hypertension, use of an ergot compound or other triptan within 24 hours, pregnancy.
• Use caution in the presence of liver or renal dysfunction, risk factors for CAD, lactation.

Available forms
Tablets—6.25, 12.5 mg

Dosages
Adults
6.25–12.5 mg PO as a single dose at first sign of migraine; if headache returns, may be repeated after 2 hr; do not use more than 2 doses/24 hr.
Pediatric patients
Safety and efficacy not established for patients < 18 yr.

Pharmacokinetics

Route	Onset	Peak
Oral	Varies	1–3 hr

Metabolism: Hepatic; $T_{1/2}$: 3–4 hr
Distribution: Crosses placenta; may pass into breast milk
Excretion: Urine and feces

Adverse effects
• **CNS:** *Dizziness,* headache, anxiety, malaise or fatigue, weakness, myalgia
• **CV:** *Blood pressure alterations, tightness or pressure in chest,* arrhythmias
• **GI:** *Nausea, dry mouth,* abdominal discomfort, dysphagia
• **Other:** Tingling, warm/hot sensations, burning sensation, feeling of heaviness, pressure sensation, numbness, feeling of tightness, feeling strange, cold sensation

Interactions
✳ **Drug-drug** • Prolonged vasoactive reactions when taken concurrently with ergot-containing drugs • Risk of severe effects if taken with or ≤ 2 wk of discontinuation of an MAO inhibitor • Increased effects and possible toxicity if taken with ketoconazole; monitor patient closely if this combination is used

■ Nursing considerations
Assessment
• **History:** Allergy to almotriptan, active coronary artery disease, Printzmetal's angina, pregnancy, lactation, peripheral vascular syndromes, uncontrolled hypertension, use of an ergot compound or other triptan within 24 hr, risk factors for CAD
• **Physical:** Skin color and lesions; orientation, reflexes, peripheral sensation; P, BP; renal and liver function tests

Interventions
• Administer to relieve acute migraine, not as a prophylactic measure.
• Ensure that the patient has not taken an ergot-containing compound or other triptan within 24 hr.
• Do not administer more than 2 doses in a 24-hr period.
• Establish safety measures if CNS, visual disturbances occur.
• Provide environmental control as appropriate to help relieve migraine (lighting, temperature, etc.).
• Monitor BP of patients with possible coronary artery disease; discontinue at any sign of angina, prolonged high blood pressure, etc.

Teaching points

- Take drug exactly as prescribed, at the onset of headache or aura. Do not take this drug to prevent a migraine, it is only used to treat migraines that are occurring. If the headache remains after you take this drug, you may repeat the dose after 2 hr have passed.
- Do not take more than 2 doses in a 24-hr period. Do not take any other migraine medication while you are taking this drug. If the headache is not relieved, call your health care provider.
- Be aware that this drug should not be taken during pregnancy; if you suspect that you are pregnant, contact physician and refrain from using drug.
- Be aware that these side effects may occur: dizziness, drowsiness (avoid driving or the use of dangerous machinery while on this drug), numbness, tingling, feelings of tightness or pressure.
- Maintain any procedures you usually use during a migraine: controlled lighting, noise reduction, etc.
- Contact health care provider immediately if you experience chest pain or pressure that is severe or does not go away.
- Report: feelings of heat, flushing, tiredness, feelings of sickness, swelling of lips or eyelids.

▽alosetron hydrochloride

*(ah **loss'** e tron)*

Lotronex

PREGNANCY CATEGORY B

Drug class
5-HT₃ antagonist

Therapeutic actions
Blocks 5-HT₃ (serotonin) receptors in the enteric nervous system of the gastrointestinal tract; interacting with these receptors blocks visceral sensitivity, increases colonic transit time, decreases GI motility, may also decrease the perception of abdominal pain and discomfort.

Indications
- Treatment of severe diarrhea-predominant irritable bowel syndrome (IBS) in women who have chronic IBS (longer than 6 mo), have no anatomic or biochemical abnormalities of the GI tract, and who have failed to respond to conventional therapy.

Contraindications and cautions
- Contraindicated with hypersensitivity to the drug, history of chronic or severe constipation or sequelae from constipation; history of intestinal obstruction, stricture, toxic megacolon, GI perforation or adhesions; history of ischemic colitis, impaired intestinal circulation, thrombophlebitis, or hypercoagulable state; history of or current Crohn's disease, ulcerative colitis, diverticulitis; inability to understand or comply with the Physician–Patient Agreement.
- Use cautiously with pregnancy, lactation, and elderly patients.

Available forms
Tablets—1 mg

Dosages
Adults
1 mg/day PO for 4 wk; may be continued if drug is tolerated and symptoms of IBS are under adequate control. Dose may be increased up to 1 mg bid PO after 4 wk if well tolerated.
Pediatric patients
Safety and efficacy not established for patients < 18 yr.
Geriatric patients or patients with hepatic impairment
These patients may be at increased risk for toxicity; monitor very closely.

Pharmacokinetics

Route	Onset	Peak
Oral	Rapid	1 hr

Metabolism: Hepatic; T₁/₂: 1.5 hr
Distribution: Crosses placenta; enters into breast milk
Excretion: Urine and bile

Adverse effects

- **CNS:** Anxiety, tremors, dreams, headache
- **Dermatologic:** sweating, urticaria
- **GI:** Abdominal pain, nausea, *constipation, ischemic colitis*
- **Other:** Malaise, fatigue, pain

Interactions

✳ Drug-drug • Increased risk of constipation if taken with other drugs that cause decreased GI motility. If this combination cannot be avoided, monitor patient very carefully and discontinue drug at first sign of constipation or ischemic colitis.

■ Nursing considerations
Assessment

- **History:** Presence of hypersensitivity to the drug, history of chronic or severe constipation or sequelae from constipation; history of intestinal obstruction, stricture, toxic megacolon, GI perforation or adhesions; history of ischemic colitis, impaired intestinal circulation, thrombophlebitis, or hypercoagulable state; history of Crohn's disease, ulcerative colitis, diverticulitis; inability to understand or comply with the Physician–Patient Agreement, pregnancy, lactation, elderly patients.
- **Physical:** Skin lesions; body temperature; reflexes, affect; urinary output, abdominal exam; bowel patterns

Interventions

- Ensure that the patient has read and understands the Physician–Patient Agreement outlining the risks associated with the use of the drug and warning signs to report.
- Ensure that the Physician–Patient Agreement is in the patient's permanent record.
- Administer drug without regard to food.
- Arrange for further evaluation of patient after 4 wk of therapy to determine effectiveness of drug.
- Encourage the use of barrier contraceptives to prevent pregnancy while on this drug.
- Maintain supportive treatment as appropriate for underlying problem.
- Provide additional comfort measures to alleviate discomfort from GI effects, headache, etc.
- Monitor patient for any signs of constipation; discontinue drug at first sign of constipation or ischemic colitis and alert the prescribing physician.

Teaching points

- Read and sign the Physician–Patient Agreement, which outlines the risks and benefits of therapy with this drug.
- Arrange to have regular medical follow-up while you are on this drug.
- Use barrier contraceptives while on this drug; serious adverse effects could occur during pregnancy; if you become or wish to become pregnant, consult with your physician.
- Be aware that these side effects may occur: headache (consult with your health care provider if these become bothersome, medications may be available to help); nausea, vomiting (proper nutrition is important, consult with your dietician to maintain nutrition).
- Maintain all of the usual activities and restrictions that apply to your condition. If this becomes difficult, consult with your health care provider.
- Report: constipation, signs of ischemic colitis—worsening abdominal pain, bloody diarrhea, blood in the stool; continuation of IBS symptoms without relief.

▷ alpha₁-proteinase inhibitor

See *Less Commonly Used Drugs*, p. 1336.

▷ alprazolam
*(al **prah'** zoe lam)*

Apo-Alpraz (CAN), Novo-Alprazol (CAN), Nu-Alpraz (CAN), Xanax, Xanax TS (CAN)

PREGNANCY CATEGORY D

C-IV CONTROLLED SUBSTANCE

Drug classes

Benzodiazepine
Antianxiety drug

Therapeutic actions

Exact mechanisms of action not understood; main sites of action may be the limbic system and reticular formation; increases the effects of gamma-aminobutyrate, an inhibitory neurotransmitter; anxiety blocking effects occur at doses well below those necessary to cause sedation, ataxia.

Indications

- Management of anxiety disorders, short-term relief of symptoms of anxiety; anxiety associated with depression.
- Treatment of panic attacks with or without agoraphobia
- *Unlabeled uses:* social phobia, premenstrual syndrome, depression

Contraindications and cautions

- Contraindicated with hypersensitivity to benzodiazepines, psychoses, acute narrow-angle glaucoma, shock, coma, acute alcoholic intoxication with depression of vital signs, pregnancy (crosses the placenta; risk of congenital malformations, neonatal withdrawal syndrome), labor and delivery ("floppy infant" syndrome), lactation (secreted in breast milk; infants become lethargic and lose weight).
- Use cautiously with impaired liver or kidney function, debilitation.

Available forms

Tablets—0.25, 0.5, 1, 2 mg; oral solution—0.5 mg/5 mL; intensol solution—1 mg/mL

Dosages

Individualize dosage; increase dosage gradually to avoid adverse effects.

Adults

- *Anxiety disorders:* Initially, 0.25–0.5 mg PO tid; adjust to maximum daily dose of 4 mg/day in divided doses.
- *Panic disorder:* Initially 0.5 mg PO tid; increase dose at 3- to 4-day intervals in increments of no more than 1 mg/day; ranges of 1–10 mg/day have been needed.
- *Social phobia:* 2–8 mg/day PO.
- *Premenstrual syndrome:* 0.25 mg PO tid.

Geriatric patients or patients with debilitating disease

Initially 0.25 mg bid–tid PO; gradually increase if needed and tolerated.

Pharmacokinetics

Route	Onset	Peak	Duration
Oral	30 min	1–2 hr	4–6 hr

Metabolism: Hepatic; $T_{1/2}$: 6.3–26.9 hr
Distribution: Crosses placenta; passes into breast milk
Excretion: Urine

Adverse effects

- **CNS:** *Transient, mild drowsiness initially; sedation, depression, lethargy, apathy, fatigue, light-headedness, disorientation, anger, hostility,* episodes of mania and hypomania, *restlessness, confusion, crying,* delirium, *headache,* slurred speech, dysarthria, stupor, rigidity, tremor, dystonia, vertigo, euphoria, nervousness, difficulty in concentration, vivid dreams, psychomotor retardation, extrapyramidal symptoms; *mild paradoxical excitatory reactions during first 2 weeks of treatment*
- **CV:** Bradycardia, tachycardia, cardiovascular collapse, hypertension, hypotension, palpitations, edema
- **Dermatologic:** Urticaria, pruritus, rash, dermatitis
- **EENT:** Visual and auditory disturbances, diplopia, nystagmus, depressed hearing, nasal congestion
- **GI:** *Constipation, diarrhea, dry mouth,* salivation, *nausea,* anorexia, vomiting, difficulty in swallowing, gastric disorders, hepatic dysfunction
- **GU:** Incontinence, changes in libido, urinary retention, menstrual irregularities
- **Hematologic:** Elevations of blood enzymes—LDH, alkaline phosphatase, AST, ALT; blood dyscrasias—agranulocytosis, leukopenia
- **Other:** Hiccups, fever, diaphoresis, paresthesias, muscular disturbances, gynecomastia. *Drug dependence with withdrawal syndrome when drug is discontinued; more common with abrupt discontinuation of higher dosage used for longer than 4 mo*

Interactions

✳ Drug-drug • Increased CNS depression with alcohol, other CNS depressants, propoxyphene • Increased effect with cimetidine, disulfiram, omeprazole, isoniazid, oral contraceptives, valproic acid • Decreased effect with carbamazepine, rifampin, theophylline • Possible increased risk of digitalis toxicity with digoxin • Decreased antiparkinson effectiveness of levodopa with benzodiazepines • Contraindicated with ketoconazole, itraconazole; serious toxicity can occur

✻ Drug-food • Decreased metabolism and risk of toxic effects if combined with grapefruit juice; avoid this combination.

✻ Drug-alternative therapy • Risk of coma if combined with kava therapy

■ Nursing considerations

 CLINICAL ALERT!
Name confusion has occurred among Xanax (alprazolam), Celexa (citalopram), and Cerebyx (fosphenytoin), and between alprazolam and lorazepam; use caution.

Assessment
• **History:** Hypersensitivity to benzodiazepines; psychoses; acute narrow-angle glaucoma; shock; coma; acute alcoholic intoxication with depression of vital signs; labor and delivery; lactation; impaired liver or kidney function; debilitation
• **Physical:** Skin color, lesions; T; orientation, reflexes, affect, ophthalmologic exam; P, BP; liver evaluation, abdominal exam, bowel sounds, normal output; CBC, liver and renal function tests

Interventions
• Arrange to taper dosage gradually after longterm therapy, especially in epileptic patients.

Teaching points
• Take this drug exactly as prescribed.
• Do not drink grapefruit juice while on this drug.
• Do not stop taking drug (long-term therapy) without consulting health care provider.
• Avoid alcohol, sleep-inducing, or OTC drugs.
• These side effects may occur: drowsiness, dizziness (less pronounced after a few days, avoid driving a car or engaging in other dangerous activities if these occur); GI upset (take drug with food); fatigue; depression; dreams; crying; nervousness.

• Report severe dizziness, weakness, drowsiness that persists, rash or skin lesions, difficulty voiding, palpitations, swelling in the extremities.

▷ alprostadil
(al pross' ta dil)

IV: Prostin VR Pediatric
Intracavernous: Caverject, Edex, Muse

PREGNANCY CATEGORY
(NOT APPLICABLE)

Drug class
Prostaglandin

Therapeutic actions
Relaxes vascular smooth muscle; the smooth muscle of the ductus arteriosus is especially sensitive to this action and will relax and stay open; this is beneficial in infants who have congenital defects that restrict pulmonary or systemic blood flow and who depend on a patent ductus arteriosus for adequate blood oxygenation and lower body perfusion. Treatment of erectile dysfunction due to neurogenic, vasculogenic, psychogenic, or mixed etiology.

Indications
• Palliative therapy to temporarily maintain the patency of the ductus arteriosus until corrective or palliative surgery can be performed in neonates with congenital heart defects who depend on a patent ductus (eg, pulmonary atresia or stenosis, tetralogy of Fallot, coarctation of the aorta)
• Treatment of erectile dysfunction (intracavernous injection)
• Unlabeled use: treatment of atherosclerosis, gangrene, and pain of peripheral vascular disease

Contraindications and cautions
• Contraindicated with respiratory distress syndrome; conditions that might predispose to priapism, deformation of the penis, penile implants (intracavernous injection), known hypersensitivity.

- Use cautiously with patients with bleeding tendencies (drug inhibits platelet aggregation).

Available forms
Powder for injection—6.15, 11.9, 23.2 mcg; pellets—125, 250, 500, 1,000 mcg; injection (IV)—500 mcg/mL; injection (penile)—5, 10, 20, 40 mcg/vial

Dosages
Adults
Intracavernous injection
0.2–140 mcg by intracavernous injection using 0.5-in 27–30 gauge needle; may be repeated up to 3 times weekly. Self injection over 6-mo period has been successful. Reduce dose if erection lasts > 1 hr.
Pediatric patients
Preferred administration is through a continuous IV infusion into a large vein; may be administered through an umbilical artery catheter placed at the ductal opening. Begin infusion with 0.1 mcg/kg/min. After an increase in pO_2 or in systemic BP and blood pH is achieved, reduce infusion to the lowest possible dosage that maintains the response (often achieved by reducing dosage from 0.1–0.05 to 0.025–0.01 mcg/kg/min). Up to 0.4 mcg/kg/min may be used for maintenance if required; higher dosage rates are not more effective.

Pharmacokinetics

Route	Onset	Peak
IV	5–25 min	—
Intracavernous	10 min	30–60 min

Metabolism: Lungs; $T_{1/2}$: 5–10 min
Excretion: Urine

▼IV facts
Preparation: Prepare solution by diluting 500 mcg alprostadil with sodium chloride injection or dextrose injection; dilute to volumes required for pump delivery system. Discard and prepare fresh infusion solutions q 24 hr; refrigerate drug ampules.

Infusion:

Add 500 mg Alprostadil to	Approximate Concentration of Resulting Solution	Infusion Rate (mL/kg/min)
250 mL	2 mcg/mL	0.05
100 mL	5 mcg/mL	0.02
50 mL	10 mcg/mL	0.01
25 mL	20 mcg/mL	0.005

Adverse effects
- **CNS:** *Seizures,* cerebral bleeding, hypothermia, jitteriness, lethargy, stiffness
- **CV:** *Bradycardia, flushing, tachycardia, hypotension,* cardiac arrest, heart block, CHF
- **GI:** Diarrhea
- **GU (with intracavernous injection):** Penile pain, rash, **fibrosis,** erection, priapism
- **Hematologic:** Inhibited platelet aggregation, bleeding, anemia, DIC, hypokalemia
- **Respiratory:** *Apnea,* respiratory distress
- **Other:** Cortical proliferation of the long bones (with prolonged use, regresses after treatment is stopped), sepsis

■ Nursing considerations

CLINICAL ALERT!
Confusion has been reported with Prostin VR Pediatric (alprostadil), Prostin F_2 (dinoprost—available outside US), Prostin E_2 (dinoprostone), Prostin 15M (carboprost in Europe); use extreme caution.

Assessment
- **History:** Respiratory distress, bleeding tendencies
- **Physical:** T; cyanosis; skeletal development, reflexes, state of agitation, arterial pressure (using auscultation or Doppler), P, auscultation, peripheral perfusion; R, adventitious sounds, bleeding times, arterial blood gases, blood pH

Interventions
IV
- Constantly monitor arterial pressure; decrease infusion rate immediately if any fall in arterial pressure occurs.

- Regularly monitor arterial blood gases to determine efficacy of alprostadil (pO_2 in infants with restricted pulmonary flow; pH and systemic blood pressure in infants with restricted systemic flow).

Intracavernous
- Reconstitute vial with 1 mL diluent. 1 mL of solution will contain 5.4–41.1 mcg of alprostadil.
- Use solution immediately after reconstitution; do not store or freeze.
- Inject along dorsal-lateral aspect of proximal third of penis using sterile technique.

Teaching points
IV
- Teaching about this drug should be incorporated into a total teaching program for the parent(s) of the infant with a cyanotic congenital heart defect; specifics about the drug that they will need to know include:
- Your infant will be continually monitored and have frequent blood tests to follow the effects of the drug.
- The infant may look better, breathe easier, become fussy, and so forth, but the drug treatment is only a temporary solution, and the baby will require corrective surgery.

Intracavernous
- Learn and repeat self-injection technique. Do not self-inject > 3 times per week; wait at least 24 hr between injections.
- Return for regular medical follow-up and evaluation.
- These side effects may occur: penile pain, swelling, rash.
- Report prolonged erection, swelling, or pain.

▽**alteplase, recombinant (recombinant tissue-type plasminogen activator, rt-PA)**
(al ti plaze')

T-PA, Activase, Cathflo Activase

PREGNANCY CATEGORY C

Drug class
Thrombolytic enzyme

Therapeutic actions
Human tissue enzyme produced by recombinant DNA techniques; converts plasminogen to the enzyme plasmin (fibrinolysin), which degrades fibrin clots; lyses thrombi and emboli; is most active at the site of the clot and causes little systemic fibrinolysis.

Indications
- Treatment of coronary artery thrombosis associated with acute MI
- Treatment of acute, massive pulmonary embolism in adults
- Treatment of acute ischemic stroke
- Restoration of function to central venous access devices occluded as assessed by the ability to withdraw blood
- Unlabeled use: treatment of unstable angina

Contraindications and cautions
- Contraindicated with allergy to TPA; active internal bleeding; recent (within 2 mo) CVA; intracranial or intraspinal surgery or neoplasm; recent major surgery, obstetric delivery, organ biopsy, or rupture of a non-compressible blood vessel; recent serious GI bleed; recent serious trauma, including CPR; SBE; hemostatic defects; cerebrovascular disease; early-onset, insulin-dependent diabetes; septic thrombosis; severe uncontrolled hypertension.
- Use cautiously with liver disease in elderly (> 75 yr—risk of bleeding may be increased).

Available forms
Powder for injection—50, 100 mg; single use vial for injection (*Cathflo Activase*)—2 mg

Dosages
Careful patient assessment and evaluation are needed to determine the appropriate dose of this drug. Because experience is limited with this drug, careful monitoring is essential.
Adults
- *Acute MI:* Total dose of 100 mg IV given as follows: 60 mg the first hour, with an initial bolus of 6–10 mg given over 1–2 min and the rest infused slowly over the rest of the hour; then 20 mg infused slowly over the second hour and 20 mg more infused slowly over the third hour. For patients weighing less than 65 kg, decrease total dose to

1.25 mg/kg. Do not use a total dose of 150 mg because of the increased risk of intracranial bleeding.

- *Pulmonary embolism:* 100 mg administered by IV infusion over 2 hr, followed immediately by heparin therapy.
- *Acute ischemic stroke:* 0.9 mg/kg (not to exceed 90 mg total dose) infused over 60 min with 10% given as an IV bolus over the first 1 min.
- *Restoration of function of central venous access devices:* 2 mg from single use vial injected into device.

Pharmacokinetics

Route	Onset	Peak	Duration
IV	Immediate	5–10 min	2.5–3 hr

Metabolism: Hepatic; $T_{1/2}$: 26 min
Distribution: Crosses placenta
Excretion: Cleared by the liver

▼ IV facts

Preparation: Do not use if vacuum is not present; add volume of the sterile water for injection provided with vial using a large bore needle and directing stream into the cake; slight foaming may occur but will dissipate after standing undisturbed for several minutes; reconstitute immediately before use. Refrigerate reconstituted solution and use within 3 hr. Do not use bacteriostatic water for injection. Reconstituted solution should be colorless or pale yellow and transparent; contains 1 mg/mL with a pH of 7.3.

Infusion: Administer as reconstituted or further dilute with an equal volume of 0.9% sodium chloride injection or 5% dextrose injection to yield 0.5 mg/mL; stable for up to 8 hr in these solutions. Avoid excessive agitation; mix by gentle swirling or slow inversion. Discard unused solution.

Incompatibilities: Do not add other medications to infusion solution; use 0.9% sodium chloride injection or 5% dextrose injection and no other solutions.

Y-site compatibility: lidocaine.

Y-site incompatibility: dobutamine, dopamine, heparin, nitroglycerin.

Adverse effects

- **CV:** Cardiac arrhythmias with coronary reperfusion, hypotension
- **Hematologic:** *Bleeding*—particularly at venous or arterial access sites, GI bleeding, **intracranial hemorrhage**
- **Other:** Urticaria, nausea, vomiting, fever

Interactions

✳ **Drug-drug** • Increased risk of hemorrhage if used with heparin or oral anticoagulants, aspirin, dipyridamole

■ Nursing considerations

 CLINICAL ALERT!
Confusion has been reported between alteplase and Altace (ramipril); use caution.

Assessment

- **History:** Allergy to TPA; active internal bleeding; recent (within 2 mo) obstetric delivery, organ biopsy, or rupture of a non-compressible blood vessel; recent serious GI bleed; recent serious trauma, including CPR; SBE; hemostatic defects; cerebrovascular disease; early-onset insulin-dependent diabetes; septic thrombosis; severe uncontrolled hypertension; liver disease
- **Physical:** Skin color, temperature, lesions; orientation, reflexes; P, BP, peripheral perfusion, baseline ECG; R, adventitous sounds; liver evaluation, Hct, platelet count, TT, APTT, PT

Interventions

- Discontinue heparin and alteplase if serious bleeding occurs.
- Monitor coagulation studies; PT or APPT should be less than 2 times control.
- Apply pressure or pressure dressings to control superficial bleeding (at invaded or disturbed areas).
- Avoid arterial invasive procedures.
- Type and cross-match blood in case serious blood loss occurs and whole-blood transfusions are required.
- Institute treatment within 6 hr of onset of symptoms for evolving myocardial infarction, within 3 hr of onset of stroke.

Teaching points
- This drug can only be given IV. You will be closely monitored during drug treatment.
- Report difficulty breathing, dizziness, disorientation, headache, numbness, tingling.

▽**altretamine**
(al tret' a meen)

Hexalen

PREGNANCY CATEGORY D

Drug class
Antineoplastic

Therapeutic actions
Cytotoxic; mechanisms by which it is able to cause cell death are not known.

Indications
- Single agent in the palliative treatment of persistent or recurrent ovarian cancer following first-line therapy with a cisplatin or alkylating agent–based combination

Contraindications and cautions
- Hypersensitivity to altretamine, bone marrow depression, severe neurologic toxicity, lactation, pregnancy.

Available forms
Capsules—50 mg

Dosages
Adults
Dosage is determined by body surface area. 260 mg/m² per day PO given for 14 or 21 consecutive days in a 28-day cycle. Total daily dose is given as divided doses after meals and hs. Temporarily discontinue altretamine for > 14 days if GI intolerance, WBC < 2,000/mm³ or granulocytes < 1,000/mm³, platelet count < 75,000/mm³, or progressive neuropathy occurs; restart with 200 mg/m² per day.

Pharmacokinetics

Route	Onset	Peak
Oral	Rapid	0.5–3 hr

Metabolism: Hepatic; $T_{1/2}$: 4.7–10 hr

Distribution: Crosses placenta; passes into breast milk
Excretion: Urine

Adverse effects
- **CNS: Peripheral sensory neuropathy** (mild to severe); fatigue, seizures
- **GI:** *Nausea, vomiting,* increased alkaline phosphatase, anorexia
- **GU:** Increased BUN
- **Hematologic: Bone marrow depression**
- **Other:** Carcinogenesis, impairment of fertility, mutagenesis

Interactions
✳ **Drug-drug** • Increased effects with cimetidine • Increased risk of orthostatic hypotension with MAO inhibitors

■ Nursing considerations
Assessment
- **History:** Hypersensitivity to altretamine; bone marrow depression; severe neurologic toxicity; lactation
- **Physical:** Neurologic status, T, abdominal exam, kidney and liver function tests, CBC

Interventions
- Give drug with meals and at bedtime.
- Discontinue drug if GI effects are intractable; severe neuropathy occurs; bone marrow depression becomes dangerous. Reevaluate patient, and consider restarting drug after up to 14 days of rest.
- Arrange for blood counts before and at least monthly during treatment.
- Monitor neurologic status frequently.
- Consider antiemetics or decreased dose if nausea and vomiting are severe.

Teaching points
- Take drug with meals and at bedtime.
- Arrange to have regular blood tests and neurologic exams while on drug.
- These side effects may occur: nausea and vomiting (this may be severe; antiemetics may help and can be ordered for you; small, frequent meals also may help); weakness, lethargy (frequent rest periods may help); increased susceptibility to infection (avoid crowds and situations that might involve exposure to many people or diseases); numb-

ness and tingling in the fingers or toes (use care to avoid injury to these areas; use care if trying to perform tasks that require precision).

- Report severe nausea and vomiting; fever, chills, sore throat; unusual bleeding or bruising; numbness or tingling in your fingers or toes.

▷ aluminum hydroxide gel

(a loo' mi num)

AlternaGEL, Alu-Cap, Alu-Tab, Amphojel, Dialume

PREGNANCY CATEGORY C

Drug class
Antacid

Therapeutic actions
Neutralizes or reduces gastric acidity, resulting in an increase in the pH of the stomach and duodenal bulb and inhibiting the proteolytic activity of pepsin, which protects the lining of the stomach and duodenum; binds with phosphate ions in the intestine to form insoluble aluminum–phosphate complexes, lowering phosphate in hyperphosphatemia and chronic renal failure; may cause hypophosphatemia in other states.

Indications
- Symptomatic relief of upset stomach associated with hyperacidity
- Hyperacidity associated with peptic ulcer, gastritis, peptic esophagitis, gastric hyperacidity, hiatal hernia
- Unlabeled uses: prophylaxis of GI bleeding, stress ulcer; reduction of phosphate absorption in hyperphosphatemia in patients with chronic renal failure

Contraindications and cautions
- Allergy to aluminum products, gastric outlet destruction, hypertension, CHF, hypophosphatemia, lactation

Available forms
Tablets—300, 500, 600 mg; capsules—400, 500 mg; suspension—320 mg/5 mL, 450 mg/5 mL, 675 mg/5 mL; liquid—600 mg/5 mL

Dosages
Adults
500–1,500 mg 3–6 times per day PO between meals and hs.
Pediatric patients
- *Hyperphosphatemia:* 50–150 mg/kg every 24 hr PO in divided doses q 4–6 hr; adjust dose to normal serum phosphorus.
- *General guidelines:* 5–15 mL PO q 3–6 hr or 1–3 hr after meals and hs.
- *Prophylaxis of GI bleeding in critically ill infants:* 2–5 mL/dose q 1–2 hr PO.
- *Prophylaxis of GI bleeding in critically ill children:* 5–15 mL/dose q 1–2 hr PO.

Pharmacokinetics

Route	Onset
Oral	Varies

Metabolism: Hepatic
Distribution: Long-term use, small amounts may be absorbed systemically and cross the placenta and enter breast milk
Excretion: GI bound in the feces

Adverse effects
- **GI:** *Constipation;* intestinal obstruction, decreased absorption of fluoride, accumulation of aluminum in serum, bone, and CNS
- **Musculoskeletal:** Osteomalacia and chronic phosphate deficiency with bone pain, malaise, muscular weakness

Interactions
❋ **Drug-drug** • Do not administer other oral drugs within 1–2 hr of antacid; change in gastric pH may interfere with absorption of oral drugs • Decreased pharmacologic effect of corticosteroids, diflunisal, digoxin, iron, isoniazid, penicillamine, phenothiazines, ranitidine, tetracyclines • Increased pharmacologic effect of benzodiazepines

---

Adverse effects in *Italics* are most common; those in **Bold** are life-threatening.

■ **Nursing considerations**
Assessment
- **History:** Allergy to aluminum products; gastric outlet obstruction; hypertension, CHF; hypophosphatemia; lactation
- **Physical:** Bone strength, muscle strength; P, auscultation, BP, peripheral edema; abdominal exam, bowel sounds; serum phosphorous, serum fluoride; bone x-ray is appropriate

Interventions
- Give hourly for first 2 wk when used for acute peptic ulcer; during the healing stage, give 1–3 hr after meals and hs.
- Do not administer oral drugs within 1–2 hr of antacid administration.
- Have patient chew tablets thoroughly; follow with a glass of water.
- Monitor serum phosphorus levels periodically during long-term therapy.

Teaching points
- Take this drug between meals and at bedtime; ulcer patients need to strictly follow prescribed dosage pattern. If tablets are being used, chew thoroughly before swallowing, and follow with a glass of water.
- Do not take maximum dosage of antacids for more than 2 weeks except under medical supervision.
- Do not take this drug with any other oral medications; absorption of those medications can be inhibited. Take other oral medications at least 1–2 hr after aluminum salt.
- Constipation may occur.
- Report constipation; bone pain, muscle weakness; coffee ground vomitus, black tarry stools; no relief from symptoms being treated.

▽ **amantadine hydrochloride**
(a **man'** ta deen)

Endantadine (CAN), Gen-Amantadine (CAN), Symmetrel

PREGNANCY CATEGORY C

Drug classes
Antiviral drug
Antiparkinsonian drug

Therapeutic actions
May inhibit penetration of influenza A virus into the host cell; may increase dopamine release in the nigostriatal pathway of patients with Parkinson's disease, relieving their symptoms.

Indications
- Prevention and treatment of influenza A virus respiratory infection, especially in high-risk patients
- Adjunct to late vaccination against influenza A virus, to provide interim coverage; supplement to vaccination in immunodeficient patients; prophylaxis when vaccination is contraindicated
- Parkinson's disease and drug-induced extrapyramidal reactions

Contraindications and cautions
- Allergy to drug product, seizures, liver disease, eczematoid rash, psychoses, CHF, renal disease, lactation.

Available forms
Tablets—100 mg; syrup—50 mg/5 mL

Dosages
Adults
- *Influenza A virus prophylaxis:* 200 mg/day PO or 100 mg bid PO for 10 days after exposure, for up to 90 days if vaccination is impossible and exposure is repeated.
- *Influenza A virus treatment:* Same dose as above; start treatment as soon after exposure as possible, continuing for 24–48 hr after symptoms are gone.
- *Parkinsonism treatment:* 100 mg bid (up to 400 mg/day) PO when used alone; reduce in patients receiving other antiparkinsonian drugs.
- *Drug-induced extrapyramidal reactions:* 100 mg bid PO, up to 300 mg/day in divided doses has been used.
Patients with seizure disorders
100 mg/day.
Patients with renal disease
For patients on hemodialysis, 200 mg PO q 7 days.
    For patients with reduced creatinine clearance, see the table on p. 100.

Creatinine Clearance (mL/min)	Dosage
< 15	200 mg PO q 7 days
15–29	200 mg PO first day, then 100 mg on alternate days
30–50	200 mg PO first day, then 100 mg/day

Pediatric patients

Not recommended for children < 1 yr.

• *Influenza A virus prophylaxis:*
1–9 yr: 4.4–8.8 mg/kg/day PO in two to three divided doses, not to exceed 150 mg/day.
9–12 yr: 100 mg PO bid.

• *Influenza A virus treatment:* As above; start as soon after exposure as possible, continuing for 24-48 hr after symptoms are gone.

Geriatric patients

• *Parkinsonism treatment:* For patients > 65 yr with no recognized renal disease, 100 mg once daily PO in parkinsonism treatment; 100 mg bid (up to 400 mg/day) when used alone; reduce dosage in patients receiving other antiparkinsonian drugs.

Pharmacokinetics

Route	Onset	Peak
Oral	36–48 hr	4 hr

Metabolism: $T_{1/2}$: 15–24 hr
Distribution: Crosses placenta; passes into breast milk
Excretion: Unchanged in the urine

Adverse effects

• **CNS:** *Light-headedness, dizziness, insomnia,* confusion, irritability, ataxia, psychosis, depression, hallucinations
• **CV:** **CHF,** orthostatic hypotension, dyspnea
• **GI:** *Nausea,* anorexia, constipation, dry mouth
• **GU:** Urinary retention

Interactions

✱ **Drug-drug** • Increased atropine-like side effects with anticholinergic drugs • Increased amantadine effects with hydrochlorothiazide, triamterene

■ Nursing considerations

Assessment

• **History:** Allergy to drug product, seizures, liver disease, eczematoid rash, psychoses, CHF, renal disease, lactation
• **Physical:** Orientation, vision, speech, reflexes; BP, orthostatic BP, P, auscultation, perfusion, edema; R, adventitious sounds; urinary output; BUN, creatinine clearance

Interventions

• Do not discontinue abruptly when treating parkinsonism syndrome; parkinsonian crisis may occur.

Teaching points

• Mark your calendar if you are on alternating dosage schedules; it is very important to take the full course of the drug.
• These may occur: drowsiness, blurred vision (use caution when driving or using dangerous equipment); dizziness, light-headedness (avoid sudden position changes); irritability or mood changes (common effect; if severe, drug may be changed).
• Report swelling of the fingers or ankles; shortness of breath; difficulty urinating, walking; tremors, slurred speech.

⟍⃝ **ambenonium chloride**
(am be noe' nee um)

Mytelase

PREGNANCY CATEGORY C

Drug classes

Cholinesterase inhibitor
Parasympathomimetic drug (indirectly acting)
Antimyasthenic drug

Therapeutic actions

Increases the concentration of acetylcholine at the sites of cholinergic transmission (parasympathetic neurons and skeletal muscles) and prolongs and exaggerates the effects of acetylcholine by inhibiting the enzyme acetylcholinesterase; this causes parasympathomimetic effects and facilitates transmission at the skeletal neuromuscular junction. Also has direct stimulating effects on skeletal muscle and has a longer duration of effect and fewer side effects than other agents.

Indications

• Symptomatic control of myasthenia gravis

Contraindications and cautions

• Contraindicated with hypersensitivity to anticholinesterases; intestinal or urogenital tract obstruction; peritonitis; lactation.
• Use cautiously with asthma, peptic ulcer, bradycardia, cardiac arrhythmias, recent coronary occlusion, vagotonia, hyperthyroidism, epilepsy.

Available forms

Tablets—10 mg

Dosages
Adults

5–25 mg PO tid–qid (5–75 mg per dose has been used). Start dosage with 5 mg, and gradually increase to determine optimum dosage based on optimal muscle strength and no GI disturbances; increase dose every 1–2 days. Dosage above 200 mg/day requires close supervision to avoid overdose.
Pediatric patients
Safety and efficacy not established.

Pharmacokinetics

Route	Onset	Peak
Oral	20–30 min	3–8 hr

Metabolism: $T_{1/2}$: Unknown
Distribution: Crosses placenta; passes into breast milk
Excretion: Unknown

Adverse effects
Parasympathomimetic effects

• **CNS:** Convulsions, dysarthria, dysphonia, drowsiness, dizziness, headache, loss of consciousness
• **CV:** *Bradycardia, cardiac arrhythmias,* AV block and nodal rhythm, cardiac arrest; decreased cardiac output, leading to hypotension, syncope
• **Dermatologic:** Diaphoresis, flushing
• **EENT:** *Lacrimation, miosis,* spasm of accommodation, diplopia, conjunctival hyperemia

• **GI:** *Salivation, dysphagia, nausea, vomiting, increased peristalsis, abdominal cramps,* flatulence, diarrhea
• **GU:** *Urinary frequency and incontinence,* urinary urgency
• **Respiratory:** *Increased pharyngeal and tracheobronchial secretions,* laryngospasm, bronchospasm, bronchiolar constriction, dyspnea
Skeletal muscle effects
• **Peripheral:** Skeletal muscle weakness, fasciculations, muscle cramps, arthralgia
• **Respiratory:** Respiratory muscle paralysis, central respiratory paralysis

Interactions

✱ **Drug-drug** • Decreased neuromuscular blockade of succinylcholine • Decreased effects of ambenonium and possible muscular depression with corticosteroids

■ Nursing considerations
Assessment

• **History:** Hypersensitivity to anticholinesterases, intestinal or urogenital tract obstruction, peritonitis, asthma, peptic ulcer, bradycardia, cardiac arrhythmias, recent coronary occlusion, vagotonia, hyperthyroidism, epilepsy, lactation
• **Physical:** Skin color, texture, lesions; reflexes, bilateral grip strength; P, auscultation, BP; R, adventitious sounds; salivation, bowel sounds, normal output; frequency, voiding pattern, normal urinary output; EEG, thyroid tests

Interventions

• Overdose can cause muscle weakness (cholinergic crisis) that is difficult to differentiate from myasthenic weakness (use of edrophonium for differential diagnosis is recommended). The administration of atropine may mask the parasympathetic effects of anticholinesterase overdose and further confound the diagnosis.
• Maintain atropine sulfate on standby as an antidote and antagonist in case of cholinergic crisis or hypersensitivity reaction.
• Monitor patient response carefully if increasing dosage.
• Discontinue drug and consult physician if excessive salivation, emesis, frequent urination, or diarrhea occurs.

- Arrange for decreased dosage of drug if excessive sweating, nausea, or GI upset occurs.

Teaching points

- Take this drug exactly as prescribed; does not need to be taken at night. Patient and home caregiver need to know about the effects of the drug, the signs and symptoms of myasthenia gravis, the fact that muscle weakness may be related to drug overdose and to exacerbation of the disease, and that it is important to report muscle weakness promptly to the nurse or physician so that proper evaluation can be made.
- These side effects may occur: blurred vision, difficulty with far vision, difficulty with dark adaptation (use caution while driving, especially at night, or performing hazardous tasks in reduced light); increased urinary frequency, abdominal cramps (if these become a problem, notify your health care provider); sweating (avoid hot or excessively humid environments).
- Report muscle weakness, nausea, vomiting, diarrhea, severe abdominal pain, excessive sweating, excessive salivation, frequent urination, urinary urgency, irregular heartbeat, difficulty breathing.

▽amifostine

See *Less Commonly Used Drugs*, p. 1336.

▽amikacin sulfate
(am i kay' sin)

Amikin

PREGNANCY CATEGORY D

Drug class
Aminoglycoside antibiotic

Therapeutic actions
Bactericidal: inhibits protein synthesis in susceptible strains of gram-negative bacteria, and the functional integrity of bacterial cell membrane appears to be disrupted, causing cell death.

Indications

- Short-term treatment of serious infections caused by susceptible strains of *Pseudomonas* species, *E. coli*, indole-positive *Proteus* species, *Providencia* species, *Klebsiella*, *Enterobacter*, and *Serratia* species, *Acinetobacter* species
- Suspected gram-negative infections before results of susceptibility studies are known (effective in infections caused by gentamicin- or tobramycin-resistant strains of gram-negative organisms)
- Initial treatment of staphylococcal infections when penicillin is contraindicated or infection may be caused by mixed organisms
- Neonatal sepsis when other antibiotics cannot be used (often used in combination with penicillin-type drug)
- Unlabeled uses: intrathecal or intraventricular administration at 8 mg/24 hr; part of a multidrug regimen for treatment of *Mycobacterium avium* complex, a common infection in AIDS patients

Contraindications and cautions

- Contraindicated with allergy to any aminoglycosides, renal or hepatic disease, preexisting hearing loss, myasthenia gravis, parkinsonism, infant botulism, lactation.
- Use cautiously with elderly patients, any patient with diminished hearing, decreased renal function, dehydration, neuromuscular disorders, pregnancy.

Available forms
Injection—50 mg/mL, 250 mg/mL

Dosages
Adults and pediatric patients
15 mg/kg/day IM or IV divided into two to three equal doses at equal intervals, not to exceed 1.5 g/day

- *UTIs:* 250 mg bid IM or IV; treatment is usually required for 7–10 days. If treatment is required for longer, carefully monitor serum levels and renal and neurologic function.

Neonatal patients
Loading dose of 10 mg/kg IM, then 7.5 mg/kg q 12 hr.

Adverse effects in *Italics* are most common; those in **Bold** are life-threatening.

Geriatric patients or patients with renal failure

Reduce dosage, and carefully monitor serum drug levels and renal function tests throughout treatment; regulate dosage based on these values. If creatinine clearance is not available and patient condition is stable, calculate a dosage interval in hours for the normal dose by multiplying patient's serum creatinine by 9. Dosage guide if creatinine clearance is known: Maintenance dose q 12 hr = observed creatinine clearance ÷ normal creatinine clearance × calculated loading dose (mg).

Pharmacokinetics

Route	Onset	Peak
IV	Immediate	30 min
IM	Varies	45–120 min

Metabolism: $T_{1/2}$: 2–3 hr
Distribution: Crosses placenta; passes into breast milk
Excretion: Unchanged in the urine

▼IV facts

Preparation: Prepare IV solution by adding the contents of a 500-mg vial to 100 or 200 mL of sterile diluent. Do not physically mix with other drugs. Administer amikacin separately. Prepared solution is stable in concentrations of 0.25 and 5 mg/mL for 24 hr at room temperature.
Infusion: Administer to adults or pediatric patients over 30–60 min; infuse to infants over 1–2 hr.
Compatibilities: Amikacin is stable in 5% dextrose injection; 5% dextrose and 0.2%, 0.45%, or 0.9% sodium chloride injection; lactated Ringer's injection; Normosol M in 5% dextrose injection; Normosol R in 5% dextrose injection; Plasma-Lyte 56 or 148 injection in 5% dextrose in water.
Y-site compatibility: May be given with enalaprilat, furosemide, magnesium sulfate, morphine, ondansetron.
Y-site incompatibility: Do not give with hetastarch.

Adverse effects

• **CNS:** *Ototoxicity,* confusion, disorientation, depression, lethargy, nystagmus, visual disturbances, headache, fever, numbness, tingling, tremor, paresthesias, muscle twitch-ing, convulsions, muscular weakness, neuromuscular blockade, apnea
• **CV:** Palpitations, hypotension, hypertension
• **GI:** *Nausea, vomiting, anorexia, diarrhea,* weight loss, stomatitis, increased salivation, splenomegaly
• **GU: Nephrotoxicity**
• **Hematologic:** Leukemoid reaction, agranulocytosis, granulocytosis, leukopenia, leukocytosis, thrombocytopenia, eosinophilia, pancytopenia, anemia, hemolytic anemia, increased or decreased reticulocyte count, electrolyte disturbances
• **Hepatic:** Hepatic toxicity; hepatomegaly
• **Hypersensitivity:** Purpura, rash, urticaria, exfoliative dermatitis, itching
• **Other:** *Superinfections, pain and irritation at IM injection sites*

Interactions

✳ **Drug-drug** • Increased ototoxic and nephrotoxic effects with potent diuretics and other similarly toxic drugs (eg, cephalosporins) • Risk of inactivation if mixed parenterally with penicillins • Increased likelihood of neuromuscular blockade if given shortly after general anesthetics, depolarizing and nondepolarizing neuromuscular junction blockers

■ Nursing considerations

CLINICAL ALERT!
Name confusion has occurred between amikacin and anakinra; use caution.

Assessment

• **History:** Allergy to any aminoglycosides, renal or hepatic disease, preexisting hearing loss, myasthenia gravis, parkinsonism, infant botulism, lactation, diminished hearing, decreased renal function, dehydration, neuromuscular disorders
• **Physical:** Arrange culture and sensitivity tests on infection prior to therapy; renal function, eighth cranial nerve function and state of hydration prior to, during, and after therapy; hepatic function tests, CBC, skin color and lesions, orientation and affect, reflexes, bilateral grip strength, weight, bowel sounds.

Interventions

• Arrange for culture and sensitivity testing of infected area before treatment.

- Monitor duration of treatment: usually 7–10 days. If clinical response does not occur within 3–5 days, stop therapy. Prolonged treatment leads to increased risk of toxicity. If drug is used longer than 10 days, monitor auditory and renal function daily.
- Give IM dosage by deep injection.
- Ensure that patient is well hydrated before and during therapy.

Teaching points
- This drug is only available for IM or IV use.
- These side effects may occur: ringing in the ears, headache, dizziness (reversible; safety measures may need to be taken if severe); nausea, vomiting, loss of appetite (small, frequent meals, frequent mouth care may help).
- Report pain at injection site, severe headache, dizziness, loss of hearing, changes in urine pattern, difficulty breathing, rash or skin lesions.

▽ **amiloride hydrochloride**
*(a **mill'** oh ride)*

Midamor

PREGNANCY CATEGORY B

Drug class
Potassium-sparing diuretic

Therapeutic actions
Inhibits sodium reabsorption in the renal distal tubule, causing loss of sodium and water and retention of potassium.

Indications
- Adjunctive therapy with thiazide or loop diuretics in edema associated with CHF and in hypertension to treat hypokalemia or to prevent hypokalemia in patients who would be at high risk if hypokalemia occurred (digitalized patients, patients with cardiac arrhythmias)
- Unlabeled uses: inhalation in the treatment of cystic fibrosis; reduction of lithium-induced polyuria without increasing lithium levels

Contraindications and cautions
- Allergy to amiloride, hyperkalemia, renal or liver disease, diabetes mellitus, metabolic or respiratory acidosis, lactation.

Available forms
Tablets—5 mg

Dosages
Adults
Add 5 mg/day PO to usual antihypertensive or dosage of kaluretic diuretic; if necessary, increase dose to 10 mg/day or to 15–20 mg/day with careful monitoring of electrolytes.
- *Single-drug therapy:* Start with 5 mg/day PO; if necessary, increase to 10 mg/day or to 15–20 mg/day with careful monitoring of electrolytes.

Pediatric patients
Safety and efficacy not established.

Pharmacokinetics

Route	Onset	Peak	Duration
Oral	2 hr	6–10 hr	24 hr

Metabolism: $T_{1/2}$: 6–9 hr
Distribution: Crosses placenta; passes into breast milk
Excretion: Unchanged in the urine

Adverse effects
- **CNS:** *Headache,* dizziness, drowsiness, fatigue, paresthesias, tremors, confusion, encephalopathy
- **GI:** *Nausea, anorexia, vomiting, diarrhea,* dry mouth, constipation, jaundice, gas pain, GI bleeding
- **GU:** *Hyperkalemia,* polyuria, dysuria, *impotence,* decreased libido
- **Musculoskeletal:** *Weakness, fatigue, muscle cramps* and muscle spasms, joint pain
- **Respiratory:** Cough, dyspnea
- **Other:** Rash, pruritus, itching, alopecia

Interactions
✳ **Drug-drug** • Increased hyperkalemia with triamterene, spironolactone, potassium sup-

---

Adverse effects in *Italics* are most common; those in **Bold** are life-threatening.

plements, diets rich in potassium, ACE inhibitors • Reduced effectiveness of digoxin with amiloride

■ Nursing considerations
Assessment
- **History:** Allergy to amiloride, hyperkalemia, renal or liver disease, diabetes mellitus, metabolic or respiratory acidosis, lactation
- **Physical:** Skin color, lesions, edema; orientation, reflexes, muscle strength; pulses, baseline ECG, BP; respiratory rate, pattern, adventitious sounds; liver evaluation, bowel sounds, urinary output patterns; CBC, serum electrolytes, blood sugar, liver and renal function tests, urinalysis

Interventions
- Administer with food or milk to prevent GI upset.
- Administer early in the day so increased urination does not disturb sleep.
- Measure and record weights to monitor mobilization of edema fluid.
- Avoid foods and salt substitutes high in potassium.
- Provide frequent mouth care, sugarless lozenges to suck.
- Arrange for regular evaluation of serum electrolytes.

Teaching points
- Take single dose early in the day so increased urination will not disturb sleep.
- Take the drug with food or meals to prevent GI upset.
- Avoid foods that are high in potassium and any flavoring that contains potassium (eg, salt substitute).
- Weigh yourself on a regular basis at the same time and in the same clothing, and record the weight on your calendar.
- These side effects may occur: increased volume and frequency of urination; dizziness, feeling faint on arising, drowsiness (avoid rapid position changes, hazardous activities like driving, and the use of alcohol which may intensify these problems); decrease in sexual function; increased thirst (sucking on sugarless lozenges may help; frequent mouth care also may help); avoid foods that are rich in potassium (eg, fruits, *Sanka*).

- Report loss or gain of more than 3 lb in 1 day; swelling in your ankles or fingers; dizziness, trembling, numbness, fatigue; muscle weakness or cramps.

▽ amino acids
(a mee' noe)

Aminess 5.2%, Aminosyn, 4% BranchAmin, FreAmine, HepatAmine, NephrAmine, Novamine, Primene (CAN), ProcalAmine, RenAmin, Travasol, TrophAmine, Vamin N (CAN)

PREGNANCY CATEGORY C

Drug classes
Protein substrate
Caloric agent

Therapeutic actions
Essential and nonessential amino acids provided in various combinations to supply calories and proteins and provide a protein-building and a protein-sparing effect for the body (a positive nitrogen balance).

Indications
- Provide nutrition to patients who are in a negative nitrogen balance when GI tract cannot absorb protein; when protein needs exceed the ability to absorb protein (burns, trauma, infections); when bowel rest is needed; when tube feeding cannot supply adequate nutrition; when health can be improved or restored by replacing lost amino acids
- Treatment of hepatic encephalopathy in patients with cirrhosis or hepatitis
- Nutritional support of uremic patients when oral nutrition is not feasible

Contraindications and cautions
- Contraindicated with hypersensitivity to any component of the solution; severe electrolyte or acid–base imbalance; inborn errors in amino acid metabolism; decreased circulating blood volume; severe kidney or liver disease; hyperammonemia; bleeding abnormalities.

- Use cautiously with liver or renal impairment; diabetes mellitus; CHF; hypertension.

Available forms
Many forms available for IV injections.

Dosages
Dosage must be individualized with careful observation of cardiac status and BUN and evaluation of metabolic needs.
Adults
1–1.7 g/kg/day amino acid injection IV into a peripheral vein; 250–500 mL/day amino acid injection IV mixed with appropriate dextrose, vitamins, and electrolytes as part of a TPN solution.
Pediatric patients
2–3 g/kg/day amino acid IV mixed with dextrose as appropriate.

Pharmacokinetics

Route	Onset
IV	Immediate

Metabolism: Part of normal anabolic processes
Distribution: Crosses placenta; passes into breast milk
Excretion: Urine as urea nitrogen

▽ IV facts
Preparation: Strict aseptic technique is required in mixing solution; use of a laminar flow hood in the pharmacy is recommended. A 0.22 mcm filter should be used to block any particulate matter and bacteria. Use mixed solution immediately. If not used within 1 hr, refrigerate solution. Mixed solutions must be used within 24 hr. Use strict aseptic technique when changing bottles, catheter tubing, and so forth. Replace all IV apparatus every 24 hr. Change dressing every 24 hr to assess insertion site.
Infusion: Use a volumetric infusion pump. Infuse only if solution is absolutely clear and without particulate matter. Infuse slowly. If infusion falls behind, do not try to speed up infusion rate; serious overload could occur. Infusion rates of 20-30 mL/hr up to a maximum of 60–100 mL/hr have been used.

Incompatibilities: Do not mix with amphotericin B, ampicillin, carbenicillin, cephradine, gentamicin, metronidazole, tetracycline, ticarcillin.

Adverse effects
- **CNS:** *Headache, dizziness,* mental confusion, **loss of consciousness**
- **CV:** Hypertension, CHF, **pulmonary edema,** tachycardia, *generalized flushing*
- **Endocrine:** Hypoglycemia, hyperglycemia, fatty acid deficiency, azotemia, hyperammonemia
- **GI:** *Nausea, vomiting,* abdominal pain, liver impairment, fatty liver
- **Hypersensitivity:** Fever, chills, rash, papular eruptions
- **Local:** *Pain, infection,* phlebitis, venous thrombosis, tissue sloughing at injection site

Interactions
✳ **Drug-drug** • Reduced protein-sparing effects of amino acids if taken with tetracyclines

■ Nursing considerations
Assessment
- **History:** Hypersensitivity to any component of the solution; severe electrolyte or acid–base imbalance; inborn errors in amino acid metabolism; decreased circulating blood volume; kidney or liver disease; hyperammonemia; bleeding abnormalities; diabetes mellitus; congestive heart failure; hypertension
- **Physical:** T, weight, height; orientation, reflexes; P, BP, edema; R, lung auscultation; abdominal exam; urinary output; CBC, platelet count, PT, electrolytes, BUN, blood glucose, uric acid, bilirubin, creatinine, plasma proteins, renal and liver function tests; urine glucose, osmolarity

Interventions
- Assess nutritional status before and frequently during treatment; weigh patient daily to monitor fluid load and nutritional status.
- Monitor vital signs frequently during infusion; monitor I&O continually during treatment.
- Observe infusion site at least daily for infection, phlebitis; change dressing using strict aseptic technique at least q 24 hr.

Adverse effects in *Italics* are most common; those in **Bold** are life-threatening.

- Arrange to give D_5W or $D_{10}W$ for injection by a peripheral line to avoid hypoglycemia rebound if TPN infusion needs to be stopped.
- Monitor urine glucose, acetone, and specific gravity q 6 hr during initial infusion period, at least bid when the infusion has stabilized; stop solution at any sign of renal failure.
- Monitor patient for vascular overload or hepatic impairment; decrease rate of infusion or discontinue.

Teaching points

- This drug can be given only through an intravenous or central line.
- This drug will help you to build new proteins and regain your strength and healing power.
- These side effects may occur: headache, dizziness (medication may be ordered to help); nausea, vomiting; pain at infusion site.
- Report fever, chills, severe pain at infusion site, changes in color of urine or stool, severe headache, rash.

▷ aminocaproic acid
(a mee noe ka proe' ik)

Amicar

PREGNANCY CATEGORY C

Drug class
Systemic hemostatic agent

Therapeutic actions
Inhibits fibrinolysis by inhibiting plasminogen activator substances and by antiplasmin activity; this action prevents the breakdown of clots.

Indications
- Treatment of excessive bleeding resulting from systemic hyperfibrinolysis and urinary fibrinolysis.
- Unlabeled uses: prevention of recurrence of subarachnoid hemorrhage; management of amegakaryocytic thrombocytopenia; to decrease the need for platelet administration; to abort and treat attacks of hereditary angioneurotic edema

Contraindications and cautions
- Contraindicated with allergy to aminocaproic acid, active intravascular clotting, cardiac disease, renal dysfunction, hematuria of upper urinary tract origin, hepatic dysfunction, lactation; use caution with hyperfibrinolysis.

Available forms
Tablets—500 mg; syrup—250 mg/mL; injection—250 mg/mL

Dosages
Adults
Initial dose of 5 g PO or IV followed by 1 g/hr to produce and sustain plasma levels of 0.13 mg/mL; do not administer more than 30 g/day.
- *Acute bleeding:* 4–5 g IV in 250 mL of diluent during the first hour of infusion; then continuous infusion of 1 g/hr in 50 mL of diluent. Continue for 8 hr or until bleeding stops.
- *Prevention of recurrence of subarachnoid hemorrhage:* 36 g/day in six divided doses, PO or IV.
- *Amegakaryocytic thrombocytopenia:* 8–24 g/day for 3 days to 13 mo.
Pediatric patients
Safety and efficacy not established.

Pharmacokinetics

Route	Onset	Peak	Duration
Oral	Rapid	2 hr	—
IV	Immediate	Minutes	2–3 hr

Distribution: Crosses placenta; may pass into breast milk
Excretion: Unchanged in the urine

▽ IV facts
Preparation: Dilute in compatible IV fluid. Rapid IV infusion undiluted is not recommended. Dilute 4 mL (1 g) of solution with 50 mL of diluent. For acute bleed, dilute 4–5 g in 250 mL diluent and give over 1 hr; then a continuous infusion of 1 g/hr given in 50 mL diluent. Store at room temperature.
Infusion: Infuse at 4–5 g the first hour of treatment, then 1 g/hr by continuous infusion; administer slowly to avoid hypotension, bradycardia, arrhythmias.

Compatibilities: Compatible with sterile water for injection, normal saline, 5% dextrose, Ringer's solution.

Adverse effects

- **CNS:** *Dizziness, tinnitus, headache,* delirium, hallucinations, psychotic reactions, weakness, conjunctival suffusion, nasal stuffiness
- **CV:** Hypotension, cardiac myopathy
- **GI:** *Nausea, cramps, diarrhea*
- **GU:** Intrarenal obstruction, renal failure, *fertility problems*
- **Hematologic:** *Elevated serum CPK,* aldolase, AST, elevated serum potassium
- **Musculoskeletal:** *Malaise,* myopathy, symptomatic weakness, fatigue
- **Other:** Rash, thrombophlebitis

Interactions

✳ **Drug-drug** • Risk of hypercoagulable state with oral contraceptives, estrogens
✳ **Drug-lab test** • Elevation of serum K+ levels, especially with impaired renal function

■ Nursing considerations
Assessment

- **History:** Allergy to aminocaproic acid, DIC, cardiac disease, renal dysfunction; hematuria of upper urinary tract origin, hepatic dysfunction, lactation, hyperfibrinolysis
- **Physical:** Skin color, lesions; muscular strength; orientation, reflexes, affect; BP, P, baseline ECG, peripheral perfusion; liver evaluation, bowel sounds, output; clotting studies, CPK, urinalysis, liver and kidney function tests

Interventions

- Patient on oral therapy may have to take up to 10 tablets the first hour of treatment and tablets around the clock during treatment.
- Orient patient and offer support if hallucinations, delirium, psychoses occur.
- Monitor patient for signs of clotting.

Teaching points

- These side effects may occur: dizziness, weakness, headache, hallucinations (avoid driving or the use of dangerous machinery; take special precautions to avoid injury); nau-

sea, diarrhea, cramps (small, frequent meals may help); infertility problems (menstrual irregularities, dry ejaculation—should go away when the drug is stopped); weakness, malaise (plan activities, take rest periods as needed).
- Report severe headache, restlessness, muscle pain and weakness, blood in the urine.

▷ aminoglutethimide
*(a meen oh gloo **teth'** i mide)*

Cytadren

PREGNANCY CATEGORY D

Drug classes
Antineoplastic
Adrenal steroid inhibitor

Therapeutic actions
Inhibits the conversion of cholesterol to the steroid base necessary for producing adrenal glucocorticoids, mineralocorticoids, estrogens, and androgens.

Indications

- Suppression of adrenal function in selected patients with Cushing's syndrome—those awaiting surgery or in whom other treatment is not appropriate
- Unlabeled use: to produce medical adrenalectomy in patients with advanced breast cancer and in patients with metastatic prostate carcinoma

Contraindications and cautions

- Hypersensitivity to glutethimide or to aminoglutethimide; hypotension; hypothyroidism; pregnancy (causes fetal harm); lactation.

Available forms
Tablets—250 mg

Dosages
Adults

- *Cushing's disease:* 250 mg PO q 6 hr; may be increased in increments of 250 mg/day at intervals of 1–2 wk to a total daily dose of 2 g.

Adverse effects in *Italics* are most common; those in **Bold** are life-threatening.

- *Cancer:* 250 mg PO bid with hydrocortisone 60 mg hs, 20 mg on arising, and 20 mg at 2 PM for 2 weeks; then 250 mg PO qid and hydrocortisone 20 mg hs, 10 mg on arising, and 10 mg at 2 PM.

Pediatric patients
Safety and efficacy not established.

Pharmacokinetics

Route	Onset	Peak
Oral	3–5 days	36–72 hr

Metabolism: $T_{1/2}$: 11–16 hr
Distribution: Crosses placenta; passes into breast milk
Excretion: Unchanged in the urine

Adverse effects

- **CNS:** *Drowsiness,* dizziness, headache
- **CV:** *Hypotension,* tachycardia
- **Dermatologic:** *Morbiliform rash,* pruritus, urticaria
- **Endocrine:** Adrenal insufficiency, **hypothyroidism,** masculinization, and hirsutism
- **GI:** *Nausea, anorexia*
- **Other:** Myalgia, fever

Interactions

✳ **Drug-drug** • Decreased therapeutic effects of warfarin • Possible decreased effectiveness of aminophylline, oxtriphylline, theophylline, medroxyprogesterone • Decreased effectiveness with dexamethasone, hydrocortisone

■ Nursing considerations
Assessment

- **History:** Hypersensitivity to glutethimide or to aminoglutethimide; hypotension; hypothyroidism; pregnancy, lactation
- **Physical:** Weight, skin condition, fever, neurologic status, reflexes, P, BP, thyroid function, renal and liver function tests, cortisol levels

Interventions

- Begin therapy in a hospital setting until response has stabilized.
- Monitor patient carefully; if extreme drowsiness, severe rash, or excessively low cortisol levels occur, reduce dose or discontinue.

- Monitor patient for signs of hypothyroidism (slow pulse, lethargy, dry skin, thick tongue), and arrange for appropriate replacement therapy.
- Discontinue drug if rash persists for longer than 5–8 days or becomes severe; it may be possible to restart therapy at a lower dose once the rash has disappeared.
- Caution patient to avoid pregnancy if taking this drug; recommend birth control.

Teaching points

- Avoid driving or dangerous activities if dizziness, weakness occur.
- These side effects may occur: dizziness, lightheadedness (change position slowly, avoid dangerous situations); loss of appetite, nausea (maintain nutrition); headache (if severe, medication may be ordered).
- A medical alert card or bracelet may help notify medical workers in an emergency situation that you are on this drug.
- Avoid pregnancy while taking this drug; it is associated with severe fetal damage; discuss contraceptive methods.
- Report rash, severe drowsiness or dizziness, headache, severe nausea.

▷ **aminolevulinic acid hydrochloride**

See *Less Commonly Used Drugs,* p. 1336.

▷ **aminophylline (theophylline ethylenediamine)**
(am in off' i lin)

Truphylline

PREGNANCY CATEGORY C

Drug classes
Bronchodilator
Xanthine

Therapeutic actions
Relaxes bronchial smooth muscle, causing bronchodilation and increasing vital capacity, which has been impaired by bronchospasm and air trapping; in higher concentrations, it

also inhibits the release of slow-reacting substance of anaphylaxis (SRS-A) and histamine.

Indications

- Symptomatic relief or prevention of bronchial asthma and reversible bronchospasm associated with chronic bronchitis and emphysema
- Unlabeled uses: respiratory stimulant in Cheyne-Stokes respiration; treatment of apnea and bradycardia in premature babies

Contraindications and cautions

- Contraindicated with hypersensitivity to any xanthine or to ethylenediamine, peptic ulcer, active gastritis; rectal or colonic irritation or infection (use rectal preparations).
- Use cautiously with cardiac arrhythmias, acute myocardial injury, CHF, cor pulmonale, severe hypertension, severe hypoxemia, renal or hepatic disease, hyperthyroidism, alcoholism, labor, lactation.

Available forms

Tablets—100, 200 mg; CR tablets—225 mg; liquid—105 mg/5 mL; injection—250 mg/10 mL; suppositories—250, 500 mg

Dosages

Individualize dosage, base adjustments on clinical responses; monitor serum theophylline levels; maintain therapeutic range of 10–20 mcg/mL; base dosage on lean body mass; 127 mg aminophylline dihydrate = 100 mg theophylline anhydrous.

Adults

- *Acute symptoms requiring rapid theophyllinization in patients not receiving theophylline:* An initial loading dose is required, as indicated below:

Patient Group	Oral Loading	Followed by	Maintenance
Young adult smokers	7.6 mg/kg	3.8 mg/kg q 6 hr × 3 doses	3.8 mg/kg q 8 hr
Adult non-smokers who are otherwise healthy	7.6 mg/kg	3.8 mg/kg q 4 hr × 2 doses	3.8 mg/kg q 6 hr

- *Long-term therapy:* Usual range is 600–1,600 mg/day PO in three to four divided doses.
- *Rectal:* 500 mg q 6–8 hr by rectal suppository or retention enema.

Pediatric patients

Use in children < 6 mo not recommended; use of timed-release products in children < 6 yr not recommended. Children are very sensitive to CNS stimulant action of theophylline; use caution in younger children who cannot complain of minor side effects.

- *Acute therapy:* For acute symptoms requiring rapid theophyllinization in patients not receiving theophylline, a loading dose is required. Dosage recommendations are as follows:

Patient Group	Oral Loading	Followed by	Maintenance
Children 6 mo–9 yr	7.6 mg/kg	5.1 mg/kg q 4 hr × 3 doses	5.1 mg/kg q 6 hr
Children 9–16 yr	7.6 mg/kg	3.8 mg/kg q 4 hr × 3 doses	3.8 mg/kg q 6 hr

- *Long-term therapy:* 12 mg/kg per 24 hr PO; slow clinical adjustment of the oral preparations is preferred; monitor clinical response and serum theophylline levels. In the absence of serum levels, adjust up to the maximum dosage shown below, providing the dosage is tolerated.

Age	Maximum Daily Dose
< 9 yr	30.4 mg/kg/day
9–12 yr	25.3 mg/kg/day
12–16 yr	22.8 mg/kg/day
> 16 yr	16.5 mg/kg/day or 1,100 mg, whichever is less

Geriatric patients or impaired adults

Use caution, especially in elderly men and in patients with cor pulmonale, CHF, liver disease (half-life of aminophylline may be markedly prolonged in CHF, liver disease). For acute symptoms requiring rapid theophyllinization in patients not receiving theophylline, a loading dose is necessary as follows:

Patient Group	Oral Loading	Followed by	Maintenance
Older patients and cor pulmonale	7.6 mg/kg	2.5 mg/kg q 6 hr × 2 doses	2.5 mg/kg q 8 hr
CHF	7.6 mg/kg	2.5 mg/kg q 8 hr × 2 doses	1.3–2.5 mg/kg q 12 hr

Pharmacokinetics

Route	Onset	Peak	Duration
Oral	1–6 hr	4–6 hr	6–8 hr
IV	Immediate	30 min	4–8 hr

Metabolism: Hepatic; $T_{1/2}$: 3–15 hr
Distribution: Crosses placenta; passes into breast milk
Excretion: Urine

▼IV facts

Preparation: May be infused in 100–200 mL of 5% dextrose injection or 0.9% sodium chloride injection.
Infusion: Do not exceed 25 mg/min infusion rate. Substitute oral therapy or IV therapy as soon as possible; administer maintenance infusions in a large volume to deliver the desired amount of drug each hour.
Adult: 6 mg/kg. For acute symptoms requiring rapid theophyllinization in patients receiving theophylline: a loading dose is required. Each 0.6 mg/kg IV administered as a loading dose will result in about a 1 mcg/mL increase in serum theophylline. Ideally, defer loading dose until serum theophylline determination is made; otherwise, base loading dose on clinical judgment and the knowledge that 3.2 mg/kg aminophylline will increase serum theophylline levels by about 5 mcg/mL and is unlikely to cause dangerous adverse effects if the patient is not experiencing theophylline toxicity before this dose. Aminophylline IV maintenance infusion rates (mg/kg/hr) are given below:

Patient Group	First 12 hr	Beyond 12 hr
Young adult smokers	1	0.8
Adult nonsmokers who are otherwise healthy	0.7	0.5

Pediatric: After an IV loading dose, these maintenance rates (mg/kg/hr) are recommended:

Patient Group	First 12 hr	Beyond 12 hr
Children 6 mo–9 yr	1.2	1
Children 9–16 yr	1	0.8

Geriatric: After a loading dose, these maintenance infusion rates (mg/kg/hr) are recommended:

Patient Group	First 12 hr	Beyond 12 hr
Other patients, cor pulmonale	0.6	0.3
CHF, liver disease	0.5	0.1–0.2

Compatibility: Aminophylline is compatible with most IV solutions, but do not mix in solution with other drugs, including vitamins.
Y-site incompatibility: dobutamine, hydralazine, ondansetron.

Adverse effects

- Serum theophylline levels < 20 mcg/mL: adverse effects uncommon
- Serum theophylline levels > 20–25 mcg/mL: nausea, vomiting, diarrhea, headache, insomnia, irritability (75% of patients)
- Serum theophylline levels > 30–35 mcg/mL: hyperglycemia, hypotension, cardiac arrhythmias, tachycardia (> 10 mcg/mL in premature newborns); **seizures, brain damage**
- **CNS:** Irritability (especially children); restlessness, dizziness, muscle twitching, convulsions, severe depression, stammering speech; abnormal behavior characterized by withdrawal, mutism, and unresponsiveness alternating with hyperactive periods
- **CV:** Palpitations, sinus tachycardia, ventricular tachycardia, life-threatening ventricular arrhythmias, circulatory failure
- **GI:** Loss of appetite, hematemesis, epigastric pain, gastroesophageal reflux during sleep, increased AST
- **GU:** Proteinuria, increased excretion of renal tubular cells and RBCs; diuresis (dehydration), urinary retention in men with prostate enlargement
- **Respiratory:** Tachypnea, respiratory arrest
- **Other:** Fever, flushing, hyperglycemia, SIADH, rash

Interactions

✳ Drug-drug • Increased effects with cimetidine, erythromycin, troleandomycin, clindamycin, lincomycin, influenza virus vaccine, oral contraceptives • Possibly increased effects with thiabendazole, rifampin, allopurinol • Increased cardiac toxicity with halothane; increased likelihood of seizures when given with ketamine; increased likelihood of adverse GI effects when given with tetracyclines • Increased or decreased effects with furosemide, levothyroxine, liothyronine, liotrix, thyroglobulin, thyroid hormones • Decreased effects in patients who are cigarette smokers (1–2 packs per day); theophylline dosage may need to be increased 50%–100% • Decreased effects with phenobarbital, aminoglutethimide • Increased effects, toxicity of sympathomimetics (especially ephedrine) with theophylline preparations • Decreased effects of phenytoin and theophylline preparations when given concomitantly • Decreased effects of lithium carbonate, nondepolarizing neuromuscular blockers given with theophylline preparations • Mutually antagonistic effects of beta-blockers and theophylline preparations

✳ Drug-food • Elimination is increased by a low-carbohydrate, high-protein diet and by charcoal broiled beef • Elimination is decreased by a high-carbohydrate, low-protein diet • Food may alter bioavailability and absorption of timed-release theophylline preparations, causing toxicity. These forms should be taken on an empty stomach

✳ Drug-lab test • Interference with spectrophotometric determinations of serum theophylline levels by furosemide, phenylbutazone, probenecid, theobromine; coffee, tea, cola beverages, chocolate, acetaminophen cause falsely high values • Alteration in assays of uric acid, urinary catecholamines, plasma free fatty acids by theophylline preparations

■ Nursing considerations
Assessment

• **History:** Hypersensitivity to any xanthine or to ethylenediamine, peptic ulcer, active gastritis, cardiac arrhythmias, acute myocardial injury, CHF, cor pulmonale, severe hypertension, severe hypoxemia, renal or hepatic disease, hyperthyroidism, alcoholism, labor, lactation, rectal or colonic irritation or infection (aminophylline rectal preparations)

• **Physical:** Bowel sounds, normal output; P, auscultation, BP, perfusion, ECG; R, adventitious sounds; frequency of urination, voiding, normal output pattern, urinalysis, renal function tests; liver palpation, liver function tests; thyroid function tests; skin color, texture, lesions; reflexes, bilateral grip strength, affect, EEG

Interventions

• Administer to pregnant patients only when clearly needed—neonatal tachycardia, jitteriness, and withdrawal apnea observed when mothers received xanthines up until delivery.
• Caution patient not to chew or crush enteric-coated timed-release forms.
• Give immediate-release, liquid dosage forms with food if GI effects occur.
• Do not give timed-release forms with food; these should be given on an empty stomach 1 hr before or 2 hr after meals.
• Maintain adequate hydration.
• Monitor results of serum theophylline levels carefully, and arrange for reduced dosage if serum levels exceed therapeutic range of 10–20 mcg/mL.
• Take serum samples to determine peak theophylline concentration drawn 15–30 min after an IV loading dose.
• Monitor for clinical signs of adverse effects, particularly if serum theophylline levels are not available.
• Maintain diazepam on standby to treat seizures.

Teaching points

• Take this drug exactly as prescribed; if a timed-release product is prescribed, take this drug on an empty stomach, 1 hr before or 2 hr after meals.
• Do not to chew or crush timed-release preparations.
• Administer rectal solution or suppositories after emptying the rectum.
• It may be necessary to take this drug around the clock for adequate control of asthma attacks.

Adverse effects in *Italics* are most common; those in **Bold** are life-threatening.

- Avoid excessive intake of coffee, tea, cocoa, cola beverages, chocolate.
- Smoking cigarettes or other tobacco products impacts the drug's effectiveness. Try not to smoke. Notify the care provider if smoking habits change while taking this drug.
- Be aware that frequent blood tests may be necessary to monitor the effect of this drug and to ensure safe and effective dosage; keep all appointments for blood tests and other monitoring.
- These side effects may occur: nausea, loss of appetite (taking this drug with food may help if taking the immediate-release or liquid dosage forms); difficulty sleeping, depression, emotional lability (reversible).
- Report nausea, vomiting, severe GI pain, restlessness, convulsions, irregular heartbeat.

▽ amiodarone hydrochloride
(a mee o' da rone)

Cordarone, Pacerone

PREGNANCY CATEGORY D

Drug classes
Antiarrhythmic
Adrenergic blocker (not used as sympatholytic agent)

Therapeutic actions
Type III antiarrhythmic: acts directly on cardiac cell membrane; prolongs repolarization and refractory period; increases ventricular fibrillation threshold; acts on peripheral smooth muscle to decrease peripheral resistance

Indications
- Only for treatment of the following documented life-threatening recurrent ventricular arrhythmias that do not respond to other antiarrhythmics or when alternative agents are not tolerated: recurrent ventricular fibrillation, recurrent hemodynamically unstable ventricular tachycardia. Serious and even fatal toxicity has been reported with this drug; use alternative agents first; very closely monitor patient receiving this drug.

- Unlabeled uses: treatment of refractory sustained or paroxysmal atrial fibrillation and paroxysmal supraventricular tachycardia; treatment of symptomatic atrial flutter.

Contraindications and cautions
- Contraindicated with hypersensitivity to amiodarone, sinus node dysfunction, heart block, severe bradycardia, hypokalemia, lactation.
- Use cautiously with thyroid dysfunction, pregnancy.

Available forms
Tablets—200, 400 mg; injection—50 mg/mL

Dosages
Careful patient assessment and evaluation with continual monitoring of cardiac response are necessary for titrating the dosage. Therapy should begin in the hospital with continual monitoring and emergency equipment on standby. The following is a guide to usual dosage.

Adults
Oral
- *Loading dose:* 800–1,600 mg/day PO in divided doses, for 1–3 wk; reduce dose to 600–800 mg/day in divided doses for 1 mo; if rhythm is stable, reduce dose to 400 mg/day in one to two divided doses for maintenance dose. Adjust to the lowest possible dose to limit side effects.

IV
1,000 mg IV over 24 hr—150 mg loading dose over 10 min, followed by 360 mg over 6 hr at rate of 1 mg/min; maintenance infusion: 540 mg at 0.5 mg/min over 18 hr. May be continued up to 96 hr or until rhythm is stable. Switch to oral form as soon as possible.

Pediatric patients
Safety and efficacy not established.

Pharmacokinetics

Route	Onset	Peak	Duration
Oral	2–3 days	3–7 hr	6–8 hr
IV	Immediate	20 min	Infusion

Metabolism: Hepatic; $T_{1/2}$: 10 days, then 40–55 days
Distribution: Crosses placenta; passes into breast milk
Excretion: Bile and feces

▼ IV facts

Preparation: Do not use PVC container. Dilute 150 mg in 100 mL D_5W for rapid loading dose (1.5 mg/mL). Dilute 900 mg in 500 mL D_5W for slow infusions (1.8 mg/mL). Store at room temperature and use within 24 hr.

Infusion: Infuse loading dose over 10 min. Immediately follow with slow infusion of 1 mg/min or 33.3 mL/hr. Maintenance infusion of 0.5 mg/min or 16.6 mL/hr can be continued up to 96 hr. Use of an infusion pump is advised.

Incompatibilities: Do not mix with aminophylline, cefamandole, cefazolin, meclocillin, heparin, sodium bicarbonate; do not mix in solution with other drugs.

Adverse effects

- **CNS:** *Malaise, fatigue, dizziness, tremors, ataxia,* paresthesias, lack of coordination
- **CV: Cardiac arrhythmias,** congestive heart failure, **cardiac arrest,** *hypotension*
- **EENT:** *Corneal microdeposits* (photophobia, dry eyes, halos, blurred vision); **ophthalmic abnormalities** including permanent blindness
- **Endocrine:** *Hypothyroidism* or *hyperthyroidism*
- **GI:** *Nausea, vomiting, anorexia, constipation, abnormal liver function tests,* **liver toxicity**
- **Respiratory: Pulmonary toxicity**—pneumonitis, infiltrates (shortness of breath, cough, rales, wheezes)
- **Other:** *Photosensitivity,* angioedema

Interactions

✳ **Drug-drug** • Increased digitalis toxicity with digoxin • Increased quinidine toxicity with quinidine • Increased procainamide toxicity with procainamide • Increased flecainide toxicity with amiodarone • Increased phenytoin toxicity with phenytoin, ethotoin, mephenytoin • Increased bleeding tendencies with warfarin • Potential sinus arrest and heart block with beta-blockers, calcium channel blockers

✳ **Drug-lab test** • Increased T_3 levels, increased serum reverse T_3 levels

■ Nursing considerations

CLINICAL ALERT!
Name confusion has occurred with amrinone (name has now been changed to inamrinone, but confusion may still occur); use caution.

Assessment

- **History:** Hypersensitivity to amiodarone, sinus node dysfunction, heart block, severe bradycardia, hypokalemia, lactation, thyroid dysfunction, pregnancy
- **Physical:** Skin color, lesions; reflexes, gait, eye exam; P, BP, auscultation, continuous ECG monitoring; R, adventitious sounds, baseline chest x-ray; liver evaluation; liver function tests, serum electrolytes, T_4, and T_3

Interventions

- Monitor cardiac rhythm continuously.
- Monitor for an extended period when dosage adjustments are made.
- Monitor for safe and effective serum levels (0.5–2.5 mcg/mL).
- Doses of digoxin, quinidine, procainamide, phenytoin, and warfarin may need to be reduced one-third to one-half when amiodarone is started.
- Give drug with meals to decrease GI problems.
- Arrange for ophthalmologic exams; reevaluate at any sign of optic neuropathy.
- Arrange for periodic chest x-ray to evaluate pulmonary status (every 3–6 mo).
- Arrange for regular periodic blood tests for liver enzymes, thyroid hormone levels.

Teaching points

- Drug dosage will be changed in relation to response of arrhythmias; you will need to be hospitalized during initiation of drug therapy; you will be closely monitored when dosage is changed.
- These side effects may occur: changes in vision (halos, dry eyes, sensitivity to light; wear sunglasses, monitor light exposure); nausea, vomiting, loss of appetite (take with meals; small, frequent meals may help); sensitivity to the sun (use a sunscreen or protective clothing when outdoors); constipa-

tion (a laxative may be ordered); tremors, twitching, dizziness, loss of coordination (do not drive, operate dangerous machinery, or undertake tasks that require coordination until drug effects stabilize and your body adjusts to it).

- Have regular medical follow-up, monitoring of cardiac rhythm, chest x-ray, eye exam, blood tests.
- Report unusual bleeding or bruising; fever, chills; intolerance to heat or cold; shortness of breath, difficulty breathing, cough; swelling of ankles or fingers; palpitations; difficulty with vision.

▷ amitriptyline hydrochloride
*(a mee **trip**' ti leen)*

Elavil, Levate (CAN), Novotriptyn (CAN)

PREGNANCY CATEGORY C

Drug class
Tricyclic antidepressant (TCA; tertiary amine)

Therapeutic actions
Mechanism of action unknown; TCAs inhibit the reuptake of the neurotransmitters norepinephrine and serotonin, leading to an increase in their effects; anticholinergic at CNS and peripheral receptors; sedative.

Indications
- Relief of symptoms of depression (endogenous most responsive); sedative effects may help when depression is associated with anxiety and sleep disturbance.
- Unlabeled uses: control of chronic pain (eg, intractable pain of cancer, central pain syndromes, peripheral neuropathies, postherpetic neuralgia, tic douloureux); prevention of onset of cluster and migraine headaches; treatment of pathologic weeping and laughing secondary to forebrain disease (due to multiple sclerosis).

Contraindications and cautions
- Contraindicated with hypersensitivity to any tricyclic drug; concomitant therapy with an MAO inhibitor; recent MI; myelography within previous 24 hr or scheduled within 48 hr; lactation.
- Use cautiously with electroshock therapy; preexisting CV disorders (severe coronary heart disease, progressive heart failure, angina pectoris, paroxysmal tachycardia); angleclosure glaucoma, increased intraocular pressure, urinary retention, ureteral or urethral spasm; seizure disorders; hyperthyroidism; impaired hepatic, renal function; psychiatric patients (schizophrenic or paranoid patients may exhibit a worsening of psychosis with TCA therapy); manicdepressive patients; elective surgery (discontinue as long as possible before surgery).

Available forms
Injection—10 mg/mL; tablets—10, 25, 50, 75, 100, 150 mg

Dosages
May be given IM if patients are unable or unwilling to take oral drug. Switch to oral drug as soon as possible.

Adults
- *Depression, hospitalized patients:* Initially, 100 mg/day PO in divided doses: gradually increase to 200–300 mg/day as required. May be given IM 20–30 mg qid, initially only in patients unable or unwilling to take drug PO. Replace with oral medication as soon as possible.
- *Outpatients:* Initially, 75 mg/day PO, in divided doses; may increase to 150 mg/day. Increases should be made in late afternoon or hs. Total daily dosage may be administered hs. Initiate single daily dose therapy with 50–100 mg hs; increase by 25–50 mg as necessary to a total of 150 mg/day. Maintenance dose is 40–100 mg/day, which may be given as a single bedtime dose. After satisfactory response, reduce to lowest effective dosage. Continue therapy for 3 mo or longer to lessen possibility of relapse.
- *Chronic pain:* 75–150 mg/day PO.
- *Prevention of cluster or migraine headaches:* 50–150 mg/day PO.
- *Prevention of weeping in MS patients with forebrain disease:* 25–75 mg PO.

Pediatric patients
Not recommended in children < 12 yr.

Children > 12 yr and geriatric patients
10 mg tid PO with 20 mg hs.

Pharmacokinetics

Route	Onset	Peak	Duration
Oral	Varies	2–4 hr	2–4 wk

Metabolism: Hepatic; $T_{1/2}$: 10–50 hr
Distribution: Crosses placenta; passes into breast milk
Excretion: Urine

Adverse effects

- **CNS:** *Disturbed concentration, sedation and anticholinergic (atropine-like) effects, confusion* (especially in elderly), hallucinations, disorientation, decreased memory, feelings of unreality, delusions, anxiety, nervousness, restlessness, agitation, panic, insomnia, nightmares, hypomania, mania, exacerbation of psychosis, drowsiness, weakness, fatigue, headache, numbness, tingling, paresthesias of extremities, incoordination, motor hyperactivity, akathisia, ataxia, tremors, peripheral neuropathy, extrapyramidal symptoms, seizures, speech blockage, dysarthria, tinnitus, altered EEG
- **CV:** *Orthostatic hypotension*, hypertension, syncope, tachycardia, palpitations, MI, arrhythmias, heart block, precipitation of CHF, stroke
- **Endocrine:** Elevated or depressed blood sugar, elevated prolactin levels, inappropriate ADH secretion
- **GI:** *Dry mouth, constipation*, paralytic ileus, *nausea*, vomiting, anorexia, epigastric distress, diarrhea, flatulence, dysphagia, peculiar taste, increased salivation, stomatitis, glossitis, parotid swelling, abdominal cramps, black tongue, hepatitis, jaundice (rare), elevated transaminase, altered alkaline phosphatase
- **GU:** Urinary retention, delayed micturition, dilation of the urinary tract, gynecomastia, testicular swelling; breast enlargement, menstrual irregularity and galactorrhea; increased or decreased libido; impotence
- **Hematologic:** Bone marrow depression, including agranulocytosis; eosinophilia, purpura, thrombocytopenia, leukopenia
- **Hypersensitivity:** Rash, pruritus, vasculitis, petechiae, photosensitization, edema (generalized, face, tongue), drug fever
- **Withdrawal:** Symptoms on abrupt discontinuation of prolonged therapy: nausea, headache, vertigo, nightmares, malaise
- **Other:** Nasal congestion, excessive appetite, weight change; sweating, alopecia, lacrimation, hyperthermia, flushing, chills

Interactions

❋ **Drug-drug** ● Increased TCA levels and pharmacologic (especially anticholinergic) effects with cimetidine, fluoxetine ● Increased TCA levels with methylphenidate, phenothiazines, hormonal contraceptives, disulfiram ● Hyperpyretic crises, severe convulsions, hypertensive episodes and deaths with MAO inhibitors, furazolidone ● Increased antidepressant response and cardiac arrhythmias with thyroid medication ● Increased or decreased effects with estrogens ● Delirium with disulfiram ● Sympathetic hyperactivity, sinus tachycardia, hypertension, agitation with levodopa ● Increased biotransformation of TCAs in patients who smoke cigarettes ● Increased sympathomimetic (especially beta-adrenergic) effects of direct-acting sympathomimetic drugs (norepinephrine, epinephrine) ● Increased anticholinergic effects of anticholinergic drugs (including anticholinergic antiparkisonian drugs) ● Increased response (especially CNS depression) to barbiturates ● Decreased antihypertensive effect of guanethidine, clonidine, other antihypertensives ● Decreased effects of indirect-acting sympathomimetic drugs (ephedrine)

■ Nursing considerations
Assessment

- **History:** Hypersensitivity to any tricyclic drug; concomitant therapy with an MAO inhibitor; recent MI; myelography within previous 24 hr or scheduled within 48 hr; lactation; EST; preexisting CV disorders; angle-closure glaucoma, increased intraocular pressure, urinary retention, ureteral or urethral spasm; seizure disorders; hyperthyroidism; impaired hepatic, renal function; psychiatric patients; manic-depressive patients; elective surgery

Adverse effects in *Italics* are most common; those in **Bold** are life-threatening.

- **Physical:** Weight; T; skin color, lesions; orientation, affect, reflexes, vision and hearing; P, BP, orthostatic BP, perfusion; bowel sounds, normal output, liver evaluation; urine flow, normal output; usual sexual function, frequency of menses, breast and scrotal exam; liver function tests, urinalysis, CBC, ECG

Interventions

- Restrict drug access for depressed and potentially suicidal patients.
- Give IM only when oral therapy is impossible.
- Do not administer IV.
- Administer major portion of dose at bedtime if drowsiness, severe anticholinergic effects occur (note that the elderly may not tolerate single daily dose therapy).
- Reduce dosage if minor side effects develop; discontinue if serious side effects occur.
- Arrange for CBC if patient develops fever, sore throat, or other sign of infection.

Teaching points

- Take drug exactly as prescribed; do not stop abruptly or without consulting health care provider.
- Avoid using alcohol, other sleep-inducing drugs, OTC drugs.
- Avoid prolonged exposure to sunlight or sunlamps; use a sunscreen or protective garments.
- These side effects may occur: headache, dizziness, drowsiness, weakness, blurred vision (reversible; if severe, avoid driving and tasks requiring alertness while these persist); nausea, vomiting, loss of appetite, dry mouth (small, frequent meals, frequent mouth care, and sucking sugarless candies may help); nightmares, inability to concentrate, confusion; changes in sexual function.
- Report dry mouth, difficulty in urination, excessive sedation.

▽ **amlodipine besylate**
(am loe' di peen)

Norvasc

PREGNANCY CATEGORY C

Drug classes
Calcium channel-blocker

Antianginal drug
Antihypertensive

Therapeutic actions

Inhibits the movement of calcium ions across the membranes of cardiac and arterial muscle cells; inhibits transmembrane calcium flow, which results in the depression of impulse formation in specialized cardiac pacemaker cells, slowing of the velocity of conduction of the cardiac impulse, depression of myocardial contractility, and dilation of coronary arteries and arterioles and peripheral arterioles; these effects lead to decreased cardiac work, decreased cardiac oxygen consumption, and in patients with vasospastic (Prinzmetal's) angina, increased delivery of oxygen to cardiac cells.

Indications

- Angina pectoris due to coronary artery spasm (Prinzmetal's variant angina)
- Chronic stable angina, alone or in combination with other agents
- Essential hypertension, alone or in combination with other antihypertensives

Contraindications and cautions

- Contraindicated with allergy to amlodipine, impaired hepatic or renal function, sick sinus syndrome, heart block (second or third degree), lactation
- Use cautiously with CHF

Available forms

Tablets—2.5, 5, 10 mg

Dosages
Adults

Initially 5 mg PO daily; dosage may be gradually increased over 10–14 days to a maximum dose of 10 mg PO daily.
Pediatric patients

Safety and efficacy not established.
Geriatric patients or patients with hepatic impairment

Initially, 2.5 mg PO daily; dosage may be gradually adjusted over 7–14 days based on clinical assessment.

Pharmacokinetics

Route	Onset	Peak
Oral	Unknown	6–12 hr

Metabolism: Hepatic; $T_{1/2}$: 30–50 hr
Distribution: Crosses placenta; may pass into breast milk
Excretion: Urine

Adverse effects

- **CNS:** *Dizziness, light-headedness, headache,* asthenia, *fatigue, lethargy*
- **CV:** *Peripheral edema,* arrhythmias
- **Dermatologic:** *Flushing,* rash
- **GI:** *Nausea,* abdominal discomfort

Interactions

✳ **Drug-drug** • Possible increased serum levels and toxicity of cyclosporine if taken concurrently

■ Nursing considerations

Assessment

- **History:** Allergy to amlodipine, impaired hepatic or renal function, sick sinus syndrome, heart block, lactation, CHF
- **Physical:** Skin lesions, color, edema; P, BP, baseline ECG, peripheral perfusion, auscultation; R, adventitious sounds; liver evaluation, GI normal output; liver and renal function tests, urinalysis

Interventions

- Monitor patient carefully (BP, cardiac rhythm, and output) while adjusting drug to therapeutic dose; use special caution if patient has CHF.
- Monitor BP very carefully if patient is also on nitrates.
- Monitor cardiac rhythm regularly during stabilization of dosage and periodically during long-term therapy.
- Administer drug without regard to meals.

Teaching points

- Take with meals if upset stomach occurs.
- These side effects may occur: nausea, vomiting (small, frequent meals may help); headache (adjust lighting, noise, and temperature; medication may be ordered).
- Report irregular heartbeat, shortness of breath, swelling of the hands or feet, pronounced dizziness, constipation.

▷ **ammonium chloride**
(ah mo' nee um)

PREGNANCY CATEGORY C

Drug classes

Electrolyte
Urinary acidifier

Therapeutic actions

Converted to urea in the liver; liberated hydrogen and chloride ions in blood and extracellular fluid lower the pH and correct alkalosis; lowers the urinary pH, producing an acidic urine that changes the excretion rate of many metabolites and drugs.

Indications

- Treatment of hypochloremic states and metabolic alkalosis
- Acidification of urine

Contraindications and cautions

- Renal function impairment; hepatic impairment; metabolic alkalosis due to vomiting of hydrochloric acid when it is accompanied by loss of sodium

Available forms

Injection—26.75% (5 mEq/mL)

Dosages

An oral dosage form of the drug is no longer commercially available in the US.
Adults
Dosage is determined by patient's condition and tolerance; monitor dosage rate and amount by repeated serum bicarbonate determinations.
Pediatric patients
Safety and efficacy for injection in children have not been established.

Pharmacokinetics

Route	Onset	Peak
IV	Rapid	1–3 hr

Metabolism: Hepatic
Distribution: Crosses placenta; passes into breast milk

Excretion: Urine

▼ IV facts
Preparation: Add contents of one or two vials (100–200 mEq) to 500 or 1,000 mL isotonic (0.9%) sodium chloride injection. Concentration should not exceed 1%–2% ammonium chloride. Avoid excessive heat; protect from freezing. If crystals do appear, warm the solution to room temperature in a water bath prior to use.
Infusion: Do not exceed rate of 5 mL/min in adults (1,000 mL infused over 3 hr). Infuse slowly. Reduce rate in infants and children.
Incompatibilities: Do not mix with codeine, levorphanol, methadone, nitrofurantoin, warfarin.

Adverse effects
- **GI: Severe hepatic impairment**
- **Local:** *Pain or irritation at injection site*, fever, venous thrombosis, phlebitis, extravasation
- **Metabolic:** Metabolic acidosis, hypervolemia, ammonia toxicity—pallor, sweating, irregular breathing, retching, bradycardia, arrhythmias, twitching, convulsion, coma

Interactions
✳ Drug-drug • Decreased therapeutic levels due to increased elimination of amphetamine, methamphetamine, dextroamphetamine, ephedrine, pseudoephedrine, methadone, mexiletine when taken with ammonium chloride • Increased effects of chlorpropamide with ammonium chloride

■ Nursing considerations
Assessment
- **History:** Renal or hepatic impairment; metabolic alkalosis due to vomiting of hydrochloric acid when it is accompanied by loss of sodium
- **Physical:** P, BP; skin color, texture; T; injection site evaluation; liver evaluation; renal and liver function tests, serum bicarbonate, urinalysis

Interventions
- Infuse by IV route slowly to avoid irritation; check infusion site frequently to monitor for reaction.

- Monitor IV doses for possible fluid overload.
- Monitor for acidosis (increased R, restlessness, sweating, increased blood pH); decrease infusion as appropriate. Maintain sodium bicarbonate or sodium lactate on standby for overdose situations.

Teaching points
- Frequent monitoring of blood tests is needed when receiving IV drugs to determine dosage and rate of drug.
- Report pain or irritation at IV site; confusion, restlessness, sweating, headache; severe GI upset, fever, chills, changes in stool or urine color (oral drug)

▽ amobarbital sodium (amylobarbitone)
(am oh bar' bi tal)

Amytal Sodium

PREGNANCY CATEGORY D

C-II CONTROLLED SUBSTANCE

Drug classes
Barbiturate (intermediate acting)
Sedative and hypnotic
Anticonvulsant

Therapeutic actions
General CNS depressant; barbiturates act on the ascending RAS, depress the cerebral cortex, alter cerebellar function, depress motor output, and can produce excitation, sedation, hypnosis, anesthesia, and deep coma; at anesthetic doses, has anticonvulsant activity.

Indications
- Sedation
- Short-term treatment of insomnia
- Preanesthetic sedative and hypnotic

Contraindications and cautions
- Contraindicated with hypersensitivity to barbiturates; manifest or latent porphyria; marked liver impairment; nephritis; severe respiratory distress, respiratory disease with dyspnea, obstruction, or cor pulmonale; previous addiction to sedative–hypnotic drugs; pregnancy.

- Use cautiously with acute or chronic pain (drug may cause paradoxical excitement or mask important symptoms); seizure disorders (abrupt discontinuation of daily doses can result in status epilepticus); lactation; fever, hyperthyroidism, diabetes mellitus, severe anemia, pulmonary or cardiac disease, status asthmaticus, shock, uremia; impaired liver or kidney function, debilitation.

Available forms
Powder for injection: 250, 500 mg/vial

Dosages
Adults
IM
Usual dose is 65–500 mg; maximum dose should not exceed 500 mg. Do not give more than 5 mL in one injection; solutions of 20% can be used to minimize volume.
- *Sedation:* 30–50 mg bid–tid
- *Hypnotic:* 65–200 mg
IV
Same dose as IM. Do not exceed a rate of 50 mg/min. Dose should not exceed 1 g. Use of the 10% solution may cause serious respiratory depression.
Pediatric patients
Use caution. Barbiturates may produce irritability, excitability, inappropriate tearfulness, and aggression. Base dosage on weight, age, and response. Because of higher metabolic rates, children tolerate comparatively higher doses; ordinarily, 65–500 mg may be given to a child 6–12 yr old. Administer by slow IV injection, and monitor response carefully.
- *Sedation:* 2 mg/kg PO in 4 equally divided doses.
Geriatric patients or patients with debilitating disease
Reduce dosage and monitor closely; may produce excitement, depression, confusion.

Pharmacokinetics

Route	Onset	Peak	Duration
IV	5 min	15 min	3–6 hr

Metabolism: Hepatic; $T_{1/2}$: 16–40 hr
Distribution: Crosses placenta; passes into breast milk
Excretion: Urine

▼IV facts
Preparation: Add sterile water for injection to the vial, then rotate it to dissolve the powder. Do not shake the vial. Use only a solution that is absolutely clear after 5 min. Inject contents within 30 min of opening the vial. Amobarbital is unstable on exposure to air.
Infusion: Infuse slowly. Do not give intra-arterially; can cause severe spasm. Do not exceed rate of 50 mg/min. Monitor patient continually during infusion.
Incompatibilities: Incompatible with many other drugs in solution; **do not mix in solution with any drugs.**

Adverse effects
- **CNS:** *Somnolence, agitation, confusion, hyperkinesia, ataxia, vertigo, CNS depression, nightmares, lethargy, residual sedation (hangover),* paradoxical excitement, nervousness, psychiatric disturbance, hallucinations, insomnia, anxiety, dizziness, thinking abnormality
- **CV:** Bradycardia, hypotension, syncope
- **GI:** *Nausea, vomiting, constipation, diarrhea,* epigastric pain
- **Hypersensitivity:** Rashes, angioneurotic edema, serum sickness, morbilliform rash, urticaria; rarely, exfoliative dermatitis, **Stevens-Johnson syndrome**
- **Injection site:** *Local pain,* tissue necrosis, gangrene; arterial spasm with inadvertent intra-arterial injection; thrombophlebitis; permanent neurologic deficit if injected near a nerve
- **Respiratory:** *Hypoventilation,* **apnea, respiratory depression,** laryngospasm, bronchospasm, circulatory collapse
- **Other:** *Tolerance, psychological and physical dependence;* withdrawal syndrome

Interactions
✳ **Drug-drug** • Increased CNS depression with alcohol, other CNS depressants, phenothiazines, antihistamines, tranquilizers • Increased blood levels and pharmacologic effects of barbiturates with MAO inhibitors • Increased renal toxicity if taken with methoxyflurane • Decreased effects of the following: oral anticoagulants, tricyclic antidepressants, corticosteroids, oral contraceptives and estrogens,

acetaminophen, metronidazole, phenmetrazine, carbamazepine, beta blockers, griseofulvin, phenylbutazones, theophyllines, quinidine, doxycycline ● Altered effectiveness of phenytoin with barbiturates

■ Nursing considerations
Assessment
- **History:** Hypersensitivity to barbiturates; manifest or latent porphyria; marked liver impairment; nephritis; severe respiratory distress, respiratory disease with dyspnea, obstruction or cor pulmonale; previous addiction to sedative-hypnotic drugs; acute or chronic pain; seizure disorders; lactation; fever, hyperthyroidism, diabetes mellitus, severe anemia, pulmonary or cardiac disease, status asthmaticus, shock, uremia; debilitation.
- **Physical:** Weight; T; skin color, lesions; orientation, affect, reflexes; P, BP, orthostatic BP; R, adventitious sounds; bowel sounds, normal output, liver evaluation; liver and kidney function tests, blood and urine glucose, BUN.

Interventions
- Monitor patient responses, blood levels if any of the above interacting drugs are given with amobarbital; suggest alternative contraceptives to oral ones if amobarbital is used.
- Do not give intra-arterially (may produce arteriospasm, thrombosis, gangrene).
- Give IM doses deep in a muscle mass.
- Monitor sites carefully for irritation, extravasation with IV use (alkaline solutions are irritating to tissues).
- Monitor P, BP, respiration carefully during IV administration.
- Have resuscitative facilities on standby in case of respiratory depression, hypersensitivity reaction.
- Taper dosage gradually after repeated use, especially in epileptic patients.

Teaching points
Incorporate teaching about the drug with the general teaching about the procedure for patients receiving this drug as preanesthetic medication; include the following:
- This drug will make you drowsy and less anxious.

- Do not try to get up after you have received this drug (request assistance if you feel you must sit up or move around).
- These side effects may occur: drowsiness, dizziness, hangover, impaired thinking (these effects may become less pronounced after a few days; avoid driving or dangerous activities); GI upset (taking the drug with food may help); dreams, nightmares, difficulty concentrating, fatigue, nervousness (reversible; will go away when drug is discontinued).
- Report severe dizziness, weakness, drowsiness that persists; rash or skin lesions; pregnancy.

▽ amoxapine
(a mox' a peen)

Asendin

PREGNANCY CATEGORY C

Drug classes
Tricyclic antidepressant (TCA)
Antianxiety drug

Therapeutic actions
Mechanism of action unknown; TCAs inhibit the reuptake of the neurotransmitters norepinephrine and serotonin, leading to an increase in their effects; anticholinergic at CNS and peripheral receptors; sedative.

Indications
- Relief of symptoms of depression (endogenous depression most responsive)
- Treatment of depression accompanied with anxiety or agitation

Contraindications and cautions
- Contraindicated with hypersensitivity to any tricyclic drug; concomitant therapy with an MAO inhibitor; recent MI; myelography within previous 24 hr or scheduled within 48 hr; lactation.
- Use cautiously with EST; preexisting CV disorders (severe coronary heart disease, progressive heart failure, angina pectoris, paroxysmal tachycardia); angle-closure glaucoma, increased intraocular pressure, urinary retention, ureteral or urethral spasm; seizure

disorders; hyperthyroidism; impaired hepatic, renal function; psychiatric patients (schizophrenic or paranoid patients may exhibit a worsening of psychosis); manic-depressive patients; elective surgery (discontinue as soon as possible before surgery).

Available forms
Tablets—25, 50, 100, 150 mg

Dosages
Adults
Initially, 50 mg PO bid–tid; gradually increase to 100 mg bid–tid by end of first week if tolerated; increase above 300 mg/day only if this dosage ineffective for at least 2 wk. Hospitalized patients refractory to antidepressant therapy and with no history of convulsive seizures may be given up to 600 mg/day in divided doses; after effective dosage is established, drug may be given in single hs dose (up to 300 mg).
Pediatric patients
Not recommended for patients < 16 yr.
Geriatric patients
Initially, 25 mg bid–tid; if tolerated, dosage may be increased by end of first week to 50 mg bid–tid. For many elderly patients, 100–150 mg/day may be adequate; some may require up to 300 mg/day.

Pharmacokinetics

Route	Onset	Peak	Duration
Oral	Varies	2–4 hr	2–4 wk

Metabolism: Hepatic; $T_{1/2}$: 8–30 hr
Distribution: Crosses placenta; passes into breast milk
Excretion: Urine

Adverse effects
- **CNS:** *Disturbed concentration, sedation and anticholinergic (atropine-like) effects, confusion* (especially in elderly), hallucinations, disorientation, decreased memory, feelings of unreality, delusions, anxiety, nervousness, restlessness, agitation, panic, insomnia, nightmares, hypomania, mania, exacerbation of psychosis, drowsiness, weakness, fatigue, headache, numbness, tingling, paresthesias of extremities, incoordination, motor hyperactivity, akathisia, ataxia, tremors, peripheral neuropathy, extrapyramidal symptoms, seizures, speech blockage, dysarthria, tinnitus, altered EEG
- **CV:** *Orthostatic hypotension,* hypertension, syncope, tachycardia, palpitations, MI, arrhythmias, heart block, precipitation of CHF, stroke
- **Endocrine:** Elevated or depressed blood sugar, elevated prolactin levels, inappropriate ADH secretion
- **GI:** *Dry mouth, constipation,* paralytic ileus, *nausea,* vomiting, anorexia, epigastric distress, diarrhea, flatulence, dysphagia, peculiar taste, increased salivation, stomatitis, glossitis, parotid swelling, abdominal cramps, black tongue, hepatitis, jaundice (rare); elevated transaminase, altered alkaline phosphatase
- **GU:** Urinary retention, delayed micturition, dilation of the urinary tract, gynecomastia, testicular swelling in men; breast enlargement, menstrual irregularity, and galactorrhea in women; changes in libido; impotence
- **Hematologic:** Bone marrow depression
- **Hypersensitivity:** Rash, pruritus, vasculitis, petechiae, photosensitization, edema (generalized, facial, tongue), drug fever
- **Withdrawal:** Symptoms on abrupt discontinuation of prolonged therapy: nausea, headache, vertigo, nightmares, malaise
- **Other:** Nasal congestion, excessive appetite, weight gain or loss, sweating, alopecia, lacrimation, hyperthermia, flushing, chills

Interactions
✳ **Drug-drug** ● Increased TCA levels and pharmacologic (especially anticholinergic) effects with cimetidine, fluoxetine ● Increased TCA levels with methylphenidate, phenothiazines, hormonal contraceptives, disulfiram, cimetidine, ranitidine ● Hyperpyretic crises, severe seizures, hypertensive episodes, and deaths with MAOIs, furazolidone ● Increased antidepressant response and cardiac arrhythmias with thyroid medication ● Increased or decreased effects with estrogens ● Delirium with disulfiram ● Sympathetic hyperactivity, sinus tachycardia, hypertension, agitation with levodopa ● Increased biotransformation of TCAs in patients who smoke cigarettes ● Increased sym-

pathomimetic (especially alpha-adrenergic) effects of direct-acting sympathomimetic drugs (norepinephrine, epinephrine) • Increased anticholinergic effects of anticholinergic drugs (including anticholinergic antiparkinsonian drugs) • Increased response (especially CNS depression) to barbiturates • Decreased antihypertensive effect of guanethidine, clonidine, other antihypertensives

■ **Nursing considerations**
Assessment
• **History:** Hypersensitivity to any tricyclic drug; concomitant therapy with an MAO inhibitor; recent MI; myelography within previous 24 hr or scheduled within 48 hr; lactation; EST; preexisting CV disorders; angle-closure glaucoma, increased intraocular pressure; urinary retention, ureteral or urethral spasm; seizure disorders; hyperthyroidism; impaired hepatic, renal function; psychiatric patients; manic-depressive patients; elective surgery
• **Physical:** Weight; T; skin color, lesions; orientation, affect, reflexes, vision and hearing; P, BP, orthostatic BP, perfusion; bowel sounds, normal output, liver evaluation; urine flow, normal output; usual sexual function, frequency of menses, breast and scrotal exam; liver function tests, urinalysis, CBC, ECG

Interventions
Restrict drug access for depressed and potentially suicidal patients.
• Give major portion of dose hs if drowsiness, severe anticholinergic effects occur (the elderly may not tolerate single daily dose).
• Reduce dosage if minor side effects develop; discontinue if serious side effects occur.
• Arrange for CBC if patient develops fever, sore throat, or other sign of infection.
• Encourage elderly men or men with prostate problems to void before taking drug.

Teaching points
• Do not stop taking this drug abruptly or without consulting health care provider.
• Avoid using alcohol, other sleep-inducing drugs, OTC drugs.
• Avoid prolonged exposure to sunlight or sunlamps; use a sunscreen or protective garments.

• These side effects may occur: headache, dizziness, drowsiness, weakness, blurred vision (reversible; safety measures may need to be taken if severe; avoid driving or tasks requiring alertness); nausea, vomiting, loss of appetite, dry mouth (small, frequent meals, frequent mouth care, and sucking sugarless candies may help); nightmares, inability to concentrate, confusion; changes in sexual function.
• Report dry mouth, difficulty in urination, excessive sedation.

▽ **amoxicillin trihydrate**
(a mox i sill' in)

Amoxil, Amoxil Pediatric Drops, Apo-Amoxi (CAN), Novamoxin (CAN), Nu-Amoxi (CAN), Trimox, Trimox Pediatric Drops, Wymox

PREGNANCY CATEGORY B

Drug class
Antibiotic, penicillin–ampicillin type

Therapeutic actions
Bactericidal: inhibits synthesis of cell wall of sensitive organisms, causing cell death.

Indications
• Infections due to susceptible strains of *Haemophilus influenzae, E. coli, Proteus mirabilis, Neisseria gonorrhoeae, Streptococcus pneumoniae,* streptococci, non-penicillinase-producing staphylococci
• *Helicobacter pylori* infection in combination with other agents
• Post-exposure prophylaxis against *Bacillus anthracis*
• Unlabeled use: *Chlamydia trachomatis* in pregnancy

Contraindications and cautions
• Contraindicated with allergies to penicillins, cephalosporins, or other allergens.
• Use cautiously with renal disorders, lactation.

Available forms
Chewable tablets—125, 250 mg; tablets—500, 875 mg; capsules—250, 500 mg; pow-

der for oral suspension—50 mg/mL; 125 mg/ 5 mL, 200 mg/5 mL, 250 mg/5 mL, 400 mg/ 5 mL
Available in oral preparations only.

Dosages
Adults and pediatric patients > 20 kg
- *URIs, GU infections, skin and soft-tissue infections:* 250–500 mg PO q 8 hr or 875 mg PO bid.
- *Post-exposure anthrax prophylaxis:* 500 mg PO tid.
- *Lower respiratory infections:* 500 mg PO q 8 hr or 875 mg PO bid.
- *Uncomplicated gonococcal infections:* 3 g amoxicillin with 1 g probenecid PO.
- *C. trachomatis in pregnancy:* 500 mg PO tid for 7 days or 875 mg PO bid.
- *Prevention of SBE: Dental, oral, or upper respiratory procedures:* 2 g 1 hr before procedure.
- *GI or GU procedures:* 2 g ampicillin plus 1.5 mg/kg gentamicin IM or IV 30 min before procedure, followed by 1 g amoxicillin; for low-risk patients, 2 g 1 hr before procedure.
- *H. pylori:* 1 g bid with clarithromycin 500 mg bid and lansoprazole 30 mg bid for 14 days.

Pediatric patients < 20 kg
- *URIs, GU infections, skin, and soft-tissue infections:* 20–40 mg/kg/day PO in divided doses q 8 hr.
- *Post-exposure anthrax prophylaxis:* 80 mg/ kg/day PO divided into 3 doses.
- *Lower respiratory infections:* 40 mg/kg/day PO in divided doses q 8 hr.
- *Prevention of SBE: Dental, oral, or upper respiratory procedures:* 50 mg/kg 1 hr before procedure.
- *GI or GU procedures:* 50 mg/kg ampicillin plus 2 mg/kg gentamicin IM or IV 30 min before procedure followed by 25 mg/kg amoxicillin. For moderate-risk patients, 50 mg/kg PO 1 hr before procedure.

Pharmacokinetics

Route	Onset	Peak	Duration
Oral	Varies	1 hr	6–8 hr

Metabolism: $T_{1/2}$: 1–1.4 hr
Distribution: Crosses placenta; passes into breast milk
Excretion: Unchanged in the urine

Adverse effects
- **CNS:** Lethargy, hallucinations, seizures
- **GI:** *Glossitis, stomatitis, gastritis, sore mouth,* furry tongue, black "hairy" tongue, *nausea, vomiting, diarrhea, abdominal pain,* bloody diarrhea, enterocolitis, pseudomembranous colitis, nonspecific hepatitis
- **GU:** Nephritis
- **Hematologic:** Anemia, thrombocytopenia, leukopenia, neutropenia, prolonged bleeding time
- **Hypersensitivity:** *Rash, fever, wheezing,* **anaphylaxis**
- **Other:** *Superinfections*—oral and rectal moniliasis, vaginitis

Interactions
✳ **Drug-drug** • Increased effect with probenecid • Decreased effectiveness with tetracyclines, chloramphenicol • Decreased efficacy of oral contraceptives
✳ **Drug-food** • Delayed or reduced GI absorption with food

■ Nursing considerations
Assessment
- **History:** Allergies to penicillins, cephalosporins, or other allergens; renal disorders; lactation
- **Physical:** Culture infected area; skin color, lesion; R, adventitious sounds; bowel sounds; CBC, liver and renal function tests, serum electrolytes, Hct, urinalysis

Interventions
- Culture infected area prior to treatment; reculture if response is not as expected.
- Give in oral preparations only; absorption may be affected by presence of food; drug should be taken 1 hr before or 2 hr after meals.
- Continue therapy for at least 2 days after signs of infection have disappeared; continuation for 10 full days is recommended.
- Use corticosteroids, antihistamines for skin reactions.

Adverse effects in *Italics* are most common; those in **Bold** are life-threatening.

Teaching points

- Take this drug around the clock. The drug should be taken on an empty stomach, 1 hr before or 2 hr after meals.
- Take the full course of therapy; do not stop because you feel better.
- This antibiotic is specific for this problem and should not be used to self-treat other infections.
- These side effects may occur: nausea, vomiting, GI upset (small frequent meals may help); diarrhea; sore mouth (frequent mouth care may help).
- Report unusual bleeding or bruising, sore throat, fever, rash, hives, severe diarrhea, difficulty breathing.

▽ **amphotericin B**
*(am foe **ter'** i sin)*

amphotericin B
Fungizone

amphotericin B desoxycholate
Amphocin, Fungizone Intravenous

amphotericin B, lipid-based
Abelcet, AmBisome, Amphotec

PREGNANCY CATEGORY B

Drug class
Antifungal agent

Therapeutic actions
Binds to sterols in the fungal cell membrane with a resultant change in membrane permeability, an effect that can destroy fungal cells and prevent their reproduction; fungicidal or fungistatic depending on concentration and organism.

Indications

- Reserve use for patients with progressive, potentially fatal infections: cryptococcosis; North American blastomycosis; disseminated moniliasis; coccidioidomycosis and histoplasmosis; mucormycosis caused by species of *Mucor, Rhizopus, Absidia, Entomoph-*

thora, Basidiobolus; sporotrichosis; aspergillosis
- Adjunct treatment of American mucocutaneous leishmaniasis (not choice in primary therapy)
- Treatment of aspergillosis in patients refractory to conventional therapy (*Abelcet, Amphotec*)
- Treatment of cryptococcal meningitis in HIV-infected patients (*AmBisome*)
- Treatment of cutaneous and mucocutaneous mycotic infections caused by *Candida* species (topical application)
- Treatment of invasive aspergillosis where renal toxicity precludes use of conventional amphotericin B (*Amphotec*)
- Treatment of presumed fungal infections in febrile, neutropenic patients (*AmBisome*)
- Treatment of *Aspergillis, Candida,* or *Cryptococcus* infections in patients intolerant to or refractory to *Fungizone* (*AmBisome*)
- Treatment of any type of progressive fungal infection that does not respond to conventional therapy
- Treatment of oral candidiasis caused by *C. albicans*
- Unlabeled use: prophylactic use to prevent fungal infections in bone marrow transplants

Contraindications and cautions

- Allergy to amphotericin B, renal dysfunction, lactation (except when life-threatening and treatable only with this drug).

Available forms
Injection—50 mg; suspension for injection—100 mg/20 mL; powder for injection—50, 100 mg; powder for infusion 50 mg/vial; topical—3% cream, ointment, lotion; oral suspension—100 mg/mL.

Dosages
Adults and pediatric patients
For test dose, give 1 mg slowly IV to determine patient tolerance. Administer by slow IV infusion over 6 hr at a concentration of 0.1 mg/mL. Increase daily dose based on patient tolerance and response. Usual dose is 0.25 mg/kg/day; do not exceed 1.5 mg/kg/day. Check manufacturer's guidelines for specifics.
Fungizone
- *Sporotrichosis:* 0.5 mg/kg/day to a total dose of 2.5 g.

- *Aspergillosis:* Treat up to 11 mo, with a total dose of 3.6 g.
- *Rhinocerebral phycomycosis:* Control diabetes; amphotericin B cumulative dose of 3 g; disease is usually rapidly fatal; treatment must be aggressive.
- *Bladder irrigation (adults):* 50 mg/1,000 mL sterile water instilled intermittently or continuously.
- *Candidiasis:* 1 mL (100 mg) oral suspension qid; instruct patient to swish and hold in mouth before swallowing. Use for 2 wk.

For topical application
Liberally apply to candidal lesions bid to qid; treatment ranges from 2–4 wk based on response.

Abelcet
- *Aspergillosis:* 5 mg/kg/day given as a single infusion at 2.5 mg/kg/hr.

Amphotec
- *Aspergillosis:* Initially 3–4 mg/kg/day, may increase to 6 mg/kg/day IV. Infuse at 1 mg/kg/hr over at least 2 hr.

AmBisome
- *Aspergillosis:* 3–5 mg/kg/day IV, give over > 2 hr.
- *Leishmaniasis:* 3 mg/kg/day IV, days 1–5, 14, and 21.

Pharmacokinetics

Route	Onset	Peak	Duration
IV	20–30 min	1–2 hr	20–24 hr

Metabolism: $T_{1/2}$: 24 hr initially and then 15 days; 173.4 hr (*Abelcet*)
Distribution: Crosses placenta; may pass into breast milk
Excretion: Urine

▽IV facts

Preparation: *Fungizone:* 5 mg/mL: rapidly inject 10 mL sterile water for injection without a bacteriostatic agent directly into the lyophilized cake using a sterile needle (minimum diameter, 20 gauge); shake vial until clear; 0.1 mg/mL solution is obtained by further dilution with 5% dextrose injection of pH above 4.2; use strict aseptic technique. Do not dilute with saline; do not use if any precipitation is found. Refrigerate vials and protect from exposure to light; store in dark at room temperature for 24 hr or refrigerated for 1 wk. Discard any unused material. Use solutions prepared for IV infusion promptly.
Abelcet: Shake vial gently until no yellow sediment is seen. Withdraw dose, replace needle with a 5-micron filter needle. Inject into bag containing 5% dextrose injection to a concentration of 1 mg/mL. May be further diluted. Store vials in refrigerator; stable for 15 hr once prepared if refrigerated, for 6 hr at room temperature.
Amphotec: Reconstitute with sterile water for injection. 10 mL to 50 mg/vial or 20 mL to 100 mg/vial. Dilute to 0.06 mg/mL. Refrigerate after reconstitution; use within 24 hr.

Infusion: *Fungizone:* protect from exposure to light if not infused within 8 hr of preparation. Infuse slowly over 6 hr.
Abelcet: Infuse at rate of 2.5 mg/kg/hr. If infusion takes > 2 hr, remix bag by shaking.
Amphotec: Infuse at 1 mg/kg/hr over at least 2 hr; do *not* use an in-line filter.
AmBisome: Infuse over > 2 hr if tolerated; stop immediately at any sign of anaphylactic reaction.

Incompatibilities: Do not mix with saline-containing solution, parenteral nutrional solutions, aminoglycosides, penicillins, phenothiazines, calcium preparations, cimetidine, metaraminol, methyldopa, polymyxin, potassium chloride, ranitidine, verapamil, clindamycin, cotrimoxazole, dopamine, dobutamine, tetracycline, vitamins, lidocaine, procaine, or heparin. **If line must be flushed, do not use heparin or saline; use D_5W.**
Y-site incompatibility: foscarnet, ondansetron

Adverse effects
Systemic administration
- **CNS:** *Fever (often with shaking chills), headache, malaise,* generalized pain
- **GI:** *Nausea, vomiting, dyspepsia, diarrhea,* cramping, epigastric pain, anorexia
- **GU:** Hypokalemia, azotemia, hyposthenuria, renal tubular acidosis, nephrocalcinosis
- **Hematologic:** Normochromic, normocytic anemia
- **Local:** *Pain at the injection site* with phlebitis and thrombophlebitis
- **Other:** Weight loss

Topical application
- **Dermatologic:** *Drying effect on skin, local irritation* (cream); *pruritus,* allergic contact dermatitis (lotion); *local irritation* (ointment)

Interactions

✳ **Drug-drug** • Do not administer with corticosteroids unless these are needed to control symptoms • Increased risk of nephrotoxicity with other nephrotoxic antibiotics, antineoplastics • Increased effects and risk of toxicity of digitalis, skeletal muscle relaxants, flucytosine • Increased nephrotoxic effects with cyclosporine

■ Nursing considerations
Assessment
- **History:** Allergy to amphotericin B, renal dysfunction, lactation
- **Physical:** Skin color, lesions; T; weight; injection site; orientation, reflexes, affect; bowel sounds, liver evaluation; renal function tests; CBC and differential; culture of area involved

Interventions
- Arrange for immediate culture of infection but begin treatment before lab results are returned.
- Monitor injection sites and veins for signs of phlebitis.
- Cleanse affected lesions before applying topical drug; apply liberally to lesions and rub in gently; do not cover with plastic wrap.
- Use soap and water to wash hands, fabrics, skin areas that may discolor as a result of topical application.
- Shake bottle before use and apply oral solution to the tongue; encourage patient to swish solution and retain in mouth as long as possible before swallowing; use between meals.
- Provide aspirin, antihistamines, antiemetics, maintain sodium balance to ease drug discomfort. Minimal use of IV corticosteroids may decrease febrile reactions. Meperidine has been used to relieve chills and fever.
- Monitor renal function tests weekly; discontinue or decrease dosage of drug at any sign of increased renal toxicity.

- Continue topical administration for long-term therapy until infection is eradicated, usually 2–4 wk.
- Discontinue topical application if hypersensitivity reaction occurs.

Teaching points
- Be aware that long-term use of this drug will be needed; beneficial effects may not be seen for several weeks; the systemic form of the drug can only be given IV.
- For topical application, apply topical drug liberally to affected area after first cleansing area.
- Oral solution—apply to tongue, swish around mouth, and retain as long as possible before swallowing.
- Use hygiene measures to prevent reinfection or spread of infection.
- Know that these side effects may occur: nausea, vomiting, diarrhea (small, frequent meals may help); discoloring, drying of the skin, staining of fabric with topical forms (washing with soap and water or cleaning fabric with standard cleaning fluid should remove stain); stinging, irritation with local application; fever, chills, muscle aches and pains, headache (medications may be ordered to help you to deal with these discomforts of the drug).
- Report pain, irritation at injection site; GI upset, nausea, loss of appetite; difficulty breathing; local irritation, burning (topical application).

▽ **ampicillin**
*(am pi **sill'** in)*

ampicillin sodium
Oral: Ampicin (CAN), Apo-Ampi (CAN), Marcillin, Novo-Ampicillin (CAN), Nu-Ampi (CAN), Omnipen, Penbritin (CAN), Principen, Totacillin

ampicillin sodium
Parenteral: Omnipen-N

PREGNANCY CATEGORY B

Drug classes
Antibiotic
Penicillin

Therapeutic actions

Bactericidal action against sensitive organisms; inhibits synthesis of bacterial cell wall, causing cell death.

Indications

- Treatment of infections caused by susceptible strains of *Shigella, Salmonella, E. coli, H. influenzae, P. mirabilis, N. gonorrhoeae,* enterococci, gram-positive organisms (penicillin G–sensitive staphylococci, streptococci, pneumococci)
- Meningitis caused by *Neisseria meningitidis*
- Unlabeled use: prophylaxis in cesarean section in certain high-risk patients

Contraindications and cautions

- Contraindicated with allergies to penicillins, cephalosporins, or other allergens.
- Use cautiously with renal disorders.

Available forms

Capsules—250, 500 mg; powder for oral suspension—125 mg/5 mL, 250 mg/5 mL; powder for injection—125, 250, 500 mg, 1, 2, 10 g

Dosages

Maximum recommended dosage: 8 mg/day; may be given IV, IM, or PO. Use parenteral routes for severe infections, and switch to oral route as soon as possible.

- *Respiratory and soft-tissue infections:*
Patients weighing ≥ 40 kg: 250–500 mg IV or IM q 6 hr.
Patients weighing < 40 kg: 25–50 mg/kg/day IM or IV in equally divided doses at 6–8 hr intervals.
Patients weighing ≥ 20 kg: 250 mg PO q 6 hr.
Patients weighing < 20 kg: 50 mg/kg/day PO in equally divided doses q 6–8 hr.
- *GI and GU infections, including women with N. gonorrhoeae:*
Patients weighing > 40 kg: 500 mg IM or IV q 6 hr.
Patients weighing ≤ 40 kg: 50–100 mg/kg/day IM or IV in equally divided doses q 6–8 hr.
Patients weighing ≥ 20 kg: 500 mg PO q 6 hr.
Patients weighing < 20 kg: 100 mg/kg/day PO in equally divided doses q 6–8 hr.

- *Gonococcal infections:* 500 mg q 6 hr for penicillin-sensitive organism or single dose of 3.5 g PO with 1 g probenecid for patients ≥ 45 kg.
- *Bacterial meningitis (adult and pediatric):* 150–200 mg/kg/day by continuous IV drip and then IM injections in equally divided doses q 3–4 hr.
- *Prevention of bacterial endocarditis for GI or GU surgery or instrumentation:*
Adults: 2 g ampicillin IM or IV with gentamicin 1.5 mg/kg IM or IV within 30 minutes of starting procedure. Six hours later give 1 g ampicillin IM or IV or 1 g amoxicillin PO.
Pediatric patients: 50 mg/kg ampicillin IM or IV with 1.5 mg/kg gentamicin IM or IV within 30 minutes of procedure. Six hours later give 25 mg/kg ampicillin IM or IV or 25 mg/kg amoxicillin PO.
- *Prevention of bacterial endocarditis for dental, oral, or upper respiratory procedures*
Adults: 2 g ampicillin IM or IV within 30 minutes of procedure.
Pediatric patients: 50 mg/kg ampicillin IM or IV within 30 minutes of procedure.
- *Septicemia (adult and pediatric):* 150–200 mg/kg/day IV for at least 3 days, then IM q 3–4 hr.
- *Sexually transmitted diseases (adult):*
Rape victims: Prophylaxis against infection.
Pregnant women and patients allergic to tetracycline: 3.5 g ampicillin PO with 1 g probenecid.
Prophylaxis in cesarean section: Single IV or IM dose of 25–100 mg/kg immediately after cord is clamped.

Pharmacokinetics

Route	Onset	Peak	Duration
Oral	30 min	2 hr	6–8 hr
IM	15 min	1 hr	6–8 hr
IV	Immediate	5 min	6–8 hr

Metabolism: $T_{1/2}$: 1–2 hr
Distribution: Crosses placenta; passes into breast milk
Excretion: Unchanged in the urine

▼ IV facts

Preparation: Reconstitute with sterile or bacteriostatic water for injection; piggyback vials may be reconstituted with sodium chloride injection; use reconstituted solution within 1 hr. Do not mix in the same IV solution as other antibiotics. Use within 1 hr after preparation because potency may decrease significantly after that.

Infusion: Direct IV administration; give slowly over 3–5 min. *Rapid administration can lead to convulsions.*

IV drip: *dilute as above before further dilution.*

IV piggyback: *administer alone or further dilute with compatible solution.*

Compatibility: Ampicillin is compatible with 0.9% sodium chloride, 5% dextrose in water, or 0.45% sodium chloride solution, 10% invert sugar water, M/6 sodium lactate solution, lactated Ringer's solution, sterile water for injection. Diluted solutions are stable for 2–8 hr; check manufacturer's inserts for specifics. Discard solution after allotted time period.

Incompatibility: Do not mix with lidocaine, verapamil, other antibiotics, dextrose solutions.

Y-site incompatibility: Do not give with epinephrine, hydralazine, ondansetron.

Adverse effects

- **CNS:** Lethargy, hallucinations, seizures
- **CV:** CHF
- **GI:** *Glossitis, stomatitis, gastritis, sore mouth,* furry tongue, black "hairy" tongue, *nausea, vomiting, diarrhea,* abdominal pain, bloody diarrhea, enterocolitis, pseudomembranous colitis, nonspecific hepatitis
- **GU: Nephritis**
- **Hematologic:** Anemia, thrombocytopenia, leukopenia, neutropenia, prolonged bleeding time
- **Hypersensitivity:** *Rash, fever, wheezing,* **anaphylaxis**
- **Local:** *Pain, phlebitis,* thrombosis at injection site (parenteral)
- **Other:** *Superinfections*—oral and rectal moniliasis, vaginitis

Interactions

❋ **Drug-drug** • Increased ampicillin effect with probenecid • Increased risk of rash with allopurinol • Increased bleeding effect with heparin, oral anticoagulants • Decreased effectiveness with tetracyclines, chloramphenicol • Decreased efficacy of oral contraceptives, atenolol with ampicillin

❋ **Drug-food** • Oral ampicillin may be less effective with food; take on an empty stomach

❋ **Drug-lab test** • False-positive Coombs' test if given IV • Decrease in plasma estrogen concentrations in pregnant women • False-positive urine glucose tests if *Clinitest*, Benedict's solution, or Fehling's solution is used; enzymatic glucose oxidase methods (*Clinistix, Tes-Tape*) should be used to check urine glucose

■ Nursing considerations
Assessment

- **History:** Allergies to penicillins, cephalosporins, or other allergens; renal disorders; lactation
- **Physical:** Culture infected area; skin color, lesion; R, adventitious sounds; bowel sounds; CBC, liver and renal function tests, serum electrolytes, hematocrit, urinalysis.

Interventions

- Culture infected area before treatment; reculture area if response is not as expected.
- Check IV site carefully for signs of thrombosis or drug reaction.
- Do not give IM injections in the same site; atrophy can occur. Monitor injection sites.
- Administer oral drug on an empty stomach, 1 hr before or 2 hr after meals with a full glass of water—no fruit juice or soft drinks.

Teaching points

- Take this drug around the clock.
- Take the full course of therapy; do not stop taking the drug if you feel better.
- Take the oral drug on an empty stomach, 1 hr before or 2 hr after meals; the oral solution is stable for 7 days at room temperature.
- This antibiotic is specific to your problem and should not be used to self-treat other infections.
- These side effects may occur: nausea, vomiting, GI upset (small frequent meals may help), diarrhea.

• Report pain or discomfort at sites, unusual bleeding or bruising, mouth sores, rash, hives, fever, itching, severe diarrhea, difficulty breathing.

▷ amprenavir
(am pren' ah ver)

Agenerase

PREGNANCY CATEGORY C

Drug class
Antiviral drug

Therapeutic actions
Antiviral activity; inhibits HIV protease activity, leading to the formation of immature, non-infectious virus particles

Indications
• Treatment of HIV infection, in combination with other antiretroviral agents

Contraindications and cautions
• Contraindicated in the presence of allergy to any component of the drug.
• Use cautiously with pregnancy, hepatic impairment, lactation, diabetes mellitus, hemophilia, sulfonamide allergy.

Available forms
Capsules—50, 150 mg; oral solution—15 mg/mL

Dosages
Adults and children ≥ 50 kg and ≥ 13 yr
1,200 mg PO bid (eight 150 mg capsules) with other antiretroviral agents or 1,400 mg bid oral solution with other antiretroviral agents.
Pediatric patients
Capsules
4–12 yr or 13–16 yr weighing < 50 kg: 20 mg/kg bid PO or 15 mg/kg tid PO (to max. daily dose of 2,400 mg) with other antiretroviral agents.
Oral solution
4–12 yr or 13–16 yr weighing < 50 kg: 22.5 mg/kg bid PO or 17 mg/kg tid PO (to max. daily dose of 2,800 mg) with other antiretroviral agents.
Patients with hepatic impairment
Child–Pugh score 5–8: 450 mg bid PO; Child–Pugh score 9–12: 300 mg bid PO.

Pharmacokinetics

Route	Onset	Peak
Oral	Varies	1.1 hr

Metabolism: Hepatic; $T_{1/2}$: 7.1–10.6 hr
Distribution: Crosses placenta; may pass into breast milk
Excretion: Feces and urine

Adverse effects
• **CNS:** *Asthenia, peripheral and circumoral paresthesias,* anxiety, dreams, headache, dizziness, *depression*
• **Dermatologic:** *Rash* to **Stevens-Johnson syndrome**
• **GI:** *Nausea, vomiting, diarrhea, anorexia, abdominal pain, taste perversion,* dry mouth, hepatitis, liver dysfunction, dehydration
• **Hematologic:** *Hyperglycemia,* hypercholesterolemia, *hypertriglyceridemia*

Interactions
✷ **Drug-drug** • Potentially large increase in the serum concentration of amiodarone, bepridil, bupropion, cisapride, cloxapine, encainide, flecainide, meperidine, piroxicam, propafenone, propoxyphene, quinidine, rifabutin, when taken with amprenavir. Potential for serious arrhythmias, seizure, and fatal reactions. Do not administer amprenavir with any of these drugs • Potentially large increases in the serum concentration of these sedatives and hypnotics: alprazolam, clorazepam, diazepam, estazolam, flurazepam, midazolam, triazolam, zolpidem. Extreme sedation and respiratory depression could occur. Do not administer amprenavir with any of these drugs • Risk of vitamin E intoxication if taken with amprenavir; caution patient to avoid products containing vitamin E • Risk of decreased effectiveness of hormonal contraceptives; advise the use of barrier contraceptives • Risk of increased adverse ef-

fects with sildenafil; use caution, report any adverse effects

✻ Drug-food • Absorption of amprenavir is decreased by the presence of high-fat food; avoid taking the drug with high-fat meals • Decreased metabolism and risk of toxic effects if combined with grapefruit juice; avoid this combination.

✻ Drug-alternative therapy • Decreased effectiveness if combined with St. John's wort

■ Nursing considerations
Assessment
- **History:** Allergy to amprenavir, sulfonamides; hepatic dysfunction; pregnancy; lactation; diabetes; hemophilia
- **Physical:** T; orientation, affect, reflexes; bowel sounds; skin color, perfusion; liver function tests, CBC, serum triglycerides, and cholesterol

Interventions
- Do not administer with high-fat meals, absorption may be decreased.
- Use caution with any history of sulfonamide allergy, cross-reactivity may occur.
- Ensure that patient is not receiving supplemental vitamin E preparations.
- Administer this drug with other antiretroviral agents.
- Monitor liver function and blood glucose levels prior to and periodically during therapy.
- Carefully screen drug history to avoid potentially dangerous drug–drug interactions.

Teaching points
- Do not take this drug with a high-fat meal. Do not drink grapefruit juice while on this drug.
- Take the full course of therapy as prescribed; do not double up doses if one is missed; do not change dosage without consulting your health care provider. Take this drug with other antiviral agents.
- This drug does not cure HIV infection; long-term effects are not yet known; continue to take precautions as the risk of transmission is not reduced by this drug.
- Do not take supplemental vitamin E preparations while you are on this drug; serious reactions could occur.

- Do not take any other drug, prescription or OTC, or St. John's wort without consulting with your health care provider; this drug interacts with many other drugs and serious problems can occur.
- Consider the use of barrier contraceptives while on this drug; oral contraceptives may not be effective.
- Use caution if taking sildenafil (*Viagra*); there is an increased risk of adverse effects; consult with your prescriber if adverse effects occur.
- These side effects may occur: nausea, vomiting, loss of appetite, diarrhea, abdominal pain (small, frequent meals may help); headache, dizziness, numbness and tingling (use caution if driving or operating dangerous machinery).
- Report severe diarrhea, severe nausea, personality changes, changes in the color of urine or stool; increased thirst or urination.

▷amyl nitrite
(am' il)

Amyl Nitrate Aspirols, Amyl Nitrate Vaporole

PREGNANCY CATEGORY C

Drug classes
Antianginal drug
Nitrate

Therapeutic actions
Relaxes vascular smooth muscle, which results in a decrease in venous return and arterial blood pressure; this reduces left ventricular workload and decreases myocardial oxygen consumption.

Indications
- Relief of angina pectoris

Contraindications and cautions
- Allergy to nitrates, severe anemia, head trauma, cerebral hemorrhage, hypertrophic cardiomyopathy, lactation.

Available forms
Inhalation—0.3 mL

Dosages
Adults
0.3 mL by inhalation of vapor from crushed capsule; may repeat in 3–5 min for relief of angina. 1–6 inhalations are usually sufficient to produce desired effect.
Pediatric patients
Safety and efficacy not established.

Pharmacokinetics

Route	Onset	Peak	Duration
Inhalation	30 sec	3 min	3–5 min

Metabolism: Hepatic; $T_{1/2}$: 1–4 min
Distribution: Crosses placenta; may pass into breast milk
Excretion: Urine

Adverse effects
- **CNS:** *Headache, apprehension, restlessness, weakness,* vertigo, dizziness, faintness, euphoria
- **CV:** *Tachycardia,* retrosternal discomfort, palpitations, *hypotension,* syncope, collapse, orthostatic hypotension, angina
- **Dermatologic:** Rash, exfoliative dermatitis, *cutaneous vasodilation with flushing*
- **Drug abuse:** Abused for sexual stimulation and euphoria, effects of inhalation are instantaneous
- **GI:** *Nausea,* vomiting, incontinence of urine and feces, abdominal pain
- **Other:** Muscle twitching, pallor, perspiration, cold sweat

Interactions
✱ **Drug-drug** • Increased risk of severe hypotension and CV collapse if used with alcohol • Increased risk of hypotension with antihypertensive drugs, beta-adrenergic blockers, phenothiazines
✱ **Drug-lab test** • False report of decreased serum cholesterol if done by the Zlatkis–Zak color reaction

■ Nursing considerations
Assessment
- **History:** Allergy to nitrates, severe anemia, head trauma, cerebral hemorrhage, hypertrophic cardiomyopathy, lactation
- **Physical:** Skin color, temperature, lesions; orientation, reflexes, affect; P, BP, orthostatic BP, baseline ECG, peripheral perfusion; R, adventitious sounds; liver evaluation; normal urinary output; CBC, hemoglobin

Interventions
- Crush the capsule and wave under the patient's nose; 2–6 inhalations are usually sufficient; may repeat every 3–5 min.
- Protect the drug from light; store in a cool place.
- Gradually reduce dose if anginal treatment is being terminated; rapid discontinuation can cause withdrawal.

Teaching points
- Crush the capsule, and inhale 2–6 times by waving under your nose; repeat in 3–5 min if necessary.
- Do not use where vapors may ignite; vapors are highly flammable.
- Protect the drug from light; store in a cool place.
- Avoid alcohol while on amyl nitrite.
- These side effects may occur: dizziness, lightheadedness (transient; use care to change positions slowly; lie or sit down when taking dose); headache (lie down and rest in a cool environment; OTC preparations may not help); flushing of the neck or face (transient).
- Report blurred vision, persistent or severe headache, rash, more frequent or more severe angina attacks, fainting.

▽ anagrelide hydrochloride
(an agb' rah lide)

Agrylin

PREGNANCY CATEGORY C

Drug class
Antiplatelet agent

Therapeutic actions
Reduces platelet production by decreasing megakaryocyte hypermaturation; inhibits cyclic

AMP and ADP collagen-induced platelet aggregation. At therapeutic doses has no effect on WBC counts or coagulation parameters; may affect RBC parameters.

Indications

- Treatment of essential thrombocythemia to reduce elevated platelet count and the risk of thrombosis

Contraindications and cautions

- Use cautiously with renal or hepatic disorders, pregnancy, lactation, known heart disease, thrombocytopenia.

Available forms

Capsules—0.5, 1 mg

Dosages

Adults

Initially 0.5 mg PO qid or 1 mg PO bid. After 1 wk, reevaluate and adjust the dosage as needed; do not increase by more than 0.5 mg/day each week. Maximum dose 10 mg/day or 2.5 mg as a single dose.

Pediatric patients

Safety and efficacy not established.

Pharmacokinetics

Route	Onset	Peak
Oral	Rapid	1 hr

Metabolism: Hepatic; $T_{1/2}$: 1.3 hr
Distribution: Crosses placenta; may pass into breast milk
Excretion: Urine and feces

Adverse effects

- **CNS:** Dizziness, *headaches, asthenia,* paresthesias
- **CV: CHF,** tachycardia, **MI, complete heart block,** atrial fibrillation, hypertension, *palpitations,* **CVA**
- **GI:** *Diarrhea, nausea, vomiting, abdominal pain,* flatulence, dyspepsia, anorexia, **pancreatitis,** ulcer
- **Hematologic:** *Thrombocytopenia*
- **Other:** Rash, purpura, edema

Interactions

✳ **Drug-food •** Reduced availability of anagrelide if taken with food

■ Nursing considerations

⬥ **CLINICAL ALERT!**
Confusion has been reported with Agrylin and Aggrastat (tirofiban); use caution.

Assessment

- **History:** Allergy to anagrelide, thrombocytopenia, hemostatic disorders, bleeding ulcer, intracranial bleeding, severe liver disease, lactation, renal disorders, pregnancy, known heart disease
- **Physical:** Skin color, lesions; orientation; bowel sounds, normal output; CBC, liver and renal function tests

Interventions

- Perform platelet counts q 2 days during the first week of therapy and at least weekly thereafter; if thrombocytopenia occurs, decrease dosage of drug and arrange for supportive therapy.
- Administer drug on an empty stomach if at all tolerated.
- Establish safety precautions to prevent injury and bleeding (electric razor, no contact sports, etc.).
- Advise patient to use barrier contraceptives while receiving this drug; it may harm the fetus.
- Monitor patient for any sign of excessive bleeding—bruises, dark stools, etc.—and monitor bleeding times.
- Mark chart of any patient receiving anagrelide to alert medical personnel of potential for increased bleeding in cases of surgery or dental surgery, invasive procedures.

Teaching points

- Take drug on an empty stomach.
- You will require frequent and regular blood tests to monitor your response to this drug.
- It may take longer than normal to stop bleeding while on this drug; avoid contact sports, use electric razors, etc.; apply pressure for extended periods to bleeding sites.
- Avoid pregnancy while on this drug; it could harm the fetus; use of barrier contraceptives is suggested.
- These side effects may occur: upset stomach, nausea, diarrhea, loss of appetite (small, frequent meals may help).

- Notify any dentist or surgeon that you are on this drug before invasive procedures.
- Report fever, chills, sore throat, rash, bruising, bleeding, dark stools or urine, palpitations, chest pain.

▽anakinra
*(ann **ack'** in rah)*

Kineret

PREGNANCY CATEGORY B

Drug classes
Interleukin-1 receptor antagonist
Antiarthritis drug

Therapeutic actions
A recombinant human interleukin-1 receptor antagonist; blocks the activity of interleukin 1 that is elevated in response to inflammatory and immune stimulation and is responsible for the degradation of cartilage due to the rapid loss of proteoglycans in rheumatoid arthritis.

Indications
- Reduction of the signs and symptoms of moderately to severely active rheumatoid arthritis in patients ≥ 18 years of age who have failed on one or more disease-modifying antirheumatic drugs (methotrexate, sulfasalazine, hydrochloroquine, gold, penicillamine, leflunomide, azathioprine)

Contraindications and cautions
- Contraindicated with allergy to anakinra or proteins produced by *Escherichia coli*.
- Use cautiously with immunosuppression, active infection, pregnancy, lactation, renal impairment.

Available forms
Prefilled glass syringes—100 mg

Dosages
Adults
- 100 mg/day SC at approximately the same time each day.

Pediatric patients
- Safety and efficacy not established.

Pharmacokinetics

Route	Onset	Peak
SC	Slow	3–7 hr

Metabolism: Tissue; $T_{1/2}$: 4–6 hr
Distribution: May cross placenta; may enter breast milk
Excretion: Urine

Adverse effects
- **CNS:** Headache
- **GI:** Nausea, diarrhea, abdominal pain
- **Hematologic:** Neutropenia, thrombocytopenia
- **Respiratory:** *URI, sinusitis*
- **Other:** *Injection site reactions, infections,* influenza-like symptoms

Interactions
✴ **Drug-drug** • Increased risk of serious infections if combined with etanercept or other tumor necrosis factor blocking drugs; avoid this combination (if no alternative is available, use extreme caution and monitor patient closely) • Immunizations given while on anakinra may be less effective

■ Nursing considerations

CLINICAL ALERT!
Name confusion has occurred between anakinra and amikacin; use caution.

Assessment
- **History:** Allergy to anakinra or proteins produced by *E. coli*, immunosuppression, renal dysfunction, pregnancy, lactation
- **Physical:** Body temperature, body weight, P, BP, R, adventitious sounds, CBC, renal function tests

Interventions
- Make sure that patient does not have an active infection before administering.
- Store the drug in the refrigerator, protected from light; use by expiration date, because solution contains no preservatives.

- Administer the subcutaneous injection at about the same time each day.
- Inspect solution before injection. Do not use solution if it is discolored or contains particulate matter.
- Discard any unused portion of the drug; do not store for later use.
- Provide analgesics if headache, muscle pain are a problem.
- Monitor injection sites for erythema, ecchymosis, inflammation, and pain. Rotating sites may help to decrease severe reactions.
- Advise women of childbearing age to use a barrier form of contraception while taking this drug.
- Monitor CBC before and periodically during therapy; drug should not be given during active infections.

Teaching points

- This drug must be injected subcutaneously once each day at approximately the same time each day.
- The drug must be stored in the refrigerator, protected from light. Use the drug by the expiration date on the box; the drug contains no preservatives and will not be effective after that date. Do not use any drug that is discolored or contains particulate matter.
- You and a family member or significant other should learn the proper way to administer a subcutaneous injection, including the proper disposal of needles and syringes. Prepare a chart of injection sites to ensure that you rotate the sites.
- Avoid infection while you are on this drug; avoid crowded areas or people with known infections.
- Know that these side effects may also occur: reactions at the injection site (rotating sites and applying heat may help); headache, pain (use of an analgesic may help; consult with your health care provider); increased risk of infection (contact your health care provider at any sign of infection [fever, muscles aches and pains, respiratory problems] because it may be necessary to stop the drug during the infection).
- This drug does not cure your rheumatoid arthritis, and appropriate therapies to deal with the disease should be followed.

- Report: fever, chills, difficulty breathing, severe discomfort at injection site.

anastrozole
(an abs' troh zol)

Arimidex

PREGNANCY CATEGORY D

Drug class
Antiestrogen

Therapeutic actions
Selective nonsteroidal aromatase inhibitor that significantly reduces serum estradiol levels with no significant effect on adrenocortical steroids or aldosterone.

Indications
- Treatment of advanced breast cancer in postmenopausal women with disease progression following tamoxifen therapy
- Adjuvant treatment of postmenopausal women with hormone receptor positive or hormone receptor unknown locally advanced or metastatic breast cancer

Contraindications and cautions
- Contraindicated with allergy to anastrazole, pregnancy, lactation.
- Use cautiously with hepatic or renal impairment, high cholesterol states.

Available forms
Tablets—1 mg

Dosages
Adults
1 mg PO daily.
Pediatric patients
Not recommended.
Patients with hepatic or renal impairment
No change in dosage is recommended.

Pharmacokinetics

Route	Onset	Peak
Oral	Varies	10–12 hr

Metabolism: Hepatic; $T_{1/2}$: 50 hr

Distribution: Crosses placenta; enters breast milk

Excretion: Feces and urine

Adverse effects

- **CNS:** Depression, light-headedness, dizziness, asthenia
- **Dermatologic:** *Hot flashes, rash*
- **GI: Nausea, vomiting,** food distaste, dry mouth, *pharyngitis*
- **GU:** Vaginal bleeding, vaginal pain, UTIs
- **Other:** Peripheral edema, *bone pain, back pain*; increased HDL, LDL levels

■ Nursing considerations

Assessment

- **History:** Allergy to anastrozole, hepatic or renal dysfunction, pregnancy, lactation, treatment profile for breast cancer, hypercholesterolemia
- **Physical:** Skin lesions, color, turgor; pelvic exam; orientation, affect, reflexes; peripheral pulses, edema; liver and renal function tests

Interventions

- Administer once daily without regard to meals.
- Arrange for periodic lipid profiles during therapy.
- Arrange for appropriate analgesic measures if pain and discomfort become severe.

Teaching points

- Take the drug once a day without regard to meals.
- These side effects may occur: bone pain; hot flashes (staying in cool temperatures may help); nausea, vomiting (small, frequent meals may help); dizziness, headache, light-headedness (use caution if driving or performing tasks that require alertness); birth defects (avoid pregnancy).
- Report changes in color of stool or urine, severe vomiting, or inability to eat.

▷ **anistreplase (anisoylated plasminogen streptokinase activator complex, APSAC)**

*(an is tre **plaze'**)*

Eminase

PREGNANCY CATEGORY C

Drug class

Thrombolytic enzyme

Therapeutic actions

A complex of streptokinase with human plasminogen, which is activated to plasmin in the body; plasmin lyses formed thrombi.

Indications

- Management of acute MI for the lysis of thrombi obstructing coronary arteries, the reduction of infarct size, the improvement of ventricular function following acute MI, and the reduction of mortality associated with acute MI

Contraindications and cautions

- Allergic reactions to anistreplase or streptokinase, active internal bleeding, CVA within 2 mo, intracranial or intraspinal surgery or neoplasm, arteriovenous malformation, aneurysm, recent major surgery, obstetric delivery, organ biopsy, rupture of a noncompressible blood vessel, recent serious GI bleed, recent serious trauma, including CPR, hemostatic defects, cerebrovascular disease, SBE, severe uncontrolled hypertension, liver disease, old age (> 75 yr), lactation

Available forms

Powder for injection—30 units/vial

Dosages

Give as soon as possible after the onset of symptoms.

Adults

30 units given only by IV injection over 2–5 min into an IV line or directly into vein.

Adverse effects in *Italics* are most common; those in **Bold** are life-threatening.

Pharmacokinetics

Route	Onset	Peak	Duration
IV	Immediate	45 min	4–6 hr

Metabolism: Plasma; $T_{1/2}$: 2 hr
Distribution: Crosses placenta; may pass into breast milk

▽ IV facts

Preparation: Reconstitute by slowly adding 5 mL of sterile water for injection to the vial. Gently roll the vial, mixing the dry powder and fluid; reconstituted solution should be colorless to a pale yellow transparent solution. Withdraw the entire contents of the vial. Reconstitute immediately before use. Must be used within 30 min of reconstitution. Discard any unused solution. Avoid excess agitation during dilution. Swirl gently to mix. *Do not shake.* Minimize foaming.
Infusion: Give as soon as possible after onset of symptoms. Administer over 2–5 min into an IV line or directly into a vein.
Compatibilities: Do not further dilute before administration; do not add to any infusion fluids. Do not add any other medications to the vial or to the syringe or the Y-site.

Adverse effects

- **CV: Cardiac arrhythmias with coronary reperfusion, hypotension**
- **Hematologic:** *Bleeding,* particularly at venous or arterial access sites, gastrointestinal bleeding, intracranial hemorrhage
- **Hypersensitivity:** Anaphylactic and anaphylactoid reactions, bronchospasm, itching, flushing, rash
- **Other:** Urticaria, nausea, vomiting, fever, chills, headache

Interactions

✳ **Drug-drug** • Increased risk of hemorrhage if used with heparin or oral anticoagulants, aspirin, dipyridamole
✳ **Drug-lab test** • Decrease in plasminogen and fibrinogen results in increases in thrombin time, APTT, PT, tests may be unreliable

■ Nursing considerations
Assessment

- **History:** Allergic reactions to anistreplase or streptokinase, active internal bleeding, CVA within 2 mo, intracranial or intraspinal

surgery or neoplasm, arteriovenous malformation, aneurysm, recent major surgery, obstetric delivery, organ biopsy, rupture of a noncompressible blood vessel, recent serious GI bleed, recent serious trauma, including CPR, hemostatic defects, cerebrovascular disease, SBE, severe uncontrolled hypertension, liver disease, old age (> 75 yr), lactation
- **Physical:** Skin color, temperature, lesions; orientation, reflexes; P, BP, peripheral perfusion, baseline ECG; R, adventitious sounds; liver evaluation; Hct, platelet count, TT, APTT, PT

Interventions

- Discontinue heparin and alteplase if serious bleeding occurs.
- Regularly monitor coagulation studies.
- Apply pressure or pressure dressings to control superficial bleeding.
- Avoid any arterial invasive procedures during therapy.
- Arrange for typing and cross-matching of blood in case serious blood loss occurs and whole blood transfusions are required.
- Institute treatment as soon as possible after onset of symptoms for evolving MI.

Teaching points

- Report difficulty breathing, dizziness, disorientation, headache, numbness, tingling.

▽ antihemophilic factor (AHF, Factor VIII)
(an tee hee moe fill' ik)

Alphanate, Bioclate, Helixate FS, Hemofil M, Humate-P, Hyate:C, Kogenate FS, Monoclate-P, Recombinate, ReFacto

PREGNANCY CATEGORY C

Drug class
Antihemophilic agent

Therapeutic actions
A normal plasma protein that is needed for the transformation of prothrombin to thrombin, the final step of the intrinsic clotting pathway.

Indications

- Treatment of classical hemophilia (hemophilia A), in which there is a demonstrated deficiency of factor VIII; provides a temporary replacement of clotting factors to correct or prevent bleeding episodes or to allow necessary surgery
- Short-term prophylaxis (*ReFacto*) to reduce frequency of spontaneous bleeding
- Treatment and prevention of bleeding in congenital hemophilia A patients with antibodies to factor VIII (*Hyate:C*)

Contraindications and cautions

- Antibodies to mouse protein.

Available forms

IV injection—250, 500, 1,000, 1,500 IU/vial in numerous preparations

Dosages

Administer IV using a plastic syringe; dose depends on weight, severity of deficiency, and severity of bleeding. Follow treatment carefully with factor VIII level assays.
Formulas used as a guide for dosage are:

$$\text{Expected Factor VHI increase}$$
$$(\% \text{ of normal}) = \frac{\text{AHF/IU given} \times 2}{\text{weight in kg}}$$

$$\text{AHF/IU required} = \text{weight (kg)}$$
$$\times \text{ desired Factor VIII increase}$$
$$(\% \text{ of normal}) \times 0.5$$

- *Prophylaxis of spontaneous hemorrhage:* Level of factor VIII required to prevent spontaneous hemorrhage is 5% of normal; 30% of normal is the minimum required for hemostasis following trauma or surgery; smaller doses may be needed if treated early.
- *Mild hemorrhage:* Do not repeat therapy unless further bleeding occurs.
- *Moderate hemorrhage or minor surgery:* 30%–50% of normal is desired for factor VIII levels; initial dose of 15–25 AHF/IU/kg with maintenance dose of 10–15 AHF/IU/kg is usually sufficient.
- *Severe hemorrhage:* Factor VIII level of 80%–100% normal is desired; initial dose of 40–50 AHF/IU/kg and a maintenance dose of 20–25 AHF/IU/kg is given q 8–12 hr.

- *Major surgery:* Dose of AHF to achieve factor VIII levels of 80%–100% of normal given an hour before surgery; second dose of half the size about 5 hr later. Maintain factor VIII levels at least 30% normal for a healing period of 10–14 days.

Pharmacokinetics

Route	Onset
IV	Immediate

Metabolism: $T_{1/2}$: 12 hr
Distribution: Does not readily cross placenta
Excretion: Cleared from the body by normal metabolism

▼ IV facts

Preparation: Reconstitute using solution provided. Refrigerate unreconstituted preparations. Before reconstitution, warm diluent and dried concentrate to room temperature. Add diluent and rotate vial, or shake gently, until completely dissolved. Do not refrigerate reconstituted preparations; give within 3 hr of reconstitution.

Infusion: Give by IV only; use a plastic syringe; solutions may stick to glass. Give preparations containing 34 AHF or more units/mL at a maximum rate of 2 mL/min; give preparations containing < 34 AHF units/mL at a rate of 10–20 mL over 3 min.

Adverse effects

- **Allergic reactions:** Erythema, hives, fever, backache, bronchospasm, urticaria, chills, nausea, *stinging at the infusion site*, vomiting, headache
- **Hematologic:** Hemolysis with large or frequently repeated doses
- **Other: Hepatitis, AIDS**—risks associated with repeated use of blood products

■ Nursing considerations
Assessment

- **History:** Antibodies to mouse protein
- **Physical:** Skin color, lesions; P, peripheral perfusion; R, adventitious sounds; factor VIII levels, Hct, direct Coombs' test, HIV screening, hepatitis screening

Interventions

- Monitor pulse during administration; if a significant increase occurs, reduce the rate or discontinue and consult physician.
- Monitor patient's clinical response and factor VIII levels regularly; if no response is noted with large doses, consider the presence of factor VIII inhibitors and need for anti-inhibitor complex therapy.

Teaching points

- Dosage is highly variable. All known safety precautions are taken to ensure that this blood product is pure and the risk of AIDS and hepatitis is as minimal as possible.
- Wear or carry a medical alert ID tag to alert medical emergency personnel that you require this treatment.
- Report headache; rash; itching; backache; difficulty breathing.

▷ antithrombin III

See *Less Commonly Used Drugs,* p. 1336.

▷ aprotinin
(ab pro' tin in)

Trasylol

PREGNANCY CATEGORY B

Drug class
Systemic hemostatic

Therapeutic actions
Derived from bovine lung, aprotinin forms complexes with plasmin, kallikreins, and other factors to block activation of the kinin and fibrinolytic systems.

Indications

- Prophylactic use: to reduce blood loss and the need for transfusion in patients undergoing cardiopulmonary bypass in the course of repeat coronary artery bypass graft surgery
- Prophylactic use: to reduce blood loss in select first-time coronary bypass surgery when the patient is at special risk for bleeding

Contraindications and cautions

- Contraindicated with allergy to aprotinin, first time CABG surgery (except in rare cases).
- Use cautiously with pregnancy, lactation.

Available forms
Injection—10,000 kallikrein inhibitor units (KIU)/mL

Dosages
Provided in a solution containing 1.4 mg/mL or 10,000 KIU/mL.
Adults
Test dose of 1 mL IV 10 min before loading dose. 1–2 million KIU IV loading dose, 1–2 million KIU into pump prime, 250,000–500,000 KIU/hr of operation as continuous IV infusion.

Pharmacokinetics

Route	Peak
IV	Immediately

Metabolism: $T_{1/2}$: 150 min
Distribution: Crosses placenta; passes into breast milk
Excretion: Urine

▽ IV facts
Preparation: No further preparation is required.
Infusion: Give loading dose over 20–30 min, then continuous infusion of 25–50 mL/hr through a central line.
Incompatibilities: Do not give in solution with corticosteroids, heparin, tetracyclines, fat emulsions, amino acids. Give all other drugs through a separate line.

Adverse effects

- **CV:** *Atrial fibrillation, MI,* CHF, atrial flutter, ventricular tachycardia, heart block, shock, hypotension
- **Respiratory:** Asthma, dyspnea, respiratory distress
- **Other:** Anaphylactic reactions

Interactions
* **Drug-drug** • Increased bleeding tendencies with heparin • Blocked antihypertensive effect with captopril

■ Nursing considerations
Assessment
- **History:** Allergy to aprotinin, first time CABG surgery, pregnancy
- **Physical:** Skin lesions, color, temperature; P, BP, peripheral perfusion, baseline ECG; R, adventitious sounds; PTT, renal and hepatic function tests

Interventions
- Give test dose of 1 mL before any administration.
- Give loading dose slowly with patient in the supine position; sudden drops in BP may occur.
- Evaluate patient regularly for signs of CV effects.

Teaching points
- Patients receiving this drug will be unaware of its effects; information about this drug can be incorporated into the general teaching about CABG.

▽ argatroban

See *Less Commonly Used Drugs*, p. 1338.

▽ aripiprazole
*(air eb **pip'** rah zole)*

Abilify

PREGNANCY CATEGORY C

Drug classes
Psychotropic drug
Dopamine, serotonin agonist and antagonist

Therapeutic actions
Acts as an agonist at dopamine and serotonin sites and antagonist at other serotonin receptor sites; this combination of actions is thought to be responsible for the drug's effectiveness in treating schizophrenia, though the mechanism of action is not understood.

Indications
- Short-term treatment of schizophrenia

Contraindications and cautions
- Contraindicated in the presence of allergy to aripiprazole, lactation.
- Use cautiously in the presence of suicidal ideation, pregnancy, cerebral vascular disease or other conditions causing hypotension, known cardiovascular disease, seizure disorders, exposure to extreme heat, patients with Alzheimer's disease, dysphagia (risk for aspiration pneumonia)

Available forms
Tablets—10, 15, 20, 30 mg

Dosages
Adults
10–15 mg/day PO.
Pediatric patients
Safety and efficacy not established.

Pharmacokinetics

Route	Onset	Peak
Oral	Slow	3–5 hr

Metabolism: Hepatic; $T_{1/2}$: 75 hr for extensive metabolizers and 146 hr for poor metabolizers
Distribution: May cross placenta; may pass into breast milk
Excretion: Urine and feces

Adverse effects
- **CNS:** headache, anxiety, insomnia, lightheadedness, somnolence, tremor, asthenia, tardive dyskinesia, blurred vision, **seizures** (potentially life-threatening), akathisia
- **CV:** orthostatic hypotension
- **Dermatologic:** rash
- **GI:** nausea, vomiting, constipation, diarrhea, abdominal pain, esophageal dysmotility
- **Respiratory:** rhinitis, cough
- **Other:** fever, **neuroleptic malignant syndrome, increased suicide risk**

Interactions
❋ **Drug-drug** • Risk of serious toxic effects if combined with strong inhibitors of the CYP3A4 system (such as ketoconazole), if any of these drug are being used, initiate treatment with one-half the usual dose of aripiprazole

---

Adverse effects in *Italics* are most common; those in **Bold** are life-threatening.

and monitor patient closely • Potential for increased serum levels and toxicity if taken with potential CYP2D6 inhibitors—quinidine, fluoxetine, paroxetine; reduce the dose of aripiprazole to one-half the normal dose • Decreased serum levels and loss of effectiveness if combined with CYP3A4 inducers such as carbamazepine—dosage of aripiprazole should be doubled and the patient monitored closely

■ Nursing considerations
Assessment
History: Allergy to aripiprazole, lactation, suicidal ideation, pregnancy, hypotension or known cardiovascular disease, seizure disorders, exposure to extreme heat, patients with Alzheimer's disease, dysphagia
Physical: Temperature, orientation, reflexes, vision; BP; R; abdominal exam

Interventions
- Dispense the least amount of drug possible to patients with suicidal ideation.
- Protect patient from extremes of heat, monitor BP if overheating occurs
- Administer drug once a day without regard to food.
- Establish baseline orientation and affect before beginning therapy.
- Assure that patient is well hydrated while on this drug.
- Establish appropriate safety precautions if patient experiences adverse CNS effects.
- Suggest another method of feeding the baby if the drug is needed in a lactating woman.
- Advise women of child-bearing age to use contraceptive measures while on this drug.

Teaching points
- Take this drug once a day as prescribed. If you forget a dose, take the next dose as soon as you remember and then resume taking the drug the next day. Do not take more than one dose in any 24-hr period.
- Know that these side effects may occur: dizziness, impaired thinking and motor coordination (use caution and avoid driving a car or performing other tasks that require alertness if you experience these effects); inability to cool body effectively (avoid extremes of heat, heavy exercise, dehydration while using this drug).

- This drug may interact with many other medications and with alcohol. Alert any health care provider caring for you that you taking this drug.
- Be aware that this drug should not be taken during pregnancy or when nursing a baby; use of barrier contraceptives is suggested.
- Make sure that you are well hydrated while taking this drug.
- Report severe dizziness, trembling, light headedness, suicidal thoughts, blurred vision.

▷ arsenic trioxide
See *Less Commonly Used Drugs*, p. 1338.

▷ asparaginase
(a spare' a gi nase)

Elspar, Kidrolase (CAN)

PREGNANCY CATEGORY C

Drug class
Antineoplastic agent

Therapeutic actions
Asparaginase is an enzyme that hydrolyzes the amino acid asparagine, which is needed by some malignant cells (but not normal cells) for protein synthesis; it inhibits malignant cell proliferation by interruption of protein synthesis; maximal effect in G1 phase of the cell cycle.

Indications
- Acute lymphocytic leukemia as part of combination therapy to induce remissions in children

Contraindications and cautions
- Allergy to asparaginase, pancreatitis or history of pancreatitis, impaired hepatic function, bone marrow depression, lactation.

Available forms
Powder for injection—10,000 IU

Dosages

Pediatric patients

• *Induction regimen I:* Prednisone 40 mg/m^2 per day PO in three divided doses for 15 days, followed by tapering of dosage as follows: 20 mg/m^2 for 2 days, 10 mg/m^2 for 2 days, 5 mg/m^2 for 2 days, 2.5 mg/m^2 for 2 days, and then discontinue. Vincristine sulfate 2 mg/m^2 IV once weekly on days 1, 8, 15; maximum dose should not exceed 2 mg. Asparaginase 1,000 IU/kg/day IV for 10 successive days beginning on day 22.

• *Induction regimen II:* Prednisone 40 mg/m^2 per day PO in three divided doses for 28 days, then gradually discontinue over 14 days. Vincristine sulfate 1.5 mg/m^2 IV weekly for four doses on days 1, 8, 15, 22; maximum dose should not exceed 2 mg. Asparaginase 6,000 IU/m^2 IM on days 4, 7, 10, 13, 16, 19, 22, 25, 28.

• *Maintenance:* When remission is obtained, institute maintenance therapy; do not use asparaginase in maintenance regimen.

• *Single-agent induction therapy:* Used only when combined therapy is inappropriate or when other therapies fail; 200 IU/kg/day IV for 28 days (children or adults).

Pharmacokinetics

Route	Onset
IM	Varies
IV	30–40 min

Metabolism: T$_{1/2}$: 8–30 hr
Distribution: Crosses placenta; may pass into breast milk
Excretion: Urine

▽ IV facts

Preparation: Reconstitute vial with 5 mL of sterile water for injection or sodium chloride injection. Ordinary shaking does not inactivate the drug. May be used for direct IV injection or further diluted with sodium chloride injection or 5% dextrose injection. Stable for 8 hr once reconstituted; use only when clear. Discard any cloudy solution.

Infusion: Infuse over not less than 30 min into an already running IV infusion of sodium chloride injection or 5% dextrose injection.

Adverse effects

• **CNS:** CNS depression
• **Endocrine:** Hyperglycemia—glucosuria, polyuria
• **GI:** *Hepatotoxicity, nausea, vomiting, anorexia,* abdominal cramps, pancreatitis
• **GU:** Uric acid nephropathy, **renal toxicity**
• **Hematologic:** Bleeding problems, **bone marrow depression**
• **Hypersensitivity:** *Rashes, urticaria, arthralgia,* respiratory distress to anaphylaxis
• **Other:** Chills, fever, weight loss; **hyperthermia**

Interactions

❋ **Drug-drug** • Increased toxicity if given IV with or immediately before vincristine or prednisone • Diminished or decreased effect of methotrexate on malignant cells if given with or immediately after asparaginase

❋ **Drug-lab test** • Inaccurate interpretation of thyroid-function tests because of decreased serum levels of thyroxine-binding globulin; levels usually return to pretreatment levels within 4 wk of the last dose of asparaginase

■ Nursing considerations

Assessment

• **History:** Allergy to asparaginase, pancreatitis or history of pancreatitis, impaired hepatic function, bone marrow depression, lactation
• **Physical:** Weight; T; skin color, lesions; orientation, reflexes; liver evaluation, abdominal exam; CBC, blood sugar, liver and renal function tests, serum amylase, clotting time, urinalysis, serum uric acid levels

Interventions

• Perform an intradermal skin test prior to initial administration and if there is a week or more between doses because of risk of severe hypersensitivity reactions. Prepare skin test solution as follows: reconstitute 10,000-IU vial with 5 mL of diluent; withdraw 0.1 mL (200 IU/mL), and inject it into a vial containing 9.9 mL of diluent, giving a solution of 20 IU/mL. Use 0.1 mL of this solution (2 IU) for the skin test. Observe site for 1 hr for a wheal or erythema that indicates allergic reaction.

- Arrange for desensitization to hypersensitivity reaction. Check manufacturer's literature for desensitization dosages, or arrange for patient to receive *Erwinia* asparaginase (available from the National Cancer Institute).
- Arrange for lab tests (CBC, serum amylase, blood glucose, liver function tests, uric acid) prior to therapy and frequently during therapy; arrange to decrease dose or stop drug if severe adverse effects occur.
- For IM administration, reconstitute by adding 2 mL of sodium chloride injection to the 10,000-IU vial. Stable for 8 hr once reconstituted; use only if clear. Limit injections at each site to 2 mL; if more is required use two injection sites.
- Monitor for signs of hypersensitivity (eg, rash, difficulty breathing). If any occur, discontinue drug and consult with physician.
- Monitor for pancreatitis; if serum amylase levels rise, discontinue drug and consult with physician.
- Monitor for hyperglycemia—reaction may resemble hyperosmolar, nonketotic hyperglycemia. If present, discontinue drug and be ready to use IV fluids and insulin.

Teaching points

- Prepare a calendar for patients who must return for specific treatments and additional therapy. Drug can be given only in the hospital under the direct supervision of physician.
- These side effects may occur: loss of appetite, nausea, vomiting (frequent mouth care, small, frequent meals may help; good nutrition is important; dietary services are available; antiemetic may be ordered); fatigue, confusion, agitation, hallucinations, depression (reversible; use special precautions to avoid injury).
- Have regular blood tests to monitor the drug's effects.
- Report fever, chills, sore throat; unusual bleeding or bruising; yellow skin or eyes; light-colored stools, dark urine; thirst, frequent urination.

▽ aspirin
(ass' pir in)

Apo-ASA (CAN), Aspergum, Bayer, Easprin, Ecotrin, Empirin, Entrophen (CAN), Genprin, Halfprin 81, 1/2 Halfprin, Heartline, Norwich, Novasen (CAN), PMS-ASA (CAN), ZORprin

Buffered aspirin products:
Alka-Seltzer, Ascriptin, Asprimox, Bufferin, Buffex, Magnaprin

PREGNANCY CATEGORY D

Drug classes

Antipyretic
Analgesic (non-narcotic)
Anti-inflammatory
Antirheumatic
Antiplatelet
Salicylate
NSAID

Therapeutic actions

Analgesic and antirheumatic effects are attributable to aspirin's ability to inhibit the synthesis of prostaglandins, important mediators of inflammation. Antipyretic effects are not fully understood, but aspirin probably acts in the thermoregulatory center of the hypothalamus to block effects of endogenous pyrogen by inhibiting synthesis of the prostaglandin intermediary. Inhibition of platelet aggregation is attributable to the inhibition of platelet synthesis of thromboxane A_2, a potent vasoconstrictor and inducer of platelet aggregation. This effect occurs at low doses and lasts for the life of the platelet (8 days). Higher doses inhibit the synthesis of prostacyclin, a potent vasodilator and inhibitor of platelet aggregation.

Indications

- Mild to moderate pain
- Fever
- Inflammatory conditions—rheumatic fever, rheumatoid arthritis, osteoarthritis
- Reduction of risk of recurrent TIAs or stroke in males with history of TIA due to fibrin platelet emboli

- Reduction of risk of death or nonfatal MI in patients with history of infarction or unstable angina pectoris
- MI prophylaxis
- Unlabeled use: prophylaxis against cataract formation with long-term use

Contraindications and cautions

- Allergy to salicylates or NSAIDs (more common with nasal polyps, asthma, chronic urticaria); allergy to tartrazine (cross-sensitivity to aspirin is common); hemophilia, bleeding ulcers, hemorrhagic states, blood coagulation defects, hypoprothrombinemia, vitamin K deficiency (increased risk of bleeding); impaired renal function; chickenpox, influenza (risk of Reye's syndrome in children and teenagers); children with fever accompanied by dehydration; surgery scheduled within 1 wk; pregnancy (maternal anemia, antepartal and postpartal hemorrhage, prolonged gestation, and prolonged labor have been reported; readily crosses the placenta; possibly teratogenic; maternal ingestion of aspirin during late pregnancy has been associated with the following adverse fetal effects: low birth weight, increased intracranial hemorrhage, stillbirths, neonatal death); lactation.

Available forms

Tablets—325, 500, 650, 975 mg; SR tablets—650, 800 mg; suppositories: 120, 200, 300, 600 mg

Dosages

Available in oral and suppository forms. Also available as chewable tablets, gum; enteric coated, sustained-release, and buffered preparations (sustained-release aspirin is not recommended for antipyresis, short-term analgesia, or children < 12 yr).

Adults

- *Minor aches and pains:* 325–650 mg q 4 hr.
- *Arthritis and rheumatic conditions:* 3.2–6 g/day in divided doses.
- *Acute rheumatic fever:* 5–8 g/day; modify to maintain serum salicylate level of 15–30 mg/dL.
- *TIAs in men:* 1,300 mg/day in divided doses (650 mg bid or 325 mg qid).

- *MI prophylaxis:* 75–325 mg/day.

Pediatric patients

- *Analgesic and antipyretic:* 65 mg/kg per 24 hr in four to six divided doses, not to exceed 3.6 g/day. Dosage recommendations by age:

Age (yr)	Dosage (mg q 4 hr)
2–3	162
4–5	243
6–8	324
9–10	405
11	486
≥ 12	648

- *Juvenile rheumatoid arthritis:* 60–110 mg/kg per 24 hr in divided doses at 4– to 6–hr intervals. Maintain a serum level of 200–300 mcg/mL.
- *Acute rheumatic fever:* 100 mg/kg/day initially, then decrease to 75 mg/kg/day for 4–6 wk. Therapeutic serum salicylate level is 15–30 mg/dL.
- *Kawasaki disease:* 80–180 mg/kg/day; very high doses may be needed during acute febrile period; after fever resolves, dosage may be adjusted to 10 mg/kg/day.

Pharmacokinetics

Route	Onset	Peak	Duration
Oral	5–30 min	0.25–2 hr	3–6 hr
Rectal	1–2 hr	4–5 hr	6–8 hr

Metabolism: Hepatic (salicylate); $T_{1/2}$: 15 min–12 hr
Distribution: Crosses placenta; passes into breast milk
Excretion: Urine

Adverse effects

- **Acute aspirin toxicity:** Respiratory alkalosis, hyperpnea, tachypnea, hemorrhage, excitement, confusion, asterixis, pulmonary edema, convulsions, tetany, metabolic acidosis, **fever, coma, cardiovascular collapse,** renal and respiratory failure (dose related 20–25 g in adults, 4 g in children)
- **Aspirin intolerance:** Exacerbation of bronchospasm, rhinitis (with nasal polyps, asthma, rhinitis)

Adverse effects in *Italics* are most common; those in **Bold** are life-threatening.

- **GI:** *Nausea, dyspepsia, heartburn, epigastric discomfort,* anorexia, hepatotoxicity
- **Hematologic:** *Occult blood loss, hemostatic defects*
- **Hypersensitivity:** Anaphylactoid reactions to **anaphylactic shock**
- **Salicylism:** *Dizziness, tinnitus, difficulty hearing, nausea,* vomiting, diarrhea, mental confusion, lassitude (dose related)

Interactions

✴ **Drug-drug** • Increased risk of bleeding with oral anticoagulants, heparin • Increased risk of GI ulceration with steroids, phenylbutazone, alcohol, NSAIDs • Increased serum salicylate levels due to decreased salicylate excretion with urine acidifiers (ammonium chloride, ascorbic acid, methionine) • Increased risk of salicylate toxicity with carbonic anhydrase inhibitors, furosemide • Decreased serum salicylate levels with corticosteroids • Decreased serum salicylate levels due to increased renal excretion of salicylates with acetazolamide, methazolamide, certain antacids, alkalinizers • Decreased absorption of aspirin with nonabsorbable antacids • Increased methotrexate levels and toxicity with aspirin • Increased effects of valproic acid secondary to displacement from plasma protein sites • Greater glucose lowering effect of sulfonylureas, insulin with large doses (> 2 g/day) of aspirin • Decreased antihypertensive effect of captopril, beta-adrenergic blockers with salicylates; consider discontinuation of aspirin • Decreased uricosuric effect of probenecid, sulfinpyrazone • Possible decreased diuretic effects of spironolactone, furosemide (in patients with compromised renal function) • Unexpected hypotension may occur with nitroglycerin

✴ **Drug-lab test** • Decreased serum protein bound iodine (PBI) due to competition for binding sites • False-negative readings for urine glucose by glucose oxidase method and copper reduction method with moderate to large doses of aspirin • Interference with urine 5-HIAA determinations by fluorescent methods but not by nitrosonaphthol colorimetric method • Interference with urinary ketone determination by the ferric chloride method • Falsely elevated urine VMA levels with most tests;

a false decrease in VMA using the Pisano method

■ Nursing considerations

Assessment

- **History:** Allergy to salicylates or NSAIDs; allergy to tartrazine; hemophilia, bleeding ulcers, hemorrhagic states, blood coagulation defects, hypoprothrombinemia, vitamin K deficiency; impaired hepatic function; impaired renal function; chickenpox, influenza; children with fever accompanied by dehydration; surgery scheduled within 1 wk; pregnancy; lactation
- **Physical:** Skin color, lesions; temperature; eighth cranial nerve function, orientation, reflexes, affect; P, BP, perfusion; R, adventitious sounds; liver evaluation, bowel sounds; CBC, clotting times, urinalysis, stool guaiac, renal and liver function tests

Interventions

- Give drug with food or after meals if GI upset occurs.
- Give drug with full glass of water to reduce risk of tablet or capsule lodging in the esophagus.
- Do not crush, and ensure that patient does not chew sustained-release preparations.
- Do not use aspirin that has a strong vinegar-like odor.
- Institute emergency procedures if overdose occurs: gastric lavage, induction of emesis, activated charcoal, supportive therapy.

Teaching points

- OTC aspirins are equivalent. Price does not reflect effectiveness.
- Use the drug only as suggested; avoid overdose. Take the drug with food or after meals if GI upset occurs.
- Do not cut, crush, or chew sustained-release products.
- These side effects may occur: nausea, GI upset, heartburn (take drug with food); easy bruising, gum bleeding (related to aspirin's effects on blood clotting)
- Avoid the use of other OTC drugs while taking this drug. Many of these drugs contain aspirin, and serious overdose can occur.
- Report ringing in the ears; dizziness, confusion; abdominal pain; rapid or difficult breathing; nausea, vomiting.

- Take extra precautions to keep this drug out of the reach of children; this drug can be very dangerous for children.

▷atenolol
(a ten' o lole)

Apo-Atenolol (CAN), Gen-Atenolol (CAN), Novo-Atenol (CAN), Tenolin (CAN), Tenormin

PREGNANCY CATEGORY D

Drug classes
Beta$_1$-selective adrenergic blocking agent
Antianginal drug
Antihypertensive drug

Therapeutic actions
Blocks beta-adrenergic receptors of the sympathetic nervous system in the heart and juxtaglomerular apparatus (kidney), thus decreasing the excitability of the heart, decreasing cardiac output and oxygen consumption, decreasing the release of renin from the kidney, and lowering blood pressure.

Indications
- Treatment of angina pectoris due to coronary atherosclerosis
- Hypertension, as a step 1 agent, alone or with other drugs, especially diuretics
- Treatment of myocardial infarction
- Unlabeled uses: prevention of migraine headaches; alcohol withdrawal syndrome, treatment of ventricular and supraventricular arrhythmias

Contraindications and cautions
- Contraindicated with sinus bradycardia, second- or third-degree heart block, cardiogenic shock, CHF.
- Use cautiously with renal failure, diabetes or thyrotoxicosis (atenolol can mask the usual cardiac signs of hypoglycemia and thyrotoxicosis), lactation.

Available forms
Tablets—25, 50, 100 mg; injection—5 mg/ 10 mL

Dosages
Adults
- *Hypertension:* Initially 50 mg PO once a day; after 1–2 wk, dose may be increased to 100 mg/day
- *Angina pectoris:* Initially 50 mg PO daily. If optimal response is not achieved in 1 wk, increase to 100 mg daily; up to 200 mg/day may be needed.
- *Acute MI:* Initially 5 mg IV given over 5 min as soon as possible after diagnosis; follow with IV injection of 5 mg 10 min later. Switch to 50 mg PO 10 min after the last IV dose; follow with 50 mg PO 12 hr later. Thereafter, administer 100 mg PO daily or 50 mg PO bid for 6–9 days or until discharge from the hospital.

Pediatric patients
Safety and efficacy not established.

Geriatric patients or patients with renal impairment
Dosage reduction is required because atenolol is excreted through the kidneys. The following dosage is suggested:

Creatinine Clearance mL/min	Half-life (hr)	Maximum Dosage
15–35	16–27	50 mg/day
< 15	> 27	25 mg/day

For patients on hemodialysis, give 50 mg after each dialysis; give only in hospital setting; severe hypotension can occur.

Pharmacokinetics

Route	Onset	Peak	Duration
Oral	Varies	2–4 hr	24 hr
IV	Immediate	5 min	24 hr

Metabolism: $T_{1/2}$: 6–7 hr
Distribution: Crosses placenta; passes into breast milk
Excretion: Urine (40%–50%) and bile, feces (50%–60%)

▼IV facts
Preparation: May be diluted in dextrose injection, sodium chloride injection, or sodium chloride and dextrose injection. Stable for 48 hr after mixing.

Infusion: Initiate treatment as soon as possible after admission to the hospital; inject 5 mg over 5 min; follow with another 5-mg IV injection 10 min later.

Adverse effects

- **Allergic reactions:** Pharyngitis, erythematous rash, fever, sore throat, laryngospasm, respiratory distress
- **CNS:** Dizziness, vertigo, tinnitus, fatigue, emotional depression, paresthesias, sleep disturbances, hallucinations, disorientation, memory loss, slurred speech
- **CV:** *Bradycardia, CHF, cardiac arrhythmias, sinoatrial or AV nodal block, tachycardia,* peripheral vascular insufficiency, claudication, CVA, pulmonary edema, hypotension
- **Dermatologic:** Rash, pruritus, sweating, dry skin
- **EENT:** Eye irritation, dry eyes, conjunctivitis, blurred vision
- **GI:** *Gastric pain, flatulence, constipation, diarrhea, nausea, vomiting,* anorexia, ischemic colitis, renal and mesenteric arterial thrombosis, retroperitoneal fibrosis, hepatomegaly, acute pancreatitis
- **GU:** *Impotence, decreased libido,* Peyronie's disease, dysuria, nocturia, frequent urination
- **Musculoskeletal:** Joint pain, arthralgia, muscle cramp
- **Respiratory:** Bronchospasm, dyspnea, cough, bronchial obstruction, nasal stuffiness, rhinitis, pharyngitis (less likely than with propranolol)
- **Other:** *Decreased exercise tolerance, development of antinuclear antibodies,* hyperglycemia or hypoglycemia, elevated serum transaminase, alkaline phosphatase, and LDH

Interactions

✹ **Drug-drug** • Increased effects with verapamil, anticholinergics, quinidine • Increased risk of orthostatic hypotension with prazosin • Increased risk of lidocaine toxicity with atenolol • Possible increased blood pressure-lowering effects with aspirin, bismuth subsalicylate, magnesium salicylate, sulfinpyrazone, oral contraceptives • Decreased antihypertensive effects with NSAIDs, clonidine • Decreased antihypertensive and antianginal effects of atenolol with ampicillin, calcium salts • Possible increased hypoglycemic effect of insulin
✹ **Drug-lab test** • Possible false results with glucose or insulin tolerance tests

■ Nursing considerations
Assessment

- **History:** Sinus bradycardia, second- or third-degree heart block, cardiogenic shock, CHF, renal failure, diabetes or thyrotoxicosis, lactation
- **Physical:** Baseline weight, skin condition, neurologic status, P, BP, ECG, respiratory status, kidney and thyroid function, blood and urine glucose

Interventions

- Do not discontinue drug abruptly after long-term therapy (hypersensitivity to catecholamines may have developed, causing exacerbation of angina, MI, and ventricular arrhythmias). Taper drug gradually over 2 wk with monitoring.
- Consult physician about withdrawing drug if patient is to undergo surgery (withdrawal is controversial).

Teaching points

- Take drug with meals if GI upset occurs.
- Do not stop taking this drug unless told to by a health care provider.
- Avoid driving or dangerous activities if dizziness, weakness occur.
- These side effects may occur: dizziness, lightheadedness, loss of appetite, nightmares, depression, sexual impotence.
- Report difficulty breathing, night cough, swelling of extremities, slow pulse, confusion, depression, rash, fever, sore throat.

▽**atomoxetine hydrochloride**
*(at oh **mox'** ah teen)*

Strattera

PREGNANCY CATEGORY C

Drug class
Selective norepinephrine reuptake inhibitor

Therapeutic actions

Selectively blocks the reuptake of norepinephrine at the neuronal synapse. The mechanism by which this action has a therapeutic effect in attention deficit hyperactivity disorder (ADHD) is not understood.

Indications

- Treatment of ADHD as part of a total treatment program

Contraindications and cautions

- Contraindicated with hypersensitivity to atomoxetine or constituents of Strattera; use of MAO inhibitors within the past 14 days; narrow-angle glaucoma
- Use cautiously with hypertension, tachycardia, cardiovascular or cerebrovascular disease, pregnancy, lactation

Pharmacokinetics

Route	Onset	Peak
Oral	Rapid	1-2 hr

Metabolism: Hepatic; $T_{1/2}$: 5 hr
Distribution: May cross placenta; may pass into breast milk
Excretion: Urine and feces

Available forms

Capsules—5, 10, 18, 25, 40, 60 mg

Dosages

Adults and children > 70 kg
40 mg/day PO, increase after a minimum of 3 days to a target total daily dose of 80 mg PO given as a single dose in the morning or two evenly divided doses, in the morning and late afternoon or early evening; after 2-4 wk, total dosage may be increase to a maximum of 100 mg/day if needed.
Pediatric patients < 70 kg
Initial dose 0.5 mg/kg/day PO, increase after a minimum of 3 days to a target total daily dose of approximately 1.2 mg/kg/day PO as a single daily dose in the morning; may be given in two evenly divided doses in the morning and late afternoon or early evening. Do not exceed 1.4 mg/kg or 100 mg/day, whichever is less.

Patients with hepatic impairment
For moderate hepatic impairment, reduce dosage to 50% of the normal dose; for severe hepatic impairment, reduce dosage to 25% of the normal dose.

Adverse effects

- **CNS:** aggression, irritability, crying, somnolence, dizziness, *headache*, mood swings, *insomnia*
- **CV:** palpitations
- **Dermatologic:** dermatitis, increased sweating
- **GI:** *dry mouth, nausea,* dyspepsia, flatulence, *decreased appetite, constipation, upper abdominal pain, vomiting*
- **GU:** urinary hesitation, urinary retention, dysmenorrhea, erectile problems
- **Respiratory:** *cough,* rhinorrhea, sinusitis
- **Other:** fever, rigors, sinusitis, weight loss, myalgia

Interactions

✳ **Drug-drug** ● Possible increased serum levels if combined with potent CYP2D6 inhibitors—paroxetine, fluoxetine, quinidine; monitor and adjust dosage of atomoxetine to 0.5 mg/kg/day with a target dose of 1.2 mg/kg/day for children < 70 kg or 40 mg/day with a target dose of 80 mg/day for children > 70 kg or adults ● Risk of neuroleptic malignant syndrome if combined with MAO inhibitors; do not combine with an MAO inhibitor and do not give atomoxetine within 14 days of using an MAO inhibitor

■ Nursing considerations
Assessment

History: Hypersensitivity to atomoxetine or constituents of *Strattera*; use of MAO inhibitors within the past 14 days; narrow-angle glaucoma, hypertension, tachycardia, cardiovascular or cerebrovascular disease, pregnancy, lactation
Physical: T; skin color, lesions; orientation, affect; P, BP, auscultation; R, adventitious sounds; bowel sounds, normal output

Implementation

- Ensure proper diagnosis before administering to children for behavioral syndromes:

Adverse effects in *Italics* are most common; those in **Bold** are life-threatening.

A

drug should not be used until other causes and concomitants of abnormal behavior (learning disability, EEG abnormalities, neurological deficits) are ruled out.

- Ensure that drug is being used as part of an overall treatment program including education and psychosocial interventions.
- Arrange to interrupt drug dosage periodically in children being treated for behavioral disorders to determine if symptoms recur at an intensity that warrants continued drug therapy.
- Monitor growth of children on long-term atomoxetine therapy.
- Administer drug before 6 PM to prevent insomnia if that is a problem.
- Monitor blood pressure early in treatment, particularly with adult patients.
- Arrange for consult with school nurse for school age patients receiving this drug.
- Suggest the use of contraceptives for women of childbearing age who are using this drug.

Teaching points

- Take this drug exactly as prescribed. It can be taken once a day in the morning, if adverse effects are a problem, the drug can be taken in two evenly divided doses in the morning and in the late afternoon or early evening.
- Take drug before 6 PM to avoid night-time sleep disturbance.
- Avoid the use of alcohol and over-the-counter (OTC) drugs, including nose drops, cold remedies, and herbal therapies while taking this drug; some of these products cause dangerous effects. If you feel that you need one of these preparations, consult your health care provider.
- Know that these side effects may occur: dizziness, insomnia, moodiness (these effects may become less pronounced after a few days, avoid driving a car or engaging in activities that require alertness if these occur, notify your health care provider if these are pronounced or bothersome); headache (analgesics may be available to help) loss of appetite, dry mouth (small frequent meals, sucking on sugarless lozenges have been known to help).
- Know that the effects of this drug on the unborn baby are not known, women of child-

bearing age are advised to use contraceptives.
- Report palpitations, dizziness, weight loss, severe dry mouth and difficulty swallowing, pregnancy.

⚗ atorvastatin calcium
(ah tor' va stah tin)

Lipitor

PREGNANCY CATEGORY X

Drug classes
Antihyperlipidemic
HMG CoA inhibitor

Therapeutic actions
Inhibits HMG co-enzyme A, the enzyme that catalyzes the first step in the cholesterol synthesis pathway, resulting in a decrease in serum cholesterol, serum LDLs (associated with increased risk of CAD), and increases serum HDLs (associated with decreased risk of CAD); increases hepatic LDL recapture sites, enhances reuptake and catabolism of LDL; lowers triglyceride levels.

Indications
- Adjunct to diet in treatment of elevated total cholesterol, serum triglycerides, and LDL cholesterol in patients with primary hypercholesterolemia (types IIa and IIb) and mixed dyslipidemia, primary dysbetalipoproteinemia, and homozygous familial hypercholesterolemia whose response to dietary restriction of saturated fat and cholesterol and other nonpharmacologic measures has not been adequate
- To increase HDL-C in patients with primary hypercholesterolemia and mixed dyslipidemia
- Adjunct to diet in treatment of boys and postmenarchal girls ages 10–17, with heterozygous familial cholesterolemia if diet alone is not adequate to control lipid levels and LDL-C levels are > 190 mg/dL or if LDL-C level is > 60 mg/dL and there is a family history of premature cardiovascular disease or the child has two or more risk factors for the development of coronary disease.

Contraindications and cautions

- Contraindicated with allergy to atorvastatin, fungal byproducts, active liver disease or unexplained and persistent elevations of transaminase levels, pregnancy, lactation
- Use cautiously with impaired endocrine function

Available forms

Tablets—10, 20, 40, 80 mg

Dosages

Adults

Initial: 10 mg PO once daily without regard to meals; maintenance: 10–80 mg PO daily. May be combined with bile acid–binding resin.

Pediatric patients 10–17 yr

Starting dose: 10 mg PO daily. Maximum dose: 20 mg/day.

Pharmacokinetics

Route	Onset	Peak
Oral	Slow	1–2 hr

Metabolism: Hepatic and cellular; $T_{1/2}$: 14 hr
Distribution: Crosses placenta; passes into breast milk
Excretion: Bile

Adverse effects

- **CNS:** *Headache,* asthenia
- **GI:** *Flatulence, abdominal pain, cramps, constipation, nausea,* dyspepsia, heartburn, **liver failure**
- **Respiratory:** Sinusitis, pharyngitis
- **Other: Rhabdomyolysis with acute renal failure,** arthralgia, myalgia

Interactions

✳ **Drug-drug** • Possible severe myopathy or rhabdomyolysis with erythromycin, cyclosporine, niacin, antifungals, other HMG-CoA reductase inhibitors • Increased digoxin levels with possible toxicity if taken together; monitor digoxin levels • Increased estrogen levels with oral contraceptives; monitor patients on this combination

✳ **Drug-food** • Decreased metabolism and risk of toxic effects if combined with grapefruit juice; avoid this combination.

■ Nursing considerations

Assessment

- **History:** Allergy to atorvastatin, fungal byproducts; active hepatic disease; acute serious illness; pregnancy, lactation
- **Physical:** Orientation, affect, muscle strength; liver evaluation, abdominal exam; lipid studies, liver and renal function tests

Interventions

- Obtain liver function tests as a baseline and periodically during therapy; discontinue drug if AST or ALT levels increase to 3 times normal levels.
- Withhold atorvastatin in any acute, serious condition (severe infection, hypotension, major surgery, trauma, severe metabolic or endocrine disorder, seizures) that may suggest myopathy or serve as risk factor for development of renal failure.
- Ensure that patient has tried cholesterol-lowering diet regimen for 3–6 mo before beginning therapy.
- Administer drug without regard to food, but at same time each day.
- Atorvastatin may be combined with a bile acid binding agent. Do not combine with other HMG-CoA reductase inhibitors or fibrates.
- Consult dietitian regarding low-cholesterol diets.
- Ensure that patient is not pregnant and has appropriate contraceptives available during therapy; serious fetal damage has been associated with this drug.

Teaching points

- Take this drug once a day, at about the same time each day; may be taken with food. Do not drink grapefruit juice while on this drug.
- Institute appropriate dietary changes that need to be made.
- These side effects may occur: nausea (eat small, frequent meals); headache, muscle and joint aches and pains (may lessen over time).
- Arrange to have periodic blood tests while you are on this drug.
- Alert any health care provider that you are on this drug; it will need to be discontinued if acute injury or illness occurs.

Adverse effects in *Italics* are most common; those in **Bold** are life-threatening.

- Do not become pregnant while you are on this drug; use barrier contraceptives. If you wish to become pregnant or think you are pregnant, consult your health care provider.
- Report muscle pain, weakness, tenderness; malaise; fever; changes in color of urine or stool; swelling.

▷ atovaquone
(a toe' va kwon)

Mepron

PREGNANCY CATEGORY C

Drug class
Antiprotozoal

Therapeutic actions
Directly inhibits enzymes required for nucleic acid and ATP synthesis in protozoa; effective against *Pneumocystis carinii.*

Indications
- Prevention and acute oral treatment of mild to moderate *P. carinii* pneumonia (PCP) in patients who are intolerant to trimethoprim-sulfamethoxazole.

Contraindications and cautions
- Contraindicated with development or history of potentially life-threatening allergic reactions to any of the components of the drug.
- Use cautiously with severe PCP infections, the elderly, lactation.

Available forms
Suspension—750 mg/5 mL

Dosages
Adults and patients 13–16 yr
- *Prevention of PCP:* 1,500 mg PO daily with a meal
- *Treatment of PCP:* 750 mg PO bid with food for 21 days
Pediatric patients
Safety and efficacy not established.
Geriatric patients
Use caution, and evaluate patient response regularly.

Pharmacokinetics

Route	Onset	Peak	Duration
Oral	Varies	1–8 hr	3–5 days

Metabolism: $T_{1/2}$: 2.2–2.9 days
Distribution: Crosses placenta; may pass into breast milk
Excretion: Feces

Adverse effects
- **CNS:** Dizziness, *insomnia, headache*
- **Dermatologic:** *Rash,* pruritus, sweating, dry skin
- **GI:** Constipation, *diarrhea, nausea, vomiting,* anorexia, abdominal pain, oral monilia infections
- **Other:** *Fever,* elevated liver enzymes, hyponatremia

Interactions
✳ **Drug-drug** • Decreased effects if taken with rifamycin
✳ **Drug-food** • Markedly increased absorption of atovaquone when taken with food

■ Nursing considerations
Assessment
- **History:** History of potentially life-threatening allergic reactions to any components of the drug, severe PCP infections, elderly, lactation
- **Physical:** T, skin condition, neurologic status, abdominal evaluation, serum electrolytes, liver function tests

Interventions
- Give drug with meals.
- Ensure that this drug is taken for 21 days as treatment.

Teaching points
- Take drug with food; food increases the absorption of the drug.
- These side effects may occur: dizziness, insomnia, headache (medication may be ordered); nausea, vomiting (small, frequent meals may help); diarrhea or constipation (consult your health care provider for appropriate treatment); superinfections (therapy may be ordered); rash (good skin care may help).
- Report fever, mouth infection, severe headache, severe nausea or vomiting, rash.

atropine sulfate

(a' troe peen)

Parenteral and oral preparations: Minims (CAN), Sal-Tropine

Ophthalmic solution: Atropine Sulfate S.O.P., Atropisol, Isopto-Atropine Ophthalmic

PREGNANCY CATEGORY C

Drug classes

Anticholinergic
Antimuscarinic
Parasympatholytic
Antiparkinsonism drug
Antidote
Diagnostic agent (ophthalmic preparations)
Belladonna alkaloid

Therapeutic actions

Competitively blocks the effects of acetylcholine at muscarinic cholinergic receptors that mediate the effects of parasympathetic postganglionic impulses, depressing salivary and bronchial secretions, dilating the bronchi, inhibiting vagal influences on the heart, relaxing the GI and GU tracts, inhibiting gastric acid secretion (high doses), relaxing the pupil of the eye (mydriatic effect), and preventing accommodation for near vision (cycloplegic effect); also blocks the effects of acetylcholine in the CNS.

Indications

Systemic administration

- Antisialagogue for preanesthetic medication to prevent or reduce respiratory tract secretions
- Treatment of parkinsonism; relieves tremor and rigidity
- Restoration of cardiac rate and arterial pressure during anesthesia when vagal stimulation produced by intra-abdominal traction causes a decrease in pulse rate, lessening the degree of AV block when increased vagal tone is a factor (eg, some cases due to digitalis)
- Relief of bradycardia and syncope due to hyperactive carotid sinus reflex

- Relief of pylorospasm, hypertonicity of the small intestine, and hypermotility of the colon
- Relaxation of the spasm of biliary and ureteral colic and bronchospasm
- Relaxation of the tone of the detrusor muscle of the urinary bladder in the treatment of urinary tract disorders
- Control of crying and laughing episodes in patients with brain lesions
- Treatment of closed head injuries that cause acetylcholine release into CSF, EEG abnormalities, stupor, neurologic signs
- Relaxation of uterine hypertonicity
- Management of peptic ulcer
- Control of rhinorrhea of acute rhinitis or hay fever
- Antidote (with external cardiac massage) for CV collapse from overdose of parasympathomimetic (cholinergic) drugs (choline esters, pilocarpine), or cholinesterase inhibitors (eg, physostigmine, isoflurophate, organophosphorus insecticides)
- Antidote for poisoning by certain species of mushroom (eg, *Amanita muscaria*)

Ophthalmic preparations

- Diagnostically to produce mydriasis and cycloplegia-pupillary dilation in acute inflammatory conditions of the iris and uveal tract

Contraindications and cautions

- Contraindicated with hypersensitivity to anticholinergic drugs.

Systemic administration

- Contraindicated with glaucoma, adhesions between iris and lens, stenosing peptic ulcer, pyloroduodenal obstruction, paralytic ileus, intestinal atony, severe ulcerative colitis, toxic megacolon, symptomatic prostatic hypertrophy, bladder neck obstruction, bronchial asthma, COPD, cardiac arrhythmias, tachycardia, myocardial ischemia, impaired metabolic, liver, or kidney function, myasthenia gravis.
- Use cautiously with Down syndrome, brain damage, spasticity, hypertension, hyperthyroidism, lactation.

Ophthalmic solution

- Contraindicated with glaucoma or tendency to glaucoma.

Available forms

Tablets—0.4 mg; injection—0.05, 0.1, 0.3, 0.4, 0.5, 0.8, 1 mg/mL; ophthalmic ointment—1%; ophthalmic solution—0.5%, 1%, 2%

Dosages
Adults
Systemic administration
0.4–0.6 mg PO, IM, SC, IV.
- *Hypotonic radiography:* 1 mg IM.
- *Surgery:* 0.5 mg (0.4–0.6 mg) IM (or SC, IV) prior to induction of anesthesia; during surgery, give IV; reduce dose to < 0.4 mg with cyclopropane anesthesia.
- *Bradyarrhythmias:* 0.4–1 mg (up to 2 mg) IV every 1–2 hr as needed.
- *Antidote:* For poisoning due to cholinesterase inhibitor insecticides, give large doses of at least 2–3 mg parenterally, and repeat until signs of atropine intoxication appear; for rapid type of mushroom poisoning, give in doses sufficient to control parasympathetic signs before coma and CV collapse intervene.

Ophthalmic solution
- *For refraction:* Instill 1–2 drops into eye(s) 1 hr before refracting.
- *For uveitis:* Instill 1–2 drops into eye(s) qid.

Pediatric patients
Systemic administration
Refer to the following table:

Weight	Dose (mg)
7–16 lb (3.2–7.3 kg)	0.1
16–24 lb (7.3–10.9 kg)	0.15
24–40 lb (10.9–18.1 kg)	0.2
40–65 lb (18.1–29.5 kg)	0.3
65–90 lb (29.5–40.8 kg)	0.4
> 90 lb (> 40.8 kg)	0.4–0.6

- *Surgery:* 0.1 mg (newborn) to 0.6 mg (12 yr) injected SC 30 min before surgery.

Geriatric patients
More likely to cause serious adverse reactions, especially CNS reactions, in elderly patients; use with caution.

Pharmacokinetics

Route	Onset	Peak	Duration
IM	10–15 min	30 min	4 hr
IV	Immediate	2–4 min	4 hr
SC	Varies	1–2 hr	4 hr
Topical	5–10 min	30–40 min	7–14 days

Metabolism: Hepatic; $T_{1/2}$: 2.5 hr
Distribution: Crosses placenta; passes into breast milk
Excretion: Urine

▼ IV facts
Preparation: Give undiluted or dilute in 10 mL sterile water.
Infusion: Give direct IV; administer 1 mg or less over 1 min.

Adverse effects
Systemic administration
- **CNS:** *Blurred vision, mydriasis, cycloplegia, photophobia,* increased intraocular pressure, headache, flushing, nervousness, weakness, dizziness, insomnia, mental confusion or excitement (after even small doses in the elderly), nasal congestion
- **CV:** *Palpitations, bradycardia* (low doses), *tachycardia* (higher doses)
- **GI:** *Dry mouth, altered taste perception, nausea,* vomiting, dysphagia, heartburn, constipation, bloated feeling, **paralytic ileus,** gastroesophageal reflux
- **GU:** *Urinary hesitancy and retention;* impotence
- **Other:** *Decreased sweating and predisposition to heat prostration,* suppression of lactation

Ophthalmic preparations
- **Local:** *Transient stinging*
- **Systemic:** Systemic adverse effects, depending on amount absorbed

Interactions
✱ Drug-drug • Increased anticholinergic effects with other drugs that have anticholinergic activity: certain antihistamines, certain antiparkinsonian drugs, TCAs, MAO inhibitors • Decreased antipsychotic effectiveness of haloperidol with atropine • Decreased effectiveness of phenothiazines, but increased incidence of paralytic ileus

■ Nursing considerations
Assessment
- **History:** Hypersensitivity to anticholinergic drugs; glaucoma; adhesions between iris and lens; stenosing peptic ulcer, pyloroduodenal obstruction, paralytic ileus, intestinal atony, severe ulcerative colitis, toxic megacolon, symptomatic prostatic hypertrophy,

bladder neck obstruction, bronchial asthma, COPD, cardiac arrhythmias, myocardial ischemia, impaired metabolic, liver, or kidney function, myasthenia gravis, Down syndrome, brain damage, spasticity, hypertension, hyperthyroidism, lactation
- **Physical:** Skin color, lesions, texture; T; orientation, reflexes, bilateral grip strength; affect; ophthalmic exam; P, BP; R, adventitious sounds; bowel sounds, normal GI output; normal urinary output, prostate palpation; liver and kidney function tests, ECG

Interventions
- Ensure adequate hydration; provide environmental control (temperature) to prevent hyperpyrexia.
- Have patient void before taking medication if urinary retention is a problem.

Teaching points
- When used preoperatively or in other acute situations, incorporate teaching about the drug with teaching about the procedure; the ophthalmic solution is used mainly acutely and will not be self-administered by the patient; the following apply to oral medication for outpatients:
- Take as prescribed, 30 min before meals; avoid excessive dosage.
- Avoid hot environments; you will be heat intolerant, and dangerous reactions may occur.
- These side effects may occur: dizziness, confusion (use caution driving or performing hazardous tasks); constipation (ensure adequate fluid intake, proper diet); dry mouth (sugarless lozenges, frequent mouth care may help; may be transient); blurred vision, sensitivity to light (reversible; avoid tasks that require acute vision; wear sunglasses in bright light); impotence (reversible); difficulty in urination (empty the bladder prior to taking drug).
- Report rash; flushing; eye pain; difficulty breathing; tremors, loss of coordination; irregular heartbeat, palpitations; headache; abdominal distention; hallucinations; severe or persistent dry mouth; difficulty swallowing; difficulty in urination; constipation; sensitivity to light.

▷ **auranofin**
(au rane' oh fin)

Ridaura

PREGNANCY CATEGORY C

Drug classes
Antirheumatic agent
Gold compound

Therapeutic actions
Suppresses and prevents arthritis and synovitis; taken up by macrophages with resultant inhibition of phagocytosis and inhibition of activities of lysosomal enzymes; decreases concentrations of rheumatoid factor and immunoglobulins; mechanisms not known; no substantial evidence of remission induction.

Indications
- Management of adults with active classic or definite rheumatoid arthritis who have insufficient response or are intolerant to NSAIDs (given only orally)
- Unlabeled use: alternative or adjuvant to corticosteroids in treatment of pemphigus, SLE; for psoriatic arthritis in patients who do not tolerate or respond to NSAIDs

Contraindications and cautions
- Contraindicated with allergy to gold preparations; history of gold-induced disorders, necrotizing enterocolitis, pulmonary fibrosis, exfoliative dermatitis, bone marrow aplasia, severe hematologic disorders, lactation.
- Use cautiously with diabetes mellitus, CHF, hypertension, compromised liver or renal function, compromised cerebral or CV circulation, inflammatory bowel disease, blood dyscrasias.

Available forms
Capsules—3 mg

Dosages

Contains approximately 29% gold

Adults

6 mg/day PO, either as 3 mg bid or 6 mg daily. If response is not adequate after 6 mo, dosage may be increased to 9 mg/day (3 mg tid). If response is not adequate after another 3 mo, discontinue drug; do not exceed 9 mg/day.

- *Transfer from injectable gold:* Discontinue injectable agent, and start auranofin 6 mg/day PO.

Pediatric patients

0.1 mg/kg/day PO initially; titrate up to 0.15 mg/kg/day; do not exceed 0.2 mg/kg/day.

Geriatric patients

Monitor patients carefully; tolerance to gold decreases with age.

Pharmacokinetics

Route	Onset	Peak
Oral	Varies	1–2 hr

Metabolism: $T_{1/2}$: 26 days
Distribution: Crosses placenta; passes into breast milk
Excretion: Urine and feces

Adverse effects

- **Allergic reactions:** Nitroid reactions: flushing, fainting, dizziness, sweating, nausea, vomiting, malaise, weakness
- **Dermatologic:** *Dermatitis, pruritus, erythema,* exfoliative dermatitis, chrysiasis (gray-blue color to the skin due to gold deposition)
- **GI:** *Nausea, vomiting, anorexia, abdominal cramps, diarrhea, stomatitis, glossitis,* gingivitis, metallic taste, pharyngitis, gastritis, colitis, hepatitis with jaundice
- **GU:** Nephrotic syndrome or glomerulitis with proteinuria and hematuria; **acute tubular necrosis and renal failure;** vaginitis
- **Hematologic:** *Anemias,* granulocytopenia, thrombocytopenia, leukopenia, eosinophilia
- **Respiratory:** Gold bronchitis, **interstitial pneumonitis and fibrosis,** cough, shortness of breath, tracheitis

Interactions

✴ **Drug-drug** • Do not use with penicillamine, antimalarials, cytotoxic drugs, immunosuppressive agents other than low doses of corticosteroids

■ Nursing considerations

Assessment

- **History:** Allergy to gold preparations, history of gold-induced disorders, diabetes mellitus, CHF, hypertension, compromised liver or renal function, compromised cerebral or CV circulation, inflammatory bowel disease, blood dyscrasias, lactation
- **Physical:** Skin color, lesions; T; edema; R, adventitious sounds; GI mucous membranes, bowel sounds, liver evaluation; CBC, renal and liver function tests, chest x-ray

Interventions

- Do not give to patients with idiosyncratic or severe reactions to gold therapy.
- Monitor hematologic status, liver and kidney function, respiratory status regularly during the course of drug therapy.
- Discontinue at first sign of toxic reaction.
- Use low-dose systemic corticosteroids for treatment of severe stomatitis, dermatitis, renal, hematologic, pulmonary, enterocolitic complications.
- Protect patient from sunlight or ultraviolet light to decrease risk of chrysiasis.

Teaching points

- Take this drug as prescribed; do not take more. Drug's effects are not seen immediately; several months of therapy are needed.
- This drug does not cure the disease but stops its effects.
- These side effects may occur: diarrhea; mouth sores, metallic taste (frequent mouth care will help); rash, gray-blue color to the skin (avoid exposure to the sun or ultraviolet light); nausea, loss of appetite (small, frequent meals may help).
- Avoid pregnancy while using this drug; if you decide to become pregnant, consult with physician about discontinuing drug.
- Report unusual bleeding or bruising; sore throat, fever; severe diarrhea; rash; mouth sores.

▽ aurothioglucose
*(aur oh thye oh **gloo**' kose)*

Solganal

PREGNANCY CATEGORY C

Drug classes
Antirheumatic agent
Gold compound

Therapeutic actions
Suppresses and prevents arthritis and synovitis; taken up by macrophages with resultant inhibition of phagocytosis and inhibition of activities of lysosomal enzymes; decreases concentrations of rheumatoid factor and immunoglobulins; no substantial evidence of remission induction.

Indications
• Treatment of selected cases of adult and juvenile rheumatoid arthritis; most effective early in disease; later, when damage has occurred, gold only prevents further damage.

Contraindications and cautions
• Allergy to gold preparations; history of gold-induced disorders—necrotizing enterocolitis, pulmonary fibrosis, exfoliative dermatitis, bone marrow aplasia, severe hematologic disorders; uncontrolled diabetes mellitus; CHF; SLE; marked hypertension, compromised liver or renal function, compromised cerebral or CV circulation, inflammatory bowel disease, blood dyscrasias, recent radiation treatments; lactation.

Available forms
Injection suspension—50 mg/mL

Dosages
Contains approximately 50% gold. Give by IM injection only, preferably intragluteally.
Adults
• *Weekly injections:* First dose: 10 mg IM; second and third doses: 25 mg IM; fourth and subsequent doses: 50 mg IM until 0.8–1 g has been given. If patient improves without toxicity, continue 50-mg dose at 3- to 4-wk intervals.

Pediatric patients 6–12 yr
Administer one-fourth the adult dose governed by body weight; do not exceed 25 mg/dose.
Geriatric patients
Monitor patients carefully; tolerance to gold decreases with age.

Pharmacokinetics

Route	Onset	Peak
IM	Slow	4–6 hr

Metabolism: $T_{1/2}$: 3–7 days
Distribution: Crosses placenta; passes into breast milk
Excretion: Urine and feces

Adverse effects
• **Allergic reactions:** Nitroid reactions: flushing, fainting, dizziness, sweating, nausea, vomiting, malaise, weakness
• **Dermatologic:** *Dermatitis; pruritus, erythema,* exfoliative dermatitus, chrysiasis (gray-blue color to the skin due to gold deposition)
• **GI:** *Nausea, vomiting, anorexia,* abdominal cramps, diarrhea, *stomatitis, glossitis,* gingivitis, metallic taste, pharyngitis, gastritis, colitis, hepatitis with jaundice
• **GU:** Nephrotic syndrome or glomerulitis with proteinuria and hematuria, **acute tubular necrosis** and renal failure, vaginitis
• **Hematologic:** *Anemias,* granulocytopenia, thrombocytopenia, leukopenia, eosinophilia
• **Immediate postinjection effects: Anaphylactic shock,** syncope, bradycardia, thickening of the tongue, dysphagia, dyspnea, angioneurotic edema
• **Nonvasomotor postinjection reaction:** Arthralgia for 1–2 days after the injection; usually subsides after the first few injections
• **Respiratory:** Gold bronchitis, **interstitial pneumonitis and fibrosis,** cough, shortness of breath, tracheitis

Interactions
✳ **Drug-drug** • Do not use with penicillamine, antimalarials, cytotoxic drugs, immunosuppressive agents other than low doses of corticosteroids

---

Adverse effects in *Italics* are most common; those in **Bold** are life-threatening.

■ Nursing considerations
Assessment
- **History:** Allergy to gold preparations; history of gold-induced disorders; uncontrolled diabetes mellitus; CHF; SLE; marked hypertension; compromised liver or renal function; compromised cerebral or CV circulation; inflammatory bowel disease; blood dyscrasias; recent radiation treatments; lactation
- **Physical:** Skin color, lesions; T; edema; P, BP; R, adventitious sounds; GI mucous membranes, bowel sounds, liver evaluation; CBC, renal and liver function tests, chest x-ray

Interventions
- Do not give drug to patients with history of idiosyncratic or severe reactions to gold therapy.
- Monitor hematologic status, liver and kidney function, respiratory status regularly during the course of drug therapy.
- Give by intragluteal IM injection.
- Monitor patient carefully at time of injection for possible postinjection reaction.
- Discontinue at first sign of toxic reaction.
- Use low-dose systemic corticosteroids for treatment of severe stomatitis, dermatitis, renal, hematologic, pulmonary, enterocolitic complications.
- Protect patient from sunlight or ultraviolet light to decrease risk of chrysiasis.

Teaching points
- Prepare a calendar of projected injection dates. Drug's effects are not seen immediately; several months of therapy are needed.
- These side effects may occur: increased joint pain for 1–2 days after injection (usually subsides after the first few injections); diarrhea; mouth sores, metallic taste (frequent mouth care will help); rash, gray-blue color or to the skin (avoid exposure to sun or ultraviolet light); nausea, loss of appetite (small, frequent meals may help).
- Avoid pregnancy while on this drug. If you decide to become pregnant, consult with physician about discontinuing drug.
- Report unusual bleeding or bruising; sore throat, fever; severe diarrhea; rash; mouth sores.

▽ azatadine maleate A
(a za' te deen)

Optimine

PREGNANCY CATEGORY C

Drug class
Antihistamine (piperidine type)

Therapeutic actions
Competitively blocks the effects of histamine at H_1 receptor sites; has anticholinergic (atropine-like), antiserotonin, antipruritic, sedative, and appetite-stimulating effects.

Indications
- Relief of symptoms associated with perennial and seasonal allergic rhinitis; vasomotor rhinitis; allergic conjunctivitis; mild, uncomplicated urticaria and angioedema; amelioration of allergic reactions to blood or plasma; dermatographism; adjunctive therapy in anaphylactic reactions
- Treatment of chronic urticaria

Contraindications and cautions
- Contraindicated with allergy to any antihistamines, lactation, third trimester of pregnancy.
- Use cautiously with narrow-angle glaucoma, stenosing peptic ulcer, symptomatic prostatic hypertrophy, asthmatic attack, bladder neck obstruction, pyloroduodenal obstruction.

Available forms
Tablets—1 mg

Dosages
Adults and patients ≥ 12 yr
1–2 mg PO bid.
Pediatric patients
Safety and efficacy not established in children < 12 yr.
Geriatric patients
More likely to cause dizziness, sedation, syncope, toxic confusional states, and hypotension in elderly patients; use with caution.

Pharmacokinetics

Route	Onset	Peak
Oral	Varies	4 hr

Metabolism: Hepatic; $T_{1/2}$: 12 hr
Distribution: Crosses placenta; passes into breast milk
Excretion: Urine

Adverse effects

- **CNS:** *Drowsiness, sedation, dizziness, disturbed coordination,* fatigue, confusion, restlessness, excitation, nervousness, tremor, headache, blurred vision, diplopia, vertigo, tinnitus, acute labyrinthitis, hysteria, tingling, heaviness and weakness of the hands
- **CV:** Hypotension, palpitations, bradycardia, tachycardia, extrasystoles
- **GI:** *Epigastric distress,* anorexia, increased appetite and weight gain, nausea, vomiting, diarrhea or constipation
- **GU:** Urinary frequency, dysuria, urinary retention, early menses, decreased libido, impotence
- **Hematologic:** Hemolytic anemia, hypoplastic anemia, thrombocytopenia, leukopenia, agranulocytosis, pancytopenia
- **Respiratory:** *Thickening of bronchial secretions,* chest tightness, wheezing, nasal stuffiness, dry mouth, dry nose, dry throat, sore throat
- **Other:** Urticaria, rash, **anaphylactic shock,** photosensitivity, excessive perspiration

Interactions

✳ **Drug-drug** • Increased and prolonged anticholinergic (drying) effects with MAO inhibitors

✳ **Drug-lab test** • Increase in PBI not attributable to an increase in thyroxine • False-positive pregnancy test (less likely if serum test is used)

■ Nursing considerations
Assessment

- **History:** Allergy to antihistamines; narrow-angle glaucoma, stenosing peptic ulcer, symptomatic prostatic hypertrophy, asthmatic attack, bladder neck obstruction, pyloroduodenal obstruction; lactation
- **Physical:** Skin color, lesions, texture; orientation, reflexes, affect; vision exam; P, BP; R, adventitious sounds; bowel sounds; prostate palpation; CBC with differential

Interventions

- Administer with food if GI upset occurs.
- Monitor patient response. Maintain at lowest possible effective dosage.

Teaching points

- Take as prescribed; avoid excessive dosage.
- Take with food if GI upset occurs.
- These side effects may occur: dizziness, sedation, drowsiness (use caution driving or performing tasks that require alertness); epigastric distress, diarrhea or constipation (take drug with meals; consult health care provider about diarrhea or constipation); dry mouth (use frequent mouth care, suck sugarless lozenges); thickening of bronchial secretions, dryness of nasal mucosa (use humidifier).
- Avoid alcohol; serious sedation could occur.
- Report difficulty breathing, hallucinations, tremors, loss of coordination, unusual bleeding or bruising, visual disturbances, irregular heartbeat.

▷ **azathioprine**
*(ay za **thye'** oh preen)*

Imuran

PREGNANCY CATEGORY D

Drug class
Immunosuppressive

Therapeutic actions
Suppresses cell-mediated hypersensitivities and alters antibody production; exact mechanisms of action in increasing homograft survival and affecting autoimmune diseases not clearly understood.

Indications

- Renal homotransplantation: adjunct for prevention of rejection
- Rheumatoid arthritis: use only with adults meeting criteria for classic rheumatoid arthritis and not responding to conventional management
- Unlabeled use: treatment of chronic ulcerative colitis, myasthenia gravis, Behçet's syndrome, Crohn's disease

---

Adverse effects in *Italics* are most common; those in **Bold** are life-threatening.

Contraindications and cautions

- Allergy to azathioprine; rheumatoid arthritis patients previously treated with alkylating agents, increasing their risk for neoplasia; pregnancy.

Available forms

Tablets—50, 75, 100 mg; injection—100 mg/vial

Dosages
Adults

- *Renal homotransplantation:* Initial dose of 3–5 mg/kg/day PO or IV as a single dose on the day of transplant; maintenance levels are 1–3 mg/kg/day PO. Do not increase dose to decrease risk of rejection.
- *Rheumatoid arthritis:* Usually given daily; initial dose of 1 mg/kg PO given as a single dose or bid. Dose may be increased at 6–8 wk and thereafter by steps at 4-wk intervals. Dose increments should be 0.5 mg/kg/day up to a maximum dose of 2.5 mg/kg/day. Once patient is stabilized, dose should be decreased to lowest effective dose; decrease in 0.5-mg/kg increments. Patients who do not respond in 12 wk are probably refractory.

Pediatric patients

- *Renal homotransplantation:* Initial dose of 3–5 mg/kg/day IV or PO followed by a maintenance dose of 1–3 mg/kg/day.

Geriatric patients or patients with renal impairment

Lower doses may be required because of decreased rate of excretion and increased sensitivity to the drug.

Route	Onset	Peak
Oral	Varies	1–2 hr
IV	Immediate	30–45 min

Metabolism: Hepatic; $T_{1/2}$: 5 hr
Distribution: Crosses placenta; may pass into breast milk
Excretion: Urine

▽IV facts

Preparation: Add 10 mL sterile water for injection and swirl until a clear solution results; use within 24 hr. Further dilution into sterile saline or dextrose is usually made for infusion.
Infusion: Infuse over 30–60 min; can range from 5 min to 8 hr for the daily dose.

Adverse effects

- **GI:** *Nausea, vomiting,* hepatotoxicity (especially in homograft patients)
- **Hematologic:** *Leukopenia, thrombocytopenia, macrocytic anemia*
- **Other: Serious infections** (fungal, bacterial, protozoal infections secondary to immunosuppression), *carcinogenesis* (increased risk of neoplasia, especially in homograft patients)

Interactions

✳ **Drug-drug** • Increased effects with allopurinol; reduce azathioprine to one-third to one-fourth the usual dose • Reversal of the neuromuscular blockade of nondepolarizing neuromuscular junction blockers (atracurium, pancuronium, tubocurarine, vecuronium) with azathioprine

■ Nursing considerations
Assessment

- **History:** Allergy to azathioprine; rheumatoid arthritis patients previously treated with alkylating agents; pregnancy or male partners of women trying to become pregnant; lactation
- **Physical:** T; skin color, lesions; liver evaluation, bowel sounds; renal and liver function tests, CBC

Interventions

- Give drug IV if oral administration is not possible; switch to oral route as soon as possible.
- Administer in divided daily doses or with food if GI upset occurs.
- Monitor blood counts regularly; severe hematologic effects may require the discontinuation of therapy.

Teaching points

- Take drug in divided doses with food if GI upset occurs.
- Avoid infections; avoid crowds or people who have infections. Notify your physician at once if injured.
- Notify your physician if you think you are pregnant or if you wish to become pregnant (also applies to men whose sexual partners wish to become pregnant).

- These side effects may occur: nausea, vomiting (take drug in divided doses or with food); diarrhea; rash.
- Report unusual bleeding or bruising; fever, sore throat, mouth sores; signs of infection; abdominal pain; severe diarrhea; darkened urine or pale stools; severe nausea and vomiting.

▽ azithromycin
(ay zi thro my' sin)

Zithromax

PREGNANCY CATEGORY B

Drug class
Macrolide antibiotic

Therapeutic actions
Bacteriostatic or bactericidal in susceptible bacteria.

Indications
- Treatment of lower respiratory tract infections: acute bacterial exacerbations of COPD due to *H. influenzae, Moraxella catarrhalis, S. pneumoniae;* community-acquired pneumonia due to *S. pneumoniae, H. influenzae*
- Treatment of lower respiratory tract infections: streptococcal pharyngitis and tonsillitis due to *Streptococcus pyogenes* in those who cannot take penicillins
- Treatment of uncomplicated skin infections due to *Staphylococcus aureus, S. pyogenes, Streptococcus agalactiae*
- Treatment of nongonococcal urethritis and cervicitis due to *C. trachomatis;* treatment of PID
- Treatment of otitis media caused by *H. influenzae, M. catarrhalis, S. pneumoniae* in children > 6 mo
- Treatment of pharyngitis and tonsillitis in children > 2 yr who cannot use first-line therapy
- Prevention and treatment of disseminated *Mycobacterium avium* complex (MAC) in patients with advanced AIDS

- Unlabeled uses: uncomplicated gonococcal infections caused by *N. gonorrhoeae;* gonococcal pharyngitis caused by *N. gonorrhoeae;* chlamydial infections caused by *C. trachomatis;* prophylaxis after sexual attack

Contraindications and cautions
- Contraindicated with hypersensitivity to azithromycin, erythromycin, or any macrolide antibiotic.
- Use cautiously with gonorrhea or syphilis, pseudomembranous colitis, hepatic or renal impairment, lactation.

Available forms
Tablets–250, 600 mg; powder for injection–500 mg; powder for oral suspension–100 mg/5 mL, 200 mg/5 mL, 1 g/packet

Dosages
Adults
- *Mild to moderate acute bacterial exacerbations of COPD, pneumonia, pharyngitis and tonsillitis (as second-line):* 500 mg PO single dose on first day, followed by 250 mg PO daily on days 2–5 for a total dose of 1.5 g or 500 mg/day PO for 3 days.
- *Nongonococcal urethritis and cervicitis due to* C. trachomati: A single 1-g PO dose.
- *Gonococcal urethritis and cervicitis:* A single dose of 2 g PO.
- *Disseminated MAC infections:* Prevention, 1,200 mg PO taken once weekly. Treatment, 600 mg/day PO with etambutol.

Pediatric patients
- *Otitis media:* Initially 10 mg/kg PO as a single dose, then 5 mg/kg on days 2–5 or 30 mg/kg PO as a single dose.
- *Community-acquired pneumonia:* 10 mg/kg PO as a single dose on first day, then 5 mg/kg PO on days 2–5.
- *Pharyngitis or tonsillitis:* 12 mg/kg/day PO on days 1–5.

Pharmacokinetics

Route	Onset	Peak	Duration
Oral	Varies	2.5–3.2 hr	24 hr

Metabolism: $T_{1/2}$: 11–48 hr
Distribution: Crosses placenta; passes into breast milk

A

Excretion: Unchanged in biliary excretion and urine

Adverse effects
- **CNS:** Dizziness, headache, vertigo, somnolence, fatigue
- **GI:** *Diarrhea, abdominal pain, nausea,* dyspepsia, flatulence, vomiting, melena, pseudomembranous colitis
- **Other:** *Superinfections,* **angioedema,** rash, photosensitivity, vaginitis

Interactions
✹ **Drug-drug** • Decreased serum levels and effectiveness of azithromycin with aluminum and magnesium-containing antacids • Possible increased effects of theophylline • Possible increased anticoagulant effects of warfarin
✹ **Drug-food** • Food greatly decreases the absorption of azithromycin

■ Nursing considerations
Assessment
- **History:** Hypersensitivity to azithromycin, erythromycin, or any macrolide antibiotic; gonorrhea or syphilis, pseudomembranous colitis, hepatic or renal impairment, lactation
- **Physical:** Site of infection; skin color, lesions; orientation, GI output, bowel sounds, liver evaluation; culture and sensitivity tests of infection, urinalysis, liver and renal function tests

Interventions
- Culture site of infection before therapy.
- Administer on an empty stomach–1 hr before or 2–3 hr after meals. Food affects the absorption of this drug.
- Counsel patients being treated for STDs about appropriate precautions and additional therapy.

Teaching points
- Take this drug on an empty stomach–1 hr before or 2–3 hr after meals; it should never be taken with food. Take the full course prescribed. Do not take with antacids.
- These side effects may occur: stomach cramping, discomfort, diarrhea; fatigue, headache (medication may help); additional infections in the mouth or vagina (consult with health care provider for treatment).

- Report severe or watery diarrhea, severe nausea or vomiting, rash or itching, mouth sores, vaginal sores.

▽ aztreonam
(az' tree oh nam)

Azactam

PREGNANCY CATEGORY B

Drug class
Monobactam antibiotic

Therapeutic actions
Bactericidal: interferes with bacterial cell wall synthesis, causing cell death in susceptible gram-negative bacteria, ineffective against gram-positive and anaerobic bacteria.

Indications
- Treatment of UTIs, LRIs, skin and skin-structure infections, septicemia, intra-abdominal infections and gynecologic infections caused by susceptible strains of *E. coli, Enterobacter, Serratia, Proteus, Salmonella, Providencia, Pseudomonas, Citrobacter, Haemophilus, Neisseria, Klebsiella*
- Unlabeled use: 1 g IM for treatment of acute uncomplicated gonorrhea as alternative to spectinomycin in penicillin-resistant gonococci

Contraindications and cautions
- Contraindicated with allergy to aztreonam.
- Use cautiously with immediate hypersensitivity reaction to penicillins or cephalosporins, renal and hepatic disorders, lactation.

Available forms
Powder for injection—500 mg, 1 g, 2 g

Dosages
Available for IV and IM use only; maximum recommended dose, 8 g/day.
Adults
- *UTIs:* 500 mg–1 g q 8–12 hr.
- *Moderately severe systemic infection:* 1–2 g q 8–12 hr.
- *Severe systemic infection:* 2 g q 6–8 hr.

Pediatric patients
- *Mild to moderate infections:* 30 mg/kg q 8 hr
- *Moderate to severe infections:* 30 mg/kg q 6–8 hr

Geriatric patients or patients with renal impairment
Reduce dosage by one-half in patients with estimated creatinine clearances between 10 and 30 mL/min/1.73m^2 after an initial loading dose of 1 or 2 g. *Patients on hemodialysis:* give 500 mg, 1 g, or 2 g initially; maintenance dose should be one-fourth the usual initial dose at fixed intervals of 6, 8, or 12 hr.

Pharmacokinetics

Route	Onset	Peak	Duration
IM	Varies	60–90 min	6–8 hr
IV	Immediate	30 min	6–8 hr

Metabolism: $T_{1/2}$: 1.5–2 hr
Distribution: Crosses placenta; passes into breast milk
Excretion: Urine

▼ IV facts
Preparation: After adding diluent to container, shake immediately and vigorously. Constituted solutions are not for multiple-dose use; discard any unused solution. Solution should be colorless to light straw yellow, which may develop a slight pink tint on standing.
IV injection: Reconstitute contents of 15-mL vial with 6–10 mL sterile water for injection.
IV infusion: Reconstitute contents of 100-mL bottle to make a final concentration of 20 mg/mL or less (add at least 50 mL of one of the following solutions per gram of aztreonam): 0.9% sodium chloride injection, Ringer's injection, lactated Ringer's injection, 5% or 10% dextrose injection, 5% dextrose and 0.2%, 0.45%, or 0.09% sodium chloride, sodium lactate injection, Ionosol B with 5% Dextrose, Isolyte E, Isolyte E with 5% Dextrose, Isolyte M with 5% Dextrose, Normosol-R, Normosol-R and 5% Dextrose, Normosol-M and 5% Dextrose, 5% and 10% mannitol injection, lactated Ringer's and 5% dextrose injection, Plasma-Lyte M and 5% Dextrose, 10% Travert Injection, 10% Travert and Electrolyte no. 1, 2, or 3 Injection. Use reconstituted solutions promptly after preparation; those prepared with sterile water for injection or sodium chloride injection should be used within 48 hr if stored at room temperature and within 7 days if refrigerated.
Infusion: IV injection: Inject slowly over 3–5 min directly into vein or into IV tubing of compatible IV infusion.
IV infusion: Administer over 20–60 min. If giving into IV tubing that is used to administer other drugs, flush tubing with delivery solution before and after aztreonam administration.
Incompatibilities: Do not mix with nafcillin sodium, cephradine, metronidazole; other admixtures are not recommended because data are not available.
Y-site incompatibilities: Vancomycin.

Adverse effects
- **Dermatologic:** *Rash, pruritus*
- **GI:** *Nausea, vomiting, diarrhea,* transient elevation of AST, ALT, LDH
- **Hypersensitivity: Anaphylaxis**
- **Local:** *Local phlebitis or thrombophlebitis* at IV injection site, *swelling or discomfort* at IM injection site
- **Other:** Superinfections

Interactions
✳ **Drug-drug** • Incompatible in solution with nafcillin sodium, cephradine, metronidazole

■ Nursing considerations
Assessment
- **History:** Allergy to aztreonam, immediate hypersensitivity reaction to penicillins or cephalosporins, renal and hepatic disorders, lactation
- **Physical:** Skin color, lesions; injection sites; T; GI mucous membranes, bowel sounds, liver evaluation; GU mucous membranes; culture and sensitivity tests of infected area; liver and renal function tests

Interventions
- Arrange for culture and sensitivity tests of infected area before therapy. In acutely ill patients, therapy may begin before test results are known. If therapeutic effects are not noted, reculture area.

• *IM administration:* Reconstitute contents of 15-mL vial with at least 3 mL of diluent per gram of aztreonam. Appropriate diluents are sterile water for injection, bacteriostatic water for injection, 0.9% sodium chloride injection, bacteriostatic sodium chloride injection. Inject deeply into a large muscle mass. Do not mix with any local anesthetic.

• Discontinue drug and provide supportive measures if hypersensitivity reaction, anaphylaxis occurs.

• Monitor injection sites and provide comfort measures.

• Provide treatment and comfort measures if superinfections occur.

• Monitor patient's nutritional status, and provide small, frequent meals, mouth care if GI effects, superinfections interfere with nutrition.

Teaching points
• This drug can only be given IM or IV.
• These side effects may occur: nausea, vomiting, diarrhea.
• Report pain, soreness at injection site; difficulty breathing; mouth sores.

▽bacitracin
(bass i tray' sin)

Oral: Altracin
Powder for injection: Baci-IM
Ophthalmic: AK-Tracin
Topical ointment: Baciguent

PREGNANCY CATEGORY C

Drug class
Antibiotic

Therapeutic actions
Antibacterial: Inhibits cell wall synthesis of susceptible bacteria, primarily staphylococci, causing cell death.

Indications
• *IM:* Pneumonia and empyema caused by susceptible strains of staphylococci in infants

• *Ophthalmic preparations:* Infections of the eye caused by susceptible strains of staphylococci

• *Topical ointment:* Prophylaxis of minor skin abrasions; treatment of superficial infections of the skin caused by susceptible staphylococci

• *Orphan drug use (oral preparation):* Antibiotic-associated pseudomembranous enterocolitis

Contraindications and cautions
• Allergy to bacitracin, renal disease (IM use), lactation

Available forms
Powder for injection—50,000 units; ophthalmic ointment—500 units/g; topical ointment—500 units/g

Dosages
IM
Infants < 2.5 kg
900 units/kg/day IM in two to three divided doses.
Infants > 2.5 kg
1,000 units/kg/day IM in two to three divided doses.

Ophthalmic
Half-inch ribbon in the infected eye bid to q 3–4 hr as directed.

Topical
Apply to affected area one to five times per day; cover with sterile bandage if needed.

Pharmacokinetics

Route	Onset	Peak	Duration
IM	Rapid	1–2 hr	12–14 hr

Metabolism: Hepatic; $T_{1/2}$: 6 hr
Distribution: Crosses placenta; passes into breast milk
Excretion: Urine

Adverse effects
• **GI:** Nausea, vomiting
• **GU:** *Nephrotoxicity*
• **Local:** *Pain at injection site* (IM); *contact dermatitis* (topical ointment); *irritation, burning, stinging, itching, blurring of vision* (ophthalmic preparations)
• **Other:** Superinfections

Interactions

* Drug-drug • Increased neuromuscular blockade and muscular paralysis with anesthetics, nondepolarizing neuromuscular blocking drugs, drugs with neuromuscular blocking activity • Increased risk of respiratory paralysis and renal failure with aminoglycosides

■ Nursing considerations
Assessment

- **History:** Allergy to bacitracin, renal disease, lactation
- **Physical:** Site of infection; skin color, lesions; normal urinary output; urinalysis, serum creatinine, renal function tests

Interventions

- *For IM use:* Reconstitute 50,000-unit vial with 9.8 mL 0.9% sodium chloride injection with 2% procaine hydrochloride; reconstitute the 10,000-unit vial with 2 mL of diluent (resulting concentration of 5,000 units/mL). Refrigerate unreconstituted vials. Reconstituted solutions are stable for 1 wk, refrigerated.
- *Topical application:* Cleanse the area before applying new ointment.
- Culture infected area before therapy.
- Ensure adequate hydration to prevent renal toxicity.
- Monitor renal function tests daily during therapy (IM use).

Teaching points

- Give ophthalmic preparation as follows: tilt head back; place medication into eyelid and close eyes; gently hold the inner corner of the eye for 1 min. Do not touch tube to eye. For topical application, cleanse area being treated before applying new ointment; cover with sterile bandage (if possible).
- These side effects may occur: superinfections (frequent hygiene measures, medications may help); burning, stinging, blurring of vision with ophthalmic use (transient).
- Report rash or skin lesions; change in urinary voiding patterns; changes in vision, severe stinging, or itching (ophthalmic).

▽**baclofen**
(**bak'** loe fen)

Apo-Baclofen (CAN), Gen-Baclofen (CAN), Lioresal, Lioresal Intrathecal, Novo-Baclofen (CAN)

PREGNANCY CATEGORY C

Drug class
Centrally acting skeletal muscle relaxant

Therapeutic actions
Precise mechanism not known; GABA analog but does not appear to produce clinical effects by actions on GABA-minergic systems; inhibits both monosynaptic and polysynaptic spinal reflexes; CNS depressant.

Indications

- Alleviation of signs and symptoms of spasticity resulting from multiple sclerosis, particularly for the relief of flexor spasms and concomitant pain, clonus, muscular rigidity (for patients with reversible spasticity to aid in restoring residual function); treatment of central spasticity (via *SynchroMed* pump)
- Spinal cord injuries and other spinal cord diseases—may be of some value
- Unlabeled uses: trigeminal neuralgia (tic douloureux); may be beneficial in reducing spasticity in cerebral palsy in children (intrathecal use)

Contraindications and cautions

- Contraindicated with hypersensitivity to baclofen; skeletal muscle spasm resulting from rheumatic disorders.
- Use cautiously with stroke, cerebral palsy, Parkinson's disease, seizure disorders, lactation.

Available forms
Tablets—10, 20 mg; intrathecal—10 mg/20 mL, 10 mg/5 mL

Dosages
Adults
Oral
Individualize dosage; start at low dosage and increase gradually until optimum effect is

---

Adverse effects in *Italics* are most common; those in **Bold** are life-threatening.

achieved (usually 40–80 mg/day). The following dosage schedule is suggested: 5 mg PO tid for 3 days; 10 mg tid for 3 days; 15 mg tid for 3 days; 20 mg tid for 3 days. Thereafter, additional increases may be needed, but do not exceed 80 mg/day (20 mg qid); use lowest effective dose. If benefits are not evident after a reasonable trial period, gradually withdraw the drug.

Intrathecal

Refer to manufacturer's instructions on pump implantation and initiation of long-term infusion. Testing is usually done with 50 mcg/mL injected into intrathecal space over 1 min. Patient is observed for 24 hr, then dose of 75 mcg/ 1.5 mL is given; final screening bolus of 100 mcg/2 mL is given 24 hr later. Patients who do not respond to this dose are not candidates for the implant. Maintenance dose is determined by monitoring patient response and ranges from 12–1,500 mcg/day. Smallest dose possible to achieve muscle tone without adverse effects is desired.

Pediatric patients

Safety for use in children < 12 yr not established; orphan drug use to decrease spasticity in children with cerebral palsy is being studied.

Geriatric patients or patients with renal impairment

Dosage reduction may be necessary; monitor closely (drug is excreted largely unchanged by the kidneys).

Pharmacokinetics

Route	Onset	Peak	Duration
Oral	1 hr	2 hr	4–8 hr
Intrathecal	30–60 min	4 hr	4–8 hr

Metabolism: Hepatic; $T_{1/2}$: 3–4 hr
Distribution: Crosses placenta; passes into breast milk
Excretion: Urine

Adverse effects

- **CNS:** *Transient drowsiness, dizziness, weakness, fatigue, confusion, headache, insomnia*
- **CV:** *Hypotension*, palpitations
- **GI:** *Nausea, constipation*
- **GU:** *Urinary frequency*, dysuria, enuresis, impotence
- **Other:** Rash, pruritus, ankle edema, excessive perspiration, weight gain, nasal con-

gestion, increased AST, elevated alkaline phosphatase, elevated blood sugar

Interactions

✳ **Drug-drug** • Increased CNS depression with alcohol, other CNS depressants

■ Nursing considerations
Assessment

- **History:** Hypersensitivity to baclofen, skeletal muscle spasm resulting from rheumatic disorders, stroke, cerebral palsy, Parkinson's disease, seizure disorders, lactation
- **Physical:** Weight; T; skin color, lesions; orientation, affect, reflexes, bilateral grip strength; visual exam; P, BP; bowel sounds, normal GI output, liver evaluation; normal urinary output; liver and kidney function tests, blood and urine glucose

Interventions

- Patients given implantable device for intrathecal delivery need to learn about the programmable delivery system, frequent checks; how to adjust dose and programming.
- Give with caution to patients whose spasticity contributes to upright posture or balance in locomotion or whenever spasticity is used to increase function.
- Taper dosage gradually to prevent hallucinations, possible psychosis, or other serious effects.

Teaching points

- Take this drug exactly as prescribed. Do not stop taking this drug without consulting your health care provider; abrupt discontinuation may cause hallucinations or other serious effects.
- Avoid alcohol, sleep-inducing, or OTC drugs because these could cause dangerous effects.
- These side effects may occur: drowsiness, dizziness, confusion (avoid driving or engaging in activities that require alertness); nausea (frequent small meals may help); insomnia, headache, painful or frequent urination (effects reversible; will go away when the drug is discontinued).
- Do not take this drug during pregnancy. If you decide to become pregnant or find that you are pregnant, consult your health care provider.

- Report frequent or painful urination, constipation, nausea, headache, insomnia, confusion that persist or are severe.

▷balsalazide disodium
(bal sal' a zyde)

Colazal

PREGNANCY CATEGORY B

Drug class
Antiflammatory

Therapeutic actions
Mechanism of action is unknown; thought to be direct, delivered intact to the colon; a local anti-inflammatory effect occurs in the colon where balsalazide is converted to mesalamine (5-ASA), which blocks cyclooxygenase and inhibits prostaglandin production in the colon.

Indications
- Treatment of mildly to moderately active ulcerative colitis

Contraindications and cautions
- Contraindicated in the presence of hypersensitivity to salicylates or mesalamine.
- Use cautiously in the presence of renal dysfunction, pregnancy, lactation.

Available forms
Capsules—750 mg

Dosages
Adults
Three 750 mg capsules PO tid for a total daily dose of 6.75 g. Continue for 8 wk.
Pediatric patients
Safety and efficacy not established.

Pharmacokinetics

Route	Onset	Peak
Oral	Varies	1–2 hr

Metabolism: Hepatic; $T_{1/2}$: unknown
Distribution: Crosses placenta; may pass into breast milk
Excretion: Feces and urine

Adverse effects
- **CNS:** *Headache, fatigue, malaise, depression,* dizziness, asthenia, insomnia
- **GI:** *Abdominal pain, cramps, vomiting, discomfort; gas; flatulence; nausea; diarrhea, dyspepsia,* bloating, hemorrhoids, rectal pain, constipation, diarrhea, dry mouth
- **Other:** *Flu-like symptoms, rash,* fever, cold, back pain, peripheral edema, *arthralgia*

■ Nursing considerations

 CLINICAL ALERT!
Name confusion has occurred between Colazal (balsalazide) and Clozaril (clozapine). Serious effects have occurred; use extreme caution.

Assessment
- **History:** Hypersensitivity to salicylates; renal dysfunction; pregnancy, lactation.
- **Physical:** Temperature, hair status; reflexes, affect; abdominal exam, rectal exam; urinary output, renal function tests

Interventions
- Administer with meals. May be given for up to 8 wk.
- Monitor patients with renal impairment for possible adverse effects.
- Ensure ready access to bathroom facilities if diarrhea occurs.
- Offer support and encouragement to deal with GI discomfort, CNS effects.
- Arrange for appropriate measures to deal with headache, arthralgia, GI problems.
- Provide small, frequent meals if GI upset is severe.
- Maintain all therapy (dietary restrictions, reduced stress, etc.) necessary to support remission of the ulcerative colitis.

Teaching points
- Take the drug with meals in evenly divided doses.
- Know that these side effects may occur: abdominal cramping, discomfort, pain, diarrhea (ensure ready access to bathroom facilities, taking the drug with meals may help), headache, fatigue, fever, flu-like symptoms (consult with health care provider if

these become bothersome, medications may be available to help); rash, itching (skin care may help; consult your health care provider if this becomes a problem).
- Report: severe diarrhea, malaise, fatigue, fever, blood in the stool.
- Maintain all of the usual restrictions and therapy that apply to your colitis. If this becomes difficult, consult with your health care provider.

▽ basiliximab

See *Less Commonly Used Drugs,* p. 1338.

▽ BCG intravesical

See *Less Commonly Used Drugs,* p. 1338.

▽ beclomethasone dipropionate
(be kloe meth' a sone)

Apo-Beclomethasone (CAN), Beclodisk (CAN), Becloforte Inhaler (CAN), Beclovent Rotacaps (CAN), Beconase Inhalation, Beconase AQ Nasal Spray, Propaderm (CAN), QVAR, Vancenase, Vancenase AQ, Vancenase AQ Nasal, Vancenase Pockethaler, Vanceril, Vanceril Double Strength

PREGNANCY CATEGORY C

Drug classes
Corticosteroid
Glucocorticoid
Hormonal agent

Therapeutic actions
Anti-inflammatory effects; local administration into lower respiratory tract or nasal passages maximizes beneficial effects on these tissues while decreasing the likelihood of adverse corticosteroid effects from systemic absorption.

Indications
- *Respiratory inhalant use:* Control of bronchial asthma that requires corticosteroids along with other therapy

- *Intranasal use:* Relief of symptoms of seasonal or perennial rhinitis that respond poorly to other treatments; prevention of recurrence of nasal polyps following surgical removal

Contraindications and cautions
- *Respiratory inhalant therapy:* Acute asthmatic attack, status asthmaticus, systemic fungal infections (may cause excerbations), allergy to any ingredient, lactation
- *Intranasal therapy:* Untreated local infections (may cause exacerbations); nasal septal ulcers, recurrent epistaxis, nasal surgery or trauma (interferes with healing); lactation

Available forms
Aerosol—42 mcg/actuation, 84 mcg/actuation; nasal spray—0.042%, 0.084%

Dosages
Respiratory inhalant use
50 mcg released at the valve delivers 42 mcg to the patient.
Adults
Two inhalations (84–168 mcg) tid or qid. In severe asthma, start with 12 to 16 inhalations per day, and adjust dosage downward. Do not exceed 20 inhalations (840 mcg/day).
Pediatric patients 5–11 yr
1 or 2 inhalations tid or qid, not to exceed 10 inhalations (420 mcg/day). Do not use in children < 5 yr.
Intranasal therapy
Each actuation delivers 42 or 84 mcg. Discontinue therapy after 3 wk if no significant symptomatic improvement.
Adults
One inhalation (42–84 mcg) in each nostril bid–qid (total dose 168–336 mcg/day).
Pediatric patients 6–11 yr
One inhalation in each nostril bid–qid.

Pharmacokinetics

Route	Onset	Peak
Inhalation	Rapid	1–2 wk

Metabolism: Lungs, GI, and liver; $T_{1/2}$: 3–15 hr
Distribution: Crosses placenta; may pass into breast milk
Excretion: Feces

Adverse effects
Respiratory inhalant use
- **Endocrine:** Cushing's syndrome with overdose, suppression of hypothalamic-pituitary-adrenal (HPA) function due to systemic absorption
- **Local:** *Oral, laryngeal, pharyngeal irritation,* fungal infections
Intranasal use
- **Local:** *Nasal irritation,* fungal infections
- **Respiratory:** *Epistaxis, rebound congestion,* perforation of the nasal septum, anosmia
- **Other:** *Headache, nausea,* urticaria

■ Nursing considerations
Assessment
- **History:** Acute asthmatic attack, status asthmaticus; systemic fungal infections; allergy to any ingredient; lactation; untreated local infections, nasal septal ulcers, recurrent epistaxis, nasal surgery or trauma
- **Physical:** Weight; T; P, BP, auscultation; R, adventitious sounds; chest x-ray before respiratory inhalant therapy; exam of nares before intranasal therapy

Interventions
- Taper systemic steroids carefully during transfer to inhalational steroids; deaths resulting from adrenal insufficiency have occurred during and after transfer from systemic to aerosol steroids.
- Use decongestant nose drops to facilitate penetration of intranasal steroids if edema, excessive secretions are present.

Teaching points
- This respiratory inhalant has been prescribed to prevent asthmatic attacks, not for use during an attack.
- Allow at least 1 min between puffs (respiratory inhalant); if you also are using an inhalational bronchodilator (isoproterenol, metaproterenol, epinephrine), use it several minutes before using the steroid aerosol.
- Rinse your mouth after using the respiratory inhalant aerosol.
- Use a decongestant before the intranasal steroid, and clear your nose of all secretions if nasal passages are blocked; intranasal

steroids may take several days to produce full benefit.
- Use this product exactly as prescribed; do not take more than prescribed, and do not stop taking the drug without consulting your health care provider. The drug must not be stopped abruptly but must be slowly tapered.
- These side effects may occur: local irritation (use the device correctly), headache (consult your health care provider for treatment).
- Report sore throat or sore mouth.

▷ benazepril hydrochloride
(ben a' za pril)

Lotensin

PREGNANCY CATEGORY C (FIRST TRIMESTER)

PREGNANCY CATEGORY D (SECOND, THIRD TRIMESTERS)

Drug classes
Antihypertensive
Angiotensin-converting enzyme (ACE) inhibitor

Therapeutic actions
Blocks ACE from converting angiotensin I to angiotensin II, a potent vasoconstrictor, leading to decreased BP, decreased aldosterone secretion, a small increase in serum potassium levels, and sodium and fluid loss; increased prostaglandin synthesis also may be involved in the antihypertensive action.

Indications
- Treatment of hypertension alone or in combination with thiazide-type diuretics

Contraindications and cautions
- Contraindicated with allergy to benazepril or other ACE inhibitors.
- Use cautiously with impaired renal function, CHF, salt or volume depletion, lactation.

Available forms
Tablets—5, 10, 20, 40 mg

Adverse effects in *Italics* are most common; those in **Bold** are life-threatening.

Dosages

Adults
Initial dose: 10 mg PO daily. Maintenance dose: 20–40 mg/day PO, single or two divided doses. Patients using diuretics should discontinue them 2–3 days prior to benazepril therapy. If BP is not controlled, add diuretic slowly. If diuretic cannot be discontinued, begin benazepril therapy with 5 mg.

Pediatric patients
Safety and efficacy not established.

Patients with renal impairment
Creatinine clearance < 30 mL/min (serum creatinine > 3 mg/dL): 5 mg PO daily. Dosage may be titrated upward until blood pressure is controlled up to a maximum of 40 mg/day.

Pharmacokinetics

Route	Onset	Peak	Duration
Oral	0.5–1 hr	3–4 hr	24 hr

Metabolism: Hepatic; $T_{1/2}$: 10–11 hr
Distribution: Crosses placenta; passes into breast milk
Excretion: Urine

Adverse effects

- **CV:** Angina pectoris, hypotension in salt or volume-depleted patients, palpitations
- **Dermatologic:** Rash, pruritus, diaphoresis, flushing
- **GI:** *Nausea,* abdominal pain, vomiting, constipation
- **Respiratory:** *Cough,* asthma, bronchitis, dyspnea, sinusitis
- **Other:** Angioedema, impotence, decreased libido, asthenia, myalgia, arthralgia

Interactions

✳ **Drug-drug** ● Increased risk of hypersensitivity reactions with allopurinal ● Increased coughing with capsaicin ● Decreased antihypertensive effects with indomethacin ● Increased lithium levels and neurotoxicity may occur if combined ● Increased risk of hyperkalemia with potassium-sparing diuretics or potassium supplements

■ Nursing considerations
Assessment

- **History:** Allergy to benazepril or other ACE inhibitors, impaired renal function, CHF, salt or volume depletion, lactation, pregnancy
- **Physical:** Skin color, lesions, turgor; T; P, BP, peripheral perfusion; mucous membranes, bowel sounds, liver evaluation; urinalysis, renal and liver function tests, CBC and differential

Interventions

- Alert surgeon: Note use of benazepril on patient's chart; the angiotensin II formation subsequent to compensatory renin release during surgery will be blocked; hypotension may be reversed with volume expansion.
- Monitor patient for possible fall in BP secondary to reduction in fluid volume (excessive perspiration and dehydration, vomiting, diarrhea) because excessive hypotension may occur.
- Reduce dosage in patients with impaired renal function.

Teaching points

- Do not stop taking the medication without consulting your health care provider.
- These side effects may occur: GI upset, loss of appetite (transient effects; if persistent consult health care provider); light-headedness (transient; change position slowly, and limit activities to those that do not require alertness and precision); dry cough (irritating but not harmful; consult health care provider).
- Be careful in any situation that may lead to a drop in blood pressure (diarrhea, sweating, vomiting, dehydration); if light-headedness or dizziness occurs, consult your health care provider.
- Report mouth sores; sore throat, fever, chills; swelling of the hands, feet; irregular heartbeat, chest pains; swelling of the face, eyes, lips, tongue, difficulty breathing, persistent cough.

▽ **bendroflumethiazide**
*(ben droe floo meh **thye'** a zide)*

Naturetin

PREGNANCY CATEGORY C

Drug class
Thiazide diuretic

Therapeutic actions

Inhibits reabsorption of sodium and chloride in distal renal tubule, increasing the excretion of sodium, chloride, and water by the kidney.

Indications

- Adjunctive therapy in edema associated with CHF
- Hypertension, as sole therapy or in combination with other antihypertensives
- Unlabeled uses: calcium nephrolithiasis alone or with amiloride or allopurinal to prevent recurrences in hypercalciuric or normal calciuric patients; diabetes insipidus, especially nephrogenic diabetes insipidus

Contraindications and cautions

- Contraindicated with allergy to thiazides, sulfonamides; fluid or electrolyte imbalance; renal disease (risk of azotemia with thiazides); liver disease (thiazide-induced alterations in fluid and electrolyte balance may precipitate hepatic coma); gout (risk of precipitation of attack).
- Use cautiously with SLE; glucose tolerance abnormalities, diabetes mellitus; hyperparathyroidism; manic-depressive disorders aggravated by hypercalcemia; lactation.

Available forms

Tablets—5, 10 mg

Dosages

Adults
- *Edema:* 5 mg PO daily, best in the morning. Up to 20 mg once a day or divided into two doses.
- *Maintenance:* 2.5–5 mg PO daily. Intermittent therapy may be best for some patients; every other day or a 3- to 5-day/wk schedule.
- *Hypertension:* Initial: 5–20 mg/day PO. Maintenance: 2.5–15 mg/day PO.

Pediatric patients
Safety and efficacy not established.

Pharmacokinetics

Route	Onset	Peak	Duration
Oral	2 hr	4 hr	6–12 hr

Metabolism: Hepatic; T$_{1/2}$: 3–4 hr
Distribution: Crosses placenta; passes into breast milk
Excretion: Unchanged in the urine

Adverse effects

- **CNS:** *Dizziness, vertigo,* paresthesias, weakness, headache, blurred vision
- **CV:** Orthostatic hypotension
- **Dermatologic:** Photosensitivity, rash, purpura, exfoliative dermatitis, hives
- **Endocrine:** Hyperglycemia, hyperuricemia, glycosuria
- **GI:** *Nausea, anorexia, vomiting, dry mouth,* diarrhea, constipation, jaundice, hepatitis, pancreatitis
- **GU:** Impotence, loss of libido
- **Other:** Muscle cramps and muscle spasms, fever, gouty attacks, flushing, weight loss, rhinorrhea

Interactions

✳ **Drug-drug** • Increased thiazide effects with diazoxide • Decreased absorption with cholestyramine, colestipol • Increased risk of cardiac glycoside toxicity if hypokalemia occurs • Increased risk of lithium toxicity • Decreased effectiveness of antidiabetic agents with bendroflumethiazide

✳ **Drug-lab test** • Decreased PBI levels without clinical signs of thyroid disturbance • Increased creatinine, BUN

■ Nursing considerations

Assessment

- **History:** Allergy to thiazides, sulfonamides; fluid or electrolyte imbalance, renal or liver disease; gout; SLE; glucose tolerance abnormalities, diabetes mellitus; hyperparathyroidism; manic-depressive disorders; lactation
- **Physical:** Skin color, lesions, edema; orientation, reflexes, muscle strength; pulses, baseline ECG, BP, orthostatic BP, perfusion; R, pattern, adventitious sounds; liver evaluation, bowel sounds; urinary output patterns; CBC, serum electrolytes, blood glucose, liver and renal function tests, serum uric acid, urinalysis

Interventions

- Give with food or milk for GI upset.

B

- Mark calendars or use other reminders of drug days if every other day or 3–5 days/wk therapy is best for treating edema.
- Reduce dosage of other antihypertensive drugs by at least 50% if given with thiazides; readjust dosages gradually as BP responds.
- Give early in the day so increased urination will not disturb sleep; monitor weight.

Teaching points
- Record dates on a calendar or dated envelopes for use as intermittent therapy.
- Take the drug early in the day so increased urination will not disturb sleep.
- Take with food or meals if GI upset occurs.
- Weigh yourself on a regular basis at the same time of the day and in the same clothing, and record the weight on your calendar.
- These side effects may occur: increased volume and frequency of urination; dizziness, feeling faint on arising, drowsiness (avoid rapid position changes, hazardous activities: driving a car and using alcohol); sensitivity to sunlight (use sunglasses, wear protective clothing, or use a sunscreen); decrease in sexual function; increased thirst (sucking on sugarless lozenges, frequent mouth care may help).
- Report change of more than 3 lb in 1 day, swelling in your ankles or fingers, unusual bleeding or bruising, dizziness, trembling, numbness, fatigue, muscle weakness or cramps.

▽benzonatate
(ben zoe' na tate)

Benzonatate Softgels, Tessalon Perles

PREGNANCY CATEGORY C

Drug class
Antitussive (non-narcotic)

Therapeutic actions
Related to the local anesthetic tetracaine; anesthetizes the stretch receptors in the respiratory passages, lungs, and pleura, hampering their activity and reducing the cough reflex at its source.

Indications
- Symptomatic relief of nonproductive cough

Contraindications and cautions
- Allergy to benzonatate or related compounds (tetracaine); lactation

Available forms
Capsules—100 mg

Dosages
Adult and patients > 10 yr
100–200 mg PO tid; up to 600 mg/day may be used.

Pharmacokinetics

Route	Onset	Duration
Oral	15–20 min	3–8 hr

Metabolism: Hepatic
Distribution: Crosses placenta; may pass into breast milk
Excretion: Urine

Adverse effects
- **CNS:** *Sedation, headache, mild dizziness,* nasal congestion, sensation of burning in the eyes
- **Dermatologic:** Pruritus, skin eruptions
- **GI:** *Constipation, nausea,* GI upset
- **Other:** Vague "chilly" feeling, numbness in the chest

■ Nursing considerations
Assessment
- **History:** Allergy to benzonatate or related compounds (tetracaine); lactation
- **Physical:** Nasal mucous membranes; skin color, lesions; orientation, affect; adventitious sounds

Interventions
- Administer orally; caution patient not to chew or break capsules but to swallow them whole.

Teaching points
- Swallow the capsules whole; do not chew or break capsules because numbness of the throat and mouth could occur, and swallowing could become difficult.
- These side effects may occur: rash, itching (skin care may help); constipation, nausea,

upset; sedation, dizziness (avoid driving or tasks that require alertness).
- Report restlessness, tremor, difficulty breathing, constipation, rash.

▷ benzthiazide
(benz thye' a zide)

Exna

PREGNANCY CATEGORY C

Drug class
Thiazide diuretic

Therapeutic actions
Inhibits reabsorption of sodium and chloride in distal renal tubule, increasing excretion of sodium, chloride, and water by the kidney.

Indications
- Adjunctive therapy in edema associated with CHF, cirrhosis, corticosteroid and estrogen therapy, renal dysfunction
- *Hypertension:* alone or with other antihypertensives
- Unlabeled use: diabetes insipidus, especially nephrogenic diabetes insipidus

Contraindications and cautions
- Contraindicated with allergy to thiazides, sulfonamides; fluid or electrolyte imbalance; renal disease (risk of azotemia with thiazides); liver disease (thiazide-induced alterations in fluid and electrolyte balance may precipitate hepatic coma); gout (risk of attack).
- Use cautiously with SLE; glucose tolerance abnormalities, diabetes mellitus; hyperparathyroidism; manic-depressive disorders aggravated by hypercalcemia; lactation.

Available forms
Tablets—50 mg

Dosages
Adults
- *Edema:* Initially 50–200 mg PO daily for several days. Administer dosages > 100 mg/day in two divided doses. Maintenance: 50–150 mg daily.

- *Hypertension:* Initially 50–100 mg PO daily in two doses of 25 or 50 mg each after breakfast and after lunch. Maintenance: individualize to patient's response; maximum dose of 200 mg/day.

Pharmacokinetics

Route	Onset	Peak	Duration
Oral	2 hr	4–6 hr	6–18 hr

Metabolism: Hepatic; $T_{1/2}$: unknown
Distribution: Crosses placenta; passes into breast milk
Excretion: Urine

Adverse effects
- **CNS:** *Dizziness, vertigo,* paresthesias, weakness, headache, blurred vision
- **CV:** Orthostatic hypotension
- **Dermatologic:** Photosensitivity, rash, purpura, exfoliative dermatitis, hives
- **Endocrine:** Hyperglycemia, hyperuricemia, glycosuria
- **GI:** *Nausea, anorexia, vomiting, dry mouth,* diarrhea, constipation, jaundice, hepatitis, pancreatitis
- **GU:** Impotence, loss of libido
- **Other:** Muscle cramps and muscle spasms, fever, gouty attacks, flushing, weight loss, rhinorrhea

Interactions
✷ **Drug-drug** • Increased thiazide effects if taken with diazoxide • Decreased absorption with cholestyramine, colestipol • Increased risk of cardiac glycoside toxicity if hypokalemia occurs • Increased risk of lithium toxicity • Decreased effectiveness of antidiabetic agents when taken concurrently with benzthiazide
✷ **Drug-lab test** • Decreased PBI levels without clinical signs of thyroid disturbance • Increased creatinine, BUN

■ Nursing considerations
Assessment
- **History:** Allergy to thiazides, sulfonamides; fluid or electrolyte imbalance, renal or liver disease; gout; SLE; glucose tolerance abnormalities, diabetes mellitus; hyperpara-

thyroidism; manic-depressive disorders; lactation
- **Physical:** Skin color, lesions, edema; orientation, reflexes, muscle strength; pulses, baseline ECG, BP, orthostatic BP, perfusion; R, pattern, adventitious sounds; liver evaluation, bowel sounds; urinary output patterns; CBC, serum electrolytes, blood glucose, liver and renal function tests, serum uric acid, urinalysis

Interventions

- Administer early in the day so increased urination will not disturb sleep; administer with food or milk if GI upset occurs.

Teaching points

- Take the drug early in the day so increased urination will not disturb sleep. May be taken with food or meals if GI upset occurs.
- Weigh yourself on a regular basis, at the same time and in the same clothing, and record the weight on calendar.
- These side effects may occur: increased volume and frequency of urination; dizziness, feeling faint on arising, drowsiness (avoid rapid position changes; hazardous activities, such as driving and alcohol); sensitivity to sunlight (use sunglasses, wear protective clothing, or use a sunscreen); decrease in sexual function; increased thirst (suck sugarless lozenges, use frequent mouth care).
- Report weight change of more than 3 lb in 1 day, swelling in ankles or fingers, unusual bleeding or bruising, dizziness, trembling, numbness, fatigue, muscle weakness or cramps.

▷benztropine mesylate
(benz' troe peen)

Apo-Benztropine (CAN), Cogentin, PMS Benztropine (CAN)

PREGNANCY CATEGORY C

Drug class

Antiparkinsonian drug (anticholinergic type)

Therapeutic actions

Has anticholinergic activity in the CNS that is believed to help normalize the hypothesized imbalance of cholinergic and dopaminergic neurotransmission in the basal ganglia of the brain of a parkinsonism patient. Reduces severity of rigidity and, to a lesser extent, akinesia and tremor; less effective overall than levodopa; peripheral anticholinergic effects suppress secondary symptoms of parkinsonism, such as drooling.

Indications

- Adjunct in the therapy of parkinsonism (postencephalitic, arteriosclerotic, and idiopathic types)
- Control of extrapyramidal disorders (except tardive dyskinesia) due to neuroleptic drugs (phenothiazines)

Contraindications and cautions

- Contraindicated with hypersensitivity to benztropine; glaucoma, especially angle-closure glaucoma; pyloric or duodenal obstruction, stenosing peptic ulcers, achalasia (megaesophagus); prostatic hypertrophy or bladder neck obstructions; myasthenia gravis.
- Use cautiously with tachycardia, cardiac arrhythmias, hypertension, hypotension, hepatic or renal dysfunction, alcoholism, chronic illness, work in hot environments; hot weather; lactation.

Available forms

Tablets—0.5, 1, 2 mg; injection—1 mg/mL

Dosages
Adults

- *Parkinsonism:* Initially 0.5–1 mg PO hs; a total daily dose of 0.5–6 mg given hs or in two to four divided doses is usual. Increase initial dose in 0.5-mg increments at 5- to 6-day intervals to the smallest amount necessary for optimal relief. Maximum daily dose is 6 mg. May be given IM or IV in same dosage as oral. When used with other drugs, gradually substitute benztropine for all or part of them and gradually reduce dosage of the other drug.
- *Drug-induced extrapyramidal symptoms:* Acute dystonic reactions: Initially 1–2 mg IM (preferred) or IV to control condition; may repeat if parkinsonian effect begins to

1–2 mg PO bid to prevent

*...idal disorders occurring ear-
...roleptic treatment:* 1–2 mg PO
...d. Withdraw drug after 1 or 2 wk to determine its continued need; reinstitute if disorder reappears.

B

Pediatric patients
Safety and efficacy not established.

Geriatric patients
Strict dosage regulation may be necessary; patients > 60 yr often develop increased sensitivity to the CNS effects of anticholinergic drugs.

Pharmacokinetics

Route	Onset	Duration
Oral	1 hr	6–10 hr
IM, IV	15 min	6–10 hr

Metabolism: Hepatic
Distribution: Crosses placenta; passes into
breast milk

▼IV facts
Preparation: Give undiluted. Store in tightly covered, light-resistant container. Store at
room temperature.
Infusion: Administer direct IV at a rate of
1 mg over 1 min.

Adverse effects
Peripheral anticholinergic effects
- **CV:** Tachycardia, palpitations, hypotension,
orthostatic hypotension
- **Dermatologic:** Rash, urticaria, other dermatoses
- **EENT:** *Blurred vision,* mydriasis, diplopia, increased intraocular tension, angle-
closure glaucoma
- **GI:** *Dry mouth, constipation,* dilation of
the colon, paralytic ileus, *nausea,* vomiting, epigastric distress
- **GU:** *Urinary retention, urinary hesitancy,* dysuria, difficulty achieving or maintaining an erection
- **Other:** Flushing, decreased sweating, elevated temperature
*CNS effects, characteristic of centrally
acting anticholinergic drugs*
- **CNS:** *Disorientation, confusion,* memory
loss, hallucinations, psychoses, agitation,

nervousness, delusions, delirium, paranoia,
euphoria, excitement, light-headedness,
dizziness, depression, drowsiness, weakness, giddiness, paresthesia, heaviness of the
limbs
- **Other:** Muscular weakness, muscular
cramping; inability to move certain muscle
groups (high doses), numbness of fingers

Interactions
✳ **Drug-drug** • Paralytic ileus, sometimes
fatal, when given with other anticholinergic
drugs, or drugs that have anticholinergic properties (phenothiazines, TCAs) • Additive adverse CNS effects (toxic psychosis) with other
drugs that have CNS anticholinergic properties (TCAs, phenothiazines) • Possible masking of the development of persistent extrapyramidal symptoms, tardive dyskinesia, in
patients on long-term therapy with antipsychotic drugs (phenothiazines, haloperidol)
• Decreased therapeutic efficacy of antipsychotic drugs (phenothiazines, haloperidol),
possibly due to central antagonism

■ Nursing considerations
Assessment
- **History:** Hypersensitivity to benztropine;
glaucoma; pyloric or duodenal obstruction,
stenosing peptic ulcers, achalasia; prostatic
hypertrophy or bladder neck obstructions;
myasthenia gravis; cardiac arrhythmias, hypertension, hypotension; hepatic or renal
dysfunction; alcoholism, chronic illness,
people who work in hot environments; lactation
- **Physical:** Weight; T; skin color, lesions; orientation, affect, reflexes, bilateral grip
strength, visual exam including tonometry;
P, BP, orthostatic BP; adventitious sounds;
bowel sounds, normal output, liver evaluation; normal urinary output, voiding pattern, prostate palpation; liver and kidney
function tests

Interventions
- Decrease dosage or discontinue temporarily if dry mouth makes swallowing or speaking difficult.
- Give with caution and reduce dosage in hot
weather. Drug interferes with sweating and

Adverse effects in *Italics* are most common; those in **Bold** are life-threatening.

body's ability to maintain heat equilibrium; provide sugarless lozenges, ice chips to suck for dry mouth.

- Give with meals if GI upset occurs; give before meals for dry mouth; give after meals if drooling or nausea occur.
- Ensure patient voids before receiving each dose if urinary retention is a problem.

Teaching points

- Take this drug exactly as prescribed.
- Avoid alcohol, sedatives, and OTC drugs (could cause dangerous effects).
- These side effects may occur: drowsiness, dizziness, confusion, blurred vision (avoid driving, engaging in activities that require alertness and visual acuity); nausea (try frequent small meals); dry mouth (suck sugarless lozenges or ice chips); painful or difficult urination (empty bladder immediately before each dose); constipation (maintain adequate fluid intake and exercise regularly); use caution in hot weather (you are susceptible to heat prostration).
- Report difficult or painful urination; constipation; rapid or pounding heartbeat; confusion, eye pain, or rash.

---

bepridil hydrochloride
(beh' pri dil)

Vascor

PREGNANCY CATEGORY C

Drug classes
Calcium channel-blocker
Antianginal drug

Therapeutic actions
Inhibits the movement of calcium ions across the membranes of cardiac and arterial muscle cells; inhibition of transmembrane calcium flow results in the depression of impulse formation in specialized cardiac pacemaker cells, slowing of the velocity of conduction of the cardiac impulse, depression of myocardial contractility, and dilation of coronary arteries and arterioles and peripheral arterioles; these effects lead to decreased cardiac work, decreased cardiac energy consumption, and

bepridil hydro~~~

176

in patients with va~~~ angina, increased de~~~ diac cells.

Indications
- Chronic stable angina in those~~~ sive to or intolerant of other antia~~~ can cause serious arrhythmias and a~~~ ulocytosis

Contraindications and cautions
- Allergy to bepridil, sick sinus syndrome, heart block (second or third degree), hypotension, history of serious ventricular arrhythmias, uncompensated CHF, congenital QT interval prolongation, lactation.

Available forms
Tablets—200, 300 mg

Dosages
Adults
Individualize dosage. Initially 200 mg/day PO. After 10 days, dosage may be adjusted upward. Maintenance: 300 mg/day PO. Maximum daily dose is 400 mg.
Pediatric patients
Safety and efficacy not established.
Geriatric patients
Same starting dose as adult dosage; monitor more closely for adverse effects.

Pharmacokinetics

Route	Onset	Peak
Oral	60 min	2–3 hr

Metabolism: Hepatic; $T_{1/2}$: 24 hr
Distribution: Crosses placenta; passes into breast milk
Excretion: Urine

Adverse effects
- **CNS:** *Dizziness, light-headedness, nervousness, headache, asthenia,* fatigue
- **CV:** *Peripheral edema,* hypotension, arrhythmias, *bradycardia, AV block,* **ventricular tachycardia, asystole**
- **Dermatologic:** *Rash*
- **GI:** *Nausea,* hepatic injury, *constipation*
- **Hematologic: Agranulocytosis**

■ **beractant**

actions

rug-drug • Cumulative negative chronotropic effects and decreased heart rate with goxin

■ Nursing considerations

CLINICAL ALERT!
Name confusion has occurred between bepridil and Prepidil (dinoprostone); use extreme caution.

Assessment
- **History:** Allergy to bepridil, sick sinus syndrome, heart block, hypotension, history of serious ventricular arrhythmias, uncompensated CHF, congenital QT interval prolongation, lactation
- **Physical:** Skin lesions, color, edema; P, BP, baseline ECG, peripheral perfusion, auscultation, R, adventitious sounds; liver evaluation, GI normal output; liver and renal function tests, CBC

Interventions
- Give only if unresponsive to or intolerant of other antianginal drugs.
- Monitor patient carefully (BP, cardiac rhythm, and output) during adjustment to therapeutic dose; dosage may be increased more rapidly in hospital under close supervision.
- Monitor BP carefully if patient is also on nitrates.
- Monitor cardiac rhythm and CBC regularly during stabilization of dosage and periodically during long-term therapy.

Teaching points
- Take this drug exactly as prescribed.
- These side effects may occur: nausea, vomiting (small, frequent meals may help); headache (adjust lighting, noise, and temperature; medication may be ordered if this becomes severe); dizziness, shakiness (avoid driving or operating dangerous machinery).
- Report irregular heartbeat, shortness of breath, swelling of the hands or feet, pronounced dizziness, constipation, unusual bleeding or bruising.

▷ **beractant (natural lung surfactant)**
(ber ak' tant)

Survanta

Drug class
Lung surfactant

Therapeutic actions
A natural bovine compound containing lipids and apoproteins that reduce surface tension and allow expansion of the alveoli; replaces the surfactant missing in the lungs of neonates suffering from respiratory distress syndrome (RDS).

Indications
- Prophylactic treatment of infants at risk of developing RDS; infants with birth weights < 1,250 g or infants with birth weights > 1,250 g who have evidence of pulmonary immaturity
- Rescue treatment of infants who have developed RDS

Contraindications and cautions
- Because beractant is used as an emergency drug in acute respiratory situations, the benefits usually outweigh any possible risks.

Available forms
Suspension—25 mg/mL suspended in 0.9% sodium chloride injection

Dosages
Accurate determination of birth weight is essential for correct dosage. Beractant is instilled into the trachea using a catheter inserted into the endotracheal tube.
- *Prophylactic treatment:* Give first dose of 100 mg phospholipids/kg birth weight (4 mL/kg) soon after birth. Four doses can be administered in the first 48 hr of life. Give no more frequently than q 6 hr.
- *Rescue treatment:* Administer 100 mg phospholipids/kg birth weight (4 mL/kg) intratracheally. Administer the first dose as soon as possible after the diagnosis of RDS is made and patient is on the ventilator. Repeat doses can be given based on clinical improve-

Adverse effects in *Italics* are most common; those in **Bold** are life-threatening.

ment and blood gases. Administer subsequent doses no sooner than q 6 hr.

Pharmacokinetics

Route	Onset	Peak
Intratracheal	Immediate	Hrs

Metabolism: Normal surfactant metabolic pathways; $T_{1/2}$: unknown
Distribution: Lung tissue

Adverse effects

- **CNS:** Seizures
- **CV:** *Patent ductus arteriosus,* **intraventricular hemorrhage, hypotension, bradycardia**
- **Hematologic:** Hyperbilirubinemia, thrombocytopenia
- **Respiratory: Pneumothorax, pulmonary air leak, pulmonary hemorrhage,** apnea, pneumomediastinum, emphysema
- **Other:** *Sepsis, nonpulmonary infections*

■ Nursing considerations
Assessment

- **History:** Time of birth, exact birth weight
- **Physical:** Skin temperature, color; R, adventitious sounds, oximeter, endotracheal tube position and patency, chest movement; ECG, P, BP, peripheral perfusion, arterial pressure (desirable); oxygen saturation, blood gases, CBC; muscular activity, facial expression, reflexes

Interventions

- Monitor ECG and transcutaneous oxygen saturation continually during administration.
- Ensure that endotracheal tube is in the correct position, with bilateral chest movement and lung sounds.
- Have staff view manufacturer's teaching video before regular use to cover all the technical aspects of administration.
- Suction the infant immediately before administration, but do not suction for 2 hr after administration unless clinically necessary.
- Visually inspect vial for discoloration. Color should be off-white to brown liquid. Gentle mixing should be attempted. Warm to room temperature before using—20 min or 8 min by hand. Do not use other warming methods.

- Store drug in refrigerator. Protect from light. Enter drug vial only once. Discard remaining drug after use.
- Insert 5 French catheter into the endotracheal tube; do not instill into the mainstem bronchus.
- Instill dose slowly; inject one-fourth dose over 2–3 sec; remove catheter and reattach infant to ventilator for at least 30 sec or until stable; repeat procedure administering one-fourth dose at a time.
- Do not suction infant for 1 hr after completion of full dose; do not flush catheter.
- Continually monitor patient's color, lung sounds, ECG, oximeter, and blood gas readings during administration and for at least 30 min after.

Teaching points

- Details of drug effects and administration are best incorporated into parents' comprehensive teaching program.

▽betaine anhydrous

See *Less Commonly Used Drugs,* p. 1338.

▽betamethasone
*(bay ta **meth'** a sone)*

betamethasone benzoate
Topical dermatologic ointment, cream, lotion, gel: Bepen (CAN), Uticort

betamethasone dipropionate
Topical dermatologic ointment, cream, lotion, aerosol: Alphatrex, Diprolene, Diprolene AF, Diprosone, Maxivate, Occlucort (CAN), Taro-Sone (CAN), Teladar

betamethasone sodium phosphate
Systemic, including IV and local injection: Betnesol (CAN), Celestone Phosphate

betamethasone sodium phosphate and acetate
Systemic, IM, and local intra-articular, intralesional, intradermal injection: Celestone Soluspan

betamethasone valerate
Topical dermatologic ointment, cream, lotion: Betacort (CAN), Betaderm (CAN), Betatrex, Beta-Val, Betnovate (CAN), Celestoderm (CAN), Luxiq, Prevex B (CAN), Psorlon Cream, Valisone

PREGNANCY CATEGORY C

Drug classes
Corticosteroid (long acting)
Glucocorticoid
Hormonal agent

Therapeutic actions
Binds to intracellular corticosteroid receptors, thereby initiating many natural complex reactions that are responsible for its anti-inflammatory and immunosuppressive effects.

Indications
- *Systemic administration:* Hypercalcemia associated with cancer
- Short-term management of inflammatory and allergic disorders, such as rheumatoid arthritis, collagen diseases (eg, SLE), dermatologic diseases (eg, pemphigus), status asthmaticus, and autoimmune disorders
- *Hematologic disorders:* Thrombocytopenia purpura, erythroblastopenia
- Ulcerative colitis, acute exacerbations of multiple sclerosis, and palliation in some leukemias and lymphomas
- Trichinosis with neurologic or myocardial involvement
- Unlabeled use: Prevention of respiratory distress syndrome in premature neonates
- *Intra-articular or soft-tissue administration:* Arthritis, psoriatic plaques, and so forth

- *Dermatologic preparations:* Relief of inflammatory and pruritic manifestations of steroid-responsive dermatoses

Contraindications and cautions
- *Systemic (oral and parenteral) administration:* Contraindicated with infections, especially tuberculosis, fungal infections, amebiasis, vaccinia and varicella, and antibiotic-resistant infections, lactation.
- Use cautiously with kidney or liver disease, hypothyroidism, ulcerative colitis with impending perforation, diverticulitis, active or latent peptic ulcer, inflammatory bowel disease, CHF, hypertension, thromboembolic disorders, osteoporosis, convulsive disorders, diabetes mellitus.

Available forms
Tablets—0.6 mg; syrup—0.6 mg/5 mL; injection—4 mg, 3 mg betamethasone sodium phosphate with 3 mg betamethasone acetate; ointment—0.1%, 0.05%; cream—0.01%, 0.05%, 0.1%; lotion—0.1%, 0.05%; gel—0.05%

Dosages
Adults
Systemic administration
Individualize dosage, based on severity and response. Give daily dose before 9 AM to minimize adrenal suppression. Reduce initial dose in small increments until the lowest dose that maintains satisfactory clinical response is reached. If long-term therapy is needed, alternate-day therapy with a short-acting corticosteroid should be considered. After long-term therapy, withdraw drug slowly to prevent adrenal insufficiency.
- *Oral (betamethasone):* Initial dosage 0.6–7.2 mg/day.
- *IV (betamethasone sodium phosphate):* Initial dosage up to 9 mg/day.
- *IM (betamethasone sodium phosphate; betamethasone sodium phosphate and acetate):* Initial dosage 0.5–9 mg/day. Dosage range: one-third to one-half oral dose given q 12 hr. In life-threatening situations, dose can be in multiples of the oral dose.
- *Intrabursal, intra-articular, intradermal, intralesional (betamethasone sodium phos-*

Adverse effects in *Italics* are most common; those in **Bold** are life-threatening.

phate and acetate): 0.25–2 mL intra-articular, depending on joint size; 0.2 mL/cm³ intradermally, not to exceed 1 mL/wk; 0.25–1 mL at 3- to 7-day intervals for disorders of the foot.

• *Topical dermatologic cream, ointment (betamethasone dipropionate):* Apply sparingly to affected area bid–qid.

Pediatric patients
Individualize dosage on the basis of severity and response rather than by formulae that correct adult doses for age or weight. Carefully observe growth and development in infants and children on prolonged therapy.

Pharmacokinetics

Route	Onset	Duration
Systemic	Varies	3 days

Metabolism: Hepatic; $T_{1/2}$: 36–54 hr
Distribution: Crosses placenta; passes into breast milk
Excretion: Unchanged in the urine

▼ IV facts
Preparation: No further preparation needed.
Infusion: Infuse by direct IV injection over 1 min or into the tubing of running IV of dextrose or saline solutions.

Adverse effects
• **CNS:** *Vertigo, headache,* paresthesias, insomnia, convulsions, psychosis, cataracts, increased intraocular pressure, glaucoma (long-term therapy)
• **CV:** Hypotension, shock, hypertension, and CHF secondary to fluid retention, thromboembolism, thrombophlebitis, fat embolism, cardiac arrhythmias
• **Electrolyte imbalance:** *Na⁺ and fluid retention,* hypokalemia, hypocalcemia
• **Endocrine:** Amenorrhea, irregular menses, growth retardation, decreased carbohydrate tolerance, diabetes mellitus, cushingoid state (long-term effect), increased blood sugar, increased serum cholesterol, decreased T_3 and T_4 levels, hypothalamic-pituitary-adrenal (HPA) suppression with systemic therapy longer than 5 days
• **GI:** Peptic or esophageal ulcer, pancreatitis, abdominal distention, nausea, vomiting, *increased appetite, weight gain (long-term therapy)*

• **Musculoskeletal:** Muscle weakness, steroid myopathy, loss of muscle mass, osteoporosis, spontaneous fractures (long-term therapy)
• **Other:** *Immunosuppression, aggravation, or masking of infections; impaired wound healing;* thin, fragile skin; petechiae, ecchymoses, purpura, striae; subcutaneous fat atrophy; hypersensitivity or anaphylactoid reactions

The following effects are related to various local routes of steroid administration:
• **Intra-articular:** Osteonecrosis, tendon rupture, infection
• **Intralesional therapy:** Blindness when applied to face and head
• **Topical dermatologic ointments, creams, sprays:** *Local burning, irritation,* acneiform lesions, striae, skin atrophy

Interactions
✱ **Drug-drug** • Risk of severe deterioration of muscle strength in myasthenia gravis patients receiving ambenonium, edrophonium, neostigmine, pyridostigmine • Decreased steroid blood levels with barbiturates, phenytoin, rifampin • Decreased effectiveness of salicylates with betamethasone
✱ **Drug-lab test** • False-negative nitroblue-tetrazolium test for bacterial infection • Suppression of skin test reactions

■ Nursing considerations
Assessment
• **History (systemic administration):** Infections, fungal infections, amebiasis, vaccinia and varicella, and antibiotic-resistant infections; kidney or liver disease; hypothyroidism; ulcerative colitis with impending perforation; diverticulitis; active or latent peptic ulcer; inflammatory bowel disease; CHF; hypertension; thromboembolic disorders; osteoporosis; convulsive disorders; diabetes mellitus; lactation
• **Physical:** Baseline weight, T, reflexes and grip strength, affect and orientation, P, BP, peripheral perfusion, prominence of superficial veins, R and adventitious sounds, serum electrolytes, blood glucose

Interventions
Systemic use
• Give daily dose before 9 AM to mimic normal peak corticosteroid blood levels.

- Increase dosage when patient is subject to stress.
- Taper doses when discontinuing high-dose or long-term therapy.
- Do not give live virus vaccines with immunosuppressive doses of corticosteroids.

Topical dermatologic preparations

- Examine area for infections, skin integrity before application.
- Administer cautiously to pregnant patients; topical corticosteroids have caused teratogenic effects and can be absorbed from systemic site.
- Use caution when occlusive dressings, tight diapers cover affected area; these can increase systemic absorption of the drug.
- Avoid prolonged use near eyes, in genital and rectal areas, and in skin creases.

Teaching points
Systemic use

- Do not stop taking the drug (oral) without consulting health care provider.
- Take single dose or alternate-day doses before 9 AM.
- Avoid exposure to infections; ability to fight infections is reduced.
- Wear a medical alert tag so emergency care providers will know that you are on this medication.
- These side effects may occur: increase in appetite, weight gain (counting calories may help); heartburn, indigestion (try small, frequent meals, antacids); poor wound healing (consult with your care provider); muscle weakness, fatigue (frequent rest periods will help).
- Report unusual weight gain, swelling of the extremities, muscle weakness, black or tarry stools, fever, prolonged sore throat, colds or other infections, worsening of original disorder.

Intrabursal, intra-articular therapy

- Do not overuse joint after therapy, even if pain is gone.

Topical dermatologic preparations

- Apply sparingly; do not cover with tight dressings.
- Avoid contact with the eyes.
- Report irritation or infection at the site of application.

▷**betaxolol hydrochloride**
(beh tax' oh lol)

Ophthalmic: Betoptic, Betoptic S
Oral: Kerlone

PREGNANCY CATEGORY C

Drug classes
Beta$_1$-selective adrenergic blocking agent
Antihypertensive
Antiglaucoma agent

Therapeutic actions
Blocks beta-adrenergic receptors of the sympathetic nervous system in the heart and juxtaglomerular apparatus (kidney), decreasing the excitability of the heart, decreasing cardiac output and oxygen consumption, decreasing the release of renin from the kidney, and lowering blood pressure. Decreases intraocular pressure by decreasing the secretion of aqueous humor.

Indications
- Hypertension, used alone or with other antihypertensive agents, particularly thiazide-type diuretics (oral)
- Treatment of ocular hypertension and open-angle glaucoma (ophthalmic)

Contraindications and cautions
- Contraindicated with sinus bradycardia, second- or third-degree heart block, cardiogenic shock, CHF.
- Use cautiously with renal failure, diabetes, or thyrotoxicosis (betaxolol masks the cardiac signs of hypoglycemia and thyrotoxicosis), lactation.

Available forms
Tablets—10, 20 mg; ophthalmic solution—5.6 mg/mL; ophthalmic suspension—2.8 mg/mL

Dosages
Adults
Oral
Initially 10 mg PO daily, alone or added to diuretic therapy. Full antihypertensive effect is

usually seen in 7–14 days. If desired response is not achieved, dose may be doubled.

Ophthalmic
One drop bid to affected eye(s).

Pediatric patients
Safety and efficacy not established.

Geriatric patients
Oral
Consider reducing initial dose to 5 mg PO daily.

Pharmacokinetics

Route	Onset	Peak	Duration
Oral	30–60 min	2 hr	12–15 hr

Metabolism: Hepatic; $T_{1/2}$: 14–22 hr
Distribution: Crosses placenta; passes into breast milk
Excretion: Urine

Adverse effects

- **Allergic reactions:** Pharyngitis, erythematous rash, fever, sore throat, laryngospasm, respiratory distress
- **CNS:** Dizziness, vertigo, tinnitus, fatigue, emotional depression, paresthesias, sleep disturbances, hallucinations, disorientation, memory loss, slurred speech
- **CV:** *Bradycardia, CHF, cardiac arrhythmias, sinoatrial or AV nodal block, tachycardia,* peripheral vascular insufficiency, claudication, CVA, pulmonary edema, hypotension
- **Dermatologic:** Rash, pruritus, sweating, dry skin
- **EENT:** Eye irritation, dry eyes, conjunctivitis, blurred vision
- **GI:** *Gastric pain, flatulence, constipation, diarrhea, nausea, vomiting,* anorexia, ischemic colitis, renal and mesenteric arterial thrombosis, retroperitoneal fibrosis, hepatomegaly, acute pancreatitis
- **GU:** *Impotence, decreased libido,* Peyronie's disease, dysuria, nocturia, frequent urination
- **Musculoskeletal:** Joint pain, arthralgia, muscle cramp
- **Respiratory:** Bronchospasm, dyspnea, cough, bronchial obstruction, nasal stuffiness, rhinitis, pharyngitis (less likely than with propranolol)
- **Other:** *Decreased exercise tolerance, development of antinuclear antibodies (ANA),* hyperglycemia or hypoglycemia, el-

evated serum transaminase, alkaline phosphatase, and LDH

Betaxolol ophthalmic solution
- **CNS:** Insomnia, depressive neurosis
- **Local:** *Brief ocular discomfort, occasional tearing, itching, decreased corneal sensitivity,* corneal staining, keratitis, photophobia

Interactions

✳ **Drug-drug** • Increased effects with verapamil, anticholinergics • Increased risk of orthostatic hypotension with prazosin • Possible increased antihypertensive effects with aspirin, bismuth subsalicylate, magnesium salicylate, sulfinpyrazone, oral contraceptives • Decreased antihypertensive effects with NSAIDs • Possible increased hypoglycemic effect of insulin with betaxolol

✳ **Drug-lab test** • Possible false results with glucose or insulin tolerance tests

■ Nursing considerations
Assessment

- **History:** Sinus bradycardia, second- or third-degree heart block, cardiogenic shock, CHF, renal failure, diabetes or thyrotoxicosis, lactation
- **Physical:** Baseline weight, skin condition, neurologic status, P, BP, ECG, R, kidney and thyroid function tests, blood and urine glucose

Interventions

- Do not discontinue drug abruptly after long-term therapy (hypersensitivity to catecholamines may develop, exacerbating angina, MI, and ventricular arrhythmias). Taper drug gradually over 2 wk with monitoring.
- Consult with physician about withdrawing drug if patient is to undergo surgery (withdrawal is controversial).
- Protect eye from injury if corneal sensitivity is lost (ophthalmic).

Teaching points

- Administer eye drops as instructed to minimize systemic absorption of the drug.
- Do not stop taking unless told to do so by a health care provider.
- Avoid driving or dangerous activities if dizziness, weakness occur.

- These side effects may occur: dizziness, light-headedness, loss of appetite, nightmares, depression, sexual impotence.
- Report difficulty breathing, night cough, swelling of extremities, slow pulse, confusion, depression, rash, fever, sore throat, eye pain or irritation (ophthalmic).

▽bethanechol chloride
*(beh **than' e kole**)*

Duvoid, Myotonachol, PMS-Bethanechol Chloride (CAN)

PREGNANCY CATEGORY C

Drug class
Parasympathomimetic drug

Therapeutic actions
Acts at cholinergic receptors in the urinary bladder (and GI tract) to mimic the effects of acetylcholine and parasympathetic stimulation; increases the tone of the detrusor muscle and causes the emptying of the urinary bladder; not destroyed by the enzyme acetylcholinesterase, so effects are more prolonged than those of acetylcholine.

Indications
- Acute postoperative and postpartum nonobstructive urinary retention and neurogenic atony of the urinary bladder with retention
- Unlabeled use: reflux esophagitis, gastroesophageal reflux (pediatric use)

Contraindications and cautions
- Contraindicated with unusual sensitivity to bethanechol, hyperthyroidism, peptic ulcer, latent or active asthma, bradycardia, vasomotor instability, coronary artery disease, epilepsy, parkinsonism, hypotension, obstructive uropathies or intestinal obstruction, recent surgery on GI tract or bladder.
- Use cautiously with lactation.

Available forms
Tablets—5, 10, 25, 50 mg

Dosages
Determine and use the minimum effective dose; larger doses may increase side effects.
Adults
10–50 mg PO bid–qid. Initial dose of 5–10 mg with gradual increases hourly until desired effect is seen; do not exceed single dose of 50 mg. Alternatively, give 10 mg initially, then 25 and 50 mg at 6-hr intervals.
Pediatric patients
Safety and efficacy not established for children < 8 yr.

Pharmacokinetics

Route	Onset	Peak	Duration
Oral	30–90 min	60–90 min	1–6 hr

Metabolism: Unknown
Distribution: Crosses placenta; may pass into breast milk

Adverse effects
- **CV: Transient heart block, cardiac arrest,** dyspnea, orthostatic hypotension (with large doses)
- **GI:** *Abdominal discomfort, salivation, nausea, vomiting,* involuntary defecation, abdominal cramps, diarrhea, belching
- **GU:** Urinary urgency
- **Other:** Malaise, headache, *sweating, flushing*

Interactions
✳ **Drug-drug** • Increased cholinergic effects with other cholinergic drugs, cholinesterase inhibitors • Critical fall in BP may occur if taken with ganglionic blockers

■ Nursing considerations
Assessment
- **History:** Unusual sensitivity to bethanechol, hyperthyroidism, peptic ulcer, latent or active asthma, bradycardia, vasomotor instability, CAD, epilepsy, parkinsonism, hypotension, obstructive uropathies or intestinal obstruction, recent surgery on GI tract or bladder, lactation
- **Physical:** Skin color, lesions; T; P, rhythm, BP; bowel sounds, urinary bladder palpation; bladder tone evaluation, urinalysis

Adverse effects in *Italics* are most common; those in **Bold** are life-threatening.

Interventions

- Administer on an empty stomach to avoid nausea and vomiting.
- Monitor response to establish minimum effective dose.
- Have atropine on standby to reverse overdose or severe response.
- Monitor bowel function, especially in elderly patients who may become impacted or develop serious intestinal problems.

Teaching points

- Take this drug on an empty stomach to avoid nausea and vomiting.
- Dizziness, light-headedness, fainting may occur when getting up from sitting or lying position.
- These side effects may occur: increased salivation, sweating, flushing, abdominal discomfort.
- Report diarrhea, headache, belching, substernal pressure or pain, dizziness.

▷bexarotene

See *Less Commonly Used Drugs*, p. 1338.

▷bicalutamide

See *Less Commonly Used Drugs*, p. 1338.

▷biperiden
(bye per' i den)

biperiden hydrochloride (oral)

biperiden lactate (injection)

Akineton

PREGNANCY CATEGORY C

Drug class

Antiparkinsonism drug (anticholinergic type)

Therapeutic actions

Anticholinergic activity in the CNS that is believed to help normalize the hypothesized imbalance of cholinergic and dopaminergic neurotransmission in the basal ganglia in the brain of a parkinsonism patient. Reduces severity of rigidity, and to a lesser extent akinesia and tremor characterizing parkinsonism; less effective overall than levodopa; peripheral anticholinergic effects suppress secondary symptoms of parkinsonism, such as drooling.

Indications

- Adjunct in the therapy of parkinsonism (postencephalitic, arteriosclerotic, and idiopathic types)
- Relief of symptoms of extrapyramidal disorders that accompany phenothiazine therapy

Contraindications and cautions

- Contraindicated with hypersensitivity to benztropine; glaucoma, especially angle-closure glaucoma; pyloric or duodenal obstruction, stenosing peptic ulcers, achalasia (megaesophagus); prostatic hypertrophy or bladder neck obstructions; myasthenia gravis.
- Use cautiously with tachycardia, cardiac arrhythmias, hypertension, hypotension, hepatic or renal dysfunction, alcoholism, chronic illness, people who work in hot environment; hot weather; lactation.

Available forms

Tablets—2 mg; injection—5 mg/mL

Dosages
Adults
- *Parkinsonism:* 2 mg PO tid–qid; individualize dosage with a maximum dose of 16 mg/day.
- *Drug-induced extrapyramidal disorders:* Oral: 2 mg PO daily to tid.
Parenteral: 2 mg IM or IV; repeat q 30 min until symptoms are resolved, do not give more than 4 consecutive doses per 24 hr.
Pediatric patients
Safety and efficacy not established.
Geriatric patients
Strict dosage regulation may be necessary; patients > 60 yr often develop increased sensitivity to the CNS effects of anticholinergic drugs.

Pharmacokinetics

Route	Onset	Peak
Oral	1 hr	1–1.5 hr
IM	15 min	Unknown

Metabolism: Hepatic; $T_{1/2}$: 18.4–24.3 hr
Distribution: Crosses placenta; passes into breast milk

▼ IV facts

Preparation: Give undiluted. Store in tightly covered, light-resistant container. Store at room temperature.
Infusion: Administer direct IV slowly; do not give more than four consecutive doses per 24 hr.

Adverse effects

- **CNS:** Some are characteristic of centrally acting anticholinergic drugs: *disorientation, confusion,* memory loss, hallucinations, psychoses, agitation, *nervousness,* delusions, delirium, paranoia, euphoria, excitement, *light-headedness, dizziness,* depression, drowsiness, weakness, giddiness, paresthesia, heaviness of the limbs
Peripheral anticholinergic effects
- **CV:** Tachycardia, palpitations, hypotension, orthostatic hypotension
- **Dermatologic:** Rash, urticaria, other dermatoses
- **EENT:** *Blurred vision, mydriasis,* diplopia, increased intraocular tension, angle-closure glaucoma
- **GI:** *Dry mouth, constipation,* dilation of the colon, paralytic ileus, acute suppurative parotitis, nausea, vomiting, epigastric distress
- **GU:** *Urinary retention, urinary hesitancy,* dysuria, difficulty achieving or maintaining an erection
- **Other:** *Flushing, decreased sweating,* elevated temperature, muscular weakness, muscular cramping

Interactions

✳ **Drug-drug** • Paralytic ileus, sometimes fatal, with other anticholinergic drugs, with drugs that have anticholinergic properties (phenothiazines, tricyclic antidepressants) • Additive adverse CNS effects (toxic psychosis) with drugs that have CNS anticholinergic properties (TCAs, phenothiazines) • Possible masking of extrapyramidal symptoms, tardive dyskinesia, in long-term therapy with antipsychotic drugs (phenothiazines, haloperidol) • Decreased therapeutic efficacy of antipsychotic drugs (phenothiazines, haloperidol), possibly due to central antagonism

■ Nursing considerations
Assessment

- **History:** Hypersensitivity to benztropine; glaucoma; pyloric or duodenal obstruction, stenosing peptic ulcers, achalasia; prostatic hypertrophy or bladder neck obstructions; myasthenia gravis; cardiac arrhythmias, hypertension, hypotension; hepatic or renal dysfunction; alcoholism, chronic illness, work in hot environment; lactation
- **Physical:** Body weight; T; skin color, lesions; orientation, affect, reflexes, bilateral grip strength, visual exam, including tonometry; P, BP, orthostatic BP; adventitious sounds; bowel sounds, normal output, liver evaluation; normal urinary output, voiding pattern, prostate palpation; liver and kidney function tests

Interventions

- Decrease dosage or discontinue temporarily if dry mouth makes swallowing or speaking difficult.
- Give with caution, and reduce dosage in hot weather. Drug interferes with sweating and ability of body to maintain heat equilibrium; anhidrosis and fatal hyperthermia have occurred.
- Give with meals if GI upset occurs; give before meals to patients with dry mouth; give after meals if drooling or nausea occurs.
- Ensure that patient voids just before receiving each dose of drug if urinary retention is a problem.

Teaching points

- Take this drug exactly as prescribed.
- Avoid the use of alcohol, sedative, and OTC drugs (can cause dangerous effects).
- These side effects may occur: drowsiness, dizziness, confusion, blurred vision (avoid driving or engaging in activities that require alertness and visual acuity); nausea (try frequent small meals); dry mouth (suck sugarless lozenges or ice chips); painful or difficult urination (empty the bladder immediately before each dose); constipation (maintain adequate fluid intake and exer-

cise regularly); use caution in hot weather (you are susceptible to heat prostration).
- Report difficult or painful urination; constipation; rapid or pounding heartbeat; confusion, eye pain, or rash.

▷bismuth subsalicylate
(*bis' mith*)

Bismatrol, Bismatrol Extra Strength, Pepto-Bismol, Pepto-Bismol Maximum Strength, Pink Bismuth

PREGNANCY CATEGORY C

Drug class
Antidiarrheal agent

Therapeutic actions
Adsorbent actions remove irritants from the intestine; forms a protective coating over the mucosa and soothes the irritated bowel lining.

Indications
- Indigestion, nausea, and control of traveler's diarrhea within 24 hr
- Relief of gas pains and abdominal cramps
- Unlabeled use: prevention of traveler's diarrhea; treatment of chronic infantile diarrhea

Contraindications and cautions
- Allergy to any components

Available forms
Caplets—262 mg; chewable tablets—262 mg; liquid—130 mg/15 mL, 262 mg/15 mL, 524 mg/15 mL

Dosages
Adults
2 tablets or 30 mL PO, repeat q 30 min–1 hr as needed, up to eight doses/24 hr.
- *Traveler's diarrhea:* Tablets/caplets—524 mg PO qid; suspension—4.2 g/day PO in divided doses.
Pediatric patients
9–12 yr: 1 tablet or 15 mL PO.
6–9 yr: two-thirds tablet or 10 mL PO.
3–6 yr:> one-third tablet or 5 mL PO.
< 3 yr: Dosage not established.

Repeat q 30 min–1 hr as needed, up to eight doses in 24 hr.

Pharmacokinetics

Route	Onset
Oral	Varies

Metabolism: Hepatic; $T_{1/2}$: unknown
Distribution: Crosses placenta
Excretion: Urine

Adverse effects
- **GI:** *Darkening of the stool,* impaction in infants or debilitated patients
- **Salicylate toxicity:** Ringing in the ears, rapid respirations

Interactions
✳ **Drug-drug** • Increased risk of salicylate toxicity with aspirin-containing products • Increased toxic effects of methotrexate, valproic acid if taken concurrently with salicylates • Use caution with drugs used for diabetes • Decreased effectiveness with corticosteroids • Decreased absorption of oral tetracyclines • Decreased effectiveness of sulfinpyrazone with salicylates
✳ **Drug-lab test** • May interfere with radiologic exams of GI tract; bismuth is radiopaque

■ Nursing considerations
Assessment
- **History:** Allergy to any components
- **Physical:** T; orientation, reflexes; R and depth of respirations; abdominal exam, bowel sounds; serum electrolytes; acid–base levels

Interventions
- Shake liquid well before administration; have patient chew tablets thoroughly or dissolve in mouth; do not swallow whole.
- Discontinue drug if any sign of salicylate toxicity occurs (ringing in the ears).

Teaching points
- Take this drug as prescribed; do not exceed prescribed dosage. Shake liquid well before using. Chew tablets thoroughly or dissolve in your mouth; do not swallow whole.
- Darkened stools may occur.

- Do not take this drug with other drugs containing aspirin or aspirin products; serious overdose can occur.
- Report fever, diarrhea that does not stop after 2 days, ringing in the ears, rapid respirations.

▷ bisoprolol fumarate
(bis ob' pro lole)

Zebeta

PREGNANCY CATEGORY C

Drug classes
Beta-selective adrenergic blocking agent
Antihypertensive

Therapeutic actions
Blocks beta-adrenergic receptors of the sympathetic nervous system in the heart and juxtaglomerular apparatus (kidney), thus decreasing the excitability of the heart, decreasing cardiac output and oxygen consumption, decreasing the release of renin from the kidney, and lowering blood pressure.

Indications
- Management of hypertension, used alone or with other antihypertensive agents

Contraindications and cautions
- Contraindicated with sinus bradycardia, second- or third-degree heart block, cardiogenic shock, CHF.
- Use cautiously with renal failure, diabetes or thyrotoxicosis (bisoprolol can mask the usual cardiac signs of hypoglycemia and thyrotoxicosis), pregnancy, lactation.

Available forms
Tablets—5, 10 mg

Dosages
Adults
Initially 5 mg PO daily, alone or added to diuretic therapy; 2.5 mg may be appropriate; up to 20 mg PO daily has been used.
Pediatric patients
Safety and efficacy not established.

Patients with renal or hepatic impairment
Initially 2.5 mg PO; adjust, and use extreme caution.

Pharmacokinetics

Route	Onset	Peak	Duration
Oral	30–60 min	2 hr	12–15 hr

Metabolism: Hepatic; $T_{1/2}$: 9–12 hr
Distribution: Crosses placenta; may pass into breast milk
Excretion: Urine

Adverse effects
- **Allergic reactions:** Pharyngitis, erythematous rash, fever, sore throat, laryngospasm, respiratory distress
- **CNS:** Dizziness, vertigo, tinnitus, fatigue, emotional depression, paresthesias, sleep disturbances, hallucinations, disorientation, memory loss, slurred speech
- **CV:** *Bradycardia, CHF, cardiac arrhythmias, sinoatrial or AV nodal block, tachycardia,* peripheral vascular insufficiency, claudication, CVA, pulmonary edema, hypotension
- **Dermatologic:** Rash, pruritus, sweating, dry skin
- **EENT:** Eye irritation, dry eyes, conjunctivitis, blurred vision
- **GI:** *Gastric pain, flatulence, constipation, diarrhea, nausea, vomiting,* anorexia, ischemic colitis, renal and mesenteric arterial thrombosis, retroperitoneal fibrosis, hepatomegaly, acute pancreatitis
- **GU:** *Impotence, decreased libido,* Peyronie's disease, dysuria, nocturia, frequent urination
- **Musculoskeletal:** Joint pain, arthralgia, muscle cramp
- **Respiratory:** Bronchospasm, dyspnea, cough, bronchial obstruction, nasal stuffiness, rhinitis, pharyngitis (less likely than with propranolol)
- **Other:** *Decreased exercise tolerance, development of antinuclear antibodies,* hyperglycemia or hypoglycemia, elevated serum transaminase, alkaline phosphatase, and LDH

Adverse effects in *Italics* are most common; those in **Bold** are life-threatening.

Interactions

❋ **Drug-drug** • Increased effects with verapamil, anticholinergics • Increased risk of orthostatic hypotension with prazosin • Possible increased BP-lowering effects with aspirin, bismuth subsalicylate, magnesium salicylate, sulfinpyrazone, oral contraceptives • Decreased antihypertensive effects with NSAIDs • Possible increased hypoglycemic effect of insulin

❋ **Drug-lab test** • Possible false results with glucose or insulin tolerance tests

■ Nursing considerations

 CLINICAL ALERT!
Name confusion has occurred between Zebeta (bisoprolol) and DiaBeta (glyburide); use caution.

Assessment

• **History:** Sinus bradycardia, cardiac arrhythmias, cardiogenic shock, CHF, renal failure, diabetes or thyrotoxicosis, pregnancy, lactation
• **Physical:** Baseline weight, skin condition, neurologic status, P, BP, ECG, R, kidney and liver function tests, blood and urine glucose

Interventions

• Do not discontinue drug abruptly after long-term therapy (hypersensitivity to catecholamines may have developed, causing exacerbation of angina, MI, and ventricular arrhythmias). Taper drug gradually over 2 wk with monitoring.
• Consult with physician about withdrawing drug if patient is to undergo surgery (withdrawal is controversial).

Teaching points

• Do not stop taking this drug unless instructed to do so by a health care provider.
• Avoid OTC medications.
• Avoid driving or dangerous activities if dizziness, weakness occur.
• These side effects may occur: dizziness, lightheadedness, loss of appetite, nightmares, depression, sexual impotence.
• Report difficulty breathing, night cough, swelling of extremities, slow pulse, confusion, depression, rash, fever, sore throat.

▽bitolterol mesylate
(bye tole' ter ole)

Tornalate

PREGNANCY CATEGORY C

Drug classes

Sympathomimetic drug
Beta$_2$-selective adrenergic agonist
Bronchodilator
Antiasthmatic drug

Therapeutic actions

Prodrug that is converted by tissue and blood enzymes to active metabolite (colterol); in low doses, acts relatively selectively at beta$_2$-adrenergic receptors to cause bronchodilation (and vasodilation); at higher doses, beta$_2$ selectivity is lost, and the drug acts at beta$_1$ receptors to cause typical sympathomimetic cardiac effects.

Indications

• Prophylaxis and treatment of bronchial asthma and reversible bronchospasm; may be used with concurrent theophylline or steroid therapy

Contraindications and cautions

• Hypersensitivity to bitolterol; tachyarrhythmias, tachycardia caused by digitalis intoxication; general anesthesia with halogenated hydrocarbons or cyclopropane, which sensitize the myocardium to catecholamines; unstable vasomotor system disorders; hypertension; coronary insufficiency, CAD; history of stroke; COPD patients with degenerative heart disease; hyperthyroidism; history of seizure disorders; psychoneurotic individuals; labor and delivery (parenteral use of beta$_2$-adrenergic agonists can accelerate fetal heartbeat; cause hypoglycemia, hypokalemia, pulmonary edema in the mother, and hypoglycemia in the neonate; systemic absorption after inhalation may be less than with systemic administration, but use only if potential benefit to mother justifies risk to mother and fetus); lactation

Available forms

Solution for inhalation—0.2%

Dosages

Adults and patients > 12 yr

- 1.5–3.5 mg over 10–15 min with continuous flow system or 0.5–1.5 mg with intermittent flow system. Usual frequency of treatment is 3 times per day; do not exceed 8 mg/day with intermittent system or 14 mg/day with continuous flow system.

Pediatric patients

Safety and efficacy not established for children < 12 yr.

Geriatric patients

Patients > 60 yr more risk of adverse effects; use extreme caution.

Pharmacokinetics

Route	Onset	Peak	Duration
Inhalation	3–4 min	0.5–2 hr	5–8 hr

Metabolism: Hepatic; $T_{1/2}$: 3 hr
Distribution: Crosses placenta; may pass into breast milk
Excretion: Lungs

Adverse effects

- **CNS:** *Restlessness, apprehension,* anxiety, fear, CNS stimulation, hyperkinesia, *insomnia,* tremor, drowsiness, *irritability,* weakness, vertigo, headache
- **CV: Cardiac arrhythmias,** tachycardia, palpitations, PVCs (rare), anginal pain (less likely with bronchodilator doses than with bronchodilator doses of a nonselective beta-agonist, ie, isoproterenol), changes in BP, sweating, pallor, flushing
- **GI:** *Nausea,* vomiting, heartburn, unusual or bad taste
- **Hypersensitivity:** Immediate hypersensitivity (allergic) reactions
- **Respiratory:** Respiratory difficulties, **pulmonary edema,** coughing, bronchospasm, paradoxical airway resistance with repeated use of inhalation preparations

Interactions

✳ **Drug-drug** • Increased sympathomimetic effects with other sympathomimetic drugs
• Enhanced toxicity, especially cardiotoxicity, with aminophylline, oxtriphylline, theophylline

■ Nursing considerations

Assessment

- **History:** Hypersensitivity to bitolterol; tachyarrhythmias; general anesthesia with halogenated hydrocarbons or cyclopropane; unstable vasomotor system disorders; hypertension; coronary insufficiency; history of stroke; COPD patients with degenerative heart disease; hyperthyroidism; history of seizure disorders; psychoneurotic individuals; labor or delivery; lactation
- **Physical:** Weight, skin color, temperature, turgor; orientation, reflexes, affect; P, BP; R, adventitious sounds; blood and urine glucose, serum electrolytes, thyroid function tests, ECG, CBC, liver function tests (AST)

Interventions

- Use minimal doses for minimum time; drug tolerance can occur with prolonged use.
- Maintain a beta-adrenergic blocker (a cardioselective beta blocker, such as atenolol should be used for respiratory distress) on standby in case cardiac arrhythmias occur.
- Do not exceed recommended dosage.

Teaching points

- Do not exceed recommended dosage; adverse effects or loss of effectiveness may result. Read product instructions, and ask health care provider or pharmacist any questions.
- These side effects may occur: drowsiness, dizziness, fatigue, apprehension (use caution if driving or performing tasks that require alertness); nausea, heartburn, change in taste (small, frequent meals may help); sweating, flushing, rapid heart rate.
- Avoid OTC drugs; they can interfere with or cause serious side effects when used with this drug. If you need one of these products, consult health care provider.
- Report chest pain, dizziness, insomnia, weakness, tremor or irregular heart beat, difficulty breathing, productive cough, failure to respond to usual dosage.

▽ **bivalirudin**

See *Less Commonly Used Drugs,* p. 1338.

▽bleomycin sulfate
*(blee oh **mye'** sin)*

BLM, Blenoxane

PREGNANCY CATEGORY D

Drug classes
Antibiotic
Antineoplastic agent

Therapeutic actions
Inhibits DNA, RNA, and protein synthesis in susceptible cells, preventing cell division; cell cycle phase-specific agent with major effects in G2 and M phases.

Indications
- Palliative treatment of squamous cell carcinoma, lymphomas, testicular carcinoma, alone or with other drugs
- Treatment of malignant pleural effusion and prevention of recurrent pleural effusions

Contraindications and cautions
- Allergy to bleomycin sulfate; lactation, pregnancy

Available forms
Powder for injection—15, 30 units

Dosages
Adults
Treat lymphoma patients with 2 units or less for the first two doses; if no acute anaphylactoid reaction occurs, use the regular dosage schedule:
- *Squamous cell carcinoma, lymphosarcoma, reticulum cell sarcoma, testicular carcinoma:* 0.25–0.5 unit/kg IV, IM, or SC, once or twice weekly.
- *Hodgkin's disease:* 0.25–0.5 unit/kg IV, IM, or SC once or twice weekly. After a 50% response, give maintenance dose of 1 unit/day or 5 unit/wk, IV or IM. Response should be seen within 2 wk (Hodgkin's disease, testicular tumors) or 3 wk (squamous cell cancers). If no improvement is seen by then, it is unlikely to occur.
- *Malignant pleural effusion:* 60 units dissolved in 50–100 mg 0.9% saline solution, given via thoracostomy tube.

Pharmacokinetics

Route	Onset	Peak
IV	Immediate	10–20 min
IM, SC	15–20 min	30–60 min

Metabolism: Hepatic; $T_{1/2}$: 2 hr
Distribution: May cross placenta; may pass into breast milk
Excretion: Urine

▽IV facts
Preparation: Dissolve contents of 15- or 30-unit vial with 5 or 10 mL physiologic saline or glucose; stable for 24 hr at room temperature in saline solution. Powder should be refrigerated.
Infusion: Infuse slowly over 10 min.
Incompatibilities: Incompatible in solution with aminophylline, ascorbic acid, carbenicillin, diazepam, hydrocortisone, methotrexate, mitomycin, nafcillin, penicillin G, terbutaline.

Adverse effects
- **Dermatologic:** *Rash, striae, vesiculation, hyperpigmentation, skin tenderness, hyperkeratosis, nail changes, alopecia, pruritus*
- **GI:** Hepatic toxicity, *stomatitis, vomiting,* anorexia, weight loss
- **GU:** Renal toxicity
- **Hypersensitivity:** Idiosyncratic reaction similar to anaphylaxis: hypotension, mental confusion, fever, chills, wheezing (lymphoma patients, 1% occurrence)
- **Respiratory:** *Dyspnea, rales, pneumonitis,* **pulmonary fibrosis**
- **Other:** *Fever, chills*

Interactions
✳ **Drug-drug** • Decreased serum levels and effectiveness of digoxin and phenytoin

■ Nursing considerations
Assessment
- **History:** Allergy to bleomycin sulfate, pregnancy, lactation
- **Physical:** T; skin color, lesions; weight; R, adventitious sounds; liver evaluation, abdominal status; pulmonary function tests, urinalysis, liver and renal function tests, chest x-ray

Interventions

- Reconstitute for IM, SC use by dissolving contents of 15-unit vial in 1–5 mL, 30-unit vial with 5–10 mL of sterile water for injection, sodium chloride for injection, 5% dextrose injection, bacteriostatic water for injection.
- Label drug solution with date and hour of preparation; check label before use. Stable at room temperature for 24 hr in sodium chloride, 5% dextrose solution, 5% dextrose containing heparin 100 or 1,000 units/mL; discard after that time.
- Monitor pulmonary function regularly and chest x-ray weekly or biweekly to monitor onset of pulmonary toxicity; consult physician immediately if changes occur.
- Arrange for periodic monitoring of renal and liver function tests.
- Advise women of child-bearing age to avoid pregnancy while on this drug.

Teaching points

- This drug has to be given by injection. Mark calendar with dates for injection.
- This drug may cause fetal harm; use of a barrier contraceptive is advised.
- These side effects may occur: rash, skin lesions, loss of hair, changes in nails (you may want to invest in a wig, skin care may help); loss of appetite, nausea, mouth sores (try frequent mouth care, small frequent meals may help; maintain good nutrition).
- Report difficulty breathing, cough, yellowing of skin or eyes, severe GI upset, fever, chills.

▷bosentan
*(bow **sen**' tan)*

Tracleer

PREGNANCY CATEGORY X

Drug classes
Endothelin receptor antagonist
Antihypertensive

Therapeutic actions
Specifically blocks receptor sites for endothelin ET_A and ET_B in the endothelium and vascular smooth muscles; these endothelins are elevated in plasma and lung tissue of patients with pulmonary arterial hypertension.

Indications
- Treatment of pulmonary arterial hypertension in patients with class III or class IV symptoms, to improve exercise ability and to decrease the rate of clinical worsening

Contraindications and cautions
- Contraindicated with allergy to bosentan, severe liver impairment, pregnancy, lactation.
- Use cautiously with liver dysfunction, anemia.

Available forms
Tablets—62.5, 125 mg

Dosages
Adults
62.5 mg PO bid for 4 wk; then increase to a maintenance dose of 125 mg PO bid. Patients < 40 kg should use a maintenance dose of 62.5 mg PO bid. Administer in the morning and evening.
Pediatric patients
Safety and efficacy not established.
Patients with hepatic impairment
Avoid use in moderate to severe hepatic dysfunction; reduce dosage and monitor patients closely with mild hepatic dysfunction.

Pharmacokinetics

Route	Onset	Peak
Oral	Varies	3–5 hr

Metabolism: Hepatic; $T_{1/2}$: 5 hr
Distribution: Crosses placenta; may pass into breast milk
Excretion: Bile

Adverse effects
- **CNS:** *Headache,* fatigue
- **CV:** *Flushing, edema, hypotension,* palpitations
- **EENT:** *Nasopharyngitis*
- **GI: Liver injury,** dyspepsia
- **Hematologic:** Decreased hemoglobin levels, decreased hematocrit
- **Skin:** Pruritus

Adverse effects in *Italics* are most common; those in **Bold** are life-threatening.

Interactions

✳ **Drug-drug** • Potential for decreased effectiveness of hormonal contraceptives; advise the use of barrier contraceptives • Bosentan serum concentrations increased with cyclosporin A, and cyclosporin A concentrations decrease by 50% with bosentan; avoid this combination • Decreased serum levels of statins if combined with bosentan; if the combination is used, patients should have serum cholesterol levels monitored regularly • Increased risk of liver damage if combined with glyburide; avoid this combination • Increased bosentan concentrations with ketoconazole; monitor patients for adverse effects

■ Nursing considerations
Assessment

- **History:** Allergy to bosentan, severe liver impairment, anemia, pregnancy, lactation
- **Physical:** Skin color and lesions, orientation, BP, liver function tests, CBC, hemoglobin levels, pregnancy test

Interventions

- Make sure that the patient is not pregnant before initiating therapy and that patient will conform to use of a nonhormonal barrier form of contraception while using this drug.
- Obtain baseline and then monthly liver enzyme levels; dosage reduction or drug withdrawal is indicated at signs of elevated liver enzymes.
- Obtain baseline hemoglobin levels and repeat at 1 and 3 mo, then every 3 mo. If hemoglobin drops, the situation should be evaluated and appropriate action taken.
- Do not administer to any patient taking cyclosporine or glyburide.
- Administer in the morning and in the evening without regard to food.
- Monitor patients who are discontinuing bosentan; tapering of dose may be needed to avoid sudden worsening of disease.
- Provide analgesics as appropriate for patients who develop headache.
- Monitor patient's functional level to note improvement in exercise tolerance.
- Maintain other measures used to treat pulmonary arterial hypertension.

Teaching points

- Take drug exactly as prescribed, in the morning and the evening.
- Be aware that this drug should not be taken during pregnancy; serious fetal abnormalities have occurred. A negative pregnancy test will be required before the drug is started. The use of barrier contraceptives is advised; hormonal contraceptives may not be effective.
- Keep a chart of your exercise tolerance to help monitor improvement in your condition.
- Be aware that these side effects may occur: headache (analgesics may be available that will help); stomach upset (taking the drug with food may help).
- Maintain any procedures you usually use for treating your pulmonary arterial hypertension.
- Know that you will need monthly blood tests to evaluate the effect of this drug on your liver and your hemoglobin.
- Report: swelling, changes in color of urine or stool, yellowing of the eyes or skin.

▷botulinum toxin type A
(bot' you lin um)

Botox Cosmetic

PREGNANCY CATEGORY C

Drug class

Neurotoxin

Therapeutic actions

Blocks neuromuscular transmission by binding to receptor sites on the motor nerve terminals and inhibiting the release of acetylcholine; this blocking results in localized muscle denervation, which causes local muscle paralysis; this denervation can lead to muscle atrophy and reinnervation if the muscle develops new acetylcholine receptors.

Indications

- Temporary improvement in the appearance of moderate to severe glabellar lines associated with corrugator or procerus muscle activity in adult patients 65 years of age or younger.

Contraindications and cautions
- Contraindicated with hypersensitivity to any component of the drug; active infection at the injection site area.
- Use cautiously with peripheral neuropathic diseases (ALS, motor neuropathies), neuromuscular disorders such as myasthenia gravis, inflammation in the injection area, lactation, pregnancy, known cardiovascular disease.

Available forms
Powder for injection—100 units/vial

Dosages
Adults
Total of 20 units (0.5 mL solution) injected as divided doses of 0.1 mL into each of five sites—two in each corrugator muscle, and one in the procerus muscle; injections usually need to be repeated every 3–4 months to maintain effect.

Pharmacokinetics
Not absorbed systemically

Adverse effects
- **CNS:** *Headache,* blepharoptosis, transient ptosis, *dizziness*
- **CV:** Arrhythmias, MI (patients with preexisting disease), hypertension
- **GI:** Nausea, difficulty swallowing, dyspepsia, tooth disorder
- **Respiratory:** Pneumonia, bronchitis, sinusitis, pharyngitis, UTI
- **Other:** Redness, edema, and pain at injection site, *flu-like syndrome,* paralysis of facial muscles, facial pain, infection, skin tightness, ecchymosis, **anaphylactic reactions**

Interactions
✳ **Drug-drug** • Risk for additive effects if combined with aminoglycosides or other drugs that interfere with neuromuscular transmission—NMJ blockers, lincosamides, quinidine, magnesium sulfate, anticholinesterases, succinylcholine, polymyxin; use extreme caution if this combination is used.

■ Nursing considerations
Assessment
- **History:** Hypersensitivity to any component of the drug; active infection in the injection site area, pregnancy, peripheral neuropathic diseases (ALS, motor neuropathies), neuromuscular disorders such as myasthenia gravis, inflammation in the injection area, lactation, known cardiovascular disease.
- **Physical:** T; reflexes; R, respiratory auscultation, assessment of injection site and muscle function.

Interventions
- Store vials in the freezer before reconstitution.
- Reconstitute with 2.5 mL 0.9% sterile, preservative-free saline (100 units in 2.5 mL) using a 21-gauge needle. Inject saline into vial; gently rotate vial to reconstitute and label vial with time and date of reconstitution. Reconstituted solution may be refrigerated but must be used within 4 hours. Discard after that time.
- Inspect vial for particulate matter or discoloration before use.
- Withdraw each 0.5 mL dose using a tuberculin syringe. A 30-gauge needle should be used for injection.
- Ensure that epinephrine is readily available in case of anaphylactic reaction to the drug.
- Inform the patient that the effect of the drug may not be seen for 1 or 2 days, with the full effect taking up to a week. The effect usually lasts 3–4 months. Do not administer the drug more often than every 3–4 months.
- Advise patient not to become pregnant while this drug is being used; advise the use of contraceptives.

Teaching points
- This drug will be injected into 5 areas in the muscles to block the furrowing of your brow.
- Be aware that the effects of the drug may not be apparent for 1–2 days and may not be fully apparent for a week. The effects of the drug persist for 3–4 months.
- Avoid pregnancy while using this drug, the effects on the fetus are not known. If you become pregnant or desire to become pregnant, consult with your health care provider. Use of contraceptive measures is advised.

- Know that these side effects may occur: pain, redness at injection site and headache (analgesics may be helpful), drooping of the eyelid (this usually is transient), nausea, flu-like syndrome.
- Report: difficulty swallowing, facial paralysis; difficulty speaking; difficulty breathing; persistent pain, redness, or swelling at injection site.

▷botulinum toxin type B

See *Less Commonly Used Drugs*, p. 1338.

▷bretylium tosylate

See *Less Commonly Used Drugs*, p. 1338.

▷bromocriptine mesylate
(broe moe krip' teen)

Apo-Bromocriptine (CAN), Parlodel, Parlodel SnapTabs

PREGNANCY CATEGORY B

Drug classes
Antiparkinsonian agent
Dopamine receptor agonist
Semisynthetic ergot derivative

Therapeutic actions
Parkinsonism: Acts as an agonist directly on postsynaptic dopamine receptors of neurons in the brain, mimicking the effects of the neurotransmitter dopamine, which is deficient in parkinsonism. Unlike levodopa, bromocriptine does not require biotransformation by the nigral neurons that are deficient in parkinsonism patients; thus, bromocriptine may be effective when levodopa has begun to lose its efficacy.
Hyperprolactinemia: Acts directly on postsynaptic dopamine receptors of the prolactin-secreting cells in the anterior pituitary, mimicking the effects of prolactin inhibitory factor, inhibiting the release of prolactin and galactorrhea. Also restores normal ovulatory menstrual cycles in patients with amenorrhea or galactorrhea, and inhibits the release of growth hormone in patients with acromegaly.

Indications
- Treatment of postencephalitic or idiopathic Parkinson's disease; may provide additional benefit in patients currently maintained on optimal dosages of levodopa with or without carbidopa, beginning to deteriorate or develop tolerance to levodopa, and experiencing "end of dose failure" on levodopa therapy; may allow reduction of levodopa dosage and decrease the dyskinesias and "on-off" phenomenon associated with long-term levodopa therapy
- Short-term treatment of amenorrhea or galactorrhea associated with hyperprolactinemia due to various etiologies, excluding demonstrable pituitary tumors
- Treatment of hyperprolactinemia associated with pituitary adenomas to reduce elevated prolactin levels, cause shrinkage of macroprolactinomas; may be used to reduce the tumor mass before surgery
- Female infertility associated with hyperprolactinemia in the absence of a demonstrable pituitary tumor
- Acromegaly: used alone or with pituitary irradiation or surgery to reduce serum growth hormone level
- Unlabeled uses: neuroleptic malignant syndrome, cocaine addiction, cyclical mastalgia

Contraindications and cautions
- Contraindicated with hypersensitivity to bromocriptine or any ergot alkaloid; severe ischemic heart disease or peripheral vascular disease; pregnancy, lactation.
- Use cautiously with history of MI with residual arrhythmias (atrial, nodal, or ventricular); renal, hepatic disease; history of peptic ulcer (fatal bleeding ulcers have occurred in patients with acromegaly treated with bromocriptine).

Available forms
Capsules—5 mg; tablets—2.5 mg

Dosages
Adults
Give drug with food; individualize dosage; increase dosage gradually to minimize side ef-

fects; adjust dosage carefully to optimize benefits and minimize side effects.

- *Hyperprolactinemia:* Initially, one-half to one 2.5-mg tablet PO daily; an additional 2.5-mg tablet may be added as tolerated q 3–7 days until optimal response is achieved; usual dosage is 5–7.5 mg/day; range is 2.5–15 mg/day. Treatment should not exceed 6 mo.
- *Acromegaly:* Initially, 1.25–2.5 mg PO for 3 days at bedtime; add 1.25–2.5 mg as tolerated q 3–7 days until optimal response is achieved. Evaluate patient monthly, and adjust dosage based on growth hormone levels. Usual dosage range is 20–30 mg/day; do not exceed 100 mg/day; withdraw patients treated with pituitary irradiation for a yearly 4- to 8-wk reassessment period.
- *Parkinson's disease:* 1.25 mg PO bid; assess every 2 wk, and adjust dosage carefully to ensure lowest dosage producing optimal response. If needed, increase dosage by increments of 2.5 mg/day q 14–28 days; usual range 10–40 mg/day; do not exceed 100 mg/day. Efficacy for > 2 yr not established.

Pediatric patients
Safety for use in patients < 15 yr not established.

Pharmacokinetics

Route	Onset	Peak	Duration
Oral	Varies	1–3 hr	14 hr

Metabolism: Hepatic; $T_{1/2}$: 3 hr initial phase, 45–50 hr terminal phase
Excretion: Bile

Adverse effects
Hyperprolactinemic indications
- **CNS:** *Dizziness, fatigue, light-headedness, nasal congestion, drowsiness,* cerebrospinal fluid rhinorrhea in patients who have had transsphenoidal surgery, pituitary radiation
- **CV:** Hypotension
- **GI:** *Nausea, vomiting, abdominal cramps, constipation, diarrhea, headache*

Physiologic lactation
- **CNS:** *Headache, dizziness, nausea, vomiting,* fatigue, syncope
- **CV:** Hypotension

- **GI:** Diarrhea, cramps

Acromegaly
- **CNS:** Nasal congestion, digital vasospasm, drowsiness
- **CV:** Exacerbation of Raynaud's syndrome, *orthostatic hypotension*
- **GI:** *Nausea, constipation, anorexia,* indigestion, dry mouth, vomiting, GI bleeding

Parkinson's disease
- **CNS:** *Abnormal involuntary movements, hallucinations, confusion, "on-off" phenomenon, dizziness, drowsiness, faintness, asthenia, visual disturbance, ataxia, insomnia, depression, vertigo*
- **CV:** *Hypotension, shortness of breath*
- **GI:** *Nausea, vomiting, abdominal discomfort, constipation*

Interactions
✳ **Drug-drug** • Increased serum bromocriptine levels and increased pharmacologic and toxic effects with erythromycin • Decreased effectiveness with phenothiazines for treatment of prolactin-secreting tumors • Increased bromocriptine adverse effects if combined with sympathomimetics

■ Nursing considerations
Assessment
- **History:** Hypersensitivity to bromocriptine or any ergot alkaloid; severe ischemic heart disease or peripheral vascular disease; pregnancy; history of MI with residual arrhythmias; renal, hepatic disease; history of peptic ulcer, lactation
- **Physical:** Skin temperature (especially fingers), color, lesions; nasal mucous membranes; orientation, affect, reflexes, bilateral grip strength, vision exam, including visual fields; P, BP, orthostatic BP, auscultation; R, depth, adventitious sounds; bowel sounds, normal output, liver evaluation; liver and kidney function tests, CBC with differential

Interventions
- Evaluate patients with amenorrhea or galactorrhea before drug therapy begins; syndrome may result from pituitary adenoma that requires surgical or radiation procedures.
- Arrange to administer drug with food.

- Taper dosage in patients with Parkinson's disease if drug must be discontinued.
- Monitor hepatic, renal, hematopoietic function periodically during therapy.

Teaching points

- Take drug exactly as prescribed with food; take the first dose at bedtime while lying down.
- Do not discontinue drug without consulting health care provider (patients with macroadenoma may experience rapid growth of tumor and recurrence of original symptoms).
- Use barrier contraceptives while taking this drug (amenorrhea or galactorrhea); pregnancy may occur before menses, and the drug is contraindicated in pregnancy (estrogen contraceptives may stimulate a prolactinoma).
- These side effects may occur: drowsiness, dizziness, confusion (avoid driving or engaging in activities that require alertness); nausea (take the drug with meals, eat frequent small meals); dizziness or faintness when getting up (change position slowly, be careful climbing stairs); headache, nasal stuffiness (medication may help).
- Report fainting; light-headedness; dizziness; uncontrollable movements of the face, eyelids, mouth, tongue, neck, arms, hands, or legs; mental changes; irregular heartbeat or palpitations; severe or persistent nausea or vomiting; coffee-ground vomitus; black tarry stools; vision changes (macroadenoma); any persistent watery nasal discharge (hyperprolactinemic).

▽brompheniramine maleate (parabromdylamine maleate)

(brome fen ir' a meen)

PREGNANCY CATEGORY C

Drug class

Antihistamine (alkylamine type)

Therapeutic actions

Competitively blocks the effects of histamine at H_1-receptor sites; has anticholinergic (atropine-like), antipruritic, and sedative effects.

Indications

- Symptomatic relief of symptoms associated with perennial and seasonal allergic rhinitis—runny nose, sneezing, itching nose and throat, watery eyes

Contraindications and cautions

- Contraindicated with allergy to any antihistamines, third trimester of pregnancy (newborn or premature infants may have severe reactions).
- Use cautiously with lactation, narrow-angle glaucoma, stenosing peptic ulcer, symptomatic prostatic hypertrophy, asthma attack, bladder neck obstruction, pyloroduodenal obstruction.

Available forms

Combination products

Dosages

Adults and children ≥ 12 yr
6–12 mg PO q 12 hr. Usual dose: 5–20 mg PO bid; maximum dose is 40 mg/24 hr.
Pediatric patients 6– < 12 yr
6 mg/day PO.
Geriatric patients
More likely to cause dizziness, sedation, syncope, toxic confusional states, and hypotension in elderly patients; use with caution.

Pharmacokinetics

Route	Onset	Peak	Duration
Oral	15–30 min	1–2 hr	4–6 hr

Metabolism: Hepatic; $T_{1/2}$: 12–35 hr
Distribution: Crosses placenta; passes into breast milk
Excretion: Urine

Adverse effects

- **CNS:** *Drowsiness, sedation, dizziness, faintness, disturbed coordination,* fatigue, confusion, restlessness, excitation, nervousness, tremor, headache, blurred vision, diplopia, vertigo, tinnitus, acute labyrinthitis, hysteria, tingling, heaviness and weakness of the hands
- **CV:** Hypotension, palpitations, bradycardia, tachycardia, extrasystoles
- **GI:** *Epigastric distress,* anorexia, increased appetite and weight gain, nausea, vomiting, diarrhea or constipation

- **GU:** Urinary frequency, dysuria, urinary retention, early menses, decreased libido, impotence
- **Hematologic:** Hemolytic anemia, hypoplastic anemia, thrombocytopenia, leukopenia, agranulocytosis, pancytopenia
- **Hypersensitivity:** Urticaria, rash, **anaphylactic shock,** photosensitivity
- **Respiratory:** *Thickening of bronchial secretions,* chest tightness, wheezing, nasal stuffiness, dry mouth, dry nose, dry throat, sore throat

Interactions

✳ **Drug-drug** • Increased sedation with alcohol, other CNS depressants • Increased and prolonged anticholinergic (drying) effects with MAO inhibitors.

■ Nursing considerations
Assessment

- **History:** Allergy to any antihistamines, narrow-angle glaucoma, stenosing peptic ulcer, symptomatic prostatic hypertrophy, asthmatic attack, bladder neck obstruction, pyloroduodenal obstruction, third trimester of pregnancy, lactation
- **Physical:** Skin color, lesions, texture; orientation, reflexes, affect; vision exam; P, BP; R, adventitious sounds; bowel sounds; prostate palpation; CBC with differential

Interventions

- Give orally with food if GI upset occurs.

Teaching points

- Take as prescribed; avoid excessive dosage; take with food if GI upset occurs.
- These side effects may occur: dizziness, sedation, drowsiness (use caution if driving or performing tasks that require alertness); epigastric distress, diarrhea or constipation (take with meals); dry mouth (frequent mouth care, sucking sugarless lozenges may help); thickening of bronchial secretions, dryness of nasal mucosa (try a humidifier).
- Avoid alcohol while on this drug; serious sedation could occur.
- Report difficulty breathing, hallucinations, tremors, loss of coordination, unusual bleeding or bruising, visual disturbances, irregular heartbeat.

▽**buclizine hydrochloride**
(byoo' kli zeen)

Bucladin-S Softabs

PREGNANCY CATEGORY C

Drug classes
Antiemetic
Anti-motion sickness drug
Antihistamine
Anticholinergic drug

Therapeutic actions
Reduces sensitivity of the labyrinthine apparatus; probably acts partly by blocking cholinergic synapses in the vomiting center, which receives input from the chemoreceptor trigger zone and from peripheral nerve pathways; peripheral anticholinergic effects may contribute to efficacy; mechanism not totally understood.

Indications
- Control of nausea, vomiting, and dizziness of motion sickness

Contraindications and cautions
- Contraindicated with allergy to buclizine; allergy to tartrazine (more common in patients who are allergic to aspirin); lactation, pregnancy.
- Use cautiously with narrow-angle glaucoma, stenosing peptic ulcer, symptomatic prostatic hypertrophy, bronchial asthma, bladder neck obstruction, pyloroduodenal obstruction, cardiac arrhythmias (conditions that may be aggravated by anticholinergic therapy).

Available forms
Tablets—50 mg

Dosages
Adults
50 mg PO usually alleviates nausea. Up to 150 mg/day may be used. Prevention: 50 mg

PO at least 30 min before travel; for extended travel, a second tablet may be taken in 4–6 hr. Usual maintenance dose is 50 mg bid; up to 150 mg/day may be given.

Pediatric patients
Safety and efficacy not established.

Geriatric patients
More likely to cause dizziness, sedation in elderly patients; use with caution.

Pharmacokinetics

Route	Onset	Duration
Oral	1 hr	4–6 hr

Metabolism: Hepatic
Distribution: Crosses placenta; passes into breast milk
Excretion: Urine

Adverse effects
- **CNS:** *Drowsiness, dry mouth, headache, jitteriness*

Interactions
✳ **Drug-drug** • Increased sedation if taken with alcohol or other CNS depressants

■ Nursing considerations
Assessment
- **History:** Allergy to buclizine; allergy to tartrazine; lactation; narrow-angle glaucoma, stenosing peptic ulcer, symptomatic prostatic hypertrophy, bronchial asthma, bladder neck obstruction, pyloroduodenal obstruction, cardiac arrhythmias
- **Physical:** Orientation, reflexes, affect; vision exam; P, BP; R, adventitious sounds; bowel sounds, normal GI output; prostate palpation, normal urinary output

Interventions
- Arrange for analgesics if needed for headache.

Teaching points
- Take this drug as prescribed. Tablets can be taken without water; place tablet in mouth and dissolve, chew, or swallow whole. Avoid excessive dosage.
- Works best if used before motion sickness occurs.
- These side effects may occur: dizziness, sedation, drowsiness (use caution if driving or

performing tasks that require alertness); dry mouth (use frequent mouth care, suck sugarless lozenges); headache (consult health care provider for analgesic); jitteriness (reversible, will stop when you discontinue the drug).
- Avoid OTC drugs; many of them contain ingredients that cause serious reactions with this drug.
- Avoid alcohol; serious sedation could occur.
- Report difficulty breathing; hallucinations, tremors, loss of coordination; visual disturbances; irregular heartbeat.

▷ budesonide
(bue des' oh nide)

Inhalation: Entocort (CAN), Pulmicort Respules: Pulmicort Turbuhaler, Rhinocort, Rhinocort Aqua, Rhinocort Turbuhaler (CAN)
Oral: Entocort EC

PREGNANCY CATEGORY C

Drug class
Corticosteroid

Therapeutic actions
Anti-inflammatory effect; local administration into nasal passages maximizes beneficial effects on these tissues, while decreasing the likelihood of adverse effects from systemic absorption.

Indications
- Management of symptoms of seasonal or perennial allergic rhinitis in adults and children; nonallergic perennial rhinitis in adults
- Maintenance treatment of asthma as prophylactic therapy in adults and children ≥ 6 yr and for patients requiring corticosteroids for asthma (*Turbuhaler*)
- Maintenance treatment and prophylaxis therapy of asthma in children 12 mo–8 yr (inhalation suspension)
- Treatment of mild to moderate active Crohn's disease involving the ileum or ascending colon (oral)

Contraindications and cautions
Inhalation
- Contraindicated with hypersensitivity to drug or for relief of acute asthma or broncho-spasm.
- Use cautiously with TB, systemic infections, lactation.

Oral
- Contraindicated with hypersensitivity to drug, lactation.
- Use cautiously with TB, hypertension, diabetes mellitus, osteoporosis, peptic ulcer disease, glaucoma, cataracts, family history of diabetes or glaucoma, other conditions in which glucocorticosteroids may have unwanted effects.

Nasal
- Contraindicated with hypersensitivity to drug, nasal infections, nasal trauma, nasal septal ulcers, recent nasal surgery.
- Use cautiously with lactation, TB, systemic infection.

Available forms
Aerosol—32 mcg/actuation; dry powder for inhalation—200 mcg (each actuation delivers 160 mcg); inhalation suspension—0.25 mg/2 mL, 0.5 mg/2 mL; capsules—3 mg

Dosages
Inhalation
Adults and children ≥ 6 yr
Initial dose 256 mcg/day given as 2 sprays in each nostril morning and evening or 4 sprays in each nostril in the morning. After desired clinical effect is achieved, reduce dose to the smallest dose possible to maintain the control of symptoms. Generally takes 3–7 days to achieve maximum clinical effect.

Pulmicort Turbuhaler:
Previously on inhaled corticosteroids—initially 200–400 mcg twice daily, maximum dose 800 mcg bid (4 inhalations), 200 mcg bid for children > 6 yr; previously on bronchodilators alone—200–400 mcg bid, 200 mcg bid for children > 6 yr; previously on oral corticosteroids—400–800 mcg bid, 400 mcg bid for children ≥ 6 yr.

Pediatric patients 12 mo–8 yr
0.25–1 mg once daily or in two divided doses of Respules, using jet nebulizer.

Oral
Adults
9 mg/day PO taken in the morning for up to 8 wk. Recurrent episodes may be retreated for 8-wk periods.

Pediatric patients
Safety and efficacy not established.

Patients with hepatic impairment
Monitor patients very closely for signs of hypercorticism; reduced dosage should be considered with these patients.

Pharmacokinetics

Route	Onset	Peak	Duration
Intranasal	Immediate	Rapid	8–12 hr
Oral	Slow	0.5–10 hr	Unknown

Metabolism: Hepatic; $T_{1/2}$: 2–3.6 hr (oral); unknown (inhalation)
Distribution: Crosses placenta; may pass into breast milk
Excretion: Urine

Adverse effects
- **CNS:** *headache, dizziness,* lethargy, *fatigue,* paresthesias, nervousness
- **Dermatologic:** Rash, edema, pruritis, alopecia
- **Endocrine:** HPA suppression, Cushing's syndrome with overdosage and systemic absorption
- **GI:** Nausea, dyspepsia, dry mouth
- **Local:** *Nasal irritation,* fungal infection
- **Respiratory:** Epistaxis, rebound congestion, *pharyngitis, cough*
- **Other:** chest pain, asthenia, moon face, acne, bruising, *back pain*

Interactions
Oral use
✴ **Drug-drug** • Increased risk of corticosteroid toxic effects if combined with ketoconazole, itraconazole, ritonavir, indinavir, saquinavir, erythromycin, or other known CYP3A4 inhibitors; if drugs must be used together, decrease dosage of budesonide and monitor patient closely

✴ **Drug-food** • Risk of increased toxic effects if combined with grapefruit juice; avoid this combination.

Adverse effects in *Italics* are most common; those in **Bold** are life-threatening.

■ Nursing considerations
Assessment
- **History:** Untreated local nasal infections, nasal trauma, septal ulcers, recent nasal surgery, lactation
- **Physical:** BP, P, auscultation; R, adventitious sounds; exam of nares

Interventions
Inhalation
- Taper systemic steroids carefully during transfer to inhalational steroids; deaths from adrenal insufficiency have occurred.
- Arrange for use of decongestant nose drops to facilitate penetration if edema, excessive secretions are present.
- Prime unit before use for *Pulmicort Turbuhaler;* have patient rinse mouth after each use.
- Use aerosol within 6 mo of opening. Shake well before each use.
- Store *Respules* upright and protected from light; gently shake before use; open envelopes should be discarded after 2 wk.

Oral
- Make sure patient does not cut, crush, or chew capsules; they must be swallowed whole.
- Administer the drug once each day, in the morning; do not administer with grapefruit juice.
- Encourage patient to complete full 8 wk of drug therapy.
- Monitor patient for signs of hypercorticism—acne, bruising, moon face, swollen ankles, hirsutism, skin striae, buffalo hump—which could indicate need to decrease dosage.

Teaching points
Inhalation
- Do not use more often than prescribed; do not stop without consulting your health care provider.
- It may take several days to achieve good effects; do not stop if effects are not immediate.
- Use decongestant nose drops first if nasal passages are blocked.
- These side effects can occur: local irritation (use your device correctly), dry mouth (suck sugarless lozenges).

- Prime unit before use for *Pulmicort Turbuhaler;* rinse mouth after each use.
- Store *Respules* upright, protect from light; discard open envelopes after 2 wk; gently shake before use.
- Report sore mouth, sore throat, worsening of symptoms, severe sneezing, exposure to chickenpox or measles, eye infections.

Oral
- Take the drug once a day in the morning. Do not cut, crush, or chew the capsules, they must be swallowed whole.
- If you miss a day, take the capsules as soon as you remember them. Take the next day's capsules at the regular time. Do not take more that 3 capsules in a day.
- Take the full course of the drug therapy (8 wk in most cases).
- Do not take this drug with grapefruit juice; avoid grapefruit juice entirely while using this drug.
- These side effects may occur: dizziness, headache (avoid driving or operating dangerous machinery if these effects occur); nausea, flatulence (small, frequent meals may help, try to maintain your fluid and food intake).
- Store *Respules* upright, protected from light; discard open envelopes after 2 wk. Shake before use.
- Report: chest pain, ankle swelling, respiratory infections, increased bruising

▽ bumetanide
(byoo met' a nide)
Bumex, Burinex (CAN)

PREGNANCY CATEGORY C

Drug class
Loop (high ceiling) diuretic

Therapeutic actions
Inhibits the reabsorption of sodium and chloride from the proximal and distal renal tubules and the loop of Henle, leading to a natriuretic diuresis.

Indications
- Edema associated with CHF, cirrhosis, renal disease
- Acute pulmonary edema (IV)

- Unlabeled use: treatment of adult nocturia (not effective in men with BPH)

Contraindications and cautions
- Allergy to bumetanide; electrolyte depletion; anuria, severe renal failure; hepatic coma; SLE; gout; diabetes mellitus; lactation.

Available forms
Tablets—0.5, 1, 2 mg; injection—0.25 mg/mL

Dosages
Adults
0.5–2 mg/day PO in a single dose; may repeat at 4- to 5-hr intervals up to a maximum daily dose of 10 mg. Intermittent dosage schedule of drug and rest days: 3–4 on/1–2 off is most effective with edema.
Parenteral therapy
0.5–1 mg IV or IM. Give over 1–2 min. Dose may be repeated at intervals of 2–3 hr. Do not exceed 10 mg/day.
Pediatric patients
Not recommended for patients < 18 yr.
Geriatric patients or patients with renal impairment
A continuous infusion of 12 mg over 12 hr may be more effective and less toxic than intermittent bolus therapy.

Pharmacokinetics

Route	Onset	Peak	Duration
Oral	30–60 min	60–120 min	4–6 hr
IV	Minutes	15–30 min	30–60 min

Metabolism: $T_{1/2}$: 60–90 min
Distribution: Crosses placenta; may pass into breast milk
Excretion: Urine

▽ IV facts
Preparation: May be given direct IV or diluted in solution with 5% dextrose in water, 0.9% sodium chloride, or lactated Ringer's solution. Discard unused solution after 24 hr.
Infusion: Give by direct injection slowly, over 1–2 min. Further diluted in solution; give slowly; do not exceed 10 mg/day.

Adverse effects
- **CNS:** *Asterixis, dizziness,* vertigo, paresthesias, confusion, fatigue, nystagmus, *weakness, headache, drowsiness,* fatigue, blurred vision, tinnitus, irreversible hearing loss
- **CV:** *Orthostatic hypotension,* volume depletion, cardiac arrhythmias, thrombophlebitis
- **GI:** *Nausea, anorexia, vomiting, diarrhea,* gastric irritation and pain, dry mouth, acute pancreatitis, jaundice
- **GU:** *Polyuria, nocturia,* glycosuria, renal failure
- **Hematologic:** *Hypokalemia,* leukopenia, anemia, thrombocytopenia
- **Local:** *Pain, phlebitis at injection site*
- **Other:** Muscle cramps and muscle spasms, weakness, arthritic pain, fatigue, hives, photosensitivity, rash, pruritus, sweating, nipple tenderness

Interactions
✳ **Drug-drug** • Decreased diuresis and natriuresis with NSAIDs • Increased risk of cardiac glycoside toxicity (secondary to hypokalemia) • Increased risk of ototoxicity if taken with aminoglycoside antibiotics, cisplatin

■ Nursing considerations
Assessment
- **History:** Allergy to bumetanide, electrolyte depletion, anuria, severe renal failure, hepatic coma, SLE, gout, diabetes mellitus, lactation
- **Physical:** Skin color, lesions; edema; orientation, reflexes, hearing; pulses, baseline ECG, BP, orthostatic BP, perfusion; R, pattern, adventitious sounds; liver evaluation, bowel sounds; urinary output patterns; CBC, serum electrolytes (including calcium), blood sugar, liver and renal function tests, uric acid, urinalysis

Interventions
- Give with food or milk to prevent GI upset.
- Mark calendars or use reminders if intermittent therapy is best for treating edema.
- Give single dose early in day so increased urination will not disturb sleep.
- Avoid IV use if oral use is possible.

- Arrange to monitor serum electrolytes, hydration, liver function during long-term therapy.
- Provide diet rich in potassium or supplemental potassium.

Teaching points

- Record alternate day or intermittent therapy on a calendar or dated envelopes.
- Take the drug early in day so increased urination will not disturb sleep; take with food or meals to prevent GI upset.
- Weigh yourself on a regular basis, at the same time, and in the same clothing; record the weight on your calendar.
- These side effects may occur: increased volume and frequency of urination; dizziness, feeling faint on arising, drowsiness (avoid rapid position changes; hazardous activities, such as driving; and alcohol consumption); sensitivity to sunlight (use sunglasses, sunscreen, wear protective clothing); increased thirst (suck sugarless lozenges; use frequent mouth care); loss of body potassium (a potassium-rich diet, or supplement will be needed).
- Report weight change of more than 3 lb in 1 day; swelling in ankles or fingers; unusual bleeding or bruising; nausea, dizziness, trembling, numbness, fatigue; muscle weakness or cramps.

▷buprenorphine hydrochloride

(byoo pre nor' feen)

Buprenex, Subutex

PREGNANCY CATEGORY C

C-V CONTROLLED SUBSTANCE

Drug class

Narcotic agonist-antagonist analgesic

Therapeutic actions

Acts as an agonist at specific opioid receptors in the CNS to produce analgesia; also acts as an opioid antagonist; exact mechanism of action not understood.

Indications

- Relief of moderate-to-severe pain

- Treatment of opioid dependence, preferably used as induction treatment

Contraindications and cautions

- Contraindicated with hypersensitivity to buprenorphine.
- Use cautiously with physical dependence on narcotic analgesics (withdrawal syndrome may occur); compromised respiratory function; increased intracranial pressure (buprenorphine may elevate CSF pressure; may cause miosis and coma, which could interfere with patient evaluation), myxedema, Addison's disease, toxic psychosis, prostatic hypertrophy or urethral stricture, acute alcoholism, delirium tremens, kyphoscoliosis, biliary tract dysfunction (may cause spasm of the sphincter of Oddi), hepatic or renal dysfunction, lactation.

Available forms

Injection—0.324 mg/mL (equivalent to 0.3 mg); sublingual tablets *(Subutex)*—2, 8 mg

Dosages

Adults

0.3 mg IM or by slow (over 2 min) IV injection. May repeat once, 30–60 min after first dose; repeat q 6 hr prn. If necessary, nonrisk patients may be given up to 0.6 mg by deep IM injection.

- *Opioid dependence:* 12–16 mg/day sublingually *(Subutex),* used as induction with switch to *Suboxone* for maintenance

Pediatric patients < 13 yr

Safety and efficacy not established.

Geriatric or debilitated patients

Reduce dosage to one-half usual adult dose.

Pharmacokinetics

Route	Onset	Peak	Duration
Oral	15 min	1 hr	6 hr
IV	10 min	30–45 min	6 hr

Metabolism: Hepatic; $T_{1/2}$: 2–3 hr
Distribution: Crosses placenta; may pass into breast milk
Excretion: Feces

▽IV facts

Preparation: May be diluted with isotonic saline, lactated Ringer's solution, 5% dextrose and 0.9% saline, 5% dextrose. Protect from light and excessive heat.

Infusion: Administer slowly over 2 min.

Compatibilities: Compatible IV with scopolamine HBr, haloperidol, glycopyrrolate, droperidol and hydroxyzine HCl.

Incompatibilities: Do not mix with diazepam and lorazepam.

Adverse effects

- **CNS:** *Sedation, dizziness or vertigo, headache,* confusion, dreaming, psychosis, euphoria, weakness, fatigue, nervousness, slurred speech, paresthesia, depression, malaise, hallucinations, depersonalization, coma, tremor, dysphoria, agitation, convulsions, tinnitus
- **CV:** *Hypotension,* hypertension, tachycardia, bradycardia, Wenckebach's block
- **Dermatologic:** *Sweating,* pruritus, rash, pallor, urticaria
- **EENT:** *Miosis,* blurred vision, diplopia, conjunctivitis, visual abnormalities, amblyopia
- **GI:** *Nausea, vomiting,* dry mouth, constipation, flatulence
- **Local:** Injection site reaction
- **Respiratory:** *Hypoventilation,* dyspnea, cyanosis, apnea

Interactions

✴ **Drug-drug** • Potentiation of effects of buprenorphine with other narcotic analgesics, phenothiazines, tranquilizers, barbiturates, general anesthetics

■ Nursing considerations
Assessment

- **History:** Hypersensitivity to buprenorphine, physical dependence on narcotic analgesics, compromised respiratory function, increased intracranial pressure, myxedema, Addison's disease, toxic psychosis, prostatic hypertrophy or urethral stricture, acute alcoholism, delirium tremens, kyphoscoliosis, biliary tract dysfunction, hepatic or renal dysfunction, lactation
- **Physical:** Skin color, texture, lesions; orientation, reflexes, bilateral grip strength, affect; pupil size, vision; pulse, auscultation, BP; R, adventitious sounds; bowel sounds, normal output, liver palpation; prostate palpation, normal urine output; liver, kidney, thyroid, adrenal function tests

Interventions

- Provide narcotic antagonist, facilities for assisted or controlled respiration on standby in case respiratory depression occurs.
- Have the patient hold sublingual tablets *(Subutex)* beneath the tongue until they dissolve; these tablets should not be swallowed.
- Instruct patient being treated for opioid dependence that CNS depression and death can occur with overdose of these drugs, or if this drug is combined with sedatives, alcohol, tranquilizers, antidepressants, benzodiazepines.
- Manage overdose by providing ventilation and support.

Teaching points

- These side effects may occur: dizziness, sedation, drowsiness, impaired visual acuity (avoid driving, performing other tasks that require alertness); nausea, loss of appetite (lying quietly, eating frequent small meals may help).
- Report severe nausea, vomiting, palpitations, shortness of breath or difficulty breathing, urinary difficulty.
- Hold sublingual tablets under the tongue until they dissolve. Do not swallow these tablets.
- Inform all health care or emergency workers that you are opioid dependent and using this drug for maintenance; serious effects could occur if certain drugs are used with this drug.
- Avoid combining *Subutex* with any alcohol, antidepressants, sedatives, benzodiazepines, tranquilizers; serious CNS depression could occur. Do not crush and inject these tablets.
- Be aware that overdose with *Subutex* can result in coma and death; use this drug exactly as prescribed.

Adverse effects in *Italics* are most common; those in **Bold** are life-threatening.

▷bupropion hydrochloride
*(byoo **proe'** pee on)*

Wellbutrin, Wellbutrin SR, Zyban

PREGNANCY CATEGORY B

Drug classes
Antidepressant
Smoking deterrent

Therapeutic actions
The neurochemical mechanism of the antidepressant effect of bupropion is not understood; it is chemically unrelated to other antidepressant agents; it is a weak blocker of neuronal uptake of serotonin and norepinephrine and inhibits the reuptake of dopamine to some extent.

Indications
- Treatment of depression (effectiveness if used > 6 wk is unknown)
- Aid to smoking cessation treatment (*Zyban*)

Contraindications and cautions
- Contraindicated with hypersensitivity to bupropion; history of seizure disorder, bulimia or anorexia, head trauma, CNS tumor (increased risk of seizures); treatment with MAOIs; lactation.
- Use cautiously with renal or liver disease; heart disease, history of MI.

Available forms
Tablets—75, 100 mg; SR tablets—100, 150, 200 mg

Dosages
Adults
- *Depression:* 300 mg PO given as 100 mg tid; begin treatment with 100 mg PO bid; if clinical response warrants, increase 3 days after beginning treatment. If 4 wk after treatment, no clinical improvement is seen, dose may be increased to 150 mg PO tid (450 mg/day). Do not exceed 150 mg in any one dose. Discontinue drug if no improvement occurs at the 450 mg/day level. *Sustained release:* 150 mg PO bid; allow at least 8 hr between doses.

- *Smoking cessation:* 150 mg PO daily for 3 days, then increase to 300 mg/day in 2 divided doses at least 8 hr apart. Treat for 7–12 weeks.

Pediatric patients
Safety and efficacy in patients < 18 yr not established.

Geriatric patients
Bupropion is excreted through the kidneys; use with caution, and monitor older patients carefully.

Pharmacokinetics

Route	Onset	Peak	Duration
Oral	Varies	2 hr	8–12 hr

Metabolism: Hepatic; $T_{1/2}$: 8–24 hr
Distribution: May cross placenta; may pass into breast milk
Excretion: Urine and feces

Adverse effects
- **CNS:** *Agitation, insomnia, headache, migraine, tremor,* ataxia, incoordination, **seizures,** mania, increased libido, hallucinations, visual disturbances
- **CV:** *Dizziness, tachycardia,* edema, ECG abnormalities, chest pain, shortness of breath
- **Dermatologic:** Rash, alopecia, dry skin
- **GI:** *Dry mouth, constipation,* nausea, vomiting, stomatitis
- **GU:** Nocturia, vaginal irritation, testicular swelling
- **Other:** *Weight loss,* flulike symptoms

Interactions
✳ **Drug-drug** • Increased risk of adverse effects with levodopa • Increased risk of toxicity with MAO inhibitors • Increased risk of seizures with drugs that lower seizure threshold, including alcohol

■ Nursing considerations
Assessment
- **History:** Hypersensitivity to bupropion, history of seizure disorder, bulimia or anorexia, head trauma, CNS tumor, treatment with MAO inhibitor, renal or liver disease, heart disease, lactation
- **Physical:** Skin, weight; orientation, affect, vision, coordination; P, rhythm, auscultation; R, adventitious sounds; bowel sounds, condition of mouth

Interventions

- Administer drug tid for depression; do not administer more than 150 mg in any one dose. Administer sustained-release forms bid with at least 8 hr between doses.
- Increase dosage slowly to reduce the risk of seizures.
- Administer 100-mg tablets qid for depression, with at least 4 hr between doses, if patient is receiving > 300 mg/day; use combinations of 75-mg tablets to avoid giving > 150 mg in any single dose.
- Arrange for patient evaluation after 6 wk; effects of drug after 6 wk are not known.
- Discontinue MAO inhibitor therapy for at least 14 days before beginning bupropion.
- Monitor liver and renal function tests in patients with a history of liver or renal impairment.
- Have patient quit smoking within first 2 wk of treatment for smoking cessation; may be used with transdermal nicotine.
- Monitor response and behavior; suicide is a risk in depressed patients.

Teaching points

- Take this drug in equally divided doses tid to qid as prescribed for depression. Take sustained-release forms bid, at least 8 hr apart. Do not combine doses or make up missed doses. Take once a day, or divided into 2 doses at least 8 hr apart for smoking cessation.
- These side effects may occur: dizziness, lack of coordination, tremor (avoid driving or performing tasks that require alertness); dry mouth (use frequent mouth care, suck sugarless lozenges); headache, insomnia (consult with care provider if these become a problem; do not self-medicate); nausea, vomiting, weight loss (small, frequent meals may help).
- Avoid or limit the use of alcohol while on this drug. Seizures can occur if these are combined.
- May be used with transdermal nicotine; most effective for smoking cessation if combined with behavioral support program.
- Report dark urine, light-colored stools; rapid or irregular heart beat; hallucinations; severe headache or insomnia; fever, chills, sore throat.

▽ buspirone hydrochloride
(byoo spye' rone)

BuSpar

PREGNANCY CATEGORY B

Drug class
Antianxiety agent

Therapeutic actions
Mechanism of action not known; lacks anticonvulsant, sedative, or muscle relaxant properties; binds serotonin receptors, but the clinical significance is unclear.

Indications
- Management of anxiety disorders or short-term relief of symptoms of anxiety
- Unlabeled use: decreasing the symptoms (aches, pains, fatigue, cramps, irritability) of PMS

Contraindications and cautions
- Hypersensitivity to buspirone; marked liver or renal impairment; lactation.

Available forms
Tablets—5, 7.5, 10, 15, 30 mg

Dosages
Adults
Initially 15 mg/day PO (5 mg tid). Increase dosage 5 mg/day at intervals of 2–3 days to achieve optimal therapeutic response. Do not exceed 60 mg/day. Divided doses of 20–30 mg/day have been used.
Pediatric patients
Safety and efficacy for patients < 18 yr not established.

Pharmacokinetics

Route	Onset	Peak
Oral	7–10 days	40–90 min

Metabolism: Hepatic; $T_{1/2}$: 3–11 hr
Distribution: May pass into breast milk
Excretion: Urine

Adverse effects in *Italics* are most common; those in **Bold** are life-threatening.

Adverse effects

- **CNS:** *Dizziness, headache, nervousness, insomnia, light-headedness,* excitement, dream disturbances, drowsiness, decreased concentration, anger, hostility, confusion, depression, tinnitus, blurred vision, numbness, paresthesia, incoordination, tremor, depersonalization, dysphoria, noise intolerance, euphoria, akathisia, fearfulness, loss of interest, disassociative reaction, hallucinations, suicidal ideation, seizures, altered taste and smell, involuntary movements, slowed reaction time
- **CV:** Nonspecific chest pain, tachycardia or palpitations, syncope, hypotension, hypertension
- **GI:** *Nausea, dry mouth, vomiting, abdominal or gastric distress, diarrhea,* constipation, flatulence, anorexia, increased appetite, salivation, irritable colon and rectal bleeding
- **GU:** Urinary frequency, urinary hesitancy, dysuria, increased or decreased libido, menstrual irregularity, spotting
- **Respiratory:** Hyperventilation, shortness of breath, chest congestion
- **Other:** Musculoskeletal aches and pains, sweating, clamminess, sore throat, nasal congestion

Interactions

✳ **Drug-drug** • Give with caution to patients taking alcohol, other CNS depressants • Decreased effects with fluoxetine • Increased serum levels of buspirone if taken with erythromycin, itraconazole, netazodone; decrease buspirone dose to 2.5 mg and monitor closely if these combinations are used • Risk of increased haloperidol levels if combined.

■ Nursing considerations
Assessment

- **History:** Hypersensitivity to buspirone, marked liver or renal impairment, lactation
- **Physical:** Weight; T; skin color, lesions; mucous membranes, throat color, lesions, orientation, affect, reflexes, vision exam; P, BP; R, adventitious sounds; bowel sounds, normal GI output, liver evaluation; normal urinary output, voiding pattern; liver and kidney function tests, urinalysis, CBC and differential

Interventions

- Provide sugarless lozenges, ice chips, if dry mouth, altered taste occur.
- Arrange for analgesic for headache, musculoskeletal aches.

Teaching points

- Take this drug exactly as prescribed.
- Avoid the use of alcohol, sleep-inducing, or OTC drugs; these could cause dangerous effects.
- These side effects may occur: drowsiness, dizziness, light-headedness (avoid driving or operating complex machinery); GI upset (frequent small meals may help); dry mouth (suck ice chips or sugarless candies); dreams, nightmares, difficulty concentrating or sleeping, confusion, excitement (reversible; will stop when the drug is discontinued).
- Report abnormal involuntary movements of facial or neck muscles; motor restlessness; sore or cramped muscles; abnormal posture; yellowing of the skin or eyes.

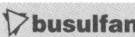

▽ busulfan
*(byoo **sul' fan**)*

Busulfex, Myleran

PREGNANCY CATEGORY D

Drug classes

Alkylating agent
Antineoplastic drug

Therapeutic actions

Cytotoxic: interacts with cellular thiol groups causing cell death; cell cycle nonspecific.

Indications

- Tablets: Palliative treatment of chronic myelogenous leukemia; less effective in patients without the Philadelphia chromosome (Ph1); ineffective in the blastic stage
- Injection: In combination with cyclophosphamide as conditioning regimen prior to allogenic hematopoietic progenitor cell transplant for CML

Contraindications and cautions

- Allergy to busulfan, history of resistance to busulfan, chronic lymphocytic leukemia, acute leukemia, blastic phase of chronic myelogenous leukemia, hematopoietic depression, pregnancy, lactation.

Available forms

Tablets—2 mg; injection—6 mg/mL

Dosages
Adults

- *Remission induction:* 4–8 mg total dose PO daily. Continue until WBC has dropped to 15,000/mm³; WBC may continue to fall for 1 mo after drug is discontinued. Normal WBC count is usually achieved in approximately 12–20 wk in most cases.
- *Maintenance therapy:* Resume treatment with induction dosage when WBC reaches 50,000/mm³. If remission is shorter than 3 mo, maintenance therapy of 1–3 mg PO daily is advised to keep hematologic status under control.
- *Conditioning regimen:* 0.8 mg/kg as a 2-hr infusion q 6 hr for 4 consecutive days (16 doses) via central venous catheter.

Pharmacokinetics

Route	Onset	Peak	Duration
Oral, IV	0.5–2 hr	2–3 hr	4 hr

Metabolism: Hepatic; $T_{1/2}$: 2.5 hr
Distribution: Crosses placenta; passes into breast milk
Excretion: Urine

▼IV facts

Preparation: Dilute to 10 times the busulfan volume using 0.9% sodium chloride injection or D_5W. Use enclosed filter when withdrawing drug from ampule. Final concentration should be greater than or equal to 0.5 mg/mL. Use strict aseptic technique. Always add busulfan to the diluent. Mix by inverting bag several times. Stable at room temperature for 8 hr, then discard.
Infusion: Use an infusion pump to deliver total dose over 2 hr. Flush catheter with 5 mL D_5W or 0.9% sodium chloride before and after each dose. Infusion must be completed within 8 hr.
Incompatibility: Do not infuse with any other solution or drugs.

Adverse effects

- **CNS: Seizures**
- **Dermatologic:** *Hyperpigmentation,* urticaria, **Stevens-Johnson syndrome,** erythema nodosum, alopecia, porphyria cutanea tarda, excessive dryness and fragility of the skin with anhidrosis
- **EENT:** Cataracts (with prolonged use)
- **Endocrine:** *Amenorrhea, ovarian suppression, menopausal symptoms,* interference with spermatogenesis, testicular atrophy, syndrome resembling adrenal insufficiency (weakness, fatigue, anorexia, weight loss, nausea, vomiting, melanoderma)
- **GI:** Dryness of the oral mucous membranes and cheilosis; *nausea, vomiting*
- **GU:** Hyperuricemia
- **Hematologic:** *Leukopenia, thrombocytopenia, anemia,* **pancytopenia** (prolonged)
- **Other:** Cancer

■ Nursing considerations
Assessment

- **History:** Allergy to or history of resistance to busulfan, chronic lymphocyctic leukemia, acute leukemia, blastic phase of chronic myelogenous leukemia, hematopoietic depression, pregnancy, lactation
- **Physical:** Weight; skin color, lesions, turgor; earlobe tophi; eye exam; bilateral hand grip; R, adventitious sounds; mucous membranes; CBC, differential; urinalysis; serum uric acid; pulmonary function tests; bone marrow exam if indicated

Interventions

- Arrange for blood tests to evaluate bone marrow function prior to, weekly during, and for at least 3 wk after therapy has ended.
- Arrange for respiratory function tests before beginning therapy, periodically during therapy, and periodically after busulfan therapy has ended.
- Reduce dosage in cases of bone marrow depression.
- Give at the same time each day.
- Suggest barrier contraceptive use during therapy.

- Ensure patient is hydrated before and during therapy; alkalinization of the urine or allopurinol may be needed to prevent adverse effects of hyperuricemia.
- Monitor patient for cataracts.
- Administer IV busulfan through a central venous catheter.
- Premedicate patient receiving IV busulfan with phenytoin to decrease occurrence of seizures.
- Medicate patient receiving IV busulfan with antiemetics prior to the first dose and on a fixed schedule through the administration regimen.

Teaching points
Oral drug

- Take drug at the same time each day.
- Drink 10–12 glasses of fluid each day.
- These side effects may occur: darkening of the skin, rash, dry and fragile skin (skin care suggestions will be outlined for you to help to prevent skin breakdown); weakness, fatigue (consult with care provider if pronounced); loss of appetite, nausea, vomiting, weight loss (try frequent small meals); amenorrhea in women, change in sperm production in men (may affect fertility).
- Have regular medical follow up, including blood tests, to monitor effects of the drug.
- Consider using barrier contraceptives. This drug has been known to cause fetal damage.
- Report unusual bleeding or bruising; fever, chills, sore throat; stomach, flank, or joint pain; cough, shortness of breath.

▷butabarbital sodium
*(byoo ta **bar'** bi tal)*

secbutabarbital

secbutobarbitone
Busodium (CAN), Butalan (CAN), Butisol Sodium, Sarisol #2 (CAN)

PREGNANCY CATEGORY D

C-III CONTROLLED SUBSTANCE

Drug classes
Barbiturate (intermediate acting)
Sedative and hypnotic

Therapeutic actions
General CNS depressant; barbiturates inhibit impulse conduction in the ascending reticular activating system, depress the cerebral cortex, alter cerebellar function, depress motor output, and can produce excitation (especially with subanesthetic doses in the presence of pain), sedation, hypnosis, anesthesia, deep coma.

Indications
- Short-term use as a sedative and hypnotic

Contraindications and cautions
- Contraindicated with hypersensitivity to barbiturates, tartrazine (in 30-, 50-mg tablets, and elixir marketed as *Butisol Sodium*); manifest or latent porphyria; marked liver impairment; nephritis; severe respiratory distress, respiratory disease with dyspnea, obstruction, or cor pulmonale; previous addiction to sedative-hypnotic drugs.
- Use cautiously with acute or chronic pain (may cause paradoxical excitement or mask important symptoms); seizure disorders (abrupt discontinuation of daily doses can result in status epilepticus); lactation (can cause drowsiness in nursing infants); fever, hyperthyroidism, diabetes mellitus, severe anemia, pulmonary or cardiac disease, status asthmaticus, shock, uremia; impaired liver or kidney function, debilitation, pregnancy.

Available forms
Tablets—15, 30, 50, 100 mg; elixir—30 mg/ 5 mL

Dosages
Adults

- *Daytime sedation:* 15–30 mg PO tid–qid.
- *Hypnotic:* 50–100 mg PO at hs. Drug loses effectiveness within 2 wk and should not be used longer than that.
- *Preanesthetic sedation:* 50–100 mg PO 60–90 min before surgery. *Note:* It is not considered safe to administer oral medication when a patient is NPO for surgery or anesthesia.

Pediatric patients
Use caution: barbiturates may produce irritability, excitability, inappropriate tearfulness, and aggression.

- *Preanesthetic sedation:* 2–6 mg/kg; maximum dose 100 mg (see note above).

Geriatric patients or patients with debilitating disease or hepatic or renal dysfunction

Reduce dosage and monitor closely; may produce excitement, depression, confusion.

Pharmacokinetics

Route	Onset	Peak	Duration
Oral	45–60 min	3–4 hr	6–8 hr

Metabolism: Hepatic; $T_{1/2}$: 50–100 hr
Distribution: Crosses placenta; passes into breast milk
Excretion: Urine

Adverse effects

- **CNS:** *Somnolence, agitation, confusion, hyperkinesia, ataxia, vertigo, CNS depression, nightmares, lethargy, residual sedation (hangover), paradoxical excitement, nervousness, psychiatric disturbance, hallucinations, insomnia, anxiety, dizziness, thinking abnormality*
- **CV:** *Bradycardia, hypotension, syncope*
- **GI:** *Nausea, vomiting, constipation, diarrhea, epigastric pain*
- **Hypersensitivity:** Rashes, angioneurotic edema, serum sickness, morbiliform rash, urticaria; rarely, exfoliative dermatitis, **Stevens-Johnson syndrome**
- **Respiratory:** *Hypoventilation, apnea, respiratory depression,* laryngospasm, bronchospasm, **circulatory collapse**
- **Other:** Tolerance, psychological and physical dependence; **withdrawal syndrome**

Interactions

✻ Drug-drug • Increased CNS depression with alcohol • Increased risk of nephrotoxicity with methoxyflurane • Decreased effects of: theophyllines, oral anticoagulants, beta-blockers, doxycycline, griseofulvin, corticosteroids, oral contraceptives and estrogens, metronidazole, phenylbutazones, quinidine, carbamazepine

■ Nursing considerations

Assessment

- **History:** Hypersensitivity to barbiturates, tartrazine, manifest or latent porphyria; marked liver impairment, nephritis, respiratory disease; previous addiction to sedative-hypnotic drugs, acute or chronic pain, seizure disorders, fever, hyperthyroidism, diabetes mellitus, severe anemia, cardiac disease, shock, uremia, debilitation, pregnancy, lactation
- **Physical:** Weight; T; skin color, lesions; orientation, affect, reflexes; P, BP, orthostatic BP; R, adventitious sounds; bowel sounds, normal output, liver evaluation; liver and kidney function tests, blood and urine glucose, BUN

Interventions

- Monitor responses, blood levels if any of the above interacting drugs are given with butabarbital; suggest alternatives to oral contraceptives.
- Provide resuscitative equipment on standby in case of respiratory depression, hypersensitivity reaction.
- Taper dosage gradually after repeated use, especially in epileptic patients.

Teaching points

- This drug will make you drowsy and less anxious.
- Try not to get up after you have received this drug (request assistance to sit up or move about).

Outpatients taking this drug

- Take this drug exactly as prescribed.
- This drug is habit-forming; its effectiveness in facilitating sleep disappears after a short time. Do not take this drug longer than 2 wk (for insomnia), and do not increase the dosage without consulting the physician.
- Consult the care provider if the drug appears to be ineffective.
- Avoid alcohol, sleep-inducing, or OTC drugs; they could cause dangerous effects.
- Use an alternative to oral contraceptives; avoid becoming pregnant while taking this drug.
- These side effects may occur: drowsiness, dizziness, hangover, impaired thinking (less

pronounced after a few days; avoid driving or engaging in dangerous activities); GI upset (take the drug with food); dreams, nightmares, difficulty concentrating, fatigue, nervousness (reversible, will go away when the drug is discontinued).
- Report severe dizziness, weakness, drowsiness that persists, rash or skin lesions, pregnancy.

▷ butorphanol tartrate
(byoo tor' fa nole)

Stadol, Stadol NS

PREGNANCY CATEGORY C (DURING PREGNANCY)

PREGNANCY CATEGORY D (DURING LABOR AND DELIVERY)

C-IV CONTROLLED SUBSTANCE

Drug class
Narcotic agonist-antagonist analgesic

Therapeutic actions
Acts as an agonist at opioid receptors in the CNS to produce analgesia, sedation (therapeutic effects), but also acts to cause hallucinations (adverse effect); has low abuse potential.

Indications
- Relief of moderate to severe pain
- Relief of migraine headache pain (nasal spray)
- For preoperative or preanesthetic medication, to supplement balanced anesthesia, and to relieve prepartum pain

Contraindications and cautions
- Contraindicated with hypersensitivity to butorphanol, physical dependence on a narcotic analgesic, pregnancy, lactation.
- Use cautiously with bronchial asthma, COPD, respiratory depression, anoxia, increased intracranial pressure, acute MI, ventricular failure, coronary insufficiency, hypertension, biliary tract surgery, renal or hepatic dysfunction.

Available forms
Injection—1 mg/mL, 2 mg/mL; nasal spray—10 mg/mL

Dosages
Adults
IM
Usual single dose is 2 mg q 3–4 hr. Dosage range is 1–4 mg q 3–4 hr; single doses should not exceed 4 mg.
- *Preoperative:* 2 mg IM, 60–90 min before surgery.
- *IV:* Usual single dose is 1 mg q 3–4 hr. Dosage range is 0.5–2 mg q 3–4 hr.
- *Balanced anesthesia:* 2 mg IV shortly before induction or 0.5–1 mg IV in increments during anesthesia.
- *Labor:* 1–2 mg IV or IM at full term during early labor; repeat q 4 hr.
- *Nasal:* 1 mg (1 spray per nostril). May repeat in 60–90 min if adequate relief is not achieved. May repeat two-dose sequence q 3–4 hr.

Pediatric patients
Not recommended for patients < 18 yr.
Geriatric patients or patients with renal or hepatic impairment
- *Parenteral:* Use one-half the usual dose at twice the usual interval. Monitor patient response.
- *Nasal:* 1 mg initially. Allow 90–120 min to elapse before a second dose is given.

Pharmacokinetics

Route	Onset	Peak	Duration
IV	Rapid	0.5–1 hr	3–4 hr
IM	10–15 min	0.5–1 hr	3–4 hr
Nasal	15 min	1–2 hr	4–5 hr

Metabolism: Hepatic; $T_{1/2}$: 2.1–9.2 hr
Distribution: Crosses placenta; passes into breast milk
Excretion: Urine and feces

▽ IV facts
Preparation: May be given undiluted. Store at room temperature. Protect from light.
Infusion: Administer direct IV at rate of 2 mg every 3–5 min.
Compatibilities: Do not mix in solution with dimenhydrinate, pentobarbital.
Y-site compatible: Enalaprilat.

Adverse effects

- **CNS:** *Sedation, clamminess, sweating, headache, vertigo, floating feeling, dizziness, lethargy, confusion, light-headedness,* nervousness, unusual dreams, agitation, euphoria, hallucinations
- **CV:** Palpitation, increase or decrease in blood pressure
- **Dermatologic:** Rash, hives, pruritus, flushing, warmth, sensitivity to cold
- **EENT:** Diplopia, blurred vision
- **GI:** *Nausea,* dry mouth
- **Respiratory:** Slow, shallow respiration

Interactions

✳ **Drug-drug** • Potentiation of effects of butorphanol when given with barbiturate anesthetics

■ Nursing considerations

Assessment

- **History:** Hypersensitivity to butorphanol, physical dependence on a narcotic analgesic, pregnancy, lactation, bronchial asthma, COPD, increased intracranial pressure, acute MI, ventricular failure, coronary insufficiency, hypertension, biliary tract surgery, renal or hepatic dysfunction
- **Physical:** Orientation, reflexes, bilateral grip strength, affect; pupil size, vision; pulse, auscultation, BP; R, adventitious sounds; bowel sounds, normal output; liver, kidney function tests

Interventions

- Provide narcotic antagonist, facilities for assisted or controlled respiration on standby during parenteral administration.

Teaching points

- These side effects may occur: dizziness, sedation, drowsiness, impaired visual acuity (avoid driving, performing other tasks that require alertness); nausea, loss of appetite (lying quietly, eating frequent small meals may help).
- Report severe nausea, vomiting, palpitations, shortness of breath or difficulty breathing, nasal lesions or discomfort (nasal spray).

▷ cabergoline

See *Less Commonly Used Drugs,* p. 1340.

▷ caffeine
(kaf een')

caffeine
Caffedrine, Enerjets, Keep Alert, NoDoz, Overtime, Stay Awake, Vivarin

caffeine citrate
CAFCIT

PREGNANCY CATEGORY C

Drug classes
Analeptic
Xanthine

Therapeutic actions
Increases calcium permeability in sarcoplasmic reticulum, promotes the accumulation of cAMP, and blocks adenosine receptors; stimulates the CNS, cardiac activity, gastric acid secretion, and diuresis.

Indications

- An aid in staying awake and restoring mental awareness
- Adjunct to analgesic formulations
- Possibly an analeptic in conjunction with supportive measures to treat respiratory depression associated with overdose with CNS depressants (IM)
- Short-term treatment of apnea of prematurity in infants between 28 and 33 wk gestation (caffeine citrate)
- Unlabeled uses: headache, alcoholism, asthma, orthostatic hypotension

Contraindications and cautions

- Depression, duodenal ulcers, diabetes mellitus, lactation.

Available forms
Tablets—200 mg; capsules—200 mg; lozenges—75 mg; injection—250 mg/mL;

---

caffeine citrate injection/oral solution—20 mg/mL

Dosages
20 mg caffeine citrate = 10 mg caffeine base; use caution.
Adults
100–200 mg PO q 3–4 hr as needed.
- *Respiratory depression:* 500 mg–1 g caffeine and sodium benzoate (250–500 mg caffeine) IM; do not exceed 2.5 g/day; may be given IV in severe emergency situation.
Pediatric patients
- *Neonatal apnea:* 20 mg/kg IV followed 24 hours later by 5 mg/kg/day as maintenance (*CAFCIT*).

Pharmacokinetics

Route	Onset	Peak
Oral	15 min	15–45 min

Metabolism: Hepatic; $T_{1/2}$: 3–7.5 hr, 100 hr (neonates)
Distribution: Crosses placenta; passes into breast milk
Excretion: Urine

▼ IV facts
Preparation: Dissolve 10 g caffeine citrate powder in 250 mL sterile water for injection USP to 500 mL; filter and autoclave. Final concentration is 10 mg/mL caffeine base (20 mg/mL caffeine citrate). Stable for 3 mo. Or dissolve 10 mg caffeine powder and 10.9 g citric acid powder in bacteriostatic water for injection, USP to 1 L. Sterilize by filtration. *CAFCIT:* 60 mg/3 mL vial may be diluted to achieve desired dose.
Infusion: IV single dose of 500 mg caffeine may be given slowly over 2 min in emergency situations; not recommended. *CAFCIT:* Give 20 mg/kg as a single dose over 30 min; maintain with infusion of 5 mg/kg/day.

Adverse effects
- **CNS:** *Insomnia, restlessness, excitement,* nervousness, tinnitus, muscular tremor, headaches, light-headedness
- **CV:** *Tachycardia,* extrasystoles, palpitations
- **GI:** Nausea, vomiting, diarrhea, stomach pain
- **GU:** *Diuresis*

- **Other:** Withdrawal syndrome: headache, anxiety, muscle tension

Interactions
✳ **Drug-drug** ● Increased CNS effects of caffeine with cimetidine, oral contraceptives, disulfiram, ciprofloxacin, mexiletine ● Decreased effects of caffeine while smoking ● Increased serum levels of theophylline, clozapine with caffeine
✳ **Drug-food** ● Decreased absorption of iron if taken with or 1 hr after coffee or tea
✳ **Drug-lab test** ● Possible false elevations of serum urate, urine VMA, resulting in false-positive diagnosis of pheochromocytoma or neuroblastoma

■ Nursing considerations
Assessment
- **History:** Depression, duodenal ulcer, diabetes mellitus, lactation
- **Physical:** Neurologic status, P, BP, ECG, normal urinary output, abdominal exam, blood glucose

Interventions
- Do not stop the drug abruptly after long-term use.
- Monitor diet for presence of caffeine-containing foods that may contribute to overdose.

Teaching points
- Do not stop taking this drug abruptly; withdrawal symptoms may occur.
- Avoid foods high in caffeine (coffee, tea, cola, chocolate), which may cause symptoms of overdose.
- Avoid driving or dangerous activities if dizziness, tremors, restlessness occur.
- Consult with your health care provider if fatigue continues.
- These side effects may occur: diuresis, restlessness, insomnia, muscular tremors, light-headedness; nausea, abdominal pain.
- Report abnormal heart rate, dizziness, palpitations.
- Caffeine citrate—parents of infants being treated for apnea should have drug information incorporated into the overall teaching plan.

▷ calcitonin
(kal si toe' nin)

calcitonin, human
Cibacalcin

calcitonin, salmon
Calcimar, Caltine (CAN), Miacalcin, Miacalcin Nasal Spray, Osteocalcin, Salmonine

PREGNANCY CATEGORY C
(HUMAN)

PREGNANCY CATEGORY B
(SALMON)

Drug classes
Hormonal agent
Calcium regulator

Therapeutic actions
The calcitonins are polypeptide hormones secreted by the thyroid; human calcitonin is a synthetic product classified as an orphan drug; salmon calcitonin appears to be a chemically identical polypeptide but with greater potency per milligram and longer duration; inhibits bone resorption; lowers elevated serum calcium in children and patients with Paget's disease; increases the excretion of filtered phosphate, calcium, and sodium by the kidney.

Indications
- Paget's disease (human and salmon calcitonin)
- Postmenopausal osteoporosis in conjunction with adequate calcium and vitamin D intake to prevent loss of bone mass (salmon calcitonin)
- Hypercalcemia, emergency treatment (salmon calcitonin)

Contraindications and cautions
- Contraindicated with allergy to salmon calcitonin or fish products, lactation.
- Use cautiously with renal insufficiency, osteoporosis, pernicious anemia.

Available forms
Injection (human)—1 mg/mL; injection (salmon)—200 IU/mL; nasal spray (salmon)—200 IU/actuation

Dosages
Adults
Calcitonin, human
- *Paget's disease:* Starting dose of 0.5 mg/day SC; some patients may respond to 0.5 mg two to three times per week or 0.25 mg/day. Severe cases may require up to 1 mg/day for 6 mo. Discontinue therapy when symptoms are relieved.

Calcitonin, salmon
- *Skin testing:* 0.1 mL of a 10 IU/mL solution injected SC.
- *Paget's disease:* Initial dose 100 IU/day SC or IM. *Maintenance dose:* 50 IU/day or every other day. Actual dose should be determined by patient response.
- *Postmenopausal osteoporosis:* 100 IU/day SC or IM, with supplemental calcium (calcium carbonate, 1.5 g/day) and vitamin D (400 units/day) *or* 200 IU intranasally daily.
- *Hypercalcemia:* Initial dose: 4 IU/kg q 12 hr SC or IM. If response is not satisfactory after 1–2 days, increase to 8 IU/kg q 12 hr; if response remains unsatisfactory after 2 more days, increase to 8 IU/kg q 6 hr.

Pediatric patients
Safety and efficacy not established.

Pharmacokinetics

Route	Onset	Peak	Duration
IM, SC	15 min	3–4 hr	8–24 hr

Metabolism: Renal; $T_{1/2}$: 1.2 hr (salmon), 1 hr (human)
Distribution: May pass into breast milk
Excretion: Urine

Adverse effects
- **Dermatologic:** *Flushing of face or hands,* rash
- **GI:** *Nausea, vomiting*
- **GU:** *Urinary frequency* (calcitonin-human)
- **Local:** *Local inflammatory reactions at injection site* (salmon), nasal irritation (nasal spray)

Adverse effects in *Italics* are most common; those in **Bold** are life-threatening.

■ Nursing considerations
Assessment
- **History:** Allergy to salmon calcitonin or fish products, lactation, osteoporosis, pernicious anemia, renal disease
- **Physical:** Skin lesions, color, T; muscle tone; urinalysis, serum calcium, serum alkaline phosphatase and urinary hydroxyproline excretion

Interventions
- Give skin test to patients with any history of allergies; salmon calcitonin is a protein, and risk of allergy is significant. Prepare solution for skin test as follows: withdraw 0.05 mL of the 200 IU/mL solution or 0.1 mL of the 100 IU/mL solution into a tuberculin syringe. Fill to 1 mL with sodium chloride injection. Mix well. Discard 0.9 mL, and inject 0.1 mL (approximately 1 IU) SC into the inner aspect of the forearm. Observe after 15 min; the presence of a wheal or more than mild erythema indicates a positive response. Risk of allergy is less in patients being treated with human calcitonin.
- Use reconstituted human calcitonin within 6 hr.
- Maintain parenteral calcium on standby in case of development of hypocalcemic tetany.
- Monitor serum alkaline phosphatase and urinary hydroxyproline excretion prior to therapy and during first 3 mo and q 3–6 mo during long-term therapy.
- Inject doses of more than 2 mL IM, not SC; use multiple injection sites.
- Refrigerate nasal spray until activated, then store at room temperature.

Teaching points
- This drug is given SC or IM; you or a significant other must learn how to do this at home. Refrigerate the drug vials.
- For intranasal use, alternate nostrils daily; notify health care provider if significant nasal irritation occurs.
- These side effects may occur: nausea, vomiting (this passes); irritation at injection site (rotate sites); flushing of the face or hands, rash.
- Report twitching, muscle spasms; dark urine; hives, rash; difficulty breathing.

▷ calcium salts

calcium carbonate
Apo-Cal (CAN), Calcite 500 (CAN), Calsan (CAN), Caltrate, Chooz, Equilet, Os-Cal, Oyst-Cal, Oystercal, Tums

calcium chloride
calcium gluceptate
calcium gluconate
calcium lactate
PREGNANCY CATEGORY C

Drug classes
Electrolyte
Antacid

Therapeutic actions
Essential element of the body; helps maintain the functional integrity of the nervous and muscular systems; helps maintain cardiac function, blood coagulation; is an enzyme cofactor and affects the secretory activity of endocrine and exocrine glands; neutralizes or reduces gastric acidity (oral use).

Indications
- Dietary supplement when calcium intake is inadequate
- Treatment of calcium deficiency in tetany of the newborn, acute and chronic hypoparathyroidism, pseudohypoparathyroidism, postmenopausal and senile osteoporosis, rickets, osteomalacia
- Prevention of hypocalcemia during exchange transfusions
- Adjunctive therapy for insect bites or stings, such as black widow spider bites; sensitivity reactions, particularly when characterized by urticaria; depression due to overdose of magnesium sulfate; acute symptoms of lead colic
- Combats the effects of hyperkalemia as measured by ECG, pending correction of increased potassium in the extracellular fluid (calcium chloride)

- Improves weak or ineffective myocardial contractions when epinephrine fails in cardiac resuscitation, particularly after open heart surgery
- Symptomatic relief of upset stomach associated with hyperacidity; hyperacidity associated with peptic ulcer, gastritis, peptic esophagitis, gastric hyperacidity, hiatal hernia (calcium carbonate)
- Prophylaxis of GI bleeding, stress ulcers, and aspiration pneumonia; possibly useful (calcium carbonate)
- Unlabeled use: treatment of hypertension in some patients with indices suggesting calcium "deficiency"

Contraindications and cautions

- Allergy to calcium, renal calculi, hypercalcemia, ventricular fibrillation during cardiac resuscitation and patients with the risk of existing digitalis toxicity.

Available forms

Tablets—250, 500, 650, 975 mg, 1 g, 1.25 g, 1.5 g; powder—2,400 mg; injection—10%, 1.1 g/5 mL

Dosages
Adults
Calcium carbonate or lactate

- *RDA:* 0–24 yr: 1,200 mg; 25–49 yr: 800 mg; > 50 yr: 1,000–1,200 mg
- *Dietary supplement:* 500 mg–2 g PO, bid–qid.
- *Antacid:* 0.5-2 g PO calcium carbonate as needed.

Calcium chloride
For IV use only: 1 g contains 272 mg (13.6 mEq) calcium.

- *Hypocalcemic disorders:* 500 mg–1 g at intervals of 1–3 days.
- *Magnesium intoxication:* 500 mg promptly. Observe patient for signs of recovery before giving another dose.
- *Hyperkalemic ECG disturbances of cardiac function:* Adjust dose according to ECG response.
- *Cardiac resuscitation:* 500 mg–1 g IV or 200–800 mg into the ventricular cavity.

Calcium gluconate
- *IV infusion preferred:* 1 g contains 90 mg (4.5 mEq) calcium. 0.5–2 g as required; daily dose 1–15 g.

Calcium glucceptate
- *IM or IV use:* 1.1 g contains 90 mg (4.5 mEq) calcium; solution for injection contains 1.1 g/5 mL. 2–5 mL IM; 5–20 mL IV.

Pediatric patients
Calcium gluconate
500 mg/kg/day IV given in divided doses.

Calcium glucceptate
- *Exchange transfusions in newborns:* 0.5 mL after every 100 mL of blood exchanged.

Pharmacokinetics

Route	Onset	Peak
Oral	3–5 min	N/A
IV	Immediate	3–5 min

Metabolism: Hepatic; $T_{1/2}$: 1–3 hr
Distribution: Crosses placenta; passes into breast milk
Excretion: Feces, urine

▼IV facts
Preparation: Warm solutions to body temperature; use a small needle inserted into a large vein to decrease irritation.

Infusion: Infuse slowly, 0.5-2 mL/min. Stop infusion if patient complains of discomfort; resume when symptoms disappear. Repeated injections are often necessary.

Incompatibilities: Avoid mixing calcium salts with carbonates, phosphates, sulfates, tartrates, amphotericin, cefamandole, cephalothin, cefazolin, clindamycin, dobutamine, prednisolone.

Adverse effects

- **CV:** *Slowed heart rate, tingling, "heat waves"* (rapid IV administration); *peripheral vasodilation, local burning,* fall in blood pressure (calcium chloride injection)
- **Local:** *Local irritation,* severe necrosis, sloughing and abscess formation (IM, SC use of calcium chloride)
- **Metabolic:** Hypercalcemia (*anorexia, nausea, vomiting, constipation,* abdominal pain, dry mouth, thirst, polyuria), *re-*

bound hyperacidity and milk-alkali syndrome (hypercalcemia, alkalosis, renal damage with calcium carbonate used as an antacid)

Interactions

✳ **Drug-drug** • Decreased serum levels of oral tetracyclines, salicylates, iron salts with oral calcium salts. Give these drugs at least 1 hr apart. • Increased serum levels of quinidine and possible toxicity with calcium salts • Antagonism of effects of verapamil with calcium

✳ **Drug-food** • Decreased absorption of oral calcium when taken concurrently with oxalic acid (found in rhubarb and spinach), phytic acid (bran and whole cereals), phosphorus (milk and dairy products)

✳ **Drug-lab test** • False-negative values for serum and urinary magnesium

■ Nursing considerations
Assessment

• **History:** Allergy to calcium; renal calculi; hypercalcemia; ventricular fibrillation during cardiac resuscitation; digitalis toxicity
• **Physical:** Injection site; P, auscultation, BP, peripheral perfusion, ECG; abdominal exam, bowel sounds, mucous membranes; serum electrolytes, urinalysis

Interventions

• Give drug hourly for first 2 wk when treating acute peptic ulcer. During healing stage, administer 1-3 hr after meals and hs.
• Do not administer oral drugs within 1–2 hr of antacid administration.
• Have patient chew antacid tablets thoroughly before swallowing; follow with a glass of water or milk.
• Give calcium carbonate antacid 1 and 3 hr after meals and hs.
• Avoid extravasation of IV injection; it irritates the tissues and can cause necrosis and sloughing. Use a small needle in a large vein.
• Have patient remain recumbent for a short time after IV injection.
• Administer into ventricular cavity during cardiac resuscitation, not into myocardium.
• Warm calcium gluconate if crystallization has occurred.
• Monitor serum phosphorus levels periodically during long-term oral therapy.

• Monitor cardiac response closely during parenteral treatment with calcium.

Teaching points
Parenteral
• Report any pain or discomfort at the injection site as soon as possible.
Oral
• Take drug between meals and at bedtime. Ulcer patients must take drug as prescribed. Chew tablets thoroughly before swallowing, and follow with a glass of water or milk.
• Do not take with other oral drugs. Absorption of those medications can be blocked; take other oral medications at least 1–2 hr after calcium carbonate.
• These side effects may occur: constipation (can be medicated), nausea, GI upset, loss of appetite (special dietary consultation may be necessary).
• Report loss of appetite; nausea, vomiting, abdominal pain, constipation; dry mouth, thirst, increased voiding.

▷calfactant (DDPC, natural lung surfactant)
*(cal **fak'** tant)*
Infasurf

Drug class
Lung surfactant

Therapeutic actions
A natural bovine compound containing lipids and apoproteins that reduce surface tension, allowing expansion of the alveoli; replaces the surfactant missing in the lungs of neonates suffering from respiratory distress syndrome (RDS).

Indications
• Prophylactic treatment of infants at risk of developing RDS; infants < 29 wk gestation
• Rescue treatment of premature infants ≤ 72 hr of age who have developed RDS and require endotracheal intubation; best if started ≤ 30 min after birth

Contraindications and cautions

- Because calfactant is used as an emergency drug in acute respiratory situations, the benefits usually outweigh any possible risks.

Available forms

Dosages

- *Intratracheal suspension*—35 mg/mL
Infants
Accurate determination of birth weight is essential for determining appropriate dosage. Calfactant is instilled into the trachea using a catheter inserted into the endotracheal tube.
- *Prophylactic treatment:* Instill 3 mL/kg of birth weight as soon after birth as possible, administered as 2 doses of 1.5 mg/kg each.
- *Rescue treatment:* Instill 3 mL/kg of birth weight in two doses of 1.5 mg/kg each. Repeat doses of 3 mL/kg of birth weight up to a total of 3 doses 12 hr apart.

Pharmacokinetics

Route	Onset	Peak
Intratracheal	Immediate	Hours

Metabolism: Normal surfactant metabolic pathways; $T_{1/2}$: < 24 hr
Distribution: Lung tissue

Adverse effects

- **CNS: Seizures, intracranial hemorrhage**
- **CV: Patent ductus arteriosus, intraventricular hemorrhage,** *hypotension, bradycardia*
- **Hematologic:** *Hyperbilirubinemia, thrombocytopenia*
- **Respiratory: Pneumothorax,** *pulmonary air leak,* **pulmonary hemorrhage** (more often seen with infants < 700 g), *apnea,* pneumomediastinum, emphysema
- **Other:** *Sepsis, non-pulmonary infections*

■ Nursing considerations
Assessment

- **History:** Time of birth, exact birth weight
- **Physical:** Temperature, color; R, adventitious sounds, oximeter, endotracheal tube position and patency, chest movement; ECG, P, BP, peripheral perfusion, arterial pressure (desirable); oxygen saturation, blood gases, CBC; muscular activity, facial expression, reflexes

Interventions

- Arrange for appropriate assessment and monitoring of critically ill infant.
- Monitor ECG and transcutaneous oxygen saturation continually during administration.
- Ensure that endotracheal tube is in the correct position, with bilateral chest movement and lung sounds.
- Do not dilute or mix calfactant with any other drugs or solutions. Administer as provided. Warm unopened vials to room temperature. Gently swirl to mix contents.
- Suction the infant immediately before administration; but do not suction for 2 hr after administration unless clinically necessary.
- Store drug in refrigerator. Protect from light. Enter drug vial only once. Discard remaining drug after use. Avoid repeated warmings to room temperature.
- Insert 5 French catheter into the endotracheal tube; do not instill into the mainstream bronchus.
- Instill dose slowly; inject one-quarter dose over 2–3 seconds; remove catheter and reattach infant to ventilator for at least 30 sec or until stable; repeat procedure administering one-quarter dose at a time.
- Do not suction infant for 1 hr after completion of full dose; do not flush catheter.
- Continually monitor patient color, lung sounds, ECG, oximeter and blood gas readings during administration and for at least 30 min following administration.
- Maintain appropriate interventions for critically ill infant.
- Offer support and encouragement to parents.

Teaching points

- Parents of the critically ill infant will need a comprehensive teaching and support program. Details of drug effects and administration are best incorporated into the comprehensive program.

Adverse effects in *Italics* are most common; those in **Bold** are life-threatening.

▷ candesartan cilexetil
*(can dah **sar'** tan)*

Atacand

PREGNANCY CATEGORY C (FIRST TRIMESTER)

PREGNANCY CATEGORY D (SECOND AND THIRD TRIMESTERS)

Drug classes
Angiotensin II receptor antagonist
Antihypertensive

Therapeutic actions
Selectively blocks the binding of angiotensin II to specific tissue receptors found in vascular smooth muscle and adrenal gland; this action blocks the vasoconstriction effect of the renin–angiotensin system as well as the release of aldosterone leading to decreased blood pressure.

Indications
- Treatment of hypertension, alone or in combination with other antihypertensive agents
- Unlabeled uses: treatment of CHF

Contraindications and cautions
- Contraindicated with hypersensitivity to candesartan, pregnancy (use during the second or third trimester can cause injury or even death to the fetus), lactation.
- Use cautiously with renal dysfunction, hypovolemia.

Available forms
Tablets—4, 8, 16, 32 mg

Dosages
Adults
Usual starting dose—16 mg PO daily. Can be administered in divided doses bid with a total daily dose of 32 mg/day.
Pediatric patients
Safety and efficacy not established.

Pharmacokinetics

Route	Onset	Peak
Oral	Rapid	1–3 hr

Metabolism: Hepatic metabolism; $T_{1/2}$: 9 hr
Distribution: Crosses placenta; passes into breast milk
Excretion: Feces and urine

Adverse effects
- **CNS:** *Headache, dizziness,* syncope, muscle weakness
- **CV:** Hypotension
- **Dermatologic:** Rash, inflammation, urticaria, pruritus, alopecia, dry skin
- **GI:** *Diarrhea, abdominal pain, nausea,* constipation, dry mouth, dental pain
- **Respiratory:** *URI symptoms,* cough, sinus disorders
- **Other:** Cancer in preclinical studies, back pain, fever, gout

■ Nursing considerations
Assessment
- **History:** Hypersensitivity to candesartan, pregnancy, lactation, renal dysfunction, hypovolemia
- **Physical:** Skin lesions, turgor; body temperature; reflexes, affect; BP; R, respiratory auscultation; kidney function tests

Interventions
- Administer without regard to meals.
- Ensure that patient is not pregnant before beginning therapy, suggest the use of barrier birth control while using candesartan; fetal injury and deaths have been reported.
- Find an alternate method of feeding the baby if given to a nursing mother. Depression of the renin–angiotensin system in infants is potentially very dangerous.
- Alert surgeon and mark patient's chart with notice that candesartan is being taken. The blockage of the renin–angiotensin system following surgery can produce problems. Hypotension may be reversed with volume expansion.
- If blood pressure control does not reach desired levels, diuretics or other antihypertensives may be added to candesartan. Monitor patient's blood pressure carefully.
- Monitor patient closely in any situation that may lead to a decrease in blood pressure secondary to reduction in fluid volume—excessive perspiration, dehydration, vomiting, diarrhea—excessive hypotension can occur.

Teaching points

- Take drug without regard to meals. Do not stop taking this drug without consulting your health care provider.
- Use a barrier method of birth control while on this drug; if you become pregnant or desire to become pregnant, consult with your physician.
- Try to maintain your fluid intake, especially in situations that could cause loss of fluids—diarrhea, vomiting, excessive sweating.
- Know that These side effects may occur: dizziness (avoid driving a car or performing hazardous tasks); headache (medications may be available to help); nausea, vomiting, diarrhea (proper nutrition is important, consult with your dietitian to maintain nutrition); symptoms of upper respiratory tract infection, cough (do not self-medicate, consult with your nurse or physician if this becomes uncomfortable).
- Report: fever, chills, dizziness, pregnancy.

▷ capecitabine
(kap ah seat' ah been)

Xeloda

PREGNANCY CATEGORY D

Drug classes
Antimetabolite
Antineoplastic drug

Therapeutic actions
A prodrug of 5-fluorourdine that is readily converted to 5-fluorouracil; inhibits thymidylate synthetase, leading to inhibition of DNA and RNA synthesis and cell death.

Indications
- Treatment of breast cancer in patients with metastatic breast cancer resistant to both paclitaxel and doxorubicin or doxorubicin-equivalent chemotherapy
- Treatment of metastatic colorectal cancer as first-time treatment when treatment with fluoropyrimidine therapy is preferred.

Contraindications and cautions
- Contraindicated with allergy to fluorouracil; pregnancy; lactation; severe renal impairment
- Use cautiously with renal or hepatic impairment; severe diarrhea or intestinal disease; coronary artery disease (adverse cardiac effects are more common).

Available forms
Tablets—150, 500 mg

Dosages
Adults
- *Breast and colorectal cancer:* Starting dose—2,500 mg/m²/day PO in two divided doses 12 hr apart at the end of a meal for 2 wk followed by a 1 wk rest period; given in 3-wk cycles.

Pediatric patients
Safety and efficacy not established.

Geriatric patients or patients with hepatic impairment
These populations may be more sensitive to the toxic effects of the drug. Monitor closely and decrease dosage as needed to avoid toxicity.

Patients with renal impairment
Creatinine clearance < 30 mL/min, contraindicated; creatinine clearance 30–50 mL/min, reduce dosage by 75%; creatinine clearance 51–80 mL/min, no adjustment recommended, monitor carefully.

Pharmacokinetics

Route	Onset	Peak
Oral	Rapid	1.5 hr

Metabolism: Hepatic and cellular; $T_{1/2}$: 45 min
Distribution: Crosses placenta; may pass into breast milk
Excretion: Urine and lungs

Adverse effects
- **CNS:** Fatigue, paresthesias, headache, dizziness, insomnia
- **CV:** MI, angina, arrhythmias, ECG changes
- **Dermatologic:** *Hand and foot syndrome* (numbness, dysesthesias, tingling, pain, swelling, blisters, pain), *dermatitis,* nail disorders

---

Adverse effects in *Italics* are most common; those in **Bold** are life-threatening.

- **GI: Diarrhea,** *anorexia, nausea, vomiting, cramps,* constipation, *stomatitis*
- **Hematologic:** *Leukopenia, thrombocytopenia,* anemia
- **Other:** Fever, edema, myalgia

Interactions

✳ **Drug-drug** • Increased capecitabine levels when taken with antacids • Increased capecitabine levels and toxicity, including death when combined with leucovorin; avoid this combination • Increased risk of excessive bleeding and even death if combined with warfarin anticoagulants; avoid this combination. If the combination must be used, INR and prothrombin levels should be monitored very closely and anticoagulant dose adjusted as needed.

■ Nursing considerations
Assessment

- **History:** Allergy to fluorouracil; impaired liver or renal function; pregnancy; lactation; diarrhea, intestinal disease, coronary disease
- **Physical:** Weight; temperature; skin lesions, color; orientation, reflexes, affect, sensation; P, BP, cardiac rhythm, peripheral perfusion; mucous membranes, liver evaluation, abdominal exam; CBC, differential; renal and liver function tests

Interventions

- Evaluate renal function before starting therapy to ensure accurate dosage.
- Always administer drug with food, within 30 min of a meal. Have patient swallow drug with water.
- Arrange for discontinuation of drug therapy if any sign of toxicity occurs—severe nausea, vomiting, diarrhea, hand and foot syndrome, stomatitis.
- Monitor nutritional status and fluid and electrolyte balance when GI effects occur; provide supportive care and fluids as needed; loperamide may be helpful for severe diarrhea.
- Provide frequent mouth care for stomatitis, mouth sores.
- Arrange for small, frequent meals and dietary consultation to maintain nutrition when GI effects are severe.
- Protect patient from exposure to infection; monitor T and CBC regularly.

- Suggest use of barrier contraceptives while patient is using this drug; serious birth defects can occur.

Teaching points

- Take this drug every 12 hr, within 30 min of a meal; always take the drug after you have eaten and have food in your stomach. Swallow the tablets with water.
- Prepare a calendar of treatment days to follow. The drug is given in 3-wk cycles.
- These side effects may occur: nausea, vomiting, loss of appetite (medication may be ordered to help, small frequent meals may also help; it is very important to maintain your nutrition while you are on this drug); mouth sores (frequent mouth care will be needed); diarrhea (have ready access to bathroom facilities if this occurs).
- Arrange to have frequent, regular medical follow-up, including frequent blood tests to follow the effects of the drug on your body.
- Avoid pregnancy while on this drug; use of barrier-type contraceptives is advised. This drug can cause serious birth defects if taken during pregnancy.
- Report fever, chills, sore throat; chest pain; mouth sores; pain or tingling in hands or feet; severe nausea, vomiting or diarrhea (more than 5 episodes of any of these per day); dizziness.

▷ capreomycin sulfate
(kap ree oh mye' sin)

Capastat Sulfate

PREGNANCY CATEGORY C

Drug classes

Antituberculous drug ("third line")
Antibiotic

Therapeutic actions

Polypeptide antibiotic; mechanism of action against *Mycobacterium tuberculosis* unknown.

Indications

- Treatment of pulmonary tuberculosis that is not responsive to first-line antituberculosis agents but is sensitive to capreomycin in conjunction with other antituberculosis agents

Contraindications and cautions
- Contraindicated with allergy to capreomycin; renal insufficiency; preexisting auditory impairment.
- Use cautiously with lactation.

Available forms
Powder for injection—1 g/10 mL

Dosages
Always give in combination with other antituberculosis drugs.
Adults
1 g daily (not to exceed 20 mg/kg/day) IM for 60–120 days, followed by 1 g IM two to three times weekly for 12–24 mo.
Pediatric patients
15 mg/kg/day IM (maximum 1 g) has been recommended.
Geriatric patients or patients with renal impairment

Creatinine Clearance (mL/min)	Dose (mg/kg) at these intervals		
	24 hr	48 hr	72 hr
0 1.29	2.58	3.87	
10	2.43	4.87	7.3
20	3.58	7.16	10.7
30	4.72	9.45	14.2
40	5.87	11.7	
50	7.01	14	
60	8.16		
80	10.4		
100	12.7		
110	13.9		

Pharmacokinetics

Route	Onset	Peak	Duration
IM	20–30 min	1–2 hr	8–12 hr

Metabolism: $T_{1/2}$: 4–6 hr
Distribution: Crosses placenta; may pass into breast milk
Excretion: Urine

Adverse effects
- **CNS:** *Ototoxicity*
- **GI:** Hepatic dysfunction
- **GU:** *Nephrotoxicity*
- **Hematologic:** Leukocytosis, leukopenia, eosinophilia, hypokalemia
- **Hypersensitivity:** Urticaria, rashes, fever
- **Local:** Pain, induration at injection sites, sterile abscesses

Interactions
✻ **Drug-drug** • Increased nephrotoxicity and ototoxicity if used with similarly toxic drugs
• Increased risk of peripheral neuromuscular blocking action with nondepolarizing muscle relaxants (atracurium, gallamine, pancuronium, tubocurarine, vecuronium)

■ Nursing considerations
Assessment
- **History:** Allergy to capreomycin; renal insufficiency; auditory impairment; lactation
- **Physical:** Skin color, lesions; T; orientation, reflexes, affect, audiometric measurement, vestibular function tests; liver evaluation; liver and renal function tests, CBC, serum K+

Interventions
- Arrange for culture and sensitivity studies before use.
- Administer this drug only when other forms of therapy have failed.
- Administer only in conjunction with other antituberculous agents to which the mycobacteria are susceptible.
- Prepare solution by dissolving in 2 mL of 0.9% sodium chloride injection or sterile water for injection; allow 2–3 min for dissolution. To administer 1 g, use entire vial—if less than 1 g is needed, see the manufacturer's instructions for dilution. Reconstituted solution may be stored for 48 hr at room temperature or 14 days refrigerated. Solution may acquire a straw color and darken with time; this is not associated with loss of potency.
- Administer by deep IM injection into a large muscle mass.
- Arrange for audiometric testing and assessment of vestibular function, renal function tests, and serum potassium before and at regular intervals during therapy.

Adverse effects in *Italics* are most common; those in **Bold** are life-threatening.

Teaching points

- This drug must be given by IM injection.
- Take this drug regularly; avoid missing doses. *Do not* discontinue this drug without first consulting your physician.
- These side effects may occur: dizziness, vertigo, loss of hearing (avoid injury).
- Arrange to have regular, periodic medical checkups, including blood.
- Report rash, loss of hearing, decreased urine output, palpitations.

▽ **captopril**

(kap' toe pril)

Apo-Capto (CAN), Capoten, Gen-Captopril (CAN), Novo-Captopril (CAN), Nu-Capto (CAN)

PREGNANCY CATEGORY C (FIRST TRIMESTER)

PREGNANCY CATEGORY D (SECOND, THIRD TRIMESTERS)

Drug classes

Angiotensin-converting enzyme (ACE) inhibitor
Antihypertensive

Therapeutic actions

Blocks ACE from converting angiotensin I to angiotensin II, a powerful vasoconstrictor, leading to decreased blood pressure, decreased aldosterone secretion, a small increase in serum potassium levels, and sodium and fluid loss; increased prostaglandin synthesis also may be involved in the antihypertensive action.

Indications

- Treatment of hypertension alone or in combination with thiazide-type diuretics
- Treatment of CHF in patients unresponsive to conventional therapy; used with diuretics and digitalis
- Treatment of diabetic nephropathy
- Treatment of left ventricular dysfunction after MI
- Unlabeled uses: management of hypertensive crises; treatment of rheumatoid arthritis; diagnosis of anatomic renal artery stenosis, hypertension related to scleroderma renal crisis; diagnosis of primary aldosteronism, idiopathic edema; Bartter's syndrome; Raynaud's syndrome

Contraindications and cautions

- Allergy to captopril; impaired renal function; CHF; salt or volume depletion, lactation, pregnancy.

Available forms

Tablets—12.5, 25, 50, 100 mg

Dosages

Adults

- *Hypertension:* 25 mg PO bid or tid; if satisfactory response is not noted within 1–2 wk, increase dosage to 50 mg bid–tid; usual range is 25–150 mg bid–tid PO with a mild thiazide diuretic. Do not exceed 450 mg/day.
- *CHF:* 6.25–12.5 mg PO tid in patients who may be salt or volume depleted. Usual initial dose is 25 mg PO tid; maintenance dose of 50–100 mg PO tid. Do not exceed 450 mg/day. Use in conjunction with diuretic and digitalis therapy.
- *Left ventricular dysfunction after MI:* 50 mg PO tid, starting as early as 3 days post MI. Initial dose of 6.25 mg, then 12.5 mg tid, increasing slowly to 50 mg tid.
- *Diabetic nephropathy:* 25 mg PO tid.

Pediatric patients

Safety and efficacy not established.

Geriatric patients and patients with renal impairment

Excretion is reduced in renal failure; use smaller initial dose; adjust at smaller doses with 1- to 2-wk intervals between increases; slowly adjust to smallest effective dose. Use a loop diuretic with renal dysfunction.

Pharmacokinetics

Route	Onset	Peak
Oral	15 min	30–90 min

Metabolism: $T_{1/2}$: 2 hr
Distribution: Crosses placenta; passes into breast milk
Excretion: Urine

Adverse effects

- **CV:** *Tachycardia,* angina pectoris, **MI,** Raynaud's syndrome, CHF, hypotension in salt- or volume-depleted patients

- **Dermatologic:** *Rash, pruritus,* pemphigoid-like reaction, scalded mouth sensation, exfoliative dermatitis, photosensitivity, alopecia
- **GI:** *Gastric irritation, aphthous ulcers, peptic ulcers, dysgeusia,* cholestatic jaundice, hepatocellular injury, anorexia, constipation
- **GU:** *Proteinuria,* renal insufficiency, renal failure, polyuria, oliguria, urinary frequency
- **Hematologic:** Neutropenia, agranulocytosis, thrombocytopenia, hemolytic anemia, **pancytopenia**
- **Other:** *Cough,* malaise, dry mouth, lymphadenopathy

Interactions

✱ **Drug-drug** • Increased risk of hypersensitivity reactions with allopurinol • Decreased antihypertensive effects with indomethacin • Increased captopril effects with probenecid
✱ **Drug-food** • Decreased absorption of captopril with food
✱ **Drug-lab test** • False-positive test for urine acetone

■ Nursing considerations
Assessment
- **History:** Allergy to captopril, impaired renal function, CHF, salt or volume depletion, pregnancy, lactation
- **Physical:** Skin color, lesions, turgor; T; P; BP, peripheral perfusion; mucous membranes, bowel sounds, liver evaluation; urinalysis, renal and liver function tests, CBC and differential

Interventions
- Administer 1 hr before or 2 hr after meals.
- Alert surgeon and mark patient's chart with notice that captopril is being taken; the angiotensin II formation subsequent to compensatory renin release during surgery will be blocked; hypotension may be reversed with volume expansion.
- Monitor patient closely for fall in BP secondary to reduction in fluid volume (excessive perspiration and dehydration, vomiting, diarrhea); excessive hypotension may occur.
- Reduce dosage in patients with impaired renal function.

Teaching points
- Take drug 1 hr before or 2 hr after meals; do not take with food. Do not stop without consulting your health care provider.
- These side effects may occur: GI upset, loss of appetite, change in taste perception (limited effects, will pass); mouth sores (frequent mouth care may help); rash; fast heart rate; dizziness, light-headedness (usually passes after the first few days; change position slowly, and limit your activities to those that do not require alertness and precision).
- Be careful of drop in blood pressure (occurs most often with diarrhea, sweating, vomiting, dehydration); if light-headedness or dizziness occurs, consult your health care provider.
- Avoid OTC medications, especially cough, cold, allergy medications that may contain ingredients that will interact with it. Consult your health care provider.
- Report mouth sores; sore throat, fever, chills; swelling of the hands, feet; irregular heartbeat, chest pains; swelling of the face, eyes, lips, tongue, difficulty breathing.

▽ carbamazepine
(kar ba maz' e peen)

Apo-Carbamazepine (CAN), Atretol, Carbatrol, Epitol, Novo-Carbamaz (CAN), Tegretol, Tegretol-XR

PREGNANCY CATEGORY D

Drug class
Antiepileptic agent

Therapeutic actions
Mechanism of action not understood; antiepileptic activity may be related to its ability to inhibit polysynaptic responses and block post-tetanic potentiation. Drug is chemically related to the tricyclic antidepressants (TCAs).

Indications
- Refractory seizure disorders: partial seizures with complex symptoms (psychomotor, temporal lobe epilepsy), generalized tonic-clonic (grand mal) seizures, mixed seizure patterns

or other partial or generalized seizures. Reserve for patients unresponsive to other agents with seizures difficult to control or who are experiencing marked side effects, such as excessive sedation

- Trigeminal neuralgia (tic douloureux): treatment of pain associated with true trigeminal neuralgia; also beneficial in glossopharyngeal neuralgia
- Unlabeled uses: neurogenic diabetes insipidus (200 mg bid–tid); certain psychiatric disorders, including bipolar disorders, schizoaffective illness, resistant schizophrenia, and dyscontrol syndrome associated with limbic system dysfunction; alcohol withdrawal (800–1,000 mg/day); restless leg syndrome (100–300 mg/day hs); non-neuritic pain syndrome (600–1,400 mg/day); hereditary or nonhereditary chorea in children (15–25 mg/kg/day).

Contraindications and cautions

- Contraindicated with hypersensitivity to carbamazepine or TCAs; history of bone marrow depression; concomitant use of MAOIs, lactation, pregnancy.
- Use cautiously with history of adverse hematologic reaction to any drug (increased risk of severe hematologic toxicity); glaucoma or increased intraocular pressure; history of cardiac, hepatic, or renal damage; psychiatric patients (may activate latent psychosis).

Available forms

Tablets—200 mg; chewable tablets—100 mg; ER tablets—100, 200, 400 mg; ER capsules—200, 300 mg; suspension—100 mg/5 mL

Dosages

Individualize dosage; a low initial dosage with gradual increase is advised.

Adults

- Epilepsy: Initial dose of 200 mg PO bid on the first day; increase gradually by up to 200 mg/day in divided doses q 6–8 hr, until best response is achieved. Suspension—100 mg PO qid. Do not exceed 1,200 mg/day in patients > 15 yr; doses up to 1,600 mg/day have been used in adults (rare). Maintenance: adjust to minimum effective level, usually 800–1,200 mg/day.

- Trigeminal neuralgia: Initial dose of 100 mg PO bid on the first day; may increase by up to 200 mg/day, using 100-mg increments q 12 hr as needed. Do not exceed 1,200 mg/day. Maintenance: control of pain can usually be maintained with 400–800 mg/day (range 200–1,200 mg/day). Attempt to reduce the dose to the minimum effective level or to discontinue the drug at least once every 3 mo.
- Combination therapy: When added to existing antiepileptic therapy, do so gradually while other antiepileptics are maintained or discontinued.

Pediatric patients

> 12 yr: Use adult dosage. Do not exceed 1,000 mg/day in patients 12–15 yr; 1,200 mg/day in patients > 15 yr.

6–12 yr: Initial dose is 100 mg PO bid on the first day. Increase gradually by adding 100 mg/day at 6- to 8-hr intervals until best response is achieved. Do not exceed 1,000 mg/day. Dosage also may be calculated on the basis of 20–30 mg/kg/day in divided doses tid–qid.

< 6 yr: Optimal daily dose < 35 mg/kg/day.

Geriatric patients

Use caution; drug may cause confusion, agitation.

Pharmacokinetics

Route	Onset	Peak
Oral	Slow	4–5 hr

Metabolism: Hepatic; $T_{1/2}$: 25–65 hr, then 12–17 hr
Distribution: Crosses placenta; passes into breast milk
Excretion: Urine and feces

Adverse effects

- **CNS:** *Dizziness, drowsiness, unsteadiness,* disturbance of coordination, confusion, headache, fatigue, visual hallucinations, depression with agitation, behavioral changes in children, talkativeness, speech disturbances, abnormal involuntary movements, paralysis and other symptoms of cerebral arterial insufficiency, peripheral neuritis and paresthesias, tinnitus, hyperacusis, blurred vision, transient diplopia and oculomotor disturbances, nystagmus, scattered punctate cortical lens opacities, conjunctivitis, ophthalmoplegia, fever, chills; SIADH

- **CV:** CHF, aggravation of hypertension, hypotension, syncope and collapse, edema, primary thrombophlebitis, recurrence of thrombophlebitis, aggravation of CAD, arrhythmias and AV block; **CV complications**
- **Dermatologic:** Pruritic and erythematous rashes, urticaria, **Stevens-Johnson syndrome,** photosensitivity reactions, alterations in pigmentation, exfoliative dermatitis, alopecia, diaphoresis, erythema multiforme and nodosum, purpura, aggravation of lupus erythematosus
- **GI:** *Nausea, vomiting,* gastric distress, abdominal pain, diarrhea, constipation, anorexia, dryness of mouth or pharynx, glossitis, stomatitis; abnormal liver function tests, cholestatic and hepatocellular jaundice, **hepatitis, massive hepatic cellular necrosis with total loss of intact liver tissue**
- **GU:** Urinary frequency, acute urinary retention, oliguria with hypertension, renal failure, azotemia, impotence, proteinuria, glycosuria, elevated BUN, microscopic deposits in urine
- **Hematologic: Hematologic disorders**
- **Respiratory:** Pulmonary hypersensitivity characterized by fever, dyspnea, pneumonitis or pneumonia

Interactions
✳ Drug-drug • Increased serum levels and manifestations of toxicity with erythromycin, troleandomycin, cimetidine, danazol, isoniazid, propoxyphene, verapamil; dosage of carbamazepine may need to be reduced (reductions of about 50% recommended with erythromycin) • Increased CNS toxicity with lithium • Increased risk of hepatotoxicity with isoniazid (MAOI); because of the chemical similarity of carbamazepine to the TCAs and because of the serious adverse interaction of TCAs and MAOIs, discontinue MAOIs for minimum of 14 days before carbamazepine administration • Decreased absorption with charcoal • Decreased serum levels and decreased effects of carbamazepine with barbiturates • Increased metabolism but no loss of seizure control with phenytoin, primidone • Increased metabolism of phenytoin, valproic acid • Decreased anticoagulant effect of warfarin, oral anticoagulants; dosage of warfarin may need to be increased during concomitant therapy but decreased if carbamazepine is withdrawn • Decreased effects of nondepolarizing muscle relaxants, haloperidol • Decreased antimicrobial effects of doxycycline

■ Nursing considerations
Assessment
- **History:** Hypersensitivity to carbamazepine or TCAs; history of bone marrow depression; concomitant use of MAOIs; history of adverse hematologic reaction to any drug; glaucoma or increased intraocular pressure; history of cardiac, hepatic, or renal damage; psychiatric history; lactation; pregnancy
- **Physical:** Weight; T; skin color, lesions; palpation of lymph glands; orientation, affect, reflexes; ophthalmologic exam (including tonometry, funduscopy, slit lamp exam); P, BP, perfusion; auscultation; peripheral vascular exam; R, adventitious sounds; bowel sounds, normal output; oral mucous membranes; normal urinary output, voiding pattern; CBC including platelet, reticulocyte counts and serum iron; hepatic function tests, urinalysis, BUN, thyroid function tests, EEG

Interventions
- Use only for classifications listed. Do not use as a general analgesic. Use only for epileptic seizures that are refractory to other safer agents.
- Give drug with food to prevent GI upset.
- Do not mix suspension with other medications or elements—precipitation may occur.
- Reduce dosage, discontinue, or substitute other antiepileptic medication gradually. Abrupt discontinuation of all antiepileptic medication may precipitate status epilepticus.
- Suspension will produce higher peak levels than tablets—start with a lower dose given more frequently.
- Ensure that patient swallows ER tablets whole—do not cut, crush, or chew.

- Arrange for frequent liver function tests; discontinue drug immediately if hepatic dysfunction occurs.
- Arrange for patient to have CBC, including platelet, reticulocyte counts, and serum iron determination, before initiating therapy; repeat weekly for the first 3 mo of therapy and monthly thereafter for at least 2–3 yr. Discontinue drug if there is evidence of marrow suppression, as follows:

Erythrocytes	< 4 million/mm^3
Hematocrit	< 32%
Hemoglobin	< 11 gm/dL
Leukocytes	< 4,000/mm^3
Platelets	< 100,000/mm^3
Reticulocytes	< 0.3% (20,000/mm^2)
Serum iron	150 g/100 mL

- Arrange for frequent eye exams, urinalysis, and BUN determinations.
- Arrange for frequent monitoring of serum levels of carbamazepine and other antiepileptic drugs given concomitantly, especially during the first few weeks of therapy. Adjust dosage on basis of data and clinical response.
- Counsel women who wish to become pregnant; advise the use of barrier contraceptives.
- Evaluate for therapeutic serum levels (usually 4–12 mcg/mL).

Teaching points

- Take drug with food as prescribed. Swallow extended-release tablets whole, do not cut, crush, or chew.
- Do not discontinue this drug abruptly or change dosage, except on the advice of your physician.
- Avoid alcohol, sleep-inducing, or OTC drugs; these could cause dangerous effects.
- Arrange for frequent checkups, including blood tests, to monitor your response to this drug. Keep all appointments for checkups.
- Use contraceptives at all times; if you wish to become pregnant, you should consult your physician.
- These side effects may occur: drowsiness, dizziness, blurred vision (avoid driving or performing other tasks requiring alertness or visual acuity); GI upset (take the drug with food or milk, eat frequent small meals).

- Wear a medical alert tag at all times so that any emergency medical personnel will know that you are an epileptic taking antiepileptic medication.
- Report bruising, unusual bleeding, abdominal pain, yellowing of the skin or eyes, pale feces, darkened urine, impotence, CNS disturbances, edema, fever, chills, sore throat, mouth ulcers, rash, pregnancy.

▷ carbenicillin indanyl sodium

(kar ben i sill' in)

Geocillin

PREGNANCY CATEGORY B

Drug classes
Antibiotic
Penicillin with extended spectrum

Therapeutic actions
Bactericidal: inhibits synthesis of cell wall of sensitive organisms, causing cell death.

Indications

- UTIs caused by susceptible strains of *Escherichia coli, Proteus mirabilis, Morganella morganii, Providencia rettgeri, Proteus vulgaris, Pseudomonas, Enterobacter,* and enterococci
- Treatment of prostatitis due to susceptible strains of *E. coli, Streptococcus faecalis, P. mirabilis, Clostridium, Enterobacter*

Contraindications and cautions

- Contraindicated with allergies to penicillins, cephalosporins, or other allergens.
- Use cautiously with renal disorders, lactation (may cause diarrhea or candidiasis in the infant).

Available forms
Tablets—382 mg

Dosages
Adults

- *UTIs caused by* E. coli, Proteus, Enterobacter: 382–764 mg PO qid.
- *UTIs caused by* Pseudomonas, *enterococci:* 764 mg qid PO.

Pediatric patients
Safety and efficacy not established.

Pharmacokinetics

Route	Onset	Peak
Oral	Varies	1 hr

Metabolism: $T_{1/2}$: 60–70 min
Distribution: Crosses placenta; passes into breast milk
Excretion: Urine

Adverse effects

- **CNS:** Lethargy, hallucinations, seizures, decreased reflexes
- **GI:** *Glossitis, stomatitis, gastritis, sore mouth,* furry tongue, black "hairy" tongue, *nausea, vomiting, diarrhea,* abdominal pain, bloody diarrhea, enterocolitis, **pseudomembranous colitis,** nonspecific hepatitis
- **GU:** Nephritis: oliguria, proteinuria, hematuria, casts, azotemia, pyuria
- **Hematologic:** Anemia, thrombocytopenia, leukopenia, neutropenia, prolonged bleeding time, hemorrhagic episodes at high doses
- **Hypersensitivity:** *Rash, fever, wheezing,* anaphylaxis
- **Other:** *Superinfections:* oral and rectal moniliasis, vaginitis

Interactions

✳ Drug-drug • Increased bleeding effects if taken in high doses with heparin, oral anticoagulants • Decreased effectiveness with tetracyclines • Decreased activity of gentamicin, tobramycin, kanamycin, neomycin, amikacin, netilimicin, streptomycin • Decreased efficacy of oral contraceptives is possible
✳ Drug-food • Decreased absorption and decreased serum levels with food

■ Nursing considerations
Assessment
- **History:** Allergies to penicillins, cephalosporins, or other allergens; renal disorders; lactation
- **Physical:** Culture infected area; skin color, lesion; R, adventitious sounds; bowel

sounds; CBC, liver and renal function tests, serum electrolytes, hematocrit, urinalysis

Interventions
- Give on an empty stomach, 1 hr before or 2 hr after meals, with a full glass of water. Do not give with fruit juice or soft drinks.
- Continue treatment for 10 days.

Teaching points
- Take drug around the clock as prescribed; take the full course of therapy, usually 10 days.
- Take the drug on an empty stomach, 1 hr before or 2 hr after meals, with a full glass of water.
- This antibiotic is specific for this infection and should not be used to self-treat other infections.
- These side effects may occur: stomach upset, nausea, diarrhea, mouth sores.
- Report unusual bleeding or bruising, fever, chills, sore throat, hives, rash, severe diarrhea, difficulty breathing.

▽**carboplatin**
(***kar' boe pla tin***)

Paraplatin

PREGNANCY CATEGORY D

Drug classes
Alkylating agent
Antineoplastic

Therapeutic actions
Cytotoxic: heavy metal that produces cross-links within and between strands of DNA, thus preventing cell replication; cell cycle nonspecific.

Indications
- Initial treatment of advanced ovarian carcinoma in combination with other antineoplastics
- Palliative treatment of patients with ovarian carcinoma recurrent after prior chemotherapy, including patients who have been treated with cisplatin

Adverse effects in *Italics* are most common; those in **Bold** are life-threatening.

- *Unlabeled uses:* alone or with other agents to treat small-cell lung cancer, squamous cell cancer of the head and neck, endometrial cancer, relapsed or refractory acute leukemia, seminoma of testicular cancer

Contraindications and cautions
- Contraindicated with history of severe allergic reactions to carboplatin, cisplatin, platinum compounds, mannitol; severe bone marrow depression; lactation.
- Use cautiously in renal impairment, pregnancy.

Available forms
Powder for injection—50, 150, 450 mg

Dosages
Adults
- *As a single agent:* 360 mg/m² IV on day 1 every 4 wk. Do not repeat single doses of carboplatin until the neutrophil count is at least 2,000/mm³ and the platelet count is at least 100,000/mm³. These adjustment of dosage can be used: platelets > 100,000 and neutrophils > 2,000—dosage 125% prior course; platelets < 50,000–100,000 and neutrophils < 500–2,000—no adjustment in dosage; platelets < 50,000 and neutrophils < 500—dosage 75% of previous course. Doses > 125% are not recommended.

Pediatric patients
Safety and efficacy not established.

Geriatric patients and patients with renal impairment
Increased risk of bone marrow depression with renal impairment. Use caution.

Creatinine Clearance (mL/min)	Dose (mg/m² on day 1)
41–59	250
16–40	200
≤ 15	No data available

Pharmacokinetics

Route	Onset	Duration
IV	Rapid	48–96 hr

Metabolism: $T_{1/2}$: 1.2–2 hr, then 2.6–5.9 hr
Distribution: Crosses placenta; may pass into breast milk
Excretion: Urine

▼ IV facts
Preparation: Immediately before use, reconstitute the contents of each vial with sterile water for injection, 5% dextrose in water, or sodium chloride injection. For a concentration of 10 mg/mL, combine 50-mg vial with 5 mL of diluent, 150-mg vial with 15 mL of diluent, or 450-mg vial with 45 mL of diluent. Carboplatin can be further diluted using 5% dextrose in water or sodium chloride injection. Store unopened vials at room temperature. Protect from exposure to light. Reconstituted solution is stable for 8 hr at room temperature. Discard after 8 hr. Do not use needles of IV administration sets that contain aluminum; carboplatin can precipitate and lose effectiveness when in contact with aluminum.
Infusion: Administer by slow infusion lasting > 15 min.

Adverse effects
- **CNS:** *Peripheral neuropathies,* ototoxicity, visual disturbances, change in taste perception
- **GI:** *Vomiting, nausea, abdominal pain, diarrhea, constipation*
- **GU:** *Increased BUN or serum creatinine*
- **Hematologic: Bone marrow depression;** *decreased serum sodium, magnesium, calcium, potassium*
- **Hypersensitivity:** *Anaphylactic-like reaction,* rash, urticaria, erythema, pruritus, bronchospasm
- **Other:** *Pain, alopecia, asthenia,* cancer

Interactions
✳ Drug-drug • Decreased potency of carboplatin and precipitate formation in solution using needles or administration sets containing aluminum

■ Nursing considerations
Assessment
- **History:** Severe allergic reactions to carboplatin, cisplatin, platinum compounds, mannitol; severe bone marrow depression; renal impairment; pregnancy, lactation
- **Physical:** Weight, skin, and hair evaluation; eighth cranial nerve evaluation; reflexes; sensation; CBC, differential; renal function tests; serum electrolytes; serum uric acid; audiogram

Interventions

- Evaluate bone marrow function before and periodically during therapy. Do not give next dose if bone marrow depression is marked. Consult physician for dosage.
- Maintain epinephrine, corticosteroids, and antihistamines on standby in case of anaphylactic-like reactions, which may occur within minutes of administration.
- Arrange for an antiemetic if nausea and vomiting are severe.

Teaching points

- This drug can only be given IV. Prepare a calendar of treatment days.
- These side effects may occur: nausea, vomiting (medication may be ordered; small, frequent meals also may help); numbness, tingling, loss of taste, ringing in ears, dizziness, loss of hearing; rash, loss of hair (obtain a wig).
- Use birth control while on this drug. This drug may cause birth defects or miscarriages.
- Have frequent, regular medical follow-up, including frequent blood tests to monitor drug effects.
- Report loss of hearing, dizziness; unusual bleeding or bruising; fever, chills, sore throat; leg cramps, muscle twitching; changes in voiding patterns; difficulty breathing.

▷ **carboprost tromethamine**

(kar' boe prost)

Hemabate

PREGNANCY CATEGORY C

Drug classes

Prostaglandin
Abortifacient

Therapeutic actions

Stimulates the myometrium of the gravid uterus to contract in a manner that is similar to the contractions of the uterus during labor, thus evacuating the contents of the gravid uterus.

Indications

- Termination of pregnancy 13–20 wk from the first day of the last menstrual period
- Evacuation of the uterus in instance of missed abortion or intrauterine fetal death in the second trimester
- Postpartum hemorrhage due to uterine atony unresponsive to conventional methods

Contraindications and cautions

- Contraindicated with allergy to prostaglandin preparations; acute PID; active cardiac, hepatic, pulmonary, renal disease.
- Use cautiously with history of asthma; hypotension; hypertension; cardiovascular, adrenal, renal, or hepatic disease; anemia; jaundice; diabetes; epilepsy; scarred uterus; cervicitis, infected endocervical lesions; acute vaginitis.

Available forms

Injection—250 mcg/mL

Dosages
Adults

- *Abortion:* 250 mcg (1 mL) IM; give 250 mcg IM at 1.5- to 3.5-hr intervals, depending on uterine response; may be increased to 500 mcg if uterine contractility is inadequate after several 250-mcg doses; do not exceed 12 mg total dose or continuous administration over 2 days.
- *Refractory postpartum uterine bleeding:* 250 mcg IM as one dose; in some cases, multiple doses at 15- to 90-min intervals may be used; do not exceed a total dose of 2 mg (8 doses)

Pharmacokinetics

Route	Onset	Peak
IM	15 min	2 hr

Metabolism: Hepatic and lung; $T_{1/2}$: 8 hr
Distribution: Crosses placenta; may pass into breast milk
Excretion: Urine

Adverse effects

- **CNS:** Headache, paresthesias, *flushing,* anxiety, weakness, syncope, dizziness
- **CV:** *Hypotension,* arrhythmias, chest pain

Adverse effects in *Italics* are most common; those in **Bold** are life-threatening.

- **GI:** Vomiting, diarrhea, *nausea*
- **GU:** Endometritis, perforated uterus, uterine rupture, uterine or vaginal pain, incomplete abortion
- **Respiratory:** Coughing, dyspnea
- **Other:** Chills, diaphoresis, backache, breast tenderness, eye pain, skin rash, pyrexia

■ Nursing considerations
Assessment
- **History:** Allergy to prostaglandin preparations; acute PID; active cardiac, hepatic, pulmonary, renal disease; history of asthma; hypotension; hypertension; anemia; jaundice; diabetes; epilepsy; scarred uterus; cervicitis, infected endocervical lesions; acute vaginitis
- **Physical:** T; BP, P, auscultation; R, adventitious sounds; bowel sounds, liver evaluation; vaginal discharge, pelvic exam, uterine tone; liver and renal function tests, WBC, urinalysis, CBC

Interventions
- Refrigerate unopened vials. Stable at room temperature for 9 days.
- Administer a test dose of 100 mcg (0.4 mL) prior to abortion if indicated.
- Administer by deep IM injection.
- Arrange for pretreatment or concurrent treatment with antiemetic and antidiarrheal drugs to decrease the incidence of GI side effects.
- Ensure that abortion is complete or that other measures are used to complete the abortion if drug effects are not sufficient.
- Monitor T, using care to differentiate prostaglandin-induced pyrexia from postabortion endometritis pyrexia.
- Monitor uterine tone and vaginal discharge during procedure and several days after to assess drug effects and recovery.
- Ensure adequate hydration throughout procedure.

Teaching points
- Several IM injections may be required to achieve desired effect.
- These side effects may occur: nausea, vomiting, diarrhea, uterine or vaginal pain, fever, headache, weakness, dizziness.
- Report severe pain, difficulty breathing, palpitations, eye pain, rash.

▽ carisoprodol (isomeprobamate)
*(kar eye soe **proe**' dol)*

Soma

PREGNANCY CATEGORY C

C

Drug class
Centrally acting skeletal muscle relaxant

Therapeutic actions
Precise mechanism not known; chemically related to meprobamate, an antianxiety drug; has sedative properties; also found in animal studies to inhibit interneuronal activity in descending reticular formation and spinal cord; does not directly relax tense skeletal muscles.

Indications
- Relief of discomfort associated with acute, painful musculoskeletal conditions as an adjunct to rest, physical therapy, and other measures

Contraindications and cautions
- Allergic or idiosyncratic reactions to carisoprodol, meprobamate (reported cross-reactions with meprobamate); acute intermittent porphyria, suspected porphyria, lactation.

Available forms
Tablets—350 mg

Dosages
Adults
350 mg PO tid–qid; take last dose hs.
Pediatric patients
Not recommended for children < 12 yr.
Geriatric patients or patients with hepatic or renal impairment
Dosage reduction may be necessary; monitor closely.

Pharmacokinetics

Route	Onset	Peak	Duration
Oral	30 min	1–2 hr	4–6 hr

Metabolism: Hepatic; $T_{1/2}$: 8 hr
Distribution: May cross placenta; passes into breast milk
Excretion: Urine

Adverse effects

- **CNS:** *Dizziness, drowsiness, vertigo, ataxia, tremor, agitation, irritability*
- **CV:** Tachycardia, orthostatic hypotension, facial flushing
- **GI:** Nausea, vomiting, hiccups, epigastric distress
- **Hypersensitivity: Allergic or idiosyncratic reactions** (seen with first to fourth dose in patients new to drug): rash, erythema multiforme, pruritus, eosinophilia, fixed drug eruption; asthmatic episodes, fever, weakness, dizziness, angioneurotic edema, smarting eyes, hypotension, **anaphylactoid shock**

■ Nursing considerations

Assessment

- **History:** Allergic or idiosyncratic reactions to carisoprodol, meprobamate; acute intermittent porphyria, suspected porphyria; lactation
- **Physical:** T; skin color, lesions; orientation, affect; P, BP, orthostatic BP; bowel sounds, liver evaluation; liver and kidney function tests, CBC

Interventions

- Reduce dose with liver dysfunction.

Teaching points

- Take this drug exactly as prescribed; do not take a higher dosage; take with food if GI upset occurs.
- Avoid alcohol, sleep-inducing, or OTC drugs; these could cause dangerous effects; if you feel you need one of these preparations, consult your health care provider.
- These side effects may occur: drowsiness, dizziness, vertigo (avoid driving or activities that require alertness); dizziness when you get up or climb stairs (avoid sudden changes in position, use caution climbing stairs); nausea (take drug with food, eat frequent small meals); insomnia, headache, depression (transient effects).
- Report rash, severe nausea, dizziness, insomnia, fever, difficulty breathing.

▽carmustine (BCNU)
*(car **mus'** teen)*

BiCNU, Gliadel

PREGNANCY CATEGORY D

Drug classes

Alkylating agent, nitrosourea
Antineoplastic

Therapeutic actions

Cytotoxic: alkylates DNA and RNA and inhibits several enzymatic processes, leading to cell death.

Indications

Palliative therapy alone or with other agents for the following:

- Brain tumors: glioblastomas, brainstem glioma, medullablastoma, astrocytoma, ependymoma, metastatic brain tumors
- Hodgkin's disease and non-Hodgkin's lymphomas (as secondary therapy)
- Multiple myeloma (with prednisone)
- Adjunct to surgery for the treatment of recurrent glioblastoma as implantable wafer after removal of tumor (*Gliadel*)
- Unlabeled use: Treatment of mycosis fungoides (topical)

Contraindications and cautions

- Allergy to carmustine; radiation therapy; chemotherapy; hematopoietic depression; impaired renal or hepatic function; pregnancy (teratogenic and embryotoxic); lactation.

Available forms

Powder for injection—100 mg; wafer (*Gliadel*)—7.7 mg

Dosages

Do not give doses more often than every 6 wk because of delayed bone marrow toxicity.

Adults and pediatric patients
As single agent in untreated patients:
150–200 mg/m^2 IV every 6 wk as a single dose or in divided daily injections (75–100 mg/m^2 on 2 successive days). Do not repeat dose until platelets > 100,000/mm^3, leukocytes

---

Adverse effects in *Italics* are most common; those in **Bold** are life-threatening.

> 4,000/mm^3. Adjust dosage after initial dose based on hematologic response, as follows:

Leukocytes	Platelets	Percentage of Prior Dose to Give
> 4,000	> 100,000	100%
3,000–3,999	75,000–99,999	100%
2,000–2,999	25,000–74,999	70%
< 2,000	< 25,000	50%

Wafer: Implanted in brain as part of a surgical procedure; up to 8 wafers at a time.

Pharmacokinetics

Route	Onset	Peak
IV	Immediate	15 min

Metabolism: Hepatic; T$_{1/2}$: 15–30 min
Distribution: Crosses placenta; may pass into breast milk
Excretion: Urine and lungs (10%)

▼ IV facts

Preparation: Reconstitute with 3 mL of supplied sterile diluent, then add 27 mL of sterile water for injection to the alcohol solution; resulting solution contains 3.3 mg/mL of carmustine in 10% ethanol, pH is 5.6–6; may be further diluted with sodium chloride injection or 5% dextrose injection. Refrigerate unopened vials. Protect reconstituted solution from light; lacking preservatives, solution decomposes with time. Check vials before use for absence of oil film residue; if present, discard vial.
Infusion: Administer reconstituted solution by IV drip over 1–2 hr; shorter infusion time may cause intense pain and burning.
Incompatibility: Do not add to sodium bicarbonate.

Adverse effects

- **CNS:** Ocular toxicity: nerve fiber-layer infarcts, retinal hemorrhage
- **GI:** *Nausea, vomiting, stomatitis,* hepatotoxicity
- **GU:** Renal toxicity: decreased renal size, azotemia, renal failure
- **Hematologic:** *Myelosuppression, leukopenia, thrombocytopenia, anemia* (delayed for 4–6 wk)
- **Respiratory:** *Pulmonary infiltrates,* fibrosis

- **Other:** *Local burning at site of injection;* intense flushing of the skin, suffusion of the conjunctiva with rapid IV infusion; cancer

Interactions

✳ Drug-drug • Increased toxicity and myelosuppression with cimetidine • Decreased serum levels of digoxin, phenytoin • Risk of corneal and epithelial damage with mitomycin

■ Nursing considerations
Assessment

- **History:** Allergy to carmustine; radiation therapy; chemotherapy; hematopoietic depression; impaired renal or hepatic function; pregnancy; lactation
- **Physical:** T; weight; ophthamologic exam; R, adventitious sounds; mucous membranes, liver evaluation; CBC, differential; urinalysis, liver and renal function tests; pulmonary function tests

Interventions

- Evaluate hematopoietic function before therapy and weekly during and for at least 6 wk after therapy.
- Do not give full dosage within 2–3 wk after a full course of radiation therapy or chemotherapy because of the risk of severe bone marrow depression; reduced dosage may be needed.
- Reduce dosage in patients with depressed bone marrow function.
- Arrange for pretherapy medicating with antiemetic to decrease the severity of nausea and vomiting.
- Monitor injection site for any adverse reaction; accidental contact of carmustine with the skin can cause burning and hyperpigmentation of the area.
- Monitor ophthalmologic status.
- Monitor urine output for volume and any sign of renal failure.
- Monitor liver, renal, and pulmonary function tests.

Teaching points

- This drug can only be given IV.
- These side effects may occur: nausea, vomiting, loss of appetite (an antiemetic may be ordered; eat small frequent meals); increased susceptibility to infection (avoid exposure to

infection by avoiding crowded places, avoid injury).
- Maintain your fluid intake and nutrition.
- Use birth control; this drug can cause severe birth defects.
- Report unusual bleeding or bruising; fever, chills, sore throat; stomach or flank pain; changes in vision; difficulty breathing, shortness of breath; burning or pain at IV injection site.

▷ carteolol hydrochloride
(kar' tee oh lole)
Cartrol, Ocupress

PREGNANCY CATEGORY C

Drug classes
Beta-adrenergic blocker
Antihypertensive

Therapeutic actions
Blocks beta-adrenergic receptors of the sympathetic nervous system in the heart and juxtaglomerular apparatus (kidney), thus decreasing the excitability of the heart, decreasing cardiac output and oxygen consumption, decreasing the release of renin from the kidney, and lowering blood pressure.

Indications
- Management of hypertension, alone or with other drugs
- Reduction of intraocular pressure in chronic open-angle glaucoma
- *Unlabeled use:* prophylaxis for angina attacks

Contraindications and cautions
- Contraindicated with sinus bradycardia (HR ≤ 45 beats per minute), second- or third-degree heart block (PR interval > 0.24 sec), cardiogenic shock, CHF, asthma, COPD, lactation, hypersensitivity to beta blockers.
- Use cautiously with diabetes or thyrotoxicosis, hepatic impairment, renal failure.

Available forms
Tablets—2.5, 5 mg; solution—1%

Dosages
Adults
Oral
Initially 2.5 mg as a single daily oral dose, alone or with a diuretic. If inadequate, gradually increase to 5–10 mg as a single daily dose. Doses > 10 mg are not likely to produce further benefit and may decrease response. Maintenance: 2.5–5 mg PO daily.
Ophthalmic
1 drop in affected eye(s) tid.
Pediatric patients
Safety and efficacy not established.
Geriatric patients or patients with impaired renal function
Because bioavailability increases twofold, lower doses may be required. Creatinine clearance of > 60 mL/min, administer q 24 hr; creatinine clearance of 20–60 mL/min, administer q 48 hr; creatinine clearance of < 20 mL/min, administer q 72 hr.

Pharmacokinetics

Route	Onset	Peak	Duration
Oral	Varies	1–3 hr	24–48 hr

Metabolism: Hepatic; $T_{1/2}$: 6 hr
Distribution: Crosses placenta; may pass into breast milk
Excretion: Urine

Adverse effects
- **Allergic:** Pharyngitis, erythematous rash, fever, sore throat, **laryngospasm, respiratory distress**
- **CNS:** Dizziness, vertigo, tinnitus, fatigue, emotional depression, paresthesias, sleep disturbances, hallucinations, disorientation, memory loss, slurred speech (carteolol is less lipid-soluble than propranolol; it is less likely to penetrate the blood–brain barrier and cause CNS effects)
- **CV:** *Bradycardia, CHF, cardiac arrhythmias, sinoatrial or AV nodal block, tachycardia,* peripheral vascular insufficiency, claudication, CVA, pulmonary edema, hypotension

- **Dermatologic:** Rash, pruritus, sweating, dry skin
- **EENT:** Eye irritation, dry eyes, conjunctivitis, blurred vision
- **GI:** *Gastric pain, flatulence, constipation, diarrhea, nausea, vomiting,* anorexia
- **GU:** *Impotence, decreased libido,* Peyronie's disease, dysuria, nocturia, frequent urination
- **Musculoskeletal:** Joint pain, arthralgia, muscle cramp
- **Respiratory: Bronchospasm,** dyspnea, cough, bronchial obstruction, nasal stuffiness, rhinitis
- **Other:** *Decreased exercise tolerance, development of antinuclear antibodies,* hyperglycemia or hypoglycemia, elevated serum transaminase

Interactions

✴ Drug-drug • Increased effects with verapamil • Decreased effects of theophyllines and carteolol if taken concurrently • Increased risk of orthostatic hypotension with prazosin • Possible increased blood pressure-lowering effects with aspirin, bismuth subsalicylate, magnesium salicylate, sulfinpyrazone • Decreased antihypertensive effects with NSAIDs, clonidine • Possible increased hypoglycemic effect of insulin • Initial hypertensive episode followed by bradycardia if combined with epinephrine • Peripheral ischemia and possible gangrene if combined with ergot alkaloids

✴ Drug-lab test • Monitor for possible false results with glucose or insulin tolerance tests.

■ Nursing considerations
Assessment

- **History:** Arrhythmias, cardiogenic shock, CHF, asthma, COPD, pregnancy, lactation, diabetes or thyrotoxicosis
- **Physical:** Weight, skin condition, neurologic status, P, BP, ECG, respiratory status, kidney and thyroid function, blood and urine glucose

Interventions

- Give carteolol once a day. Monitor response and maintain at lowest possible dose.
- Do not discontinue drug abruptly after long-term therapy (hypersensitivity to catecholamines may have developed, causing exacerbation of angina, MI, and ventricular arrhythmias); taper drug gradually over 2 wk with monitoring.
- Consult with physician about withdrawing drug if patient is to undergo surgery (withdrawal is controversial).
- Monitor IOP of patients receiving eye drops; if pressure not controlled, institute concomitant therapy.

Teaching points

- Take oral drug with meals.
- Follow instructions for instillation of eyedrops carefully.
- Do not stop taking this drug unless told to by a health care provider.
- Avoid driving or dangerous activities if dizziness, weakness occur.
- These side effects may occur: dizziness, lightheadedness, loss of appetite, nightmares, depression, sexual impotence.
- Report difficulty breathing, night cough, swelling of extremities, slow pulse, confusion, depression, rash, fever, sore throat.

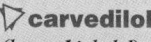

▽ carvedilol
(kar vah' da lol)

Coreg

PREGNANCY CATEGORY C

Drug classes

Alpha- and beta-adrenergic blocker
Antihypertensive

Therapeutic actions

Competitively blocks alpha and beta- and beta$_2$-adrenergic receptors, and has some sympathomimetic activity at beta$_2$-receptors. Both alpha and beta blocking actions contribute to the BP-lowering effect; beta blockade prevents the reflex tachycardia seen with most alpha-blocking drugs and decreases plasma renin activity. Significantly reduces plasma renin activity.

Indications

- Hypertension, alone or with other oral drugs, especially diuretics
- Treatment of mild to severe CHF of ischemic or cardiomyopathic origin with digitalis, diuretics, ACE inhibitors

- Unlabeled uses: angina (25–50 mg bid), idiopathic cardiomyopathy (6.25–25 mg bid)

Contraindications and cautions

- Contraindicated with decompensated CHF, bronchial asthma, heart block, cardiogenic shock, hypersensitivity to carvedilol, pregnancy, lactation.
- Use cautiously with hepatic impairment, peripheral vascular disease, thyrotoxicosis, diabetes, anesthesia or major surgery.

Available forms

Tablets–3.125, 6.25, 12.5, 25 mg

Dosages

Adults

- *Hypertension:* 6.25 mg PO bid; maintain for 7–14 days, then increase to 12.5 mg PO bid if needed to control BP. Do not exceed 50 mg/day.
- *CHF:* Monitor patient very closely, individualize dose based on patient response. Initial dose: 3.125 mg PO bid for 2 wk, may then be increased to 6.25 mg PO bid. Maximum dose: 25 mg PO bid in patients < 85 kg or 50 mg PO bid in patients > 85 kg.

Pediatric patients

Safety and efficacy not established.

Patients with hepatic impairment

Do not administer to any patient with severe hepatic impairment.

Pharmacokinetics

Route	Onset	Peak	Duration
Oral	Rapid	30 min	8–10 hr

Metabolism: Hepatic; $T_{1/2}$: 7–10 hr
Distribution: Crosses placenta; may enter breast milk
Excretion: Bile, feces

Adverse effects

- **CNS:** *Dizziness, vertigo, tinnitus, fatigue,* emotional depression, paresthesias, sleep disturbances
- **CV:** *Bradycardia, orthostatic hypertension,* CHF, cardiac arrhythmias, pulmonary edema, hypotension
- **GI:** *Gastric pain, flatulence, constipation, diarrhea,* **hepatic failure**

- **Respiratory:** *Rhinitis,* pharyngitis, dyspnea
- **Other:** *Fatigue,* back pain, infections

Interactions

✴ **Drug-drug** • Increased effectiveness of antidiabetic agents; monitor blood glucose and adjust dosages appropriately • Increased effectiveness of clonidine; monitor patient for potential severe bradycardia and hypotension • Increased serum levels of digoxin; monitor serum levels and adjust dose accordingly • Increased plasma levels of carvedilol with rifampin • Potential for dangerous conduction system disturbances with verapamil or diltiazem; if this combination is used, closely monitor ECG and BP

✴ **Drug-food** • Slowed rate of absorption, but not decreased effectiveness with food

■ Nursing considerations

Assessment

- **History:** CHF, bronchial asthma, heart block, cardiogenic shock, hypersensitivity to carvedilol, pregnancy, lactation, hepatic impairment, peripheral vascular disease, thyrotoxicosis, diabetes, anesthesia or major surgery
- **Physical:** Baseline weight, skin condition, neurologic status, P, BP, ECG, respiratory status, kidney and thyroid function, blood and urine glucose, liver function tests

Interventions

- Do not discontinue drug abruptly after chronic therapy (hypersensitivity to catecholamines may have developed, causing exacerbation of angina, MI, and ventricular arrhythmias); taper drug gradually over 2 wk with monitoring.
- Consult with physician about withdrawing drug if patient is to undergo surgery (withdrawal is controversial).
- Give with food to decrease orthostatic hypotension and adverse effects.
- Monitor for orthostatic hypotension and provide safety precautions.
- Monitor patient for any sign of liver dysfunction (pruritus, dark urine or stools, anorexia, jaundice, pain); arrange for liver

---

Adverse effects in *Italics* are most common; those in **Bold** are life-threatening.

function tests and discontinue drug if tests indicate liver injury. Do not restart carvedilol.

Teaching points

- Take drug with meals.
- Do not stop taking drug unless instructed to do so by a health care provider.
- Avoid use of OTC medications.
- These side effects may occur: dizziness, light-headedness, depression (avoid driving or performing dangerous activities; getting up and changing positions slowly may help ease dizziness).
- Report difficulty breathing, swelling of extremities, changes in color of stool or urine, very slow heart rate, continued dizziness.

▷ caspofungin acetate

See *Less Commonly Used Drugs*, p. 1340.

▷ cefaclor
(sef' a klor)

Apo-Cefaclor (CAN), Ceclor, Ceclor CD, Ceclor Pulvules, PMS-Cefaclor (CAN)

PREGNANCY CATEGORY B

Drug classes
Antibiotic
Cephalosporin (second generation)

Therapeutic actions
Bactericidal: inhibits synthesis of bacterial cell wall, causing cell death.

Indications

- Lower respiratory tract infections caused by *Streptococcus pneumoniae, Haemophilus influenzae, S. pyogenes*
- Upper respiratory infections caused by *S. pyogenes*
- Dermatologic infections caused by *Staphylococcus aureus, S. pyogenes*
- UTIs caused by *E. coli, P. mirabilis, Klebsiella,* coagulase-negative staphylococci
- Otitis media caused by *S. pneumoniae, H. influenzae, S. pyogenes,* staphylococci
- Extended-release tablets: acute exacerbations of chronic bronchitis, secondary infections of acute bronchitis, pharyngitis, and tonsilitis due to *S. pyogenes;* uncomplicated skin infections
- Unlabeled use: acute uncomplicated UTI in select patients, single 2-g dose

Contraindications and cautions

- Allergy to cephalosporins or penicillins, renal failure, lactation

Available forms
Capsules—250, 500 mg; ER tablets—375, 500 mg; powder for suspension—125 mg/5 mL, 187 mg/5 mL, 250 mg/5 mL, 375 mg/5 mL

Dosages
Adults
250 mg PO q 8 hr; dosage may be doubled in severe cases. Do not exceed 4 g/day. ER tablets—375–500 mg PO q 12 hr for 7–10 days.
Pediatric patients
20 mg/kg per day PO in divided doses q 8 hr; in severe cases 40 mg/kg/day may be given. Do not exceed 1 g/day.
- *Otitis media and pharyngitis:* Total daily dosage may be divided and administered q 12 h.

Pharmacokinetics

Route	Peak	Duration
Oral	30–60 min	8–10 hr

Metabolism: $T_{1/2}$: 30–60 min
Distribution: Crosses the placenta; enters breast milk
Excretion: Renal, unchanged

Adverse effects

- **CNS:** Headache, dizziness, lethargy, paresthesias
- **GI:** *Nausea, vomiting, diarrhea, anorexia, abdominal pain, flatulence,* **pseudomembranous colitis,** liver toxicity
- **GU:** Nephrotoxicity
- **Hematologic:** Bone marrow depression
- **Hypersensitivity:** *Ranging from rash to fever* to **anaphylaxis;** serum sickness reaction
- **Other:** *Superinfections*

Interactions

✳ **Drug-drug** • Increased nephrotoxicity with aminoglycosides • Increased bleeding effects with oral anticoagulants

✳ **Drug-lab test** • Possibility of false results on tests of urine glucose using Benedict's solution, Fehling's solution, *Clinitest* tablets; urinary 17-ketosteroids; direct Coombs' test.

■ Nursing considerations

Assessment

- **History:** Penicillin or cephalosporin allergy, pregnancy or lactation
- **Physical:** Kidney function, respiratory status, skin status, culture and sensitivity tests of infected area

Interventions

- Culture infection before drug therapy.
- Give drug with meals or food to decrease GI discomfort.
- Refrigerate suspension after reconstitution, and discard after 14 days.
- Instruct patient to swallow ER tablet whole—do not cut, crush, or chew.
- Discontinue drug if hypersensitivity reaction occurs.
- Give patient yogurt or buttermilk in case of diarrhea.
- Arrange for oral vancomycin for serious colitis that fails to respond to discontinuation of drug.

Teaching points

- Take this drug with meals or food. Swallow ER tablets whole; do not cut, crush, or chew.
- Complete the full course of this drug, even if you feel better.
- This drug is prescribed for this particular infection; do not self-treat any other infection.
- These side effects may occur: stomach upset, loss of appetite, nausea (take drug with food); diarrhea; headache, dizziness.
- Report severe diarrhea with blood, pus, or mucus; rash or hives; difficulty breathing; unusual tiredness, fatigue; unusual bleeding or bruising.

▷ **cefadroxil**
(sef a drox' ill)

Duricef, Novo-Cefadroxil (CAN)

PREGNANCY CATEGORY B

Drug classes

Antibiotic
Cephalosporin (first generation)

Therapeutic actions

Bactericidal: inhibits the formation of bacterial cell wall, causing the cell's death.

Indications

- UTIs caused by *E. coli, P. mirabilis, Klebsiella*
- Pharyngitis, tonsillitis caused by group A beta-hemolytic streptococci
- Dermatologic infections caused by staphylococci, streptococci

Contraindications and cautions

- Allergy to cephalosporins or penicillins, renal failure, lactation

Available forms

Capsules—500 mg; tablets—1 g; powder for oral suspension—125, 250, 500 mg/5 mL

Dosages

Adults

- *UTIs:* 1–2 g/day PO in single or two divided doses for uncomplicated lower UTIs. For all other UTIs, 2 g/day in two divided doses.
- *Dermatologic infections:* 1 g/day PO in single or two divided doses.
- *Pharyngitis, tonsillitis caused by group A beta-hemolytic streptococci:* 1 g/day PO in single or two divided doses for 10 days.

Pediatric patients

- *UTIs, dermatologic infections:* 30 mg/kg per day PO in divided doses q 12 hr.
- *Pharyngitis, tonsillitis caused by group A beta-hemolytic streptococci:* 30 mg/kg/day in single or two divided doses, continue for 10 days.

Geriatric patients or patients with impaired renal function

1 g PO loading dose, followed by 500 mg PO at these intervals:

Creatinine Clearance (mL/min)	Interval (hr)
0–10	36
10–25	24
25–50	12

Pharmacokinetics

Route	Peak	Duration
Oral	1.5–2 hr	20–22 hr

Metabolism: $T_{1/2}$: 78–96 min
Distribution: Crosses the placenta; enters breast milk
Excretion: Renal

Adverse effects

- **CNS:** Headache, dizziness, lethargy, paresthesias
- **GI:** *Nausea, vomiting, diarrhea, anorexia, abdominal pain, flatulence,* **pseudomembranous colitis,** liver toxicity
- **GU:** Nephrotoxicity
- **Hematologic:** Bone marrow depression
- **Hypersensitivity:** *Ranging from rash to fever to* **anaphylaxis;** serum sickness reaction
- **Other:** *Superinfections*

Interactions

✳ **Drug-drug** • Decreased bactericidal activity if used with bacteriostatic agents • Increased serum levels of cephalosporins if used with probenecid

✳ **Drug-lab test** • False-positive urine glucose using Benedict's solution, Fehling's solution, *Clinitest* tablets • False-positive direct Coombs' test • Falsely elevated urinary 17-ketosteroids

■ Nursing considerations

Assessment

- **History:** Penicillin or cephalosporin allergy, pregnancy or lactation
- **Physical:** Kidney function, respiratory status, skin status, culture and sensitivity tests of infected area

Interventions

- Culture infection before drug therapy.
- Give drug with meals or food to decrease GI discomfort.
- Refrigerate suspension after reconstitution, and discard after 14 days; shake refrigerated suspension well before using.
- Discontinue if hypersensitivity reaction occurs.
- Give the patient yogurt or buttermilk in case of diarrhea.
- Arrange for oral vancomycin for serious colitis that fails to respond to discontinuation of drug.

Teaching points

- Take this drug only for this infection; do not use to self-treat other problems.
- Refrigerate the suspension, and discard unused portion after 14 days; shake suspension well before each use.
- These side effects may occur: stomach upset, loss of appetite, nausea (take drug with food), diarrhea, headache, dizziness.
- Report severe diarrhea with blood, pus, or mucus; rash; difficulty breathing; unusual tiredness, fatigue; unusual bleeding or bruising.

▽ cefazolin sodium
(sef a' zoe lin)

Ancef, Kefzol, Zolicef

PREGNANCY CATEGORY B

Drug classes

Antibiotic
Cephalosporin (first generation)

Therapeutic actions

Bactericidal: inhibits synthesis of bacterial cell wall and causes cell death.

Indications

- Respiratory tract infections caused by *S. pneumoniae, S. aureus,* group A beta-hemolytic streptococci, *Klebsiella, H. influenzae*
- Dermatologic infections caused by *S. aureus,* group A beta-hemolytic streptococci, other strains of streptococci

- GU infections caused by *E. coli, P. mirabilis, Klebsiella,* sensitive strains of *Enterobacter,* and enterococci
- Biliary tract infections caused by *E. coli,* streptococci, *P. mirabilis, Klebsiella, S. aureus*
- Septicemia caused by *S. pneumoniae, S. aureus, E. coli, P. mirabilis, Klebsiella*
- Bone and joint infections caused by *S. aureus*
- Endocarditis caused by *S. aureus,* group A beta-hemolytic streptococci
- Perioperative prophylaxis

Contraindications and cautions
- Allergy to cephalosporins or penicillins, renal failure, lactation

Available forms
Powder for injection—250, 500 mg; 1, 5, 10, 20 g; Injection—500 mg, 1 g

Dosages
Adults
250–500 mg IM or IV q 6–12 hr.
- *Mild infections:* 250–500 mg IV or IM q 8 hr.
- *Moderate to severe infections:* 500 mg–1 g IM or IV q 6–8 hr.
- *Life-threatening infections:* 1–1.5 g IM or IV q 6 hr.
- *Acute UTI:* 1 g IM or IV q 12 hr.
- *Pneumoccocal pneumonia:* 500 mg IV or IM q 12 hr.
- *Perioperative prophylaxis:* 1 g IV 30–60 min prior to initial incision; 0.5–1 g IV or IM during surgery at appropriate intervals; 0.5–1 g IV or IM q 6–8 hr for 24 hr after surgery. Prophylactic treatment may be continued for 3–5 days.

Pediatric patients
- *Mild infections:* 25–50 mg/kg/day IM or IV in three to four equally divided doses.
- *Severe infections:* Increase total daily dose to 100 mg/kg IM or IV. Adjust dosage for impaired renal function (see package insert for details).
- *Perioperative prophylaxis:* Adjust dose according to body weight or age (see Appendix A, Alternative and Complementary Therapies for formulas).

Premature infants and infants < 1 mo
Safety and efficacy not established.

Geriatric patients or patients with impaired renal function
IV or IM loading dose of 500 mg; maximum maintenance dosages are as follows:

Creatinine Clearance (mL/min)	Mild to Moderate Infection	Severe Infection
≥ 55	250–500 mg q 6–8 hr	500–1,000 mg q 6–8 hr
35–54	250–500 mg q 8 hr	500–1,000 mg q 12 hr
11–34	125–250 mg q 12 hr	250–500 mg q 12 hr
≤ 10	125–250 mg q 18–24 hr	250–500 mg q 18–24 hr

Pharmacokinetics

Route	Onset	Peak	Duration
IM	30 min	1.5–2 hr	6–8 hr
IV	Immediate	5 min	6–8 hr

Metabolism: $T_{1/2}$: 90–120 min
Distribution: Crosses the placenta; enters breast milk
Excretion: Renal, unchanged

▼IV facts
Preparation: Use a volume control set or separate piggy-back container. Dilute reconstituted 500 mg–1 g of cefazolin in 50–100 mL of 0.9% sodium chloride injection; 5% or 10% dextrose injection; 5% dextrose in lactated Ringer's injection; 5% dextrose and 0.2%, 0.45%, or 0.9% sodium chloride injection; lactated Ringer's injection; 5% or 10% invert sugar in sterile water for injection; 5% sodium bicarbonate in sterile water for injection; Ringer's injection; *Normosol-M in D_5W; Ionosol B with Dextrose 5%; Plasma-Lyte and 5% Dextrose.* For direct IV injection as follows: dilute reconstituted 500 mg–1 g cefazolin with at least 10 mL of sterile water for injection. Shake well until dissolved. Stable for 24 hr at room temperature.
Infusion: By direct IV injection, inject slowly over 3–5 min; by infusion give each g over at least 5 min.

Adverse effects in *Italics* are most common; those in **Bold** are life-threatening.

Incompatibilities: If given as part of combination therapy with aminoglycosides, give each antibiotic at a different site. *Do not mix aminoglycosides and cefazolin in the same IV solution.*

Adverse effects

- **CNS:** Headache, dizziness, lethargy, paresthesias
- **GI:** *Nausea, vomiting, diarrhea, anorexia, abdominal pain, flatulence,* **pseudomembranous colitis,** liver toxicity
- **GU:** Nephrotoxicity
- **Hematologic:** Bone marrow depression
- **Hypersensitivity:** *Ranging from rash* to *fever* to **anaphylaxis,** serum sickness reaction
- **Other:** *Superinfections, pain,* abscess (redness, tenderness, heat, tissue sloughing), inflammation at injection site, *phlebitis, disulfiram-like reaction with alcohol*

Interactions

✳ **Drug-drug** • Increased nephrotoxicity with aminoglycosides • Increased bleeding effects with oral anticoagulants • Disulfiram-like reaction may occur if alcohol is taken within 72 hr of cefazolin administration.

✳ **Drug-lab test** • False results of urine glucose using Benedict's solution, Fehling's solution, *Clinitest* tablets; urinary 17-ketosteroids; direct Coombs' test.

■ Nursing considerations
Assessment

- **History:** Penicillin or cephalosporin allergy, pregnancy or lactation
- **Physical:** Kidney function, respiratory status, skin status; culture and sensitivity tests of infected area, injection site

Interventions

- Culture infection, arrange for sensitivity tests before drug therapy.
- Reconstitute for IM use using sterile water for injection, bacteriostatic water for injection, or 0.9% sodium chloride injection as follows:

Vial Size	Diluent to Add	Available Volume	Concentration
250 mg	2 mL	2 mL	125 mg/mL
500 mg	2 mL	2.2 mL	225 mg/mL
1 g	2.5 mL	3 mL	330 mg/mL

- Inject IM doses deeply into large muscle group.
- Solution is stable for 24 hr at room temperature or 4 days if refrigerated; redissolve by warming to room temperature and agitating slightly.
- Have vitamin K available in case hypoprothrombinemia occurs.

Teaching points

- Do not use alcohol while on this drug and for 3 days after because severe reactions often occur.
- These side effects may occur: stomach upset, loss of appetite, nausea (take drug with food); diarrhea; headache, dizziness.
- Report severe diarrhea, difficulty breathing, unusual tiredness or fatigue, pain at injection site.

▽ **cefdinir**
(sef′ din er)

Omnicef

PREGNANCY CATEGORY B

Drug classes
Antibiotic
Cephalosporin (third generation)

Therapeutic actions
Bactericidal: inhibits synthesis of bacterial cell wall, causing cell death.

Indications
Adults and adolescents

- Community-acquired pneumonia caused by *H. influenzae, H. parainfluenzae, Streptococcus pneumoniae, Moraxella catarrhalis*
- Acute exacerbations of chronic bronchitis caused by *H. influenzae, H. parainfluenzae, S. pneumoniae, M. catarrhalis*
- Acute maxillary sinusitis caused by *H. influenzae, S. pneumoniae, M. catarrhalis*
- Pharyngitis and tonsillitis caused by *S. pyogenes*
- Uncomplicated skin and skin structure infections caused by *Staphylococcus aureus, S. pyogenes*

Pediatric patients

- Acute bacterial otitis media caused by *H. influenzae, S. pneumoniae, M. catarrhalis*
- Pharyngitis and tonsillitis caused by *S. pyogenes*
- Uncomplicated skin and skin structure infections caused by *Staphylococcus aureus, S. pyogenes*

Contraindications and cautions

- Allergy to cephalosporins or penicillins; renal failure; lactation.

Available forms

Capsules—300 mg; oral suspension—125 mg/5 mL

Dosages
Adults and adolescents

- *Community-acquired infection, uncomplicated skin, or skin structure infections:* 300 mg PO q 12 hr for 10 days
- *Acute exacerbation of chronic bronchitis, acute maxillary sinusitis, pharyngitis, or tonsillitis:* 300 mg q 12 hr PO for 10 days or 600 mg q 24 hr PO for 10 days

Pediatric patients 6 mo–12 yr

- *Otitis media, acute maxillary sinusitis, pharyngitis, tonsillitis:* 7 mg/kg q 12 hr PO or 14 mg/kg q 24 hr PO for 10 days
- *Skin and skin structure infections:* 7 mg/kg PO q 12 hr for 10 days

Patients with renal impairment

Creatinine clearance < 30 mL/min—300 mg PO daily; on dialysis—300 mg PO every other day; start with 300 mg PO at the end of dialysis and then every other day.

Pharmacokinetics

Route	Peak	Duration
Oral	60 min	8–10 hr

Metabolism: $T_{1/2}$: 100 min
Distribution: Crosses the placenta, enters breast milk
Excretion: Renal, unchanged

Adverse effects

- **CNS:** Headache, dizziness, lethargy, paresthesias
- **GI:** *Nausea, vomiting, diarrhea, anorexia, abdominal pain, flatulence,* **pseudomembranous colitis,** liver toxicity
- **GU:** Nephrotoxicity
- **Hematologic:** Bone marrow depression
- **Hypersensitivity:** *Ranging from rash* to *fever* to **anaphylaxis;** serum sickness reaction
- **Other:** *Superinfections*

Interactions

✳ **Drug-drug** ● Increased nephrotoxicity with aminoglycosides ● Increased bleeding effects if taken with oral anticoagulants ● Interferes with absorption of cefdinir if taken with antacids containing magnesium or aluminum or with iron supplements; separate by at least 2 hr

✳ **Drug-lab test** ● Possibility of false results on tests of urine glucose using Benedict's solution, Fehling's solution, *Clinitest* tablets; urinary 17-ketosteroids; direct Coombs' test

■ Nursing considerations
Assessment

- **History:** Penicillin or cephalosporin allergy; pregnancy or lactation
- **Physical:** Kidney function, respiratory status, skin status; culture and sensitivity tests of infected area

Interventions

- Arrange for culture and sensitivity tests of infected area before beginning drug therapy and during therapy if infection does not resolve.
- Reconstitute oral suspension by adding 39 mL water to the 60 mL bottle, 65 mL water to the 120 mL bottle; shake well before each use. Store at room temperature. Discard after 10 days.
- Give drug with meals; arrange for small, frequent meals if GI complications occur. Separate antacids or iron supplements by 2 hr from the cefdinir dose.
- Arrange for treatment of superinfections if they occur.

Adverse effects in *Italics* are most common; those in **Bold** are life-threatening.

Teaching points
- Take this drug with meals or food. Store suspension at room temperature, shake well before each use; discard any drug after 10 days.
- Complete the full course of this drug, even if you feel better before the course of treatment is over.
- Be aware that this drug is prescribed for this particular infection; do not self-treat any other infection with this drug.
- Know that these side-effects may occur: stomach upset, loss of appetite, nausea (taking the drug with food may help); diarrhea (stay near bathroom facilities); headache, dizziness.
- Report: severe diarrhea with blood, pus, or mucus; rash or hives; difficulty breathing; unusual tiredness, fatigue; unusual bleeding or bruising.

▷ cefditoren pivoxil
(*sef' di tore en*)

Spectracef

PREGNANCY CATEGORY B

Drug classes
Antibiotic
Cephalosporin

Therapeutic actions
Bactericidal. Inhibits synthesis of susceptible gram-negative and gram-positive bacterial cell wall, causing cell death. Effective in the presence of beta-lactamases, including penicillinases and cephalosporinases.

Indications
- Acute exacerbations of chronic bronchitis caused by *Haemophilus influenzae, H. parainfluenzae, Streptococcus pneumoniae, Moraxella catarrhalis*
- Pharyngitis and tonsillitis caused by *Streptococcus pyogenes*
- Uncomplicated skin and skin structure infections caused by *Staphylococcus aureus, S. pyogenes*

Contraindications and cautions
- Contraindicated with allergy to cephalosporins or penicillins, carnitine deficiencies,

milk protein hypersensitivities, renal failure, lactation.
- Use cautiously with renal or hepatic impairment, pregnancy.

Available forms
Tablets—200 mg

Dosages
Adults and patients > 12 yr
- *Uncomplicated skin or skin structure infections:* 200 mg PO bid for 10 days.
- *Acute exacerbation of chronic bronchitis, pharyngitis, or tonsillitis:* 400 mg PO bid for 10 days.
Patients with renal impairment
Creatinine clearance 30–49 ml/min—200 mg PO bid; creatinine clearance > 50—200 mg PO daily.

Pharmacokinetics
Route	Peak	Duration
Oral	1.5–3 hr	8–10 hr

Metabolism: $T_{1/2}$: 100–115 minutes
Distribution: Crosses the placenta; enters breast milk
Excretion: Renal, primarily unchanged

Adverse effects
- **CNS:** Headache, dizziness, lethargy, paresthesias, nervousness
- **GI:** *Nausea, vomiting, diarrhea,* anorexia, *abdominal pain,* **pseudomembranous colitis,** liver toxicity
- **GU:** Nephrotoxicity, vaginitis, urinary frequency
- **Hematologic:** Bone marrow depression, carnitine deficiency with long-term use
- **Hypersensitivity:** *Ranging from rash* to *fever* to **anaphylaxis;** serum sickness reaction
- **Other:** *Superinfections*

Interactions
✳ **Drug-drug** • Increased bleeding effects if taken with oral anticoagulants • Interference with absorption of cefditoren if taken with antacids containing magnesium or aluminum or with histamine₂-receptor antagonists; separate by at least 2 hr if concomitant use is necessary

✳ Drug-lab test ● Possibility of false results on tests of urine glucose using Benedict's solution, Fehling's solution, *Clinitest* tablets; urinary 17-ketosteroids; direct Coombs' test

■ Nursing considerations
Assessment
- **History:** Penicillin or cephalosporin allergy, carnitine deficiency, milk protein hypersensitivity, renal or hepatic impairment, pregnancy, lactation
- **Physical:** Kidney function, respiratory status, skin status, culture and sensitivity tests of infected area, GI function, orientation, affect

Interventions
- Arrange for culture and sensitivity tests of infected area before therapy and during therapy if infection does not resolve.
- Do not administer for longer than 10 days; risk of carnitine deficiency with prolonged use.
- Do not administer to patients with hypersensitivities to sodium caseinate, milk protein; this is not lactose intolerance.
- Give drug with meals; arrange for small, frequent meals if GI complications occur. Separate antacids or histamine$_2$-receptor antagonists by 2 hr from the cefditoren dose.
- Arrange for treatment of superinfections if they occur.

Teaching points
- Take this drug with meals or food.
- Complete the full course of this drug, even if you feel better before the course of treatment is over.
- Be aware that this drug is prescribed for this particular infection; do not self-treat any other infection with this drug.
- Know that these side-effects may occur: stomach upset, loss of appetite, nausea (taking the drug with food may help); diarrhea (stay near bathroom facilities); headache, dizziness.
- Report: severe diarrhea with blood, pus, or mucus; rash or hives; difficulty breathing; unusual tiredness, fatigue; unusual bleeding or bruising.

▽ cefepime hydrochloride
(sef' ah peem)

Maxipime

PREGNANCY CATEGORY B

Drug classes
Antibiotic
Cephalosporin (third generation)

Therapeutic actions
Bactericidal: inhibits synthesis of bacterial cell wall, causing cell death.

Indications
- Urinary tract infections caused by *E. coli, P. mirabilis, Klebsiella, K. pneumoniae*
- Pneumonia caused by *S. pneumoniae, Pseudomonas aeruginosa, K. pneumoniae, Enterobacter*
- Dermatologic infections caused by *S. aureus,* group or *S. pyogenes*
- Empiric therapy for febrile neutropenic patients
- Complicated intra-abdominal infections in combination with metronidazole

Contraindications and cautions
- Contraindicated with allergy to cephalosporins or penicillins; renal failure; lactation.

Available forms
Powder for injection—500 mg; 1, 2 g

Dosages
Adults
0.5–2 g IV or IM q 12 hr.
- *Mild to moderate UTI:* 0.5–1 g IM or IV q 12 hr for 7–10 days.
- *Severe UTI:* 2 g IV q 12 hr for 10 days.
- *Moderate to severe pneumonia:* 1–2 g IV q 12 hr for 10 days.
- *Moderate to severe skin infections:* 2 g IV q 12 hr for 10 days.
- *Empiric therapy for febrile neutropenic patients:* 2 g IV q 8 hr for 7 days.
- *Complicated intra-abdominal infections:* 2 g IV q 12 hr for 7–10 days.

Adverse effects in *Italics* are most common; those in **Bold** are life-threatening.

Pediatric patients 2 mo–16 yr
50 mg/kg/day dose IV or IM q 12 hr for 7–10 days depending on severity of infection.

Geriatric patients or patients with impaired renal function
Recommended starting dose as adult, then maintenance dose as follows:

Creatinine Clearance (mL/min)	Mild Infection	Moderate Infection	Severe Infection
> 60	500 mg q 12 hr	1 g q 12 hr	2 g q 12 hr
30–60	500 mg q 24 hr	1 g q 24 hr	2 g q 24 hr
11–29	500 mg q 24 hr	500 mg q 24 hr	1 g q 24 hr
< 11	250 mg q 24 hr	250 mg q 24 hr	500 mg q 24 hr

Pharmacokinetics

Route	Onset	Peak	Duration
IM	30 min	1.5–2 hr	10–12 hr
IV	Immediate	5 min	10–12 hr

Metabolism: $T_{1/2}$: 102–138 min
Distribution: Crosses placenta; enters breast milk
Excretion: Renal, unchanged

▽IV facts

Preparation: Dilute with 50–100 mL 0.9% sodium chloride, 5% and 10% dextrose injection, M/6 sodium lactate injection, 5% dextrose and 0.9% sodium chloride injection, lactated Ringer's and 5% dextrose injection, *Normosol-R, Normosol-M and D5W* injection. Diluted solution is stable for 24 hr at room temperature or up to 7 days if refrigerated. Protect from light.
Infusion: Infuse slowly over 30 min.
Incompatibilities: Do not mix with ampicillin, metronidazole, vancomycin, gentamicin, tobramycin, netilmicin, or aminophylline. If concurrent therapy is needed, administer each drug separately. If possible, do not give any other drug in same solution as cefepime.

Adverse effects

- **CNS:** Headache, dizziness, lethargy, paresthesias
- **GI:** *Nausea, vomiting, diarrhea, anorexia, abdominal pain, flatulence,* **pseudomembranous colitis,** liver toxicity

- **GU:** Nephrotoxicity
- **Hematologic:** Bone marrow depression
- **Hypersensitivity:** Ranging from *rash* to *fever* to **anaphylaxis;** serum sickness reaction
- **Other:** *Superinfections, pain,* abscess (redness, tenderness, heat, tissue sloughing), inflammation at injection site, *phlebitis, disulfiram-like reaction with alcohol*

Interactions

✱ **Drug-drug** • Increased nephrotoxicity with aminoglycosides; monitor renal function tests
• Increased bleeding effects with oral anticoagulants; reduced dosage may be needed
✱ **Drug-lab test** • False reports of urine glucose using Benedict's solution, Fehling's solution, *Clinitest* tablets; urinary 17-ketosteroids; direct Coombs' test

■ Nursing considerations

Assessment

- **History:** Penicillin or cephalosporin allergy; pregnancy, lactation
- **Physical:** Kidney function, respiratory status, skin status; culture and sensitivity tests of infection area, injection site

Interventions

- Culture infected area and arrange for sensitivity tests before beginning therapy.
- Reconstitute for IM use with 0.9% sodium chloride, 5% dextrose injection, 0.5% or 1% lidocaine HCl or bacteriostatic water with parabens or benzyl alcohol. Reserve IM use for mild to moderate UTIs due to *E. coli.*
- Have vitamin K available in case hypoprothrombinemia occurs.

Teaching points

- Do not use alcohol while on this drug and for 3 days after drug has been stopped; severe reactions may occur.
- These side effects may occur: stomach upset, loss of appetite, nausea (take drug with food); diarrhea (stay near bathroom); headache, dizziness.
- Report severe diarrhea, difficulty breathing, unusual tiredness or fatigue, pain at injection site.

▽cefmetazole sodium

*(sef **met'** a zol)*

Zefazone

PREGNANCY CATEGORY B

Drug classes

Antibiotic
Cephalosporin (second generation)

Therapeutic actions

Bactericidal: inhibits the formation of bacterial cell wall, causing cell death.

Indications

- UTIs caused by *E. coli*
- Lower respiratory tract infections caused by *S. aureus, S. pneumoniae, E. coli, H. influenzae*
- Dermatologic infections caused by *S. aureus, S. epidermidis, S. pyogenes, Streptococcus agalactiae, E. coli, P. mirabilis, P. vulgaris, M. morganii, Proteus stuartii, Klebsiella pneumoniae, Klebsiella oxytoca, Bacteroides fragilis, Bacteroides melaninogenicus*
- Intra-abdominal infections caused by *E. coli, K. pneumoniae, K. oxytoca, B. fragilis, Clostridium perfringens*
- Perioperative prophylaxis for cesarean section, abdominal or vaginal hysterectomy, cholecystectomy, colorectal surgery

Contraindications and cautions

- Allergy to cephalosporins or penicillins, renal failure, lactation, pregnancy

Available forms

Powder for injection—1, 2 g; injection—1 g or 2 g/50 mL

Dosages

Adults

General guidelines, 2 g IV q 6–12 hr for 5–14 days.

Perioperative prophylaxis

- *Vaginal hysterectomy:* 2-g single dose 30–90 min before surgery or 1-g doses 30–90 min before surgery and repeated 8 and 16 hr later.

- *Abdominal hysterectomy:* 1-g doses 30–90 min before surgery and repeated 8 and 16 hr later.
- *Cesarean section:* 2-g single dose after clamping cord or 1-g doses after clamping cord; repeated at 8 and 16 hr later.
- *Colorectal surgery:* 2-g single dose 30–90 min before surgery or 2-g doses 30–90 min before surgery and repeated 8 and 16 hr later.
- *Cholecystectomy (high risk):* 1-g doses 30–90 min before surgery and repeated 8 and 16 hr later.

Pediatric patients

Safety and efficacy not established.

Geriatric patients or patients with impaired renal function

Creatinine Clearance (mL/min)	Dose (g)	Frequency
50–90	1–2	q 12 hr
30–49	1–2	q 16 hr
10–29	1–2	q 24 hr
< 10	1–2	q 48 hr

Pharmacokinetics

Route	Onset	Peak
IV	Rapid	End of infusion

Metabolism: $T_{1/2}$: 1.2 hr
Distribution: Enters breast milk; crosses placenta
Excretion: Urine

▽IV facts

Preparation: Use sterile water for injection, bacteriostatic water for injection, or 0.9% sodium chloride injection. Dilute 1 g with 3.7 mL to yield 250 mg/mL or 1 g with 10 mL to yield 100 mg/mL; 2 g diluted with 7 mL will yield 250 mg/mL, or 2 g with 15 mL yields 125 mg/mL. Primary solutions may be further diluted to concentrations of 1–20 mg/mL in 0.9% sodium chloride injection, 5% dextrose injection, or lactated Ringer's injection. Stable for 24 hr at room temperature, 7 days if refrigerated, or 6 wk if frozen. Do not refreeze thawed solutions; discard any unused solution.
Infusion: If using a piggy-back IV setup, discontinue the other solution while cefmetazole

---

Adverse effects in *Italics* are most common; those in **Bold** are life-threatening.

is being given. If given as part of combination therapy with aminoglycosides, give each antibiotic at a different site. Do not mix aminoglycosides and cefmetazole in the same IV solution. Direct IV infusion over 3–5 min; slow infusion over 10–60 min.

Incompatibility: Do not mix in solution with aminoglycosides.

Adverse effects

- **CNS:** Headache, dizziness, lethargy, paresthesias
- **GI:** *Nausea, vomiting, diarrhea, anorexia, abdominal pain, flatulence,* **pseudomembranous colitis,** liver toxicity
- **GU:** Nephrotoxicity
- **Hematologic: Bone marrow depression:** decreased WBC, decreased platelets, decreased Hct
- **Hypersensitivity:** *Ranging from rash* to *fever* to **anaphylaxis,** serum sickness reaction
- **Local:** *Pain,* abscess at injection site, *phlebitis,* inflammation at IV site
- **Other:** *Superinfections, disulfiram-like reaction with alcohol*

Interactions

✱Drug-drug • Increased nephrotoxicity with aminoglycosides • Increased bleeding effects with oral anticoagulants • Disulfiram-like reaction may occur if alcohol is taken within 72 hr after cefmetazole administration.

✱Drug-lab test • Possibility of false results on tests of urine glucose using Benedict's solution, Fehling's solution, *Clinitest* tablets; urinary 17-ketosteroids; direct Coombs' test.

■ Nursing considerations
Assessment

- **History:** Liver and kidney dysfunction, lactation, pregnancy
- **Physical:** Skin status, liver and kidney function test, culture of affected area, sensitivity tests

Interventions

- Have vitamin K available in case hypoprothrombinemia occurs.
- Discontinue drug if hypersensitivity reaction occurs.

Teaching points

- These side effects may occur: stomach upset, diarrhea.
- Avoid alcohol while on this drug and for 3 days after because severe reactions often occur.
- Report severe diarrhea, difficulty breathing, unusual tiredness or fatigue, pain at injection site.

▷**cefonicid**
(se fon' i sid)

Monocid

PREGNANCY CATEGORY B

Drug classes
Antibiotic
Cephalosporin (second generation)

Therapeutic actions
Bactericidal: inhibits synthesis of bacterial cell wall, causing cell death.

Indications

- Lower respiratory tract infections caused by *S. pneumoniae, K. pneumoniae, H. influenzae, E. coli*
- UTIs caused by *E. coli, Proteus species, K. pneumoniae*
- Dermatologic infections caused by *S. aureus, S. pyogenes, S. epidermidis, S. agalactiae*
- Septicemia caused by *S. pneumoniae, E. coli*
- Bone and joint infections caused by *S. aureus*
- Perioperative prophylaxis

Contraindications and cautions

- Allergy to cephalosporins or penicillins, renal failure, lactation.

Available forms
Powder for injection—1, 10 g (bulk vials)

Dosages
Adults

- *Uncomplicated UTI:* 0.5 g IV or IM q 24 hr.
- *Mild-to-moderate infection:* 1 g IV or IM q 24 hr.
- *Severe infection:* 2 g IV or IM q 24 hr.

- *Perioperative prophylaxis:* 1 g IV 1 hr prior to initial incision; 1 g/day for up to 2 days.
- *Cesarean section:* Give after the cord is clamped, 1 g IV.

Pediatric patients

Safety and efficacy not established.

Geriatric patients or patients with impaired renal function

Initial dose of 7.5 mg/kg IV or IM followed by:

Creatinine Clearance (mL/min)	Moderate Infections	Severe Infections
60–79	10 mg/kg q 24 hr	25 mg/kg q 24 hr
40–59	8 mg/kg q 24 hr	20 mg/kg q 24 hr
20–39	4 mg/kg q 24 hr	15 mg/kg q 24 hr
10–19	4 mg/kg q 48 hr	15 mg/kg q 48 hr
5–9	4 mg/kg q 3–5 days	15 mg/kg q 3–5 days
< 5	3 mg/kg q 3–5 days	4 mg/kg q 3–5 days

Pharmacokinetics

Route	Onset	Peak	Duration
IV	Immediate	5 min	24 hr
IM	1 hr	1 hr	24 hr

Metabolism: $T_{1/2}$: 4.5–5.8 hr
Distribution: Crosses placenta; enters breast milk
Excretion: Urine

▼IV facts

Preparation: Reconstitute single-dose vials as follows: 500-mg vial, add 2 mL sterile water for injection (220 mg/mL concentration); 1-g vial, add 2.5 mL sterile water for injection (325 mg/mL concentration). For IV infusion, add reconstituted solution to 50–100 mL of one of the following: 0.9% sodium chloride; 5% or 10% dextrose injection; 5% dextrose and 0.2%, 0.45%, or 0.9% sodium chloride injection; Ringer's injection; lactated Ringer's injection; 5% dextrose and lactated Ringer's injection; 10% invert sugar in sterile water for injection; 5% dextrose and 0.15% potassium chloride injection; sodium lactate injection. Reconstituted or diluted solution is stable for up to 24 hr

at room temperature, 72 hr if refrigerated; discard unused solutions within the allotted time period.
Infusion: Give bolus injections slowly over 3–5 min into vein or IV tubing; for infusion, give over 30 min. If given as part of combination therapy with aminoglycosides, give each antibiotic at a different site: do not mix aminoglycosides and cefonicid in the same IV solution.
Incompatibilities: Incompatible in solution with aminoglycosides.

Adverse effects

- **CNS:** Headache, dizziness, lethargy, paresthesias
- **GI:** *Nausea, vomiting, diarrhea, anorexia, abdominal pain, flatulence,* **pseudomembranous colitis,** liver toxicity
- **GU:** Nephrotoxicity
- **Hematologic: Bone marrow depression:** decreased WBC, decreased platelets, decreased Hct
- **Hypersensitivity:** *Ranging from rash to fever to* **anaphylaxis;** serum sickness reaction
- **Local:** *Pain,* abscess at injection site, *phlebitis,* inflammation at IV site
- **Other:** *Superinfections, disulfiram-like reaction with alcohol*

Interactions

✳ **Drug-drug** • Increased nephrotoxicity with aminoglycosides • ncreased bleeding effects with oral anticoagulants
✳ **Drug-lab test** • Possibility of false results on tests of urine glucose using Benedict's solution, Fehling's solution, *Clinitest* tablets; urinary 17-ketosteroids; direct Coombs' test.

■ Nursing considerations
Assessment

- **History:** Liver and kidney dysfunction, lactation, pregnancy
- **Physical:** Skin status, liver and kidney function test, culture of affected area, sensitivity tests

Interventions
- Culture infection, arrange for sensitivity tests before and during therapy if expected response is not seen.
- Divide IM doses of 2 g once daily and give as two equal doses deeply into two different large muscles.
- Have vitamin K available in case hypoprothrombinemia occurs.
- Discontinue drug if hypersensitivity reaction occurs.

Teaching points
- These side effects may occur: stomach upset, diarrhea.
- Avoid alcohol while on this drug and for 3 days after because severe reactions often occur.
- Report severe diarrhea, difficulty breathing, unusual tiredness or fatigue, pain at injection site.

▷ cefoperazone sodium
(sef oh per' a zone)

Cefobid

PREGNANCY CATEGORY B

Drug classes
Antibiotic
Cephalosporin (third generation)

Therapeutic actions
Bactericidal: inhibits synthesis of bacterial cell wall, causing cell death.

Indications
- Respiratory tract infections caused by *S. pneumoniae, S. aureus, S. pyogenes, Pseudomonas aeruginosa, K. pneumoniae, H. influenzae, E. coli, Proteus, Enterobacter*
- Dermatologic infections caused by *S. aureus, S. pyogenes, P. aeruginosa*
- UTIs caused by *E. coli, P. aeruginosa*
- Septicemia caused by *S. pneumoniae, S. aureus, S. agalactiae, enterococci, H. influenzae, P. aeruginosa, E. coli, Klebsiella, Proteus, Clostridium,* anaerobic grampositive cocci
- Peritonitis and intra-abdominal infections caused by *E. coli, P. aeruginosa,* anaerobic gram-positive cocci, anaerobic grampositive and gram-negative bacilli
- Pelvic inflammatory disease, endometritis caused by *N. gonorrhoeae, S. epidermidis, S. agalactiae, E. coli, Clostridium, Bacteroides,* and anaerobic gram-positive cocci

Contraindications and cautions
- Allergy to cephalosporins or penicillins, hepatic failure, lactation.

Available forms
Powder for injection—1, 2 g; injection—1, 2 g

Dosages
Adults
2–4 g/day IM or IV in equal divided doses q 12 hr; up to 6–12 g/day if severe.
Pediatric patients
Safety and efficacy not established.
Patients with hepatic impairment
Total daily dose of 4 g. Monitor patient carefully.
Patients with renal impairment on hemodialysis
Do not exceed 1–2 g/day.

Pharmacokinetics

Route	Onset	Peak	Duration
IV	5–10 min	15–20 min	6–12 hr
IM	1 hr	1–2 hr	6–12 hr

Metabolism: $T_{1/2}$: 1.75–2.5 hr
Distribution: Crosses placenta; enters breast milk
Excretion: Bile

▽ IV facts
Preparation: For IV infusion; concentrations of 2–50 mg/mL are recommended. Reconstitute powder for IV use in 5% or 10% dextrose injection; 5% dextrose and 0.2% or 0.9% sodium chloride injection; 5% dextrose and lactated Ringer's injection; lactated Ringer's injection; 0.9% sodium chloride injection; *Normosol M and 5% Dextrose* injection; *Normosol R.* After reconstituting, allow to stand until all foaming is gone; vigorous agitation may be necessary. Reconstituted solution is sta-

ble for 24 hr at room temperature or up to 5 days if refrigerated.

Vial Dose	Desired Concentration	Diluent to Add	Resulting Volume
1 g	333 mg/mL	2.6 mL	3 ml
	250 mg/mL	3.8 mL	4 mL
2 g	333 mg/mL	5 mL	6 mL
	250 mg/mL	7.2 mL	8 mL

Infusion: Administer single dose over 15–30 min, continuous infusion over 6–24 hr. If using a piggy-back IV setup, discontinue the other solution while cefoperazone is being given. If given with aminoglycosides, give each at a different site.

Incompatibilities: Do not mix aminoglycosides and cefoperazone in the same IV solution.

Y-site incompatibilities: Hetastarch, labetalol, meperidine, ondansetron, perphenazine, promethazine.

Adverse effects

- **CNS:** Headache, dizziness, lethargy, paresthesias
- **GI:** *Nausea, vomiting, diarrhea, anorexia, abdominal pain, flatulence,* **pseudomembranous colitis,** liver toxicity
- **GU:** Nephrotoxicity
- **Hematologic: Bone marrow depression:** decreased WBC, decreased platelets, decreased Hct
- **Hypersensitivity:** *Ranging from rash* to *fever* to **anaphylaxis;** serum sickness reaction
- **Local:** *Pain,* abscess at injection site; *phlebitis,* inflammation at IV site
- **Other:** *Superinfections, disulfiram-like reaction with alcohol*

Interactions

✳ **Drug-drug** ● Increased nephrotoxicity with aminoglycosides ● Increased bleeding effects with oral anticoagulants ● Disulfiram-like reaction may occur if alcohol is taken within 72 hr after cefoperazone administration.

✳ **Drug-lab test** ● Possibility of false results on tests of urine glucose sing Benedict's solution, Fehling's solution, *Clinitest* tablets; urinary 17-ketosteroids; direct Coombs' test.

■ Nursing considerations

Assessment

- **History:** Liver and kidney dysfunction, lactation, pregnancy
- **Physical:** Skin status, liver and kidney function tests, culture of affected area, sensitivity tests

Interventions

- Culture infection, arrange for sensitivity tests before and during therapy if expected response is not seen.
- Keep dosage under 4 g/day, or monitor serum concentrations in patients with liver disease or biliary obstruction.
- To prepare drug for IM use: reconstitute powder in bacteriostatic water for injection, sterile water for injection, or 0.5% lidocaine HCl injection (concentrations > 250 mg/mL).
- Maintain vitamin K on standby in case hypoprothrombinemia occurs.
- Discontinue drug if hypersensitivity reaction occurs.

Teaching points

- These side effects may occur: stomach upset, diarrhea.
- Avoid alcohol while on this drug and for 3 days after because severe reactions often occur.
- Report severe diarrhea, difficulty breathing, unusual tiredness or fatigue, pain at injection site.

▽ **cefotaxime sodium**
(sef oh taks' eem)

Claforan

PREGNANCY CATEGORY B

Drug classes

Antibiotic
Cephalosporin (third generation)

Therapeutic actions

Bactericidal: inhibits synthesis of bacterial cell wall, causing cell death.

Indications

- LRIs caused by *S. pneumoniae, S. aureus, Klebsiella, H. influenzae, E. coli, P. mirabilis, Enterobacter, Serratia marcescens, S. pyogenes*
- UTIs caused by *Enterococcus, S. epidermidis, S. aureus, Citrobacter, Enterobacter, E. coli, Klebsiella, P. mirabilis, Proteus, S. marcescens*
- Gynecologic infections caused by *S. epidermidis, Enterococcus, E. coli, P. mirabilis, Bacteroides, Clostridium, Peptococcus, Peptostreptococcus,* streptococci; and uncomplicated gonorrhea caused by *N. gonorrhoeae*
- Dermatologic infections caused by *S. aureus, E. coli, Serratia, Proteus, Klebsiella, Enterobacter, Pseudomonas, S. marcescens, Bacteroides, Peptococcus, Peptostreptococcus, P. mirabilis, S. epidermidis, S. pyogenes, Enterococcus*
- Septicemia caused by *E. coli, Klebsiella, S. marcescens*
- Peritonitis and intra-abdominal infections caused by *E. coli, Peptostreptococcus, Bacteroides, Peptococcus, Klebsiella*
- CNS infections caused by *E. coli, H. influenzae, Neisseria meningitidis, S. pneumoniae, K. pneumoniae*
- Bone and joint infections caused by *S. aureus*
- Perioperative prophylaxis

Contraindications and cautions

- Allergy to cephalosporins or penicillins, renal failure, lactation, pregnancy.

Available forms

Powder for injection—500 mg, 1, 2 g; injection—1, 2 g

Dosages
Adults
2–8 g/day IM or IV in equally divided doses q 6–8 hr. Do not exceed 12 g/day.
- *Gonorrhea:* 1 g IM in a single injection.
- *Disseminated infection:* 1 g IV q 8 hr.
- *Gonococcal ophthalmia:* 500 mg IV qid.
- *Perioperative prophylaxis:* 1 g IV or IM 30–90 min before surgery.
- *Cesarean section:* 1 g IV after cord is clamped and then 1 g IV or IM at 6 and 12 hr.

Pediatric patients
0–1 wk: 50 mg/kg IV q 12 hr.
1–4 wk: 50 mg/kg IV q 8 hr.
1 mo–12 yr (< 50 kg): 50–180 mg/kg/day IV or IM in four to six divided doses.
Geriatric patients or patients with reduced renal function
If creatinine clearance is < 20 mL/min, reduce dosage by half.

Pharmacokinetics

Route	Onset	Peak	Duration
IV	Immediate	5 min	18–24 hr
IM	5–10 min	30 min	18–24 hr

Metabolism: $T_{1/2}$: 1 hr
Distribution: Crosses the placenta; enters breast milk
Excretion: Urine

▽ IV facts

Preparation: Reconstitute for intermittent IV injection with 1 or 2 g with 10 mL sterile water for injection. Reconstitute vials for IV infusion with 10 mL of sterile water for injection. Reconstitute infusion bottles with 50 or 100 mL of 0.9% sodium chloride injection or 5% dextrose injection. Drug solution may be further diluted with 50–100 mL of 5% or 10% dextrose injection; 5% dextrose and 0.2%, 0.45%, or 0.9% sodium chloride injection; lactated Ringer's solution; 0.9% sodium chloride injection; sodium lactate injection (M/6); 10% invert sugar. Reconstituted solution is stable for 24 hr at room temperature or 5 days if refrigerated. Powder and reconstituted solution darken with storage.

Infusion: Inject slowly into vein over 3–5 min or over a longer time through IV tubing; give continuous infusion over 6–24 hr. If administered with aminoglycosides, administer at different sites.

Incompatibilities: Do not mix in solutions with aminoglycoside solutions.

Y-site incompatibility: Hetastarch.

Adverse effects

- **CNS:** Headache, dizziness, lethargy, paresthesias
- **GI:** *Nausea, vomiting, diarrhea, anorexia, abdominal pain, flatulence,* **pseudomembranous colitis,** liver toxicity
- **GU:** Nephrotoxicity

- **Hematologic: Bone marrow depression:** decreased WBC, decreased platelets, decreased Hct
- **Hypersensitivity:** *Ranging from rash* to *fever* to **anaphylaxis;** serum sickness reaction
- **Local:** *Pain,* abscess at injection site, *phlebitis,* inflammation at IV site
- **Other:** *Superinfections, disulfiram-like reaction with alcohol*

Interactions
✳ **Drug-drug** • Increased nephrotoxicity with aminoglycosides • Increased bleeding effects with oral anticoagulants
✳ **Drug-lab test** • Possibility of false results on tests of urine glucose using Benedict's solution, Fehling's solution, *Clinitest* tablets; urinary 17-ketosteroids; direct Coombs' test.

■ Nursing considerations
Assessment
- **History:** Liver and kidney dysfunction, lactation, pregnancy
- **Physical:** Skin status, liver and kidney function test, culture of affected area, sensitivity tests

Interventions
- Culture infection, arrange for sensitivity tests before and during therapy if expected response is not seen.
- Reconstitution of drug varies by size of package; see manufacturer's directions for details.
- Reconstitute drug for IM use with sterile water or bacteriostatic water for injection; divide doses of 2 g and administer at two different sites by deep IM injection.
- Discontinue if hypersensitivity reaction occurs.

Teaching points
- These side effects may occur: stomach upset, diarrhea.
- Avoid alcohol while on this drug and for 3 days after because severe reactions often occur.
- Report severe diarrhea, difficulty breathing, unusual tiredness or fatigue, pain at injection site.

▽ **cefotetan disodium**
(sef' oh tee tan)
Cefotan

PREGNANCY CATEGORY B

Drug classes
Antibiotic
Cephalosporin (second generation)

Therapeutic actions
Bactericidal: inhibits synthesis of bacterial cell wall, causing cell death.

Indications
- LRIs caused by *S. pneumoniae, S. aureus, Klebsiella, H. influenzae, E. coli*
- UTIs caused by *E. coli, Klebsiella, P. vulgaris, P. mirabilis, Morganella morganii, Providencia rettgeri*
- Intra-abdominal infections caused by *E. coli, K. pneumoniae, Klebsiella, Streptococcus* (excluding enterococci), *Bacteroides*
- Gynecologic infections caused by *S. aureus, S. epidermidis, Streptococcus* (excluding enterococci), *E. coli, P. mirabilis, N. gonorrhoeae, Bacteroides, Fusobacterium, Peptococcus, Peptostreptococcus*
- Dermatologic infections caused by *S. aureus, S. pyogenes, S. epidermidis, Streptococcus* (excluding enterococci), *E. coli*
- Bone and joint infections caused by *S. aureus*
- Perioperative prophylaxis

Contraindications and cautions
- Allergy to cephalosporins or penicillins, renal failure, lactation.

Available forms
Powder for injection—1, 2, 10 g; injection—1 g/50 mL, 2 g/50 mL.

Dosages
Adults
1–2 g/day IM or IV in equally divided doses q 12 hr for 5–10 days. Do not exceed 6 g/day.
- *UTI:* 1–4 g/day given as 500 mg q 12 hr IV, IM or 1–2 g q 24 hr IV or IM, or 1–2 g q 12 hr IV or IM.

Adverse effects in *Italics* are most common; those in **Bold** are life-threatening.

- *Other infections:* 2–4 g/day given as 1–2 g q 12 hr IV or IM.
- *Severe infections:* 4 g/day given as 2 g q 12 hr IV.
- *Life-threatening infections:* 6 g/day given as 3 g q 12 hr IV.
- *Perioperative prophylaxis:* 1–2 g IV 30–60 min before surgery.
- *Cesarean section:* Administer 1–2 g IV as soon as the cord is clamped.

Pediatric patients
Safety and efficacy not established.

Geriatric patients or patients with impaired renal function

Creatinine Clearance (mL/min)	Dosage
> 30	1–2 g q 12 hr
10–30	1–2 g q 24 hr
< 10	1–2 g q 48 hr

Pharmacokinetics

Route	Onset	Peak	Duration
IV	15–20 min	30 min	18–24 hr
IM	30–60 min	1.5–3 hr	18–24 hr

Metabolism: $T_{1/2}$: 3–4.5 hr
Distribution: Crosses the placenta; enters breast milk
Excretion: Urine, bile

▽ IV facts

Preparation: Reconstitute for IV use with sterile water for injection.
1-g vial: Add 10 mL diluent; withdraw 10.5 mL; concentration is 95 mg/mL.
2-g vial: Add 10–20 mL diluent; withdraw 11–21 mL; concentration is 182–195 mg/mL. Reconstituted solution is stable for 24 hr at room temperature or 4 days if refrigerated. Protect drug from light.
Infusion: Inject slowly over 3–5 min into vein or over a longer time into IV tubing. Discontinue infusion of other solutions temporarily while cefotetan is running. If given with aminoglycosides, give each antibiotic at a different site.
Incompatibilities: Do not mix aminoglycosides and cefotetan in the same IV solution.

Adverse effects

- **CNS:** Headache, dizziness, lethargy, paresthesias
- **GI:** *Nausea, vomiting, diarrhea, anorexia, abdominal pain, flatulence,* **pseudomembranous colitis,** liver toxicity
- **GU:** Nephrotoxicity
- **Hematologic: Bone marrow depression:** decreased WBC, decreased platelets, decreased Hct
- **Hypersensitivity:** *Ranging from rash to fever* **to anaphylaxis,** serum sickness reaction
- **Local:** *Pain,* abscess at injection site, *phlebitis,* inflammation at IV site
- **Other:** *Superinfection, disulfiram-like reaction with alcohol*

Interactions

✳ **Drug-drug** • Increased nephrotoxicity with aminoglycosides • Increased bleeding effects with oral anticoagulants • Disulfiram-like reaction may occur if alcohol is used within 72 hr after cefotetan administration.

✳ **Drug-lab test** • Possibility of false results on tests of urine glucose using Benedict's solution, Fehling's solution, *Clinitest* tablets; urinary 17-ketosteroids; direct Coombs' test.

■ Nursing considerations
Assessment

- **History:** Liver and kidney dysfunction, lactation, pregnancy
- **Physical:** Skin status, liver and kidney function test, culture of affected area, sensitivity tests

Interventions

- Culture infection, arrange for sensitivity tests before and during therapy if expected response is not seen.
- Reconstitute for IM use with sterile water for injection, 0.9% sodium chloride solution, bacteriostatic water for injection, 0.5% or 1% lidocaine HCl; inject deeply into large muscle group.
- Protect drug from light.
- Have vitamin K available in case hypoprothrombinemia occurs.
- Discontinue if hypersensitivity reaction occurs.

Teaching points

- These side effects may occur: stomach upset, diarrhea.

- Avoid alcohol while on this drug and for 3 days after because severe reactions often occur.
- Report severe diarrhea, difficulty breathing, unusual tiredness or fatigue, pain at injection site.

▷ **cefoxitin sodium**
(se fox' i tin)

Mefoxin

PREGNANCY CATEGORY B

Drug classes
Antibiotic
Cephalosporin (second generation)

Therapeutic actions
Bactericidal: inhibits synthesis of bacterial cell wall, causing cell death.

Indications
- LRIs caused by *S. pneumoniae, S. aureus, streptococci, E. coli, Klebsiella, H. influenzae, Bacteroides*
- Dermatologic infections caused by *S. aureus, S. epidermidis, streptococci, E. coli, P. mirabilis, Klebsiella, Bacteroides, Clostridium, Peptococcus, Peptostreptococcus*
- UTIs caused by *E. coli, P. mirabilis, Klebsiella, M. morganii, P. rettgeri, P. vulgaris, Providencia,* uncomplicated gonorrhea caused by *N. gonorrhoeae*
- Intra-abdominal infections caused by *E. coli, Klebsiella, Bacteroides, Clostridium*
- Gynecologic infections caused by *E. coli, N. gonorrhoeae, Bacteroides, Clostridium, Peptococcus, Peptostreptococcus,* group B streptococci
- Septicemia caused by *S. pneumoniae, S. aureus, E. coli, Klebsiella, Bacteroides*
- Bone and joint infections caused by *S. aureus*
- Perioperative prophylaxis
- Treatment of oral bacterial *Eikenella corrodens*

Contraindications and cautions
- Allergy to cephalosporins or penicillins, renal failure, lactation.

Available forms
Powder for injection—1, 2 g; injection—1, 2 g in 5% dextrose in water

Dosages
Adults
1–2 g IM or IV q 6–8 hr, depending on the severity of the infection.
- *Uncomplicated gonorrhea:* 2 g IM with 1 g oral probenecid.
- *Uncomplicated LRIs, UTIs, skin infections:* 1 g q 6–8 hr IV.
- *Moderate to severe infections:* 1 g q 4 hr IV to 2 g q 6–8 hr IV.
- *Severe infections:* 2 g q 4 hr IV or 3 g q 6 hr IV.
- *Perioperative prophylaxis:* 2 g IV or IM 30–60 min prior to initial incision and q 6 hr for 24 hr after surgery.
- *Cesarean section:* 2 g IV as soon as the umbilical cord is clamped, followed by 2 g IM or IV at 4 and 8 hr, then q 6 hr for up to 24 hr.
- *Transurethral prostatectomy:* 1 g prior to surgery and then 1 g q 8 hr for up to 5 days.
Pediatric patients ≥ 3 mo
80–160 mg/kg/day IM or IV in divided doses q 4–6 hr. Do not exceed 12 g/day.
- *Prophylactic use:* 30–40 mg/kg per dose IV or IM q 6 hr.
Geriatric patients or patients with impaired renal function
IV loading dose of 1–2 g. Maintenance dosages are as follows:

Creatinine Clearance (mL/min)	Maintenance Dosage
30–50	1–2 g q 8–12 hr
10–29	1–2 g q 12–24 hr
5–9	0.5–1 g q 12–24 hr
< 5	0.5–1 g q 24–48 hr

Pharmacokinetics

Route	Onset	Peak	Duration
IV	Immediate	5 min	6–8 hr
IM	5–10 min	20–30 min	6–8 hr

Metabolism: $T_{1/2}$: 45–60 min
Distribution: Crosses the placenta; enters breast milk
Excretion: Urine

Adverse effects in *Italics* are most common; those in **Bold** are life-threatening.

▼ IV facts

Preparation: For IV intermittent administration, reconstitute 1 or 2 g with 10–20 mL sterile water for injection. For continuous IV infusion, add reconstituted solution to 5% dextrose injection, 0.9% sodium chloride injection, 5% dextrose and 0.9% sodium chloride injection, or 5% dextrose injection with 0.02% sodium bicarbonate solution. Store dry powder in cool, dry area. Powder and reconstituted solution darken with storage. Stable for 24 hr at room temperature.

Infusion: Intermittent administration: Slowly inject over 3–5 min, or give over longer time through IV tubing; discontinue other solutions temporarily. If given with aminoglycosides, give each at a different site.

Incompatibilities: Do not mix aminoglycosides and cefoxitin in the same IV solution.

Y-site incompatability: Hetastarch.

Adverse effects

- **CNS:** Headache, dizziness, lethargy, paresthesias
- **GI:** *Nausea, vomiting, diarrhea, anorexia, abdominal pain, flatulence,* **pseudomembranous colitis,** liver toxicity
- **GU:** Nephrotoxicity
- **Hematologic: Bone marrow depression:** decreased WBC, decreased platelets, decreased Hct
- **Hypersensitivity:** *Ranging from rash* to *fever* to **anaphylaxis,** serum sickness reaction
- **Local:** *Pain,* abscess at injection site, *phlebitis,* inflammation at IV site
- **Other:** *Superinfections, disulfiram-like reaction with alcohol*

Interactions

✳ **Drug-drug** ● Increased nephrotoxicity with aminoglycosides ● Increased bleeding effects with oral anticoagulants ● Disulfiram-like reaction may occur if alcohol is taken within 72 hr after cefoxitin administration

✳ **Drug-lab test** ● Possibility of false results on tests of urine glucose using Benedict's solution, Fehling's solution, *Clinitest* tablets; urinary 17-ketosteroids; direct Coombs' test.

■ Nursing considerations

Assessment

- **History:** Liver and kidney dysfunction, lactation, pregnancy
- **Physical:** Skin status, liver and kidney function test, culture of affected area, sensitivity tests

Interventions

- Culture infection, arrange for sensitivity tests before and during therapy if expected response is not seen.
- Reconstitute each gram for IM use with 2 mL sterile water for injection or with 2 mL of 0.5% lidocaine HCl solution (without epinephrine) to decrease pain at injection site. Inject deeply into large muscle group.
- Dry powder and reconstituted solutions darken slightly at room temperature.
- Have vitamin K available in case hypoprothrombinemia occurs.
- Discontinue if hypersensitivity reaction occurs.

Teaching points

- These side effects may occur: stomach upset or diarrhea.
- Avoid alcohol while on this drug and for 3 days after because severe reactions often occur.
- Report severe diarrhea, difficulty breathing, unusual tiredness or fatigue, pain at injection site.

▽ **cefpodoxime proxetil**
*(sef poe **docks' eem**)*

Vantin

PREGNANCY CATEGORY B

Drug classes

Antibiotic
Cephalosporin (third generation)

Therapeutic actions

Bactericidal: inhibits synthesis of bacterial cell wall, causing cell death.

Indications

- LRIs caused by *S. pneumoniae, H. influenzae*

- Upper respiratory infections caused by *S. pyogenes, H. influenzae, Moraxella catarrhalis*
- Dermatologic infections caused by *S. aureus, S. pyogenes*
- UTIs caused by *E. coli, P. mirabilis, Klebsiella, Staphylococcus saprophyticus*
- Otitis media caused by *S. pneumoniae, H. influenzae, M. catarrhalis*
- Sexually transmitted disease caused by *N. gonorrhoeae*

Contraindications and cautions
- Allergy to cephalosporins or penicillins, renal failure, lactation, pregnancy.

Available forms
Tablets—100, 200 mg; granules for suspension—50, 100 mg/5 mL

Dosages
Adults
100–400 mg q 12 hr PO depending on severity of infection; continue for 7–14 days.
Pediatric patients
5 mg/kg per dose PO q 12 hr; do not exceed 100–200 mg per dose; continue for 10 days.
- *Acute otitis media:* 10 mg/kg/day PO; do not exceed 400-mg dose; continue for 10 days.
Geriatric patients or patients with renal impairment
Creatinine clearance < 30 mL/min: increase dosing interval to q 24 hr.

Pharmacokinetics

Route	Peak	Duration
Oral	30–60 min	16–18 hr

Metabolism: $T_{1/2}$: 120–180 min
Distribution: Crosses the placenta; enters breast milk
Excretion: Renal, unchanged

Adverse effects
- **CNS:** Headache, dizziness, lethargy, paresthesias
- **GI:** *Nausea, vomiting, diarrhea, anorexia, abdominal pain, flatulence,* **pseudomembranous colitis,** liver toxicity
- **GU:** Nephrotoxicity

- **Hematologic: Bone marrow depression**
- **Hypersensitivity:** *Ranging from rash* to *fever* to **anaphylaxis;** serum sickness reaction
- **Other:** *Superinfections*

Interactions
✱**Drug-drug** • Increased nephrotoxicity with aminoglycosides • Increased bleeding effects with oral anticoagulants

✱**Drug-food** • Increased absorption and increased effects of cefpodoxime if taken with food

✱**Drug-lab test** • Possibility of false results on tests of urine glucose using Benedict's solution, Fehling's solution, *Clinitest* tablets; urinary 17-ketosteroids; direct Coombs' test.

■ Nursing considerations
Assessment
- **History:** Penicillin or cephalosporin allergy, pregnancy or lactation
- **Physical:** Kidney function, respiratory status, skin status; culture and sensitivity tests of infected area

Interventions
- Culture infection before drug therapy.
- Give drug with meals or food to enhance absorption.
- Prepare suspension as follows: suspend 50 mg/5 mL strength in a total of 58 mL distilled water. Gently tap the bottle to loosen the powder. Add 25 mL distilled water and shake vigorously for 15 seconds. Add 33 mL distilled water, and shake vigorously for 3 min or until all particles are suspended. Suspend 100 mg/5 mL strength in a total of 57 mL distilled water. Proceed as above, adding 25 mL distilled water and 32 mL distilled water, respectively.
- Refrigerate suspension after reconstitution; shake vigorously before use, and discard after 14 days.
- Discontinue drug if hypersensitivity reaction occurs.
- Give the patient yogurt or buttermilk in case of diarrhea.
- Arrange for oral vancomycin for serious colitis that fails to respond to discontinuation.

Adverse effects in *Italics* are most common; those in **Bold** are life-threatening.

Teaching points
- Take this drug with food.
- Complete the full course of this drug even if you feel better.
- This drug is prescribed for this particular infection; do not self-treat any other infection.
- These side effects may occur: stomach upset, loss of appetite, nausea (take drug with food); diarrhea; headache, dizziness.
- Report severe diarrhea with blood, pus, or mucus; rash or hives; difficulty breathing; unusual tiredness, fatigue; unusual bleeding or bruising.

▷ cefprozil
(sef pro' zil)

Cefzil

PREGNANCY CATEGORY B

Drug classes
Antibiotic
Cephalosporin (second generation)

Therapeutic actions
Bactericidal: inhibits synthesis of bacterial cell wall, causing cell death.

Indications
- Pharyngitis or tonsillitis caused by *S. pyogenes*
- Secondary bacterial infection of acute bronchitis and exacerbation of chronic bronchitis caused by *S. pneumoniae, H. influenzae, M. catarrhalis*
- Dermatologic infections caused by *S. aureus, S. pyogenes*
- Otitis media caused by *S. pneumoniae, H. influenzae, M. catarrhalis*
- Acute sinusitis caused by *S. pneumoniae, S. aureus, H. influenzae, M. catarrhalis*

Contraindications and cautions
- Allergy to cephalosporins or penicillins, renal failure, lactation, pregnancy.

Available forms
Tablets—250, 500 mg; powder for suspension—125, 250 mg/5 mL

Dosages
Adults
250–500 mg PO q 12–24 hr. Continue treatment for 10 days.
Pediatric patients
2–12 yr: 7.5–20 mg/kg PO q 12 hr; continue treatment for 10 days.
6 mo–2 yr: 7.5–15 mg/kg PO q 12 hr for 10 days.
Geriatric patients or patients with renal impairment
Creatinine clearance 30–120 mL/min, use standard dose; creatinine clearance 0–30 mL/min, use 50% of standard dose.

Pharmacokinetics

Route	Peak	Duration
Oral	6–10 hr	24–28 hr

Metabolism: $T_{1/2}$: 78 min
Distribution: Crosses the placenta, enters breast milk
Excretion: Renal, unchanged

Adverse effects
- **CNS:** Headache, dizziness, lethargy, paresthesias
- **GI:** *Nausea, vomiting, diarrhea, anorexia, abdominal pain, flatulence,* **pseudomembranous colitis,** liver toxicity
- **GU:** Nephrotoxicity
- **Hematologic: Bone marrow depression**
- **Hypersensitivity:** *Ranging from rash* to *fever* to **anaphylaxis;** serum sickness reaction
- **Other:** *Superinfections*

Interactions
✳ **Drug-drug** • Increased nephrotoxicity with aminoglycosides • Increased bleeding effects if taken with oral anticoagulants
✳ **Drug-lab test** • Possibility of false results on tests of urine glucose using Benedict's solution, Fehling's solution, *Clinitest* tablets; urinary 17-ketosteroids; direct Coombs' test.

■ Nursing considerations
Assessment
- **History:** Penicillin or cephalosporin allergy, pregnancy or lactation

- **Physical:** Kidney function, respiratory status, skin status, culture and sensitivity tests of infected area

Interventions
- Culture infection before drug therapy.
- Give drug with food to decrease GI discomfort.
- Refrigerate suspension after reconstitution, and discard after 14 days.
- Discontinue if hypersensitivy reaction occurs.
- Give the patient yogurt or buttermilk in case of diarrhea.
- Arrange for oral vancomycin for serious colitis that fails to respond to discontinuation.

Teaching points
- Take this drug with food.
- Complete the full course of this drug, even if you feel better.
- This drug is prescribed for this particular infection; do not use it to self-treat any other infection.
- These side effects may occur: stomach upset, loss of appetite, nausea (take drug with food); diarrhea; headache, dizziness.
- Report severe diarrhea with blood, pus, or mucus; rash or hives; difficulty breathing; unusual tiredness, fatigue; unusual bleeding or bruising.

▽ ceftazidime
*(sef **taz'** i deem)*

Ceptaz, Fortaz, Tazicef, Tazidime

PREGNANCY CATEGORY B

Drug classes
Antibiotic
Cephalosporin (third generation)

Therapeutic actions
Bactericidal: inhibits synthesis of bacterial cell wall, causing cell death.

Indications
- Lower respiratory tract infections caused by *P. aeruginosa*, other *Pseudomonas, S. pneumoniae, S. aureus, Klebsiella, H. in-* *fluenzae, P. mirabilis, E. coli, Enterobacter, Serratia, Citrobacter*
- UTIs caused by *P. aeruginosa, Enterobacter, E. coli, Klebsiella, P. mirabilis, Proteus*
- Gynecologic infections caused by *E. coli*
- Dermatologic infections caused by *P. aeruginosa, S. aureus, E. coli, Serratia, Proteus, Klebsiella, Enterobacter, S. pyogenes*
- Septicemia caused by *P. aeruginosa, E. coli, Klebsiella, H. influenzae, Serratia, S. pneumoniae, S. aureus*
- Intra-abdominal infections caused by *E. coli, S. aureus, Bacteroides, Klebsiella*
- CNS infections caused by *H. influenzae, N. meningitidis*
- Bone and joint infections caused by *P. aeruginosa, Klebsiella, Enterobacter, S. aureus*

Contraindications and cautions
- Allergy to cephalosporins or penicillins, renal failure, lactation.

Available forms
Powder for injection—500 mg, 1, 2, 6 g; injection—1, 2 g

Dosages
Adults
Usual dose: 1 g (range 250 mg–2 g) q 8–12 hr IM or IV. Do not exceed 6 g/day. Dosage will vary with infection.
- *UTI:* 250–500 mg IV or IM q 8–12 hr.
- *Pneumonia, dermatologic infections:* 500 mg–1 g IV or IM q 8 hr.
- *Bone and joint infections:* 2 g IV q 12 hr.
- *Gynecologic, intra-abdominal, life-threatening infections, meningitis:* 2 g IV q 8 hr.

Pediatric patients
0–4 wk: 30 mg/kg IV q 12 hr.
1 mo–12 yr: 30–50 mg/kg IV q 8 hr. Do not exceed 6 g/day.

Geriatric patients or patients with reduced renal function
Loading dose of 1 g IV, followed by:

Creatinine Clearance (mL/min)	Dosage
50–31	1 g q 12 hr
30–16	1 g q 24 hr
15–6	500 mg q 24 hr
≤ 5	500 mg q 48 hr

Pharmacokinetics

Route	Onset	Peak	Duration
IV	Rapid	1 hr	24–28 hr
IM	30 min	1 hr	24–28 hr

Metabolism: $T_{1/2}$: 114–120 min
Distribution: Crosses the placenta; enters breast milk
Excretion: Urine

▽ IV facts

Preparation: Reconstitute drug for direct IV injection with sterile water for injection. Reconstituted solution is stable for 18 hr at room temperature or 7 days if refrigerated. **500-mg vial:** mix with 5 mL diluent; resulting concentration, 11 mg/mL. **1-g vial:** mix with 5 (10) mL diluent; resulting concentration, 180 (100) mg/mL. **2-g vial:** mix with 10 mL diluent; resulting concentration, 170–180 mg/mL.
Infusion: For IV, reconstitute 1- or 2-g infusion pack with 100 mL sterile water for injection; infuse slowly. Direct injection: slowly over 3–5 min. Infusion: over 30 min. If patient is also receiving aminoglycosides, administer at separate sites.
Incompatibilities: Do not mix with sodium bicarbonate injection and aminoglycoside solutions.

Adverse effects

- **CNS:** Headache, dizziness, lethargy, paresthesias
- **GI:** *Nausea, vomiting, diarrhea, anorexia, abdominal pain, flatulence,* **pseudomembranous colitis,** liver toxicity
- **GU:** Nephrotoxicity
- **Hematologic: Bone marrow depression:** decreased WBC, decreased platelets, decreased Hct
- **Hypersensitivity:** *Ranging from rash to fever to* **anaphylaxis,** serum sickness reaction
- **Local:** *Pain,* abscess at injection site; *phlebitis,* inflammation at IV site
- **Other:** *Superinfections, disulfiram-like reaction with alcohol*

Interactions

✳ **Drug-drug** • Increased nephrotoxicity with aminoglycosides • Increased bleeding effects with oral anticoagulants

✳ **Drug-lab test** • Possibility of false results on tests of urine glucose using Benedict's solution, Fehling's solution, *Clinitest* tablets; urinary 17-ketosteroids; direct Coombs' test.

■ Nursing considerations
Assessment

- **History:** Liver and kidney dysfunction, lactation, pregnancy
- **Physical:** Skin status, liver and kidney function test, culture of affected area, sensitivity tests

Interventions

- Culture infection, arrange for sensitivity tests before and during therapy if expected response is not seen.
- Reconstitute drug for IM use with sterile water or bacteriostatic water for injection or with 0.5% or 1% lidocaine HCl injection to reduce pain; inject deeply into large muscle group.
- Do not mix with aminoglycoside solutions. Administer these drugs separately.
- Powder and reconstituted solution darken with storage.
- Have vitamin K available in case hypoprothrombinemia occurs.
- Discontinue if hypersensitivity reaction occurs.

Teaching points

- These side effects may occur: stomach upset or diarrhea.
- Avoid alcohol while on this drug and for 3 days after because severe reactions often occur.
- Report severe diarrhea, difficulty breathing, unusual tiredness or fatigue, pain at injection site.

▽ ceftibuten hydrochloride
*(sef ta **byoo**' ten)*

Cedax

PREGNANCY CATEGORY B

Drug classes
Antibiotic
Cephalosporin (third generation)

Therapeutic actions

Bactericidal: inhibits synthesis of bacterial cell wall, causing cell death.

Indications

- Acute bacterial exacerbations of chronic bronchitis due to *H. influenzae, Moraxella catarrhalis, Streptococcus pneumonia*
- Acute bacterial otitis media due to *H. influenzae, M. catarrhalis, Streptococcus pyogenes*
- Pharyngitis and tonsillitis due to *S. pyogenes*

Contraindications and cautions

- Allergy to cephalosporins or penicillins; renal failure; lactation, pregnancy.

Available forms

Capsules—400 mg; oral suspension—90, 180 mg/5 mL

Dosages
Adults
400 mg PO daily for 10 days.
Pediatric patients
9 mg/kg/day PO for 10 days to a maximum daily dose of 400 mg/day.
Patients with renal impairment

Creatinine Clearance (mL/min)	Dose
> 50	9 mg/kg or 400 mg PO in 24 hr
30–49	4.5 mg/kg or 200 mg PO in 24 hr
5–29	2.25 mg/kg or 100 mg PO in 24 hr

Pharmacokinetics

Route	Peak	Duration
Oral	30–60 min	8–10 hr

Metabolism: $T_{1/2}$: 30–60 min
Distribution: Crosses placenta; enters breast milk
Excretion: Renal, unchanged

Adverse effects

- **CNS:** Headache, dizziness, lethargy, paresthesias
- **GI:** *Nausea, vomiting, diarrhea, anorexia, abdominal pain, flatulence,* **pseudomembranous colitis,** liver toxicity
- **GU:** Nephrotoxicity
- **Hematologic:** Bone marrow depression
- **Hypersensitivity:** *Ranging from rash* to *fever* to **anaphylaxis,** serum sickness reaction
- **Other:** *Superinfections*

Interactions

✳ **Drug-drug** • Increased nephrotoxicity with aminoglycosides • Increased bleeding effects with oral anticoagulants • Disulfiram-like reaction may occur if alcohol is taken within 72 hr after administration

✳ **Drug-lab test** • Possibility of false results on tests of urine glucose using Benedict's solution, Fehling's, *Clinitest* tablets; urinary 17-ketosteroids; direct Coombs' test

■ Nursing considerations
Assessment

- **History:** Allergy to penicillin or cephalosporin; pregnancy, lactation
- **Physical:** Kidney function, respiratory status, skin status; culture and sensitivity tests of infection

Interventions

- Culture infection before beginning drug therapy.
- Give capsules with meals to decrease GI discomfort; suspension must be given on an empty stomach at least 1 hr before or 2 hr after meals.
- Refrigerate suspension after reconstitution; shake vigorously before use and discard after 14 days.
- Discontinue drug if hypersensitivity reaction occurs.
- Give patient yogurt or buttermilk in case of diarrhea.
- Arrange for treatment of superinfections.
- Reculture infection if patient fails to respond.

Teaching points

- Take capsules with meals or food; suspension must be taken on an empty stomach, at least 1 hr before or 2 hr after meals.
- Refrigerate suspension; shake vigorously after use and discard after 14 days.

- Complete the full course of this drug, even if you feel better before the course of treatment is over.
- This drug is prescribed for this particular infection; do not use it to self-treat any other infection.
- These side effects may occur: stomach upset, loss of appetite, nausea (take drug with food); diarrhea; headache, dizziness.
- Report severe diarrhea with blood, pus, or mucus; rash or hives; difficulty breathing; unusual tiredness, fatigue; unusual bleeding or bruising.

▽ceftizoxime sodium
(sef ti zox' eem)

Cefizox

PREGNANCY CATEGORY B

Drug classes
Antibiotic
Cephalosporin (third generation)

Therapeutic actions
Bactericidal: inhibits synthesis of bacterial cell wall, causing cell death.

Indications
- LRIs caused by *S. pneumoniae, S. aureus, Klebsiella, H. influenzae, E. coli, P. mirabilis, Enterobacter, Serratia, Bacteroides*
- UTIs caused by *S. aureus, Citrobacter, Enterobacter, E. coli, Klebsiella, P. aeruginosa, P. vulgaris, P. rettgeri, P. mirabilis, M. morganii, S. marcescens, Enterobacter*
- Uncomplicated cervical and urethral gonorrhea caused by *N. gonorrhoeae*
- PID caused by *N. gonorrhoeae, E. coli, S. agalactiae*
- Intra-abdominal infections caused by *E. coli, S. epidermidis, Streptococcus* (except enterococci), *Enterobacter, Klebsiella, Bacteroides, Peptococcus, Peptostreptococcus*
- Dermatologic infections caused by *S. aureus, E. coli, Klebsiella, Enterobacter, Bacteroides, Peptococcus, Peptostreptococcus, P. mirabilis, S. epidermidis, S. pyogenes*
- Septicemia caused by *E. coli, Klebsiella, S. pneumoniae, S. aureus, Bacteroides, Serratia*
- Bone and joint infections caused by *S. aureus,* streptococci (excluding enterococci), *P. mirabilis, Bacteroides, Peptococcus, Peptostreptococcus*
- Meningitis caused by *H. influenzae,* some cases caused by *S. pneumoniae*

Contraindications and cautions
- Allergy to cephalosporins or penicillins, renal failure, lactation, pregnancy

Available forms
Powder for injection—500 mg, 1, 2, 10 g; injection in D_5W—1, 2 g

Dosages
Adults
Usual dose: 500 mg–2 g (range 500 mg–4 g) IM or IV q 8–12 hr. Do not exceed 12 g/day. Dosage will vary with infection.
- *Gonorrhea:* Single 1-g IM dose.
- *Uncomplicated UTIs:* 500 mg q 12 hr IM or IV.
- *PID:* 2 g q 8 hr IV.
- *Life-threatening infections:* 3–4 g q 8 hr IV.
Pediatric patients ≥ 6 mo
50 mg/kg q 6–8 hr; up to 200 mg/kg/day in severe infections.
Geriatric patients or patients with reduced renal function
Initial dose of 500 mg–1 g IM or IV followed by:

Creatinine Clearance (mL/min)	Usual Dosage	Maximum Dosage
79–80	500 mg q 8 hr	0.75–1.5 g q 8 hr
49–5	250–500 mg q 12 hr	0.5–1 g q 12 hr
4–0	500 mg q 48 hr or 250 mg q 24 hr	0.5–1 g q 48 hr or 0.5 g q 24 hr

Pharmacokinetics

Route	Onset	Peak	Duration
IV	Rapid	1 hr	18–24 hr
IM	30 min	1 hr	18–24 hr

Metabolism: $T_{1/2}$: 84–114 min
Distribution: Crosses the placenta; enters breast milk
Excretion: Urine

▽IV facts

Preparation: Dilute reconstituted solution for IV infusion with 50–100 mL of 5% or 10% dextrose injection; 5% dextrose and 0.2%, 0.45%, or 0.9% sodium chloride injection; lactated Ringer's injection; Ringer's injection; 0.9% sodium chloride injection; invert sugar 10% in sterile water for injection; 5% sodium bicarbonate in sterile water for injection; or 5% dextrose in lactated Ringer's injection if reconstituted with 4% sodium bicarbonate injection.

Package Size	Diluent to Add	Volume	Resulting Concentration
1-g vial	10 mL	10.7 mL	95 mg/mL
2-g vial	20 mL	21.4 mL	95 mg/mL
10-g vial	30 mL	37 mL	1 g/3.5 mL
	45 mL	51 mL	1 g/5 mL

Piggy-back vials should be reconstituted with 50–100 mL of any of the above solutions. Shake well, and administer as a single dose with primary IV fluids. Reconstituted solution is stable for 24 hr at room temperature or 4 days if refrigerated; discard solution after allotted time.
Infusion: If given with aminoglycosides, give each antibiotic at a different site. Direct injection: administer slowly over 3–5 min directly or through tubing. Infusion: over 30 min.
Incompatibilities: Do not mix aminoglycosides and ceftizoxime in the same IV solution.

Adverse effects

- **CNS:** Headache, dizziness, lethargy, paresthesias
- **GI:** *Nausea, vomiting, diarrhea, anorexia, abdominal pain, flatulence,* **pseudomembranous colitis,** liver toxicity
- **GU:** Nephrotoxicity
- **Hematologic: Bone marrow depression:** decreased WBC, decreased platelets, decreased Hct
- **Hypersensitivity:** *Ranging from rash* to *fever* to **anaphylaxis;** serum sickness reaction
- **Local:** *Pain,* abscess at injection site, *phlebitis,* inflammation at IV site
- **Other:** *Superinfections, disulfiram-like reaction with alcohol*

Interactions

✱ **Drug-drug** • Increased nephrotoxicity with aminoglycosides • Increased bleeding effects with oral anticoagulants
✱ **Drug-lab test** • Possibility of false results on tests of urine glucose using Benedict's solution, Fehling's solution, *Clinitest* tablets; urinary 17-ketosteroids; direct Coombs' test.

■ Nursing considerations
Assessment

- **History:** Liver and kidney dysfunction, lactation, pregnancy
- **Physical:** Skin status, liver and kidney function test, culture of affected area, sensitivity tests

Interventions

- Culture infection, arrange for sensitivity tests before and during therapy if expected response is not seen.
- Divide and administer IM doses of 2 g at two different sites by deep IM injection.
- Give each antibiotic at a different site, if given as part of combination therapy with aminoglycosides.
- Discontinue if hypersensitivity reaction occurs.
- Have vitamin K available in case hypoprothrombinemia occurs.

Teaching points

- These side effects may occur: stomach upset or diarrhea.
- Avoid alcohol while on this drug and for 3 days after because severe reactions often occur.
- Report severe diarrhea, difficulty breathing, unusual tiredness or fatigue, pain at injection site.

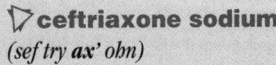

▽ceftriaxone sodium
*(sef try **ax'** ohn)*

Rocephin

PREGNANCY CATEGORY B

Drug classes

Antibiotic
Cephalosporin (third generation)

Adverse effects in *Italics* are most common; those in **Bold** are life-threatening.

Therapeutic actions
Bactericidal: inhibits synthesis of bacterial cell wall, causing cell death.

Indications
- Lower respiratory tract infections caused by *S. pneumoniae, S. aureus, Klebsiella, H. influenzae, E. coli, P. mirabilis, E. aerogens, Serratia marcescens, Haemophilus parainfluenzae, Streptococcus* (excluding enterococci)
- UTIs caused by *E. coli, Klebsiella, P. vulgaris, P. mirabilis, M. morganii*
- Gonorrhea caused by *N. gonorrhoeae*
- Intra-abdominal infections caused by *E. coli, K. pneumoniae*
- PID caused by *N. gonorrhoeae*
- Dermatologic infections caused by *S. aureus, Klebsiella, Enterobacter cloacae, P. mirabilis, S. epidermidis, P. aeruginosa, Streptococcus* (excluding enterococci)
- Septicemia caused by *E. coli, S. pneumoniae, H. influenzae, S. aureus, K. pneumoniae*
- Bone and joint infections caused by *S. aureus,* streptococci (excluding enterococci), *P. mirabilis, S. pneumoniae, E. coli, K. pneumoniae, Enterobacter*
- Meningitis caused by *H. influenzae, S. pneumoniae, N. meningitidis*
- Perioperative prophylaxis for patients undergoing coronary artery bypass surgery
- Unlabeled use: treatment of Lyme disease in doses of 2 g IV bid for 14 days

Contraindications and cautions
- Allergy to cephalosporins or penicillins, renal failure, lactation, pregnancy

Available forms
Powder for injection—250, 500 mg, 1, 2 g; injection—1, 2 g

Dosages
Adults
1–2 g/day IM or IV once a day or in equal divided doses bid. Do not exceed 4 g/day.
- *Gonorrhea:* Single 250 mg IM dose.
- *Meningitis:* 100 mg/kg/day IV or IM in divided doses q 12 hr. Do not exceed 4 g/day.
- *Perioperative prophylaxis:* 1 g IV 30–60 min before surgery.

Pediatric patients
50–75 mg/kg/day IV or IM in divided doses q 12 hr. Do not exceed 2 g/day.
- *Meningitis:* 100 mg/kg/day IV or IM in divided doses q 12 hr. Loading dose of 80–100 mg/kg may be used.

Pharmacokinetics

Route	Onset	Peak	Duration
IV	Rapid	Immediate	15–18 hr
IM	30 min	1.5–4 hr	15–18 hr

Metabolism: $T_{1/2}$: 5–10 hr
Distribution: Crosses the placenta; enters breast milk
Excretion: Urine and bile

▽IV facts
Preparation: Dilute reconstituted solution for IV infusion with 50–100 mL of 5% or 10% dextrose injection, 5% dextrose and 0.45% or 0.9% sodium chloride injection, 0.9% sodium chloride injection, 10% invert sugar, 5% sodium bicarbonate, *FreAmine 111, Normosol-M in 5% Dextrose, Ionosol-B in 5% Dextrose,* 5% or 10% mannitol, sodium lactate.

Package Size	Diluent to Add	Resulting Concentration
250-mg vial	2.4 mL	100 mg/mL
500-mg vial	4.8 mL	100 mg/mL
1-g vial	9.6 mL	100 mg/mL
2-g vial	19.2 mL	100 mg/mL
Piggyback 1 g	10 mL	
Piggyback 2 g	20 mL	

Stability of reconstituted and diluted solution depends on diluent, concentration and type of container (eg, glass, PVC); check manufacturer's inserts for specific details. Protect drug from light.
Infusion: Administer by intermittent infusion over 15–30 min. Do not mix ceftriaxone with any other antimicrobial drug.
Incompatibilities: Do not mix aminoglycosides and ceftriaxone in the same IV solution.

Adverse effects
- **CNS:** Headache, dizziness, lethargy, paresthesias
- **GI:** *Nausea, vomiting, diarrhea, anorexia, abdominal pain, flatulence,* **pseudomembranous colitis,** liver toxicity

- **GU:** Nephrotoxicity
- **Hematologic: Bone marrow depression:** decreased WBC, decreased platelets, decreased Hct
- **Hypersensitivity:** *Ranging from rash* to *fever* to **anaphylaxis;** serum sickness reaction
- **Local:** *Pain,* abscess at injection site; *phlebitis,* inflammation at IV site
- **Other:** *Superinfections, disulfiram-like reaction with alcohol*

Interactions
✳ **Drug-drug** ● Increased nephrotoxicity with aminoglycosides ● Increased bleeding effects with oral anticoagulants ● Disulfiram-like reaction may occur if alcohol is taken within 72 hr after ceftriaxone administration.

✳ **Drug-lab test** ● Possibility of false results on tests of urine glucose using Benedict's solution, Fehling's solution, *Clinitest* tablets; urinary 17-ketosteroids; direct Coombs' test.

■ Nursing considerations
- **History:** Liver and kidney dysfunction, lactation, pregnancy
- **Physical:** Skin status, liver and kidney function test, culture of affected area, sensitivity tests

Interventions
- Culture infection, arrange for sensitivity tests before and during therapy if expected response is not seen.
- Reconstitute for IM use with sterile water for injection, 0.9% sodium chloride solution, 5% dextrose solution, bacteriostatic water with 0.9% benzyl alcohol, or 1% lidocaine solution (without epinephrine); inject deeply into a large muscle group.
- Check manufacturer's inserts for specific details. Stability of reconstituted and diluted solution depends on diluent, concentration and type of container (eg, glass, PVC).
- Protect drug from light.
- Do not mix ceftriaxone with any other antimicrobial drug.
- Monitor ceftriaxone blood levels in patients with severe renal impairment and in patients with renal and hepatic impairment.

- Have vitamin K available in case hypoprothrombinemia occurs.
- Discontinue if hypersensitivity reaction occurs.

Teaching points
- These side effects may occur: stomach upset or diarrhea.
- Avoid alcohol while on this drug and for 3 days after because severe reactions often occur.
- Report severe diarrhea, difficulty breathing, unusual tiredness or fatigue, pain at injection site.

▽**cefuroxime**
(se fyoor ox' eem)

cefuroxime axetil
Ceftin

cefuroxime sodium
Kefurox, Zinacef

PREGNANCY CATEGORY B

Drug classes
Antibiotic
Cephalosporin (second generation)

Therapeutic actions
Bactericidal: inhibits synthesis of bacterial cell wall, causing cell death.

Indications
Oral (cefuroxime axetil)
- Pharyngitis, tonsillitis caused by *S. pyogenes*
- Otitis media caused by *S. pneumoniae, H. influenzae, M. catarrhalis, S. pyogenes*
- Lower respiratory tract infections caused by *S. pneumoniae, H. parainfluenzae, H. influenzae*
- UTIs caused by *E. coli, K. pneumoniae*
- Dermatologic infections, including impetigo caused by *S. aureus, S. pyogenes*
- Treatment of early Lyme disease

Parenteral (cefuroxime sodium)
- Lower respiratory tract infections caused by *S. pneumoniae, S. aureus, E. coli, Klebsiella, H. influenzae, S. pyogenes*

- Dermatologic infections caused by *S. aureus, S. pyogenes, E. coli, Klebsiella, Enterobacter*
- UTIs caused by *E. coli, Klebsiella*
- Uncomplicated and disseminated gonorrhea caused by *N. gonorrhoea*
- Septicemia caused by *S. pneumoniae, S. aureus, E. coli, Klebsiella, H. influenzae*
- Meningitis caused by *S. pneumoniae, H. influenzae, S. aureus, N. meningitidis*
- Bone and joint infections caused by *S. aureus*
- Perioperative prophylaxis
- Treatment of acute bacterial maxillary sinusitis in patients 3 mo–12 yr

Contraindications and cautions

- Allergy to cephalosporins or penicillins, renal failure, lactation, pregnancy

Available forms

Tablets—125, 250, 500 mg; suspension—125, 250 mg/5 mL; powder for injection—750 mg, 1.5, 7.5 g; injection—750 mg, 1.5 g

Dosages
Oral
Adults and patients > 12 yr
250 mg bid. For severe infections, may be increased to 500 mg bid.
- *Uncomplicated UTIs:* 125 mg bid. Increase to 250 mg bid in severe cases.

Pediatric patients < 12 yr
125 mg bid.
- *Otitis media:* < 2 yr: 125 mg bid. >2 yr: 250 mg bid or 30 mg/kg/day in divided doses bid (suspension).
- *Pharyngitis or tonsillitis:* 125 mg bid or 20 mg/kg/day in divided doses (suspension).
- *Impetigo:* 30 mg/kg/day in divided doses bid (suspension).

Parenteral
Adults
750 mg–1.5 g IM or IV q 8 hr, depending on severity of infection.
- *Uncomplicated gonorrhea:* 1.5 g IM (at two different sites) with 1 g of oral probenecid.
- *Perioperative prophylaxis:* 1.5 g IV 30–60 min prior to initial incision; then 750 mg IV or IM q 8 hr for 24 hr after surgery.

Pediatric patients > 3 mo
50–100 mg/kg/day IM or IV in divided doses q 6–8 hr.
- *Bacterial meningitis:* 200–240 mg/kg/day IV in divided doses q 6–8 hr.
- *Impaired renal function:* Adjust adult dosage for renal impairment by weight or age of child.

Geriatric patients or adults with impaired renal function

Creatinine Clearance (mL/min)	Dosage
> 20	750 mg–1.5 g q 8 hr
10–20	750 mg q 12 hr
< 10	750 mg q 24 hr

Pharmacokinetics

Route	Onset	Peak	Duration
IV	Rapid	Immediate	18–24 hr
IM	20 min	30 min	18–24 hr
Oral	Varies	2 hr	18–24 hr

Metabolism: $T_{1/2}$: 1–2 hr
Distribution: Crosses the placenta; enters breast milk
Excretion: Urine

▼ IV facts

Preparation: Preparation of parenteral drug solutions and suspensions differs for different starting preparations and different brand names; check the manufacturer's directions carefully. Reconstitute parenteral drug with sterile water for injection, 5% dextrose in water, 0.9% sodium chloride, or any of the following, which also may be used for further dilution: 0.9% sodium chloride, 5% or 10% dextrose injection, 5% dextrose and 0.45% or 0.9% sodium chloride injection, or M/6 sodium lactate injection. Stability of solutions depends on diluent and concentration: Check manufacturer's specifications. Do not mix with IV solutions containing aminoglycosides. Powder form, solutions, and suspensions darken during storage.
Infusion: Inject slowly over 3–5 minutes directly into vein for IV administration, or infuse over 30 min, 6–24 hr if by continuous infusion. Give aminoglycosides and cefuroxime at different sites.
Incompatibilities: Do not mix aminoglycosides and cefuroxime in the same IV solution.

Adverse effects

- **CNS:** Headache, dizziness, lethargy, paresthesias
- **GI:** *Nausea, vomiting, diarrhea, anorexia, abdominal pain, flatulence,* **pseudomembranous colitis,** liver toxicity
- **GU:** Nephrotoxicity
- **Hematologic: Bone marrow depression,** decreased WBC, decreased platelets, decreased Hct
- **Hypersensitivity:** *Ranging from rash to fever to* **anaphylaxis,** serum sickness reaction
- **Local:** *Pain,* abscess at injection site, *phlebitis,* inflammation at IV site
- **Other:** *Superinfections, disulfiram-like reaction with alcohol*

Interactions

※ **Drug-drug** • Increased nephrotoxicity with aminoglycosides • Increased bleeding effects with oral anticoagulants

※ **Drug-lab test** • Possibility of false results on tests of urine glucose using Benedict's solution, Fehling's solution, *Clinitest* tablets; urinary 17-ketosteroids; direct Coombs' test.

■ Nursing considerations

Assessment

- **History:** Liver and kidney dysfunction, lactation, pregnancy
- **Physical:** Skin status, liver and kidney function test, culture of affected area, sensitivity tests

Interventions

- Culture infection, arrange for sensitivity tests before and during therapy if expected response is not seen.
- Give oral drug with food to decrease GI upset and enhance absorption.
- Give oral drug to children who can swallow tablets; crushing the drug results in a bitter, unpleasant taste.
- Have vitamin K available in case hypoprothrombinemia occurs.
- Discontinue if hypersensitivity reaction occurs.

Teaching points

Oral drug

- Take full course of therapy.
- This drug is specific for this infection and should not be used to self-treat other problems.
- Swallow tablets whole; do not crush. Take the drug with food.
- These side effects may occur: stomach upset or diarrhea.
- Report severe diarrhea with blood, pus, or mucus; rash; difficulty breathing; unusual tiredness, fatigue; unusual bleeding or bruising; unusual itching or irritation.

Parenteral drug

- These side effects may occur: stomach upset or diarrhea.
- Avoid alcohol while on this drug and for 3 days after because severe reactions often occur.
- Report severe diarrhea, difficulty breathing, unusual tiredness or fatigue, pain at injection site.

▷ **celecoxib**
(sell ah cocks' ib)

Celebrex

PREGNANCY CATEGORY

Drug classes

NSAID (nonsteroidal anti-inflammatory drug)
Analgesic (non-narcotic)
Specific COX-2 enzyme blocker

Therapeutic actions

Analgesic and anti-inflammatory activities related to inhibition of the COX-2 enzyme, which is activated in inflammation to cause the signs and symptoms associated with inflammation; does not affect the COX-1 enzyme, which protects the lining of the GI tract and has blood clotting and renal functions.

Indications

- Acute and long-term treatment of signs and symptoms of rheumatoid arthritis and osteoarthritis

- Reduction of the number of colorectal polyps in familial adenomatous polyposis (FAP)
- Management of acute pain
- Treatment of primary dysmenorrhea

Contraindications and cautions

- Contraindicated with allergies to sulfonamides, celecoxib, NSAIDs, or aspirin; significant renal impairment; pregnancy; lactation.
- Use cautiously with impaired hearing, hepatic and cardiovascular conditions.

Available forms

Capsules—100, 200 mg

Dosages

Adults

Initially, 100 mg PO bid; may increase to 200 mg/day PO bid as needed.

- *Acute pain, dysmenorrhea:* 400 mg, then 200 mg PO bid.
- *FAP:* 400 mg PO bid.

Patients with hepatic impairment

Reduce dosage by 50%.

Pediatric patients

Safety and efficacy have not been established.

Pharmacokinetics

Route	Onset	Peak
Oral	Slow	3 hr

Metabolism: Hepatic; $T_{1/2}$: 11 hours
Distribution: Crosses placenta; may pass into breast milk
Excretion: Urine and bile

Adverse effects

- **CNS:** *Headache, dizziness, somnolence, insomnia,* fatigue, tiredness, dizziness, tinnitus, ophthamologic effects
- **Dermatologic:** *Rash,* pruritus, sweating, dry mucous membranes, stomatitis
- **GI:** Nausea, abdominal pain, *dyspepsia,* flatulence, GI bleed
- **Hematologic:** Neutropenia, eosinophilia, leukopenia, pancytopenia, thrombocytopenia, agranulocytosis, granulocytopenia, aplastic anemia, decreased hemoglobin or hematocrit, bone marrow depression, menorrhagia
- **Other:** Peripheral edema, **anaphylactoid reactions to anaphylactic shock**

Interactions

✳ **Drug-drug** • Increased risk of bleeding if taken concurrently with warfarin. Monitor patient closely and reduce warfarin dose as appropriate

■ Nursing considerations

CLINICAL ALERT!

Name confusion has occurred between Celebrex (celecoxib), Celexa (citalopram), Xanax (alprazolam), and Cerebyx (fosphenytoin); use caution.

Assessment

- **History:** Renal impairment, impaired hearing, allergies, hepatic and cardiovascular conditions, lactation
- **Physical:** Skin color and lesions; orientation, reflexes, ophthalmologic and audiometric evaluation, peripheral sensation; P, edema; R, adventitious sounds; liver evaluation; CBC, renal and liver function tests; serum electrolytes

Interventions

- Administer drug with food or after meals if GI upset occurs.
- Establish safety measures if CNS, visual disturbances occur.
- Arrange for periodic ophthalmologic examination during long-term therapy.
- Institute emergency procedures if overdose occurs—gastric lavage, induction of emesis, supportive therapy.
- Provide further comfort measures to reduce pain (positioning, environmental control, etc), and to reduce inflammation (warmth, positioning, rest, etc).

Teaching points

- Take drug with food or meals if GI upset occurs.
- Take only the prescribed dosage.
- Know that dizziness, drowsiness can occur (avoid driving or the use of dangerous machinery while on this drug).
- Report: sore throat, fever, rash, itching, weight gain, swelling in ankles or fingers; changes in vision.

▽cellulose sodium phosphate (CSP)
(sell' u lohs)

Calcibind

PREGNANCY CATEGORY C

Drug classes
Antilithic agent
Resin exchange agent
Cation

Therapeutic actions
Binds calcium and magnesium in the bowel; promotes the excretion of calcium and reduces serum calcium levels, decreasing the formation of renal calculi.

Indications
• Absorptive hypercalciuria type I (recurrent passage or formation of calcium oxalate or calcium phosphate renal stones not eliminated by diet)

Contraindications and cautions
• Contraindicated with primary or secondary hyperparathyroidism; high fasting urinary calcium or hypophosphatemia; pregnancy; children.
• Use cautiously with CHF, ascites, nephrotic syndrome.

Available forms
Powder—300 g bulk

Dosages
Adults
Initial dose of 15 g/day PO (5 g with each meal) in patients with urinary calcium > 300 mg/day; when urinary calcium declines to < 150 mg/day, reduce to 10 g/day (5 g with supper and 2.5 g with two other meals). Patients with urinary calcium < 300 mg/day but > 200 mg/day, 10 g/day.
Pediatric patients
Safety and efficacy not established.

Pharmacokinetics
Not absorbed systemically.

Adverse effects
• **GI:** *Bad taste, loose stools, diarrhea, dyspepsia*
• **Other:** *Decreased magnesium levels*

■ Nursing considerations
Assessment
• **History:** Primary or secondary hyperparathyroidism; high fasting urinary calcium or hypophosphatemia; lactation; CHF, ascites, nephrotic syndrome
• **Physical:** Weight, skin condition, neurologic status, abdominal exam, urinary calcium, serum electrolytes

Interventions
• Give drug with meals.
• Arrange for supplemental magnesium gluconate with this drug. Those receiving 15 g CSP/day should receive 1.5 g magnesium gluconate before breakfast and again hs. Those receiving 10 g CSP/day should receive 1 g magnesium gluconate twice a day. Give magnesium 1 hr before or 2 hr after CSP to prevent binding.
• Suspend each dose of CSP powder in a glass of water, soft drink, or fruit juice. Give 1 hr before meal.
• Monitor 24-hr urinary calcium levels periodically during therapy; adjust dosage accordingly.
• Arrange for dietary consultation to help patient moderate calcium and dietary oxalate intake.
• Increase fluid intake each day.

Teaching points
• Take drug 1 hr before meals as ordered. Take magnesium supplement 1 hr before the CSP; suspend each dose in a glass of water, soft drink, or juice.
• Avoid vitamin C supplements.
• Drink as much fluid as tolerable.
• Moderate your calcium intake (dairy products), oxalate intake (spinach, rhubarb, chocolate, brewed tea), salt intake.
• These side effects may occur: bad taste, loose stools, diarrhea, indigestion.
• Report swelling of extremities, tremors, palpitations.

Adverse effects in *Italics* are most common; those in **Bold** are life-threatening.

▷cephalexin
(sef a lex' in)

cephalexin
Apo-Cephalex (CAN), Biocef, Keflex, Novo-Lexin (CAN), Nu-Cephalex (CAN), PMS-Cephalexin (CAN)

cephalexin hydrochloride monohydrate
Biocef, Keftab

PREGNANCY CATEGORY B

Drug classes
Antibiotic
Cephalosporin (first generation)

Therapeutic actions
Bactericidal: inhibits synthesis of bacterial cell wall, causing cell death.

Indications
- Respiratory tract infections caused by *S. pneumoniae,* group A beta-hemolytic streptococci
- Dermatologic infections caused by staphylococci, streptococci
- Otitis media caused by *S. pneumoniae, H. influenzae,* streptococci, staphylococci, *M. catarrhalis*
- Bone infections caused by staphylococci, *P. mirabilis*
- GU infections caused by *E. coli, P. mirabilis, Klebsiella*

Contraindications and cautions
- Allergy to cephalosporins or penicillins; renal failure; lactation, pregnancy

Available forms
Capsules—250, 500 mg; tablets—250, 500 mg, 1 g; oral suspension—125, 250 mg/5 mL

Dosages
Adults
1–4 g/day in divided dose; 250 mg PO q 6 hr usual dose.
- *Skin and skin-structure infections:* 500 mg PO q 12 hr. Larger doses may be needed in severe cases; do not exceed 4 g/day.

Pediatric patients
25–50 mg/kg/day PO in divided doses.
- *Skin and skin-structure infections:* Divide total daily dose, and give q 12 hr. Dosage may be doubled in severe cases.
- *Otitis media:* 75–100 mg/kg/day PO in four divided doses.

Pharmacokinetics

Route	Peak	Duration
Oral	60 min	8–10 hr

Metabolism: $T_{1/2}$: 50–80 min
Distribution: Crosses the placenta, enters breast milk
Excretion: Renal

Adverse effects
- **CNS:** Headache, dizziness, lethargy, paresthesias
- **GI:** *Nausea, vomiting, diarrhea, anorexia, abdominal pain, flatulence,* **pseudomembranous colitis,** liver toxicity
- **GU:** Nephrotoxicity
- **Hematologic:** Bone marrow depression
- **Hypersensitivity:** *Ranging from rash* to *fever* to **anaphylaxis;** serum sickness reaction
- **Other:** *Superinfections*

Interactions
✳ Drug-drug • Increased nephrotoxicity with aminoglycosides • Increased bleeding effects with oral anticoagulants • Disulfiram-like reaction may occur if alcohol is taken within 72 hr after cephalexin administration.

✳ Drug-lab test • Possibility of false results on tests of urine glucose using Benedict's solution, Fehling's solution, *Clinitest* tablets; urinary 17-ketosteroids; direct Coombs' test.

■ Nursing considerations
Assessment
- **History:** Penicillin or cephalosporin allergy, pregnancy, or lactation
- **Physical:** Kidney function, respiratory status, skin status; culture and sensitivity tests of infected area

Interventions
- Arrange for culture and sensitivity tests of infection before and during therapy if infection does not resolve.

- Give drug with meals; arrange for small, frequent meals if GI complications occur.
- Refrigerate suspension, discard after 14 days.

Teaching points
- Take this drug with food. Refrigerate suspension; discard any drug after 14 days.
- Complete the full course of this drug even if you feel better.
- This drug is prescribed for this particular infection; do not self-treat any other infection.
- These side effects may occur: stomach upset, loss of appetite, nausea (take drug with food); diarrhea; headache, dizziness.
- Report severe diarrhea with blood, pus, or mucus; rash or hives; difficulty breathing; unusual tiredness, fatigue; unusual bleeding or bruising.

▷cephapirin sodium
(sef a pye' rin)

Cefadyl

PREGNANCY CATEGORY B

Drug classes
Antibiotic
Cephalosporin (first generation)

Therapeutic actions
Bactericidal: inhibits synthesis of bacterial cell wall, causing cell death.

Indications
- Respiratory tract infections caused by *S. pneumoniae, S. aureus,* group A beta-hemolytic streptococci, *Klebsiella, H. influenzae*
- Dermatologic infections caused by *S. aureus,* group A beta-hemolytic streptococci, *E. coli, P. mirabilis, Klebsiella, S. epidermidis*
- GU infections caused by *S. aureus, E. coli, P. mirabilis, Klebsiella*
- Septicemia caused by *S. aureus,* group A beta-hemolytic streptococci, *S. viridans, E. coli, Klebsiella*
- Endocarditis caused by *S. viridans, S. aureus*

- Osteomyelitis caused by *S. aureus, Klebsiella, P. mirabilis,* group A beta-hemolytic streptococci
- Perioperative prophylaxis

Contraindications and cautions
- Allergy to cephalosporins or penicillins, renal failure, lactation, pregnancy

Available forms
Powder for injection—1 g

Dosages
Adults
500 mg–1 g IM or IV q 4–6 hr, depending on severity of infection; up to 12 g daily in severe cases.
- *Perioperative prophylaxis:* 1–2 g 30–60 min before initial incision; 1–2 g during surgery; 1–2 g q 6 hr for 24 hr after surgery or up to 3–5 days.

Pediatric patients
40–80 mg/kg/day IM or IV in four divided doses. Do not use in infants < 3 mo.
- *Perioperative prophylaxis:* Reduce adult dose according to weight or age (see Appendix K for formulas).

Geriatric patients or patients with renal impairment
Serum creatinine > 5 mg/100 mL, 7.5–15 mg/kg q 12 hr.

Pharmacokinetics

Route	Onset	Peak	Duration
IV	Rapid	5 min	6–8 hr
IM	10 min	30 min	6–8 hr

Metabolism: $T_{1/2}$: 24–36 min
Distribution: Crosses the placenta; enters breast milk
Excretion: Urine

▽IV facts
Preparation: Prepare IV intermittent doses, reconstituting 500 mg or 1- to 2-g vial with 10 mL diluent. Stability of diluted IV solutions varies: See manufacturer's inserts. Prepare IV doses with compatible solutions: sodium chloride injection; 5% sodium chloride in water; 5%, 10%, 20% dextrose in water; sodium lactate injection; 10% invert sugar in normal

---

Adverse effects in *Italics* are most common; those in **Bold** are life-threatening.

saline or water; 5% lactated Ringer's injection; lactated Ringer's with 5% dextrose; Ringer's injection; sterile water for injection; 5% dextrose in Ringer's injection; *Normosol R; Normosol R in 5% Dextrose* injection; *Ionosol D-CM; Ionosol G in 10% Dextrose* injection.

Infusion: Inject intermittent dose slowly over 3–5 min. If giving cephapirin IV piggyback, stop other infusion while cephapirin is being infused; infuse 1 g over 5 min or longer. Give aminoglycosides and cephapirin at different sites.

Incompatibilities: Do not mix aminoglycosides and cephapirin in the same IV solution.

Adverse effects

- **CNS:** Headache, dizziness, lethargy, paresthesias
- **GI:** *Nausea, vomiting, diarrhea, anorexia, abdominal pain, flatulence,* **pseudomembranous colitis,** liver toxicity
- **GU:** Nephrotoxicity
- **Hematologic: Bone marrow depression:** decreased WBC, decreased platelets, decreased Hct
- **Hypersensitivity:** *Ranging from rash* to *fever* to **anaphylaxis;** serum sickness reaction
- **Local:** *Pain,* abscess at injection site; *phlebitis,* inflammation at IV site
- **Other:** *Superinfections, disulfiram-like reaction with alcohol*

Interactions

✳ **Drug-drug** • Increased nephrotoxicity with aminoglycosides • Increased bleeding effects with oral anticoagulants • Disulfiram-like reaction if alcohol is taken within 72 hr after cephapirin administration

✳ **Drug-lab test** • Possibility of false results on tests of urine glucose using Benedict's solution, Fehling's solution, *Clinitest* tablets; urinary 17-ketosteroids; direct Coombs' test.

■ Nursing considerations
Assessment

- **History:** Liver and kidney dysfunction, lactation, pregnancy
- **Physical:** Skin status, liver and kidney function test, culture of affected area, sensitivity tests

Interventions

- Culture infection, arrange for sensitivity tests before and during therapy if expected response is not seen.
- Prepare IM solution as follows: reconstitute 500-mg vials with 1 mL of sterile water for injection or bacteriostatic water for injection; reconstitute 1-g vials with 2 mL of diluent; each 1.2 mL contains 500 mg cephapirin.
- Give IM injections deeply into large muscle mass.
- Have vitamin K available in case hypoprothrombinemia occurs.
- Discontinue if hypersensitivity reaction occurs.

Teaching points

- These side effects may occur: stomach upset or diarrhea.
- Avoid alcohol while on this drug and for 3 days after because severe reactions often occur.
- Report severe diarrhea, difficulty breathing, unusual tiredness or fatigue, pain at injection site.

▽ cephradine
(sef' ra deen)

Velosef

PREGNANCY CATEGORY B

Drug classes
Antibiotic
Cephalosporin (first generation)

Therapeutic actions
Bactericidal: inhibits synthesis of bacterial cell wall, causing cell death.

Indications
Oral use

- Respiratory tract infections caused by group A beta-hemolytic streptococci, *S. pneumonia*
- Otitis media caused by group A beta-hemolytic streptococci, *S. pneumoniae, H. influenzae,* and staphylococci
- Dermatologic infections caused by staphylococci and beta-hemolytic streptococci
- UTIs caused by *E. coli, P. mirabilis, Klebsiella,* enterococci

Parenteral use

- Respiratory tract infections caused by *S. pneumoniae, Klebsiella, H. influenzae, S. aureus,* and group A beta-hemolytic streptococci
- UTIs caused by *E. coli, P. mirabilis, Klebsiella*
- Dermatologic infections caused by *S. aureus,* group A beta-hemolytic streptococci
- Bone infections caused by *S. aureus*
- Septicemia caused by *S. pneumoniae, S. aureus, P. mirabilis, E. coli*
- Perioperative prophylaxis

Contraindications and cautions

- Allergy to cephalosporins or penicillins, renal failure, lactation

Available forms

Capsules—250, 500 mg; oral suspension—125, 250 mg/5 mL; powder for injection—250, 500 mg, 1, 2 g

Dosages
Adults

250–500 mg PO q 6–12 hr (dose depends on the severity of infection); 2–4 g/day IV or IM in equal divided doses qid.

- *Perioperative prophylaxis:* 1 g IV or IM 30–90 min before surgery; then 1 g q 4–6 hr for up to 24 hr.
- *Cesarean section:* 1 g IV as soon as cord is clamped; then 1 g IM or IV at 6 and 12 hr.

Pediatric patients > 9 mo

25–50 mg/kg/day in equally divided doses PO q 6–12 hr.

- *Otitis media:* 75–100 mg/kg/day PO in equal divided doses q 6–12 hr. Do not exceed 4 g/day. 50–100 mg/kg/day IV or IM in four equally divided doses.

Geriatric patients or patients with reduced renal function

Creatinine Clearance (mL/min)	Dosage
> 20	500 mg q 6 hr
5–20	250 mg q 6 hr
< 5	250 mg q 12 hr

Dialysis: 250 mg initially, repeat at 12 hr and again 36–48 hr after

Pharmacokinetics

Route	Onset	Peak	Duration
IV	Rapid	5 min	6–8 hr
IM	20 min	1–2 hr	6–8 hr
Oral	Varies	1 hr	6–8 hr

Metabolism: $T_{1/2}$: 48–80 min
Distribution: Crosses the placenta; enters breast milk
Excretion: Urine

▼ IV facts

Preparation: Prepare for direct IV injections by diluting drug with sterile water for injection, 5% dextrose injection, or sodium chloride injection using 5 mL with the 250- to 500-mg vials, 10 mL with the 1-g vial, or 20 mL with the 2-g vial. Prepare for IV infusion as follows: add 10, 20, or 40 mL sterile water for injection to 1-, 2-, or 4-g preparations; withdraw and dilute further with 5% or 10% dextrose injection, sodium chloride injection, M/6 sodium lactate, dextrose and sodium chloride injection, 10% invert sugar in water, *Normosol-R,* or *Ionosol B with 5% Dextrose.* Use direct IV solutions within 2 hr at room temperature. IV infusion solution is stable for 10 hr at room temperature or 48 hr if refrigerated; for prolonged infusions replace solution every 10 hr. Protect solutions from light or direct sunlight.
Infusion: Inject direct IV slowly over 3–5 min, or give through IV tubing; infuse 1 g over 5 min or longer.
Incompatibilities: Do not mix cephradine with any other antibiotic. Do not use with lactated Ringer's injection.

Adverse effects

- **CNS:** Headache, dizziness, lethargy, paresthesias
- **GI:** *Nausea, vomiting, diarrhea, anorexia, abdominal pain, flatulence,* **pseudomembranous colitis,** liver toxicity
- **GU:** Nephrotoxicity
- **Hematologic: Bone marrow depression:** decreased WBC, decreased platelets, decreased Hct
- **Hypersensitivity:** *Ranging from rash* to *fever* to **anaphylaxis;** serum sickness reaction

Adverse effects in *Italics* are most common; those in **Bold** are life-threatening.

- **Local:** *Pain,* abscess at injection site, *phlebitis,* inflammation at IV site
- **Other:** *Superinfections, disulfiram-like reaction with alcohol*

Interactions

* **Drug-drug** • Increased nephrotoxicity with aminoglycosides • Increased bleeding effects with oral anticoagulants • Disulfiram-like reaction if alcohol is taken within 72 hr after cephradine administration

* **Drug-lab test** • Possibility of false results on tests of urine glucose using Benedict's solution, Fehling's solution, *Clinitest* tablets; urinary 17-ketosteroids; direct Coombs' test.

■ Nursing considerations

Assessment

- **History:** Liver and kidney dysfunction, lactation, pregnancy
- **Physical:** Skin status, liver and kidney function test, culture of affected area, sensitivity tests

Interventions

- Culture infection, arrange for sensitivity tests before and during therapy if expected response is not seen.
- Prepare for IM use by reconstituting drug with sterile water or bacteriostatic water for injection; inject deeply into large muscle group.
- Use IM solution within 2 hr if stored at room temperature.
- Protect solutions from light or direct sunlight.
- Do not mix cephradine with any other antibiotic.
- Give oral drug with meals.
- Have vitamin K available in case hypoprothrombinemia occurs.
- Discontinue if hypersensitivity reaction occurs.

Teaching points
Parenteral drug

- These side effects may occur: stomach upset or diarrhea.
- Avoid alcohol while on this drug and for 3 days after because severe reactions often occur.

- Report severe diarrhea, difficulty breathing, unusual tiredness or fatigue, pain at injection site.

Oral drug

- Take full course of therapy.
- This drug is specific for this infection and should not be used to self-treat other problems.
- Take drug with food.
- Avoid alcohol while on this drug and for 3 days after because severe reactions often occur.
- These side effects may occur: stomach upset or diarrhea.
- Report severe diarrhea with blood, pus, or mucus; rash; difficulty breathing; unusual tiredness, fatigue; unusual bleeding or bruising; unusual itching or irritation.

▷ **cetirizine hydrochloride**
*(se **teer'** i zeen)*

Reactine (CAN), Zyrtec

PREGNANCY CATEGORY B

Drug class
Antihistamine

Therapeutic actions
Potent histamine (H_1) receptor antagonist; inhibits histamine release and eosinophil chemotaxis during inflammation, leading to reduced swelling and decreased inflammatory response

Indications

- Management of seasonal and perennial allergic rhinitis
- Treatment of chronic, idiopathic urticaria
- Treatment of year-round allergic rhinitis and chronic idiopathis urticaria in infants ≥ 6 mo

Contraindications and cautions

- Contraindicated with allergy to any antihistamines, hydroxyzine; narrow-angle glaucoma, stenosing peptic ulcer, symptomatic prostatic hypertrophy, asthmatic attack, bladder neck obstruction, pyloroduodenal obstruction (avoid use or use with caution as condition may be exacerbated by drug effects); lactation

Available forms
Tablets—5, 10 mg; syrup—5 mg/5 mL

Dosages
Adults and patients ≥ 12 yr
5–10 mg daily PO; maximum dose 20 mg/day.
Pediatric patients
6–11 yr: 5 or 10 mg daily PO.
6 mo–5 yr: 2.5 mg (one-half teaspoon) PO once daily. In children 1 yr and older, may increase to maximum 5 mg daily given as one-half teaspoon q 12 hr.
Patients with hepatic or renal impairment
5 mg PO daily.

Pharmacokinetics

Route	Onset	Peak	Duration
Oral	Rapid	1 hr	24 hr

Metabolism: Hepatic; $T_{1/2}$: 7–10 hr
Distribution: Crosses placenta; enters breast milk
Excretion: Urine and feces

Adverse effects
- **CNS:** *Somnolence, sedation*
- **CV:** Palpitation, edema
- **GI:** Nausea, diarrhea, abdominal pain, constipation
- **Respiratory:** Bronchospasm, pharyngitis
- **Other:** Fever, photosensitivity, rash, myalgia, arthralgia, angioedema

■ Nursing considerations

CLINICAL ALERT!
Name confusion has occurred between Zyrtec (cetirizine) and Zyprexa (olanzapine); use caution.

Assessment
- **History:** Allergy to any antihistamines, hydroxyzine; narrow-angle glaucoma, stenosing peptic ulcer, symptomatic prostatic hypertrophy, asthmatic attack, bladder neck obstruction, pyloroduodenal obstruction; lactation

- **Physical:** Skin color, lesions, texture; orientation, reflexes, affect; vision exam; R, adventitious sounds; prostate palpation; renal function tests

Interventions
- Give without regard to meals.
- Provide syrup form for pediatric use if needed.
- Arrange for use of humidifier if thickening of secretions, nasal dryness become bothersome; encourage adequate intake of fluids.
- Provide skin care for urticaria.

Teaching points
- Take this drug without regard to meals.
- These side effects may occur: dizziness, sedation, drowsiness (use caution if driving or performing tasks that require alertness); thickening of bronchial secretions, dryness of nasal mucosa (humidifier may help).
- Report difficulty breathing, hallucinations, tremors, loss of coordination, irregular heartbeat.

▽ cetrorelix acetate
See *Less Commonly Used Drugs,* p. 1340.

▽ cevimeline hydrochloride
See *Less Commonly Used Drugs,* p. 1340.

▽ charcoal, activated
(char' kole)

OTC: Actidose-Aqua, Actidose with Sorbitol, CharcoAid, Charcodote (Can), Liqui-Char

PREGNANCY CATEGORY C

Drug class
Antidote

Therapeutic actions
Adsorbs toxic substances swallowed into the GI tract, inhibiting GI absorption; maximum amount of toxin absorbed is 100–1,000 mg/g charcoal.

Adverse effects in *Italics* are most common; those in **Bold** are life-threatening.

Indications
- Emergency treatment in poisoning by most drugs and chemicals

Contraindications and cautions
- Poisoning or overdosage of cyanide, mineral acids, alkalies, ethanol, methanol, and iron salts

Available forms
Powder—15, 30, 40, 120, 240 g; liquid—208 mg/mL; suspension—15, 30 g; granules—15 g

Dosages
Adults
25–100 g or 1 g/kg PO or approximately 5–10 times the amount of poison ingested, as an oral suspension; administer as soon as possible after poisoning.
- *Gastric dialysis:* 20–40 g q 6 hr for 1–2 days for severe poisonings; for optimum effect, administer within 30 min of poisoning.

Pharmacokinetics
Not absorbed systemically. Excreted in feces.

Adverse effects
- **GI:** *Vomiting* (related to rapid ingestion of high doses), *constipation, diarrhea,* black stools

Interactions
✳ **Drug-drug** • Adsorption and inactivation of syrup of ipecac, laxatives with activated charcoal • Decreased effectiveness of other medications because of adsorption by activated charcoal

✳ **Drug-food** • Decreased adsorptive capacity if taken with milk, ice cream, or sherbet

■ Nursing considerations
Assessment
- **History:** Poisoning or overdosage of cyanide, mineral acids, alkalies, ethanol, methanol, and iron salts
- **Physical:** Stools, bowel sounds

Interventions
- Induce emesis before giving activated charcoal.
- Give drug to conscious patients only.
- Give drug as soon after poisoning as possible; most effective results are seen if given within 30 min.
- Prepare suspension of powder in 6–8 oz of water; taste may be gritty and disagreeable. Sorbitol is added to some preparations to improve taste; diarrhea more likely with these preparations.
- Store in closed containers; activated charcoal adsorbs gases from the air and will lose its effectiveness with prolonged exposure to air.
- Maintain life-support equipment on standby for poisoning and overdose.

Teaching points
- These side effects may occur: black stools, diarrhea or constipation.

▷ chenodiol
See *Less Commonly Used Drugs,* p. 1340.

▷ chloral hydrate
(klor' al hye' drate)

Aquachloral Supprettes, PMS-Chloral Hydrate (CAN)

PREGNANCY CATEGORY C

C-IV CONTROLLED SUBSTANCE

Drug class
Sedative and hypnotic (nonbarbiturate)

Therapeutic actions
Mechanism by which CNS is affected is not known; hypnotic dosage produces mild cerebral depression and quiet, deep sleep; does not depress REM sleep, produces less hangover than most barbiturates and benzodiazepines.

Indications
- Nocturnal sedation
- Preoperative sedation to lessen anxiety and induce sleep without depressing respiration or cough reflex
- Adjunct to opiates and analgesics in postoperative care and control of pain

Contraindications and cautions

- Contraindicated with hypersensitivity to chloral derivatives; allergy to tartrazine (in 324-mg suppositories marketed as *Aquachloral Supprettes*); severe cardiac disease, gastritis; hepatic or renal impairment; lactation.
- Use cautiously with acute intermittent porphyria (may precipitate attacks).

Available forms

Capsules—500 mg; syrup—250, 500 mg/5 mL; suppositories—324, 500, 648 mg

Dosages
Adults
Single doses or daily dosage should not exceed 2 g.
- *Hypnotic:* 500 mg–1 g PO or rectally 15–30 min before bedtime or 30 min before surgery (*Note:* it is not usually considered safe practice to give oral medication to patients who are NPO for anesthesia or surgery).
- *Sedative:* 250 mg PO or rectally tid after meals.

Pediatric patients
- *Hypnotic:* 50 mg/kg/day PO up to 1 g per single dose; may be given in divided doses.
- *Sedative:* 25 mg/kg/day PO up to 500 mg per single dose; may be given in divided doses.

Pharmacokinetics

Route	Onset	Peak	Duration
Oral, PR	30–60 min	1–3 hr	4–8 hr

Metabolism: Hepatic; $T_{1/2}$: 7–10 hr
Distribution: Crosses placenta; passes into breast milk
Excretion: Urine and bile

Adverse effects

- **CNS:** *Somnambulism, disorientation, incoherence, paranoid behavior,* excitement, delirium, drowsiness, staggering gait, ataxia, light-headedness, vertigo, nightmares, malaise, mental confusion, headache, hallucinations

- **Dermatologic:** *Skin irritation;* allergic rashes including hives, erythema, eczematoid dermatitis, urticaria
- **GI:** Gastric irritation, nausea, vomiting, **gastric necrosis** (following intoxicating doses), flatulence, diarrhea, unpleasant taste
- **Hematologic:** *Leukopenia, eosinophilia*
- **Other:** Physical, psychological dependence; tolerance; withdrawal reaction

Interactions

✳ **Drug-drug** • Additive CNS depression with alcohol, other CNS depressants • Mutual inhibition of metabolism with alcohol (possible vasodilation reaction characterized by tachycardia, palpitations, and facial flushing)
• Complex effects on oral (coumarin) anticoagulants given with chloral hydrate (monitor prothrombin levels and adjust coumarin dosage whenever chloral hydrate is instituted or withdrawn from drug regimen)
✳ **Drug-lab test** • Interference with the copper sulfate test for glycosuria, fluorometric tests for urine catecholamines, and urinary 17-hydroxycorticosteroid determinations (when using the Reddy, Jenkins, and Thorn procedure)

■ Nursing considerations
Assessment

- **History:** Hypersensitivity to chloral derivatives, allergy to tartrazine, severe cardiac disease, gastritis, hepatic or renal impairment, acute intermittent porphyria, lactation
- **Physical:** Skin color, lesions; orientation, affect, reflexes; P, BP, perfusion; bowel sounds, normal output, liver evaluation; liver and kidney function tests, CBC and differential, stool guaiac test

Interventions

- Give capsules with a full glass of liquid; ensure that patient swallows capsules whole; give syrup in half glass of water, fruit juice, or ginger ale.
- Supervise dose and amount of drug prescribed for patients who are addiction prone or alcoholic; give least amount feasible to patients who are depressed or suicidal.

Adverse effects in *Italics* are most common; those in **Bold** are life-threatening.

- Withdraw gradually over 2 wk if patient has been maintained on high doses for weeks or months; if patient has built up high tolerance, withdrawal should occur in a hospital, using supportive therapy similar to that for barbiturate withdrawal; fatal withdrawal reactions have occurred.
- Reevaluate patients with prolonged insomnia; therapy for the underlying cause (eg, pain, depression) is preferable to prolonged use of sedative–hypnotic drugs.

Teaching points
- Take this drug exactly as prescribed: Swallow capsules whole with a full glass of liquid (take syrup in half glass of water, fruit juice, or ginger ale).
- Do not discontinue the drug abruptly. Consult your care provider if you wish to discontinue the drug.
- Avoid alcohol, sleep-inducing, or OTC drugs; these could cause dangerous effects.
- These side effects may occur: drowsiness, dizziness, light-headedness (avoid driving or performing tasks requiring alertness); GI upset (frequent small meals may help); sleep-walking, nightmares, confusion (use caution: close doors, keep medications out of reach so inadvertent overdose does not occur while confused).
- Report rash, coffee ground vomitus, black or tarry stools, severe GI upset, fever, sore throat.

▷ chlorambucil
(klor am' byoo sil)

Leukeran

PREGNANCY CATEGORY D

Drug classes
Alkylating agent, nitrogen mustard
Antineoplastic

Therapeutic actions
Cytotoxic: alkylates cellular DNA, interfering with the replication of susceptible cells.

Indications
- Palliative treatment of chronic lymphocytic leukemia; malignant lymphomas, including lymphosarcoma; giant follicular lymphoma; and Hodgkin's disease
- Unlabeled uses: treatment of uveitis and meningoencephalitis associated with Behçet's disease; treatment of idiopathic membranous nephropathy; treatment of rheumatoid arthritis

Contraindications and cautions
- Allergy to chlorambucil; cross-sensitization with melphalen; radiation therapy, chemotherapy; hematopoietic depression; pregnancy, lactation.

Available forms
Tablets—2 mg; individualize dosage based on hematologic profile and response

Dosages
Adults
- *Initial dose and short-course therapy:* 0.1–0.2 mg/kg per day PO for 3–6 wk; single daily dose may be given.
- *Chronic lymphocytic leukemia (alternate regimen):* 0.4 mg/kg PO q 2 wk, increasing by 0.1 mg/kg with each dose until therapeutic or toxic effect occurs.
- *Maintenance dose:* 0.03–0.1 mg/kg/day PO. Do not exceed 0.1 mg/kg/day. Short courses of therapy are safer than continuous maintenance therapy; base dosage and duration on patient response and bone marrow status.
Pediatric patients
Safety and efficacy not established.

Pharmacokinetics
Route	Onset	Peak	Duration
Oral	Varies	1 hr	15–20 hr

Metabolism: Hepatic; $T_{1/2}$: 60–90 min
Distribution: Crosses placenta; passes into breast milk
Excretion: Urine

Adverse effects
- **CNS:** *Tremors, muscular twitching, confusion,* agitation, ataxia, flaccid paresis, hallucinations, seizures
- **Dermatologic:** Rash, urticaria, alopecia, keratitis
- **GI:** Nausea, vomiting, anorexia, **hepatotoxicity,** jaundice (rare)

- **GU:** *Sterility* (especially in prepubertal or pubertal males and adult men; amenorrhea can occur in females)
- **Hematologic: Bone marrow depression,** hyperuricemia
- **Respiratory:** Bronchopulmonary dysplasia, pulmonary fibrosis
- **Other:** *Cancer, acute leukemia*

■ Nursing considerations

 CLINICAL ALERT!
Name confusion has occurred between Leukeran (chlorambucil) and leucovorin; use caution.

Assessment
- **History:** Allergy to chlorambucil, cross-sensitization with melphalen (rash), radiation therapy, chemotherapy, hematopoietic depression, pregnancy, lactation
- **Physical:** T; weight; skin color, lesions; R, adventitious sounds; liver evaluation; CBC, differential, hemoglobin, uric acid, liver function tests

Interventions
- Arrange for blood tests to evaluate hematopoietic function before and weekly during therapy.
- Do not give full dosage within 4 wk after a full course of radiation therapy or chemotherapy because of risk of severe bone marrow depression.
- Ensure that patient is well hydrated before treatment.
- Ensure that patient is not pregnant before beginning therapy; encourage use of barrier contraceptives.
- Monitor uric acid levels; ensure adequate fluid intake, and prepare for appropriate treatment of hyperuricemia if it occurs.
- Divide single daily dose if nausea and vomiting occur with large single dose.

Teaching points
- Take this drug once a day. If nausea and vomiting occur, consult health care provider about dividing the dose.
- These side effects may occur: nausea, vomiting, loss of appetite (dividing dose, small

frequent meals also may help; maintain your fluid intake and nutrition; drink at least 10–12 glasses of fluid each day); infertility (from irregular menses to complete amenorrhea; men may stop producing sperm—may be irreversible; discuss with health care provider); severe birth defects—use barrier contraceptives.
- Report unusual bleeding or bruising; fever, chills, sore throat; cough, shortness of breath; yellow color of the skin or eyes; flank or stomach pain.

▷ **chloramphenicol**
(klor am fen' i kole)

chloramphenicol
Ophthalmic solutions: Ak-Chlor, Chloromycetin Ophthalmic, Chloroptic Ophthalmic
Otic solution: Chloromycetin Otic

chloramphenicol sodium succinate
PREGNANCY CATEGORY C

Drug class
Antibiotic

Therapeutic actions
Bacteriostatic effect against susceptible bacteria; prevents cell replication.

Indications
Systemic
- Serious infections for which no other antibiotic is effective
- Acute infections caused by *Salmonella typhi*
- Serious infections caused by *Salmonella, H. influenzae,* rickettsiae, lymphogranuloma—psittacosis group
- Cystic fibrosis regimen

Ophthalmic
- Treatment of superficial ocular infections caused by susceptible microorganisms

Adverse effects in *Italics* are most common; those in **Bold** are life-threatening.

Otic

- Treatment of superficial infections of the external auditory canal (inner ear infections should be treated with systemic antibiotics)

Contraindications and cautions

- Allergy to chloramphenicol, renal failure, hepatic failure, G-6-PD deficiency, intermittent porphyria, pregnancy (may cause gray syndrome), lactation

Available forms

Capsules—250 mg; powder for injection—100 mg/mL; ophthalmic solution—5 mg/5 mL; ophthalmic ointment—10 mg/g; ophthalmic powder for solution—25 mg vial; otic solution—0.5%

Dosages
Systemic

Severe and sometimes fatal blood dyscrasias (adults) and severe and sometimes fatal gray syndromes (in newborns and premature infants) may occur. Use should be restricted to situations in which no other antibiotic is effective. Serum levels should be monitored at least weekly to minimize risk of toxicity (therapeutic concentrations: peak, 10–20 mcg/mL; trough, 5–10 mcg/mL).

Adults

50 mg/kg/day PO or IV in divided doses q 6 hr up to 100 mg/kg/day in severe cases.

Pediatric patients

50–75 mg/kg/day PO or IV in divided doses q 6 hr.

- *Meningitis:* 50–100 mg/kg/day PO or IV in divided doses q 6 hr.

Newborns

25 mg/kg PO or IV per day in four doses q 6 hr; after 2 weeks of age, full-term infants usually tolerate 50 mg/kg/day in four doses q 6 hr (dosage should be monitored using serum concentrations of the drug as a guide).

Infants and children with immature metabolic processes

25 mg/kg/day PO or IV (monitor serum concentration carefully).

Geriatric patients or patients with renal or hepatic failure

Use serum concentration of the drug to adjust dosage.

Otic

Instill 2–3 drops into the ear tid.

Ophthalmic

Instill ointment or solution as prescribed.

Pharmacokinetics

Route	Onset	Peak	Duration
Oral	Varies	1–3 hr	48–72 hr
IV	20–30 min	1 hr	48–72 hr

Metabolism: Hepatic; $T_{1/2}$: 1.5–4 hr
Distribution: Crosses placenta; passes into breast milk
Excretion: Urine

▽ IV facts

Preparation: Dilute with 10 mL of sterile water for injection, or 5% dextrose injection.
Infusion: Administer as a 10% solution over 3–5 min, single-dose infusion over 30–60 min. Substitute oral dosage as soon as possible.

Adverse effects
Systemic

- **CNS:** *Headache,* mild depression, mental confusion, delirium
- **GI:** *Nausea, vomiting, glossitis, stomatitis, diarrhea*
- **Hematologic:** *Blood dyscrasias*
- **Other:** Fever, macular rashes, urticaria, **anaphylaxis; gray baby syndrome** (seen in neonates and premature babies: abdominal distension, pallid cyanosis, vasomotor collapse, irregular respirations), superinfections

Ophthalmic solution, otic solution, dermatologic cream

- **Hematologic:** Bone marrow hypoplasia and aplastic anemia with prolonged or frequent intermittent ocular use
- **Hypersensitivity:** *Irritation, burning, itching,* angioneurotic edema, urticaria, dermatitis
- **Other:** Superinfections

Interactions

✳ **Drug-drug** • Increased serum levels and drug effects of warfarin, phenytoins, tolbutamide, acetohexamide, glipizide, glyburide, tolazamide with chloramphenicol • Decreased hematologic response to iron salts, vitamin B_{12} with chloramphenicol

■ Nursing considerations

Assessment

- **History:** Allergy to chloramphenicol, renal or hepatic failure, G-6-PD deficiency, intermittent porphyria, pregnancy, lactation
- **Physical:** Culture infection; orientation, reflexes, sensation; R, adventitious sounds; bowel sounds, output, liver function; urinalysis, BUN, CBC, liver function tests, renal function tests

Interventions

Systemic administration

- Culture infection before beginning therapy.
- Give drug on an empty stomach, 1 hr before or 2 hr after meals. If severe GI upset occurs, give drug with meals.
- Do not give this drug IM because it is ineffective.
- Monitor hematologic data carefully, especially with long-term therapy by any route of administration.
- Reduce dosage in patients with renal or hepatic disease.
- Monitor serum levels periodically as indicated in dosage section.

Ophthalmic and otic solution

- Topical preparations of the drug should be used only when necessary. Sensitization from the topical use of this drug may preclude its later use in serious infections. Topical preparations that contain antibiotics that are not ordinarily given systemically are preferable.

Teaching points

- Never use any leftover medication to self-treat any other infection.

Oral therapy

- Take this drug q 6 hr around the clock; schedule doses to minimize sleep disruption. Take drug on an empty stomach, 1 hr before or 2 hr after meals. Take the full course of this medication.
- These side effects may occur: nausea, vomiting (if this becomes severe, the drug can be taken with food); diarrhea (reversible); headache (request medication); confusion (avoid driving or operating delicate machinery); superinfections (frequent hygiene measures may help; medications are available if severe).

- Report sore throat, tiredness; unusual bleeding or bruising (even as late as several weeks after you finish the drug); numbness, tingling, pain in the extremities; pregnancy.

Ophthalmic solution

- Give eye drops as follows: lie down or tilt head backward, and look at ceiling. Drop solution inside lower eyelid while looking up. After instilling eye drops, close eyes, and apply gentle pressure to the inside corner of the eye for 1 min.
- These side effects may occur: temporary stinging or blurring of vision after administration (notify health care provider if pronounced).

Otic solution

- Give as follows: lie on side or tilt head so that ear to be treated is uppermost. Grasp ear and gently pull up and back (adults) or down and back (children); drop medication into the ear canal. Stay in this position for 2–3 min. Solution should be warmed to near body temperature before use; do not use cold or hot solutions.

▽ chlordiazepoxide hydrochloride (metaminodiazepoxide hydrochloride)
(klor dye az e pox' ide)

Apo-Chlordiazepoxide (CAN), Librium, Libritabs, Mitran, Reposans-10

PREGNANCY CATEGORY D

C-IV CONTROLLED SUBSTANCE

Drug classes

Benzodiazepine
Antianxiety agent

Therapeutic actions

Exact mechanisms of action not understood; acts mainly at subcortical levels of the CNS; main sites of action may be the limbic system and reticular formation; potentiates the effects of gamma-aminobutyric acid (GABA).

Indications

- Management of anxiety disorders or for short-term relief of symptoms of anxiety
- Acute alcohol withdrawal; may be useful in symptomatic relief of acute agitation, tremor, delirium tremens, hallucinosis
- Preoperative relief of anxiety and tension

Contraindications and cautions

- Contraindicated with hypersensitivity to benzodiazepines, psychoses, acute narrow-angle glaucoma, shock, coma, acute alcoholic intoxication with depression of vital signs, pregnancy (increased risk of congenital malformations, neonatal withdrawal syndrome), labor and delivery ("floppy infant" syndrome reported), lactation (infants may become lethargic and lose weight).
- Use cautiously with impaired liver or kidney function, debilitation.

Available forms

Capsules—5, 10, 25 mg; tablets—10, 25 mg; powder for injection—100 mg/amp

Dosages
Adults
Individualize dosage; increase dosage cautiously to avoid adverse effects.
Oral
- *Anxiety disorders:* 5 or 10 mg, up to 20 or 25 mg, tid–qid, depending on severity of symptoms.
- *Preoperative apprehension:* 5–10 mg tid–qid on days preceding surgery.
- *Alcohol withdrawal:* Parenteral form usually used initially. If given orally, initial dose is 50–100 mg, followed by repeated doses as needed up to 300 mg/day; then reduce to maintenance levels.
Parenteral
- *Severe anxiety:* 50–100 mg IM or IV initially; then 25–50 mg tid–qid if necessary, or switch to oral dosage form.
- *Preoperative apprehension:* 50–100 mg IM 1 hr prior to surgery.
- *Alcohol withdrawal:* 50–100 mg IM or IV initially; repeat in 2–4 hr if necessary. Up to 300 mg may be given in 6 hr; do not exceed 300 mg/24 hr.

Pediatric patients
Oral
> *6 yr:* 5 mg bid–qid initially; may be increased in some children to 10 mg bid–tid.
< *6 yr:* Not recommended.
Parenteral
12–18 yr: 25–50 mg IM or IV.
Geriatric patients or patients with debilitating disease
5 mg PO bid–qid; 25–50 mg IM or IV.

Pharmacokinetics

Route	Onset	Peak	Duration
Oral	Varies	1–4 hr	48–72 hr
IM	10–15 min	15–30 min	48–72 hr
IV	Immediate	3–30 min	48–72 hr

Metabolism: Hepatic; $T_{1/2}$: 5–30 hr
Distribution: Crosses placenta; passes into breast milk
Excretion: Urine

▽IV facts
Preparation: Add 5 mL sterile physiologic saline or sterile water for injection to contents of ample; agitate gently until drug is dissolved.
Infusion: Administer IV doses slowly over 1 min. Change patients on IV therapy to oral therapy as soon as possible.

Adverse effects
- **CNS:** *Transient, mild drowsiness initially; sedation, depression, lethargy, apathy, fatigue, light-headedness, disorientation, restlessness, confusion,* crying, delirium, headache, slurred speech, dysarthria, stupor, rigidity, tremor, psychomotor retardation, extrapyramidal symptoms; mild *paradoxical excitatory reactions during first 2 wk of treatment* (especially in psychiatric patients, aggressive children, and those with high dosage), visual and auditory disturbances, diplopia, nystagmus, depressed hearing, nasal congestion
- **CV:** *Bradycardia, tachycardia,* CV collapse, hypertension and hypotension, palpitations, edema
- **Dependence:** *Drug dependence with withdrawal syndrome* when drug is discontinued (more common with abrupt discontinuation of higher dosage used for longer than 4 mo)

- **Dermatologic:** Urticaria, pruritus, skin rash, dermatitis
- **GI:** *Constipation, diarrhea,* dry mouth, salivation, nausea, anorexia, vomiting, difficulty in swallowing, gastric disorders, hepatic dysfunction, jaundice
- **GU:** *Incontinence, urinary retention, changes in libido,* menstrual irregularities
- **Hematologic:** Decreased hematocrit, blood dyscrasias
- **Other:** Phlebitis and thrombosis at IV injection sites, hiccups, fever, diaphoresis, paresthesias, muscular disturbances, gynecomastia, pain, burning, and redness after IM injection

Interactions

✳ **Drug-drug** • Increased CNS depression with alcohol, omeprazole • Increased pharmacologic effects with cimetidine, disulfiram, oral contraceptives • Decreased sedative effects with theophylline, aminophylline, dyphylline, oxitriphylline

■ Nursing considerations
Assessment

- **History:** Hypersensitivity to benzodiazepines; psychoses; acute narrow-angle glaucoma; shock; coma; acute alcoholic intoxication; pregnancy; lactation; impaired liver or kidney function, debilitation
- **Physical:** Skin color, lesions; T; orientation, reflexes, affect, ophthalmologic exam; P, BP; R, adventitious sounds; liver evaluation, abdominal exam, bowel sounds, normal output; CBC, liver and renal function tests

Interventions

- Do not administer intra-arterially; arteriospasm, gangrene may result.
- Reconstitute solutions for IM injection only with special diluent provided; do not use diluent if it is opalescent or hazy; prepare injection immediately before use, and discard any unused solution.
- Do not use drug solutions made with physiologic saline or sterile water for injection for IM injections because of pain.

- Give IM injection slowly into upper outer quadrant of the gluteus muscle; monitor injection sites.
- Do not use small veins (dorsum of hand or wrist) for IV injection.
- Monitor P, BP, R carefully during IV administration.
- Keep patients receiving parenteral benzodiazepines in bed for 3 hr; do not permit ambulatory patients to drive following an injection.
- Reduce dosage of narcotic analgesics in patients receiving IV benzodiazepines; doses should be reduced by at least one-third or totally eliminated.
- Monitor liver and kidney function, CBC at intervals during long-term therapy.
- Taper dosage gradually after long-term therapy, especially in epileptic patients.

Teaching points

- Take drug exactly as prescribed.
- Do not stop taking this drug (long-term therapy) without consulting health care provider. Avoid alcohol, sleep-inducing, or OTC drugs.
- Avoid pregnancy while on this drug; serious adverse effects could occur. Use of barrier contraceptives is suggested.
- These side effects may occur: drowsiness, dizziness (transient; avoid driving or engaging in other dangerous activities); GI upset (take drug with water); depression, dreams, emotional upset, crying.
- Report severe dizziness, weakness, drowsiness that persists, rash or skin lesions, palpitations, swelling of the extremities, visual changes, difficulty voiding.

▷**chloroquine phosphate**

(klo' ro kwin)

Aralen Phosphate

PREGNANCY CATEGORY NOT ESTABLISHED

Drug classes
Amebicide

Adverse effects in *Italics* are most common; those in **Bold** are life-threatening.

Antimalarial
4-aminoquinoline

Therapeutic actions
Inhibits protozoal reproduction and protein synthesis. Mechanism of anti-inflammatory action in rheumatoid arthritis is not known.

Indications
- Treatment of extraintestinal amebiasis
- Prophylaxis and treatment of acute attacks of malaria caused by susceptible strains of *Plasmodia*
- Unlabeled uses: treatment of rheumatoid arthritis and discoid lupus erythematosus

Contraindications and cautions
- Allergy to chloroquine and other 4-amino-quinolines, porphyria, psoriasis, retinal disease, hepatic disease, G-6-PD deficiency, alcoholism, lactation.

Available forms
Tablets—250, 500 mg

Dosages
Adults
- *Amebicide:* 1 g (600 mg base)/day PO for 2 days; then 500 mg (300 mg base)/day for 2–3 wk.
- *Antimalarial: Suppression:* 300 mg base PO once a week on the same day for 2 wk before exposure and continuing until 6–8 wk after exposure. *Acute attack:* 600 mg base PO initially; then 300 mg 6 hr later and on days 2 and 3.
- *Antirheumatoid:* 200 mg (160 mg base) PO qid or bid.

Pediatric patients
- *Amebicide:* Not recommended.
- *Antimalarial:* Suppression: 5 mg base/kg PO once a week on the same day for 2 wk before exposure and continuing until 6–8 wk after exposure.
- *Acute attack:* 10 mg base/kg PO initially; then 5 mg base/kg 6 hr later and on days 2 and 3. Do not exceed 10 mg base/kg/day or 300 mg/base/day.

Pharmacokinetics

Route	Onset	Peak	Duration
Oral	Varies	1–2 hr	1 wk

Metabolism: Hepatic; $T_{1/2}$: 70–1.
Distribution: May cross placenta; p̶̶̶s̶ into breast milk
Excretion: Urine

Adverse effects
- **CNS:** *Visual disturbances,* retinal changes (blurring of vision, difficulty in focusing), ototoxicity, muscle weakness
- **CV:** *Hypotension, ECG changes*
- **GI:** *Nausea, vomiting, diarrhea,* loss of appetite, abdominal pain
- **Hematologic:** Blood dyscrasias, hemolysis in patients with G-6-PD deficiency

Interactions
✳ **Drug-drug** • Increased effects of chloroquine with cimetidine • Decreased GI absorption of both drugs with magnesium trisilicate

■ Nursing considerations
Assessment
- **History:** Allergy to chloroquine and other 4-aminoquinolines, porphyria, psoriasis, retinal disease, hepatic disease, G-6-PD deficiency, alcoholism, lactation
- **Physical:** Reflexes, muscle strength, auditory and ophthalmologic screening; BP, ECG; liver palpation; CBC, G-6-PD in deficient patients, liver function tests

Interventions
- Administer with meals if GI upset occurs.
- Schedule weekly, same-day therapy on a calendar.
- Double check pediatric doses; children are very susceptible to overdosage.
- Arrange for ophthalmologic exams during long-term therapy.

Teaching points
- Take full course of drug therapy. Take drug with meals if GI upset occurs. Mark your calendar with the drug days for malarial prophylaxis.
- These side effects may occur: stomach pain, loss of appetite, nausea, vomiting, or diarrhea.
- Arrange to have regular ophthalmologic exams if long-term use is indicated.

• Report blurring of vision, loss of hearing, ringing in the ears, muscle weakness, fever.

▷ **chlorothiazide**
(klor oh thye' a zide)

chlorothiazide
Diurigen, Diuril

chlorothiazide sodium
Sodium Diuril

PREGNANCY CATEGORY B

Drug class
Thiazide diuretic

Therapeutic actions
Inhibits reabsorption of sodium and chloride in distal renal tubule, increasing the excretion of sodium, chloride, and water by the kidney.

Indications
• Adjunctive therapy in edema associated with CHF, cirrhosis, corticosteroid, and estrogen therapy, renal dysfunction
• Treatment of hypertension, alone or with other antihypertensives
• Unlabeled uses: treatment of diabetes insipidus, especially nephrogenic diabetes insipidus; reduction of incidence of osteoporosis in postmenopausal women

Contraindications and cautions
• Fluid or electrolyte imbalances, renal or liver disease, gout, SLE, glucose tolerance abnormalities, hyperparathyroidism, manic-depressive disorders, lactation

Available forms
Tablets—250, 500 mg; oral suspension—250 mg/5 mL; powder for injection—500 mg

Dosages
Adults
• *Edema:* 0.5–2 g PO or IV (if patient unable to take PO) daily or bid.
• *Hypertension:* 0.5–2 g/day PO as a single or divided dose; adjust dose to BP response,

giving up to 2 g/day in divided doses. IV use is not recommended.
Pediatric patients
22 mg/kg/day PO in two doses.
< 6 mo: up to 33 mg/kg per day PO in two doses. IV use not recommended.
≤ 2 yr: 125–375 mg PO in two divided doses.
2–12 yr: 375 mg–1 g PO in two divided doses.

Pharmacokinetics

Route	Onset	Peak	Duration
Oral	2 hr	3–6 hr	6–12 hr
IV	15 min	30 min	2 hr

Metabolism: $T_{1/2}$: 45–120 min
Distribution: Crosses placenta; passes into breast milk
Excretion: Urine

▽ IV facts
Preparation: Dilute vial for parenteral solution with 18 mL sterile water for injection. Never add less than 18 mL. Discard diluted solution after 24 hr.
Infusion: Administer slowly. Switch to oral drug as soon as possible.
Compatibilities: Compatible with dextrose and sodium chloride solutions.
Incompatibilities: Do not give parenteral solution with whole blood or blood products.

Adverse effects
• **CNS:** *Dizziness, vertigo,* paresthesias, weakness, headache, drowsiness, fatigue
• **CV:** Orthostatic hypotension, venous thrombosis, volume depletion, cardiac arrhythmias, chest pain
• **Dermatologic:** Photosensitivity, rash, purpura, exfoliative dermatitis
• **GI:** *Nausea, anorexia, vomiting, dry mouth, diarrhea, constipation,* jaundice, hepatitis, pancreatitis
• **GU:** *Polyuria, nocturia, impotence,* loss of libido
• **Hematologic:** Leukopenia, thrombocytopenia, agranulocytosis, aplastic anemia, neutropenia, fluid and electrolyte imbalances
• **Other:** Muscle cramps and muscle spasms, fever, hives, gouty attacks, flushing, weight loss, rhinorrhea

Interactions

⁜ Drug-drug • Increased thiazide effects and chance of acute hyperglycemia with diazoxide • Decreased absorption with cholestyramine • Increased risk of cardiac glycoside toxicity if hypokalemia occurs • Increased risk of lithium toxicity • Increased dosage of antidiabetic agents may be needed

⁜ Drug-lab test • Monitor for decreased PBI levels without clinical signs of thyroid disturbances.

■ Nursing considerations
Assessment

- **History:** Fluid or electrolyte imbalances, renal or liver disease, gout, SLE, glucose tolerance abnormalities, hyperparathyroidism, manic-depressive disorders, lactation
- **Physical:** Orientation, reflexes, muscle strength; pulses, BP, orthostatic BP, perfusion, edema, baseline ECG; R, adventitious sounds; liver evaluation, bowel sounds; CBC, serum electrolytes, blood glucose, liver and renal function tests, serum uric acid, urinalysis

Interventions

- Administer with food or milk if GI upset occurs.
- Administer early in the day, so increased urination will not disturb sleep.
- Measure and record weight to monitor fluid changes.

Teaching points

- Take drug early in the day, so sleep will not be disturbed by increased urination.
- Weigh yourself daily, and record weights.
- Protect skin from exposure to the sun or bright lights.
- Increased urination will occur.
- Use caution if dizziness, drowsiness, feeling faint occur.
- Report rapid weight change, swelling in ankles or fingers, unusual bleeding or bruising, muscle cramps.

<hr>

▷ chlorphenesin carbamate
(klor fen' e sin)

Maolate, Mycil (CAN)

PREGNANCY CATEGORY C

Drug class
Skeletal muscle relaxant, centrally acting

Therapeutic actions
Precise mechanism not known; has sedative properties; does not directly relax tense skeletal muscles; does not directly affect the motor endplate or motor nerves.

Indications
- Relief of discomfort from acute, painful musculoskeletal conditions, as an adjunct to rest, physical therapy, and other measures

Contraindications and cautions
- Allergic or idiosyncratic reactions to chlorphenesin, tartrazine; lactation, pregnancy

Available forms
Tablets—400 mg

Dosages
Adults
Initially, 800 mg PO tid until desired effect is obtained; reduce maintenance dosage to 400 mg qid or less. Do not use for > 8 wk.
Pediatric patients
Safety and efficacy not established for children < 12 yr.
Geriatric patients or patients with hepatic impairment
Dosage reduction may be necessary; monitor closely.

Pharmacokinetics

Route	Onset	Peak	Duration
Oral	Varies	1–3 hr	8–12 hr

Metabolism: Hepatic; $T_{1/2}$: 3.5 hr
Distribution: Crosses placenta; may pass into breast milk
Excretion: Urine

Adverse effects

- **CNS:** *Dizziness, drowsiness, confusion,* paradoxical stimulation, insomnia, headache
- **GI:** *Nausea, epigastric distress*
- **Hematologic:** Leukopenia, thrombocytopenia, agranulocytosis, pancytopenia
- **Hypersensitivity: Anaphylactoid reactions,** drug fever

■ Nursing considerations
Assessment

- **History:** Allergic or idiosyncratic reactions to chlorphenesin, tartrazine, lactation
- **Physical:** Skin color, lesions; orientation, affect; liver evaluation; liver function tests, CBC with differential

Interventions
- Reduce dosage with liver dysfunction.

Teaching points
- Take this drug exactly as prescribed; do not take a higher dosage.
- Avoid alcohol, sleep-inducing, or OTC drugs; these could cause dangerous effects.
- These side effects may occur: drowsiness, dizziness, confusion (avoid driving or engaging in activities that require alertness); nausea (take with food and eat frequent small meals); insomnia, headache (reversible).
- Report rash, severe nausea, dizziness, insomnia, fever, difficulty breathing.

▽chlorpheniramine maleate
*(klor fen **ir**' a meen)*

Aller-Chlor; Allergy; Chlo-Amine; Chlor-Trimeton Allergy 4 hr, 8 hr, and 12 hr; Chlor-Tripolon (CAN)

PREGNANCY CATEGORY B

Drug class
Antihistamine (alkylamine type)

Therapeutic actions
Competitively blocks the effects of histamine at H_1-receptor sites; has atropine-like, antipruritic, and sedative effects.

Indications
- Symptomatic relief of symptoms associated with perennial and seasonal allergic rhinitis; vasomotor rhinitis; allergic conjunctivitis.

Contraindications and cautions
- Contraindicated with allergy to any antihistamines, narrow-angle glaucoma, stenosing peptic ulcer, symptomatic prostatic hypertrophy, asthmatic attack, bladder neck obstruction, pyloroduodenal obstruction, third trimester of pregnancy, lactation.
- Use cautiously in pregnancy.

Available forms
Chewable tablets—2 mg; tablets—4 mg; ER tablets—8, 12 mg; syrup—2 mg/5 mL; SR capsules—8, 12 mg

Dosages
Adults and patients > 12 yr
Tablets or syrup
4 mg PO q 4–6 hr; do not exceed 24 mg in 24 hr.
Sustained-release
8–12 mg PO hs or q 8–12 hr during the day; do not exceed 24 mg in 24 hr.
Pediatric patients
Tablets or syrup
6–12 yr: 2 mg q 4–6 hr PO; do not exceed 12 mg in 24 hr.
2–6 yr: 1 mg q 4–6 hr PO; do not exceed 4 mg in 24 hr.
Sustained-release
6–12 yr: 8 mg PO hs or during the day.
< 6 yr: Not recommended.
Geriatric patients
More likely to cause dizziness, sedation, syncope, toxic confusional states, and hypotension in elderly patients; use with caution.

Pharmacokinetics

Route	Onset	Peak
Oral	0.5–6 hr	2–6 hr

Metabolism: Hepatic; $T_{1/2}$: 12–15 hr
Distribution: Crosses placenta; may enter breast milk
Excretion: Urine

Adverse effects in *Italics* are most common; those in **Bold** are life-threatening.

Adverse effects

- **CNS:** *Drowsiness, sedation, dizziness, disturbed coordination,* fatigue, confusion, restlessness, excitation, nervousness, tremor, headache, blurred vision, diplopia, vertigo, tinnitus, acute labyrinthitis, hysteria, tingling, heaviness and weakness of the hands
- **CV:** Hypotension, palpitations, bradycardia, tachycardia, extrasystoles
- **GI:** *Epigastric distress,* anorexia, increased appetite and weight gain, nausea, vomiting, diarrhea or constipation
- **GU:** Urinary frequency, dysuria, urinary retention, early menses, decreased libido, impotence
- **Hematologic:** Hemolytic anemia, hypoplastic anemia, thrombocytopenia, leukopenia, agranulocytosis, pancytopenia
- **Respiratory:** *Thickening of bronchial secretions,* chest tightness, wheezing, nasal stuffiness, dry mouth, dry nose, dry throat, sore throat
- **Other:** Urticaria, rash, anaphylactic shock, photosensitivity, excessive perspiration, chills

Interactions

✴ **Drug-drug** • Increased depressant effects with alcohol, other CNS depressants

■ Nursing considerations
Assessment

- **History:** Allergy to any antihistamines; narrow-angle glaucoma, stenosing peptic ulcer, symptomatic prostatic hypertrophy, asthmatic attack, bladder neck obstruction, pyloroduodenal obstruction, pregnancy, lactation
- **Physical:** Skin color, lesions, texture; orientation, reflexes, affect; vision exam; P, BP ; R, adventitious sounds; bowel sounds; prostate palpation; CBC with differential

Interventions

- Administer with food if GI upset occurs.
- Caution patient not to crush or chew sustained-release preparations.
- Arrange for periodic blood tests during prolonged therapy.

Teaching points

- Take as prescribed; avoid excessive dosage. Take with food if GI upset occurs; do not cut,

crush, or chew the sustained-release preparations.
- These side effects may occur: dizziness, sedation, drowsiness (use caution driving or performing tasks that require alertness); epigastric distress, diarrhea, or constipation (take with meals; consult care provider if severe); dry mouth (frequent mouth care, sucking sugarless lozenges may help); thickening of bronchial secretions, dryness of nasal mucosa (use a humidifier).
- Avoid OTC drugs; many contain ingredients that could cause serious reactions if taken with this antihistamine.
- Avoid alcohol; serious sedation may occur.
- Report difficulty breathing; hallucinations, tremors, loss of coordination; unusual bleeding or bruising; visual disturbances; irregular heartbeat.

▷ chlorpromazine hydrochloride
(klor proe' ma zeen)

Chlorpromanyl (CAN), Largactil (CAN), Thorazine, Thorazine Spansules

PREGNANCY CATEGORY C

Drug classes

Phenothiazine
Dopaminergic blocking agent
Antipsychotic
Antiemetic
Antianxiety agent

Therapeutic actions

Mechanism not fully understood; antipsychotic drugs block postsynaptic dopamine receptors in the brain; depress those parts of the brain involved with wakefulness and emesis; anticholinergic, antihistaminic (H_1), and alpha-adrenergic blocking.

Indications

- Management of manifestations of psychotic disorders; control of manic phase of manic-depressive illness
- Relief of preoperative restlessness and apprehension
- Adjunct in treatment of tetanus

- Acute intermittent porphyria therapy
- Severe behavioral problems in children: therapy for combativeness, hyperactivity
- Control of nausea and vomiting and intractable hiccups
- Possibly effective in the treatment of nonpsychotic anxiety (not drug of choice)

Contraindications and cautions

- Allergy to chlorpromazine; comatose or severely depressed states; bone marrow depression; circulatory collapse; subcortical brain damage, Parkinson's disease; liver damage; cerebral or coronary arteriosclerosis; severe hypotension or hypertension; respiratory disorders; glaucoma; epilepsy or history of epilepsy; peptic ulcer or history of peptic ulcer; decreased renal function; prostate hypertrophy; breast cancer; thyrotoxicosis; myelography within 24 hr or scheduled within 48 hr; lactation; exposure to heat, phosphorous insecticides; children with chickenpox, CNS infections (makes children more susceptible to dystonias, confounding the diagnosis of Reye's syndrome or other encephalopathy; antiemetic effects of drug may mask symptoms of Reye's syndrome, encephalopathies)

Available forms

Tablets—10, 25, 50, 100, 200 mg; SR capsules—30, 75, 150 mg; syrup—10 mg/5 mL; concentrate—30, 100 mg/mL; suppositories—25, 100 mg; injection—25 mg/mL

Dosages

Full clinical antipsychotic effects may require 6 wk to 6 mo of therapy.

Adults

- *Excessive anxiety, agitation in psychiatric patients:* 25 mg IM; may repeat in 1 hr. Increase dosage gradually in inpatients, up to 400 mg q 4–6 hr. Switch to oral dosage as soon as possible: 25–50 mg PO tid for outpatients; up to 2,000 mg/day PO for inpatients. Initial oral dosage: 10 mg tid–qid PO or 25 mg PO bid–tid; increase daily dosage by 20–50 mg semiweekly until optimum dosage is reached (maximum response may require months); doses of 200–800 mg/day

PO are not uncommon in discharged mental patients.

- *Surgery:* Preoperatively, 25–50 mg PO 2–3 hr before surgery or 12.5–25 mg IM 1–2 hr before surgery; intraoperatively, 12.5 mg IM, repeated in 30 min or 2 mg IV repeated q 2 min up to 25 mg total to control vomiting (if no hypotension occurs); postoperatively, 10–25 mg PO q 4–6 hr or 12.5–25 mg IM repeated in 1 hr (if no hypotension occurs).
- *Acute intermittent porphyria:* 25–50 mg PO or 25 mg IM tid–qid.
- *Tetanus:* 25–50 mg IM tid–qid, usually with barbiturates, or 25–50 mg IV diluted and infused at rate of 1 mg/min.
- *Antiemetic:* 10–25 mg PO q 4–6 hr; 50–100 mg rectally q 6–8 hr; 25 mg IM. If no hypotension, give 25–50 mg q 3–4 hr. Switch to oral dose when vomiting ends.
- *Intractable hiccups:* 25–50 mg PO tid–qid. If symptoms persist for 2–3 days, give 25–50 mg IM; if inadequate response, give 25–50 mg IV in 500–1,000 mL of saline with BP monitoring.

Pediatric patients

Generally not used in children < 6 mo.

- *Psychiatric outpatients:* 0.5 mg/kg PO q 4–6 hr; 1 mg/kg rectally q 6–8 hr; 0.5 mg/kg IM q 6–8 hr, not to exceed 40 mg/day (up to 5 yr) or 75 mg/day (5–12 yr).
- *Surgery:* Preoperatively, 0.5 mg/kg PO 2–3 hr before surgery or 0.5 mg/kg IM 1–2 hr before surgery; intraoperatively, 0.25 mg/kg IM or 1 mg (diluted) IV, repeated at 2-min intervals up to total IM dose; postoperatively, 0.5 mg/kg PO q 4–6 hr or 0.5 mg/kg IM, repeated in 1 hr if no hypotension.
- *Psychiatric inpatients:* 50–100 mg/day PO; maximum of 40 mg/day IM for children up to 5 yr; maximum of 75 mg/day IM for children 5–12 yr.
- *Tetanus:* 0.5 mg/kg IM q 6–8 hr or 0.5 mg/ min IV, not to exceed 40 mg/day for children up to 23 kg; 75 mg/day for children 23–45 kg.
- *Antiemetic:* 0.55 mg/kg PO q 4–6 hr; 1.1 mg/kg rectally q 6–8 hr or 0.55 mg/kg IM q 6–8 hr. Maximum IM dosage 40 mg/day for children up to 5 yr or 75 mg/day for children 5–12 yr.

Geriatric patients

Start dosage at one-fourth to one-third that given in younger adults and increase more gradually.

Pharmacokinetics

Route	Onset	Peak	Duration
Oral	30–60 min	2–4 hr	4–6 hr
IM	10–15 min	15–20 min	4–6 hr

Metabolism: Hepatic, $T_{1/2}$: 2 hr, then 30 hr
Distribution: Crosses placenta; enters breast milk
Excretion: Urine

▼ IV facts

Preparation: Dilute drug for IV injection to a concentration of 1 mg/mL or less.
Infusion: Reserve IV injections for hiccups, tetanus, or use during surgery. Administer at a rate of 1 mg/2 min.
Incompatibilities: Precipitate or discoloration may occur when mixed with morphine, meperidine, cresols.

Adverse effects

- **CNS:** *Drowsiness, insomnia, vertigo,* headache, weakness, tremors, ataxia, slurring, cerebral edema, seizures, exacerbation of psychotic symptoms, *extrapyramidal syndromes,* neuroleptic malignant syndrome
- **CV:** *Hypotension, orthostatic hypotension,* hypertension, tachycardia, bradycardia, cardiac arrest, CHF, cardiomegaly, refractory arrhythmias, pulmonary edema
- **EENT:** Nasal congestion, glaucoma, *photophobia, blurred vision,* miosis, mydriasis, deposits in the cornea and lens, pigmentary retinopathy
- **Endocrine:** Lactation, breast engorgement in females, galactorrhea, SIADH, amenorrhea, menstrual irregularities, gynecomastia, changes in libido, hyperglycemia, inhibition of ovulation, infertility, pseudopregnancy, reduced urinary levels of gonadotropins, estrogens, and progestins
- **GI:** *Dry mouth, salivation, nausea, vomiting, anorexia, constipation,* paralytic ileus, incontinence
- **GU:** *Urinary retention,* polyuria, incontinence, priapism, ejaculation inhibition, male impotence, urine discolored pink to red-brown
- **Hematologic:** Eosinophilia, leu. leukocytosis, *anemia,* aplastic anemia, hemolytic anemia, thrombocytopenic or nonthrombocytopenic purpura, pancytopenia, elevated serum cholesterol
- **Hypersensitivity:** Jaundice, *urticaria,* angioneurotic edema, laryngeal edema, photosensitivity, eczema, asthma, anaphylactoid reactions, exfoliative dermatitis, contact dermatitis
- **Respiratory:** Bronchospasm, laryngospasm, dyspnea, suppression of cough reflex and potential aspiration
- **Other:** Fever, heat stroke, pallor, flushed facies, sweating, *photosensitivity*

Interactions

✳ Drug-drug • Additive anticholinergic effects and possibly decreased antipsychotic efficacy with anticholinergic drugs • Additive CNS depression, hypotension if given preoperatively with barbiturate anesthetics, alcohol, meperidine • Additive effects of both drugs if taken concurrently with beta-blockers • Increased risk of tachycardia, hypotension with epinephrine, norepinephrine • Decreased hypotension effect with guanethidine

✳ Drug-lab test • False-positive pregnancy tests (less likely if serum test is used) • Increase in protein-bound iodine, not attributable to an increase in thyroxine

■ Nursing considerations

 CLINICAL ALERT!
Name confusion has occurred between chlorpromazine and chlorpropamide; use caution.

Assessment

- **History:** Allergy to chlorpromazine; comatose or severely depressed states; bone marrow depression; circulatory collapse; subcortical brain damage, Parkinson's disease; liver damage; cerebral or coronary arteriosclerosis; severe hypotension or hypertension; respiratory disorders; glaucoma; epilepsy or history of epilepsy; peptic ulcer or history of peptic ulcer; decreased renal function; prostate hypertrophy; breast cancer; thyrotoxicosis; myelography within 24 hr or scheduled within 48 hr; lactation; exposure to heat, phosphorous insecticides; children with chickenpox; CNS infections

- **Physical:** T, weight; skin color, turgor; reflexes, orientation, intraocular pressure, ophthalmologic exam; P, BP, orthostatic BP, ECG; R, adventitious sounds; bowel sounds, normal output, liver evaluation; prostate palpation, normal urine output; CBC; urinalysis; thyroid, liver, and kidney function tests; EEG

Interventions

- Do not change brand names of oral dosage forms or rectal suppositories; bioavailability differs.
- Dilute the oral concentrate just before administration in 60 mL or more of tomato or fruit juice, milk, simple syrup, orange syrup, carbonated beverage, coffee, tea, or water, or in semisolid foods (soup, puddings).
- Protect oral concentrate from light.
- Do not allow the patient to crush or chew the sustained-release capsules.
- Do not give by SC injection; give slowly by deep IM injection into upper outer quadrant of buttock.
- Keep recumbent for 30 min after injection to avoid orthostatic hypotension.
- Avoid skin contact with oral concentrates and parenteral drug solutions due to possible contact dermatitis.
- Patient or the patient's guardian should be advised about the possibility of tardive dyskinesias.
- Be alert to potential for aspiration because of suppressed cough reflex.
- Monitor renal function tests, discontinue if serum creatinine, BUN become abnormal.
- Monitor CBC, discontinue if WBC count is depressed.
- Consult with physician about dosage reduction or use of anticholinergic antiparkinsonian drugs (controversial) if extrapyramidal effects occur.
- Withdraw drug gradually after high-dose therapy; possible gastritis, nausea, dizziness, headache, tachycardia, insomnia after abrupt withdrawal.
- Monitor elderly patients for dehydration; sedation and decreased sensation of thirst; CNS effects can lead to dehydration, hemoconcentration, and reduced pulmonary ventilation; promptly institute remedial measures.
- Avoid epinephrine as vasopressor if drug-induced hypotension occurs.

Teaching points

- Take drug exactly as prescribed. Avoid OTC drugs and alcohol unless you have consulted your health care provider.
- Do not cut, crush, or chew sustained-release capsules.
- Do not change brand names without consulting your health care provider.
- Learn how to dilute oral drug concentrate; how to use rectal suppository.
- Do not get oral concentrate on your skin or clothes; contact dermatitis can occur.
- These side effects may occur: drowsiness (avoid driving or operating dangerous machinery; avoid alcohol, increases drowsiness); sensitivity to the sun (avoid prolonged sun exposure, wear protective garments or use a sunscreen); pink or reddish-brown urine (expected effect); faintness, dizziness (change position slowly; use caution climbing stairs; usually transient).
- Use caution in hot weather; risk of heat stroke; keep up fluid intake, and do not overexercise in a hot climate.
- Report sore throat, fever, unusual bleeding or bruising, rash, weakness, tremors, impaired vision, dark urine, pale stools, yellowing of the skin and eyes.

▽ **chlorpropamide**
*(klor **proe'** pa mide)*

Apo-Chlorpropamide (CAN),
Diabinese

PREGNANCY CATEGORY C

Drug classes

Antidiabetic agent
Sulfonylurea, first generation

Therapeutic actions

Stimulates insulin release from functioning beta cells in the pancreas; may improve binding between insulin and insulin receptors or increase the number of insulin receptors; can increase the effect of ADH (antidiuretic hormone).

Indications

- Adjunct to diet to lower blood glucose in patients with non–insulin-dependent diabetes mellitus (type 2)
- Unlabeled uses: treatment of neurogenic diabetes insipidus at doses of 200–500 mg/day; temporary adjunct to insulin therapy in type 2 diabetes to improve diabetic control

Contraindications and cautions

- Allergy to sulfonylureas; diabetes complicated by fever, severe infections, severe trauma, major surgery, ketosis, acidosis, coma; type 1 or juvenile diabetes, serious hepatic impairment, serious renal impairment, uremia, thyroid or endocrine impairment, glycosuria, hyperglycemia associated with primary renal disease; pregnancy, lactation

Available forms

Tablets—100, 250 mg

Dosages

Adults

- *Initial therapy:* 250 mg/day PO. *Maintenance therapy:* 100–250 mg/day PO. Up to 500 mg/day may be needed; do not exceed 750 mg/day.
- *Transfer of type 2 diabetics from insulin to chlorpropamide:* ≤ 40 units insulin—250 mg/day with abrupt withdrawal of insulin; > 40 units insulin—250 mg/day, reduce insulin dose by 50%, reduce dose as response is observed.

Pediatric patients

Safety and efficacy not established.

Geriatric patients

Greater sensitivity to drug; start with initial dose of 100–125 mg/day PO; monitor for 24 hr, and gradually increase as needed.

Pharmacokinetics

Route	Onset	Peak	Duration
Oral	1 hr	3–4 hr	60 hr

Metabolism: Hepatic, $T_{1/2}$: 36 hr
Distribution: Crosses placenta; enters breast milk
Excretion: Urine and bile

Adverse effects

- **CV:** Possible increased risk of CV mortality
- **Endocrine:** SIADH
- **GI:** *Anorexia, nausea, vomiting, epigastric discomfort, heartburn*
- **Hematologic:** *Hypoglycemia,* leukopenia, thrombocytopenia, anemia
- **Hypersensitivity:** Allergic skin reactions, eczema, pruritus, erythema, urticaria, photosensitivity, fever, jaundice

Interactions

✳ **Drug-drug** • Increased risk of hypoglycemia if chlorpropamide combined with sulfonamides, urine acidifiers, chloramphenicol, oxyphenbutazone, phenylbutazone, salicylates, monoamine oxidase inhibitors, clofibrate, rifampin • Decreased effectiveness of chlorpropamide and diazoxide if taken concurrently • Increased risk of hyperglycemia if chlorpropamide taken with urine alkalinizers, thiazides, other diuretics • Risk of hypoglycemia and hyperglycemia if chlorpropamide combined with ethanol; disulfiram reaction also has been reported

✳ **Drug-alternative therapy** • Increased risk of hypogylcemia if taken with juniper berries, ginseng, garlic, fenugreek, coriander, dandelion root, celery.

■ Nursing considerations

 CLINICAL ALERT!
Name confusion has occurred between chlorpropamide and chlorpromazine; use caution.

Assessment

- **History:** Allergy to sulfonylureas; diabetes complicated by fever, severe infections, severe trauma, major surgery, ketosis, acidosis, coma; type 1 or juvenile diabetes, serious hepatic or renal impairment, uremia, thyroid or endocrine impairment, glycosuria, hyperglycemia associated with primary renal disease; pregnancy, lactation
- **Physical:** Skin color, lesions; T; orientation, reflexes, peripheral sensation; R, adventitious sounds; liver evaluation, bowel sounds; urinalysis, BUN, serum creatinine, liver function tests, blood glucose, CBC

Interventions

- Give drug before breakfast; if severe GI upset occurs, divide dose—one before breakfast and one before evening meal.
- Monitor urine or serum glucose levels often to determine efficacy and dosage.
- Transfer to insulin therapy during periods of high stress (infections, surgery, trauma).
- Use IV glucose if severe hypoglycemia occurs due to overdose; support and monitoring may be prolonged for 3–5 days because of the long half-life of chlorpropamide.

Teaching points

- Do not discontinue this medication without consulting health care provider.
- Maintain diet and exercise program to control diabetes.
- Monitor urine or blood for glucose and ketones.
- Do not use this drug during pregnancy.
- Avoid OTC drugs and alcohol.
- Report fever, sore throat, unusual bleeding or bruising, rash, dark urine, light-colored stools, hypoglycemic or hyperglycemic reactions.

▷ chlorthalidone

*(klor **thal**' i done)*

Apo-Chlorthalidone (CAN), Hygroton, Thalitone

PREGNANCY CATEGORY B

Drug class

Thiazide-like diuretic

Therapeutic actions

Inhibits reabsorption of sodium and chloride in distal renal tubule, increasing excretion of sodium, chloride, and water by the kidney.

Indications

- Adjunctive therapy in edema associated with CHF, cirrhosis, corticosteroid and estrogen therapy, renal dysfunction
- Hypertension, alone or with other antihypertensives

Contraindications and cautions

- Fluid or electrolyte imbalances, renal or liver disease, gout, SLE, glucose tolerance abnormalities, hyperparathyroidism, manic-depressive disorders, lactation, pregnancy

Available forms

Tablets—15, 25, 50, 100 mg

Dosages

Adults

- *Edema:* 50–100 mg/day PO (30–60 mg *Thalitone*) or 100 mg every other day: up to 200 mg/day (120 mg *Thalitone*).
- *Hypertension:* 25–100 mg/day PO (15–50 mg *Thalitone*) based on patient response (doses > 25 mg/day are likely to increase K^+ excretion, but provide no further increase in Na^+ excretion or decrease in BP).

Pediatric patients

Safety and efficacy not established.

Pharmacokinetics

Route	Onset	Peak	Duration
Oral	2 hr	3–6 hr	24–72 hr

Metabolism: Hepatic, $T_{1/2}$: 54 hr
Distribution: Crosses placenta; enters breast milk
Excretion: Urine

Adverse effects

- **CNS:** *Dizziness, vertigo,* paresthesias, weakness, headache, drowsiness, fatigue
- **CV:** Orthostatic hypotension, venous thrombosis, volume depletion, cardiac arrhythmias, chest pain
- **Dermatologic:** Photosensitivity, rash, purpura, exfoliative dermatitis
- **GI:** *Nausea, anorexia, vomiting, dry mouth, diarrhea, constipation,* jaundice, hepatitis, pancreatitis
- **GU:** *Polyuria, nocturia, impotence,* loss of libido
- **Hematologic:** Leukopenia, thrombocytopenia, agranulocytosis, aplastic anemia, neutropenia, fluid and electrolyte imbalances
- **Other:** Muscle cramps and muscle spasms, fever, hives, gouty attacks, flushing, weight loss

---

Adverse effects in *Italics* are most common; those in **Bold** are life-threatening.

Interactions

✳ Drug-drug • Increased thiazide effects and chance of acute hyperglycemia with diazoxide • Decreased absorption with cholestyramine, colestipol • Increased risk of cardiac glycoside toxicity if hypokalemia occurs • Increased risk of lithium toxicity • Increased dosage of antidiabetic agents may be needed

✳ Drug-lab test • Decreased PBI levels without clinical signs of thyroid disturbances

■ Nursing considerations
Assessment

- **History:** Fluid or electrolyte imbalances, renal or liver disease, gout, SLE, glucose tolerance abnormalities, hyperparathyroidism, manic-depressive disorders, lactation
- **Physical:** Skin color and lesions; orientation, reflexes, muscle strength; pulses, BP, orthostatic BP, perfusion, edema, baseline ECG; R, adventitious sounds; liver evaluation, bowel sounds; CBC, serum electrolytes, blood glucose, liver and renal function tests, serum uric acid, urinalysis

Interventions

- Differentiate between *Thalitone* and other preparations; dosage varies.
- Give with food or milk if GI upset occurs.
- Administer early in the day, so increased urination will not disturb sleep.
- Mark calendars or other reminders of drug days for outpatients on every other day or 3- to 5-day/wk therapy.
- Measure and record weight to monitor fluid changes.

Teaching points

- Take drug early in the day, so sleep will not be disturbed by increased urination.
- Weigh yourself daily, and record weights.
- Protect skin from exposure to the sun or bright lights.
- Increased urination will occur.
- Use caution if dizziness, drowsiness, feeling faint occur.
- Report rapid weight change, swelling in ankles or fingers, unusual bleeding or bruising, muscle cramps.

▽ chlorzoxazone
(klor zox' a zone)

Paraflex, Parafon Forte DSC, Remular-S

PREGNANCY CATEGORY C

Drug class
Skeletal muscle relaxant, centrally acting

Therapeutic actions
Precise mechanism not known; has sedative properties; acts at spinal and supraspinal levels of the CNS to depress reflex arcs involved in producing and maintaining skeletal muscle spasm.

Indications
- Relief of discomfort associated with acute, painful musculoskeletal conditions, adjunct to rest, physical therapy, and other measures

Contraindications and cautions
- Contraindicated with allergic or idiosyncratic reactions to chlorzoxazone.
- Use cautiously with history of allergies or allergic drug reactions, lactation.

Available forms
Tablets—250, 500 mg; caplets—250, 500 mg

Dosages
Adults
Usual dose: 250 mg PO tid–qid; painful conditions may require 500 mg PO tid–qid; may increase to 750 mg tid–qid; reduce dosage as improvement occurs.
Pediatric patients
Safety and efficacy not established.

Pharmacokinetics

Route	Onset	Peak	Duration
Oral	30–60 min	1–2 hr	3–4 hr

Metabolism: Hepatic; $T_{1/2}$: 60 min
Distribution: Crosses placenta; may enter breast milk
Excretion: Urine

Adverse effects
- **CNS:** *Dizziness, light-headedness, drowsiness,* malaise, overstimulation

- **GI:** *GI disturbances,* GI bleeding (rare)
- **GU:** Urine discoloration—orange to purple-red
- **Hypersensitivity:** Rashes, petechiae, ecchymoses, angioneurotic edema, **anaphylaxis** (rare)

Interactions

✱ **Drug-drug** • Additive CNS effects with alcohol, other CNS depressants

■ Nursing considerations
Assessment

- **History:** Allergic or idiosyncratic reactions to chlorzoxazone; history of allergies or allergic drug reactions; lactation
- **Physical:** Skin color, lesions; orientation; liver evaluation; liver function tests

Interventions

- Discontinue if signs or symptoms of liver dysfunction or allergic reaction (urticaria, redness, or itching) occur.

Teaching points

- Take this drug exactly as prescribed; do not take a higher dosage.
- Avoid alcohol, sleep-inducing, or OTC drugs; these could cause dangerous effects.
- These side effects may occur: drowsiness, dizziness, light-headedness (avoid driving or engaging in activities that require alertness); nausea (take with food and eat frequent small meals); discolored urine (expected effect).
- Report rash, severe nausea, coffee-ground vomitus, black or tarry stools, pale stools, yellow skin or eyes, difficulty breathing.

▽ cholestyramine
*(koe **less'** tir a meen)*

LoCHOLEST, LoCHOLEST Light, Novo-Cholamine (CAN), Novo-Cholamine Light (CAN), Prevalite, Questran, Questran Light

PREGNANCY CATEGORY NOT ESTABLISHED

Drug classes
Antihyperlipidemic agent
Bile acid sequestrant

Therapeutic actions
Binds bile acids in the intestine, allowing excretion in the feces; as a result, cholesterol is oxidized in the liver to replace the bile acids lost; serum cholesterol and LDL are lowered.

Indications

- Adjunctive therapy: reduction of elevated serum cholesterol in patients with primary hypercholesterolemia (elevated LDL)
- Pruritus associated with partial biliary obstruction
- Unlabeled uses: antibiotic-induced pseudomembranous colitis; chlordecone *(Kepone)* pesticide poisoning to bind the poison in the intestine; treatment of thyroid hormone overdose, treatment of digitalis toxicity

Contraindications and cautions

- Allergy to bile acid sequestrants, tartrazine (tartrazine sensitivity occurs often with allergies to aspirin); complete biliary obstruction; abnormal intestinal function; pregnancy; lactation.

Available forms
Powder—4 g/6.4 g powder; powder for suspension—4 g/5.5, 5.7 or 9 g powder

Dosages
Adults
4 g one to two times per day PO. Individualize dose based on response.

- *Maintenance:* 8–16 g/day divided into 2 doses.

Pediatric patients
Safety and efficacy not established.

Pharmacokinetics
Not absorbed systemically; excreted in the feces.

Adverse effects

- **CNS:** Headache, anxiety, vertigo, dizziness, fatigue, syncope, drowsiness
- **Dermatologic:** Rash and irritation of skin, tongue, perianal area

Adverse effects in *Italics* are most common; those in **Bold** are life-threatening.

- **GI:** *Constipation to fecal impaction, exacerbation of hemorrhoids,* abdominal cramps, pain, flatulence, anorexia, heartburn, nausea, vomiting, steatorrhea
- **GU:** Hematuria, dysuria, diuresis
- **Hematologic:** *Increased bleeding tendencies related to vitamin K malabsorption,* vitamins A and D deficiencies, reduced serum and red cell folate, hyperchloremic acidosis
- **Other:** Osteoporosis, backache, muscle and joint pain, arthritis, fever

Interactions
✱ **Drug-drug** • Decreased or delayed absorption with warfarin, thiazide diuretics, digitalis preparations, thyroid, corticosteroids
• Malabsorption of fat-soluble vitamins with cholestyramine

■ Nursing considerations
Assessment
- **History:** Allergy to bile acid sequestrants, tartrazine; complete biliary obstruction; abnormal intestinal function; lactation
- **Physical:** Skin lesions, color, temperature; orientation, affect, reflexes; P, auscultation, baseline ECG, peripheral perfusion; liver evaluation, bowel sounds; lipid studies, liver function tests, clotting profile

Interventions
- Mix contents of one packet or one level scoop of powder with 2–6 fluid oz of beverage (water, milk, fruit juices, noncarbonates), highly fluid soup, pulpy fruits (applesauce, pineapple); do not give drug in dry form.
- Administer drug before meals.
- Monitor intake of other oral drugs due to risk of binding in the intestine and delayed or decreased absorption; give oral medications 1 hr before or 4–6 hr after the cholestyramine.
- Alert patient and concerned others about high cost of drug.

Teaching points
- Take drug before meals; do not take the powder in the dry form; mix one packet or one scoop with 2–6 oz of fluid—water, milk, juice, noncarbonates, highly fluid soups, cereals, pulpy fruits.

- Take other medications 1 hr before or 4–6 hr after cholestyramine.
- These side effects may occur: constipation (consult about measures that may help); nausea, heartburn, loss of appetite (small, frequent meals may help); dizziness, drowsiness, vertigo, fainting (avoid driving and operating dangerous machinery); headache, muscle and joint aches and pains (may lessen with time).
- Report unusual bleeding or bruising, severe constipation, severe GI upset, chest pain, difficulty breathing, rash, fever.

▷ **choline magnesium trisalicylate**
(ko' leen mag nee' see um tri sal' i ci late)

Tricosal, Trilisate

PREGNANCY CATEGORY C

Drug classes
Nonsteroidal anti-inflammatory drug (NSAID)
Salicylate
Analgesic–antipyretic

Therapeutic actions
Inhibits prostaglandin synthesis; action lowers fever, decreases inflammation.

Indications
- Treatment of osteoarthritis, rheumatoid arthritis
- Relief of moderate pain, fever

Contraindications and cautions
- Contraindicated with allergy to salicylates, NSAIDs.
- Use cautiously with chronic renal failure, peptic ulcer, hepatic failure, children with chickenpox or CNS symptoms, lactation.

Available forms
Tablets—500, 750, 1,000 mg; liquid—500 mg/5 mL

Dosages
Adults
- *Arthritis:* 1.5–2.5 g/day PO in 1 to 3 divided doses. Do not exceed 4.5 g/day.

• *Pain, fever:* 2–3 g/day PO in 2 divided doses.
Pediatric patients
• *Pain, fever:* 50 mg/kg/day PO in two divided doses.

Pharmacokinetics

Route	Onset	Peak
Oral	30 min	1–3 hr

Metabolism: Hepatic; $T_{1/2}$: 2–3 hr
Distribution: Crosses placenta; passes into breast milk
Excretion: Urine

Adverse effects

• **CNS:** Dizziness, vertigo, confusion, drowsiness, headache, tinnitus
• **GI:** *Diarrhea, nausea,* GI lesion, GI bleed

Interactions

✳ **Drug-drug** • Increased risk of salicylate toxicity with aminosalicylic acid, ammonium chloride, acidifying agents, carbonic anhydrase inhibitors • Increased risk of bleeding with oral anticoagulants • Increased risk of toxicity of methotrexate with choline magnesium trisalicylate • Decreased effectiveness of probenecid, sulfinpyrazone

■ Nursing considerations
Assessment

• **History:** Allergy to salicylates or NSAIDs, peptic ulcer disease, hepatic failure, chronic renal failure, lactation
• **Physical:** Skin condition, T, neurologic status, abdominal exam, kidney and liver function tests, urinalysis, bleeding times

Interventions

• Give with meals to decrease GI effects.

Teaching points

• Take drug with meals; use the drug only as prescribed.
• Know that these side effects may occur: dizziness, light-headedness, drowsiness (avoid driving or operating dangerous machinery if this occurs); nausea, diarrhea.
• Report sore throat, fever, rash, itching, black or tarry stools.

<hr>

▷ **choline salicylate**
(ko' leen sal' i ci late)

Teejel (CAN)
OTC:Arthropan

PREGNANCY CATEGORY C

Drug classes

Nonsteroidal anti-inflammatory drug (NSAID)
Salicylate
Analgesic–antipyretic

Therapeutic actions

Inhibits prostaglandin synthesis, which lowers fever, decreases inflammation.

Indications

• Treatment of osteoarthritis, rheumatoid arthritis
• Relief of moderate pain, fever

Contraindications and cautions

• Contraindicated with allergy to salicylates, NSAIDs.
• Use cautiously with chronic renal failure, peptic ulcer, hepatic failure, children with chickenpox or CNS symptoms, lactation.

Available forms

Liquid—870 mg/5 mL

Dosages
Adults and patients > 12 yr
870 mg PO q 3–4 hr; do not exceed 6 doses per day. Patients with rheumatoid arthritis may start with 5–10 mL, up to qid.

Pharmacokinetics

Route	Onset	Peak
Oral	5–10 min	10–30 min

Metabolism: Hepatic; $T_{1/2}$: 2–3 hr
Distribution: Crosses placenta; enters breast milk
Excretion: Urine

Adverse effects

• **CNS:** Dizziness, vertigo, confusion, drowsiness, headache, tinnitus, sweating
• **GI:** *Diarrhea, nausea,* hepatotoxicity

<hr>

Adverse effects in *Italics* are most common; those in **Bold** are life-threatening.

Interactions

✳ **Drug-drug** • Increased risk of salicylate toxicity with aminosalicylic acid, ammonium chloride, acidifying agents, carbonic anhydrase inhibitors • Increased risk of bleeding with oral anticoagulants • Increased risk of toxicity of methotrexate with choline magnesium trisalicylate • Decreased effectiveness of probenecid, sulfinpyrazone

■ Nursing considerations

Assessment

- **History:** Allergy to salicylates or NSAIDs, peptic ulcer disease, hepatic or chronic renal failure, lactation
- **Physical:** Skin condition, T, neurologic status, abdominal exam, kidney and liver function tests, urinalysis, bleeding times

Interventions

- Give with meals to decrease GI effects; may be mixed with fruit juice or carbonated beverage to improve taste.

Teaching points

- Take drug with meals; use as prescribed. May take with fruit juice, carbonated beverages to improve taste. Store drug at room temperature.
- These side effects may occur: dizziness, lightheadedness, drowsiness (avoid driving or operating dangerous machinery); nausea, diarrhea.
- Report sore throat, fever, rash, itching, black or tarry stools.

▷chorionic gonadotropin (human chorionic gonadotropin, HCG)

*(goe **nad'** oh troe pin)*

Chorex-5, Chorex-10, Choron 10, Gonic, Pregnyl, Profasi HP

PREGNANCY CATEGORY X

Drug class

Hormone

Therapeutic actions

A human placental hormone with actions identical to pituitary leutenizing hormone (LH); stimulates production of testosterone and progesterone.

Indications

- Prepubertal cryptorchidism not due to anatomic obstruction
- Treatment of selected cases of hypogonadotropic hypogonadism in males
- Induction of ovulation in the anovulatory, infertile woman in whom the cause of anovulation is secondary and not due to primary ovarian failure and who has been pretreated with human menotropins

Contraindications and cautions

- Contraindicated with known sensitivity to chorionic gonadotropin, precocious puberty, prostatic carcinoma or androgen-dependent neoplasm, pregnancy.
- Use cautiously with epilepsy, migraine, asthma, cardiac or renal disease, lactation.

Available forms

Powder for injection—5,000, 10,000, 20,000 units/vial with 10 mL diluent

Dosages

For IM use only; individualize dosage; the following dosage regimens are suggested:

- *Prepubertal cryptorchidism not due to anatomic obstruction:* 4,000 USP units IM, 3 times per week for 3 wk; 5,000 USP units IM, every second day for 4 injections; 15 injections of 500–1,000 USP units over 6 wk; 500 USP units 3 times per week for 4–6 wk; if not successful, start another course 1 mo later, giving 1,000 USP units/injection.
- *Hypogonadotropic hypogonadism in males:* 500–1,000 USP units, IM 3 times per week for 3 wk; followed by the same dose twice a week for 3 wk; 1,000–2,000 USP units IM 3 times per week; 4,000 USP units 3 times per week for 6–9 mo; reduce dosage to 2,000 USP units 3 times per week for an additional 3 mo.
- *Induction of ovulation and pregnancy:* 5,000–10,000 units IM, 1 day following the last dose of menotropins.

Pharmacokinetics

Route	Onset	Peak
IM	2 hr	6 hr

Metabolism: Hepatic; $T_{1/2}$: 23 hr
Distribution: Crosses placenta; may enter breast milk
Excretion: Urine

Adverse effects

- **CNS:** *Headache, irritability, restlessness,* depression, fatigue
- **CV:** Edema, **arterial thromboembolism**
- **Endocrine:** *Precocious puberty, gynecomastia,* ovarian hyperstimulation (sudden ovarian enlargement, ascites, rupture of ovarian cysts, multiple births)
- **Other:** *Pain at injection site*

■ Nursing considerations
Assessment

- **History:** Sensitivity to chorionic gonadotropin, precocious puberty, prostatic carcinoma or androgen-dependent neoplasm, epilepsy, migraine, asthma, cardiac or renal disease, lactation, pregnancy
- **Physical:** Skin texture, edema; prostate exam; injection site; sexual development; orientation, affect, reflexes; R, adventitious sounds; P, auscultation, BP, peripheral edema; liver evaluation; renal function tests

Interventions

- Prepare solution for injection using manufacturers' instructions; brand and concentrations vary.
- Discontinue at any sign of ovarian overstimulation, and have patient admitted to the hospital for observation and supportive measures.
- Provide comfort measures for CNS effects, pain at injection site.

Teaching points

- This drug can only be given IM. Prepare a calendar with treatment schedule.
- These side effects may occur: headache, irritability, restlessness, depression, fatigue (reversible; if uncomfortable, consult health care provider).

- Report pain at injection site, severe headache, restlessness, swelling of ankles or fingers, difficulty breathing, severe abdominal pain.

▽ chorionic gonadotropin alfa

See *Less Commonly Used Drugs*, p. 1340.

▽ chymopapain

See *Less Commonly Used Drugs*, p. 1340.

▽ cidofovir
*(si **dob'** foh ver)*

Vistide

PREGNANCY CATEGORY C

Drug class
Antiviral

Therapeutic actions
Antiviral activity; selectively inhibits CMV replication by inhibition of viral DNA synthesis.

Indications
- Treatment of CMV retinitis in AIDS patients

Contraindications and cautions
- Contraindicated with allergy to cidofovir, probenecid, or sulfa; pregnancy, lactation; severe renal impairment
- Use cautiously with renal impairment and in elderly

Available forms
Injection—75 mg/mL

Dosages
Adults
5 mg/kg IV infused over 1 hr once per wk for 2 consecutive wk during induction; 5 mg/kg IV once every 2 wk for maintenance. Probenecid must be administered orally with each dose, 2 g PO 3 hr before cidofovir and 1 g at 2 hr and 8 hr after completion of infusion.

Pediatric patients
Safety and efficacy not established in children < 12 yr.

Patients with renal impairment
If patients have an increase in serum creatinine of 0.3–0.4 mg/dL, reduce dose to 3 mg/kg; discontinue drug if serum creatinine increases ≥ 0.5 mg/dL above baseline or if ≥ 3+ proteinuria develops.

Pharmacokinetics

Route	Onset	Peak
IV	Rapid	15 min

Metabolism: $T_{1/2}$: 1 hr
Distribution: Crosses placenta; may enter breast milk
Excretion: Renal

▽ IV facts

Preparation: Patient should receive 2 g probenecid before starting infusion and 1 g at 2 and 8 hr after infusion; patient should be hydrated with 1 L normal saline before each dose. A second liter can be given over 1–3 hr after dose, if tolerated. Dilute in 100 mL 0.9% saline solution before administration. Store at room temperature; mixtures may be stored up to 24 hr refrigerated; warm to room temperature before using.
Infusion: Infuse over 1 hr.
Incompatibilities: Do not mix in solution with any other drugs.

Adverse effects

- **CNS:** *Headache,* ocular hypotony, asthenia
- **CV:** Palpitations
- **Dermatologic:** Alopecia, rash
- **GI:** *Nausea, vomiting, diarrhea,* anorexia, dry mouth
- **GU: Nephrotoxicity,** proteinuria
- **Hematologic: Neutropenia,** metabolic acidosis, elevated serum creatinine
- **Respiratory:** Dyspnea, sinusitis
- **Other:** Infection, chills, fever

Interactions

✳ **Drug-drug** • Avoid other nephrotoxic drugs (amphotericin B, aminoglycosides, foscarnet, IV pentamidine) • Risk of increased serum levels of zidovudine when probenecid (required pretreatment with cidofovir) is given concurrently; reduce dosage of zidovudine by up to 50% on day of cidofovir therapy or discontinue for that day

■ Nursing considerations
Assessment

- **History:** Allergy to cidofovir, probenecid, sulfa drugs; renal dysfunction, pregnancy, lactation
- **Physical:** T; orientation, reflexes; BP, P, peripheral perfusion; R, adventitious sounds; bowel sounds; urinary output; skin color, perfusion, hydration; renal function tests

Interventions

- Medicate patient with 2 g probenecid PO 3 hr before starting cidofovir infusion and 1 g at 2 and 8 hr after infusion; patient should be hydrated with 1 L normal saline before each dose and 2 L after dose, if tolerated.
- Monitor renal function carefully before and during therapy; dosage must be adjusted based on renal function. For serum creatinine increase of 0.3–0.4 mg/dL, reduce dose from 5 mg/kg to 3 mg/kg. Discontinue drug and notify physician if serum creatinine > 0.5 mg/dL or 3+ proteinuria.
- Monitor hydration carefully; increase fluids as tolerated.

Teaching points

- This drug can only be given IV. You will need to receive normal saline IV before drug is given. Mark calendar with dates to return for subsequent doses.
- This drug does not cure your CMV retinitis; other AIDS therapy should be continued. If on zidovudine, dosage adjustments will be needed when probenecid is taken.
- Return for medical follow-up, including blood tests to monitor kidney function; decreases in kidney function may require discontinuation of this drug.
- These side effects may occur: nausea, vomiting, loss of appetite, diarrhea, abdominal pain; headache, dizziness, insomnia.
- Report severe diarrhea, severe nausea, flank pain, discomfort at IV site.

▽ cilostazol
(sill abs' tab zoll)

Pletal

PREGNANCY CATEGORY C

Drug class
Antiplatelet agent

Therapeutic actions
Reversibly inhibits platelet aggregation induced by a variety of stimuli including ADP, thrombin, collagen, shear stress, epinephrine, and arachidonic acid by inhibiting cAMP phosphodiesterase III (PDE III); produces vascular dilation in vascular beds with a specificity for femoral beds; seems to have no effect on renal arteries.

Indications
• Reduction of symptoms of intermittent claudication allowing increased walking distance

Contraindications and cautions
• Contraindicated with allergy to cilostazol; in the presence of CHF (decreased survival rates have occurred), pregnancy, and lactation.
• Use cautiously with CV disorders.

Available forms
Tablets—50, 100 mg

Dosages
Adults
100 mg PO bid taken ≥ 30 min before or 2 hr after breakfast and dinner. Response may not be noted for 2–4 wk and may take up to 12 wk.
Pediatric patients
Safety and efficacy not established.

Pharmacokinetics

Route	Onset	Peak
Oral	Gradual	4–6 hr

Metabolism: Hepatic; $T_{1/2}$: 11–13 hr
Distribution: Crosses placenta; may pass into breast milk
Excretion: Urine

Adverse effects
• **CNS:** *Dizziness, headaches,* asthenia, paresthesias, **CVA**
• **CV: CHF,** tachycardia, complete heart block, **MI,** hypertension, *palpitations*
• **GI:** *Diarrhea, nausea, flatulence, dyspepsia,* anorexia
• **Respiratory:** Cough, pharyngitis, *rhinitis*
• **Other:** Peripheral edema, infection, back pain

Interactions
✳ **Drug-drug** • Increased serum levels and risk of toxic effects of cilostazol if combined with macrolide antibiotics, diltiazem; if this combination is used, consider decreasing cilostazol dose to 50 mg bid and monitor patient closely
✳ **Drug-food** • Increased absorption if taken with high-fat meal; administer drug ≥ 30 min before or 2 hr after meals • Increased serum levels and risk of adverse effects if combined with grapefruit juice; avoid grapefruit juice if taking this drug

■ Nursing considerations
Assessment
• **History:** Allergy to cilostazol, CHF, lactation, cardiovascular disorders, pregnancy
• **Physical:** Skin color, lesions; orientation; bowel sounds, normal output; P, BP; R, adventitious sounds; CBC, liver and renal function tests

Interventions
• Monitor blood clotting studies prior to and periodically during therapy.
• Administer drug on an empty stomach, ≥ 30 min before or 2 hr after breakfast and dinner.
• Encourage patient to avoid the use of grapefruit juice.
• Establish baseline walking distance to monitor drug effectiveness.
• Establish safety precautions to prevent injury and bleeding (electric razor, no contact sports, etc).
• Advise patient to use barrier contraceptives while receiving this drug, it may harm the fetus.

- Encourage patient to continue therapy; results may not be seen for 2–4 wk and in some cases may take up to 12 wk.
- Advise patient that the cardiovascular risks associated with this drug are not known; potentially serious cardiovascular effects have occurred in laboratory animals.

Teaching points

- Take drug on an empty stomach ≥ 30 min before or 2 hr after breakfast and dinner.
- Avoid the use of grapefruit juice while you are taking this drug.
- Be aware that the therapeutic effects of this drug may not be seen for 2–4 wk and may take up to 12 wk.
- Avoid pregnancy while on this drug; it could cause harm to the fetus. Use barrier contraceptives; notify physician immediately if you think you are pregnant.
- Upset stomach, nausea, diarrhea, loss of appetite (small, frequent meals may help) may occur.
- Report fever, chills, sore throat, palpitations, chest pain, edema or swelling, difficulty breathing, fatigue.

▽ cimetidine
*(sye **met' i** deen)*

Apo-Cimetidine (CAN), Gen-Cimetidine (CAN), Novo-Cimetine (CAN), Nu-Cimet (CAN), Peptol (CAN), Tagamet, Tagamet HB, Tagamet HB Suspension

PREGNANCY CATEGORY B

Drug class
Histamine$_2$ (H$_2$) antagonist

Therapeutic actions
Inhibits the action of histamine at the histamine$_2$ (H$_2$) receptors of the stomach, inhibiting gastric acid secretion and reducing total pepsin output.

Indications

- Short-term treatment of active duodenal ulcer
- Short-term treatment of benign gastric ulcer
- Treatment of pathologic hypersecretory conditions (Zollinger-Ellison syndrome)
- Prophylaxis of stress-induced ulcers and acute upper GI bleeding in critical patients
- Treatment of erosive gastroesophageal reflux
- Relief of symptoms of heartburn, acid indigestion, sour stomach (OTC use)

Contraindications and cautions
- Allergy to cimetidine, impaired renal or hepatic function, lactation.

Available forms
Tablets—100, 200, 300, 400, 800 mg; liquid—300 mg/5 mL; injection 150 mg/mL, 300 mg/2 mL

Dosages
Adults
- *Active duodenal ulcer:* 800 mg PO hs or 300 mg PO qid at meals and hs or 400 mg PO bid; continue for 4–6 wk. For intractable ulcers, 300 mg IM or IV q 6–8 hr.
- *Maintenance therapy for duodenal ulcer:* 400 mg PO hs.
- *Active gastric ulcer:* 300 mg PO qid at meals and hs or 800 mg hs.
- *Pathologic hypersecretory syndrome:* 300 mg PO qid at meals and hs, or 300 mg IV or IM q 6 hr. Individualize doses as needed; do not exceed 2,400 mg/day.
- *Erosive gastroesophageal reflux disease:* 1,600 mg PO in divided doses bid–qid for 12 wk.
- *Prevention of upper GI bleeding:* Continuous IV infusion of 50 mg/hr. Do not treat beyond 7 days.
- *Heartburn, acid indigestion:* 200 mg as symptoms occur: up to 4 tablets/24 hr.

Pediatric patients
Not recommended for children < 12 yr.

Geriatric patients or patients with impaired renal function
Accumulation may occur. Use lowest dose possible: 300 mg PO or IV q 12 hr; may be increased to q 8 hr if patient tolerates it, and levels are monitored.

Pharmacokinetics

Route	Onset	Peak
Oral	Varies	1–1.5 hr
IV, IM	Rapid	1–1.5 hr

Metabolism: Hepatic; $T_{1/2}$: 2 hr
Distribution: Crosses placenta; enters breast milk
Excretion: Urine

▽IV facts

Preparation: *IV injections:* Dilute in 0.9% sodium chloride injection, 5% or 10% dextrose injection, lactated Ringer's solution, 5% sodium bicarbonate injection to a volume of 20 mL. Solution is stable for 48 hr at room temperature. *IV infusions:* Dilute 300 mg in at least 50 mL of 5% dextrose injection or one of above listed solutions.

Infusion: Inject by direct injection over not less than 2 min; by infusion, slowly over 15–20 min.

Incompatibilities: Incompatible with aminophylline, barbiturate in IV solutions; pentobarbital sodium and pentobarbital sodium and atropine in the same syringe.

Adverse effects

- **CNS:** *Dizziness, somnolence, headache, confusion, hallucinations,* peripheral neuropathy; symptoms of brain stem dysfunction (dysarthria, ataxia, diplopia)
- **CV:** Cardiac arrhythmias, **cardiac arrest,** hypotension (IV use)
- **GI:** *Diarrhea*
- **Hematologic:** Increases in plasma creatinine, serum transaminase
- **Other:** *Impotence* (reversible), gynecomastia (in long-term treatment), rash, vasculitis, pain at IM injection site

Interactions

✳ Drug-drug • Increased risk of decreased white blood cell counts with antimetabolites, alkylating agents, other drugs known to cause neutropenia • Increased serum levels and risk of toxicity of warfarin-type anticoagulants, phenytoin, beta-adrenergic blocking agents, alcohol, quinidine, lidocaine, theophylline, chloroquine, certain benzodiazepines (alprazolam, chlordiazepoxide, diazepam, flurazepam, triazolam), nifedipine, pentoxifylline, tricyclic antidepressants, procainamide, carbamazepine when taken with cimetidine

■ Nursing considerations

Assessment

- **History:** Allergy to cimetidine, impaired renal or hepatic function, lactation
- **Physical:** Skin lesions; orientation, affect; pulse, baseline ECG (continuous with IV use); liver evaluation, abdominal exam, normal output; CBC, liver and renal function tests

Interventions

- Give drug with meals and at hs.
- Decrease doses in renal and liver dysfunction.
- Administer IM dose undiluted deep into large muscle group.
- Arrange for regular follow-up, including blood tests to evaluate effects.

Teaching points

- Take drug with meals and at bedtime; therapy may continue for 4–6 wk or longer.
- Take antacids as prescribed, and at recommended times.
- Inform your health care provider about your cigarette smoking habits. Cigarette smoking decreases drug efficacy.
- Have regular medical follow-ups to evaluate your response to drug.
- Report sore throat, fever, unusual bruising or bleeding, tarry stools, confusion, hallucinations, dizziness, muscle or joint pain.

▽ **cinoxacin**
(sin ox' a sin)

Cinobac

PREGNANCY CATEGORY B

Drug classes

Urinary tract anti-infective
Antibacterial

Therapeutic actions

Bactericidal; interferes with DNA replication in susceptible gram-negative bacteria, preventing cell division.

Indications
- Urinary tract infections caused by susceptible gram-negative bacteria, including *E.
coli, P. mirabilis, P. vulgaris, K. pneumoniae, Klebsiella* species, *Enterobacter*
species
- Effective in preventing UTIs for up to 5 mo
in women with recurrent UTIs.

Contraindications and cautions
- Allergy to cinoxacin; renal dysfunction (do
not use with anuric patients); liver dysfunction; pregnancy; lactation

Available forms
Capsules—250, 500 mg

Dosages
Adults
1 g/day in two to four divided doses PO for
7–14 days. *Preventive therapy:* 250 mg PO hs
for up to 5 mo.
Pediatric patients
Not recommended for children < 12 yr.
**Patients with impaired renal
function**
Initial dose of 500 mg PO, then the following
maintenance schedule is suggested:

Creatinine Clearance (mL/min)	Dosage
> 80	500 mg bid
80–50	250 mg tid
50–20	250 mg bid
< 20	250 mg daily

Pharmacokinetics

Route	Onset	Peak	Duration
Oral	2 hr	2–4 hr	10–12 hr

Metabolism: Hepatic; $T_{1/2}$: 1–1.5 hr
Distribution: Crosses placenta; may enter
breast milk
Excretion: Urine

Adverse effects
- **CNS:** *Headache, dizziness,* insomnia, nervousness, confusion
- **GI:** *Nausea,* abdominal cramps, vomiting,
diarrhea, anorexia, perineal burning
- **Hematologic:** Elevated BUN, AST, ALT,
serum creatinine, alkaline phosphatase

- **Hypersensitivity:** *Rash, urticaria, pruritus,* edema

Interactions
✳ **Drug-drug** • Lowered urine concentrations of cinoxacin if pretreated with probenecid

■ Nursing considerations
Assessment
- **History:** Allergy to cinoxacin, renal or liver dysfunction, pregnancy, lactation
- **Physical:** Skin color, lesions; orientation,
reflexes; liver and renal function tests

Interventions
- Arrange for culture and sensitivity tests.
- Administer drug with food if GI upset occurs.
- Arrange for periodic renal and liver function
tests during prolonged therapy.
- Monitor clinical response; if no improve-
ment is seen or a relapse occurs, send urine
for repeat culture and sensitivity.
- Encourage patient to complete full course
of therapy.

Teaching points
- Take drug with food. Complete full course
of therapy.
- Know that these side effects may occur: nausea, vomiting, abdominal pain (try small,
frequent meals); diarrhea; drowsiness, blurring of vision, dizziness (use caution driving or using dangerous equipment).
- Report rash, visual changes, severe GI problems, weakness, tremors.

▽ **ciprofloxacin**
*(si proe **flox**' a sin)*

Ciloxan (CAN), Cipro, Cipro HC Otic,
Cipro I.V.

PREGNANCY CATEGORY C

Drug class
Antibacterial

Therapeutic actions
Bactericidal; interferes with DNA replication
in susceptible gram-negative bacteria preventing cell reproduction.

Indications

- For the treatment of infections caused by susceptible gram-negative bacteria, including *E. coli, P. mirabilis, K. pneumoniae, Enterobacter cloacae, P. vulgaris, P. rettgeri, M. morganii, P. aeruginosa, Citrobacter freundii, S. aureus, S. epidermidis,* group D streptococci
- Treatment of acute otitis externa (otic)
- Treatment of chronic bacterial prostatitis
- Treatment of nosocomial pneumonia caused by *Haemophilus influenzae, K. pneumoniae* (IV)
- Typhoid fever (oral)
- Sexually transmitted diseases caused by *N. gonorrhea* (oral)
- Prevention of anthrax following exposure to anthrax bacilla (prophylactic use in regions suspected of using germ warfare)
- Unlabeled use: effective in patients with cystic fibrosis who have pulmonary exacerbations

Contraindications and cautions

- Contraindicated with allergy to ciprofloxacin, norfloxacin, pregnancy, lactation.
- Use cautiously with renal dysfunction, seizures, tendinitis or tendon rupture associated with fluoroquinolone use.

Available forms

Tablets—100, 250, 500, 750 mg; oral suspension—5, 10 g/100 ml; injection—200, 400 mg; ophthalmic solution—3.5 mg/mL; otic suspension—2 mg/mL

Dosages
Adults

- *Uncomplicated urinary tract infections:* 100–250 mg PO q 12 hr for 3 days.
- *Mild to moderate UTI:* 250 mg q 12 hr PO for 7–14 days or 200 mg IV q 12 hr for 7–14 days.
- *Complicated urinary tract infections:* 500 mg bid PO for 10–21 days or 400 mg IV.
- *Infectious diarrhea:* 500 mg q 12 hr PO for 5–7 days.
- *Anthrax postexposure:* 500 mg PO q 12 hr for 60 days or 400 mg IV q 12 hr for 60 days.
- *Respiratory infections* 500–750 mg PO or 400 mg IV q 12 hr for 7–14 days.

- *Bone, joint, skin infections:* 500–750 mg PO or 400 mg IV q 12 hr for 4–6 wk.
- *Nosocomial pneumonia:* 400 mg IV q 8 hr.
- *Ophthalmic infections caused by susceptible organisms not responsive to other therapy:* 1 or 2 drops/eye daily or bid.
- *Acute otitis externa:* 4 drops in infected ear, tid–qid.

Pediatric patients

Not recommended; produced lesions of joint cartilage in immature experimental animals.

- *Inhalational anthrax:* 15 mg/kg/dose PO q 12 hr for 60 days *or* 10 mg/kg/dose IV q 12 hr for 60 days; do not exceed 500 mg/dose PO or 400 mg/dose IV.

Geriatric patients or patients with impaired renal function

- *Creatinine clearance:* 30–50 mL/min, give 250 to 500 mg PO q 12 hr. If creatinine clearance 5–29 mL/min, give 250 to 500 mg PO q 18 hr or 200 to 400 mg IV q 18–24 hr.
- *Hemodialysis:* 250–500 mg q 24 hr, after dialysis.

Pharmacokinetics

Route	Onset	Peak	Duration
Oral	Varies	60–90 min	4–5 hr
IV	10 min	30 min	4–5 hr

Metabolism: Hepatic; T$_{1/2}$: 3.5–4 hr
Distribution: Crosses placenta; enters breast milk
Excretion: Urine and bile

▽ IV facts

Preparation: Dilute to a final concentration of 1–2 mg/mL with 0.9% NaCl injection or 5% dextrose injection. Stable up to 14 days refrigerated or at room temperature.
Infusion: Administer slowly over 60 min.
Incompatibilities: Discontinue the administration of any other solutions during ciprofloxacin infusion. Incompatible with aminophylline, amoxicillin, clindamycin, floxacillin, heparin, mezlocillin in solution.

Adverse effects

- **CNS:** *Headache,* dizziness, insomnia, fatigue, somnolence, depression, blurred vision
- **CV:** Arrhythmias, hypotension, angina

- **GI:** *Nausea,* vomiting, dry mouth, *diarrhea,* abdominal pain
- **Hematologic:** Elevated BUN, AST, ALT, serum creatinine and alkaline phosphatase; decreased WBC, neutrophil count, Hct
- **Other:** Fever, rash

Interactions

✳ **Drug-drug** • Decreased therapetic effect with iron salts, sucralfate • Decreased absorption with antacids, didanosine • Increased serum levels and toxic effects of theophyllines if taken concurrently with ciprofloxacin

✳ **Drug-alternative therapy** • Increased risk of severe photosensitivity reactions if combined with St. John's wort therapy.

■ Nursing considerations
Assessment

- **History:** Allergy to ciprofloxacin, norfloxacin; renal dysfunction; seizures; lactation
- **Physical:** Skin color, lesions; T; orientation, reflexes, affect; mucous membranes, bowel sounds; renal and liver function tests

Interventions

- Arrange for culture and sensitivity tests before beginning therapy.
- Continue therapy for 2 days after signs and symptoms of infection are gone.
- Give oral drug 1 hr before or 2 hr after meals with a glass of water.
- Ensure that patient is well hydrated.
- Give antacids at least 2 hr after dosing.
- Monitor clinical response; if no improvement is seen or a relapse occurs, repeat culture and sensitivity.
- Encourage patient to complete full course of therapy.

Teaching points

- Take oral drug on an empty stomach—1 hr before or 2 hr after meals. If an antacid is needed take it at least 2 hr before or after dose.
- Drink plenty of fluids while you are on this drug.
- Know that these side effects may occur: nausea, vomiting, abdominal pain (small, frequent meals may help); diarrhea or constipation; drowsiness; blurring of vision,

dizziness (observe caution if driving or using dangerous equipment).
- Report rash, visual changes, severe GI problems, weakness, tremors.

> ▷ **cisplatin (CDDP)**
> *(sis' pla tin)*
>
> Platinol-AQ
>
> **PREGNANCY CATEGORY D**

Drug classes
Alkylating agent
Antineoplastic

Therapeutic actions
Cytotoxic: heavy metal that inhibits cell replication; cell cycle nonspecific.

Indications

- Metastatic testicular tumors: combination therapy with bleomycin sulfate and vinblastine sulfate after surgery or radiotherapy
- Metastatic ovarian tumors: as single therapy in resistant patients or in combination therapy with doxorubicin or cyclophosphamide after surgery or radiotherapy
- Advanced bladder cancer: single agent for transitional cell bladder cancer no longer amenable to surgery or radiotherapy

Contraindications and cautions

- Allergy to cisplatin, platinum-containing products; hematopoietic depression; impaired renal function; hearing impairment; pregnancy; lactation

Available forms
Injection—1 mg/mL

Dosages
Adults
Metastatic testicular tumors

- *Remission induction:* Cisplatin: 20 mg/m^2 per day IV for 5 consecutive days (days 1–5) every 3 wk for three courses of therapy. Bleomycin: 30 units IV weekly (day 2 of each wk) for 12 consecutive doses. Vinblastine: 0.15–0.2 mg/kg IV twice weekly (days 1 and 2) every 3 wk for four courses.

- *Maintenance:* Vinblastine: 0.3 mg/kg IV every 4 wk for 2 yr.

Metastatic ovarian tumors
100 mg/m^2 IV once every 4 wk

- *Combination therapy:* Administer sequentially: cisplatin: 50–100 mg/m^2 IV once every 3–4 wk; cyclophosphamide: 600 mg/m^2 IV once every 4 wk

Advanced bladder cancer
50–70 mg/m^2 IV once every 3–4 wk; in heavily pretreated (radiotherapy or chemotherapy) patients, give an initial dose of 50 mg/m^2 repeated every 4 wk. Do not give repeated courses until serum creatinine is < 1.5 mg/100 mL or BUN is > 25 mg/100 mL or until platelets > 100,000/mm^3 and WBC > 4,000/mm^3. Do not give subsequent doses until audiometry indicates hearing is within normal range.

Pharmacokinetics

Route	Onset	Peak	Duration
IV	8–10 hr	18–23 days	30–35 days

Metabolism: Hepatic; T$_{1/2}$: 25–49 min, then 58–73 hr
Distribution: Crosses placenta; enters breast milk
Excretion: Urine

▽**IV facts**
Preparation: Dissolve the powder in the 10-mg and 50-mg vials with 10 or 50 mL of sterile water for injection respectively; resulting solution contains 1 mg/mL cisplatin; stable for 20 hr at room temperature—do not refrigerate. Dilute reconstituted drug in 1–2 L of 5% dextrose in one-half or one-third normal saline containing 37.5 g mannitol.
Infusion: Hydrate patient with 1–2 L of fluid infused for 8–12 hr before drug therapy; infuse dilute drug over 6–8 hr.

Adverse effects

- **CNS:** *Ototoxicity,* peripheral neuropathies, seizures, loss of taste
- **GI:** *Nausea, vomiting, anorexia,* liver impairment
- **GU:** *Nephrotoxicity,* dose limiting
- **Hematologic:** *Leukopenia, thrombocytopenia, anemia,* hypomagnesemia, hypo-

calcemia, hypokalemia, hypophosphatemia, hyperuricemia

- **Hypersensitivity:** Anaphylactic-like reactions, facial edema, bronchoconstriction, tachycardia, hypotension (treat with epinephrine, corticosteroids, antihistamines)

Interactions

✴ **Drug-drug** • Additive ototoxicity with furosemide, bumetanide, ethacrynic acid • Decreased serum levels of phenytoins with cisplatin

■ Nursing considerations
Assessment

- **History:** Allergy to cisplatin, platinum-containing products; hematopoietic depression; impaired renal function; hearing impairment; pregnancy; lactation
- **Physical:** Weight; eighth cranial nerve evaluation; reflexes; sensation; CBC, differential; renal function tests; serum electrolytes; serum uric acid; audiogram

Interventions

- Arrange for tests to evaluate serum creatinine, BUN, creatinine clearance, magnesium, calcium, potassium levels before initiating therapy and before each subcourse of therapy. Do not give if there is evidence of nephrotoxicity.
- Arrange for audiometric testing before beginning therapy and prior to subsequent doses. Do not give dose if audiometric acuity is outside normal limits.
- Do not use needles of IV sets containing aluminum parts; can cause precipitate and loss of drug potency. Use gloves while preparing drug to prevent contact with the skin or mucosa; contact can cause skin reactions. If contact occurs, wash area immediately with soap and water.
- Maintain adequate hydration and urinary output for the 24 hr following drug therapy.
- Use an antiemetic if nausea and vomiting are severe (metoclopramide).
- Monitor uric acid levels; if markedly increased, allopurinol may be ordered.
- Monitor electrolytes and maintain by supplements.

Adverse effects in *Italics* are most common; those in **Bold** are life-threatening.

Teaching points

- This drug can only be given IV. Prepare a calendar of treatment days.
- These side effects may occur: nausea, vomiting (medication may be ordered; small frequent meals also may help); numbness, tingling, loss of taste, ringing in the ears, dizziness, loss of hearing (reversible).
- Use birth control; drug may cause birth defects or miscarriages.
- Have frequent, regular medical follow-up, including frequent blood tests to monitor drug effects.
- Report loss of hearing, dizziness; unusual bleeding or bruising, fever, chills, sore throat, leg cramps, muscle twitching, changes in voiding patterns.

▽ citalopram hydrobromide
(si tal' oh pram)

Celexa

PREGNANCY CATEGORY C

Drug classes
Antidepressant
SSRI

Therapeutic actions
Potentiates serotonergic activity in the CNS by inhibiting neuronal reuptake of serotonin, resulting in antidepressant effect, with little effect on norepinephrine or dopamine reuptake.

Indications
- Treatment of depression, particularly effective in major depressive disorders
- Unlabeled uses: Treatment of alcoholism, panic disorder, PMDD, social phobia, trichotillomania.

Contraindications and cautions
- Contraindicated with MAO inhibitor use; allergy to drug or any component of the drug or other SSRIs.
- Use cautiously with renal or hepatic impairment, the elderly, pregnancy, lactation, suicidal patients.

Available forms
Tablets—20, 40 mg; oral solution—10 mg/5 mL

Dosages
Adults
Initially 20 mg/day PO as a single daily dose. May be increased to 40 mg/day if needed.
Pediatric patients
Safety and efficacy not established.
Geriatric patients or patients with renal or hepatic impairment
20 mg/day PO as a single dose; increase to 40 mg/day only if clearly needed and patient is not responding.

Pharmacokinetics

Route	Onset	Peak
Oral	Slow	2–4 hr

Metabolism: Hepatic; $T_{1/2}$: 35 hr
Distribution: Crosses placenta; passes into breast milk
Excretion: Urine

Adverse effects
- **CNS:** *Somnolence, dizziness, insomnia, tremor,* nervousness, headache, anxiety, paresthesia, blurred vision
- **CV:** Palpitations, vasodilation, orthostatic hypotension, hypertension
- **Dermatologic:** *Sweating,* rash, redness
- **GI:** *Nausea, dry mouth,* constipation, diarrhea, anorexia, flatulence, vomiting
- **GU:** *Ejaculatory disorders*
- **Respiratory:** Sinusitis, URI, cough, rhinitis

Interactions
✳ **Drug-drug** ● Increased citalopram levels and toxicity if taken with MAOIs; ensure that patient has been off the MAOI for at least 14 days before administering citalopram ● Increased citalopram levels with azole antifungals ● Possible severe adverse effects if combined with tricyclic antidepressants, erythromycin; use caution ● Possible increased effects of beta blockers; monitor patient and reduce beta blocker dose as needed ● Possible increased bleeding with warfarin, monitor patient carefully

✳ **Drug-alternative therapy** ● Increased risk of severe reaction if combined with St. John's wort therapy.

■ Nursing considerations

 CLINICAL ALERT!
Name confusion has occurred between Celexa (citalopram), Celebrex (celecoxib), Xanax (alprazolam), and Cerebyx (fosphenytoin); use caution.

Assessment
- **History:** MAO inhibitor use; allergy to drug or any component of the drug; renal or hepatic impairment, the elderly, pregnancy, lactation, suicidal tendencies
- **Physical:** Orientation, reflexes; P, BP, perfusion; bowel sounds, normal output; urinary output; liver evaluation; liver and renal function tests

Interventions
- Administer once a day, in the morning; may be taken with food if desired.
- Encourage patient to continue use for 4–6 wk, as directed, to ensure adequate levels to affect depression.
- Limit amount of drug given in prescription to potentially suicidal patients.
- Establish appropriate safety precautions if patient experiences adverse CNS effects.
- Institute appropriate therapy for patient suffering from depression.

Teaching points
- Take this drug exactly as directed, and as long as directed; it may take a few weeks to realize the benefits of the drug. The drug may be taken with food if desired.
- These side effects may occur: drowsiness, dizziness, tremor (use caution and avoid driving a car or performing other tasks that require alertness if you experience daytime drowsiness); GI upset (small, frequent meals, frequent mouth care may help); alterations in sexual function (it may help to know that this is a drug effect, and will pass when drug therapy is ended).
- Be aware that this drug should not be taken during pregnancy or when nursing a baby; use of barrier contraceptives is suggested.
- Report severe nausea, vomiting; palpitations; blurred vision; excessive sweating.

▽ cladribine (CdA, 2-chlorodeoxyadenosine)
(kla' dri been)

Leustatin

PREGNANCY CATEGORY D

Drug class
Antineoplastic

Therapeutic actions
Blocks DNA synthesis and repair, causing cell death in active and resting lymphocytes and monocytes.

Indications
- Treatment of active hairy cell leukemia
- Unlabeled uses: advanced cutaneous T-cell lymphomas, chronic lymphocytic leukemia, non-Hodgkin's lymphomas, acute myeloid leukemia, autoimmune hemolytic anemia, mycosis fungoides, Sezary syndrome

Contraindications and cautions
- Contraindicated with hypersensitivity to cladribine or any components, pregnancy, lactation.
- Use cautiously with active infection, myelosuppression, debilitating illness, renal or hepatic impairment.

Available forms
IV solution—1 mg/mL

Dosages
Adults
Single course given by continuous IV infusion of 0.09 mg/kg/day for 7 days.
Pediatric patients
Safety and efficacy not established.

Pharmacokinetics

Route	Onset	Peak
IV	Rapid	8–10 hr

Metabolism: Hepatic; $T_{1/2}$: 5.4 hr
Distribution: Crosses placenta; may enter breast milk
Excretion: Urine

Adverse effects in *Italics* are most common; those in **Bold** are life-threatening.

▽IV facts

Preparation: Prepare daily dose by adding calculated dose to 500-mL bag of 0.9% sodium chloride injection. Stable for 24 hr at room temperature. Prepare 7-day infusion using aseptic technique, and add calculated dose to 100 mL bacteriostatic, 0.9% sodium chloride injection (0.9% benzyl alcohol preserved) through a sterile 0.22-µm filter. Store unopened vials in refrigerator, and protect from light. Vials are single-use only, discard after use.

Infusion: Infuse daily dose slowly over 24 hr. 7-day dose should be infused continuously over the 7-day period.

Incompatibilities: Do not mix with any other solutions, drugs, or additives. Do not infuse through IV line with any other drug or additive.

Adverse effects

- **CNS:** *Fatigue, headache,* dizziness, insomnia, **neurotoxicity**
- **CV:** Tachycardia, edema
- **Dermatologic:** *Rash,* pruritus, pain, erythema, petechiae, purpura
- **GI:** *Nausea, anorexia, vomiting, diarrhea,* constipation, abdominal pain
- **GU:** *Nephrotoxicity*
- **Hematologic:** *Neutropenia,* **myelosuppression,** anemia, thrombocytopenia
- **Local:** *Injection site redness, swelling, pain;* thrombosis, phlebitis
- **Respiratory:** *Cough, abnormal breath sounds,* shortness of breath
- **Other:** *Fever, chills,* asthenia, diaphoresis, myalgia, arthralgia, **infection,** cancer

■ Nursing considerations
Assessment

- **History:** Allergy to cladribine or any component, renal or hepatic impairment, myelosuppression, infection, pregnancy, lactation
- **Physical:** Weight, skin condition, neurologic status, abdominal exam, P, respiratory status, kidney and liver function tests, CBC, uric acid levels

Interventions

- Use disposable gloves and protective garments when handling cladribine. If drug contacts skin or mucous membranes, wash

immediately with copious amounts of water.

- Ensure continuous infusion of drug over 7 days.
- Alert child-bearing–age patients to drug's severe effects on fetus; advise using birth control during and for several weeks after treatment.
- Monitor complete hematologic profile, renal and liver function tests before and frequently during treatment. Consult with physician at first sign of toxicity; consider delaying or discontinuing dose if neurotoxicity or renal toxicity occur.

Teaching points

- This drug must be given continuously for 7 days.
- Frequent monitoring of blood tests is needed during the treatment and for several weeks thereafter to assess the drug's effect.
- Use of barrier contraceptives is advised during therapy and for several weeks following therapy.
- These side effects may occur: fever, headache, rash, nausea, vomiting, fatigue, pain at injection site.
- Report numbness or tingling, severe headache, nausea, rash, extreme fatigue, edema, pain or swelling at injection site.

▽ clarithromycin
*(klar **ith'** ro my sin)*

Biaxin, Biaxin XL

PREGNANCY CATEGORY B

Drug class
Macrolide antibiotic

Therapeutic actions
Inhibits protein synthesis in susceptible bacteria, causing cell death.

Indications

- Treatment of upper respiratory infections caused by *S. pyogenes, S. pneumoniae*
- Treatment of lower respiratory infections caused by *Mycoplasma pneumoniae, S. pneumoniae, H. influenzae, M. catarrhalis*

- Treatment of skin and structure infections caused by *S. aureus, S. pyogenes*
- Treatment of disseminated mycobacterial infections due to *M. avium* and *M. intracellular*
- Treatment of active duodenal ulcer with *H. pylori* in combination with proton pump inhibitor
- Treatment of acute otitis media, acute maxillary sinusitis due to *H. influenzae, M. cararrhalis, S. pneumoniae*
- Treatment of mild to moderate community-acquired pneumonia in adults (ER tablets)

Contraindications and cautions

- Contraindicated with hypersensitivity to clarithromycin, erythromycin, or any macrolide antibiotic.
- Use cautiously with colitis, hepatic or renal impairment, pregnancy, lactation.

Available forms

Tablets—250, 500 mg; granules for suspension—125, 250 mg/5 mL; ER tablets–500 mg

Dosages
Adults

- *Pharyngitis, tonsillitis; pneumonia due to* S. pneumoniae, M. pneumoniae; *skin or skin-structure infections; lower respiratory infections due to* S. pneumoniae, M. catarrhalis: 250 mg PO q 12 hr for 7–14 days.
- *Acute maxillary sinusitis, lower respiratory infection caused by* H. influenzae: 500 mg PO q 12 hr for 7–14 days.
- *Mycobacterial infections:* 500 mg PO bid.
- *Treatment of duodenal ulcers:* 500 mg PO tid plus omeprazole 40 mg PO q AM for 14 days, then omeprazole 20 mg PO q morning for 14 days.
- *Treatment of community-acquired pneumonia:* 500 mg/day PO of ER tablet for 7 days.

Pediatric patients

Usual dosage 15 mg/kg/day PO q 12 hr for 10 days.

- *Mycobacterial infections:* 7.5 mg/kg PO bid.

Geriatric patients or patients with impaired renal function

Decrease dosage or prolong dosing intervals as appropriate.

Pharmacokinetics

Route	Onset	Peak
Oral	Varies	2 hr

Metabolism: Hepatic; $T_{1/2}$: 3–7 hr
Distribution: Crosses placenta; enters breast milk
Excretion: Urine

Adverse effects

- **CNS:** Dizziness, headache, vertigo, somnolence, fatigue
- **GI:** *Diarrhea, abdominal pain, nausea,* dyspepsia, flatulence, vomiting, melena, **pseudomembranous colitis**
- **Other:** *Superinfections,* increased PT, decreased WBC

Interactions

✴ **Drug-drug** ● Increased serum levels and effects of carbamazepine, theophylline, lovastatin, phenytoin

✴ **Drug-food** ● Food decreases the rate of absorption of clarithromycin but does not alter effectiveness ● Decreased metabolism and risk of toxic effects if combined with grapefruit juice; avoid this combination.

■ Nursing considerations
Assessment

- **History:** Hypersensitivity to clarithromycin, erythromycin, or any macrolide antibiotic; pseudomembranous colitis, hepatic or renal impairment, lactation, pregnancy
- **Physical:** Site of infection; skin color, lesions; orientation, GI output, bowel sounds, liver evaluation; culture and sensitivity tests of infection, urinalysis, liver and renal function tests

Interventions

- Culture infection before therapy.
- Do not cut or crush, and ensure that patient does not chew ER tablets.
- Monitor patient for anticipated response.

Adverse effects in *Italics* are most common; those in **Bold** are life-threatening.

- Administer without regard to meals; administer with food if GI effects occur.

Teaching points

- Take drug with food if GI effects occur. Take the full course of therapy. Do not drink grapefruit juice while on this drug.
- Shake suspension before use; do not refrigerate; do not cut, crush, or chew ER tablets; swallow whole.
- These side effects may occur: stomach cramping, discomfort, diarrhea; fatigue, headache (medication may be ordered); additional infections in the mouth or vagina (consult with care provider for treatment).
- Report severe or watery diarrhea, severe nausea or vomiting, rash or itching, mouth sores, vaginal sores.

▽ clemastine fumarate

(klem' as teen)

Antihist-1, Tavist

PREGNANCY CATEGORY B

Drug class

Antihistamine

Therapeutic actions

Blocks the effects of histamine at H_1-receptor sites; has atropine-like, antipruritic, and sedative effects.

Indications

- Symptomatic relief of symptoms associated with perennial and seasonal allergic rhinitis; vasomotor rhinitis; allergic conjunctivitis
- Mild, uncomplicated urticaria and angioedema

Contraindications and cautions

- Contraindicated with allergy to any antihistamines, third trimester of pregnancy, lactation.
- Use cautiously in the presence of narrow-angle glaucoma, stenosing peptic ulcer, symptomatic prostatic hypertrophy, asthmatic attack, bladder neck obstruction, pyloroduodenal obstruction.

Available forms

Tablets—1.34, 2.68 mg; syrup—0.67 mg/ 5 mL

Dosages

Adults and patients > 12 yr

- *Allergic rhinitis:* 1.34 mg PO bid. Do not exceed 8.04 mg/day.
- *Urticaria or angioedema:* 2.68 mg PO daily–tid. Do not exceed 8.04 mg/day.

Pediatric patients 6–12 yr

- *Allergic rhinitis:* 0.67 mg PO as syrup bid. Do not exceed 4.02 mg/day.
- *Urticaria or angioedema:* 1.34 mg PO as syrup bid. Do not exceed 4.02 mg/day.

Pediatric patients < 6 yr

Safety and efficacy not established.

Geriatric patients

More likely to cause dizziness, sedation, syncope, toxic confusional states, and hypotension in elderly patients; use with caution.

Pharmacokinetics

Route	Onset	Peak	Duration
Oral	15–30 min	1–2 hr	12 hr

Metabolism: Hepatic; $T_{1/2}$: 3–4 hr
Distribution: Crosses placenta; enters breast milk
Excretion: Urine

Adverse effects

- **CNS:** *Drowsiness, sedation, dizziness, disturbed coordination,* fatigue, confusion, restlessness, excitation, nervousness, tremor, headache, blurred vision, diplopia, vertigo, tinnitus, acute labyrinthitis, hysteria, tingling, heaviness and weakness of the hands
- **CV:** Hypotension, palpitations, bradycardia, tachycardia, extrasystoles
- **GI:** *Epigastric distress,* anorexia, increased appetite and weight gain, nausea, vomiting, diarrhea or constipation
- **GU:** Urinary frequency, dysuria, urinary retention, early menses, decreased libido, impotence
- **Hematologic:** Hemolytic anemia, hypoplastic anemia, thrombocytopenia, leukopenia, agranulocytosis, pancytopenia
- **Respiratory:** *Thickening of bronchial secretions,* chest tightness, wheezing, nasal stuffiness, dry mouth, dry nose, dry throat, sore throat

- **Other:** Urticaria, rash, **anaphylactic shock,** photosensitivity, excessive perspiration, chills

Interactions
✳ **Drug-drug** • Increased depressant effects with alcohol, other CNS depressants • Increased and prolonged anticholinergic (drying) effects with MAO inhibitors; avoid this combination.

■ Nursing considerations
Assessment
- **History:** Allergy to any antihistamines; narrow-angle glaucoma, stenosing peptic ulcer, symptomatic prostatic hypertrophy, asthmatic attack, bladder neck obstruction, pyloroduodenal obstruction; lactation
- **Physical:** Skin color, lesions, texture; orientation, reflexes, affect; vision exam; P, BP; R, adventitious sounds; bowel sounds; prostate palpation; CBC with differential

Interventions
- Administer with food if GI upset occurs.
- Administer syrup form if patient is unable to take tablets; children 6–12 yr should only receive syrup form.
- Monitor patient response, adjust to lowest possible effective dose.

Teaching points
- Take drug as prescribed; avoid excessive dosage.
- Take with food if GI upset occurs.
- These side effects may occur: dizziness, sedation, drowsiness (use caution if driving or performing tasks that require alertness); epigastric distress, diarrhea, or constipation (take with meals; consult care provider); dry mouth (frequent mouth care, sucking sugarless lozenges may help); thickening of bronchial secretions, dryness of nasal mucosa (use a humidifier).
- Avoid alcohol; serious sedation could occur.
- Report difficulty breathing, hallucinations, tremors, loss of coordination, unusual bleeding or bruising, visual disturbances, irregular heartbeat.

▷**clindamycin**
(klin da mye' sin)

clindamycin hydrochloride
Oral: Cleocin, Cleocin Suppository, Dalacin C (CAN)

clindamycin palmitate hydrochloride
Oral: Cleocin Pediatric

clindamycin phosphate
Oral, parenteral, topical dermatologic solution for acne, vaginal preparation: Cleocin Phosphate, Cleocin T, Clinda-Derm (CAN), Dalacin C (CAN), Cleocin Vaginal Ovules

PREGNANCY CATEGORY B

Drug class
Lincosamide antibiotic

Therapeutic actions
Inhibits protein synthesis in susceptible bacteria, causing cell death.

Indications
- *Systemic administration:* Serious infections caused by susceptible strains of anaerobes, streptococci, staphylococci, pneumococci; reserve use for penicillin-allergic patients or when penicillin is inappropriate; less toxic antibiotics (erythromycin) should be considered
- *Parenteral form:* Treatment of septicemia caused by staphylococci, streptococci; acute hematogenous osteomyelitis; adjunct to surgical treatment of chronic bone and joint infections due to susceptible organisms; do not use to treat meningitis; does not cross the blood–brain barrier.
- *Topical dermatologic solution:* Treatment of acne vulgaris
- *Vaginal preparation:* Treatment of bacterial vaginosis

Contraindications and cautions

- *Systemic administration:* Allergy to clindamycin, history of asthma or other allergies, tartrazine (in 75- and 150-mg capsules); hepatic or renal dysfunction; lactation. Use caution in newborns and infants due to benzyl alcohol content; associated with gasping syndrome.
- *Topical dermatologic solution, vaginal preparation:* Allergy to clindamycin or lincomycin; history of regional enteritis or ulcerative colitis; history of antibiotic-associated colitis.

Available forms

Capsules—75, 150, 300 mg; granules for oral solution—75 mg/5 mL; injection—150 mg/mL; topical gel—10 mg; topical lotion—10 mg; topical solution—10 mg; vaginal cream—2%; vaginal suppository—100 mg

Dosages
Adults
Oral
150–300 mg q 6 hr, up to 300–450 mg q 6 hr in more severe infections.
Parenteral
600–2,700 mg/day in two to four equal doses; up to 4.8 g/day IV or IM may be used for life-threatening situations.
Vaginal preparations
One applicator (100 mg clindamycin phosphate) intravaginally, preferably at hs for 7 consecutive days; or insert vaginal suppository, preferably at hs for 7 consecutive days, 3 days for Cleocin Vaginal Ovules.
Topical
Apply a thin film to affected area bid.
Pediatric patients
Oral
- *Clindamycin HCl:* 8–20 mg/kg/day in three or four equal doses.
- *Clindamycin palmitate HCl:* 8–25 mg/kg/day in three or four equal doses.; children weighing < 10 kg—use 37.5 mg tid as the minimum dose.
Parenteral
> *1 mo:* 15–40 mg/kg/day in three or four equal doses or 300 mg/m²/day to 400 mg/m²/day; in severe infections, give 300 mg/day regardless of weight.
Neonates: 15–20 mg/kg/day in three or four equal doses.

Geriatric patients or patients with renal failure
Reduce dose, and monitor patient's serum levels carefully.

Pharmacokinetics

Route	Onset	Peak	Duration
Oral	Varies	1–2 hr	8–12 hr
IM	20–30 min	1–3 hr	8–12 hr
IV	Immediate	Minutes	8–12 hr
Topical	Minimal systemic absorption		

Metabolism: Hepatic; $T_{1/2}$: 2–3 hr
Distribution: Crosses placenta; enters breast milk
Excretion: Urine and feces

▽ IV facts

Preparation: Store unreconstituted product at room temperature. Reconstitute by adding 75 mL of water to 100-mL bottle of palmitate in two portions. Shake well; do not refrigerate reconstituted solution. Reconstituted solution is stable for 2 wk at room temperature. Dilute reconstituted solution to a concentration of 300 mg/50 mL or more of diluent using 0.9% sodium chloride injection, 5% dextrose injection, or lactated Ringer's solution. Solution is stable for 16 days at room temperature.

Infusion: Do not administer more than 1,200 mg in a single 1-hr infusion. Infusion rates: 300 mg in 50 mL diluent, 10 min; 600 mg in 50 mL diluent, 20 min; 900 mg in 50–100 mL diluent, 30 min; 1,200 mg in 100 mL diluent, 40 min.

Incompatibilities: Do not mix with calcium gluconate, ampicillin, phenytoin, barbiturates, aminophylline, and magnesium sulfate. May be mixed with sodium chloride, dextrose, calcium, potassium, vitamin B complex, cephalothin, kanamycin, gentamicin, penicillin, carbenicillin. Incompatible in syringe with tobramycin.

Adverse effects
Systemic administration
- **CV:** Hypotension, **cardiac arrest** (with rapid IV infusion)
- **GI:** Severe colitis, including **pseudomembranous colitis**, *nausea, vomiting, diarrhea, abdominal pain, esophagi-*

tis, anorexia, jaundice, liver function changes
- **Hematologic:** Neutropenia, leukopenia, agranulocytosis, eosinophilia
- **Hypersensitivity:** *Rashes,* urticaria to anaphylactoid reactions
- **Local:** *Pain following injection,* induration and sterile abscess after IM injection, thrombophlebitis after IV use

Topical dermatologic solution
- **CNS:** *Fatigue, headache*
- **Dermatologic:** *Contact dermatitis, dryness,* gram-negative folliculitis
- **GI: Pseudomembranous colitis,** diarrhea, bloody diarrhea; abdominal pain, sore throat
- **GU:** Urinary frequency

Vaginal preparation
- **GU:** *Cervicitis, vaginitis,* vulvar irritation

Interactions
Systemic administration
❋ **Drug-drug** • Increased neuromuscular blockade with neuromuscular blocking agents
• Decreased GI absorption with kaolin, aluminum salts

■ Nursing considerations
Assessment
- **History:** Allergy to clindamycin, history of asthma or other allergies, allergy to tartrazine (in 75- and 150-mg capsules); hepatic or renal dysfunction; lactation; history of regional enteritis or ulcerative colitis; history of antibiotic associated colitis
- **Physical:** Site of infection or acne; skin color, lesions; BP; R, adventitious sounds; bowel sounds, output, liver evaluation; complete blood count, renal and liver function tests

Interventions
Systemic administration
- Administer oral drug with a full glass of water or with food to prevent esophageal irritation.
- Do not give IM injections of more than 600 mg; inject deep into large muscle to avoid serious problems.
- Culture infection before therapy.
- Do not use for minor bacterial or viral infections.

- Monitor renal and liver function tests, and blood counts with prolonged therapy.

Topical dermatologic administration
- Keep solution away from eyes, mouth, and abraded skin or mucous membranes; alcohol base will cause stinging. Shake well before use.
- Keep cool tap water available to bathe eye, mucous membranes, abraded skin inadvertently contacted by drug solution.

Vaginal preparation
- Give intravaginally, preferably at hs.

Teaching points
Systemic administration
- Take oral drug with a full glass of water or with food.
- Take full prescribed course of oral drug. Do not stop taking without notifying health care provider.
- Report severe or watery diarrhea, abdominal pain, inflamed mouth or vagina, skin rash or lesions.
- These side effects may occur: nausea, vomiting (small frequent meals may help); superinfections in the mouth, vagina (use frequent hygiene measures, request treatment if severe).

Topical dermatologic administration
- Apply thin film of acne solution to affected area twice daily, being careful to avoid eyes, mucous membranes, abraded skin; if solution contacts one of these areas, flush with copious amounts of cool water.
- Report abdominal pain, diarrhea.

Vaginal preparation
- Use vaginal preparation for 7 or 3 consecutive days, preferably at bedtime. Refrain from sexual intercourse during treatment with this product.
- Report vaginal irritation, itching; diarrhea, no improvement in complaint being treated.

▷ clofazimine

See *Less Commonly Used Drugs,* p. 1340.

Adverse effects in *Italics* are most common; those in **Bold** are life-threatening.

▽clofibrate
(kloe fye' brate)

Atromid-S, Claripex (CAN)

PREGNANCY CATEGORY C

Drug class
Antihyperlipidemic

Therapeutic actions
Stimulates the liver to increase breakdown of VLDL to LDL; decreases liver synthesis of VLDL; inhibits cholesterol formation, lowering serum lipid levels; has antiplatelet effect.

Indications
- Primary dysbetalipoproteinemia (type III hyperlipidemia) that does not respond to diet
- Very high serum triglycerides (type IV and V hyperlipidemia) with abdominal pain and pancreatitis that does not respond to diet

Contraindications and cautions
- Allergy to clofibrate, hepatic or renal dysfunction, primary biliary cirrhosis, peptic ulcer, pregnancy, lactation.

Available forms
Capsules—500 mg

Dosages
Adults
2 g/day PO in divided doses. Caution: use this drug only if strongly indicated, and lipid studies show a definite response; hepatic tumorigenicity occurs in lab animals.
Pediatric patients
Safety and efficacy not established.

Pharmacokinetics

Route	Onset	Peak	Duration
Oral	Varies	3–6 hr	Weeks

Metabolism: Hepatic; $T_{1/2}$: 15 hr
Distribution: Crosses placenta; enters breast milk
Excretion: Urine

Adverse effects
- **CV:** Angina, arrhythmias, swelling, phlebitis, thrombophlebitis, pulmonary emboli
- **Dermatologic:** *Rash,* alopecia, dry skin, dry and brittle hair, pruritus, urticaria
- **GI:** *Nausea,* vomiting, diarrhea, dyspepsia, flatulence, bloating, stomatitis, gastritis, gallstones (with long-term therapy), peptic ulcer, GI hemorrhage, **hepatic tumors**
- **GU:** *Impotence, decreased libido,* dysuria, hematuria, proteinuria, decreased urine output
- **Hematologic:** Leukopenia, anemia, eosinophilia, increased AST and ALT, increased thymol turbidity, increased CPK, BSP retention
- **Other:** *Myalgia, flu-like syndromes,* arthralgia, weight gain, polyphagia, increased perspiration, systemic lupus erythematosus, blurred vision, gynecomastia

Interactions
✳ **Drug-drug** • Increased bleeding tendencies if oral anticoagulants are also given; reduce dosage of anticoagulant, usually by 50% • Increased pharmacologic effects of sulfonylureas, insulin, with resultant increased risk of hypoglycemia • Increased risk of rhabdomyolysis with HMG-CoA reductase inhibitors • Increased clofibrate effects with probenecid

■ Nursing considerations
Assessment
- **History:** Allergy to clofibrate, hepatic or renal dysfunction, primary biliary cirrhosis, peptic ulcer, lactation, pregnancy
- **Physical:** Skin lesions, color, T; P, BP, auscultation, baseline ECG, peripheral perfusion, edema; bowel sounds, normal output, liver evaluation; normal output; lipid studies, CBC, clotting profile, liver and renal function tests, urinalysis

Interventions
- Administer drug with meals or milk if GI upset occurs.
- Arrange for regular follow-up including blood tests for lipids, liver function, CBC during long-term therapy.
- Monitor urine output.

Teaching points
- Take the drug with meals or with milk if GI upset occurs.
- These side effects may occur: diarrhea, loss of appetite (eat small frequent meals); dry

skin, dry and brittle hair, excessive sweating (frequent skin care, use of nonabrasive lotion may help); loss of libido, impotence.
- Have regular follow-ups for blood tests.
- Report chest pain, shortness of breath, palpitations, severe stomach pain with nausea and vomiting, fever and chills or sore throat, blood in the urine, little urine output, swelling of the ankles or legs, unusual weight gain.

▷clomiphene citrate
(kloe' mi feen)

Clomid, Milophene, Serophene

PREGNANCY CATEGORY X

Drug classes
Hormone
Fertility drug

Therapeutic actions
Binds to estrogen receptors, decreasing the number of available estrogen receptors, which gives the hypothalamus the false signal to increase FSH and LH secretion, resulting in ovarian stimulation.

Indications
- Treatment of ovarian failure in patients with normal liver function and normal endogenous estrogen levels, whose partners are fertile and potent
- Unlabeled use: treatment of male infertility

Contraindications and cautions
- Known sensitivity to clomiphene, liver disease, abnormal bleeding of undetermined origin, ovarian cyst, lactation, pregnancy

Available forms
Tablets—50 mg

Dosages
- *Treatment of ovarian failure:*
Initial therapy: 50 mg/day PO for 5 days started anytime there has been no recent uterine bleeding or about the fifth day of the cycle if uterine bleeding does occur.

Second course: If ovulation does not occur after the first course, administer 100 mg/day PO for 5 days; start this course as early as 30 days after the previous one.
Third course: Repeat second course regimen; if patient does not respond to three courses of treatment, further treatment is not recommended.
- *Male sterility:* 50–400 mg/day PO for 2–12 mo (controversial).

Pharmacokinetics

Route	Onset	Duration
Oral	5–8 days	6 wk

Metabolism: Hepatic; $T_{1/2}$: 5 days
Distribution: Crosses placenta
Excretion: Feces

Adverse effects
- **CNS:** Visual symptoms (blurring, spots, flashes), nervousness, insomnia, dizziness, light-headedness
- **CV:** *Vasomotor flushing*
- **GI:** *Abdominal discomfort, distention, bloating, nausea, vomiting*
- **GU:** Uterine bleeding, *ovarian enlargement*, **ovarian overstimulation,** birth defects in resulting pregnancies
- **Other:** *Breast tenderness*

Interactions
✳ **Drug-lab test** • Increased levels of serum thyroxine, thyroxine-binding globulin

■ Nursing considerations

 CLINICAL ALERT!
Name confusion has occurred between Serophene (clomiphene) and Sarafem (fluoxetine); use caution.

Assessment
- **History:** Sensitivity to clomiphene, liver disease, abnormal bleeding of undetermined origin, ovarian cyst, pregnancy
- **Physical:** Skin color, T; affect, orientation, ophthalmologic exam; abdominal exam, pelvic exam, liver evaluation; urinary estrogens and estriol levels (women); liver function tests

Interventions

- Complete a pelvic exam before each treatment to rule out ovarian enlargement, pregnancy, other uterine difficulties.
- Check urine estrogen and estriol levels before therapy; normal levels indicate appropriate patient selection.
- Refer for complete ophthalmic exam; if visual symptoms occur, discontinue drug.
- Discontinue drug at any sign of ovarian overstimulation, admit patient to hospital for observation and supportive measures.
- Provide women with calendar of treatment days and explanations about signs of estrogen and progesterone activity; caution patient that 24-hr urine collections will be needed periodically; timing of intercourse is important for achieving pregnancy.
- Alert to risks and hazards of multiple births.
- Explain failure to respond after 3 courses of therapy probably means drug will not help, and treatment will be discontinued.

Teaching points

- Prepare a calendar showing the treatment schedule, plotting ovulation.
- These side effects may occur: abdominal distention; flushing; breast tenderness; dizziness, drowsiness, light-headedness, visual disturbances (use caution driving or performing tasks that require alertness).
- There is an increased incidence of multiple births in women using this drug.
- Report bloating, stomach pain, blurred vision, yellow skin or eyes, unusual bleeding or bruising, fever, chills, visual changes.

▽clomipramine hydrochloride

(kloe mi' pra meen)

Anafranil, Apo-Clomipramine (CAN), Gen-Clomipramine (CAN), Novo-Clopamine (CAN)

PREGNANCY CATEGORY C

Drug class

Tricyclic antidepressant (TCA; tertiary amine)

Therapeutic actions

Mechanism unknown; inhibits the presynaptic reuptake of the neurotransmitters norepinephrine and serotonin; anticholinergic at CNS and peripheral receptors; sedative.

Indications

- Treatment of obsessions and compulsions in patients with obsessive-compulsive disorder (OCD), whose obsessions or compulsions cause marked distress, are time-consuming, or interfere with social or occupational functioning.
- Unlabeled uses: panic disorders, PMS, depression.

Contraindications and cautions

- Contraindicated with hypersensitivity to any tricyclic drug, concomitant therapy with an MAO inhibitor, recent MI, myelography within previous 24 hr or scheduled within 48 hr, lactation.
- Use cautiously with allergy to dibenzazepines, EST, preexisting CV disorders (eg, severe coronary heart disease, progressive heart failure, angina pectoris, paroxysmal tachycardia); angle-closure glaucoma, increased intraocular pressure, urinary retention, ureteral or urethral spasm; seizure disorders; hyperthyroidism; impaired hepatic, renal function; psychiatric patients (schizophrenic or paranoid patients may exhibit a worsening of psychosis with TCA therapy); manic-depressive patients; elective surgery.

Available forms

Capsules—25, 50, 75 mg

Dosages
Adults

Initial: 25 mg PO daily; gradually increase as tolerated to approximately 100 mg during the first 2 wk. Then increase gradually over the next several weeks to a maximum dose of 250 mg/day. At maximum dose, give once a day hs to minimize sedation.
Maintenance: Adjust to maintain the lowest effective dosage, and periodically assess need for treatment. Effectiveness after 10 wk has not been documented.
Pediatric patients
Initial: 25 mg PO daily; gradually increase as tolerated during the first 2 wk to a maximum

of 3 mg/kg or 100 mg, whichever is smaller. Then increase dosage to a daily maximum of 3 mg/kg or 200 mg, whichever is smaller. At maximum give once a day hs to minimize sedation.

Maintenance: Adjust dosage to maintain lowest effective dosage, and periodically assess patient to determine the need for treatment. Effectiveness after 10 wk has not been documented.

Pharmacokinetics

Route	Onset	Duration
Oral	Slow	1–6 wk

Metabolism: Hepatic; $T_{1/2}$: 21–31 hr
Distribution: Crosses placenta; enters breast milk
Excretion: Bile, feces

Adverse effects

- **CNS:** *Sedation and anticholinergic (atropine-like) effects; confusion* (especially in elderly), *disturbed concentration,* hallucinations, disorientation, decreased memory, feelings of unreality, delusions, anxiety, nervousness, restlessness, agitation, panic, insomnia, nightmares, hypomania, mania, *asthenia, aggressive reaction*
- **CV:** *Orthostatic hypotension,* hypertension, syncope, tachycardia, palpitations, MI, arrhythmias, heart block, precipitation of CHF, stroke
- **Endocrine:** Elevated or depressed blood sugar; elevated prolactin levels; SIADH secretion
- **GI:** *Dry mouth, constipation,* paralytic ileus, *nausea,* vomiting, anorexia, epigastric distress, diarrhea, flatulence, dysphagia, peculiar taste, increased salivation, stomatitis, parotid swelling, abdominal cramps, black tongue, *eructation*
- **GU:** Urinary retention, delayed micturition, dilation of the urinary tract, gynecomastia, testicular swelling; breast enlargement, *menstrual irregularity* and galactorrhea in women; increased or decreased libido; *impotence*
- **Hematologic:** Bone marrow depression, including agranulocytosis; eosinophilia, purpura, thrombocytopenia, leukopenia, *anemia*
- **Hypersensitivity:** Skin rash, pruritus, vasculitis, petechiae, photosensitization, edema (generalized, facial, tongue), drug fever
- **Withdrawal:** Symptoms on abrupt discontinuation of prolonged therapy: nausea, headache, vertigo, nightmares, malaise
- **Other:** *Nasal congestion, laryngitis,* excessive appetite, weight change; sweating hyperthermia, flushing, chills

Interactions

✳ Drug-drug • Increased TCA levels and pharmacologic effects with cimetidine • Increased TCA levels with fluoxetine, methylphenidate, phenothiazines, oral contraceptives, disulfiram • Hyperpyretic crises, severe convulsions, hypertensive episodes and deaths when MAO inhibitors, furazolidone, clonidine are given with TCAs • Increased antidepressant response and cardiac arrhythmias when given with thyroid medication • Increased anticholinergic effects of anticholinergic drugs when given with TCAs • Increased response to alcohol, barbiturates, benzodiazepines, other CNS depressants with TCAs • Decreased effects of indirect-acting sympathomimetic drugs (ephedrine) with TCAs • Risk of arrhythmias if combined with fluoroquinolones

■ Nursing considerations
Assessment

- **History:** Hypersensitivity to any tricyclic drug; concomitant therapy with an MAO inhibitor; recent MI; myelography within previous 24 hr or scheduled within 48 hr; lactation; EST; preexisting CV disorders; angle-closure glaucoma, increased intraocular pressure, urinary retention, ureteral or urethral spasm; seizure disorders; hyperthyroidism, impaired hepatic, renal function; psychiatric patients; elective surgery, pregnancy.
- **Physical:** Weight; T; skin color, lesions; orientation, affect, reflexes, vision and hearing; P, BP, orthostatic BP, perfusion; bowel sounds, normal output, liver evaluation; urine flow, normal output; usual sexual function, frequency of menses, breast and

---

Adverse effects in *Italics* are most common; those in **Bold** are life-threatening.

scrotal exam; liver function tests, urinalysis, CBC, ECG.

Interventions

- Limit depressed and potentially suicidal patients' access to drug.
- Administer in divided doses with meals to reduce GI side effects while increasing dosage to therapeutic levels.
- Give maintenance dose once daily hs to decrease daytime sedation.
- Reduce dose if minor side effects develop; discontinue drug if serious side effects occur.
- Arrange for CBC if patient develops fever, sore throat, or other signs of infection.

Teaching points

- Take this drug as prescribed; do not to stop taking abruptly or without consulting health care provider.
- Avoid alcohol, sleep-inducing drugs, OTC drugs.
- Avoid prolonged exposure to sun or sunlamps; use a sunscreen or protective garments if exposure to sun is unavoidable.
- These side effects may occur: headache, dizziness, drowsiness, weakness, blurred vision (reversible; take safety measures if severe; avoid driving or performing tasks that require alertness); nausea, vomiting, loss of appetite, dry mouth (small, frequent meals; frequent mouth care; and sucking sugarless candies may help); nightmares, inability to concentrate, confusion; changes in sexual function.
- Report dry mouth, difficulty urinating, excessive sedation.

▽clonazepam

*(kloe **na' ze pam**)*

Apo-Clonazepam (CAN), Clonapam (CAN), Gen-Clonazepam (CAN), Klonopin, Rivotril (CAN)

PREGNANCY CATEGORY D

C-IV CONTROLLED SUBSTANCE

Drug classes

Benzodiazepine
Antiepileptic agent

Therapeutic actions

Exact mechanisms not understood; benzodiazepines potentiate the effects of GABA, an inhibitory neurotransmitter.

Indications

- Used alone or as adjunct in treatment of Lennox-Gastaut syndrome (petit mal variant), akinetic and myoclonic seizures; may be useful in patients with absence (petit mal) seizures who have not responded to succinimides; up to 30% of patients show loss of effectiveness of drug, often within 3 mo of therapy (may respond to dosage adjustment)
- Unlabeled uses: treatment of panic attacks, periodic leg movements during sleep, hypokinetic dysarthria, acute manic episodes, multifocal tic disorders, adjunct treatment of schizophrenia, neuralgias

Contraindications and cautions

- Contraindicated with hypersensitivity to benzodiazepines, psychoses, acute narrow-angle glaucoma, shock, coma, acute alcoholic intoxication with depression of vital signs; pregnancy (risk of congenital malformations, neonatal withdrawal syndrome), labor and delivery ("floppy infant" syndrome), lactation (infants become lethargic and lose weight).
- Use cautiously with impaired liver or kidney function, debilitation.

Available forms

Tablets—0.5, 1, 2 mg

Dosages

Individualize dosage; increase dosage gradually to avoid adverse effects; drug is available only in oral dosage forms.

Adults

Initial dose should not exceed 1.5 mg/day PO divided into 3 doses; increase in increments of 0.5–1 mg PO every 3 days until seizures are adequately controlled or until side effects preclude further increases. Maximum recommended dosage is 20 mg/day.

Pediatric patients ≤ 10 yr or 30 kg

0.01–0.03 mg/kg/day PO initially; do not exceed 0.05 mg/kg/day PO, given in 2 to 3 doses. Increase dosage by not more than 0.25–0.5 mg every third day until a daily maintenance dose of 0.1–0.2 mg/kg has been reached, unless seizures are controlled by lower dosage or side effects preclude increases. Whenever possible, divide daily dose into three equal doses, or give largest dose hs.

Pharmacokinetics

Route	Onset	Peak	Duration
Oral	Varies	1–2 hr	Weeks

Metabolism: Hepatic; $T_{1/2}$: 18–50 hr
Distribution: Crosses placenta; enters breast milk
Excretion: Urine

Adverse effects

- **CNS:** *Transient, mild drowsiness initially; sedation, depression, lethargy, apathy, fatigue, light-headedness, disorientation, anger, hostility,* episodes of mania and hypomania, *restlessness, confusion, crying,* delirium, *headache,* slurred speech, dysarthria, stupor, rigidity, tremor, dystonia, vertigo, euphoria, nervousness, difficulty in concentration, vivid dreams, psychomotor retardation, extrapyramidal symptoms; *mild paradoxical excitatory reactions during first 2 weeks of treatment*
- **CV:** Bradycardia, tachycardia, CV collapse, hypertension and hypotension, palpitations, edema
- **Dermatologic:** Urticaria, pruritus, rash, dermatitis
- **EENT:** Visual and auditory disturbances, diplopia, nystagmus, depressed hearing, nasal congestion
- **GI:** *Constipation, diarrhea, dry mouth,* salivation, *nausea,* anorexia, vomiting, difficulty in swallowing, gastric disorders, hepatic dysfunction, encoporesis
- **GU:** Incontinence, urinary retention, changes in libido, menstrual irregularities
- **Hematologic:** Elevations of blood enzymes: LDH, alkaline phosphatase, AST, ALT; **blood dyscrasias: agranulocytosis, leukopenia**
- **Other:** Hiccups, fever, diaphoresis, paresthesias, muscular disturbances, gynecomastia. Drug dependence with withdrawal syndrome when drug is discontinued; more common with abrupt discontinuation of higher dosage used for longer than 4 mo.

Interactions

✳ **Drug-drug** • Increased CNS depression with alcohol • Increased effect with cimetidine, disulfiram, omeprazole, oral contraceptives • Decreased effect with theophylline • Risk of increased digoxin levels and toxicity; monitor patient carefully

■ Nursing considerations

 CLINICAL ALERT!
Name confusion has occurred between Klonopin (clonazepam) and clonidine; use caution.

Assessment

- **History:** Hypersensitivity to benzodiazepines; psychoses; acute narrow-angle glaucoma; shock; coma; acute alcoholic intoxication; pregnancy; lactation; impaired liver or kidney function, debilitation
- **Physical:** Skin color, lesions; T; orientation, reflexes, affect, ophthalmologic exam; P, BP; R, adventitious sounds; liver evaluation, abdominal exam, bowel sounds, normal output; CBC, liver and renal function tests

Interventions

- Monitor addiction-prone patients carefully because of their predisposition to habituation and drug dependence.
- Monitor liver function, blood counts periodically in patients on long-term therapy.
- Taper dosage gradually after long-term therapy, especially in epileptic patients; substitute another antiepileptic drug.
- Monitor patient for therapeutic drug levels: 20–80 ng/mL.
- Arrange for patient to wear medical alert ID indicating epilepsy and drug therapy.

Teaching points

- Take drug exactly as prescribed; do not stop taking drug (long-term therapy) without consulting health care provider.
- Avoid alcohol, sleep-inducing, or OTC drugs.
- These side effects may occur: drowsiness, dizziness (may become less pronounced; avoid driving or engaging in other dangerous activities); GI upset (take drug with

food); fatigue; dreams; crying; nervousness; depression, emotional changes; bed-wetting, urinary incontinence.
- Avoid pregnancy; serious adverse effects can occur. Use of barrier contraceptives is advised while taking this drug.
- Report severe dizziness, weakness, drowsiness that persists, rash or skin lesions, difficulty voiding, palpitations, swelling in the extremities.

▷clonidine hydrochloride
(kloe' ni deen)

Antihypertensives: Apo-Clonidine (CAN), Catapres, Catapres-TTS (transdermal preparation), Dixarit (CAN), Nu-Clonidine (CAN)
Analgesic: Duraclon

PREGNANCY CATEGORY C

Drug classes
Antihypertensive
Sympatholytic, centrally acting
Central analgesic

Therapeutic actions
Stimulates CNS alpha$_2$-adrenergic receptors, inhibits sympathetic cardioaccelerator and vasoconstrictor centers, and decreases sympathetic outflow from the CNS.

Indications
- Hypertension, used alone or as part of combination therapy
- Treatment of severe pain in cancer patients in combination with opiates; epidural more effective with neuropathic pain (*Duraclon*)
- Unlabeled uses: Tourette's syndrome; migraine, decreases severity and frequency; menopausal flushing, decreases severity and frequency of episodes; chronic methadone detoxification; rapid opiate detoxification (in doses up to 17 mcg/kg/day); alcohol and benzodiazepine withdrawal treatment; management of hypertensive "urgencies"; (oral clonidine "loading" is used; initial dose of 0.2 mg then 0.1 mg every hour until a dose of 0.7 mg is reached or until BP is controlled)

Contraindications and cautions
- Contraindicated with hypersensitivity to clonidine or any adhesive layer components of the transdermal system.
- Use cautiously with severe coronary insufficiency, recent MI, cerebrovascular disease; chronic renal failure; pregnancy, lactation.

Available forms
Tablets—0.1, 0.2, 0.3 mg; transdermal—0.1, 0.2, 0.3 mg/24 hr; epidural injection—100 mcg/mL

Dosages
Adults
Oral therapy
Individualize dosage. Initial dose: 0.1 mg bid; maintenance dose: increase in increments of 0.1 or 0.2 mg to reach desired response. Common range is 0.2–0.6 mg/day, in divided doses; maximum dose is 2.4 mg/day. Minimize sedation by slowly increasing daily dosage; giving majority of daily dose hs.
Transdermal system
Apply to a hairless area of intact skin of upper arm or torso once every 7 days. Change skin site for each application. If system loosens while wearing, apply adhesive overlay directly over the system to ensure adhesion. Start with the 0.1-mg system (releases 0.1 mg/24 hr); if, after 1–2 wk, desired BP reduction is not achieved, add another 0.1-mg system, or use a larger system. Dosage of more than two 0.3-mg systems does not improve efficacy. Antihypertensive effect may only begin 2–3 days after application; therefore, when substituting transdermal systems, a gradual reduction of prior dosage is advised. Previous antihypertensive medication may have to be continued, particularly with severe hypertension.
- *Pain management:* 30 mcg/hr by continuous epidural infusion.
Pediatric patients
Safety and efficacy not established.

Pharmacokinetics

Route	Onset	Peak	Duration
Oral	30–60 min	3–5 hr	24 hr
Transdermal	Slow	2–3 days	7 days
Epidural	Rapid	19 min	Variable

Metabolism: Hepatic; $T_{1/2}$: 12–16 hr, 19 hr (transdermal system); 48 hr (epidural)

Distribution: Crosses placenta; enters breast milk
Excretion: Urine

Adverse effects

- **CNS:** *Drowsiness, sedation, dizziness,* headache, fatigue that tend to diminish within 4–6 wk, dreams, nightmares, insomnia, hallucinations, delirium, nervousness, restlessness, anxiety, depression, retinal degeneration
- **CV:** CHF, orthostatic hypotension, palpitations, tachycardia, bradycardia, Raynaud's phenomenon, ECG abnormalities manifested as Wenckebach period or ventricular trigeminy
- **Dermatologic:** Rash, angioneurotic edema, hives, urticaria, hair thinning and alopecia, pruritus, dryness, itching or burning of the eyes, pallor
- **GI:** *Dry mouth, constipation,* anorexia, malaise, nausea, vomiting, parotid pain, parotitis, mild transient abnormalities in liver function tests
- **GU:** Impotence, decreased sexual activity, diminished libido, nocturia, difficulty in micturition, urinary retention
- **Other:** Weight gain, transient elevation of blood glucose or serum creatine phosphokinase, gynecomastia, weakness, muscle or joint pain, cramps of the lower limbs, dryness of the nasal mucosa, fever

Transdermal system

- **CNS:** *Drowsiness,* fatigue, headache, lethargy, sedation, insomnia, nervousness
- **GI:** *Dry mouth,* constipation, nausea, change in taste, dry throat
- **GU:** Impotence, sexual dysfunction
- **Local:** *Transient localized skin reactions,* pruritus, erythema, allergic contact sensitization and contact dermatitis, localized vesiculation, hyperpigmentation, edema, excoriation, burning, papules, throbbing, blanching, generalized macular rash

Interactions

✳ **Drug-drug** • Decreased antihypertensive effects with TCAs (imipramine) • Paradoxical hypertension with propranolol; also greater withdrawal hypertension when abruptly discontinued and patient is taking beta-adrenergic blocking agents

■ Nursing considerations

> **⚠ CLINICAL ALERT!**
> Name confusion has occurred between clonidine and Klonopin (clonazepam); use caution.

Assessment

- **History:** Hypersensitivity to clonidine or adhesive layer components of the transdermal system; severe coronary insufficiency, recent MI, cerebrovascular disease; chronic renal failure; lactation, pregnancy
- **Physical:** Body weight; body temperature; skin color, lesions, temperature; mucous membranes—color, lesion; breast exam; orientation, affect, reflexes; ophthalmologic exam; P, BP, orthostatic BP, perfusion, edema, auscultation; bowel sounds, normal output, liver evaluation, palpation of salivary glands; normal urinary output, voiding pattern; liver function tests, ECG

Interventions

- Do not discontinue abruptly; discontinue therapy by reducing the dosage gradually over 2–4 days to avoid rebound hypertension, tachycardia, flushing, nausea, vomiting, cardiac arrhythmias (hypertensive encephalopathy and death have occurred after abrupt cessation of clonidine).
- Do not discontinue prior to surgery; monitor BP carefully during surgery; have other BP-controlling drugs on standby.
- Store epidural injection at room temperature; discard any unused portions.
- Reevaluate therapy if clonidine tolerance occurs; giving concomitant diuretic increases the antihypertensive efficacy of clonidine.
- Monitor BP carefully when discontinuing clonidine; hypertension usually returns within 48 hr.
- Assess compliance with drug regimen in a supportive manner with pill counts, or other methods.

Adverse effects in *Italics* are most common; those in **Bold** are life-threatening.

Teaching points

- Take this drug exactly as prescribed. Do not miss doses. Do not discontinue the drug unless so instructed. Do not discontinue abruptly; life-threatening adverse effects may occur. If you travel, take an adequate supply of drug.
- Use the transdermal system as prescribed; refer to directions in package insert, or contact your health care provider with questions.
- Attempt lifestyle changes that will reduce your BP: stop smoking and alcohol use; lose weight; restrict intake of sodium (salt); exercise regularly.
- Use caution with alcohol. Your sensitivity may increase while using this drug.
- These side effects may occur: drowsiness, dizziness, light-headedness, headache, weakness (often transient; observe caution driving or performing other tasks that require alertness or physical dexterity); dry mouth (sucking on sugarless lozenges or ice chips may help); GI upset (eat frequent small meals); dreams, nightmares (reversible); dizziness, light-headedness when you change position (get up slowly; use caution climbing stairs); impotence, other sexual dysfunction, decreased libido (discuss with care providers); breast enlargement, sore breasts; palpitations.
- Report urinary retention, changes in vision, blanching of fingers, rash.

▷clopidogrel
(cloe **pid'** oh grel)

Plavix

PREGNANCY CATEGORY B

Drug classes
Adenosine diphosphate (ADP) receptor antagonist
Antiplatelet agent

Therapeutic actions
Inhibits platelet aggregation by blocking ADP receptors on platelets, preventing clumping of platelets.

Indications
- Treatment of patients at risk for ischemic events—history of MI, ischemic stroke, peripheral artery disease
- Treatment of patients with acute coronary syndrome

Contraindications and cautions
- Contraindicated with allergy to clopidogrel, lactation.
- Use cautiously with bleeding disorders, recent surgery, closed head injury, pregnancy.

Available forms
Tablets—75 mg

Dosages
Adults
- *Recent MI or stroke:* 75 mg PO daily.
- *Acute coronary syndrome:* 300 mg PO loading dose, then 75 mg/day PO with aspirin.

Pharmacokinetics

Route	Onset	Peak	Duration
Oral	Varies	75 min	3–4 hr

Metabolism: Hepatic; $T_{1/2}$: 8 hr
Distribution: Crosses placenta; passes into breast milk
Excretion: Feces, bile, and urine

Adverse effects
- **CNS:** *Headache, dizziness,* weakness, syncope, flushing
- **CV:** Hypertension, edema
- **Dermatologic:** *Rash,* pruritus
- **GI:** Nausea, GI distress, constipation, diarrhea, GI bleed
- **Other:** Increased bleeding risk

Interactions
✳ **Drug-drug** ● Potential increased risk of GI bleeding with NSAIDs, monitor patient carefully ● Potential increased bleeding with warfarin; monitor carefully

■ Nursing considerations
Assessment
- **History:** Allergy to clopidogrel, pregnancy, lactation, bleeding disorders, recent surgery, closed head injury
- **Physical:** Skin color, temperature, lesions; orientation, reflexes, affect; P, BP, orthosta-

tic BP, baseline ECG, peripheral perfusion; R, adventitious sounds

Interventions
• Provide small, frequent meals if GI upset occurs (not as common as with aspirin).
• Provide comfort measures and arrange for analgesics if headache occurs.

Teaching points
• Take daily as prescribed. May be taken with meals.
• These side effects may occur: dizziness, lightheadedness (this may pass as you adjust to the drug); headache (lie down in a cool environment and rest; OTC preparations may help); nausea, gastric distress (eat small, frequent meals); prolonged bleeding (alert doctors, dentists of this drug use).
• Report skin rash, chest pain, fainting, severe headache, abnormal bleeding.

▽ clorazepate dipotassium
(klor az' e pate)

Apo-Clorazepate (CAN), Gen-Xene, Novo-Clopate (CAN), Tranxene-SD, Tranxene-SD Half Strength, Tranxene-T

PREGNANCY CATEGORY D

C-IV CONTROLLED SUBSTANCE

Drug classes
Benzodiazepine
Antianxiety agent
Antiepileptic agent

Therapeutic actions
Exact mechanisms not understood; benzodiazepines potentiate the effects of GABA, an inhibitory neurotransmitter; anxiolytic effects occur at doses well below those necessary to cause sedation, ataxia.

Indications
• Management of anxiety disorders or for short-term relief of symptoms of anxiety

• Symptomatic relief of acute alcohol withdrawal
• Adjunctive therapy for partial seizures

Contraindications and cautions
• Contraindicated with hypersensitivity to benzodiazepines; psychoses; acute narrow-angle glaucoma; shock; coma; acute alcoholic intoxication with depression of vital signs; pregnancy (risk of congenital malformations, neonatal withdrawal syndrome); labor and delivery ("floppy infant" syndrome); lactation (infants tend to become lethargic and lose weight).
• Use cautiously with impaired liver or kidney function, debilitation.

Available forms
Tablets—3.75, 7.5, 15 mg; single-dose tablets—11.25, 22.5 mg. Capsules—3.75, 7.5, 15 mg. Individualize dosage; increase dosage gradually to avoid adverse effects. Drug is available only in oral forms.

Dosages
Adults
• *Anxiety:* Usual dose is 30 mg/day PO in divided doses tid; adjust gradually within the range of 15–60 mg/day; also may be given as a single daily dose hs; start with a dose of 15 mg. Maintenance: give the 22.5-mg PO tablet in a single daily dose as an alternate form for patients stabilized on 7.5 mg PO tid; do not use to initiate therapy; the 11.5-mg tablet may be given as a single daily dose.
• *Adjunct to antiepileptic medication:* Maximum initial dose is 7.5 mg PO tid. Increase dosage by no more than 7.5 mg every wk, do not exceed 90 mg/day.
• *Acute alcohol withdrawal:* Day 1: 30 mg PO initially, then 30–60 mg in divided doses. Day 2: 45–90 mg PO in divided doses. Day 3: 22.5–45 mg PO in divided doses. Day 4: 15–30 mg PO in divided doses. Thereafter, gradually reduce dose to 7.5–15 mg/day PO, and stop as soon as condition is stable.
Pediatric patients
• *Adjunct to antiepileptic medication:*
> *12 yr:* Same as adult.

Adverse effects in *Italics* are most common; those in **Bold** are life-threatening.

9–12 yr: Maximum initial dose is 7.5 mg PO bid; increase dosage by no more than 7.5 mg every wk, and do not exceed 60 mg/day.
< 9 yr: Not recommended.

Geriatric patients or patients with debilitating disease
- *Anxiety:* Initially, 7.5–15 mg/day PO in divided doses. Adjust as needed and tolerated.

Pharmacokinetics

Route	Onset	Peak	Duration
Oral	Fast	1–2 hr	Days

Metabolism: Hepatic; $T_{1/2}$: 30–100 hr
Distribution: Crosses placenta; enters breast milk
Excretion: Urine

Adverse effects

- **CNS:** *Transient, mild drowsiness initially; sedation, depression, lethargy, apathy, fatigue, light-headedness, disorientation, anger, hostility,* episodes of mania and hypomania, *restlessness, confusion, crying,* delirium, *headache,* slurred speech, dysarthria, stupor, rigidity, tremor, dystonia, vertigo, euphoria, nervousness, difficulty in concentration, vivid dreams, psychomotor retardation, extrapyramidal symptoms; *mild paradoxical excitatory reactions, during first 2 wk of treatment*
- **CV:** Bradycardia, tachycardia, CV collapse, hypertension and hypotension, palpitations, edema
- **Dermatologic:** Urticaria, pruritus, rash, dermatitis
- **EENT:** Visual and auditory disturbances, diplopia, nystagmus, depressed hearing, nasal congestion
- **GI:** *Constipation, diarrhea, dry mouth,* salivation, *nausea,* anorexia, vomiting, difficulty in swallowing, gastric disorders, hepatic dysfunction, encopresis
- **GU:** Incontinence, urinary retention, changes in libido, menstrual irregularities
- **Hematologic:** Elevations of blood enzymes—LDH, alkaline phosphatase, AST, ALT; blood dyscrasias—agranulocytosis, leukopenia
- **Other:** Hiccups, fever, diaphoresis, paresthesias, muscular disturbances, gynecomastia. Drug dependence with withdrawal syndrome is common with abrupt discontinuation of higher dosage used for longer than 4 mo.

Interactions

✴ **Drug-drug** • Increased CNS depression with alcohol • Increased effect with cimetidine, disulfiram, omeprazole, oral contraceptives • Decreased effect with theophylline • Risk of increased digoxin levels and toxicity; monitor patient carefully

■ Nursing considerations
Assessment

- **History:** Hypersensitivity to benzodiazepines; psychoses; acute narrow-angle glaucoma; shock; coma; acute alcoholic intoxication; pregnancy; lactation; impaired liver or kidney function; debilitation
- **Physical:** Skin color, lesions; T; orientation, reflexes, affect, ophthalmologic exam; P, BP; R, adventitious sounds; liver evaluation, abdominal exam, bowel sounds, normal output; CBC, liver and renal function tests

Interventions

- Taper dosage gradually after long-term therapy, especially in epileptics.
- Arrange for epileptics to wear medical alert ID, indicating disease and medication usage.

Teaching points

- Take drug exactly as prescribed; do not stop taking drug (long-term therapy) without consulting health care provider.
- Avoid alcohol, sleep-inducing, or OTC drugs.
- Avoid pregnancy while taking this drug; use of barrier contraceptives is advised.
- These side effects may occur: drowsiness, dizziness (may be transient; avoid driving a car or engaging in other dangerous activities); GI upset (take with food); fatigue; depression; dreams; crying; nervousness; depression, emotional changes; bed-wetting, urinary incontinence.
- Report severe dizziness, weakness, drowsiness that persists, rash or skin lesions, difficulty voiding, palpitations, swelling in the extremities.

▷ clotrimazole
*(kloe **trim'** a zole)*

Vaginal preparations: Canesten Vaginal (CAN), Gyne-Lotrimin-3 and -7, Mycelex-7, Mycelex-7 Combination Pack, Myclo (CAN)

Topical preparations: Clotrimaderm (CAN), Lotrimin, Lotrimin AF, Mycelex, Mycelex OTC

PREGNANCY CATEGORY C (TROCHE)

PREGNANCY CATEGORY B (TOPICAL, VAGINAL FORMS)

Drug class
Antifungal

Therapeutic actions
Fungicidal and fungistatic: binds to fungal cell membrane with a resultant change in membrane permeability, allowing leakage of intracellular components, causing cell death.

Indications
- Treatment of oropharyngeal candidiasis (troche)
- Prevention of oropharyngeal candidiasis in patients receiving radiation or chemotherapy
- Local treatment of vulvovaginal candidiasis (moniliasis; vaginal preparations)
- Topical treatment of tinea pedia, tinea cruris, tinea corporis due to *Trichophyton rubrum, Trichophyton mentagrophytes, Epidermophyton floccosum, Microsporum canis*; candidiasis due to *Candida albicans*; tinea versicolor due to *Microsporum furfur* (topical preparations)

Contraindications and cautions
- Allergy to clotrimazole or components used in preparation

Available forms
Vaginal suppositories—100, 200 mg; vaginal cream, solution, lotion—1%, 2%; topical cream, solution, lotion—1%; oral troche—10 mg

Vaginal preparation, cream: One applicator (5 g/day), preferably hs for 3–7 consecutive days.

Dosages
Oral troche
Dissolve slowly in the mouth 5 times/day for 14 days for treatment; tid for prevention.
Topical
Gently massage into affected and surrounding skin areas bid in the morning and evening for 7 days. Relief is usually noted during first wk of therapy; therapy 2–4 wk.
Vaginal suppository
Insert one suppository intravaginally at bedtime for 3 consecutive nights.

Pharmacokinetics
Action is primarily local; pharmacokinetics are not known.

Adverse effects
Troche
- **GI:** *Nausea, vomiting, abnormal liver function tests*
Vaginal
- **Dermatologic:** Rash
- **GI:** *Lower abdominal cramps,* bloating
- **GU:** *Slight urinary frequency; burning or irritation in the sexual partner*
Topical
- **Local:** *Erythema, stinging,* blistering, peeling, edema, pruritus, urticaria, general skin irritation

■ Nursing considerations
Assessment
- **History:** Allergy to clotrimazole or components used in preparation, pregnancy
- **Physical:** Skin color, lesions, area around lesions; bowel sounds; culture of area involved, liver function tests

Interventions
- Culture fungus involved before therapy.
- Have patient dissolve troche slowly in mouth.
- Insert vaginal suppository into vagina at bedtime for 3–7 consecutive nights. Provide sanitary napkin to protect clothing from stains.
- Administer vaginal cream high into vagina using the applicator supplied with the prod-

uct. Administer for 3–7 consecutive nights, even during menstrual period.
- Cleanse affected area before topical application. Do not apply to eyes or eye areas.
- Monitor response to drug therapy. If no response is noted, arrange for more cultures to determine causative organism.
- Ensure that patient receives full course of therapy to eradicate the fungus and prevent recurrence.
- Discontinue topical or vaginal administration if rash or sensitivity occurs.

Teaching points
- Take the full course of drug therapy, even if symptoms improve. Continue during menstrual period if vaginal route is being used. Long-term use of the drug may be needed; beneficial effects may not be seen for several weeks. Vaginal creams should be inserted high into the vagina. Troche preparation should be allowed to dissolve slowly in the mouth. Apply topical preparation by gently massaging into the affected area.
- Use hygiene measures to prevent reinfection or spread of infection.
- Vaginal use: Refrain from sexual intercourse, or advise partner to use a condom to avoid reinfection. Use a sanitary napkin to prevent staining of clothing.
- These side effects may occur: nausea, vomiting, diarrhea (oral use); irritation, burning, stinging (local).
- Report worsening of the condition being treated, local irritation, burning (topical), rash, irritation, pelvic pain (vaginal), nausea, GI distress (oral administration).

▽cloxacillin sodium
(klox a sill' in)

Apo-Cloxi (CAN), Cloxapen, Novo-Cloxin (CAN), Nu-Cloxi (CAN), Orbenin (CAN)

PREGNANCY CATEGORY B

Drug classes
Antibiotic
Penicillinase-resistant pencillin

Therapeutic actions
Bactericidal: inhibits cell wall synthesis of sensitive organisms, causing cell death.

Indications
- Infections due to penicillinase-producing staphylococci.
- May be used to initiate therapy when a staphylococci infection is suspected.

Contraindications and cautions
- Contraindicated with allergies to penicillins, cephalosporins, or other allergens.
- Use cautiously with renal disorders, lactation (causes diarrhea or candidiasis in infants).

Available forms
Capsules—250, 500 mg; powder for oral solution—125 mg/5 mL

Dosages
Adults
250 mg q 6 hr PO; up to 500 mg q 6 hr PO in severe infections.
Pediatric patients < 20 kg
50 mg/kg/day PO in equally divided doses q 6 hr; up to 100 mg/kg/day PO in equally divided doses q 6 hr in severe infections.

Pharmacokinetics
Route	Onset	Peak
Oral	Varies	1 hr

Metabolism: $T_{1/2}$: 30–90 min
Distribution: Crosses placenta; enters breast milk
Excretion: Urine

Adverse effects
- **CNS:** Lethargy, hallucinations, seizures, decreased reflexes
- **CV:** Tachycardia, pulmonary hypertension, hypotension, pulmonary embolism
- **GI:** Glossitis, stomatitis, gastritis, sore mouth, furry tongue, black "hairy" tongue, nausea, vomiting, diarrhea, abdominal pain, bloody diarrhea, enterocolitis, **pseudomembranous colitis,** nonspecific hepatitis
- **GU:** Nephritis—oliguria, proteinuria, hematuria, casts, azotemia, pyuria

- **Hematologic:** Anemia, thrombocytopenia, leukopenia, neutropenia, prolonged bleeding time, hemorrhagic episodes at high doses
- **Hypersensitivity:** *Rash, fever, wheezing,* **anaphylaxis**
- **Other:** *Superinfections*—oral and rectal moniliasis, vaginitis

Interactions

✳ **Drug-drug** • Decreased effectiveness with tetracyclines • Decreased efficacy of oral contraceptives is possible • Increased half-life of penicillins with probenecid; often used for synergy

✳ **Drug-food** • Decreased absorption and decreased serum levels if taken with food

■ Nursing considerations
Assessment
- **History:** Allergies to penicillins, cephalosporins, or other allergens; renal disorders, lactation
- **Physical:** Culture infected area; skin color, lesion; R, adventitious sounds; bowel sounds; CBC, liver and renal function tests, serum electrolytes, Hct, urinalysis

Interventions
- Administer on an empty stomach, 1 hr before or 2 hr after meals, with a full glass of water. Do not give with fruit juice or soft drinks.
- Continue treatment for 10 full days.

Teaching points
- Take around the clock; take the full course of therapy, usually 10 days. Take on an empty stomach, 1 hr before or 2 hr after meals, with a full glass of water.
- This antibiotic is for this infection and should not be used to self-treat other infections.
- These side effects may occur: stomach upset, nausea, diarrhea, mouth sores (if severe, consult health care provider for treatment).
- Report unusual bleeding or bruising, fever, chills, sore throat, hives, rash, severe diarrhea, difficulty breathing.

▽ **clozapine**
(kloe' za peen)

Clozaril

PREGNANCY CATEGORY B

Drug classes
Antipsychotic
Dopaminergic blocking agent

Therapeutic actions
Mechanism not fully understood: blocks dopamine receptors in the brain, depresses the RAS; anticholinergic, antihistaminic (H_1), and alpha-adrenergic blocking activity may contribute to some of its therapeutic (and adverse) actions. Clozapine produces fewer extrapyramidal effects than other antipsychotics.

Indications
- Management of severely ill schizophrenics who are unresponsive to standard antipsychotic drugs.
- Reduction of the risk of recurrent suicidal behavior in patients with schizophrenia or schizoaffective disorder.

Contraindications and cautions
- Contraindicated with allergy to clozapine, myeloproliferative disorders, history of clozapine-induced agranulocytosis or severe granulocytopenia, severe CNS depression, comatose states, history of seizure disorders, lactation.
- Use cautiously with CV disease, prostate enlargement, narrow-angle glaucoma, pregnancy.

Available forms
Tablets—25, 100 mg

Dosages
Adults
Initial: 25 mg PO daily or bid; then gradually increase with daily increments of 25–50 mg/day, if tolerated, to a dose of 300–450 mg/day by the end of second week. Adjust later dosage no more often than twice weekly in increments < 100 mg. Do not exceed 900 mg/day.

Maintenance: Maintain at the lowest effective dose for remission of symptoms.

Discontinuation: Gradual reduction over a 2-wk period is preferred. If abrupt discontinuation is required, carefully monitor patient for signs of acute psychotic symptoms.

Reinitiation of treatment: Follow initial dosage guidelines, use extreme care; increased risk of severe adverse effects with re-exposure.

Pediatric patients
Safety and efficacy in patients < 16 yr not established.

Pharmacokinetics

Route	Onset	Peak	Duration
Oral	Varies	1–6 hr	Weeks

Metabolism: Hepatic; $T_{1/2}$: 4–12 hr
Distribution: Crosses placenta; enters breast milk
Excretion: Urine and feces

Adverse effects

- **CNS:** *Drowsiness, sedation, seizures, dizziness, syncope, headache,* tremor, disturbed sleep, nightmares, restlessness, agitation, increased salivation, sweating, tardive dyskinesia, **neuroleptic malignant syndrome**
- **CV:** *Tachycardia, hypotension,* ECG changes, hypertension
- **GI:** *Nausea, vomiting, constipation,* abdominal discomfort, dry mouth
- **GU:** Urinary abnormalities
- **Hematologic:** Leukopenia, granulocytopenia, agranulocytopenia
- **Other:** *Fever,* weight gain, rash

Interactions

✴ **Drug-drug** • Increased therapeutic and toxic effects with cimetidine • Decreased therapeutic effect with phenytoin, mephenytoin, ethotoin

■ Nursing considerations

CLINICAL ALERT!
Name confusion has occurred with Clozaril (clozapine) and Colazal (balsalazide); dangerous effects could occur. Use extreme caution.

Assessment

- **History:** Allergy to clozapine, myeloproliferative disorders, history of clozapine-induced agranulocytosis or severe granulocytopenia, severe CNS depression, comatose states, history of seizure disorders, CV disease, prostate enlargement, narrow-angle glaucoma, lactation, pregnancy
- **Physical:** T, weight; reflexes, orientation, intraocular pressure, ophthalmologic exam; P, BP, orthostatic BP, ECG; R, adventitious sounds; bowel sounds, normal output, liver evaluation; prostate palpation, normal urine output; CBC, urinalysis, liver and kidney function tests, EEG

Interventions

- Use only when unresponsive to conventional antipsychotic drugs.
- Obtain clozapine through the Clozaril Patient Management System.
- Dispense only 1 wk supply at a time.
- Monitor WBC carefully prior to first dose.
- Weekly monitoring of WBC during treatment and for 4 wk thereafter. Dosage may be adjusted based on WBC count.
- Monitor T. If fever occurs, rule out underlying infection, and consult physician for comfort measures.
- Monitor elderly patients for dehydration. Institute remedial measures promptly; sedation and decreased thirst related to CNS effects can lead to dehydration.
- Encourage voiding before taking drug to decrease anticholinergic effects of urinary retention.
- Follow guidelines for discontinuation or reinstitution of the drug.

Teaching points

- Weekly blood tests will be taken to determine safe dosage; dosage will be increased gradually to achieve most effective dose. Only 1 wk of medication can be dispensed at a time. Do not take more than your prescribed dosage. Do not make up missed doses, instead contact care provider. Do not stop taking this drug suddenly; gradual reduction of dosage is needed to prevent side effects.
- These effects may occur as a result of drug therapy: drowsiness, dizziness, sedation, seizures (avoid driving or performing tasks that require concentration); dizziness, faint-

ness on arising (change positions slowly); increased salivation (reversible); constipation (consult care provider for correctives); fast heart rate (rest, take your time).

- This drug cannot be taken during pregnancy. If you think you are pregnant or wish to become pregnant, contact your care provider.
- Report lethargy, weakness, fever, sore throat, malaise, mouth ulcers, and flu-like symptoms.

▽coagulation factor VIIa

See *Less Commonly Used Drugs,* p. 1340.

▽codeine phosphate
(koe' deen)

PREGNANCY CATEGORY C
(DURING PREGNANCY)

PREGNANCY CATEGORY D
(DURING LABOR)

C-II CONTROLLED SUBSTANCE

Drug classes
Narcotic agonist analgesic
Antitussive

Therapeutic actions
Acts at opioid receptors in the CNS to produce analgesia, euphoria, sedation; acts in medullary cough center to depress cough reflex.

Indications
- Relief of mild to moderate pain in adults and children
- Coughing induced by chemical or mechanical irritation of the respiratory system

Contraindications and cautions
- Contraindicated with hypersensitivity to narcotics, physical dependence on a narcotic analgesic (drug may precipitate withdrawal).
- Use cautiously with pregnancy, labor, lactation, bronchial asthma, COPD, respiratory depression, anoxia, increased intracranial pressure, acute MI, ventricular failure, coro-

nary insufficiency, hypertension, biliary tract surgery, renal or hepatic dysfunction.

Available forms
Tablets—15, 30, 60 mg; oral solution—15 mg/5 mL; injection—30, 60 mg; soluble tablets—30, 60 mg

Dosages
Adults
Analgesic
15–60 mg PO, IM, IV or SC q 4–6 hr; do not exceed 360 mg/24 hr.
Antitussive
10–20 mg PO q 4–6 hr; do not exceed 120 mg/24 hr.
Pediatric patients
Contraindicated in premature infants.
Analgesic
≥ *1 yr:* 0.5 mg/kg SC, IM or PO q 4–6 hr.
Antitussive
6–12 yr: 5–10 mg PO q 4–6 hr; do not exceed 60 mg/24 hr.
2–6 yr: 2.5–5 mg PO q 4–6 hr; do not exceed 30 mg/24 hr.
Geriatric patients or impaired adults
Use caution; respiratory depression may occur in elderly, the very ill, those with respiratory problems. Reduced dosage may be necessary.

Pharmacokinetics

Route	Onset	Peak	Duration
Oral, IM, IV	10–30 min	30–60 min	4–6 hr

Metabolism: Hepatic; $T_{1/2}$: 2.5–4 hr
Distribution: Crosses placenta; enters breast milk
Excretion: Urine

▼IV facts
Preparation: Protect vials from light.
Infusion: Administer slowly over 5 min by direct injection or into running IV tubing.

Adverse effects
- **CNS:** *Sedation, clamminess, sweating, headache, vertigo, floating feeling, dizziness, lethargy, confusion, light-headedness,* nervousness, unusual dreams, agitation, eu-

Adverse effects in *Italics* are most common; those in **Bold** are life-threatening.

phoria, hallucinations, delirium, insomnia, anxiety, fear, disorientation, impaired mental and physical performance, coma, mood changes, weakness, headache, tremor, **seizures**
- **CV:** Palpitation, increase or decrease in BP, circulatory depression, **cardiac arrest, shock,** tachycardia, bradycardia, arrhythmia, palpitations
- **Dermatologic:** Rash, hives, pruritus, flushing, warmth, sensitivity to cold
- **EENT:** Diplopia, blurred vision
- **GI:** *Nausea, vomiting,* dry mouth, anorexia, *constipation,* biliary tract spasm
- **GU:** Ureteral spasm, spasm of vesical sphincters, urinary retention or hesitancy, oliguria, antidiuretic effect, reduced libido or potency
- **Local:** Phlebitis following IV injection, pain at injection site; tissue irritation and induration (SC injection)
- **Respiratory:** Slow, shallow respiration; apnea; suppression of cough reflex; laryngospasm; bronchospasm
- **Other:** Physical tolerance and dependence, psychological dependence

Interactions
✳ **Drug-drug** • Potentiation of effects of codeine with barbiturate anesthetics; decrease dose of codeine when coadministering
✳ **Drug-lab test** • Elevated biliary tract pressure may increase plasma amylase, lipase; determinations of these levels may be unreliable for 24 hr after administration of narcotics

■ Nursing considerations

CLINICAL ALERT!
Name confusion has occurred between codeine and Cardene (nicardipine) and Lodine (etodolac); use caution.

Assessment
- **History:** Hypersensitivity to codeine, physical dependence on a narcotic analgesic, pregnancy, labor, lactation, bronchial asthma, COPD, increased intracranial pressure, acute MI, ventricular failure, coronary insufficiency, hypertension, biliary tract surgery, renal or hepatic dysfunction
- **Physical:** Orientation, reflexes, bilateral grip strength, affect; pupil size, vision; pulse,

auscultation, BP; R, adventitious sounds; bowel sounds, normal output; liver and kidney function tests

Interventions
- Give to nursing women 4–6 hr before scheduled feeding to minimize drug in milk.
- Provide narcotic antagonist, facilities for assisted or controlled respirations on standby during parenteral administration.
- Use caution when injecting SC into chilled body areas or in patients with hypotension or in shock; impaired perfusion may delay absorption; with repeated doses, an excessive amount may be absorbed when circulation is restored.
- Instruct postoperative patients in pulmonary toilet; drug suppresses cough reflex.
- Monitor bowel function, arrange for laxatives (especially senna compounds—approximate dose of 187 mg senna concentrate per 120 mg codeine equivalent), bowel training program if severe constipation occurs.

Teaching points
- Take drug exactly as prescribed.
- These side effects may occur: dizziness, sedation, drowsiness, impaired visual acuity (avoid driving and performing other tasks that require alertness); nausea, loss of appetite (lie quietly, eat frequent, small meals); constipation (use a laxative).
- Do not take any leftover drug for other disorders, and do not let anyone else take it.
- Report severe nausea, vomiting, palpitations, shortness of breath or difficulty breathing.

▽ colchicine
(*kol' chi seen*)

PREGNANCY CATEGORY C
(ORAL)

PREGNANCY CATEGORY D
(PARENTERAL)

Drug class
Antigout drug

Therapeutic actions
Exact mechanism unknown; decreases deposition of uric acid; inhibits kinin formation

and phagocytosis, and decreases inflammatory reaction to urate crystal deposition.

Indications
- Pain relief of acute gout attack; also used between attacks as prophylaxis; IV use reserved for rapid response or when GI side effects interfere with use
- Orphan drug use: arrest progression of neurologic disability caused by chronic progressive multiple sclerosis
- Unlabeled uses: hepatic cirrhosis (1 mg/day), familial Mediterranean fever (1–3 mg/day), skin manifestations of scleroderma (1 mg/day), psoriasis (0.02 mg/kg/day), dermatitis herpetiformis (0.6 mg bid–tid), treatment of Behçet's disease (0.5–1.5 mg/day)

Contraindications and cautions
- Allergy to colchicine, blood dyscrasias, serious GI disorders, liver, renal or cardiac disorders, pregnancy, lactation

Available forms
Tablets—0.5, 0.6 mg; injection—1 mg

Dosages
Adults
- *Acute gouty arthritis:* 1–1.2 mg PO followed by 0.5–1.2 mg q 1–2 hr until pain is relieved or nausea, vomiting, or diarrhea occurs. IV dose: 2 mg followed by 0.5 mg q 6 hr until desired effect is achieved. Do not exceed 4 mg/24 hr. Do not repeat dosing in < 7 days.
- *Prophylaxis in intercritical periods:* For < 1 attack per year: 0.5–0.6 mg/day PO for 3–4 days/wk. For > 1 attack per year: 0.5–0.6 mg/day; up to 1.8 mg/day PO may be needed in severe cases. IV dose: 0.5–1 mg once or twice daily; change to oral therapy as soon as possible.
- *Prophylaxis for patients undergoing surgery:* 0.5–0.6 mg tid PO for 3 days before and 3 days after the procedure.
Pediatric patients
Safety and efficacy not established.
Geriatric patients or patients with renal impairment
Use with caution; reduce dosage if weakness, anorexia, nausea, vomiting, or diarrhea occurs.

Pharmacokinetics

Route	Onset	Peak
Oral	0.5–2 hr	12 hr
IV	30–50 min	6–12 hr

Metabolism: Hepatic; $T_{1/2}$: 20–60 min
Distribution: Crosses placenta; enters breast milk
Excretion: Urine and bile

▽▼ IV facts
Preparation: Use undiluted or diluted in 0.9% sodium chloride injection that does not have a bacteriostatic agent. Do not dilute with 5% dextrose in water. Do not use solutions that have become turbid.
Infusion: Infuse slowly over 2–5 min by direct injection or into tubing of running IV.
Incompatibilities: Do not use with dextrose solutions.

Adverse effects
- **CNS:** Peripheral neuritis, purpura, myopathy
- **Dermatologic:** Dermatoses, loss of hair
- **GI:** *Diarrhea, vomiting,* abdominal pain, nausea
- **GU:** Azoospermia (reversible)
- **Hematologic:** Bone marrow depression, elevated alkaline phosphatase, AST levels
- **Local:** Thrombophlebitis at IV sites

Interactions
✳ Drug-drug • Decreased absorption of vitamin B_{12} when taken with colchicine
✳ Drug-lab test • False-positive results for urine RBC, urine hemoglobin • Decreased thrombocyte levels

■ Nursing considerations
Assessment
- **History:** Allergy to colchicine, blood dyscrasias, serious GI, liver, renal or cardiac disorders, pregnancy, lactation
- **Physical:** Skin lesions, color; orientation, reflexes; P, cardiac auscultation, BP; liver evaluation, normal bowel output; normal urinary output; CBC, renal and liver function tests, urinalysis

Adverse effects in *Italics* are most common; those in **Bold** are life-threatening.

Interventions

- Monitor for relief of pain, signs and symptoms of gout attack; usually abate within 12 hr and are gone within 24–48 hr.
- Parenteral drug is to be used IV only; SC or IM use causes severe irritation.
- Monitor total dose received.
- Arrange for opiate antidiarrheal medication if diarrhea is severe.
- Discuss the dosage regimen with patients who have been using colchicine; these patients know when to stop the medication before GI side effects occur.
- Administration should begin at the first sign of an acute attack; delay can decrease drug's effectiveness in alleviating symptoms of gout.
- Have regular medical follow-ups and blood tests.

Teaching points

- Take this drug at the first warning of an acute attack; delay will impair the drug's effectiveness in relieving your symptoms. Stop drug at the first sign of nausea, vomiting, stomach pain, or diarrhea.
- These side effects may occur: nausea, vomiting, loss of appetite (take drug following meals or eat small, frequent meals); loss of fertility (reversible); loss of hair (reversible).
- Report severe diarrhea, rash, sore throat, fever, unusual bleeding or bruising, fever, chills, sore throat, persistence of gout attack, numbness or tingling, tiredness, weakness.

▷ colesevelam
*(koe leh **seve' eh** lam)*

Welchol

PREGNANCY CATEGORY NOT ESTABLISHED

Drug classes
Antihyperlipidemic agent
Bile acid sequestrant

Therapeutic actions
Binds bile acids in the intestine allowing excretion in the feces; as a result, cholesterol is oxidized in the liver to replace the bile acids lost; serum cholesterol and low density lipoproteins (LDL) are lowered.

Indications
- Reduction of elevated LDLs as adjunct to diet and exercise in patients with primary hypercholesterolemia; used alone or in conjunction with an HCG-CoA reductase inhibitor

Contraindications and cautions
- Contraindicated with allergy to bile acid sequestrants; complete biliary obstruction; intestinal obstruction; pregnancy; lactation.
- Use cautiously with difficulty swallowing; GI motility disorders; major GI tract surgery; patients susceptible to fat-soluble vitamin deficiency.

Available forms
Tablets—625 mg

Dosages
Adults
- *Monotherapy:* 3 tablets bid PO with meals or 6 tablets daily PO with a meal; do not exceed 7 tablets/day
- *Combination therapy with an HCG-CoA inhibitor:* 3 tablets PO bid with meals or 6 tablets once a day PO with a meal; do not exceed 6 tablets/day

Pediatric patients
Safety and efficacy not established.

Pharmacokinetics
Not absorbed systemically; excreted in the feces.

Adverse effects
- **CNS:** Headache, anxiety, vertigo, dizziness, fatigue, syncope, drowsiness
- **GI:** *Constipation to fecal impaction,* exacerbation of hemorrhoids, abdominal cramps, pain, flatulence, nausea, vomiting, diarrhea, heartburn
- **GU:** Hematuria, dysuria, diuresis
- **Hematologic:** *Increased bleeding tendencies related to vitamin K malabsorption,* vitamin A and D deficiencies, reduced serum and red cell folate, hyperchloremic acidosis
- **Other:** Osteoporosis, backache, muscle and joint pain, arthritis, fever, pharyngitis

Interactions
* **Drug-drug** ● Malabsorption of fat-soluble vitamins if taken concurrently with cholestyramine ● Decreased absorption of oral

drugs; take other oral drugs 1 hr before or 4–6 hr after colesevelam

■ Nursing considerations
Assessment
- **History:** Allergy to bile acid sequestrants; complete biliary obstruction; intestinal obstruction; pregnancy; lactation; difficulty swallowing, GI motility disorders; major GI tract surgery; susceptibility to fat-soluble vitamin deficiency
- **Physical:** Skin lesions, color, temperature; orientation, affect, reflexes; P, auscultation, baseline ECG, peripheral perfusion; liver evaluation, bowel sounds; lipid studies, liver function tests, clotting profile

Interventions
- Monitor serum cholesterol, LDLs, triglycerides before starting treatment and periodically during treatment.
- Administer drug with meals.
- Store at room temperature; protect from moisture.
- Establish bowel program to deal with constipation.
- Monitor nutritional status and arrange for consults if needed.
- Consult with dietitian regarding low-cholesterol diets and provide information regarding exercise programs.
- Arrange for regular follow-up during long-term therapy.

Teaching points
- Take drug with meals.
- Continue to follow your low-fat diet and participate in an exercise program.
- Plan to return for periodic blood tests to evaluate the effectiveness of this drug.
- These side effects may occur: constipation (this may resolve, or other measures may need to be taken to alleviate this problem); nausea, heartburn, loss of appetite (small frequent meals may help); dizziness, drowsiness, vertigo, fainting (avoid driving and operating dangerous machinery until you know how this drug affects you); headache, muscle and joint aches and pains (this may lessen over time; if it becomes bothersome, consult with your nurse or physician).

- Report unusual bleeding or bruising, severe constipation, severe GI upset, chest pain, difficulty breathing, rash, fever.

▽ **colestipol hydrochloride**
(koe les' ti pole)

Colestid

PREGNANCY CATEGORY C

Drug classes
Antihyperlipidemic
Bile acid sequestrant

Therapeutic actions
Binds bile acids in the intestine to form a complex that is excreted in the feces; as a result, cholesterol is lost, oxidized in the liver, and serum cholesterol and LDL are lowered.

Indications
- Reduction of elevated serum cholesterol in patients with primary hypercholesterolemia (elevated LDL) (adjunctive therapy)

Contraindications and cautions
- Allergy to bile acid sequestrants, complete biliary obstruction, abnormal intestinal function, pregnancy, lactation

Available forms
Tablets—1 g; granules—5 g packets, 5 g/7.5 g powder

Dosages
Adults
- Granules: 5–30 g/day PO in divided doses 2–4 times/day. Start with 5 g daily or bid PO, and increase in 5-g/day increments at 1- to 2-mo intervals; tablets: 2–16 g/day PO in 1–2 divided doses; initially 2 g once or twice daily; increasing 2 g increments at 1- to 2-mo intervals.

Pediatric patients
Safety and efficacy not established.

Pharmacokinetics
Not absorbed systemically. Eliminated in the feces.

Adverse effects
- **CNS:** *Headache,* anxiety, vertigo, dizziness, fatigue, syncope, drowsiness
- **Dermatologic:** Rash and irritation of skin, tongue, perianal area
- **GI:** *Constipation* to fecal impaction, *exacerbation of hemorrhoids,* abdominal cramps, *abdominal pain,* flatulence, anorexia, heartburn, nausea, vomiting, steatorrhea
- **GU:** Hematuria, dysuria, diuresis
- **Hematologic:** Increased bleeding tendencies related to vitamin K malabsorption, vitamin A and D deficiencies, hyperchloremic acidosis
- **Other:** Osteoporosis, chest pain, backache, muscle and joint pain, arthritis, fever

Interactions
✳ **Drug-drug** • Decreased serum levels or delayed absorption of thiazide diuretics, digitalis preparations • Malabsorption of fat-soluble vitamins • Decreased absorption of oral drugs; administer 1 hr before or 4–6 hr after colestipol

■ Nursing considerations
Assessment
- **History:** Allergy to bile acid sequestrant, complete biliary obstruction, abnormal intestinal function, pregnancy, lactation
- **Physical:** Skin lesions, color, temperature; orientation, affect, reflexes; P, auscultation, baseline ECG, peripheral perfusion; liver evaluation, bowel sounds; lipid studies, liver function tests, clotting profile

Interventions
- Do not administer drug in dry form. Mix in liquids, soups, cereals, or pulpy fruits; add the prescribed amount to a glassful (90 mL) of liquid; stir until completely mixed. The granules will not dissolve. May be mixed with carbonated beverages, slowly stirred in a large glass. Rinse the glass with a small amount of additional beverage to ensure all of the dose has been taken.
- Ensure that patient swallows tablets whole; do not cut, crush, or chew. Tablets should be taken with plenty of fluids.
- Administer drug before meals.

- Monitor administration of other oral drugs for binding in the intestine and delayed or decreased absorption. Give them 1 hr before or 4–6 hr after the colestipol.
- Arrange for regular follow-up during long-term therapy.
- Alert patient and concerned others about the high cost of drug.

Teaching points
- Take drug before meals. Do not take the powder in the dry form. Mix in liquids, soups, cereals, or pulpy fruit; add the prescribed amount to a glassful of the liquid; stir until completely mixed. The granules will not dissolve; rinse the glass with a small amount of additional liquid to ensure that you receive the entire dose of the drug; carbonated beverages may be used; mix by slowly stirring in a large glass. If taking tablet form, swallow whole with plenty of fluids; do not cut, crush, or chew.
- This drug may interfere with the absorption of other oral medications. Take other oral medications 1 hr before or 4–6 hr after colestipol.
- These side effects may occur: constipation (transient, if it persists, request correctives); nausea, heartburn, loss of appetite (small, frequent meals may help); dizziness, drowsiness, vertigo, fainting (avoid driving and operating dangerous machinery); headache, muscle and joint aches and pains (may lessen in time).
- Report unusual bleeding or bruising, severe constipation, severe GI upset, chest pain, difficulty breathing, rash, fever.

▽ colfosceril palmitate (synthetic lung surfactant, dipalmitoylphosphatidylcholine)
(kole fos' seer el)

Exosurf Neonatal

Drug class
Lung surfactant

Therapeutic actions

A natural compound that reduces surface tension in the alveoli, allowing expansion of the alveoli; replaces the surfactant missing in the lungs of neonates suffering from RDS.

Indications

- Prophylactic treatment of infants at risk of developing RDS; infants with birth weights < 1,350 g or infants with birth weights > 1,350 g who have evidence of pulmonary immaturity
- Rescue treatment for infants with RDS
- Orphan drug use: prevention of RDS in infants ≤ 32 wk gestation; treatment of hyaline membrane disease; treatment of adult RDS

Contraindications and cautions

- Colfosceril is used as an emergency drug in acute respiratory situations; benefits outweigh any potential risks of therapy.

Available forms

Powder for injection—108 mg

Dosages

Accurate birth weight is necessary for determing correct dosage. Colfosceril is instilled into the trachea using the endotracheal tube adapter that comes with the product.

- *Prophylactic treatment:* Give drug in a single 5-mL/kg intratracheal dose as soon as possible after birth. Give second (12 hr) and third (24 hr) doses to all infants who remain on mechanical ventilation.
- *Rescue treatment:* Administer in two 5-mL/kg doses. Give first dose as soon as possible after the diagnosis of RDS is made. The second dose should be given in 12 hr, if the infant remains on mechanical ventilation. Data on safety and efficacy of rescue treatment with more than two doses are not available.

Pharmacokinetics

Route	Onset	Duration
Intratracheal	Rapid	12 hr

Metabolism: Lung, $T_{1/2}$: 12 hr
Excretion: Respiratory

Adverse effects

- **CNS: Seizures**
- **CV:** *Patent ductus arteriosus, intraventricular hemorrhage, hypotension*
- **Hematologic:** *Hyperbilirubinemia, thrombocytopenia*
- **Respiratory:** *Pneumothorax, pulmonary air leak,* **pulmonary hemorrhage,** *apnea,* pneumomediastinum, emphysema
- **Other:** *Sepsis, nonpulmonary infections*

■ Nursing considerations

Assessment

- **History:** Time of birth, history of gestation
- **Physical:** T, color; R, adventitious sounds, oximeter, endotracheal tube position and patency, chest movement; ECG, P, BP, peripheral perfusion, arterial pressure (desirable); oxygen saturation, blood gases, CBC; motor activity, facial expression, reflexes

Interventions

- Monitor ECG and transcutaneous oxygen saturation continually during administration.
- Ensure that endotracheal tube is in the correct position, with bilateral chest movement and lung sounds.
- Arrange for staff to preview teaching videotape, available from the manufacturer, before regular use to cover all the technical aspects of administration.
- Suction the infant immediately before administration; do not suction for 2 hr after administration unless clinically necessary.
- Reconstitute immediately before use with the 8 mL of diluent that comes with the product; do not use bacteriostatic water for injection. Reconstitute using the manufacturer's directions to ensure proper mixing and dilution.
- Check reconstituted vial, it should look like a milky liquid; if flakes or precipitates appear, attempt gentle mixing. If precipitate remains, do not use.
- Insert correct size endotracheal adapter into the endotracheal tube; attach the breathing circuit to the adapter; remove cap from the sideport of the adapter; attach syringe containing the drug into the sideport and administer correct dose.

Adverse effects in *Italics* are most common; those in **Bold** are life-threatening.

- Instill dose slowly over 1–2 min, 30–50 ventilations, moving infant after each half dose to ensure adequate instillation into both lungs.
- Continually monitor color, lung sounds, ECG, oximeter, and blood gas readings during administration and for at least 30 min following administration.

Teaching points
- Parents of the critically ill infant will need a comprehensive teaching and support program, including details of drug effects.

▷corticotropin (ACTH, adrenocorticotropin, corticotrophin)
*(kor ti koe **troe'** pin)*

Injection: Acthar
Repository injection: H.P. Acthar Gel, ACTH-80

PREGNANCY CATEGORY C

Drug classes
Anterior pituitary hormone
Diagnostic agent

Therapeutic actions
Stimulates the adrenal cortex to synthesize and secrete adrenocortical hormones.

Indications
- Diagnostic tests of adrenal function
- Therapy of some glucocorticoid-sensitive disorders
- Nonsuppurative thyroiditis
- Hypercalcemia associated with cancer
- Acute exacerbations of multiple sclerosis
- Tuberculous meningitis with subarachnoid block
- Trichinosis with neurologic or myocardial involvement
- Rheumatic, collagen, dermatologic, allergic, ophthalmologic, respiratory, hematologic, edematous, and GI diseases
- Unlabeled use: treatment of infantile spasms

Contraindications and cautions
- Adrenocortical insufficiency or hyperfunction; infections, especially systemic fungal infections, ocular herpes simplex; scleroderma; osteoporosis; recent surgery; CHF, hypertension; allergy to pork or pork products (corticotropin is isolated from porcine pituitaries); liver disease; ulcerative colitis with impending perforation; diverticulitis; recent GI surgery; active or latent peptic ulcer; inflammatory bowel disease; diabetes mellitus; hypothyroidism; pregnancy, lactation

Available forms
Powder for injection—25, 40 units/vial; repository injection—40, 80 units/mL

Dosages
Adults
- *Diagnostic tests:* 10–25 units dissolved in 500 mL of 5% dextrose injection infused IV over 8 hr.
- *Therapy:* 20 units IM or SC qid; when indicated, gradually reduce dosage by increasing intervals between injections or decreasing the dose injected, or both.
- *Acute exacerbations of multiple sclerosis:* 80–120 units/day IM for 2–3 wk.
- *Repository injection:* 40–80 units IM or SC q 24–72 hr.

Pediatric patients
Use only if necessary, and only intermittently and with careful observation. Prolonged use will inhibit skeletal growth.
- *Infantile spasms:* 20–40 units/day or 80 units every other day IM for 3 mo or 1 mo after cessation of seizures.

Pharmacokinetics

Route	Onset	Peak	Duration
IM, IV	Rapid	1 hr	2–4 hr

Metabolism: $T_{1/2}$: 15 min
Distribution: Does not cross placenta; may enter breast milk

▽IV facts
Preparation: Reconstitute powder by dissolving in sterile water for injection or sodium chloride injection. Total volume will be 1–2 mL. Refrigerate reconstituted solution. Stable for 24 hr.
Infusion: 10–25 units dissolved in 500 mL of 5% dextrose injection infused over 8 hr.
Incompatibilities: Do not mix with aminophylline or sodium bicarbonate.

Adverse effects

- **CNS:** Convulsions, vertigo, *headaches, pseudotumor cerebri, euphoria, insomnia, mood swings, depression,* psychosis, intracerebral hemorrhage, reversible cerebral atrophy in infants, cataracts, increased intraocular pressure, glaucoma
- **CV:** *Hypertension,* CHF, necrotizing angiitis
- **Endocrine:** Growth retardation, decreased carbohydrate tolerance, diabetes mellitus, cushingoid state, *secondary adrenocortical and pituitary unresponsiveness*
- **GI:** Peptic or esophageal ulcer, pancreatitis, abdominal distention
- **GU:** *Amenorrhea, irregular menses*
- **Hematologic:** *Fluid and electrolyte disturbances,* negative nitrogen balance
- **Hypersensitivity: Anaphylactoid** or hypersensitivity reactions
- **Musculoskeletal:** *Muscle weakness,* steroid myopathy, loss of muscle mass, osteoporosis, spontaneous fractures
- **Other:** *Impaired wound healing, petechiae, ecchymoses, increased sweating, thin and fragile skin, acne, immunosuppression and masking of signs of infection,* activation of latent infections, including tuberculosis, fungal, and viral eye infections, pneumonia, abscess, septic infection, GI and GU infections

Interactions

✹ **Drug-drug** • Decreased effects with barbiturates • Decreased effects of anticholinesterases with corticotropin; profound muscular depression is possible • Decreased effectiveness of insulin, antidiabetic agents; monitor patient closely and increase dosage as needed

✹ **Drug-lab test** • Suppression of skin test reactions

■ Nursing considerations
Assessment

- **History:** Adrenocortical insufficiency or hyperfunction; infections, ocular herpes simplex; scleroderma, osteoporosis; recent surgery; CHF, hypertension; allergy to pork or pork products; liver disease: cirrhosis; ulcerative colitis; diverticulitis; active or latent peptic ulcer; inflammatory bowel disease; lactation; diabetes mellitus; hypothyroidism; pregnancy
- **Physical:** Weight, T; skin color, integrity; reflexes, bilateral grip strength, ophthalmologic exam, affect, orientation; P, BP, auscultation, peripheral perfusion, status of veins; R, adventitious sounds, chest x-ray; upper GI x-ray (peptic ulcer symptoms), liver palpation; CBC, serum electrolytes, 2-hr postprandial blood glucose, thyroid function tests, urinalysis

Interventions

- Verify adrenal responsiveness (increased urinary and plasma corticosteroid levels) to corticotropin before therapy, use the administrative route proposed for treatment.
- Administer corticotropin repository injection only by IM or SC injection.
- Administer IV injections only for diagnostic purposes or to treat thrombocytopenic purpura.
- Prepare solutions for IM and SC injections: Reconstitute powder by dissolving in sterile water for injection or sodium chloride injection so that the individual dose will be contained in 1–2 mL of solution. Refrigerate reconstituted solutions, and use within 24 hr.
- Use minimal doses for minimal duration to minimize adverse effects.
- Taper doses when discontinuing high-dose or long-term therapy.
- Administer a rapidly acting corticosteroid before, during, and after stress when patients are on long-term therapy.
- Do not give patients receiving corticotropins live virus vaccines.

Teaching points

- Avoid immunizations with live vaccines.
- Diabetics may require an increased dosage of insulin or oral hypoglycemic drug; consult your health care provider.
- Take antacids between meals to reduce heartburn.
- Avoid exposure to people and contagious diseases. This drug masks signs of infection and decreases resistance to infection; wash hands

---

Adverse effects in *Italics* are most common; those in **Bold** are life-threatening.

carefully after touching contaminated surfaces.
• Report unusual weight gain, swelling of lower extremities, muscle weakness, abdominal pain, seizures, headache, fever, prolonged sore throat, cold or other infection, worsening of symptoms for which drug is being taken.

▷ cortisone acetate
(kor' ti sone)

Cortone Acetate

PREGNANCY CATEGORY C

Drug classes
Adrenal cortical hormone
Corticosteroid, short acting
Hormone

Therapeutic actions
Enters target cells where it has anti-inflammatory and immunosuppressive (glucocorticoid) and salt-retaining (mineralocorticoid) effects.

Indications
• Replacement therapy in adrenal cortical insufficiency
• Hypercalcemia associated with cancer
• Short-term management of various inflammatory and allergic disorders: rheumatoid arthritis, collagen diseases (SLE), dermatologic diseases (pemphigus), status asthmaticus, and autoimmune disorders
• Hematologic disorders: thrombocytopenic purpura, erythroblastopenia
• Trichinosis with neurologic or myocardial involvement
• Ulcerative colitis, acute exacerbations of multiple sclerosis, and palliation in some leukemias and lymphomas

Contraindications and cautions
• Contraindicated with infections, especially tuberculosis, fungal infections, amebiasis, vaccinia and varicella, and antibiotic-resistant infections, pregnancy, lactation.
• Use cautiously with renal or hepatic disease; hypothyroidism, ulcerative colitis with impending perforation; diverticulitis; active or latent peptic ulcer; inflammatory bowel disease; CHF, hypertension, thromboembolic disorders; osteoporosis; convulsive disorders; diabetes mellitus, pregnancy, lactation.

Available forms
Tablets—5, 10, 25 mg; injection—50 mg/mL

Dosages
• *Physiologic replacement:* 0.5–0.75 mg/kg/day PO or 25 mg/m² per day PO divided into equal doses q 8 hr; 0.25–0.35 mg/kg/day or 12–15 mg/m² per day IM.
Adults
Individualize dosage based on severity and response. In long-term therapy, alternate-day therapy should be considered. After long-term therapy, withdraw drug slowly to avoid adrenal insufficiency.
Initial: 25–300 mg/day PO; 20–330 mg/day IM.
Maintenance: Reduce dose in small increments at intervals until the lowest dose that maintains satisfactory clinical response is reached.
Pediatric patients
Individualize dosage on the basis of severity and response, rather than by adherence to formulas that correct adult doses for age or weight. Carefully observe growth and development in infants and children on prolonged therapy.

Pharmacokinetics

Route	Onset	Peak	Duration
Oral	Rapid	2 hr	1–1.5 days
IM	Slow	20–40 hr	1–1.5 days

Metabolism: Hepatic; $T_{1/2}$: 30 min
Distribution: Crosses placenta; enters breast milk
Excretion: Urine

Adverse effects
• **CNS:** Convulsions, *vertigo, headaches,* pseudotumor cerebri, *euphoria, insomnia, mood swings, depression,* psychosis, **intracerebral hemorrhage,** reversible cerebral atrophy in infants, cataracts, increased intraocular pressure, glaucoma
• **CV:** *Hypertension,* CHF, necrotizing angiitis
• **Endocrine:** Growth retardation, decreased carbohydrate tolerance, diabetes mellitus,

cushingoid state, *secondary adrenocortical and pituitary unresponsiveness*

- **GI:** Peptic or esophageal ulcer, pancreatitis, abdominal distention
- **GU:** *Amenorrhea, irregular menses*
- **Hematologic:** *Fluid and electrolyte disturbances,* negative nitrogen balance, increased blood sugar, glycosuria, increased serum cholesterol, decreased serum T_3 and T_4 levels
- **Hypersensitivity: Anaphylactoid** or hypersensitivity reactions
- **Musculoskeletal:** *Muscle weakness,* steroid myopathy, loss of muscle mass, osteoporosis, spontaneous fractures
- **Other:** *Impaired wound healing, petechiae, ecchymoses, increased sweating, thin and fragile skin, acne, immunosuppression and masking of signs of infection,* activation of latent infections including tuberculosis, fungal and viral eye infections, pneumonia, abscess, septic infection, GI and GU infections

Interactions

✳ **Drug-drug** • Increased therapeutic and toxic effects of cortisone if taken concurrently with troleandomycin • Decreased effects of anticholinesterases if taken concurrently with corticotropin; profound muscular depression is possible • Decreased steroid blood levels if taken concurrently with phenytoin, phenobarbital, rifampin • Decreased serum levels of salicylates if taken concurrently with cortisone

✳ **Drug-lab test** • False-negative nitrobluetetrazolium test for bacterial infection • Suppression of skin test reactions

■ Nursing considerations
Assessment

- **History:** Infections, hypothyroidism, ulcerative colitis; diverticulitis; active or latent peptic ulcer; inflammatory bowel disease; CHF, hypertension, thromboembolic disorders; osteoporosis; convulsive disorders; diabetes mellitus, lactation
- **Physical:** Baseline body weight, T; reflexes, and grip strength, affect, and orientation; P, BP, peripheral perfusion, prominence of superficial veins; R and adventitious sounds; serum electrolytes, blood glucose

Interventions

- Give daily doses before 9 AM to mimic peak corticosteroid blood levels.
- Increase dosage when patient is subject to stress.
- Taper doses when discontinuing high-dose or long-term therapy.
- Do not give live virus vaccines with immunosuppressive doses of corticosteroids.

Teaching points

- Take drug before 9 AM each day.
- Do not stop taking the drug (oral) without consulting health care provider.
- Avoid exposure to infection.
- Report unusual weight gain, swelling of the extremities, muscle weakness, black or tarry stools, fever, prolonged sore throat, colds or other infections, worsening of this disorder.

▽**cosyntropin**

See *Less Commonly Used Drugs,* p. 1340.

▽**cromolyn sodium (disodium cromoglycate, cromoglicic acid, cromoglycic acid)**

(*kroe' moe lin*)

Oral concentrate: Gastrocrom
Respiratory inhalant, nasal solution, ophthalmic solution: Intal, Nalcrom (CAN), Nasalcrom, Rynacrom (CAN)

PREGNANCY CATEGORY B

Drug classes
Antiasthmatic drug (prophylactic)
Antiallergic agent

Therapeutic actions
Inhibits the allergen-triggered release of histamine and slow-releasing substance of anaphylaxis, leukotriene, from mast cells; decreases the overall allergic response and inflammatory reaction.

Indications

- Respiratory inhalant: Prophylaxis of severe bronchial asthma; prevention of exercise-induced bronchospasm
- Nasal preparations: Prevention and treatment of allergic rhinitis
- Ophthalmic solution: Treatment of allergic disorders (vernal keratoconjunctivitis and conjunctivitis, giant papillary conjunctivitis, vernal keratitis, allergic keratoconjunctivitis)
- Oral use: orphan drug use—mastocytosis
- Unlabeled uses: prevention of GI and systemic reactions to food allergies; treatment of eczema, dermatitis, ulcerations, urticaria pigmentosa, chronic urticaria, hay fever, postexercise bronchospasm

Contraindications and cautions

- Contraindicated with allergy to cromolyn.
- Use cautiously with pregnancy, lactation.

Available forms

Nebulizer solution—20 mg/2 mL ampule; aerosol spray—800 mcg/actuation; nasal solution—40 mg/mL; ophthalmic solution—4%; oral concentrate—5 mL/100 mg

Dosages
Adults and pediatric patients
Respiratory inhalant product used in spinhaler
Adults and children > 5 yr: Initially 20 mg (contents of 1 capsule) inhaled qid at regular intervals.
Children < 5 yr: Safety and efficacy not established; use of capsule product not recommended.
Nebulizer solution for oral inhalation
Adults and children > 2 yr: Initially 20 mg qid at regular intervals, administered from a power-operated nebulizer with an adequate flow rate and equipped with a suitable face mask; do not use a hand-operated nebulizer.
Children < 2 yr: Safety and efficacy not established.
Children > 2 yr:
- *Prevention of exercise-induced bronchospasm:* Inhale 20 mg no more than 1 hr before anticipated exercise; during prolonged exercise, repeat as needed for protection.

Nasal solution used with nasalmatic metered-spray device
Adults and children > 6 yr: 1 spray in each nostril three to six times per day at regular intervals.
Children < 6 yr: Safety and efficacy not established.
- *Seasonal (pollenotic) rhinitis and prevention of rhinitis caused by exposure to other specific inhalant allergens:* Begin use before exposure, and continue during exposure.

Ophthalmic solution
Adults and children > 4 yr: 1–2 drops in each eye from four to six times per day at regular intervals.
Children < 4 yr: Safety and efficacy not established.

Oral concentrate
Adults
2 ampules qid. Open ampule and squeeze liquid contents into a glass of water at least 30 min before meals and hs.

Pediatric patients
< 2 yr: Not recommended.
2–12 yr: One ampule PO qid 30 min before meals and hs. Dosage may be increased if satisfactory results are seen within 2–3 wk. Do not exceed 40 mg/kg/day (30 mg/kg/day in children 6 mo–2 yr).

Pharmacokinetics

Route	Onset	Peak	Duration
All	1 wk	15 min	6–8 hr

Metabolism: Hepatic; $T_{1/2}$: 80 min
Distribution: Crosses placenta; may enter breast milk
Excretion: Urine and bile; respiratory (inhalation)

Adverse effects
Respiratory inhalant product
- **CNS:** *Dizziness, headache,* lacrimation
- **Dermatologic:** Urticaria, rash, angioedema, joint swelling and pain
- **GI:** *Nausea, dry and irritated throat,* swollen parotid glands
- **GU:** Dysuria, frequency
Nebulizer solution
- **GI:** Abdominal pain

- **Respiratory:** *Cough, nasal congestion, wheezing, sneezing,* nasal itching, epistaxis, nose burning

Nasal solution

- **CNS:** *Headache*
- **Dermatologic:** Rash
- **GI:** Bad taste in mouth
- **Respiratory:** *Sneezing, nasal stinging or burning, nasal irritation,* epistaxis, postnasal drip

Ophthalmic solution

- **Local:** *Transient ocular stinging or burning on instillation*

Oral

- **CNS:** *Dizziness, fatigue, paresthesia, headache,* migraine, psychosis, anxiety, depression, insomnia, behavior change, hallucinations, lethargy
- **Dermatologic:** *Flushing,* urticaria, angioedema, skin erythema and burning
- **GI:** *Taste perversion, diarrhea,* esophagospasm, flatulence, dysphagia, hepatic function tests abnormality, burning in the mouth and throat

■ Nursing considerations
Assessment

- **History:** Allergy to cromolyn, impaired renal or hepatic function, lactation
- **Physical:** Skin color, lesions; palpation of parotid glands; joint size, overlying color and T; orientation; R, auscultation, patency of nasal passages (with respiratory inhalant and nasal products); liver evaluation; normal output; renal and liver function tests, urinalysis

Interventions
Respiratory inhalant products

- Do not use during acute asthma attack; begin therapy when acute episode is over and patient can inhale.
- Arrange for continuation of treatment with bronchodilators and corticosteroids during initial cromolyn therapy, tapering corticosteroids or reinstituting them based on patient stress.
- Use caution if cough or bronchospasm occurs after inhalation; this may (rarely) preclude continuation of treatment.

- Discontinue therapy if eosinophilic pneumonia occurs.
- Taper cromolyn if withdrawal is desired.
- Mix cromolyn solution only with compatible solutions: compatible with metaproterenol sulfate, isoproterenol HCl, 0.25% isoetharine HCl, epinephrine HCl, terbutaline sulfate, and 20% acetylcysterine solution for at least 1 hr after their admixture.
- Store nebulizer solution below 30° C; protect from light.

Nasal solution

- Have patient clear nasal passages before use.
- Have patient inhale through nose during administration.
- Observable response to treatment may require 2–4 wk (perennial allergic rhinitis); continued use of antihistamines and nasal decongestants may be necessary.
- Replace *Nasalmatic* pump device every 6 mo.

Ophthalmic solution

- Instruct patients not to wear soft contact lenses.
- Although symptomatic response is usually evident within a few days, up to 6 wk of treatment may be needed.

All

- Give corticosteroids as needed.
- Carefully teach patients how to use the specialized *Spinhaler, Nasalmatic,* or power nebulizer devices.

Oral concentrate

- Give drug 30 min before meals and hs.
- Open ampule and pour contents into glass of water; stir until completely dissolved. Do not mix with fruit juice, milk, or foods. Drink all of the liquid.
- Do not give oral capsules for inhalation.

Teaching points

- Take drug at regular intervals. When drug is used to prevent specific allergen exposure reactions or to prevent exercise-induced bronchospasm, instruct patient about the best time to take drug.
- Take drug as follows: *Respiratory inhalant and nasal solution:* See manufacturer's insert; do not swallow capsule used in *Spinhaler. Ophthalmic solution:* Lie down or tilt head back, and look at ceiling; drop solu-

tion inside lower eyelid while looking up. After instilling eye drops, close eyes; apply gentle pressure to inside corner of eye for 1 min. *Oral solution:* Break ampule and squeeze contents into a glass of water. Stir. Drink all of liquid. Do not mix with fruit juice, milk, or food.

- Do not discontinue abruptly except on advice of your health care provider (respiratory inhalant and nasal products).
- Do not wear soft contact lenses while using cromolyn eye drops.
- Be aware that you may experience transient stinging or burning in your eyes on instillation of the eye drops.
- These side effects may occur (oral): dizziness, drowsiness, fatigue. If this occurs, avoid driving or operating dangerous machinery.
- Report coughing, wheezing (respiratory products); change in vision (ophthalmic products); swelling, difficulty swallowing, depression (oral product).

▷cyanocobalamin, nasal
(sigh' an oh cob ball' a min)

Nascobal

PREGNANCY CATEGORY C

Drug class
Vitamin

Therapeutic actions
Intranasal gel that allows absorption of vitamin B_{12} which is essential to cell growth and reproduction, hematopoiesis, and nucleoprotein and myelin synthesis, and has been associated with fat and carbohydrate metabolism and protein synthesis.

Indications
- Maintenance of patients in hematologic remission after IM vitamin B_{12} therapy for pernicious anemia, inadequate secretion of intrinsic factor, dietary deficiency, malabsorption, competition by intestinal bacteria or parasites, or inadequate utilization of vitamin B_{12}

- Maintenance of effective therapeutic levels of vitamin B_{12} in patients with HIV, AIDS, MS, and Crohn's disease.

Contraindications and cautions
- Contraindicated with hypersensitivity to cobalt, vitamin B_{12}, or any component of drug.
- Use cautiously with pregnancy or lactation, Leber's disease, nasal lesions, or upper respiratory infections.

Available forms
Intranasal gel—500 mcg/0.1 mL

Dosages
Adults
One spray (500 mcg) in one nostril, once/wk.
Pediatric patients
Safety and efficacy not established.

Pharmacokinetics

Route	Onset	Peak
Nasal	Slow	1–2 hr

Metabolism: $T_{1/2}$: unknown
Distribution: May cross placenta, may enter breast milk
Excretion: Urine

Adverse effects
- **CNS:** *Headache*
- **Hematologic:** Bone marrow suppression
- **Local:** *Rhinitis, nasal congestion*
- **Other:** Fever, pain, local irritation

Interactions
＊**Drug-drug** ● Decreased effectiveness may be seen with antibiotics, methotrexate, pyrimethamine, colchicine, para-aminosalicylic acid, heavy alcohol use

■ Nursing considerations
Assessment
- **History:** Pregnancy or lactation, Leber's disease, nasal lesions or upper respiratory infections; history of pernicious anemia, vitamin B_{12} deficiency, dates of IM cyanocobalamin therapy
- **Physical:** State of nasal mucous membranes; serum vitamin B_{12} levels, CBC, potassium level

Interventions

- Confirm diagnosis before administering; ensure that patient is hemodynamically stable after IM therapy.
- Teach patient proper technique for administering nasal gel.
- Monitor serum vitamin B_{12} levels before starting, 1 mo after starting, and every 3–6 mo during therapy.
- Do not administer if nasal congestion, rhinitis, or upper respiratory infection is present.
- Evaluate patient response and consider need for folate or iron replacement.

Teaching points

- Learn the proper technique for administering nasal gel. Mark calendar with date for weekly dose.
- Periodic blood tests will be needed to monitor your response to this drug.
- Do not administer if you have nasal congestion, rhinitis, or upper respiratory infection; consult with your health care provider.
- These side effects may occur: headache (analgesics may help), nausea (take small, frequent meals).
- Report nasal pain, nasal sores, fatigue, weakness, easy bruising.

▽cyclizine hydrochloride

(sye' kli zeen)

Marezine

PREGNANCY CATEGORY B

Drug classes

Antiemetic
Anti-motion sickness agent
Antihistamine
Anticholinergic

Therapeutic actions

Reduces sensitivity of the labyrinthine apparatus; peripheral anticholinergic effects may contribute to efficacy.

Indications

- Prevention and treatment of nausea, vomiting, dizziness associated with motion sickness

Contraindications and cautions

- Contraindicated with allergy to cyclizine.
- Use cautiously with pregnancy, lactation, narrow-angle glaucoma, stenosing peptic ulcer, symptomatic prostatic hypertrophy, bronchial asthma, bladder neck obstruction, pyloroduodenal obstruction, cardiac arrhythmias; postoperative patients (hypotensive effects may be confusing and dangerous).

Available forms

Tablets—50 mg

Dosages

Adults

50 mg PO 30 min before exposure to motion; repeat q 4–6 hr. Do not exceed 200 mg in 24 hr.

Pediatric patients 6–12 yr

25 mg PO up to three times a day.

Geriatric patients

More likely to cause dizziness, sedation, syncope, toxic confusional states, and hypotension in elderly patients; use with caution.

Pharmacokinetics

Route	Onset	Peak	Duration
Oral	30–60 min	60–90 min	4–6 hr

Metabolism: Hepatic; $T_{1/2}$: 2–3 hr
Distribution: Crosses placenta; enters breast milk
Excretion: Unknown

Adverse effects

- **CNS:** *Drowsiness, confusion,* euphoria, nervousness, restlessness, insomnia and excitement, convulsions, vertigo, tinnitus, blurred vision, diplopia, auditory and visual hallucinations
- **CV:** Hypotension, palpitations, tachycardia
- **Dermatologic:** Urticaria, drug rash
- **GI:** *Dry mouth, anorexia, nausea,* vomiting, diarrhea or constipation, cholestatic jaundice

Adverse effects in *Italics* are most common; those in **Bold** are life-threatening.

- **GU:** *Urinary frequency, difficult urination,* urinary retention
- **Respiratory:** Respiratory depression, dry nose and throat

Interactions

❋ **Drug-drug** • Increased depressant effects with alcohol, other CNS depressants

■ Nursing considerations
Assessment

- **History:** Allergy to cyclizine, narrow-angle glaucoma, stenosing peptic ulcer, symptomatic prostatic hypertrophy, bronchial asthma, bladder neck obstruction, pyloroduodenal obstruction, cardiac arrhythmias, recent surgery, lactation
- **Physical:** Skin color, lesions, texture; orientation, reflexes, affect; vision exam; P, BP; R, adventitious sounds; bowel sounds; prostate palpation; CBC

Interventions

- Monitor elderly patients carefully for adverse effects
- Be aware that IM form is available for use in adults only as 50 mg q 4–6 hr. Switch to oral form as soon as possible.

Teaching points

- Take drug as prescribed; avoid excessive dosage.
- Use before motion sickness occurs; antimotion sickness drugs work best if used prophylactically.
- These side effects may occur: dizziness, sedation, drowsiness (use caution driving or performing tasks that require alertness); epigastric distress, diarrhea or constipation (take drug with food); dry mouth (use frequent mouth care, suck sugarless lozenges); thickening of bronchial secretions, dryness of nasal mucosa (consider another type of motion sickness remedy).
- Avoid alcohol; serious sedation could occur.
- Report difficulty breathing, hallucinations, tremors, loss of coordination, unusual bleeding or bruising, visual disturbances, irregular heartbeat.

▷ cyclobenzaprine hydrochloride
(sye kloe ben' za preen)

Apo-Cyclobenzaprine (CAN), Flexeril, Novo-Cycloprine (CAN)

PREGNANCY CATEGORY B

Drug class
Skeletal muscle relaxant, centrally acting

Therapeutic actions
Precise mechanism not known; does not directly relax tense skeletal muscles but appears to act mainly at brain stem levels or in the spinal cord.

Indications
- Relief of discomfort associated with acute, painful musculoskeletal conditions, as adjunct to rest, physical therapy
- Unlabeled use: adjunct in the management of fibrositis syndrome

Contraindications and cautions
- Contraindicated with hypersensitivity to cyclobenzaprine, acute recovery phase of MI, arrhythmias, heart block or conduction disturbances, CHF, hyperthyroidism.
- Use cautiously with urinary retention, angle-closure glaucoma, increased intraocular pressure, lactation.

Available forms
Tablets—10 mg

Dosages
Adults
10 mg PO tid (range 20–40 mg/day in divided doses); do not exceed 60 mg/day; do not use longer than 2 or 3 wk.
Pediatric patients
Safety and efficacy in patients < 15 yr not established.

Pharmacokinetics

Route	Onset	Peak	Duration
Oral	1 hr	4–6 hr	12–24 hr

Metabolism: Hepatic; $T_{1/2}$: 1–3 days

Distribution: Crosses placenta; may enter breast milk
Excretion: Urine

Adverse effects
- **CNS:** *Drowsiness, dizziness,* fatigue, tiredness, asthenia, blurred vision, headache, nervousness, confusion
- **CV:** Arrhythmias, **MI**
- **GI:** *Dry mouth,* nausea, constipation, dyspepsia, unpleasant taste, liver toxicity
- **GU:** Frequency, urinary retention

Interactions
✳ **Drug-drug** • Additive CNS effects with alcohol, barbiturates, other CNS depressants, MAOIs, TCAs; avoid concomitant use

■ Nursing considerations
Assessment
- **History:** Hypersensitivity to cyclobenzaprine, acute recovery phase of MI, arrhythmias, CHF, hyperthyroidism, urinary retention, angle-closure glaucoma, increased intraocular pressure, lactation
- **Physical:** Orientation, affect, ophthalmic exam (tonometry); bowel sounds, normal GI output; prostate palpation, normal voiding pattern; thyroid function tests

Interventions
- Arrange for analgesics if headache occurs (possible adjunct for relief of muscle spasm).

Teaching points
- Take this drug exactly as prescribed. Do not take a higher dosage.
- Avoid alcohol, sleep-inducing, or OTC drugs; these may cause dangerous effects.
- These side effects may occur: drowsiness, dizziness, blurred vision (avoid driving or engaging in activities that require alertness); dyspepsia (take drug with food, eat frequent small meals); dry mouth (suck sugarless lozenges or ice chips).
- Report urinary retention or difficulty voiding, pale stools, yellow skin or eyes.

▷ cyclophosphamide
*(sye kloe **foss'** fa mide)*
Cytoxan, Neosar, Procytox (CAN)
PREGNANCY CATEGORY D

Drug classes
Alkylating agent
Nitrogen mustard
Antineoplastic

Therapeutic actions
Cytotoxic: interferes with the replication of susceptible cells. Immunosuppressive: lymphocytes are especially sensitive to drug effects.

Indications
- Treatment of malignant lymphomas, multiple myeloma, leukemias, mycosis fungoides, neuroblastoma, adenocarcinoma of the ovary, retinoblastoma, carcinoma of the breast; used concurrently or sequentially with other antineoplastic drugs
- Treatment of minimal change nephrotic syndrome in children
- Unlabeled uses: severe rheumatologic conditions, Wegener's granulomatosis, steroid-resistant vasculitis, SLE

Contraindications and cautions
- Contraindicated with allergy to cyclophosphamide, allergy to tartrazine (in tablets marketed as *Cytoxan*), pregnancy, lactation.
- Use cautiously with radiation therapy; chemotherapy; tumor cell infiltration of the bone marrow; adrenalectomy with steroid therapy; infections, especially varicella-zoster; hematopoietic depression, impaired hepatic or renal function.

Available forms
Tablets—25, 50 mg; powder for injection—75 mg mannitol/100 mg cyclophosphamide, 82 mg sodium bicarbonate/100 mg cyclophosphamide

Dosages
Individualize dosage based on hematologic profile and response.

Adverse effects in *Italics* are most common; those in **Bold** are life-threatening.

Adults
- *Induction therapy:* 40–50 mg/kg (1.5–1.8 g/m²) IV given in divided doses over 2–5 days or 1–5 mg/kg/day PO.
- *Maintenance therapy:* 1–5 mg/kg/day PO, 10–15 mg/kg (350–530 mg/m²) IV every 7–10 days, or 3–5 mg/kg (110–185 mg/m²) IV twice weekly.

Pediatric patients
- *Minimal change nephrotic syndrome:* 2.5–3 mg/day PO for 60–90 days.

Patients with hepatic dysfunction
Bilirubin of 3.1–5 mg/dL or AST > 180: reduce dose by 25%. Bilirubin > 5 mg/dL: omit dose.

Patients with renal dysfunction
Glomerular filtration rate < 10 mL/min: decrease dose by 50%.

Pharmacokinetics

Route	Onset	Peak
Oral	Varies	1 hr
IV	Rapid	15–30 min

Metabolism: Hepatic; $T_{1/2}$: 3–12 hr
Distribution: Crosses placenta; enters breast milk
Excretion: Urine

▽ IV facts

Preparation: Add sterile water for injection or bacteriostatic water for injection to the vial, and shake gently. Use 5 mL for 100-mg vial, 10 mL for 200-mg vial, 25 mL for 500-mg vial, 50 mL for 1-g vial. Prepared solutions may be injected IV, IM, intraperitoneally, intrapleurally. Use within 24 hr if stored at room temperature or within 6 days if refrigerated. If bacteriostatic water for injection is not used, use within 6 hr.

Infusion: Infuse in 5% dextrose injection, 5% dextrose and 0.9% sodium chloride injection; each 100 mg infused over 15 min.

Adverse effects

- **CV:** Cardiotoxicity
- **Dermatologic:** *Alopecia,* darkening of skin and fingernails
- **GI:** *Anorexia, nausea, vomiting, diarrhea,* stomatitis
- **GU:** *Hemorrhagic cystitis,* bladder fibrosis, hematuria to potentially fatal **hemorrhagic cystitis,** increased urine uric acid levels, gonadal suppression
- **Hematologic:** *Leukopenia,* thrombocytopenia, anemia (rare), increased serum uric acid levels
- **Respiratory:** Interstitial pulmonary fibrosis
- **Other:** SIADH, immunosuppression secondary to neoplasia

Interactions

✱ **Drug-drug** • Prolonged apnea with succinylcholine: metabolism is inhibited by cyclophosphamide • Decreased serum levels and therapeutic acitivity of digoxin

✱ **Drug-food** • Decreased metabolism and risk of toxic effects if combined with grapefruit juice; avoid this combination

■ Nursing considerations
Assessment

- **History:** Allergy to cyclophosphamide, allergy to tartrazine, radiation therapy, chemotherapy, tumor cell infiltration of the bone marrow, adrenalectomy with steroid therapy, infections, hematopoietic depression, impaired hepatic or renal function, pregnancy, lactation
- **Physical:** T; weight; skin color, lesions; hair; P, auscultation, baseline ECG; R, adventitious sounds; mucous membranes, liver evaluation; CBC, differential; urinalysis; liver and renal function tests

Interventions

- Arrange for blood tests to evaluate hematopoietic function before therapy and weekly during therapy.
- Do not give full dosage within 4 wk after a full course of radiation therapy or chemotherapy due to the risk of severe bone marrow depression; reduced dosage may be needed.
- Arrange for reduced dosage in patients with impaired renal or hepatic function.
- Ensure that patient is well hydrated before treatment to decrease risk of cystitis.
- Prepare oral solution by dissolving injectable cyclophosphamide in aromatic elixir. Refrigerate and use within 14 days.
- Give tablets on an empty stomach. If severe GI upset occurs, tablet may be given with food.
- Counsel male patients not to father a child during or immediately after therapy; infant

cardiac and limb abnormalities have occurred.

Teaching points
- Take drug on an empty stomach. If severe GI upset occurs, the tablet may be taken with food. Do not drink grapefruit juice while on this drug.
- These side effects may occur: nausea, vomiting, loss of appetite (take drug with food, eat small frequent meals); darkening of the skin and fingernails; loss of hair (obtain a wig or other head covering prior to hair loss; head must be covered in extremes of temperature).
- Try to maintain your fluid intake and nutrition (drink at least 10–12 glasses of fluid each day).
- Use birth control during drug use and for a time thereafter (male and female); this drug can cause severe birth defects.
- Report unusual bleeding or bruising, fever, chills, sore throat, cough, shortness of breath, blood in the urine, painful urination, rapid heart beat, swelling of the feet or hands, stomach or flank pain.

▷cycloserine
(sye kloe ser' een)

Seromycin Pulvules

PREGNANCY CATEGORY C

Drug classes
Antituberculous drug (third line)
Antibiotic

Therapeutic actions
Inhibits cell wall synthesis in susceptible strains of gram-positive and gram-negative bacteria and in *Mycobacterium tuberculosis,* causing cell death.

Indications
- Treatment of active pulmonary and extrapulmonary (including renal) tuberculosis that is not responsive to first-line antituberculous drugs in conjunction with other antituberculous drugs

- UTIs caused by susceptible bacteria

Contraindications and cautions
- Allergy to cycloserine, epilepsy, depression, severe anxiety or psychosis, severe renal insufficiency, excessive concurrent use of alcohol, lactation.

Available forms
Capsules—250 mg

Dosages
Adults
- *Initial dose:* 250 mg bid PO at 12-hr intervals for first 2 wk; monitor serum levels (above 30 mcg/mL is generally toxic).
- *Maintenance dose:* 500 mg–1 g/day PO in divided doses. Do not exceed 1 g/day.
Pediatric patients
Safety and dosage not established.

Pharmacokinetics

Route	Onset	Peak	Duration
Oral	Varies	4–8 hr	48–72 hr

Metabolism: $T_{1/2}$: 10 hr
Distribution: Crosses placenta; enters breast milk
Excretion: Urine and feces

Adverse effects
- **CNS:** *Convulsions, drowsiness, somnolence, headache, tremor, vertigo, confusion,* disorientation, loss of memory, **psychoses** (possibly with suicidal tendencies), hyperirritability, aggression, paresis, hyperreflexia, paresthesias, seizures, coma
- **Dermatologic:** Rash
- **Hematologic:** Elevated serum transaminase levels

■ Nursing considerations
Assessment
- **History:** Allergy to cycloserine, epilepsy, depression, severe anxiety or psychosis, severe renal insufficiency, excessive concurrent use of alcohol, lactation
- **Physical:** Skin color, lesions; orientation, reflexes, affect, EEG; liver evaluation; liver function tests

Interventions

- Arrange for culture and sensitivity studies before use.
- Give this drug only when other therapy has failed, and only in conjunction with other antituberculosis agents when treating tuberculosis.
- Arrange for follow-up of liver and renal function tests, hematologic tests, and serum drug levels.
- Consult with physician regarding the use of anticonvulsants, sedatives, or pyridoxine if CNS effects become severe.
- Discontinue drug, and notify physician if rash, severe CNS reactions occur.

Teaching points

- Avoid excessive alcohol consumption.
- Take this drug regularly; avoid missing doses. Do not discontinue this drug without first consulting your health care provider.
- These side effects may occur: drowsiness, tremor, disorientation (use caution operating a car or dangerous machinery); depression, personality change, numbness and tingling.
- Have regular, periodic medical checkups, that include blood tests to evaluate the drug effects.
- Report rash, headache, tremors, shaking, confusion, dizziness.

cyclosporine (cyclosporin A)
(sye' kloe spor een)

Neoral, Sandimmune, SangCya

PREGNANCY CATEGORY C

Drug class
Immunosuppressant

Therapeutic actions

Exact mechanism of immunosuppressant is not known; specifically and reversibly inhibits immunocompetent lymphocytes in the G_0 or G_1 phase of the cell cycle; inhibits T-helper and T-suppressor cells, lymphokine production, and release of interleukin-2 and T-cell growth factor.

Indications

- Prophylaxis for organ rejection in kidney, liver, and heart transplants in conjunction with adrenal corticosteroids
- Treatment of chronic rejection in patients previously treated with other immunosuppressive agents
- Alone, or in combination with methotrexate for treatment of patients with severe active rheumatoid arthritis (*Neoral*)
- Treatment of recalcitrant, plaque psoriasis in non-immune-compromised adults (*Neoral*)
- Unlabeled use: limited but successful use in other procedures, including pancreas, bone marrow, heart and lung transplants; Crohn's disease, SLE

Contraindications and cautions

- Contraindicated with allergy to cyclosporine or polyoxyethylated castor oil (oral preparation), pregnancy, lactation.
- Use cautiously with impaired renal function, malabsorption.

Available forms

Capsules (*Sandimmune*)—25, 50, 100 mg; soft gel capsules for microemulsion (*Neoral*)—25, 100 mg; oral solution—100 mg/mL; oral solution for microemulsion—100 mg/mL; IV solution (*Sandimmune*)—50 mg/mL

Dosages
Adults and pediatric patients
Neoral and *Sandimmune* are not bioequivalent—do not interchange.
Oral

- *Organ rejection:* 15 mg/kg/day PO (*Sandimmune*) initially given 4–12 hr prior to transplantation; continue dose postoperatively for 1–2 wk, then taper by 5%/wk to a maintenance level of 5–10 mg/kg/day.
- *Rheumatoid arthritis:* 2.5 mg/kg/day (*Neoral*) PO in divided doses; may increase up to 4 mg/kg/day.
- *Psoriasis:* 2.5 mg/kg/day PO (*Neoral*) for 4 wk, then may increase up to 4 mg/kg/day.

Parenteral
Patients unable to take oral solution preoperatively or postoperatively may be given IV infusion (*Sandimmune*) at one-third the oral dose (ie, 5–6 mg/kg/day given 4–12 hr prior to transplantation, administered as a slow in-

fusion over 2–6 hr). Continue this daily dose postoperatively. Switch to oral drug as soon as possible.

Pharmacokinetics

Route	Onset	Peak
Oral	Varies	3.5 hr
IV	Rapid	1–2 hr

Metabolism: Hepatic; $T_{1/2}$: 19–27 hr (*Sandimmune*), 5–8 hr (*Neoral*)
Distribution: Crosses placenta; enters breast milk
Excretion: Bile and urine

▽ IV facts

Preparation: Dilute IV solution immediately before use. Dilute 1 mL concentrate in 20–100 mL of 0.9% sodium chloride injection or 5% dextrose injection. Protect from exposure to light.
Infusion: Give in a slow IV infusion over 2–6 hr.
Incompatibilities: Do not mix with magnesium sulfate.

Adverse effects

- **CNS:** *Tremor,* convulsions, headache, paresthesias
- **CV:** *Hypertension*
- **GI: Hepatotoxicity,** *gum hyperplasia, diarrhea,* nausea, vomiting, anorexia
- **GU:** *Renal dysfunction,* nephrotoxicity
- **Hematologic:** Leukopenia, hyperkalemia, hypomagnesemia, hyperuricemia
- **Other:** *Hirsutism, acne,* lymphomas, infections

Interactions

✳ **Drug-drug** • Increased risk of nephrotoxicity with other nephrotoxic agents (aminoglycosides, amphotericin B, acyclovir) • Increased risk of digoxin toxicity • Risk of severe myopathy or rhabdomyolysis with lovastatin • Increased risk of toxicity if taken with diltiazem, metoclopramide, nicardipine, amiodarone, androgens, azole antifungals, colchicine, oral contraceptives, foscarnet, macrolides, metoclopramide • Increased plasma concentration of cyclosporine with ketoconazole • Decreased therapeutic effect with hydantoins, rifampin, phenobarbital, carbamazepine
✳ **Drug-food** • Increased serum levels and adverse effects if combined with grapefruit juice

■ Nursing considerations

Assessment

- **History:** Allergy to cyclosporine or polyoxyethylated castor oil, impaired renal function, malabsorption, lactation
- **Physical:** T; skin color, lesions; BP, peripheral perfusion; liver evaluation, bowel sounds, gum evaluation; renal and liver function tests, CBC

Interventions

- Mix oral solution with milk, chocolate milk or orange juice at room temperature. Stir well, and administer at once. Do not allow mixture to stand before drinking. Use a glass container, and rinse with more diluent to ensure that the total dose is taken.
- Use parenteral administration only if patient is unable to take the oral solution; transfer to oral solution as soon as possible. *Sandimmune* must be taken with corticosteroids.
- Do not refrigerate oral solution; store at room temperature and use within 2 mo after opening.
- Monitor renal and liver function tests prior to and during therapy; marked decreases in function may require dosage adjustment or discontinuation.
- Monitor BP; heart transplant patients may require concomitant antihypertensive therapy.

Teaching points

- Dilute solution with milk, chocolate milk or orange juice at room temperature; drink immediately after mixing. Rinse the glass with the solution to ensure that all the dose is taken. Store solution at room temperature. Use solution within 2 mo of opening the bottle.
- Do not drink grapefruit juice while on this drug.
- Avoid infection; avoid crowds or people who have infections. Notify your health care provider at once if you injure yourself.

Adverse effects in *Italics* are most common; those in **Bold** are life-threatening.

- These side effects may occur: nausea, vomiting (take the drug with food); diarrhea; rash; mouth sores (frequent mouth care may help).
- This drug should not be taken during pregnancy. Use of barrier contraceptives is advised. If you think that you are pregnant or you want to become pregnant, discuss this with your health care provider.
- Have periodic blood tests to monitor your response to drug effects.
- Do not discontinue this medication without your health care provider's advice.
- Report unusual bleeding or bruising, fever, sore throat, mouth sores, tiredness.

▽cyproheptadine hydrochloride

*(si proe **hep'** ta deen)*

Periactin, PMS-Cyproheptadine (CAN)

PREGNANCY CATEGORY B

Drug class
Antihistamine (piperidine type)

Therapeutic actions
Blocks the effects of histamine at H_1 receptor sites; has atropine-like, antiserotonin, antipruritic, sedative, and appetite-stimulating effects.

Indications
- Relief of symptoms associated with perennial and seasonal allergic rhinitis; vasomotor rhinitis; allergic conjunctivitis; mild, uncomplicated urticaria and angioedema; amelioraton of allergic reactions to blood or plasma; dermatographism; adjunctive therapy in anaphylactic reactions
- Treatment of cold urticaria
- Unlabeled uses: treatment of vascular cluster headaches

Contraindications and cautions
- Contraindicated with allergy to any antihistamines, third trimester of pregnancy, newborns, premature infants.
- Use cautiously with narrow-angle glaucoma, stenosing peptic ulcer, symptomatic pro-

static hypertrophy, asthmatic attack, bladder neck obstruction, pyloroduodenal obstruction, lactation.

Available forms
Tablets—4 mg; syrup—2 mg/5 mL

Dosages
Adults
- *Initial therapy:* 4 mg tid PO.
- *Maintenance therapy:* 4–20 mg/day in three divided doses PO; do not exceed 0.5 mg/kg/day.

Pediatric patients
0.25 mg/kg/day PO or 8 mg/m².
7–14 yr: 4 mg PO bid or tid; do not exceed 16 mg/day.
2–6 yr: 2 mg PO bid or tid; do not exceed 12 mg/day.

Geriatric patients
More likely to cause dizziness, sedation, syncope, toxic confusional states, and hypotension in elderly patients; use with caution.

Pharmacokinetics

Route	Onset	Peak	Duration
Oral	15–30 min	1–2 hr	4–6 hr

Metabolism: Hepatic; $T_{1/2}$: 3–4 hr
Distribution: Crosses placenta; enters breast milk
Excretion: Urine

Adverse effects
- **CNS:** *Drowsiness, sedation, dizziness, disturbed coordination,* fatigue, confusion, restlessness, excitation, nervousness, tremor, headache, blurred vision, diplopia, vertigo, tinnitus, acute labyrinthitis, hysteria, tingling, heaviness and weakness of the hands
- **CV:** Hypotension, palpitations, bradycardia, tachycardia, extrasystoles
- **GI:** *Epigastric distress,* anorexia, increased appetite and weight gain, nausea, vomiting, diarrhea or constipation
- **GU:** Urinary frequency, dysuria, urinary retention, early menses, decreased libido, impotence
- **Hematologic:** Hemolytic anemia, hypoplastic anemia, thrombocytopenia, leukopenia, agranulocytosis, pancytopenia
- **Respiratory:** *Thickening of bronchial secretions,* chest tightness, wheezing, nasal

stuffiness, dry mouth, dry nose, dry throat, sore throat

- **Other:** Urticaria, rash, **anaphylactic shock,** photosensitivity, excessive perspiration, chills

Interactions

✳ **Drug-drug** • Subnormal pituitary-adrenal response to metyrapone • Decreased effects of fluoxetine • Increased and prolonged anticholinergic (drying) effects if taken with MAO inhibitors

■ Nursing considerations
Assessment

- **History:** Allergy to any antihistamines; narrow-angle glaucoma, stenosing peptic ulcer, symptomatic prostatic hypertrophy, asthmatic attack, bladder neck obstruction, pyloroduodenal obstruction; lactation, pregnancy
- **Physical:** Skin color, lesions, texture; orientation, reflexes, affect; vision exam; P, BP; R, adventitious sounds; bowel sounds; prostate palpation; CBC with differential

Interventions

- Administer with food if GI upset occurs.
- Give syrup form if unable to take tablets.
- Monitor patient response, and adjust dosage to lowest possible effective dose.

Teaching points

- Take as prescribed; avoid excessive dosage.
- Take drug with food if GI upset occurs.
- These side effects may occur: dizziness, sedation, drowsiness (use caution if driving or performing tasks that require alertness); epigastric distress, diarrhea, or constipation (take drug with meals); dry mouth (use frequent mouth care, suck sugarless lozenges); thickening of bronchial secretions, dryness of nasal mucosa (use humidifier).
- Avoid alcohol, serious sedation could occur.
- Report difficulty breathing, hallucinations, tremors, loss of coordination, unusual bleeding or bruising, visual disturbances, irregular heartbeat.

▷ cysteamine bitartrate

See *Less Commonly Used Drugs,* p. 1340.

▷ cytarabine (cytosine arabinoside)
(sye tare′ a been)

Cytosar-U, DepoCyt, Tarabine PFS

PREGNANCY CATEGORY D

Drug classes
Antimetabolite
Antineoplastic

Therapeutic actions
Inhibits DNA polymerase; cell cycle phase specific—S phase (stage of DNA synthesis); also blocks progression of cells from G_1 to S.

Indications

- Induction and maintenance of remission in acute myelocytic leukemia (higher response rate in children than in adults)
- Treatment of acute lymphocytic leukemia in adults and children; treatment of chronic myelocytic leukemia and erythroleukemia
- Treatment of meningeal leukemia (intrathecal use)
- Treatment of lymphomatous meningitis (liposomal)
- Treatment of non-Hodgkin's lymphoma in children (in combination therapy)

Contraindications and cautions

- Contraindicated with allergy to cytarabine, active meningeal infection (liposomal).
- Use cautiously with hematopoietic depression secondary to radiation or chemotherapy; impaired liver function, pregnancy, lactation, premature infants.

Available forms
Powder for injection—100, 500 mg, 1, 2 g; injection—10 mg/mL (liposomal), 20 mg/mL. Given by IV infusion or injection or SC.

Dosages
Adults
- *Acute myelocytic leukemia (AML) induction of remission:* 200 mg/m² per day by continuous infusion for 5 days for a total dose of 1,000 mg/m²; repeat every 2 wk. Individualize dosage based on hematologic response.
- *Maintenance of AML:* Use same dosage and schedule as induction; often a longer rest period is allowed.
- *Acute lymphocytic leukemia (ALL):* Dosage similar to AML.
- *Intrathecal use for meningeal leukemia:* 5 mg/m² to 75 mg/m² once daily for 4 days or once every 4 days. Most common dose is 30 mg/m² every 4 days until CSF is normal, followed by one more treatment.
- *Treatment of lymphomatous meningitis:* 50 mg liposomal cytarabine intrathecal q 14 days for two doses; then q 14 days for three doses; repeat q 28 days for four doses.
Pediatric patients
- *Remission induction and maintenance of AML:* Calculate dose by body weight or surface area.
- *ALL:* Same dosage as AML.
Intrathecal use
(Has been used as treatment of meningeal leukemia and prophylaxis in newly diagnosed patients): Cytarabine, 30 mg/m² every 4 days until CSF is normal; hydrocortisone sodium succinate, 15 mg/m²; methotrexate, 15 mg/m².
Combination therapies
For persistent leukemias—give at 2- to 4-wk intervals.
Cytarabine: 100 mg/m²/day by continuous IV infusion, days 1–10. *Doxorubicin:* 30 mg/m²/day by IV infusion over 30 min, days 1–3. *Cytarabine:* 100 mg/m²/day by IV infusion over 30 min q 12 hr, days 1–7. *Thioguanine:* 100 mg/m² PO q 12 hr, days 1–7. *Daunorubicin:* 60 mg/m²/day by IV infusion, days 5–7. *Cytarabine:* 100 mg/m²/day by continuous infusion, days 1–7. *Doxorubicin:* 30 mg/m²/day by IV infusion, days 1–3. *Vincristine:* 1.5 mg/m²/day by IV infusion, days 1 and 5. *Prednisone:* 40 mg/m²/day by IV infusion q 12 hr, days 1–5. *Cytarabine:* 100 mg/m²/day IV q 12 hr, days 1–7. *Daunorubicin:* 70 mg/m²/day by infusion, days 1–3. *Thioguanine:* 100 mg/m²/day PO q 12 hr, days 1–7. *Prednisone:* 40 mg/m²/

day PO, days 1–7. *Vincristine:* 1 mg/m²/day by IV infusion, days 1 and 7.
Cytarabine: 100 mg/m²/day by continuous infusion, days 1–7. *Daunorubicin:* 45 mg/m²/day by IV push, days 1–3.

Pharmacokinetics

Route	Onset	Peak	Duration
IV	Rapid	20–60 min	12–18 hr

Metabolism: Hepatic; T₁/₂: 1–3 hr
Distribution: Crosses placenta; enters breast milk
Excretion: Urine

▽IV facts
Preparation: Reconstitute 100-mg vial with 5 mL of bacteriostatic water for injection with benzyl alcohol 0.9%; resultant solution contains 20 mg/mL cytarabine. Reconstitute 500-mg vial with 10 mL of the above; resultant solution contains 50 mg/mL cytarabine. Store at room temperature for up to 48 hr. Discard solution if a slight haze appears. Can be further diluted with water for injection, 5% dextrose in water, or sodium chloride injection; stable for 8 days.
Infusion: Administer by IV infusion over at least 30 min, IV injection over 1–3 min for each 100 mg, or SC; patients can usually tolerate higher doses when given by rapid IV injection. There is no clinical advantage to any particular route.
Incompatibilities: Do not mix with insulin, heparin, penicillin G, oxacillin, nafcillin, fluorouracil.

Adverse effects
- **CNS:** Neuritis, neural toxicity
- **Dermatologic:** Fever, rash, urticaria, freckling, skin ulceration, pruritus, conjunctivitis, alopecia
- **GI:** *Anorexia, nausea, vomiting, diarrhea, oral and anal inflammation or ulceration;* esophageal ulcerations, esophagitis, abdominal pain, *hepatic dysfunction (jaundice),* acute pancreatitis
- **GU:** Renal dysfunction, urinary retention
- **Hematologic:** Bone marrow depression, hyperuricemia
- **Local:** Thrombophlebitis, cellulitis at injection site

- **Other:** Cytarabine syndrome (fever, myalgia, bone pain, occasional chest pain, maculopapular rash, conjunctivitis, malaise, which is sometimes responsive to corticosteroids), *fever, rash,* arachnoiditis (liposomal preparation)

Interactions
✳ **Drug-drug** • Decreased therapeutic action of digoxin if taken with cytarabine

■ Nursing considerations
Assessment
- **History:** Allergy to cytarabine, hematopoietic depression, impaired liver function, lactation, pregnancy
- **Physical:** Weight; T; skin lesions, color; hair; orientation, reflexes; R, adventitious sounds; mucous membranes, liver evaluation, abdominal exam; CBC, differential; renal and liver function tests; urinalysis

Interventions
- Evaluate hematopoietic status before and frequently during therapy.
- Discontinue drug therapy if platelet count < 50,000/mm^3, polymorphonuclear granulocyte count < 1,000/mm^3; consult physician for dosage adjustment.
- Use Elliott's B solution for diluent, similar to CSF, for intrathecal use. Administer within 4 hr after withdrawal from vial; contains no preservatives. Do not use in-line filters; inject directly into CSF.
- Use caution to avoid skin contact with liposomal form; use liposomal form within 4 hr of withdrawing from vial.
- Give comfort measures for anal inflammation, headache, other pain associated with cytarabine syndrome.

Teaching points
- Prepare a calendar of treatment days. Drug must be given IV, SC, or intrathecally.
- These side effects may occur: nausea, vomiting, loss of appetite (medication may be ordered; eat small frequent meals; maintain nutrition); malaise, weakness, lethargy (reversible; avoid driving or operating dangerous machinery); mouth sores (use frequent mouth care); diarrhea; loss of hair (obtain

a wig or other head covering; keep the head covered in extreme temperatures); anal inflammation (use comfort measures).
- Use birth control; this drug may cause birth defects or miscarriages.
- Have frequent, regular medical follow-ups, including blood tests to assess drug effects.
- Report black, tarry stools, fever, chills, sore throat, unusual bleeding or bruising, shortness of breath, chest pain, difficulty swallowing.

▷ dacarbazine (DTIC, imidazole carboxamide)
*(da **kar'** ba zeen)*

DTIC-Dome

PREGNANCY CATEGORY C

Drug class
Antineoplastic

Therapeutic actions
Cytotoxic: exact mechanism of action unknown; inhibits DNA and RNA synthesis, causing cell death; cell cycle nonspecific.

Indications
- Metastatic malignant melanoma
- Hodgkin's disease—second-line therapy in combination with other drugs
- Unlabeled uses: malignant pheochromocytoma with cyclophosphamide and vincristine; metastatic malignant melanoma with tamoxifen

Contraindications and cautions
- Contraindicated with allergy to dacarbazine, pregnancy, lactation.
- Use cautiously with impaired hepatic function, bone marrow depression.

Available forms
Injection—10 mg/mL

Dosages
- *Adult and pediatric malignant melanoma:* 2–4.5 mg/kg/day IV for 10 days, re-

peated at 4-wk intervals or 250 mg/m² per day IV for 5 days, repeated every 3 wk.

- *Hodgkin's disease:* 150 mg/m²/day for 5 days with other drugs, repeated every 4 wk or 375 mg/m² on day 1 with other drugs, repeated every 15 days.

Pharmacokinetics

Route	Onset	Duration
IV	15–20 min	6–8 hr

Metabolism: Hepatic; $T_{1/2}$: 19 min then 5 hr
Distribution: Crosses placenta; enters breast milk
Excretion: Urine

▽ IV facts
Preparation: Reconstitute 100-mg vials with 9.9 mL and the 200-mg vials with 19.7 mL of sterile water for injection; the resulting solution contains 10 mg/mL of dacarbazine. Reconstituted solution may be further diluted with 5% dextrose injection or sodium chloride injection and administered as an IV infusion. Reconstituted solution is stable for 72 hr if refrigerated, 8 hr at room temperature. If further diluted, solution is stable for 24 hr if refrigerated or 8 hr at room temperature.
Infusion: Infuse slowly over 30–60 min; avoid extravasation.
Incompatibilities: Do not combine with hydrocortisone sodium succinate.

Adverse effects
- **Dermatologic:** *Photosensitivity,* erythematous and urticarial rashes, alopecia
- **GI:** *Anorexia, nausea, vomiting,* hepatotoxicity, **hepatic necrosis**
- **Hematologic:** *Hemopoietic depression*
- **Hypersensitivity: Anaphylaxis**
- **Local:** *Local tissue damage and pain if extravasation occurs*
- **Other:** Facial paresthesias, flulike syndrome, cancer

∎ Nursing considerations
Assessment
- **History:** Allergy to dacarbazine, impaired hepatic function, bone marrow depression, lactation, pregnancy

- **Physical:** Weight; temperature; skin color, lesions; hair; mucous membranes, liver evaluation; CBC, liver and renal function tests

Interventions
- Arrange for lab tests (liver and renal function, WBC, RBC, platelets) before and frequently during therapy.
- Give IV only; avoid extravasation into the subcutaneous tissues during administration because tissue damage and severe pain may occur.
- Apply hot packs to relieve pain locally if extravasation occurs.
- Restrict oral intake of fluid and foods for 4–6 hr before therapy to alleviate nausea and vomiting.
- Consult with physician for antiemetic if severe nausea and vomiting occur. Phenobarbital and prochlorperazine may be used. Assure patient that nausea usually subsides after 1–2 days.

Teaching points
- Prepare a calendar for treatment days and additional therapy.
- These side effects may occur: loss of appetite, nausea, vomiting (frequent mouth care, small frequent meals may help; maintain good nutrition; consult dietitian; antiemetic available); rash; loss of hair (reversible; obtain a wig or other suitable head covering; keep head covered in extreme temperature); sensitivity to ultraviolet light (use a sunscreen and protective clothing).
- Have regular blood tests to monitor drug's effects.
- Report fever, chills, sore throat, unusual bleeding or bruising, yellow skin or eyes, light-colored stools, dark urine, pain or burning at IV injection site.

▽ daclizumab
See *Less Commonly Used Drugs,* p. 1340.

▷dactinomycin
(actinomycin D, ACT)
*(dak ti noe **mye**' sin)*

Cosmegen

PREGNANCY CATEGORY C

Drug classes
Antibiotic
Antineoplastic

Therapeutic actions
Cytotoxic: inhibits synthesis of messenger RNA, causing cell death; cell cycle nonspecific.

Indications
- Wilms' tumor, rhabdomyosarcoma, metastatic and nonmetastatic choriocarcinoma, Ewing's sarcoma, sarcoma botryoides, in combination therapy
- Nonseminomatous testicular carcinoma
- Potentiation of effects of radiation therapy
- Palliative treatment or adjunct to tumor resection via isolation-perfusion technique

Contraindications and cautions
- Contraindicated with allergy to dactinomycin; chickenpox, herpes zoster (severe, generalized disease and death could result); pregnancy; lactation.
- Use cautiously with bone marrow suppression, radiation therapy, and patients with reduced renal and hepatic function.

Available forms
Powder for injection—0.5 mg

Dosages
Individualize dosage. Toxic reactions are frequent, limiting the amount of the drug that can be given. Give drug in short courses.
Adults
IV
0.5 mg/day for up to 5 days. Give a second course after at least 3 wk. Do not exceed 15 mcg/kg/day for 5 days. Calculate dosage for obese or edematous patients on the basis of surface area as an attempt to relate dosage to lean body mass. Do not exceed 400–600 mcg/m² per day.

- *Isolation-perfusion technique:* 0.05 mg/kg for lower extremity or pelvis; 0.035 mg/kg for upper extremity. Use lower dose for obese patients or when previous therapy has been used.
Pediatric patients
Do not give to children < 6–12 mo.
IV
0.015 mg/kg/day for 5 days or a total dose of 2.5 mg/m² over 1 wk; give a second course after at least 3 wk.

Pharmacokinetics

Route	Onset	Duration
IV	Rapid	9 days

Metabolism: Hepatic; $T_{1/2}$: 36 hr
Distribution: Crosses placenta; may enter breast milk
Excretion: Urine and bile

▽IV facts
Preparation: Reconstitute by adding 1.1 mL of sterile water for injection (without preservatives) to vial, creating a 0.5 mg/mL concentration solution. Discard any unused portion.
Infusion: Add to IV infusions of 5% dextrose or to sodium chloride, or inject into IV tubing of a running IV infusion. Direct drug injection without infusion requires 2 needles, one sterile needle to remove drug from vial and another for the direct IV injection. Do not inject into IV lines with cellulose ester membrane filters; drug may be partially removed by filter. Inject over 2–3 min; infuse slowly over 20–30 min. Protect from light.

Adverse effects
- **Dermatologic:** *Alopecia, skin eruptions,* acne, erythema, increased pigmentation of previously irradiated skin
- **GI:** *Cheilitis, dysphagia, esophagitis,* ulcerative stomatitis, pharyngitis, *anorexia, abdominal pain, diarrhea,* GI ulceration, proctitis, nausea, vomiting, hepatic toxicity
- **GU:** Renal abnormalities
- **Hematologic:** *Anemia,* **aplastic anemia, agranulocytosis, leukopenia, thrombocytopenia, pancytopenia, reticulopenia**

Adverse effects in Italics are most common; those in Bold are life-threatening.

- **Local:** *Tissue necrosis at sites of extravasation*
- **Other:** *Malaise, fever, fatigue, lethargy, myalgia,* hypocalcemia, **death,** increased incidence of second primary tumors with radiation

Interactions
✳ **Drug-lab test** • Inaccurate bioassay procedure results for determination of antibacterial drug levels

■ Nursing considerations
Assessment
- **History:** Allergy to dactinomycin; chickenpox, herpes zoster; bone marrow suppression, radiation therapy; pregnancy, lactation
- **Physical:** Temperature; skin color, lesions; weight; hair; local injection site; mucous membranes, abdominal exam; CBC, hepatic and renal function tests, urinalysis

Interventions
- Do not give IM or SC; severe local reaction and tissue necrosis occur; IV use only.
- Monitor injection site for extravasation, burning, or stinging. Discontinue infusion immediately, apply cold compresses to the area, and restart in another vein. Local infiltration with injectable corticosteroid and flushing with saline may lessen reaction.
- Monitor response, including CBC, often at start of therapy; adverse effects may require a decrease in dose or discontinuation of the drug; consult physician.
- Adverse effects may not occur immediately, may be maximal 1–2 wk after therapy.

Teaching points
- Prepare a calendar for therapy days.
- These side effects may occur: rash, skin lesions, loss of hair (obtain a wig; use skin care); loss of appetite, nausea, mouth sores (frequent mouth care, small frequent meals may help; maintain good nutrition; consult a dietitian; antiemetic may be ordered).
- Adverse effects of the drug may not occur immediately; may be 1 wk after therapy before maximal effects.
- Have regular medical follow-up, including blood tests to monitor the drug's effects.

- Report severe GI upset, diarrhea, vomiting, burning or pain at injection site, unusual bleeding or bruising, severe mouth sores, GI lesions.

▽ dalteparin
(*dahl' tep ah rin*)

Fragmin

PREGNANCY CATEGORY B

Drug classes
Antithrombotic
Low-molecular-weight heparin

Therapeutic actions
Low-molecular-weight heparin that inhibits thrombus and clot formation by blocking factor Xa, factor IIa, preventing the formation of clots.

Indications
- Treatment of unstable angina and non–Q-wave MI for the prevention of complications in patients on aspirin therapy
- Prevention of deep vein thrombosis, which may lead to pulmonary embolism, following abdominal or hip replacement surgery
- Unlabeled use: systemic anticoagulation in venous and arterial thromboembolic complications

Contraindications and cautions
- Contraindicated with hypersensitivity to dalteparin, heparin, pork products; severe thrombocytopenia; uncontrolled bleeding.
- Use cautiously with pregnancy or lactation, history of GI bleed.

Available forms
Injection—2,500, 5,000, 10,000 IU

Dosages
Adults
- *Unstable angina:* 120 IU/kg SC q 12 hr with aspirin therapy for 5–8 days
- *DVT prophylaxis, abdominal surgery:* 2,500 IU SC each day starting 1–2 hr before surgery and repeating once daily for 5–10 days post-op; high risk patients, 5,000 IU

SC starting the evening before surgery; then daily for 5–10 days

- *Hip replacement surgery:* 5,000 IU SC the evening before surgery *or* 2,500 IU ≤ 2 hr before surgery *or* 2,500 IU 4–8 hr after surgery; then, 5,000 IU SC each day for 5–10 days or up to 14 days.
- *Systemic anticoagulation:* 200 IU/kg SC daily or 100 IU/kg SC bid

Pediatric patients

Safety and efficacy not established.

Pharmacokinetics

Route	Onset	Peak	Duration
SC	20–60 min	3–5 hr	2–12 hr

Metabolism: $T_{1/2}$: 4.5 hr
Distribution: May cross placenta, may enter breast milk
Excretion: Urine

Adverse effects

- **Hematologic: Hemorrhage;** *bruising;* thrombocytopenia; elevated AST, ALT levels; hyperkalemia
- **Hypersensitivity:** Chills, fever, urticaria, asthma
- **Other:** Fever; pain; local irritation, hematoma, erythema at site of injection
- **Treatment of overdose:** Protamine sulfate (1% solution). Each mg of protamine neutralizes 1 mg dalteparin. Give very slowly IV over 10 min.

Interactions

✳ **Drug-drug** • Increased bleeding tendencies with oral anticoagulants, salicylates, penicillins, cephalosporins
✳ **Drug-lab test** • Increased AST, ALT levels
✳ **Drug-alternative therapy** • Increased risk of bleeding if combined with chamomile, garlic, ginger, ginkgo, and ginseng therapy, high-dose vitamin E

■ Nursing considerations
Assessment

- **History:** Recent surgery or injury; sensitivity to heparin, pork products, enoxaparin; lactation, pregnancy; history of GI bleed

- **Physical:** Peripheral perfusion, R, stool guaiac test, PTT or other tests of blood coagulation, platelet count, kidney function tests

Interventions

- Give 1–2 hr before abdominal surgery.
- Give deep SC injections; do not give dalteparin by IM injection.
- Administer by deep SC injection; patient should be lying down; alternate administration between the left and right anterolateral and left and right posterolateral abdominal wall. Introduce the whole length of the needle into a skin fold held between the thumb and forefinger; hold the skin fold throughout the injection.
- Apply pressure to all injection sites after needle is withdrawn; inspect injection sites for signs of hematoma.
- Do not massage injection sites.
- Do not mix with other injections or infusions.
- Store at room temperature; fluid should be clear, colorless to pale yellow.
- Alert all health care providers that patient is on dalteparin.
- If thromboembolic episode should occur despite therapy, discontinue and initiate appropriate therapy.
- Have protamine sulfate (dalteparin antidote) on standby in case of overdose.

Teaching points

- This drug must be given by a parenteral route (not orally). You and a significant other may need to learn to administer the drug subcutaneously.
- Periodic blood tests are needed to monitor response.
- Avoid injury while on this drug: use an electric razor, avoid potentially injurious activities.
- Report nose bleed, bleeding of the gums, unusual bruising, black or tarry stools, cloudy or dark urine, abdominal or lower back pain, severe headache.

▷ danaparoid sodium
*(dah **nap'** a royed)*

Orgaran

PREGNANCY CATEGORY B

Drug classes
Antithrombotic
Low-molecular-weight heparin (heparinoid)

Therapeutic actions
Low-molecular-weight heparinoid that inhibits thrombus and clot formation by blocking factor Xa and factor IIa, accelerating the activity of antithrombin III, and inhibiting the binding of heparin cofactor II. Danaparoid is derived from porcine intestinal mucosa.

Indications
- Prevention of deep vein thrombosis, which may lead to pulmonary embolism, following elective hip replacement surgery
- Unlabeled uses: treatment of thromboembolism, anticoagulation during hemodialysis, hemofiltration, in pregnant patients at high risk for thromboembolism

Contraindications and cautions
- Contraindicated with hypersensitivity to danaparoid, heparin, or pork products; severe thrombocytopenia; uncontrolled bleeding.
- Use cautiously with pregnancy or lactation, severe liver or renal disease, recent brain surgery, retinopathy, asthma, history of GI bleed, sulfite sensitivity.

Available forms
Injection—750 anti-Xa units/0.6 mL

Dosages
Adults
750 anti-Xa units SC bid with the initial dose given 1–4 hr before surgery and then no sooner than 2 hr after surgery. Continue for at least 7–10 days; up to 14 days may be necessary.
Pediatric patients
Safety and efficacy not established.
Patients with renal impairment
Reduce maintenance dose and monitor very closely if serum creatinine ≥ 2 mg/dL.

Pharmacokinetics

Route	Onset	Peak	Duration
SC	20–60 min	2–5 hr	12 hr

Metabolism: $T_{1/2}$: 24 hr
Distribution: May cross placenta, may enter breast milk
Excretion: Urine

Adverse effects
- **CV:** Chest pain, dizziness, CVA
- **GI:** *Nausea, constipation*
- **Hematologic: Hemorrhage;** *bruising;* thrombocytopenia; elevated AST, ALT levels; hyperkalemia
- **Hypersensitivity:** Chills, fever, urticaria, asthma
- **Other:** *Fever,* pain, local irritation, hematoma, erythema at site of injection
- **Treatment of overdose:** No known agent is effective for the treatment of overdose; protamine sulfate may have some effect. If overdose occurs, discontinue danaparoid and administer whole blood or blood products.

Interactions
✳ **Drug-drug** • Increased bleeding tendencies with drugs that affect hemostasis (anticoagulants, platelet inhibitors, etc.)
✳ **Drug-alternative therapy** • Increased risk of bleeding if combined with chamomile, garlic, ginger, ginkgo, and ginseng therapy, high-dose vitamin E

■ Nursing considerations
Assessment
- **History:** Recent surgery or injury; sensitivity to heparin, pork products, danaparoid; lactation; renal or liver disease; retinopathy; history of GI bleed; pregnancy
- **Physical:** Peripheral perfusion, R, stool guaic test, partial thromboplastin time (PTT) or other tests of blood coagulation, platelet count, kidney and liver function tests

Interventions
- Arrange to give drug 1–4 hr before surgery and no sooner than 2 hr post-op.
- Give deep SC injection; do not give danaparoid by IM injection.
- Administer by deep SC injection; patient should be lying down; alternate administration between the left and right anterolat-

eral and the left and right posterolateral abdomen. Introduce the whole length of the needle into a skin fold held between the thumb and forefinger; hold the skin fold throughout the injection.

- Apply pressure to all injection sites after needle is withdrawn; inspect injection sites for signs of hematoma.
- Do not massage injection sites.
- Provide for safety measures (electric razor, soft toothbrush) to prevent injury to patient who is at risk for bleeding.
- Check patient for signs of bleeding; monitor blood tests.
- Alert all health care providers that patient is on danaparoid.

Teaching points

- This drug must be given by subcutaneous injection into your abdomen.
- Periodic blood tests will be needed to monitor your response to this drug.
- Be careful to avoid injury while you are on this drug; use an electric razor, avoid activities that might lead to injury.
- Report nose bleed, bleeding of the gums, unusual bruising, black or tarry stools, cloudy or dark urine, abdominal or lower back pain, severe headache.

▽ **danazol**
(da′ na zole)

Cyclomen (CAN), Danocrine

PREGNANCY CATEGORY X

Drug classes
Androgen
Hormone

Therapeutic actions
Synthetic androgen that suppresses the release of the pituitary gonadotropins FSH and LH, which inhibits ovulation and decreases estrogen and progesterone levels; inhibits sex steroid synthesis and binds to steroid receptors in cells of target tissues. Therapeutic effects in hereditary angioedema are probably due to drug effects in the liver; danazol partially or com-

pletely corrects the primary defect in this disorder.

Indications

- Treatment of endometriosis amenable to hormonal management
- Treatment of fibrocystic breast disease; decreases nodularity, pain, and tenderness; symptoms return after therapy
- Prevention of attacks of hereditary angioedema
- Unlabeled uses: treatment of precocious puberty, gynecomastia, menorrhagia, immune thrombocytopenia, hemolytic anemia

Contraindications and cautions

- Known sensitivity to danazol; undiagnosed abnormal genital bleeding; impaired hepatic, renal, or cardiac function; pregnancy; porphyria; lactation.

Available forms
Capsules—50, 100, 200 mg

Dosages
Adults

- *Endometriosis:* Begin during menstruation, or ensure patient is not pregnant; 800 mg/day PO, in two divided doses; downward adjustment to a dose sufficient to maintain amenorrhea may be considered. For mild cases, give 200–400 mg PO, in 2 divided doses. Continue for 3–6 mo or up to 9 mo. Reinstitute if symptoms recur after termination.
- *Fibrocystic breast disease:* Begin therapy during menstruation, or ensure that patient is not pregnant; 100–400 mg/day PO in two divided doses; 2–6 mo of therapy may be required to alleviate all signs and symptoms. Treatment may be restarted if symptoms recur after discontinuation.
- *Hereditary angioedema:* Individualize dosage; starting dose of 200 mg PO bid or tid. After favorable response, decrease dose by 50% or less at 1- to 3-mo intervals. If an attack occurs, increase dose to 200 mg/day; monitor response closely during adjustment of dose.

Adverse effects in *Italics* are most common; those in **Bold** are life-threatening.

Pharmacokinetics

Route	Peak	Duration
Oral	6–8 wk	3–6 mo

Metabolism: Hepatic; $T_{1/2}$: 4.5 hr
Distribution: Crosses placenta; enters breast milk
Excretion: Unknown

Adverse effects

- **CNS:** Dizziness, headache, sleep disorders, fatigue, tremor, pseudotumor cerebri
- **Endocrine:** *Androgenic effects* (acne, edema, mild hirsutism, decrease in breast size, deepening of the voice, oily skin or hair, weight gain, menstrual disturbances, clitoral hypertrophy or testicular atrophy), *hypoestrogenic effects* (flushing, sweating, vaginitis, nervousness, emotional lability)
- **GI:** Hepatic dysfunction, **peliosis hepatitis**
- **GU:** Fluid retention
- **Hematologic:** Thromboembolism, **thrombophlebitis**

Interactions

✳ **Drug-drug** • Prolongation of PT in patients stabilized on oral anticoagulants • Increased carbamazepine and cyclosporine toxicity; monitor patient and adjust dosages as needed

✳ **Drug-lab test** • Interferes with testosterone levels. • Abnormalities in CPK, glucose, thyroid tests, lipids and protein tests, sex-binding globulins

■ Nursing considerations

Assessment

- **History:** Known sensitivity to danazol; undiagnosed abnormal genital bleeding; impaired hepatic, renal or cardiac function; pregnancy; lactation
- **Physical:** Weight; hair distribution pattern; skin color, texture, lesions; breast exam; orientation, affect, reflexes; P, auscultation, BP, peripheral edema; liver evaluation; liver and renal function tests, semen and sperm evaluation

Interventions

- Ensure patient is not pregnant before therapy; begin therapy for endometriosis and fibrocystic breast disease during menstruation.
- Ensure there is no carcinoma of the breast before therapy for fibrocystic breast disease; rule out carcinoma if nodule persists or enlarges.
- Alert patient that androgenic effects may not be reversible.
- Arrange for periodic liver function tests during therapy; hepatic dysfunction occurs with long-term use.
- Periodic tests of semen and sperm, especially in adolescents; marked changes may indicate need to discontinue therapy.
- Encourage patient to use barrier contraceptives during therapy; pregnancy should be avoided.

Teaching points

- These side effects may occur: masculinizing effects (acne, hair growth, deepening of voice, oily skin or hair; may not be reversible), low-estrogen effects (flushing, sweating, vaginal irritation, mood changes, nervousness).
- Use a nonhormonal form of birth control during therapy. If you become pregnant, discontinue the drug, and consult with your physician immediately. This drug is contraindicated during pregnancy.
- Report abnormal growth of facial hair, deepening of the voice, unusual bleeding or bruising, fever, chills, sore throat, vaginal itching or irritation.

▽ dantrolene sodium
(dan' troe leen)

Dantrium, Dantrium Intravenous

PREGNANCY CATEGORY C

Drug class

Skeletal muscle relaxant, direct acting

Therapeutic actions

Relaxes skeletal muscle within the skeletal muscle fiber, probably by interfering with the release of calcium from the sarcoplasmic reticulum; does not interfere with neuromuscular transmission or affect the surface membrane of skeletal muscle

Indications

- Oral: Control of clinical spasticity resulting from upper motor neuron disorders, such as spinal cord injury, stroke, cerebral palsy, or multiple sclerosis; not indicated for relief of skeletal muscle spasm resulting from rheumatic disorders; continued long-term administration is justified if use significantly reduces painful or disabling spasticity (clonus); significantly reduces the intensity or degree of nursing care required; rids the patient of problematic manifestation of spasticity
- Preoperatively to prevent or attenuate the development of malignant hyperthermia in susceptible patients who must undergo surgery or anesthesia; after a malignant hyperthermia crisis to prevent recurrence
- Unlabeled use: exercise-induced muscle pain
- Parenteral (IV): management of the fulminant hypermetabolism of skeletal muscle characteristic of malignant hyperthermia crisis; preoperative prevention of malignant hyperthermia

Contraindications and cautions

- Contraindicated with active hepatic disease; spasticity used to sustain upright posture, balance in locomotion or to gain or retain increased function; lactation.
- Use cautiously with female patients and patients > 35 yr (increased risk for potentially fatal, hepatocellular disease); impaired pulmonary function; severely impaired cardiac function due to myocardial disease; history of previous liver disease or dysfunction.
- See discussion above on chronic use of drug; malignant hyperthermia is a medical emergency that would override contraindications and cautions.

Available forms

Capsules—25, 50, 100 mg; powder for injection—20 mg/vial

Dosages
Adults
Oral
- *Chronic spasticity:* Titrate and individualize dosage; establish a therapeutic goal before therapy, and increase dosage until max-

imum performance compatible with the dysfunction is achieved. Initially, 25 mg daily; increase to 25 mg bid–qid; then increase in increments of 25 mg up to as high as 100 mg bid–qid if necessary. Most patients will respond to 400 mg/day or less; maintain each dosage level for 4–7 days to evaluate response. Discontinue drug after 45 days if benefits are not evident.
- *Preoperative prophylaxis of malignant hyperthermia:* 4–8 mg/kg/day PO in three to four divided doses for 1–2 days prior to surgery; give last dose about 3–4 hr before scheduled surgery with a minimum of water. Adjust dosage to the recommended range to prevent incapacitation due to drowsiness and excessive GI irritation.
- *Postcrisis follow-up:* 4–8 mg/kg/day PO in four divided doses for 1–3 days to prevent recurrence.

Parenteral
- *Treatment of malignant hyperthermia:* Discontinue all anesthetics as soon as problem is recognized. Give dantrolene by continuous rapid IV push beginning at a minimum dose of 1 mg/kg and continuing until symptoms subside or a maximum cumulative dose of 10 mg/kg has been given. If physiologic and metabolic abnormalities reappear, repeat regimen. Give continuously until symptoms subside.
- *Preoperative prophylaxis of malignant hyperthermia:* 2.5 mg/kg IV 1 hr before surgery infused over 1 hr.

Pediatric patients
Safety for use in children < 5 yr not established. Since adverse effects may appear only after many years, weigh benefits and risks of long-term use carefully.
Oral
- *Chronic spasticity:* Use an approach similar to that described above for the adult. Initially, 0.5 mg/kg bid PO. Increase to 0.5 mg/kg tid–qid; then increase by increments of 0.5 mg/kg up to 3 mg/kg, bid–qid if necessary. Do not exceed dosage of 100 mg qid.
- *Malignant hyperthermia:* Dosage orally and IV is same as adult.

Pharmacokinetics

Route	Onset	Peak	Duration
Oral	Slow	4–6 hr	8–10 hr
IV	Rapid	5 hr	6–8 hr

Metabolism: Hepatic; $T_{1/2}$: 9 hr (oral), 4–8 hr (IV)
Distribution: Crosses placenta; enters breast milk
Excretion: Urine

▼ IV facts

Preparation: Add 60 mL of sterile water for injection (without bacteriostatic agents); shake until solution is clear. Protect from light, and use within 6 hr. Store at room temperature, protected from light.
Infusion: Administer by rapid continuous IV push. Administer continuously until symptoms subside; prophylactic doses infused over 1 hr.

Adverse effects
Oral

- **CNS:** *Drowsiness, dizziness, weakness, general malaise, fatigue,* speech disturbance, seizure, headache, light-headedness, visual disturbance, diplopia, alteration of taste, insomnia, mental depression, mental confusion, increased nervousness
- **CV:** Tachycardia, erratic BP, phlebitis, effusion with pericarditis
- **Dermatologic:** Abnormal hair growth, acnelike rash, pruritus, urticaria, eczematoid eruption, sweating, photosensitivity
- **GI:** *Diarrhea,* constipation, GI bleeding, anorexia, dysphagia, gastric irritation, abdominal cramps, **hepatitis**
- **GU:** Increased urinary frequency, hematuria, crystalluria, difficult erection, urinary incontinence, nocturia, dysuria, urinary retention
- **Other:** Myalgia, backache, chills and fever, feeling of suffocation

Parenteral

- None of the above reactions with short-term IV therapy for malignant hyperthermia

Interactions

✳ **Drug-drug** • Risk of hyperkalemia, myocardial depression if combined with verapamil

■ Nursing considerations
Assessment

- **History:** Active hepatic disease; spasticity used to sustain upright posture and balance in locomotion or to gain and retain increased function; female patient and patients > 35 yr; impaired pulmonary function; severely impaired cardiac function; history of previous liver disease; lactation, pregnancy
- **Physical:** T; skin color, lesions; orientation, affect, reflexes, bilateral grip strength, vision; P, BP, auscultation; adventitious sounds; bowel sounds, normal GI output; prostate palpation, normal output, voiding pattern; urinalysis, liver function tests (AST, ALT, alkaline phosphatase, total bilirubin)

Interventions

- Monitor IV injection sites, and ensure that extravasation does not occur—drug is very alkaline and irritating to tissues.
- Ensure that other measures are used to treat malignant hyperthermia: discontinuation of triggering agents, monitoring and providing for increased oxygen requirements, managing metabolic acidosis and electrolyte imbalance, cooling if necessary.
- Establish a therapeutic goal before beginning long-term oral therapy to gain or enhance ability to engage in therapeutic exercise program, use of braces, transfer maneuvers.
- Withdraw drug for 2–4 days to confirm therapeutic benefits; clinical impression of exacerbation of spasticity would justify use of this potentially dangerous drug.
- Discontinue if diarrhea is severe; it may be possible to reinstitute it at a lower dose.
- Monitor liver function tests periodically; arrange to discontinue at first sign of abnormality; early detection of liver abnormalities may permit reversion to normal function.

Teaching points
Preoperative prophylaxis of malignant hyperthermia

- Call for assistance if you wish to get up; do not move about alone; this drug can cause drowsiness.
- Report GI upset; a dosage change is possible; eat small frequent meals.

Long-term oral therapy for spasticity

- Take this drug exactly as prescribed; do not take a higher dosage.
- Avoid alcohol, sleep-inducing, or OTC drugs; these could cause dangerous effects.
- These side effects may occur: drowsiness, dizziness, blurred vision (avoid driving or engaging in activities that require alertness); diarrhea; nausea (take with food, eat frequent small meals); difficulty urinating, increased urinary frequency, urinary incontinence (empty bladder just before taking medication); headache, malaise (an analgesic may be allowed); photosensitivity (avoid sun and ultraviolet light or use sunscreens, protective clothing).
- Report rash, itching, bloody or black tarry stools, pale stools, yellowish discoloration of the skin or eyes, severe diarrhea.

▷dapsone

See *Less Commonly Used Drugs*, p. 1342.

▷darbepoetin alfa
(dar bah poe e' tin)

Aranesp

PREGNANCY CATEGORY C

Drug class

Erythropoiesis-stimulating protein

Therapeutic actions

An erythropoetin-like protein produced in Chinese hamster ovary cells by recombinant DNA technology; stimulates red blood cell production in the bone marrow in the same manner as naturally occurring erythropoetin, a hormone released into the bloodstream in response to renal hypoxia.

Indications

- Treatment of anemia associated with chronic renal failure, including during dialysis
- Treatment of chemotherapy-induced anemia in patients with nonmyeloid malignancies

Contraindications and cautions

- Contraindicated with uncontrolled hypertension or hypersensitivity to any component of the drug.
- Use cautiously with hypertension, pregnancy, lactation.

Available forms

Polysorbate solution for injection—25, 40, 60, 100, 200 mcg/mL

Dosages
Adults

- *Starting dose:* 0.45 mcg/kg IV or SC once per wk. Dosage may be adjusted no more frequently than once per mo. Target hemoglobin level is 12 g/dL. Adjust dosage by 25% at a time to achieve that level. Avoid rapid increase in hemoglobin.
- *Switching from epoetin alfa:*

Epoetin alfa dose in units/wk	Darbepoetin alfa dose in mcg/wk
< 2,500	6.25
2,500–4,999	12.5
5,000–10,999	25
11,000–17,999	40
18,000–33,999	60
34,000–89,999	100
≥ 90,000	200

Patients who were receiving epoetin 2 to 3 times per week should receive darbepoetin once per wk. Patients who were receiving epoetin once per wk should receive darbepoetin once every 2 wk.

- *Chemotherapy-induced anemia:* 2.25 mg/kg SC once per wk; adjust to maintain acceptable hemoglobin levels.

Pediatric patients

Safety and efficacy not established.

Pharmacokinetics

Route	Peak	Duration
SC	34 hr	24–72 hr
IV	1.4 hr	24–72 hr

Metabolism: Serum; $T_{1/2}$: 21 hr (IV), 49 hr (SC)

Distribution: Crosses placenta; passes into breast milk

Excretion: Urine

▼IV facts

Preparation: Administer as provided; no additional preparation needed. Enter vial only once; discard any unused solution. Refrigerate. Do not shake vial. Inspect for any discoloring or precipitates before use.

Infusion: Administer by direct IV injection or into tubing of running IV.

Incompatibilities: Do not mix with any other drug solution.

Adverse effects

- **CNS:** *Headache, fatigue, asthenia,* dizziness, seizure, CVA, TIA
- **CV:** *Hypertension, edema,* chest pain, arrhythmias, chest pain, **MI, stroke**
- **GI:** *Nausea, vomiting, diarrha, abdominal pain*
- **Respiratory:** *Upper respiratory infection, dyspnea, cough*
- **Other:** *Arthralgias, myalgias,* limb pain, clotting of access line, pain at injection site

■ Nursing considerations
Assessment

- **History:** Hypertension; hypersensitivity to any component of product, pregnancy, lactation
- **Physical:** Reflexes, affect, BP, P, R, adventitious sounds, urinary output, renal function, renal function tests, CBC, Hct, iron levels, electrolytes

Interventions

- Ensure chronic, renal nature of anemia. Darbepoetin is not intended as a treatment of severe anemia and is not a substitute for emergency transfusion.
- Prepare solution by gently mixing. Do not shake; shaking may denature the glycoprotein. Use only one dose per vial; do not reenter the vial. Discard unused portions.
- Do not administer with any other drug solution.
- Administer dose once weekly. If administered independent of dialysis, administer into venous access line. If patient is not on dialysis, administer IV or SC.
- Monitor access lines for signs of clotting.
- Arrange for Hct reading before administration of each dose to determine appropriate dosage. If patient fails to respond within 4 wk

of therapy, evaluate patient for other causes of the problem.

- Evaluate iron stores before and periodically during therapy. Supplemental iron may be needed.
- Monitor diet and assess nutrition; arrange for nutritional consult as necessary.
- Establish safety precautions (side rails, environmental control, lighting, etc.) if CNS effects occur.
- Maintain seizure precautions on standby during administration.
- Provide additional comfort measures, as necessary, to alleviate discomfort from GI effects, headache, etc.
- Offer support and encouragement to deal with chronic disease and need for prolonged therapy and testing.

Teaching points

- The drug will need to be given once a week and can only be given IV or SC or into a dialysis access line. Prepare a schedule of administration dates.
- Keep appointments for blood tests; frequent blood tests will be needed to determine the effects of the drug on your blood count and to determine the appropriate dosage needed.
- These side effects may occur: dizziness (avoid driving a car or performing hazardous tasks); headache, fatigue, joint pain (consult with your health care provider if these become bothersome; medications may be available to help); nausea, vomiting, diarrhea (proper nutrition is important; consult with your dietitian to maintain nutrition and ensure ready access to bathroom facilities); upper respiratory infection, cough (consult with your health care provider if this occurs).
- Maintain all of the usual activities and restrictions that apply to your chronic renal failure. If this becomes difficult, consult with your health care provider.
- Report difficulty breathing, numbness or tingling, chest pain, seizures, severe headache.

▷ daunorubicin citrate liposomal

*(daw noe **roo'** bi sin)*

DNR, DaunoXome

PREGNANCY CATEGORY D

Drug classes
Antibiotic
Antineoplastic

Therapeutic actions
Cytotoxic, antimiotic, immunosuppressive: binds to DNA and inhibits DNA synthesis, causing cell death; encapsulated in lipid to increase selectivity to tumor cells.

Indications
- First-line treatment for advanced HIV-associated Kaposi's sarcoma

Contraindications and cautions
- Contraindicated with allergy to daunorubicin; systemic infections; myelosuppression; cardiac disease; pregnancy; lactation.
- Use cautiously with impaired hepatic or renal function.

Available forms
Injection—2 mg/mL

Dosages
Adults
40 mg/m^2 IV infused over 1 hr; repeat q 2 wk.
Pediatric patients
Safety and efficacy not established.
Patients with impaired hepatic or renal function

Serum Bilirubin (mg/dL)	Serum Creatinine (mg/dL)	Dose
1.2–3		3/4 normal dose
> 3	> 3	1/2 normal dose

Pharmacokinetics

Route	Onset
IV	Slow

Metabolism: Hepatic; T$_{1/2}$: 4.4 hr
Distribution: Crosses placenta; enters breast milk
Excretion: Bile and urine

▽ IV facts
Preparation: Dilute 1:1 with 5% dextrose injection before administration. Do not use an in-line filter. Refrigerate. Store reconstituted solution up to 6 hr. Protect from light.
Infusion: Infuse over 1 hr.
Incompatibilities: Do not mix with any other drugs or heparin.

Adverse effects
- **CNS:** Depression, dizziness, *fatigue, headache, neuropathy*
- **CV: Cardiac toxicity,** CHF, palpitations, hypertension
- **Dermatologic:** *Complete but reversible alopecia,* rash
- **GI:** *Nausea, vomiting,* mucositis, diarrhea
- **GU:** *Hyperuricemia* due to cell lysis, *red urine*
- **Hematologic:** *Myelosuppression*
- **Local:** *Local tissue necrosis if extravasation occurs*
- **Respiratory:** *Cough, dyspnea, rhinitis,* sinusitis
- **Other:** Fever, chills, cancer

■ Nursing considerations
Assessment
- **History:** Allergy to daunorubicin; systemic infections; myelosuppression; cardiac disease; impaired hepatic or renal function; lactation, pregnancy
- **Physical:** T; skin color, lesions; weight; hair; local injection site; auscultation, peripheral perfusion, pulses, ECG; R, adventitious sounds; liver evaluation, mucous membranes; CBC, liver and renal function tests, serum uric acid

Interventions
- Do not give IM or SC; severe local reaction and tissue necrosis occur.
- Monitor injection site for extravasation: reports of burning or stinging. Discontinue infusion immediately, and restart in another vein. Local SC extravasation: local infiltra-

tion with corticosteroid may be ordered, flood area with normal saline; apply cold compress to area. If ulceration begins, arrange consultation with plastic surgeon.
• Monitor patient's response, frequently at beginning of therapy: serum uric acid level, cardiac output (listen for S_3), ECG, CBC. Changes may require a decrease in dose; consult physician. Drug therapy for hyperuricemia, CHF may be advisable.
• Caution patient of the risk for fetal damage; advise use of barrier contraceptives.

Teaching points
• Prepare a calendar of dates for therapy.
• These side effects may occur: rash, skin lesions, loss of hair, changes in nails (obtain a wig; use good skin care); loss of appetite, nausea, mouth sores (frequent mouth care, small frequent meals may help; maintain good nutrition; consult a dietitian; antiemetics may be helpful).
• Have regular medical follow-ups, including blood tests to monitor effects.
• Use barrier contraceptives while on drug; drug can cause fetal harm.
• Report difficulty breathing, sudden weight gain, swelling, burning or pain at injection site, unusual bleeding or bruising.

▽deferoxamine mesylate
See *Less Commonly Used Drugs,* p. 1342.

▽delavirdine mesylate
(dell ah vur' den)
Rescriptor
PREGNANCY CATEGORY C

Drug class
Antiviral

Therapeutic actions
Non-nucleoside inhibitor of HIV reverse transcriptase; binds directly to HIV's reverse transcriptase and blocks RNA-dependent and DNA-dependent DNA polymerase activities.

Indications
• Treatment of HIV-1 infection in combination with other appropriate retroviral agents when therapy is warranted; not intended as a monotherapy—resistant virus emerges rapidly

Contraindications and cautions
• Contraindicated with life-threatening allergy to any component.
• Use cautiously with compromised impaired liver function, pregnancy, lactation.

Available forms
Tablets—100, 200 mg

Dosages
Adults and patients > 16 yr
400 mg PO tid used in combination with appropriate agents.
Pediatric patients
Not recommended for patients < 16 yr.

Pharmacokinetics

Route	Onset	Peak
Oral	Rapid	1 hr

Metabolism: Hepatic; $T_{1/2}$: 2–11 hr
Distribution: Crosses placenta; passes into breast milk
Excretion: Urine

Adverse effects
• **CNS:** *Headache,* insomnia, myalgia, *asthenia,* malaise, dizziness, paresthesia, somnolence, fatigue
• **GI:** *Nausea,* GI pain, *diarrhea,* anorexia, vomiting, dyspepsia, increased liver enzymes
• **Skin:** *Rash,* pruritus, maculopapular rash, nodules, urticaria
• **Other:** Anemia, arthralgia, breast enlargement

Interactions
✳**Drug-drug** • Potentially serious or life-threatening adverse effects may occur in combination with clarithromycin, dapsone, rifabutin, benzodiazepines, calcium channel blockers, ergot derivatives, indinavir, saquinavir, quinidine or warfarin; avoid these combinations if at all possible; if the combination cannot be avoided, monitor patient very closely and decrease dosage as appropriate

■ Nursing considerations

Assessment

- **History:** Life-threatening allergy to any component, impaired liver function, pregnancy, lactation
- **Physical:** Skin rashes, lesions, texture; T; affect, reflexes, peripheral sensation; bowel sounds, liver function tests, CBC and differential

Interventions

- Arrange to monitor hematologic indices and liver function periodically during therapy.
- Monitor patient for signs of opportunistic infections that will need to be treated appropriately.
- Administer the drug concurrently with appropriate antiretroviral agents.
- Disperse tablets in water before administration; add 4 tablets to at least 3 oz water; allow to stand for a few minutes, stir until a uniform dispersion occurs; have patient drink immediately. Rinse glass and have patient drink rinse.
- Offer support and encouragement to deal with the diagnosis; explain that this drug must be taken in combination with other agents and that the long-term effects of the use of this drug are not known.

Teaching points

- Take drug as prescribed; take concurrently with other prescribed drugs; do not change dose or alter routine without checking with your health care provider.
- Disperse 4 tablets in 3 oz water; let stand, then stir and drink immediately, rinse glass with water and drink rinse.
- These drugs are not a cure for AIDS or ARC; opportunistic infections may occur and regular medical care should be sought to deal with the disease.
- Frequent blood tests are needed during the course of treatment; results of blood counts may indicate a need for decreased dosage or discontinuation of the drug for a period of time.
- This drug may interact with several other drugs; alert any health care provider that you are on this drug. If you are taking

antacids, take them at least 1 hr apart from delavirdine.

- The following side effects may occur: nausea, loss of appetite, change in taste (small, frequent meals may help); headache, fever, muscle aches (an analgesic may help; consult with your care provider); rash (skin care will be important).
- Delavirdine does not reduce the risk of transmission of HIV to others by sexual contact or blood contamination; use appropriate precautions.
- Report rash, severe headache, severe nausea, vomiting, changes in color of urine or stool, fatigue.

▷ demeclocycline hydrochloride (demethylchlortetracycline hydrochloride)

(dem e kloe sye' kleen)

Declomycin

PREGNANCY CATEGORY D

Drug classes

Antibiotic
Tetracycline antibiotic

Therapeutic actions

Bacteriostatic: inhibits protein synthesis of susceptible bacteria, preventing cell reproduction.

Indications

- Infections caused by rickettsiae; *Mycoplasma pneumoniae;* agents of psittacosis, ornithosis, lymphogranuloma venereum, and granuloma inguinale; *Borrelia recurrentis; Haemophilus ducreyi; Pasteurellia pestis; Pasteurellia tularensis; Bartonella bacilliformis; Bacteroides; Vibrio comma; Vibrio fetus; Brucella; Escherichia coli; Enterobacter aerogenes; Shigella; Acinetobacter calcoaceticus; Haemophilus influenzae; Klebsiella; Diplococcus pneumoniae; Staphylococcus aureus*
- When penicillin is contraindicated, infections caused by *Neisseria gonorrhoeae, Treponema pallidum, Treponema pertenue,*

Listeria monocytogenes, Clostridium, Bacillus anthracis, Fusobacterium fusiforme, Actinomyces, Neisseria meningitidis
- As an adjunct to amebicides in acute intestinal amebiasis
- Treatment of acne, uncomplicated urethral, endocervical, or rectal infections in adults caused by *Chlamydia trachomatis*
- Unlabeled use: management of the chronic form of SIADH

Contraindications and cautions
- Allergy to tetracyclines, renal or hepatic dysfunction, pregnancy, lactation; with children, in tooth-forming years.

Available forms
Capsules—150 mg; tablets—150, 300 mg

Dosages
Adults
150 mg qid PO or 300 mg bid PO.
- *Gonococcal infection:* 600 mg PO then 300 mg q 12 hr for 4 days to a total of 3 g.
Pediatric patients
- *> 8 yr:* 6–12 mg/kg/day PO in two to four divided doses.
- *< 8 yr:* Not recommended.

Pharmacokinetics

Route	Onset	Peak	Duration
Oral	Varies	3–4 hr	18–20 hr

Metabolism: Hepatic; $T_{1/2}$: 12–16 hr
Distribution: Crosses placenta; enters breast milk
Excretion: Urine and feces

Adverse effects
- **Dental:** *Discoloring and inadequate calcification of primary teeth of fetus if used by pregnant women, discoloring and inadequate calcification of permanent teeth if used during period of dental development*
- **Dermatologic:** *Phototoxic reactions, rash,* exfoliative dermatitis (especially frequent and severe with this tetracycline)
- **GI:** *Fatty liver,* **liver failure,** *anorexia, nausea, vomiting, diarrhea, glossitis,* dysphagia, enterocolitis, esophageal ulcer

- **Hematologic:** Hemolytic anemia, thrombocytopenia, neutropenia, eosinophilia, leukocytosis, leukopenia
- **Other:** Superinfections, nephrogenic diabetes insipidus syndrome (polyuria, polydipsia, weakness) in patients being treated for SIADH

Interactions
✷ Drug-drug • Decreased absorption with antacids, iron, alkali • Increased digoxin toxicity • Increased nephrotoxicity with methoxyflurane • Decreased activity of penicillin • Possibly decreased effectiveness of hormonal contraceptives
✷ Drug-food • Decreased effectiveness of demeclocycline if taken with food, dairy products
✷ Drug-lab test • Interference with culture studies for several days following therapy

■ Nursing considerations
Assessment
- **History:** Allergy to tetracyclines, renal or hepatic dysfunction, pregnancy, lactation
- **Physical:** Skin status, R and sounds, GI function and liver evaluation, urinary output and concentration, urinalysis and BUN, liver and renal function tests; culture infected area before beginning therapy

Interventions
- Give oral form on an empty stomach; if severe GI upset occurs, give with food.
- Discontinue drug if diabetes insipidus occurs in SIADH patients.

Teaching points
- Take drug throughout the day for best results; take on an empty stomach, 1 hr before or 1 hr after meals, unless GI upset occurs; then it can be taken with food.
- These side effects may occur: sensitivity to sunlight (use protective clothing and sunscreen), diarrhea.
- Report rash, itching; difficulty breathing; dark urine or light-colored stools; severe cramps; increased thirst, increased urination, weakness (SIADH patients).

▽ denileukin diftitox
See *Less Commonly Used Drugs,* p. 1342.

▷ desipramine hydrochloride

(dess ip' ra meen)

Apo-Desipramine (CAN), Norpramin, Novo-Desipramine (CAN), PMS-Desipramine (CAN)

PREGNANCY CATEGORY C

Drug class
Tricyclic antidepressant (TCA) (secondary amine)

Therapeutic actions
Mechanism of action unknown; inhibits the presynaptic reuptake of the neurotransmitters norepinephrine and serotonin; anticholinergic at CNS and peripheral receptors; sedating.

Indications
- Relief of symptoms of depression (endogenous depression most responsive)
- Unlabeled uses: facilitation of cocaine withdrawal (50–200 mg/day), treatment of eating disorders, premenstrual symptoms, chronic urticaria

Contraindications and cautions
- Contraindicated with hypersensitivity to any tricyclic drug, concomitant therapy with an MAO inhibitor, recent MI, myelography within previous 24 hr or scheduled within 48 hr.
- Use cautiously with EST; preexisting CV disorders (eg, severe coronary heart disease, progressive heart failure, angina pectoris, paroxysmal tachycardia; possibly increased risk of serious CVS toxicity with TCAs); angle-closure glaucoma, increased intraocular pressure, urinary retention, ureteral or urethral spasm (anticholinergic effects of TCAs may exacerbate these conditions); seizure disorders (TCAs lower the seizure threshold); hyperthyroidism (predisposes to CVS toxicity, including cardiac arrhythmias); impaired hepatic, renal function; psychiatric patients (schizophrenic or paranoid patients may exhibit a worsening of psychosis with TCA therapy); manic-depressive patients (may shift to hypomanic or manic phase); elective surgery (TCAs should be discontinued as long

as possible before surgery), pregnancy, lactation.

Available forms
Tablets—10, 25, 50, 75, 100, 150 mg

Dosages
Adults
- *Depression:* 100–200 mg/day PO as single dose or in divided doses initially. May gradually increase to 300 mg/day. Do not exceed 300 mg/day. Patients requiring 300 mg/day should generally have treatment initiated in a hospital. Continue a reduced maintenance dosage for at least 2 mo after a satisfactory response has been achieved.

Pediatric patients
Not recommended in children < 12 yr.

Geriatric patients and adolescents
Initially 25–100 mg/day PO; dosages more than 150 mg are not recommended.

Pharmacokinetics

Route	Onset	Peak	Duration
Oral	Varies	2–4 hr	3–4 days

Metabolism: Hepatic; $T_{1/2}$: 12–24 hr
Distribution: Crosses placenta; enters breast milk
Excretion: Urine

Adverse effects
- **CNS:** *Sedation and anticholinergic effects, confusion* (especially in elderly), *disturbed concentration,* hallucinations, disorientation, decreased memory, feelings of unreality, delusions, anxiety, nervousness, restlessness, agitation, panic, insomnia, nightmares, hypomania, mania, exacerbation of psychosis, drowsiness, weakness, fatigue, headache, numbness, tingling, paresthesias of extremities, incoordination, motor hyperactivity, akathisia, ataxia, tremors, peripheral neuropathy, extrapyramidal symptoms, *seizures,* speech blockage, dysarthria, tinnitus, altered EEG
- **CV:** *Orthostatic hypotension,* hypertension, syncope, tachycardia, palpitations, MI, arrhythmias, heart block, precipitation of CHF, stroke

Adverse effects in *Italics* are most common; those in **Bold** are life-threatening.

- **Endocrine:** Elevated or depressed blood sugar; elevated prolactin levels; SIADH secretion
- **GI:** *Dry mouth, constipation,* paralytic ileus, *nausea,* vomiting, anorexia, epigastric distress, diarrhea, flatulence, dysphagia, peculiar taste, increased salivation, stomatitis, glossitis, parotid swelling, abdominal cramps, black tongue
- **GU:** Urinary retention, delayed micturition, dilation of the urinary tract, gynecomastia, testicular swelling in men; breast enlargement, menstrual irregularity and galactorrhea in women; increased or decreased libido; impotence
- **Hematologic:** Bone marrow depression
- **Hypersensitivity:** Rash, pruritus, vasculitis, petechiae, photosensitization, edema (generalized or of face and tongue), drug fever
- **Withdrawal:** Symptoms on abrupt discontinuation of prolonged therapy: nausea, headache, vertigo, nightmares, malaise
- **Other:** Nasal congestion, excessive appetite, weight gain or loss; sweating (paradoxical effect in a drug with prominent anticholinergic effects), alopecia, lacrimation, hyperthermia, flushing, chills

Interactions

✳ Drug-drug • Increased TCA levels and pharmacologic (especially anticholinergic) effects with cimetidine, fluoxetine, ranitidine • Increased serum levels and risk of bleeding with oral anticoagulants • Altered response, including arrhythmias and hypertension with sympathomimetics, quinolones • Risk of severe hypertension with clonidine • Hyperpyretic crises, severe convulsions, hypertensive episodes, and deaths when MAO inhibitors are given with TCAs • Decreased hypotensive activity of guanethidine

■ Nursing considerations
Assessment

- **History:** Hypersensitivity to any tricyclic drug; concomitant therapy with an MAO inhibitor; recent MI; myelography within previous 24 hr or scheduled within 48 hr; lactation; EST; preexisting CV disorders; angle-closure glaucoma, increased intraocular pressure, urinary retention, ureteral or urethral spasm; seizure disorders; hyperthy-

roidism; impaired hepatic, renal function; psychiatric patients; elective surgery; pregnancy, lactation
- **Physical:** Body weight; temperature; skin color, lesions; orientation, affect, reflexes, vision and hearing; P, BP, orthostatic BP, perfusion; bowel sounds, normal output, liver evaluation; urine flow, normal output; usual sexual function, frequency of menses, breast and scrotal exam; liver function tests, urinalysis, CBC, ECG

Interventions

- Limit access of depressed and potentially suicidal patients to drug.
- Give major portion of dose hs if drowsiness, severe anticholinergic effects occur.
- Reduce dosage if minor side effects develop; discontinue if serious side effects occur.
- Arrange for CBC if patient develops fever, sore throat, or other sign of infection.

Teaching points

- Take drug exactly as prescribed; do not stop taking this drug abruptly or without consulting the health care provider.
- Avoid alcohol, other sleep-inducing drugs, OTC drugs while on this drug.
- Avoid prolonged exposure to sunlight or sunlamps; use a sunscreen or protective garments with prolonged exposure to sunlight.
- These side effects may occur: headache, dizziness, drowsiness, weakness, blurred vision (reversible; if severe, avoid driving or performing tasks that require alertness); nausea, vomiting, loss of appetite, dry mouth (small frequent meals, frequent mouth care, and sucking sugarless candies may help); nightmares, inability to concentrate, confusion; changes in sexual function.
- Report dry mouth, difficulty in urination, excessive sedation.

▷ desloratadine
(dess lor at' a deen)

Clarinex, Clarinex Reditabs

PREGNANCY CATEGORY C

Drug class
Antihistamine (non-sedating type)

Therapeutic actions
Competitively blocks the effects of histamine at peripheral H_1-receptor sites

Indications
- Relief of nasal and non-nasal symptoms of seasonal allergic rhinitis in patients ≥ 12 yr
- Treatment of chronic idiopathic urticaria and allergies caused by indoor and outdoor allergens in patients ≥ 12 yr

Contraindications and cautions
- Contraindicated with allergy to desloratadine, loratadine, or any components of the product; lactation.
- Use cautiously with hepatic or renal impairment or pregnancy.

Available forms
Tablets—5 mg; rapidly disintegrating tablets—5 mg

Dosages
Adults and patients ≥ 12 yr
5 mg/day PO.
Pediatric patients < 12 yr
Safety and efficacy not established.
Patients with hepatic or renal impairment
5 mg PO every other day.

Pharmacokinetics

Route	Onset	Peak	Duration
Oral	1 hr	3 hr	24 hr

Metabolism: Hepatic; $T_{1/2}$: 27 hr
Distribution: Crosses placenta; passes into breast milk
Excretion: Urine and feces

Adverse effects
- **CNS:** Somnolence, nervousness, dizziness, fatigue
- **CV:** Tachycardia
- **GI:** *Dry mouth,* nausea
- **Respiratory:** Bronchospasm, pharyngitis, dry throat
- **Other:** Flulike symptoms, hypersensitivity

■ Nursing considerations
Assessment
- **History:** Allergy to desloratadine, loratadine, other antihistamines; hepatic or renal impairment; pregnancy; lactation
- **Physical:** T, orientation, reflexes, affect, R, adventitious sounds, renal and hepatic function tests

Interventions
- Administer without regard to meals.
- Arrange for use of humidifier if thickening of secretions, throat dryness become bothersome; encourage adequate intake of fluids.
- Provide sugarless lozenges to suck and regular mouth care if dry mouth is a problem.
- Provide safety measures if CNS effects occur.

Teaching points
- Take this drug exactly as prescribed, with or without food.
- These side effects may occur: dizziness, fatigue (use caution if driving or performing tasks that require alertness); dry throat, thickening of bronchial secretions, dryness of nasal mucosa (use of a humidifier may help if this becomes a problem); dry mouth (sucking on sugarless lozenges and frequent mouth care may help).
- Report difficulty breathing, tremors, palpitations.

▽**desmopressin acetate (1-deamino-8-D-arginine vasopressin)**
*(des moe **press'** in)*

DDAVP, Octostim (CAN), Stimate

PREGNANCY CATEGORY B

Drug class
Hormone

Therapeutic actions
Synthetic analog of human ADH; promotes resorption of water in the renal tubule; increases levels of clotting factor VIII.

Indications

- DDAVP: neurogenic diabetes insipidus (not nephrogenic in origin; intranasal and parenteral); hemophilia A (with factor VIII levels > 5%; parenteral); von Willebrand's disease (type I; parenteral); primary nocturnal enuresis (intranasal)
- Stimate: treatment of hemophilia A, von Willebrand's disease
- Unlabeled use: treatment of chronic autonomic failure (intranasal)

Contraindications and cautions

- Contraindicated with allergy to desmopressin acetate; type II von Willebrand's disease.
- Use cautiously with vascular disease or hypertension, lactation, water intoxication, fluid and electrolyte imbalance.

Available forms

Tablets—0.1, 0.2 mg; nasal solution—0.1 mg/mL, 1.5 mg/mL; injection—4 mcg/mL

Dosages
Adults

- *Diabetes insipidus:* 0.1–0.4 mL/day intranasally as a single dose or divided into two to three doses; 1 spray/nostril for total of 300 mg; 0.5–1 mL/day SC or IV, divided into two doses, adjusted to achieve a diurnal water turnover pattern, or 0.05 mg PO bid—adjust according to water turnover pattern.
- *Hemophilia A or von Willebrand's disease:* 0.3 mcg/kg diluted in 50 mL sterile physiologic saline; infuse IV slowly over 15–30 min. If needed preoperatively, infuse 30 min before the procedure. Determine need for repeated administration based on patient reponse. Intranasal—1 spray per nostril, 2 hr pre-op for a total dose of 300 mcg.

Adults and children > 6 yr

- *Primary nocturnal enuresis:* 20 mcg (0.2 mL) intranasal hs. Up to 40 mcg may be needed.

Pediatric patients

- *Diabetes insipidus (3 mo–12 yr):* 0.05–0.3 mL/day intranasally as a single dose or divided into two doses; 1 spray/nostril for total of 300 mg; or 0.05 mg PO daily—adjust according to water turnover pattern.
- *Hemophilia A or von Willebrand's disease (10 kg or less):* 0.3 mcg/kg diluted in 10 mL of sterile physiologic saline. Infuse IV slowly over 15–30 min.

Pharmacokinetics

Route	Onset	Peak	Duration
Oral	1 hr	60–90 min	7 hr
IV, SC	30 min	90–120 min	Varies
Nasal	15–60 min	1–5 hr	5–21 hr

Metabolism: $T_{1/2}$: 7.8 min then 75.5 min (IV); 1.5–2.5 hr (oral); 3.3–3.5 hr (nasal)
Distribution: Crosses placenta; enters breast milk

▼ IV facts

Preparation: Use drug as provided; refrigerate vial.
Infusion: Administer by direct IV injection over 1 min; infuse for hemophilia A or von Willebrand's disease over 15–30 min. May dilute in normal saline solution.

Adverse effects

- **CNS:** Transient headache
- **CV:** Slight elevation of BP, facial flushing (with high doses)
- **GI:** Nausea, mild abdominal cramps
- **GU:** Vulval pain, fluid retention, water intoxication, hyponatremia (high doses)
- **Local:** *Local erythema, swelling, burning pain* (parenteral injection)

Interactions

＊ **Drug-drug** • Risk of increased antidiuretic effects if combined with carbamazepine, chlorpropamide

■ Nursing considerations
Assessment

- **History:** Allergy to desmopressin acetate; type II von Willebrand's disease; vascular disease or hypertension; lactation
- **Physical:** Nasal mucous membranes; skin color; P, BP, edema; R, adventitious sounds; bowel sounds, abdominal exam; urine volume and osmolality, plasma osmolality; factor VIII coagulant activity, skin bleeding times, factor VIII coagulant levels, factor VIII

antigen and ristocetin cofactor levels (as appropriate)

Interventions
- Refrigerate nasal solution and injection.
- Administer intranasally by drawing solution into the rhinyle or flexible calibrated plastic tube supplied with preparation. Insert one end of tube into nostril; blow on the other end to deposit solution deep into nasal cavity. Administer to infants, young children, or obtunded adults by using an air-filled syringe attached to the plastic tube. Spray form also available (1 spray/nostril).
- Monitor condition of nasal passages during long-term therapy; inappropriate administration can lead to nasal ulcerations.
- Monitor patients with CV diseases very carefully for cardiac reactions.
- Arrange to individualize dosage to establish a diurnal pattern of water turnover; estimate response by adequate duration of sleep and adequate, not excessive, water turnover.
- Monitor P and BP during infusion for hemophilia A or von Willebrand's disease. Monitor clinical response and lab reports to determine effectiveness of therapy and need for more desmopressin or use of blood products.

Teaching points
- Administer intranasally by drawing solution into the rhinyle or flexible calibrated plastic tube supplied with preparation. Insert one end of tube into nostril; blow on the other end to deposit solution deep into nasal cavity. Review proper administration technique for nasal use.
- These side effects may occur: GI cramping, facial flushing, headache, nasal irritation (proper administration may decrease these problems).
- Report drowsiness, listlessness, headache, shortness of breath, heartburn, abdominal cramps, vulval pain, severe nasal congestion or irritation.

▷ dexamethasone
*(dex a **meth**' a sone)*

dexamethasone
Oral, topical dermatologic aerosol and gel, ophthalmic suspension: Aeroseb-Dex, Decadron, Dexameth, Dexasone (CAN), Dexone, Hexadrol, Maxidex Ophthalmic

dexamethasone acetate
IM, intra-articular, or soft-tissue injection: Cortastat LA, Dalalone L.A., Decaject LA, Dexasone-L.A., Dexone LA, Solurex LA

dexamethasone sodium phosphate
IV, IM, intra-articular, intralesional injection; respiratory inhalant; intranasal steroid; ophthalmic solution and ointment; topical dermatologic cream: Cortastat, Dalalone, Decadron Phosphate, Decadron Phosphate Ophthalmic, Decadron Phosphate Turbinaire, Decaject, Dexasone, Dexone, Hexadrol Phosphate, Solurex, Turbinaire Decadron Phosphate

PREGNANCY CATEGORY C

Drug classes
Corticosteroid
Glucocorticoid
Hormone

Therapeutic actions
Enters target cells and binds to specific receptors, initiating many complex reactions that are responsible for its anti-inflammatory and immunosuppressive effects.

Indications
- Hypercalcemia associated with cancer

- Short-term management of various inflammatory and allergic disorders, such as rheumatoid arthritis, collagen diseases (SLE), dermatologic diseases (pemphigus), status asthmaticus, and autoimmune disorders
- Hematologic disorders: thrombocytopenic purpura, erythroblastopenia
- Trichinosis with neurologic or myocardial involvement
- Ulcerative colitis, acute exacerbations of multiple sclerosis, and palliation in some leukemias and lymphomas
- Cerebral edema associated with brain tumor, craniotomy, or head injury
- Testing adrenocortical hyperfunction
- Unlabeled uses: Antiemetic for cisplatin-induced vomiting, diagnosis of depression
- Intra-articular or soft-tissue administration: Arthritis, psoriatic plaques
- Respiratory inhalant: Control of bronchial asthma requiring corticosteroids in conjunction with other therapy
- Intranasal: Relief of symptoms of seasonal or perennial rhinitis that responds poorly to other treatments
- Dermatologic preparations: Relief of inflammatory and pruritic manifestations of dermatoses that are steroid-responsive
- Ophthalmic preparations: Inflammation of the lid, conjunctiva, cornea, and globe

Contraindications and cautions

- Contraindicated with infections, especially tuberculosis, fungal infections, amebiasis, vaccinia and varicella, and antibiotic-resistant infections.
- Use cautiously with renal or hepatic disease; hypothyroidism, ulcerative colitis with impending perforation; diverticulitis; active or latent peptic ulcer; inflammatory bowel disease; CHF, hypertension, thromboembolic disorders; osteoporosis; convulsive disorders; diabetes mellitus; lactation.

Available forms

Tablets—0.25, 0.5, 0.75, 1, 1.5, 2, 4, 6 mg; elixir—0.5 mg/5 mL; oral solution—0.5 mg/5 mL; injection—8 mg/mL, 16 mg/mL, 4 mg/mL, 10 mg/mL, 20 mg/mL, 24 mg/mL; aerosol—84 mcg/actuation; ophthalmic solution—0.1%; ophthalmic suspension—0.1%; ophthalmic ointment—0.05%; topical ointment—0.05%; topical cream—0.05%, 0.1%; topical aerosol—0.01%, 0.04%

Dosages
Systemic administration
Adults
Individualize dosage based on severity of condition and response. Give daily dose before 9 AM to minimize adrenal suppression. If long-term therapy is needed, alternate-day therapy with a short-acting steroid should be considered. After long-term therapy, withdraw drug slowly to avoid adrenal insufficiency. For maintenance therapy, reduce initial dose in small increments at intervals until the lowest clinically satisfactory dose is reached.
Pediatric patients
Individualize dosage based on severity of condition and response, rather than by strict adherence to formulas that correct adult doses for age or body weight. Carefully observe growth and development in infants and children on long-term therapy.
Oral (dexamethasone)
0.75–9 mg/day.
- Suppression tests:
For Cushing's syndrome: 1 mg at 11 PM; assay plasma cortisol at 8 PM the next day. For greater accuracy, give 0.5 mg q 6 hr for 48 hr, and collect 24-hr urine to determine 17-OH-corticosteroid excretion.
Test to distinguish Cushing's syndrome due to ACTH excess from that resulting from other causes: 2 mg q 6 hr for 48 hr. Collect 24-hr urine to determine 17-OH-corticosteroid excretion.
IM (dexamethasone acetate)
8–16 mg; may repeat in 1–3 wk. Dexamethasone phosphate: 0.5–0.9 mg/day; usual dose range is one-third to one-half the oral dose.
IV (dexamethasone sodium phosphate)
0.5–9 mg/day.
- Cerebral edema: 10 mg IV and then 4 mg IM q 6 hr; change to oral therapy, 1–3 mg tid, as soon as possible and taper over 5–7 days.
Pediatric patients
- Unresponsive shock: 1–6 mg/kg as a single IV injection (as much as 40 mg initially followed by repeated injections q 2–6 hr has been reported).

Dexamethasone acetate
4–16 mg intra-articular, soft tissue; 0.8–1.6 mg intralesional.

Dexamethasone sodium phosphate
0.4–6 mg (depending on joint or soft-tissue injection site).

Respiratory inhalant (dexamethasone sodium phosphate)
84 mcg released with each actuation.

Adults
3 inhalations tid–qid, not to exceed 12 inhalations/day.

Pediatric patients
2 inhalations tid–qid, not to exceed 8 inhalations/day.

Intranasal (dexamethasone sodium phosphate)
Each spray delivers 84 mcg dexamethasone.

Adults
2 sprays (168 mcg) into each nostril bid–tid, not to exceed 12 sprays (1,008 mcg)/day.

Pediatric patients
1 or 2 sprays (84–168 mcg) into each nostril bid, depending on age, not to exceed 8 sprays (672 mcg). Arrange to reduce dose and discontinue therapy as soon as possible.

Topical dermatologic preparations
Apply sparingly to affected area bid–qid.

Ophthalmic solutions, suspensions
Instill 1 or 2 drops into the conjunctival sac q 1 hr during the day and q 2 hr during the night; after a favorable response, reduce dose to 1 drop q 4 hr and then 1 drop tid–qid.

Ophthalmic ointment
Apply a thin coating in the lower conjunctival sac tid–qid; reduce dosage to bid and then qid after improvement.

Pharmacokinetics

Route	Onset	Peak	Duration
Oral	Slow	1–2 hr	2–3 days
IM	Rapid	30–60 min	2–3 days
IV	Rapid	30–60 min	2–3 days

Metabolism: Hepatic; $T_{1/2}$: 110–210 min
Distribution: Crosses placenta; enters breast milk
Excretion: Urine

▼**IV facts**
Preparation: No preparation required.

Infusion: Administer by slow, direct IV injection over 1 min.
Incompatibilities: Do not combine with daunorubicin, doxorubicin, metaraminol, vancomycin.

Adverse effects

Adverse effects depend on dose, route, and duration of therapy. The first list is primarily associated with absorption; the list following is related to specific routes of administration.

- **CNS:** Convulsions, *vertigo, headaches,* pseudotumor cerebri, *euphoria, insomnia, mood swings, depression,* psychosis, intracerebral hemorrhage, reversible cerebral atrophy in infants, cataracts, increased intraocular pressure, glaucoma
- **CV:** *Hypertension,* CHF, necrotizing angiitis
- **Endocrine:** Growth retardation, decreased carbohydrate tolerance, diabetes mellitus, cushingoid state, *secondary adrenocortical and pituitary unresponsiveness*
- **GI:** Peptic or esophageal ulcer, pancreatitis, abdominal distention
- **GU:** *Amenorrhea, irregular menses*
- **Hematologic:** *Fluid and electrolyte disturbances,* negative nitrogen balance, increased blood sugar, glycosuria, increased serum cholesterol, decreased serum T_3 and T_4 levels
- **Hypersensitivity:** Anaphylactoid or hypersensitivity reactions
- **Musculoskeletal:** *Muscle weakness,* steroid myopathy, loss of muscle mass, osteoporosis, spontaneous fractures
- **Other:** *Impaired wound healing; petechiae; ecchymoses; increased sweating; thin and fragile skin; acne; immunosuppression and masking of signs of infection;* activation of latent infections, including tuberculosis, fungal, and viral eye infections; pneumonia; abscess; septic infection; GI and GU infections

Intra-articular
- **Musculoskeletal:** Osteonecrosis, tendon rupture, infection

Intralesional therapy
- **CNS:** Blindness (when used on face and head—rare)

Adverse effects in *Italics* are most common; those in **Bold** are life-threatening.

Respiratory inhalant
- **Endocrine:** Suppression of HPA function due to systemic absorption
- **Respiratory:** Oral, laryngeal, pharyngeal irritation
- **Other:** Fungal infections

Intranasal
- **CNS:** Headache
- **Dermatologic:** Urticaria
- **Endocrine:** Suppression of HPA function due to systemic absorption
- **GI:** Nausea
- **Respiratory:** Nasal irritation, fungal infections, epistaxis, rebound congestion, perforation of the nasal septum, anosmia

Topical dermatologic ointments, creams, sprays
- **Endocrine:** Suppression of HPA function due to systemic absorption, growth retardation in children (children may be at special risk for systemic absorption because of their large skin surface area to body weight ratio)
- **Local:** Local burning, irritation, acneiform lesions, striae, skin atrophy

Ophthalmic preparations
- **Endocrine:** Suppression of HPA function due to systemic absorption; more common with long-term use
- **Local:** Infections, especially fungal; glaucoma, cataracts with long-term use

Interactions
❋ Drug-drug • Increased therapeutic and toxic effects of dexamethasone with troleandomycin • Decreased effects of anticholinesterases with corticotropin; profound muscular depression is possible • Decreased steroid blood levels with phenytoin, phenobarbital, rifampin • Decreased serum levels of salicylates with dexamethasone
❋ Drug-lab test • False-negative nitrobluetetrazolium test for bacterial infection • Suppression of skin test reactions

■ Nursing considerations
Assessment
- **History for systemic administration:** Active infections; renal or hepatic disease; hypothyroidism, ulcerative colitis; diverticulitis; active or latent peptic ulcer; inflammatory bowel disease; CHF, hypertension, thromboembolic disorders; osteoporosis; convulsive disorders; diabetes mellitus; lactation

For ophthalmic preparations, acute superficial herpes simplex keratitis, fungal infections of ocular structures; vaccinia, varicella, and other viral diseases of the cornea and conjunctiva; ocular tuberculosis
- **Physical:** For systemic administration: Baseline body weight, temperature; reflexes, and grip strength, affect, and orientation; P, BP, peripheral perfusion, prominence of superficial veins; R and adventitious sounds; serum electrolytes, blood glucose

For topical dermatologic preparations, affected area for infections, skin injury

Interventions
- *For systemic administration:* Do not give drug to nursing mothers; drug is secreted in breast milk.
- Give daily doses before 9 AM to mimic normal peak corticosteroid blood levels.
- Increase dosage when patient is subject to stress.
- Taper doses when discontinuing high-dose or long-term therapy.
- Do not give live virus vaccines with immunosuppressive doses of corticosteroids.
- *For respiratory inhalant, intranasal preparation:* Do not use respiratory inhalant during an acute asthmatic attack or to manage status asthmaticus.
- Do not use intranasal product with untreated local nasal infections, epistaxis, nasal trauma, septal ulcers, or recent nasal surgery.
- Taper systemic steroids carefully during transfer to inhalational steroids; adrenal insufficiency deaths have occurred.
- *For topical dermatologic preparations:* Use caution when occlusive dressings, tight diapers cover affected area; these can increase systemic absorption.
- Avoid prolonged use near the eyes, in genital and rectal areas, and in skin creases.

Teaching points
Systemic administration
- Do not stop taking the oral drug without consulting health care provider.
- Avoid exposure to infection.
- Report unusual weight gain, swelling of the extremities, muscle weakness, black or tarry stools, fever, prolonged sore throat, colds or other infections, worsening of this disorder.

Intra-articular administration
- Do not overuse joint after therapy, even if pain is gone.

Respiratory inhalant, intranasal preparation
- Do not use more often than prescribed.
- Do not stop using this drug without consulting health care provider.
- Use the inhalational bronchodilator drug before using the oral inhalant product when using both.
- Administer decongestant nose drops first if nasal passages are blocked.

Topical
- Apply the drug sparingly.
- Avoid contact with eyes.
- Report any irritation or infection at the site of application.

Ophthalmic
- Administer as follows: Lie down or tilt head backward and look at ceiling. Warm tube of ointment in hand for several minutes. Apply one-fourth–one-half–inch of ointment, or drop suspension inside lower eyelid while looking up. After applying ointment, close eyelids and roll eyeball in all directions. After instilling eye drops, release lower lid, but do not blink for at least 30 sec; apply gentle pressure to the inside corner of the eye for 1 min. Do not close eyes tightly, and try not to blink more often than usual; do not touch ointment tube or dropper to eye, fingers, or any surface.
- Wait at least 10 min before using any other eye preparations.
- Eyes will become more sensitive to light (use sunglasses).
- Report worsening of the condition, pain, itching, swelling of the eye, failure of the condition to improve after 1 wk.

▽ **dexchlorpheniramine maleate**

(dex klor fen ir' a meen)

Polaramine, Polaramine Repetabs

PREGNANCY CATEGORY B

Drug class
Antihistamine (alkylamine type)

Therapeutic actions
Blocks the effects of histamine at H_1-receptor sites, has atropine-like, antipruritic, and sedative effects.

Indications
- Relief of symptoms associated with perennial and seasonal allergic rhinitis; vasomotor rhinitis; allergic conjunctivitis; mild, uncomplicated urticaria and angioedema; amelioration of allergic reactions to blood or plasma; dermatographism; adjunctive therapy in anaphylactic reactions

Contraindications and cautions
- Contraindicated with allergy to any antihistamines, narrow-angle glaucoma, stenosing peptic ulcer, symptomatic prostatic hypertrophy, asthmatic attack, bladder neck obstruction, pyloroduodenal obstruction, MAOI use, third trimester of pregnancy, lactation.
- Use cautiously with pregnancy.

Available forms
Tablets—2 mg; TR tablets—4, 6 mg; syrup—2 mg/5 mL

Dosages
Adults and patients ≥ 12 yr
2 mg q 4–6 hr PO, or 4–6 mg repeat-action tablets at bedtime PO or q 8–10 hr PO during the day.

Pediatric patients < 12 yr
6–11 yr: 1 mg q 4–6 hr PO or 4 mg repeat-action tablet once daily hs.
2–5 yr: 0.5 mg q 4–6 hr PO; do not use repeat-action tablets.

Geriatric patients
More likely to cause dizziness, sedation, syncope, toxic confusional states, and hypotension in elderly patients; use with caution.

Pharmacokinetics

Route	Onset	Peak
Oral	15–30 min	3 hr

Metabolism: Hepatic; $T_{1/2}$: 12–15 hr
Distribution: Crosses placenta; enters breast milk
Excretion: Urine

Adverse effects in *Italics* are most common; those in **Bold** are life-threatening.

Adverse effects

- **CNS:** *Drowsiness, sedation, dizziness, disturbed coordination,* fatigue, confusion, restlessness, excitation, nervousness, tremor, headache, blurred vision, diplopia, vertigo, tinnitus, acute labyrinthitis, hysteria, tingling, heaviness and weakness of the hands
- **CV:** Hypotension, palpitations, bradycardia, tachycardia, extrasystoles
- **GI:** *Epigastric distress,* anorexia, increased appetite and weight gain, nausea, vomiting, diarrhea or constipation
- **GU:** Urinary frequency, dysuria, urinary retention, early menses, decreased libido
- **Hematologic:** Hemolytic anemia, hypoplastic anemia, thrombocytopenia, leukopenia, agranulocytosis, pancytopenia
- **Respiratory:** *Thickening of bronchial secretions,* chest tightness, wheezing, nasal stuffiness, dry mouth, dry nose, dry throat, sore throat
- **Other:** Urticaria, rash, anaphylactic shock, photosensitivity, excessive perspiration

Interactions

✳**Drug-drug** • Increased depressant effects with alcohol, other CNS depressants

■ Nursing considerations
Assessment

- **History:** Allergy to any antihistamines; narrow-angle glaucoma, stenosing peptic ulcer, symptomatic prostatic hypertrophy, asthmatic attack, bladder neck obstruction, pyloroduodenal obstruction, pregnancy, lactation
- **Physical:** Skin color, lesions, texture; orientation, reflexes, affect; vision exam; P, BP; R, adventitious sounds; bowel sounds; prostate palpation; CBC with differential

Interventions

- Administer with food if GI upset occurs.
- Have patient swallow timed release tablets whole—do not cut, crush, or chew.
- Administer syrup form if patient is unable to take tablets.
- Monitor patient response, and adjust dosage to lowest possible effective dose.

Teaching points

- Take as prescribed; avoid excessive dosage. Take with food if GI upset occurs; do not crush or chew the sustained-release preparations.
- These side effects may occur: dizziness, sedation, drowsiness (use caution driving or performing tasks that require alertness); epigastric distress, diarrhea, or constipation (take with meals); dry mouth (frequent mouth care, sucking sugarless lozenges may help); thickening of bronchial secretions, dryness of nasal mucosa (use a humidifier).
- Avoid alcohol; serious sedation can occur.
- Report difficulty breathing; hallucinations, tremors, loss of coordination; unusual bleeding or bruising; visual disturbances; irregular heartbeat.

▽ dexmedetomidine hydrochloride

See *Less Commonly Used Drugs*, p. 1342.

▽ dexmethylphenidate hydrochloride
(decks meth ill fen' i date)

Focalin

PREGNANCY CATEGORY C

C-II CONTROLLED SUBSTANCE

Drug class
CNS stimulant

Therapeutic actions
Mild cortical stimulant with CNS actions similar to those of the amphetamines; is thought to block the reuptake of norephinephrine and dopamine, increasing their concentration in the synaptic cleft; mechanism of effectiveness in hyperkinetic syndromes is not understood.

Indications

- Treatment of attention deficit-hyperactivity disorder in patients ≥ 6 yr as part of a total treatment program

Contraindications and cautions

- Contraindicated with hypersensitivity to dexmethylphenidate or methylphenidate; marked anxiety, tension, and agitation; glaucoma; motor tics, family history or diagnosis of Tourette's syndrome; use of MAO inhibitors within the past 14 days.

- Use cautiously with psychosis, seizure disorders; CHF, recent MI, hyperthyroidism; drug dependence, alcoholism, severe depression of endogenous or exogenous origin; as treatment of normal fatigue states; pregnancy, lactation.

Available forms

Tablets—2.5, 5, 10 mg

Dosages

Adults and children ≥ 6 yr

Individualize dosage. Administer orally twice a day, at least 4 hr apart, without regard to meals. Starting dose: 2.5 mg PO bid; may increase as needed in 2.5- to 5-mg increments to a maximum dose of 10 mg PO bid.

- *Patients already on methylphenidate:* Start dose at one-half the methylphenidate dose with a maximum dose of 10 mg PO bid.

Pediatric patients

Safety and efficacy not established for children < 6 yr.

Pharmacokinetics

Route	Onset	Peak
Oral	Varies	1–1.5 hr

Metabolism: Hepatic; $T_{1/2}$: 2.2 hr
Distribution: Crosses placenta; may pass into breast milk
Excretion: Urine

Adverse effects

- **CNS:** *Nervousness, insomnia,* dizziness, headache, dyskinesia, chorea, drowsiness, Tourette's syndrome, toxic psychosis, blurred vision, accommodation difficulties
- **CV:** Increased or decreased pulse and blood pressure; *tachycardia,* angina, arrhythmias, palpitations
- **Dermatologic:** Skin rash, loss of scalp hair
- **GI:** *Anorexia, nausea, abdominal pain;* weight loss, abnormal liver function
- **Hematologic:** Leukopenia, anemia
- **Other:** Fever, tolerance, psychological dependence, abnormal behavior with abuse

Interactions

✳ **Drug-drug** ● Possible increased serum levels of coumarin anticoagulants, phenobarbital, phenytoin, primidone, TCAs, some SSRIs; if any of these drugs are used with dexmethylphenidate, monitor the patient closely and decrease dose of the other drugs as needed ● Risk of severe hypertensive crisis if combined with MAOIs; do not administer dexmethylphenidate with or within 14 days of an MAOI ● Risk of adverse effects if combined with pressor agents (dopamine, epinephrine) or antihypertensives; monitor patients closely

■ Nursing considerations

Assessment

- **History:** Hypersensitivity to dexmethylphenidate or methylphenidate; marked anxiety, tension, and agitation; glaucoma; motor tics, family history or diagnosis of Tourette's syndrome; severe depression of endogenous or exogenous origin; seizure disorders; hypertension; drug dependence, alcoholism, emotional instability; pregnancy, lactation
- **Physical:** Body weight, height, body temperature, skin color, lesions, orientation, affect, ophthalmic exam (tonometry), P, BP, auscultation, R, adventitious sounds, bowel sounds, normal output, CBC with differential, platelet count, baseline ECG (as indicated)

Interventions

- Ensure proper diagnosis before administering to children for behavioral syndromes. Drug should not be used until other causes and concomitants of abnormal behavior (learning disability, EEG abnormalities, neurologic deficits) are ruled out.
- Arrange to interrupt drug dosage periodically in children being treated for behavioral disorders to determine if symptoms recur at an intensity that warrants continued drug therapy.
- Monitor growth of children on long-term dexmethylphenidate therapy.
- Arrange to dispense the least feasible amount of drug at any one time to minimize risk of overdose.

- Administer drug before 6 PM to prevent insomnia if that is a problem.
- Arrange to monitor CBC, platelet counts periodically in patients on long-term therapy.
- Monitor blood pressure frequently early in treatment.
- Arrange for consult with school nurse of school-age patients receiving this drug.

Teaching points
- Take this drug exactly as prescribed. It is taken two times a day, at least 4 hr apart.
- Take drug before 6 PM to avoid night-time sleep disturbance.
- Store this drug in a safe place, out of the reach of children.
- Avoid the use of alcohol and OTC drugs, including nose drops, cold remedies, while taking this drug; some OTC drugs could cause dangerous effects. If you feel that you need one of these preparations, consult your health care provider.
- These side effects may occur: nervousness, restlessness, dizziness, insomnia, impaired thinking (these effects may become less pronounced after a few days, avoid driving a car or engaging in activities that require alertness if these occur, notify your health care provider if these are pronounced or bothersome); headache, loss of appetite, dry mouth.
- Report nervousness, insomnia, palpitations, vomiting, skin rash, depression.

▽**dexpanthenol (dextro-pantothenyl alcohol)**

(dex **pan'** the nole)

Ilopan, Panthoderm

PREGNANCY CATEGORY C

Drug class
GI stimulant

Therapeutic actions
Mechanism is unknown; is the alcohol analog of pantothenic acid, a cofactor in the synthesis of the neurotransmitter acetylcholine; acetylcholine is the transmitter released by parasympathetic postganglionic nerves; the parasympathetic nervous system provides stimulation to maintain intestinal function.

Indications
- Prophylactic use immediately after major abdominal surgery to minimize paralytic ileus, intestinal atony causing abdominal distention
- Treatment of intestinal atony causing abdominal distention; postoperative or postpartum retention of flatus; postoperative delay in resumption of intestinal motility; paralytic ileus
- Topical treatment of mild eczema, dermatosis, bee stings, diaper rash, chafing

Contraindications and cautions
- Contraindicated with allergy to dexpanthenol, hemophilia, ileus due to mechanical obstruction.
- Use cautiously in pregnancy, lactation.

Available forms
Injection—250 mg/mL; topical cream—2%

Dosages
Adults
IM
- *Prevention of postoperative adynamic ileus:* 250–500 mg IM; repeat in 2 hr, then q 6 hr until danger of adynamic ileus has passed.
- *Treatment of adynamic ileus:* 500 mg IM; repeat in 2 hr, then q 6 hr as needed.
IV
500 mg diluted in IV solutions.
Topical
Apply once or twice daily to affected areas.
Pediatric patients
Safety and efficacy not established.

Pharmacokinetics

Route	Onset	Peak
IM	Rapid	4 hr

Metabolism: Hepatic; $T_{1/2}$: unknown
Distribution: Crosses placenta; enters breast milk
Excretion: Urine and feces

▽**IV facts**
Preparation: Dilute with bulk solutions of glucose or lactated Ringer's.

Infusion: Infuse slowly over 3–6 hr. Do not administer by direct IV injection.

Adverse effects
- **CV:** *Slight drop in blood pressure*
- **Dermatologic:** Itching, tingling, red patches of skin, generalized dermatitis, urticaria
- **GI:** *Intestinal colic* (30 min after administration), *nausea, vomiting; diarrhea*
- **Respiratory:** Dyspnea

■ Nursing considerations
Assessment
- **History:** Allergy to dexpanthenol, hemophilia, ileus due to mechanical obstruction, lactation
- **Physical:** Skin color, lesions, texture; P, BP; bowel sounds, normal output

Interventions
- Monitor BP carefully during IV administration.

Teaching points
Teaching about this drug should be incorporated into the overall postoperative or postpartum teaching. Intestinal colic may occur within 30 min of administration.
- These side effects may occur: nausea, vomiting, diarrhea, itching, rash.
- Report difficulty breathing, severe itching, or rash.

▷ dextran, high-molecular-weight
(dex' tran)

Dextran 70, Dextran 75, Gendex 75, Gentran 70, Macrodex

PREGNANCY CATEGORY C

Drug class
Plasma volume expander nonbacteriostatic

Therapeutic actions
Synthetic polysaccharide used to approximate the colloidal properties of albumin.

Indications
- Adjunctive therapy for treatment of shock or impending shock due to hemorrhage, burns, surgery, or trauma; to be used only in emergency situations when blood or blood products are not available

Contraindications and cautions
- Contraindicated with allergy to dextran (dextran 1 can be used prophylactically in patients known to be allergic to clinical dextran); marked hemostatic defects (risk for increased bleeding effects); severe cardiac congestion; renal failure, anuria, or oliguria.
- Use cautiously in pregnancy and lactation.

Available forms
Injection—6% dextran 75 in 0.9% sodium chloride, 6% dextran 70 in 0.9% sodium chloride, 6% dextran 75 in 5% dextrose, 6% dextran 70 in 5% dextrose

Dosages
Adults
500–1,000 mL, given at a rate of 24–40 mL/min IV as an emergency procedure. Do not exceed 20 mL/kg the first 24 hr of treatment.
Pediatric patients
Determine dosage by body weight or surface area of the patient. Do not exceed 20 mL/kg IV.

Pharmacokinetics

Route	Onset	Peak	Duration
IV	Minutes	Minutes	12 hr

Metabolism: Hepatic; $T_{1/2}$: 24 hr
Distribution: Crosses placenta; enters breast milk
Excretion: Urine

▼ IV facts
Preparation: Administer in unit provided. Discard any partially used containers. Do not use unless the solution is clear.
Infusion: Infuse at rate of 20–40 mL/min.

Adverse effects
- **GI:** Nausea, vomiting

- **Hematologic:** *Hypervolemia, coagulation problems*
- **Hypersensitivity:** Urticaria, nasal congestion, wheezing, tightness of chest, mild hypotension (antihistamines may be helpful in relieving these symptoms)
- **Local:** Infection at injection site, extravasation
- **Other:** Fever, joint pains

Interactions

✳ **Drug-lab test** • Falsely elevated blood glucose assays • Interference with bilirubin assays in which alcohol is used, with total protein assays using biuret reagent • Blood typing and cross-matching procedures using enzyme techniques may give unreliable readings; draw blood samples before giving infusion of dextran

■ Nursing considerations
Assessment

- **History:** Allergy to dextran; marked hemostatic defects; severe cardiac congestion; renal failure or anuria; pregnancy
- **Physical:** T; skin color, lesions; P, BP, adventitious sounds, peripheral edema; R, adventitious sounds; urinalysis, renal and liver function tests, clotting times, PT, PTT, Hgb, Hct, urine output

Interventions

- Administer by IV infusion only; monitor rates based on patient response.
- Do not give more than recommended dose.
- Use only clear solutions. Discard partially used containers; solution contains no bacteriostat.
- Monitor patients carefully for any sign of hypervolemia or the development of CHF; supportive measures may be needed.

Teaching points

- Report difficulty breathing, rash, unusual bleeding or bruising, pain at IV site.

▽ dextran, low-molecular-weight
(dex' tran)

Dextran 40, Gentran 40, 10% LMD, Rheomacrodex

PREGNANCY CATEGORY C

Drug class
Plasma volume expander nonbacteriostatic

Therapeutic actions
Synthetic polysaccharide used to approximate the colloidal properties of albumin.

Indications

- Adjunctive therapy for treatment of shock or impending shock due to hemorrhage, burns, surgery, or trauma
- Priming fluid in pump oxygenators during extracorporeal circulation
- Prophylaxis against deep vein thrombosis (DVT) and pulmonary emboli (PE) in patients undergoing procedures known to be associated with a high incidence of thromboembolic complications, such as hip surgery

Contraindications and cautions

- Allergy to dextran (dextran 1 can be used prophylactically in patients known to be allergic to clinical dextran); marked hemostatic defects; severe cardiac congestion; renal failure, anuria, or oliguria.

Available forms
Injection—10% Dextran 40 in 0.9% sodium chloride, 10% Dextran 40 in 5% dextrose

Dosages
Adults

- *Adjunctive therapy in shock:* Total dosage of 20 mL/kg IV in first 24 hr. The first 10 mL/kg should be infused rapidly, the remaining dose administered slowly. Beyond 24 hr, total daily dosage should not exceed 10 mL/kg. Do not continue therapy for more than 5 days.
- *Hemodiluent in extracorporeal circulation:* Generally 10—20 mL/kg are added to perfusion circuit. Do not exceed a total dosage of 20 mL/kg.

- *Prophylaxis therapy for DVT, PE:* 500–1,000 mL IV on day of surgery, continue treatment at dose of 500 mL/day for an additional 2–3 days. Thereafter, based on procedure and risk, 500 mL may be administered every second to third day for up to 2 wk.

Pediatric patients
Total dose should not exceed 20 mL/kg.

Pharmacokinetics

Route	Onset	Peak	Duration
IV	Immediate	Minutes	12 hr

Metabolism: Hepatic; $T_{1/2}$: 3 hr
Distribution: Crosses placenta; enters breast milk
Excretion: Urine

▽IV facts
Preparation: Protect from freezing. Use in bottles provided, no further preparation necessary.
Infusion: Administer first 10 mL rapidly, remainder of solution slowly over 8–24 hr, monitoring patient response.

Adverse effects
- **CV:** Hypotension, anaphylactoid shock, *hypervolemia*
- **GI:** Nausea, vomiting
- **Hypersensitivity:** Ranging from mild cutaneous eruptions to generalized urticaria
- **Local:** Infection at site of injection, extravasation, venous thrombosis or phlebitis
- **Other:** Headache, fever, wheezing

Interactions
✳Drug-lab test ● Falsely elevated blood glucose assays ● Interference with bilirubin assays in which alcohol is used, with total protein assays using biuret reagent ● Blood typing and cross-matching procedures using enzyme techniques may give unreliable readings; draw blood samples before giving infusion of dextran

■ Nursing considerations
Assessment
- **History:** Allergy to dextran; marked hemostatic defects; severe cardiac congestion; renal failure or anuria; lactation, pregnancy

- **Physical:** T; skin color, lesions; P, BP, adventitious sounds, peripheral edema; R, adventitious sounds; urinalysis, renal and liver function tests, clotting times, PT, PTT, Hgb, Hct, urine output

Interventions
- Administer by IV infusion only; monitor rates based on patient response.
- Do not administer more than recommended dose.
- Monitor urinary output carefully; if no increase in output is noted after 500 mL of dextran, discontinue drug until diuresis can be induced by other means.
- Monitor patients carefully for signs of hypervolemia or development of CHF; slow rate or discontinue drug if rapid CVP increase occurs.

Teaching points
- Report difficulty breathing, rash, unusual bleeding or bruising, pain at IV site.

▽**dextroamphetamine sulfate**
(dex troe am fet' a meen)

Dexedrine, Dexedrine Spansule, DextroStat

PREGNANCY CATEGORY C

C-II CONTROLLED SUBSTANCE

Drug classes
Amphetamine
Central nervous system stimulant

Therapeutic actions
Acts in the CNS to release norepinephrine from nerve terminals; in higher doses also releases dopamine; suppresses appetite; increases alertness, elevates mood; often improves physical performance, especially when fatigue and sleep-deprivation have caused impairment; efficacy in hyperkinetic syndrome, attention-deficit disorders in children appears paradoxical and is not understood.

Adverse effects in *Italics* are most common; those in **Bold** are life-threatening.

Indications

- Narcolepsy
- Adjunct therapy for abnormal behavioral syndrome in children (attention-deficit disorder, hyperkinetic syndrome) that includes psychological, social, educational measures

Contraindications and cautions

- Hypersensitivity to sympathomimetic amines, tartrazine (*Dexedrine*); advanced arteriosclerosis, symptomatic CV disease, moderate to severe hypertension, hyperthyroidism, glaucoma, agitated states, history of drug abuse; pregnancy; lactation.

Available forms

Tablets—5, 10 mg; SR capsules—5, 10, 15 mg

Dosages
Adults

- *Narcolepsy:* Start with 10 mg/day PO in divided doses; increase in increments of 10 mg/day at weekly intervals. If insomnia, anorexia occur, reduce dose. Usual dosage is 5–60 mg/day PO in divided doses. Give first dose on awakening, additional doses (1 or 2) q 4–6 hr; long-acting forms can be given once a day.

Pediatric patients

- *Narcolepsy:*

6–12 yr: Condition is rare in children < 12 yr; when it does occur, initial dose is 5 mg/day PO. Increase in increments of 5 mg at weekly intervals until optimal response is obtained. ≥ *12 yr:* Use adult dosage.

- *Attention-deficit disorder:*

< *3 yr:* Not recommended.

3–5 yr: 2.5 mg/day PO. Increase in increments of 2.5 mg/day at weekly intervals until optimal response is obtained.

≥ *6 yr:* 5 mg PO daily–bid. Increase in increments of 5 mg/day at weekly intervals until optimal response is obtained. Dosage will rarely exceed 40 mg/day. Give first dose on awakening, additional doses (1 or 2) q 4–6 hr. Long-acting forms may be used once a day.

Pharmacokinetics

Route	Onset	Peak	Duration
Oral	Rapid	1–5 hr	8–10 hr

Metabolism: Hepatic; $T_{1/2}$: 10–30 hr

Distribution: Crosses placenta; enters breast milk

Excretion: Urine

Adverse effects

- **CNS:** *Overstimulation, restlessness, dizziness, insomnia,* dyskinesia, euphoria, dysphoria, tremor, headache, psychotic episodes
- **CV:** *Palpitations, tachycardia, hypertension*
- **Dermatologic:** Urticaria
- **Endocrine:** Reversible elevations in serum thyroxine with heavy use
- **GI:** *Dry mouth, unpleasant taste, diarrhea,* constipation, anorexia and weight loss
- **GU:** Impotence, changes in libido
- **Other:** Tolerance, psychological dependence, social disability with abuse

Interactions

✳ **Drug-drug** • Hypertensive crisis and increased CNS effects if given within 14 days of monoamine oxidase inhibitors (MAOIs); do not give dextroamphetamine to patients who are taking or who have recently taken MAOIs • Increased duration of effects if taken with urinary alkalinizers (acetazolamide, sodium bicarbonate), furazolidone • Decreased effects if taken with urinary acidifiers • Decreased efficacy of antihypertensive drugs (guanethidine) given with amphetamines

■ Nursing considerations
Assessment

- **History:** Hypersensitivity to sympathomimetic amines, tartrazine; advanced arteriosclerosis, symptomatic CV disease, moderate to severe hypertension, hyperthyroidism, glaucoma, agitated states, history of drug abuse; lactation, pregnancy
- **Physical:** Weight; T; skin color, lesions; orientation, affect, ophthalmic exam (tonometry); P, BP, auscultation; R, adventitious sounds; bowel sounds, normal output; thyroid function tests, blood and urine glucose, baseline ECG

Interventions

- Ensure proper diagnosis before administering to children for behavioral syndromes: drug should not be used until other causes (learning disability, EEG abnormalities, neurologic deficits) are ruled out.

- Interrupt drug dosage periodically in children being treated for behavioral disorders to determine if symptomatic response still validates drug therapy.
- Monitor growth of children on long-term amphetamine therapy.
- Dispense the lowest feasible dose to minimize risk of overdosage; should be in a light-resistant container.
- Ensure that patient swallows SR tablets whole; do not cut, crush, or chew.
- Give drug early in the day to prevent insomnia.
- Monitor BP frequently early in therapy.

Teaching points

- Take this drug exactly as prescribed. Do not increase the dosage without consulting your physician. If the drug appears ineffective, consult your health care provider.
- Do not crush or chew sustained-release or long-acting tablets.
- Take drug (especially sustained-release preparations) early in the day to avoid insomnia.
- Avoid pregnancy while on this drug. This drug can cause harm to the fetus.
- These side effects may occur: nervousness, restlessness, dizziness, insomnia, impaired thinking (may diminish in a few days; avoid driving or engaging in activities that require alertness); headache, loss of appetite, dry mouth.
- Report nervousness, insomnia, dizziness, palpitations, anorexia, GI disturbances.

▷ dextromethorphan hydrobromide
(dex troe meth or' fan)

Balminil DM (CAN), Benylin Adult, Benylin DM, Benylin Pediatric, Children's Hold, Creo-Terpin, Delsym, Diabetes CF, Drixoral Cough Liquid Caps, Hold DM, Koffex (CAN), Novahistex DM (CAN), Novahistine DM (CAN), Pertussin CS, Pertussin ES, Robidex, Robitussin Pediatric (CAN), Scot Tussin Cough Chaser,

St. Joseph Cough Suppressant, Sucrets Cough Control, Sucrets 4-Hour Cough, Suppress, Trocal, Vicks Dry Hacking Cough

PREGNANCY CATEGORY C

Drug class
Non-narcotic antitussive

Therapeutic actions
Lacks analgesic and addictive properties; controls cough spasms by depressing the cough center in the medulla; analog of codeine.

Indications
- Control of nonproductive cough

Contraindications and cautions
- Hypersensitivity to any component (check label of products for flavorings, vehicles); sensitivity to bromides; cough that persists for more than 1 wk, tends to recur, is accompanied by excessive secretions, high fever, rash, nausea, vomiting, or persistent headache (dextromethorphan should not be used; patient should consult a physician); lactation, pregnancy.

Available forms
Capsules—30 mg; lozenges—2.5, 5, 7.5 mg; liquid—3.5, 7.5, 15 mg/5 mL; 10 mg/15 mL; syrup—10 mg/5 mL; 15 mg/15 mL; sustained action liquid—30 mg/5 mL

Dosages
Adults
Lozenges, syrup, and chewy squares
10–30 mg q 4–8 hr PO. Do not exceed 120 mg/24 hr.
Sustained-action liquid
60 mg bid PO.
Pediatric patients
>12 yr: As for adults.
Lozenges, syrup, and chewy squares
6–12 yr: 5–10 mg q 4 hr PO or 15 mg q 6–8 hr. Do not exceed 60 mg/24 hr.
Sustained-action liquid
30 mg bid PO.

Adverse effects in *Italics* are most common; those in **Bold** are life-threatening.

Syrup and chewy squares
2–6 yr: 2.5–7.5 mg q 4–8 hr PO. Do not exceed 30 mg/24 hr. Do not give lozenges to this age group.
Sustained-action liquid
15 mg bid PO.
< 2 yr: Use only as directed by a physician.

Pharmacokinetics

Route	Onset	Peak	Duration
Oral	15–30 min	2 hr	3–6 hr

Metabolism: Hepatic; $T_{1/2}$: 2–4 hr
Distribution: Crosses placenta; enters breast milk
Excretion: Urine

Adverse effects

- **Respiratory:** Respiratory depression (with overdose)

Interactions

❋ **Drug-drug** • Concomitant MAOI use may cause hypotension, fever, nausea, myoclonic jerks and coma; avoid this combination

■ Nursing considerations
Assessment

- **History:** Hypersensitivity to any component; sensitivity to bromides; cough that persists for more than 1 wk or is accompanied by excessive secretions, high fever, rash, nausea, vomiting, or persistent headache; lactation, pregnancy
- **Physical:** T; R, adventitious sounds

Interventions

- Ensure drug is used only as recommended. Coughs may be symptomatic of a serious underlying disorder that should be diagnosed and properly treated; drug may mask symptoms of serious disease.

Teaching points

- Take this drug exactly as prescribed. Do not take more than or for longer than recommended.
- Report continued or recurring cough, cough accompanied by fever, rash, persistent headache, nausea, vomiting.

▽ diazepam
(dye az' e pam)

Apo-Diazepam (CAN), Diastat, Diazemuls (CAN), Diazepam Intensol, Valium, Vivol (CAN)

PREGNANCY CATEGORY D

C-IV CONTROLLED SUBSTANCE

Drug classes

Benzodiazepine
Antianxiety agent
Antiepileptic agent
Skeletal muscle relaxant, centrally acting

Therapeutic actions

Exact mechanisms of action not understood; acts mainly at the limbic system and reticular formation; may act in spinal cord and at supraspinal sites to produce skeletal muscle relaxation; potentiates the effects of GABA, an inhibitory neurotransmitter; anxiolytic effects occur at doses well below those necessary to cause sedation, ataxia; has little effect on cortical function.

Indications

- Management of anxiety disorders or for short-term relief of symptoms of anxiety
- Acute alcohol withdrawal; may be useful in symptomatic relief of acute agitation, tremor, delirium tremens, hallucinosis
- Muscle relaxant: adjunct for relief of reflex skeletal muscle spasm due to local pathology (inflammation of muscles or joints) or secondary to trauma; spasticity caused by upper motoneuron disorders (cerebral palsy and paraplegia); athetosis, stiff-man syndrome
- Treatment of tetanus (parenteral)
- Antiepileptic: adjunct in status epilepticus and severe recurrent convulsive seizures (parenteral); adjunct in convulsive disorders (oral)
- Preoperative: relief of anxiety and tension and to lessen recall in patients prior to surgical procedures, cardioversion, and endoscopic procedures (parenteral)
- Management of selected, refractory patients with epilepsy who require intermittent use

to control bouts of increased seizure activity (rectal)
- Unlabeled use: treatment of panic attacks

Contraindications and cautions
- Contraindicated with hypersensitivity to benzodiazepines; psychoses, acute narrow-angle glaucoma, shock, coma, acute alcoholic intoxication; pregnancy (cleft lip or palate, inguinal hernia, cardiac defects, microcephaly, pyloric stenosis when used in first trimester; neonatal withdrawal syndrome reported in newborns); lactation.
- Use cautiously with elderly or debilitated patients; impaired liver or kidney function.

Available forms
Tablets—2, 5, 10 mg; SR capsule—15 mg; oral solution—1 mg/mL, 5 mg/5 mL; rectal pediatric gel—2.5, 5, 10 mg; rectal adult gel—10, 15, 20 mg; injection—5 mg/mL

Dosages
Individualize dosage; increase dosage cautiously to avoid adverse effects.
Adults
Oral
- *Anxiety disorders, skeletal muscle spasm, convulsive disorders:* 2–10 mg bid–qid.
- *Alcohol withdrawal:* 10 mg tid–qid first 24 hr; reduce to 5 mg tid–qid, as needed.
Oral sustained-release
- *Anxiety disorders:* 15–30 mg/day.
- *Alcohol withdrawal:* 30 mg first 24 hr; reduce to 15 mg/day as needed.
Rectal
0.2 mg/kg PR; treat no more than one episode q 5 days. May be given a second dose in 4–12 hr.
Parenteral
Usual dose is 2–20 mg IM or IV. Larger doses may be required for some indications (tetanus). Injection may be repeated in 1 hr.
- *Anxiety:* 2–10 mg IM or IV; repeat in 3–4 hr if necessary.
- *Alcohol withdrawal:* 10 mg IM or IV initially, then 5–10 mg in 3–4 hr if necessary.
- *Endoscopic procedures:* 10 mg or less, up to 20 mg IV just before procedure or 5–10 mg IM 30 min prior to procedure. Reduce or omit dosage of narcotics.

- *Muscle spasm:* 5–10 mg IM or IV initially, then 5–10 mg in 3–4 hr if necessary.
- *Status epilepticus:* 5–10 mg, preferably by slow IV. May repeat q 5–10 min up to total dose of 30 mg. If necessary, repeat therapy in 2–4 hr; other drugs are preferable for long-term control.
- *Preoperative:* 10 mg IM.
- *Cardioversion:* 5–15 mg IV 5–10 min before procedure.
Pediatric patients
Oral
> 6 mo: 1–2.5 mg PO tid–qid initially. Gradually increase as needed and tolerated. Can be given rectally if needed.
Rectal
> 2 yr: Not recommended.
2–5 yr: 0.5 mg/kg.
6–11 yr: 0.3 mg/kg.
>12 yr: adult dose; may give a second dose in 4–12 hr.
Parenteral
Maximum dose of 0.25 mg/kg IV administered over 3 min; may repeat after 15–30 min. If no relief of symptoms after 3 doses, adjunctive therapy is recommended.
- *Tetanus (> 1 mo):* 1–2 mg IM or IV slowly q 3–4 hr as necessary.
- *Tetanus (≥ 5 yr):* 5–10 mg q 3–4 hr.
- *Status epilepticus (> 1 mo– < 5 yr):* 0.2–0.5 mg slowly IV q 2–5 min up to a maximum of 5 mg.
- *Status epilepticus (≥ 5 yr):* 1 mg IV q 2–5 min up to a maximum of 10 mg; repeat in 2–4 hr if necessary.
Geriatric patients or patients with debilitating disease
2–2.5 mg PO daily–bid or 2–5 mg parenteral initially; reduce rectal dose. Gradually increase as needed and tolerated; use cautiously.

Pharmacokinetics

Route	Onset	Peak	Duration
Oral	30–60 min	1–2 hr	3 hr
IM	15–30 min	30–45 min	3 hr
IV	1–5 min	30 min	15–60 min
Rectal	Rapid	1.5 hr	3 hr

Metabolism: Hepatic; $T_{1/2}$: 20–80 hr
Distribution: Crosses placenta; enters breast milk

Excretion: Urine

▼IV facts

Preparation: Do not mix with other solutions; do not mix in plastic bags or tubing.

Infusion: Inject slowly into large vein, 1 mL/min at most; for children do not exceed 3 min; do not inject intra-arterially; if injected into IV tubing, inject as close to vein insertion as possible.

Incompatibilities: Do not mix with other solutions; do not mix with any other drugs.

Y-site Incompatibilities: Atracurium, heparin, foscarnet, pancuronium, potassium, vecuronium.

Adverse effects

- **CNS:** *Transient, mild drowsiness initially; sedation, depression, lethargy, apathy, fatigue, light-headedness, disorientation, restlessness, confusion,* crying, delirium, headache, slurred speech, dysarthria, stupor, rigidity, tremor, dystonia, vertigo, euphoria, nervousness, difficulty in concentration, vivid dreams, psychomotor retardation, extrapyramidal symptoms; *mild paradoxical excitatory reactions, during first 2 wk of treatment,* visual and auditory disturbances, diplopia, nystagmus, depressed hearing, nasal congestion
- **CV:** *Bradycardia, tachycardia,* CV collapse, hypertension and hypotension, palpitations, edema
- **Dependence:** *Drug dependence with withdrawal syndrome* when drug is discontinued (common with abrupt discontinuation of higher dosage used for longer than 4 mo); IV diazepam: 1.7% incidence of fatalities; oral benzodiazepines ingested alone; no well-documented fatal overdoses
- **Dermatologic:** Urticaria, pruritus, skin rash, dermatitis
- **GI:** *Constipation; diarrhea,* dry mouth; salivation; nausea; anorexia; vomiting; difficulty in swallowing; gastric disorders; elevations of blood enzymes—LDH, alkaline phosphatase, AST, ALT; hepatic dysfunction; jaundice
- **GU:** *Incontinence, urinary retention, changes in libido,* menstrual irregularities
- **Hematologic:** Decreased hematocrit, blood dyscrasias
- **Other:** Phlebitis and thrombosis at IV injection sites, hiccups, fever, diaphoresis, paresthesias, muscular disturbances, gynecomastia; pain, burning, and redness after IM injection

Interactions

✳ **Drug-drug** • Increased CNS depression with alcohol, omeprazole • Increased pharmacologic effects of diazepam if combined with cimetidine, disulfiram, hormonal contraceptives • Decreased effects of diazepam with theophyllines, ranitidine

■ Nursing considerations
Assessment

- **History:** Hypersensitivity to benzodiazepines; psychoses, acute narrow-angle glaucoma, shock, coma, acute alcoholic intoxication; elderly or debilitated patients; impaired liver or kidney function; pregnancy, lactation
- **Physical:** Weight; skin color, lesions; orientation, affect, reflexes, sensory nerve function, ophthalmologic exam; P, BP; R, adventitious sounds; bowel sounds, normal output, liver evaluation; normal output; liver and kidney function tests, CBC

Interventions

- Do not administer intra-arterially; may produce arteriospasm, gangrene.
- Change from IV therapy to oral therapy as soon as possible.
- Do not use small veins (dorsum of hand or wrist) for IV injection.
- Reduce dose of narcotic analgesics with IV diazepam; dose should be reduced by at least one-third or eliminated.
- Carefully monitor P, BP, respiration during IV administration.
- Maintain patients receiving parenteral benzodiazepines in bed for 3 hr; do not permit ambulatory patients to operate a vehicle following an injection.
- Monitor EEG in patients treated for status epilepticus; seizures may recur after initial control, presumably because of short duration of drug effect.
- Monitor liver and kidney function, CBC during long-term therapy.
- Taper dosage gradually after long-term therapy, especially in epileptic patients.

- Arrange for epileptic patients to wear medical alert ID indicating that they are epileptics taking this medication.
- Discuss risk of fetal abnormalities with patients desiring to become pregnant.

Teaching points

- Take this drug exactly as prescribed. Do not stop taking this drug (long-term therapy, antiepileptic therapy) without consulting your health care provider.
- Caregiver should learn to assess seizures, administer rectal form, and monitor patient.
- These side effects may occur: drowsiness, dizziness (may lessen; avoid driving or engaging in other dangerous activities); GI upset (take drug with food); dreams, difficulty concentrating, fatigue, nervousness, crying (reversible).
- Use of barrier contraceptives is advised while on this drug; if you become or wish to become pregnant, consult with your health care provider.
- Report severe dizziness, weakness, drowsiness that persists, rash or skin lesions, palpitations, swelling of the ankles, visual or hearing disturbances, difficulty voiding.

▷ diazoxide
(di az ok' side)

Oral: Proglycem
Parenteral: Hyperstat IV

PREGNANCY CATEGORY C

Drug classes
Glucose-elevating agent (oral)
Antihypertensive
Thiazide diuretic

Therapeutic actions
Increases blood glucose by decreasing insulin release and decreasing glucose. Decreases BP by relaxing arteriolar smooth muscle.

Indications
- Oral: management of hypoglycemia due to hyperinsulinism in infants and children and to inoperable pancreatic islet cell malignancies
- Parenteral: short-term use in malignant and nonmalignant hypertension, used primarily in hospital

Contraindications and cautions
- Contraindicated with allergy to thiazides or other sulfonamide derivatives; pregnancy, lactation, functional hypoglycemia.
- Use extreme caution with decreased cardiac reserve, decreased renal function, gout or hyperurecemia when using oral diazoxide; compensatory hypertension, dissecting aortic aneurysm, pheochromocytoma, decreased cerebral or cardiac circulation, labor and delivery (IV use may stop uterine contractions and cause neonatal hyperbilirubinemia, thrombocytopenia) when using parenteral diazoxide.

Available forms
Capsules—50 mg; oral suspension—50 mg/mL; injection—15 mg/mL

Dosages
Adults
Oral diazoxide
3–8 mg/kg/day PO in 2–3 doses q 8–12 hr. *Starting dose:* 3 mg/kg/day in 3 equal doses q 8 hr.
Parenteral diazoxide
1–3 mg/kg (maximum dose 150 mg) undiluted and rapidly by IV injection in a bolus dose within 30 sec; repeat bolus doses q 5–15 min until desired decrease in BP is achieved. Repeat doses q 4–24 hr until oral antihypertensive medications can be started. Treatment is seldom needed for longer than 4–5 days and should not be continued for more than 10 days.
Pediatric patients
Oral diazoxide
Infants and newborns: 8–15 mg/kg/day PO in 2–3 doses q 8–12 hr. *Starting dose:* 10 mg/kg/day in 3 equal doses q 8 hr.
Children: 3–8 mg/kg/day PO in 2–3 doses q 8–12 hr. *Starting dose:* 3 mg/kg/day in 3 equal doses q 8 hr.

Pharmacokinetics

Route	Onset	Peak	Duration
Oral	1 hr	8 hr	N/A
IV	30–60 sec	5 min	2–12 hr

Metabolism: Hepatic; $T_{1/2}$: 21–45 hr
Distribution: Crosses placenta; enters breast milk
Excretion: Urine

▼ IV facts
Preparation: Do not mix or dilute solution. Protect from light.
Infusion: Inject directly as rapid bolus, over 30 sec or less; maximum of 150 mg in one injection.
Y-site Incompatibilities: Do not give with hydralazine, propranolol.

Adverse effects
- **CNS:** Cerebral ischemia, headache, hearing loss, blurred vision, apprehension, cerebral infarction, coma, convulsions, paralysis, *dizziness, weakness,* altered taste sensation
- **CV:** *Hypotension* (managed by Trendelenburg position or sympathomimetics), occasional hypertension, angina, MI, cardiac arrhythmias, palpitations, *CHF secondary to fluid and sodium retention*
- **Dermatologic:** Hirsutism, rash
- **GI:** *Nausea, vomiting,* hepatotoxicity, anorexia, parotid swelling, constipation, diarrhea, acute pancreatitis
- **GU:** Renal toxicity
- **Hematologic:** Thrombocytopenia, decreased Hgb, decreased Hct, hyperuricemia
- **Local:** Pain at IV injection site
- **Metabolic:** Hyperglycemia, glycosuria, ketoacidosis, and nonketotic hyperosmolar coma
- **Respiratory:** Dyspnea, choking sensation

Interactions
✳ Drug-drug • Increased therapeutic and toxic effects of diazoxide if taken concurrently with thiazides • Increased risk of hyperglycemia if taken concurrently with acetohexamide, chlorpropamide, glipizide, glyburide, tolazamide, tolbutamide • Decreased serum levels and effectiveness of hydantoins taken concurrently with diazoxide

✳ Drug-lab test • Hyperglycemic and hyperuricemic effects of diazoxide prevent testing for disorders of glucose and xanthine metabolism • False-negative insulin response to glucagon

■ Nursing considerations
Assessment
- **History:** Allergy to thiazides or other sulfonamide derivatives; pregnancy; lactation; functional hypoglycemia, decreased cardiac reserve, decreased renal function, gout or hyperurecemia; compensatory hypertension, dissecting aortic aneurysm, pheochromocytoma; decreased cerebral or cardiac circulation; pregnancy
- **Physical:** Body weight, skin integrity, swelling or limited motion in joints, earlobes; P, BP, edema, peripheral perfusion; R, pattern, adventitious sounds; intake and output; CBC, blood glucose, serum electrolytes and uric acid, urinalysis, urine glucose and ketones, kidney and liver function tests

Interventions
- Monitor intake and output and weigh patient daily at the same time to check for fluid retention.
- Check urine glucose and ketones daily.
- Have insulin and tolbutamide on standby in case hyperglycemic reaction occurs.
- Have dopamine, norepinephrine on standby in case of severe hypotensive reaction.

Oral diazoxide
- Decrease dose in renal disease.
- Protect oral drug suspensions from light.
- Reassure patient that hirsutism will resolve when drug is discontinued.

Parenteral diazoxide
- Monitor BP closely during administration until stable and then q 30 min–1 hr.
- Protect drug from freezing and light.
- Patient should remain supine for 1 hr after last injection.

Teaching points
Oral diazoxide
- Check urine or blood daily for glucose and ketones; report elevated levels.
- Weigh yourself daily at the same time and with the same clothes, and record the results.

- Excessive hair growth may appear on your forehead, back, or limbs; growth will end after drug is stopped.
- Report weight gain of more than 5 lb in 2–3 days, increased thirst, nausea, vomiting, confusion, fruity odor on breath, abdominal pain, swelling of extremities, difficulty breathing, bruising, bleeding.

Parenteral diazoxide

- Report increased thirst, nausea, headache, dizziness, hearing or vision changes, difficulty breathing, pain at injection site.

▷ **diclofenac**
(dye kloe' fen ak)

diclofenac potassium
Cataflam, Voltaren Rapide (CAN)

diclofenac sodium
Novo-Difenac (CAN), Nu-Diclo (CAN), Solaraze, Voltaren, Voltaren Ophtha (CAN), Voltaren-XR

PREGNANCY CATEGORY B

Drug classes
Anti-inflammatory agent
Nonsteroidal anti-inflammatory drug (NSAID)

Therapeutic actions
Inhibits prostaglandin synthetase to cause antipyretic and anti-inflammatory effects; the exact mechanism is unknown.

Indications
- Acute or long-term treatment of mild to moderate pain, including dysmenorrhea
- Rheumatoid arthritis
- Osteoarthritis
- Ankylating spondylitis
- Treatment of actinic keratosis in conjunction with sun avoidance
- Post-op inflammation from cataract extraction (ophthalmic)

Contraindications and cautions
- Contraindicated with allergy to NSAIDs, significant renal impairment, pregnancy, lactation.

- Use cautiously with impaired hearing, allergies, hepatic, cardiovascular, and GI conditions.

Available forms
Tablets—50 mg; DR tablets—25, 50, 75 mg; ER tablets—100 mg; topical gel—30 mg/g; ophthalmic solution—0.1%

Dosages
Adults
- *Pain, including dysmenorrhea:* 50 mg tid PO; initial dose of 100 mg may help some patients (*Cataflam*).
- *Osteoarthritis:* 100–150 mg/day PO in divided doses (*Voltaren*); 50 mg bid–tid PO (*Cataflam*).
- *Rheumatoid arthritis:* 150–200 mg/day PO in divided doses (*Voltaren*); 50 mg bid–tid PO (*Cataflam*).
- *Ankylosing spondylitis:* 100–125 mg/day PO. Give as 25 mg qid, with an extra 25-mg dose hs (*Voltaren*); 25 mg qid PO with an additional 25 mg hs if needed (*Cataflam*).
- *Actinic keratosis:* Cover lesion with gel and smooth into skin; do not cover with dressings or cosmetics.

Ophthalmic use
1 drop to affected eye qid starting 24 hr post-op for 2 wk

Pediatric patients
Safety and efficacy not established.

Pharmacokinetics

Route	Onset	Peak	Duration
Oral (sodium)	Varies	2–3 hr	12–15 hr
Oral (potassium)	Rapid	20–120 min	12–15 hr

Metabolism: Hepatic; $T_{1/2}$: 1.5–2 hr
Distribution: Crosses placenta; enters breast milk
Excretion: Urine and feces

Adverse effects
- **CNS:** *Headache, dizziness,* somnolence, insomnia, fatigue, tiredness, dizziness, tinnitus, ophthalmologic effects

---

Adverse effects in *Italics* are most common; those in **Bold** are life-threatening.

- **Dermatologic:** Rash, pruritus, sweating, dry mucous membranes, stomatitis
- **GI:** *Nausea, dyspepsia, GI pain, diarrhea,* vomiting, *constipation,* flatulence
- **GU:** Dysuria, renal impairment
- **Hematologic:** Bleeding, platelet inhibition with higher doses
- **Other:** Peripheral edema, anaphylactoid reactions to fatal anaphylactic shock

Interactions
✳ Drug-drug • Increased serum levels and increased risk of lithium toxicity • Increased risk of bleeding with anticoagulants; monitor patient closely

■ Nursing considerations
Assessment
- **History:** Renal impairment; impaired hearing; allergies; hepatic, CV, and GI conditions; lactation
- **Physical:** Skin color and lesions; orientation, reflexes, ophthalmologic and audiometric evaluation, peripheral sensation; P, edema; R, adventitious sounds; liver evaluation; CBC, clotting times, renal and liver function tests; serum electrolytes, stool guaiac

Interventions
- Administer drug with food or after meals if GI upset occurs.
- Arrange for periodic ophthalmologic exam during long-term therapy.
- Institute emergency procedures if overdose occurs (gastric lavage, induction of emesis, supportive therapy).

Teaching points
- Take drug with food or meals if GI upset occurs.
- Take only the prescribed dosage.
- Dizziness, drowsiness can occur (avoid driving or using dangerous machinery while on this drug).
- Report sore throat, fever, rash, itching, weight gain, swelling in ankles or fingers, changes in vision; black, tarry stools.

▷ dicloxacillin sodium
*(dye klox a **sill'** in)*

Dycill, Dynapen, Pathocil

PREGNANCY CATEGORY B

D

Drug classes
Antibiotic
Penicillinase-resistant penicillin

Therapeutic actions
Bactericidal: inhibits cell wall synthesis of sensitive organisms, causing cell death.

Indications
- Infections due to penicillinase-producing staphylococci; may be used to initiate therapy if staphylococcal infection is suspected

Contraindications and cautions
- Contraindicated with allergies to penicillins, cephalosporins, or other allergens.
- Use cautiously with renal disorders, lactation (may cause diarrhea or candidiasis in the infant), pregnancy.

Available forms
Capsules—125, 250, 500 mg; powder for oral suspension—62.5 mg/5 mL

Dosages
Adults
125 mg q 6 hr PO. Up to 250 mg q 6 hr PO in severe infections.
Pediatric patients
< 40 kg: 12.5 mg/kg/day PO in equally divided doses q 6 hr. Up to 25 mg/kg/day PO in equally divided doses q 6 hr in severe infections.

Pharmacokinetics

Route	Onset	Peak	Duration
Oral	Varies	0.5–1 hr	4–6 hr

Metabolism: Hepatic; $T_{1/2}$: 30–60 min
Distribution: Crosses placenta; enters breast milk
Excretion: Urine

Adverse effects
- **CNS:** Lethargy, hallucinations, seizures, decreased reflexes

- **GI:** *Glossitis, stomatitis, gastritis, sore mouth,* black and furry tongue
- **GU:** Nephritis: oliguria, proteinuria, hematuria, casts, azotemia, pyuria
- **Hematologic:** Anemia, thrombocytopenia, leukopenia, neutropenia, prolonged bleeding time, hemorrhagic episodes at high doses
- **Hypersensitivity:** *Rash, fever, wheezing,* **anaphylaxis**
- **Other:** *Superinfections:* oral and rectal moniliasis, vaginitis

Interactions
✳ **Drug-drug** • Decreased effectiveness if taken with tetracyclines • Possible decreased effectiveness of hormonal contraceptives
✳ **Drug-food** • Decreased absorption and decreased serum levels if taken with food

■ Nursing considerations
Assessment
- **History:** Allergies; renal disorders; lactation, pregnancy
- **Physical:** Culture infected area; skin color, lesion; R, adventitious sounds; bowel sounds; CBC, liver and renal function tests, serum electrolytes, Hct, urinalysis

Interventions
- Culture infection before treatment; reculture if response is not as expected.
- Administer by oral route only.
- Continue oral treatment for 10 full days.
- Administer on an empty stomach, 1 hr before or 2 hr after meals.
- Do not administer with fruit juices or soft drinks; a full glass of water is preferable.

Teaching points
- Take drug around the clock; take the full course of therapy, usually 10 days.
- Take the drug on an empty stomach, 1 hr before or 2 hr after meals, with a full glass of water.
- This antibiotic is only for this infection; do not use it to self-treat other infections.
- These side effects may occur: stomach upset, nausea, diarrhea, mouth sores.

- Report unusual bleeding or bruising, fever, chills, sore throat, hives, rash, severe diarrhea, difficulty breathing.

> ▽ **dicyclomine hydrochloride**
> *(dye sye' kloe meen)*
>
> Antispas, Bentyl, Bentylol (CAN), Byclomine, Dibent, Dilomine, Di-Spasz, Formulex (CAN), Or-Tyl
>
> **PREGNANCY CATEGORY C**

Drug classes
Antispasmodic
Anticholinergic
Antimuscarinic agent
Parasympatholytic

Therapeutic actions
Direct GI smooth muscle relaxant; competitively blocks the effects of acetylcholine at muscarinic cholinergic receptors that mediate the effects of parasympathetic postganglionic impulses, thus relaxing the GI tract.

Indications
- Treatment of functional bowel or irritable bowel syndrome (irritable colon, spastic colon, mucous colitis)

Contraindications and cautions
- Contraindicated with glaucoma; adhesions between iris and lens, stenosing peptic ulcer, pyloroduodenal obstruction, paralytic ileus, intestinal atony, severe ulcerative colitis, toxic megacolon, symptomatic prostatic hypertrophy, bladder neck obstruction, bronchial asthma, COPD, cardiac arrhythmias, tachycardia, myocardial ischemia; impaired metabolic, liver, or kidney function, myasthenia gravis; lactation.
- Use cautiously with Down's syndrome, brain damage, spasticity, hypertension, hyperthyroidism.

Available forms
Capsules—10, 20 mg; tablets—20 mg; syrup—10 mg/5 mL; injection—10 mg/mL

Dosages

Adults
Oral
The only effective dose is 160 mg/day PO divided into four equal doses; however, begin with 80 mg/day divided into four equal doses; increase to 160 mg/day unless side effects limit dosage.

Parenteral
80 mg/day IM in four divided doses; do not give IV.

Pediatric patients
Not recommended.

Geriatric patients
Use caution; more prone to side effects.

Pharmacokinetics

Route	Onset	Duration
Oral	1–2 hr	4 hr

Metabolism: Hepatic; $T_{1/2}$: 9–10 hr
Distribution: Crosses placenta; enters breast milk
Excretion: Urine

Adverse effects
- **CNS:** *Blurred vision,* mydriasis, cycloplegia, photophobia, increased intraocular pressure
- **CV:** Palpitations, tachycardia
- **GI:** *Dry mouth, altered taste perception, nausea, vomiting, dysphagia,* heartburn, constipation, bloated feeling, paralytic ileus, gastroesophageal reflux
- **GU:** *Urinary hesitancy and retention,* impotence
- **Local:** *Irritation at site of IM injection*
- **Other:** Decreased sweating and predisposition to heat prostration, suppression of lactation

Interactions
✳ **Drug-drug** • Decreased effectiveness of all antipsychotic medications when used in combination with dicyclomine • Increased anticholinergic effects when administered with TCAs, amantadine • Possible increased effect of atenolol and digoxin

■ Nursing considerations
Assessment
- **History:** Glaucoma; adhesions between iris and lens, stenosing peptic ulcer, pyloroduo-denal obstruction, paralytic ileus, intestinal atony, severe ulcerative colitis, toxic megacolon, symptomatic prostatic hypertrophy, bladder neck obstruction, bronchial asthma, COPD, cardiac arrhythmias, myocardial ischemia; impaired metabolic, liver, or kidney function, myasthenia gravis; Down's syndrome, brain damage, spasticity, hypertension, hyperthyroidism; lactation, pregnancy
- **Physical:** Bowel sounds, normal output; normal urinary output, prostate palpation; R, adventitious sounds; pulse; BP; intraocular pressure, vision; bilateral grip strength, reflexes; liver palpation, liver and renal function tests; skin color, lesions, texture

Interventions
- Ensure adequate hydration; provide environmental control (temperature) to prevent hyperpyrexia.
- Have patient void before each drug dose if urinary retention is a problem.
- Monitor lighting to minimize discomfort of photophobia.

Teaching points
- Take drug exactly as prescribed.
- Avoid hot environments while taking this drug (heat intolerance may lead to dangerous reactions).
- These side effects may occur: constipation (ensure adequate fluid intake, proper diet); dry mouth (sugarless lozenges, frequent mouth care may help; may lessen with time); blurred vision, sensitivity to light (transient effects; avoid tasks that require acute vision; wear sunglasses); impotence (reversible); difficulty in urination (empty bladder immediately before taking drug).
- Report rash, flushing, eye pain, difficulty breathing, tremors, loss of coordination, irregular heartbeat, palpitations, headache, abdominal distention, hallucinations, severe or persistent dry mouth, difficulty swallowing, difficulty in urination, severe constipation, sensitivity to light.

■ didanosine

▽ didanosine (ddl, dideoxyinosine)
*(dye **dan**' oh seen)*

Videx, Videx EC

PREGNANCY CATEGORY B

Drug class
Antiviral

Therapeutic actions
A synthetic nucleoside that inhibits replication of HIV, leading to viral death.

Indications
- Treatment of patients with HIV infection in combination with other antiretroviral drugs (*Videx*)
- Treatment of adults with advanced HIV infection who would require once-daily therapy with didanosine (*Videx EC*)

Contraindications and cautions
- Contraindicated with allergy to any component of the formulation, lactation.
- Use cautiously with impaired hepatic or renal function; history of alcohol abuse.

Available forms
Tablets—25, 50, 100, 150, 200 mg tablets; DR capsules—125, 200, 250, 400 mg; powder for oral solution—100, 167, 250 mg; powder for pediatric solution—2, 4 g

Dosages
Adults
125–200 mg PO bid or 250–400 mg/day as one dose; buffered powder: 167–250 mg PO bid; DR capsules—250–400 mg PO daily (*Videx EC*). Dosage based on weight.
Pediatric patients

Body Surface (m²)	Tablets (bid)	Pediatric Powder (m²)
1.1–1.4	100 mg	125 mg bid (12.5 mL)
0.8–1	75 mg	94 mg bid (9.5 mL)
0.5–0.7	50 mg	62 mg bid (6 mL)
< 0.4	25 mg	31 mg bid (3 mL)

Patients with renal impairment
Creatinine clearance ≥ 60 mL/min: Usual dose. Creatinine clearance 30–59 mL/min: 150–200 mg daily or 75–100 mg bid or 100–200 mg buffered powder bid *or* > 125–200 mg/day. Creatinine clearance 10–29 mL/min: ER capsules 100–150 mg daily tablets *or* 100–167 mg/day; buffered powder *or* 125 mg/day ER capsules. Creatinine clearance < 10 mL/min: 75–100 mg/day tablets *or* 100 mg/day buffered powder *or* (> 60 kg) 125 mg/day ER tablets.

Pharmacokinetics

Route	Peak	Onset
Oral	0.25–1.5 hr	Varies

Metabolism: Hepatic; $T_{1/2}$: 1.6 hr
Distribution: Crosses placenta; enters breast milk
Excretion: Urine

Adverse effects
- **CNS:** Headache, pain, anxiety, confusion, nervousness, twitching, depression, peripheral neuropathy
- **Dermatologic:** Rash, pruritus
- **GI:** *Nausea, vomiting, hepatotoxicity, abdominal pain,* diarrhea, **pancreatitis,** stomatitis, oral thrush, melena, dry mouth
- **Hematologic:** *Hemopoietic depression,* elevated bilirubin, elevated uric acid
- **Other:** Chills, fever, infections, dyspnea, myopathy, lactic acidosis

Interactions
✷ Drug-drug • Decreased effectiveness of tetracycline, fluoroquinolone antibiotics • Increased effect of *Videx* when combined with allopurinol • Changed concentrations for either drug when combined with ganciclovir • Decreased effect of *Videx* when combined with methadone • Decreased effect of azole antifungal agents
✷ Drug-food • Decreased absorption and effectiveness of didanosine if taken with food

■ Nursing considerations
Assessment
- **History:** Allergy to any components of formulation, impaired hepatic or renal func-

Adverse effects in *Italics* are most common; those in **Bold** are life-threatening.

tion, lactation, history of alcohol abuse, pregnancy
- **Physical:** Weight; T; skin color, lesions; orientation, reflexes, muscle strength, affect; abdominal exam; CBC, pancreatic enzymes, renal and liver function tests

Interventions
- Arrange for lab tests (CBC, SMA 12) before and frequently during therapy; monitor for bone marrow depression.
- Administer drug on an empty stomach, 1 hr before or 2 hr after meals.
- Instruct patient to chew tablets thoroughly or crush tablets and disperse 2 tablets in at least 1 oz of water; stir until a uniform dispersion forms. For buffered powder, pour contents of packet into 4 oz of water. Do not mix with fruit juice or acid-containing liquid. Stir until powder completely dissolves; have patient drink entire solution immediately. Pediatric solution should be reconstituted by the pharmacy. Shake admixture thoroughly. Store tightly closed in the refrigerator.
- Avoid generating dust. When cleaning up powdered products, use a wet mop or damp sponge. Clean surface with soap and water. Contain large spills. Avoid inhaling dust.
- Monitor patient for signs of pancreatitis—abdominal pain, elevated enzymes, nausea, vomiting. Stop drug, resume only if pancreatitis has been ruled out.
- Monitor patients with hepatic or renal impairment; decreased doses may be needed if toxicity occurs.

Teaching points
- Take drug on an empty stomach, 1 hr before or 2 hr after meals.
- Chew tablets thoroughly, or crush tablets and disperse 2 tablets in at least 1 oz of water; stir until a uniform dispersion forms. For buffered powder, pour contents of packet into 4 oz of water. Do not mix with fruit juice or acid-containing liquid. Stir until powder completely dissolves; drink entire solution immediately. Pediatric solution should be reconstituted by the pharmacy. Shake admixture thoroughly. Store tightly closed in the refrigerator.
- These side effects may occur: loss of appetite, nausea, vomiting (frequent mouth care,

small frequent meals may help); rash; chills, fever; headache.
- Have regular blood tests and physical exams to monitor drug's effects and progress of disease.
- Report abdominal pain, nausea, vomiting, cough, sore throat, change in color of urine or stools.

▽ diflunisal
(dye floo' ni sal)

Apo-Diflunisal (CAN), Dolobid, Novo-Diflunisal (CAN), Nu-Diflunisal (CAN)

PREGNANCY CATEGORY C

Drug classes
Analgesic (non-narcotic)
Antipyretic
Anti-inflammatory agent
Nonsteroidal anti-inflammatory drug (NSAID)

Therapeutic actions
Exact mechanism of action not known: inhibition of prostaglandin synthetase, the enzyme that breaks down prostaglandins, may account for its antipyretic and anti-inflammatory effects.

Indications
- Acute or long-term treatment of mild to moderate pain
- Rheumatoid arthritis
- Osteoarthritis

Contraindications and cautions
- Contraindicated with allergy to diflunisal, salicylates or other NSAIDs, pregnancy, lactation.
- Use cautiously with CV dysfunction, peptic ulceration, GI bleeding, impaired hepatic or renal function.

Available forms
Tablets—250, 500 mg

Dosages
Adults
- *Mild to moderate pain:* 1,000 mg PO initially, followed by 500 mg q 8–12 hr PO.

- *Osteoarthritis or rheumatoid arthritis:* 500–1,000 mg/day PO in two divided doses; maintenance dosage should not exceed 1,500 mg/day.

Pediatric patients
Safety and efficacy has not been established.

Pharmacokinetics

Route	Onset	Peak	Duration
Oral	30–60 min	2–3 hr	12 hr

Metabolism: Hepatic; $T_{1/2}$: 8–12 hr
Distribution: Crosses placenta; enters breast milk
Excretion: Urine

Adverse effects

- **CNS:** *Headache, dizziness, somnolence, insomnia,* fatigue, tiredness, dizziness, tinnitus, ophthamologic effects
- **Dermatologic:** *Rash,* pruritus, sweating, dry mucous membranes, stomatitis
- **GI:** *Nausea, dyspepsia, GI pain, diarrhea,* vomiting, constipation, flatulence
- **GU:** Dysuria, renal impairment
- **Hematologic:** Bleeding, platelet inhibition with higher doses
- **Other:** Peripheral edema, **anaphylactoid reactions to anaphylactic shock**

Interactions

✳ **Drug-drug** • Decreased absorption with antacids (especially aluminum salts) • Decreased serum diflunisal levels with multiple doses of aspirin • Possible increased acetaminophen levels if combined

■ Nursing considerations
Assessment

- **History:** Allergy to diflunisal, salicylates or other NSAIDs, CV dysfunction, peptic ulceration, GI bleeding, impaired hepatic or renal function, lactation, pregnancy
- **Physical:** Skin color, lesions; T; orientation, reflexes, ophthalmologic evaluation; P, BP, edema; R, adventitious sounds; liver evaluation, bowel sounds; CBC, clotting times, urinalysis, renal and liver function tests

Interventions

- Give drug with food or after meals if GI upset occurs.
- Do not crush, and ensure that patient does not chew tablets.
- Institute emergency procedures if overdose occurs—gastric lavage, induction of emesis, supportive therapy.
- Arrange for ophthalmologic exam if patient offers any eye complaints.

Teaching points

- Take the drug only as recommended to avoid overdose.
- Take the drug with food or after meals if GI upset occurs. Swallow the tablet whole; do not cut, chew, or crush it.
- These side effects may occur: nausea, GI upset, dyspepsia (take drug with food); diarrhea or constipation; dizziness, vertigo, insomnia (use caution if driving or operating dangerous machinery).
- Report eye changes, unusual bleeding or bruising, swelling of the feet or hands, difficulty breathing, severe GI pain.

▽ **digoxin**
(di jox' in)

Lanoxicaps, Lanoxin, Novo-Digoxin (CAN)

PREGNANCY CATEGORY C

Drug classes
Cardiac glycoside
Cardiotonic agent

Therapeutic actions
Increases intracellular calcium and allows more calcium to enter the myocardial cell during depolarization via a sodium–potassium pump mechanism; this increases force of contraction (positive inotropic effect), increases renal perfusion (seen as diuretic effect in patients with CHF), decreases heart rate (negative chronotropic effect), and decreases AV node conduction velocity.

Adverse effects in *Italics* are most common; those in **Bold** are life-threatening.

Indications
- CHF
- Atrial fibrillation

Contraindications and cautions
- Contraindicated with allergy to digitalis preparations, ventricular tachycardia, ventricular fibrillation, heart block, sick sinus syndrome, IHSS, acute MI, renal insufficiency and electrolyte abnormalities (decreased K^+, decreased Mg^{++}, increased Ca^{++}).
- Use cautiously with pregnancy and lactation.

Available forms
Lanoxicaps capsules—0.05, 0.1, 0.2 mg; tablets—0.125, 0.25, mg, elixir—0.05 mg/mL; injection—0.25 mg/mL; pediatric injection—0.1 mg/mL

Dosages
Patient response is quite variable. Evaluate patient carefully to determine the appropriate dose.
Adults
- *Loading dose:* 0.75–1.25 mg PO or 0.125–0.25 mg IV. *Maintenance dose:* 0.125–0.25 mg/day PO.
- *Lanoxicaps capsules:* 0.4–0.6 mg PO; maintenance dose: 0.5–0.1 mg/day PO.
Pediatric patients
- *Loading dose:*

	Oral (mcg/kg)	IV (mcg/kg)
Premature	20–30	15–25
Neonate	25–35	20–30
1–24 mo	35–60	30–50
2–5 yr	30–40	25–35
5–10 yr	20–35	15–30
> 10 yr	10–15	8–12

- *Maintenance dose:* 25%–35% of loading dose in divided daily doses. Usually 0.125–0.5 mg/day PO.
Geriatric patients with impaired renal function

Creatinine Clearance (mL/min)	Dose
10–25	0.125 mg/day
26–49	0.1875 mg/day
50–79	0.25 mg/day

Pharmacokinetics

Route	Onset	Peak	Duration
Oral	30–120 min	2–6 hr	6–8 days
IV	5–30 min	1–5 hr	4–5 days

Metabolism: Some hepatic; $T_{1/2}$: 30–40 hr
Distribution: May cross placenta; enters breast milk
Excretion: Largely unchanged in the urine

▽ IV facts
Preparation: Give undiluted or diluted in fourfold or greater volume of sterile water for injection, 0.9% sodium chloride injection, 5% dextrose injection, or lactated Ringer's injection. Use diluted product promptly. Do not use if solution contains precipitates.
Infusion: Inject slowly over 5 min or longer.
Incompatibility: Do not mix with dobutamine.

Adverse effects
- **CNS:** *Headache, weakness,* drowsiness, visual disturbances, mental status change
- **CV:** *Arrhythmias*
- **GI:** *GI upset,* anorexia

Interactions
✳ **Drug-drug** • Increased therapeutic and toxic effects of digoxin with thioamines, verapamil, amiodarone, quinidine, quinine, erythromycin, cyclosporine (a decrease in digoxin dosage may be necessary to prevent toxicity; when the interacting drug is discontinued, an increase in the digoxin dosage may be necessary) • Increased incidence of cardiac arrhythmias with potassium-losing (loop and thiazide) diuretics • Increased absorption or increased bioavailability of oral digoxin, leading to increased effects with tetracyclines, erythromycin • Decreased therapeutic effects with thyroid hormones, metoclopramide, penicillamine • Decreased absorption of oral digoxin if taken with cholestyramine, charcoal, colestipol, antineoplastic agents (bleomycin, cyclophosphamide, methotrexate) • Increased or decreased effects of oral digoxin (adjust the dose of digoxin during concomitant therapy) with oral aminoglycosides

✳ **Drug-alternative therapy** • Increased risk of digoxin toxicity if taken with ginseng, hawthorn, or licorice therapy • Decreased absorption with psyllium • Decreased serum levels with St. John's wort

■ Nursing considerations
Assessment
- **History:** Allergy to digitalis preparations, ventricular tachycardia, ventricular fibrillation, heart block, sick sinus syndrome, IHSS, acute MI, renal insufficiency, decreased K^+, decreased Mg^{++} increased Ca^{++}
- **Physical:** Weight; orientation, affect, reflexes, vision; P, BP, baseline ECG, cardiac auscultation, peripheral pulses, peripheral perfusion, edema; R, adventitious sounds; abdominal percussion, bowel sounds, liver evaluation; urinary output; electrolyte levels, liver and renal function tests

Interventions
- Monitor apical pulse for 1 min before administering; hold dose if pulse < 60 in adult or < 90 in infant; retake pulse in 1 hr. If adult pulse remains < 60 or infant < 90, hold drug and notify prescriber. Note any change from baseline rhythm or rate.
- Take care to differentiate *Lanoxicaps* from *Lanoxin;* dosage is very different.
- Check dosage and preparation carefully.
- Avoid IM injections, which may be very painful.
- Follow diluting instructions carefully, and use diluted solution promptly.
- Avoid giving with meals; this will delay absorption.
- Have emergency equipment ready; have K^+ salts, lidocaine, phenytoin, atropine, cardiac monitor on standby in case toxicity develops.
- Monitor for therapeutic drug levels: 0.5–2 ng/mL.

Teaching points
- Do not stop taking this drug without notifying your health care provider.
- Take pulse at the same time each day, and record it on a calendar (normal pulse for you is___); call your health care provider if your pulse rate falls below ___.
- Weigh yourself every other day with the same clothing and at the same time. Record this on the calendar.

- Wear or carry a medical alert tag stating that you are on this drug.
- Have regular medical checkups, which may include blood tests, to evaluate the effects and dosage of this drug.
- Report unusually slow pulse, irregular pulse, rapid weight gain, loss of appetite, nausea, vomiting, blurred or "yellow" vision, unusual tiredness and weakness, swelling of the ankles, legs or fingers, difficulty breathing.

▽**digoxin immune fab (ovine; digoxin-specific antibody fragments)**
(di jox' in)

Digibind, Digifab

PREGNANCY CATEGORY C

Drug class
Antidote

Therapeutic actions
Antigen-binding fragments (fab) derived from specific antidigoxin antibodies; binds molecules of digoxin, making them unavailable at the site of action; fab-fragment complex accumulates in the blood and is excreted by the kidneys.

Indications
- Treatment of life-threatening digoxin intoxication (serum digoxin levels >10 ng/mL, serum K^+ > 5 mEq/L in setting of digitalis intoxication)

Contraindications and cautions
- Contraindicated with allergy to sheep products.
- Use cautiously with pregnancy or lactation.

Available forms
Powder for injection—38 mg/vial (*Digibind*), 40 mg/vial (*Digifab*)

Dosages
Adults and pediatric patients
Dosage is determined by serum digoxin level or estimate of the amount of digoxin ingested. If no estimate is available and serum digoxin levels cannot be obtained, use 800 mg (20 vials), which should treat most life-threatening ingestions in adults and children.

- *Estimated fab fragment dose based on amount of digoxin ingested:*

Digibind

Estimated Number of
0.25-mg Tablets or
0.2-mg Capsules
Ingested

Estimated Number of 0.25-mg Tablets or 0.2-mg Capsules Ingested	Dose of Fab Fragments
25	340 mg (8.5 vials)
50	680 mg (17 vials)
75	1,000 mg (25 vials)
100	1,360 mg (34 vials)
150	2,000 mg (50 vials)
200	2,680 mg (67 vials)

- *Estimated fab fragments dose based on serum digoxin concentration:*

Wt (kg)	Serum Digoxin Concentration (ng/mL)						
	1	2	4	8	12	16	20
Pediatric patients (dose in mg)							
1	0.4	1	1.5	3	5	6	8
3	1	2	5	9	14	18	23
5	2	4	8	15	23	30	38
10	4	8	15	30	46	61	76
20	8	15	30	61	91	122	152
Adults (dose in mg)							
40	0.5	1	2	3	5	7	8
60	0.5	1	3	5	7	10	12
70	1	2	3	6	9	11	14
80	1	2	3	7	10	13	16
100	1	2	4	8	12	16	20

Digifab
- *Estimated fab fragment dose based on amount of digoxin ingested:*

Estimated Number of 0.25-mg Tablets or 0.2-mg Capsules Ingested	Dose (Number of Vials of Digifab)
25	10
50	20
75	30
100	40
150	60
200	80

- *Estimated fab fragments dose based on serum digoxin concentration:*

Wt (kg)	Serum Digoxin Concentration (ng/mL)						
	1	2	4	8	12	16	20
Pediatric patients (dose in mg)*							
1	0.4	1	1.5	3	5	6.5	8
3	1	2.5	5	10	14	19	24
5	2	4	8	16	24	32	40
10	4	8	16	32	48	64	80
20	8	16	32	64	96	128	160
Adults (dose in vials)							
40	0.5	1	2	3	5	7	8
60	0.5	1	3	5	7	10	12
70	1	2	3	6	9	11	14
80	1	2	3	7	10	13	16
100	1	2	4	8	12	16	20

*Dilution of reconstituted vial to 1 mg/mL is desirable.

Equations also are available for calculating exact dosage from serum digoxin concentrations.

Pharmacokinetics

Route	Onset	Duration
IV	15–30 min	4–6 hr

Metabolism: $T_{1/2}$: 15–20 hr
Distribution: Crosses placenta; may enter breast milk
Excretion: Urine

▼ IV facts
Preparation: Dissolve the contents in each vial with 4 mL of sterile water for injection. Mix gently to give an approximate isosmotic solution with a protein concentration of 10 mg/mL. Use reconstituted solution promptly. Store in refrigerator for up to 4 hr. Discard after that time. Reconstituted solution may be further diluted with sterile isotonic saline.
Infusion: Administer IV over 30 min through a 0.22-mcm filter; administer as a bolus injection if cardiac arrest is imminent.

Adverse effects
- **CV:** *Low cardiac output states,* CHF, rapid ventricular response in patients with atrial fibrillation
- **Hematologic:** Hypokalemia due to reactivation of Na^+, K^+, ATPase
- **Hypersensitivity:** Allergic reactions: drug fever to **anaphylaxis**

■ Nursing considerations
Assessment
- **History:** Allergy to sheep products, digoxin drug history, lactation
- **Physical:** P, BP, auscultation, baseline ECG, serum digoxin levels, serum electrolytes

Interventions
- Check dosage carefully before administering. The two available brand names have slightly different recommended doses. Distinguish between *Digibind* and *Digifab*.
- Arrange for serum digoxin concentration determinations before administration.
- Monitor patient's cardiac response to digoxin overdose and therapy—cardiac rhythm, serum electrolytes, T, BP.
- Maintain life-support equipment and emergency drugs (IV inotropes) on standby for severe overdose.
- Do not redigitalize patient until digoxin immune-fab has been cleared from the body; several days to a week or longer in cases of renal insufficiency. Serum digoxin levels will be very high and will be unreliable for up to 3 days after administration.

Teaching points
- Report muscle cramps, dizziness, palpitations.

▽ **dihydroergotamine mesylate**

(dye hye droe er got' a meen)

D.H.E. 45, Dihydroergotamine-Sandoz (CAN), Migranal

PREGNANCY CATEGORY X

Drug classes
Ergot derivative
Antimigraine agent

Therapeutic actions
Mechanism of action not understood; constricts cranial blood vessels; decreases pulsation in cranial arteries and decreases hyperperfusion of basilar artery vascular bed.

Indications
- Rapid control of vascular headaches (parenteral)
- Prevention or abortion of vascular headaches when other routes of administration are not feasible (parenteral)
- Acute treatment of migraine headaches with or without aura (nasal spray)

Contraindications and cautions
- Contraindicated with allergy to ergot preparations, peripheral vascular disease, severe hypertension, coronary artery disease, impaired liver or renal function, sepsis, pruritus, malnutrition, pregnancy.
- Use extreme caution with lactation.

Available forms
Injection—1 mg/mL; nasal spray—4 mg/mL (0.5 mg/spray)

Dosages
Adults
1 mg IM at first sign of headache; repeat at 1-hr intervals to a total of 3 mg. Use the minimum effective dose based on patient's experience. For IV use, up to a maximum of 2 mg; do not exceed 6 mg/wk.
Nasal spray
2 mg dose given as one spray in each nostril; may be repeated in 15–30 min as needed at first sign of headache or aura.
Pediatric patients
Safety and efficacy not established.

Pharmacokinetics

Route	Onset	Peak	Duration
IM	15–30 min	2 hr	3–4 hr
IV	Immediate	1–2 hr	3–4 hr
Nasal	Immediate	0.9 hr	2–4 hr

Metabolism: Hepatic; $T_{1/2}$: 21–32 hr
Distribution: Crosses placenta; enters breast milk
Excretion: Bile

▼ IV facts
Preparation: No preparation necessary.
Infusion: Give by direct injection, or into running IV, each 1 mg over 1 min; administer a maximum of 2 mg.

Adverse effects in *Italics* are most common; those in **Bold** are life-threatening.

Adverse effects
- **CNS:** *Numbness, tingling of fingers and toes*
- **CV:** Pulselessness, weakness in the legs; precordial distress and pain; transient tachycardia, bradycardia; localized edema and itching; increased arterial pressure, arterial insufficiency, coronary vasoconstriction, bradycardia; hypoperfusion, chest pain, BP changes, confusion
- **GI:** *Nausea, vomiting*
- **Nasal spray:** Nasal congestion, rhinorrhea, sneezing, throat discomfort
- **Other:** Muscle pain in the extremities; ergotism (nausea, vomiting, diarrhea, severe thirst); drug dependency and abuse with extended use

Interactions
✳ Drug-drug • Increased bioavailability with nitroglycerin, nitrates • Increased risk of peripheral ischemia with beta blockers, macrolides

■ Nursing considerations
Assessment
- **History:** Allergy to ergot preparations, peripheral vascular disease, severe hypertension, CAD, impaired liver or renal function, sepsis, pruritus, malnutrition, pregnancy, lactation
- **Physical:** Skin color, edema, lesions; peripheral sensation; P, BP, peripheral pulses, peripheral perfusion; liver evaluation, bowel sounds; CBC, liver and renal function tests

Interventions
- Avoid prolonged administration or excessive dosage.
- Use atropine or phenothiazine antiemetics if nausea and vomiting are severe.
- Examine extremities carefully for gangrene or decubitus ulcer formation.

Teaching points
- Take this drug as soon as possible after the first symptoms of an attack.
- Prime the pump prior to nasal spray administration by squeezing pump 4 times. Once prepared, discard unused portion within 8 hr.
- These side effects may occur: nausea, vomiting (if severe, medication may be ordered); numbness, tingling, loss of sensation in the extremities (use caution to avoid injury, and examine extremities daily for injury).
- Do not take during pregnancy; if you become or desire to become pregnant, consult with your physician.
- Report irregular heartbeat, pain or weakness of extremities, severe nausea or vomiting, numbness or tingling of fingers or toes.

▷diltiazem hydrochloride
(dil tye' a zem)

Alti-Diltiazem (CAN), Apo-Diltiaz (CAN), Cardizem, Cardizem CD, Cardizem SR, Cartia XT, Dilacor XR, Diltia XT, Gen-Diltiazem (CAN), Novo-Diltiazem (CAN), Nu-Diltiaz (CAN), Tiamate, Tiazac

PREGNANCY CATEGORY C

Drug classes
Calcium channel-blocker
Antianginal agent
Antihypertensive

Therapeutic actions
Inhibits the movement of calcium ions across the membranes of cardiac and arterial muscle cells, resulting in the depression of impulse formation in specialized cardiac pacemaker cells, slowing of the velocity of conduction of the cardiac impulse, depression of myocardial contractility, and dilation of coronary arteries and arterioles and peripheral arterioles; these effects lead to decreased cardiac work, decreased cardiac energy consumption, and in patients with vasospastic (Prinzmetal's) angina, increased delivery of oxygen to myocardial cells.

Indications
- Angina pectoris due to coronary artery spasm (Prinzmetal's variant angina)
- Effort-associated angina; chronic stable angina in patients not controlled by beta-adrenergic blockers, nitrates
- Essential hypertension (sustained release)
- Paroxysmal supraventricular tachycardia, atrial fibrillation, atrial flutter (parenteral)

Contraindications and cautions

- Allergy to diltiazem, impaired hepatic or renal function, sick sinus syndrome, heart block (second or third degree), lactation.

Available forms

Tablets—30, 60, 90, 120 mg; ER capsules—60, 90, 120, 180, 240, 300, 360, 420 mg; injection— 5 mg/mL; powder for injection—25, 100 mg; SR tablets—60, 90, 120 mg

Dosages

Evaluate patient carefully to determine the appropriate dose of this drug.

Adults

Initially 30 mg PO qid before meals and hs; gradually increase dosage at 1- to 2-day intervals to 180–360 mg PO in 3–4 divided doses.

Sustained and extended release

Cardizem SR: Initially 60–120 mg PO bid; adjust dosage when maximum antihypertensive effect is achieved (around 14 days); optimum range is 240–360 mg/day.

Cardizem CD and Cartia XT: 180–240 mg daily PO for hypertension; 120–180 mg daily PO for angina.

Dilacor XR and Diltia XT: 180–240 mg daily PO as needed; up to 480 mg has been used.

Tiazac: 120–240 mg daily PO for hypertension—once daily dose; 120–180 mg PO once daily for angina.

IV

Direct IV bolus: 0.25 mg/kg (20 mg for the average patient); second bolus of 0.35 mg/kg.

Continuous IV infusion: 5–10 mg/hr with increases up to 15 mg/hr; may be continued for up to 24 hr.

Pediatric patients

Safety and efficacy not established.

Pharmacokinetics

Route	Onset	Peak
Oral	30–60 min	2–3 hr
SR, ER	30–60 min	6–11 hr
IV	Immediate	2–3 min

Metabolism: Hepatic; $T_{1/2}$: 3.5–6 hr; 5–7 hr (SR)

Distribution: Crosses placenta; enters breast milk

Excretion: Urine

▼IV facts

Preparation: For continuous infusion, transfer to normal saline, D_5W, $D_5W/0.45\%$ NaCl as below. Mix thoroughly. Use within 24 hr. Keep refrigerated.

Diluent Volume mL)	Quantity of Injection	Final Concentration (mg/mL)	Dose (mg/hr)	Infusion Rate (mL/hr)
100	125 mg	1	10	10
	(25 mL)	—	15	15
250	250 mg	0.83	10	12
	(50 mL)	—	15	18
500	250 mg	0.45	10	22
	(50 mL)	—	15	33

Infusion: Administer bolus dose over 2 min. For continuous infusion, rate of 10 mL/hr is the recommended rate. Do not use continuous infusion longer than 24 hr.

Incompatibilities: Do not mix in the same solution with furosemide solution.

Adverse effects

- **CNS:** *Dizziness, light-headedness, headache, asthenia,* fatigue
- **CV:** *Peripheral edema,* hypotension, arrhythmias, *bradycardia, AV block,* asystole
- **Dermatologic:** *Flushing,* rash
- **GI:** *Nausea,* hepatic injury, reflux

Interactions

✳ Drug-drug • Increased serum levels and toxicity of cyclosporine if taken concurrently with diltiazem • Possible depression of myocardial contractility, AV conduction if combined with beta blockers; use caution and monitor patient closely

✳ Drug-food • Decreased metabolism and increased risk of toxic effects if taken with grapefruit juice; avoid this combination

■ Nursing considerations

Assessment

- **History:** Allergy to diltiazem, impaired hepatic or renal function, sick sinus syndrome, heart block, lactation, pregnancy
- **Physical:** Skin lesions, color, edema; P, BP, baseline ECG, peripheral perfusion, auscultation; R, adventitious sounds; liver evalu-

ation, normal output; liver and renal function tests, urinalysis

Interventions

- Monitor patient carefully (BP, cardiac rhythm, and output) while drug is being titrated to therapeutic dose; dosage may be increased more rapidly in hospitalized patients under close supervision.
- Monitor BP carefully if patient is on concurrent doses of nitrates.
- Monitor cardiac rhythm regularly during stabilization of dosage and periodically during long-term therapy.
- Ensure patient swallows ER and SR preparations whole; do not cut, crush, or chew.

Teaching points

- Swallow SR and ER preparations whole; do not cut, crush, or chew; do not drink grapefruit juice while using this drug.
- These side effects may occur: nausea, vomiting (small, frequent meals may help); headache (regulate light, noise, and temperature; medicate if severe).
- Report irregular heart beat, shortness of breath, swelling of the hands or feet, pronounced dizziness, constipation.

▷dimenhydrinate
(dye men hye' dri nate)

Oral preparations: Apo-Dimenhydrinate (CAN), Calm-X, Children's Dramamine, Dimetabs, Dramamine, Gravol (CAN), Traveltabs (CAN), Triptone
Parenteral preparations: Dinate, Dramanate, Dymenate, Hydrate

PREGNANCY CATEGORY B

Drug classes
Anti-motion sickness agent
Antihistamine
Anticholinergic

Therapeutic actions
Antihistamine with antiemetic and anticholinergic activity; depresses hyperstimulated labyrinthine function; may block synapses in the vomiting center; peripheral anticholinergic effects may contribute to antimotion sickness efficacy.

Indications
- Prevention and treatment of nausea, vomiting, or vertigo of motion sickness

Contraindications and cautions
- Contraindicated with allergy to dimenhydrinate or its components, lactation.
- Use cautiously with narrow-angle glaucoma, stenosing peptic ulcer, symptomatic prostatic hypertrophy, bronchial asthma, bladder neck obstruction, pyloroduodenal obstruction, cardiac arrhythmias, pregnancy.

Available forms
Tablets—50 mg; chewable tablets—50 mg; injection—50 mg/mL; liquid—12.5 mg/4 mL, 15.62 mg/5 mL

Dosages
Adults
Oral
50–100 mg q 4–6 hr PO; for prophylaxis, first dose should be taken 30 min before exposure to motion. Do not exceed 400 mg in 24 hr.
Parenteral
50 mg IM as needed; 50 mg in 10 mL sodium chloride injection given IV over 10 min.
Pediatric patients
6–12 yr: 25–50 mg PO q 6–8 hr, not to exceed 150 mg/24 hr.
2–6 yr: Up to 25 mg PO q 6–8 hr, not to exceed 75 mg/24 hr.
< 2 yr: Only on advice of physician; 1.25 mg/kg IM qid, not to exceed 30 mg/24 hr.
Neonates: Contraindicated.
Geriatric patients
Can cause dizziness, sedation, syncope, confusion, and hypotension in elderly patients; use with caution.

Pharmacokinetics

Route	Onset	Peak	Duration
Oral	15–30 min	2 hr	3–6 hr
IM	20–30 min	1–2 hr	3–6 hr
IV	Immediate	1–2 hr	3–6 hr

Metabolism: Hepatic; $T_{1/2}$: unknown

Distribution: Crosses placenta; enters breast milk
Excretion: Urine

▼IV facts

Preparation: Dilute 50 mg in 10 mL sodium chloride injection.
Infusion: Administer by direct IV injection over 2 min.
Incompatibilities: Do not combine with tetracycline, thiopental.
Y-site incompatibilities: Do not mix with aminophylline, heparin, hydrocortisone, hydroxyzine, phenobarbital, phenytoin, prednisolone, promethazine.

Adverse effects

- **CNS:** *Drowsiness, confusion, nervousness, restlessness, headache, dizziness, vertigo, lassitude, tingling, heaviness and weakness of hands; insomnia* and excitement (especially in children), hallucinations, convulsions, **death,** blurring of vision, diplopia
- **CV:** Hypotension, palpitations, tachycardia
- **Dermatologic:** Urticaria, drug rash, photosensitivity
- **GI:** Epigastric distress, anorexia, nausea, vomiting, diarrhea or constipation; dryness of mouth, nose, and throat
- **GU:** Urinary hesitancy, urinary retention
- **Respiratory:** Nasal stuffiness, chest tightness, thickening of bronchial secretions, **anaphylaxis**

Interactions

✳ Drug-drug • Increased depressant effects with alcohol, other CNS depressants

■ Nursing considerations
Assessment

- **History:** Allergy to dimenhydrinate or its components, lactation, narrow-angle glaucoma, stenosing peptic ulcer, symptomatic prostatic hypertrophy, bronchial asthma, bladder neck obstruction, pyloroduodenal obstruction, cardiac arrhythmias
- **Physical:** Skin color, lesions, texture; orientation, reflexes, affect; vision exam; P, BP; R, adventitious sounds; bowel sounds; prostate palpation; CBC

Interventions

- Maintain epinephrine 1:1,000 readily available when using parenteral preparations; hypersensitivity reactions, including anaphylaxis, have occurred.

Teaching points

- Take drug as prescribed; avoid excessive dosage.
- Drug works best if taken before motion sickness occurs.
- These side effects may occur: dizziness, sedation, drowsiness (use caution if driving or performing tasks that require alertness); epigastric distress, diarrhea or constipation (take drug with food); dry mouth (use frequent mouth care, suck sugarless lozenges); thickening of bronchial secretions, dryness of nasal mucosa (try another motion sickness remedy).
- Avoid alcohol; serious sedation could occur.
- Report difficulty breathing, hallucinations, tremors, loss of coordination, unusual bleeding or bruising, visual disturbances, irregular heartbeat.

▽dimercaprol

See *Less Commonly Used Drugs,* p. 1342.

▽dinoprostone (prostaglandin E₂)

(dye noe prost' ohn)

Cervidil, Prepidil, Prostin E₂

PREGNANCY CATEGORY C

Drug classes
Prostaglandin
Abortifacient

Therapeutic actions
Stimulates the myometrium of the pregnant uterus to contract, similar to the contractions of the uterus during labor, thus evacuating the contents of the uterus.

Indications

- Termination of pregnancy 12–20 wk from the first day of the last menstrual period
- Evacuation of the uterus in the management of missed abortion or intrauterine fetal death up to 28 wk gestational age
- Management of nonmetastatic gestational trophoblastic disease (benign hydatidiform mole)
- Initiation of cervical ripening before induction of labor

Contraindications and cautions

- Contraindicated with allergy to prostaglandin preparations; acute PID; active cardiac, hepatic, pulmonary, renal disease; women in whom prolonged uterine contractions are inappropriate (c-section, uterine surgery, fetal distress, obstetric emergency, etc.).
- Use cautiously with history of asthma; hypotension; hypertension; CV, adrenal, renal, or hepatic disease; anemia; jaundice; diabetes; epilepsy; scarred uterus; cervicitis, infected endocervical lesions, acute vaginitis.

Available forms

Vaginal suppository—20 mg; vaginal gel—0.5 mg; vaginal insert—10 mg

Dosages
Adults

- *Termination of pregnancy:* Insert one suppository (20 mg) high into the vagina; keep supine for 10 min after insertion. Additional suppositories may be given at 3- to 5-hr intervals based on uterine response and tolerance. Do not give longer than 2 days.
- *Cervical ripening:* Give 0.5 mg gel via cervical catheter provided with patient in the dorsal position and cervix visualized using a speculum. Repeat dose may be given if no response in 6 hr. Wait 6–12 hr before beginning oxytocin IV to initiate labor. Insert: Place one insert transversely in the posterior fornix of the vagina. Keep patient supine for 2 hr; one insert delivers 0.3 mg/hr over 12 hr. Remove, using retrieval system, at onset of active labor or 12 hr post insertion.

Pharmacokinetics

Route	Onset	Peak	Duration
Intravaginal	10 min	15 min	2–3 hr

Metabolism: Tissue; $T_{1/2}$: 5–10 hr
Distribution: Crosses placenta; enters breast milk
Excretion: Urine

Adverse effects

- **CNS:** *Headache,* paresthesias, anxiety, weakness, syncope, dizziness
- **CV:** *Hypotension,* arrhythmias, chest pain
- **Fetal:** Abnormal heart rates
- **GI:** *Vomiting, diarrhea, nausea*
- **GU:** Endometritis, perforated uterus, uterine rupture, uterine or vaginal pain, incomplete abortion
- **Respiratory:** Coughing, dyspnea
- **Other:** Chills, diaphoresis, backache, breast tenderness, eye pain, skin rash, pyrexia

■ Nursing considerations

 CLINICAL ALERT!
Name confusion has occurred among Prostin VR Pediatric (alprostadil), Prostin FZ (dinoprost—available outside the U.S.), Prostin E₂ (dinoprostone), and Prostin 15 (carboprost in Europe). Confusion has also been reported with Prepidil (dinoprostone) and bepridil. Use extreme caution.

Assessment

- **History:** Allergy to prostaglandin preparations; acute PID; active cardiac, hepatic, pulmonary, renal disease; history of asthma; hypotension; hypertension; anemia; jaundice; diabetes; epilepsy; scarred uterus; cervicitis, infected endocervical lesions, acute vaginitis
- **Physical:** T; BP, P, auscultation; R, adventitious sounds; bowel sounds, liver evaluation; vaginal discharge, pelvic exam, uterine tone; liver and renal function tests, WBC, urinalysis, CBC

Interventions

- Store suppositories in freezer; bring to room temperature before insertion.
- Arrange for pre- or concurrent treatment with antiemetic and antidiarrheal drugs to decrease the incidence of GI side effects.

- Ensure that abortion is complete or that other measures are used to complete the abortion if drug effects are not sufficient.
- Monitor T, using care to differentiate prostaglandin-induced pyrexia from post-abortion endometritis pyrexia.
- Give gel using aseptic technique via cervical catheter to patient in dorsal position. Patient should remain in this position 15–30 min.
- Monitor uterine tone and vaginal discharge throughout procedure and several days after the procedure.
- Ensure adequate hydration throughout procedure.
- Be prepared to support patient through labor (cervical ripening). Give oxytocin infusion 6–12 hr after dinoprostone.

Teaching points
Teaching about dinoprostone should be incorporated into the total teaching plan, including the following:
- If the patient has never had a vaginal suppository, explain the procedure and that she will need to lie down for 10 min after insertion.
- You will need to stay on your side for 15–30 min after injection of gel.
- These side effects may occur: nausea, vomiting, diarrhea, uterine or vaginal pain, fever, headache, weakness, dizziness.
- Report severe pain, difficulty breathing, palpitations, eye pain, rash.

---

diphenhydramine hydrochloride
(dye fen hye' dra meen)

Oral: Allerdryl (CAN), Allergy Medication, AllerMax Caplets, Banophen, Banophen Caplets, Benadryl Allergy, Benadryl Allergy Kapseals, Benadryl Allergy Ultratabs, Benadryl Dye-Free Allergy LiquiGels, Diphen AF, Diphen Cough, Diphenhist, Diphenhist Captabs, Genahist, Siladryl, Silphen Cough, Uni-Bent Cough

Oral prescription preparations: Benadryl, Tusstat

Parenteral preparations: Benadryl, Hyrexin-50

PREGNANCY CATEGORY B

Drug classes
Antihistamine
Anti-motion sickness agent
Sedative and hypnotic
Antiparkinsonian agent
Cough suppressant

Therapeutic actions
Competitively blocks the effects of histamine at H_1-receptor sites, has atropine-like, antipruritic, and sedative effects.

Indications
- Relief of symptoms associated with perennial and seasonal allergic rhinitis; vasomotor rhinitis; allergic conjunctivitis; mild, uncomplicated urticaria and angioedema; amelioration of allergic reactions to blood or plasma; dermatographism; adjunctive therapy in anaphylactic reactions
- Active and prophylactic treatment of motion sickness
- Nighttime sleep aid
- Parkinsonism (including drug-induced parkinsonism and extrapyramidal reactions), in the elderly intolerant of more potent agents, for milder forms of the disorder in other age groups, and in combination with centrally acting anticholinergic antiparkinsonian drugs
- Suppression of cough due to colds or allergy (syrup formulation)

Contraindications and cautions
- Contraindicated with allergy to any antihistamines, third trimester of pregnancy, lactation.
- Use cautiously with narrow-angle glaucoma, stenosing peptic ulcer, symptomatic prostatic hypertrophy, asthmatic attack, bladder neck obstruction, pyloroduodenal ob-

struction, pregnancy; elderly patients who may be sensitive to anticholinergic effects.

Available forms

Capsule soft gels—25 mg; capsules—25, 50 mg; tablets—25, 50 mg; chewable tablets—12.5 mg; elixir—12.5 mg/5 mL; syrup—12.5 mg/5 mL; liquid—6.25, 12.5 mg/5 mL; injection—10, 50 mg/mL; solution—12.5 mg/5 mL

Dosages
Adults
Oral
25–50 mg q 4–8 hr PO.
- *Motion sickness:* Give full dose prophylactically 30 min before exposure to motion, and repeat before meals and at bedtime.
- *Nighttime sleep aid:* 25–50 mg PO at bedtime.
- *Cough suppression:* 25 mg q 4 hr PO, not to exceed 150 mg in 24 hr.
Parenteral
10–50 mg IV or deep IM or up to 100 mg if required. Maximum daily dose is 400 mg.
Pediatric patients > 10 kg or 20 lb
Oral
12.5–25 mg tid–qid PO or 5 mg/kg/day PO or 150 mg/m² per day PO. Maximum daily dose 300 mg.
- *Motion sickness:* Give full dose prophylactically 30 min before exposure to motion and repeat before meals and at bedtime.
- *Cough suppression:*
6–12 yr: 12.5 mg q 4 hr PO, not to exceed 75 mg in 24 hr.
2–6 yr: 6.25 mg q 4 hr, not to exceed 25 mg in 24 hr.
Parenteral
5 mg/kg/day or 150 mg/m² per day IV or by deep IM injection. Maximum daily dose is 300 mg divided into four doses.
Geriatric patients
More likely to cause dizziness, sedation, syncope, toxic confusional states, and hypotension in elderly patients; use with caution.

Pharmacokinetics

Route	Onset	Peak	Duration
Oral	15–30 min	1–4 hr	4–7 hr
IM	20–30 min	1–4 hr	4–8 hr
IV	Rapid	30–60 min	4–8 hr

Metabolism: Hepatic; $T_{1/2}$: 2.5–7 hr
Distribution: Crosses placenta; enters breast milk
Excretion: Urine

▼IV facts
Preparation: No additional preparation required.
Infusion: Administer slowly each 25 mg over 1 min by direct injection or into tubing of running IV.
Incompatibilities: Do not combine with amobarbital, amphotericin B, cephalothin, hydrocortisone, phenobarbital, phenytoin, thiopental.
Y-site incompatibilities: Do not mix with foscarnet.

Adverse effects
- **CNS:** *Drowsiness, sedation, dizziness, disturbed coordination,* fatigue, confusion, restlessness, excitation, nervousness, tremor, headache, blurred vision, diplopia
- **CV:** Hypotension, palpitations, bradycardia, tachycardia, extrasystoles
- **GI:** *Epigastric distress,* anorexia, increased appetite and weight gain, nausea, vomiting, diarrhea or constipation
- **GU:** Urinary frequency, dysuria, urinary retention, early menses, decreased libido, impotence
- **Hematologic:** Hemolytic anemia, hypoplastic anemia, thrombocytopenia, leukopenia, agranulocytosis, pancytopenia
- **Respiratory:** *Thickening of bronchial secretions,* chest tightness, wheezing, nasal stuffiness, dry mouth, dry nose, dry throat, sore throat
- **Other:** Urticaria, rash, **anaphylactic shock,** photosensitivity, excessive perspiration

Interactions
✳ **Drug-drug** • Possible increased and prolonged anticholinergic effects with MAO inhibitors

■ Nursing considerations
Assessment
- **History:** Allergy to any antihistamines, narrow-angle glaucoma, stenosing peptic ulcer, symptomatic prostatic hypertrophy, asthmatic attack, bladder neck obstruction,

pyloroduodenal obstruction, third trimester of pregnancy, lactation
- **Physical:** Skin color, lesions, texture; orientation, reflexes, affect; vision exam; P, BP; R, adventitious sounds; bowel sounds; prostate palpation; CBC with differential

Interventions
- Administer with food if GI upset occurs.
- Administer syrup form if patient is unable to take tablets.
- Monitor patient response, and arrange for adjustment of dosage to lowest possible effective dose.

Teaching points
- Take as prescribed; avoid excessive dosage.
- Take with food if GI upset occurs.
- These side effects may occur: dizziness, sedation, drowsiness (use caution driving or performing tasks requiring alertness); epigastric distress, diarrhea or constipation (take drug with meals); dry mouth (use frequent mouth care, suck sugarless lozenges); thickening of bronchial secretions, dryness of nasal mucosa (use a humidifier).
- Avoid alcohol; serious sedation could occur.
- Report difficulty breathing, hallucinations, tremors, loss of coordination, unusual bleeding or bruising, visual disturbances, irregular heartbeat.

▽ dipyridamole
(dye peer id' a mole)

Apo-Dipyridamole (CAN), Dipridacot (CAN), Persantine, Persantine IV

PREGNANCY CATEGORY B

Drug classes
Antianginal agent
Antiplatelet agent
Diagnostic agent

Therapeutic actions
Decreases coronary vascular resistance and increases coronary blood flow without increasing myocardial oxygen consumption; inhibits platelet aggregation.

Indications
- With warfarin to prevent thromboembolism in patients with prosthetic heart valves
- IV use: diagnostic aid in evaluation of CAD in patients who cannot exercise, as an alternative to exercise in thallium myocardial perfusion imaging studies
- Unlabeled uses: prevention of MI or reduction of mortality post-MI; with aspirin to prevent coronary bypass graft occlusion

Contraindications and cautions
- Contraindicated with allergy to dipyridamole, pregnancy, lactation.
- Use cautiously with hypotension (drug can cause peripheral vasodilation that could exacerbate hypotension).

Available forms
Tablets—25, 50, 75 mg; injection—10 mg

Dosages
Adults
- *Prophylaxis in thromboembolism following cardiac valve surgery:* 75–100 mg qid PO as an adjunct to warfarin therapy.
- *Diagnostic agent in thallium myocardial perfusion imaging:* 0.142 mg/kg/min (0.57 mg total) infused over 4 min. Inject thallium-201 within 5 min following the 4-min infusion of dipyridamole.

Pharmacokinetics

Route	Onset	Peak	Duration
Oral	Varies	75 min	3–4 hr
IV	Rapid	6.5 min	30 min

Metabolism: Hepatic; $T_{1/2}$: 40 min, then 10 hr
Distribution: Crosses placenta; enters breast milk
Excretion: Bile

▼IV facts
Preparation: Dilute dose based on weight in at least a 1:2 ratio with 0.5N sodium chloride injection, 1N sodium chloride injection, or 5% dextrose injection for a total volume of about 20–50 mL. Protect from direct light.

Adverse effects in *Italics* are most common; those in **Bold** are life-threatening.

Infusion: Infuse slowly over 4 min. Do not infuse undiluted drug; local irritation can occur.

Adverse effects

- **CNS:** *Headache, dizziness,* weakness, syncope, flushing
- **CV: MI, ventricular fibrillation** (IV)
- **Dermatologic:** *Rash,* pruritus
- **GI:** Nausea, *GI distress,* constipation, diarrhea
- **GU:** Possible decreased fertility and loss of eggs in women
- **Local:** Pain and burning at injection site
- **Respiratory: Bronchospasm** (IV)

Interactions

✴ **Drug-drug** • Decreased coronary vasodilation effects if IV use with theophylline

■ Nursing considerations
Assessment

- **History:** Allergy to dipyridamole, hypotension, lactation, pregnancy
- **Physical:** Skin color, temperature, lesions; orientation, reflexes, affect; P, BP, orthostatic BP, baseline ECG, peripheral perfusion; R, adventitious sounds

Interventions

- Provide continual monitoring of ECG, BP, and orientation during administration of IV dipyridamole.
- Administer oral drug at least 1 hr before meals with a full glass of fluid.

Teaching points

- Take dipyridamole at least 1 hr before meals with a full glass of fluid.
- These side effects may occur: dizziness, lightheadedness (transient; change positions slowly; lie or sit down when you take your dose to decrease the risk of falling); headache (lie down and rest in a cool environment; OTC drugs may help); flushing of the neck or face (transient); nausea, gastric distress (small, frequent meals may help).
- Report rash, chest pain, fainting, severe headache; pain at injection site (IV).

▽ dirithromycin
(dir ith' ro my sin)

Dynabac

PREGNANCY CATEGORY C

Drug class
Macrolide antibiotic

Therapeutic actions
Inhibits protein synthesis in susceptible bacteria, causing cell death.

Indications

- Acute bacterial exacerbations of chronic bronchitis caused by *Streptococcus pneumoniae, Moraxella catarrhalis, Haemophilus influenzae*
- Secondary bacterial infections of acute bronchitis caused by *M. catarrhalis, S. pneumoniae*
- Community-acquired pneumonia caused by *Legionella pneumophila, Mycoplasma pneumoniae, S. pneumoniae*
- Treatment of pharyngitis and tonsillitis caused by *Streptococcus pyogenes*
- Treatment of skin and skin-structure infections caused by *Staphylococcus aureus, Streptococcus pyogenes*

Contraindications and cautions

- Contraindicated with hypersensitivity to dirithromycin, erythromycin, or any macrolide antibiotic, bacteremia, coadministration with pimozide.
- Use cautiously with colitis, hepatic or renal impairment, pregnancy, lactation.

Available forms
Delayed-release tablets—250 mg

Dosages
Adults
500 mg PO daily. Skin and skin-structure infections—treat for 5–7 days; pharyngitis or tonsillitis—treat for 10 days; community-acquired pneumonia—treat for 14 days; chronic bronchitis—treat for 5–7 days.
Pediatric patients
Safety and efficacy not established in children < 12 yr.

Pharmacokinetics

Route	Onset	Peak
Oral	Slow	4 hr

Metabolism: Hepatic metabolism, $T_{1/2}$: 44 hr
Distribution: Crosses placenta; passes into breast milk
Excretion: Feces, bile

Adverse effects

- **CNS:** Dizziness, headache, vertigo, somnolence, fatigue
- **GI:** *Diarrhea, abdominal pain, nausea,* dyspepsia, flatulence, vomiting, melena, **pseudomembranous colitis**
- **Other:** *Superinfections,* cough, rash, **electrolyte imbalance**

■ Nursing considerations
Assessment

- **History:** Hypersensitivity to erythromycin or any macrolide antibiotic; pseudomembranous colitis, hepatic or renal impairment, bacteremia, lactation, pregnancy
- **Physical:** Site of infection, skin color, lesions; orientation, GI output, bowel sounds, liver evaluation; culture and sensitivity tests of infection, urinalysis, liver and renal function tests

Interventions

- Culture site of infection before beginning therapy.
- Give with food to increase GI effects and absorption.
- Ensure that patient swallows tablet whole; continue therapy for complete course.
- Institute appropriate hygiene measures and arrange treatment if superinfections occur.
- Provide small, frequent meals and good mouth care if GI problems occur.

Teaching points

- Drug should be taken once a day with food. Swallow tablet whole; do not cut or crush. Take full course of therapy prescribed.
- These side effects may occur: stomach cramping, discomfort, diarrhea; fatigue, headache (medication may help); additional infections in mouth or vagina (consult with

health care provider for appropriate treatment).
- Report severe or watery diarrhea, severe nausea or vomiting, rash or itching, mouth or vaginal sores.

▷ disopyramide phosphate
*(dye soe **peer'** a mide)*

Norpace, Norpace CR, Rythmodan (CAN)

PREGNANCY CATEGORY C

Drug class
Antiarrhythmic

Therapeutic actions
Type 1a antiarrhythmic: decreases rate of diastolic depolarization, decreases automaticity, decreases the rate of rise of the action potential, prolongs the refractory period of cardiac muscle cells.

Indications
- Treatment of ventricular arrhythmias considered to be life threatening
- Unlabeled use: treatment of paroxysmal supraventricular tachycardia

Contraindications and cautions
- Contraindicated with cardiogenic shock, allergy to disopyramide, cardiac conduction abnormalities (eg, Wolff-Parkinson-White syndrome, sick sinus syndrome, heart block, prolonged QT interval); use caution with CHF, hypotension, cardiac myopathies, urinary retention, glaucoma, myasthenia gravis, renal or hepatic disease, potassium imbalance, pregnancy, lactation.

Available forms
Capsules—100, 150 mg; ER capsules—100, 150 mg

Dosages
Evaluate patient carefully and monitor cardiac response closely to determine the correct dosage for each patient.

Adults

400–800 mg/day PO given in divided doses q 6 hr or q 12 hr if using the controlled-release products.

- *Rapid control of ventricular arrhythmias:* 300 mg PO (immediate release). If no response within 6 hr, give 200 mg PO q 6 hr; may increase to 250–300 mg q 6 hr if no response in 48 hr.
- *Cardiomyopathy:* No loading dose, 100 mg PO q 6–8 hr immediate release.

Pediatric patients

Give in equal, divided doses q 6 hr PO, adjusting the dose to the patient's need.

Age	Daily Dosage (mg/kg)
< 1 yr	10–30
1–4 yr	10–20
4–12 yr	10–15
12–18 yr	6–15

Patients with renal impairment

Loading dose of 150 mg PO may be given, followed by 100 mg at the intervals shown.

Creatinine Clearance (mL/min)	Interval
30–40	q 8 hr
15–30	q 12 hr
< 15	q 24 hr

Pharmacokinetics

Route	Onset	Peak	Duration
Oral	30–60 min	2 hr	1.5–8.5 hr

Metabolism: Hepatic; $T_{1/2}$: 4–10 hr
Distribution: Crosses placenta; enters breast milk
Excretion: Urine

Adverse effects

- **CNS:** Dizziness, fatigue, headache, *blurred vision*
- **CV:** CHF, hypotension, cardiac conduction disturbances
- **GI:** *Dry mouth, constipation,* nausea, abdominal pain, gas
- **GU:** *Urinary hesitancy and retention, impotence*
- **Other:** *Dry nose, eyes, and throat; rash;* itching; *muscle weakness; malaise; aches and pains.*

Interactions

✳ **Drug-drug** • Decreased disopyramide plasma levels if used with phenytoins, rifampin
• Risk of increased disopyramide effects with antiarrhythmics, erythromycin, quinidine

■ Nursing considerations

Assessment

- **History:** Allergy to disopyramide, CHF, hypotension, Wolff-Parkinson-White syndrome, sick sinus syndrome, heart block, cardiac myopathies, urinary retention, glaucoma, myasthenia gravis, renal or hepatic disease, potassium imbalance, labor or delivery, lactation, pregnancy
- **Physical:** Weight; orientation, reflexes; P, BP, auscultation, ECG, edema; R, adventitious sounds; bowel sounds, liver evaluation; urinalysis, renal and liver function tests, blood glucose, serum K+

Interventions

- Check that patients with supraventricular tachyarrhythmias have been digitalized before starting disopyramide.
- Reduce dosage in patients < 110 lb.
- Reduce dosage in patients with hepatic or renal failure.
- Monitor patients with severe refractory tachycardia who may be given up to 1,600 mg/day continuously.
- Make a pediatric suspension form (1–10 mg/mL) by adding the contents of the immediate release capsule to cherry syrup, NF if desired. Store in dark bottle, and refrigerate. Shake well before using. Stable for 1 mo.
- Take care to differentiate the controlled release form from the immediate-release preparation. Ensure that patient swallows CR form whole; do not cut, crush, or chew.
- Monitor BP, orthostatic pressure.
- Evaluate for safe and effective serum levels (2–8 mcg/mL).

Teaching points

- You will require frequent monitoring of cardiac rhythm, BP.
- Swallow CR capsules whole; do not cut, crush, or chew tablets.
- These side effects may occur: dry mouth (try frequent mouth care, suck sugarless lozenges); constipation (laxatives may be ordered); difficulty voiding (empty the blad-

der before taking drug); muscle weakness or aches and pains.
- Do not stop taking this drug for any reason without checking with your health care provider.
- Return for regular follow-up visits to check your heart rhythm and blood pressure.
- Report swelling of fingers or ankles, difficulty breathing, dizziness, urinary retention, severe headache or visual changes.

▷ disulfiram
(dye sul' fi ram)

Antabuse

PREGNANCY CATEGORY C

Drug classes
Antialcoholic agent
Enzyme inhibitor

Therapeutic actions
Inhibits the enzyme aldehyde dehydrogenase, blocking oxidation of alcohol and allowing acetaldehyde to accumulate to concentrations in the blood 5–10 times higher than normally achieved during alcohol metabolism; accumulation of acetaldehyde produces the highly unpleasant reaction described below that deters consumption of alcohol.

Indications
- Aids in the management of selected chronic alcoholics who want to remain in a state of enforced sobriety

Contraindications and cautions
- Contraindicated with allergy to disulfiram or other thiuram derivatives used in pesticides and rubber vulcanization, severe myocardial disease or coronary occlusion; psychoses, current or recent treatment with metronidazole, paraldehyde, alcohol, alcohol-containing preparations (eg, cough syrups, tonics), pregnancy.
- Use cautiously with diabetes mellitus, hypothyroidism, epilepsy, cerebral damage, chronic and acute nephritis, hepatic cirrhosis or dysfunction.

Available forms
Tablets—250, 500 mg

Dosages
Never administer to an intoxicated patient or without patient's knowledge. Do not administer until patient has abstained from alcohol for at least 12 hr.
Adults
- *Initial dosage:* Administer maximum of 500 mg/day PO in a single dose for 1–2 wk. If a sedative effect occurs, administer at bedtime or decrease dosage.
- *Maintenance regimen:* 125–500 mg/day PO. Do not exceed 500 mg/day. Continue use until patient is fully recovered socially and a basis for permanent self-control is established.
- *Trial with alcohol (do not administer to anyone > 50 yr):* After 1–2 wk of therapy with 500 mg/day PO, a drink of 15 mL of 100 proof whiskey or its equivalent is taken slowly. Dose may be repeated once, if patient is hospitalized and supportive facilities are available.

Pharmacokinetics

Route	Onset	Peak	Duration
Oral	Slow	12 hr	1–2 wk

Metabolism: Hepatic; $T_{1/2}$: unclear
Distribution: Crosses placenta; enters breast milk
Excretion: Feces, lungs

Adverse effects
Disulfiram with alcohol
- Flushing, throbbing in head and neck, throbbing headaches, respiratory difficulty, nausea, copious vomiting, sweating, thirst, chest pain, palpitations, dyspnea, hyperventilation, tachycardia, hypotension, syncope, weakness, vertigo, blurred vision, confusion; severe reactions may include arrhythmias, CV collapse, acute CHF, unconsciousness, **convulsions, MI, death**
Disulfiram alone
- **CNS:** *Drowsiness, fatigability, headache,* restlessness, peripheral neuropathy, optic or retrobulbar neuritis

---

Adverse effects in *Italics* are most common; those in **Bold** are life-threatening.

- **Dermatologic:** *Skin eruptions,* acneiform eruptions, allergic dermatitis
- **GI:** *Metallic or garliclike aftertaste,* hepatotoxicity

Interactions
* Drug-drug • Increased serum levels and risk of toxicity of phenytoin and its congeners, diazepam, chlordiazepoxide • Increased therapeutic and toxic effects of theophyllines • Increased PT caused by disulfiram may lead to a need to adjust dosage of oral anticoagulants • Severe alcohol-intolerance reactions with any alcohol-containing liquid medications (eg, elixirs, tinctures) • Acute toxic psychosis with metronidazole

Nursing considerations
Assessment
- **History:** Allergy to disulfiram or other thiuram derivatives; severe myocardial disease or coronary occlusion; psychoses; current or recent treatment with metronidazole, paraldehyde, alcohol, alcohol-containing preparations (eg, cough syrups, tonics); diabetes mellitus, hypothyroidism, epilepsy, cerebral damage, chronic and acute nephritis, hepatic cirrhosis or dysfunction; pregnancy
- **Physical:** Skin color, lesions; thyroid palpation; orientation, affect, reflexes; P, auscultation, BP; R, adventitious sounds; liver evaluation; renal and liver function tests, CBC, SMA-12

Interventions
- Do not administer until patient has abstained from alcohol for at least 12 hr.
- Administer orally; tablets may be crushed and mixed with liquid beverages.
- Monitor liver function tests before, in 10–14 days, and every 6 mo during therapy to evaluate for hepatic dysfunction.
- Monitor CBC, SMA-12 before and every 6 mo during therapy.
- Inform patient about the seriousness of disulfiram-alcohol reaction and the potential consequences of alcohol use: disulfiram should not be taken for at least 12 hr after alcohol ingestion, and a reaction may occur up to 2 wk after disulfiram therapy is stopped; all forms of alcohol must be avoided.
- Arrange for treatment with antihistamines if skin reaction occurs.

Teaching points
- Take drug daily; if drug makes you dizzy or tired, take it at bedtime. Tablets may be crushed and mixed with liquid.
- Abstain from forms of alcohol (beer, wine, liquor, vinegars, cough mixtures, sauces, aftershave lotions, liniments, colognes). Taking alcohol while on this drug can cause severe, unpleasant reactions—flushing, copious vomiting, throbbing headache, difficulty breathing, even death.
- Wear or carry a medical ID while you are on this drug to alert any medical emergency personnel that you are on this drug.
- Have periodic blood tests while on drug to evaluate its effects on the liver.
- These side effects may occur: drowsiness, headache, fatigue, restlessness, blurred vision (use caution driving or performing tasks that require alertness); metallic aftertaste (transient).
- Report unusual bleeding or bruising, yellowing of skin or eyes, chest pain, difficulty breathing, ingestion of any alcohol.

▷ dobutamine hydrochloride
(doe' byoo ta meen)

Dobutrex

PREGNANCY CATEGORY B

Drug classes
Sympathomimetic
Beta₁-selective adrenergic agonist

Therapeutic actions
Positive inotropic effects are mediated by $beta_1$-adrenergic receptors in the heart; increases the force of myocardial contraction with relatively minor effects on heart rate, arrhythmogenesis; has minor effects on blood vessels.

Indications
- For inotropic support in the short-term treatment of adults with cardiac decompensation due to depressed contractility, resulting from either organic heart disease or from cardiac surgical procedures
- Investigational use in children with congenital heart disease undergoing diagnos-

tic cardiac catheterization, to augment CV function

Contraindications and cautions

- Contraindicated with IHSS; hypovolemia (dobutamine is not a substitute for blood, plasma, fluids, electrolytes, which should be restored promptly when loss has occurred and in any case before treatment with dobutamine); acute MI (may increase the size of an infarct by intensifying ischemia); general anesthesia with halogenated hydrocarbons or cyclopropane, which sensitize the myocardium to catecholamines; pregnancy.
- Use cautiously with diabetes, lactation.

Available forms

Injection—12.5 mg/mL

Dosages

Administer only by IV infusion. Titrate on the basis of the patient's hemodynamic and renal response. Close monitoring is necessary.

Adults

2.5–10 mcg/kg/min IV is usual rate to increase cardiac output; rarely, rates up to 40 mcg/kg/min are needed.

Pediatric patients

Safety and efficacy not established. When used investigationally in children undergoing cardiac catheterization (see above), doses of 2 and 7.75 mcg/kg/min were infused for 10 min.

Pharmacokinetics

Route	Onset	Peak	Duration
IV	1–2 min	10 min	Length of infusion

Metabolism: Hepatic; $T_{1/2}$: 2 min
Distribution: Crosses placenta; enters breast milk
Excretion: Urine

▽ IV facts

Preparation: Reconstitute by adding 10 mL sterile water for injection or 5% dextrose injection to 250-mg vial. If material is not completely dissolved, add 10 mL of diluent. Further dilute to at least 50 mL with 5% dextrose injection, 0.9% sodium chloride injection, or sodium lactate injection. Store reconstituted solution under refrigeration for 48 hr or at room temperature for 6 hr. Store final diluted solution in glass or Viaflex container at room temperature. Stable for 24 hr. Do not freeze. (Note: drug solutions may exhibit a color that increases with time; this indicates oxidation of the drug, not a loss of potency.)

Infusion: May be administered through common IV tubing with dopamine, lidocaine, tobramycin, nitroprusside, potassium chloride, or protamine sulfate. Titrate rate based on patient response—P, BP, rhythm; use of an infusion pump is suggested.

Incompatibilities: Do not mix drug with alkaline solutions, such as 5% sodium bicarbonate injection; do not mix with hydrocortisone sodium succinate, cefazolin, cefamandole, neutral cephalothin, penicillin, sodium ethacrynate; sodium heparin.

Y-site incompatibilities: Do not mix with acyclovir, alteplase, aminophylline, foscarnet.

Adverse effects

- **CNS:** *Headache*
- **CV:** *Increase in heart rate, increase in systolic blood pressure, increase in ventricular ectopic beats (PVCs),* anginal pain, palpitations, shortness of breath
- **GI:** *Nausea*

Interactions

✳ Drug-drug • Increased effects with TCAs (eg, imipramine), furazolidone, methyldopa • Decreased effects of guanethidine with dobutamine • Increased risk of arrhythmias with bretylium

■ Nursing considerations

Assessment

- **History:** IHSS, hypovolemia, acute MI, general anesthesia with halogenated hydrocarbons or cyclopropane, diabetes, lactation, pregnancy
- **Physical:** Weight, skin color, T; P, BP, pulse pressure, auscultation; R, adventitious sounds; urine output; serum electrolytes, Hct, ECG

Interventions

- Arrange to digitalize patients who have atrial fibrillation with a rapid ventricular rate

before giving dobutamine—dobutamine facilitates AV conduction.
- Monitor urine flow, cardiac output, pulmonary wedge pressure, ECG, and BP closely during infusion; adjust dose and rate accordingly.

Teaching points
- Used only in acute emergencies; teaching depends on patient's awareness and emphasizes need for the drug.

▽**docetaxel**

*(dobs eh **tax**' ell)*

Taxotere

PREGNANCY CATEGORY D

Drug class
Antineoplastic

Therapeutic actions
Inhibits the normal dynamic reorganization of the microtubule network that is essential for dividing cells; leads to cell death in rapidly dividing cells.

Indications
- Treatment of patients with locally advanced or metastatic breast cancer who have progressed during anthracycline therapy or relapsed during anthracycline adjuvant therapy or after other chemotherapy failure
- Treatment of non–small-cell lung cancer after failure with platinum-based chemotherapy, with metastases
- First-line treatment of unresectable, locally advanced, or metastatic non–small-cell lung cancer in patients who have not received prior chemotherapy when used in combination with cisplatin
- Unlabeled uses: gastric, head-and-neck, ovarian, pancreatic, prostate, small-cell lung, urothelial cancers; melanoma; soft-tissue sarcoma; non-Hodgkin's lymphoma

Contraindications and cautions
- Contraindicated with hypersensitivity to docetaxel or drugs using polysorbate 80; bone marrow depression with neutrophil counts < 1,500 cells/mm^2.
- Use cautiously with hepatic dysfunction, pregnancy, lactation; history of treatment with platinum-based chemotherapy.

Available forms
Injection—20, 80 mg

Dosages
Adults
- *Breast cancer:* 60–100 mg/m^2 IV infused over 1 hr every 3 wk.
- *Non–small-cell lung cancer:* 75 mg/m^2 IV over 1 hr every 3 wk.
- *First-line treatment of non–small-cell lung cancer:* 75 mg/m^2 of *Taxotere* given over 1 hr followed by 75 mg/m^2 cisplatin IV given over 30–60 min every 3 wk.

Pediatric patients
Safety and efficacy not established.

Pharmacokinetics

Route	Onset	Duration
IV	Slow	20–24 hr

Metabolism: Hepatic; T$_{1/2}$: 36 min and 11.1 hr
Distribution: Crosses placenta; enters breast milk
Excretion: Feces and urine

▽**IV facts**
Preparation: Dilute concentrate with provided diluent; resultant concentration is 10 mg/mL. Stand vials at room temperature for 5 min before diluting; stable at room temperature for 8 hr; refrigerate unopened vials, protect from light; avoid use of PVC infusion bags and tubing. Final dilution: add to 250 mL normal saline solution or 5% dextrose injection; final concentration is 0.3–0.9 mg/mL. Premedicate patient with oral corticosteroids before beginning infusion.
Infusion: Administer over 1 hr.

Adverse effects
- **CNS:** Neurosensory disturbances including paresthesias, pain, *asthenia*
- **CV:** Sinus tachycardia, hypotension, arrhythmias, **fluid retention**
- **GI:** *Nausea, vomiting, diarrhea, stomatitis,* constipation
- **Hematologic: Bone marrow depression,** *infection*

- **Other:** *Hypersensitivity reactions, myalgia, arthralgia, alopecia*

Interactions

✳ **Drug-drug** ● Possible increase in effectiveness and toxicity with cyclosporine, ketoconazole, erthyromycin, troleandomycin; avoid these combinations

■ Nursing considerations

CLINICAL ALERT!
Name confusion has occurred between Taxotere (docetaxel) and Taxol (paclitaxel). Serious adverse effects can occur; use extreme caution.

Assessment

- **History:** Hypersensitivity to docetaxel, polysorbate 80; bone marrow depression; hepatic impairment, pregnancy, lactation
- **Physical:** Neurologic status; T; P, BP, peripheral perfusion; abdominal exam, mucous membranes; liver function tests, CBC

Interventions

- Do not give drug unless blood counts are within acceptable parameters (neutrophils > 1,500 cells/m²).
- Handle drug with great care; use of gloves is recommended; if drug comes into contact with skin, wash immediately with soap and water.
- Premedicate patient before administration with oral corticosteroids (eg, dexamethasone 16 mg/day PO for 5 days starting 1 day before docetaxel administration) to reduce severity of fluid retention.
- Monitor BP and P during administration.
- Arrange for blood counts before and regularly during therapy.
- Monitor patient's neurologic status frequently during treatment; provide safety measures as needed.

Teaching points

- This drug is given once every 3 wk; mark calendar with days to return for treatment.
- These side effects may occur: nausea and vomiting (if severe, antiemetics may be helpful; eat small, frequent meals); weakness,

lethargy (take frequent rest periods); increased susceptibility to infection (avoid crowds, exposure to many people or diseases); numbness and tingling in fingers or toes (avoid injury to these areas; use care if performing tasks that require precision); loss of hair (arrange for a wig or other head covering; keep the head covered at extremes of temperature).
- Report severe nausea and vomiting; fever, chills, sore throat; unusual bleeding or bruising; numbness or tingling in fingers or toes; fluid retention or swelling.

▽ **dofetilide**
(doe fe' ti lyed)

Tikosyn

PREGNANCY CATEGORY C

Drug class

Antiarrhythmic

Therapeutic actions

Selectively blocks potassium channels, widening the QRS complex and prolonging the action potential; has no effect on calcium channels or cardiac contraction.

Indications

- Conversion of atrial fibrillation or flutter to normal sinus rhythm
- Maintenance of normal sinus rhythm in patients with atrial fibrillation or flutter of more than 1 wk's duration who have been converted to sinus rhythm

Contraindications and cautions

- Contraindicated with hypersensitivity to dofetilide, ibutilide; second- or third-degree AV heart block, prolonged QT intervals; pregnancy; lactation.
- Use cautiously with ventricular arrhythmias, renal impairment, severe liver dysfunction.

Available forms

Capsules—125, 250, 500 mcg

Dosages
Adults
Dosage is based on ECG response and creatinine clearance. Creatinine clearance > 60 mL/min: 500 mcg bid PO; creatinine clearance 40–60 mL/min: 250 mcg bid PO; creatinine clearance 20–< 40 mL/min: 125 mcg bid PO; creatinine clearance < 20 mL/min: contraindicated
Pediatric patients
Not recommended.

Pharmacokinetics

Route	Onset	Peak
Oral	Varies	2–3 hr

Metabolism: Hepatic; T$_{1/2}$: 10 hr
Distribution: Crosses placenta, may be excreted in breast milk
Excretion: Urine and feces

Adverse effects
- **CNS:** *Headache, fatigue,* light-headedness, dizziness, tingling in arms, numbness
- **CV: Ventricular arrhythmias,** hypotension, hypertension
- **GI:** Nausea

Interactions
✳ **Drug-drug** • Increased risk of serious to life-threatening arrhythmias with disopyramide, quinidine, procainamide, amiodarone, sotalol; do not give together • Increased risk of proarrhythmias if given with phenothiazines, TCAs, antihistamines

■ Nursing considerations
Assessment
- **History:** Hypersensitivity to dofetilide, ibutilide; second- or third-degree AV heart block, time of onset of atrial arrhythmia; prolonged QT intervals; pregnancy; lactation; ventricular arrhythmias
- **Physical:** Orientation, BP, P, auscultation, ECG, R, adventitious sounds, renal function tests

Interventions
- Be aware that dofetilide is only available to those who have completed a *Tikosyn* education program.

- Determine time of onset of arrhythmia and timing of conversion to sinus rhythm before beginning therapy (for maintenance).
- Monitor patient's ECG before and periodically during administration. Dosage may be adjusted based on the maintenance of sinus rhythm.
- Do not attempt electroconversion within 24 hr of starting therapy; if then successful, closely monitor patient for 3 days.
- Provide appointments for continued follow-up including ECG monitoring; tendency to revert to the atrial arrhythmia after conversion increases with length of time patient was in the abnormal rhythm.

Teaching points
- This drug should be taken twice a day. It will help to keep your heart in a normal rhythm.
- Arrange for follow-up medical evaluation, including ECG, which is important to monitor the effect of this drug on your heart.
- These side effects may occur: headache, fatigue, dizziness, light-headedness (avoid driving a car or operating dangerous equipment if these effects occur).
- Report chest pain, difficulty breathing, numbness or tingling, palpitations.

▷**dolasetron mesylate**
(doe laz' e tron)
Anzemet
PREGNANCY CATEGORY B

Drug class
Antiemetic

Therapeutic actions
Selectively binds to serotonin receptors in the CTZ, blocking the nausea and vomiting caused by the release of serotonin by mucosal cells during chemotherapy, radiotherapy, or surgical invasion (an action that stimulates the CTZ and causes nausea and vomiting).

Indications
- Prevention and treatment of nausea and vomiting associated with emetogenic chemotherapy

- Prevention of postoperative nausea and vomiting
- Treatment of postoperative nausea and vomiting (injection only)
- Unlabeled use: treatment and prevention of radiotherapy-induced nausea and vomiting

Contraindications and cautions

- Contraindicated with allergy to dolasetron or any of its components; markedly prolonged QTc interval, second- or third-degree AV block.
- Use cautiously in any patient at risk of developing prolongation of cardiac conduction intervals, especially QT interval (congenital QT syndrome, hypokalemia, hypomagnesemia), pregnancy, lactation.

Available forms

Tablets—50, 100 mg; injection—20 mg/mL

Dosages

Adults

100 mg PO within 1 hr before chemotherapy or within 2 hr before surgery; or 1.8 mg/kg IV about 30 min before chemotherapy or 100 mg IV injection; prevention of post-op nausea and vomiting—12.5 mg IV about 15 min before stopping anesthesia; treatment of post-op nausea and vomiting—12.5 mg IV as soon as needed.

Pediatric patients

< 2 yr: Not recommended.
2–16 yr: 1.8 mg/kg PO tablets or injection diluted in apple or apple-grape juice within 1 hr before chemotherapy; or 1.2 mg/kg PO tablets or injection diluted in apple or apple-grape juice within 2 hr before surgery; or 1.8 mg/kg IV for chemotherapy-induced nausea and vomiting about 30 min before chemotherapy; 1.2 mg/kg IV about 15 min before stopping anesthesia to prevent post-op nausea and vomiting; 0.35 mg/kg IV as soon as needed to treat post-op nausea and vomiting; up to a maximum of 100 mg.

Pharmacokinetics

Route	Onset	Peak
Oral	Rapid	1–2 hr
IV	Immediate	End of infusion

Metabolism: Hepatic; $T_{1/2}$: 3.5–5 hr
Distribution: Crosses placenta; passes into breast milk
Excretion: Urine, feces

▼ IV facts

Preparation: Dilute in 50 mL 5% dextrose injection, 0.9% sodium chloride injection, 5% dextrose and 0.9% sodium chloride injection, 5% dextrose and 0.45% sodium chloride injection, lactated Ringer's, 10% mannitol; 3% sodium chloride injection; do not mix in any alkaline solution, precipitates may form. Stable at room temperature for 48 hr after dilution.
Infusion: Inject 100 mg undiluted over 30 sec, or infuse diluted over up to 15 min.
Incompatibilities: Dilute only in recommended solutions.

Adverse effects

- **CNS:** *Headache, dizziness,* somnolence, drowsiness, sedation, *fatigue*
- **CV:** *Tachycardia,* EKG changes
- **GI:** *Diarrhea,* constipation, abdominal pain
- **Other:** Fever, pruritus, injection site reaction

Interactions

✷ Drug-drug • Possible cardiac arrhythmias with drugs which cause EKG interval prolongation • Potential for severe toxic reaction with high-dose anthracycline therapy • Decreased levels if combined with rifampin

■ Nursing considerations

Assessment

- **History:** Allergy to dolasetron, pregnancy, lactation, QTc prolongation
- **Physical:** Orientation, reflexes, affect; BP; P, baseline EKG

Interventions

- Dilute injection in apple or apple-grape juice if patient is unable to swallow tablets; dosage remains the same.
- Provide mouth care, sugarless lozenges to suck to help alleviate nausea.
- Obtain baseline EKG and periodically monitor EKG in any patient at risk for QTc prolongation.

Adverse effects in *Italics* are most common; those in **Bold** are life-threatening.

- Provide appropriate analgesics for headache.

Teaching points

- This drug may be given IV or orally when you are receiving your chemotherapy; it will help decrease nausea and vomiting.
- These side effects may occur: dizziness, drowsiness (use caution if driving or performing tasks that require alertness), diarrhea; headache (appropriate medication will be arranged to alleviate this problem).
- Report severe headache, fever, numbness or tingling, palpitations, fainting episodes, change in color of stools or urine.

▽ donepezil hydrochloride

*(doe **nep'** ah zill)*

Aricept

PREGNANCY CATEGORY C

Drug classes

Cholinesterase inhibitor
Alzheimer's drug

Therapeutic actions

Centrally acting reversible cholinesterase inhibitor leading to elevated acetylcholine levels in the cortex, which slows the neuronal degradation that occurs in Alzheimer's disease.

Indications

- Treatment of mild to moderate dementia of the Alzheimer's type

Contraindications and cautions

- Contraindicated with allergy to donepezil, pregnancy, lactation.
- Use cautiously with sick sinus syndrome, GI bleeding, seizures, asthma.

Available forms

Tablets—5, 10 mg

Dosages

Adults

5 mg PO daily hs. May be increased to 10 mg daily after 4–6 wk.

Pediatric patients

Safety and efficacy not established.

Pharmacokinetics

Route	Onset	Peak
Oral	Varies	2–4 hr

Metabolism: Hepatic; $T_{1/2}$: 70 hr
Distribution: Crosses placenta; may enter breast milk
Excretion: Urine

Adverse effects

- **CNS:** *Insomnia, fatigue,* dizziness, confusion, ataxia, somnolence, tremor, agitation, depression, anxiety, abnormal thinking
- **Dermatologic:** *Rash,* flushing, purpura
- **GI:** *Nausea, vomiting, diarrhea, dyspepsia, anorexia, abdominal pain,* flatulence, constipation, **hepatotoxicity**
- **Other:** *Muscle cramps*

Interactions

✳ **Drug-drug** • Increased effects and risk of toxicity with theophylline, cholinesterase inhibitors • Decreased effects of anticholinergics
- Increased risk of GI bleeding with NSAIDs
- Decreased efficacy with anticholinergics

■ Nursing considerations

CLINICAL ALERT!
Name confusion has occurred between Aricept (donepezil) and Aciphex (rabeprazole); use caution.

Assessment

- **History:** Allergy to donepezil, pregnancy, lactation, sick sinus syndrome, GI bleeding, seizures, asthma
- **Physical:** Orientation, affect, reflexes; BP, P; abdominal exam; renal and liver function tests

Interventions

- Administer hs each day.
- Provide small, frequent meals if GI upset is severe.
- Notify surgeons that patient is on donepezil; exaggerated muscle relaxation may occur if succinylcholine-type drugs are used.

Teaching points

- Take this drug exactly as prescribed, at bedtime.

- This drug does not cure the disease but is thought to slow down the degeneration associated with the disease.
- Arrange for regular blood tests and follow-up visits while adjusting to this drug.
- These side effects may occur: nausea, vomiting (eat small, frequent meals); insomnia, fatigue, confusion (use caution if driving or performing tasks that require alertness).
- Report severe nausea, vomiting, changes in stool or urine color, diarrhea, changes in neurologic functioning, yellowing of eyes or skin.

▷ dopamine hydrochloride
(doe' pa meen)

Intropin, Revimine (CAN)

PREGNANCY CATEGORY C

Drug classes
Sympathomimetic
Alpha adrenergic agonist
Beta$_1$-selective adrenergic agonist
Dopaminergic agent

Therapeutic actions
Drug acts directly and by the release of norepinephrine from sympathetic nerve terminals; dopaminergic receptors mediate dilation of vessels in the renal and splanchnic beds, which maintains renal perfusion and function; alpha receptors, which are activated by higher doses of dopamine, mediate vasoconstriction, which can override the vasodilating effects; beta$_1$ receptors mediate a positive inotropic effect on the heart.

Indications
- Correction of hemodynamic imbalances present in the shock syndrome due to MI, trauma, endotoxic septicemia, open heart surgery, renal failure, and chronic cardiac decompensation in CHF

Contraindications and cautions
- Contraindicated with pheochromocytoma, tachyarrhythmias, ventricular fibrillation,

hypovolemia (dopamine is not a substitute for blood, plasma, fluids, electrolytes, which should be restored promptly when loss has occurred), general anesthesia with halogenated hydrocarbons or cyclopropane, which sensitize the myocardium to catecholamines.
- Use cautiously with atherosclerosis, arterial embolism, Reynaud's disease, cold injury, frostbite, diabetic endarteritis, Buerger's disease (monitor color and temperature of extremities), pregnancy, lactation.

Available forms
Injection—40, 80, 160 mg/mL; injection in 5% dextrose—80, 160, 320 mg/100 mL

Dosages
Dilute before using; administer only by IV infusion, using a metering device to control the rate of flow. Titrate on the basis of patient's hemodynamic and renal response. Close monitoring is necessary. In titrating to desired systolic BP response, optimum administration rate for renal response may be exceeded, thus necessitating a reduction in rate after hemodynamic stabilization.
Adults
- *Patients likely to respond to modest increments of cardiac contractility and renal perfusion:* Initially, 2–5 mcg/kg/min IV.
- *Patients who are more seriously ill:* Initially, 5 mcg/kg/min IV. Increase in increments of 5–10 mcg/kg/min up to a rate of 20–50 mcg/kg/min. Check urine output frequently if doses > 16 mcg/kg/min.
Pediatric patients
Safety and efficacy not established.

Pharmacokinetics

Route	Onset	Peak	Duration
IV	1–2 min	10 min	Length of infusion

Metabolism: Hepatic; T$_{1/2}$: 2 min
Distribution: Crosses placenta; enters breast milk
Excretion: Urine

▼IV facts

Preparation: Prepare solution for IV infusion as follows: Add 200–400 mg dopamine to 250–500 mL of one of the following IV solutions: sodium chloride injection; 5% dextrose injection; 5% dextrose and 0.45% or 0.9% sodium chloride solution; 5% dextrose in lactated Ringer's solution; sodium lactate (1/5 Molar) injection; lactated Ringer's injection. Commonly used concentrations are 800 mcg/mL (200 mg in 250 mL) and 1,600 mcg/mL (400 mg in 250 mL). The 160 mg/mL concentrate may be preferred in patients with fluid retention. Protect drug solutions from light; drug solutions should be clear and colorless.

Infusion: Determine infusion rate based on patient response.

Incompatibilities: Do not mix with other drugs; do not add to 5% sodium bicarbonate or other alkaline IV solutions, oxidizing agents, or iron salts because drug is inactivated in alkaline solution (solutions become pink to violet).

Y-site incompatibilities: Do not give with acyclovir, alteplase.

Adverse effects

- **CV:** *Ectopic beats, tachycardia, anginal pain, palpitations, hypotension, vasoconstriction, dyspnea,* bradycardia, hypertension, widened QRS
- **GI:** *Nausea, vomiting*
- **Other:** Headache, piloerection, azotemia, gangrene with prolonged use

Interactions

✳ **Drug-drug** • Increased effects with MAOIs, TCAs (imipramine) • Increased risk of hypertension with deserpidine, furazolidone, methyldopa • Seizures, hypotension, bradycardia when infused with phenytoin • Decreased cardiostimulating effects with guanethidine

■ Nursing considerations
Assessment

- **History:** Pheochromocytoma, tachyarrhythmias, ventricular fibrillation, hypovolemia, general anesthesia with halogenated hydrocarbons or cyclopropane, occlusive vascular disease, pregnancy, labor, and delivery

- **Physical:** Body weight; skin color; T; P, BP, pulse pressure; R, adventitious sounds; urine output; serum electrolytes, Hct, ECG

Interventions

- Exercise extreme caution in calculating and preparing doses; dopamine is a very potent drug; small errors in dosage can cause serious adverse effects. Drug should always be diluted before use if not prediluted.
- Arrange to reduce initial dosage by one-tenth in patients who have been on MAO inhibitors.
- Administer into large veins of the antecubital fossa in preference to veins in hand or ankle.
- Provide phentolamine on standby in case extravasation occurs (infiltration with 10–15 mL saline containing 5–10 mg phentolamine is effective).
- Monitor urine flow, cardiac output, and BP closely during infusion.

Teaching points

- Used only in acute emergency; teaching will depend on patient's awareness and will relate mainly to patient's status, monitors, rather than to drug. Instruct patient to report any pain at injection site.

▷dornase alfa (recombinant human deoxyribonuclease, DNase)
(door' nace)

Pulmozyme

PREGNANCY CATEGORY B

Drug class

Cystic fibrosis drug

Therapeutic actions

Breaks down DNA molecules in sputum, resulting in a break up of thick, sticky mucus that clogs airways.

Indications

- Management of respiratory symptoms associated with cystic fibrosis in conjunction with standard therapies
- Treatment of advanced cystic fibrosis

Contraindications and cautions
- Contraindicated with allergy to dornase, Chinese hamster ovary products.
- Use cautiously with lactation.

Available forms
Solution for inhalation—1 mg/mL

Dosages
Adults and pediatric patients
2.5 mg daily inhaled through nebulizer for adults and children > 5 yr with cystic fibrosis; may increase to 2.5 mg bid.

Pharmacokinetics

Route	Onset	Peak	Duration
Inhalation	15 min	3–4 hr	Up to 1 wk

Metabolism: Tissue; $T_{1/2}$: unknown

Adverse effects
- **Respiratory:** Increased cough, dyspnea, hemoptysis, *pharyngitis*, rhinitis, sputum increase, wheezes, voice changes
- **Other:** Conjunctivitis, chest pain

■ Nursing considerations
Assessment
- **History:** Diagnosis of cystic fibrosis, allergy to dornase, Chinese hamster ovary cell products; lactation
- **Physical:** R, auscultation

Interventions
- Store drug in refrigerator and protect from light.
- Monitor patient closely.
- Ensure proper use of inhalation device.

Teaching points
- This drug does not cure the disease but improves the respiratory symptoms.
- Review the use of nebulizer with health care provider; store in refrigerator and protect from light.
- Report worsening of disease, difficulty breathing, increased productive cough.

▷doxapram hydrochloride
(docks' a pram)

Dopram

PREGNANCY CATEGORY B

Drug class
Analeptic

Therapeutic actions
Stimulates the peripheral carotid chemoreceptors to cause an increase in tidal volume and slight increase in respiratory rate; this stimulation also has a pressor effect.

Indications
- To stimulate respiration in patients with drug-induced postanesthesia respiratory depression or apnea; also used to "stir up" patients in combination with oxygen postoperatively
- To stimulate respiration, hasten arousal in patients experiencing drug-induced CNS depression
- As a temporary measure in hospitalized patients with acute respiratory insufficiency superimposed on COPD
- Unlabeled use: treatment of apnea of prematurity when methylxanthines have failed, obstructive sleep apnea, laryngospasm secondary to tracheal extubation

Contraindications and cautions
- Contraindicated with newborns (contains benzyl alcohol), epilepsy, incompetence of the ventilatory mechanism, flail chest, hypersensitivity to doxapram, head injury, pneumothorax, acute bronchial asthma, pulmonary fibrosis, severe hypertension, CVA.
- Use cautiously with pregnancy, lactation.

Available forms
Injection—20 mg/mL

Dosages
Adults
- *Postanesthetic use:* Single injection of 0.5–1 mg/kg IV; do not exceed 1.5 mg/kg as a total single injection or 2 mg/kg when giv-

en as mutiple injections at 5-min intervals.
Infusion: 250 mg in 250 mL of dextrose or
saline solution; initiate at 5 mg/min until
response is seen; maintain at 1–3 mg/min;
recommended total dose is 300 mg.

• *Chronic obstructive pulmonary disease associated with acute hypercapnia:* Mix 400 mg in 180 mL of IV infusion; start infusion at 1–2 mg/min (0.5–1 mL/min); check blood gases, and adjust rate accordingly. Do not use for longer than 2 hr.

• *Management of drug-induced CNS depression:*

Intermittent injection

Priming dose of 2 mg/kg IV; repeat in 5 min.
Repeat every 1–2 hr until patient awakens; if
relapse occurs, repeat at 1–2 hr intervals.

Intermittent IV infusion

Priming dose of 2 mg/kg IV; if no response, infuse 250 mg in 250 mL of dextrose or saline solution at a rate of 1–3 mg/min, discontinue at end of 2 hr if patient awakens; repeat in 30 min–2 hr if relapse occurs; do not exceed 3 g/day.

Pediatric patients

Do not give to children < 12 yr.

Pharmacokinetics

Route	Onset	Peak	Duration
IV	20–40 sec	1–2 min	5–12 min

Metabolism: Hepatic; $T_{1/2}$: 2.4–4.1 hr
Distribution: May cross placenta; may enter breast milk
Excretion: Urine

▽ IV facts

Preparation: Add 250 mg doxapram to
250 mL of 5 or 10% DW or normal saline.
Infusion: Initiate infusion at 5 mg/min; once
response is seen, 1–3 mg/min is satisfactory.
Incompatibilities: Do not mix in alkaline
solutions—precipitate or gas may form;
aminophylline, sodium bicarbonate, thiopental.

Adverse effects

• **CNS:** Headache, dizziness, apprehension, disorientation, pupillary dilation, *increased reflexes,* hyperactivity, **convulsions,** muscle spasticity, clonus, pyrexia, flushing, sweating

• **CV:** Arrhythmias, chest pain, tightness in the chest, *increased blood pressure*
• **GI:** Nausea, vomiting, diarrhea
• **GU:** Urinary retention, spontaneous voiding, proteinuria
• **Hematologic:** Decreased hemoglobin, hematocrit
• **Respiratory:** Cough, dyspnea, tachypnea, laryngospasm, **bronchospasm,** hiccups, rebound hyperventilation

Interactions

✳ **Drug-drug** • Increased pressor effect with
sympathomimetics, MAO inhibitors • Increased
effects with halothane, cyclopropane, enflurane (delay treatment for at least 10 min after discontinuance of anesthesia) • Possible
masked residual effects of muscle relaxants if
combined with doxapram

■ Nursing considerations
Assessment

• **History:** Epilepsy, incompetence of the ventilatory mechanism, flail chest, hypersensitivity to doxapram, head injury, pneumothorax, acute bronchial asthma, pulmonary fibrosis, severe hypertension, CVA, lactation, pregnancy
• **Physical:** T; skin color; weight; R, adventitious sounds; P, BP, ECG; reflexes; urinary output; arterial blood gases, CBC

Interventions

• Administer IV only.
• Monitor injection site for extravasation. Discontinue, and restart in another vein; apply cold compresses.
• Monitor patient carefully until fully awake—P, BP, ECG, reflexes and respiratory status. Patients with COPD should have arterial blood gases monitored during drug use.
• Do not use longer than 2 hr.
• Discontinue drug and notify physician if deterioration, sudden hypotension, dyspnea occur.

Teaching points

• Used in emergency; patient teaching should be general and include procedure and drug.

▽ doxazosin mesylate
(dox ay' zoe sin)

Cardura

PREGNANCY CATEGORY C

Drug classes
Alpha-adrenergic blocker
Antihypertensive

Therapeutic actions
Reduces total peripheral resistance through alpha-blockade; does not affect cardiac output or heart rate; increases HDL and the HDL to cholesterol ratio, while lowering total cholesterol and LDL, making it desirable for patients with atherosclerosis or hyperlipidemia.

Indications
• Treatment of mild-to-moderate hypertension, alone or as part of combination therapy
• Benign prostatic hyperplasia (BPH)

Contraindications and cautions
• Contraindicated with lactation.
• Use cautiously with allergy to doxazosin, CHF, renal failure, pregnancy, hepatic impairment.

Available forms
Tablets—1, 2, 4, 8 mg

Dosages
Adults
• *Hypertension:* Initially 1 mg daily PO, given once daily. Maintenance: 2, 4, 8, or 16 mg daily PO, given once a day.
• *BPH:* Initially: 1 mg PO daily; maintenance: may increase to 2 mg, 4 mg, and 8 mg daily, adjust at 1–2 wk intervals.
Pediatric patients
Safety and efficacy not established.

Pharmacokinetics

Route	Onset	Peak
Oral	Varies	2–3 hr

Metabolism: Hepatic; $T_{1/2}$: 22 hr

Distribution: Crosses placenta; enters breast milk
Excretion: Bile, feces, and urine

Adverse effects
• **CNS:** *Headache, fatigue, dizziness, postural dizziness, lethargy, vertigo,* rhinitis, asthenia, anxiety, parasthesia, increased sweating, muscle cramps, insomnia, eye pain, conjunctivitis
• **CV:** *Tachycardia, palpitations, edema, orthostatic hypotension,* chest pain
• **GI:** *Nausea, dyspepsia, diarrhea,* abdominal pain, flatulence, constipation
• **GU:** *Sexual dysfunction,* increased urinary frequency
• **Other:** Dyspnea, increased sweating, rash

Interactions
✴ **Drug-drug** • Increased hypotensive effects if taken with alcohol, nitrates, other antihypertensives

■ Nursing considerations
Assessment
• **History:** Allergy to doxazosin, CHF, renal failure, hepatic impairment, lactation
• **Physical:** Weight; skin color, lesions; orientation, affect, reflexes; ophthalmologic exam; P, BP, orthostatic BP, supine BP, perfusion, edema, auscultation; R, adventitious sounds, status of nasal mucous membranes; bowel sounds, normal output; voiding pattern, normal output; kidney function tests, urinalysis

Interventions
• Monitor edema, weight in patients with incipient cardiac decompensation, and arrange to add a thiazide diuretic to the drug regimen if sodium and fluid retention, signs of impending CHF occur.
• Monitor patient carefully with first dose; chance of orthostatic hypotension, dizziness and syncope are great with the first dose. Establish safety precautions.
• Monitor signs and symptoms of BPH to adjust dosage.

Adverse effects in *Italics* are most common; those in **Bold** are life-threatening.

Teaching points

- Take this drug exactly as prescribed, once a day. Dizziness, syncope may occur at beginning of therapy. Change position slowly to avoid increased dizziness.
- These side effects may occur: dizziness, weakness (when changing position, in the early morning, after exercise, in hot weather, and after consuming alcohol; some tolerance may occur after a while; avoid driving or engaging in tasks that require alertness; change position slowly, use caution in climbing stairs, lie down if dizziness persists); GI upset (frequent, small meals may help); impotence; stuffy nose; most of these effects gradually disappear with continued therapy.
- Report frequent dizziness or fainting.

▽ doxepin hydrochloride
(dox' e pin)

Alti-Doxepin (CAN), Apo-Doxepin (CAN), Novo-Doxepin (CAN), Sinequan, Triadapin (CAN), Zonalon (CAN)

PREGNANCY CATEGORY C

Drug classes
Tricyclic antidepressant (TCA) (tertiary amine)
Antianxiety agent

Therapeutic actions
Mechanism of action unknown; TCAs inhibit the reuptake of the neurotransmitters norepinephrine and serotonin, leading to an increase in their effects; anticholinergic at CNS and peripheral receptors; sedative.

Indications
- Relief of symptoms of depression (endogenous depression most responsive); sedative effects may help depression associated with anxiety and sleep disturbance
- Treatment of depression in patients with manic-depressive illness
- Antianxiety agent
- Unlabeled uses: neuropathy, neurogenic pain

Contraindications and cautions
- Contraindicated with hypersensitivity to any tricyclic drug; concomitant therapy with an MAO inhibitor; recent MI; myelography within previous 24 hr or scheduled within 48 hr; lactation, pregnancy.
- Use cautiously with EST; preexisting CV disorders (severe coronary heart disease, progressive heart failure, angina pectoris, paroxysmal tachycardia); angle-closure glaucoma, increased intraocular pressure, urinary retention, ureteral or urethral spasm; seizure disorders; hyperthyroidism; impaired hepatic, renal function; psychiatric patients (schizophrenic or paranoid patients may exhibit a worsening of psychosis); manic-depressive patients; elective surgery (TCAs should be discontinued as long as possible before surgery).

Available forms
Capsules—10, 25, 50, 75, 100, 150 mg; oral concentrate—10 mg/mL

Dosages
Adults
- *Mild to moderate anxiety or depression:* Initially 25 mg tid PO; individualize dosage. Usual optimum dosage is 75–150 mg/day; alternatively, total daily dosage, up to 150 mg, may be given at bedtime.
- *More severe anxiety or depression:* Initially 50 mg tid PO; if needed, may gradually increase to 300 mg/day.
- *Mild symptomatology or emotional symptoms accompanying organic disease:* 25–50 mg PO is often effective.

Pediatric patients
Not recommended for children < 12 yr.

Pharmacokinetics

Route	Onset	Peak
Oral	Varies	4 hr

Metabolism: Hepatic; $T_{1/2}$: 8–25 hr
Distribution: Crosses placenta; enters breast milk
Excretion: Urine

Adverse effects
- **CNS:** *Sedation and anticholinergic (atropine-like) effects; confusion* (especially in elderly), *disturbed concentration,*

hallucinations, disorientation, decreased memory, feelings of unreality, delusions, anxiety, nervousness, restlessness, agitation, panic, insomnia, nightmares, hypomania, mania, exacerbation of psychosis, drowsiness, weakness, fatigue, headache, numbness, tingling, paresthesias of extremities, incoordination, motor hyperactivity, akathisia, ataxia, tremors, peripheral neuropathy, extrapyramidal symptoms, seizures, speech blockage, dysarthria, tinnitus, altered EEG
- **CV:** *Orthostatic hypotension,* hypertension, syncope, tachycardia, palpitations, MI, arrhythmias, heart block, precipitation of CHF, stroke
- **Endocrine:** Elevated or depressed blood sugar; elevated prolactin levels; inappropriate ADH secretion
- **GI:** *Dry mouth, constipation,* paralytic ileus, *nausea,* vomiting, anorexia, epigastric distress, diarrhea, flatulence, dysphagia, peculiar taste, increased salivation, stomatitis, glossitis, parotid swelling, abdominal cramps, black tongue, hepatitis, jaundice (rare); elevated transaminase, altered alkaline phosphatase
- **GU:** Urinary retention, delayed micturition, dilation of the urinary tract, gynecomastia, testicular swelling; breast enlargement, menstrual irregularity and galactorrhea; changes in libido; impotence
- **Hematologic:** Bone marrow depression, including agranulocytosis; eosinophilia, purpura, thrombocytopenia, leukopenia
- **Hypersensitivity:** Rash, pruritus, vasculitis, petechiae, photosensitization, edema (generalized or of face and tongue), drug fever
- **Withdrawal:** Symptoms on abrupt discontinuation of prolonged therapy: nausea, headache, vertigo, nightmares, malaise
- **Other:** Nasal congestion, excessive appetite, weight gain or loss; sweating (paradoxical effect in a drug with prominent anticholinergic effects), alopecia, lacrimation, hyperthermia, flushing, chills

Interactions

❋ **Drug-drug** • Increased TCA levels and pharmacologic (especially anticholinergic) effects with cimetidine, fluoxetine • Increased TCA levels (due to decreased metabolism) with methylphenidate, phenothiazines, hormonal contraceptives, disulfiram • Hyperpyretic crises, severe convulsions, hypertensive episodes and deaths with MAO inhibitors • Increased antidepressant response and cardiac arrhythmias with thyroid medication • Increased or decreased effects with estrogens • Delirium with disulfiram • Sympathetic hyperactivity, sinus tachycardia, hypertension, agitation with levodopa • Increased biotransformation of TCAs in patients who smoke cigarettes • Increased sympathomimetic (especially alpha-adrenergic) effects of direct-acting sympathomimetic drugs (norepinephrine, epinephrine), due to inhibition of uptake into adrenergic nerves • Increased anticholinergic effects of anticholinergic drugs (including anticholinergic antiparkinsonian drugs) • Increased response (especially CNS depression) to barbiturates • Increased effects of dicumarol (oral anticoagulant) • Decreased antihypertensive effect of guanethidine, clonidine, other antihypertensives (because the uptake of the antihypertensive drug into adrenergic neurons is inhibited) • Decreased effects of indirect-acting sympathomimetic drugs (ephedrine) because of inhibition of uptake into adrenergic nerves

■ Nursing considerations

 CLINICAL ALERT!
Name confusion has occurred between Sinequan (doxepin) and saquinavir; use caution.

Assessment
- **History:** Hypersensitivity to any tricyclic drug; concomitant therapy with an MAO inhibitor; recent MI; myelography within previous 24 hr or scheduled within 48 hr; lactation; EST; preexisting CV disorders; angle-closure glaucoma, increased intraocular pressure, urinary retention, ureteral or urethral spasm; seizure disorders; hyperthyroidism; impaired hepatic, renal function; psychiatric patients; manic-depressive patients; elective surgery; pregnancy
- **Physical:** Weight; T; skin color, lesions; orientation, affect, reflexes, vision and hearing; P, BP, orthostatic BP, perfusion; bowel

sounds, normal output, liver evaluation; urine flow, normal output; usual sexual function, frequency of menses, breast and scrotal exam; liver function tests, urinalysis, CBC, ECG

Interventions

- Limit drug access to depressed and potentially suicidal patients.
- Give major portion of dose hs if drowsiness, severe anticholinergic effects occur.
- Dilute oral concentrate with approximately 120 mL of water, milk, or fruit juice just prior to administration; do not prepare or store bulk dilutions.
- Expect clinical antianxiety response to be rapidly evident, although antidepressant response may require 2–3 wk.
- Reduce dosage if minor side effects develop; discontinue the drug if serious side effects occur.
- Arrange for CBC if patient develops fever, sore throat, or other sign of infection during therapy.

Teaching points

- Take drug exactly as prescribed; do not stop abruptly or without consulting the health care provider.
- Avoid alcohol, sleep-inducing drugs, OTC drugs.
- Avoid prolonged exposure to sunlight or sunlamps; use a sunscreen or protective garments for exposure to sunlight.
- These side effects may occur: headache, dizziness, drowsiness, weakness, blurred vision (reversible; safety measures will be needed if severe; avoid driving or performing tasks that require alertness while these persist); nausea, vomiting, loss of appetite, dry mouth (small frequent meals, frequent mouth care, and sucking sugarless candies may help); nightmares, inability to concentrate, confusion; changes in sexual function.
- Report dry mouth, difficulty in urination, excessive sedation.

▷ doxercalciferol

See *Less Commonly Used Drugs,* p. 1342.

▷ doxorubicin hydrochloride
*(dox oh **roo'** bi sin)*

Adriamycin PFS, Adriamycin RDF, Doxil, Rubex

PREGNANCY CATEGORY D

Drug classes
Antibiotic
Antineoplastic

Therapeutic actions
Cytotoxic: binds to DNA and inhibits DNA synthesis in susceptible cells, causing cell death.

Indications

- To produce regression in the following neoplasms: acute lymphoblastic leukemia, acute myeloblastic leukemia, Wilm's tumor, neuroblastoma, soft tissue and bone sarcoma, breast carcinoma, ovarian carcinoma, transitional cell bladder carcinoma, thyroid carcinoma, Hodgkin's and non-Hodgkin's lymphomas, bronchogenic carcinoma
- Liposomal form: treatment of AIDS-related Kaposi's sarcoma

Contraindications and cautions

- Contraindicated with allergy to doxorubicin hydrochloride, malignant melanoma, kidney carcinoma, large bowel carcinoma, brain tumors, CNS metastases, myelosuppression, cardiac disease (may predispose to cardiac toxicity), pregnancy, lactation.
- Use cautiously with impaired hepatic function, previous courses of doxorubicin or daunorubicin therapy (may predispose to cardiac toxicity), prior mediastinal irradiation, concurrent cyclophosphamide therapy (predispose to cardiac toxicity).

Available forms
Powder for injection—10, 20, 50, 100 mg; injection (aqueous)—2 mg/mL; preservative-free injection—2 mg/mL; injection (lipid)—20 mg

Dosages
Adults
60–75 mg/m^2 as a single IV injection administered at 21-day intervals. Alternate schedule:

30 mg/m^2 IV on each of 3 successive days, repeated every 4 wk.

Liposomal form

20 mg/m^2 IV over 30 min once every 3 wk.

Patients with elevated bilirubin

Serum bilirubin 1.2–3 mg/100 mL: 50% of normal dose. Serum bilirubin > 3 mg/100 mL: 25% of normal dose.

Liposomal form

Serum bilirubin 1.2–3 mg/100 mL: 50% of normal dose. Serum bilirubin > 3 mg/100 mL: 25% of normal dose.

Pharmacokinetics

Route	Onset	Peak	Duration
IV	Rapid	2 hr	24–36 hr

Metabolism: Hepatic; T$_{1/2}$: 12 min, then 3.3 hr, then 29.6 hr

Distribution: Crosses placenta; enters breast milk

Excretion: Bile, feces, and urine

▽ IV facts

Preparation: Reconstitute the 10-mg vial with 5 mL, the 50-mg vial with 25 mL of 0.9% sodium chloride or sterile water for injection to give a concentration of 2 mg/mL doxorubicin. Reconstituted solution is stable for 24 hr at room temperature or 48 hr if refrigerated. Protect from sunlight. *Liposomal form:* dilute dose to maximum of 90 mg in 250 mL of 5% dextrose injection; do not use in-line filters; refrigerate and use within 24 hr.

Infusion: Administer slowly into tubing of a freely running IV infusion of sodium chloride injection or 5% dextrose injection; attach the tubing to a butterfly needle inserted into a large vein; avoid veins over joints or in extremities with poor perfusion. Rate of administration will depend on the vein and dosage; do not give in less than 3–5 min; red streaking over the vein and facial flushing are often signs of too rapid administration. Liposomal form: single dose infused over 30 min; rapid infusion increases risk of reaction.

Incompatibilities: Do not mix with heparin, cephalothin, dexamethasone sodium phosphatase (a precipitate forms and the IV solution must not be used), aminophylline, and 5–fluorouracil (doxorubicin decomposes)

denoted by a color change from red to blue-purple.

Y-site incompatibilities: Do not give with furosemide, heparin.

Adverse effects

- **CV: Cardiac toxicity,** CHF, phlebosclerosis
- **Dermatologic:** *Complete but reversible alopecia,* hyperpigmentation of nailbeds and dermal creases, facial flushing
- **GI:** *Nausea, vomiting, mucositis,* anorexia, diarrhea
- **GU:** *Red urine*
- **Hematologic:** *Myelosuppression,* hyperuricemia due to cell lysis
- **Hypersensitivity:** Fever, chills, urticaria, **anaphylaxis**
- **Local: Severe local cellulitis,** vesication and tissue necrosis if extravasation occurs
- **Other:** Carcinogenesis (documented in experimental models)

Interactions

✳ **Drug-drug** • Decreased serum levels and actions of digoxin if taken concurrently with doxorubicin

■ Nursing considerations

Assessment

- **History:** Allergy to doxorubicin hydrochloride, malignant melanoma, kidney carcinoma, large bowel carcinoma, brain tumors, CNS metastases, myelosuppression, cardiac disease, impaired hepatic function, previous courses of doxorubicin or daunorubicin therapy, prior mediastinal irradiation, concurrent cyclophosphamide therapy, lactation, pregnancy
- **Physical:** T; skin color, lesions; weight; hair; nailbeds; local injection site; auscultation, peripheral perfusion, pulses, ECG; R, adventitious sounds; liver evaluation, mucous membranes; CBC, liver function tests, uric acid levels.

Interventions

- Do not give IM or SC because severe local reaction and tissue necrosis occur.
- Monitor injection site for extravasation: reports of burning or stinging. Discontinue,

and restart in another vein. Local SC extravasation: local infiltration with corticosteroid may be ordered; flood area with normal saline; apply cold compress to area. If ulceration begins, arrange consultation with plastic surgeon.

- Monitor patient's response frequently at beginning of therapy: serum uric acid level, cardiac output (listen for S_3); CBC changes may require a decrease in the dose; consult with physician.
- Record doses received to monitor total dosage; toxic effects are often dose related, as total dose approaches 550 mg/m^2.
- Ensure adequate hydration during the course of therapy to prevent hyperuricemia.

Teaching points

- Prepare a calendar of days to return for drug therapy.
- Avoid pregnancy while on this drug; use of barrier contraceptives is advised.
- These side effects may occur: rash, skin lesions, loss of hair, changes in nails (you may want to invest in a wig before hair loss occurs; skin care may help); loss of appetite, nausea, mouth sores (frequent mouth care, small frequent meals may help; try to maintain good nutrition; a dietitian may be able to help; an antiemetic may be ordered); red urine (transient).
- Arrange for regular medical followup, including blood tests.
- Report difficulty breathing, sudden weight gain, swelling, burning or pain at injection site, unusual bleeding or bruising.

▽doxycycline
(dox i sye' kleen)

Apo-Doxy (CAN), Doryx, Doxy- Caps, Doxycin (CAN), Doxychel Hyclate, Doxytec (CAN), Novo-Doxylin (CAN), Nu-Doxycycline (CAN), Periostat, Vibra-Tabs, Vibramycin

PREGNANCY CATEGORY D

Drug classes
Antibiotic
Tetracycline antibiotic

Therapeutic actions
Bacteriostatic: inhibits protein synthesis of susceptible bacteria, causing cell death.

Indications

- Infections caused by rickettsiae; *M. pneumoniae;* agents of psittacosis, ornithosis, lymphogranuloma venereum and granuloma inguinale; *B. recurrentis; H. ducreyi; P. pestis; P. tularensis; B. bacilliformis; Bacteroides; V. comma; V. fetus; Brucella; E. coli; E. aerogenes; Shigella; A. calcoaceticus; H. influenzae; Klebsiella; D. pneumoniae; S. aureus*
- When penicillin is contraindicated, infections caused by *N. gonorrhoeae, T. pallidum, T. pertenue, L. monocytogenes, Clostridium, B. anthracis;* adjunct to amebicides in acute intestinal amebiasis
- Oral tetracyclines used for acne, uncomplicated adult urethral, endocervical, or rectal infections caused by *C. trachomatis*
- Malaria prophylaxis for malaria due to plasmodium falciparum for short-term use in travelers
- Treatment of periodontal disease as an adjunct to scaling and root planing
- Unlabeled use: prevention of "traveler's diarrhea" commonly caused by enterotoxigenic *E. coli*

Contraindications and cautions
- Allergy to tetracyclines, renal or hepatic dysfunction, pregnancy, lactation.

Available forms
Tablets—20, 50, 100 mg; capsules—20, 50, 100 mg; powder for oral suspension—25 mg; syrup—50 mg; powder for injection—100, 200 mg

Dosages
Adults
200 mg IV in one or two infusions (each over 1–4 hr) on the first treatment day, followed by 100–200 mg/day IV, depending on the severity of the infection.

- *Primary or secondary syphilis:* 300 mg/day IV for 10 days; or 100 mg q 12 hr PO on the first day, followed by 100 mg/day as one dose or 50 mg q 12 hr PO.
- *Acute gonococcal infection:* 200 mg PO, then 100 mg at bedtime, followed by 100 mg

bid for 3 days; or 300 mg PO followed by 300 mg in 1 hr.

- *Primary and secondary syphilis:* 300 mg/day PO in divided doses for at least 10 days.
- *Traveler's diarrhea:* 100 mg/day PO as prophylaxis.
- *Malaria prophylaxis:* 100 mg PO daily.
- *Anthrax prophylaxis:* 100 mg PO bid.
- *CDC recommendations for STDs:* 100 mg bid PO for 7–10 days.
- *Periodontal disease:* 20 mg PO bid, following scaling and root planing.

Pediatric patients

> 8 yr and < 100 lb: 4.4 mg/kg, IV in one or two infusions, followed by 2.2–4.4 mg/kg/day IV in one or two infusions; or 4.4 mg/kg, PO in two divided doses the first day of treatment, followed by 2.2–4.4 mg/kg/day on subsequent days.

> 8 yr and > 100 lb: Give adult dose.

- *Malaria prophylaxis:* 2 mg/kg/day PO, up to 100 mg/day.
- *Anthrax prophylaxis:* 2.2 mg/kg PO bid; switch to amoxicillin as soon as susceptibility is established.

Geriatric patients or patients with renal failure

IV doses of doxycycline are not as toxic as other tetracyclines in these patients.

Pharmacokinetics

Route	Onset	Peak
Oral	Varies	1.5–4 hr
IV	Rapid	End of infusion

Metabolism: $T_{1/2}$: 15–25 hr
Distribution: Crosses placenta; enters breast milk
Excretion: Urine and feces

▽IV facts

Preparation: Prepare solution of 10 mg/mL, reconstitute with 10 mL (100-mg vial): 20 mL (200 mg vial) of sterile water for injection; dilute further with 100–1,000 mL (100-mg vial) or 200–2,000 mL (200-mg vial) of sodium chloride injection, 5% dextrose injection, Ringer's injection, 10% invert sugar in water, lactated Ringer's injection, 5% dextrose in lactated Ringer's, *Normosol-M* in D_5W,

Normosol-R in D_5W, or *Plasma-Lyte 56 or 148 in 5% Dextrose.* If mixed in lactated Ringer's or 5% dextrose in lactated Ringer's, infusion must be completed within 6 hr after reconstitution; otherwise, may be stored up to 72 hr if refrigerated and protected from light, but infusion should then be completed within 12 hr; discard solution after that time.
Infusion: Infuse slowly over 1–4 hr.

Adverse effects

- **Dental:** *Discoloring and inadequate calcification of primary teeth of fetus if used by pregnant women, discoloring and inadequate calcification of permanent teeth if used during period of dental development*
- **Dermatologic:** *Phototoxic reactions, rash,* **exfoliative dermatitis** (more frequent and more severe with this tetracycline than with any others)
- **GI:** Fatty liver, liver failure, *anorexia, nausea, vomiting, diarrhea, glossitis,* dysphagia, enterocolitis, esophageal ulcer
- **Hematologic:** Hemolytic anemia, thrombocytopenia, neutropenia, eosinophilia, leukocytosis, leukopenia
- **Local:** Local irritation at injection site
- **Other:** Superinfections, nephrogenic diabetes insipidus syndrome

Interactions

✳ **Drug-drug** • Decreased absorption with antacids, iron, alkali • Decreased therapeutic effects with barbiturates, carbamazepine, phenytoins • Increased digoxin toxicity with doxycycline • Increased nephrotoxicity with methoxyflurane • Decreased activity of penicillins

✳ **Drug-food** • Decreased effectiveness of doxycycline if taken with food, dairy products

✳ **Drug-lab test** • Interference with culture studies for several days following therapy

■ Nursing considerations
Assessment

- **History:** Allergy to tetracyclines, renal or hepatic dysfunction, pregnancy, lactation
- **Physical:** Skin status, R and sounds, GI function and liver evaluation, urinary output and concentration, urinalysis and BUN,

liver and renal function tests; culture infected area before beginning therapy

Interventions
- Administer the oral medication without regard to food or meals; if GI upset occurs, give with meals; patients being treated for periodontal disease should receive tablet at least 1 hr before morning and evening meals.
- Protect patient from light and sun exposure.

Teaching points
- Take drug throughout the day for best results; if GI upset occurs, take drug with food. If being treated for periodontal disease, take at least 1 hr before morning and evening meals.
- Avoid pregnancy while on this drug; use of barrier contraceptives is advised.
- These side effects may occur: sensitivity to sunlight (wear protective clothing, use sunscreen), diarrhea.
- Report rash, itching; difficulty breathing; dark urine or light-colored stools; pain at injection site.

▷dronabinol (delta-9-tetrahydrocannabinol, delta-9-THC)
(droe **nab**' i nol)

Marinol

PREGNANCY CATEGORY B

C-IV CONTROLLED SUBSTANCE

Drug class
Antiemetic

Therapeutic actions
Principal psychoactive substance in marijuana; has complex CNS effects; mechanism of action as antiemetic is not understood.

Indications
- Treatment of nausea and vomiting associated with cancer chemotherapy in patients who have failed to respond adequately to conventional antiemetic treatment (should be used only under close supervision by a responsible individual because of potential to alter the mental state)
- Treatment of anorexia associated with weight loss in patients with AIDS

Contraindications and cautions
- Contraindicated with allergy to dronabinol or sesame oil vehicle in capsules, nausea and vomiting arising from any cause other than cancer chemotherapy, lactation.
- Use cautiously with hypertension; heart disease; manic, depressive, schizophrenic patients (dronabinol may unmask symptoms of these disease states), pregnancy.

Available forms
Capsules—2.5, 5, 10 mg

Dosages
Adults and pediatric patients
- *Antiemetic:* Initially, 5 mg/m^2 PO 1–3 hr prior to the administration of chemotherapy. Repeat dose q 2–4 hr after chemotherapy is given, for a total of 4–6 doses per day. If the 5 mg/m^2 dose is ineffective and there are no significant side effects, increase dose by 2.5 mg/m^2 increments to a maximum of 15 mg/m^2 per dose.
- *Appetite stimulation:* Initially give 2.5 mg PO bid before lunch and supper. May reduce dose to 2.5 mg/day as a single evening or bedtime dose; up to 10 mg PO bid (not recommended for pediatric use).

Pharmacokinetics
Route	Onset	Peak	Duration
Oral	30–60 min	2–4 hr	4–6 hr

Metabolism: Hepatic; $T_{1/2}$: 25–36 hr
Distribution: Crosses placenta; enters breast milk
Excretion: Bile, feces, and urine

Adverse effects
- *CNS: Drowsiness; elation, laughing easily, heightened awareness, often termed a "high" dizziness; anxiety; muddled thinking; perceptual difficulties; impaired coordination; irritability, depression; weird feeling, weakness, sluggishness, headache; unsteadiness, hallucinations, memory lapse;* paresthesia, visual distortions; ataxia; paranoia, depersonalization; disorientation,

confusion; tinnitus, nightmares, speech difficulty
- **CV:** Tachycardia, orthostatic hypotension; syncope
- **Dependence:** Psychological and physical dependence; tolerance to CVS and subjective effects after 30 days of use; withdrawal syndrome (irritability, insomnia, restlessness, hot flashes, sweating, rhinorrhea, loose stools, hiccups, anorexia) beginning 12 hr and ending 96 hr after discontinuation of high doses of the drug
- **Dermatologic:** Facial flushing, perspiring
- **GI:** *Dry mouth*
- **GU:** Decrease in pregnancy rate, spermatogenesis when doses higher than those used clinically were given in preclinical studies

Interactions
❋ **Drug-drug** • Do not give with alcohol, sedatives, hypnotics, other psychotomimetic substances • Increased tachycardia, hypertension, drowsiness with anticholinergics, antihistamines, TCAs

■ Nursing considerations
Assessment
- **History:** Allergy to dronabinol or sesame oil vehicle in capsules, nausea and vomiting arising from any cause other than cancer chemotherapy, hypertension, heart disease, manic, depressive, schizophrenic patients, lactation, pregnancy
- **Physical:** Skin color, texture; orientation, reflexes, bilateral grip strength, affect; P, BP, orthostatic BP; status of mucous membranes

Interventions
- Store capsules in refrigerator.
- Limit prescriptions to the minimum necessary for a single cycle of chemotherapy because of abuse potential.
- Warn patient about drug's profound effects on mental status, abuse potential before giving drug; patient needs full information regarding the use of this drug.
- Warn patient about drug's potential effects on mood and behavior to prevent panic in case these occur.

- Patient should be supervised by a responsible adult while on drug; monitor during the first cycle of chemotherapy in which dronabinol is used to determine how long patient will need supervision.
- Discontinue drug if psychotic reaction occurs; observe patient closely until evaluated and counseled; patient should participate in decision about further use of drug, perhaps at lower dosage.

Teaching points
- Take drug exactly as prescribed; a responsible adult should be with you at all times while you are taking this drug.
- Avoid alcohol, sedatives, OTC drugs, including nose drops, cold remedies, while you are taking this drug.
- These side effects may occur: mood changes (euphoria, laughing, feeling "high," anxiety, depression, weird feeling, hallucinations, memory lapse, impaired thinking); weakness, faintness (change position slowly to avoid injury); dizziness, drowsiness (do not drive or perform tasks that require alertness if you experience these effects).
- Report bizarre thoughts, uncontrollable behavior or thought processes, fainting, dizziness, irregular heartbeat.

▷ drotrecogin alfa (activated)
(drow tra cob' gin)

Xigris

PREGNANCY CATEGORY C

Drug classes
Human activated protein
Sepsis agent

Therapeutic actions
A human activated protein C that exerts an antithrombotic effect by inhibiting factors Va and VIIIa; may also have indirect profibrinolytic activity. May exert an anti-inflammatory effect by inhibiting human necrosis factor production by monocytes, blocking leukocyte adhesion to cells, and limiting thrombin induced

inflammatory responses within the microvascular endothelium. Mechanism of action in severe sepsis is not completely understood but thought to be a combination of the above effects leading to a decrease in the complex organ failure associated with sepsis.

Indications

- Reduction of mortality in adult patients with severe sepsis (sepsis with acute organ dysfunction) who have a high risk of death

Contraindications and cautions

- Contraindicated with allergy to drotrecogin, active internal bleeding, hemorrhagic stroke within the last 3 mo; intracranial or intraspinal surgery or severe head trauma within the last 2 mo; trauma with an increased risk of life-threatening bleeding; presence of an epidural catheter; intracranial neoplasm or mass lesion or evidence of cerebral herniation.
- Use cautiously with known bleeding disorders; recent use of thrombolytic (within 3 days) or anticoagulant (within 7 days) therapy; GI bleeding within the last 6 wk; recent use of aspirin (> 650 mg/day) or other platelet inhibitors (within 7 days); chronic, severe hepatic disease; pregnancy; lactation.

Available forms

Single-use vials—5, 20 mg

Dosages

Adults
- 24 mcg/kg/hr by IV infusion for a total of 96 hr; do not exceed 24 mcg/kg/hr.

Pediatric patients
- Safety and efficacy not established for patients < 18 yr.

Pharmacokinetics

Route	Onset	Peak
IV	Minutes	Length of infusion

Metabolism: Plasma; $T_{1/2}$: unknown
Distribution: Crosses placenta; may enter breast milk

▽▼ IV facts

Preparation: Protect from heat and light. Reconstitute 5-mg vial with 2.5 mL sterile water for injection; 20-mg vials with 10 mL sterile water for injection (resulting solution contains 2 mg/mL). Add the diluent slowly and avoid shaking or inverting the vial; gently swirl until the powder is completely dissolved. Dilute reconstituted solution with 0.9% sodium chloride injection; inject solution slowly against the side of the infusion bag. Avoid agitation. Gently invert bag to mix; do not transport in a mechanical delivery system. Reconstituted solution must be used within 3 hr; diluted solution must be used within 12 hr. If particulate matter is present or solution is discolored, discard solution.

Infusion: Infuse via a dedicated line at a rate of 24 mcg/kg/hr; do not administer by bolus or IV push injection.

Incompatibilities: Do not mix with any other drug solution; can be mixed in solution only with 0.9% sodium chloride injection, lactated Ringer's injection, dextrose or dextrose and saline mixtures. Always administer via a separate line.

Adverse effects

- **CNS:** Intracranial bleeding
- **GI:** GI bleeding, intra-abdominal bleeding, retroperitoneal bleeding
- **GU:** Genitourinary bleeding
- **Hematologic:** *Bleeding*
- **Other:** Skin-soft tissue bleeding, intrathoracic bleeding

Interactions

✳ **Drug-drug** • Increased risk for bleeding to severe bleeding if combined with other drugs that affect coagulation (platelet inhibitors, anticoagulants, etc); if this combination is used, monitor patient very closely for hemorrhagic effects and discontinue drug as appropriate

✳ **Drug-lab test** • False low clotting factor values using APTT assay; avoid this test, and use PT for monitoring drug effects

■ Nursing considerations
Assessment

- **History:** Allergy to drotrecogin, active internal bleeding, hemorrhagic stroke within the last 3 mo, intracranial or intraspinal surgery or severe head trauma within the last 2 mo, trauma with an increased risk of life-threatening bleeding, presence of an epidural catheter, intracranial neoplasm or mass lesion or evidence of cerebral herniation, known bleeding disorders, recent thrombolytic (3 days) or anticoagulant (7 days) therapy, GI bleeding within the last 6 wk, recent use of aspirin or other platelet inhibitors (7 days), chronic severe hepatic disease, pregnancy, lactation

• **Physical:** Body temperature, body weight, skin color, lesions, P, R, BP, GI, cardiac and respiratory evaluation, prothrombin time (PT)

Interventions

• Obtain a baseline and regular PT level to evaluate effects of drug on coagulopathy; do not rely on aPPT assays.
• Arrange for packed red blood cell availability when drug is started.
• Discontinue drug 2 hr before any invasive procedure with inherent bleeding risk; once hemostasis has been achieved, restarting of drug may be considered—12 hr after major invasive procedure or immediately if uncomplicated, minor procedure.
• Stop drotrecogin immediately if clinically significant bleeding occurs. Reevaluate use of this and other drugs that affect coagulation before resuming therapy.
• Continue monitoring and other supportive measures being used to treat the sepsis.
• Ensure that IV bag is covered with UV protectant bag.
• Do not administer longer than 96 hr.
• Monitor patient closely for any signs of bleeding and take appropriate steps to limit blood loss.

Teaching points

Many patients with severe sepsis are not cognizant; patients should be told what they are being given and what effects they may experience.

• This drug must be given IV; you will be monitored very closely.
• Bleeding may occur as a result of this drug.
• You will be closely followed with blood tests to monitor the effects of this drug on your blood.

▽ dutasteride
*(du **tas**' teh ride)*

Avodart

PREGNANCY CATEGORY X

Drug classes
Androgen hormone inhibitor
BPH drug

Therapeutic actions
Inhibits the intracellular enzyme (5 alpha-reductase) that converts testosterone into a potent androgen (DHT); does not affect androgen receptors in the body; the prostate gland is dependent on DHT for its development and maintenance

Indications
• Treatment of symptomatic benign prostatic hyperplasia (BPH) in men with an enlarged prostate gland

Contraindications and cautions
• Contraindicated with allergy to any component of the product, other 5-alpha-reductase inhibitors, women, children, pregnancy, lactation.
• Use cautiously with hepatic impairment.

Available forms
Capsule—0.5 mg

Dosages
Adults
0.5 mg/day PO. Swallow whole.
Pediatric patients
Contraindicated in pediatric patients.

Pharmacokinetics

Route	Peak	Duration
Oral	Rapid	2–3 hr

Metabolism: Hepatic; $T_{1/2}$: 5 wk
Distribution: Crosses placenta; may pass into breast milk (but not indicated for use in women)
Excretion: Feces

Adverse effects

- **GI:** Abdominal upset
- **GU:** Impotence, decreased libido, decreased volume of ejaculation
- **Other:** Breast enlargement, breast tenderness

Interactions

✳ **Drug-drug** • Possible increased serum levels with ketoconazole, ritonavir, verapamil, diltiazem, cimetidine, ciprofloxacin

✳ **Drug-lab test** • Decreased PSA levels; false decrease in PSA does not mean that patient is free of risk of prostate cancer

■ Nursing considerations
Assessment

- **History:** Allergy to any component of the product or other 5 alpha-reductase inhibitors, hepatic impairment, pregnancy, lactation
- **Physical:** Liver evaluation, abdominal exam; renal and liver function tests, normal urine output, prostate exam

Interventions

- Assess patient to ensure that problem is BPH and that other disorders—prostate cancer, infection, strictures, hypotonic bladder, etc—have been ruled out.
- Administer without regard to meals; ensure that the patient swallows capsules whole; do not cut, crush, or chew capsules.
- Arrange for regular follow-up including prostate exam, PSA levels, and evaluation of urine flow.
- Monitor urine flow and output, increase in urine flow may not occur in all patients.
- Do not allow pregnant women to handle dutasteride capsules because of risk of absorption, which could adversely affect the fetus.
- Caution patient that if his sexual partner is or may become pregnant, she should be protected from his semen, which contains dutasteride and could adversely affect the fetus. The patient should use a condom or discontinue dutasteride therapy.
- Caution patient that he will not be able to donate blood until at least 6 months after the last dose of dutasteride.
- Alert patient that libido may be decreased as well as volume of ejaculate; these effects

are usually reversible wl
stopped.
- Provide counseling to help p.
effects on sexuality.

Teaching points

- Take this drug without regard to meals. Swallow the capsule whole; do not cut, crush, or chew capsules. If you miss a dose, take the capsule as soon as you remember and take the next dose the following day. Do not take more than one capsule each day.
- Arrange to have regular medical follow-up while you are on this drug to evaluate your response.
- These side effects may occur: loss of libido, impotence, decreased amount of ejaculate (these effects are usually reversible when the drug is stopped).
- Be aware that this drug has serious adverse effects on unborn babies; do not allow a pregnant woman to handle the drug; if your sexual partner is or may become pregnant, protect her from exposure to your semen by using a condom; you may need to discontinue the drug if this is not acceptable.
- Be aware that you will not be able to donate blood until at least 6 months after your last dose of dutasteride to prevent inadvertently giving dutasteride to a pregnant woman in a blood transfusion.
- Report inability to void, groin pain, sore throat, fever, weakness.

▷ dyphylline (dihydroxypropyl theophyllin)
(dye' fi lin)

Dilor, Lufyllin

PREGNANCY CATEGORY C

Drug classes
Bronchodilator
Xanthine

Therapeutic actions
A theophylline derivative that is not metabolized to theophylline; relaxes bronchial smooth muscle, causing bronchodilation and increasing vital capacity, which has been im-

paired by bronchospasm and air trapping; at high doses it also inhibits the release of slow-reacting substance of anaphylaxis and histamine.

Indications
- Symptomatic relief or prevention of bronchial asthma and reversible bronchospasm associated with chronic bronchitis and emphysema

Contraindications and cautions
- Contraindicated with hypersensitivity to any xanthine or to ethylenediamine, peptic ulcer, active gastritis.
- Use cautiously with cardiac arrhythmias, acute myocardial injury, CHF, cor pulmonale, severe hypertension, severe hypoxemia, renal or hepatic disease, hyperthyroidism, alcoholism, labor, pregnancy, lactation.

Available forms
Tablets—200, 400 mg; elixir—100, 160 mg/15 mL; injection—250 mg/mL

Dosages
Individualize dosage based on clinical responses with monitoring of serum dyphylline levels; serum theophylline levels do not measure dyphylline; equivalence of dyphylline to theophylline is not known.

Adults
Up to 15 mg/kg, PO qid or 250–500 mg injected slowly IM (not for IV use); do not exceed 15 mg/kg per 6 hr.

Pediatric patients
Safety and efficacy not established.

Geriatric patients or impaired adults
Use cautiously in elderly men and with cor pulmonale, CHF, kidney disease.

Pharmacokinetics

Route	Peak	Duration
Oral	1 hr	6 hr
IM	30–45 min	6 hr

Metabolism: Hepatic; $T_{1/2}$: 2 hr
Distribution: Crosses placenta; enters breast milk
Excretion: Urine

Adverse effects
- **CNS:** *Headache, insomnia,* irritability; restlessness, dizziness, muscle twitching, convulsions, severe depression, stammering speech; abnormal behavior: withdrawal, mutism, and unresponsiveness alternating with hyperactivity; brain damage, **death**
- **CV:** Palpitations, sinus tachycardia, ventricular tachycardia, life-threatening ventricular arrhythmias, circulatory failure, hypotension
- **GI:** *Nausea, vomiting, diarrhea,* loss of appetite, hematemesis, epigastric pain, gastroesophageal reflux during sleep, increased AST
- **GU:** Proteinuria, increased excretion of renal tubular cells and RBCs; diuresis (dehydration), urinary retention in men with prostate enlargement
- **Respiratory:** Tachypnea, respiratory arrest
- **Other:** Fever, flushing, hyperglycemia, SIADH, rash

Interactions
✳ **Drug-drug** • Increased effects with probenecid, mexiletine • Increased cardiac toxicity with halothane • Decreased effects of benzodiazepines, nondepolarizing neuromuscular blockers • Mutually antagonistic effects of beta blockers and dyphylline

■ Nursing considerations
Assessment
- **History:** Hypersensitivity to any xanthine or to ethylenediamine, peptic ulcer, active gastritis, cardiac arrhythmias, acute myocardial injury, CHF, cor pulmonale, severe hypertension, severe hypoxemia, renal or hepatic disease, hyperthyroidism, alcoholism, labor, lactation
- **Physical:** Bowel sounds, normal output; P, auscultation, BP, perfusion, ECG; R, adventitious sounds; frequency, voiding, normal output pattern, urinalysis, renal function tests; liver palpation, liver function tests; thyroid function tests; skin color, texture, lesions; reflexes, bilateral grip strength, affect, EEG

Interventions

- Give oral dosage forms with food if GI effects occur.
- Monitor patient carefully for clinical signs of adverse effects.
- Maintain diazepam on standby to treat seizures.
- Monitor for therapeutic serum level: 12 mcg/mL.

Teaching points

- Take this drug exactly as prescribed (around the clock for adequate control of asthma attacks).
- Avoid excessive intake of coffee, tea, cocoa, cola beverages, chocolate.
- Keep all appointments for monitoring of response to this drug.
- These side effects may occur: nausea, loss of appetite (take with food); difficulty sleeping, depression, emotional lability.
- Report nausea, vomiting, severe GI pain, restlessness, convulsions, irregular heartbeat.

▷ edetate
(ed' e tate)

edetate calcium disodium (calcium EDTA)
Calcium Disodium Versenate

edetate disodium
Endrate

PREGNANCY CATEGORY C

Drug class
Antidote

Therapeutic actions
Calcium in this compound is easily displaced by heavy metals, such as lead, to form stable complexes that are excreted in the urine; edetate disodium has strong affinity to calcium, lowering calcium levels and pulling calcium out of extracirculatory stores during slow infusion.

Indications

- Acute and chronic lead poisoning and lead encephalopathy (edetate calcium disodium)
- Emergency treatment of hypercalcemia (edetate disodium)
- Control of ventricular arrhythmias associated with digitalis toxicity (edetate disodium)

Contraindications and cautions

- Contraindicated with sensitivity to EDTA preparations, anuria, increased intracranial pressure (rapid IV infusion).
- Use cautiously with cardiac disease, CHF, lactation, renal impairment, pregnancy.

Available forms
Injection—150 mg/mL (edetate disodium), 200 mg/mL (edetate calcium disodium)

Dosages
Effective by IM, SC, IV routes. IM route is safest in children and patients with lead encephalopathy.
Adults
- *Lead poisoning:* Edetate calcium disodium.
IV
- *Asymptomatic patients:* 5 mL diluted IV bid for up to 5 days. Interrupt therapy for 2 days; follow with another 5 days of treatment if indicated. Do not exceed 50 mg/kg/day. *Symptomatic adults:* Keep fluids to basal levels; administer above dilution over 2 hr. Give second daily infusion 6 hr or more after the first.
IM
Do not exceed 35 mg/kg bid, total of approximately 75 mg/kg/day.
- *Hypercalcemia, treatment of ventricular arrhythmias due to digitalis toxicity:* Edetate disodium: Administer 50 mg/kg/day IV to a maximum dose of 3 g in 24 hr. A suggested regimen includes five consecutive daily doses followed by 2 days without medication. Repeat courses as necessary to a total of 15 doses.
Pediatric patients
- *Lead poisoning:* Edetate calcium disodium.
IM
Do not exceed 35 mg/kg bid, total of approximately 75 mg/kg/day. In mild cases do not exceed 50 mg/kg/day. For younger children, give total daily dose in divided doses q 8–12 hr

for 3–5 days. Give a second course after a rest period of 4 days or more.

- *Lead encephalopathy:* Use above IM dosage. If used in combination with dimercaprol, give at separate deep IM sites.
- *Hypercalcemia, treatment of ventricular arrhythmias due to digitalis toxicity:* Edetate disodium. Administer 40 mg/kg/day IV to a maximum dose of 70 mg/kg/day, or give 15–50 mg/kg/day to a maximum of 3 g/day, allowing 5 days between courses of therapy.

Pharmacokinetics

Route	Onset	Peak
IM, IV	1 hr	24–48 hr

Metabolism: $T_{1/2}$: 20–60 min (IV), 90 min (IM)
Excretion: Urine

▼ IV facts

Preparation: Lead poisoning: Dilute the 5-mL ampule with 250–500 mL of normal saline or 5% dextrose solution. Hypercalcemia: Dissolve dose in 500 mL of 5% dextrose injection or 0.9% sodium chloride injection. Pediatric: Dissolve dose in a sufficient volume of 5% dextrose injection or 0.9% sodium chloride injection to bring the final concentration to not more than 3%.

Infusion: Lead poisoning: Administer prepared solution over at least 1 hr. Hypercalcemia: Infuse over 3 hr or more, and do not exceed the patient's cardiac reserve. Pediatric: Infuse over 3 hr or more. Do not exceed the patient's cardiac reserve.

Adverse effects

- **CNS:** Headache, transient circumoral paresthesia, numbness
- **CV:** CHF, blood pressure changes, thrombophlebitis
- **GI:** *Nausea, vomiting, diarrhea* (edetate disodium)
- **GU:** Renal tubular necrosis
- **Hematologic:** *Electrolyte imbalance* (hypocalcemia, hypokalemia, hypomagnesemia, altered blood sugar)

■ Nursing considerations
Assessment

- **History:** Sensitivity to EDTA preparations; anuria; increased intracranial pressure; cardiac disease, CHF, lactation
- **Physical:** Pupillary reflexes, orientation; P, BP; urinalysis, BUN, serum electrolytes

Interventions

- Administer edetate calcium disodium IM.
- Avoid rapid IV infusion, which can cause fatal increases in intracranial pressure or fatal hypocalcemia with edetate disodium.
- Avoid excess fluids in patients with lead encephalopathy and increased intracranial pressure; for these patients, mix edetate calcium disodium 20% solution with procaine to give a final concentration of 0.5% procaine, and administer IM.
- Monitor patient response and electrolytes carefully during slow IV infusion of edetate disodium.
- Establish urine flow by IV infusion prior to first dose to those dehydrated from vomiting. Once urine flow is established, restrict further IV fluid. Stop EDTA when urine flow ceases.
- Arrange for periodic BUN and serum electrolyte determinations before and during each course of therapy. Stop drug if signs of increasing renal damage occur.
- Do not administer in larger than recommended doses.
- Arrange for cardiac monitoring if edetate disodium is being used to treat digitalis-induced ventricular arrhythmias. Patient should be carefully monitored for signs of CHF and other adverse effects as digitalis is withdrawn.
- Keep patient supine for a short period because of the possibility of orthostatic hypotension.
- Do not administer edetate disodium as a chelating agent for treatment of atherosclerosis; such therapy is not approved and is suspect.

Teaching points

- Prepare a schedule of rest and drug days.
- Arrange for periodic blood tests during the course of therapy.

Adverse effects in *Italics* are most common; those in **Bold** are life-threatening.

- Constant monitoring of heart rhythm may be needed during drug administration.
- Report pain at injection site, difficulty voiding.

▷ edrophonium chloride
(ed roe foe' nee um)

Enlon, Reversol, Tensilon

PREGNANCY CATEGORY C

Drug classes
Cholinesterase inhibitor (anticholinesterase)
Diagnostic agent
Antidote
Muscle stimulant

Therapeutic actions
Increases the concentration of acetylcholine at the sites of cholinergic transmission; prolongs and exaggerates the effects of acetylcholine by reversibly inhibiting the enzyme acetylcholinesterase, facilitating transmission at the skeletal neuromuscular junction.

Indications
- Differential diagnosis and adjunct in evaluating treatment of myasthenia gravis
- Antidote for nondepolarizing neuromuscular junction blockers (curare, tubocurarine, gallamine) after surgery

Contraindications and cautions
- Contraindicated with hypersensitivity to anticholinesterases, intestinal or urogenital tract obstruction, peritonitis, sulfite sensitivity, lactation.
- Use cautiously with asthma, peptic ulcer, bradycardia, cardiac arrhythmias, recent coronary occlusion, vagotonia, hyperthyroidism, epilepsy, pregnancy near term.

Available forms
Injection—10 mg/mL

Dosages
Adults
- *Differential diagnosis of myasthenia gravis:*

IV
Prepare tuberculin syringe containing 10 mg edrophonium with IV needle. Inject 2 mg IV in 15–30 sec; leave needle in vein. If no reaction occurs after 45 sec, inject the remaining 8 mg. If a cholinergic reaction (parasympathomimetic effects, muscle fasciculations, or increased muscle weakness) occurs after 2 mg, discontinue the test, and administer atropine sulfate 0.4–0.5 mg IV. May repeat test after 30 min.

IM
If veins are inaccessible, inject 10 mg IM. Patients who demonstrate cholinergic reaction (see below) should be retested with 2 mg IM after 30 min to rule out false-negative results.

- *Evaluation of treatment requirements in myasthenia gravis:* 1–2 mg IV 1 hr after oral intake of the treatment drug. Responses are summarized below:

Response to Edrophonium Test	Myasthenia (Under-treated)	Cholinergic (Over-treated)
Muscle strength: ptosis, diplopia, respiration, limb strength	Increased	Decreased
Fasciculations: orbicularis oculi, facial and limb muscles	Absent	Present or absent
Side reactions: lacrimation, sweating, salivating, nausea, vomiting, diarrhea, abdominal cramps	Absent	Severe

- *Edrophonium test in crisis:* Secure controlled respiration immediately if patient is apneic, then administer test. If patient is in cholinergic crisis, administration of edrophonium will increase oropharyngeal secretions and further weaken respiratory muscles. If crisis is myasthenic, administration of edrophonium will improve respiration, and patient can be treated with longer-acting IV anticholinesterase medication. To administer the test, draw up no more than 2 mg edrophonium into the syringe. Give 1 mg IV initially. Carefully observe cardiac response. If after 1 min this dose does not further impair the patient, inject the remaining 1 mg. If after a 2-mg dose no clear improvement in respiration occurs, discontinue all anticholinesterase drug therapy, and control ventilation by tracheostomy and assisted respiration.

• *Antidote for curare:* 10 mg given slowly IV over 30–45 sec so that onset of cholinergic reaction can be detected; repeat when necessary. Maximal dose for any patient is 40 mg.

Pediatric patients

• *Differential diagnosis of myasthenia gravis*

IV

≤ *75 lb (34 kg):* 1 mg.

Children > 75 lb: 2 mg.

Infants: 0.5 mg.

If children do not respond in 45 sec, dose may be titrated up to 5 mg in children < 75 lb, up to 10 mg in children > 75 lb, given in increments of 1 mg q 30–45 sec.

IM

≤ *75 lb (34 kg):* 2 mg.

> *75 lb:* 5 mg. A delay of 2–10 min occurs until reaction.

Pharmacokinetics

Route	Onset	Duration
IM	2–10 min	5–30 min
IV	30–60 sec	5–10 min

Metabolism: $T_{1/2}$: 5–10 min

Distribution: Crosses placenta; enters breast milk

Excretion: Unknown

▼IV facts

Preparation: Drug is used directly; no preparation is required.

Infusion: Rate of infusion varies with reason for administration; see Dosages section above.

Adverse effects

Parasympathomimetic effects

• **CV:** *Bradycardia, cardiac arrhythmias,* AV block and nodal rhythm, cardiac arrest; decreased cardiac output, leading to hypotension, syncope

• **Dermatologic:** Diaphoresis, flushing

• **EENT:** *Lacrimation, miosis,* spasm of accommodation, diplopia, conjunctival hyperemia

• **GI:** *Salivation, dysphagia, nausea, vomiting, increased peristalsis, abdominal cramps,* flatulence, diarrhea

• **GU:** *Urinary frequency and incontinence,* urinary urgency

• **Respiratory:** *Increased pharyngeal and tracheobronchial secretions,* laryngospasm, bronchospasm, bronchiolar constriction, dyspnea

Skeletal muscle effects

• **CNS:** Convulsions, dysarthria, dysphonia, drowsiness, dizziness, headache, loss of consciousness

• **Peripheral:** Skeletal muscle weakness, fasciculations, muscle cramps, arthralgia

• **Respiratory:** Respiratory muscle paralysis, central respiratory paralysis

Other

• **Dermatologic:** Rash, urticaria, **anaphylaxis**

• **Local:** Thrombophlebitis after IV use

Interactions

❋ **Drug-drug** • Risk of profound muscular depression refractory to anticholinesterases if given concurrently with corticosteroids, succinylcholine

■ Nursing considerations

Assessment

Note: The administration of edrophonium for diagnostic purposes would generally be supervised by a neurologist or other physician skilled and experienced in dealing with myasthenic patients; the administration of edrophonium to reverse neuromuscular blocking agents would generally be supervised by an anesthesiologist. The following are points that any nurse participating in the care of a patient receiving anticholinesterases should keep in mind.

• **History:** Hypersensitivity to anticholinesterases; intestinal or urogenital tract obstruction, peritonitis, lactation, asthma, peptic ulcer, cardiac arrhythmias, recent coronary occlusion, vagotonia, hyperthyroidism, epilepsy, pregnancy near term

• **Physical:** Bowel sounds, normal output; frequency, voiding pattern, normal output; R, adventitious sounds; P, auscultation, blood pressure; reflexes, bilateral grip strength,

---

Adverse effects in *Italics* are most common; those in **Bold** are life-threatening.

EEG; thyroid function tests; skin color, texture, lesions

Interventions
- Administer IV slowly with constant monitoring of patient's response.
- Be aware that overdosage with anticholinesterase drugs can cause muscle weakness (cholinergic crisis) that is difficult to differentiate from myasthenic weakness; edrophonium is used to help make this diagnostic distinction. The administration of atropine may mask the parasympathetic effects of anticholinesterases and confound the diagnosis.
- Maintain atropine sulfate on standby as an antidote and antagonist to edrophonium.

Teaching points
- The patient should know what to expect during diagnostic test with edrophonium (patients receiving drug to reverse neuromuscular blockers will not be aware of drug effects and do not require specific teaching about the drug).

▽ efavirenz
(eff ah vye' renz)

Sustiva

PREGNANCY CATEGORY C

Drug class
Antiviral drug

Therapeutic actions
A non-nucleoside, reverse transcriptase inhibitor shown to be effective in suppressing the HIV virus in adults and children.

Indications
- Treatment of HIV and AIDS in adults and children when used in combination with other retroviral agents

Contraindications and cautions
- Contraindicated with life-threatening allergy to any component, pregnancy, lactation.
- Use cautiously with impaired hepatic function, hypercholesterolemia.

Available forms
Capsules—50, 100, 200 mg; tablets—600 mg

Dosages
Adults
600 mg PO daily in conjunction with a protease inhibitor or other nucleoside reverse transcriptase inhibitor.
Pediatric patients
< 3 yr: Not recommended.
≥ 3 yr: 10 kg to < 15 kg: 200 mg daily PO; 15 kg to < 20 kg: 250 mg daily PO; 20 kg to < 25 kg: 300 mg daily PO; 25 kg to < 32.5 kg: 350 mg daily PO; 32.5 kg to < 40 kg: 400 mg daily PO; ≥ 40 kg: 600 mg daily PO.

Pharmacokinetics

Route	Onset	Peak
Oral	Varies	3–5 hr

Metabolism: Hepatic metabolism; $T_{1/2}$: 52–76 hr
Distribution: Crosses placenta; may pass into breast milk
Excretion: Urine

Adverse effects
- **CNS:** *Headache,* insomnia, *drowsiness, asthenia,* malaise, *dizziness,* paresthesia, somnolence, impaired concentration, depression
- **GI:** *Nausea, diarrhea,* anorexia, vomiting, dyspepsia, liver impairment
- **Other:** Increased cholesterol, *rash*

Interactions
✳ **Drug-drug** • Possible severe adverse effects if taken with cisapride, midazolam, rifabutin, triazolam, ergot derivatives; avoid these combinations • Possible increased hepatic dysfunction if combined with alcohol or hepatotoxic drugs; avoid this combination • Decreased effectiveness of indinavir, saquinavir; dosage adjustments should be considered.
✳ **Drug-food** • Decreased absorption and therapeutic effects if taken with a high-fat meal; avoid high-fat meals
✳ **Drug-lab test** • False-positive urine cannabinoid test
✳ **Drug-alternative therapy** • Decreased effectiveness of efavirenz with St. John's wort; avoid this combination

■ Nursing considerations
Assessment
- **History:** Life-threatening allergy to any component, impaired hepatic function, pregnancy, lactation, hypercholesterolemia
- **Physical:** Skin rashes, lesions, texture; body temperature; affect, reflexes, peripheral sensation; bowel sounds, liver evaluation; hepatic function tests, CBC and differential, serum cholesterol

Interventions
- Arrange to monitor hematologic indices every 2 wk during therapy.
- Ensure that patient is taking this drug as part of a combination therapy program.
- Administer the drug at bedtime for the first 2–4 wk of therapy to minimize the CNS effects of the drug.
- Monitor patient for signs of opportunistic infections that will need to be treated appropriately.
- Administer the drug once a day, with meals if GI effects occur. Avoid high-fat meals.
- Provide comfort measures to help patient to cope with drug's effects—environmental control: temperature, lighting, etc.; back rubs; mouth care; etc.
- Recommend the use of barrier contraceptives while on this drug; serious fetal deformities have occurred.
- Establish safety precautions if CNS effects occur, especially likely during the first few days of treatment.
- Offer support and encouragement to the patient to deal with the diagnosis as well as the effects of drug therapy.

Teaching points
- Take drug once a day. Take the drug at bedtime for the first 2–4 wk to cut down some of the unpleasant effects of the drug. You may take the drug with meals if GI upset is a problem. Avoid taking this drug with high-fat meals. Be sure to take your other drugs regularly along with the efavirenz.
- Be aware that efavirenz is not a cure for AIDS or HIV; opportunistic infections may occur and regular medical care should be sought to deal with the disease.

- These side effects may occur: nausea, loss of appetite, GI upset (small, frequent meals may help; consult with your nurse or physician if this becomes severe); dizziness, drowsiness (this is more likely at the beginning of drug therapy; avoid driving and operating machinery if these occur).
- Be aware that efavirenz does not reduce the risk of transmission of HIV to others by sexual contact or blood contamination—use appropriate precautions.
- Use barrier contraceptives while you are taking this drug; serious fetal deformities can occur. If you wish to become pregnant, consult with your health care provider.
- Report extreme fatigue, lethargy, severe headache, severe nausea, vomiting, difficulty breathing, rash, depression, changes in color or of stools.

▷**enalapril maleate**
(*e* **nal'** *a pril*)
Vasotec

enalaprilat
Vasotec I.V.

PREGNANCY CATEGORY C

Drug classes
Antihypertensive
ACE inhibitor

Therapeutic actions
Renin, synthesized by the kidneys, is released into the circulation where it acts on a plasma precursor to produce angiotensin I, which is converted by angiotensin-converting enzyme to angiotensin II, a potent vasoconstrictor that also causes release of aldosterone from the adrenals; both of these actions increase BP. Enalapril blocks the conversion of angiotensin I to angiotensin II, decreasing BP, decreasing aldosterone secretion, slightly increasing serum K^+ levels, and causing Na^+ and fluid loss; increased prostaglandin synthesis also may be involved in the antihypertensive action. In patients with heart failure, peripheral resistance, afterload, preload, and heart size are decreased.

Indications
- Treatment of hypertension alone or in combination with other antihypertensives, especially thiazide-type diuretics
- Treatment of acute and chronic CHF
- Treatment of asymptomatic left ventricular dysfunction (LVD)
- Unlabeled use: diabetic nephropathy

Contraindications and cautions
- Contraindicated with allergy to enalapril.
- Use cautiously with impaired renal function; salt or volume depletion (hypotension may occur); lactation, pregnancy.

Available forms
Tablets—2.5, 5, 10, 20 mg; injection—1.25 mg/mL

Dosages
Adults
Oral
- *Hypertension:*
Patients not taking diuretics: Initial dose is 5 mg/day PO. Adjust dosage based on patient response. Usual range is 10–40 mg/day as a single dose or in two divided doses.
Patients taking diuretics: Discontinue diuretic for 2–3 days if possible. If it is not possible to discontinue diuretic, give initial dose of 2.5 mg, and monitor for excessive hypotension.
Converting to oral therapy from IV therapy: 5 mg daily with subsequent doses based on patient response.
Parenteral
Give IV only. 1.25 mg q 6 hr given IV over 5 min. A response is usually seen within 15 min, but peak effects may not occur for 4 hr.
- *Hypertension:*
Converting to IV therapy from oral therapy: 1.25 mg q 6 hr; monitor patient response.
Patients taking diuretics: 0.625 mg IV over 5 min. If adequate response is not seen after 1 hr, repeat the 0.625-mg dose. Give additional doses of 1.25 mg q 6 hr.
- *Heart failure:* 2.5 mg PO daily or bid in conjunction with diuretics and digitalis. Maintenance dose is 5–20 mg/day given in two divided doses. Maximum daily dose is 40 mg.
- *Asymptomatic LVD:* 2.5 mg PO bid; target maintenance dose 20 mg/day in two divided doses.

Pediatric patients 1 mo–16 yr
- *Hypertension:* Initial dose is 0.08 mg/kg PO once daily; maximum dose is 5 mg.
Geriatric patients and patients with renal impairment
Excretion is reduced in renal failure; use smaller initial dose, and adjust upward to a maximum of 40 mg/day PO. For patients on dialysis, use 2.5 mg on dialysis days.

Creatinine Clearance (mL/min)	Serum Creatinine	Initial Dose
> 80		5 mg/day
≤ 80 to > 30	< 3 mg/dL	5 mg/day
≤ 30	> 3 mg/dL	2.5 mg/day

IV
If creatinine clearance ≥ 30 mL/min, the initial dose is 0.625 mg, which may be repeated. Additional doses of 1.25 mg q 6 hr may be given with careful patient monitoring; if creatinine clearance < 30 mL/min, drug is not recommended.

Pharmacokinetics

Route	Onset	Peak	Duration
Oral	60 min	4–6 hr	24 hr
IV	15 min	3–4 hr	6 hr

Metabolism: $T_{1/2}$: 11 hr
Distribution: Crosses placenta; enters breast milk
Excretion: Urine

▼IV facts
Preparation: Enalaprilat can be given as supplied or mixed with up to 50 mL of 5% dextrose injection, 0.9% sodium chloride injection, 0.9% sodium chloride injection in 5% dextrose, 5% dextrose in lactated Ringer's, *Isolyte E.* Stable at room temperature for 24 hr.
Infusion: Give by slow IV infusion over at least 5 min.

Adverse effects
- **CNS:** *Headache, dizziness, fatigue,* insomnia, paresthesias
- **CV:** Syncope, chest pain, palpitations, hypotension in salt- or volume-depleted patients
- **GI:** Gastric irritation, *nausea,* vomiting, *diarrhea,* abdominal pain, dyspepsia, elevated liver enzymes

- **GU:** Proteinuria, renal insufficiency, renal failure, polyuria, oliguria, urinary frequency, impotence
- **Hematologic:** *Decreased hematocrit and hemoglobin*
- **Other:** *Cough,* muscle cramps, hyperhidrosis

Interactions

✳ **Drug-drug •** Decreased hypotensive effect if taken concurrently with indomethacin, rifampin

■ Nursing considerations
Assessment

- **History:** Allergy to enalapril, impaired renal function, salt or volume depletion, lactation, pregnancy
- **Physical:** Skin color, lesions, turgor; T; orientation, reflexes, affect, peripheral sensation; P, BP, peripheral perfusion; mucous membranes, bowel sounds, liver evaluation; urinalysis, renal and liver function tests, CBC, and differential

Interventions

- Alert surgeon, and mark patient's chart with notice that enalapril is being taken; the angiotensin II formation subsequent to compensatory renin release during surgery will be blocked; hypotension may be reversed with volume expansion.
- Monitor patients on diuretic therapy for excessive hypotension following the first few doses of enalapril.
- Monitor patient closely in any situation that may lead to a fall in BP secondary to reduced fluid volume (excessive perspiration and dehydration, vomiting, diarrhea) because excessive hypotension may occur.
- Arrange for reduced dosage in patients with impaired renal function.
- Monitor patient carefully because peak effect may not be seen for 4 hr. Do not administer second dose until checking BP.

Teaching points

- Do not stop taking the medication without consulting your nurse or physician.
- These side effects may occur: GI upset, loss of appetite, change in taste perception (will

pass with time); mouth sores (frequent mouth care may help); rash; fast heart rate; dizziness, light-headedness (usually passes in a few days; change position slowly, limit activities to those not requiring alertness and precision).
- Be careful in any situation that may lead to a drop in blood pressure (diarrhea, sweating, vomiting, dehydration).
- Avoid OTC medications, especially cough, cold, allergy medications that may interact with this drug.
- Report mouth sores; sore throat, fever, chills; swelling of the hands, feet; irregular heartbeat, chest pains; swelling of the face, eyes, lips, tongue, difficulty breathing.

▷ **enoxaparin**
*(en **ocks'** a par in)*

Lovenox

PREGNANCY CATEGORY B

Drug classes
Low-molecular-weight heparin
Antithrombotic agent

Therapeutic actions
Low-molecular-weight heparin that inhibits thrombus and clot formation by blocking factor Xa, factor IIa, preventing the formation of clots.

Indications

- Prevention of deep vein thrombosis, which may lead to pulmonary embolism following hip replacement, knee replacement surgery, abdominal surgery
- Prevention of ischemic complications of unstable angina and non–Q-wave MI
- Treatment of deep vein thrombosis (DVT), pulmonary embolus with warfarin
- Prevention of deep vein thrombosis in medical patients who are at risk for thromboembolic complications due to severely restricted mobility during acute illnesses

---

Adverse effects in *Italics* are most common; those in **Bold** are life-threatening.

Contraindications and cautions

- Contraindicated with hypersensitivity to enoxaparin, heparin, pork products; severe thrombocytopenia; uncontrolled bleeding.
- Use cautiously with pregnancy or lactation, history of GI bleed.

Available forms

Injection—30 mg/0.3 mL; 40 mg/0.4 mL; 60 mg/0.6 mL; 80 mg/0.8 mL; 100 mg/1 mL; 90 mg/0.6 mL; 120 mg/0.8 mL; 150 mg/mL

Dosages
Adults

- *DVT prophylaxis:* 30 mg SC bid initial dose soon as possible after surgery, not more than 24 hr. Continue throughout the postoperative period for 7–10 days; then 40 mg daily SC for up to 3 wk may be used.
- *Patients undergoing abdominal surgery:* 40 mg/day SC begun within 2 hr preop and continued for 7–10 days.
- *Outpatient DVT treatment:* 1 mg/kg SC q 12 hr.
- *Unstable angina and non–Q-wave MI:* 1 mg/kg SC q 12 hr for 2–8 days.
- *Prevention of DVT in high-risk medical patients:* 40 mg/day SC for 6–11 days, has been used up to 14 days.
Pediatric patients
Safety and efficacy not established.

Pharmacokinetics

Route	Onset	Peak	Duration
SC	20–60 min	3–5 hr	12 hr

Metabolism: $T_{1/2}$: 4 1/2 hr
Distribution: May cross placenta; may enter breast milk
Excretion: Urine

Adverse effects

- **Hematologic: Hemorrhage;** *bruising;* thrombocytopenia; elevated AST, ALT levels; hyperkalemia
- **Hypersensitivity:** Chills, fever, urticaria, asthma
- **Other:** Fever; pain; local irritation, hematoma, erythema at site of injection

Interactions

✴ **Drug-drug** • Increased bleeding tendencies with oral anticoagulants, salicylates, NSAIDs, penicillins, cephalosporins
✴ **Drug-lab test** • Increased AST, ALT levels
✴ **Drug-alternative therapy** • Increased risk of bleeding if combined with chamomile, garlic, ginger, ginkgo, and ginseng therapy

■ Nursing considerations
Assessment

- **History:** Recent surgery or injury; sensitivity to heparin, pork products, enoxaparin; lactation; history of GI bleed; pregnancy
- **Physical:** Peripheral perfusion, R, stool guaiac test, PTT or other tests of blood coagulation, platelet count, kidney function tests

Interventions

- Give drug as soon as possible after hip surgery, within 12 hr of knee surgery, and within 2 hr preop for abdominal surgery.
- Give deep SC injections; do not give enoxaparin by IM injection.
- Administer by deep SC injection; patient should be lying down. Alternate between the left and right anterolateral and posterolateral abdominal wall. Introduce the whole length of the needle into a skin fold held between the thumb and forefinger; hold the skin fold throughout the injection.
- Apply pressure to all injection sites after needle is withdrawn; inspect injection sites for signs of hematoma; do not massage injection sites.
- Do not mix with other injections or infusions.
- Store at room temperature; fluid should be clear, colorless to pale yellow.
- Provide for safety measures (electric razor, soft toothbrush) to prevent injury to patient who is at risk for bleeding.
- Check patient for signs of bleeding; monitor blood tests.
- Alert all health care providers that patient is on enoxaparin.
- Discontinue and initiate appropriate therapy if thromboembolic episode occurs despite enoxaparin therapy.
- Have protamine sulfate (enoxaparin antidote) on standby in case of overdose.

- Treat overdose as follows: Protamine sulfate (1% solution). Each mg of protamine neutralizes 1 mg enoxaparin. Give very slowly IV over 10 min.

Teaching points

- Have periodic blood tests needed to monitor your response to this drug.
- You and a significant other may need to learn to give the drug by subcutaneous injection and how to properly dispose of needles and syringes.
- Avoid injury while you are on this drug: Use an electric razor; avoid activities that might lead to injury.
- Report nose bleed, bleeding of the gums, unusual bruising, black or tarry stools, cloudy or dark urine, abdominal or lower back pain, severe headache.

▽ entacapone
*(en tah **kap**' own)*

Comtan

PREGNANCY CATEGORY C

Drug class
Antiparkinsonian drug

Therapeutic actions
Selectively and reversibly inhibits COMT, an enzyme that eliminates biologically active catecholamines, including dopa, dopamine, norepinephrine, epinephrine; when given with levodopa, entacapone's inhibition of COMT is believed to increase the plasma concentrations and duration of action of levodopa.

Indications
- Adjunct with levodopa and carbidopa in the treatment of the signs and symptoms of idiopathic Parkinson's disease in patients who are experiencing "wearing off" of drug effects

Contraindications and cautions
- Contraindicated with hypersensitivity to drug or its component, pregnancy, lactation.

- Use cautiously with hypertension, hypotension, hepatic or renal dysfunction.

Available forms
Tablets—200 mg

Dosages
Adults
200 mg PO taken concomitantly with the dose of levodopa–carbidopa, a maximum of 8 times/day.
Pediatric patients
Safety and efficacy not established.

Pharmacokinetics

Route	Onset	Peak
Oral	Varies	1 hr

Metabolism: Hepatic metabolism; $T_{1/2}$: 0.4–0.7 hr then 2.4 hr
Distribution: Crosses placenta; passes into breast milk
Excretion: Feces and urine

Adverse effects
- **CNS:** *Disorientation, confusion,* memory loss, **hallucinations,** psychoses, agitation, nervousness, delusions, delirium, paranoia, euphoria, excitement, *light-headedness, dizziness,* depression, drowsiness, weakness, giddiness, paresthesias, heaviness of the limbs, numbness of fingers, *dyskinesias, hyperkinesia*
- **CV:** Hypotension, orthostatic hypotension
- **Dermatologic:** Rash, urticaria, other dermatoses
- **GI:** *Nausea, vomiting,* epigastric distress, flatulence
- **Respiratory:** URIs, dyspnea, sinus congestion
- **Other:** *Fever*

Interactions
＊ **Drug-drug** • Increased toxicity and serum levels if combined with MAO inhibitors. Avoid this combination • Possible decreased excretion if combined with probenecid, cholestyramine, erythromycin, rifampin, ampicillin, chloramphenicol; if this combination is used, monitor patient closely • Risk of increased heart rate, arrhythmias, excessive BP changes

if combined with norepinephrine, dopamine, dobutamine, methyldopa, isoetherine, bitolterol, epinephrine; administer with extreme caution and monitor patient closely

■ Nursing considerations
Assessment
- **History:** Hypersensitivity to drug or its components, hypertension, hypotension, hepatic or renal dysfunction, pregnancy, lactation
- **Physical:** Body weight; body temperature; skin color, lesions; orientation, affect, reflexes, bilateral grip strength, visual exam; P, BP, orthostatic BP, auscultation; bowel sounds, normal output, liver evaluation; urinary output, voiding pattern, liver and kidney function tests

Interventions
- Administer only in conjunction with levodopa and carbidopa. Monitor patient response, customary levodopa dosage may need to be decreased.
- Provide sugarless lozenges, ice chips to suck if dry mouth is a problem.
- Give with meals if GI upset occurs; give before meals to patients bothered by dry mouth; give after meals if drooling is a problem or if drug causes nausea.
- Advise patient to use barrier contraceptives, serious birth defects can occur while using this drug; advise nursing mothers to use another means of feeding the baby as drug can enter breast milk and adversely affect the infant.
- Establish safety precautions if CNS, vision changes, hallucinations, hypotension occur (side rails, accompany patient when ambulating, etc.).
- Provide additional comfort measures appropriate to patient with parkinsonism.

Teaching points
- Take this drug exactly as prescribed. Always take in conjunction with your levodopa and carbidopa.
- Know that the following side effects may occur: drowsiness, dizziness, confusion, blurred vision (avoid driving a car or engaging in activities that require alertness and visual acuity; if these occur, rise slowly when changing positions to help decrease dizziness); nausea (frequent small meals may help);

dry mouth (sucking sugarless lozenges or ice chips may help); hallucinations (it may help to know that this is a side effect of the drug; use care and have someone stay with you if this occurs); constipation (if maintaining adequate fluid intake and exercising regularly do not help, consult your nurse or physician).
- Use barrier contraceptives while on this drug, serious birth defects can occur. Do not nurse while on this drug, the drug passes into breast milk and can adversely affect the baby.
- Report constipation, rapid or pounding heartbeat, confusion, eye pain, hallucinations, rash.

▽ ephedrine sulfate
(e fed' rin)

Nasal decongestant: Pretz-D

PREGNANCY CATEGORY C

Drug classes
Sympathomimetic drug
Vasopressor
Bronchodilator drug
Nasal decongestant

Therapeutic actions
Peripheral effects are mediated by receptors in target organs and are due in part to the release of norepinephrine from nerve terminals. Effects mediated by these receptors include vasoconstriction (increased BP, decreased nasal congestion alpha receptors), cardiac stimulation (beta$_1$), and bronchodilation (beta$_2$). Longer acting but less potent than epinephrine; also has CNS stimulant properties.

Indications
- Treatment of hypotensive states, especially those associated with spinal anesthesia; Stokes-Adams syndrome with complete heart block; CNS stimulant in narcolepsy and depressive states; acute bronchospasm (parenteral)
- Pressor agent in hypotensive states following sympathectomy, overdosage with ganglionic-blocking agents, antiadrenergic agents, or other drugs used for lowering BP (parenteral)

- Relief of acute bronchospasm (parenteral; epinephrine is the preferred drug)
- Treatment of allergic disorders, such as bronchial asthma, and local treatment of nasal congestion in acute coryza, vasomotor rhinitis, acute sinusitis, hay fever (oral)
- Symptomatic relief of nasal and nasopharyngeal mucosal congestion due to the common cold, hay fever, or other respiratory allergies (topical)
- Adjunctive therapy of middle ear infections by decreasing congestion around the eustachian ostia (topical)

Contraindications and cautions
- Contraindicated with allergy to ephedrine, angle-closure glaucoma, anesthesia with cyclopropane or halothane, thyrotoxicosis, diabetes, hypertension, CV disorders, women in labor whose BP < 130/80.
- Use cautiously with angina, arrhythmias, prostatic hypertrophy, unstable vasomotor syndrome, lactation.

Available forms
Nasal spray—0.25%; capsules—25 mg; injection—50 mg/mL

Dosages
May be given orally, IM, SC, or slow IV; nasally.
Adults
- *Hypotensive episodes, allergic disorders:* 25–50 mg IM (fast absorption), SC (slower absorption), or 10–20 mg IV (emergency administration) to a maximum 150 mg/day.
- *Labor:* Titrate parenteral doses to maintain BP at or below 130/80.
- *Acute asthma:* Administer the smallest effective dose (0.25–0.5 mL or 12.5–25 mg). If oral drug is used 12.5–25 mg q 4 hr.
- *Topical nasal decongestant:* Instill solution in each nostril q 4 hr. Do not use longer than 3–4 consecutive days.
Pediatric patients
0.5–0.75 mg/kg IM, SC, or IV q 4–6 hr. Oral route not recommended for children < 12 yr.
- *Topical nasal decongestant (> 6 yr):* Instill solution in each nostril q 4 hr. Do not use for longer than 3–4 consecutive days. Do not use in children < 6 yr unless directed by physician.

Geriatric patients
More likely to experience adverse reactions; use with caution.

Pharmacokinetics

Route	Onset	Duration
Oral	30–40 min	1 hr
IM	10–20 min	1 hr
IV	Instant	1 hr
Nasal	Rapid	4–6 hr

Metabolism: Hepatic; $T_{1/2}$: 3–6 hr
Distribution: Crosses placenta; enters breast milk
Excretion: Urine

▼ IV facts
Preparation: Administer as provided; no preparation required.
Infusion: Administer directly into vein or tubing of running IV; administer slowly, each 10 mg over at least 1 min.

Adverse effects
Systemic effects are less likely with topical administration, but can take place, and should be considered.
- **CNS:** *Fear, anxiety, tenseness, restlessness, headache, light-headedness, dizziness,* drowsiness, tremor, insomnia, hallucinations, psychological disturbances, convulsions, CNS depression, weakness, blurred vision, ocular irritation, tearing, photophobia, symptoms of paranoid schizophrenia
- **CV:** Arrhythmias, hypertension resulting in intracranial hemorrhage, CV collapse with hypotension, palpitations, tachycardia, precordial pain in patients with ischemic heart disease
- **GI:** *Nausea,* vomiting, anorexia
- **GU:** Constriction of renal blood vessels and *decreased urine formation* (initial parenteral administration), *dysuria, vesical sphincter spasm* resulting in difficult and painful urination, urinary retention in males with prostatism
- **Local:** *Rebound congestion* with topical nasal application
- **Other:** *Pallor,* respiratory difficulty, orofacial dystonia, sweating

---

Adverse effects in *Italics* are most common; those in **Bold** are life-threatening.

Interactions

* Drug-drug * Severe hypertension with MAO-inhibitors, TCAs, furazolidone • Additive effects and increased risk of toxicity with urinary alkalinizers • Decreased vasopressor response with reserpine, methyldopa, urinary acidifiers • Decreased hypotensive action of guanethidine with ephedrine

* Drug-alternative therapy * Coadministration with ephedra, ma huang, guarana, and caffeine leads to additive effects and may lead to overstimulation, increased blood pressure, stroke, and death

■ Nursing considerations
Assessment
- **History:** Allergy to ephedrine; angle-closure glaucoma; anesthesia with cyclopropane or halothane; thyrotoxicosis, diabetes, hypertension, CV disorders; prostatic hypertrophy, unstable vasomotor syndrome; lactation
- **Physical:** Skin color, temperature; orientation, reflexes, peripheral sensation, vision; P, BP, auscultation, peripheral perfusion; R, adventitious sounds; urinary output pattern, bladder percussion, prostate palpation

Interventions
- Protect solution from light; give only if clear; discard any unused portion.
- Monitor urine output with parenteral administration; initially renal blood vessels may be constricted and urine formation decreased.
- Do not use nasal decongestant for longer than 3–5 days.
- Avoid prolonged use of systemic ephedrine (a syndrome resembling an anxiety effect may occur); temporary cessation of the drug usually reverses this syndrome.
- Monitor CV effects carefully; patients with hypertension may experience changes in BP because of the additional vasoconstriction. If a nasal decongestant is needed, give pseudoephedrine.

Teaching points
- Do not exceed recommended dose. Demonstrate proper topical nasal application. Avoid prolonged use because underlying medical problems can be disguised. Use nasal decongestant no longer than 3–5 days.

- Avoid OTC medications. Many of them contain the same or similar drugs and serious overdosage can occur.
- These side effects may occur: dizziness, weakness, restlessness, light-headedness, tremor (avoid driving or operating dangerous equipment); urinary retention (empty the bladder before taking drug).
- Report nervousness, palpitations, sleeplessness, sweating.

▷ epinephrine (adrenaline)
(ep i nef' rin)

epinephrine bitartrate
Aerosols: Bronkaid Mist, Primatene Mist

epinephrine borate
Ophthalmic solution: Epinal

epinephrine hydrochloride
Injection, OTC nasal solution: Adrenalin Chloride

Ophthalmic solution: Epifrin, Glaucon

Insect-sting emergencies: EpiPen Auto-Injector (delivers 0.3 mg IM adult dose), EpiPen Jr. Auto-Injector (delivers 0.15 mg IM for children)

OTC solutions for nebulization: AsthmaNefrin, microNefrin, Nephron, S-2

PREGNANCY CATEGORY C

Drug classes
Sympathomimetic drug
Alpha-adrenergic agonist
Beta$_1$ and beta$_2$-adrenergic agonist
Cardiac stimulant
Vasopressor
Bronchodilator
Antiasthmatic drug
Nasal decongestant
Mydriatic
Antiglaucoma drug

Therapeutic actions

Naturally occurring neurotransmitter, the effects of which are mediated by alpha or beta receptors in target organs. Effects on alpha receptors include vasoconstriction, contraction of dilator muscles of iris. Effects on beta receptors include positive chronotropic and inotropic effects on the heart (beta$_1$ receptors); bronchodilation, vasodilation, and uterine relaxation (beta$_2$ receptors); decreased production of aqueous humor.

Indications

- *Intravenous:* In ventricular standstill after other measures have failed to restore circulation, given by trained personnel by intracardiac puncture and intramyocardial injection; treatment and prophylaxis of cardiac arrest and attacks of transitory AV heart block with syncopal seizures (Stokes-Adams syndrome); syncope due to carotid sinus syndrome; acute hypersensitivity (anaphylactoid) reactions, serum sickness, urticaria, angioneurotic edema; in acute asthmatic attacks to relieve bronchospasm not controlled by inhalation or SC injection; relaxation of uterine musculature; additive to local anesthetic solutions for injection to prolong their duration of action and limit systemic absorption
- *Injection:* Relief from respiratory distress of bronchial asthma, chronic bronchitis, emphysema, other COPDs
- *Aerosols and solutions for nebulization:* Temporary relief from acute attacks of bronchial asthma, COPD
- *Topical nasal solution:* Temporary relief from nasal and nasopharyngeal mucosal congestion due to a cold, sinusitis, hay fever, or other upper respiratory allergies; adjunctive therapy in middle ear infections by decreasing congestion around eustachian ostia
- *0.25%–2% ophthalmic solutions:* Management of open-angle (chronic simple) glaucoma, often in combination with miotics or other drugs
- *0.1% ophthalmic solution:* Conjunctivitis, during eye surgery to control bleeding, to produce mydriasis

Contraindications and cautions

- Contraindicated with allergy or hypersensitivity to epinephrine or components of preparation (many of the inhalant and ophthalmic products contain sulfites: sodium bisulfite, sodium or potassium metabisulfite; check label before using any of these products in a sulfite-sensitive patient); narrow-angle glaucoma; shock other than anaphylactic shock; hypovolemia; general anesthesia with halogenated hydrocarbons or cyclopropane; organic brain damage, cerebral arteriosclerosis; cardiac dilation and coronary insufficiency; tachyarrhythmias; ischemic heart disease; hypertension; renal dysfunction (drug may initially decrease renal blood flow); COPD patients who have developed degenerative heart disease; diabetes mellitus; hyperthyroidism; lactation.
- Use cautiously with prostatic hypertrophy (may cause bladder sphincter spasm, difficult and painful urination), history of seizure disorders, psychoneurotic individuals, labor and delivery (may delay second stage of labor; can accelerate fetal heart beat; may cause fetal and maternal hypoglycemia), children (syncope has occurred when epinephrine has been given to asthmatic children).
- Route-specific contraindications for ophthalmic preparations: wearing contact lenses (drug may discolor the contact lens), aphakic patients (maculopathy with decreased visual acuity may occur).

Available forms

Solution for inhalation—1:100, 1:1,000, 1.125%, 1%; aerosol—0.35 mg, 0.5%, 0.22 mg; injection—1, 5 mg/mL; solution for injection—1:1,000, 1:2,000, 1:10,000, 1:100,000; suspension for injection—1:200; ophthalmic solution—0.1%, 0.5%, 1%, 2%

Dosages
Adults
Epinephrine injection

- *Cardiac arrest:* 0.5–1 mg (5–10 mL of 1:10,000 solution) IV or by intracardiac injection into left ventricular chamber; during resuscitation, 0.5 mg q 5 min.

Intraspinal

0.2–0.4 mL of a 1:1,000 solution added to anesthetic spinal fluid mixture.

- *Other use with local anesthetic:* Concentrations of 1:100,000–1:20,000 are usually used.

1:1,000 solution

- *Respiratory distress:* 0.3–0.5 mL of 1:1,000 solution (0.3–0.5 mg), SC or IM, q 20 min for 4 hr.

1:200 suspension (for SC administration only)

- *Respiratory distress:* 0.1–0.3 mL (0.5–1.5 mg) SC.

Inhalation (aerosol)

Begin treatment at first symptoms of bronchospasm. Individualize dosage. Wait 1–5 min between inhalations to avoid overdose.

Inhalation (nebulization)

Place 8–15 drops into the nebulizer reservoir. Place nebulizer nozzle into partially opened mouth. Patient inhales deeply while bulb is squeezed one to three times. If no relief in 5 min, give 2–3 additional inhalations. Use 4–6 times per day usually maintains comfort.

Topical nasal solution

Apply locally as drops or spray or with a sterile swab, as required.

Ophthalmic solution for glaucoma

Instill 1–2 drops into affected eye(s) daily–bid. May be given as infrequently as every 3 days; determine frequency by tonometry. When used in conjunction with miotics, instill miotic first.

Ophthalmic solution for vasoconstriction, mydriasis

Instill 1–2 drops into the eye(s); repeat once if necessary.

Pediatric patients

Epinephrine injection

1:1,000 solution, children and infants except premature infants and full-term newborns: 0.01 mg/kg or 0.3 mL/m^2 (0.01 mg/kg or 0.3 mg/m^2) SC q 20 min (or more often if needed) for 4 hr. Do not exceed 0.5 mL (0.5 mg) in a single dose. *1:200 suspension, infants and children (1 mo–1 yr):* 0.005 mL/kg (0.025 mg/kg) SC. *Children ≤ 30 kg:* Maximum single dose is 0.15 mL (0.75 mg). Administer subsequent doses only when necessary and not more often than q 6 hr.

Topical nasal solution (children > 6 yr)

Apply locally as drops or spray or with a sterile swab, as required.

Ophthalmic solutions

Safety and efficacy for use in children not established.

Geriatric patients or patients with renal failure

Use with caution; patients > 60 yr are more likely to develop adverse effects.

Pharmacokinetics

Route	Onset	Peak	Duration
SC	5–10 min	20 min	20–30 min
IM	5–10 min	20 min	20–30 min
IV	instant	20 min	20–30 min
Inhalation	3–5 min	20 min	1–3 hr
Eye	< 1 hr	4–8 hr	24 hr

Metabolism: Neural

Distribution: Crosses placenta; passes into breast milk

▼ IV facts

Preparation: 0.5 mL dose may be diluted to 10 mL with sodium chloride injection for direct injection; prepare infusion by mixing 1 mg in 250 mL D$_5$W (4 mcg/mL).

Infusion: Administer by direct IV injection or into the tubing of a running IV, each 1 mg over 1 min, or run infusion at 1–4 mcg/min (15–60 mL/hr).

Adverse effects

Systemic administration

- **CNS:** *Fear, anxiety, tenseness, restlessness, headache, light-headedness, dizziness,* drowsiness, tremor, insomnia, hallucinations, psychological disturbances, convulsions, CNS depression, weakness, blurred vision, ocular irritation, tearing, photophobia, symptoms of paranoid schizophrenia
- **CV:** Arrhythmias, hypertension resulting in intracranial hemorrhage, cardiovascular collapse with hypotension, palpitations, tachycardia, precordial pain in patients with ischemic heart disease
- **GI:** *Nausea,* vomiting, anorexia
- **GU:** Constriction of renal blood vessels and *decreased urine formation* (initial parenteral administration), *dysuria, vesical sphincter spasm* resulting in difficult and

painful urination, urinary retention in males with prostatism
- **Other:** *Pallor,* respiratory difficulty, orofacial dystonia, sweating

Local injection
- **Local:** Necrosis at sites of repeat injections (due to intense vasoconstriction)

Nasal solution
- **Local:** Rebound congestion, local burning and stinging

Ophthalmic solutions
- **CNS:** *Headache, browache, blurred vision,* photophobia, difficulty with night vision, pigmentary (adrenochrome) deposits in the cornea, conjunctiva, or lids with prolonged use
- **Local:** *Transitory stinging on initial instillation,* eye pain or ache, conjunctival hyperemia

Interactions

✳ Drug-drug • Increased sympathomimetic effects with other TCAs (eg, imipramine) • Excessive hypertension with propranolol, beta-blockers, furazolidone • Decreased cardiostimulating and bronchodilating effects with beta-adrenergic blockers (eg, propranolol) • Decreased vasopressor effects with chlorpromazine, phenothiazines • Decreased antihypertensive effect of guanethidine, methyldopa

■ Nursing considerations
Assessment

- **History:** Allergy or hypersensitivity to epinephrine or components of drug preparation; narrow-angle glaucoma; shock other than anaphylactic shock; hypovolemia; general anesthesia with halogenated hydrocarbons or cyclopropane; organic brain damage, cerebral arteriosclerosis; cardiac dilation and coronary insufficiency; tachyarrhythmias; ischemic heart disease; hypertension; renal dysfunction; COPD; diabetes mellitus; hyperthyroidism; prostatic hypertrophy; history of seizure disorders; psychoneuroses; labor and delivery; lactation; contact lens use, aphakic patients (ophthalmic prep)
- **Physical:** Weight; skin color, temperature, turgor; orientation, reflexes, intraocular pressure; P, BP; R, adventitious sounds; prostate palpation, normal urine output; urinalysis, kidney function tests, blood and urine glucose, serum electrolytes, thyroid function tests, ECG

Interventions

- Use extreme caution when calculating and preparing doses; epinephrine is a very potent drug; small errors in dosage can cause serious adverse effects. Double-check pediatric dosage.
- Use minimal doses for minimal periods of time; "epinephrine-fastness" (a form of drug tolerance) can occur with prolonged use.
- Protect drug solutions from light, extreme heat, and freezing; do not use pink or brown solutions. Drug solutions should be clear and colorless (does not apply to suspension for injection).
- Shake the suspension for injection well before withdrawing the dose.
- Rotate SC injection sites to prevent necrosis; monitor injection sites frequently.
- Maintain a rapidly acting alpha-adrenergic blocker (phentolamine) or a vasodilator (a nitrate) on standby in case of excessive hypertensive reaction.
- Maintain an alpha-adrenergic blocker or facilities for intermittent positive pressure breathing on standby in case pulmonary edema occurs.
- Maintain a beta-adrenergic blocker (propranolol; a cardioselective beta-blocker, such as atenolol, should be used in patients with respiratory distress) on standby in case cardiac arrhythmias occur.
- Do not exceed recommended dosage of inhalation products; administer pressurized inhalation drug forms during second half of inspiration, because the airways are open wider and the aerosol distribution is more extensive. If a second inhalation is needed, administer at peak effect of previous dose, 3–5 min.
- Use topical nasal solutions only for acute states; do not use for longer than 3–5 days, and do not exceed recommended dosage. Rebound nasal congestion can occur after vasoconstriction subsides.

Teaching points

- Do not exceed recommended dosage; adverse effects or loss of effectiveness may result. Read the instructions that come with respiratory inhalant products, and consult your health care provider or pharmacist if you have any questions.
- To give eye drops: Lie down or tilt head backward, and look up. Hold dropper above eye; drop medicine inside lower lid while looking up. Do not touch dropper to eye, fingers, or any surface. Release lower lid; keep eye open, and do not blink for at least 30 sec. Apply gentle pressure with fingers to inside corner of the eye for about 1 min; wait at least 5 min before using other eye drops.
- These side effects may occur: dizziness, drowsiness, fatigue, apprehension (use caution if driving or performing tasks that require alertness); anxiety, emotional changes; nausea, vomiting, change in taste (small, frequent meals may help); fast heart rate. *Nasal solution:* burning or stinging when first used (transient). *Ophthalmic solution:* slight stinging when first used (transient); headache or browache (only during the first few days).
- Report chest pain, dizziness, insomnia, weakness, tremor or irregular heart beat (respiratory inhalant, nasal solution); difficulty breathing, productive cough, failure to respond to usual dosage (respiratory inhalant), decrease in visual acuity (ophthalmic).

▽ epirubicin hydrochloride

(ep ee roo' bi sin)

Ellence

PREGNANCY CATEGORY D

Drug classes

Antibiotic
Antineoplastic agent

Therapeutic actions

Cytotoxic anthracycline: binds to DNA and inhibits DNA and protein synthesis in susceptible cells causing cell death; interferes with replication and transcription by inhibiting DNA helicase and generates cytotoxic free radicals. Closely related to doxorubicin and daunorubicin.

Indications

- Adjunctive therapy in patients with evidence of axillary node tumor involvement after resection of primary breast cancer

Contraindications and cautions

- Contraindicated with allergy to anthracyclines, myelosuppression, cardiac disease (may predispose to cardiac toxicity), recent MI, severe hepatic dysfunction, pregnancy, lactation.
- Use cautiously with impaired hepatic function, previous maximum dose courses of doxorubicin or daunorubicin therapy (may predispose to cardiac toxicity).

Available forms

Solution for injection—2 mg/mL

Dosages

Adults

- *Starting dose:* 100–120 mg/m^2 IV given in repeated 3- to 4-wk cycles, all on day 1 or divided on days 1 and 8.
- *Adjunctive therapy:* 5-FU 500 mg/m^2, cyclophosphamide 500 mg/m^2, and epirubicin 100 mg/m^2; all given IV on day 1 and repeated q 21 days for 6 cycles. Alternatively, cyclophosphamide 75 mg/m^2 PO day 1–14, epirubicin 60 mg/m^2 IV days 1, 8 and 5-FU 500 mg/m^2 IV days 1, 8 repeated q 28 days for 6 cycles.

Pediatric patients

Safety and efficacy not established.

Geriatric patients

Not recommended.

Pharmacokinetics

Route	Onset	Peak
IV	Rapid	2 hr

Metabolism: Hepatic; $T_{1/2}$: 12 min, then 3.3 hr, then 29.6 hr

Distribution: Crosses placenta; passes into breast milk

Excretion: Bile, feces, and urine

▽ IV facts

Preparation: Reconstitute the 50 mg vial with 0.9% sodium chloride or sterile water for injection. Reconstituted solution is stable for 24 hr at room temperature or 48 hr if refrigerated. Protect from sunlight. Handle and dispose of vials properly.

Infusion: Administer slowly into tubing of a freely running IV infusion of sodium chloride injection or 5% dextrose injection; attach the tubing to a butterfly needle inserted into a large vein; avoid veins over joints or in extremities with poor perfusion. Rate of administration will depend on the vein and dosage; do not give in less than 3–5 minutes—red streaking over the vein and facial flushing are often signs of too rapid administration.

Incompatibilities: Do not mix with heparin, cephalothin, dexamethasone sodium phosphatase (a precipitate forms and the IV solution must not be used), aminophylline, and 5-fluorouracil.

Adverse effects

- **CV: Cardiac toxicity,** CHF, phlebosclerosis, delayed cardiomyopathy
- **Dermatologic:** *Complete but reversible alopecia;* hyperpigmentation of nailbeds and dermal creases, facial flushing
- **GI:** *Nausea, vomiting, mucositis,* anorexia, diarrhea
- **Hematologic:** *Myelosuppression,* hyperuricemia due to cell lysis
- **Hypersensitivity:** Fever, chills, urticaria, anaphylaxis
- **Local: Severe local cellulitis,** vesiccation and tissue necrosis if extravasation occurs
- **Other:** Carcinogenesis including leukemia

Interactions

✴ **Drug-drug** • Increased toxicity if given with cardiotoxic, hepatotoxic, or cytotoxic drugs; avoid this combination • Risk of severe toxicity if given with cimetidine. Discontinue cimetidine before administering

■ Nursing considerations
Assessment

- **History:** Allergy to anthracyclines, myelosuppression, cardiac disease, recent MI, severe hepatic dysfunction, pregnancy, lactation, impaired hepatic function, previous maximum dose courses of doxorubicin or daunorubicin therapy
- **Physical:** Temperature; skin color, lesions; weight; hair; nailbeds; local injection site; auscultation, peripheral perfusion, pulses, ECG; R, adventitious sounds; liver evaluation, mucous membranes; CBC, liver function tests, uric acid levels

Interventions

- Do baseline monitoring for cardiac status, bone marrow function, renal and hepatic function.
- Do not administer if neutrophil count is < 1,500 cells/mm3.
- Monitor injection site for extravasation, reports of burning or stinging. Discontinue infusion immediately and restart in another vein. Local SC extravasation: local infiltration with corticosteroid may be ordered; flood area with normal saline, apply cold compress to area. If ulceration begins, arrange consult with plastic surgeon.
- Monitor patient's response to therapy, frequently at beginning of therapy: serum uric acid level, cardiac output (listen for S_3), CBC changes may require a decrease in the dose; consult with physician.
- Alert patient that drug may induce inflammatory recall at irradiation sites.
- Premedicate patient with antiemetics, allopurinol, trimethoprim-sulfamethoxazole, or a fluoroquinolone before beginning therapy.
- Ensure adequate hydration during the course of therapy to prevent hyperuricemia; alkalinize urine.
- Monitor nutritional status and weight loss; consult with dietitian to ensure nutritional meals.
- Provide skin care as needed for cutaneous effects.
- Arrange for wig or other acceptable head covering before total alopecia occurs; stress importance of keeping head covered in extremes of temperatures.

Teaching points

- Prepare a calendar for outpatients who will need to return for drug therapy.

Adverse effects in *Italics* are most common; those in **Bold** are life-threatening.

- Use of barrier contraceptives is advised; this drug can have serious effects on the fetus. Nursing mothers should find an alternative method of feeding the baby.
- Know that the following side effects may occur: rash, skin lesions, loss of hair, changes in nails (you may want to invest in a wig before hair loss occurs, skin care may help somewhat); loss of appetite, nausea, mouth sores (frequent mouth care, small frequent meals may help, you will need to try to maintain good nutrition if at all possible, a dietitian may be able to help, an antiemetic may also be ordered).
- Arrange for regular medical follow-up which will include blood tests to monitor the drug's effects.
- Report difficulty breathing, sudden weight gain, swelling, burning or pain at injection site, unusual bleeding or bruising.

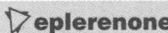

eplerenone
(ep ler' eh nown)

Inspra

PREGNANCY CATEGORY B

Drug classes
Antihypertensive
Aldosterone receptor blocker

Therapeutic actions
Binds to aldosterone receptors, blocking the binding of aldosterone, leading to increased loss of sodium and water and lowering of blood pressure

Indications
- Treatment of hypertension, alone or in combination with other antihypertensive drugs

Contraindications and cautions
- Contraindicated with allergy to eplerenone, hyperkalemia (> 5.5 mEq/L), type 2 diabetes with microalbuminuria, severe renal impairment (creatinine clearance < 50 mL/min) or serum creatinine > 2 mg/dL in males or > 1.8 mg/dL in females, lactation.
- Use cautiously with hepatic impairment, pregnancy, concurrent treatment with potas-

sium supplements, CYP450 inhibitors (eg, ketoconazole).

Available forms
Tablets—25, 50, 100 mg

Dosages
Adults
Initially 50 mg/day PO as a single daily dose; if necessary, may be increased to 50 mg PO bid after a minimum of a 4-wk trial period. Maximum, 100 mg/day.
Pediatric patients
Safety and efficacy not established.

Pharmacokinetics

Route	Onset	Peak
Oral	Slow	1.5 hr

Metabolism: Hepatic; $T_{1/2}$: 4-6 hr
Distribution: May cross placenta; may pass into breast milk
Excretion: Urine and feces

Adverse effects
CNS: Headache, dizziness, fatigue
CV: Angina, MI
GI: Diarrhea, abdominal pain
GU: Abnormal vaginal bleeding, albuminuria, changes in sexual function
Metabolic: Hypercholesterolemia, **hyperkalemia**
Respiratory: Cough
Other: Gynecomastia and breast pain in men, flulike symptoms

Interactions
✳ **Drug–drug** • Risk of serious toxic effects if combined with strong inhibitors of the CYP450 system (ketoconazole, itraconazole, erythromycin, verapamil, saquinavir, fluconazole); if any of these drugs are being used, initiate treatment with 25 mg eplerenone and monitor patient closely • Increased risk of hyperkalemia if combined with ACE inhibitors and ARBs, monitor patient closely • Possible risk of lithium toxicity if combined with lithium; monitor serum lithium levels closely if this combination is necessary • Possible risk of decreased antihypertensive effect if combined with NSAIDs; monitor BP carefully

■ Nursing considerations
Assessment
- **History:** Allergy to eplerenone, hyperkalemia, type 2 diabetes, severe renal impairment, lactation, hepatic impairment, pregnancy, concurrent treatment with potassium supplements, CYP450 inhibitors
- **Physical:** Orientation, reflexes; BP; R; urinary output; liver and renal function tests, serum potassium levels, serum cholesterol

Interventions
- Arrange for pretreatment and periodic evaluation of serum potassium and renal function.
- Establish baseline patient weight to monitor drug effect.
- Administer once a day, in the morning, so increased urination will not interrupt sleep.
- Avoid giving patient any foods rich in potassium (see Appendix N for a complete list).
- Establish appropriate safety precautions if patient experiences adverse CNS effects.
- Suggest another method of feeding the baby if the drug is needed in a lactating woman.

Teaching points
- Take this drug early in the morning so any increase in urination will not affect sleep.
- Weigh yourself on a regular basis, at the same time of day and in the same clothes, and record this weight on your calendar.
- These side effects may occur: dizziness (use caution and avoid driving a car or performing other tasks that require alertness if you experience dizziness); enlargement or pain of the breasts (it may help to know that this is a drug effect and will pass when drug therapy is ended).
- This drug may interact with many other medications. Alert any health care provider caring for you that you taking this drug.
- Be aware that this drug should not be taken during pregnancy or when nursing a baby; use of barrier contraceptives is suggested.
- You will need periodic blood tests to evaluate the effect of this drug on your serum potassium level and cholesterol level.
- Avoid foods that are high in potassium (fruits, Sanka coffee).

- Report weight change of more than 3 pounds in one day, severe dizziness, trembling, numbness, muscle weakness or cramps, palpitations.

▽ **epoetin alfa (EPO, erythropoietin)**
(e poe e' tin)

Epogen, Eprex (CAN), Procrit

PREGNANCY CATEGORY C

Drug class
Recombinant human erythropoietin

Therapeutic actions
A natural glycoprotein produced in the kidneys, which stimulates red blood cell production in the bone marrow.

Indications
- Treatment of anemia associated with chronic renal failure, including patients on dialysis
- Treatment of anemia of renal failure requiring dialysis ages 1 mo–16 yr; not recommended for < 1 mo
- Treatment of anemia related to therapy with AZT in HIV-infected patients
- Treatment of anemia related to chemotherapy in cancer patients
- Reduction of allogenic blood transfusions in surgical patients
- Unlabeled use: pruritus associated with renal failure

Contraindications and cautions
- Uncontrolled hypertension; hypersensitivity to mammalian cell-derived products or to albumin human; lactation.

Available forms
Injection—2,000, 3,000, 4,000, 10,000, 20,000 units/mL

Dosages
Adults
- *Anemia of chronic renal failure:* Starting dose: 50–100 units/kg three times weekly, IV for dialysis patients and IV or SC for non-

---

Adverse effects in *Italics* are most common; those in **Bold** are life-threatening.

dialysis patients. Reduce dose if Hct increases > 4 points in any 2-wk period. Increase dose if Hct does not increase by 5–6 points after 8 wk of therapy. Maintenance dose: individualize based on Hct, generally 25 units/kg three times weekly. Target Hct range 30%–36%.

- *HIV-infected patients on AZT therapy:* Patients receiving AZT dose ≤ 4,200 mg/wk with serum erythropoietin levels ≤ 500 mU/mL: 100 units/kg IV or SC 3 times/wk for 8 wk; when desired response is achieved, titrate dose to maintain Hct with lowest possible dose.
- *Cancer patients on chemotherapy (*Procrit *only):* 150 units/kg SC 3 times/wk; after 8 wk, can be increased to 300 units/kg.
- *Surgery:* 300 units/kg/day SC for 10 days before surgery, on day of surgery, and 4 days after surgery. Ensure Hgb is > 10– < 13 g/dL.

Pediatric patients 1 mo–16 yr
- *Chronic renal failure on dialysis:* 50 mcg/ kg IV or SC 3 times/wk.

Pharmacokinetics

Route	Onset	Peak	Duration
SC	7–14 days	5–24 hr	24 hr

Metabolism: Serum; $T_{1/2}$: 4–13 hr
Distribution: Crosses placenta; enters breast milk
Excretion: Urine

▽ IV facts

Preparation: As provided; no additional preparation. Enter vial only once; do not shake vial. Discard any unused solution. Refrigerate.
Infusion: Administer by direct IV injection or into tubing of running IV.
Incompatibilities: Do not mix with any other drug solution.

Adverse effects
- **CNS:** *Headache, arthralgias, fatigue, asthenia, dizziness,* seizure, CVA/TIA
- **CV:** *Hypertension, edema, chest pain*
- **GI:** *Nausea, vomiting, diarrhea*
- **Other:** Clotting of access line

■ Nursing considerations
Assessment
- **History:** Uncontrolled hypertension, hypersensitivity to mammalian cell-derived products or to albumin human, lactation

- **Physical:** Reflexes, affect; BP, P; urinary output, renal function; renal function tests; CBC, Hct, iron levels, electrolytes

Interventions
- Confirm chronic, renal nature of anemia; not intended as a treatment of severe anemia or substitute for emergency transfusion.
- Gently mix; do not shake, shaking may denature the glycoprotein. Use only one dose per vial; do not reenter the vial. Discard unused portions.
- Do not give with any other drug solution.
- Administer dose 3 times/wk. If administered independent of dialysis, administer into venous access line. If patient is not on dialysis, administer IV or SC.
- Monitor access lines for signs of clotting.
- Arrange for Hct reading before administration of each dose to determine dosage. If patient fails to respond within 8 wk of therapy, evaluate patient for other etiologies of the problem.
- Evaluate iron stores prior to and periodically during therapy. Supplemental iron may need to be ordered.
- Maintain seizure precautions on standby.

Teaching points
- Drug will need to be given 3 times/wk and can only be given IV or SC or into a dialysis access line. Prepare a schedule of administration dates.
- Keep appointments for blood tests necessary to determine the effects of the drug on your blood count and to determine dosage.
- These side effects may occur: dizziness, headache, seizures (avoid driving or performing hazardous tasks); fatigue, joint pain (may be medicated); nausea, vomiting, diarrhea (proper nutrition is important).
- Report difficulty breathing, numbness or tingling, chest pain, seizures, severe headache.
- Maintain all of the usual activities and restrictions that apply to your chronic renal failure. If this becomes difficult, consult with your health care provider.

▽ epoprostenol sodium

See *Less Commonly Used Drugs,* p. 1342.

▽ eprosartan mesylate
*(ep row **sar'** tan)*

Teveten

PREGNANCY CATEGORY C (FIRST TRIMESTER)

PREGNANCY CATEGORY D (SECOND AND THIRD TRIMESTERS)

Drug classes
Angiotensin II receptor antagonist (ARB)
Antihypertensive

Therapeutic actions
Selectively blocks the binding of angiotensin II to specific tissue receptors found in the vascular smooth muscle and adrenal gland; this action blocks the vasoconstriction effect of the renin–angiotensin system as well as the release of aldosterone leading to decreased blood pressure.

Indications
- Treatment of hypertension, alone or in combination with other antihypertensive agents, particularly diuretics and calcium channel blockers
- Unlabeled use: CHF

Contraindications and cautions
- Contraindicated with hypersensitivity to any ARB, pregnancy (use during the second or third trimester can cause injury or even death to the fetus), lactation.
- Use cautiously with renal dysfunction, hypovolemia.

Available forms
Tablets—400, 600 mg

Dosages
Adults
Usual starting dose is 600 mg PO daily. Can be administered in divided doses bid with a total daily dose of 400–800 mg/day being effective. If used as part of combination therapy, eprosartan should be added to established dose of other antihypertensive, starting at the lowest dose

and increasing dosage based on patient response.
Pediatric patients
Safety and efficacy not established.

Pharmacokinetics

Route	Onset	Peak
Oral	Rapid	1–2 hr

Metabolism: Hepatic; $T_{1/2}$: 5–9 hr
Distribution: Crosses placenta; passes into breast milk
Excretion: Feces and urine

Adverse effects
- **CNS:** Headache, dizziness, syncope, muscle weakness, *fatigue, depression*
- **CV:** Hypotension
- **Dermatologic:** Rash, inflammation, urticaria, pruritus, alopecia, dry skin
- **GI:** Diarrhea, *abdominal pain,* nausea, constipation
- **Respiratory:** *URI symptoms,* cough, sinus disorders
- **Other:** Cancer in preclinical studies, UTIs

■ Nursing considerations
Assessment
- **History:** Hypersensitivity to any ARB, pregnancy, lactation, renal dysfunction, hypovolemia
- **Physical:** Skin lesions, turgor; body temperature; reflexes; affect; BP; R, respiratory auscultation; kidney function tests

Interventions
- Administer without regard to meals.
- Ensure that patient is not pregnant before beginning therapy, suggest the use of barrier birth control while using eprosartan; fetal injury and deaths have been reported.
- Find an alternate method of feeding the infant if given to a nursing mother. Depression of the renin–angiotensin system in infants is potentially very dangerous.
- Alert surgeon and mark patient's chart with notice that eprosartan is being taken. The blockage of the renin–angiotensin system following surgery can produce problems. Hypotension may be reversed with volume expansion.

- If blood pressure control does reach desired levels, diuretics or other antihypertensives may be added to the drug regimen. Monitor patient's blood pressure carefully.
- Monitor patient closely in any situation that may lead to a decrease in blood pressure secondary to reduction in fluid volume—excessive perspiration, dehydration, vomiting, diarrhea—excessive hypotension can occur.

Teaching points

- Take drug without regard to meals. Do not stop taking this drug without consulting your health care provider.
- Use a barrier method of birth control while on this drug; if you become pregnant or desire to become pregnant, consult with your health care provider.
- Know that the following side effects may occur: dizziness (avoid driving a car or performing hazardous tasks); nausea, abdominal pain (proper nutrition is important, consult with your dietitian to maintain nutrition); symptoms of upper respiratory tract or urinary tract infection, cough (do not self-medicate, consult with your nurse or physician if this becomes uncomfortable).
- Report fever, chills, dizziness, pregnancy.

▷ eptifibatide
(ep tiff ib' ah tide)

Integrilin

PREGNANCY CATEGORY B

Drug class
Antiplatelet drug

Therapeutic actions
Inhibits platelet aggregation by binding to the platelet receptor glycoprotein, which prevents the binding of fibrinogen and other adhesive ligands to the platelet.

Indications
- Treatment of acute coronary syndrome
- Prevention of cardiac ischemic complications in patients undergoing elective, emergency, or urgent percutaneous coronary intervention

Contraindications and cautions
- Contraindicated with allergy to eptifibatide, bleeding diathesis, hemorrhagic stroke, active, abnormal bleeding or stroke within 30 days, uncontrolled or severe hypertension, major surgery within 6 wk, dialysis, low platelet count.
- Use cautiously with pregnancy, lactation, renal insufficiency, the elderly.

Available forms
Injection—0.75, 2 mg/mL

Dosages
Adults
- *Acute coronary syndrome:* 180 mcg/kg IV (maximum of 22.6 mg) over 1–2 min as soon as possible after diagnosis, then 2 mcg/kg/min (maximum 15 mg/hr) by continuous IV infusion for up to 72 hr. If patient is to undergo percutaneous coronary intervention, reduce infusion to 0.5 mcg/kg/min and continue for 20–24 hr after the procedure, up to 96 hr of therapy.
- *Percutaneous coronary intervention:* 180 mcg/kg IV as a bolus immediately before the procedure, then 2 mcg/kg/min by continuous IV infusion for 20–24 hr.

Pediatric patients
Not recommended.

Pharmacokinetics

Route	Onset	Peak	Duration
IV	15 min	45 min	2–4 hr

Metabolism: Tissue; $T_{1/2}$: 50–60 min
Distribution: Crosses placenta; may pass into breast milk
Excretion: Urine

▽ IV facts
Preparation: Withdraw bolus from 10 mL vial. No preparation needed for continuous infusion. Spike the 100 mL vial with a vented infusion set. Protect from light.
Infusion: Infuse bolus quickly; infuse as continuous infusion using guidelines under Dosages section.
Compatibilities: May be given with alteplase, atropine, dobutamine, heparin, lidocaine, meperidine, metoprolol, morphine, nitroglycerin, verapamil.

Incompatibilities: Do not mix with furosemide.

Adverse effects

- **CNS:** *Headache, dizziness,* weakness, syncope, flushing
- **Dermatologic:** *Rash,* pruritus
- **GI:** Nausea, GI distress, constipation, diarrhea
- **Other:** *Bleeding, hypotension*

Interactions

✻ **Drug-drug** • Use caution when combining with other drugs that affect blood clotting—thrombolytics, anticoagulants, ticlopidine, dipyridamole, clopidogrel, NSAIDs: increased risk of bleeding or hemorrhage

■ Nursing considerations
Assessment

- **History:** Allergy to eptifibatide; bleeding diathesis; hemorrhagic stroke; active, abnormal bleeding or stroke within 30 days; uncontrolled or severe hypertension; major surgery within 6 wk; dialysis; low platelet count; pregnancy, lactation
- **Physical:** Skin color, temperature, lesions; orientation, reflexes, affect; P, BP, orthostatic BP, baseline ECG, peripheral perfusion; respiratory rate, adventitious sounds, aPTT, PT, active clotting time

Interventions

- Use eptifibatide in conjunction with heparin and aspirin.
- Minimize arterial and venous punctures, IM injections, catheterizations, intubations while using this drug to minimize blood loss.
- Avoid the use of non-compressible IV access sites to prevent excessive, uncontrollable bleeding.
- Do baseline and periodic CBC, PT, aPTT, and active clotting time. Maintain aPTT between 50–70 sec; and active bleeding time between 300–350 sec.
- Properly care for femoral access site to minimize bleeding. Document aPTT of < 45 sec and stop heparin for 3–4 hr before pulling sheath.
- Provide comfort measures and arrange for analgesics if headache occurs.

Teaching points

- This drug is given to minimize blood clotting and cardiac damage. It must be given IV.
- Know that you will be monitored closely and periodic blood tests will be done to monitor the effects of this drug on your body.
- Know that the following side effects may occur: dizziness, light-headedness, bleeding.
- Report light-headedness, palpitations, pain at IV site, bleeding.

▽ ergonovine maleate
(er goe noe' veen)

Ergotrate Maleate

PREGNANCY CATEGORY UNKNOWN

Drug class
Oxytocic

Therapeutic actions
Increases the strength, duration, and frequency of uterine contractions, and decreases postpartum uterine bleeding by direct effects at neuroreceptor sites.

Indications

- Prevention and treatment of postpartum and postabortal hemorrhage due to uterine atony
- Unlabeled use: diagnostic test for Printzmetal's angina; doses of 0.05–0.2 mg IV during coronary arteriography provoke coronary artery spasm (reversible with nitroglycerin; arrhythmias, ventricular tachycardia, MI have occurred)

Contraindications and cautions

- Contraindicated with allergy to ergonovine, induction of labor, threatened spontaneous abortion.
- Use cautiously with hypertension, heart disease, venoatrial shunts, mitral-valve stenosis, obliterative vascular disease, sepsis, hepatic or renal impairment, lactation.

Available forms
Injection—0.2 mg/mL

Adverse effects in *Italics* are most common; those in **Bold** are life-threatening.

Dosages

Adults

0.2 mg IM (IV in emergency situations). Severe bleeding may require repeat doses q 2–4 hr for no more than 5 doses.

Diagnostic

0.1–0.4 mg IV.

Pharmacokinetics

Route	Onset	Duration
IM	2–5 min	3 hr
IV	Immediate	45 min

Metabolism: Hepatic; $T_{1/2}$: 0.5–2 hr
Distribution: Crosses placenta; enters breast milk
Excretion: Feces, urine

▽ IV facts

Preparation: No preparation required.
Infusion: Administer by direct IV or into tubing of running IV; reserve IV use for emergency situation or diagnostic test, 0.2 mg over 1 min.

Adverse effects

- **CNS:** *Dizziness, headache,* ringing in the ears
- **CV:** Elevation of BP—more common with ergonovine than other oxytocics
- **GI:** *Nausea, vomiting,* diarrhea
- **Hypersensitivity:** Allergic response, including shock
- **Other:** Ergotism—nausea, BP changes, weak pulse, dyspnea, chest pain, numbness and coldness of the extremities, confusion, excitement, delirium, hallucinations, convulsions, coma

■ Nursing considerations

Assessment

- **History:** Allergy to ergonovine, induction of labor, threatened spontaneous abortion, hypertension, heart disease, venoatrial shunts, obliterative vascular disease, sepsis, hepatic or renal impairment, lactation
- **Physical:** Uterine tone; orientation, reflexes, affect; P, BP, edema; R, adventitious sounds; CBC, renal and liver function tests

Interventions

- Administer by IM injection unless emergency requires IV use; complications are more frequent with IV use.
- Monitor postpartum women for BP changes and amount and character of vaginal bleeding.
- Arrange for discontinuation of drug if signs of ergotism occur.
- Avoid prolonged use of the drug.

Teaching points

- Usually part of an immediate medical situation. Teaching about the complication of delivery or abortion should include drug. The patient needs to know the name of the drug and what she can expect once it is administered.
- These side effects may occur: nausea, vomiting, dizziness, headache, ringing in the ears.
- Report difficulty breathing, headache, numb or cold extremities, severe abdominal cramping.

▷ ergotamine tartrate

(er got' a meen)

Sublingual preparation:
Ergomar

PREGNANCY CATEGORY X

Drug classes

Ergot derivative
Antimigraine drug

Therapeutic actions

Mechanism of action not understood; constricts cranial blood vessels; decreases pulsation in cranial arteries, and decreases hyperperfusion of basilar artery vascular bed.

Indications

- Prevention or abortion of vascular headaches, such as migraine, migraine variant, cluster headache

Contraindications and cautions

- Allergy to ergot preparations; peripheral vascular disease, severe hypertension, CAD, impaired liver or renal function, sepsis, pruritus, malnutrition; pregnancy; lactation (can cause ergotism—vomiting, diarrhea, seizures—in infant).

Available forms
Sublingual tablets—2 mg

Dosages
Adults
1 tablet under the tongue soon after the first symptoms of an attack; take subsequent doses at 30-min intervals if necessary. Do not exceed 3 tablets/day; do not exceed 10 mg/wk.
Pediatric patients
Safety and efficacy not established.

Pharmacokinetics

Route	Onset	Peak
Sublingual	Rapid	0.5–3 hr

Metabolism: Hepatic; $T_{1/2}$: 2.7 hr, then 21 hr
Distribution: Crosses placenta; enters breast milk
Excretion: Feces

Adverse effects
- **CNS:** *Numbness, tingling of fingers and toes, muscle pain in the extremities*
- **CV:** *Pulselessness, weakness in the legs; precordial distress and pain, transient tachycardia, bradycardia, localized edema and itching;* increased arterial pressure, arterial insufficiency, coronary vasoconstriction, bradycardia
- **GI:** *Nausea, vomiting* (drug stimulates CTZ)
- **Other:** Ergotism—nausea, vomiting, diarrhea, severe thirst, hypoperfusion, chest pain, BP changes, confusion (with prolonged use); drug dependency and abuse (extended use); may require increasing doses for relief of headaches and for prevention of dysphoric effects of drug withdrawal

Interactions
✳ **Drug-drug** • Peripheral ischemia manifested by cold extremities; possible peripheral gangrene if taken concurrently with beta blockers

■ Nursing considerations
Assessment
- **History:** Allergy to ergot preparations, peripheral vascular disease, severe hypertension, coronary artery disease, impaired liver or renal function, sepsis, pruritus, malnutrition, pregnancy, lactation
- **Physical:** Skin color, edema, lesions; T; peripheral sensation; P, BP, peripheral pulses, peripheral perfusion; liver evaluation, bowel sounds; CBC, liver and renal function tests

Interventions
- Avoid prolonged administration or excessive dosage.
- Arrange for use of atropine or phenothiazine antiemetics if nausea and vomiting are severe.
- Check extremities carefully for gangrene or decubitus ulcer formation.
- Provide supportive measures if acute overdose occurs.

Teaching points
- Take the drug soon after the first symptoms of an attack. Do not exceed the recommended dosage; if relief is not obtained, contact your physician.
- These side effects may occur: vomiting (if severe, may be medicated); numbness, tingling, loss of sensation in the extremities (avoid injury and examine extremities daily for injury).
- Do not take this drug during pregnancy. If you become or desire to become pregnant, consult with your health care provider.
- Report irregular heartbeat, pain or weakness of extremities, severe nausea or vomiting, numbness or tingling of fingers or toes.

▷ **ertapenem**
*(er tah **pen' em**)*

Invanz

PREGNANCY CATEGORY B

Drug classes
Antibiotic
Methyl-carbapenem

Therapeutic actions
Bactericidal. Inhibits synthesis of susceptible bacterial cell wall causing cell death.

Adverse effects in *Italics* are most common; those in **Bold** are life-threatening.

Indications

- Community-acquired pneumonia caused by *Streptococcus pneumoniae* (penicillin-resistant strains only), *Haemophilus influenzae* (beta-lactamase–negative strains only), *Moraxella catarrhalis*
- Skin and skin structure infections caused by *Staphylococcus aureus* (methicillin-resistant strains only), *Streptococcus pyogenes*, *Escherichia coli*, *Peptostreptococcus* species
- Complicated GU infections, including pyelonephritis caused by *E. coli* or *Klebsiella pneumoniae*
- Complicated intra-abdominal infections due to *E. coli*, *Clostridium clostridioforme*, *Eubacterium lentum*, *Peptostreptococcus* species, *Bacteroides fragilis*, *Bacteroides distasonis*, *Bacteroides ovatus*, *Bacteroides thetaiotaomicron*, *Bacteroides uniformis*
- Acute pelvic infections, including postpartum endomyometritis, septic abortion, postsurgical gynecologic infections due to *Streptococcus agalactiae*, *E. coli*, *B. fragilis*, *Porphyromonas asaccharolytica*, *Peptostreptococcus* species, *Prevotella bivia*

Contraindications and cautions

- Contraindicated with allergies to any component of the drug and to beta lactam antibiotics; allergy to amide-type local anesthetics (IM use).
- Use cautiously with allergy to penicillins, cephalosporins, other allergens; pregnancy; lactation, seizure disorder.

Available forms

Vials for reconstitution—1 g/vial

Dosages

Adults

1 g IM or IV each day; length of treatment varies with infection—intra-abdominal, 5–14 days; urinary tract, 10–14 days; skin and skin structure, 7–14 days; community-acquired pneumonia, 10–14 days; acute pelvic infections, 3–10 days.

Pediatric patients

Not recommended for patients < 18 yr.

Pharmacokinetics

Route	Onset	Peak
IV	Rapid	30 min
IM	10 min	2.3 hr

Metabolism: $T_{1/2}$: 4 hr
Distribution: Crosses the placenta; enters breast milk
Excretion: Unchanged in the urine

▼ IV facts

Preparation: Reconstitute 1-g vial with 10 mL of water for injection, 0.9% sodium chloride injection or bacteriostatic water for injection; do not dilute with diluents containing dextrose. Shake well to dissolve and transfer to 50 mL of 0.9% sodium chloride injection; use within 6 hr of reconstitution, or store refrigerated for up to 24 hr, but use within 4 hr of removal from refrigeration; inspect solution for particulate matter.
Infusion: Infuse over 30 min.
Incompatibilites: Do not mix in solution or in the same line as any other medications or any solution containing dextrose.

Adverse effects

- **CNS:** *Headache,* dizziness, asthenia, fatigue, insomnia, altered mental status, anxiety, **seizures**
- **CV:** CHF, arrhythmias, edema, swelling, hypotension, hypertension, chest pain
- **GI:** *Nausea,* vomiting, *diarrhea,* abdominal pain, constipation, dyspepsia, **pseudomembranous colitis,** liver toxicity, GERD
- **GU:** Vaginitis
- **Hypersensitivity:** *Ranging from rash* to *fever* to **anaphylaxis;** serum sickness reaction
- **Local:** *Pain, phlebitis,* thrombophlebitis, inflammation at IV site
- **Respiratory:** Pharyngitis, rales, respiratory distress, cough, dyspnea, ronchi
- **Other:** Fever, rash

■ Nursing considerations

 CLINICAL ALERT!
Name confusion has occurred between Avinza (extended-release morphine) and Invanz (ertapenem); use extreme caution.

Assessment

- **History:** Allergies to any component of the drug and to beta-lactam antibiotics; allergy to amide-type local anesthetics (IM use), penicillins, cephalosporins, other allergens; pregnancy, lactation, seizures
- **Physical:** T, skin status, swelling, orientation, reflexes, R, adventitious sounds, P, BP, peripheral perfusion, culture of affected area, sensitivity tests

Interventions

- Culture infected area and arrange for sensitivity tests before beginning drug therapy and during therapy if expected response is not seen.
- Prepare IM solution as follows: Reconstitute 1-g vials with 3.2 mL of 1% lidocaine injection without epinephrine; shake to form solution; immediately withdraw contents for injection.
- Administer IM injections deeply into large muscle mass within 1 hr of reconstitution.
- Have emergency and life support equipment on standby in case of severe hypersensitivity reaction.
- Discontinue drug if hypersensitivity reaction occurs.
- Monitor injection site for adverse reactions.
- Ensure ready access to bathroom facilities and provide small, frequent meals if GI complications occur.
- Arrange for treatment of superinfections if they occur.

Teaching points

- The following side effects may occur: nausea, diarrhea, dizziness, headache (consult with your health care provider if any of these are severe).
- Report severe diarrhea, difficulty breathing, unusual tiredness or fatigue, pain at injection site.

▷ **erythromycin**
(er ith roe mye' sin)

erythromycin base

Oral, ophthalmic ointment, topical dermatologic solution for acne, topical dermatologic ointment: Akne-mycin, A/T/S, Apo-Erythro (CAN), Diomycin (CAN), E-Mycin, Erybid (CAN), Eryc, EryDerm, Erygel, Erymax, Ery-Tab, Erythra-Derm, Erythromid (CAN), Erythromycin Film-tabs, Ilotycin, Novo-Rythro (CAN), PCE (CAN), PCE Dispertab, Staticin

erythromycin estolate

Oral: Ilosone, Ilosone Pulvules, Novo-Rythro (CAN)

erythromycin ethylsuccinate

Oral: Apo-Erythro ES (CAN), E.E.S., E.E.S. 200, E.E.S. 400, E.E.S. Granules, E-Mycin, EryPed, EryPed 200, EryPed 400, EryPed Drops

erythromycin glucoeptate

Parenteral, IV: Ilotycin Gluceptate

erythromycin lactobionate

Erythrocin I.V. (CAN)

erythromycin stearate

Apo-Erythro-S (CAN), Erythrocin (CAN), Nu-Erythromycin-S (CAN)

PREGNANCY CATEGORY B

Drug class

Macrolide antibiotic

Therapeutic actions

Bacteriostatic or bactericidal in susceptible bacteria; binds to cell membrane, causing change in protein function, leading to cell death.

Adverse effects in *Italics* are most common; those in **Bold** are life-threatening.

Indications
Systemic administration
- Acute infections caused by sensitive strains of *Streptococcus pneumoniae, Mycoplasma pneumoniae, Listeria monocytogenes, Legionella pneumophila*
- URIs, LRIs, skin and soft-tissue infections caused by group A beta-hemolytic streptococci when oral treatment is preferred to injectable benzathine penicillin
- PID caused by *N. gonorrhoeae* in patients allergic to penicillin
- In conjunction with sulfonamides in URIs caused by *Haemophilus influenzae*
- As an adjunct to antitoxin in infections caused by *Corynebacterium diphtheriae* and *Corynebacterium minutissimum*
- Prophylaxis against alpha-hemolytic streptococcal endocarditis before dental or other procedures in patients allergic to penicillin who have valvular heart disease

Oral erythromycin
- Treatment of intestinal amebiasis caused by *Entamoeba histolytica*; infections in the newborn and in pregnancy that are caused by *Chlamydia trachomatis* and in adult chlamydial infections when tetracycline cannot be used; primary syphilis (*Treponema pallidum*) in penicillin-allergic patients; eliminating *Bordetella pertussis* organisms from the nasopharynx of infected individuals and as prophylaxis in exposed and susceptible individuals
- Unlabeled uses: erythromycin base is used with neomycin before colorectal surgery to reduce wound infection; treatment of severe diarrhea associated with *Campylobacter* enteritis or enterocolitis; treatment of genital, inguinal, or anorectal lymphogranuloma venereum infection; treatment of *Haemophilus ducreyi* (chancroid)

Ophthalmic ointment
- Treatment of superficial ocular infections caused by susceptible strains of microorganisms; prophylaxis of ophthalmia neonatorum caused by *N. gonorrhoeae* or *C. trachomatis*

Topical dermatologic solutions for acne
- Treatment of acne vulgaris

Topical dermatologic ointment
- Prophylaxis against infection in minor skin abrasions

- Treatment of skin infections caused by sensitive microorganisms

Contraindications and cautions
Systemic administration
- Contraindicated with allergy to erythromycin.
- Use cautiously with hepatic dysfunction, lactation (secreted and may be concentrated in breast milk; may modify bowel flora of nursing infant and interfere with fever workups).

Ophthalmic ointment
- Contraindicated with allergy to erythromycin; viral, fungal, mycobacterial infections of the eye.

Available forms
Base: Tablets—250, 333, 500 mg; DR capsules—250 mg; ophthalmic ointment—5 mg/g. Estolate: Tablets—500 mg; capsules—250 mg; suspension—125, 250 mg/5 mL. Stearate tablets—250, 500 mg ethylsuccinate: Ethylsuccinate tablets—200, 400 mg; suspension—200, 400 mg/5 mL, 100 mg/2–5 mL; powder for suspension—200 mg/5 mL; granules for suspension—400 mg/5 mL; topical solution—1.5%, 2%; topical gel, ointment—2%. Lactobionate injection: 500, 1,000 mg.

Dosages
Systemic administration
Oral preparations of the different erythromycin salts differ in pharmacokinetics: 400 mg erythromycin ethylsuccinate produces the same free erythromycin serum levels as 250 mg of erythromycin base, stearate, or estolate.

Adults
15–20 mg/kg/day in continuous IV infusion or up to 4 g/day in divided doses q 6 hr; 250 mg (400 mg of ethylsuccinate) q 6 hr PO or 500 mg q 12 hr PO or 333 mg q 8 hr PO, up to 4 g/day, depending on the severity of the infection.

- *Streptococcal infections:* 20–50 mg/kg/day PO in divided doses (for group A beta-hemolytic streptococcal infections, continue therapy for at least 10 days).
- *Legionnaire's disease:* 1–4 g/day PO or IV in divided doses (ethylsuccinate 1.6 g/day; optimal doses not established).
- *Dysenteric amebiasis:* 250 mg (400 mg of ethylsuccinate) PO qid or 333 mg q 8 hr for 10–14 days.
- *Acute pelvic inflammatory disease* (N. gonorrhoeae): 500 mg of lactobionate or glu-

E

ceptate IV q 6 hr for 3 days and then 250 mg stearate or base PO q 6 hr or 333 mg q 8 hr for 7 days.

- *Prophylaxis against bacterial endocarditis before dental or upper respiratory procedures:* 1 g (1.6 g of ethylsuccinate) 2 hr before procedure and 500 mg (800 mg ethylsuccinate) 6 hr later.
- *Chlamydial infections:* Urogenital infections during pregnancy: 500 mg PO qid or 666 mg q 8 hr for at least 7 days, one-half this dose q 8 hr for at least 14 days if intolerant to first regimen. Urethritis in males: 800 mg of ethylsuccinate PO tid for 7 days.
- *Primary syphilis:* 30–40 g (48–64 g of ethylsuccinate) in divided doses over 10–15 days.
- *CDC recommendations for STDs:* 500 mg PO qid for 7–30 days, depending on the infection.

Pediatric patients
30–50 mg/kg/day PO in divided doses. Specific dosage determined by severity of infection, age and weight.

- *Dysenteric amebiasis:* 30–50 mg/kg/day in divided doses for 10–14 days.
- *Pertussis:* 1 g PO daily in divided doses for 14 days.
- *Prophylaxis against bacterial endocarditis:* 20 mg/kg before procedure and then 10 mg/kg 6 hr later.
- *Chlamydial infections:* 50 mg/kg/day PO in divided doses, for at least 2 (conjunctivitis of newborn) or 3 (pneumonia of infancy) wk.

Ophthalmic ointment
One-half–inch ribbon instilled into conjunctival sac of affected eye two to six times per day, depending on severity of infection.

Topical
- *Dermatologic solution for acne:* Apply to affected areas morning and evening.
- *Topical dermatologic ointment:* Apply to affected area 1–5 times/day.

Pharmacokinetics

Route	Onset	Peak
Oral	1–2 hr	1–4 hr
IV	Rapid	1 hr

Metabolism: Hepatic; $T_{1/2}$: 3–5 hr

Distribution: Crosses placenta; enters breast milk

Excretion: Bile and urine

▽ IV facts

Preparation: Reconstitute powder for IV infusion only with sterile water for injection without preservatives—10 mL for 250- and 500-mg vials, 20 mL for 1-g vials. Prepare intermittent infusion as follows: Dilute 250–500 mg in 100–250 mL of 0.9% sodium chloride injection or 5% dextrose in water. Prepare for continuous infusion by adding reconstituted drug to 0.9% sodium chloride injection, lactated Ringer's injection, or D_5W that will make a solution of 1 g/L.

Infusion: Intermittent infusion: administer over 20–60 min qid; infuse slowly to avoid vein irritation. Administer continuous infusion within 4 hr, or buffer the solution to neutrality if administration is prolonged.

Incompatibilities: *Gluceptate*—do not add to aminophylline, oxytetracycline, pentobarbital, secobarbital, tetracycline. *Lactobionate*—do not mix with cephalothin, heparin, metoclopramide, tetracycline.

Y-site incompatibilities: Avoid chloramphenicol, heparin, phenobarbital, phenytoin.

Adverse effects
Systemic administration
- **CNS:** Reversible hearing loss, confusion, uncontrollable emotions, abnormal thinking
- **GI:** *Abdominal cramping, anorexia, diarrhea, vomiting,* **pseudomembranous colitis,** hepatotoxicity
- **Hypersensitivity:** Allergic reactions ranging from rash to **anaphylaxis**
- **Other:** *Superinfections*

Ophthalmic ointment
- **Dermatologic:** Edema, urticaria, dermatitis, angioneurotic edema
- **Local:** *Irritation, burning, itching* at site of application

Topical dermatologic preparations
- **Local:** *Superinfections,* particularly with long-term use

---

Adverse effects in *Italics* are most common; those in **Bold** are life-threatening.

Interactions
Systemic administration
❋ **Drug-drug** • Increased serum levels of digoxin • Increased effects of oral anticoagulants, theophyllines, carbamazepine, ergot derivatives, disopyramide, calcium blockers, fluoroquinolones, HMG CoA reductase inhibitors, proton pump inhibitors • Increased therapeutic and toxic effects of corticosteroids • Increased levels of cyclosporine and risk of renal toxicity
❋ **Drug-food** • Decreased metabolism and increased risk of toxic effects if taken with grapefruit juice; avoid this combination
Topical dermatologic solution for acne
❋ **Drug-drug** • Increased irritant effects with peeling, desquamating, or abrasive agents
Systemic administration
❋ **Drug-lab test** • Interferes with fluorometric determination of urinary catecholamines • Decreased urinary estriol levels due to inhibition of hydrolysis of steroids in the gut

■ Nursing considerations
Assessment
• **History:** Allergy to erythromycin, hepatic dysfunction, lactation; viral, fungal, mycobacterial infections of the eye (ophthalmologic)
• **Physical:** Site of infection; skin color, lesions; orientation, affect, hearing tests; R, adventitious sounds; GI output, bowel sounds, liver evaluation; culture and sensitivity tests of infection, urinalysis, liver function tests

Interventions
Systemic administration
• Culture site of infection before therapy.
• Administer oral erythromycin base or stearate on an empty stomach, 1 hr before or 2–3 hr after meals, with a full glass of water (oral erythromycin estolate, ethylsuccinate, and certain enteric-coated tablets [see manufacturer's instructions] may be given without regard to meals).
• Administer around the clock to maximize effect; adjust schedule to minimize sleep disruption.
• Monitor liver function in patients on prolonged therapy.

• Give some preparations (see above) with meals, or substitute one of these preparations, if GI upset occurs with oral therapy.
Topical dermatologic solution for acne
• Wash affected area, rinse well, and dry before application.
Ophthalmic and topical dermatologic preparation
• Use topical products only when needed. Sensitization produced by the topical use of an antibiotic may preclude its later systemic use in serious infections. Topical antibiotic preparations not normally used systemically are best.
• Culture site before beginning therapy.
• Cover the affected area with a sterile bandage if needed (topical).

Teaching points
Systemic administration
• Take oral drug on an empty stomach, 1 hr before or 2–3 hr after meals, with a full glass of water; some forms may be taken without regard to meals. Do not drink grapefruit juice while on this drug. The drug should be taken around the clock; schedule to minimize sleep disruption. Finish the full course of the drug therapy.
• These side effects may occur: stomach cramping, discomfort (take the drug with meals, if appropriate); uncontrollable emotions, crying, laughing, abnormal thinking (reversible).
• Report severe or watery diarrhea, severe nausea or vomiting, dark urine, yellowing of the skin or eyes, loss of hearing, rash or itching.
Ophthalmic ointment
• Pull the lower eyelid down gently and squeeze a one-half–inch ribbon of the ointment into the sac, avoid touching the eye or lid. A mirror may be helpful. Gently close the eye, and roll the eyeball in all directions.
• Drug may cause temporary blurring of vision, stinging, or itching.
• Report stinging or itching that becomes pronounced.
Topical dermatologic solution for acne
• Wash and rinse area, and pat it dry before applying solution.

• Use fingertips or an applicator to apply; wash hands thoroughly after application.

escitalopram oxalate
(ess si tal' oh pram)

Lexapro

PREGNANCY CATEGORY C

Drug classes
Antidepressant
SSRI

Therapeutic actions
Potentiates serotonergic activity in the CNS by inhibiting reuptake of serotonin resulting in antidepressant effect with little effect on norepinephrine or dopamine; an isomer of citalopram.

Indications
• Treatment of major depressive disorder
• Maintenance treatment for patients with major depressive disorder

Contraindications and cautions
• Contraindicated with MAO inhibitor use; with allergy to drug or to citalopram or any component of the drug.
• Use cautiously with renal or hepatic impairment, the elderly, illnesses of metabolism or hemodynamic response, pregnancy, lactation, suicidal patients.

Available forms
Tablets—5, 10, 20 mg; oral solution—5 mg/5 mL

Dosages
Adults
Initially 10 mg/day PO as a single daily dose; if necessary, may be increased to 20 mg/day after a minimum of 1-wk trial period.
Pediatric patients
Safety and efficacy not established.
Geriatric patients or adults with hepatic impairment
10 mg/day PO as a single dose; do not increase dose.

Pharmacokinetics

Route	Onset	Peak
Oral	Slow	3.5-6.5 hr

Metabolism: Hepatic metabolism; $T_{1/2}$: 27–32 hour
Distribution: Crosses placenta; passes into breast milk
Excretion: Urine

Adverse effects
• **CNS:** *Somnolence, dizziness,* insomnia, fatigue
• **Dermatological:** Sweating
• **GI:** *Nausea,* dry mouth, constipation, diarrhea, indigestion, abdominal pain, decreased appetite
• **GU:** *Ejaculatory disorders,* impotence, anorgasmia in females, decreased libido
• **Respiratory:** Rhinitis, sinusitis, flulike symptoms

Interactions
✳ **Drug-drug** • Risk of serious toxic effects if combined with citalopram; do not use these drugs concomitantly • Increased escitalopram levels and toxicity if taken with MAOIs; ensure that patient has been off the MAOI for at least 14 days before administering escitalopram • Possible severe adverse effects if combined with other centrally acting CNS drugs; use caution • Possible decreased effects of escitalopram if combined with carbamazepine, lithium; monitor patient closely

✳ **Drug-alternative therapy** • Increased risk of severe reaction if combined with St. John's wort; avoid this combination

■ Nursing considerations

CLINICAL ALERT!
There is potential for name confusion between escitalopram and citalopram; use caution.

Assessment
• **History:** MAO inhibitor use; allergy to drug, citalopram, or any component of the drug; renal or hepatic impairment; the elderly; pregnancy; lactation; suicidal tendencies;

metabolic illnesses or problems with hemo-dynamic response; alcoholism
- **Physical:** Orientation, reflexes; P, BP, per-fusion; R, bowel sounds, normal output; uri-nary output; liver evaluation; liver and re-nal function tests

Interventions
- Administer once a day, in the morning or the evening; may be taken with food if de-sired.
- Encourage patient to continue use for 4-6 weeks, as directed, to ensure adequate levels to affect depression.
- Limit amount of drug given in prescription to potentially suicidal patients.
- Advise any depressed patients to avoid the use of alcohol while being treated with an-tidepressive drugs.
- Establish appropriate safety precautions if patient experiences adverse CNS effects.
- Institute appropriate therapy for patient suf-fering from depression.

Teaching points
- Take this drug exactly as directed, and as long as directed; it may take a few weeks to realize the benefits of the drug. The drug may be taken with food if desired.
- These side effects may occur: drowsiness, dizziness, tremor (use caution and avoid driving a car or performing other tasks that require alertness if you experience daytime drowsiness); GI upset (small, frequent meals, frequent mouth care may help); alterations in sexual function (it may help to know that this is a drug effect and will pass when drug therapy is ended).
- Avoid the use of alcohol while you are tak-ing this drug.
- This drug should not be taken during preg-nancy or when nursing a baby; use of bar-rier contraceptives is suggested.
- Report severe nausea, vomiting; blurred vi-sion; excessive sweating, suicidal ideation, sexual dysfunction, insomnia.

▽ **esmolol hydrochloride**
(*ess' moe lol*)

Brevibloc

PREGNANCY CATEGORY C

E

Drug class
Beta$_1$-selective adrenergic blocking agent

Therapeutic actions
Blocks beta-adrenergic receptors in the heart and juxtaglomerular apparatus, reducing the influence of the sympathetic nervous system on these tissues; decreasing the excitability of the heart, cardiac output, and release of renin; and lowering BP. At low doses, acts relatively selectively at the beta$_1$-adrenergic receptors of the heart; has very rapid onset and short du-ration.

Indications
- Supraventricular tachycardia, when rapid but short-term control of ventricular rate is desirable (atrial fibrillation, flutter, periop-erative or postoperative situations)
- Noncompensatory tachycardia when heart rate requires specific intervention
- Intraoperative and postoperative tachycardia and hypertension when intervention is needed

Contraindications and cautions
- Because this drug is reserved for emergency situations, there are no contraindications to its use.

Available forms
Injection—10 mg/mL, 250 mg/mL

Dosages
Adults
Individualize dosage by titration (loading dose followed by a maintenance dose): initial load-ing dose of 500 mcg/kg/min IV for 1 min fol-lowed by a maintenance dose of 50 mcg/kg/min for 4 min. If adequate response is not ob-served in 5 min, repeat loading dose and fol-low with maintenance infusion of 100 mcg/kg/min. Repeat titration as necessary, in-creasing rate of maintenance dose in incre-ments of 50 mcg/kg/min. As desired heart rate or safe end point is approached, omit loading

infusion and decrease incremental dose in maintenance infusion to 25 mcg/kg/min (or less), or increase interval between titration steps from 5 to 10 min. Usual range is 50–200 mcg/kg/min. Infusions for up to 24 hr have been used; up to 48 hr may be well tolerated. Dosage should be individualized based on patient response; do not exceed 300 mcg/kg/min.

Pediatric patients
Safety and efficacy not established.

Pharmacokinetics

Route	Onset	Peak	Duration
IV	< 5 min	10–20 min	10–30 min

Metabolism: RBC esterases; $T_{1/2}$: 9 min
Distribution: Crosses placenta; enters breast milk
Excretion: Urine

▽IV facts

Preparation: Dilute drug before infusing as follows: Add the contents of 2 ampuls of esmolol (2.5 g) to a compatible diluent: 5% dextrose injection; 5% dextrose in Ringer's injection; 5% dextrose and 0.9% or 0.45% sodium chloride injection; lactated Ringer's injection; 0.9% or 0.45% sodium chloride injection after removing 20 mL from a 500 mL bottle, to make a drug solution with a concentration of 10 mg/mL. Diluted solution is stable for 24 hr at room temperature.
Infusion: Rate of infusion is determined by patient response; see Dosage section above.
Incompatibility: Do not mix in solution with other drugs or sodium bicarbonate.

Adverse effects

- **CNS:** *Light-headedness, speech disorder, midscapular pain, weakness, rigors,* somnolence, confusion
- **CV:** *Hypotension,* pallor
- **GI:** *Taste perversion*
- **GU:** *Urinary retention*
- **Local:** *Inflammation,* induration, edema, erythema, burning at the site of infusion
- **Other:** Fever, rhonchi, flushing

Interactions

✳ **Drug-drug** • Increased therapeutic and toxic effects with verapamil • Impaired anti-

hypertensive effects with ibuprofen, indomethacin, piroxicam

■ Nursing considerations
Assessment
- **History:** Cardiac, cerebrovascular disease
- **Physical:** P, BP, ECG; orientation, reflexes; R, adventitious sounds; urinary output

Interventions
- Ensure that drug is not used in chronic settings when transfer to another agent is anticipated.
- Do not give undiluted drug.
- Do not mix with sodium bicarbonate; do not mix undiluted esmolol with other drug solutions.
- Monitor BP closely.

Teaching points
- This drug is reserved for emergency use; incorporate information about this drug into an overall teaching plan.

▷**esomeprazole magnesium (perprazole, S-omeprazole)**
*(ess oh **me'** pray zol)*

Nexium

PREGNANCY CATEGORY C

Drug classes
Antisecretory agent
Proton pump inhibitor

Therapeutic actions
Gastric acid-pump inhibitor: suppresses gastric acid secretion by specific inhibition of the hydrogen–potassium ATPase enzyme system at the secretory surface of the gastric parietal cells; blocks the final step of acid production; is broken down less in the first pass through the liver than the parent compound omeprazole, allowing for increased serum levels.

Indications
- Gastroesophageal reflux disease—treatment of heartburn and other related symptoms

Adverse effects in *Italics* are most common; those in **Bold** are life-threatening.

- Erosive esophagitis—short-term treatment for healing and symptom relief
- As part of combination therapy for the treatment of duodenal ulcer associated with *H. Pylori*

Contraindications and cautions
- Contraindicated with hypersensitivity to omeprazole, esomeprazole, or other proton pump inhibitor.
- Use cautiously with hepatic dysfunction, pregnancy, lactation.

Available forms
Delayed-release capsules—20, 40 mg

Dosages
Adults
- *Acute treatment:* 20–40 mg PO daily for 4–8 wk.
- *Maintenance:* 20 mg daily, may be used with antacids for 4 wk.
- *Duodenal ulcer:* 40 mg/day PO for 10 days with 1,000 mg PO bid ampicillin and 500 mg PO bid clarithromycin.

Pediatric patients
Safety and efficacy not established.

Patients with hepatic dysfunction
Reduce dose and monitor patient carefully in cases of severe hepatic dysfunction.

Pharmacokinetics

Route	Onset	Peak	Duration
Oral	1–2 hr	1.4–5.1 hr	17 hr

Metabolism: Hepatic; $T_{1/2}$: 0.8–1.2 hr
Distribution: Crosses placenta; may pass into breast milk
Excretion: Urine and bile

Adverse effects
- **CNS:** *Headache, dizziness,* asthenia, vertigo, insomnia, apathy, anxiety, paresthesias, dream abnormalities
- **Dermatologic:** Rash, inflammation, urticaria, pruritus, alopecia, dry skin
- **GI:** *Diarrhea, abdominal pain, nausea, vomiting,* constipation, dry mouth, tongue atrophy, flatulence
- **Respiratory:** *URI symptoms, sinusitis,* cough, epistaxis

Interactions
✳ **Drug-drug interactions** • Increased serum levels and potential increase in toxicity of benzodiazepines and phenytoin when taken concurrently

■ Nursing considerations

 CLINICAL ALERT!
Potential for name confusion exists between esomeprazole and omeprazole; use caution.

E

Assessment
- **History:** Hypersensitivity to any proton pump inhibitor; hepatic dysfunction; pregnancy, lactation
- **Physical:** Skin lesions; body temperature; reflexes, affect; urinary output, abdominal exam; respiratory auscultation, liver function tests

Interventions
- Arrange for further evaluation of patient after 4 wk of therapy for gastroesophageal reflux disorders. Symptomatic improvement does not rule out gastric cancer.
- If administering antacids, they may be administered concomitantly with esomeprazole.
- Ensure that the patient swallows capsule whole; do not crush, or chew; patients having difficulty swallowing may open capsule and sprinkle in applesauce; do not crush or chew pellets.
- Obtain baseline liver function tests and monitor periodically during therapy.
- Maintain supportive treatment as appropriate for underlying problem.
- Provide additional comfort measures to alleviate discomfort from GI effects, headache, and so on.
- Establish safety precautions if dizziness, CNS effects occur (side rails, accompany patient, etc).

Teaching points
- Take the drug before meals. Swallow the capsules whole; do not chew or crush. If you cannot swallow the capsule, it can be opened and sprinkled in applesauce; do not crush or chew the pellets. This drug will need to be taken for 4–8 wk, at which time your condition will be reevaluated.

- Arrange to have regular medical follow-up while you are on this drug.
- These side effects may occur: dizziness (avoid driving a car or performing hazardous tasks); headaches (consult with your health care provider if these become bothersome; medications may be available to help); nausea, vomiting, diarrhea (proper nutrition is important; consult with your dietitian to maintain nutrition; ensure ready access to bathroom); symptoms of upper respiratory tract infection, cough (it may help to know that this is a drug effect; do not self-medicate; consult with your health care provider if this becomes uncomfortable).
- Report severe headache, worsening of symptoms, fever, chills, darkening of the skin, changes in color of urine or stool.
- Maintain all of the usual activities and restrictions that apply to your condition. If this becomes difficult, consult with your nurse or physician.

▽estazolam
(es taz' e lam)

ProSom

PREGNANCY CATEGORY X

C-IV CONTROLLED SUBSTANCE

Drug classes
Benzodiazepine
Sedative and hypnotic

Therapeutic actions
Exact mechanisms of action not understood; acts mainly at subcortical levels of the CNS, leaving the cortex relatively unaffected; potentiates the effects of GABA, an inhibitory neurotransmitter.

Indications
- Insomnia characterized by difficulty in falling asleep, frequent nocturnal awakenings, or early morning awakening
- Recurring insomnia or poor sleeping habits
- Acute or chronic medical situations requiring restful sleep

Contraindications and cautions
- Contraindicated with hypersensitivity to benzodiazepines, psychoses, acute narrow-angle glaucoma, shock, coma, acute alcoholic intoxication with depression of vital signs, pregnancy (increased risk of congenital malformations, neonatal withdrawal syndrome; labor and delivery ("floppy infant" syndrome reported), lactation (secreted in breast milk; chronic administration of diazepam, another benzodiazepine, to nursing mothers has caused infants to become lethargic and lose weight).
- Use cautiously with impaired liver or kidney function, debilitation, depression, suicidal tendencies.

Available forms
Tablets—1, 2 mg

Dosages
Individualize dosage.
Adults
1 mg PO before bedtime; up to 2 mg may be needed.
Pediatric patients
Not for use in patients < 15 yr.
Geriatric patients or patients with debilitating disease
1 mg PO if healthy; start with 0.5 mg in debilitated patients.

Pharmacokinetics

Route	Onset	Peak
Oral	45–60 min	2 hr

Metabolism: Hepatic; $T_{1/2}$: 10–24 hr
Distribution: Crosses placenta; enters breast milk
Excretion: Urine

Adverse effects
- **CNS:** *Transient, mild drowsiness initially; sedation, depression, lethargy, apathy, fatigue, light-headedness, disorientation, restlessness, asthenia,* crying, delirium, headache, slurred speech, dysarthria, stupor, rigidity, tremor, dystonia, vertigo, euphoria, nervousness, difficulty in concentration, vivid dreams, psychomotor retardation, extrapyramidal symptoms, *mild paradoxical*

excitatory reactions during first 2 wk of treatment (especially in psychiatric patients, aggressive children, and with high dosage), visual and auditory disturbances, diplopia, nystagmus, depressed hearing, nasal congestion
- **CV:** *Bradycardia, tachycardia,* cardiovascular collapse, hypertension and hypotension, palpitations, edema
- **Dependence:** *Drug dependence with withdrawal syndrome* when drug is discontinued (more common with abrupt discontinuation of higher dosage used for longer than 4 mo)
- **Dermatologic:** Urticaria, pruritus, skin rash, dermatitis
- **GI:** *Constipation, diarrhea, dyspepsia,* dry mouth, salivation, nausea, anorexia, vomiting, difficulty in swallowing, gastric disorders, elevations of blood enzymes: LDH, alkaline phosphatase, AST, ALT; hepatic dysfunction, jaundice
- **GU:** *Incontinence, urinary retention, changes in libido,* menstrual irregularities
- **Hematologic:** Decreased hematocrit, blood dyscrasias
- **Other:** Hiccups, fever, diaphoresis, paresthesias, muscular disturbances, gynecomastia

Interactions
✻ **Drug-drug** • Increased CNS depression when taken with alcohol, omeprazole • Increased pharmacologic effects of estazolam when given with cimetidine • Decreased sedative effects of estazolam if taken concurrently with theophylline, aminophylline, dyphylline, oxitriphylline

■ Nursing considerations
Assessment
- **History:** Hypersensitivity to benzodiazepines; psychoses; acute narrow-angle glaucoma; shock; coma; acute alcoholic intoxication; pregnancy; labor; lactation; impaired liver or kidney function, debilitation, depression, suicidal tendencies
- **Physical:** Skin color, lesions; T, orientation, reflexes, affect, ophthalmologic exam; P, BP; R, adventitious sounds; liver evaluation, abdominal exam, bowel sounds, normal output; CBC, liver and renal function tests

Interventions
- Arrange to monitor liver and kidney function, CBC during long-term therapy.
- Taper dosage gradually after long-term therapy, especially in epileptic patients.

Teaching points
- Take drug exactly as prescribed; do not stop taking this drug without consulting your health care provider.
- Avoid alcohol, sleep-inducing, or OTC drugs while on this drug.
- These side effects may occur: transient drowsiness, dizziness (avoid driving or engaging in dangerous activities); GI upset (take the drug with water); depression, dreams, emotional upset, crying; sleep may be disturbed for several nights after discontinuing the drug.
- Report severe dizziness, weakness, drowsiness that persists, rash or skin lesions, palpitations, swelling of the extremities, visual changes, difficulty voiding.

▷ **estradiols**
(ess tra dye' ole)

estradiol
Oral: Estrace, Gynodiol
Transdermal system: Alora, Climara, Climara 25, Estraderm, FemPatch, Vivelle, Vivelle Dot
Topical vaginal cream: Estrace
Vaginal ring: Estring

estradiol cypionate
Injection in oil: Depo-Estradiol Cypionate, depGynogen, Depogen

estradiol hemihydrate
Vaginal tablet: Vagifem

estradiol valerate
Injection in oil: Delestrogen, Estra-L 40, Gynogen L.A. 20, Valergen 20

PREGNANCY CATEGORY X

Drug classes
Hormone
Estrogen

Therapeutic actions

Estradiol is the most potent endogenous female sex hormone. Estrogens are important in the development of the female reproductive system and secondary sex characteristics; affect the release of pituitary gonadotropins; cause capillary dilatation, fluid retention, protein anabolism and thin cervical mucus; conserve calcium and phosphorus and encourage bone formation; inhibit ovulation and prevent postpartum breast discomfort. They are responsible for the proliferation of the endometrium; absence or decline of estrogen produces signs and symptoms of menopause on the uterus, vagina, breasts, cervix; relief in androgen-dependent prostatic carcinoma is attributable to competition with androgens for receptor sites, decreasing the influence of androgens.

Indications

- Palliation of moderate to severe vasomotor symptoms, atrophic vaginitis or kraurosis vulvae associated with menopause; prevention of postmenopausal osteoporosis (estradiol oral, transdermal, cream, estradiol valerate)
- Treatment of female hypogonadism, female castration, primary ovarian failure (estradiol oral, transdermal, estradiol cypionate, valerate)
- Palliation of inoperable prostatic cancer (estradiol oral, estradiol valerate)
- Palliation of inoperable, progressing breast cancer (estradiol oral)

Contraindications and cautions

- Contraindicated with allergy to estrogens, allergy to tartrazine (in 2-mg oral tablets), breast cancer (with exceptions), estrogen-dependent neoplasm, undiagnosed abnormal genital bleeding, active or past history of thrombophlebitis or thromboembolic disorders (potential serious fetal defects; women of childbearing age should be advised of risks and birth control measures suggested).
- Use cautiously with metabolic bone disease, renal insufficiency, CHF, lactation.

Available forms

Transdermal—release rates of 0.025, 0.0375, 0.05, 0.075, 0.1 mg/24 hr; tablets—0.5, 1,

2 mg; injection—10, 20, 40 mg/mL; vaginal cream—0.1 mg; vaginal ring—2 mg; vaginal tablet—25 mcg

Dosages
Adults

- *Moderate to severe vasomotor symptoms, atrophic vaginitis, kraurosis vulvae associated with menopause:* 1–2 mg/day PO. Adjust dose to control symptoms. Cyclic therapy (3 wk on/1 wk off) is recommended, especially in women who have not had a hysterectomy. 1–5 mg estradiol cypionate in oil IM every 3–4 wk. 10–20 mg estradiol valerate in oil IM, every 4 wk. 0.025–0.05-mg system applied to the skin weekly or twice weekly. If oral estrogens have been used, start transdermal system 1 wk after withdrawal of oral form. Given on a cyclic schedule (3 wk on/1wk off). Attempt to taper or discontinue medication every 3–6 mo.

Vaginal

- *Vaginal cream:* 2–4 g intravaginally daily for 1–2 wk, then reduce to one-half dosage for similar period followed by maintenance doses of 1 g 1–3 times/wk thereafter. Discontinue or taper at 3- to 6-mo intervals.
- *Vaginal ring:* Insert one ring high into vagina. Replace every 90 days.
- *Vaginal tablet:* 1 tablet inserted vaginally daily for 2 wk; then twice weekly.
- *Female hypogonadism, female castration, primary ovarian failure:* 1–2 mg/day PO. Adjust dose to control symptoms. Cyclic therapy (3 wk on/1 wk off) is recommended. 1.5–2 mg estradiol cypionate in oil IM at monthly intervals. 10–20 mg estradiol valerate in oil IM every 4 wk. 0.05-mg system applied to skin twice weekly as above.

Oral

- *Prostatic cancer (inoperable):* 1–2 mg PO tid. Administer long-term. 30 mg or more estradiol valerate in oil IM every 1–2 wk.
- *Breast cancer (inoperable, progressing):* 10 mg tid PO for at least 3 mo.
- *Prevention of postpartum breast engorgement:* 10–25 mg estradiol valerate in oil IM as a single injection at the end of the first stage of labor.
- *Osteoporosis prevention:* 0.5 mg/day PO given cyclically—23 days on, 5 days rest—

starting as soon after menopause as possible *or* 0.05 mg/24 hr applied to skin once or twice weekly.

Pediatric patients
Not recommended due to effect on the growth of the long bones.

Pharmacokinetics

Route	Onset	Peak
Oral	Slow	Days

Metabolism: Hepatic; $T_{1/2}$: not known
Distribution: Crosses placenta; enters breast milk
Excretion: Urine

Adverse effects

- **CNS:** Steepening of the corneal curvature with a resultant change in visual acuity and intolerance to contact lenses, *headache*, migraine, dizziness, mental depression, chorea, convulsions
- **CV:** Increased blood pressure, thromboembolic and thrombotic disease
- **Dermatologic:** *Photosensitivity, peripheral edema, chloasma,* erythema nodosum or multiforme, hemorrhagic eruption, loss of scalp hair, hirsutism, urticaria, dermatitis
- **GI:** Gallbladder disease (in postmenopausal women), **hepatic adenoma,** *nausea, vomiting, abdominal cramps, bloating,* **cholestatic jaundice, colitis, acute pancreatitis**
- **GU:** Increased risk of postmenopausal endometrial cancer, *breakthrough bleeding, change in menstrual flow, dysmenorrhea, premenstrual-like syndrome,* amenorrhea, vaginal candidiasis, cystitis-like syndrome, endometrial cystic hyperplasia
- **Hematologic:** Hypercalcemia, decreased glucose tolerance
- **Local:** *Pain at injection site,* sterile abscess, postinjection flare
- **Other:** Weight changes, reduced carbohydrate tolerance, aggravation of porphyria, edema, changes in libido, breast tenderness

Topical vaginal cream
Systemic absorption may cause uterine bleeding in menopausal women and may cause serious bleeding of remaining endometrial foci in sterilized women with endometriosis.

Interactions

* **Drug-drug** • Increased therapeutic and toxic effects of corticosteroids • Decreased serum levels of estradiol with drugs that enhance hepatic metabolism of the drug: barbiturates, phenytoin, rifampin

* **Drug-lab test** • Increased sulfobromophthalein retention; prothrombin and factors VII, VIII, IX, and X; thyroid-binding globulin with increased PBI, T_4, increased uptake of free T_3 resin (free T_4 is unaltered), serum triglycerides and phospholipid concentration • Decreased antithrombin III, pregnanediol excretion, response to metyrapone test, serum folate concentration • Impaired glucose tolerance

■ Nursing considerations
Assessment

- **History:** Allergy to estrogens, tartrazine; breast cancer, estrogen-dependent neoplasm; undiagnosed abnormal genital bleeding; active or previous thrombophlebitis or thromboembolic disorders; pregnancy; lactation; metabolic bone disease; renal insufficiency; CHF
- **Physical:** Skin color, lesions, edema; breast exam; injection site; orientation, affect, reflexes; P, auscultation, BP, peripheral perfusion; R, adventitious sounds; bowel sounds, liver evaluation, abdominal exam; pelvic exam; serum calcium, phosphorus; liver and renal function tests; Pap smear; glucose tolerance test

Interventions

- Arrange for pretreatment and periodic (at least annual) history and physical, which should include BP, breasts, abdomen, pelvic organs, and a Pap smear.
- Caution patient of the risks of estrogen use, the need to prevent pregnancy during treatment, for frequent medical follow-up, and for periodic rests from drug treatment.
- Administer cyclically for short-term only when treating postmenopausal conditions because of the risk of endometrial neoplasm; taper to the lowest effective dose, and provide a drug-free week each month.
- Apply transdermal system to a clean, dry area of skin on the trunk of the body, preferably the abdomen; do not apply to breasts; rotate the site at least 1 wk between applications;

avoid the waistline because clothing may rub the system off; apply immediately after opening and compress for about 10 sec to attach.

- Insert vaginal ring as deeply as possible into upper one-third of vagina. Ring will remain in place for 3 months. Then, remove and evaluate need for continued therapy. If a ring falls out during 3 mo, rinse with warm water and reinsert.

- Arrange for the concomitant use of progestin therapy during long-term estrogen therapy; this will mimic normal physiologic cycling and allow for a cyclic uterine bleeding that may decrease the risk of endometrial cancer.

- Administer parenteral preparations by deep IM injection only. Monitor injection sites and rotate with each injection to decrease development of abscesses.

Teaching points

- Use this drug in cycles or short term; prepare a calendar of drug days, rest days, and drug-free periods.

- Apply transdermal system and vaginal cream properly; insert vaginal tablet as high into the vagina as is comfortable.

- Insert vaginal ring high in vagina; it should remain in place for 3 months. If it falls out before that time, rinse with warm water and reinsert.

- Potentially serious side effects: cancers, blood clots, liver problems; it is very important to have periodic medical exams throughout therapy.

- This drug cannot be given to pregnant women because of serious toxic effects to the baby.

- These side effects may occur: nausea, vomiting, bloating, headache, dizziness, mental depression (use caution if driving or performing tasks that require alertness); sensitivity to sunlight (use a sunscreen and wear protective clothing); rash, loss of scalp hair, darkening of the skin on the face; changes in menstrual patterns.

- Report pain in the groin or calves of the legs, chest pain or sudden shortness of breath, abnormal vaginal bleeding, lumps in the breast, sudden severe headache, dizziness or

fainting, changes in vision or speech, weakness or numbness in the arm or leg, severe abdominal pain, yellowing of the skin or eyes, severe mental depression, pain at injection site.

▷ **estramustine phosphate sodium**
(ess tra muss' teen)

Emcyt

PREGNANCY CATEGORY X

Drug classes
Hormonal agent
Estrogen
Antineoplastic agent

Therapeutic actions
Estradiol and an alkylating agent are linked in each molecule of drug; the drug binds preferentially to cells with estrogen (steroid) receptors, where alkylating effect is enhanced and cell death occurs.

Indications
- Palliative treatment of metastatic or progressive carcinoma of the prostate

Contraindications and cautions
- Contraindicated with allergy to estradiol or nitrogen mustard; active thrombophlebitis or thromboembolic disorders (except when the tumor mass is the cause of the thromboembolic phenomenon, and the benefits outweigh the risks); pregnancy.
- Use cautiously with cerebral vascular and coronary artery disorders; epilepsy, migraine, renal dysfunction, CHF; impaired hepatic function; metabolic bone diseases with hypercalcemia; diabetes mellitus.

Available forms
Capsules—140 mg

Dosages
Adults
10–16 mg/kg/day PO in 3–4 divided doses. Treat for 30–90 days before assessing benefits.

Adverse effects in *Italics* are most common; those in **Bold** are life-threatening.

Continue therapy as long as response is favorable.

Pharmacokinetics

Route	Onset	Peak
Oral	Varies	2–3 hr

Metabolism: Hepatic; $T_{1/2}$: 20 hr
Excretion: Feces

Adverse effects

- **CNS:** *Lethargy, emotional lability, insomnia, headache, anxiety,* chest pain, tearing of the eyes
- **CV:** CVA, MI, thrombophlebitis, **pulmonary emboli,** *CHF, edema, dyspnea, elevated blood pressure, leg cramps*
- **Dermatologic:** *Rash, pruritus, dry skin, peeling skin or fingertips,* easy bruising, flushing, thinning hair
- **GI:** *Nausea, vomiting, diarrhea, anorexia,* flatulence, GI bleeding, burning throat, thirst, hepatic impairment
- **Hematologic:** Leukopenia, thrombopenia, abnormalities in bilirubin, LDH, AST; decreased glucose tolerance
- **Respiratory:** Upper respiratory discharge, hoarseness
- **Other:** *Breast tenderness, mild to moderate breast enlargement,* carcinoma of the liver, breast

■ Nursing considerations

Assessment

- **History:** Allergy to estradiol or nitrogen mustard; active thrombophlebitis or thromboembolic disorder; cerebrovascular and coronary artery disorders; epilepsy, migraine, renal dysfunction, CHF; impaired hepatic function; metabolic bone diseases with hypercalcemia; diabetes mellitus, pregnancy
- **Physical:** Skin lesions, color, turgor; hair; breast exam; body weight; orientation, affect, reflexes; P, BP, auscultation, peripheral pulses, edema; R, adventitious sounds; liver evaluation, bowel sounds; stool guaiac, renal and liver function tests, blood glucose

Interventions

- Administer the drug for 30–90 days before assessing the possible benefits of continued therapy; therapy can be continued as long as response is favorable.

- Refrigerate capsules; capsules may be left out of the refrigerator for up to 48 hr without loss of potency.
- Monitor diabetic patients carefully, glucose tolerance may change, affecting need for insulin.
- Arrange to monitor hepatic function periodically during therapy.
- Monitor BP regularly throughout therapy.
- Caution patient to use some contraceptive method while on this drug, because mutagenesis has been reported.

Teaching points

- The effects may not be seen for several weeks. Capsules should be stored in the refrigerator; they will be stable for up to 48 hr out of the refrigerator.
- Take drug with water; avoid taking with products containing calcium.
- These side effects may occur: nausea, vomiting, diarrhea, flatulence; dry, peeling skin and rash; headache, emotional lability, lethargy (reversible).
- Use contraceptive measures; there is a risk of fetal deformity with this drug.
- Report pain or swelling in the legs, chest pain, difficulty breathing, edema, leg cramps.

▷estrogens, conjugated
(ess' troe jenz)

Oral, topical vaginal cream: C.E.S. (CAN), Congest (CAN), Premarin
Parenteral: Premarin Intravenous
Synthetic: Cenestin

PREGNANCY CATEGORY X

Drug classes
Hormone
Estrogen

Therapeutic actions
Estrogens are endogenous female sex hormones important in the development of the female reproductive system and secondary sex characteristics. They affect the release of pituitary gonadotropins; cause capillary dilatation, fluid retention, protein anabolism, and thin

cervical mucus; conserve calcium and phosphorus; encourage bone formation; inhibit ovulation and prevent postpartum breast discomfort. They are responsible for the proliferation of the endometrium; absence or decline of estrogen produces signs and symptoms of menopause on the uterus, vagina, breasts, cervix. Their efficacy as palliation in male patients with androgen-dependent prostatic carcinoma is attributable to their competition with androgens for receptor sites, thus decreasing the influence of androgens.

Indications

- Oral palliation of moderate to severe vasomotor symptoms, atrophic vaginitis, or kraurosis vulvae associated with menopause
- Treatment of female hypogonadism; female castration; primary ovarian failure
- Osteoporosis: to retard progression
- Palliation of inoperable prostatic cancer
- Palliation of mammary cancer
- Treatment of moderate to severe vasomotor symptoms associated with menopause (Cenestin)
- Unlabeled use: postcoital contraceptive
- Parenteral: treatment of uterine bleeding due to hormonal imbalance in the absence of organic pathology
- Vaginal cream: treatment of atrophic vaginitis and kraurosis vulvae associated with menopause

Contraindications and cautions

- Contraindicated with allergy to estrogens, breast cancer (with exceptions), estrogen-dependent neoplasm, undiagnosed abnormal genital bleeding, active or past thrombophlebitis or thromboembolic disorders from previous estrogen use, pregnancy (serious fetal defects; women of childbearing age should be advised of risks and birth control measures suggested).
- Use cautiously with metabolic bone disease, renal insufficiency, CHF, lactation.

Available forms

Tablets—0.3, 0.625, 0.9, 1.25, 2.5 mg; injection—25 mg; vaginal cream—0.625 mg

Dosages

Oral drug should be given cyclically (3 wk on/1 wk off) except in selected cases of carcinoma and prevention of postpartum breast engorgement.

Adults

- *Moderate to severe vasomotor symptoms associated with menopause:* 0.625 mg/day PO. If patient has not menstruated in 2 mo, start at any time. If patient is menstruating, start therapy on day 5 of bleeding; 0.625–1.25 mg Cenestin.
- *Atrophic vaginitis, kraurosis vulvae associated with menopause:* 0.3–1.25 mg/day PO or more if needed. 2–4 g vaginal cream daily intravaginally or topically, depending on severity of condition. Taper or discontinue at 3- to 6-mo intervals.
- *Female hypogonadism:* 0.3–0.625 mg/day PO in divided doses for 20 days followed by 10 days of rest. If bleeding does not appear at the end of this time, repeat course. If bleeding does occur before the end of the 10-day rest, begin a 20-day 2.5–7.5 mg estrogen cyclic regimen with oral progestin given during the last 5 days of therapy. If bleeding occurs before this cycle is finished, restart course on day 5 of bleeding.
- *Female castration, primary ovarian failure:* 1.25 mg/day PO. Adjust dosage by patient response to lowest effective dose.
- *Prostatic cancer (inoperable):* 1.25–2.5 mg tid PO. Judge effectiveness by phosphatase determinations and by symptomatic improvement.
- *Osteoporosis:* 0.625 mg/day PO.
- *Breast cancer (inoperable, progressing):* 10 mg tid PO for at least 3 mo.
- *Prevention of postpartum breast engorgement:* 3.75 mg q 4 hr PO for 5 doses, or 1.25 mg q 4 hr for 5 days.
- *Abnormal uterine bleeding due to hormonal imbalance:* 25 mg IV or IM. Repeat in 6–12 hr as needed. IV route provides a more rapid response.
- *Postcoital contraceptive:* 30 mg/day PO in divided doses for 5 consecutive days within 72 hr after intercourse.

Pediatric patients

Not recommended due to effect on the growth of the long bones.

Pharmacokinetics

Route	Onset	Peak
Oral	Slow	Days
IV	Gradual	Hours

Metabolism: Hepatic; $T_{1/2}$: not known
Distribution: Crosses placenta; enters breast milk
Excretion: Urine

▼ IV facts

Preparation: Reconstitute with provided diluent; add to normal saline, dextrose, and invert sugar solutions. Refrigerate unreconstituted parenteral solution; use reconstituted solution within a few hours. Refrigerated reconstituted solution is stable for 60 days; do not use solution if darkened or precipitates have formed.
Infusion: Inject slowly over 2–5 min.
Incompatibilities: Do not mix with protein hydrolysate, ascorbic acid, or any solution with an acid pH.

Adverse effects

- **CNS:** Steepening of the corneal curvature with a resultant change in visual acuity and intolerance to contact lenses, *headache,* migraine, dizziness, mental depression, chorea, convulsions
- **CV:** Increased blood pressure, thromboembolic and thrombotic disease
- **Dermatologic:** *Photosensitivity, peripheral edema, chloasma,* erythema nodosum or multiforme, hemorrhagic eruption, loss of scalp hair, hirsutism, urticaria, dermatitis
- **GI:** Gallbladder disease (in postmenopausal women), **hepatic adenoma,** *nausea, vomiting, abdominal cramps, bloating,* **cholestatic jaundice,** *colitis,* **acute pancreatitis**
- **GU:** Increased risk of endometrial cancer in postmenopausal women, *breakthrough bleeding, change in menstrual flow, dysmenorrhea, premenstrual-like syndrome,* amenorrhea, vaginal candidiasis, cystitis-like syndrome, endometrial cystic hyperplasia
- **Hematologic:** Hypercalcemia, decreased glucose tolerance
- **Local:** *Pain at injection site,* sterile abscess, postinjection flare

- **Other:** Weight changes, reduced carbohydrate tolerance, aggravation of porphyria, edema, changes in libido, breast tenderness

Topical vaginal cream
Systemic absorption may cause uterine bleeding in menopausal women and serious bleeding of remaining endometrial foci in sterilized women with endometriosis.

Interactions

✴ Drug-drug • Increased therapeutic and toxic effects of corticosteroids • Decreased serum levels of estrogen with drugs that enhance hepatic metabolism of the drug: barbiturates, phenytoin, rifampin
✴ Drug-lab test • Increased sulfobromophthalein retention; prothrombin and factors VII, VIII, IX, and X; thyroid-binding globulin with increased PBI, T_4, increased uptake of free T_3 resin (free T_4 is unaltered), serum triglycerides and phospholipid concentration • Decreased antithrombin III, pregnanediol excretion, response to metyrapone test, serum folate concentration • Impaired glucose tolerance

■ Nursing considerations
Assessment

- **History:** Allergy to estrogens; breast cancer, estrogen-dependent neoplasm; undiagnosed abnormal genital bleeding; active or previous thrombophlebitis or thromboembolic disorders; pregnancy; lactation; metabolic bone disease; renal insufficiency; CHF
- **Physical:** Skin color, lesions, edema; breast exam; injection site; orientation, affect, reflexes; P, auscultation, BP, peripheral perfusion; R, adventitious sounds; bowel sounds, liver evaluation, abdominal exam; pelvic exam; serum calcium, phosphorus; liver and renal function tests; Pap smear; glucose tolerance test

Interventions

- Arrange for pretreatment and periodic (at least annual) history and physical, which should include BP, breasts, abdomen, pelvic organs, and a Pap smear.
- Caution patient of the risks involved with estrogen use, the need to prevent pregnancy during treatment, for frequent medical follow-up, and periodic rests from drug treatment.

- Give cyclically for short term only when treating postmenopausal conditions because of the risk of endometrial neoplasm; taper to the lowest effective dose, and provide a drug-free week each month.
- Refrigerate unreconstituted parenteral solution; use reconstituted solution within a few hours.
- Refrigerated reconstituted solution is stable for 60 days; do not use solution if darkened or precipitates have formed.
- Arrange for the concomitant use of progestin therapy during long-term estrogen therapy in women; this will mimic normal physiologic cycling and allow for cyclic uterine bleeding, which may decrease the risk of endometrial cancer.

Teaching points
- Use this drug cyclically or short term; prepare a calendar of drug days, rest days, and drug-free periods.
- Use vaginal cream properly.
- Potentially serious side effects can occur: cancers, blood clots, liver problems; it is very important that you have periodic medical exams throughout therapy.
- This drug cannot be given to pregnant women because of serious toxic effects to the baby.
- These side effects may occur: nausea, vomiting, bloating; headache, dizziness, mental depression (use caution if driving or performing tasks that require alertness); sensitivity to sunlight (use a sunscreen and wear protective clothing); rash, loss of scalp hair, darkening of the skin on the face; changes in menstrual patterns.
- Report pain in the groin or calves of the legs, chest pain or sudden shortness of breath, abnormal vaginal bleeding, lumps in the breast, sudden severe headache, dizziness or fainting, changes in vision or speech, weakness or numbness in the arm or leg, severe abdominal pain, yellowing of the skin or eyes, severe mental depression, pain at injection site.

▽ estrogens, esterified
(ess' troe jenz)

Estratab, Estromed (CAN), Menest

PREGNANCY CATEGORY X

Drug classes
Hormone
Estrogen

Therapeutic actions
Estrogens are endogenous hormones important in the development of the female reproductive system and secondary sex characteristics. They cause capillary dilatation, fluid retention, protein anabolism, and thin cervical mucus; conserve calcium and phosphorus and encourage bone formation; inhibit ovulation and prevent postpartum breast discomfort. They are responsible for the proliferation of the endometrium; absence or decline of estrogen produces signs and symptoms of menopause on the uterus, vagina, breasts, cervix. Palliation with androgen-dependent prostatic carcinoma is attributable to competition for androgen receptor sites, decreasing the influence of androgens.

Indications
- Palliation of moderate to severe vasomotor symptoms, atrophic vaginitis, or kraurosis vulvae associated with menopause
- Treatment of female hypogonadism; female castration; primary ovarian failure
- Palliation of inoperable prostatic cancer
- Palliation of inoperable, progressing breast cancer in men, postmenopausal women
- Prevention of osteoporosis

Contraindications and cautions
- Contraindicated with allergy to estrogens, breast cancer (with exceptions), estrogen-dependent neoplasm, undiagnosed abnormal genital bleeding, active or past thrombophlebitis or thromboembolic disorders from previous estrogen use, pregnancy (serious fetal defects; women of childbearing age should be advised of the risks and birth control measures suggested).

Adverse effects in *Italics* are most common; those in **Bold** are life-threatening.

- Use cautiously with metabolic bone disease, renal insufficiency, CHF, lactation.

Available forms
Tablets—0.3, 0.625, 1.25, 2.5 mg

Dosages
Administer PO only.
Adults
- *Moderate to severe vasomotor symptoms, atrophic vaginitis, kraurosis vulvae associated with menopause:* 0.3–1.25 mg/day PO. Adjust to lowest effective dose. Cyclic therapy (3 wk of daily estrogen followed by 1 wk of rest from drug therapy) is recommended.
- *Female hypogonadism:* 2.5–7.5 mg/day PO in divided doses for 20 days on/10 days off. If bleeding does not occur by the end of that period, repeat the same dosage schedule. If bleeding does occur before the end of the 10-day rest, begin a 20-day estrogen-progestin cyclic regimen with progestin given orally during the last 5 days of estrogen therapy. If bleeding occurs before end of 10-day rest period, begin a 20-day estrogen-progestin cyclic regimen.
- *Female castration, primary ovarian failure:* Begin a 20-day estrogen-progestin regimen of 2.5–7.5 mg/day PO estrogen in divided doses for 20 days with oral progestin given during the last 5 days of estrogen therapy. If bleeding occurs before the regimen is completed, discontinue therapy and resume on the fifth day of bleeding.
- *Prostatic cancer (inoperable):* 1.25–2.5 mg tid PO. Long-term therapy: judge effectiveness by symptomatic response and serum phosphatase determinations.
- *Breast cancer (inoperable, progressing):* 10 mg tid PO for at least 3 mo in selected men and postmenopausal women.
- *Prevention of osteoporosis:* 0.3 mg/day, increase to a maximum of 1.25 mg/day.
Pediatric patients
Not recommended due to effect on the growth of the long bones.

Pharmacokinetics

Route	Onset	Peak
Oral	Slow	Days

Metabolism: Hepatic; $T_{1/2}$: not known
Distribution: Crosses placenta; enters breast milk
Excretion: Urine

Adverse effects
- **CNS:** Steepening of the corneal curvature with a resultant change in visual acuity and intolerance to contact lenses, *headache,* migraine, dizziness, mental depression, chorea, convulsions
- **CV:** Increased BP, thromboembolic and thrombotic disease (with high doses in certain groups of susceptible women and in men receiving estrogens for prostatic cancer)
- **Dermatologic:** *Photosensitivity, peripheral edema, chloasma,* erythema nodosum or multiforme, hemorrhagic eruption, loss of scalp hair, hirsutism, urticaria, dermatitis
- **GI:** Gallbladder disease (in postmenopausal women), **hepatic adenoma** (rarely occurs, but may rupture and cause death), *nausea, vomiting, abdominal cramps, bloating,* cholestatic jaundice, colitis, acute pancreatitis
- **GU:** Increased risk of endometrial cancer in postmenopausal women, *breakthrough bleeding, change in menstrual flow, dysmenorrhea, premenstrual-like syndrome,* amenorrhea, vaginal candidiasis, cystitis-like syndrome, endometrial cystic hyperplasia
- **Hematologic:** Hypercalcemia (in breast cancer patients with bone metastases), decreased glucose tolerance
- **Other:** Weight changes, reduced carbohydrate tolerance, aggravation of porphyria, edema, changes in libido, breast tenderness

Interactions
✻ **Drug-drug** • Increased therapeutic and toxic effects of corticosteroids • Decreased serum levels of estrogen if taken with drugs that enhance hepatic metabolism of the drug: barbiturates, phenytoin, rifampin

✻ **Drug-lab test** • Increased sulfobromophthalein retention; prothrombin and factors VII, VIII, IX, and X; thyroid-binding globulin with increased PBI, T_4 increased uptake of free T_3 resin (free T_4 is unaltered), serum triglycerides and phospholipid concentration • Decreased antithrombin III, pregnanediol excretion, response to metyrapone test, serum folate concentration • Impaired glucose tolerance

■ Nursing considerations
Assessment
- **History:** Allergy to estrogens; breast cancer, estrogen-dependent neoplasm; undiagnosed abnormal genital bleeding; thrombophlebitis or thromboembolic disorders; pregnancy; lactation; metabolic bone disease; renal insufficiency; CHF
- **Physical:** Skin color, lesions, edema; breast exam; injection site; orientation, affect, reflexes; P, auscultation, BP, peripheral perfusion; R, adventitious sounds; bowel sounds, liver evaluation, abdominal exam; pelvic exam; serum calcium, phosphorus; liver and renal function tests; Pap smear; glucose tolerance test

Interventions
- Arrange for pretreatment and periodic (at least annual) history and physical, which should include BP, breasts, abdomen, pelvic organs, and a Pap smear.
- Caution patient of the risks involved with estrogen use; the need to prevent pregnancy during treatment, for frequent medical follow-up, and for periodic rests from drug treatment.
- Give cyclically for short term only when treating postmenopausal conditions because of the risk of endometrial neoplasm; taper to the lowest effective dose, and provide a drug-free week each month.
- Arrange for the concomitant use of progestin therapy during long-term estrogen therapy in women; this will mimic normal physiologic cycling and allow for cyclic uterine bleeding, which may decrease the risk of endometrial cancer.

Teaching points
- Use this drug in cycles or short term; prepare a calendar of drug days, rest days, and drug-free periods (as appropriate).
- Potentially serious side effects can occur: cancers, blood clots, liver problems; it is very

important that you have periodic medical exams throughout therapy.
- This drug cannot be given to pregnant women because of serious toxic effects to the baby.
- These side effects may occur: nausea, vomiting, bloating; headache, dizziness, mental depression (use caution if driving or performing tasks that require alertness); sensitivity to sunlight (use a sunscreen and wear protective clothing); rash, loss of scalp hair, darkening of the skin on the face; changes in menstrual patterns.
- Report pain in the groin or calves of the legs, chest pain or sudden shortness of breath, abnormal vaginal bleeding, lumps in the breast, sudden severe headache, dizziness or fainting, changes in vision or speech, weakness or numbness in the arm or leg, severe abdominal pain, yellowing of the skin or eyes, severe mental depression.

▷estrone (estrogenic substance, mainly estrone)
(ess' trone)

Estrone Aqueous, Kestrone 5

PREGNANCY CATEGORY X

Drug classes
Hormone
Estrogen

Therapeutic actions
Estrogens are endogenous hormones important in the development of the female reproductive system and secondary sex characteristics. They cause capillary dilatation, fluid retention, protein anabolism, and thin cervical mucus; conserve calcium and phosphorus and encourage bone formation; inhibit ovulation and prevent postpartum breast discomfort. They are responsible for the proliferation of the endometrium; absence or decline of estrogen produces signs and symptoms of menopause on the uterus, vagina, breasts, cervix. Palliation with androgen-dependent prostatic carcinoma is attributable to compe-

tition with androgens for receptor sites, decreasing the influence of androgens.

Indications

- Palliation of moderate to severe vasomotor symptoms, atrophic vaginitis or kraurosis vulvae associated with menopause
- Treatment of female hypogonadism, female castration, primary ovarian failure
- Palliation of inoperable prostatic cancer and breast cancer
- Treatment of abnormal uterine bleeding due to hormone imbalance

Contraindications and cautions

- Contraindicated with allergy to estrogens, breast cancer (with exceptions), estrogen-dependent neoplasm, undiagnosed abnormal genital bleeding, active or previous thrombophlebitis or thromboembolic disorders from estrogen use, pregnancy (serious fetal defects; women of childbearing age should be advised of risks and birth control measures suggested).
- Use cautiously with metabolic bone disease, renal insufficiency, CHF, lactation.

Available forms

Injection—5 mg/mL

Dosages

Administer IM only.
Adults
- *Moderate to severe vasomotor symptoms, atrophic vaginitis, kraurosis vulvae associated with menopause:* 0.1–0.5 mg 2–3 times/wk IM.
- *Female hypogonadism, female castration, primary ovarian failure:* Initially, 0.1–1 mg/wk in single or divided doses IM. 0.5–2 mg/wk has been used in some cases.
- *Prostatic cancer (inoperable):* 2–4 mg 2–3 times/wk IM. Response should occur within 3 mo. If a response does occur, continue drug until disease is again progressive.
- *Breast cancer (inoperable):* 5 mg IM 3 or more times per wk based on pain.
- *Abnormal uterine bleeding due to hormone imbalance:* 2–5 mg IM for several days.
Pediatric patients
Not recommended due to effect on the growth of the long bones.

Pharmacokinetics

Route	Onset	Peak
IM	Slow	Days

Metabolism: Hepatic; $T_{1/2}$: not known
Distribution: Crosses placenta; enters breast milk
Excretion: Urine

Adverse effects

- **CNS:** Steepening of the corneal curvature with a resultant change in visual acuity and intolerance to contact lenses, *headache*, migraine, dizziness, mental depression, chorea, convulsions
- **CV:** Increased BP, thromboembolic and thrombotic disease
- **Dermatologic:** *Photosensitivity, peripheral edema, chloasma,* erythema nodosum or multiforme, hemorrhagic eruption, loss of scalp hair, hirsutism, urticaria, dermatitis
- **GI:** Gallbladder disease (in postmenopausal women), **hepatic adenoma,** *nausea, vomiting, abdominal cramps, bloating,* **cholestatic jaundice,** *colitis,* **acute pancreatitis**
- **GU:** Increased risk of endometrial cancer in postmenopausal women, *breakthrough bleeding, change in menstrual flow, dysmenorrhea, premenstrual-like syndrome,* amenorrhea, vaginal candidiasis, cystitis-like syndrome, endometrial cystic hyperplasia
- **Hematologic:** Hypercalcemia, decreased glucose tolerance
- **Local:** *Pain at injection site,* sterile abscess, postinjection flare
- **Other:** Weight changes, reduced carbohydrate tolerance, aggravation of porphyria, edema, changes in libido, breast tenderness

Interactions

✴ **Drug-drug** ● Increased therapeutic and toxic effects of corticosteroids ● Decreased serum levels of estrogens if taken with drugs that enhance hepatic metabolism of the drug: barbiturates, phenytoin, rifampin

✴ **Drug-lab test** ● Increased sulfobromophthalein retention; prothrombin and factors VII, VIII, IX, and X; thyroid-binding globulin with increased PBI, T_4, increased uptake of free T_3 resin (free T_4 is unaltered), serum triglycerides and phospholipid concentration ● Decreased antithrombin III, pregnanediol excretion, response to metyrapone test, serum folate concentration • Impaired glucose tolerance

■ Nursing considerations
Assessment
- **History:** Allergy to estrogens; breast cancer, estrogen-dependent neoplasm; undiagnosed abnormal genital bleeding; thrombophlebitis or thromboembolic disorders; pregnancy; lactation; metabolic bone disease; renal insufficiency; CHF
- **Physical:** Skin color, lesions, edema; breast exam; injection site; orientation, affect, reflexes; P, auscultation, BP, peripheral perfusion; R, adventitious sounds; bowel sounds, liver evaluation, abdominal exam; pelvic exam; serum calcium, phosphorus; liver and renal function tests; Pap smear; glucose tolerance test

Interventions
- Arrange for pretreatment and periodic (at least annual) history and physical, which should include BP, breasts, abdomen, pelvic organs, and a Pap smear.
- Caution patient of the risks involved with estrogen use, the need to prevent pregnancy during treatment, for frequent medical follow-up, and for periodic rests from drug treatment.
- Give cyclically for short term only when treating postmenopausal conditions because of the risk of endometrial neoplasm. Taper to the lowest effective dose, and provide a drug-free week each month.
- Arrange for the concomitant use of progestin therapy during long-term estrogen therapy in women; this will mimic normal physiologic cycling and allow for a cyclic uterine bleeding, which may decrease the risk of endometrial cancer.
- Administer by deep IM injection only; monitor and rotate injection sites to decrease development of abscesses.

Teaching points
- This drug can only be given IM. Keep a calendar of drug days, rest days, and drug-free periods.

- This drug has potentially serious side effects: cancers, blood clots, liver problems; it is very important that you have periodic medical exams throughout therapy.
- This drug cannot be given to pregnant women because of serious toxic effects to the baby. Use of barrier contraceptives is urged.
- These side effects may occur: nausea, vomiting, bloating; headache, dizziness, mental depression (use caution driving or performing tasks that require alertness); sensitivity to sunlight (use a sunscreen and wear protective clothing); rash, loss of scalp hair, darkening of the skin on the face; changes in menstrual patterns.
- Report pain in the groin or calves of the legs, chest pain or sudden shortness of breath, abnormal vaginal bleeding, lumps in the breast, sudden severe headache, dizziness or fainting, changes in vision or speech, weakness or numbness in the arm or leg, severe abdominal pain, yellowing of the skin or eyes, severe mental depression, pain at injection site.

▽**estropipate**
(piperazine estrone sulfate)
(ess' troe pi' pate)

Ogen, Ortho-Est

PREGNANCY CATEGORY X

Drug classes
Hormone
Estrogen

Therapeutic actions
Estrogens are endogenous female sex hormones important in the development of the female reproductive system and secondary sex characteristics. They cause capillary dilatation, fluid retention, protein anabolism, and thin cervical mucus; conserve calcium and phosphorus and encourage bone formation; inhibit ovulation and prevent postpartum breast discomfort. They are responsible for the proliferation of the endometrium; absence or decline of estrogen produces signs and symp-

---

Adverse effects in *Italics* are most common; those in **Bold** are life-threatening.

toms of menopause on the uterus, vagina, breasts, cervix. Palliation with androgen-dependent prostatic carcinoma is attributable to competition with androgens for receptor sites, decreasing the influence of androgens.

Indications
- Palliation of moderate to severe vasomotor symptoms, atrophic vaginitis, or kraurosis vulvae associated with menopause
- Treatment of female hypogonadism, female castration, primary ovarian failure
- Prevention of osteoporosis

Contraindications and cautions
- Contraindicated with allergy to estrogens, breast cancer (with exceptions), estrogen-dependent neoplasm, undiagnosed abnormal genital bleeding, active or past thrombophlebitis or thromboembolic disorders from previous estrogen use, pregnancy (serious fetal defects; women of childbearing age should be advised of the potential risks and birth control measures suggested).
- Use cautiously with metabolic bone disease, renal insufficiency, CHF, lactation.

Available forms
Tablets—0.625, 1.25, 2.5, 5 mg

Dosages
Adults
- *Moderate to severe vasomotor symptoms, atrophic vaginitis, kraurosis vulvae associated with menopause:* 0.625–5 mg/day PO given cyclically.
- *Female hypogonadism, female castration, primary ovarian failure:* 1.25–7.5 mg/day PO for the first 3 wk, followed by a rest period of 8–10 days. Repeat if bleeding does not occur at end of rest period.
- *Prevention of osteoporosis:* 0.625 mg daily PO for 25 days of a 31-day cycle per month.
Pediatric patients
Not recommended due to effect on the growth of the long bones.

Pharmacokinetics

Route	Onset	Peak
Oral	Slow	Days

Metabolism: Hepatic; $T_{1/2}$: not known

Distribution: Crosses placenta; enters breast milk
Excretion: Urine

Adverse effects
- **CNS:** Steepening of the corneal curvature with a resultant change in visual acuity and intolerance to contact lenses, *headache,* migraine, dizziness, mental depression, chorea, convulsions
- **CV:** Increased BP, thromboembolic and thrombotic disease
- **Dermatologic:** *Photosensitivity, peripheral edema, chloasma,* erythema nodosum or multiforme, hemorrhagic eruption, loss of scalp hair, hirsutism, urticaria, dermatitis
- **GI:** Gallbladder disease (in postmenopausal women), **hepatic adenoma,** *nausea, vomiting, abdominal cramps, bloating,* **cholestatic jaundice,** *colitis,* acute pancreatitis
- **GU:** Increased risk of endometrial cancer in postmenopausal women, *breakthrough bleeding, change in menstrual flow, dysmenorrhea, premenstrual-like syndrome,* amenorrhea, vaginal candidiasis, cystitis-like syndrome, endometrial cystic hyperplasia
- **Hematologic:** Hypercalcemia, decreased glucose tolerance
- **Other:** Weight changes, reduced carbohydrate tolerance, aggravation of porphyria, edema, changes in libido, breast tenderness

Interactions
✳ **Drug-drug** • Increased therapeutic and toxic effects of corticosteroids • Decreased serum levels of estrogens if taken with drugs that enhance hepatic metabolism of the drug: barbiturates, phenytoin, rifampin
✳ **Drug-lab test** • Increased sulfobromophthalein retention; prothrombin and factors VII, VIII, IX, and X; thyroid-binding globulin with increased PBI, T_4, increased uptake of free T_3 resin (free T_4 is unaltered), serum triglycerides and phospholipid concentration • Decreased antithrombin III, pregnanediol excretion, response to metyrapone test, serum folate concentration • Impaired glucose tolerance

■ Nursing considerations
Assessment
- **History:** Allergy to estrogens; breast cancer, estrogen-dependent neoplasm; undiagnosed abnormal genital bleeding; thrombophlebitis or thromboembolic disorders; pregnancy; lactation; metabolic bone disease; renal insufficiency; CHF
- **Physical:** Skin color, lesions, edema; breast exam; injection site; orientation, affect, reflexes; P, auscultation, BP, peripheral perfusion; R, adventitious sounds; bowel sounds, liver evaluation, abdominal exam; pelvic exam; serum calcium, phosphorus; liver and renal function tests; Pap smear; glucose tolerance test

Interventions
- Arrange for pretreatment and periodic (at least annual) history and physical, which should include BP, breasts, abdomen, pelvic organs, and a Pap smear.
- Caution patient of the risks involved with estrogen use, the need to prevent pregnancy during treatment, for frequent medical follow-up, and for periodic rests from drug treatment.
- Give cyclically for short term only when treating postmenopausal conditions because of the risk of endometrial neoplasm. Taper to the lowest effective dose and provide a drug-free week each month.
- Arrange for the concomitant use of progestin therapy during long-term estrogen therapy in women; this will mimic normal physiologic cycling and allow for a cyclic uterine bleeding, which may decrease the risk of endometrial cancer.

Teaching points
- Prepare a calendar of drug days, rest days, and drug-free periods.
- Potentially serious side effects can occur: cancers, blood clots, liver problems; it is very important that you have periodic medical exams throughout therapy.
- This drug cannot be given to pregnant women because of serious toxic effects to the baby.
- These side effects may occur: nausea, vomiting, bloating; headache, dizziness, mental depression (use caution driving or performing tasks that require alertness); sensitivity to sunlight (use a sunscreen and wear protective clothing); rash, loss of scalp hair, darkening of the skin on the face; changes in menstrual patterns.
- Report pain in the groin or calves of the legs, chest pain or sudden shortness of breath, abnormal vaginal bleeding, lumps in the breast, sudden severe headache, dizziness or fainting, changes in vision or speech, weakness or numbness in the arm or leg, severe abdominal pain, yellowing of the skin or eyes, severe mental depression.

▷etanercept
*(ee tah **ner'** sept)*

Enbrel

PREGNANCY CATEGORY B

Drug classes
Antiarthritis drug
Biological response modifier

Therapeutic actions
Genetically engineered tumor necrosis factor receptors from Chinese hamster ovary cells; keep inflammatory response to autoimmune disease in check by reacting with and deactivating free-floating tumor necrosis factor released by active leukocytes.

Indications
- Reduction of the signs and symptoms of moderately to severely active rheumatoid arthritis; to delay the structural damage associated with rheumatoid arthritis, or may be used in combination with methotrexate when patients do not respond to methotrexate alone
- Polyarticular-course juvenile rheumatoid arthritis in patients who have not had an adequate response to one or more antirheumatic drugs
- Reduction of signs and symptoms of psoriatic arthritis; may be used alone or in combination with methotrexate
- Unlabeled uses: psoriatic arthritis, psoriasis

Contraindications and cautions
- Contraindicated with allergy to etanercept or Chinese hamster products, lactation, pregnancy, cancer, severe infection including sepsis, CNS demyelinating disorders, myelosuppression.
- Use cautiously with renal or hepatic disorders, any infection.

Available forms
Powder for injection—25 mg

Dosages
Adults
25 mg SC 2 times/wk with 72–96 hr between doses.
Pediatric patients
4–17 yr: 0.4 mg/kg SC 2 times/wk with 72–96 hr between doses to maximum 25 mg/dose.
< 4 yr: Safety and efficacy not established.

Pharmacokinetics

Route	Onset	Peak
SC	Slow	72 hr

Metabolism: Tissue; $T_{1/2}$: 15 hr
Distribution: Crosses placenta; passes into breast milk
Excretion: Tissues

Adverse effects
- **CNS: CNS demyelinating disorders (multiple sclerosis, myelitis, optic neuritis)**
- **GI:** Abdominal pain, dyspepsia
- **Hematologic: Pancytopenia**
- **Respiratory:** *URIs*, congestion, rhinitis, cough, pharyngitis
- **Other:** *Irritation at injection site;* **increased risk of infections, cancers;** ANA development; headache; autoimmune diseases

■ Nursing considerations
Assessment
- **History:** Allergy to etanercept or Chinese hamster products; pregnancy, lactation; serious infections; cancer; CNS demyelinating disorders, myelosuppression
- **Physical:** Skin lesions, color; R, adventitious sounds; injection site evaluation; ROM to monitor drug effectiveness; CNS—neurologic evaluation, reflexes; CBC

Interventions
- Obtain a baseline and periodic CBC; discontinue drug at signs of severe bone marrow suppression.
- Obtain baseline values of neurologic function; discontinue drug at any sign of CNS demyelinating disorders.
- Advise patient that this drug does not cure the disease and appropriate therapies for rheumatoid arthritis should be used.
- Reconstitute for injection by slowly injecting 1 mL sterile bacteriostatic water provided with powder into the vial; swirl gently, do not shake; avoid foaming; liquid should be clear and free of particulate matter; use within 6 hr of reconstitution. Do not mix with any other medications.
- Rotate injection sites between abdomen, thigh, and upper arm. Maintain a chart to ensure that sites are rotated regularly.
- Teach patient and a significant other how to reconstitute and administer SC injections; observe the process periodically.
- Monitor patient for any sign of infection; discontinue drug if infection occurs.
- Evaluate drug effectiveness periodically; 1–2 wk may be required before any change is noted; if no response has occurred within 3 mo, discontinue drug.
- Do not administer drug with any vaccinations; allow at least 2–3 wk between starting this drug and a vaccination.
- Protect patient from exposure to infections and ensure routine physical examinations and monitoring for potential cancers and autoimmune diseases.

Teaching points
- Take this drug exactly as prescribed. Note that this drug does not cure rheumatoid arthritis and appropriate therapies to deal with the disease should be followed. You and a significant other should learn how to prepare the drug and to administer SC injections. Prepare a chart of injection sites to ensure that sites are rotated on a regular basis. Consult with your health care provider about proper disposal of needles and syringes.
- These side effects may occur: signs and symptoms of upper respiratory infections, cough, sore throat (consult with your health care provider for potential treatment if this becomes severe); headache (analgesics may

be available to help); increased susceptibility to infections (avoid crowded areas and people who might have infections; use strict handwashing and good hygiene).
- Arrange for frequent, regular medical follow-up, including blood tests to follow the effects of the drug on your body.
- Report fever, chills, lethargy; rash, difficulty breathing; swelling; worsening of arthritis; severe diarrhea.

▷ ethacrynic acid
(eth a krin' ik)
Edecrin

ethacrynate sodium
Edecrin Sodium

PREGNANCY CATEGORY B

Drug class
Loop (high ceiling) diuretic

Therapeutic actions
Inhibits the reabsorption of sodium and chloride from the proximal and distal renal tubules and the loop of Henle, leading to a sodium-rich diuresis.

Indications
- Edema associated with CHF, cirrhosis, renal disease
- Acute pulmonary edema (IV)
- Ascites due to malignancy, idiopathic edema, lymphedema
- Short-term management of pediatric patients with congenital heart disease

Contraindications and cautions
- Contraindicated with allergy to ethacrynic acid, electrolyte depletion, anuria, severe renal failure, hepatic coma, SLE, gout, diabetes mellitus, lactation.
- Use cautiously with hypoproteinemia (reduces response to drug).

Available forms
Tablet—25, 50 mg; powder for injection—50 mg/vial

Dosages
Adults
- *Edema:* Initial dose: 50–100 mg/day PO. Adjust dose in 25- to 50-mg intervals. Higher doses, up to 200 mg/day, may be required in refractory patients. Intermittent maintenance dosage is best. When used with other diuretics, give initial dose of 25 mg/day and adjust dosage in 25-mg increments.

Parenteral
Do not give IM or SC–causes pain and irritation. Usual adult dose is 50 mg or 0.5–1 mg/kg run slowly through IV tubing or by direct injection over several minutes. Single dose not to exceed 100 mg. *Not recommended for pediatric patients.*

Pediatric patients
Initial dose of 25 mg PO with careful adjustment of dose by 25-mg increment. Maintain at lowest effective dose. Avoid use in infants.

Pharmacokinetics

Route	Onset	Peak	Duration
Oral	30 min	2 hr	6–8 hr
IV	5 min	15–30 min	2 hr

Metabolism: Hepatic; $T_{1/2}$: 30–70 min
Distribution: Crosses placenta; enters breast milk
Excretion: Urine and bile

▼IV facts
Preparation: Add 50 mL of 5% dextrose injection or sodium chloride injection to the vial of parenteral solution; do not use solution diluted with dextrose if it appears hazy or opalescent. Dextrose solutions may have a low pH. Discard unused solution after 24 hr.
Infusion: Give slowly over several minutes by direct IV injection or into the tubing of actively running IV over 30 min.
Incompatibilities: Do not mix IV solution with whole blood or its derivatives.

Adverse effects
- **CNS:** *Dizziness, vertigo, paresthesias, confusion,* apprehension, fatigue, nystagmus, weakness, headache, drowsiness, blurred vision, tinnitus, irreversible hearing loss
- **CV:** *Orthostatic hypotension,* volume depletion, cardiac arrhythmias, thrombophlebitis

Adverse effects in *Italics* are most common; those in **Bold** are life-threatening.

- **Dermatologic:** *Photosensitivity, rash,* pruritus, urticaria, purpura
- **GI:** *Nausea, anorexia, vomiting, GI bleeding, dysphagia; sudden, profuse watery diarrhea,* acute pancreatitis, jaundice
- **GU:** *Polyuria, nocturia, glycosuria,* hematuria
- **Hematologic:** Leukopenia, anemia, thrombocytopenia, fluid and electrolyte imbalances (hyperuricemia, metabolic alkalosis, hypokalemia, hyponatremia, hypochloremia, hypocalcemia, hyperuricemia, hyperglycemia, increased serum creatinine)
- **Other:** Muscle cramps and muscle spasms

Interactions

✷ Drug-drug • Increased risk of cardiac glycoside (digitalis) toxicity (secondary to hypokalemia) • Increased risk of ototoxicity with aminoglycoside antibiotics, cisplatin • Decreased diuretic effect with NSAIDs

■ Nursing considerations
Assessment

- **History:** Allergy to ethacrynic acid; electrolyte depletion; anuria, severe renal failure; hepatic coma; SLE; gout; diabetes mellitus; hypoproteinemia; lactation
- **Physical:** Skin color, lesions, edema; orientation, reflexes, hearing; P, baseline ECG, BP, orthostatic BP, perfusion; R, pattern, adventitious sounds; liver evaluation, bowel sounds; output patterns; CBC, serum electrolytes (including calcium), blood sugar, liver and renal function tests, uric acid, urinalysis

Interventions

- Administer oral doses with food or milk to prevent GI upset.
- Mark calendars for outpatients if every other day or 3–5 days/wk therapy is the most effective for treating edema.
- Administer early in the day so that increased urination does not disturb sleep.
- Avoid IV use if oral use is at all possible.
- Change injection sites to prevent thrombophlebitis if more than one IV injection is needed.
- Measure and record regular body weights to monitor fluid changes.
- Arrange to monitor serum electrolytes, hydration, liver function during long-term therapy.

- Provide potassium-rich diet or supplemental potassium.

Teaching points

- Record alternate-day therapy on calendar or dated envelopes. Take the drug early in the day, as increased urination will occur. The drug should be taken with food or meals to prevent GI upset.
- Weigh yourself regularly at the same time and in the same clothing; record weight on calendar.
- These side effects may occur: increased volume and frequency of urination; dizziness, feeling faint on arising, drowsiness (avoid rapid position changes; hazardous activities, driving a car; and consumption of alcohol, which can intensify these problems); sensitivity to sunlight (use sunglasses, sunscreen, and wear protective clothing); increased thirst (suck on sugarless lozenges; frequent mouth care may help); loss of body potassium (a potassium-rich diet or potassium supplement will be necessary).
- Report loss or gain of more than 3 lb in 1 day, swelling in your ankles or fingers, unusual bleeding or bruising, dizziness, trembling, numbness, fatigue, muscle weakness or cramps.

▽ethambutol hydrochloride
(e tham' byoo tole)

Etibi (CAN), Myambutol

PREGNANCY CATEGORY B

Drug class
Antituberculous drug (second line)

Therapeutic actions
Inhibits the synthesis of metabolites in growing mycobacterium cells, impairing cell metabolism, arresting cell multiplication, and causing cell death.

Indications
- Treatment of pulmonary tuberculosis in conjunction with at least one other antituberculous drug

Contraindications and cautions
- Contraindicated with allergy to ethambutol; optic neuritis; pregnancy (the safest antituberculous regimen for use in pregnancy is considered to be ethambutol, isoniazid, and rifampin).
- Use cautiously with impaired renal function.

Available forms
Tablets—100, 400 mg

Dosages
Ethambutol is not administered alone; use in conjunction with four other antituberculosis agents.
Adults
- *Initial treatment:* 15 mg/kg/day PO as a single daily oral dose. Continue therapy until bacteriologic conversion has become permanent and maximal clinical improvement has occurred.
- *Retreatment:* 25 mg/kg/day as a single daily oral dose. After 60 days, reduce dose to 15 mg/kg/day as a single daily dose.
Pediatric patients
Not recommended for patients < 13 yr.

Pharmacokinetics

Route	Onset	Peak	Duration
Oral	Rapid	2–4 hr	20–24 hr

Metabolism: Hepatic; $T_{1/2}$: 3.3 hr
Distribution: Crosses placenta; enters breast milk
Excretion: Urine, feces

Adverse effects
- **CNS:** *Optic neuritis* (loss of visual acuity, changes in color perception), *fever, malaise, headache,* dizziness, mental confusion, disorientation, hallucinations, peripheral neuritis
- **GI:** *Anorexia, nausea, vomiting,* GI upset, abdominal pain, transient liver impairment
- **Hypersensitivity:** Allergic reactions—dermatitis, pruritus, anaphylactoid reaction
- **Other:** Toxic epidermal necrolysis, thrombocytopenia, joint pain, acute gout

Interactions
✳ **Drug-drug** • Decreased absorption with aluminum salts

■ Nursing considerations
Assessment
- **History:** Allergy to ethambutol, optic neuritis, impaired renal function
- **Physical:** Skin color, lesions; T, orientation, reflexes, ophthalmologic examination; liver evaluation, bowel sounds; CBC, liver and renal function tests

Interventions
- Administer with food if GI upset occurs.
- Administer in a single daily dose; must be used in combination with other antituberculous agents.
- Arrange for follow-up of liver and renal function tests, CBC, ophthalmologic examinations.

Teaching points
- Take drug in a single daily dose; it may be taken with meals if GI upset occurs.
- Take this drug regularly; avoid missing doses. Do not discontinue this drug without first consulting your health care provider.
- These side effects may occur: nausea, vomiting, epigastric distress; skin rashes or lesions; disorientation, confusion, drowsiness, dizziness (use caution if driving or operating dangerous machinery; use precautions to avoid injury).
- Arrange to have periodic medical checkups, which will include an eye examination and blood tests.
- Report changes in vision (blurring, altered color perception), rash.

▽ **ethchlorvynol**
(eth klor vi' nole)

Placidyl

PREGNANCY CATEGORY C

C-IV CONTROLLED SUBSTANCE

Drug class
Sedative and hypnotic (nonbarbiturate)

Adverse effects in *Italics* are most common; those in **Bold** are life-threatening.

Therapeutic actions

Has sedative, hypnotic, anticonvulsant, and muscle relaxant properties; produces EEG patterns similar to those produced by the barbiturates.

Indications

- Short-term hypnotic therapy for periods up to 1 wk in the management of insomnia; repeat only after drug-free interval of 1 wk or more and further evaluation of the patient
- Treatment of severe insomnia
- Unlabeled use: sedative (dosage of 100–200 mg bid–tid PO)

Contraindications and cautions

- Contraindicated with hypersensitivity to ethchlorvynol, allergy to tartrazine, acute intermittent porphyria, insomnia with pain, lactation, pregnancy.
- Use cautiously with those known to exhibit unpredictable behavior or paradoxical restlessness or excitement with barbiturates or alcohol; impaired hepatic or renal function; addiction-prone and emotionally depressed patients with or without suicidal tendencies.

Available forms

Capsules—200, 500, 750 mg

Dosages

Adults

Individualize dosage. Usual hypnotic dosage is 500 mg PO at bedtime. 750–1,000 mg may be needed for severe insomnia. May supplement with 200 mg PO to reinstitute sleep in patients who awaken during early morning hours after the original bedtime dose of 500 or 750 mg. Do not prescribe for longer than 1 wk.

Pediatric patients

Safety and efficacy not established; not recommended.

Geriatric or debilitated patients

Give the smallest effective dose.

Pharmacokinetics

Route	Onset	Peak	Duration
Oral	15–60 min	2 hr	5 hr

Metabolism: Hepatic; $T_{1/2}$: 10–20 hr
Distribution: Crosses placenta; enters breast milk
Excretion: Urine

Adverse effects

- **CNS:** *Dizziness, facial numbness, transient giddiness and ataxia*, mild hangover, blurred vision
- **Dermatologic:** Urticaria, rash
- **GI:** *Vomiting, gastric upset, nausea,* aftertaste, cholestatic jaundice
- **Hematologic:** Thrombocytopenia
- **Other:** Idiosyncratic reactions: syncope without marked hypotension; mild stimulation; marked excitement, hysteria; prolonged hypnosis; profound muscular weakness; physical, psychological dependence; tolerance; withdrawal reaction

Interactions

✱ **Drug-drug** • Decreased PT response to coumarin anticoagulants, dosage adjustment may be necessary when ethchlorvynol therapy is initiated or discontinued • Exaggerated depressant effects with alcohol, barbiturates, narcotics

■ Nursing considerations
Assessment

- **History:** Hypersensitivity to ethchlorvynol, tartrazine, acute intermittent porphyria, insomnia with unpredictable behavior or paradoxical restlessness or excitement in response to barbiturates or alcohol, impaired hepatic or renal function, addiction-prone patients, emotionally depressed patients with or without suicidal tendencies, lactation, pregnancy
- **Physical:** Skin color, lesions; orientation, affect, reflexes, vision exam; P, BP; bowel sounds, normal output, liver evaluation; CBC with differential, hepatic and renal function tests

Interventions

- Supervise prescription for patients who are addiction prone or likely to increase dosage on their own initiative.
- Dispense least effective amount of drug to patients who are depressed or suicidal.
- Withdraw drug gradually if patient has used drug long term or developed tolerance; supportive therapy similar to that for withdrawal from barbiturates may be necessary.

Teaching points

- Take this drug exactly as prescribed. Take drug with food to reduce GI upset, giddiness, ataxia. Do not exceed prescribed dosage.
- Avoid alcohol, sleep-inducing, or OTC drugs while you are on this drug.
- These side effects may occur: drowsiness, dizziness, blurred vision (avoid driving or performing tasks requiring alertness or visual acuity), GI upset (frequent small meals may help).
- Do not use this drug during pregnancy. Use of barrier contraceptives is recommended.
- Report rash, yellowing of the skin or eyes, bruising.

▽ **ethionamide**
(e thye on am' ide)

Trecator-SC

PREGNANCY CATEGORY C

Drug class

Antituberculous drug (third line)

Therapeutic actions

Bacteriostatic against *Mycobacterium tuberculosis;* mechanism of action is not known.

Indications

- Tuberculosis—any form that is not responsive to first-line antituberculous agents—in conjunction with other antituberculous agents

Contraindications and cautions

- Contraindicated with allergy to ethionamide, pregnancy.
- Use cautiously with hepatic impairment, diabetes mellitus.

Available forms

Tablets—250 mg

Dosages

Adults

Always use with at least one other antituberculous agent: 15–20 mg/kg/day PO up to a maximum 1 g/day; dosage may be divided if

GI upset is intolerable. Concomitant use of pyridoxine is recommended.

Pediatric patients

10–20 mg/kg/day PO in 2–3 divided doses or 15 mg/kg/24 hr as a single daily dose.

Pharmacokinetics

Route	Peak	Duration
Oral	3 hr	9 hr

Metabolism: Hepatic; $T_{1/2}$: 2 hr
Distribution: Crosses placenta; enters breast milk
Excretion: Urine

Adverse effects

- **CNS:** *Depression, drowsiness, asthenia,* convulsions, peripheral neuritis, neuropathy, olfactory disturbances, blurred vision, diplopia, optic neuritis, dizziness, headache, restlessness, tremors, psychosis
- **CV:** Postural hypotension
- **Dermatologic:** Rash, acne, alopecia, thrombocytopenia, pellagra-like syndrome
- **GI:** *Anorexia, nausea, vomiting, diarrhea, metallic taste,* stomatitis, hepatitis
- **Other:** Gynecomastia, impotence, menorrhagia, difficulty managing diabetes mellitus

■ Nursing considerations
Assessment

- **History:** Allergy to ethionamide; hepatic impairment, diabetes mellitus; pregnancy
- **Physical:** Skin color, lesions; orientation, reflexes, ophthalmologic exam, affect; BP, orthostatic BP; liver evaluation; liver function tests, blood and urine glucose

Interventions

- Arrange for culture and sensitivity tests before use.
- Give only with other antituberculous agent.
- Arrange for follow-up of liver function tests prior to and every 2–4 wk during therapy.
- Monitor diabetic patients carefully.
- Caution patient to avoid pregnancy.

Teaching points

- Take drug once a day; take with food if GI upset occurs. Dose may be divided if GI upset is severe.

Adverse effects in *Italics* are most common; those in **Bold** are life-threatening.

- Take this drug regularly; avoid missing doses. Do not discontinue this drug without first consulting health care provider.
- Do not use this drug during pregnancy; serious fetal abnormalities have been reported. Use of barrier contraceptives is advised.
- These side effects may occur: loss of appetite, nausea, vomiting, metallic taste in mouth, increased salivation (take the drug with food, frequent mouth care, small frequent meals may help), diarrhea; drowsiness, depression, dizziness, blurred vision (use caution operating a car or dangerous machinery; change position slowly; avoid injury); impotence, menstrual difficulties.
- Arrange to have regular, periodic medical checkups, including blood tests.
- Report unusual bleeding or bruising, severe GI upset, severe changes in vision.

▷ ethosuximide
(eth oh sux' i mide)

Zarontin

PREGNANCY CATEGORY C

Drug classes
Antiepileptic
Succinimide

Therapeutic actions
Suppresses the EEG pattern associated with lapses of consciousness in absence (petit mal) seizures; reduces frequency of attacks; mechanism of action not understood, but may act in inhibitory neuronal systems.

Indications
- Control of absence (petit mal) seizures; may be given in combination with other anticonvulsants

Contraindications and cautions
- Contraindicated with hypersensitivity to succinimides, lactation.
- Use cautiously with hepatic, renal abnormalities; pregnancy.

Available forms
Capsules—250 mg; syrup—250 mg/5 mL

Dosages
Adults
Initial dosage is 500 mg/day PO. Increase by small increments to maintenance level. One method is to increase the daily dose by 250 mg every 4–7 days until control is achieved with minimal side effects. Administer dosages > 1.5 g/day in divided doses only under strict supervision (compatible with other antiepileptics when other forms of epilepsy coexist with absence seizures).

Pediatric patients
3–6 yr: Initial dose is 250 mg/day PO. Increase as described for adults above.
≥ 6 yr: Adult dosage.

Pharmacokinetics

Route	Peak
Oral	3–7 hr

Metabolism: Hepatic; $T_{1/2}$: 30 hr in children, 60 hr in adults
Distribution: Crosses placenta; enters breast milk
Excretion: Urine, bile

Adverse effects
Succinimides
- **CNS:** *Drowsiness, ataxia, dizziness, irritability, nervousness, headache, blurred vision,* myopia, photophobia, hiccups, euphoria, dreamlike state, lethargy, hyperactivity, fatigue, insomnia, increased frequency of grand mal seizures may occur when used alone in some patients with mixed types of epilepsy, confusion, instability, mental slowness, depression, hypochondriacal behavior, sleep disturbances, night terrors, aggressiveness, inability to concentrate
- **Dermatologic: Stevens-Johnson syndrome,** *pruritus, urticaria,* pruritic erythematous rashes, skin eruptions, erythema multiforme, systemic lupus erythematosus, alopecia, hirsutism
- **GI:** *Nausea, vomiting, vague gastric upset, epigastric and abdominal pain, cramps, anorexia, diarrhea, constipation, weight loss,* swelling of tongue, gum hypertrophy
- **Hematologic:** Eosinophilia, granulocytopenia, leukopenia, agranulocytosis, aplastic anemia, monocytosis, **pancytopenia**

- **Other:** Vaginal bleeding, periorbital edema, hyperemia, muscle weakness, abnormal liver and kidney function tests

Interactions
✱ **Drug-drug** • Decreased serum levels of primidone

■ Nursing considerations
Assessment
- **History:** Hypersensitivity to succinimides; hepatic, renal abnormalities; lactation, pregnancy
- **Physical:** Skin color, lesions; orientation, affect, reflexes, bilateral grip strength, vision exam; bowel sounds, normal output, liver evaluation; liver and kidney function tests, urinalysis, CBC with differential, EEG

Interventions
- Reduce dosage, discontinue, or substitute other antiepileptic medication gradually; abrupt discontinuation may precipitate absence (petit mal) status.
- Monitor CBC and differential before and frequently during therapy.
- Discontinue drug if rash, depression of blood count, or unusual depression, aggressiveness, or behavioral alterations occur.
- Arrange counseling for women of childbearing age who need long-term maintenance therapy with antiepileptic drugs and who wish to become pregnant.
- Evaluate for therapeutic serum levels (40–100 mcg/mL).

Teaching points
- Take this drug exactly as prescribed. Do not discontinue this drug abruptly or change dosage.
- Avoid alcohol, sleep-inducing, or OTC drugs while you are on this drug.
- Arrange for frequent checkups to monitor this drug; keep all appointments for checkups.
- These side effects may occur: drowsiness, dizziness, confusion, blurred vision (avoid driving or performing tasks requiring alertness or visual acuity); GI upset (take the drug with food or milk and eat frequent small meals).

- Wear a medical ID at all times so that any emergency medical personnel will know that you are an epileptic taking antiepileptic medication.
- Report rash, joint pain, unexplained fever, sore throat, unusual bleeding or bruising, drowsiness, dizziness, blurred vision, pregnancy.

▷ **ethotoin**
(*eth' i toe in*)

Peganone

PREGNANCY CATEGORY D

Drug classes
Antiepileptic
Hydantoin

Therapeutic actions
Has antiepileptic activity without causing general CNS depression; stabilizes neuronal membranes and prevents hyperexcitability caused by excessive stimulation; limits the spread of seizure activity from an active focus.

Indications
- Control of grand mal (tonic-clonic) and psychomotor seizures; may be combined with other anticonvulsants

Contraindications and cautions
- Contraindicated with hypersensitivity to hydantoins, pregnancy, lactation, hepatic abnormalities, hematologic disorders.
- Use cautiously with acute intermittent porphyria; hypotension, severe myocardial insufficiency; diabetes mellitus, hyperglycemia.

Available forms
Tablets—250, 500 mg

Dosages
Administer in 4–6 divided doses daily. Take after eating; space as evenly as possible.
Adults
Initial dose should be ≤ 1 g/day PO. Increase gradually over several days; maintenance from

2–3 g/day PO in 4–6 divided doses; < 2 g/day is ineffective in most adults. If replacing another drug, reduce the dose of the other drug gradually as ethotoin dose is increased.

Pediatric patients
Initial dose should not exceed 750 mg/day PO in 4–6 divided doses; maintenance doses range from 500 mg/day to 1 g/day PO.

Pharmacokinetics

Route	Onset	Peak
Oral	Rapid	1–3 hr

Metabolism: Hepatic; $T_{1/2}$: 3–9 hr
Distribution: Crosses placenta; enters breast milk
Excretion: Urine

Adverse effects

- **CNS:** *Nystagmus, ataxia, dysarthria, slurred speech, mental confusion, dizziness, drowsiness, insomnia, transient nervousness, motor twitchings, fatigue, irritability, depression, numbness, tremor, headache,* photophobia, diplopia, conjunctivitis
- **Dermatologic:** Scarlatiniform, morbilliform, maculopapular, urticarial and nonspecific rashes; also serious and sometimes fatal dermatologic reactions: bullous, exfoliative, or purpuric dermatitis, lupus erythematosus, and **Stevens-Johnson syndrome;** toxic epidermal necrolysis, hirsutism, alopecia, coarsening of the facial features, enlargement of the lips, Peyronie's disease
- **GI:** *Nausea,* vomiting, diarrhea, constipation, *gingival hyperplasia,* toxic hepatitis, **liver damage,** hypersensitivity reactions with hepatic involvement, including hepatocellular degeneration and **hepatocellular necrosis**
- **GU:** Nephrosis
- **Hematologic: Thrombocytopenia, leukopenia, granulocytopenia, agranulocytosis, pancytopenia; macrocytosis and megaloblastic anemia that usually respond to folic acid therapy; eosinophilia, monocytosis, leukocytosis, simple anemia, hemolytic anemia, aplastic anemia, hyperglycemia**
- **Respiratory: Pulmonary fibrosis,** acute pneumonitis
- **Other:** Lymph node hyperplasia, sometimes progressing to frank malignant lymphoma, monoclonal gammopathy and multiple myeloma (prolonged therapy), polyarthropathy, osteomalacia, weight gain, chest pain, periarteritis nodosa

Interactions

✳ Drug-drug • Increased pharmacologic effects with chloramphenicol, cimetidine, disulfiram, isoniazid, phenacemide, phenylbutazone, sulfonamides, trimethoprim • Complex interactions and effects when hydantoins and valproic acid are given together: toxicity with apparently normal serum ethotoin levels; decreased plasma levels of valproic acid given with hydantoins; breakthrough seizures when the two drugs are given together • Decreased pharmacologic effects with antineoplastics, diazoxide, folic acid, rifampin, theophyllines • Increased pharmacologic effects and toxicity with primidone, oxyphenbutazone, fluconazole, amiodarone • Increased hepatotoxicity with acetaminophen • Decreased pharmacologic effects of the following drugs: corticosteroids, cyclosporine, disopyramide, doxycycline, estrogens, levodopa, methadone, metyrapone, mexiletine, hormonal contraceptives, carbamazepine

✳ Drug-lab test • Interference with the metyrapone and the 1-mg dexamethasone tests; avoid the use of hydantoins for at least 7 days prior to metyrapone testing

■ Nursing considerations
Assessment

- **History:** Hypersensitivity to hydantoins; hepatic abnormalities; hematologic disorders; acute intermittent porphyria; hypotension, severe myocardial insufficiency; diabetes mellitus, hyperglycemia; pregnancy; lactation
- **Physical:** T; skin color, lesions; lymph node palpation; orientation, affect, reflexes, vision exam; P, BP; R, adventitious sounds; bowel sounds, normal output, liver evaluation; periodontal exam; liver function tests, urinalysis, CBC and differential, blood proteins, blood and urine glucose, EEG and ECG

Interventions

- Give after food to enhance absorption and reduce GI upset; give in 4–6 divided doses.

- Administer with other anticonvulsants to regulate seizures; not compatible with phenacemide.
- Reduce dosage, discontinue, or substitute other antiepileptic medication gradually; abrupt discontinuation may precipitate status epilepticus.
- Discontinue drug if rash, depression of blood count, enlarged lymph nodes, hypersensitivity reaction, signs of liver damage, or Peyronie's disease (induration of the corpora cavernosa of the penis) occurs. Institute another antiepileptic drug promptly.
- Monitor hepatic function periodically during long-term therapy; monitor blood counts, urinalysis monthly.
- Monitor urine sugar of patients with diabetes mellitus regularly. Adjustment of dosage of hypoglycemic drug may be necessary because antiepileptic drug may inhibit insulin release and induce hyperglycemia.
- Arrange to have lymph node enlargement occurring during therapy evaluated carefully. Lymphadenopathy, which simulates Hodgkin's disease, has occurred. Lymph node hyperplasia may progress to lymphoma.
- Monitor blood proteins to detect early malfunction of the immune system (multiple myeloma).
- Arrange dental consultation for patients on long-term therapy; proper oral hygiene can prevent development of gum hyperplasia.
- Arrange counseling for women of childbearing age who need long-term maintenance therapy with antiepileptic drugs and who wish to become pregnant.

Teaching points
- Take this drug exactly as prescribed, after food to enhance absorption and reduce GI upset.
- Do not discontinue this drug abruptly or change dosage.
- Maintain good oral hygiene—regular brushing and flossing—to prevent gum disease while you are taking this drug.
- Arrange frequent dental checkups to prevent serious gum disease.
- Arrange for frequent checkups to monitor your response to this drug; keep all appointments for checkups.

- Monitor your urine sugar regularly, and report any abnormality if you are a diabetic.
- Use some form of contraception, other than birth control pills, while you are on this drug. This drug is not recommended for use during pregnancy. If you wish to become pregnant, discuss with health care provider.
- These side effects may occur: drowsiness, dizziness, confusion, blurred vision (avoid driving or performing tasks requiring alertness or visual acuity); GI upset (take the drug with food and eat frequent small meals).
- Wear a medical alert tag at all times so that any emergency medical personnel will know that you are an epileptic taking antiepileptic medication.
- Report rash, severe nausea or vomiting, drowsiness, slurred speech, impaired coordination, swollen glands, bleeding, swollen or tender gums, yellowish discoloration of the skin or eyes, joint pain, unexplained fever, sore throat, unusual bleeding or bruising, persistent headache, malaise, any indication of an infection or bleeding tendency, abnormal erection, pregnancy.

▷ **etidronate disodium**
(e tid' ro nate)

Didronel, Didronel IV

PREGNANCY CATEGORY C (PARENTERAL)

PREGNANCY CATEGORY B (ORAL)

Drug classes
Bisphosphonate
Calcium regulator

Therapeutic actions
Slows normal and abnormal bone resorption; reduces bone formation.

Indications
- Treatment of Paget's disease of bone (oral)
- Treatment of heterotopic ossification (oral)
- Treatment of hypercalcemia of malignancy in patients inadequately managed by diet or oral hydration (parenteral)

Adverse effects in *Italics* are most common; those in **Bold** are life-threatening.

- Treatment of hypercalcemia of malignancy which persists after adequate hydration has been restored (parenteral)
- Unlabeled use: treatment of postmenopausal osteoporosis and prevention of early menopausal bone loss

Contraindications and cautions
- Contraindicated with allergy to bisphosphonates; hypocalcemia, pregnancy, lactation, severe renal impairment.
- Use cautiously with renal dysfunction, upper GI disease.

Available forms
Tablets—200, 400 mg; injection—300 mg/amp

Dosages
Adults
- *Paget's disease:* 5–10 mg/kg/day PO for up to 6 mo; or 11–20 mg/kg/day PO for up to 3 mo. If retreatment is needed, wait at least 90 days between treatment regimens.
- *Heterotopic ossification:* 20 mg/kg/day PO for 2 wk followed by 10 mg/kg/day PO for 10 wk (following spinal cord injury); 20 mg/kg/day PO for 1 mo preoperatively if due to total hip replacement, then 20 mg/kg/day PO for 3 mo post-op.
- *Hypercalcemia of malignancy:* 7.5 mg/kg/day IV for 3 successive days.

Pediatric patients
Safety and efficacy not established.

Patients with renal impairment
Use caution and monitor patient frequently.

Pharmacokinetics

Route	Onset	Duration
Oral	Slow	90 days
IV	Rapid	Days

Metabolism: Not metabolized; $T_{1/2}$: 6 hr
Distribution: Crosses placenta; may pass into breast milk
Excretion: Urine

▼ IV facts
Preparation: Dilute daily dose in 250 mL normal saline for infusion; store at room temperature.
Infusion: Infuse over at least 2 hr.

Adverse effects
- **CNS:** *Headache*
- **GI:** *Nausea, diarrhea,* altered taste, metallic taste
- **Hematological:** Elevated BUN, serum creatinine
- **Skeletal:** *Increased or recurrent bone pain,* focal osteomalacia

Interactions
✱ **Drug-drug** • Increased risk of GI distress with aspirin • Decreased absorption with antacids, calcium, iron, multivalent cations; separate dosing by at least 30 min
✱ **Drug-food** • Significantly decreased absorption and serum levels if taken with any food; administer on an empty stomach 2 hr before meals

■ Nursing considerations
Assessment
- **History:** Allergy to bisphosphonates, renal failure, upper GI disease, lactation, pregnancy
- **Physical:** Muscle tone, bone pain; bowel sounds; urinalysis, serum calcium, renal function tests

Interventions
- Administer with a full glass of water, 2 hr before meals.
- Monitor serum calcium levels before, during, and after therapy.
- Ensure 3-mo rest period after treatment for Paget's disease if retreatment is required, 7 days between treatments for hypercalcemia of malignancy.
- Ensure adequate vitamin days and calcium intake.
- Provide comfort measures if bone pain returns.

Teaching points
- Take this drug with a full glass of water 2 hr before meals.
- Periodic blood tests may be required to monitor your calcium levels.
- These side effects may occur: nausea, diarrhea, bone pain, headache (analgesics may be available to help).
- Report twitching, muscle spasms, dark-colored urine, severe diarrhea.

▽ etodolac
*(ee toe **doe'** lak)*

Lodine, Lodine XL, Ultradol (CAN)

PREGNANCY CATEGORY C

Drug classes
Analgesic (non-narcotic)
Antipyretic
NSAID

Therapeutic actions
Inhibits prostaglandin synthetase to cause antipyretic and anti-inflammatory effects; the exact mechanism of action is not known.

Indications
- Acute or long-term use in the management of signs and symptoms of osteoarthritis and rheumatoid arthritis
- Management of pain (*Lodine*)
- Unlabeled uses: ankylosing spondylitis, tendinitis, bursitis, gout

Contraindications and cautions
- Contraindicated with significant renal impairment, pregnancy, lactation.
- Use cautiously with impaired hearing, allergies, hepatic, cardiovascular, and GI conditions.

Available forms
Capsules—200, 300 mg; tablets—400, 500 mg; ER capsules—400, 500, 600 mg

Dosages
Adults
- *Osteoarthritis, rheumatoid arthritis:* Initially 800—1,200 mg/day PO in divided doses; maintenance ranges 600—1,200 mg/day in divided doses. Do not exceed 1,200 mg/day. Patients < 60 kg: Do not exceed 20 mg/kg. Sustained release: 400—1,000 mg/day PO; adjust based on patient response.
- *Analgesia, acute pain:* 200—400 mg q 6—8 hr PO. Do not exceed 1,200 mg/day. Patients < 60 kg: Do not exceed 20 mg/kg.
Pediatric patients
Safety and efficacy not established.

Pharmacokinetics

Route	Onset	Peak
Oral	Varies	1–2 hr
Oral (SR)	Slow	7.3 hr

Metabolism: Hepatic; $T_{1/2}$: 7.3 hr, 8.3 hr (SR)
Distribution: Crosses placenta; enters breast milk
Excretion: Urine and feces

Adverse effects
- **CNS:** *Dizziness,* somnolence, insomnia, fatigue, tiredness, tinnitus, ophthalmologic effects
- **Dermatologic:** Rash, pruritus, sweating, dry mucous membranes, stomatitis
- **GI:** *Nausea, dyspepsia, GI pain, diarrhea,* vomiting, *constipation,* flatulence, **bleeding ulcers**
- **GU:** Dysuria, **renal impairment or insufficiency**
- **Hematologic:** Bleeding, platelet inhibition with higher doses
- **Other:** Peripheral edema, **anaphylactoid reactions** to fatal anaphylactic shock

Interactions
✳ **Drug-drug** ● Increased risk of bleeding if combined with anticoagulants, antiplatelet drugs ● Possible decreased effectiveness of antihypertensives if taken with etodolac

■ Nursing considerations

 CLINICAL ALERT!
Name confusion has occurred between Lodine (etodolac) and iodine and Lodine and codeine; use caution.

Assessment
- **History:** Renal impairment, impaired hearing, allergies, hepatic, CV, and GI conditions, lactation, pregnancy
- **Physical:** Skin color and lesions; orientation, reflexes, ophthalmologic and audiometric evaluation, peripheral sensation; P, edema; R, adventitious sounds; liver evaluation; CBC, clotting times, renal and liver function tests; serum electrolytes, stool guaiac

Interventions

- Give with food or after meals if GI upset occurs.
- Arrange for periodic ophthalmologic examination during long-term therapy.
- Institute emergency procedures if overdose occurs (gastric lavage, induction of emesis, supportive therapy).

Teaching points

- Take with food or meals if GI upset occurs.
- Take only the prescribed dosage.
- Dizziness, drowsiness can occur (avoid driving or the use of dangerous machinery while on this drug).
- Report sore throat, fever, rash, itching, weight gain, swelling in ankles or fingers; changes in vision; black, tarry stools.

▽ etoposide (VP-16-213)

*(e toe **poe'** side)*

Etopophos, Toposar, VePesid

PREGNANCY CATEGORY D

Drug classes

Mitotic inhibitor
Antineoplastic agent

Therapeutic actions

G_2 specific cell toxic: lyses cells entering mitosis; inhibits cells from entering prophase; inhibits DNA synthesis, leading to cell death.

Indications

- Refractory testicular tumors as part of combination therapy
- Treatment of small-cell lung carcinoma as part of combination therapy

Contraindications and cautions

- Allergy to etoposide, bone marrow suppression, pregnancy, lactation.

Available forms

Capsules—50 mg; injection—20 mg/mL; powder for injection—100 mg

Dosages

Modify dosage based on myelosuppression.

Adults

- *Testicular cancer:* 50–100 mg/m^2 per day IV on days 1 to 5 or 100 mg/m^2 per day IV on days 1, 3, and 5, every 3–4 wk in combination with other agents.
- *Small-cell lung cancer:* 35 mg/m^2 per day IV for 4 days to 50 mg/m^2 per day for 5 days; repeat every 3–4 wk after recovery from toxicity.

Oral

Two times the IV dose rounded to the nearest 50 mg.

Pediatric patients

Safety and efficacy not established.

Patients with renal impairment

If creatinine clearance is < 50 mL/mm, reduce dosage and monitor patient closely.

Pharmacokinetics

Route	Onset	Peak	Duration
Oral	30–60 min	60–90 min	20–30 hr
IV	30 min	60 min	20–30 hr

Metabolism: Hepatic; $T_{1/2}$: 4–11 hr
Distribution: Crosses placenta; enters breast milk
Excretion: Urine and bile

▼ IV facts

Preparation: Dilute with 5% dextrose injection or 0.9% sodium chloride injection to give a concentration of 0.2 or 0.4 mg/mL. Unopened vials are stable at room temperature for 2 yr; diluted solutions are stable at room temperature for 2 (0.4 mg/mL) or 4 (0.2 mg/mL) days.
Infusion: Administer slowly over 30–60 min. Do not give by rapid IV push.

Adverse effects

- **CNS:** *Somnolence, fatigue,* peripheral neuropathy
- **CV:** Hypotension (after rapid IV administration)
- **Dermatologic:** *Alopecia*
- **GI:** *Nausea, vomiting, anorexia, diarrhea,* stomatitis, aftertaste, liver toxicity
- **Hematologic:** *Myelotoxicity*
- **Hypersensitivity:** Chills, fever, tachycardia, bronchospasm, dyspnea, anaphylactic-like reaction
- **Other:** Potentially, carcinogenesis

■ Nursing considerations
Assessment
- **History:** Allergy to etoposide; bone marrow suppression; pregnancy; lactation
- **Physical:** T; weight; hair; orientation, reflexes; BP, P; mucous membranes, abdominal exam; CBC

Interventions
- Do not administer IM or SC; severe local reaction and tissue necrosis occur.
- Avoid skin contact with this drug; use rubber gloves; if contact occurs, immediately wash with soap and water.
- Monitor BP during administration; if hypotension occurs, discontinue dose and consult with physician. Fluids and other supportive therapy may be needed.
- Obtain platelet count, Hgb, WBC count, differential before starting therapy and prior to each dose. If severe response occurs, discontinue therapy and consult with physician.
- Arrange for an antiemetic for severe nausea and vomiting.
- Arrange for wig or other suitable head covering before alopecia occurs. Teach patient the importance of covering the head at extremes of temperature.

Teaching points
- Keep a calendar for specific treatment days and additional courses of therapy.
- Avoid pregnancy while on this drug; use of barrier contraceptives is advised.
- These side effects may occur: loss of appetite, nausea, vomiting, mouth sores (frequent mouth care, small frequent meals may help; try to maintain good nutrition; a dietitian may be able to help, and an antiemetic may be ordered); loss of hair (arrange for a wig or other suitable head covering before the hair loss occurs; it is important to keep the head covered at extremes of temperature).
- Have regular blood tests to monitor the drug's effects.
- Report severe GI upset, diarrhea, vomiting, unusual bleeding or bruising, fever, chills, sore throat, difficulty breathing.

▽ exemestane

See *Less Commonly Used Drugs,* p. 1342.

▽ ezetimibe
(ee zet' ah mib)

Zetia

PREGNANCY CATEGORY C

Drug classes
Cholesterol-lowering agent
Cholesterol absorption inhibitor

Therapeutic actions
Localizes in the brush border of the small intestine and inhibits the absorption of cholesterol from the small intestine; this leads to a decrease delivery of dietary cholesterol to the liver, which will then increase the clearance of cholesterol from the blood and lead to a decrease in serum cholesterol.

Indications
- As an adjunct to diet and exercise to lower the cholesterol, LDL and Apo-B levels in patients with primary hypercholesterolemia as monotherapy or in combination with HMG CoA reductase inhibitors (statins) or bile acid sequestrants
- In combination with atorvastatin or simvastatin for the treatment of homozygous familial hypercholesterolemia as adjuncts to other lipid-lowering treatments
- As adjunctive therapy to diet for the treatment of homozygous sitosterolemia to reduce elevated sitosterol and campesterol levels

Contraindications and cautions
- Contraindicated with allergy to any component of the drug. If given in combination with an HMG CoA reductase inhibitor, contraindicated with pregnancy, lactation, active liver disease, or unexplained persistent increases in serum transaminase levels.
- In monotherapy, use cautiously with liver dysfunction, pregnancy, lactation, elderly patients.

Adverse effects in *Italics* are most common; those in **Bold** are life-threatening.

Pharmacokinetics

Route	Onset	Peak
Oral	Moderate	4–12 hr

Metabolism: Small intestine and hepatic; $T_{1/2}$: 22 hr
Distribution: May cross placenta; may enter into breast milk
Excretion: Feces and urine

Available forms
Tablets—10 mg

Dosages
Adults
10 mg/day PO taken without regard to food; may be taken at the same time as an HMG CoA reductase inhibitor; if combined with a bile acid sequestrant, should be taken ≥ 2 hr before or ≥ 4 hr after the bile acid sequestrant.
Pediatric patients
Safety and efficacy not established.

Adverse effects
- **CNS:** Headache, dizziness, fatigue
- **GI:** Abdominal pain, diarrhea
- **Respiratory:** Pharyngitis, sinusitis, *upper respiratory infection, cough*
- **Other:** Back pain, myalgia, arthralgia, viral infection

Interactions
✱ **Drug-drug** • Increased serum levels and decreased effectiveness of ezetimibe if combined with cholestryamine, fenofibrate, gemfibrozil; monitor patient closely and space exetimibe dosing ≥ 2 hr before or ≥ 4 hr after the other drug • Risk of cholethiasis if combined with fibrates • Risk of increased levels and toxicity of exetimibe if combined with cyclosporine; if this combination is used; monitor patient very carefully.

■ Nursing considerations
Assessment
- **History:** Allergy to any component of the drug; pregnancy, liver dysfunction, lactation, evidence of diet and exercise program
- **Physical:** Skin lesions, color, temperature; orientation, affect; liver evaluation, bowel sounds; lipid studies, liver function tests

Interventions
- Monitor serum cholesterol, LDLs, triglycerides before starting treatment and periodically during treatment.
- Determine that patient has been on low cholesterol diet and exercise program for at least 2 wk before starting ezetimibe.
- If used as part of combination therapy; give drug at the same time as HMG CoA reductase inhibitors and ≥ 2 hr before or ≥ 4 hr after bile acid sequestrants.
- Encourage the use of barrier contraceptives if used with an HMG CoA reductase inhibitor.
- Help mother to find another method of feeding her baby if this drug is needed for a nursing woman, it is not known if the drug passes into breast milk.
- Consult with dietitian regarding low cholesterol diets and provide information about exercise programs.
- Arrange for regular follow-up during long-term therapy.

Teaching points
- Take drug once each day at a time that is easy for you to remember. Do not take more than one tablet per day.
- Continue to take any other lipid-lowering drugs that have been prescribed for you. If you are also taking a bile acid sequestrant, take this drug at least 2 hr before or at least 4 hr after the bile sequestrant.
- Continue to follow your low-fat diet and participate in an exercise program.
- Plan to return for periodic blood tests, including tests of liver function and cholesterol levels, to evaluate the effectiveness of this drug.
- These side effects may occur: abdominal pain, diarrhea (these usually pass with time, notify your health care provider if this becomes a problem); dizziness, (avoid driving and operating dangerous machinery until you know how this drug affects you); headache (analgesics may help).
- Report unusual muscle pain, weakness, or tenderness; severe diarrhea; respiratory infections.

E

▷factor IX concentrates

AlphaNine SD, BeneFix, Bepulin VH, Immunine VH (CAN), Mononine, Profilnine SD, Proplex T

PREGNANCY CATEGORY C

Drug class
Antihemophilic agent

Therapeutic actions
Human factor IX complex consists of plasma fractions involved in the intrinsic pathway of blood coagulation; causes an increase in blood levels of clotting factors II, VII, IX, and X.

Indications
- Factor IX deficiency (hemophilia B, Christmas disease) to prevent or control bleeding
- Bleeding episodes in patients with factor VII deficiency with inhibitors to factor VIII (*Proplex T* only)
- Prevention or control of bleeding episodes in patients with factor VII deficiency (*Proplex T* only)

Contraindications and cautions
- Factor VII deficiencies (except as listed above for *Proplex T*); liver disease with signs of intravascular coagulation or fibrinolysis; do not use if hypersensitive to mouse or hamster protein (*Mononine* or *Benefix*)

Available forms
Injection—varies with brand, see label

Dosages
Dosage depends on severity of deficiency and severity of bleeding; follow treatment carefully with factor IX level assays. To calculate dosage, use the following formula: Dose = 1 unit/kg × body weight (kg) × desired increase (% of normal). Administer daily–bid (once every 2–3 days may suffice to maintain lower effective levels) IV.

Adults and pediatric patients
- *Surgery:* Maintain levels > 25% for at least 1 wk. Calculate dose to raise level to 40%–60% of normal.

- *Hemarthroses:* In hemophiliacs with inhibitors to factor VIII, dosage levels approximate 75 units/kg IV. Give a second dose after 12 hr if needed.
- *Maintenance dose:* Dose is usually 10–20 units/kg/day IV. Individualize dose based on patient response.
- *Inhibitor patients (hemophilia A patients with inhibitors to factor VIII):* 75 units/kg IV; give a second dose after 12 hr if needed.
- *Reversal of coumadin effect:* 15 units/kg IV is suggested.
- *Prophylaxis:* 10–20 units/kg IV once or twice a week may prevent spontaneous bleeding in hemophilia B patients. Individualize dose. Increase dose if patient is exposed to trauma or surgery.

Pharmacokinetics

Route	Onset	Duration
IV	Immediate	1–2 days

Metabolism: Plasma; $T_{1/2}$: 24–32 hr
Distribution: Crosses placenta; enters breast milk

▽IV facts
Preparation: Prepare using diluents and needles supplied with product. Refrigerate.
Infusion: Infuse slowly. 100 units/min and 2–3 mL/min have been suggested. Do not exceed 3 mL/min, and stop or slow the infusion at any sign of headache; pulse, or BP changes.

Adverse effects
- **CNS:** *Headache,* flushing, chills, tingling, somnolence, lethargy
- **GI:** *Nausea,* vomiting, **hepatitis** (risk associated with use of blood products)
- **Hematologic:** *Thrombosis,* DIC, **AIDS** (risk associated with use of blood products; not as common with preparations treated with solvent detergents)
- **Other:** Chills, fever; blood pressure changes, urticaria

■ Nursing considerations
Assessment
- **History:** Factor VII deficiencies; liver disease with signs of intravascular coagulation or fibrinolysis

- **Physical:** Skin color, lesions; T; orientation, reflexes, affect; P, BP, peripheral perfusion; clotting factor levels, liver function tests

Interventions
- Administer by IV route only.
- Decrease rate of infusion if headache, flushing, fever, chills, tingling, urticaria occur; in some individuals, the drug will need to be discontinued.
- Monitor patient's clinical response and factors IX, II, VII, X levels regularly, and regulate dosage based on response.
- Monitor patient for any sign of thrombosis; use comfort and preventive measures when possible (exercise, support stockings, ambulation, positioning).

Teaching points
- Dosage varies widely. Safety precautions are taken to ensure that this blood product is pure and the risk of AIDS and hepatitis is minimal.
- Wear or carry a medical ID to alert emergency medical personnel that you require this treatment.
- Report headache, rash, chills, calf pain, swelling, unusual bleeding, or bruising.

▷famciclovir sodium
(fam sye' kloe vir)

Famvir

PREGNANCY CATEGORY B

Drug class
Antiviral

Therapeutic actions
Antiviral activity; inhibits viral DNA replication in acute herpes zoster.

Indications
- Management of acute herpes zoster (shingles)
- Treatment of recurrent episodes of genital herpes

Contraindications and cautions
- Contraindicated with hypersensitivity to famciclovir or acyclovir, lactation.
- Use cautiously with cytopenia, history of cytopenic reactions, pregnancy, impaired renal function.

Available forms
Tablets—125, 250, 500 mg

Dosages
Adults
- *Herpes zoster:* 500 mg q 8 hr PO for 7 days.
- *Genital herpes:* 125 mg PO bid for 5 days.
- *Suppression of recurrent genital herpes:* 250 mg PO bid for up to 1 yr.

Pediatric patients
Safety and efficacy not established.

Patients with renal impairment
- *Herpes zoster:*

Creatinine Clearance (mL/min)	Dose
≥ 60	500 mg q 8 hr
40–59	500 mg q 12 hr
20–39	500 mg q 24 hr
< 20	250 mg q 48 hr

- *Genital herpes:*

Creatinine Clearance (mL/min)	Dose
≥ 40	125 mg q 12 hr
20–39	125 mg q 24 hr
< 20	125 mg q 48 hr

Pharmacokinetics

Route	Onset	Peak
Oral	Varies	0.5–1 hr

Metabolism: $T_{1/2}$: 2 hr
Distribution: Crosses placenta; may enter breast milk
Excretion: Urine

Adverse effects
- **CNS:** Dreams, ataxia, coma, confusion, dizziness, *headache*
- **CV:** Arrhythmia, hypertension, hypotension
- **Dermatologic:** *Rash,* alopecia, pruritus, urticaria
- **GI:** Abnormal liver function tests, nausea, vomiting, anorexia, *diarrhea,* abdominal pain
- **Hematologic:** Granulocytopenia, thrombocytopenia, anemia
- **Other:** *Fever,* chills, **cancer,** sterility

Interactions

✱ Drug-drug • Increased serum concentration of famciclovir if taken with cimetidine • Increased digoxin levels if taken together

■ Nursing considerations
Assessment

• **History:** Hypersensitivity to famciclovir or acyclovir; cytopenia; impaired renal function; lactation, pregnancy
• **Physical:** Skin color, lesions; orientation; BP, P, auscultation, perfusion, edema; R, adventitious sounds; urinary output; CBC, Hct, BUN, creatinine clearance, liver function tests

Interventions

• Decrease dosage in patients with impaired renal function.
• Arrange for CBC before and every 2 days during therapy and at least weekly thereafter. Consult with physician to reduce dosage if WBCs or platelets fall.

Teaching points

• Take this drug for 5 or 7 full days as prescribed.
• These side effects may occur: decreased blood count leading to susceptibility to infection (blood tests may be needed; avoid crowds and exposure to disease), headache (analgesics may be ordered), diarrhea.
• Famciclovir is not a cure for genital herpes; use appropriate precautions to prevent transmission.
• Report bruising, bleeding, worsening of condition, fever, infection.

▽ famotidine
(fa moe' ti deen)

Apo-Famotidine (CAN), Novo-Famotidine (CAN), Pepcid, Pepcid AC, Pepcid RPD

PREGNANCY CATEGORY B

Drug class

Histamine 2 (H_2) antagonist

Therapeutic actions

Competitively blocks the action of histamine at the histamine (H_2) receptors of the parietal cells of the stomach; inhibits basal gastric acid secretion and chemically induced gastric acid secretion.

Indications

• Short-term treatment and maintenance of duodenal ulcer
• Short-term treatment of benign gastric ulcer
• Treatment of pathologic hypersecretory conditions
• Short-term treatment of gastroesophageal reflux disease (GERD), esophagitis due to GERD
• Relief of symptoms of heartburn, acid indigestion, sour stomach (OTC)

Contraindications and cautions

• Allergy to famotidine; renal failure; pregnancy; lactation.

Available forms

Tablets—10, 20, 40 mg; chewable tablets—10 mg; powder for oral suspension—40 mg/5 mL; injection—10 mg/mL; injection, premixed—20 mg/50 mL in 0.9% sodium chloride; orally disintegrating tablet—20, 40 mg

Dosages
Adults

• *Active duodenal ulcer:* 40 mg PO or IV at bedtime *or* 20 mg bid PO or IV. Therapy at full dosage should generally be discontinued after 6–8 wk.
• *Maintenance therapy, duodenal ulcer:* 20 mg PO at bedtime.
• *Benign gastric ulcer:* 40 mg PO daily at bedtime.
• *Hypersecretory syndrome:* 20 mg q 6 hr PO initially. Doses up to 160 mg q 6 hr have been administered. 20 mg IV q 12 hr in patients unable to take oral drugs.
• *GERD:* 20 mg bid PO for up to 6 wk.
• *Heartburn, acid indigestion:* 10 mg PO for relief; 10 mg PO 1 hr before eating for prevention. Do not exceed 20 mg/24 hr.

Pediatric patients

Safety and efficacy not established.

---

*Adverse effects in Italics are most common; those in **Bold** are life-threatening.*

Geriatric patients or patients with renal insufficiency
Reduce dosage to 20 mg PO at bedtime *or* 40 mg PO q 36–48 hr.

Pharmacokinetics

Route	Onset	Peak	Duration
Oral	Slow	1–3 hr	6–12 hr
IV	< 1 hr	30 min–3 hr	8–15 hr

Metabolism: Hepatic; $T_{1/2}$: 2.5–3.5 hr
Distribution: Crosses placenta; enters breast milk
Excretion: Urine

▼ IV facts
Preparation: For direct injection, dilute 2 mL (solution contains 10 mg/mL) with 0.9% sodium chloride injection, water for injection, 5% or 10% dextrose injection, lactated Ringer's injection, or 5% sodium bicarbonate injection to a total volume of 5–10 mL. For infusion, 2 mL diluted with 100 mL 5% dextrose solution or other IVs. Stable for 48 hr at room temperature, 14 days if refrigerated.
Infusion: Inject directly slowly, over not less than 2 min. Infuse over 15–30 min; continuous infusion: 40 mg/24 hr.

Adverse effects
- **CNS:** *Headache,* malaise, *dizziness,* somnolence, insomnia
- **Dermatologic:** Rash
- **GI:** *Diarrhea, constipation,* anorexia, abdominal pain
- **Other:** Muscle cramp, increase in total bilirubin, sexual impotence

■ Nursing considerations
Assessment
- **History:** Allergy to famotidine; renal failure; lactation, pregnancy
- **Physical:** Skin lesions; liver evaluation, abdominal exam, normal output; renal function tests, serum bilirubin

Interventions
- Administer drug at bedtime.
- Decrease doses with renal failure.
- Arrange for administration of concurrent antacid therapy to relieve pain.

Teaching points
- Take this drug at bedtime (or in the morning and at bedtime). Therapy may continue for 4–6 wk or longer. Place RPD tablet on tongue and swallow with or without water.
- Take antacid exactly as prescribed, being careful of the times of administration.
- Have regular medical follow-up while on this drug to evaluate your response.
- Take OTC drug 1 hr before eating to prevent indigestion. Do not take more than 2 per day.
- These side effects may occur: constipation or diarrhea; loss of libido or impotence (reversible); headache (adjust lights, temperature, noise levels).
- Report sore throat, fever, unusual bruising or bleeding, severe headache, muscle or joint pain.

▷ fat emulsion, intravenous

Intralipid 10%, 20%; Liposyn II 10%, 20%; Liposyn III 10%, 20%

PREGNANCY CATEGORY C

Drug class
Caloric agent

Therapeutic actions
A preparation from soybean or safflower oil that provides neutral triglycerides, mostly unsaturated fatty acids; these are used as a source of energy, causing an increase in heat production, decrease in respiratory quotient, and increase in oxygen consumption.

Indications
- Source of calories and essential fatty acids for patients requiring parenteral nutrition for extended periods
- Essential fatty acid deficiency

Contraindications and cautions
- Contraindicated with disturbance of normal fat metabolism (hyperlipemia, lipoid nephrosis, acute pancreatitis), allergy to eggs.
- Use cautiously with severe liver damage, pulmonary disease, anemia, blood coagulation

disorders, pregnancy, jaundiced or premature infants.

Available forms
Injection—10% (50, 100, 200, 250, 300 mL), 20% (50, 100, 200, 250, 500 mL)

Dosages
Adults
- *Parenteral nutrition:* Should not comprise more than 60% of total calorie intake. *10%:* infuse IV at 1 mL/min for the first 15–30 min; may be increased to 2 mL/min. Infuse only 500 mL the first day, and increase the following day. Do not exceed 2.5 g/kg/day. *20%:* infuse at 0.5 mL/min for the first 15–30 min; infuse only 250 mL *Liposyn II* or 500 mL *Intralipid* the first day, and increase the following day. Do not exceed 3 g/kg/day.
- *Fatty acid deficiency:* Supply 8%–10% of the caloric intake by IV fat emulsion.

Pediatric patients
- *Parenteral nutrition:* Should not comprise more than 60% of total calorie intake. *10%:* initial IV infusion rate is 0.1 mL/min for the first 10–15 min. *20%:* initial infusion rate is 0.05 mL/min for the first 10–15 min. If no untoward reactions occur, increase rate to 1 g/kg in 4 hr. Do not exceed 3 g/kg/day.

Pharmacokinetics

Route	Onset
IV	Rapid

Metabolism: Hepatic and tissue; $T_{1/2}$: varies
Distribution: Crosses placenta; may enter breast milk

▼IV facts
Preparation: Supplied in single-dose containers; do not store partially used bottles; do not resterilize for later use; do not use with filters; do not use any bottle in which there appears to be separation from the emulsion.
Infusion: Infusion rate is 1 mL/min for 10% solution, monitor for 15–30 min; if no adverse reaction occurs, may be increased to 2 mL/min; 0.5 mL/min for 20% solution, may be increased if no adverse reactions. May be infused simultaneously with amino acid-dextrose mixtures by means of Y-connector located near the in-

fusion site using separate flow rate; keep the lipid solution higher than the amino acid-dextrose line.
Incompatibilities: Do not mix or inject at Y site with amikacin, tetracycline. Monitor electrolyte and acid content; fat emulsion separates in acid solution.

Adverse effects
- **CNS:** *Headache,* flushing, fever, sweating, sleepiness, pressure over the eyes, dizziness
- **GI:** *Nausea,* vomiting
- **Hematologic:** *Thrombophlebitis,* **sepsis,** hyperlipidemia, hypercoagulability, thrombocytopenia, leukopenia, elevated liver enzymes
- **Other:** Irritation at infusion site, brown pigmentation in RES (IV fat pigment), cyanosis

■ Nursing considerations
Assessment
- **History:** Disturbance of normal fat metabolism, allergy to eggs, severe liver damage, pulmonary disease, anemia, blood coagulation disorders, pregnancy, jaundiced or premature infants
- **Physical:** Skin color, lesions; T; orientation; P, BP, peripheral perfusion; CBC, plasma lipid profile, clotting factor levels, liver function tests

Interventions
- Administer by IV route only.
- Inspect admixture for "breaking or oiling out" of the emulsion—seen as yellow streaking or accumulation of yellow droplets—or for the formation of any particulates; discard any admixture if these occur.
- Monitor patient carefully for fluid or fat overloading during infusion: diluted serum electrolytes, overhydration, pulmonary edema, elevated JVP, metabolic acidosis, impaired pulmonary diffusion capacity. Discontinue the infusion; reevaluate patient before restarting infusion at a lower rate.
- Monitor patient's clinical response, serum lipid profile, weight gain, improved nitrogen balance.

- Monitor patient for thrombosis or sepsis; use comfort and preventive measures (exercise, support stockings, ambulation, positioning).

Teaching points

- Report pain at infusion site, difficulty breathing, chest pain, calf pain, excessive sweating.

▽**felodipine**
(fell ob' di peen)

Plendil, Renedil (CAN)

PREGNANCY CATEGORY C

Drug classes

Calcium channel-blocker
Antihypertensive

Therapeutic actions

Inhibits the movement of calcium ions across the membranes of cardiac and arterial muscle cells; inhibition of transmembrane calcium flow results in the depression of impulse formation in pacemaker cells, slowing of velocity of conduction of cardiac impulse, depression of myocardial contractility, dilation of coronary arteries, arterioles and peripheral arterioles; these effects lead to decreased cardiac work, energy consumption, and decreased BP.

Indications

- Essential hypertension, alone or in combination with other antihypertensives

Contraindications and cautions

- Allergy to felodipine or other calcium channel-blockers, impaired hepatic or renal function, sick sinus syndrome, heart block (second or third degree), lactation.

Available forms

ER tablets—2.5, 5, 10 mg

Dosages
Adults

Initially 5 mg PO daily; dosage may be gradually increased over 10–14 days to an average 10–15 mg PO daily. Maximum effective dose is 20 mg daily.

Pediatric patients

Safety and efficacy not established.
Geriatric patients or patients with hepatic impairment

Carefully monitor; do not exceed 10 mg daily PO.

Pharmacokinetics

Route	Onset	Peak
Oral	120–130 min	2.5–5 hr

Metabolism: Hepatic; $T_{1/2}$: 11–16 hr
Distribution: Crosses placenta; may pass into breast milk
Excretion: Urine

Adverse effects

- **CNS:** *Dizziness, light-headedness, headache,* asthenia, *fatigue, lethargy*
- **CV:** *Peripheral edema,* arrhythmias
- **Dermatologic:** *Flushing,* rash
- **GI:** *Nausea,* abdominal discomfort, reflux

Interactions

✳ **Drug-drug** • Decreased serum levels with barbiturates, hydantoins • Increased serum levels and toxicity with erythromycin, cimetidine, ranitidine, antifungal agents

✳ **Drug-food** • Decreased metabolism and increased risk of toxic effects if taken with grapefruit juice; avoid this combination

■ Nursing considerations

CLINICAL ALERT!
Name confusion has occurred between Plendil (felodipine) and Isordil (isosorbide); use caution.

Assessment

- **History:** Allergy to felodipine, impaired hepatic or renal function, sick sinus syndrome, heart block, lactation, pregnancy
- **Physical:** Skin lesions, color, edema; P, BP, baseline ECG, peripheral perfusion, auscultation, R, adventitious sounds; liver evaluation, GI normal output; liver and renal function tests, urinalysis

Interventions

- Have patient swallow tablet whole; do not chew or crush.

- Monitor patient carefully (BP, cardiac rhythm and output) while drug is being adjusted to therapeutic dose.
- Monitor cardiac rhythm regularly during stabilization of dosage and periodically during long-term therapy.
- Administer drug without regard to meals.

Teaching points
- Take this drug with meals if upset stomach occurs; swallow tablet whole, do not cut, crush, or chew. Do not drink grapefruit juice while using this drug.
- These side effects may occur: nausea, vomiting (small, frequent meals may help); headache (adjust lighting, noise, and temperature; medication may be ordered if severe).
- Report irregular heart beat, shortness of breath, swelling of the hands or feet, pronounced dizziness, constipation.

▷**fenofibrate**
(fee no fye' brate)

Tricor

PREGNANCY CATEGORY C

Drug class
Antihyperlipidemic agent

Therapeutic actions
Inhibits triglyceride synthesis in the liver resulting in a reduction in VLDL released into circulation; may also stimulate the breakdown of triglyceride-rich lipoproteins; also increases the secretion of uric acid.

Indications
- Adjunct to diet in treating adults with primary hypercholesterolemia
- Adjunct to diet for treatment of adults with hypertriglyceridemia
- Unlabeled use: polymetabolic syndrome x

Contraindications and cautions
- Contraindicated with allergy to fenofibrate, hepatic dysfunction, primary biliary cirrhosis, gall bladder disease, pregnancy.

- Use cautiously with renal impairment, lactation.

Available forms
Tablets—54, 160 mg

Dosages
Adults
- *Hypertriglyceridemia:* Initially 160 mg/day PO with a meal. Discontinue if improvement is not seen in the first 2 mo.
- *Hypercholesterolemia:* 54–160 mg/day PO.

Pediatric patients
Safety and efficacy not established.

Elderly patients
Initial dose, 54 mg/day PO; titrate slowly with close monitoring.

Patients with renal impairment
Initiate therapy with 54 mg/day PO; monitor renal function tests carefully for 4–8 wk before increasing.

Pharmacokinetics

Route	Onset	Peak	Duration
Oral	Varies	6–8 hr	Weeks

Metabolism: Hepatic; $T_{1/2}$: 20 hours
Distribution: Crosses placenta; passes into breast milk
Excretion: Urine

Adverse effects
- **CV:** Angina, arrhythmias, swelling, phlebitis, thrombophlebitis, pulmonary emboli
- **Dermatologic:** *Rash,* alopecia, dry skin, dry and brittle hair, pruritus, urticaria
- **GI:** *Nausea,* vomiting, diarrhea, dyspepsia, flatulence, bloating, stomatitis, gastritis, **pancreatitis,** peptic ulcer, GI hemorrhage
- **GU:** *Impotence, decreased libido,* dysuria, hematuria, proteinuria, decreased urine output
- **Hematologic:** Leukopenia, anemia, eosinophilia, increased AST and ALT, increased thymol turbidity, increased CPK, BSP retention
- **Other:** *Myalgia, flulike syndromes,* arthralgia, weight gain, polyphagia, increased perspiration, systemic lupus erythematosus, blurred vision, gynecomastia

---

Adverse effects in *Italics* are most common; those in **Bold** are life-threatening.

Interactions

✳ **Drug-drug** • Increased bleeding tendencies if oral anticoagulants are given with fenofibrate—reduce dosage of anticoagulant, usually by 50% • Possible rhabdomyolysis, acute renal failure if given with any statins; avoid this combination • Decreased absorption and effectiveness if given with bile acid sequestrants; administer at least 1 hr before or 4–6 hr after these drugs • Increased risk of renal toxicity if combined with immunosuppressants or other nephrotoxic drugs; use caution and monitor patient carefully

■ Nursing considerations
Assessment

- **History:** Allergy to fenofibrate, hepatic dysfunction, primary biliary cirrhosis, gall bladder disease, pregnancy, renal impairment, lactation
- **Physical:** Skin lesions, color, temperature; P, BP, auscultation, baseline ECG, peripheral perfusion, edema; bowel sounds, normal output, liver evaluation; lipid studies, CBC, clotting profile, liver function tests, renal function tests, urinalysis

Interventions

- Administer drug with meals.
- Monitor patient carefully, if no response is noted within first 2 mo, discontinue drug.
- Ensure that patient continues strict dietary restrictions and exercise program.
- Arrange for regular follow-up including blood tests for lipids, liver function, CBC during long-term therapy.
- Give frequent skin care to deal with rashes, dryness.

Teaching points

- Take the drug with meals.
- Continue to follow strict dietary regimen and exercise program.
- These side effects may occur: diarrhea, loss of appetite (ensure ready access to the bathroom if this occurs; small frequent meals may help).
- Arrange to have regular follow-up visits to your health care provider, which will include blood tests.
- Report chest pain, shortness of breath, palpitations, myalgia, malaise, excessive fatigue, fever.

▽ fenoprofen calcium
*(fen oh **proe' fen**)*

Nalfon Pulvules

PREGNANCY CATEGORY B

Drug classes

Nonsteroidal anti-inflammatory drug (NSAID)
Analgesic (non-narcotic)
Propionic acid derivative

Therapeutic actions

Analgesic, anti-inflammatory, and antipyretic activities largely related to inhibition of prostaglandin synthesis; exact mechanisms of action are not known.

Indications

- Acute and long-term treatment of rheumatoid arthritis and osteoarthritis
- Relief of mild to moderate pain

Contraindications and cautions

- Contraindicated with significant renal impairment, pregnancy, lactation.
- Use cautiously with impaired hearing, allergies; hepatic, CV, and GI conditions.

Available forms

Capsules—200, 300 mg; tablets—600 mg

Dosages

Do not exceed 3,200 mg/day.
Adults

- *Rheumatoid arthritis or osteoarthritis:* 300–600 mg PO tid or qid. 2–3 wk may be required to see improvement.
- *Mild to moderate pain:* 200 mg q 4–6 hr PO, as needed.

Pediatric patients

Safety and efficacy have not been established.

Pharmacokinetics

Route	Onset	Peak
Oral	30–60 min	1–2 hr

Metabolism: Hepatic; $T_{1/2}$: 2–3 hr
Distribution: Crosses placenta; enters breast milk
Excretion: Urine

Adverse effects
NSAIDs
- **CNS:** *Headache, dizziness, somnolence, insomnia,* fatigue, tiredness, dizziness, tinnitus, ophthalmologic effects
- **Dermatologic:** *Rash,* pruritus, sweating, dry mucous membranes, stomatitis
- **GI:** *Nausea, dyspepsia, GI pain,* diarrhea, *vomiting, constipation,* flatulence, ulcer, **GI bleed**
- **GU:** Dysuria, **renal impairment** (fenoprofen is one of the most nephrotoxic NSAIDs)
- **Hematologic:** Bleeding, platelet inhibition with higher doses, neutropenia, eosinophilia, leukopenia, pancytopenia, thrombocytopenia, agranulocytosis, granulocytopenia, aplastic anemia, decreased hemoglobin or hematocrit, bone marrow depression, menorrhagia
- **Respiratory:** Dyspnea, hemoptysis, pharyngitis, bronchospasm, rhinitis
- **Other:** Peripheral edema, **anaphylactoid reactions to fatal anaphylactic shock**

Interactions
✳ Drug-drug • Increased risk of bleeding with anticoagulants, antiplatelet drugs

■ Nursing considerations
Assessment
- **History:** Renal impairment, impaired hearing, allergies, hepatic, cardiovascular, and GI conditions, lactation, pregnancy
- **Physical:** Skin color and lesions; orientation, reflexes, ophthalmologic and audiometric evaluation, peripheral sensation; P, edema; R, adventitious sounds; liver evaluation; CBC, clotting times, renal and liver function tests; serum electrolytes, stool guaiac

Interventions
- Administer drug with food or after meals if GI upset occurs.
- Arrange for periodic ophthalmologic examination during long-term therapy.
- Institute emergency procedures if overdose occurs—gastric lavage, induction of emesis, supportive therapy.

Teaching points
- Take drug with food or meals if GI upset occurs.
- Take only the prescribed dosage.
- Dizziness, drowsiness can occur (avoid driving or using dangerous machinery).
- Do not take this drug during pregnancy; use of contraceptives is advised.
- Report sore throat, fever, rash, itching, weight gain, swelling in ankles or fingers; changes in vision, black, tarry stools.

▽fentanyl
(fen' ta nil)

Actiq; Duragesic 25, 50, 75, 100; Fentanyl Oralet; Sublimaze

PREGNANCY CATEGORY B

C-II CONTROLLED SUBSTANCE

Drug class
Narcotic agonist analgesic

Therapeutic actions
Acts at specific opioid receptors, causing analgesia, respiratory depression, physical depression, euphoria.

Indications
- Analgesic action of short duration during anesthesia and immediate postop period
- Analgesic supplement in general or regional anesthesia
- Administration with a neuroleptic as an anesthetic premedication, for induction of anesthesia, and as an adjunct in maintenance of general and regional anesthesia
- For use as an anesthetic agent with oxygen in selected high-risk patients
- Transdermal system: management of chronic pain in patients requiring opioid analgesia
- Treatment of breakthrough pain in cancer patients being treated with narcotics (*Actiq*)

Contraindications and cautions
- Contraindicated with hypersensitivity to narcotics, diarrhea caused by poisoning, acute

---

Adverse effects in Italics are most common; those in Bold are life-threatening.

bronchial asthma, upper airway obstruction, pregnancy.
• Use cautiously with bradycardia, history of seizures, lactation.

Available forms
Lozenges—100, 200, 300, 400 mcg; sugar lozenge on a stick (*Actiq*)—200, 400, 600, 800, 1,200, 1,600 mcg; transdermal—25, 50, 75, 100 mcg/hr; injection–0.05 mg/mL

Dosages
Individualize dosage; monitor vital signs.
Adults
• *Premedication:* 0.05–0.1 mg IM 30–60 min prior to surgery.
• *Adjunct to general anesthesia:* Total dosage is 0.002 mg/kg. Maintenance dose: 0.025–0.1 mg IV or IM when changes in vital signs indicate surgical stress or lightening of analgesia.
• *With oxygen for anesthesia:* Total high dose is 0.05–0.1 mg/kg IV; up to 0.12 mg/kg may be necessary.
• *Adjunct to regional anesthesia:* 0.05–0.1 mg IM or slowly IV over 1–2 min.
• *Postoperatively:* 0.05–0.1 mg IM for the control of pain, tachypnea, or emergence delirium; repeat in 1–2 if needed.
Transdermal
Apply to nonirritated and nonirradiated skin on a flat surface of the upper torso; may require replacement in 72 hr if pain has not subsided.
Lozenges
Place in mouth and suck, 20–40 min before desired effect; *Actiq* should be sucked slowly over 15 min.
Pediatric patients 2–12 yr
2–3 mcg/kg IV as vital signs indicate.
Transdermal
Do not exceed 15 mcg/kg.
Lozenges
5–15 mcg/kg transmucosal *Oralets*.

Pharmacokinetics

Route	Onset	Duration
IM	7–8 min	1–2 hr
Transdermal	Gradual	72 hr

Metabolism: Plasma; $T_{1/2}$: 1.5–6 hr
Distribution: Crosses placenta; enters breast milk

▼ IV facts
Preparation: May be used undiluted or diluted with 250 mL of D_5W. Protect vials from light.
Infusion: Administer slowly by direct injection, each mL over at least 1 min, or into running IV tubing.
Incompatibilities: Do not mix with methohexital, pentobarbital, thiopental.

Adverse effects
• **CNS:** *Sedation, clamminess, sweating, headache, vertigo, floating feeling, dizziness, lethargy, confusion, light-headedness,* nervousness, unusual dreams, agitation, euphoria, hallucinations, delirium, insomnia, anxiety, fear, disorientation, impaired mental and physical performance, coma, mood changes, weakness, headache, tremor, convulsions
• **CV:** Palpitation, increase or decrease in BP, circulatory depression, **cardiac arrest, shock,** tachycardia, bradycardia, arrhythmia, palpitations
• **Dermatologic:** Rash, hives, pruritus, flushing, warmth, sensitivity to cold
• **EENT:** Diplopia, blurred vision
• **GI:** *Nausea, vomiting,* dry mouth, anorexia, constipation, biliary tract spasm
• **GU:** Ureteral spasm, spasm of vesical sphincters, urinary retention or hesitancy, oliguria, antidiuretic effect, reduced libido or potency
• **Local:** Phlebitis following IV injection, pain at injection site; tissue irritation and induration (SC injection)
• **Respiratory:** Slow, shallow respiration, **apnea,** suppression of cough reflex, laryngospasm, bronchospasm
• **Other:** Physical tolerance and dependence, psychological dependence; local skin irritation with transdermal system

Interactions
✱ **Drug-drug** • Potentiation of effects when given with other CNS acting drugs or barbiturate anesthetics; decrease dose of fentanyl when coadministering
✱ **Drug-food** • Decreased metabolism and risk of toxic effects if taken with grapefruit juice; avoid this combination
✱ **Drug-lab test** • Elevated biliary tract pressure may cause increases in plasma amylase, lipase; determinations of these levels may be

unreliable for 24 hr after administration of narcotics

■ Nursing considerations

CLINICAL ALERT!
Name confusion has occurred between fentanyl and sufentanil; use extreme caution.

Assessment

- **History:** Hypersensitivity to fentanyl or narcotics, physical dependence on a narcotic analgesic, pregnancy, labor, lactation, COPD, respiratory depression, anoxia, increased intracranial pressure, acute MI, ventricular failure, coronary insufficiency, hypertension, biliary tract surgery, renal or hepatic dysfunction
- **Physical:** Orientation, reflexes, bilateral grip strength, affect; pupil size, vision; P, auscultation, BP; R, adventitious sounds; bowel sounds, normal output; liver and kidney function tests

Interventions

- Administer to women who are nursing a baby 4–6 hr before the next scheduled feeding to minimize the amount in milk.
- Provide narcotic antagonist, facilities for assisted or controlled respiration on standby during parenteral administration.
- Prepare site for transdermal form by clipping (not shaving) hair at site; do not use soap, oils, lotions, alcohol; allow skin to dry completely before application. Apply immediately after removal from the sealed package; firmly press the transdermal system in place with the palm of the hand for 10–20 sec, making sure the contact is complete. Must be worn continually for 72 hr.
- Use caution with *Actiq* form to keep this drug out of the reach of children (looks like a lollipop) and follow the distribution restrictions in place with this drug very carefully.

Teaching points

- These side effects may occur: dizziness, sedation, drowsiness, impaired visual acuity (ask for assistance if you need to move); nausea, loss of appetite (lie quietly, eat frequent small meals); constipation (a laxative may help).

- Do not drink grapefruit juice while on this drug.
- Report severe nausea, vomiting, palpitations, shortness of breath, or difficulty breathing.

▷ferrous salts
(fair' us)

ferrous fumarate
Femiron, Feostat, Hemocyte, Ircon, Nephro-Fer, Palafer (CAN), Vitron-C

ferrous gluconate
Apo-Ferrous Gluconate (CAN), Fergon

ferrous sulfate
Apo-Ferrous Sulfate (CAN), ED-IN-SOL, Feosol, Fer-In-Sol, Fer-Iron, Fer-gen-sol

ferrous sulfate exsiccated
Feosol, Feratab, Ferodan (CAN), Fero-Grad (CAN), Slow Fe, FE$_{50}$

PREGNANCY CATEGORY A

Drug class
Iron preparation

Therapeutic actions
Elevates the serum iron concentration and is then converted to hemoglobin or trapped in the reticuloendothelial cells for storage and eventual conversion to a usable form of iron.

Indications
- Prevention and treatment of iron deficiency anemias
- Dietary supplement for iron
- Unlabeled use: supplemental use during epoetin therapy to ensure proper hematologic response to epoetin

Contraindications and cautions
- Allergy to any ingredient; sulfite allergy; hemochromatosis, hemosiderosis, hemolytic anemias; normal iron balance; peptic ulcer, regional enteritis, ulcerative colitis

Available forms

Tablets—sulfate, 324, 325 mg; sulfate exsiccated, 187, 200 mg; gluconate, 240, 325 mg; fumarate, 63, 200, 324, 325, 350 mg; timed-release capsules—sulfate exsiccated, 160 mg; timed-release tablets—sulfate exsiccated, 160 mg; syrup—sulfate, 90 mg/5 mL; elixir—sulfate, 220 mg/5 mL; drops—sulfate, 75 mg/0.6 mL, 125 mg/mL; fumarate, 45 mg/0.6 mL; tablet, chewable—fumarate, 100 mg; suspension—fumarate, 100 mg/5 mL

Dosages
Adults
- *Daily requirements:* Males, 10 mg/day PO; females, 18 mg/day PO; pregnancy and lactation, 30–60 mg/day PO.
- *Replacement in deficiency states:* 90–300 mg/day (6 mg/kg/day) PO for approximately 6–10 mo may be required.

Pediatric patients
Daily requirement: 10–15 mg/day PO.

Pharmacokinetics

Route	Onset	Peak	Duration
Oral	4 days	7–10 days	2–4 mo

Metabolism: Recycled for use; $T_{1/2}$: not known
Distribution: Crosses placenta; enters breast milk

Adverse effects
- **CNS:** CNS toxicity, acidosis, **coma and death**—overdose
- **GI:** *GI upset, anorexia, nausea, vomiting, constipation,* diarrhea, dark stools, temporary staining of the teeth (liquid preparations)

Interactions
✳ **Drug-drug** • Decreased anti-infective response to ciprofloxacin, norfloxacin, ofloxacin • Decreased absorption with antacids, cimetidine • Decreased effects of levodopa if taken with iron • Increased serum iron levels with chloramphenicol
✳ **Drug-food** • Decreased absorption with antacids, eggs or milk, coffee and tea; avoid concurrent administration of any of these

■ Nursing considerations
Assessment
- **History:** Allergy to any ingredient, sulfite; hemochromatosis, hemosiderosis, hemolytic anemias; normal iron balance; peptic ulcer, regional enteritis, ulcerative colitis
- **Physical:** Skin lesions, color; gums, teeth (color); bowel sounds; CBC, Hgb, Hct, serum ferritin assays

Interventions
- Confirm that patient does have iron deficiency anemia before treatment.
- Give drug with meals (avoiding milk, eggs, coffee, and tea) if GI discomfort is severe, and slowly increase to build up tolerance.
- Administer liquid preparations in water or juice to mask the taste and prevent staining of teeth; have the patient drink solution with a straw.
- Warn patient that stool may be dark or green.
- Arrange for periodic monitoring of hematocrit and hemoglobin levels.

Teaching points
- Take drug on an empty stomach with water. Take after meals if GI upset is severe (avoid milk, eggs, coffee, and tea).
- Take liquid preparations diluted in water or juice and sipped through a straw to prevent staining of the teeth.
- Treatment may not be necessary if cause of anemia can be corrected. Treatment may be needed for several months to reverse the anemia.
- Have periodic blood tests during therapy to determine the appropriate dosage.
- Do not take this preparation with antacids or tetracyclines. If these drugs are needed, they will be prescribed.
- These side effects may occur: GI upset, nausea, vomiting (take drug with meals); diarrhea or constipation; dark or green stools.
- Report severe GI upset, lethargy, rapid respirations, constipation.

▽ **fexofenadine hydrochloride**
*(fecks oh **fen'** a deen)*

Allegra

PREGNANCY CATEGORY C

Drug class
Antihistamine (nonsedating type)

Therapeutic actions

Competitively blocks the effects of histamine at peripheral H_1-receptor sites; has no anticholinergic (atropine-like) or sedating effects.

Indications

- Symptomatic relief of symptoms associated with seasonal allergic rhinitis in adults and children ≥ 6 yr
- Chronic idiopathic urticaria in adults and children ≥ 6 yr

Contraindications and cautions

- Contraindicated with allergy to any antihistamines, pregnancy, lactation
- Use cautiously with hepatic or renal impairment, geriatric patients

Available forms

Tablets—30, 60, 180 mg

Dosages

Adults and patients ≥ 12 yr
60 mg PO bid or 180 mg once/day.
Pediatric patients 6–11 yr
30 mg PO bid.
Geriatric patients or patients with renal impairment
60 mg PO daily.

Pharmacokinetics

Route	Onset	Peak
Oral	Rapid	2.6 hr

Metabolism: Hepatic; $T_{1/2}$: 14.4 hr
Distribution: Crosses placenta; may enter breast milk
Excretion: Feces and urine

Adverse effects

- **CNS:** Fatigue, drowsiness
- **GI:** Nausea, dyspepsia
- **Other:** Dysmenorrhea, flulike illness

Interactions

✻ **Drug-drug** • Increased levels and possible toxicity with ketoconazole, erythromycin; fexofenadine dose may need to be decreased

■ Nursing considerations

Assessment

- **History:** Allergy to any antihistamines, renal or hepatic impairment, pregnancy, lactation
- **Physical:** Mucous membranes, oropharynx, R, adventitious sounds; skin color, lesions; orientation, affect; renal and liver function tests

Interventions

- Arrange for use of humidifier if thickening of secretions, nasal dryness become bothersome; encourage adequate intake of fluids.
- Provide supportive care if flulike symptoms occur.

Teaching points

- Avoid excessive dosage; take only the dosage prescribed.
- These side effects may occur: dizziness, sedation, drowsiness (use caution if driving or performing tasks that require alertness); thickening of bronchial secretions, dryness of nasal mucosa (use of a humidifier may help); menstrual irregularities; flulike symptoms (medication may be helpful).
- Report difficulty breathing, severe nausea, fever.

▷ **filgrastim (granulocyte colony-stimulating factor, G-CSF)**

*(fill **grass' stim**)*

Neupogen

PREGNANCY CATEGORY C

Drug class

Colony-stimulating factor

Therapeutic actions

Human granulocyte colony-stimulating factor produced by recombinant DNA technology; increases the production of neutrophils within the bone marrow with little effect on the production of other hematopoietic cells.

Adverse effects in *Italics* are most common; those in **Bold** are life-threatening.

Indications

- To decrease the incidence of infection in patients with nonmyeloid malignancies receiving myelosuppressive anticancer drugs associated with a significant incidence of severe neutropenia with fever
- To reduce the duration of neutropenia following bone marrow transplant
- Treatment of severe chronic neutropenia
- Mobilization of hematopoietic progenitor cells into the blood for leukapheresis collection
- Orphan drug uses: treatment of myelodysplastic syndrome, aplastic anemia

Contraindications and cautions

- Contraindicated with hypersensitivity to *Escherichia coli* products, pregnancy.
- Use cautiously with lactation.

Available forms

Injection—300 mcg/mL

Dosages

Adults

Starting dose is 5 mcg/kg/day SC or IV as a single daily injection. May be increased in increments of 5 mcg/kg for each chemotherapy cycle. 4–8 mcg/kg/day is usually effective.

- *Bone marrow transplant:* 10 mcg/kg/day IV or continuous SC infusion.
- *Severe chronic neutropenia:* 6 mcg/kg SC bid.
- *Mobilization for harvesting:* 10 mcg/kg/day SC at least 4 days before first leukapheresis; continue to last leukapheresis.

Pediatric patients

Safety and efficacy not established.

Pharmacokinetics

Route	Peak	Duration
SC	8 hr	4 days
IV	2 hr	4 days

Metabolism: Unknown; $T_{1/2}$: 210–231 min
Distribution: Crosses placenta; may enter breast milk

▼ IV facts

Preparation: No special preparation required. Refrigerate; avoid shaking. Prior to injection, allow to warm to room temperature. Discard vial after one use, and do not reenter

vial; discard any vial that has been at room temperature > 6 hr.
Infusion: Inject directly IV slowly over 15–30 min, or inject slowly into tubing of running IV over 4–24 hr.
Incompatibilities: Do not mix in solutions other than D₅W. Incompatible with numerous drugs in solution; check manufacturer's details before any combination.

Adverse effects

- **CNS:** Headache, fever, generalized weakness, fatigue
- **Dermatologic:** *Alopecia,* rash, mucositis
- **GI:** *Nausea, vomiting,* stomatitis, anorexia, *diarrhea,* constipation
- **Other:** *Bone pain,* generalized pain, sore throat, cough

■ Nursing considerations
Assessment

- **History:** Hypersensitivity to *E. coli* products, pregnancy, lactation
- **Physical:** Skin color, lesions, hair; T; abdominal exam, status of mucous membranes; CBC, platelets

Interventions

- Obtain CBC and platelet count prior to and twice weekly during therapy; doses may be increased after chemotherapy cycles according to the duration and severity of bone marrow suppression.
- Do not give within 24 hr before and after chemotherapy.
- Give daily for up to 2 wk until the neutrophil count is 10,000/mm³; discontinue therapy if this number is exceeded.
- Store in refrigerator; allow to warm to room temperature before use; if vial is at room temperature for > 6 hr, discard. Use each vial for one dose; do not reenter the vial. Discard any unused drug.
- Do not shake vial before use. If SC dose exceeds 1 mL, consider using two sites.

Teaching points

- Store drug in refrigerator; do not shake vial. Each vial can be used only once; do not reuse syringes or needles (proper container for disposal will be provided). Another person should be instructed in the proper administration technique. Use sterile technique.

- Avoid exposure to infection while you are receiving this drug (eg, avoid crowds).
- These side effects may occur: bone pain (analgesia may be ordered), nausea and vomiting (eat small, frequent meals), loss of hair (it is very important to cover head in extreme temperatures).
- Keep appointments for frequent blood tests to evaluate effects of drug on your blood count.
- Report fever, chills, severe bone pain, sore throat, weakness, pain or swelling at injection site.

▷ **finasteride**

(fin as' teh ride)

Propecia, Proscar

PREGNANCY CATEGORY X

Drug class
Androgen hormone inhibitor

Therapeutic actions
Inhibits the intracellular enzyme that converts testosterone into a potent androgen (DHT); does not affect androgen receptors in the body; the prostate gland depends on DHT for its development and maintenance.

Indications
- Treatment of symptomatic benign prostatic hyperplasia (BPH); most effective with long-term use; reduces the need for prostate surgery and reduces the risk of urinary retention (*Proscar*)
- Prevention of male pattern baldness in patients with family history or early signs of loss (*Propecia*)
- Unlabeled uses: adjuvant monotherapy following radical prostatectomy; prevention of the progression of first-stage prostate cancer; treatment of acne, hirsutism

Contraindications and cautions
- Contraindicated with allergy to finasteride or any component of the product, pregnancy, lactation.
- Use cautiously with hepatic impairment.

Available forms
Tablets—1 mg (*Propecia*), 5 mg (*Proscar*)

Dosages
Adults
- *BPH:* 5 mg daily PO with or without meals; may take 6–12 mo for response.
- *Male pattern baldness:* 1 mg/day PO.

Pediatric patients
Safety and efficacy not established.

Geriatric patients or patients with renal insufficiency
No dosage adjustment is needed.

Pharmacokinetics

Route	Onset	Peak	Duration
Oral	Rapid	8 hr	24 hr

Metabolism: Hepatic; $T_{1/2}$: 6 hr
Distribution: Crosses placenta; may enter breast milk (not used in women)
Excretion: Feces and urine

Adverse effects
- **GI:** Abdominal upset
- **GU:** *Impotence, decreased libido,* decreased volume of ejaculation

Interactions
✴ **Drug-drug** • No reported drug interactions
✴ **Drug-lab test** • Decreased PSA levels when measured; false decrease does not mean patient is free of risk of prostate cancer

■ Nursing considerations
Assessment
- **History:** Allergy to finasteride or any component, hepatic impairment
- **Physical:** Liver evaluation, abdominal exam; renal function tests, normal urine output, prostate exam

Interventions
- Confirm that problem is BPH, and other disorders (prostate cancer, infection, strictures, hypotonic bladder) have been ruled out.
- Administer without regard to meals; protect container from light.

Adverse effects in *Italics* are most common; those in **Bold** are life-threatening.

- Arrange for regular follow-up, including prostate exam, PSA levels, and evaluation of urine flow.
- Monitor urine flow and output; increase in urine flow may not occur in all situations.
- Do not allow pregnant women to handle crushed or broken tablets because of risk of inadvertent absorption, adversely affecting the fetus.
- Alert patient that libido may be decreased as well as the volume of ejaculate; usually reversible when the drug is stopped.

Teaching points

- Take this drug once a day without regard to meals; protect from light.
- Have regular medical follow-up to evaluate your response. Your health care provider will monitor your liver and kidney function as well as prostate specific antigen (PSA) levels.
- These side effects may occur: loss of libido, impotence, decreased amount of ejaculate (usually reversible when the drug is stopped).
- This drug has serious adverse effects on unborn babies. Do not allow a pregnant woman to handle the tablet if it is crushed or broken.
- Report inability to void, groin pain, sore throat, fever, weakness.

▽flavoxate hydrochloride
(fla vox' ate)

Urispas

PREGNANCY CATEGORY B

Drug classes
Urinary antispasmodic
Parasympathetic blocking agent

Therapeutic actions
Counteracts smooth muscle spasm of the urinary tract by relaxing the detrusor and other muscles through action at the parasympathetic receptors; has local anesthetic and analgesic properties.

Indications
- Symptomatic relief of dysuria, urgency, nocturia, suprapubic pain, frequency and incontinence due to cystitis, prostatitis, urethritis, urethrocystitis, urethrotrigonitis

Contraindications and cautions
- Contraindicated with allergy to flavoxate, pyloric or duodenal obstruction, obstructive intestinal lesions or ileus, achalasia, GI hemorrhage, obstructive uropathies of the lower urinary tract.
- Use cautiously with glaucoma, pregnancy, lactation.

Available forms
Tablets—100 mg

Dosages
Adults and pediatric patients > 12 yr
100–200 mg PO tid or qid. Reduce dose when symptoms improve. Use up to 1,200 mg/day in severe urinary urgency following pelvic radiotherapy.
Pediatric patients < 12 yr
Safety and efficacy not established.

Pharmacokinetics

Route	Onset	Duration
Oral	Slow	6 hr

Metabolism: $T_{1/2}$: 2–3 hr
Distribution: May cross placenta
Excretion: Urine

Adverse effects
- **CNS:** *Nervousness, vertigo, headache, drowsiness,* mental confusion, hyperpyrexia, *blurred vision,* increased ocular tension, disturbance in accommodation
- **CV:** Tachycardia, palpitations
- **Dermatologic:** Urticaria, dermatoses
- **GI:** *Nausea, vomiting, dry mouth*
- **GU:** Dysuria
- **Hematologic:** Eosinophilia, leukopenia

Interactions
✱ **Drug-drug** • Risk of toxic effects if combined with anticholinergic drugs • Loss of effectiveness of cholinergic drugs such as Alzheimer's drugs if combined

■ Nursing considerations
Assessment
- **History:** Allergy to flavoxate, pyloric or duodenal obstruction, obstructive intestinal lesions or ileus, achalasia, GI hemorrhage, obstructive uropathies of the lower urinary tract, glaucoma, pregnancy, lactation
- **Physical:** Skin color, lesions; T; orientation, affect, reflexes, ophthalmic exam, ocular pressure measurement; P; bowel sounds, oral mucous membranes; CBC, stool guaiac

Interventions
- Arrange for definitive treatment of urinary tract infections causing the symptoms being managed by flavoxate.
- Arrange for ophthalmic exam before and during therapy.

Teaching points
- Take drug three to four times a day.
- This drug is meant to relieve the symptoms you are experiencing; other medications will be used to treat the cause.
- These side effects may occur: dry mouth, GI upset (suck on sugarless lozenges and use frequent mouth care); drowsiness, blurred vision (avoid driving or performing tasks requiring alertness).
- Report blurred vision, fever, rash, nausea, vomiting.

▽flecainide acetate
(fle kay' nide)

Tambocor

PREGNANCY CATEGORY C

Drug class
Antiarrhythmic

Therapeutic actions
Type 1c antiarrhythmic: acts selectively to depress fast sodium channels, decreasing the height and rate of rise of cardiac action potentials and slowing conduction in all parts of the heart.

Indications
- Treatment of life-threatening ventricular arrhythmias, such as sustained ventricular tachycardia (not recommended for less severe ventricular arrhythmias)
- Prevention of paroxysmal atrial fibrillation or flutter (PAF) associated with symptoms and paroxysmal supraventricular tachycardias (PSVT), including atrioventricular nodal and atrioventricular reentrant tachycardia; other supraventricular tachycardias of unspecified mechanism with disabling symptoms in patients without structural heart disease

Contraindications and cautions
- Contraindicated with allergy to flecainide; CHF; cardiogenic shock; cardiac conduction abnormalities (heart blocks of any kind, unless an artificial pacemaker is present to maintain heartbeat); sick sinus syndrome; lactation, pregnancy.
- Use cautiously with endocardial pacemaker (permanent or temporary—stimulus parameters may need to be increased); hepatic or renal disease; potassium imbalance.

Available forms
Tablets—50, 100, 150 mg

Dosages
Evaluation with close monitoring of cardiac response necessary for determining the correct dosage.
Adults
- *PSVT and PAF:* Starting dose of 50 mg q 12 hr PO; may be increased in increments of 50 mg bid q 4 days until efficacy is achieved; maximum dose is 300 mg/day.
- *Sustained ventricular tachycardia:* 100 mg q 12 hr PO. Increase in 50-mg increments twice a day every fourth day until efficacy is achieved. Maximum dose is 400 mg/day.
- *Recent MI or CHF:* Initial dose of no more than 100 mg q 12 hr PO. May increase in 50-mg increments bid every fourth day to a max of 200 mg/day; higher doses associated with increased CHF.
- *Transfer to flecainide:* Allow at least 2–4 plasma half-lives to elapse of drug being discontinued before starting flecainide. Con-

---

*Adverse effects in Italics are most common; those in **Bold** are life-threatening.*

sider hospitalization for withdrawal of a previous antiarrhythmic is likely to produce life-threatening arrhythmias.

Pediatric patients
Safety and efficacy in patients < 18 yr has not been established.

Geriatric patients and patients with renal impairment
- *Initial dose:* 100 mg daily PO or 50 mg q 12 hr. Wait about 4 days to reach a steady state, then increase dose cautiously. Creatinine clearance < 20 mL/min: decrease dose by 25%–50%.

Pharmacokinetics

Route	Onset	Peak	Duration
Oral	30–60 min	3 hr	24 hr

Metabolism: Hepatic; $T_{1/2}$: 20 hr
Distribution: Crosses placenta; may enter breast milk
Excretion: Urine and feces

Adverse effects

- **CNS:** *Dizziness, fatigue, drowsiness, visual changes, headache,* tinnitus, paresthesias
- **CV:** *Cardiac arrhythmias,* congestive heart failure, slowed cardiac conduction, *palpitations, chest pain*
- **GI:** *Nausea, vomiting, abdominal pain, constipation,* diarrhea
- **GU:** Polyuria, urinary retention, decreased libido
- **Other:** *Dyspnea,* sweating, hot flashes, night sweats, leukopenia

Interactions

✻ **Drug-drug** • Risk of marked drop in cardiac output if combined with disopyramide or verapamil; avoid these combinations if possible • Risk of increased flecainide levels if combined with amiodarone, cimetidine, propranolol

■ Nursing considerations
Assessment

- **History:** Allergy to flecainide, CHF, cardiogenic shock, cardiac conduction abnormalities, sick sinus syndrome, endocardial pacemaker, hepatic or renal disease, potassium imbalance, lactation, pregnancy
- **Physical:** Weight; orientation, reflexes, vision; P, BP, auscultation, ECG, edema, R, ad-

ventitious sounds; bowel sounds, liver evaluation; urinalysis, CBC, serum electrolytes, liver and renal function tests

Interventions

- Monitor patient response carefully, especially when beginning therapy.
- Reduce dosage in patients with renal disease, hepatic failure, CHF, or recent MI.
- Check serum K+ levels before giving.
- Monitor cardiac rhythm carefully.
- Evaluate for therapeutic serum levels of 0.2–1 mcg/mL.
- Provide life support equipment, including pacemaker, on standby in case serious CVS, CNS effects occur—also dopamine, dobutamine, isoproterenol, or other positive inotropic agents.

Teaching points

- You will need frequent monitoring of cardiac rhythm.
- These side effects may occur: drowsiness, dizziness, numbness, visual disturbances (avoid driving or using dangerous machinery); nausea, vomiting (small, frequent meals may help); diarrhea, polyuria; sweating, night sweats, hot flashes, loss of libido (reversible after stopping the drug).
- Do not stop taking this drug for any reason without checking with your health care provider. Drug is taken at 12-hr intervals; work out a schedule so you take the drug as prescribed without waking up at night.
- Return for regular follow-up visits to check your heart rhythm and have a blood test to check your blood levels of this drug.
- Report swelling of ankles or fingers, palpitations, fainting, chest pain.

▽**floxuridine**
(flox yoor' i deen)

FUDR

Pregnancy Category D

Drug classes
Antimetabolite
Antineoplastic

Therapeutic actions

Converted in the body to fluorouracil, another antineoplastic drug; inhibits the enzyme thymidylate synthetase, leading to inhibition of DNA synthesis.

Indications

- Palliative management of GI adenocarcinoma metastatic to the liver in patients considered to be incurable by surgery or other means (appropriate only for patients with disease limited to an area that will be reached when given only by regional intra-arterial perfusion)

Contraindications and cautions

- Allergy to floxuridine; poor nutritional status; serious infections; hematopoietic depression secondary to radiation or chemotherapy; impaired liver function; pregnancy; lactation.

Available forms

Powder for injection—500 mg

Dosages
Adults

Given by intra-arterial infusion only: continuous arterial infusion of 0.1–0.6 mg/kg/day (larger doses of 0.4–0.6 mg/kg/day are used for infusion into the hepatic artery as the liver metabolizes the drug). Continue until adverse reactions occur; resume therapy when side effects subside. Maintain use as long as patient is responding to therapy.

Pharmacokinetics

Route	Onset	Peak	Duration
Intra-arterial	Immediate	1–2 hr	3 hr

Metabolism: Hepatic; $T_{1/2}$: 20 hr
Distribution: Crosses placenta; enters breast milk
Excretion: Urine

Adverse effects

- **CNS:** *Lethargy, malaise, weakness,* euphoria, acute cerebellar syndrome, photophobia, lacrimation, decreased vision, nystagmus, diplopia, fever, epistaxis
- **CV:** Myocardial ischemia, angina

- **Dermatologic:** *Alopecia, dermatitis,* maculopapular rash, photosensitivity, nail changes, including nail loss, dry skin, fissures
- **GI:** *Diarrhea, anorexia, nausea, vomiting,* cramps, enteritis, duodenal ulcer, duodenitis, gastritis, glossitis, stomatitis, pharyngitis, esophagopharyngitis
- **Hematologic:** *Leukopenia, thrombocytopenia,* elevations of alkaline phosphatase, serum transaminase, serum bilirubin, lactic dehydrogenase
- **Regional arterial infusion:** Arterial aneurysm, arterial ischemia, arterial thrombosis, bleeding at catheter site, embolism, fibromyositis, abscesses, infection at catheter site, thrombophlebitis

Interactions

✷ Drug-lab test • 5-hydroxyindoleacetic acid (5-HIAA) urinary excretion may increase • Plasma albumin may decrease due to protein malabsorption

■ Nursing considerations
Assessment

- **History:** Allergy to floxuridine, poor nutritional status, serious infections, hematopoietic depression secondary to radiation or chemotherapy, impaired liver function, pregnancy, lactation
- **Physical:** Weight; T; skin lesions, color; hair; vision, speech, orientation, reflexes, sensation; R, adventitious sounds; mucous membranes, liver evaluation, abdominal exam; CBC, differential; renal and liver function tests; urinalysis, chest x-ray

Interventions

- Evaluate hematologic status prior to therapy and before each dose.
- Arrange for discontinuation of drug therapy if any sign of toxicity occurs (stomatitis, esophagopharyngitis, rapidly falling WBC count, intractable vomiting, diarrhea, GI ulceration and bleeding, thrombocytopenia, hemorrhage); consult with physician.
- Reconstitute with 5 mL sterile water; refrigerate no more than 2 wk.
- Administer by intra-arterial line only; use an infusion pump to ensure continual delivery and overcome pressure of arteries.

Adverse effects in *Italics* are most common; those in **Bold** are life-threatening.

Teaching points

- Prepare a calendar of treatment days.
- These side effects may occur: nausea, vomiting, loss of appetite (medication may be ordered; small, frequent meals may help; try to maintain your nutrition while you are on this drug); decreased vision, tearing, double vision, malaise, weakness, lethargy (it is advisable to avoid driving or operating dangerous machinery); mouth sores (use frequent mouth care); diarrhea; loss of hair (obtain a wig or other suitable head covering; keep head covered in extremes of temperature); rash, sensitivity of skin and eyes to sunlight and UV light (avoid exposure or use a sunscreen and protective clothing).
- Use birth control while on this drug; may cause birth defects or miscarriages.
- Arrange to have frequent, regular medical follow-up, including frequent blood tests.
- Report black, tarry stools; fever; chills; sore throat; unusual bleeding or bruising; chest pain; mouth sores.

▽ fluconazole
*(floo **kon'** a zole)*

Diflucan

PREGNANCY CATEGORY C

Drug class
Antifungal

Therapeutic actions
Binds to sterols in the fungal cell membrane, changing membrane permeability; fungicidal or fungistatic depending on concentration and organism.

Indications
- Treatment of oropharyngeal, esophageal, and vaginal candidiasis
- Treatment of cryptococcal meningitis
- Treatment of systemic fungal infections
- Prophylaxis to decrease incidence of candidiasis in bone marrow transplants

Contraindications and cautions
- Contraindicated with hypersensitivity to fluconazole, lactation.
- Use cautiously with renal impairment.

Available forms
Tablets—50, 100, 150, 200 mg; powder for oral suspension—10, 40 mg/mL; injection—2 mg/mL

Dosages
Individualize dosage; same for oral or IV routes because of rapid and almost complete absorption.

Adults
- *Oropharyngeal candidiasis:* 200 mg PO or IV on the first day, followed by 100 mg daily. Continue treatment for at least 2 wk to decrease likelihood of relapse.
- *Esophageal candidiasis:* 200 mg PO or IV on the first day, followed by 100 mg daily. Dosage up to 400 mg/day may be used in severe cases. Treat for a minimum of 3 wk; at least 2 wk after resolution.
- *Systemic candidiasis:* 400 mg PO or IV on the first day, followed by 200 mg daily. Treat for a minimum of 4 wk; at least 2 wk after resolution.
- *Vaginal candidiasis:* 150 mg PO as a single dose.
- *Cryptococcal meningitis:* 400 mg PO or IV on the first day, followed by 200 mg daily. 400 mg daily may be needed. Continue treatment for 10–12 wk.
- *Suppression of cryptococcal meningitis in AIDS patients:* 200 mg daily PO or IV.
- *Prevention of candidiasis in bone marrow transplants:* 400 mg PO daily for several days before and 7 days after neutropenia.

Pediatric patients
- *Oropharyngeal candidiasis:* 6 mg/kg PO or IV on the first day, followed by 3 mg/kg once daily for at least 2 wk.
- *Esophageal candidiasis:* 6 mg/kg PO or IV on the first day, followed by 3 mg/kg once daily. Treat for a minimum of 3 wk; at least 2 wk after resolution.
- *Systemic* Candida *infections:* Daily doses of 6–12 mg/kg/day PO or IV.
- *Cryptococcal meningitis:* 12 mg/kg PO or IV on the first day, followed by 6 mg/kg once daily. Continue treatment for 10–12 wk.

Geriatric patients or patients with renal impairment
Initial dose of 50–400 mg PO or IV. If creatinine clearance > 50 mL/min, use 100% recommended dose; creatinine clearance 21–50 mL/

min, use 50% of the recommended dose; creatinine clearance 11–20, use 25% of recommended dose; patients on hemodialysis, use one dose after each dialysis.

Pharmacokinetics

Route	Onset	Peak	Duration
Oral	Slow	1–2 hr	2–4 days
IV	Rapid	1 hr	2–4 days

Metabolism: Hepatic; $T_{1/2}$: 30 hr
Distribution: Crosses placenta; may enter breast milk
Excretion: Urine

▽ IV facts

Preparation: Do not remove overwrap until ready for use. Inner bag maintains sterility of product. Do not use plastic containers in series connections. Tear overwrap down side at slit, and remove solution container. Some opacity of plastic may occur; check for minute leaks, squeezing bag firmly. Discard solution if any leaks are found.
Infusion: Infuse at a maximum rate of 200 mg/hr given as a continuous infusion.
Incompatibilities: Do not add any supplementary medications.

Adverse effects

- **CNS:** *Headache*
- **GI:** *Nausea, vomiting, diarrhea, abdominal pain*
- **Other:** Rash

Interactions

✳ **Drug-drug** • Increased serum levels and therefore therapeutic and toxic effects of cyclosporine, phenytoin, benzodiazepines, oral hypoglycemics, warfarin anticoagulants, zidovudine • Decreased serum levels with rifampin, theophylline, TCAs, losartan

■ Nursing considerations
Assessment

- **History:** Hypersensitivity to fluconazole, renal impairment, lactation, pregnancy
- **Physical:** Skin color, lesions; T; injection site; orientation, reflexes, affect; bowel sounds; renal function tests; CBC and differential; culture of area involved

Interventions

- Culture infection prior to therapy; begin treatment before lab results are returned.
- Decrease dosage in cases of renal failure.
- Infuse IV only; not intended for IM or SC use.
- Do not add supplement medication to fluconazole.
- Administer through sterile equipment at a maximum rate of 200 mg/hr given as a continuous infusion.
- Monitor renal function tests weekly, discontinue or decrease dosage of drug at any sign of increased renal toxicity.

Teaching points

- Drug may be given orally or IV as needed. The drug will need to be taken for the full course and may need to be taken long term.
- Use hygiene measures to prevent reinfection or spread of infection.
- Arrange for frequent follow-up while you are on this drug. Be sure to keep all appointments, including blood tests.
- These side effects may occur: nausea, vomiting, diarrhea (small frequent meals may help); headache (analgesics may be ordered).
- Report rash, changes in stool or urine color, difficulty breathing, increased tears or salivation.

▽ flucytosine (5-FC, 5-fluorocytosine)
(floo sye' toe seen)

Ancobon

PREGNANCY CATEGORY C

Drug class
Antifungal

Therapeutic actions
Affects cell membranes of susceptible fungi to cause fungus death; exact mechanism of action is not understood.

Indications

- Treatment of serious infections caused by susceptible strains of *Candida, Cryptococcus*

Adverse effects in *Italics* are most common; those in **Bold** are life-threatening.

- Unlabeled use: treatment of chromomycosis

Contraindications and cautions
- Contraindicated with allergy to flucytosine, pregnancy, lactation.
- Use cautiously with renal impairment (drug accumulation and toxicity may occur), bone marrow depression.

Available forms
Capsules—250, 500 mg

Dosages
Adults
50–150 mg/kg/day PO at 6-hr intervals.
Geriatric patients or patients with renal impairment
Initial dose should be at the lower level; monitor patient very closely.

Pharmacokinetics

Route	Onset	Peak	Duration
Oral	Varies	2 hr	10–12 hr

Metabolism: $T_{1/2}$: 2–5 hr
Distribution: Crosses placenta; may enter breast milk
Excretion: Urine and feces

Adverse effects
- **CNS:** Confusion, hallucinations, headache, sedation, vertigo
- **Dermatologic:** *Rash*
- **GI:** *Nausea, vomiting, diarrhea*
- **Hematologic:** *Anemia, leukopenia, thrombopenia,* elevation of liver enzymes, BUN and creatinine

■ Nursing considerations
Assessment
- **History:** Allergy to flucytosine, renal impairment, bone marrow depression, lactation, pregnancy
- **Physical:** Skin color, lesions; orientation, reflexes, affect; bowel sounds, liver evaluation; renal and liver function tests; CBC and differential

Interventions
- Administer capsules a few at a time over a 15-min period to decrease the GI upset and diarrhea.

- Monitor hepatic and renal function tests and hematologic function periodically throughout treatment.

Teaching points
- Take the capsules a few at a time over a 15-min period to decrease GI upset.
- These side effects may occur: nausea, vomiting, diarrhea (take capsules a few at a time over 15 min); sedation, dizziness, confusion (avoid driving or performing tasks that require alertness).
- Report rash, severe nausea, vomiting, diarrhea, fever, sore throat, unusual bleeding or bruising.

▽ fludarabine phosphate
*(floo **dar**' a been)*

Fludara

PREGNANCY CATEGORY D

Drug classes
Antimetabolite
Antineoplastic

Therapeutic actions
Inhibits DNA polymerase alpha, ribonucleotid reductase and DNA primase, which inhibits DNA synthesis and prevents cell replication.

Indications
- Chronic lymphocytic leukemia (CLL); unresponsive B-cell CLL or no progress during treatment with at least one standard regimen that contains an alkylating agent
- Unlabeled uses: non-Hodgkin's lymphoma, macroglobulinemic lymphoma, prolymphocytic leukemia or prolymphocytoid variant of CLL, mycosis fungoides, hairy-cell leukemia, Hodgkin's disease

Contraindications and cautions
- Contraindicated with allergy to fludarabine or any component, lactation, pregnancy, severe bone marrow depression.
- Use cautiously with renal impairment.

Available forms
Powder for reconstitution—50 mg

F

Dosages

Adults

25 mg/m^2 IV over 30 min for 5 consecutive days. Begin each 5-day course every 28 days. It is recommended that three additional cycles follow the achievement of a maximal response, then discontinue drug.

Pharmacokinetics

Route	Onset	Peak
IV	Rapid	1–2 hr

Metabolism: Hepatic; T$_{1/2}$: 10 hr
Distribution: Crosses placenta; enters breast milk
Excretion: Urine

▼IV facts

Preparation: Reconstitute with 2 mL of sterile water for injection; the solid cake should dissolve in < 15 sec; each mL of resulting solution will contain 25 mg fludarabine, 25 mg mannitol and sodium hydroxide; may be further diluted in 100 or 125 mL of 5% dextrose injection or 0.9% sodium chloride; use within 8 hr of reconstitution; discard after that time. Store unreconstituted drug in refrigerator.
Infusion: Infuse slowly over no less than 30 min.

Adverse effects

- **CNS:** *Weakness, paresthesia, headache, visual disturbance,* hearing loss, sleep disorder, depression, **CNS toxicity**
- **CV:** *Edema,* angina
- **Dermatologic:** *Rash, pruritus,* seborrhea
- **GI:** *Diarrhea, anorexia, nausea, vomiting, stomatitis,* esophagopharyngitis, GI bleeding, mucositis
- **GU:** Dysuria, urinary infection, hematuria, **renal failure**
- **Hematologic:** *Bone marrow toxicity*
- **Respiratory:** *Cough, pneumonia, dyspnea, sinusitis,* upper respiratory infection, epistaxis, bronchitis, hypoxia
- **Other:** *Fever, chills, fatigue, infection, pain, malaise,* diaphoresis, hemorrhage, myalgia, arthralgia, osteoporosis, **tumor lysis syndrome**

■ Nursing considerations

Assessment

- **History:** Allergy to fludarabine or any component, lactation, pregnancy, severe bone marrow depression, renal impairment
- **Physical:** Weight; T; skin lesions, color, edema; hair; vision, speech, orientation, reflexes, sensation; R, adventitious sounds; mucous membranes, liver evaluation, abdominal exam; CBC, differential; renal and liver function tests; urinalysis, chest x-ray

Interventions

- Evaluate hematologic status prior to therapy and before each dose.
- Discontinue therapy if any sign of toxicity occurs (CNS complaints, stomatitis, esophagopharyngitis, rapidly falling WBC count, intractable vomiting, diarrhea, GI ulceration and bleeding, thrombocytopenia, hemorrhage); consult with physician.
- Caution patient to avoid pregnancy while on this drug.

Teaching points

- Prepare a calendar of treatment days.
- These side effects may occur: nausea, vomiting, loss of appetite (medication; small, frequent meals may help; maintain your nutrition while you are on this drug); headache, fatigue, malaise, weakness, lethargy (avoid driving or operating dangerous machinery); mouth sores (use frequent mouth care); diarrhea; increased susceptibility to infection (avoid crowds, exposure to infection; report any sign of infection, eg, fever, fatigue).
- Use birth control while on this drug; may cause birth defects or miscarriages.
- Have frequent, regular medical follow-up, including blood tests.
- Report black, tarry stools; fever; chills; sore throat; unusual bleeding or bruising; chest pain; mouth sores; changes in vision; dizziness.

Adverse effects in *Italics* are most common; those in **Bold** are life-threatening.

▽ fludrocortisone acetate

*(floo droe **kor'** ti sone)*

Florinef Acetate

PREGNANCY CATEGORY C

Drug classes
Corticosteroid
Mineralocorticoid
Hormone

Therapeutic actions
Increases sodium reabsorption in renal tubules and increases potassium and hydrogen excretion, leading to sodium and water retention.

Indications
- Partial replacement therapy in primary and secondary cortical insufficiency and for the treatment of salt-losing adrenogenital syndrome (therapy must be accompanied by adequate doses of glucocorticoids)
- Unlabeled use: management of severe orthostatic hypotension (100–400 mcg/day)

Contraindications and cautions
- Contraindicated with CHF, hypertension, cardiac disease, pregnancy.
- Use cautiously with infections, high sodium intake, lactation.

Available forms
Tablets—0.1 mg

Dosages
Adults
- *Addison's disease:* 0.1 mg/day (range 0.1 mg 3 times per wk to 0.2 mg/day) PO. Reduce dose to 0.05 mg/day if transient hypertension develops. Administration with hydrocortisone (10–30 mg/day) or cortisone (10–37.5 mg/day) is preferable.
- *Salt-losing adrenogenital syndrome:* 0.1–0.2 mg/day PO.

Pediatric patients
If infants or children are maintained on prolonged therapy, their growth and development must be carefully observed.
Children: 0.05–0.1 mg/24 hr.
Infants: 0.1–0.2 mg/24 hr.

Pharmacokinetics

Route	Onset	Peak	Duration
Oral	Gradual	1.7 hr	18–36 hr

Metabolism: Hepatic; $T_{1/2}$: 3.5 hr
Distribution: Crosses placenta; enters breast milk

Adverse effects
- **CNS:** *Frontal and occipital headaches, arthralgia,* tendon contractures, weakness of extremities with ascending paralysis
- **CV:** *Increased blood volume, edema, hypertension,* CHF, cardiac arrhythmias, enlargement of the heart
- **Hypersensitivity:** Rash to **anaphylaxis**

Interactions
✳ Drug-drug • Decreased effects with barbiturates, hydantoins, rifampin • Decreased effects of anticholinesterases with resultant muscular depression in myasthenia gravis • Decreased serum levels and effectiveness of salicylates

■ Nursing considerations
Assessment
- **History:** CHF, hypertension, cardiac disease, infections, high sodium intake, lactation, pregnancy
- **Physical:** P, BP, chest sounds, weight, T, tissue turgor, reflexes and bilateral grip strength, serum electrolytes

Interventions
- Use only in conjunction with glucocorticoid therapy and control of electrolytes and infection.
- Increase dosage during times of stress to prevent drug-induced adrenal insufficiency.
- Monitor BP and serum electrolytes regularly to prevent overdosage.
- Discontinue if signs of overdosage (hypertension, edema, excessive weight gain, increased heart size) appear.
- Treat muscle weakness due to excessive K^+ loss with supplements.
- Restrict sodium intake if edema develops.

Teaching points
- Use range-of-motion exercises, positioning to deal with musculoskeletal effects.

- Take drug exactly as prescribed; do not stop without notifying health care provider; if a dose is missed, take it as soon as possible unless it is almost time for the next dose—do not double the next dose.
- Keep appointments for frequent follow-up visits so response may be determined and dosage adjusted.
- Wear a medical alert ID so that any emergency medical personnel will know about this drug therapy.
- Report unusual weight gain, swelling of the lower extremities, muscle weakness, dizziness, and severe or continuing headache.

▷ flumazenil
(floo maz' eh nill)

Anexate (CAN), Romazicon

PREGNANCY CATEGORY C

Drug classes
Antidote
Benzodiazepine receptor antagonist

Therapeutic actions
Antagonizes the actions of benzodiazepines on the CNS and inhibits activity at GABA-benzodiazepine receptor sites.

Indications
- Complete or partial reversal of the sedative effects of benzodiazepines when general anesthesia has been induced or maintained with them, and when sedation has been produced for diagnostic and therapeutic procedures
- Management of benzodiazepine overdose

Contraindications and cautions
- Contraindicated with hypersensitivity to flumazenil or benzodiazepines; patients who have been given benzodiazepines to control potentially life-threatening conditions; patients showing signs of serious cyclic antidepressant overdose.
- Use cautiously with history of seizures, hepatic impairment, panic disorders, head

injury, history of drug or alcohol dependence.

Available forms
Injection—0.1 mg/mL

Dosages
Use smallest effective dose possible.
Adults
- *Reversal of conscious sedation or in general anesthesia:* Initial dose of 0.2 mg (2 mL) IV; wait 45 sec; if ineffectual, repeat dose at 60-sec intervals. Maximum dose of 1 mg (10 mL).
- *Management of suspected benzodiazepine overdose:* Initial dose of 0.2 mg IV; repeat with 0.3 mg IV q 30 sec, up to a maximum cumulative dose of 3 mg.
Pediatric patients
Safety and efficacy not established.
Geriatric patients
No reduction of dosage.

Pharmacokinetics

Route	Onset	Peak	Duration
IV	20–30 sec	6–10 min	72 hr

Metabolism: Hepatic; $T_{1/2}$: 7–15 min, then 41–79 min
Distribution: Crosses placenta; may enter breast milk

▽ IV facts
Preparation: Can be drawn into syringe with 5% dextrose in water, lactated Ringer's, and normal saline solutions. Discard within 24 hr if mixed in solution. Do not remove from vial until ready for use.
Infusion: Infuse slowly over 15 sec for general anesthesia, over 30 sec for overdose. To reduce pain of injection, administer through a freely running IV infusion in a large vein.
Compatibilities: Stable with aminophylline, dobutamine, cimetidine, famotidine, ranitidine, heparin, lidocaine, procainamide.

Adverse effects
- **CNS:** *Dizziness, vertigo,* agitation, nervousness, dry mouth, tremor, palpitations, emotional lability, confusion, crying, vision changes, seizures

- **CV:** Vasodilation, flushing, arrhythmias, chest pain
- **GI:** *Nausea, vomiting,* hiccups
- **Other:** *Headache, pain at injection site, increased sweating,* fatigue

Interactions
✳ **Drug-food •** Ingestion of food during IV infusion decreases serum levels and effectiveness

■ Nursing considerations
Assessment
- **History:** Hypersensitivity to flumazenil or benzodiazepines; use of benzodiazepines for control of potentially life-threatening conditions; signs of serious cyclic antidepressant overdose, history of seizures, hepatic impairment, panic disorders, head injury, history of drug or alcohol dependence
- **Physical:** Skin color, lesions; T; orientation, reflexes, affect; P, BP, peripheral perfusion; serum drug levels

Interventions
- Administer by IV route only.
- Have emergency equipment ready, secure airway during administration.
- Monitor clinical response carefully to determine effects of drug and need for repeated doses.
- Inject into running IV in a large vein to decrease pain of injection.
- Provide patient with written information after use; amnesia may be long-term, and teaching may not be remembered, including safety measures.

Teaching points
- Drug may cause changes in vision, dizziness, changes in alertness (avoid driving or operating hazardous machinery for at least 18–24 hr after drug use).
- Do not use any alcohol or OTC drugs for 18–24 hr after use of this drug.
- Report difficulty breathing, pain at IV site, changes in vision, severe headache.

▽ **flunisolide**
*(floo **niss'** oh lide)*

AeroBid, AeroBid-M, Bronalide (CAN), Nasalide, Nasarel, Rhinalar (CAN)

PREGNANCY CATEGORY C

Drug classes
Corticosteroid
Glucocorticoid
Hormone

Therapeutic actions
Anti-inflammatory effect; local administration into lower respiratory tract or nasal passages maximizes beneficial effects while decreasing possible adverse effects from systemic absorption.

Indications
- *Respiratory inhalant:* control of bronchial asthma that requires corticosteroids
- *Intranasal:* relief of symptoms of seasonal or perennial rhinitis that respond poorly to other treatments

Contraindications and cautions
- Systemic fungal infections, untreated local nasal infections, epistaxis, nasal trauma, septal ulcers, recent nasal surgery, lactation.

Available forms
Aerosol—250 mcg/actuation; spray—25 mcg/actuation

Dosages
Respiratory inhalant
Each actuation delivers 250 mcg.
Adults
Two inhalations (500 mcg) bid morning and evening (total dose 1 mg), not to exceed 4 bid (2 mg).
Pediatric patients
6–15 yr: Two inhalations bid morning and evening.
< 6 yr: Do not use.
Intranasal
Each actuation of the inhaler delivers 25 mcg.
Adults
Initial dosage 2 sprays (50 mcg) in each nostril bid (total dose 200 mcg/day); may be in-

creased to 2 sprays in each nostril tid (total dose 300 mcg/day). Maximum daily dose, 8 sprays in each nostril (400 mcg/day).

Pediatric patients 6–14 yr
- *Initial dosage:* 1 spray in each nostril tid or 2 sprays in each nostril bid (total dose 150–200 mcg/day). Maximum daily dose 4 sprays in each nostril (200 mcg/day). Not recommended for children < 6 yr.
- *Maintenance dosage:* Reduce to smallest effective dose. Discontinue therapy after 3 wk if no significant symptomatic improvement.

Pharmacokinetics

Route	Onset	Peak	Duration
Intranasal	Slow	10–30 min	4–6 hr

Metabolism: Hepatic; $T_{1/2}$: 1–2 hr
Distribution: Crosses placenta; enters breast milk
Excretion: Urine and feces

Adverse effects
Respiratory inhalant
- **Endocrine:** Suppression of hypothalamic-pituitary-adrenal (HPA) function due to systemic absorption
- **Local:** *Oral, laryngeal, pharyngeal irritation;* fungal infections

Intranasal
- **CNS:** *Headache*
- **Dermatologic:** Urticaria
- **Endocrine:** HPA suppression, Cushing's syndrome with overdosage
- **GI:** Nausea
- **Local:** *Nasal irritation, fungal infection*
- **Respiratory:** *Epistaxis, rebound congestion,* perforation of the nasal septum, anosmia

■ Nursing considerations
Assessment
- **History:** Systemic fungal infections, untreated local nasal infections, epistaxis, nasal trauma, septal ulcers, recent nasal surgery, lactation
- **Physical:** Weight, T, BP, P, auscultation, R, adventitious sounds, examination of nares

Interventions
- Do not use during an acute asthmatic attack or to manage status asthmaticus.
- Taper systemic steroids carefully during transfer to inhalational steroids; deaths from adrenal insufficiency have occurred.
- Use decongestant nose drops to facilitate penetration if edema, excessive secretions are present.

Teaching points
- Do not use this drug more often than prescribed.
- Do not stop using this drug without consulting your health care provider.
- Use inhalational bronchodilator drug before oral inhalant if receiving concomitant bronchodilator therapy. Allow at least 1 min between puffs.
- Rinse your mouth after using.
- Use decongestant nose drops first if nasal passages are blocked when using intranasal form.
- These side effects may occur: local irritation (make sure you are using your device correctly), headache.
- Report sore mouth, sore throat.

▷ fluorouracil
(5-fluorouracil, 5-F)
*(flure oh **yoor'** a sill)*

Adrucil, Efudex, Fluoroplex

PREGNANCY CATEGORY D

Drug classes
Antimetabolite
Antineoplastic

Therapeutic actions
Inhibits thymidylate synthetase, leading to inhibition of DNA synthesis and cell death.

Indications
- Palliative management of carcinoma of the colon, rectum, breast, stomach, pancreas in selected patients considered incurable by surgery or other means (parenteral)
- Topical treatment of multiple actinic or solar keratoses

- Topical treatment of superficial basal cell carcinoma
- Unlabeled use: Topical treatment of condylomata acuminata
- Orphan drug uses: In combination with interferon alfa 2-a recombinant for esophageal and advanced colorectal carcinoma; with leucovorin for colon or rectum metastatic adenocarcinoma

Contraindications and cautions

- Allergy to fluorouracil; poor nutritional status; serious infections; hematopoietic depression secondary to radiation or chemotherapy; impaired liver function; pregnancy; lactation.

Available forms

Injection—50 mg/mL; cream—1%, 5%; solution—1%, 2%, 5%

Dosages
Adults

Initial dosage: 12 mg/kg IV daily for 4 successive days; do not exceed 800 mg/day. If no toxicity occurs, give 6 mg/kg on the 6th, 8th, 10th, and 12th day with no drug therapy on days 5, 7, 9, and 11. Discontinue therapy at end of 12th day, even if no toxicity.

Patients who are poor-risk or undernourished

6 mg/kg/day IV for 3 days. If no toxicity develops, give 3 mg/kg on the 5th, 7th, and 9th days. No drug is given on days 4, 6, and 8. Do not exceed 400 mg/day.

Patients with hepatic failure

If serum bilirubin > 5 mg/dL, do not administer fluorouracil. Maintenance therapy: Continue therapy on appropriate schedules:

For patients without toxicity: Repeat dosage every 30 days after the last day of the previous treatment.

For patients with toxicity: Give 10–15 mg/kg/wk as a single dose after signs of toxicity subside. Do not exceed 1 g/wk. Adjust dosage based on patient response; therapy may be prolonged (12–60 mo).

Topical use

- *Actinic or solar keratoses:* Apply bid to cover lesions. Continue until inflammatory response reaches erosion, necrosis, and ulceration stage, then discontinue. Usual course of therapy is 2–6 wk. Complete healing may

not be evident for 1–2 mo after cessation of therapy.

- *Superficial basal cell carcinoma:* Apply 5% strength bid in an amount sufficient to cover the lesions. Continue treatment for at least 3–6 wk. Treatment may be required for 10–12 wk.

Pharmacokinetics

Route	Onset	Peak	Duration
IV	Immediate	1–2 hr	6 hr
Topical	Minimal absorption		

Metabolism: Hepatic; $T_{1/2}$: 18–20 min
Distribution: Crosses placenta; enters breast milk
Excretion: Urine and lungs

▽ IV facts

Preparation: Store vials at room temperature; solution may discolor during storage with no adverse effects. Protect ampule from light. Precipitate may form during storage, heat to 60° C, and shake vigorously to dissolve. Cool to body temperature before administration. No dilution is required.

Infusion: Infuse slowly over 24 hr; inject into tubing of running IV to avoid pain on injection; direct injection over 1–3 min.

Incompatibilities: Do not mix with IV additives or other chemotherapeutic agents.

Y-site incompatibilities: Do not inject with droperidol.

Adverse effects
Parenteral

- **CNS:** *Lethargy, malaise, weakness,* euphoria, acute cerebellar syndrome, photophobia, lacrimation, decreased vision, nystagmus, diplopia
- **CV:** Myocardial ischemia, angina
- **Dermatologic:** *Alopecia, dermatitis, maculopapular rash, photosensitivity,* nail changes including nail loss, dry skin, fissures
- **GI:** *Diarrhea, anorexia, nausea, vomiting, cramps, enteritis, duodenal ulcer, duodenitis, gastritis, glossitis, stomatitis,* pharyngitis, esophagopharyngitis
- **Hematologic:** *Leukopenia, thrombocytopenia,* elevations in alkaline phosphatase, serum transaminase, serum bilirubin, lactic dehydrogenase
- **Other:** Fever, epistaxis

Topical
- **Hematologic:** Leukocytosis, thrombocytopenia, toxic granulation, eosinophilia
- **Local:** *Local pain, pruritus, hyperpigmentation, irritation, inflammation and burning at the site of application,* allergic contact dermatitis, scarring, soreness, tenderness, suppuration, scaling and swelling

Interactions
✳ **Drug-lab test** • 5-hydroxyindoleacetic acid (5-HIAA) urinary excretion may increase
• Plasma albumin may decrease due to protein malabsorption

■ Nursing considerations
Assessment
- **History:** Allergy to fluorouracil, poor nutritional status, serious infections, hematopoietic depression, impaired liver function, pregnancy, lactation
- **Physical:** Weight; T; skin lesions; color; hair; vision, speech, orientation, reflexes, sensation; R, adventitious sounds; mucous membranes, liver evaluation, abdominal exam; CBC, differential; renal and liver function tests; urinalysis, chest x-ray

Interventions
- Evaluate hematologic status before beginning therapy and before each dose.
- Discontinue drug therapy at any sign of toxicity (stomatitis, esophagopharyngitis, rapidly falling WBC count, intractable vomiting, diarrhea, GI ulceration and bleeding, thrombocytopenia, hemorrhage); consult with physician.
- Arrange for biopsies of skin lesions to rule out frank neoplasm before beginning topical therapy and in all patients who do not respond to topical therapy.
- Wash hands thoroughly immediately after application of topical preparations. Use caution in applying near the nose, eyes, and mouth.
- Avoid occlusive dressings with topical application; the incidence of inflammatory reactions in adjacent skin areas is increased with these dressings. Use porous gauze dressings for cosmetic reasons.

Teaching points
- Prepare a calendar of treatment days. If using the topical application, wash hands thoroughly after application. Do not use occlusive dressings; a porous gauze dressing may be used for cosmetic reasons.
- These side effects may occur: nausea, vomiting, loss of appetite (request medication; small, frequent meals may help; maintain nutrition); decreased vision, tearing, double vision, malaise, weakness, lethargy (reversible; avoid driving or operating dangerous machinery); mouth sores (frequent mouth care is needed); diarrhea; loss of hair (obtain a wig or other head covering; keep the head covered in extremes of temperature); rash, sensitivity of skin and eyes to sun and ultraviolet light (avoid exposure to the sun; use a sunscreen and protective clothing; topical application: ultraviolet will increase the severity of the local reaction); birth defects or miscarriages (use birth control); unsightly local reaction to topical application (transient; use a porous gauze dressing to cover areas); pain, burning, stinging, swelling at local application.
- Have frequent, regular medical follow-up, including frequent blood tests to evaluate drug effects.
- Report black, tarry stools; fever; chills; sore throat; unusual bleeding or bruising; chest pain; mouth sores; severe pain; tenderness; scaling at sight of local application.

▷ **fluoxetine hydrochloride**
(floo ox' e teen)

Apo-Fluoxetine (CAN), Novo-Fluoxetine (CAN), PMS-Fluoxetine (CAN), Prozac, Prozac Weekly, Sarafem

PREGNANCY CATEGORY B

Drug classes
Antidepressant
Selective serotonin reuptake inhibitor (SSRI)

Therapeutic actions

Acts as an antidepressant by inhibiting CNS neuronal uptake of serotonin; blocks uptake of serotonin with little effect on norepinephrine; little affinity for muscarinic, histaminergic, and alpha$_1$-adrenergic receptors.

Indications

- Treatment of depression; most effective in patients with major depressive disorder
- Treatment of obsessive-compulsive disorder
- Treatment of bulimia
- Treatment of PMDD (pre-menstrual dysphoric disorder) (*Sarafem*)
- Treatment of panic disorder with or without agoraphobia (*Prozac*)
- Unlabeled use: treatment of obesity, alcoholism, numerous psychiatric disorders, chronic pain, various neuropathies

Contraindications and cautions

- Contraindicated with hypersensitivity to fluoxetine; pregnancy.
- Use cautiously with impaired hepatic or renal function, diabetes mellitus, lactation.

Available forms

Tablets—10 mg; pulvules—10, 20, 40 mg; liquid—20 mg/5 mL; DR capsules—90 mg

Dosages
Adults

- *Antidepressant:* The full antidepressant effect may not be seen for up to 4 wk. Initial: 20 mg/day PO in the morning. If no clinical improvement is seen, increase dose after several weeks. Administer doses > 20 mg/day on a bid schedule. Do not exceed 80 mg/day. Once stabilized, may switch to 90 mg DR capsules once a week.
- *Obsessive-compulsive disorder:* 20–60 mg/day PO; may require up to 5 wk for effectiveness.
- *Bulimia:* 60 mg/day PO in the morning.
- *PMDD (Sarafem):* 20 mg/day PO or 20 mg/day PO starting 14 days prior to the anticipated beginning of menses and continuing through the first full day of menses, then no drug until 14 days before next menses; do not exceed 80 mg/day.
- *Panic disorder (Prozac):* 10 mg/day PO for the first week, increase to 20 mg/day if needed. Maximum dose: 60 mg/day.

Pediatric patients

Safety and efficacy not established.

Geriatric patients or patients with hepatic impairment

Give a lower or less frequent dose. Monitor response to guide dosage.

Pharmacokinetics

Route	Onset	Peak
Oral	Slow	6–8 hr

Metabolism: Hepatic; $T_{1/2}$: 2–4 wk
Distribution: Crosses placenta; enters breast milk
Excretion: Urine and feces

Adverse effects

- **CNS:** *Headache, nervousness, insomnia, drowsiness, anxiety, tremor, dizziness, light-headedness,* agitation, sedation, abnormal gait, convulsions
- **CV:** Hot flashes, palpitations
- **Dermatologic:** *Sweating, rash, pruritus,* acne, alopecia, contact dermatitis
- **GI:** *Nausea, vomiting, diarrhea, dry mouth, anorexia, dyspepsia, constipation, taste changes,* flatulence, gastroenteritis, dysphagia, gingivitis
- **GU:** *Painful menstruation, sexual dysfunction, frequency,* cystitis, impotence, urgency, vaginitis
- **Respiratory:** *Upper respiratory infections, pharyngitis,* cough, dyspnea, bronchitis, rhinitis
- **Other:** *Weight loss, asthenia, fever*

Interactions

✳ **Drug-drug** • Increased therapeutic and toxic effects of TCAs • Decreased therapeutic effects if taken with cyproheptadine • Decreased effectiveness if taken while smoking • Increased toxicity of lithium; avoid this combination • Possible fatal reactions with MAOIs; do not administer together; 2-wk washout period needed • Additive CNS effects if combined with benzodiazepines, alcohol; avoid these combinations • Avoid administration with other serotonergic drugs; may lead to serotonin syndrome

✳ **Drug-alternative therapy** • Increased risk of severe reaction if combined with St. John's wort therapy.

F

■ Nursing considerations

CLINICAL ALERT!
Name confusion has occurred between Sarafem (fluoxetine) and Serophene (clomiphene); use caution.

Assessment
- **History:** Hypersensitivity to fluoxetine, impaired hepatic or renal function, diabetes mellitus, lactation, pregnancy
- **Physical:** Weight, T; skin rash, lesions; reflexes, affect; bowel sounds, liver evaluation; P, peripheral perfusion; urinary output, renal and liver function tests, CBC

Interventions
- Arrange for lower or less frequent doses in elderly patients and patients with hepatic or renal impairment.
- Establish suicide precautions for severely depressed patients. Limit quantity of capsules dispensed.
- Administer drug in the morning. If dose of > 20 mg/day is needed, administer in divided doses.
- Monitor patient for response to therapy for up to 4 wk before increasing dose.
- Switch to once a week therapy by starting weekly dose 7 days after last 20 mg/day dose. If response is not satisfactory, reconsider daily dosing.

Teaching points
- It may take up to 4 wk before the full effect occurs. Take in the morning (or in divided doses if necessary). If you are taking the once weekly capsule, mark calendar with reminders of drug day.
- These side effects may occur: dizziness, drowsiness, nervousness, insomnia (avoid driving or performing hazardous tasks); nausea, vomiting, weight loss (small, frequent meals may help; monitor your weight loss); sexual dysfunction; flulike symptoms.
- Do not take this drug during pregnancy. If you think that you are pregnant or wish to become pregnant, consult with your physician.
- Report rash, mania, seizures, severe weight loss.

- Keep this drug, and all medications, out of the reach of children.

▽ fluoxymesterone
*(floo ox i **mes'** te rone)*

Halotestin

PREGNANCY CATEGORY X

C-III CONTROLLED SUBSTANCE

Drug classes
Androgen
Hormone

Therapeutic actions
Analog of testosterone, the primary natural androgen; endogenous androgens are responsible for growth and development of male sex organs and the maintenance of secondary sex characteristics; administration of androgen analogs increases the retention of nitrogen, sodium, potassium, phosphorus, and decreases urinary excretion of calcium; increases protein anabolism and decreases protein catabolism; stimulates the production of red blood cells.

Indications
- *Male:* replacement therapy in hypogonadism—primary hypogonadism, hypogonadotropic hypogonadism, delayed puberty
- *Female:* metastatic cancer—inoperable breast cancer in women who are 1—5 years postmenopausal

Contraindications and cautions
- Contraindicated with known sensitivity to androgens, allergy to tartrazine or aspirin (in products marketed under the brand name *Halotestin*), prostate or breast cancer in males, pregnancy, lactation.
- Use cautiously with MI, liver disease.

Available forms
Tablets—2, 5, 10 mg

Dosages
Adults
- *Hypogonadism:* 5–20 mg/day PO.

- *Delayed puberty:* 2.5–20 mg/day PO, although generally 2.5–10 mg/day PO for 4–6 mo is sufficient.
- *Carcinoma of the breast:* 10–40 mg/day PO in divided doses. Continue for 1 mo for a subjective response and 2–3 mo for an objective response.

Pharmacokinetics

Route	Onset	Peak
Oral	Rapid	2 hr

Metabolism: Hepatic; T$_{1/2}$: 9.5 hr
Distribution: Crosses placenta; enters breast milk
Excretion: Urine and feces

Adverse effects

- **CNS:** *Dizziness, headache, sleep disorders, fatigue,* tremor, sleeplessness, generalized paresthesia, sleep apnea syndrome, CNS hemorrhage, nervousness, depression
- **Dermatologic:** *Rash,* dermatitis, anaphylactoid reactions
- **Endocrine:** *Androgenic effects* (acne, edema, mild hirsutism, decrease in breast size, deepening of the voice, oily skin or hair, weight gain, clitoral hypertrophy or testicular atrophy), *hypoestrogenic effects* (flushing, sweating, vaginitis, nervousness, emotional lability)
- **GI:** *Nausea,* hepatic dysfunction; hepatocellular carcinoma, **peliosis hepatitis**
- **GU:** Fluid retention, decreased urinary output
- **Hematologic:** *Polycythemia, leukopenia,* hypercalcemia, altered serum cholesterol levels; retention of sodium, chloride, water, potassium, phosphates, and calcium
- **Other:** Chills, premature closure of the epiphyses, increased libido

Interactions

✳ **Drug-drug** • Potentiation of oral anticoagulants with androgens; anticoagulant dosage may need to be decreased • May decrease insulin requirements

✳ **Drug-lab test** • Altered glucose tolerance tests • Decrease in thyroid function tests, may persist for 2–3 wk after stopping therapy • Suppression of clotting factors II, V, VII, and X • Increased creatinine, creatinine clearance, may last for 2 wk after therapy

■ Nursing considerations
Assessment

- **History:** Sensitivity to androgens, allergy to tartrazine or aspirin, prostate or breast cancer in males, MI, liver disease, pregnancy, lactation
- **Physical:** Skin color, lesions, texture; hair distribution pattern; affect, orientation, peripheral sensation; abdominal exam, liver evaluation; serum electrolytes, serum cholesterol levels, liver function tests, glucose tolerance tests, thyroid function tests, long bone x-ray (in children)

Interventions

- Administer drug with meals or snacks to decrease GI upset.
- Monitor effect on children with long bone x-rays every 3–6 mo. Stop drug well before the bone age reaches the norm for the patient's chronologic age.
- Monitor patient for occurrence of edema; arrange for diuretic therapy.
- Monitor liver function, serum electrolytes periodically, and consult with physician for corrective measures.
- Measure cholesterol levels in those at high risk for CAD.
- Monitor diabetic patients closely as glucose tolerance may change. Adjust insulin, oral hypoglycemic dosage, and diet.
- Arrange for periodic monitoring of urine and serum calcium of disseminated breast carcinoma, and arrange for treatment or stop drug.
- Monitor geriatric males for prostatic hypertrophy and carcinoma.
- Stop drug and arrange for consultation if abnormal vaginal bleeding occurs.

Teaching points

- Take drug with meals or snacks to decrease the GI upset.
- These side effects may occur: body hair growth, baldness, deepening of the voice, loss of libido, impotence (reversible); excitation, confusion, insomnia (avoid driving, performing tasks that require alertness); swelling of the ankles, fingers (request medication).
- Diabetic patients need to monitor urine or blood sugar closely as glucose tolerance may

change. Report any abnormalities to physician, for corrective action.

- Report ankle swelling, nausea, vomiting, yellowing of skin or eyes, unusual bleeding or bruising, penile swelling or pain, hoarseness, body hair growth, deepening of the voice, acne, menstrual irregularities.

▽**fluphenazine**

(floo fen' a zeen)

fluphenazine decanoate
Injection: Modecate Deconoate (CAN), Prolixin Decanoate, Rho-Fluphenazine Deconate (CAN)

fluphenazine enanthate
Injection: Moditen Enanthate (CAN), PMS-Fluphenazine (CAN)

fluphenazine hydrochloride
Oral tablets, concentrate, elixir, injection: Apo-Fluphenazine (CAN), Moditen Hydrochloride (CAN), Permitil, PMS-Fluphenazine (CAN)

PREGNANCY CATEGORY C

Drug classes
Phenothiazine
Dopaminergic blocking agent
Antipsychotic

Therapeutic actions
Mechanism not fully understood: antipsychotic drugs block postsynaptic dopamine receptors in the brain, depress the RAS, including the parts of the brain involved with wakefulness and emesis; anticholinergic, antihistaminic (H_1), and alpha-adrenergic blocking activity also may contribute to some of its therapeutic (and adverse) actions.

Indications
- Management of manifestations of psychotic disorders; the longer acting parenteral dosage forms, fluphenazine enanthate and fluphenazine decanoate, indicated for management of patients (chronic schizophren-

ics) who require prolonged parenteral therapy
- Management of behavioral complications in patients with mental retardation (fluphenazine decanoate)

Contraindications and cautions
- Contraindicated with coma or severe CNS depression, bone marrow depression, blood dyscrasia, circulatory collapse, subcortical brain damage, Parkinson's disease, liver damage, cerebral arteriosclerosis, coronary disease, severe hypotension or hypertension; pregnancy.
- Use cautiously with respiratory disorders ("silent pneumonia"); glaucoma, prostatic hypertrophy (anticholinergic effects may exacerbate glaucoma and urinary retention); epilepsy or history of epilepsy (drug lowers seizure threshold); breast cancer (elevations in prolactin may stimulate a prolactin-dependent tumor); thyrotoxicosis; peptic ulcer, decreased renal function; myelography within previous 24 hr or myelography scheduled within 48 hr; exposure to heat or phosphorous insecticides; pregnancy; lactation; children younger than 12 yr, especially those with chickenpox, CNS infections (children are especially susceptible to dystonias that may confound the diagnosis of Reye's syndrome).

Available forms
Tablets—1, 2.5, 5, 10 mg; injection—25 mg/mL

Dosages
Full clinical effects may require 6 wk–6 mo of therapy. Patients who have never taken phenothiazines, "poor-risk" patients (those disorders that predispose to undue reactions) should be treated initially with this shorter acting dosage form and then switched to the longer acting parenteral forms, fluphenazine enanthate or decanoate.

The duration of action of the esterified forms of fluphenazine is markedly longer than those of fluphenazine hydrochloride; the duration of action of fluphenazine enanthate is estimated to be 1–3 wk; the duration of action of fluphenazine decanoate is estimated to be 4 wk.

No precise formula is available for the conversion of fluphenazine hydrochloride dosage to fluphenazine decanoate dosage, but one study suggests that 20 mg of fluphenazine hydrochloride daily was equivalent to 25 mg decanoate every 3 wk.

Fluphenazine hydrochloride
Adults
Individualize dosage, begin with low dosage, gradually increase.

Oral
0.5–10 mg/day in divided doses q 6–8 hr; usual daily dose is less than 3 mg. Give daily doses greater than 20 mg with caution. When symptoms are controlled, gradually reduce dosage.

IM
Average starting dose is 1.25 mg (range 2.5–10 mg), divided and given q 6–8 hr; parenteral dose is one-third to one-half the oral dose. Give daily doses greater than 10 mg with caution.

Pediatric patients
Generally not recommended for children < 12 yr.

Geriatric patients
Initial oral dose is 1–2.5 mg/day.

Fluphenazine enanthate, fluphenazine decanoate
Adults
• *Initial dose:* 12.5–25 mg IM or SC; determine subsequent doses and dosage interval based on patient response. Dose should not exceed 100 mg.

Pharmacokinetics

Route	Onset	Peak	Duration
Oral	60 min	2 hr	6–8 hr
IM (HCl)	60 min	1–2 hr	6–8 hr
IM (enanthate)	24–72 hr		2 wk
IM (decanoate)	24–72 hr		1–6 wk

Metabolism: Hepatic; $T_{1/2}$: 4.5–15.3 hr (fluphenazine hydrochloride), 3.7 days (fluphenazine enanthate), 6.8–9.6 days (fluphenazine decanoate)
Distribution: Crosses placenta; enters breast milk
Excretion: Unchanged in the urine

Adverse effects
• **Autonomic:** Dry mouth, salivation, nasal congestion, nausea, vomiting, anorexia, fever, pallor, flushed facies, sweating, constipation, paralytic ileus, urinary retention, incontinence, polyuria, enuresis, priapism, ejaculation inhibition, male impotence
• **CNS:** *Drowsiness,* insomnia, vertigo, headache, weakness, tremor, ataxia, slurring, cerebral edema, seizures, exacerbation of psychotic symptoms, extrapyramidal syndromes *(pseudoparkinsonism); dystonias; akathisia,* tardive dyskinesias, potentially irreversible, neuroleptic malignant syndrome (extrapyramidal symptoms), hyperthermias, **autonomic disturbances** (rare, but 20% fatal)
• **CV:** Hypotension, orthostatic hypotension, hypertension, tachycardia, bradycardia, **cardiac arrest,** CHF, cardiomegaly, **refractory arrhythmias,** pulmonary edema
• **Endocrine:** Lactation, breast engorgement in females, galactorrhea; syndrome of inappropriate ADH secretion; amenorrhea, menstrual irregularities; gynecomastia in males; changes in libido; hyperglycemia or hypoglycemia; glycosuria; hyponatremia; pituitary tumor with hyperprolactinemia; inhibition of ovulation, infertility, pseudopregnancy; reduced urinary levels of gonadotropins, estrogens, progestins
• **Hematologic:** Eosinophilia, leukopenia, leukocytosis, anemia; aplastic anemia; hemolytic anemia; thrombocytopenic or nonthrombocytopenic purpura; pancytopenia
• **Hypersensitivity:** Jaundice, urticaria, angioneurotic edema, laryngeal edema, photosensitivity, eczema, asthma, anaphylactoid reactions, exfoliative dermatitis
• **Respiratory:** Bronchospasm, laryngospasm, dyspnea; suppression of cough reflex and potential for aspiration **(sudden death related to asphyxia or cardiac arrest has been reported)**

Indications
✳ **Drug-drug** • Additive CNS depression with alcohol • Additive anticholinergic effects and possibly decreased antipsychotic efficacy with anticholinergic drugs • Increased likelihood of seizures with metrizamide (contrast agent used in myelography) • Decreased antihypertensive effect of guanethidine with antipsychotic drugs

✳ **Drug-lab test** • False-positive pregnancy tests (less likely if serum test is used) • Increase in PBI, not attributable to an increase in thyroxine

■ Nursing considerations
Assessment
- **History:** Coma or severe CNS depression; bone marrow depression; blood dyscrasia; circulatory collapse; subcortical brain damage; Parkinson's disease; liver damage; cerebral arteriosclerosis; coronary disease; severe hypotension or hypertension; respiratory disorders; glaucoma, prostatic hypertrophy; epilepsy; breast cancer; thyrotoxicosis; peptic ulcer, decreased renal function; myelography within previous 24 hr or myelography scheduled within 48 hr; exposure to heat or phosphorous insecticides; children < 12 yr, chickenpox, CNS infections; pregnancy
- **Physical:** Weight, T; reflexes, orientation, intraocular pressure; P, BP, orthostatic BP; R, adventitious sounds; bowel sounds and normal output, liver evaluation; urinary output, prostate size; CBC, urinalysis, thyroid, liver and kidney function tests

Interventions
- Arrange for discontinuation of drug if serum creatinine, BUN become abnormal or if WBC count is depressed.
- Monitor elderly patients for dehydration, institute remedial measures promptly. Sedation and decreased sensation of thirst related to CNS effects can lead to severe dehydration.
- Consult physician regarding appropriate warning of patient or patient's guardian about tardive dyskinesias.
- Consult physician about dosage reduction, use of anticholinergic antiparkinsonian drugs (controversial) if extrapyramidal effects occur.

Teaching points
- Take drug exactly as prescribed.
- Avoid driving or engaging in other dangerous activities if CNS, vision changes occur.
- Avoid prolonged exposure to sun; use a sunscreen or covering garments if exposure is unavoidable.
- Maintain fluid intake, and use precautions against heatstroke in hot weather.

- Report sore throat, fever, unusual bleeding or bruising, rash, weakness, tremors, impaired vision, dark urine (pink or reddish brown urine is expected), pale stools, yellowing of skin or eyes.

▽flurazepam hydrochloride
(flur az' e pam)

Dalmane, Somnol (CAN)

PREGNANCY CATEGORY X

C-IV CONTROLLED SUBSTANCE

Drug classes
Benzodiazepine
Sedative and hypnotic

Therapeutic actions
Exact mechanisms not understood; acts mainly at subcortical levels of the CNS, leaving the cortex relatively unaffected; potentiates the effects of gamma-aminobutyate, an inhibitory neurotransmitter.

Indications
- Insomnia characterized by difficulty in falling asleep, frequent nocturnal awakenings, or early morning awakening
- Recurring insomnia or poor sleeping habits
- Acute or chronic medical situations requiring restful sleep

Contraindications and cautions
- Contraindicated with hypersensitivity to benzodiazepines, psychoses, acute narrow-angle glaucoma, shock, coma, acute alcoholic intoxication with depression of vital signs, pregnancy (risk of congenital malformations, neonatal withdrawal syndrome), labor and delivery ("floppy infant" syndrome), lactation (infants become lethargic and lose weight).
- Use cautiously with impaired liver or kidney function, debilitation, depression, suicidal tendencies, elderly.

Available forms
Capsules—15, 30 mg

Adverse effects in *Italics* are most common; those in **Bold** are life-threatening.

Dosages
Individualize dosage.
Adults
30 mg PO before hs; 15 mg may suffice.
Pediatric patients
Not for use in patients < 15 yr.
Geriatric patients or patients with debilitating disease
Initially, 15 mg PO; adjust as needed and tolerated.

Pharmacokinetics

Route	Onset	Peak
Oral	Fast	30–60 min

Metabolism: Hepatic; $T_{1/2}$: 47–100 hr
Distribution: Crosses placenta; enters breast milk
Excretion: Urine

Adverse effects
- **CNS:** *Transient, mild drowsiness initially; sedation, depression, lethargy, apathy, fatigue, light-headedness, disorientation, restlessness, asthenia,* crying, delirium, headache, slurred speech, dysarthria, stupor, rigidity, tremor, dystonia, vertigo, euphoria, nervousness, difficulty in concentration, vivid dreams, psychomotor retardation, extrapyramidal symptoms; *mild paradoxical excitatory reactions during first 2 wk of treatment* (psychiatric patients, aggressive children, with high dosage), visual and auditory disturbances, diplopia, nystagmus, depressed hearing, nasal congestion
- **CV:** *Bradycardia, tachycardia,* **CV collapse,** hypertension and hypotension, palpitations, edema
- **Dependence:** *Drug dependence with withdrawal syndrome* when drug is discontinued (common with abrupt cessation of high dosage used more than 4 mo)
- **Dermatologic:** Urticaria, pruritus, rash, dermatitis
- **GI:** *Constipation, diarrhea, dyspepsia,* dry mouth, salivation, nausea, anorexia, vomiting, difficulty in swallowing, gastric disorders, elevations of blood enzymes: LDH, alkaline phosphatase, AST, ALT, hepatic dysfunction, jaundice
- **GU:** *Incontinence, urinary retention, changes in libido,* menstrual irregularities
- **Hematologic:** Decreased hematocrit, blood dyscrasias
- **Other:** Hiccups, fever, diaphoresis, paresthesias, muscular disturbances, gynecomastia

Interactions
✳ Drug-drug • Increased CNS depression with alcohol, omeprazole • Increased pharmacologic effects of flurazepam with cimetidine, disulfiram, hormonal contraceptives, SSRIs • Decreased sedative effects of flurazepam with theophylline, aminophylline, dyphylline, oxitriphylline

■ Nursing considerations
Assessment
- **History:** Hypersensitivity to benzodiazepines; psychoses; acute narrow-angle glaucoma; shock; coma; acute alcoholic intoxication; pregnancy; labor; lactation; impaired liver or kidney function, debilitation, depression, suicidal tendencies
- **Physical:** Skin color, lesions; T; orientation, reflexes, affect, ophthalmologic exam; P, BP; R, adventitious sounds; liver evaluation, abdominal exam, bowel sounds, normal output; CBC, liver and renal function tests

Interventions
- Monitor liver and kidney function, CBC during long-term therapy.
- Taper dosage gradually after long-term therapy, especially in epileptics.
- Do not administer to pregnant women.

Teaching points
- Take drug exactly as prescribed.
- Do not stop taking (long-term therapy) without consulting the health care provider.
- Avoid pregnancy while on this drug; use of barrier contraceptives is advised.
- These side effects may occur: drowsiness, dizziness (may lessen; avoid driving or engaging in other dangerous activities); GI upset (take with water); depression, dreams, emotional upset, crying; nocturnal sleep disturbance (may be prolonged after drug cessation).
- Report severe dizziness, weakness, drowsiness that persists, rash or skin lesions, palpitations, swelling of the extremities, visual changes, difficulty voiding.

▽ flurbiprofen
(flure bi' proe fen)

Ophthalmic solution: Ocufen

Oral: Ansaid, Apo-Flurbiprofen (CAN), Froben (CAN), Froben-SR (CAN), Novo-Flurprofen (CAN)

PREGNANCY CATEGORY B

Drug classes
Nonsteroidal anti-inflammatory drug (NSAID)
Analgesic (non-narcotic)
Anti-inflammatory agent

Therapeutic actions
Analgesic, anti-inflammatory, and antipyretic activities largely related to inhibition of prostaglandin synthesis; exact mechanisms of action are not known.

Indications
- Acute or long-term treatment of the signs and symptoms of rheumatoid arthritis and osteoarthritis (oral)
- Inhibition of intraoperative miosis (ophthalmic solution)
- Unlabeled uses of ophthalmic solution: topical treatment of cystoid macular edema, inflammation after cataract surgery and uveitis syndromes

Contraindications and cautions
- Contraindicated with significant renal impairment, pregnancy, lactation.
- Use cautiously with impaired hearing, allergies, hepatic, CV, and GI conditions.

Available forms
Tablets—50, 100 mg; ophthalmic solution—0.03%

Dosages
Adults
Oral
Initial recommended daily dose of 200–300 mg PO, give in divided doses bid, tid, qid. Largest recommended single dose is 100 mg. Doses above 300 mg/day PO are not recommended. Taper to lowest possible dose.

Ophthalmic solution
Instill 1 drop approximately every 30 min, beginning 2 hr before surgery (total of 4 drops).
Pediatric patients
Safety and efficacy not established.

Pharmacokinetics

Route	Onset	Peak
Oral	30–60 min	90 min
Opthalmic	Minimal systemic absorption	

Metabolism: Hepatic; $T_{1/2}$: 5.7 hr
Distribution: Crosses placenta; enters breast milk
Excretion: Urine

Adverse effects
NSAIDs
- **CNS:** *Headache, dizziness, somnolence, insomnia,* fatigue, tiredness, dizziness, tinnitus, ophthalmologic effects
- **Dermatologic:** Rash, pruritus, sweating, dry mucous membranes, stomatitis
- **GI:** *Nausea, dyspepsia, GI pain,* diarrhea, vomiting, *constipation,* flatulence, **ulcer**
- **GU:** Dysuria, **renal impairment**
- **Hematologic:** Bleeding, platelet inhibition with higher doses, neutropenia, eosinophilia, leukopenia, pancytopenia, thrombocytopenia, agranulocytosis, granulocytopenia, aplastic anemia, decreased hemoglobin or hematocrit, bone marrow depression, menorrhagia
- **Respiratory:** Dyspnea, hemoptysis, pharyngitis, bronchospasm, rhinitis
- **Other:** Peripheral edema, **fatal anaphylactic shock**
Ophthalmic solution
- **Local:** *Transient stinging and burning on instillation, ocular irritation*

■ Nursing considerations
Assessment
- **History:** Renal impairment; impaired hearing; allergies; hepatic, CV, and GI conditions; lactation, pregnancy
- **Physical:** Skin color and lesions; orientation, reflexes, ophthalmologic and audiometric evaluation, peripheral sensation; P, edema; R, adventitious sounds; liver evaluation; CBC, clotting times, renal and liver

function tests; serum electrolytes, stool guaiac'

Interventions
- Administer drug with food or after meals if GI upset occurs.
- Assess patient receiving ophthalmic solutions for systemic effects, because absorption does occur.
- Arrange for periodic ophthalmologic examination during long-term therapy.
- Institute emergency procedures if overdose occurs: gastric lavage, induction of emesis, supportive therapy.

Teaching points
- Take drug with food or meals if GI upset occurs; take only the prescribed dosage.
- Avoid use during pregnancy, serious adverse effects could occur. Use of barrier contraceptives is advised.
- Dizziness, drowsiness can occur (avoid driving or using dangerous machinery).
- Report sore throat, fever, rash, itching, weight gain, swelling in ankles or fingers, changes in vision, black, tarry stools.

▷ flutamide
(floo' ta mide)

Euflex (CAN), Eulexin, Novo-Flutamide (CAN)

PREGNANCY CATEGORY D

Drug class
Antiandrogen

Therapeutic actions
A nonsteroidal agent, it exerts potent antiandrogenic activity by inhibiting androgen uptake or by inhibiting nuclear binding of androgen in target tissues

Indications
- Treatment of early-stage and metastatic prostatic carcinoma in combination with LHRH agonistic analogs (leuprolide acetate, goserelin)
- Unlabeled use: treatment of hirsutism in women (250 mg/day)

Contraindications and cautions
- Hypersensitivity to flutamide or any component of the preparation, pregnancy, lactation.

Available forms
Capsules—125 mg; tablets—250 mg (CAN)

Dosages
Adults
- Early-stage prostatic cancer: 250 mg PO tid.
- Metastatic prostatic cancer: Two capsules tid PO at 8-hr intervals; total daily dosage of 750 mg.
Pediatric patients
Safety and efficacy not established.

Pharmacokinetics

Route	Onset	Peak	Duration
Oral	Varies	2 hr	72 hr

Metabolism: Hepatic; $T_{1/2}$: 6 hr
Distribution: Crosses placenta; enters breast milk
Excretion: Urine

Adverse effects
- **CNS:** Drowsiness, confusion, depression, anxiety, nervousness
- **Dermatologic:** Rash, photosensitivity
- **Endocrine:** Gynecomastia, hot flashes
- **GI:** Nausea, vomiting, diarrhea, GI disturbances, jaundice, hepatitis, hepatic necrosis
- **GU:** Impotence, loss of libido
- **Hematologic:** Anemia, leukopenia, thrombocytopenia, elevated AST, ALT
- **Other:** Carcinogenesis, mutagenesis

■ Nursing considerations
Assessment
- **History:** Hypersensitivity to flutamide or any component of the preparation, pregnancy, lactation
- **Physical:** Skin color, lesions; reflexes, affect; urinary output; bowel sounds, liver evaluation; CBC, Hct, electrolytes, liver function tests

Interventions
- Give flutamide with other drugs used for medical castration.

- Arrange for periodic monitoring of liver function tests during long-term therapy.

Teaching points
- Take this drug with other drugs to treat your problem. Do not interrupt dosing or stop taking these medications without consulting your health care provider.
- Periodic blood tests will be necessary to monitor the drug effects. Keep appointments for these tests.
- These side effects may occur: dizziness, drowsiness (avoid driving or performing hazardous tasks); nausea, vomiting, diarrhea (maintain nutrition, consult dietitian); impotence, loss of libido (reversible); sensitivity to light (use sunscreen or protective clothing).
- Report change in stool or urine color, yellow skin, difficulty breathing, malaise.

▷ fluvastatin sodium
*(flue va **sta**' tin)*

Lescol, Lescol XL

PREGNANCY CATEGORY X

Drug classes
Antihyperlipidemic
Statin

Therapeutic actions
A fungal metabolite that inhibits the enzyme HMG-CoA that catalyzes the first step in the cholesterol synthesis pathway, resulting in a decrease in serum cholesterol, serum LDLs (associated with increased risk of CAD), and either an increase or no change in serum HDLs (associated with decreased risk of CAD).

Indications
- Adjunct to diet in the treatment of elevated total cholesterol and LDL cholesterol with primary hypercholesterolemia (types IIa and IIb) where response to dietary restriction of saturated fat and cholesterol and other nonpharmacologic measures has not been adequate

- To slow progression of coronary atheroscleroses in patients with CAD, along with diet and exercise

Contraindications and cautions
- Contraindicated with allergy to fluvastatin, fungal byproducts, pregnancy, lactation.
- Use cautiously with impaired hepatic function, cataracts.

Available forms
Capsules—20, 40 mg; extended-release capsules—80 mg

Dosages
Adults
- *Initial dosage:* 20 mg/day PO administered in the evening. Maintenance doses: 20–80 mg/day PO; give 80 mg/day as two 40-mg doses, or use 80-mg extended release form.
Pediatric patients
Safety and efficacy not established.

Pharmacokinetics

Route	Onset	Peak
Oral	Slow	4–6 wk

Metabolism: Hepatic; $T_{1/2}$: unknown
Distribution: Crosses placenta; enters breast milk
Excretion: Bile and feces

Adverse effects
- **CNS:** *Headache, blurred vision,* dizziness, insomnia, fatigue, muscle cramps, cataracts
- **GI:** *Flatulence, abdominal pain, cramps, constipation, nausea,* dyspepsia, heartburn
- **Hematologic:** Elevations of CPK, alkaline phosphatase and transaminases
- **Other: Rhabdomyolysis**

Interactions
✳ **Drug-drug** • Possible severe myopathy or rhabdomyolysis if taken with cyclosporine, erythromycin, gemfibrozil, niacin, other statins
✳ **Drug-food** • Decreased metabolism and increased risk of toxic effects if taken with grapefruit juice; avoid this combination

---

Adverse effects in *Italics* are most common; those in **Bold** are life-threatening.

■ Nursing considerations
Assessment
- **History:** Allergy to fluvastatin, fungal byproducts; impaired hepatic function; cataracts (use caution); pregnancy; lactation
- **Physical:** Orientation, affect, ophthalmologic exam; liver evaluation; lipid studies, liver function tests

Interventions
- Give in the evening; highest rates of cholesterol synthesis are between midnight and 5 AM. Doses of 80 mg/day should be taken as two 40-mg doses.
- Ensure that patient is not pregnant and understands need to avoid pregnancy before administering.
- Arrange for regular follow-up during long-term therapy.
- Arrange for periodic ophthalmologic exam to check for cataract development.

Teaching points
- Take drug in the evening. Do not drink grapefruit juice while on this drug.
- Institute dietary changes.
- These side effects may occur: nausea (small, frequent meals may help); headache, muscle and joint aches and pains (may lessen).
- This drug cannot be taken during pregnancy; use of barrier contraceptives is advised.
- Arrange to have periodic ophthalmic exams while you are on this drug.
- Report severe GI upset, changes in vision, unusual bleeding or bruising, dark urine or light-colored stools, muscle pain, fever.

▽fluvoxamine maleate
(floo vox' a meen)

Apo-Fluvoxamine (CAN), Luvox

PREGNANCY CATEGORY C

Drug class
Selective serotonin reuptake inhibitor (SSRI)

Therapeutic actions
Selectively inhibits CNS neuronal uptake of serotonin; blocks uptake of serotonin with weak effect on norepinephrine; little affinity for muscarinic, histaminergic, and alpha$_1$-adrenergic receptors.

Indications
- Treatment of obsessive-compulsive disorder
- Unlabeled use: treatment of depression, autism, panic disorder, social phobia, PMDD, posttraumatic stress disorder

Contraindications and cautions
- Contraindicated with hypersensitivity to fluvoxamine, lactation.
- Use cautiously with impaired hepatic or renal function, suicidal tendencies, seizures, mania, ECT therapy, CV disease, labor and delivery, pregnancy.

Available forms
Tablets—25, 50, 100 mg

Dosages
Adults
Initially 50 mg PO hs. Increase in 50 mg increments at 4–7 day intervals. Usual range 100–300 mg/day. Divide doses over 100 mg and give larger dose hs.
Pediatric patients 8–17 yr
Initially 25 mg PO hs. Increase dose by 25 mg/day every 4–7 days to achieve desired effect.
Geriatric patients or patients with hepatic impairment
Give a reduced dose, titrate more slowly.

Pharmacokinetics
Route	Onset	Peak
Oral	Rapid	2–8 hr

Metabolism: Hepatic; T$_{1/2}$: 15 hr
Distribution: Crosses placenta; passes into breast milk
Excretion: Urine

Adverse effects
- **CNS:** *Headache, nervousness, insomnia, drowsiness, anxiety, tremor, dizziness, light-headedness,* agitation, sedation, abnormal gait, convulsions
- **Dermatologic:** *Sweating, rash, pruritus,* acne, alopecia, contact dermatitis
- **GI:** *Nausea, vomiting, diarrhea, dry mouth, anorexia, dyspepsia, constipation,*

taste changes, flatulence, gastroenteritis, dysphagia, gingivitis

- **GU:** *Sexual dysfunction, frequency,* cystitis, impotence, urgency, vaginitis
- **Respiratory:** *Upper respiratory infections, pharyngitis,* cough, dyspnea, bronchitis, rhinitis

Interactions

✳ **Drug-drug** • Do not administer with MAO inhibitors (during or within 14 days) • Increased effects of triazolam, alprazolam, warfarin, carbamazepine, methadone, beta blockers, statins, diltiazem. Reduced dosages of these drugs will be needed • Decreased effects due to increased metabolism in cigarette smokers • Increased risk of serotonin syndrome if combined with other serotonergic drugs

✳ **Drug-alternative therapy** • Increased risk of severe reaction if combined with St. John's wort therapy

■ Nursing considerations

Assessment

- **History:** Hypersensitivity to fluvoxamine; lactation; impaired hepatic or renal function; suicidal tendencies; seizures; mania; ECT therapy; CV disease; labor and delivery; pregnancy
- **Physical:** Weight; T; skin rash, lesions; reflexes; affect; bowel sounds; liver evaluation; P, peripheral perfusion; urinary output; renal function; renal and liver function tests; CBC

Interventions

- Give lower or less frequent doses in elderly patients, and with hepatic or renal impairment.
- Establish suicide precautions for severely depressed patients. Limit quantity of tablets dispensed.
- Administer drug at bedtime, if dose exceeds 100 mg, divide dose and administer the largest dose at bedtime.
- Monitor patient for therapeutic response for up to 4–7 days before increasing dose.

Teaching points

- Take this drug at bedtime; if a large dose is needed, the dose may be divided, but take the largest dose at bedtime.

- Do not stop taking this drug abruptly, should be discontinued slowly.
- These side effects may occur: dizziness, drowsiness, nervousness, insomnia (avoid driving or performing hazardous tasks), nausea, vomiting, weight loss (small frequent meals may help), sexual dysfunction (reversible).
- Report rash, mania, seizures, severe weight loss.

folic acid (folacin, pteroylglutamic acid, folate)
(foe' lik)

Folvite

PREGNANCY CATEGORY A

Drug class
Folic acid

Therapeutic actions
Active reduced form of folic acid; required for nucleoprotein synthesis and maintenence of normal erythropoiesis.

Indications

- Treatment of megoblastic anemias due to sprue, nutritional deficiency, pregnancy, infancy, and childhood

Contraindications and cautions

- Contraindicated with allergy to folic acid preparations; pernicious, aplastic, normocytic anemias.
- Use cautiously during lactation.

Available forms
Tablets—0.4, 0.8, 1 mg; injection—5 mg/mL

Dosages
Administer orally unless severe intestinal malabsorption is present.
Adults
- *Therapeutic dose:* Up to 1 mg/day PO, IM, IV, or SC. Larger doses may be needed in severe cases.
- *Maintenance dose:* 0.4 mg/day.

- *Pregnancy and lactation:* 0.8 mg/day.
Pediatric patients
- *Maintenance dose:*
Infants: 0.1 mg/day.
< 4 yr: Up to 0.3 mg/day.
> 4 yr: 0.4 mg/day.

Pharmacokinetics

Route	Onset	Peak
Oral, IM, SC, IV	Varies	30–60 min

Metabolism: Hepatic; $T_{1/2}$: unknown
Distribution: Crosses placenta; enters breast milk
Excretion: Urine

▼ IV facts
Preparation: Solution is yellow to yellow-orange; may be added to hyperalimentation solution or dextrose solutions.
Infusion: Infuse at rate of 5 mg/min by direct IV injection; may be diluted in hyperalimentation for continuous infusion.

Adverse effects
- **Hypersensitivity:** Allergic reactions
- **Local:** *Pain and discomfort at injection site*

Interactions
✱ **Drug-drug** • Decrease in serum phenytoin and increase in seizure activity with folic acid preparations • Decreased absorption with sulfasalazine, aminosalicylic acid

■ Nursing considerations

CLINICAL ALERT!
Name confusion has occurred between folinic acid (leucovorin) and folic acid; use extreme caution.

Assessment
- **History:** Allergy to folic acid preparations; pernicious, aplastic, normocytic anemias; lactation
- **Physical:** Skin lesions, color; R, adventitious sounds; CBC, Hgb, Hct, serum folate levels, serum vitamin B_{12} levels, Schilling test

Interventions
- Administer orally if at all possible. With severe GI malabsorption or very severe disease, give IM, SC, or IV.
- Test using Schilling test and serum vitamin B_{12} levels to rule out pernicious anemia. Therapy may mask signs of pernicious anemia while the neurologic deterioration continues.
- Use caution when giving the parenteral preparations to premature infants. These preparations contain benzyl alcohol, may produce a fatal gasping syndrome in premature infants.
- Monitor patient for hypersensitivity reactions, especially if drug previously taken. Maintain supportive equipment and emergency drugs on standby in case of serious allergic response.

Teaching points
- When the cause of megaloblastic anemia is treated or passes (infancy, pregnancy), there may be no need for folic acid because it normally exists in sufficient quantities in the diet.
- Report rash, difficulty breathing, pain or discomfort at injection site.

▷ follitropin alfa
See *Less Commonly Used Drugs,* p. 1342.

▷ follitropin beta
See *Less Commonly Used Drugs,* p. 1342.

▷ fomepizole
See *Less Commonly Used Drugs,* p. 1344.

▷ fondaparinux
*(fon dah **pear'** ah nucks)*

Arixtra

PREGNANCY CATEGORY B

Drug classes
Antithrombotic agent
Factor Xa inhibitor

Therapeutic actions

Blocks naturally occurring factor Xa, leading to an alteration in the clot formation process; decreasing the risk of clot and thrombus formation

Indications

- Prevention of venous thromboembolic events (including deep vein thrombosis and pulmonary emboli) in patient undergoing surgery for hip fracture, hip replacement, knee replacement

Contraindications and cautions

- Contraindicated with hypersensitivity to fondaparinux, severe renal impairment, adults < 50 kg, active major bleeding, bacterial endocarditis, thrombocytopenia.
- Use cautiously with pregnancy or lactation, mild to moderate renal impairment, adults > 65 years of age, bleeding disorders, history of heparin-induced thrombocytopenia, uncontrolled arterial hypertension, GI ulcers, diabetic retinopathy, spinal puncture, neuroaxial anesthesia.

Available forms

Prefilled syringes—2.5 mg/0.5 mL

Dosages

Adults

2.5 mg/day SC starting 6–8 hr following surgical closure and continuing for 5–9 days.

Pediatric patients

Safety and efficacy not established.

Geriatric patients or patients with renal impairment

Dosage adjustment is not recommended, but increased risk of bleeding exists. Monitor patient closely and discontinue drug if renal impairment increases or severe bleeding occurs.

Pharmacokinetics

Route	Onset	Peak
SC	Rapid	3 hr

Metabolism: $T_{1/2}$: 17–21 hr
Distribution: May cross placenta; may enter breast milk
Excretion: Unchanged in the urine

Adverse effects

- **CNS:** Insomnia, dizziness, confusion, headache
- **CV:** Edema, hypotension
- **GI:** *Nausea,* constipation, diarrhea, vomiting, dyspepsia
- **GU:** UTI, urinary retention
- **Hematologic: Hemorrhage;** *bruising;* **thrombocytopenia;** *anemia*
- **Hypersensitivity:** Chills, fever, urticaria, asthma
- **Metabolic:** Elevated AST, ALT levels; hypokalemia
- **Renal:** Impaired renal functions
- **Other:** *Fever;* pain; local irritation, hematoma, erythema at site of injection, rash

Interactions

✳ **Drug-drug** • Increased bleeding tendencies with oral anticoagulants, salicylates, penicillins, cephalosporins, NSAIDs

■ Nursing considerations

Assessment

- **History:** Recent surgery or injury; sensitivity to fondaparinux; renal impairment; pregnancy, lactation; recent bleeding, thrombocytopenia, bacterial endocarditis, spinal puncture
- **Physical:** Weight, peripheral perfusion, R, stool guaiac test, PTT or other tests of blood coagulation, platelet count, CBC, renal function tests

Interventions

- Arrange to give drug 6–8 hr following surgical closure; continue for 5–9 days.
- Give deep SC injections; do not give by IM injection.
- Administer by deep SC injection; patient should be lying down; alternate administration between the left and right anterolateral and left and right posterolateral abdominal wall. Introduce the whole length of the needle into a skin fold held between the thumb and forefinger; hold the skin fold throughout the injection.
- Apply pressure to all injection sites after needle is withdrawn; inspect injection sites for signs of hematoma.
- Do not massage injection sites.

Adverse effects in *Italics* are most common; those in **Bold** are life-threatening.

- Do not mix with other injections or infusions.
- Store at room temperature; fluid should be clear, colorless to pale yellow.
- Provide for safety measures (electric razor, soft toothbrush) to prevent injury to patient who is at risk for bleeding.
- Check patient for signs of bleeding, monitor blood tests.

Teaching points
- Know that this drug must be given by a parenteral route (not orally). You and a significant other will be instructed in how to administer the drug if you are being discharged with it. Arrange for proper disposal of syringes and needles.
- Arrange for periodic blood tests that will be needed to monitor your response to this drug.
- Be careful to avoid injury while on this drug: use an electric razor, avoid activities that might lead to injury.
- Report nose bleed, bleeding of the gums, unusual bruising, black or tarry stools, cloudy or dark urine, abdominal or lower back pain, severe headache.

▽ formoterol fumarate
(for mob' te rol)

Foradil Aerolizer

PREGNANCY CATEGORY C

Drug classes
Beta₂ agonist
Asthmatic drug

Therapeutic actions
Long-acting agonist that binds to beta₂ receptors in the lungs causing bronchodilation; may also inhibit the release of inflammatory mediators in the lung, blocking swelling and inflammation.

Indications
- Long-term maintenance treatment of asthma in adults and children ≥ 5 yr
- Prevention of exercise-induced bronchospasm in adults and children ≥ 12 yr when used on an occasional, as-needed basis

- Long-term maintenance treatment of bronchoconstriction in patients with COPD

Contraindications and cautions
- Contraindicated with hypersensitivity to adrenergics, amines, or to formoterol, acute asthma attack, acute airway obstruction.
- Use cautiously with pregnancy, lactation, and the elderly.

Available forms
Inhalation powder in capsules—12 mcg

Dosages
Adults
- *Maintenance treatment of COPD:* Oral inhalation of contents of one capsule (12 mcg) using *Aerolizer Inhaler* q 12 hr. Do not exceed a total daily dose of 24 mcg.
- *Maintenance treatment of asthma:*
Adults and patients ≥ 5 yr
Oral inhalation of contents of one capsule (12 mcg) using the *Aerolizer Inhaler* every 12 hr. Do not exceed 1 capsule every 12 hr.
- *Prevention of exercise-induced bronchospasm:*
Adults and patients ≥ 12 yr
Oral inhalation of contents of one capsule (12 mcg) using the *Aerolizer Inhaler* 15 min before exercise. Use on an occasional, as-needed basis.

Pharmacokinetics

Route	Onset	Peak	Duration
Inhalation	15–20 min	1–3 hr	8–20 hr

Metabolism: Hepatic; $T_{1/2}$: 10–14 hr
Distribution: Crosses placenta; may pass into breast milk
Excretion: Feces

Adverse effects
- **CNS:** Tremor, dizziness, insomnia, dysphonia, *headache, nervousness*
- **CV:** Hypertension, tachycardia, chest pain
- **GI:** Nausea, dyspepsia, abdominal pain, *irritation of the throat and mouth*
- **Respiratory:** Bronchitis, respiratory infection, dyspnea, tonsillitis
- **Other:** *Viral infection* (most likely in children)

■ Nursing considerations

 CLINICAL ALERT!
Name confusion has occurred between Foradil (formoterol) and Toradol (ketorolac); use extreme caution.

Assessment
- **History:** Hypersensitivity to adrenergics, amines, or formoterol, acute asthma attack, acute airway obstruction, pregnancy, lactation
- **Physical:** R, adventitious sounds, P, BP, ECG, orientation, reflexes, liver function tests

Interventions
- Instruct patient in the proper use of *Aerolizer Inhaler*. Ensure that patient does not swallow the capsule.
- Monitor use of inhaler. Patient should not wash the inhaler but should keep it dry; it should not be used for delivering any other medication. If a bronchodilator is needed between doses, consult with health care provider. Do not use more often than every 12 hr.
- Encourage patients who experience exercise-induced asthma to use drug 15 min before activity, and to reserve this drug for occasional, as-needed use.
- Ensure that patient continues with appropriate use of corticosteroids or other drugs used to block bronchospasm, as appropriate.
- Arrange for periodic evaluation of respiratory condition during therapy.
- Arrange for analgesics as appropriate for headache.
- Establish safety precautions if tremor becomes a problem.

Teaching points
- Use the *Aerolizer Inhaler* as instructed. This is the only inhaler that can be used with this drug.
- Use only twice a day. Do not wash the inhaler; keep it dry at all times. Do not use this inhaler to deliver any other drugs. Check the "use by" date on your drug and discard any capsules that have expired.

- If drug is to be used periodically for exercise-induced asthma, use 15 min before activity.
- Arrange for periodic evaluation of your respiratory problem while on this drug; continue to use any other therapies that have been prescribed to control your asthma.
- These side effects can occur: headache (appropriate analgesics may be ordered); tremors (use care in performing dangerous tasks if this occurs); fast heartbeat, palpitations (monitor activity if this occurs, rest frequently).
- Report severe headache, irregular heartbeat, worsening of asthma, difficulty breathing.

▷**foscarnet sodium (phosphonoformic acid, PFA)**
(foss kar' net)

Foscavir

PREGNANCY CATEGORY C

Drug class
Antiviral

Therapeutic actions
Inhibits replication of all known herpes viruses by selectively inhibiting specific DNA and RNA enzymes.

Indications
- Treatment of CMV retinitis in patients with aids; combination therapy with ganciclovir for patients who have relapsed after monotherapy with either drug
- Treatment of acyclovir-resistant HSV infections in immunocompromised patients

Contraindications and cautions
- Contraindicated with allergy to foscarnet.
- Use cautiously during lactation.

Available forms
Injection—24 mg/ml

Adverse effects in *Italics* are most common; those in **Bold** are life-threatening.

Dosages
Adults
- *CMV retinitis:* Induction: 60 mg/kg q 8 hr IV for 2–3 wk. Maintenance: 90–120 mg/kg IV.
- *HSV infection:* Induction: 40 mg/kg q 8–12 hr IV for 2–3 wk or until healed.

Geriatric patients or patients with renal impairment
Monitor patient carefully; if creatinine clearance falls below 0.4 mL/min/kg, discontinue therapy.

Pharmacokinetics

Route	Onset
IV	Immediate

Metabolism: $T_{1/2}$: 1.4–3 hr
Distribution: Crosses placenta; enters breast milk
Excretion: Urine

▼IV facts
Preparation: Give with normal saline, 5% dextrose solution.
Infusion: Infuse slowly. Induction dose: infuse over a minimum of 1 hr using an infusion pump. Maintenance dose: infuse over 2 hr using an infusion pump to control rate.
Incompatibilities: Do not mix in the same catheter with anything but normal saline or 5% dextrose solution. Incompatible with 30% dextrose, amphotericin B, solutions containing calcium; acyclovir sodium, ganciclovir, trimetrexate, pentamidine, vancomycin, trimethoprim-sulfamethoxazole, diazepam, midazolam, digoxin, phenytoin, leucovorin, prochlorperazine.

Adverse effects
- **CNS:** *Headache, seizures,* paresthesia, tremor, ataxia, abnormal coordination, **coma, death,** depression, confusion, anxiety, insomnia, nervousness, emotional lability, vision changes, taste abnormalities
- **GI:** *Nausea, vomiting, diarrhea,* abdominal pain, dry mouth, melena, pancreatitis
- **Hematologic: Bone marrow suppression,** *anemia,* mineral and electrolyte imbalance
- **Renal: Acute renal failure, abnormal renal function,** dysuria, polyuria, urinary retention, urinary tract infections
- **Respiratory:** Cough, dyspnea, pneumonia, sinusitis, pharyngitis
- **Other:** *Fever,* fatigue, rash, pain, edema, pain at site of injection

Interactions
✳ Drug-drug • Increased risk of renal problems with other renal toxic drugs • Risk of hypocalcemia with pentamidine

■ Nursing considerations
Assessment
- **History:** Presence of allergy to foscarnet, lactation, pregnancy
- **Physical:** Skin color, lesions; T; orientation, reflexes, affect; urinary output; R, adventitious sounds; CBC, serum electrolytes, renal function tests

Interventions
- Give by IV route only; give by bolus or rapid injection.
- Monitor serum creatinine and renal function carefully during treatment; dosage adjustment may be necessary.
- Stop infusion immediately at any report of tingling, paresthesias, numbness. Monitor electrolytes.
- Ensure adequate hydration during treatment; push fluids to ensure diuresis and decrease the risk of renal impairment.
- Arrange for periodic ophthalmic exams for retinitis; foscarnet is not a cure.

Teaching points
- This drug must be given IV using a special pump.
- Foscarnet is not a cure for retinitis; symptoms may continue. Arrange for periodic ophthalmic exams.
- Drink a lot of fluids, and you may also receive a lot of IV fluids.
- Arrange for periodic medical exams, including blood tests.
- These side effects may occur: fever, headache (medication may be ordered); dizziness, fatigue, vision changes (do not drive or operate dangerous machinery); nausea, vomiting, diarrhea.
- Report tingling around the mouth, numbness, "heavy" extremities, difficulty breathing, leg cramps, tremors, pain at injection site.

▷fosfomycin tromethamine
(foss foe my' sin)

Monurol

PREGNANCY CATEGORY B

Drug classes
Antibacterial
Urinary tract anti-infective

Therapeutic actions
Bactericidal; interferes with bacterial cell wall synthesis, blocks adherence of bacteria to uroepithelial cells.

Indications
- Uncomplicated urinary tract infections in women caused by susceptible strains of *E. coli* and *E. faecalis*; not indicated for the treatment of pyelonephritis or perinephric abscess

Contraindications and cautions
- Contraindicated with allergy to fosfomycin.
- Use cautiously with pregnancy, lactation.

Available forms
Granule packet—3 g

Dosages
Adults
1 packet dissolved in water PO.
Pediatric patients < 18 yr
Not recommended.

Pharmacokinetics

Route	Onset	Peak
Oral	Rapid	2–4 hr

Metabolism: Hepatic; $T_{1/2}$: 5.7 hr
Distribution: Crosses placenta; passes into breast milk
Excretion: Urine and feces

Adverse effects
- **CNS:** *Headache, dizziness,* back pain, asthenia
- **GI:** *Nausea,* abdominal cramps, dyspepsia
- **GU:** Vaginitis, dysmenorrhea
- **Other:** Rhinitis, rash

Interactions
✳ **Drug-drug** • Lowered serum concentration and urinary tract excretion with metoclopramide

■ Nursing considerations
Assessment
- **History:** Allergy to fosfomycin, pregnancy, lactation
- **Physical:** Skin color, lesions; orientation, reflexes; urine for analysis

Interventions
- Arrange for culture and sensitivity tests.
- Administer drug with food if GI upset occurs.
- Do not administer dry; mix a single dose packet in 90–120 mL of water and stir to dissolve; do not use hot water. Administer immediately.
- Monitor clinical response; if no improvement is seen or a relapse occurs, send urine for repeat culture and sensitivity.
- Encourage patient to observe other measures (avoid bubble baths, alkaline ash foods, sexual intercourse; drink lots of fluids) to decrease risk of urinary tract infection.

Teaching points
- This drug is meant to be a one-dose treatment for urinary tract infection; improvement should be seen in 2–3 days. If no improvement occurs, consult your health care provider.
- Take drug with food if GI upset occurs. Do not take in the dry form; mix a single dose packet in 90–120 mL of water and stir to dissolve; do not use hot water. Drink immediately after mixing.
- These side effects may occur: nausea, abdominal pain (eat small, frequent meals; take the drug with meals); dizziness (observe caution if driving or using dangerous equipment).
- Report rash, visual changes, severe GI problems, weakness, tremors, worsening of urinary tract symptoms.

▷fosinopril sodium
(fob sin' ob pril)

Monopril

PREGNANCY CATEGORY C
(FIRST TRIMESTER)

PREGNANCY CATEGORY D
(SECOND AND THIRD TRIMESTERS)

Drug classes
Antihypertensive
Angiotensin-converting enzyme inhibitor (ACE inhibitor)

Therapeutic actions
Renin, synthesized by the kidneys, is released into the circulation where it acts on a plasma precursor to produce angiotensin I, which is converted by angiotensin-converting enzyme to angiotensin II, a potent vasoconstrictor that also causes release of aldosterone from the adrenals; fosinopril blocks the conversion of angiotensin I to angiotensin II, leading to decreased BP, decreased aldosterone secretion, a small increase in serum potassium levels, and sodium and fluid loss; increased prostaglandin synthesis may be involved in the antihypertensive action.

Indications
- Treatment of hypertension, alone or in combination with thiazide-type diuretics
- Management of CHF as adjunctive therapy
- Unlabeled use: diabetic nephropathy

Contraindications and cautions
- Contraindicated with allergy to fosinopril or other ACE inhibitors; pregnancy.
- Use cautiously with impaired renal function, CHF, salt or volume depletion, lactation.

Available forms
Tablets—10, 20, 40 mg

Dosages
Adults
Initial dose: 10 mg PO daily. Maintenance dose: 20–40 mg/day PO as a single dose or two divided doses. Discontinue diuretics 2–3 days before beginning fosinopril. If BP is not controlled, add diuretic slowly. If diuretic cannot be discontinued, begin fosinopril therapy with 10 mg. Do not exceed maximum dose of 80 mg.
Pediatric patients
Safety and efficacy not established.

Pharmacokinetics

Route	Onset	Peak	Duration
Oral	1 hr	3 hr	24 hr

Metabolism: Hepatic; $T_{1/2}$: 12 hr
Distribution: Crosses placenta; enters breast milk
Excretion: Urine and feces

Adverse effects
- **CV:** Angina pectoris, orthostatic hypotension in salt- or volume-depleted patients, palpitations
- **Dermatologic:** Rash, pruritus, diaphoresis, flushing
- **GI:** *Nausea,* abdominal pain, vomiting, diarrhea
- **Respiratory:** *Cough,* asthma, bronchitis, dyspnea, sinusitis
- **Other:** Angioedema, asthenia, myalgia, arthralgia

Interactions
✳ **Drug-drug** • Increased coughing if combined with capsaicin • Decreased effectiveness if combined with indomethacin or other NSAIDs • Risk of lithium toxicity if combined with ACE inhibitors • Risk of increased potassium levels if taken with potassium-sparing diuretics

■ Nursing considerations

 CLINICAL ALERT!
Name confusion has occurred between fosinopril and lisinopril; use caution.

Assessment
- **History:** Allergy to fosinopril and other ACE inhibitors, impaired renal function, CHF, salt or volume depletion, lactation, pregnancy
- **Physical:** Skin color, lesions, turgor; T; P, BP, peripheral perfusion; mucous membranes, bowel sounds, liver evaluation; uri-

nalysis, renal and liver function tests, CBC, and differential

Interventions

- Alert surgeon and mark patient's chart with notice that fosinopril is being taken; the angiotensin II formation subsequent to compensatory renin release during surgery will be blocked; hypotension may be reversed with volume expansion.
- Arrange to switch to a different drug if pregnancy occurs; suggest use of barrier contraceptives.
- Monitor patient closely for a fall in BP secondary to reduction in fluid volume (excessive perspiration and dehydration, vomiting, diarrhea) because excessive hypotension may occur.

Teaching points

- Do not stop taking the medication without consulting your prescriber.
- These side effects may occur: GI upset, loss of appetite (these may be transient); lightheadedness (transient; change position slowly and limit activities to those that do not require alertness and precision); dry cough (not harmful).
- Avoid pregnancy while on this drug; use of barrier contraceptives is advised.
- Be careful in any situation that may lead to a drop in BP (diarrhea, sweating, vomiting, dehydration); if light-headedness or dizziness occurs, consult your care provider.
- Report mouth sores; sore throat, fever, chills; swelling of the hands, feet; irregular heartbeat, chest pains; swelling of the face, eyes, lips, tongue, difficulty breathing, persistent cough.

▽fosphenytoin sodium
(faws fen' i toe in)

Cerebyx

PREGNANCY CATEGORY D

Drug classes
Antiepileptic agent
Hydantoin

Therapeutic actions
A metabolite of phenytoin that has antiepileptic activity without causing general CNS depression; stabilizes neuronal membranes and prevents hyperexcitability caused by excessive stimulation; limits the spread of seizure activity from an active focus

Indications
- Short-term control of general convulsive status epilepticus
- Prevention and treatment of seizures occurring during or following neurosurgery

Contraindications and cautions
- Contraindicated with hypersensitivity to hydantoins, sinus bradycardia, sinoatrial block, second- or third-degree AV heart block, Stokes-Adams syndrome, pregnancy (data suggest an association between use of antiepileptic drugs by women with epilepsy and an elevated incidence of birth defects in children born to these women; however, do not discontinue antiepileptic therapy in pregnant women who are receiving therapy to prevent major seizures—this is likely to precipitate status epilepticus, with attendant hypoxia and risk to both mother and unborn child); lactation
- Use cautiously with hypotension, hepatic dysfunction

Available forms
Injection—150 (100 PE), 750 (500 PE) mg/vial

Dosages
Dosage is given as phenytoin equivalents (PE) to facilitate transfer from phenytoin.
Adults
- *Status epilepticus:* Loading dose of 15–20 mg PE/kg administered at 100–150 mg PE/min.
- *Neurosurgery (prophylaxis):* Loading dose of 10–20 mg PE/kg IM or IV; maintenance dose of 4–6 mg PE/kg/day.
Pediatric patients
Not recommended.
Patients with renal or hepatic impairment
Use caution and monitor for early signs of toxicity—handling of the metabolism of the drug may result in increased risk of adverse effects.

Adverse effects in *Italics* are most common; those in **Bold** are life-threatening.

Pharmacokinetics

Route	Onset	Peak
IV	Rapid	End of infusion

Metabolism: Hepatic; $T_{1/2}$: 15 min
Distribution: Crosses placenta; enters breast milk
Excretion: Urine

▽ IV facts

Preparation: Dilute in 5% dextrose or 0.9% saline solution to a concentration of 1.5–25 mg PE/mL. Refrigerate; stable at room temperature for < 48 hr.

Infusion: Infuse for status epilepticus at rate of 100–150 mg PE/min; never administer at a rate > 150 mg PE/min.

Adverse effects

- **CNS:** *Nystagmus, ataxia, dizziness, somnolence,* drowsiness, insomnia, transient nervousness, motor twitchings, fatigue, irritability, depression, numbness, tremor, headache, photophobia, diplopia, asthenia, back pain
- **CV:** *Hypotension,* vasodilation, tachycardia
- **Dermatologic:** *Pruritus*
- **GI:** *Nausea,* vomiting, dry mouth, taste perversion
- **Other:** Lymph node hyperplasia, sometimes progressing to frank malignant lymphoma, monoclonal gammopathy and multiple myeloma (prolonged therapy), polyarthropathy, osteomalacia, weight gain, chest pain, periarteritis nodosa

Interactions

No specific drug interactions have been reported, but since fosphenytoin is a metabolite of phenytoin, documented interactions with that drug should be considered.

✳ **Drug-drug** • Increased pharmacologic effects of hydantoins with chloramphenicol, cimetidine, disulfiram, phenacemide, phenylbutazone, sulfonamides, trimethoprim; reduced fosphenytoin dose may be needed • Complex interactions and effects when phenytoin and valproic acid are given together; phenytoin toxicity with apparently normal serum phenytoin levels; decreased plasma levels of valproic acid given with phenytoin; breakthrough seizures when the two drugs are given together • Increased pharmacologic effects and toxicity when primidone, oxyphenbutazone, amiodarone, chloramphenicol, fluconazole, isoniazid are given with hydantoins • Decreased pharmacologic effects of the following with hydantoins: corticosteroids, cyclosporine, dicumarol, disopyramide, doxycycline, estrogens, furosemide, levodopa, methadone, metyrapone, mexiletine, hormonal contraceptives, quinidine, atracurium, gallamine triethiodide, pancuronium, tubocurarine, vecuronium, carbamazepine, diazoxide

✳ **Drug-lab test** • Interference with metyrapone and 1-mg dexamethasone tests for at least 7 days

■ Nursing considerations

CLINICAL ALERT!
Name confusion has occurred between Cerebyx (fosphenytoin), Celebrex (celecoxib), Celexa (citalopram), and Xanax (alprazolam); use caution.

Assessment

- **History:** Hypersensitivity to hydantoins; sinus bradycardia, sinoatrial block, second- or third-degree AV heart block, Stokes-Adams syndrome, pregnancy, lactation, hepatic failure
- **Physical:** T; skin color, lesions; orientation, affect, reflexes, vision exam; P, BP; bowel sounds, normal output, liver evaluation; liver function tests, urinalysis, CBC and differential, EEG and ECG

Interventions

- Continue supportive measures, including use of an IV benzodiazepine, until drug becomes effective against seizures.
- Administer IV slowly to prevent severe hypotension; margin of safety between full therapeutic and toxic doses is small. Continually monitor cardiac rhythm and check BP frequently and regularly during IV infusion and for 10–20 min after infusion.
- Monitor infusion site carefully—drug solutions are very alkaline and irritating.
- This drug is recommended for short-term use only (up to 5 days); switch to oral phenytoin as soon as possible.

Teaching points
- This drug can only be given IV and will be stopped as soon as you are able to take an oral drug.
- These side effects may occur: drowsiness, dizziness, GI upset.
- Report rash, severe nausea or vomiting, drowsiness, slurred speech, impaired coordination (ataxia), sore throat, unusual bleeding or bruising, persistent headache, malaise, pain at injection site.

▽frovatriptan succinate
*(frow vah **trip'** tan)*

Frova

PREGNANCY CATEGORY C

Drug classes
Antimigraine agent
Serotonin selective agonist
Triptan

Therapeutic actions
Binds to serotonin receptors to cause vascular constrictive effects on cranial blood vessels, causing the relief of migraine in selective patients.

Indications
- Treatment of acute migraines with or without aura in adults

Contraindications and cautions
- Contraindicated with allergy to frovatriptan, active coronary artery disease, ischemic heart disease, Printzmetal's angina, peripheral or cerebral vascular syndromes, uncontrolled hypertension, use of an ergot compound or other triptan within 24 hr.
- Use cautiously with liver or renal dysfunction, risk factors for CAD, lactation, pregnancy.

Available forms
Tablets—2.5 mg

Dosages
Adults
2.5 mg PO as a single dose at first sign of migraine; if headache returns, may be repeated after 2 hr. Do not use more than 3 doses/24 hr.
Pediatric patients
Safety and efficacy not established for patients < 18 yr.

Pharmacokinetics

Route	Onset	Peak
Oral	Varies	2–4 hr

Metabolism: Hepatic; $T_{1/2}$: 26 hr
Distribution: Crosses placenta; may pass into breast milk
Excretion: Urine and feces

Adverse effects
- **CNS:** Dizziness, headache, anxiety, malaise, fatigue, weakness, myalgia, somnolence, paresthesia (tingling, burning, prickling, itching sensation), loss of sensation, abnormal vision, tinnitus
- **CV:** Palpitations, tightness or pressure in chest, flushing, **MI, cerebrovascular events**
- **GI:** Vomiting, diarrhea, abdominal pain, dry mouth, dyspepsia, nausea
- **Musculoskeletal:** Skeletal pain
- **Other:** Warm or hot sensations, cold sensation, pain, increased sweating, rhinitis

Interactions
✴ **Drug-drug** • Prolonged vasoactive reactions when taken concurrently with ergot-containing drugs or other triptans; space these drugs at least 24 hr apart • Increased risk of weakness, hyperreflexia, CNS effects if combined with an SSRI (fluoxetine, fluvoxamine, paroxetine, sertraline); if combined with these drugs, appropriate safety precautions should be observed and patient monitored closely

■ Nursing considerations
Assessment
- **History:** Allergy to frovatriptan, active coronary artery disease, Printzmetal's angina, pregnancy, lactation, peripheral or cerebral vascular syndromes, uncontrolled hyper-

---

*Adverse effects in Italics are most common; those in **Bold** are life-threatening.*

tension, use of an ergot compound or other triptan within 24 hr, risk factors for CAD
- **Physical:** Skin color and lesions, orientation, reflexes, peripheral sensation, P, BP, renal and liver function tests

Interventions
- Ensure that the patient has been diagnosed with migraine headaches.
- Administer to relieve acute migraine, not as a prophylactic measure.
- Ensure that the patient has not taken an ergot-containing compound or other triptan within 24 hr.
- Do not administer more than 3 doses in a 24-hr period, space them at least 2 hr apart.
- Establish safety measures if CNS; visual disturbances occur.
- Provide environmental control as appropriate to help relieve migraine (lighting, temperature, etc.).
- Monitor BP of patients with possible coronary artery disease; discontinue at any sign of angina, prolonged high blood pressure, etc.

Teaching points
- Take drug exactly as prescribed, at the onset of headache or aura. Do not take this drug to prevent a migraine, it is only used to treat migraines that are occurring. If the headache remains after you take this drug, you may repeat the dose after 2 hr have passed.
- Do not take more than 3 doses in a 24-hr period. Do not take any other migraine medication while you are taking this drug. If the headache is not relieved, call your health care provider.
- Be aware that this drug should not be taken during pregnancy; if you suspect that you are pregnant, contact physician and refrain from using drug.
- These side effects may occur: dizziness, drowsiness can occur (avoid driving or the use of dangerous machinery while on this drug); numbness, tingling, feelings of tightness or pressure.
- Maintain any procedures you usually use during a migraine (controlled lighting, noise, etc.).
- Contact health care provider immediately if you experience chest pain or pressure which is severe or does not go away.

- Report feelings of heat, flushing, tiredness, feelings of sickness, swelling of lips or eyelids.

▷fulvestrant
(full ves' trant)

Faslodex

PREGNANCY CATEGORY D

Drug classes
Estrogen receptor antagonist
Antineoplastic agent

Therapeutic actions
Binds to estrogen receptors, has anti-estrogen effects; and inhibits growth of estrogen receptor-positive breast cancer cell lines

Indications
- Treatment of hormone receptor-positive breast cancer in postmenopausal women with disease progression following anti-estrogen therapy.

Contraindications and cautions
- Contraindicated with allergy to any component of the drug, pregnancy.
- Use cautiously with bleeding disorders, thrombocytopenia, hepatic dysfunction, lactation.

Available forms
Prefilled syringes—250 mg/5 mL, 125 mg/2.5 mL

Dosages
Adults
250 mg IM each month in the buttock as a single 5-mL injection or two concomitant 2.5-mL injections.

Pharmacokinetics

Route	Onset	Peak
IM	Slow	2–3 days

Metabolism: Hepatic; $T_{1/2}$: 40 days
Distribution: Crosses placenta; passes into breast milk
Excretion: Feces

Adverse effects

- **CNS:** Depression, lightheadedness, dizziness, *headache,* hallucinations, vertigo, insomnia, paresthesia, anxiety, *asthenia*
- **CV:** Chest pain, *vasodilation*
- **Dermatologic:** *Hot flashes,* skin rash
- **GI:** *Nausea, vomiting,* food distaste, *constipation, diarrhea,* anorexia, *abdominal pain*
- **GU:** UTI, *pelvic pain*
- **Respiratory:** *Dyspnea, increased cough*
- **Other:** Peripheral edema, fever, *pharyngitis, injection site reactions, pain,* flulike syndrome, *increased sweat, anemia, back pain, bone pain, arthritis*

Interactions

✳ **Drug-drug** • Increased risk of bleeding if taken with oral anticoagulants

■ Nursing considerations
Assessment

- **History:** Allergy to any component of the drug; pregnancy, lactation; liver dysfunction, bleeding disorders, thrombocytopenia
- **Physical:** Skin color, lesions, turgor; pelvic exam; orientation, affect, reflex; BP, peripheral pulses, edema; liver function tests

Interventions

- Ensure that the patient is not pregnant before administering drug.
- Counsel patient about the need to use contraceptives to avoid pregnancy while taking this drug. Inform patient that serious fetal harm could occur.
- Suggest an alternate method of feeding the baby if this drug is prescribed for a nursing mother.
- Mark a calendar for dates for monthly injections; periodically monitor injection sites if patient is self-administering drug.
- Provide comfort measures to help patient deal with drug effects: hot flashes (environmental temperature control); headache, depression (monitoring light and noise); vaginal bleeding (hygiene measures); nausea, food distaste (small, frequent meals).

Teaching points

- You and a significant other should learn the proper technique for administering an IM injection; proper disposal of needles and syringes is important and should be reviewed.
- Mark your calendar with the date of your injection. If you are not able to self-administer the injection, mark your calendar with the dates to return to your health care provider for injections.
- These side effects may occur: hot flashes (staying in cool temperatures may help); nausea, vomiting (small, frequent meals may help); weight gain; dizziness, headache, lightheadedness (use caution if driving or performing tasks that require alertness if these occur).
- Be aware that this drug can cause serious fetal harm and must not be taken during pregnancy. Use contraceptives while you are taking this drug. If you become pregnant or decide that you would like to become pregnant, consult with your physician immediately.
- Report marked weakness, sleepiness, mental confusion, changes in color of urine or stool, pregnancy.

▽furosemide
(fur ob' se mide)

Apo-Furosemide (CAN), Furoside (CAN), Lasix, Myrosemide (CAN)

PREGNANCY CATEGORY C

Drug class
Loop diuretic

Therapeutic actions
Inhibits the reabsorption of sodium and chloride from the proximal and distal renal tubules and the loop of Henle, leading to a sodium-rich diuresis.

Indications

- Edema associated with CHF, cirrhosis, renal disease (oral, IV)
- Acute pulmonary edema (IV)
- Hypertension (oral)

Adverse effects in *Italics* are most common; those in **Bold** are life-threatening.

Contraindications and cautions

- Contraindicated with allergy to furosemide, sulfonamides; allergy to tartrazine (in oral solution); electrolyte depletion; anuria, severe renal failure; hepatic coma; pregnancy; lactation.
- Use cautiously with SLE, gout, diabetes mellitus.

Available forms

Tablets—20, 40, 80 mg; oral solution—10 mg/mL, 40 mg/5 mL; injection—10 mg/mL

Dosages
Adults

- *Edema:* Initially, 20–80 mg/day PO as a single dose. If needed, a second dose may be given in 6–8 hr. If response is unsatisfactory, dose may be increased in 20- to 40-mg increments at 6- to 8-hr intervals. Up to 600 mg/day may be given. Intermittent dosage schedule (2–4 consecutive days/wk) is preferred for maintenance, *or* 20–40 mg IM or IV (slow IV injection over 1–2 min). May increase dose in increments of 20 mg in 2 hr. High-dose therapy should be given as infusion at rate not exceeding 4 mg/min.
- *Acute pulmonary edema:* 40 mg IV over 1–2 min. May be increased to 80 mg IV given over 1–2 min if response is unsatisfactory after 1 hr.
- *Hypertension:* 40 mg bid PO. If needed, additional antihypertensive agents may be added at 50% usual dosage.

Pediatric patients

Avoid use in premature infants: stimulates PGE_2 synthesis and may increase incidence of patent ductus arteriosus and complicate respiratory distress syndrome.

- *Edema:* Initially, 2 mg/kg/day PO. If needed, increase by 1–2 mg/kg in 6–8 hr. *Do not exceed* 6 mg/kg. Adjust maintenance dose to lowest effective level.
- *Pulmonary edema:* 1 mg/kg IV or IM. May increase by 1 mg/kg in 2 hr until the desired effect is seen. *Do not exceed* 6 mg/kg.

Geriatric patients or patients with renal impairment

Up to 2–2.5 g/day has been tolerated. IV bolus injection should not exceed 1 g/day given over 30 min.

Pharmacokinetics

Route	Onset	Peak	Duration
Oral	60 min	60–120 min	6–8 hr
IV, IM	5 min	30 min	2 hr

Metabolism: Hepatic; $T_{1/2}$: 120 min
Distribution: Crosses placenta; enters breast milk
Excretion: Urine

▼ IV facts

Preparation: Store at room temperature; exposure to light may slightly discolor solution.
Infusion: Inject directly or into tubing of actively running IV; inject slowly over 1–2 min.
Incompatibilities: Do not mix with acidic solutions. Isotonic saline, lactated Ringer's injection, and 5% dextrose injection may be used after pH has been adjusted (if necessary); precipitates form with gentamicin, netilimicin, milrinone in 5% dextrose, 0.9% sodium chloride.

Adverse effects

- **CNS:** *Dizziness, vertigo, paresthesias, xanthopsia, weakness,* headache, drowsiness, fatigue, blurred vision, tinnitus, irreversible hearing loss
- **CV:** *Orthostatic hypotension,* volume depletion, cardiac arrhythmias, *thrombophlebitis*
- **Dermatologic:** *Photosensitivity, rash, pruritus, urticaria,* purpura, exfoliative dermatitis, erythema multiforme
- **GI:** *Nausea, anorexia, vomiting, oral and gastric irritation, constipation,* diarrhea, acute pancreatitis, jaundice
- **GU:** Polyuria, nocturia, *glycosuria, urinary bladder spasm*
- **Hematologic:** *Leukopenia, anemia, thrombocytopenia,* fluid and electrolyte imbalances
- **Other:** *Muscle cramps and muscle spasms*

Interactions

✳ **Drug-drug** • Increased risk of cardiac arrhythmias with digitalis glycosides (due to electrolyte imbalance) • Increased risk of ototoxicity with aminoglycoside antibiotics, cisplatin • Decreased absorption of furosemide with phenytoin • Decreased natriuretic and antihypertensive effects with indomethacin, ibuprofen, other NSAIDs • Decreased GI absorption with charcoal

■ Nursing considerations

 CLINICAL ALERT!
Name confusion has occurred between furosemide and torsemide; use extreme caution.

Assessment

- **History:** Allergy to furosemide, sulfonamides, tartrazine; electrolyte depletion anuria, severe renal failure; hepatic coma; SLE; gout; diabetes mellitus; lactation, pregnancy
- **Physical:** Skin color, lesions, edema; orientation, reflexes, hearing; pulses, baseline ECG, BP, orthostatic BP, perfusion; R, pattern, adventitious sounds; liver evaluation, bowel sounds; urinary output patterns; CBC, serum electrolytes (including calcium), blood sugar, liver and renal function tests, uric acid, urinalysis

Interventions

- Administer with food or milk to prevent GI upset.
- Reduce dosage if given with other antihypertensives; readjust dosage gradually as BP responds.
- Give early in the day so that increased urination will not disturb sleep.
- Avoid IV use if oral use is at all possible.
- Do not mix parenteral solution with highly acidic solutions with pH below 3.5.
- Do not expose to light, may discolor tablets or solution; do not use discolored drug or solutions.
- Discard diluted solution after 24 hr.
- Refrigerate oral solution.
- Measure and record weight to monitor fluid changes.
- Arrange to monitor serum electrolytes, hydration, liver function.
- Arrange for potassium-rich diet or supplemental potassium as needed.

Teaching points

- Record intermittent therapy on a calendar or dated envelopes. When possible, take the drug early so increased urination will not disturb sleep. Take with food or meals to prevent GI upset.
- Weigh yourself on a regular basis, at the same time and in the same clothing, and record the weight on your calendar.
- These side effects may occur: increased volume and frequency of urination; dizziness, feeling faint on arising, drowsiness (avoid rapid position changes; hazardous activities, like driving; and consumption of alcohol); sensitivity to sunlight (use sunglasses, wear protective clothing, or use a sunscreen); increased thirst (suck on sugarless lozenges; use frequent mouth care); loss of body potassium (a potassium-rich diet or potassium supplement will be necessary).
- Report loss or gain of more than 3 lb in 1 day, swelling in your ankles or fingers, unusual bleeding or bruising, dizziness, trembling, numbness, fatigue, muscle weakness or cramps.

▽ gabapentin
*(gab ah **pen'** tin)*

Neurontin

PREGNANCY CATEGORY C

Drug class
Antiepileptic agent

Therapeutic actions
Mechanism of action not understood; antiepileptic activity may be related to its ability to inhibit polysynaptic responses and block post-tetanic potentiation.

Indications

- Adjunctive therapy in the treatment of partial seizures with and without secondary generalization in adults and children 3–12 yr with epilepsy
- Orphan drug use: treatment of amyotrophic lateral sclerosis
- Management of post-herpetic neuralgia or pain in the area affected by herpes zoster after the disease has been treated
- Unlabeled uses: tremors of multiple sclerosis, neuropathic pain, bipolar disorder, migraine prophylaxis

*Adverse effects in Italics are most common; those in **Bold** are life-threatening.*

Contraindications and cautions
- Hypersensitivity to gabapentin; lactation, pregnancy.

Available forms
Capsules—100, 300, 400 mg; tablets—600, 800 mg; oral solution—250 mg/5 mL

Dosages
Adults
900–1,800 mg/day PO in divided doses tid PO; maximum time between doses should not exceed 12 hr. Up to 2,400–3,600 mg/day has been used. Initial dose of 300 mg/day PO; 300 mg bid PO on day 2; 300 mg tid PO on day 3.
Pediatric patients 3–12 yr
10–15 mg/kg/day PO in 3 divided doses; adjust upward to 25–35 mg/kg/day if needed.
Geriatric patients or patients with renal impairment
Creatinine clearance > 60 mL/min: 400 mg tid PO; 30–60 mL/min: 300 mg bid PO; 15–30 mL/min: 300 mg daily PO; < 15 mL/min: 300 mg PO every other day; patients on dialysis: 200–300 mg PO following each 4 hr of dialysis.

Pharmacokinetics

Route	Onset	Duration
Oral	Varies	6–8 hr

Metabolism: Hepatic; $T_{1/2}$: 5–7 hr
Distribution: Crosses placenta; enters breast milk
Excretion: Urine

Adverse effects
- **CNS:** *Dizziness, insomnia,* nervousness, fatigue, *somnolence, ataxia,* diplopia
- **Dermatologic:** Pruritus, abrasion
- **GI:** Dyspepsia, vomiting, nausea, constipation
- **Respiratory:** Rhinitis, pharyngitis
- **Other:** Weight gain, facial edema, cancer, impotence

Interactions
✳ **Drug-drug** • Decreased serum levels with antacids

■ Nursing considerations
Assessment
- **History:** Hypersensitivity to gabapentin; lactation, pregnancy
- **Physical:** Weight; T; skin color, lesions; orientation, affect, reflexes; P; R, adventitious sounds; bowel sounds, normal output

Interventions
- Give drug with food to prevent GI upset.
- Arrange for consultation with support groups for epileptics.

Teaching points
- Take this drug exactly as prescribed; do not discontinue abruptly or change dosage, except on the advice of your health care provider.
- These side effects may occur: dizziness, blurred vision (avoid driving or performing other tasks requiring alertness or visual acuity); GI upset (take drug with food or milk, eat frequent small meals); headache, nervousness, insomnia; fatigue (periodic rest periods may help).
- Wear a medical alert tag at all times so that any emergency medical personnel will know that you are an epileptic taking antiepileptic medication.
- Report severe headache, sleepwalking, rash, severe vomiting, chills, fever, difficulty breathing.

▽ galantamine hydrobromide
(gah lan' tah meen)

Reminyl

PREGNANCY CATEGORY B

Drug classes
Cholinesterase inhibitor
Alzheimer's drug

Therapeutic actions
Centrally acting, selective, long-acting, reversible cholinesterase inhibitor; causes elevated acetylcholine levels in the cortex, which is thought to slow the neuronal degradation that occurs in Alzheimer's disease.

Indications
- Treatment of mild to moderate dementia of the Alzheimer's type
- Unlabeled use: vascular dementia

Contraindications and cautions
- Contraindicated with allergy to galantamine, severe hepatic impairment, severe renal impairment. Avoid use with pregnancy, lactation.
- Use cautiously with moderate renal or hepatic dysfunction, GI bleeding, seizures, asthma, COPD.

Available forms
Tablets—4, 8, and 12 mg; oral solution with dosing syringe—4 mg/mL

Dosages
Adults
Initially, 4 mg PO bid. If well tolerated after 4 wk, increase to 8 mg PO bid. If well tolerated, increase to 12 mg PO bid.
Patients with hepatic or renal impairment
Do not exceed 16 mg/day. Contraindicated if creatinine clearance < 9 mL/min.
Pediatric patients
Safety and efficacy not established.

Pharmacokinetics

Route	Onset	Peak	Duration
Oral	Varies	1 hr	8 hr

Metabolism: Hepatic; $T_{1/2}$: 7 hr
Distribution: Crosses placenta; may pass into breast milk
Excretion: Urine

Adverse effects
- **CNS:** *Insomnia,* tremor, *dizziness,* fatigue, sedation, somnolence, tremor, headache
- **CV:** Bradycardia, syncope
- **GI:** *Nausea, vomiting, diarrhea, dyspepsia, anorexia, abdominal pain,* weight loss
- **GU:** UTI, hematuria

Interactions
✳ **Drug-drug** • Increased effects and risk of galantamine toxicity if combined with cime-

tidine, ketoconazole, paroxetine, erythromycin, succinylcholine, or bethanechol; if any of these combinations are used, monitor patient closely and adjust dosage as needed.

■ Nursing considerations
Assessment
- **History:** Allergy to galantamine, pregnancy, lactation, impaired renal or hepatic function, GI bleeding, seizures, asthma, COPD
- **Physical:** Orientation, affect, reflexes, BP, P, abdominal exam, renal and liver function tests

Interventions
- Establish baseline functional profile to allow evaluation of drug effectiveness.
- Ensure at least 4 wk at each dosage level to establish effectiveness and tolerance of adverse effects.
- Administer with food morning and evening to decrease GI discomfort.
- Mix solution with water, fruit juice, or soda to improve compliance.
- Monitor patient for weight loss, diarrhea, arrhythmias before use and periodically with prolonged use.
- Provide small, frequent meals if GI upset is severe; antiemetics may be used if necessary.
- Provide patient safety measures if CNS effects occur.
- Notify surgeon that patient takes galantamine; exaggerated muscle relaxation may occur if succinylcholine-type drugs are used.

Teaching points
- Take drug exactly as prescribed, with food, in the morning and evening to decrease GI upset.
- Switch to oral solution if swallowing becomes difficult; mix with water, fruit juice, or soda to improve taste.
- Be aware that this drug does not cure the disease, but is thought to slow the degeneration associated with the disease.
- Be aware that dosage changes may be needed to achieve the best effects. If the drug is stopped for more than a few days, consult your health care provider; it should be restarted at the original, lower dose.

- These side effects may occur: nausea, vomiting (small, frequent meals may help); insomnia, fatigue, confusion (use caution if driving or performing tasks that require alertness).
- Report severe nausea, vomiting, changes in stool or urine color, diarrhea, changes in neurologic functioning, palpitations.

▷ganciclovir sodium (DHPG)
(gan sye' kloe vir)

Cytovene, Vitrasert

PREGNANCY CATEGORY C

Drug class
Antiviral

Therapeutic actions
Antiviral activity; inhibits viral DNA replication in CMV.

Indications
- Treatment of CMV retinitis in immunocompromised patients, including patients with AIDS (IV and implant)
- Prevention of CMV disease in transplant recipients at risk for CMV disease (IV)
- Alternative to IV for maintenance treatment of CMV retinitis (PO)
- Prevention of CMV disease in individuals with advanced HIV infection at risk of developing CMV disease (oral)
- Unlabeled use: Treatment of other CMV infections in immunocompromised patients

Contraindications and cautions
- Contraindicated with hypersensitivity to ganciclovir or acyclovir, lactation.
- Use cautiously with cytopenia, history of cytopenic reactions, impaired renal function.

Available forms
Capsules—250, 500 mg; powder for injection—500 mg/vial; ocular implant—4.5 mg

Dosages
Adults
- *CMV retinitis:* Initial dose: 5 mg/kg given IV at a constant rate over 1 hr, q 12 hr for 14–21 days. Maintenance: 5 mg/kg given by IV infusion over 1 hr once/day, 7 days/wk *or* 6 mg/kg once/day, 5 days/wk; or 1,000 mg PO tid with food or 500 mg PO 6 times/day every 3 hr with food while awake. Implant surgically placed in affected eye q 5–8 mo.
- *Prevention of CMV disease in transplant recipients:* 5 mg/kg IV over 1 hr q 12 hr for 7–14 days; then 5 mg/kg/day once daily for 7 days/wk, or 6 mg/kg/day once daily for 5 days/wk.
- *Prevention of CMV disease with advanced AIDS:* 1,000 mg PO tid with food.

Pediatric patients
Safety and efficacy not established. Use only if benefit outweighs potential carcinogenesis and reproductive toxicity.

Geriatric patients or patients with renal impairment
Reduce initial dose by up to 50%, monitoring patient response. Maintenance dose:

Creatinine Clearance	Dose IV (mg/kg)	Dosing Intervals
≥ 70	5	12 hr
50–69	2.5	12 hr
25–49	2.5	24 hr
10–24	1.25	24 hr
< 10	1.25	3 times per wk following hemodialysis

Maintenance Dose (mg/kg)	Dosing Intervals
5	24 hr
2.5	24 hr
1.25	24 hr
0.625	24 hr
0.625	3 times per wk following hemodialysis

Creatinine Clearance	Dose PO (mg)
≥ 70	1,000 tid or 500 q 3 hr 6 times per day
50–69	1,500 daily or 500 tid
25–49	1,000 daily or 500 bid
10–24	500 daily
< 10	500 3 times per wk followed by dialysis

G

Pharmacokinetics

Route	Onset	Peak
IV	Slow	1 hr
Oral	Slow	2–4 hr

Metabolism: Hepatic; $T_{1/2}$: 2–4 hr (IV), 4.8 hr (PO)
Distribution: Crosses placenta; may enter breast milk
Excretion: Urine and feces

▽ IV facts
Preparation: Reconstitute vial by injecting 10 mL of sterile water for injection into vial; do not use bacteriostatic water for injection; shake vial to dissolve the drug. Discard vial if any particulate matter or discoloration is seen. Reconstituted solution in the vial is stable at room temperature for 12 hr.
Do not refrigerate reconstituted solution.
Infusion: Infuse slowly over 1 hr.
Compatibilities: Compatible with 0.9% sodium chloride, 5% dextrose, Ringer's injection, and lactated Ringer's injection.
Y-site incompatibilities: Do not combine with foscarnet, ondansetron.

Adverse effects
- **CNS:** Dreams, ataxia, coma, confusion, dizziness, headache
- **CV:** Arrhythmia, hypertension, hypotension
- **Dermatologic:** *Rash,* alopecia, pruritus, urticaria
- **GI:** *Abnormal liver function tests,* nausea, vomiting, anorexia, diarrhea, abdominal pain
- **Hematologic:** *Granulocytopenia, thrombocytopenia, anemia*
- **Local:** *Pain, inflammation at injection site,* phlebitis
- **Other:** *Fever,* chills, **cancer,** sterility

Interactions
✳ **Drug-drug** • Increased effects if taken with probenecid • Use with extreme caution with cytotoxic drugs because the accumulation effect could cause severe bone marrow depression and other GI and dermatologic problems • Increased risk of seizures with imipenem-cilastatin • Extreme drowsiness and risk of bone marrow depression with zidovudine

■ Nursing considerations
Assessment
- **History:** Hypersensitivity to ganciclovir or acyclovir; cytopenia; impaired renal function; lactation, pregnancy
- **Physical:** Skin color, lesions; orientation; BP, P, auscultation, perfusion, edema; R, adventitious sounds; urinary output; CBC, Hct, BUN, creatinine clearance, liver function tests

Interventions
- Give by IV infusion only. Do not give IM or SC; drug is very irritating to tissues.
- Do not exceed the recommended dosage, frequency, or infusion rates.
- Monitor infusion carefully; infuse at concentrations no greater than 10 mg/mL.
- Decrease dosage in patients with impaired renal function.
- Give oral doses with food.
- Obtain CBC before therapy, every 2 days during daily dosing, and at least weekly thereafter. Consult with physician and arrange for reduced dosage if WBCs or platelets fall.
- Consult with pharmacy for proper disposal of unused solution. Precautions are required for disposal of nucleoside analogues.
- Provide patient with a calendar of drug days, and arrange convenient times for the IV infusion in outpatients.
- Advise patients having surgical implant of ganciclovir that procedure will need to be repeated q 5–8 mo.
- Arrange for periodic ophthalmic examinations. Drug is not a cure for the disease, and deterioration may occur.
- Advise patients that ganciclovir can decrease sperm production and cause birth defects in fetuses. Advise the patient to use contraception during ganciclovir therapy. Men receiving ganciclovir therapy should use barrier contraception during and for at least 90 days after ganciclovir therapy.
- Advise patient that ganciclovir has caused cancer in animals and that risk is possible in humans.

Teaching points
- Appointments will be made for outpatients on IV therapy. Long-term therapy is fre-

quently needed. Take the oral drug with food. Surgical implant of drug will need to be repeated q 5–8 mo.

- Frequent blood tests will be necessary to determine drug effects on your blood count and to adjust drug dosage. Keep appointments for these tests.
- Arrange for periodic ophthalmic examinations during therapy to evaluate progress of the disease. This drug is not a cure for your retinitis.
- If you also are receiving zidovudine, the two drugs cannot be given concomitantly; severe adverse effects may occur.
- These side effects may occur: rash, fever, pain at injection site; decreased blood count leading to susceptibility to infection (frequent blood tests will be needed; avoid crowds and exposure to disease); birth defects and decreased sperm production (drug must not be taken during pregnancy; if pregnant or intending to become pregnant, consult with your physician; use some form of contraception during therapy; male patients should use barrier contraception during therapy and for at least 90 days after therapy).
- Report bruising, bleeding, pain at injection site, fever, infection.

▽ganirelix acetate

See *Less Commonly Used Drugs,* p. 1344.

▽gatifloxacin
(ga tah flox' a sin)

Tequin

PREGNANCY CATEGORY C

Drug classes
Antibacterial drug
Fluoroquinolone

Therapeutic actions
Bactericidal; interferes with DNA replication in susceptible gram-negative and gram-positive bacteria, preventing cell reproduction.

Indications
- Treatment of adults with community-acquired pneumonia caused by susceptible strains of *Streptococcus pneumoniae, Haemophilus influenzae, Mycoplasma pneumoniae, Chlamydia pneumoniae, Moraxella catarrhalis, Haemophilus parainfluenza, Staphylococcus aureus, Legionella pneumophila*
- Treatment of bacterial sinusitis caused by *S. pneumoniae, H. influenzae*
- Treatment of acute bacterial exacerbation of chronic bronchitis caused by *S. pneumoniae, H. influenzae, H. parainfluenzae, S. aureus, M. catarrhalis*
- Treatment of uncomplicated UTIs due to *Escherichia coli, K. pneumoniae, P. mirabilis*
- Treatment of complicated UTIs due to *E. coli, K. pneumoniae, P. mirabilis*
- Treatment of pyelonephritis due to *E. coli*
- Treatment of uncomplicated urethral and cervical gonorrhea and acute, uncomplicated rectal infections in women due to *N. gonorrhoeae*
- Treatment of uncomplicated skin and skin structure infections
- Unlabeled uses: atypical pneumonia; uncomplicated soft-tissue infections; chronic prostatitis

Contraindications and cautions
- Contraindicated with allergy to fluoroquinolones, pregnancy, lactation; presence of prolonged QT interval, hypokalemia.
- Use cautiously with renal dysfunction, diabetic patients, seizures.

Available forms
Tablets—200, 400 mg; injection—200, 400 mg vials; ready to use intravenous bags—200 (100 mL) mg, 400 (200 mL) mg

Dosages
Adults
- *Community-acquired pneumonia:* 400 mg daily PO or IV for 7–14 days.
- *Sinusitis:* 400 mg daily PO or IV for 10 days.
- *Chronic bronchitis:* 400 mg daily PO or IV for 7–10 days; short course regimen—400 mg/day PO or IV for 5 days.
- *Uncomplicated UTIs:* 200 mg daily PO or IV for 3 days; or 400 mg PO or IV as a single dose.
- *Complicated UTIs, polynephritis:* 400 mg daily PO or IV for 7–10 days.

- *Skin and skin structure infections:* 400 mg daily PO or IV for 7–10 days.

Pediatric patients

Not recommended in patients < 18 yr.

Patients with renal impairment

- *Creatinine clearance:* ≥ 40 mL/min— 400 mg PO or IV as initial dose, then 400 mg daily. < 40 mL/min—400 mg PO or IV as initial dose, then 200 mg daily.
- *Dialysis:* 400 mg PO or IV as initial dose, then 200 mg every other day.

Pharmacokinetics

Route	Onset	Peak	Duration
Oral	Varies	1 hr	18–24 hr
IV	Rapid	1 hr	18–24 hr

Metabolism: Hepatic; $T_{1/2}$: 7–14 hr
Distribution: Crosses placenta; passes into breast milk
Excretion: Urine

▽IV facts

Preparation: Dilute injection to a concentration of 2 mg/mL in 5% dextrose injection, 0.9% sodium chloride injection, 5% dextrose and 0.9% sodium chloride injection, lactated Ringer's and 5% dextrose injection, 5% sodium bicarbonate injection, *Plasma-Lyte 56 and 5% Dextrose* injection, M/6 sodium lactate injection or water for injection. Discard solution if any visible particles are present. Discard after 24 hr. Discard any leftover solution.
Infusion: Administer slowly over at least 60 min.
Incompatibilities: Do not mix with any other drug or solution. Do not give through the same line with any other drug or solution; if other drugs are given through the same line, the line should be flushed before and after gatifloxacin use.

Adverse effects

- **CNS:** *Headache,* dizziness, *insomnia,* fatigue, somnolence, depression, nervousness, anxiety, paresthesias, visual changes
- **CV:** Palpitations, **prolonged QTc interval**
- **GI:** *Nausea,* vomiting, dry mouth, *diarrhea,* anorexia, gastritis, stomatitis

- **Respiratory:** Dyspnea, pharyngitis, rhinitis
- **Other:** Fever, rash, sweating, photosensitivity (less likely than with ciprofloxacin or levofloxacin), tendonitis

Interactions

✳ Drug-drug • Increased serum levels and systemic effects if combined with probenecid • Risk of severe cardiac arrhythmias if combined with any other drug known to prolong the QTc interval (quinidine, procainamide, amiodarone, sotalol)—avoid this combination • Increased risk of seizures if fluoroquinolones are combined with NSAIDs. Monitor patient closely

✳ Drug-alternative therapy • Risk of severe photosensitivity reaction if taken with St. John's wort

■ Nursing considerations

 CLINICAL ALERT!
Name confusion has occurred between Tequin (gatifloxacin) and tacrine; use caution.

Assessment

- **History:** Allergy to fluoroquinolones; pregnancy, lactation; presence of prolonged QTc interval; hypokalemia; renal dysfunction; diabetic patients; seizures
- **Physical:** Skin color, lesions; body temperature; orientation, reflexes, affect; mucous membranes; bowel sounds; P, auscultation; renal function tests, ECG

Interventions

- Arrange for culture and sensitivity tests before beginning therapy.
- Continue therapy as indicated for condition being treated.
- Administer oral drug at the same time each day; ensure that drug is swallowed whole and not crushed or chewed.
- Ensure that patient is well hydrated during course of drug therapy.
- Discontinue drug at any sign of hypersensitivity (rash, photophobia) or at complaint of tendon pain, inflammation, or rupture.

- Monitor clinical response—if no improvement is seen or a relapse occurs, repeat culture and sensitivity.

Teaching points

- Take oral drug once a day at the same time each day; swallow whole, do not chew, crush, or cut.
- These side effects may occur: nausea, vomiting, abdominal pain (small, frequent meals may help); diarrhea or constipation (consult nurse or physician if this occurs); drowsiness, blurring of vision, dizziness (observe caution if driving or using dangerous equipment); sensitivity to the sun (avoid exposure, use a sunscreen if needed).
- Report rash, visual changes, severe GI problems, weakness, tremors, sensitivity to light.

▽gemcitabine hydrochloride
*(jem **site'** ah ben)*

Gemzar

PREGNANCY CATEGORY D

Drug class
Antineoplastic

Therapeutic actions
Cytotoxic: a nucleoside analog that is cell cycle S specific; causes cell death by disrupting and inhibiting DNA synthesis

Indications

- First-line treatment of locally advanced or metastatic adenocarcinoma of pancreas; indicated for patients who have previously received 5-FU
- In combination with cisplatin as the first-line treatment of inoperable, locally advanced or metastatic non–small-cell lung cancer

Contraindications and cautions

- Contraindicated with hypersensitivity to gemcitabine.
- Use cautiously with bone marrow suppression, renal or hepatic impairment, pregnancy, lactation.

Available forms
Powder for injection—20 mg/mL

Dosages
Adults

- *Pancreatic cancer:* 1,000 mg/m^2 IV over 30 min given once weekly for up to 7 wk or until bone marrow suppression requires withholding treatment; subsequent cycles of once weekly for 3 consecutive wk out of 4 can be given after 1-wk rest from treatment. Patients who require further therapy and have not experienced severe toxicity may be given 25% larger dose with careful monitoring.
- *Non–small-cell lung cancer:* 1,000 mg/m^2 IV over 30 min days 1, 8, 15 of each 28-day cycle with 100 mg/m^2 cisplatin on day 1 after gemcitabine infusion *or* 1,250 mg/m^2 IV over 30 min days 1, 8 of each 21-day cycle with 100 mg/m^2 cisplatin on day 1 after gemcitabine infusion.

Pediatric patients
Safety and efficacy not established.

Pharmacokinetics

Route	Onset	Peak
IV	Rapid	30 min

Metabolism: Hepatic; T$_{1/2}$: 42–70 min
Distribution: Crosses placenta; may enter breast milk
Excretion: Bile and urine

▽IV facts
Preparation: Use 0.9% sodium chloride injection as diluent for reconstitution of powder, 5 mL of 0.9% sodium chloride injection added to the 200-mg vial or 25 mL added to the 1-g vial. This will yield a concentration of 40 mg/mL; higher concentrations may lead to inadequate dissolution of powder. Resultant drug can be injected as reconstituted or further diluted in 0.9% sodium chloride injection. Stable for 24 hr at room temperature after reconstitution.
Infusion: Infuse slowly over 30 min.

Adverse effects

- **CNS:** Somnolence, paresthesias
- **GI:** *Nausea, vomiting,* diarrhea, constipation, mucositis, GI bleeding, stomatitis, hepatic dysfunction

- **Hematologic: Bone marrow depression,** *infections*
- **Pulmonary:** Dyspnea
- **Renal:** Hematuria, proteinuria, elevated BUN and creatinine
- **Other:** *Fever, alopecia, pain, rash*

■ Nursing considerations
Assessment
- **History:** Hypersensitivity to gemcitabine; bone marrow depression; renal or hepatic dysfunction; pregnancy, lactation
- **Physical:** T; skin color, lesions; R, adventitious sounds; abdominal exam, mucous membranes; liver and renal function tests, CBC with differential, urinalysis

Interventions
- Follow CBC, renal and liver function tests carefully before and frequently during therapy; dosage adjustment may be needed if myelosuppression becomes severe or hepatic or renal dysfunction occurs.
- Protect patient from exposure to infection; monitor occurrence of infection at any site and arrange for appropriate treatment.
- Provide medication, frequent small meals for severe nausea and vomiting; monitor nutritional status.

Teaching points
- This drug will need to be given IV over 30 min once a wk. Mark calendar with days to return for treatment. Regular blood tests will be needed to evaluate the effects of treatment.
- These side effects may occur: nausea and vomiting (may be severe; antiemetics may be helpful; eat small, frequent meals); increased susceptibility to infection (avoid crowds and situations that may expose you to diseases); loss of hair (arrange for a wig or other head covering; keep the head covered at extremes of temperature).
- Report severe nausea and vomiting, fever, chills, sore throat, unusual bleeding or bruising, changes in color of urine or stool.

▽ gemfibrozil
(jem fi' broe zil)

Apo-Gemfibrozil (CAN), Gen-Fibro (CAN), Lopid, Novo-Gemfibrozil (CAN)

PREGNANCY CATEGORY C

Drug class
Antihyperlipidemic

Therapeutic actions
Inhibits peripheral lipolysis and decreases the hepatic excretion of free fatty acids; this reduces hepatic triglyceride production; inhibits synthesis of VLDL carrier apolipoprotein; decreases VLDL production; increases HDL concentration.

Indications
- Hypertriglyceridemia in adult patients with very high elevations of triglyceride levels (type IV and V hyperlipidemia) at risk of pancreatitis unresponsive to diet therapy
- Reduction of coronary heart disease risk in patients who have not responded to diet, exercise, and other agents

Contraindications and cautions
- Allergy to gemfibrozil, hepatic or renal dysfunction, primary biliary cirrhosis, gallbladder disease, pregnancy, lactation.

Available forms
Tablets—600 mg

Dosages
Adults
1,200 mg/day PO in two divided doses, 30 min before morning and evening meals. Caution: Use only if strongly indicated and lipid studies show a definite response; hepatic tumorigenicity occurs in laboratory animals.
Pediatric patients
Safety and efficacy not established.

Pharmacokinetics

Route	Onset	Peak
Oral	Varies	1–2 hr

Adverse effects in *Italics* are most common; those in **Bold** are life-threatening.

Metabolism: Hepatic; $T_{1/2}$: 90 min
Distribution: Crosses placenta; enters breast milk
Excretion: Urine and feces

Adverse effects

- **CNS:** *Headache, dizziness, blurred vision,* vertigo, insomnia, paresthesia, tinnitus, *fatigue,* malaise, syncope
- **Dermatologic:** *Eczema, rash,* dermatitis, pruritus, urticaria
- **GI:** *Abdominal pain, epigastric pain, diarrhea, nausea, vomiting,* flatulence, dry mouth, constipation, anorexia, *dyspepsia,* cholelithiasis
- **GU:** Impairment of fertility
- **Hematologic:** Anemia, eosinophilia, leukopenia, hypokalemia, liver function changes, hyperglycemia
- **Other:** Painful extremities, back pain, arthralgia, muscle cramps, myalgia, swollen joints

Interactions

✳ **Drug-drug** • Risk of rhabdomyolysis from 3 wk to several mo after therapy when combined with HMG-CoA inhibitors (lovastatin, simvastatin, etc.) • Risk of increased bleeding when combined with anticoagulants; monitor patient closely • Risk of hypoglycemia if combined with sulfonylureas; monitor closely

■ Nursing considerations
Assessment

- **History:** Allergy to gemfibrozil, hepatic or renal dysfunction, primary biliary cirrhosis, gallbladder disease, pregnancy, lactation
- **Physical:** Skin lesions, color, temperature; gait, range of motion; orientation, affect, reflexes; bowel sounds, normal output, liver evaluation; lipid studies, CBC, liver and renal function tests, blood glucose

Interventions

- Administer drug with meals or milk if GI upset occurs.
- Arrange for regular follow-up, including blood tests for lipids, liver function, CBC, blood glucose during long-term therapy.

Teaching points

- Take the drug with meals or with milk if GI upset occurs; diet changes will need to be made.
- These side effects may occur: diarrhea, loss of appetite, flatulence (small, frequent meals may help); muscular aches and pains, bone and joint discomfort; dizziness, faintness, blurred vision (use caution if driving or operating dangerous equipment).
- Have regular follow-up visits to your doctor for blood tests to evaluate drug effectiveness.
- Report severe stomach pain with nausea and vomiting, fever and chills or sore throat, severe headache, vision changes.

G

▽ gemtuzumab ozogamicin

See *Less Commonly Used Drugs,* p. 1344.

▽ gentamicin sulfate
(jen ta mye' sin)

Parenteral, intrathecal: Alcomicin (CAN), Cidomycin (CAN), Garamycin, Pediatric Gentamicin Sulfate

Topical dermatologic cream, ointment: Garamycin, G-myticin

Ophthalmic: Garamycin, Gentak, Gentacidin, Genoptic, Genoptic S.O.P.

Gentamicin impregnated PMMA beads: Septopal

Gentamicin Liposome injection: Maite

PREGNANCY CATEGORY C

Drug class
Aminoglycoside

Therapeutic actions
Bactericidal: inhibits protein synthesis in susceptible strains of gram-negative bacteria; appears to disrupt functional integrity of bacterial cell membrane, causing cell death.

Indications

Parenteral
- Serious infections caused by susceptible strains of *Pseudomonas aeruginosa, Proteus* species, *Escherichia coli, Klebsiella-Enterobacter-Serratia* species, *Citrobacter, Staphylococcus* species.
- In serious infections when causative organisms are not known (often in conjunction with a penicillin or cephalosporin)
- Unlabeled use: with clindamycin as alternative regimen in PID

Intrathecal
- For serious CNS infections caused by susceptible *Pseudomonas* species

Ophthalmic preparations
- Treatment of superficial ocular infections due to strains of microorganisms susceptible to gentamicin

Topical dermatologic preparation
- Infection prophylaxis in minor skin abrasions and treatment of superficial infections of the skin due to susceptible organisms amenable to local treatment

Gentamicin-impregnated PMAA beads on surgical wire
- Orphan drug use: treatment of chronic osteomyelitis of post-traumatic, postoperative, or hematogenous origin

Gentamicin liposome injection
- Orphan drug use: treatment of disseminated *Myobacterium avium-intracellulare* infection

Contraindications and cautions
- Contraindicated with allergy to any aminoglycosides; renal or hepatic disease; preexisting hearing loss; active infection with herpes, vaccinia, varicella, fungal infections, myobacterial infections (ophthalmic preparations); myasthenia gravis; parkinsonism; infant botulism; lactation.
- Use cautiously with pregnancy.

Available forms
Injection—10, 40 mg/mL; ophthalmic solution—3 mg/mL; ophthalmic ointment—3 mg/g; topical ointment—0.1%; topical cream—0.1%; ointment—1 mg; cream—1 mg

Dosages

Adults
3 mg/kg/day in 3 equal doses q 8 hr IM or IV. Up to 5 mg/kg/day in 3–4 equal doses in severe infections. For IV use, a loading dose of 1–2 mg/kg may be infused over 30–60 min, followed by a maintenance dose usually for 7–10 days.
- *PID:* 2 mg/kg IV followed by 1.5 mg/kg tid plus clindamycin 600 mg IV qid. Continue for at least 4 days and at least 48 hr after patient improves, then continue clindamycin 450 mg orally qid for 10–14 days total therapy.
- *Surgical prophylaxis regimens:* Several complex, multidrug prophylaxis regimens are available for preoperative use; consult manufacturer's instructions.

Pediatric patients
2–2.5 mg/kg q 8 hr IM or IV.
Infants and neonates: 2.5 mg/kg q 8 hr.
Premature or full-term neonates: 2.5 mg/kg q 12 hr.

Geriatric patients or patients with renal failure
Reduce dosage or extend time dosage intervals, and carefully monitor serum drug levels and renal function tests.

Ophthalmic solution
1–2 drops into affected eye(s) q 4 hr; up to 2 drops hourly in severe infections.

Ophthalmic ointment
Apply small amount to affected eye bid–tid.

Dermatologic preparations
Apply tid to qid. Cover with sterile bandage if needed.

Pharmacokinetics

Route	Onset	Peak
IM, IV	Rapid	30–90 min

Metabolism: Hepatic; $T_{1/2}$: 2–3 hr
Distribution: Crosses placenta; enters breast milk
Excretion: Urine

▼ IV facts
Preparation: Dilute single dose in 50–200 mL of sterile isotonic saline or 5% dextrose in water. Do not mix in solution with any other drugs.
Infusion: Infuse over 30-120 min.

Adverse effects in *Italics* are most common; those in **Bold** are life-threatening.

Incompatibilities: Do not mix in solution with any other drugs.

Adverse effects

- **CNS:** Ototoxicity—*tinnitus, dizziness,* vertigo, deafness (partially reversible to irreversible), vestibular paralysis, confusion, disorientation, depression, lethargy, nystagmus, visual disturbances, headache, *numbness, tingling,* tremor, paresthesias, muscle twitching, convulsions, muscular weakness, neuromuscular blockade
- **CV:** Palpitations, hypotension, hypertension
- **GI:** Hepatic toxicity, *nausea, vomiting, anorexia,* weight loss, stomatitis, increased salivation
- **GU:** Nephrotoxicity
- **Hematologic:** *Leukemoid reaction,* agranulocytosis, granulocytosis, leukopenia, leukocytosis, thrombocytopenia, eosinophilia, pancytopenia, anemia, hemolytic anemia, increased and decreased reticulocyte count, electrolyte disturbances
- **Hypersensitivity:** *Purpura, rash,* urticaria, exfoliative dermatitis, itching
- **Local:** *Pain, irritation, arachnoiditis at IM injection sites*
- **Other:** Fever, apnea, splenomegaly, joint pain, *superinfections*

Ophthalmic preparations

- **Local:** *Transient irritation, burning, stinging, itching,* angioneurotic edema, urticaria, vesicular and maculopapular dermatitis

Topical dermatologic preparations

- **Local:** *Photosensitization,* superinfections

Interactions

✳ Drug-drug • Increased ototoxic, nephrotoxic, neurotoxic effects with other aminoglycosides, cephalothin, potent diuretics • Increased neuromuscular blockade and muscular paralysis with anesthetics, nondepolarizing neuromuscular blocking drugs, succinylcholine, citrate-anticoagulated blood • Potential inactivation of both drugs if mixed with beta-lactam–type antibiotics (space doses with concomitant therapy) • Increased bactericidal effect with penicillins, cephalosporins (to treat some gram-negative organisms and enterococci), carbenicillin, ticarcillin (to treat *Pseudomonas* infections)

■ Nursing considerations
Assessment

- **History:** Allergy to any aminoglycosides; renal or hepatic disease; preexisting hearing loss; active infection with herpes, vaccinia, varicella, fungal infections, myobacterial infections (ophthalmic preparations); myasthenia gravis; parkinsonism; infant botulism; lactation, pregnancy
- **Physical:** Site of infection; skin color, lesions; orientation, reflexes, eighth cranial nerve function; P, BP; R, adventitious sounds; bowel sounds, liver evaluation; urinalysis, BUN, serum creatinine, serum electrolytes, liver function tests, CBC

Interventions

- Give by IM route if at all possible; give by deep IM injection.
- Culture infected area before therapy.
- Use 2 mg/mL intrathecal preparation without preservatives, for intrathecal use.
- Cleanse area before application of dermatologic preparations.
- Ensure adequate hydration of patient before and during therapy.
- Monitor renal function tests, complete blood counts, serum drug levels during long-term therapy. Consult with prescriber to adjust dosage.

Teaching points

- Apply ophthalmic preparations by tilting head back; place medications into conjunctival sac and close eye; apply light pressure on lacrimal sac for 1 min. Cleanse area before applying dermatologic preparations; area may be covered if necessary.
- These side effects may occur: ringing in the ears, headache, dizziness (reversible; use safety measures if severe); nausea, vomiting, loss of appetite (small frequent meals, frequent mouth care may help); burning, blurring of vision with ophthalmic preparations (avoid driving or performing dangerous activities if visual effects occur); photosensitization with dermatologic preparations (wear sunscreen and protective clothing).
- Report pain at injection site, severe headache, dizziness, loss of hearing, changes in urine pattern, difficulty breathing, rash or skin lesions; itching or irritation (ophthalmic

preparations); worsening of the condition, rash, irritation (dermatologic preparation).

▽ glatiramer acetate
*(gla **tear'** ah mer)*

Copaxone

PREGNANCY CATEGORY B

Drug class
Multiple sclerosis agent

Therapeutic actions
Mechanism of action is unknown; it is thought to modify the immune process that is thought to be responsible for the pathogenesis of multiple sclerosis.

Indications
• Reduction of the frequency of relapses in patients with relapsing or remitting multiple sclerosis

Contraindications and cautions
• Contraindicated with allergy to glatiramer or mannitol.
• Use cautiously with pregnancy and lactation.

Available forms
Injection—20 mg

Dosages
Adults
20 mg/day SC.
Pediatric patients
Safety and efficacy not established.

Pharmacokinetics

Route	Onset	Duration
SC	Slow	Unknown

Metabolism: Local; $T_{1/2}$: unknown
Distribution: May cross placenta; may pass into breast milk
Excretion: Unknown

Adverse effects
• **CNS:** *Anxiety, hypertonia,* tremor, vertigo, agitation

• **CV:** *Vasodilation, palpitations,* tachycardia
• **Dermatologic:** *Rash, pruritus, sweating,* erythema, uticaria
• **GI:** *Nausea,* GI distress, *diarrhea,* vomiting, anorexia
• **Local:** *Pain at injection site, erythema, inflammation, induration, mass*
• **Other:** *Infection, asthenia, pain, chest pain, flulike syndrome, back pain,* fever, chills, *arthralgias*

■ Nursing considerations
Assessment
• **History:** Allergy to glatiramer, mannitol; pregnancy, lactation
• **Physical:** T; orientation, affect, reflexes; skin color, lesions; P, BP, peripheral perfusion; evaluate sites for injection

Interventions
• Reconstitute with diluent supplied, sterile water for injection; gently swirl bottle and let stand at room temperature until all solid material is dissolved; use immediately. Refrigerate unreconstituted vial.
• Administer by SC injection in the arms, abdomen, hips, and thighs. Rotate sites and keep chart of areas used.
• Encourage patient to avoid pregnancy while on this drug; use of barrier contraceptives is recommended.
• Offer supportive care to deal with the unpleasant side effects of this drug.

Teaching points
• This drug must be given by SC injection; you and a significant other should learn to administer the drug. Refrigerate drug until ready to use; dilute with diluent provided, gently swirl bottle and let stand at room temperature until all solid material is dissolved. Use immediately.
• Keep chart of sites used for injection, rotate sites; abdomen, arms, thigh, and hips can be used.
• Do not become pregnant while on this drug; use of barrier contraceptives is advised. If you think that you are pregnant, consult your health care provider immediately.
• These side effects may occur: nausea, diarrhea, GI distress (take the drug with meals);

sweating, flushing, rash (temperature control and frequent skin care may help); pain and swelling at the injection site (rotate sites daily, observe sterile technique).

- Report chest pain, difficulty breathing, severe GI upset, rash, severe pain at injection site, continued swelling or hardening of injection sites.

▷glimepiride
*(glye **meh'** per ide)*

Amaryl

PREGNANCY CATEGORY C

Drug classes
Antidiabetic agent
Sulfonylurea (second generation)

Therapeutic actions
Stimulates insulin release from functioning beta cells in the pancreas; may improve binding between insulin and insulin receptors or increase the number of insulin receptors; thought to be more potent in effect than first-generation sulfonylureas

Indications
- As an adjunct to diet to lower blood glucose in patients with type 2 diabetes mellitus whose hypoglycemia cannot be controlled by diet alone.
- In combination with metformin or insulin to better control glucose as an adjunct to diet and exercise in patients with type 2 diabetes mellitus.

Contraindications and cautions
- Contraindicated with allergy to sulfonylureas; diabetes complicated by fever, severe infections, severe trauma, major surgery, ketosis, acidosis, coma (insulin is indicated in these conditions); type 1 or juvenile diabetes, serious hepatic or renal impairment, uremia, thyroid or endocrine impairment, glycosuria, hyperglycemia associated with primary renal disease; labor and delivery—if glimepiride is used during pregnancy, discontinue drug at least 1 mo before delivery; lactation, safety not established.

Available forms
Tablets—1, 2, 4 mg

Dosages
Adults
Usual starting dose is 1–2 mg PO once daily with breakfast or first meal of the day; usual maintenance dose is 1–4 mg PO once daily, depending on patient response and glucose levels. Do not exceed 8 mg/day.
- *Combination with insulin therapy:* 8 mg PO daily with first meal of the day with low-dose insulin.
- *Transfer from other hypoglycemic agents:* No transition period is necessary.

Pediatric patients
Safety and efficacy not established.

Patients with renal impairment
Usual starting dose is 1 mg PO once daily; titrate dose carefully, lower maintenance doses may be sufficient to control blood sugar.

Pharmacokinetics

Route	Onset	Peak
Oral	1 hr	2–3 hr

Metabolism: Hepatic; $T_{1/2}$: 5.5–7 hr
Distribution: Crosses placenta; enters breast milk
Excretion: Bile and urine

Adverse effects
- **CV: Increased risk of cardiovascular mortality** (possible)
- **Endocrine:** *Hypoglycemia*
- **GI:** *Anorexia, nausea,* vomiting, *epigastric discomfort, heartburn, diarrhea*
- **Hematologic:** Leukopenia, thrombocytopenia, anemia
- **Hypersensitivity:** *Allergic skin reactions,* eczema, pruritus, erythema, urticaria, photosensitivity, fever, eosinophilia, jaundice

Interactions
✳ **Drug-drug** • Increased risk of hypoglycemia with sulfonamides, chloramphenicol, oxyphenbutazone, phenylbutazone, salicylates, clofibrate • Decreased effectiveness of both glimepiride and diazoxide if taken concurrently • Increased risk of hyperglycemia with rifampin, thiazides • Risk of hypoglycemia and hyperglycemia with ethanol; "disulfiram reaction" has also been reported

✳ Drug-alternative therapy • Increased risk of hypoglycemia if taken with juniper berries, ginseng, garlic, fenugreek, coriander, dandelion root, celery

■ Nursing considerations
Assessment
- **History:** Allergy to sulfonylureas; diabetes complicated by fever, severe infections, severe trauma, major surgery, ketosis, acidosis, coma (insulin is indicated in these conditions); type 1 or juvenile diabetes, serious hepatic or renal impairment, uremia, thyroid or endocrine impairment, glycosuria, hyperglycemia associated with primary renal disease; pregnancy
- **Physical:** Skin color, lesions; T; orientation, reflexes, peripheral sensation; R, adventitious sounds; liver evaluation, bowel sounds; urinalysis, BUN, serum creatinine, liver function tests, blood glucose, CBC

Interventions
- Monitor urine or serum glucose levels frequently to determine effectiveness of drug and dosage being used.
- Transfer to insulin therapy during periods of high stress (infections, surgery, trauma, etc.).
- Use IV glucose if severe hypoglycemia occurs as a result of overdose.
- Arrange for consultation with dietitian to establish weight-loss program and dietary control.
- Arrange for thorough diabetic teaching program, including disease, dietary control, exercise, signs and symptoms of hypoglycemia and hyperglycemia, avoidance of infection, hygiene.

Teaching points
- Take this drug once a day with breakfast or the first main meal of the day.
- Do not discontinue this drug without consulting your health care provider; continue with diet and exercise program for diabetes control.
- Monitor urine or blood for glucose and ketones as prescribed.
- Do not use this drug if you are pregnant.
- Avoid alcohol while on this drug.

- Report fever, sore throat, unusual bleeding or bruising, rash, dark urine, light-colored stools, hypoglycemic or hyperglycemic reactions.

▽ glipizide
(glip' i zide)

Glucotrol, Glucotrol XL

PREGNANCY CATEGORY C

Drug classes
Antidiabetic agent
Sulfonylurea (second generation)

Therapeutic actions
Stimulates insulin release from functioning beta cells in the pancreas; may improve binding between insulin and insulin receptors or increase the number of insulin receptors; more potent in effect than first-generation sulfonylureas.

Indications
- Adjunct to diet and exercise to lower blood glucose with type 2 diabetes mellitus
- Adjunct to insulin therapy in the stabilization of certain cases of insulin-dependent maturity-onset diabetes, reducing the insulin requirement and decreasing the chance of hypoglycemic reactions

Contraindications and cautions
- Allergy to sulfonylureas; diabetes complicated by fever, severe infections, severe trauma, major surgery, ketosis, acidosis, coma (insulin is indicated); type 1 or juvenile diabetes, serious hepatic impairment, serious renal impairment, uremia, thyroid or endocrine impairment, glycosuria, hyperglycemia associated with primary renal disease; labor and delivery (if glipizide is used during pregnancy, discontinue drug at least 1 mo before delivery); lactation.

Available forms
Tablets—5, 10 mg; ER tablets—2.5, 5, 10 mg

Adverse effects in *Italics* are most common; those in **Bold** are life-threatening.

Dosages

Give approximately 30 min before meal to achieve greatest reduction in postprandial hyperglycemia.

Adults

- *Initial therapy:* 5 mg PO before breakfast. Adjust dosage in increments of 2.5–5 mg as determined by blood glucose response. At least several days should elapse between adjustments. Maximum once-daily dose should not exceed 15 mg; above 15 mg, divide dose, and administer before meals. Do not exceed 40 mg/day. ER tablets: 5 mg/day. Adjust dosage in 5-mg increments every 3 mo; maximum dose—20 mg/day.
- *Maintenance therapy:* Total daily doses above 15 mg PO should be divided; total daily doses above 30 mg are given in divided doses bid.
- *Extended release:* 5 mg/day with breakfast, may be increased to 10 mg/day after 3 mo if indicated.

Pediatric patients

Safety and efficacy not established.

Geriatric patients and patients with hepatic impairment

Geriatric patients tend to be more sensitive to the drug. Start with initial dose of 2.5 mg/day PO. Monitor for 24 hr and gradually increase dose after several days as needed.

Pharmacokinetics

Route	Onset	Peak	Duration
Oral	1–1.5 hr	1–3 hr	10–16 hr

Metabolism: Hepatic; $T_{1/2}$: 2–4 hr
Distribution: Crosses placenta; enters breast milk
Excretion: Bile and urine

Adverse effects

- **CV: Increased risk of CV mortality**
- **Endocrine:** *Hypoglycemia*
- **GI:** *Anorexia, nausea,* vomiting, *epigastric discomfort, heartburn, diarrhea*
- **Hematologic:** Leukopenia, thrombocytopenia, anemia
- **Hypersensitivity:** *Allergic skin reactions,* eczema, pruritus, erythema, urticaria, photosensitivity, fever, eosinophilia, jaundice

Interactions

✳ **Drug-drug** ● Increased risk of hypoglycemia with sulfonamides, chloramphenicol, oxyphenbutazone, phenylbutazone, salicylates, clofibrate ● Decreased effectiveness of glipizide and diazoxide if taken concurrently ● Increased risk of hyperglycemia with rifampin, thiazides ● Risk of hypoglycemia and hyperglycemia with ethanol; "disulfiram reaction" also has been reported

✳ **Drug-alternative therapy** ● Increased risk of hypoglycemia if taken with juniper berries, ginseng, garlic, fenugreek, coriander, dandelion root, celery

■ Nursing considerations

Assessment

- **History:** Allergy to sulfonylureas; diabetes with complications; type 1 or juvenile diabetes, serious hepatic or renal impairment, uremia, thyroid or endocrine impairment, glycosuria, hyperglycemia associated with primary renal disease; pregnancy
- **Physical:** Skin color, lesions; T; orientation, reflexes, peripheral sensation; R, adventitious sounds; liver evaluation, bowel sounds; urinalysis, BUN, serum creatinine, liver function tests, blood glucose, CBC

Interventions

- Give drug 30 min before breakfast; if severe GI upset occurs or more than 15 mg/day is required, dose may be divided and given before meals.
- Monitor urine or serum glucose levels frequently to determine drug effectiveness and dosage.
- Transfer to insulin therapy during periods of high stress (eg, infections, surgery, trauma).
- Use IV glucose if severe hypoglycemia occurs as a result of overdose.

Teaching points

- Take this drug 30 min before breakfast for best results.
- Do not discontinue this medication without consulting your health care provider.
- Monitor urine or blood for glucose and ketones.
- Do not use this drug during pregnancy; consult health care provider.
- Avoid alcohol while on this drug.

• Report fever, sore throat, unusual bleeding or bruising, rash, dark urine, light-colored stools, hypoglycemic or hyperglycemic reactions.

▽glucagon
(gloo' ka gon)

Glucagon Diagnostic Kit, Glucagon Emergency Kit

PREGNANCY CATEGORY B

Drug classes
Glucose elevating agent
Hormone
Diagnostic agent

Therapeutic actions
Accelerates the breakdown of glycogen to glucose (glycogenolysis) in the liver, causing an increase in blood glucose level; relaxes smooth muscle of the GI tract

Indications
• Hypoglycemia: counteracts severe hypoglycemic reactions in diabetic patients
• Diagnostic aid in the radiologic examination of the stomach, duodenum, small bowel, or colon when a hypotonic state is advantageous
• Unlabeled use: treatment of beta blocker overdose, and in cardiac emergencies

Contraindications and cautions
• Insulinoma (drug releases insulin), pheochromocytoma (drug releases catecholamines), pregnancy, lactation.

Available forms
Powder for injection—1 mg

Dosages
Adults and children > 20 kg
• *Hypoglycemia:* 0.5–1.0 mg SC, IV, or IM. Response is usually seen in 5–20 min. If response is delayed, dose may be repeated one to two times.
• *Diagnostic aid:* Suggested dose, route, and timing of dose vary with the segment of GI

tract to be examined and duration of effect needed. Carefully check manufacturer's literature before use.
Pediatric patients < 20 kg
0.5 mg SC, IM, or IV or a dose equivalent to 20–30 mcg/kg.

Pharmacokinetics

Route	Onset	Peak	Duration
IV	1 min	15 min	9–20 min
IM	8–10 min	20–30 min	19–32 min

Metabolism: Hepatic; $T_{1/2}$: 3–10 min
Distribution: Crosses placenta; enters breast milk
Excretion: Bile and urine

▽IV facts
Preparation: Reconstitute with vial provided. Use immediately; refrigerated solution stable for 48 hr. If doses higher than 2 mg, reconstitute with sterile water for injection and use immediately.
Infusion: Inject directly into the IV tubing of an IV drip infusion, each 1 mg over 1 min.
Incompatibilities: Compatible with dextrose solutions, but precipitates may form in solutions of sodium chloride, potassium chloride, or calcium chloride.

Adverse effects
• **GI:** *Nausea, vomiting*
• **Hematologic:** Hypokalemia in overdose
• **Hypersensitivity:** Urticaria, respiratory distress, hypotension

Interactions
✳ **Drug-drug** • Increased anticoagulant effect and risk of bleeding with oral anticoagulants

■ Nursing considerations
Assessment
• **History:** Insulinoma, pheochromocytoma, lactation, pregnancy
• **Physical:** Skin color, lesions, temperature; orientation, reflexes; P, BP, peripheral perfusion; R; liver evaluation, bowel sounds; blood and urine glucose, serum potassium

*Adverse effects in Italics are most common; those in **Bold** are life-threatening.*

Interventions

- Arouse hypoglycemic patient as soon as possible after drug injection, and provide supplemental carbohydrates to restore liver glycogen and prevent secondary hypoglycemia.
- Arrange for evaluation of insulin dosage in cases of hypoglycemia as a result of insulin overdosage; insulin dosage may need to be adjusted.

Teaching points

- Diabetic and significant others should learn to administer the drug SC in case of hypoglycemia. They also should learn how to administer drug and when to notify physician.

▷ glutethimide
(gloo *teth'* i mide)

PREGNANCY CATEGORY C

C-II CONTROLLED SUBSTANCE

Drug class
Sedative and hypnotic (nonbarbiturate)

Therapeutic actions
Mechanism by which CNS is affected is not known; causes CNS depression similar to barbiturates; anticholinergic.

Indications

- Short-term relief of insomnia (3–7 days); not indicated for long-term administration; allow a drug-free interval of 1 wk or more before retreatment

Contraindications and cautions

- Contraindicated with hypersensitivity to glutethimide, porphyria, lactation.
- Use cautiously with pregnancy.

Available forms
Tablets—250 mg

Dosages
Adults
Usual dosage: 250–500 mg PO hs.
Pediatric patients
Not recommended.

Geriatric or debilitated patients
Initial daily dosage should not exceed 500 mg PO hs to avoid oversedation.

Pharmacokinetics

Route	Onset	Peak
Oral	Erratic	1–6 hr

Metabolism: Hepatic; $T_{1/2}$: 10–12 hr
Distribution: Crosses placenta; enters breast milk
Excretion: Urine

Adverse effects

- **CNS:** *Drowsiness, hangover,* suppression of REM sleep; REM rebound when drug is discontinued, mydriasis
- **Dermatologic:** *Rash*
- **GI:** *Nausea,* dry mouth, decreased intestinal motility
- **Hematologic:** Porphyria, blood dyscrasias
- **Other:** Physical, psychological dependence; tolerance; withdrawal reaction

Interactions
✳ **Drug-drug** • Additive CNS depression when given with alcohol • Increased metabolism and decreased effectiveness of oral (coumarin) anticoagulants • Reduced absorption and decreased circulating levels with charcoal interactants

■ Nursing considerations
Assessment

- **History:** Hypersensitivity to glutethimide, porphyria, lactation, pregnancy
- **Physical:** Skin color, lesions; orientation, affect, reflexes; bowel sounds

Interventions

- Supervise dose and amount prescribed carefully in patients who are addiction prone or alcoholic; normally a week's supply is sufficient; patient should then be reevaluated.
- Dispense least amount of drug feasible to patients who are depressed or suicidal.
- Withdraw drug gradually in long-term use or if tolerance has developed; supportive therapy similar to that for barbiturate withdrawal may be necessary to prevent dangerous withdrawal symptoms (nausea, abdominal discomfort, tremors, convulsions, delirium).

- Arrange for reevaluation of patients with prolonged insomnia. Therapy of the underlying cause (eg, pain, depression) is preferable to prolonged therapy with sedative or hypnotic drugs.

Teaching points
- Take this drug exactly as prescribed. Do not exceed prescribed dosage; do not use for longer than 1 wk.
- Do not discontinue the drug abruptly; consult your health care provider if you wish to stop before instructed to do so.
- Avoid alcohol, sleep-inducing, or OTC drugs; these could cause dangerous effects.
- These side effects may occur: drowsiness, dizziness, blurred vision (avoid driving or performing other tasks requiring alertness or visual acuity), GI upset (frequent small meals may help).
- Report skin rash.

▽ glyburide
(glye' byoor ide)

Albert Glyburide (CAN), DiaBeta, Euglucon (CAN), Gen-Glybe (CAN), Glynase PresTab, Micronase

PREGNANCY CATEGORY B

Drug class
Antidiabetic agent

Therapeutic actions
Stimulates insulin release from functioning beta cells in the pancreas; may improve binding between insulin and insulin receptors or increase the number of insulin receptors; more potent in effect than first-generation sulfonylureas.

Indications
- Adjunct to diet to lower blood glucose with type 2 diabetes mellitus
- Adjunct to metformin when adequate results are not achieved with either drug alone
- Adjunct to insulin therapy in the stabilization of certain cases of type 2 diabetes, reducing the insulin requirement, and decreasing the chance of hypoglycemic reactions

Contraindications and cautions
- Allergy to sulfonylureas; diabetes complicated by fever, severe infections, severe trauma, major surgery, ketosis, acidosis, coma (insulin is indicated); type 1 or juvenile diabetes, serious hepatic or renal impairment, uremia, thyroid or endocrine impairment, glycosuria, hyperglycemia associated with primary renal disease; labor and delivery (if glyburide is used during pregnancy, discontinue drug at least 1 mo before delivery); lactation.

Available forms
Tablets—1.25, 1.5, 2.5, 3, 4.5, 5, 6 mg

Dosages
Adults
- Initial therapy: 2.5–5 mg PO with breakfast (DiaBeta, Micronase); 1.5–3 mg/day PO (Glynase).
- Maintenance therapy: 1.25–20 mg/day PO given as a single dose or in divided doses. Increase in increments of no more than 2.5 mg at weekly intervals based on patient's blood glucose response (DiaBeta, Micronase); 0.75–12 mg/day PO (Glynase).
Pediatric patients
Safety and efficacy not established.
Geriatric patients
Geriatric patients tend to be more sensitive to the drug; start with initial dose of 1.25 mg/day PO (DiaBeta, Micronase) 0.75 mg/day PO (Glynase). Monitor for 24 hr, and gradually increase dose after at least 1 wk as needed.

Pharmacokinetics

Route	Onset	Duration
Oral	1 hr	24 hr

Metabolism: Hepatic; $T_{1/2}$: 4 hr
Distribution: Crosses placenta; enters breast milk
Excretion: Bile and urine

Adverse effects
- **CV: Increased risk of CV mortality**
- **Endocrine:** *Hypoglycemia*

Adverse effects in *Italics* are most common; those in **Bold** are life-threatening.

- **GI:** *Anorexia, nausea,* vomiting, *epigastric discomfort, heartburn, diarrhea*
- **Hematologic:** Leukopenia, thrombocytopenia, anemia
- **Hypersensitivity:** *Allergic skin reactions,* eczema, pruritus, erythema, urticaria, photosensitivity, fever, eosinophilia, jaundice

Interactions

✳ **Drug-drug** ● Increased risk of hypoglycemia with sulfonamides, chloramphenicol, oxyphenbutazone, phenylbutazone, salicylates, clofibrate ● Decreased effectiveness of glyburide and diazoxide if taken concurrently ● Increased risk of hyperglycemia with rifampin, thiazides ● Risk of hypoglycemia and hyperglycemia with ethanol; "disulfiram reaction" has been reported

✳ **Drug-alternative therapy** ● Increased risk of hypoglycemia if taken with juniper berries, ginseng, garlic, fenugreek, coriander, dandelion root, celery

■ Nursing considerations

CLINICAL ALERT!
Name confusion has occurred between DiaBeta (glyburide) and Zebeta (bisoprolol); use caution.

Assessment

- **History:** Allergy to sulfonylureas; diabetes with complications; type 1 or juvenile diabetes, serious hepatic or renal impairment, uremia, thyroid or endocrine impairment, glycosuria, hyperglycemia associated with primary renal disease, pregnancy
- **Physical:** Skin color, lesions; T; orientation, reflexes, peripheral sensation; R, adventitious sounds; liver evaluation, bowel sounds; urinalysis, BUN, serum creatinine, liver function tests, blood glucose, CBC

Interventions

- Give drug before breakfast. If severe GI upset occurs, dose may be divided and given before meals.
- Monitor urine or serum glucose levels frequently to determine drug effectiveness and dosage.
- Monitor dosage carefully if switching to or from *Glynase*.

- Transfer to insulin therapy during periods of high stress (eg, infections, surgery, trauma).
- Use IV glucose if severe hypoglycemia occurs as a result of overdose.

Teaching points

- Do not discontinue this medication without consulting your health care provider.
- Monitor urine or blood for glucose and ketones.
- Do not use this drug during pregnancy; consult health care provider.
- Avoid alcohol while on this drug.
- Report fever, sore throat, unusual bleeding or bruising, rash, dark urine, light-colored stools, hypoglycemic or hyperglycemic reactions.

▷**glycerin (glycerol)**
(gli' ser in)

Colace Suppositories, Fleet Babylax, Osmoglyn, SaniSupp

PREGNANCY CATEGORY C

Drug classes

Osmotic diuretic
Hyperosmolar laxative

Therapeutic actions

Elevates the osmolarity of the glomerular filtrate, thereby hindering the reabsorption of water and leading to a loss of water, sodium, and chloride; creates an osmotic gradient in the eye between plasma and ocular fluids, thereby reducing intraocular pressure; causes the local absorption of sodium and water in the stool, leading to a more liquid stool and local intestinal movement.

Indications

- Glaucoma: to interrupt acute attacks, or when a temporary drop in intraocular pressure is required (*Osmoglyn*)
- Prior to ocular surgery performed under local anesthetic when a reduction in intraocular pressure is indicated (*Osmoglyn*)
- Temporary relief of constipation

- Unlabeled use: IV (with proper preparation) to lower intracranial or intraocular pressure

Contraindications and cautions
- Contraindicated with hypersensitivity to glycerin.
- Use cautiously with hypervolemia, CHF, confused mental states, severe dehydration, the elderly, senility, diabetes, lactation.

Available forms
Oral solution—50% (0.6 mg/mL); liquid—4 mL/applicator; suppositories

Dosages
Adults
- *Reduction of intraocular pressure: Osmoglyn:* Given PO only: 1–2 g/kg, 1 hr–90 min prior to surgery.
- *Laxative:* Insert one suppository high in rectum and retain 15–30 min; rectal liquid: insert stem with tip pointing toward navel; squeeze unit until nearly all liquid is expelled, then remove.
Pediatric patients
Safety and efficacy not established.

Pharmacokinetics

Route	Onset	Peak	Duration
Oral (Osmoglyn)	Varies	1 hr	5 hr

Metabolism: Hepatic; $T_{1/2}$: 2–3 hr
Distribution: Crosses placenta; may enter breast milk
Excretion: Urine

Adverse effects
- **CNS:** *Confusion, headache, syncope,* disorientation
- **CV:** Cardiac arrhythmias
- **Endocrine: Hyperosmolar nonketotic coma**
- **GI:** *Nausea, vomiting*
- **Other:** Severe dehydration, weight gain with continued use

■ Nursing considerations
Assessment
- **History:** Hypersensitivity to glycerin, hypervolemia, CHF, confused mental states, severe dehydration, elderly, senility, diabetes, lactation, pregnancy
- **Physical:** Skin color, edema; orientation, reflexes, muscle strength, pupillary reflexes; P, BP, perfusion; R, pattern, adventitious sounds; urinary output patterns; serum electrolytes, urinalysis

Interventions
- Give *Osmoglyn* orally only; not for injection.
- Give laxative as follows: Insert one suppository high in rectum, and have patient retain 15 min; rectal liquid—insert stem with tip pointing toward navel; squeeze unit until nearly all liquid is expelled, then remove.
- Monitor urinary output carefully.
- Monitor BP regularly.

Teaching points
- Take laxative as follows: Insert one suppository high in rectum and retain 15 min; rectal liquid—insert stem with tip pointing toward navel; squeeze unit until nearly all liquid is expelled, then remove.
- These side effects may occur: increased urination, GI upset (small, frequent meals may help), dry mouth (sugarless lozenges to suck may help), headache, blurred vision (use caution when moving around; ask for assistance).
- Report severe headache, chest pain, confusion, rapid respirations, violent diarrhea.

▽ **glycopyrrolate**
(glye koe pye' roe late)

Robinul, Robinul Forte

PREGNANCY CATEGORY B

PREGNANCY CATEGORY C (PARENTERAL)

Drug classes
Anticholinergic (quaternary)
Antimuscarinic agent
Parasympatholytic
Antispasmodic

Therapeutic actions

Competitively blocks the effects of acetylcholine at receptors that mediate the effects of parasympathetic postganglionic impulses; depresses salivary and bronchial secretions; dilates the bronchi; inhibits vagal influences on the heart; relaxes the GI and GU tracts; inhibits gastric acid secretion

Indications

- Adjunctive therapy in the treatment of peptic ulcer (oral)
- Reduction of salivary, tracheobronchial, and pharyngeal secretions preoperatively; reduction of the volume and free acidity of gastric secretions; and blocking of cardiac vagal inhibitory reflexes during induction of anesthesia and intubation; may be used intraoperatively to counteract drug-induced or vagal traction reflexes with the associated arrhythmias (parenteral)
- Protection against the peripheral muscarinic effects (eg, bradycardia, excessive secretions) of cholinergic agents (neostigmine, pyridostigmine) that are used to reverse the neuromuscular blockade produced by nondepolarizing neuromuscular junction blockers (parenteral)

Contraindications and cautions

- Contraindicated with glaucoma; adhesions between iris and lens; stenosing peptic ulcer; pyloroduodenal obstruction; paralytic ileus; intestinal atony; severe ulcerative colitis; toxic megacolon; symptomatic prostatic hypertrophy; bladder neck obstruction; bronchial asthma; COPD; cardiac arrhythmias; tachycardia; myocardial ischemia; lactation; impaired metabolic, liver, or kidney function; myasthenia gravis.
- Use cautiously with Down syndrome, brain damage, spasticity, hypertension, hyperthyroidism, pregnancy.

Available forms

Tablets—1, 2, mg; injection 0.2 mg/mL

Dosages
Adults
Oral

1 mg tid or 2 mg bid–tid; maintenance: 1 mg bid.

Parenteral

- Peptic ulcer: 0.1–0.2 mg IM or IV tid–qid.
- Preanesthetic medication: 0.004 mg/kg (0.002 mg/lb) IM 30–60 min prior to anesthesia.
- Intraoperative: 0.1 mg IV; repeat as needed at 2- to 3-min intervals.
- Reversal of neuromuscular blockade: With neostigmine, pyridostigmine: 0.2 mg for each 1 mg neostigmine or 5 mg pyridostigmine; administer IV simultaneously.

Pediatric patients

Not recommended for children < 12 yr for peptic ulcer.

Parenteral

- Preanesthetic medication (< 2 yr): 0.004 mg/lb IM 30 min to 1 hr prior to anesthesia. < 12 yr: 0.002–0.004 mg/lb IM.
- Intraoperative: 0.004 mg/kg (0.002 mg/lb) IV, not to exceed 0.1 mg in a single dose. May be repeated at 2- to 3-min intervals.
- Reversal of neuromuscular blockade: 0.2 mg for each 1 mg neostigmine or 5 mg pyridostigmine. Give IV simultaneously.

Pharmacokinetics

Route	Onset	Peak	Duration
Oral	60 min	60 min	8–12 hr
IM, SC	15–30 min	30–45 min	2–7 hr
IV	1 min		

Metabolism: Hepatic; $T_{1/2}$: 2.5 hr
Distribution: Crosses placenta; enters breast milk
Excretion: Urine

▼ IV facts

Preparation: No additional preparation required.
Infusion: Administer slowly into tubing of a running IV, each 0.2 mg over 1–2 min.
Incompatibilities: Do not combine with methylprednisolone; sodium succinate.

Adverse effects

- **CNS:** Blurred vision, mydriasis, cycloplegia, photophobia, increased intraocular pressure
- **CV:** Palpitations, tachycardia
- **GI:** Dry mouth, altered taste perception, nausea, vomiting, dysphagia, heartburn, constipation, bloated feeling, paralytic ileus, gastroesophageal reflux

- **GU:** *Urinary hesitancy and retention,* impotence
- **Local:** *Irritation at site of IM injection*
- **Other:** Decreased sweating and predisposition to heat prostration, suppression of lactation, nasal congestion

Interactions
✳ Drug-drug • Decreased antipsychotic effectiveness of haloperidol with anticholinergic drugs

■ Nursing considerations
Assessment
- **History:** Glaucoma; adhesions between iris and lens, stenosing peptic ulcer, pyloroduodenal obstruction, paralytic ileus, intestinal atony, severe ulcerative colitis, toxic megacolon, symptomatic prostatic hypertrophy, bladder neck obstruction, COPD, cardiac arrhythmias, myocardial ischemia, impaired metabolic, liver or kidney function, myasthenia gravis; lactation; Down syndrome, brain damage, spasticity, hypertension, hyperthyroidism, pregnancy
- **Physical:** Bowel sounds, normal output; normal urinary output, prostate palpation; R, adventitious sounds; P, BP; intraocular pressure, vision; bilateral grip strength, reflexes; hepatic palpation, liver and renal function tests; skin color, lesions, texture

Interventions
- Ensure adequate hydration; provide environmental control (temperature) to prevent hyperpyrexia.
- Have patient void before each dose if urinary retention is a problem.

Teaching points
- Take this drug exactly as prescribed.
- Avoid hot environments (you will be heat-intolerant, and dangerous reactions may occur).
- These side effects may occur: constipation (ensure adequate fluid intake, proper diet); dry mouth (sugarless lozenges, frequent mouth care may help; effect may lessen); blurred vision, sensitivity to light (reversible; avoid tasks that require acute vision; wear sunglasses in bright light); impotence (re-

versible); difficulty in urination (empty bladder immediately before taking each dose).
- Report rash, flushing, eye pain, difficulty breathing, tremors, loss of coordination, irregular heartbeat, palpitations, headache, abdominal distention, hallucinations, severe or persistent dry mouth, difficulty swallowing, difficulty urinating, severe constipation, sensitivity to light.

▽ gold sodium thiomalate (gold)

Aurolate

PREGNANCY CATEGORY C

Drug classes
Antirheumatic
Gold compound

Therapeutic actions
Suppresses and prevents arthritis and synovitis: taken up by macrophages, this results in inhibition of phagocytosis and inhibition of activities of lysosomal enzymes; decreases concentrations of rheumatoid factor and immunoglobulins.

Indications
- Treatment of selected cases of adult and juvenile rheumatoid arthritis; most effective early in disease; late in the disease when damage has occurred, gold can only prevent further damage.
- Unlabeled uses: psoriatic arthritis, discoid lupus erythematosus, pemphigus, palindromic rheumatism

Contraindications and cautions
- Allergy to gold preparations, uncontrolled diabetes mellitus, severe debilitation, renal disease, hepatic dysfunction, history of infectious hepatitis, marked hypertension, uncontrolled CHF, SLE, agranulocytosis, hemorrhagic diathesis, blood dyscrasias, recent radiation treatment, previous toxic response to gold or heavy metals (urticaria, eczema, colitis), pregnancy, lactation.

Available forms

Injection—50 mg/mL

Dosages

Contains approximately 50% gold. Administer by IM injection only, preferably intragluteally.

Adults

- *Weekly injections:* First injection, 10 mg, IM; second injection, 25 mg, IM; third and subsequent injections, 25–50 mg IM until major clinical improvement is seen, toxicity occurs, or cumulative dose reaches 1 g.
- *Maintenance:* 25–50 mg IM every other week for 2–20 wk. If clinical course remains stable, give 25–50 mg every third and then every fourth week indefinitely. Some patients require maintenance intervals of 1–3 wk. If arthritis is exacerbated, resume weekly injections. In severe cases, dosage can be increased by 10-mg increments; do not exceed 100 mg in a single injection.

Pediatric patients

Initial test dose of 10 mg IM, then give 1 mg/kg/wk, not to exceed 50 mg as a single injection. Adult guidelines for dosage apply.

Geriatric patients

Monitor patients carefully; tolerance to gold decreases with age.

Pharmacokinetics

Route	Onset	Peak
IM	Slow	3–6 hr

Metabolism: Hepatic; $T_{1/2}$: 14–40 days, then 168 days
Distribution: Crosses placenta; enters breast milk
Excretion: Urine and feces

Adverse effects

- **Dermatologic:** *Dermatitis; pruritus, erythema, exfoliative dermatitis,* chrysiasis (gray-blue color to the skin due to gold deposition), rash
- **GI:** *Stomatitis, glossitis, gingivitis,* metallic taste, pharyngitis, gastritis, colitis, tracheitis, nausea, vomiting, anorexia, abdominal cramps, *diarrhea,* hepatitis with jaundice
- **GU:** Vaginitis, nephrotic syndrome or glomerulitis with proteinuria and hematuria, acute tubular necrosis and renal failure

- **Hematologic:** Granulocytopenia, thrombocytopenia, leukopenia, eosinophilia, anemias
- **Hypersensitivity:** Nitritoid or allergic reactions: flushing, fainting, dizziness, sweating, nausea, vomiting, malaise, weakness
- **Immediate postinjection effects: Anaphylactic shock,** syncope, bradycardia, thickening of the tongue, dysphagia, dyspnea, angioneurotic edema
- **Respiratory:** Gold bronchitis, interstitial pneumonitis and fibrosis, cough, shortness of breath
- **Other:** Fever, nonvasomotor postinjection reaction: arthralgia for 1–2 days after the injection, usually subsides after the first few injections; carcinogenesis, mutagenesis, impairment of fertility (reported in preclinical studies)

■ Nursing considerations

Assessment

- **History:** Allergy to gold preparations, uncontrolled diabetes mellitus, severe debilitation, renal or hepatic dysfunction, history of infectious hepatitis, marked hypertension, uncontrolled CHF, SLE, hemorrhagic diathesis, blood dyscrasias, recent radiation treatment, previous toxic response to gold or heavy metals, lactation, pregnancy
- **Physical:** Skin color, lesions; T; edema; P, BP; R, adventitious sounds; mucous membranes, bowel sounds, liver evaluation; CBC, renal and liver function tests, chest x-ray

Interventions

- Do not give to patients with history of idiosyncratic or severe reactions to gold therapy.
- Monitor hematologic status, liver and kidney function, respiratory status regularly.
- Do not use if material has darkened; color should be a pale yellow.
- Give by intragluteal IM injection; have patient remain recumbent for 10 min after injection.
- Discontinue at first sign of toxic reaction.
- Use systemic corticosteroids for treatment of severe stomatitis, dermatitis, renal, hematologic, pulmonary, enterocolitic complications.
- Protect from sunlight or ultraviolet light to decrease risk of chrysiasis.

Teaching points

- Prepare a calendar of projected injection dates. This drug's effects are not seen immediately; several months of therapy are needed to see results. You will be asked to stay in the recumbent position for about 10 min after each injection.
- This drug does not cure the disease, but only stops its effects.
- These side effects may occur: increased joint pain for 1–2 days after injection (usually subsides after first few injections); diarrhea; mouth sores, metallic taste (frequent mouth care will help); rash, gray-blue color to the skin (avoid exposure to sun or ultraviolet light); nausea, loss of appetite (small, frequent meals may help).
- Do not become pregnant while on this drug; if you decide to become pregnant, consult with physician about discontinuing drug.
- Report unusual bleeding or bruising, sore throat, fever, severe diarrhea, rash, mouth sores.

▷ gonadorelin hydrochloride

See *Less Commonly Used Drugs*, p. 1344.

▷ goserelin acetate
(goe' se rel in)

Zoladex, Zoladex LA (CAN)

PREGNANCY CATEGORY X

Drug classes
Antineoplastic
Hormone

Therapeutic actions
An analog of LHRH or GnRH; potent inhibitor of pituitary gonadotropin secretion; initial administration causes an increase in FSH and LH and resultant increase in testosterone levels; with long-term administration, these hormone levels fall to levels normally seen with surgical castration within 2–4 wk, as pituitary is inhibited.

Indications

- Palliative treatment of advanced prostatic cancer when orchiectomy or estrogen administration is not indicated or is unacceptable
- Stage B$_2$-C prostatic cancer with flutamide
- Management of endometriosis, including pain relief and reduction of endometriotic lesions
- Palliative treatment of advanced breast cancer in premenopausal and perimenopausal women
- Endometrial thinning agent prior to endometrial ablation

Contraindications and cautions

- Pregnancy, lactation, hypersensitivity to LHRH or any component.

Available forms
Implant—3.6, 10.8 mg

Dosages
Adults
3.6 mg SC every 28 days or 10.8 mg every 3 mo into the upper abdominal wall.

- *Prostatic or breast carcinoma:* Long-term use of 3.6 mg.
- *Endometriosis:* Continue therapy with 3.6 mg for 6 mo.
- *Endometrial thinning:* One to two 3.6-mg SC depots 4 wk apart; surgery should be done 4 wk after first dose—within 2–4 wk after second depot if 2 are used.
- *Stage B$_2$-C prostatic cancer:* 10.8 mg SC implant q 12 wk into upper abdominal wall.
Pediatric patients
Safety and efficacy not established.

Pharmacokinetics

Route	Onset	Peak
SC	Slow	12–15 days

Metabolism: Hepatic; T$_{1/2}$: 4.2 hr
Distribution: Crosses placenta; may enter breast milk
Excretion: Urine

Adverse effects

- **CNS:** Insomnia, dizziness, lethargy, anxiety, depression

Adverse effects in *Italics* are most common; those in **Bold** are life-threatening.

- **CV:** CHF, edema, hypertension, arrhythmia, chest pain
- **GI:** Nausea, anorexia
- **GU:** *Hot flashes, sexual dysfunction, decreased erections, lower urinary tract symptoms*
- **Other:** Rash, sweating, cancer

■ Nursing considerations
Assessment
- **History:** Pregnancy, lactation
- **Physical:** Skin temperature, lesions; reflexes, affect; BP, P; urinary output; pregnancy test if appropriate

Interventions
- Ensure that patient is not pregnant before use; barrier contraceptives should be advised.
- Use syringe provided. Discard if package is damaged. Remove sterile syringe immediately before use. Use a local anesthetic prior to injection to decrease pain and discomfort.
- Administer using aseptic technique under the supervision of a physician familiar with the implant technique.
- Bandage area after implant has been injected.
- Repeat injection in 28 days; keep as close to this schedule as possible.

Teaching points
- This drug will be implanted into your upper abdomen every 28 days or 3 mo as appropriate. It is important to keep to this schedule. Mark a calendar of injection dates.
- These side effects may occur: hot flashes (a cool temperature may help); sexual dysfunction—regression of sex organs, impaired fertility, decreased erections; pain at injection site (a local anesthetic will be used; if discomfort is severe, analgesics may be ordered).
- Do not take this drug if pregnant; if you are pregnant or wish to become pregnant, consult with your health care provider.
- Report chest pain, increased signs and symptoms of your cancer, difficulty breathing, dizziness, severe pain at injection site.

▽ **granisetron hydrochloride**
(gran iz' e tron)

Kytril

PREGNANCY CATEGORY B

Drug class
Antiemetic

Therapeutic actions
Selectively binds to serotonin receptors in the CTZ, blocking the nausea and vomiting caused by the release of serotonin by mucosal cells during chemotherapy, which stimulates the CTZ and causes nausea and vomiting.

Indications
- Prevention and treatment of nausea and vomiting associated with emetogenic chemotherapy and radiation
- Prevention and treatment of postoperative nausea and vomiting

Contraindications and cautions
- Contraindicated with pregnancy, lactation.

Available forms
Tablets—1 mg; injection—1 mg/mL; oral solution—2 mg/10 mL

Dosages
Adults and patients > 2 yr
IV
10 mcg/kg IV over 5 min starting within 30 min of chemotherapy; only on days of chemotherapy.
Oral
1 mg PO bid or 2 mg/day as one dose, beginning up to 1 hr before chemotherapy and second dose 12 hr after chemotherapy; only on days of chemotherapy.
Pediatric patients < 2 yr
Not recommended.

Pharmacokinetics

Route	Onset	Peak
IV	Rapid	30–45 min
Oral	Moderate	60–90 min

Metabolism: Hepatic; $T_{1/2}$: 5 hr (IV), 6.2 hr (oral)

Distribution: Crosses placenta; enters breast milk
Excretion: Urine

▼IV facts
Preparation: Dilute in 0.9% sodium chloride or 5% dextrose to a total volume of 20–50 mL; stable up to 24 hr refrigerated; protect from light.
Infusion: Inject slowly over 5 min.
Incompatibility: Do not mix in solution with other drugs.

Adverse effects
- **CNS:** *Headache,* asthenia, somnolence
- **CV:** Hypertension
- **GI:** Diarrhea or constipation
- **Other:** Fever

Nursing considerations
Assessment
- **History:** Allergy to granisetron, pregnancy, lactation, liver or renal impairment
- **Physical:** Orientation, reflexes, affect; BP; bowel sounds; T

Interventions
- Provide mouth care, sugarless lozenges to suck to help alleviate nausea.
- Give drug only on days of chemotherapy.

Teaching points
- This drug may be given IV or orally when you are receiving your chemotherapy; it will help decrease nausea and vomiting.
- These side effects may occur: lack of sleep, drowsiness (use caution if driving or performing tasks that require alertness); diarrhea or constipation; headache (request medication).
- Report severe headache, fever, numbness or tingling, severe diarrhea or constipation.

▽ griseofulvin
See *Less Commonly Used Drugs,* p. 1344.

▽ guaifenesin
(gwye fen' e sin)

Anti-Tuss, Breonesin, Diabetic Tussin EX, Duratuss-G, Fenesin, Gee-Gee, Genatuss, Glyate, Glytuss, Guaifenex LA, Humibid LA, Humibid Sprinkle, Hytuss, Hytuss 2X, Liquibid, Monafed, Muco-Fen-LA, Mytussin, Naldecon Senior EX, Organidin NR, Pneumomist, Respa-GF, Robitussin, Scot-tussin Expectorant, Siltussin, Siltussin SA, Sinumist-SR Capsulets, Touro EX, Tussin

PREGNANCY CATEGORY C

Drug class
Expectorant

Therapeutic actions
Enhances the output of respiratory tract fluid by reducing adhesiveness and surface tension, facilitating the removal of viscous mucus.

Indications
- Symptomatic relief of respiratory conditions characterized by dry, nonproductive cough and in the presence of mucus in the respiratory tract.

Contraindications and cautions
- Contraindicated with allergy to guaifenesin.
- Use cautiously with pregnancy.

Available forms
Syrup—100 mg/5 mL; liquid—100, 200 mg/ 5 mL; capsules—200 mg; SR capsules— 300 mg; tablets—100, 200, 1,200 mg; SR tablets—600 mg

Dosages
Adults and patients > 12 yr
100–400 mg PO q 4 hr. Do not exceed 2.4 g/day.
Pediatric patients ≤ 12 yr
6–12 yr: 100–200 mg PO q 4 hr. Do not exceed 1.2 g/day.
2–6 yr: 50–100 mg PO q 4 hr. Do not exceed 600 mg/day.

Pharmacokinetics

Route	Onset	Duration
Oral	30 min	4–6 hr

Metabolism: Not known; $T_{1/2}$: not known
Distribution and excretion: Unknown

Adverse effects

- **CNS:** Headache, dizziness
- **Dermatologic:** Rash
- **GI:** *Nausea, vomiting*

Interactions

❊ **Drug-lab test** • Color interference and false results of 5-HIAA and VMA urinary determinations

■ Nursing considerations
Assessment

- **History:** Allergy to guaifenesin; persistent cough due to smoking, asthma, or emphysema; very productive cough; pregnancy
- **Physical:** Skin lesions, color; T; orientation, affects; R, adventitious sounds

Interventions

- Monitor reaction to drug; persistent cough for more than 1 wk, fever, rash, or persistent headache may indicate a more serious condition.

Teaching points

- Do not take for longer than 1 wk; if fever, rash, headache occur, consult health care provider.
- These side effects may occur: nausea, vomiting (small, frequent meals may help); dizziness, headache (avoid driving or operating dangerous machinery).
- Report fever, rash, severe vomiting, persistent cough.

▽ guanabenz acetate
(*gwahn' a benz*)

Wytensin

PREGNANCY CATEGORY C

Drug classes

Antihypertensive
Sympatholytic, centrally acting

Therapeutic actions

Stimulates central (CNS) alpha$_2$-adrenergic receptors, reduces sympathetic nerve impulses from the vasomotor center to the heart and blood vessels, decreases peripheral vascular resistance, and lowers systemic blood pressure.

Indications

- Management of hypertension, alone or in combination with a thiazide diuretic

Contraindications and cautions

- Contraindicated with hypersensitivity to guanabenz, lactation.
- Use cautiously with severe coronary insufficiency, recent MI, CV disease, severe renal or hepatic failure, pregnancy.

Available forms

Tablets—4, 8 mg

Dosages
Adults

Individualize dosage. Initial dose of 4 mg PO bid, alone or with a thiazide diuretic; increase in increments of 4–8 mg/day every 1–2 wk. Maximum dose 32 mg bid, but doses this high are rarely needed.

Pediatric patients

Safety and efficacy not established for children < 12 yr.

Pharmacokinetics

Route	Onset	Peak	Duration
Oral	45–60 min	2–5 hr	6–12 hr

Metabolism: Unknown; $T_{1/2}$: 6 hr
Distribution: Crosses placenta; enters breast milk
Excretion: Urine and feces

Adverse effects

- **CNS:** *Sedation, weakness, dizziness, headache*
- **CV:** Chest pain, edema, **arrhythmias**
- **GI:** *Dry mouth*

■ Nursing considerations
Assessment

- **History:** Hypersensitivity to guanabenz; severe coronary insufficiency, cerebrovascular disease, severe renal or hepatic failure; lactation, pregnancy

- **Physical:** Orientation, affect, reflexes; P, BP, orthostatic BP, perfusion, auscultation; liver and kidney function tests, ECG

Interventions

- Store tightly sealed, protected from light.
- Do not discontinue drug abruptly; discontinue therapy by reducing the dosage gradually over 2–4 days to avoid rebound hypertension, increased blood and urinary catecholamines, anxiety, nervousness, and other subjective effects.
- Assess compliance with drug regimen in a nonthreatening, supportive manner.

Teaching points

- Take this drug exactly as prescribed; do not miss doses. Do not discontinue unless instructed to do so. Do not discontinue abruptly. Store tightly sealed, protected from light.
- These side effects may occur: drowsiness, dizziness, light-headedness, headache, weakness (transient; observe caution while driving or performing other tasks that require alertness or physical dexterity).
- Report persistent or severe drowsiness, dry mouth.

▽guanadrel sulfate
(*gwahn' a drel*)

Hylorel

PREGNANCY CATEGORY B

Drug classes

Antihypertensive
Adrenergic neuron blocker

Therapeutic actions

Antihypertensive effects depend on inhibition of norepinephrine release and depletion of norepinephrine from postganglionic sympathetic adrenergic nerve terminals.

Indications

- Treatment of hypertension in patients not responding adequately to a thiazide-type diuretic

Contraindications and cautions

- Contraindicated with hypersensitivity to guanadrel; known or suspected pheochromocytoma, frank CHF not due to hypertension; lactation.
- Use cautiously with CAD with insufficiency or recent MI, CV disease (special risk if orthostatic hypotension occurs); history of bronchial asthma; active peptic ulcer, ulcerative colitis (may be aggravated by a relative increase in parasympathetic tone); renal dysfunction (drug-induced hypotension may further compromise renal function).

Available forms

Tablets—10, 25 mg

Dosages

Individualize dosage.
Adults

Usual starting dose is 10 mg/day PO. Most patients require a daily dosage of 20–75 mg, usually in twice daily doses. For larger doses, tid to qid dosing may be needed. Administer in divided doses; adjust dosage weekly or monthly until BP is controlled. In long-term therapy, some tolerance may occur, and dosage may need to be increased.

Pediatric patients

Safety and efficacy not established.

Geriatric patients or patients with renal impairment

Reduce initial dosage to 5 mg q 24 hr PO for creatinine clearance of 30–60 mL/min; creatinine clearance < 30 mL/min: give 5 mg q 48 hr PO. Cautiously adjust dosage at intervals of 7–14 days.

Pharmacokinetics

Route	Onset	Peak	Duration
Oral	1.5–2 hr	4–6 hr	4–14 hr

Metabolism: Hepatic; $T_{1/2}$: 10 hr
Distribution: May cross placenta; may enter breast milk
Excretion: Urine

Adverse effects

Incidence is higher during the first 8 wk of therapy.

Adverse effects in *Italics* are most common; those in **Bold** are life-threatening.

- **CNS:** *Fatigue, headache, faintness, drowsiness, visual disturbances, paresthesias, confusion,* psychological problems
- **CV/Respiratory:** *Shortness of breath on exertion,* **palpitations,** *chest pain, coughing,* shortness of breath at rest
- **GI:** *Increased bowel movements, gas pain/indigestion, constipation, anorexia,* glossitis
- **GU:** *Nocturia, urinary urgency or frequency, peripheral edema, ejaculation disturbances,* impotence
- **Other:** *Excessive weight loss, excessive weight gain, aching limbs,* leg cramps

■ Nursing considerations
Assessment
- **History:** Hypersensitivity to guanadrel; known or suspected pheochromocytoma; frank CHF; CAD, cerebrovascular disease; history of bronchial asthma; active peptic ulcer, ulcerative colitis; renal dysfunction; lactation
- **Physical:** Weight; skin color, lesions; orientation, affect, reflexes; P, BP, orthostatic BP, supine BP, perfusion, edema, auscultation; R, adventitious sounds, status of nasal mucous membranes; bowel sounds, normal output, palpation of salivary glands; voiding pattern, normal output; kidney function tests, urinalysis

Interventions
- Discontinue drug if diarrhea is severe.
- Discontinue guanadrel therapy 48–72 hr prior to surgery to reduce the possibility of vascular collapse and cardiac arrest during anesthesia.
- Note prominently on patient's chart that patient is receiving guanadrel if emergency surgery is needed; a reduced dosage of preanesthetic medication and anesthetics will be needed.
- Monitor patient for orthostatic hypotension, which is most marked in the morning, and is accentuated by hot weather, alcohol, exercise.
- Monitor edema, weight with incipient cardiac decompensation; arrange to add a thiazide diuretic if sodium and fluid retention, signs of impending CHF, occur.

Teaching points
- Take this drug exactly as prescribed.
- Do not get out of bed without help while dosage is being adjusted.
- These side effects may occur: dizziness, weakness (most likely to occur when you change position, in the early morning, after exercise, in hot weather, and when you have consumed alcohol; some tolerance may occur over time; avoid driving or engaging in tasks that require alertness; remember to change position slowly; use caution when climbing stairs); diarrhea; GI upset (frequent small meals may help); impotence, failure of ejaculation; emotional depression; stuffy nose.
- Report severe diarrhea, frequent dizziness or fainting.

G

▽ **guanethidine monosulfate**
*(gwahn **eth' i** deen)*

Ismelin

PREGNANCY CATEGORY C

Drug classes
Antihypertensive
Adrenergic neuron blocker

Therapeutic actions
Antihypertensive effects depend on inhibition of norepinephrine release and depletion of norepinephrine from postganglionic sympathetic adrenergic nerve terminals.

Indications
- Moderate to severe hypertension either alone or as an adjunct
- Renal hypertension, including that secondary to pyelonephritis, renal amyloidosis, and renal artery stenosis
- Orphan drug use: treatment of moderate to severe reflex sympathetic dystrophy and causalgia

Contraindications and cautions
- Contraindicated with hypersensitivity to guanethidine; known or suspected pheochromocytoma; frank CHF; lactation, pregnancy.
- Use cautiously with CAD with insufficiency or recent MI; CV disease, especially with en-

cephalopathy; history of bronchial asthma (increased likelihood to be hypersensitive to catecholamine depletion); active peptic ulcer, ulcerative colitis (may be aggravated by a relative increase in parasympathetic tone); renal dysfunction (drug-induced hypotension may further compromise renal function).

Available forms
Tablets—10, 25 mg

Dosages
Initial doses should be small, and dosage should be increased slowly. It may take 2 wk to adequately evaluate the response to daily administration.

Adults
- *Ambulatory patients:* 10 mg/day PO initially. Do not increase dosage more often than every 5–7 days. Take BP in supine position, after standing for 10 min, and immediately after exercise if feasible. Increase dosage only if there has been no decrease in standing BP from the previous levels. Average dose is 25–50 mg daily. Reduce dosage with the following: normal supine pressure, excessive orthostatic fall in pressure, severe diarrhea.
- *Hospitalized patients:* Initial dose of 25–50 mg PO. Increase by 25 or 50 mg daily or every other day as indicated.
- *Combination therapy:* Diuretics enhance guanethidine effectiveness, may reduce incidence of edema, and may allow reduction of guanethidine dosage. Withdraw MAO inhibitors at least 1 wk before starting guanethidine. May be advisable to withdraw ganglionic blockers gradually to avoid spiking BP response during transfer.

Pediatric patients
Initial dose of 0.2 mg/kg (6 mg/m^2 per 24 hr) as a single oral dose. Increase by 0.2 mg/kg per 24 hr PO every 7–10 days. Maximum dosage: 3 mg/kg per 24 hr PO.

Geriatric patients or patients with impaired renal function
Use reduced dosage.

Pharmacokinetics

Route	Onset	Peak	Duration
Oral	Slow	1–3 wk	Up to 2 wk

Metabolism: Hepatic; $T_{1/2}$: 4–8 days
Distribution: Crosses placenta; enters breast milk
Excretion: Urine

Adverse effects
- **CNS:** *Dizziness, weakness, lassitude, syncope resulting from either postural or exertional hypotension,* fatigue, myalgia, muscle tremor, emotional depression, ptosis of the lids and blurring of vision
- **CV:** *Bradycardia,* angina, chest paresthesias, *fluid retention and edema with occasional development of CHF*
- **Dermatologic:** Dermatitis, alopecia
- **GI:** *Increase in bowel movements and diarrhea,* nausea, vomiting, dry mouth, parotid tenderness
- **GU:** *Inhibition of ejaculation,* nocturia, urinary incontinence
- **Respiratory:** Dyspnea, nasal congestion, asthma

Interactions
✳ **Drug-drug** • Decreased antihypertensive effect with anorexiants (eg, amphetamines), TCAs (imipramine, etc), phenothiazines (chlorpromazine), indirect-acting sympathomimetics (ephedrine, pseudoephedrine) • Increased pressor response and arrhythmogenic potential of direct-acting sympathomimetics (epinephrine, norepinephrine, phenylephrine), metaraminol, methoxamine • Risk of severe reactions with MAO inhibitors; withdraw at least 1 wk before starting guanethidine

■ Nursing considerations
Assessment
- **History:** Hypersensitivity to guanethidine; known or suspected pheochromocytoma; frank CHF; CAD; cerebrovascular disease; history of bronchial asthma; active peptic ulcer, ulcerative colitis; renal dysfunction; lactation, pregnancy
- **Physical:** Weight; skin color, lesions; orientation, affect, reflexes; P, BP, orthostatic BP, supine BP, perfusion, edema, ausculta-

tion; R, adventitious sounds, status of nasal mucous membranes; bowel sounds, normal output, palpation of salivary glands; voiding pattern, normal output; kidney function tests, urinalysis

Interventions

• Discontinue drug if diarrhea is severe.
• Discontinue guanethidine therapy at least 2 wk prior to surgery to reduce the possibility of vascular collapse and cardiac arrest during anesthesia.
• Note prominently on patient's chart that patient is receiving guanethidine if emergency surgery is needed; a reduced dosage of preanesthetic medication and anesthetics will be needed.
• Decrease dosage during fever, which decreases drug requirements.
• Monitor patient for orthostatic hypotension, which is most marked in the morning and is accentuated by hot weather, alcohol, exercise.
• Monitor edema, weight with incipient cardiac decompensation, and arrange to add a thiazide diuretic if sodium and fluid retention, signs of impending CHF, occur.

Teaching points

• Take this drug exactly as prescribed.
• Do not get out of bed without help while dosage is being adjusted.
• These side effects may occur: dizziness, weakness (most likely to occur when you change position, in the early morning, after exercise, in hot weather, and when you have consumed alcohol; some tolerance may occur over time, but avoid driving or engaging in tasks that require alertness; remember to change positions slowly; use caution in climbing stairs); diarrhea; GI upset (frequent small meals may help); impotence, failure of ejaculation; emotional depression; stuffy nose.
• Report severe diarrhea, frequent dizziness or fainting.

▷ guanfacine hydrochloride
(gwahn' fa seen)

Tenex

PREGNANCY CATEGORY B

Drug classes
Antihypertensive
Sympatholytic, centrally acting

Therapeutic actions
Stimulates central (CNS) alpha$_2$-adrenergic receptors, reduces sympathetic nerve impulses from the vasomotor center to the heart and blood vessels, decreases peripheral vascular resistance, and lowers systemic blood pressure.

Indications
• Management of hypertension, alone or with a thiazide diuretic
• Unlabeled use: amelioration of withdrawal symptoms in heroin withdrawal

Contraindications and cautions
• Contraindicated with hypersensitivity to guanfacine, labor and delivery, lactation.
• Use cautiously with severe coronary insufficiency, recent MI, CV disease, chronic renal or hepatic failure, pregnancy.

Available forms
Tablets—1, 2 mg

Dosages
Adults
Recommended dose is 1 mg/day PO given hs to minimize somnolence. If 1 mg/day does not give a satisfactory result after 3–4 wk of therapy, doses of 2 mg and then 3 mg may be given, although most of the drug's effect is seen at 1 mg. If BP rises toward the end of the dosing interval, divided dosage should be used. Higher daily doses (rarely up to 4 mg/day in divided doses) have been used, but adverse reactions increase with doses > 3 mg/day, and there is no evidence of increased efficacy.
Pediatric patients
Safety and efficacy not established for children < 12 yr; therefore, not recommended for use in this age group.

Pharmacokinetics

Route	Onset	Peak	Duration
Oral	2 hr	1–4 hr	24 hr

Metabolism: Hepatic; $T_{1/2}$: 10–30 hr
Distribution: Crosses placenta; enters breast milk
Excretion: Urine

Adverse effects

- **CNS:** *Sedation, weakness, dizziness,* headache, insomnia, amnesia, confusion, depression, conjunctivitis, iritis, vision disturbance, malaise, paresthesia, paresis, taste perversion, tinnitus, hypokinesia
- **CV:** Bradycardia, palpitations, substernal pain
- **Dermatologic:** Dermatitis, pruritus, purpura, sweating
- **GI:** *Dry mouth, constipation,* abdominal pain, diarrhea, dyspepsia, dysphagia, nausea
- **GU:** *Impotence,* libido decrease, testicular disorder, urinary incontinence
- **Other:** Rhinitis, leg cramps

■ Nursing considerations
Assessment

- **History:** Hypersensitivity to guanfacine; severe coronary insufficiency, cerebrovascular disease; chronic renal or hepatic failure; pregnancy; lactation
- **Physical:** Skin color, lesions; orientation, affect, reflexes; ophthalmologic exam; P, BP, orthostatic BP, perfusion, auscultation; R, adventitious sounds; bowel sounds, normal output; normal urinary output, voiding pattern; liver and kidney function tests, ECG

Interventions

- Do not discontinue drug abruptly; discontinue therapy by reducing the dosage gradually over 2–4 days to avoid rebound hypertension (much less likely than with clonidine; BP usually returns to pretreatment levels in 2–4 days without ill effects).
- Assess compliance with drug regimen in a nonthreatening, supportive manner.

Teaching points

- Take this drug exactly as prescribed; it is important that you do not miss doses. Do not discontinue the drug unless instructed to do so. Do not discontinue abruptly.
- These side effects may occur: drowsiness, dizziness, light-headedness, headache, weakness (transient; observe caution while driving or performing other tasks that require alertness or physical dexterity); dry mouth (sucking on sugarless lozenges or ice chips may help); GI upset (frequent small meals may help); dizziness, light-headedness when you change position (get up slowly; use caution when climbing stairs); impotence, other sexual dysfunction, decreased libido; palpitations.
- Report urinary incontinence, changes in vision, rash.

▽**haloperidol**
(ha loe per' i dole)

haloperidol
Apo-Haloperidol (CAN), Haldol, Haldol LA (CAN), Novo-Peridol (CAN), Peridol (CAN)

haloperidol decanoate
Haldol

PREGNANCY CATEGORY C

Drug classes
Dopaminergic blocking drug
Antipsychotic drug
Butyrophenone (not a phenothiazine)

Therapeutic actions
Mechanism not fully understood: antipsychotic drugs block postsynaptic dopamine receptors in the brain, depress the RAS, including those parts of the brain involved with wakefulness and emesis; chemically resembles the phenothiazines.

Indications
- Management of manifestations of psychotic disorders
- Control of tics and vocalizations in Tourette's syndrome in adults and children
- Behavioral problems in children with combative, explosive hyperexcitability that cannot be attributed to immediate provocation

Adverse effects in *Italics* are most common; those in **Bold** are life-threatening.

- Short-term treatment of hyperactive children with excessive motor activity, mood lability
- Prolonged parenteral therapy of chronic schizophrenia (haloperidol decanoate)
- Unlabeled uses: control of nausea and vomiting, control of acute psychiatric situations (IV use), treatment of intractable hiccoughs, agitation, hyperkinesia, infantile autism

Contraindications and cautions
- Contraindicated with coma or severe CNS depression, bone marrow depression, blood dyscrasia, circulatory collapse, subcortical brain damage, Parkinson's disease, liver damage, cerebral arteriosclerosis, coronary disease, severe hypotension or hypertension, pregnancy, lactation.
- Use cautiously with respiratory disorders ("silent pneumonia"); glaucoma, prostatic hypertrophy (anticholinergic effects may exacerbate glaucoma and urinary retention); epilepsy or history of epilepsy (drug lowers seizure threshold); breast cancer (elevations in prolactin may stimulate a prolactin-dependent tumor); thyrotoxicosis; peptic ulcer, decreased renal function; myelography within previous 24 hr or scheduled within 48 hr; exposure to heat or phosphorous insecticides; lactation; children younger than 12 yr, especially those with chickenpox, CNS infections (children are especially susceptible to dystonias that may confound the diagnosis of Reye's syndrome); allergy to aspirin if giving the 1-, 2-, 5-, and 10-mg tablets (these tablets contain tartrazine).

Available forms
Tablets—0.5, 1, 2, 5, 10, 20 mg; concentrate—2 mg/mL; injection—50, 100 mg/mL as deconate, 5 mg/mL as lactate

Dosages
Full clinical effects may require 6 wk–6 mo of therapy. Children, debilitated and geriatric patients, and patients with a history of adverse reactions to neuroleptic drugs may require lower dosage.
Adults
Oral
Initial dosage range: 0.5–2 mg bid–tid PO with moderate symptoms; 3–5 mg bid–tid PO for more resistant patients. Daily dosages up to 100 mg/day (or more) have been used, but safety of prolonged use has not been demonstrated. For maintenance, reduce dosage to lowest effective level.
IM, haloperidol lactate injection
2–5 mg (up to 10–30 mg) q 60 min or q 4–8 hr IM as necessary for prompt control of acutely agitated patients with severe symptoms. Switch to oral dosage as soon as feasible, using total IM dosage in previous 24 hr as a guide to total daily oral dosage.
IV, haloperidol lactate injection
- Unlabeled use for acute situations: 2–25 mg IV q hr at a rate of 5 mg/min.
IM, haloperidol decanoate injection
Initial dose: 10–15 times the daily oral dose; do not exceed 3 mL per injection site; repeat at 4-wk intervals.
Pediatric patients
3–12 yr or 15–40 kg weight: Initial dose of 0.5 mg/day PO; may increase in increments of 0.5 mg q 5–7 days as needed. Total daily dose may be divided and given bid–tid.
- Psychiatric disorders: 0.05–0.15 mg/kg/day PO. Severely disturbed psychotic children may require higher dosage. There is little evidence that behavior is improved by doses greater than 6 mg/day.
- Nonpsychotic and Tourette's syndromes: 0.05–0.075 mg/kg/day PO.
Geriatric patients
Use lower doses (0.5–2.0 mg bid–tid), and increase dosage more gradually than in younger patients.

Pharmacokinetics

Route	Onset	Peak
Oral	Varies	3–5 hr
IM	Rapid	20 min
IM, decanoate	Slow	4–11 days

Metabolism: Hepatic; $T_{1/2}$: 21–24 hr, 3 wk for decanoate
Distribution: Crosses placenta; enters breast milk
Excretion: Urine and bile

Adverse effects
Not all effects have been reported with haloperidol; however, because haloperidol has certain pharmacologic similarities to the phenothiazine class of antipsychotic drugs, all adverse effects associated with phenothiazine

therapy should be kept in mind when haloperidol is used.

- **Autonomic:** Dry mouth, salivation, nasal congestion, nausea, vomiting, anorexia, fever, pallor, flushed facies, sweating, constipation, paralytic ileus, urinary retention, incontinence, polyuria, enuresis, priapism, ejaculation inhibition
- **CNS:** *Drowsiness,* insomnia, vertigo, headache, weakness, tremor, ataxia, slurring, cerebral edema, seizures, exacerbation of psychotic symptoms, extrapyramidal syndromes—*pseudoparkinsonism; dystonias; akathisia,* tardive dyskinesias, potentially irreversible (no known treatment), **neuroleptic malignant syndrome**—extrapyramidal symptoms, hyperthermia, autonomic disturbances
- **CV:** Hypotension, orthostatic hypotension, hypertension, tachycardia, bradycardia, **cardiac arrest,** CHF, cardiomegaly, **refractory arrhythmias,** pulmonary edema
- **Endocrine:** Lactation, breast engorgement in females, galactorrhea; SIADH; amenorrhea, menstrual irregularities; gynecomastia in males; changes in libido; hyperglycemia or hypoglycemia; glycosuria; hyponatremia; pituitary tumor with hyperprolactinemia; inhibition of ovulation, infertility, pseudopregnancy
- **Hematologic:** Eosinophilia, leukopenia, leukocytosis, anemia; aplastic anemia; hemolytic anemia; thrombocytopenic or nonthrombocytopenic purpura; pancytopenia
- **Hypersensitivity:** Jaundice, urticaria, angioneurotic edema, laryngeal edema, photosensitivity, eczema, asthma, **anaphylactoid reactions,** exfoliative dermatitis
- **Respiratory:** Bronchospasm, laryngospasm, dyspnea; **suppression of cough reflex and potential for aspiration**

Interactions

✳ Drug-drug ● Additive anticholinergic effects and possibly decreased antipsychotic efficacy with anticholinergic drugs ● Increased risk of toxic side effects with lithium ● Decreased effectiveness with carbamazepine

✳ Drug-lab test ● False-positive pregnancy tests (less likely if serum test is used) ● Increase in PBI, not attributable to an increase in thyroxine

■ Nursing considerations
Assessment

- **History:** Severe CNS depression; bone marrow depression; blood dyscrasia; circulatory collapse; subcortical brain damage; Parkinson's disease; liver damage; cerebral arteriosclerosis; coronary disease; severe hypotension or hypertension; respiratory disorders; glaucoma; prostatic hypertrophy; epilepsy or history of epilepsy; breast cancer; thyrotoxicosis; peptic ulcer, decreased renal function; myelography within previous 24 hr or scheduled within 48 hr; exposure to heat or phosphorus insecticides; children younger than 12 yr, especially those with chickenpox, CNS infections; allergy to aspirin, pregnancy, lactation
- **Physical:** Weight, T; reflexes, orientation, intraocular pressure; P, BP, orthostatic BP; R, adventitious sounds; bowel sounds and normal output, liver evaluation; urinary output, prostate size, CBC, urinalysis, thyroid, liver and kidney function tests

Interventions

- Do not give children IM injections.
- Do not use haloperidol decanoate for IV injections.
- Gradually withdraw drug when patient has been on maintenance therapy to avoid withdrawal-emergent dyskinesias.
- Discontinue drug if serum creatinine, BUN become abnormal or if WBC count is depressed.
- Monitor elderly patients for dehydration; institute remedial measures promptly; sedation and decreased thirst related to CNS effects can lead to severe dehydration.
- Consult physician regarding appropriate warning of patient or patient's guardian about tardive dyskinesias.
- Consult physician about dosage reduction, use of anticholinergic antiparkinsonian drugs (controversial) if extrapyramidal effects occur.

Teaching points

- Take this drug exactly as prescribed.

- Avoid driving or engaging in other dangerous activities if CNS, vision changes occur.
- Avoid prolonged exposure to sun, or use a sunscreen or covering garments.
- Maintain fluid intake, and use precautions against heatstroke in hot weather.
- Report sore throat, fever, unusual bleeding or bruising, rash, weakness, tremors, impaired vision, dark-colored urine (pink or reddish brown urine is to be expected), pale stools, yellowing of the skin or eyes.

▽ **heparin**
(hep' ah rin)

heparin sodium injection
Hepalean (CAN), Heparin Leo(CAN)

heparin sodium and 0.9% sodium chloride

heparin sodium lock flush solution
Hepalean-Lok (CAN), Heparin Lock Flush, Hep-Lock, Hep-Lock U/P

PREGNANCY CATEGORY C

Drug class
Anticoagulant

Therapeutic actions
Inhibits thrombus and clot formation by blocking the conversion of prothrombin to thrombin and fibrinogen to fibrin, the final steps in the clotting process.

Indications
- Prevention and treatment of venous thrombosis and pulmonary embolism
- Treatment of atrial fibrillation with embolization
- Diagnosis and treatment of DIC
- Prevention of clotting in blood samples and heparin lock sets and during dialysis procedures
- Unlabeled uses: adjunct in therapy of coronary occlusion with acute MI, prevention of left ventricular thrombi and CVA post-MI, prevention of cerebral thrombosis in the evolving stroke

Contraindications and cautions
- Hypersensitivity to heparin; severe thrombocytopenia; uncontrolled bleeding; any patient who cannot be monitored regularly with blood coagulation tests; labor and immediate postpartum period; women older than 60 yr are at high risk for hemorrhaging; dysbetalipoproteinemia; recent surgery or injury.

Available forms
Injection—1,000, 2,000, 2,500, 5,000, 7,500, 10,000, 12,500, 20,000, 40,000 units/mL; also single dose and unit-dose forms. Lock flush solution—10, 100 units/mL.

Dosages
Adjust dosage according to coagulation tests. Dosage is adequate when WBCT = 2.5–3 times control—or APTT = 1.5–3 times control value. The following are guidelines to dosage:
Adults
SC (deep SC injection)
- *For general anticoagulation:* IV loading dose of 5,000 units and then 10,000–20,000 units SC followed by 8,000–10,000 units q 8 hr or 15,000–20,000 units q 12 hr.
IV
- *Intermittent IV:* Initial dose of 10,000 units and then 5,000–10,000 units q 4–6 hr.
- *Continuous IV infusion:* Loading dose of 5,000 units and then 20,000–40,000 units/day.
- *Prophylaxis of postoperative thromboembolism:* 5,000 units by deep SC injection 2 hr before surgery and q 8–12 hr thereafter for 7 days or until patient is fully ambulatory.
- *Surgery of heart and blood vessels for patients undergoing total body perfusion:* Not less than 150 units/kg; guideline often used is 300 units/kg for procedures less than 60 min, 400 units/kg for longer procedures.
- *Clot prevention in blood samples:* 70–150 units/10–20 mL of whole blood.
- *Heparin lock and extracorporal dialysis:* See manufacturer's instructions.
Pediatric patients
Initial IV bolus of 50 units/kg and then 100 units/kg IV q 4 hr, or 20,000 units/m^2 per 24 hr by continuous IV infusion.

Pharmacokinetics

Route	Onset	Peak	Duration
IV	Immediate	Minutes	2–6 hr
SC	20–60 min	2–4 hr	8–12 hr

Metabolism: $T_{1/2}$: 30–180 min
Distribution: Does not cross placenta, does not enter breast milk; broken down in liver
Excretion: Urine

▼IV facts

Continuous infusion: Can be mixed in normal saline, D_5W, Ringer's; mix well; invert bottle numerous times to ensure adequate mixing. Monitor patient closely; infusion pump is recommended.

Single dose: Direct, undiluted IV injection of up to 5,000 units (adult) or 50 units/kg (pediatric), given over 60 seconds.

Monitoring: Blood should be drawn for coagulation testing 30 min before each intermittent IV dose or q 4 hr if patient is on continuous infusion pump.

Incompatibilities: Heparin should not be mixed in solution with any other drug unless specifically ordered; direct incompatibilities in solution and at Y-site seen with amikacin, codeine, chlorpromazine, cytarabine, diazepam, dobutamine, doxorubicin, droperidol, ergotamine, erythromycin, gentamicin, haloperidol, hydrocortisone, kanamycin, levorphanol, meperidine, methadone, methicillin, methotrimeprazine, morphine, netilimicin, pentazocine, phenytoin, polymyxin B, promethazine, streptomycin, tetracycline, tobramycin, triflupromazine, vancomycin.

Adverse effects

- **Dermatologic:** Loss of hair
- **Hematologic: Hemorrhage;** *bruising;* thrombocytopenia; elevated AST, ALT levels, hyperkalemia
- **Hypersensitivity:** Chills, fever, urticaria, asthma
- **Other:** Osteoporosis, suppression of renal function (long-term, high-dose therapy)
- **Treatment of overdose:** Protamine sulfate (1% solution). Each mg of protamine neutralizes 100 USP heparin units. Give very slowly IV over 10 min, not to exceed 50 mg.

Establish dose based on blood coagulation studies.

Interactions

✳ **Drug-drug** • Increased bleeding tendencies with oral anticoagulants, salicylates, penicillins, cephalosporins • Decreased anticoagulation effects if taken concurrently with nitroglycerin

✳ **Drug-lab test** • Increased AST, ALT levels • Increased thyroid function tests • Altered blood gas analyses, especially levels of carbon dioxide, bicarbonate concentration, and base excess

✳ **Drug-alternative therapy** • Increased risk of bleeding if combined with chamomile, garlic, ginger, ginkgo, and ginseng therapy

■ Nursing considerations
Assessment

- **History:** Recent surgery or injury; sensitivity to heparin; hyperlipidemia; pregnancy
- **Physical:** Peripheral perfusion, R, stool guaiac test, PTT or other tests of blood coagulation, platelet count, kidney function tests

Interventions

- Adjust dose according to coagulation test results performed just before injection (30 min before each intermittent dose or q 4 hr if continuous IV dose). Therapeutic range APTT: 1.5–2.5 times control.
- Use heparin lock needle to avoid repeated injections.
- Give deep SC injections; do not give heparin by IM injection.
- Do not give IM injections to patients on heparin therapy (heparin predisposes to hematoma formation).
- Apply pressure to all injection sites after needle is withdrawn; inspect injection sites for signs of hematoma; do not massage injection sites.
- Mix well when adding heparin to IV infusion.
- Do not add heparin to infusion lines of other drugs, and do not piggyback other drugs into heparin line. If this must be done, ensure drug compatibility.

Adverse effects in *Italics* are most common; those in **Bold** are life-threatening.

- Provide for safety measures (electric razor, soft toothbrush) to prevent injury from bleeding.
- Check for signs of bleeding; monitor blood tests.
- Alert all health care providers of heparin use.
- Have protamine sulfate (heparin antidote) on standby in case of overdose; each mg neutralizes 100 units of heparin.

Teaching points
- This drug must be given by a parenteral route (cannot be taken orally).
- Frequent blood tests are necessary to determine blood clotting time is within the correct range.
- Be careful to avoid injury; use an electric razor, avoid contact sports, avoid activities that might lead to injury.
- Side effects may include the loss of hair.
- Report nose bleed, bleeding of the gums, unusual bruising, black or tarry stools, cloudy or dark urine, abdominal or lower back pain, severe headache.

▽hetastarch (hydroxyethyl starch, HES)
(bet' a starch)

Hespan

PREGNANCY CATEGORY C

Drug class
Plasma expander

Therapeutic actions
Complex mixture of various molecules with colloidal properties that raise human plasma volume when administered IV; increases the erythrocyte sedimentation rate and improves the efficiency of granulocyte collection by centrifugal means.

Indications
- Adjunctive therapy for plasma volume expansion in shock due to hemorrhage, burns, surgery, sepsis, trauma
- Adjunctive therapy in leukapheresis to improve harvesting and increase the yield of granulocytes

Contraindications and cautions
- Contraindicated with allergy to hetastarch, severe bleeding disorders, severe cardiac congestion, renal failure or anuria.
- Use cautiously with liver dysfunction, pregnancy.

Available forms
Injection—6 g/100 mL in 500 mL IV infusion bottle

Dosages
Adults
- *Plasma volume expansion:* 500–1,000 mL IV. Do not usually exceed 1,500 mL/day. In acute hemorrhagic shock, rates approaching 20 mL/kg/hr are often needed.
- *Leukapheresis:* 250–700 mL hetastarch infused at a constant fixed ratio of 1:8 to 1:13 to venous whole blood. Safety of up to 2 procedures per week and a total of 7–10 procedures using hetastarch have been established.
Pediatric patients
Safety and efficacy have not been established.

Pharmacokinetics

Route	Onset	Peak	Duration
IV	Immediate	24 hr	24–36 hr

Metabolism: Hepatic; $T_{1/2}$: 17 days, then 48 days
Distribution: Crosses placenta; enters breast milk
Excretion: Urine

▼IV facts
Preparation: Use as prepared by manufacturer; store at room temperature; do not use if turbid deep brown or if crystalline precipitate forms.
Infusion: Rate of infusion should be determined by patient response; start at approximately 20 mL/kg, reduce rate to lowest possible needed to maintain hemodynamics.
Incompatibilities: Do not mix in solution with any other drug and do not add at Y-site with any other drugs.

Adverse effects
- **CNS:** *Headache,* muscle pain
- **GI:** *Vomiting, submaxillary and parotid glandular enlargement*

- **Hematologic:** Prolongation of PT, PTT; **bleeding and increased clotting times**
- **Hypersensitivity:** Periorbital edema, urticaria, wheezing
- **Other:** *Mild temperature elevations, chills, itching, mild influenza-like symptoms,* peripheral edema of the lower extremities

■ Nursing considerations
Assessment
- **History:** Allergy to hetastarch, severe bleeding disorders, severe cardiac congestion, renal failure or anuria; liver dysfunction; pregnancy
- **Physical:** T; submaxillary and parotid gland evaluation; P, BP, adventitious sounds, peripheral and periorbital edema; R, adventitious sounds; liver evaluation; urinalysis, renal and liver function tests, clotting times, PT, PTT, Hgb, Hct

Interventions
- Administer by IV infusion only; monitor rates based on patient response.
- Maintain life support equipment on standby in cases of shock.
- Ensure that no other drugs are mixed with or added to hetastarch.

Teaching points
- This drug can only be given IV.
- Report difficulty breathing, headache, muscle pain, rash, unusual bleeding or bruising.

▽**histrelin acetate**
*(his **trell'** in)*

Supprelin

PREGNANCY CATEGORY X

Drug class
Gonadotropin-releasing hormone (GnRH) agonist

Therapeutic actions
GnRH or LHRH agonist; inhibits gonadotropin secretion in long-term administration, resulting in decreased sex steroid levels and regression of secondary sexual characteristics.

Indications
- Control of the biochemical and clinical manifestations of central precocious puberty

Contraindications and cautions
- Hypersensitivity to histrelin or any of the components; pregnancy; congenital adrenal hyperplasia; steroid-secreting tumors.

Available forms
Injection—120, 300, 600 mcg/0.6 mL

Dosages
Pediatric patients
10 mcg/kg SC as a single daily injection. If response is not as anticipated within 3 mo, reevaluate therapy.

Pharmacokinetics

Route	Onset	Duration
SC	Slow	3 mo

Metabolism: Plasma; $T_{1/2}$: unknown
Distribution: Crosses placenta; may enter breast milk
Excretion: Unknown

Adverse effects
- **CNS:** *Headache*, light-headedness, mood changes, libido changes, depression, ear pain
- **CV:** *Vasodilation,* edema, palpitations
- **Endocrine:** Breast pain or discharge, goiter, tenderness of female genitalia
- **GI:** Nausea, vomiting, abdominal pain, flatulence, dyspepsia, anorexia
- **GU:** *Vaginal dryness, irritation, odor,* leukorrhea; metrorrhagia; *vaginal bleeding* (within first 1–3 wk)
- **Local:** *Inflammation, infection at injection site*
- **Respiratory:** URI, cough, asthma
- **Other:** *Chills, pyrexia, malaise,* weight gain, viral infections, joint stiffness, muscle pain

■ Nursing considerations
Assessment
- **History:** Hypersensitivity to histrelin or any of the components, pregnancy, congenital adrenal hyperplasia, steroid-secreting tumors, lactation

---

*Adverse effects in Italics are most common; those in **Bold** are life-threatening.*

- **Physical:** Height and weight; T; skin color, lesions; P; R, adventitious sounds; reflexes, affect; abdominal exam; injection site; wrist and hand x-rays; steroid levels; GnRH stimulation test; tomography of the head; pelvic, adrenal, testicular ultrasounds; beta-human chorionic gonadotropin levels; GnRH levels

Interventions

- Ensure patient has only central precocious puberty before treatment: wrist and hand x-rays; steroid levels; GnRH stimulation test; tomography of the head; pelvic, adrenal, testicular ultrasounds; beta-human chorionic gonadotropin levels to rule out other problems.
- Monitor response to drug, including GnRH levels. If desired response is not seen within 3 mo, consider alternate therapy.
- Rotate injection sites daily. Monitor sites for inflammation, pain, infection. Arrange for treatment: hot soaks, steroids.
- Instruct patient and significant others in the proper techniques for SC injection.
- Refrigerate vials; use each vial only once and discard. Allow vial to warm to room temperature before injection.
- Discontinue therapy at any sign of hypersensitivity: difficulty breathing, swallowing; rash, fever, chills; tachycardia.

Teaching points

- Histrelin must be given by single, daily SC injections. Learn the proper technique for administering this drug. Refrigerate vials. Warm vial to room temperature before injection. Use each vial only once and then discard.
- Administer drug each day. Failure to inject daily may result in failure of therapy and return to pubertal state.
- Rotate injection sites daily. Monitor sites for any sign of infection—swelling, pain, redness.
- Arrange for regular medical follow-ups: blood tests, x-rays of bones, and monitoring of sexual development.
- Possible side effects may occur: headache, abdominal discomfort (medications may be available to help); vaginal bleeding (during the first 1–3 wk of therapy); vaginal pain, irritation, odor; nausea, loss of appetite, vomiting (small, frequent meals may help); flushing, red face (cool environment, avoiding exposure to heat will help).
- Report difficulty breathing, rash, swelling, rapid heartbeat, difficulty swallowing, irritation or redness of injection sites that does not go away.

▽hydralazine hydrochloride
*(bye **dral'** a zeen)*

Apo-Hydralazine (CAN), Apresoline, Novo-Hylazin (CAN), Nu-Hydral (CAN)

PREGNANCY CATEGORY C

Drug classes
Antihypertensive drug
Vasodilator

Therapeutic actions
Acts directly on vascular smooth muscle to cause vasodilation, primarily arteriolar; maintains or increases renal and cerebral blood flow.

Indications

- Oral: essential hypertension alone or in combination with other agents
- Parenteral: severe essential hypertension when drug cannot be given orally or when need to lower blood pressure is urgent
- Unlabeled uses: reducing afterload in the treatment of CHF, severe aortic insufficiency, and after valve replacement (doses up to 800 mg tid)

Contraindications and cautions

- Contraindicated with hypersensitivity to hydralazine, tartrazine (in 100-mg tablets marketed as *Apresoline*); CAD; mitral valvular rheumatic heart disease (implicated in MI); pregnancy.
- Use cautiously with CVAs; increased intracranial pressure (drug-induced BP fall risks cerebral ischemia); severe hypertension with uremia; advanced renal damage; slow acetylators (higher plasma levels may be achieved; lower dosage may be adequate); lactation.

Available forms

Tablets—10, 25, 50, 100 mg; injection—20 mg/mL

Dosages
Adults
Oral

Initiate therapy with gradually increasing dosages. Start with 10 mg qid PO for the first 2–4 days; increase to 25 mg qid PO for the first week. Second and subsequent weeks: 50 mg qid. Maintenance: Adjust to lowest effective dosage; twice daily dosage may be adequate. Some patients may require up to 300 mg/day. Incidence of toxic reactions, particularly the LE syndrome, is high in patients receiving large doses.

Parenteral

Patient should be hospitalized. Give IV or IM. Use parenteral therapy only when drug cannot be given orally. Usual dose is 20–40 mg, repeated as necessary. Monitor BP frequently; average maximal decrease occurs in 10–80 min.

Pediatric patients

Although safety and efficacy have not been established by controlled clinical trials, there is experience with the use of hydralazine in children.

Oral

0.75 mg/kg/day PO, given in divided doses q 6–12 hr. Dosage may be gradually increased over the next 3–4 wk to a maximum of 7.5 mg/kg/day PO or 200 mg/day PO.

Parenteral

0.1–0.2 mg/kg/day IV or IM q 4–6 hr as needed.

Pharmacokinetics

Route	Onset	Peak	Duration
Oral	Varies	1–2 hr	6–12 hr
IM, IV	Rapid	10–20 min	2–4 hr

Metabolism: Hepatic; $T_{1/2}$: 3–7 hr
Distribution: Crosses placenta; may enter breast milk
Excretion: Urine

▽IV facts

Preparation: No further preparation required, use as provided.

Infusion: Inject slowly over 1 min, directly into vein or into tubing of running IV; monitor BP response continually.

Incompatibilities: Do not mix with aminophylline, ampicillin, chlorothiazide, edetate, hydrocortisone, nitroglycerin, phenobarbital, verapamil.

Y-site incompatibilities: Do not mix with aminophylline, ampicillin, diazoxide, furosemide.

Adverse effects

- **CNS:** *Headache,* lacrimation, conjunctivitis, peripheral neuritis, dizziness, tremors; psychotic reactions characterized by depression, disorientation, or anxiety
- **CV:** *Palpitations, tachycardia, angina pectoris,* hypotension, paradoxical pressor response
- **GI:** *Anorexia, nausea, vomiting, diarrhea,* constipation, paralytic ileus
- **GU:** Difficult micturition, impotence
- **Hematologic:** Blood dyscrasias
- **Hypersensitivity:** Rash, urticaria, pruritus; fever, chills, arthralgia, eosinophilia; rarely, hepatitis and obstructive jaundice
- **Other:** Nasal congestion, flushing, edema, muscle cramps, lymphadenopathy, splenomegaly, dyspnea, lupus-like (LE) syndrome, possible carcinogenesis

Interactions

＊ **Drug-drug** ● Increased bioavailability of oral hydralazine given with food ● Increased pharmacologic effects of beta-adrenergic blockers and hydralazine when given concomitantly; dosage of beta blocker may need adjusting

■ Nursing considerations
Assessment

- **History:** Hypersensitivity to hydralazine, tartrazine; heart disease; CVA; increased intracranial pressure; severe hypertension; advanced renal damage; slow acetylators; lactation, pregnancy
- **Physical:** Weight; T; skin color, lesions; lymph node palpation; orientation, affect, reflexes; exam of conjunctiva; P, BP, orthostatic BP, supine BP, perfusion, edema, auscultation; R, adventitious sounds, status of nasal mucous membranes; bowel sounds, normal output; voiding pattern, normal output; CBC with differential, LE cell prepara-

tions, antinuclear antibody (ANA) determinations, kidney function tests, urinalysis

Interventions

- Give oral drug with food to increase bioavailability (drug should be given in a consistent relationship to ingestion of food for consistent response to therapy).
- Use parenteral drug immediately after opening ampule. Use as quickly as possible after drawing through a needle into a syringe. Hydralazine changes color after contact with metal, and discolored solutions should be discarded.
- Withdraw drug gradually, especially from patients who have experienced marked blood pressure reduction. Rapid withdrawal may cause a possible sudden increase in BP.
- Arrange for CBC, LE cell preparations, ANA titers before and periodically during prolonged therapy, even in the asymptomatic patient. Discontinue if blood dyscrasias occur. Reevaluate therapy if ANA or LE tests are positive.
- Discontinue or reevaluate therapy if patient develops arthralgia, fever, chest pain, continued malaise.
- Arrange for pyridoxine therapy if patient develops symptoms of peripheral neuritis.
- Monitor patient for orthostatic hypotension; most marked in the morning and in hot weather, with alcohol or exercise.

Teaching points

- Take this drug exactly as prescribed. Take with food. Do not discontinue or reduce dosage without consulting your health care provider.
- These side effects may occur: dizziness, weakness (these are most likely when changing position, in the early morning, after exercise, in hot weather, and when you have consumed alcohol; some tolerance may occur; avoid driving or engaging in tasks that require alertness; change position slowly; use caution in climbing stairs; lie down for a while if dizziness persists); GI upset (frequent, small meals may help); constipation; impotence; numbness, tingling (vitamin supplements may ameliorate symptoms); stuffy nose.
- Report persistent or severe constipation; unexplained fever or malaise, muscle or joint aching; chest pain; rash; numbness, tingling.

▷ hydrochlorothiazide
(hye droe klor oh thye' a zide)

Apo-Hydro (CAN), Esidrix, Ezide, HydroDIURIL, Hydro-Par, Microzide Capsules, Novo-Hydrazide (CAN), Oretic, Urozide (CAN)

PREGNANCY CATEGORY B

Drug class
Thiazide diuretic

Therapeutic actions
Inhibits reabsorption of sodium and chloride in distal renal tubule, increasing the excretion of sodium, chloride, and water by the kidney.

Indications

- Adjunctive therapy in edema associated with CHF, cirrhosis, corticosteroid, and estrogen therapy; renal dysfunction
- Hypertension as sole therapy or in combination with other antihypertensives
- Unlabeled uses: calcium nephrolithiasis alone or with amiloride or allopurinol to prevent recurrences in hypercalciuric or normal calciuric patients; diabetes insipidus, especially nephrogenic diabetes insipidus; osteoporosis

Contraindications and cautions

- Contraindicated with allergy to thiazides, sulfonamides; fluid or electrolyte imbalance; renal disease (can lead to azotemia); liver disease (risk of hepatic coma); gout (risk of attack); SLE; glucose tolerance abnormalities, diabetes mellitus; hyperparathyroidism; manic-depressive disorder (aggravated by hypercalcemia); pregnancy; lactation.

Available forms
Tablets—25, 50, 100 mg; solution—50 mg/5 mL; capsules—12.5 mg

Dosages
Adults

- *Edema:* 25–200 mg daily PO until dry weight is attained. Then, 25–100 mg daily PO or intermittently, up to 200 mg/day.
- *Hypertension:* 12.5–50 mg PO as a starting dose. 25–100 mg daily, maintenance.

- *Calcium nephrolithiasis:* 50 mg daily or bid PO.

Pediatric patients
2.2 mg/kg/day PO in 2 doses.
< 6 mo: Up to 3.3 mg/kg/day in 2 doses.
6 mo–2 yr: 12.5–37.5 mg/day in 2 doses.
2–12 yr: 37.5–100.0 mg/day in 2 doses.

Pharmacokinetics

Route	Onset	Peak	Duration
Oral	2 hr	4–6 hr	6–12 hr

Metabolism: Hepatic; $T_{1/2}$: 5.6–14.8 hr
Distribution: Crosses placenta; enters breast milk
Excretion: Urine

Adverse effects

- **CNS:** *Dizziness, vertigo,* paresthesias, weakness, headache, drowsiness, fatigue, leukopenia, thrombocytopenia, agranulocytosis, aplastic anemia, neutropenia
- **CV:** Orthostatic hypotension, venous thrombosis, volume depletion, cardiac arrhythmias, chest pain
- **Dermatologic:** Photosensitivity, rash, purpura, exfoliative dermatitis, hives
- **GI:** *Nausea, anorexia, vomiting, dry mouth,* diarrhea, constipation, jaundice, hepatitis, pancreatitis
- **GU:** *Polyuria, nocturia,* impotence, loss of libido
- **Other:** Muscle cramps and muscle spasms, fever, gouty attacks, flushing, weight loss, rhinorrhea

Interactions

✷ Drug-drug • Increased thiazide effects with diazoxide • Decreased absorption with cholestyramine, colestipol • Increased risk of cardiac glycoside toxicity if hypokalemia occurs • Increased risk of lithium toxicity • Decreased effectiveness of antidiabetic agents
✷ Drug-lab test • Decreased PBI levels without clinical signs of thyroid disturbance

■ Nursing considerations
Assessment

- **History:** Allergy to thiazides, sulfonamides; fluid or electrolyte imbalance; renal or liver disease; gout; SLE; glucose tolerance abnormalities, diabetes mellitus; hyperparathyroidism; manic-depressive disorders; lactation, pregnancy
- **Physical:** Skin color, lesions, edema; orientation, reflexes, muscle strength; pulses, baseline ECG, BP, orthostatic BP, perfusion; R, pattern, adventitious sounds; liver evaluation, bowel sounds, urinary output patterns; CBC, serum electrolytes, blood glucose, liver and renal function tests, serum uric acid, urinalysis

Interventions

- Give with food or milk if GI upset occurs.
- Mark calendars or provide other reminders of drug for alternate day or 3–5 days/wk therapy.
- Reduce dosage of other antihypertensives by at least 50% if given with thiazides; readjust dosages gradually as BP responds.
- Administer early in the day so increased urination will not disturb sleep.
- Measure and record weights to monitor fluid changes.

Teaching points

- Record intermittent therapy on a calendar, or use prepared, dated envelopes. Take drug early so increased urination will not disturb sleep. Drug may be taken with food or meals if GI upset occurs.
- Weigh yourself on a regular basis, at the same time and in the same clothing; record weight on your calendar.
- These side effects may occur: increased volume and frequency of urination; dizziness, feeling faint on arising, drowsiness (avoid rapid position changes; hazardous activities, like driving; and alcohol); sensitivity to sunlight (use sunglasses, wear protective clothing, or use a sunscreen); decrease in sexual function; increased thirst (sucking on sugarless lozenges and frequent mouth care may help).
- Report weight change of more than 3 lb in 1 day, swelling in your ankles or fingers, unusual bleeding or bruising, dizziness, trembling, numbness, fatigue, muscle weakness or cramps.

▽ hydrocortisone
*(bye droe **kor**'ti zone)*

hydrocortisone acetate

Dermatologic cream, ointment:
Cortaid with Aloe, Cortef Feminine
Itch, Corticaine, Gynecort Female
Creme, Lanacort-5, Lanacort-10,
Maximum Strength Cortaid,
Maximum Strength Caldecort

hydrocortisone butyrate

**Dermatologic ointment and
cream:** Locoid

hydrocortisone cypionate

Oral suspension:
Aquacort (CAN), Cortate (CAN),
Cortef, Hycort (CAN), Texacort (CAN)

hydrocortisone sodium phosphate

IV, IM, or SC injection:
Hydrocortone phosphate

hydrocortisone sodium succinate

V, IM injection: A-hydroCort,
Solu-Cortef

hydrocortisone valerate

**Dermatologic cream, ointment,
lotion:** Westcort

PREGNANCY CATEGORY C

Drug classes
Corticosteroid, short acting
Glucocorticoid
Mineralocorticoid
Adrenal cortical hormone (hydrocortisone)
Hormonal agent

Therapeutic actions
Enters target cells and binds to cytoplasmic receptors; initiates many complex reactions that are responsible for its anti-inflammatory, immunosuppressive (glucocorticoid), and salt-retaining (mineralocorticoid) actions. Some actions may be undesirable, depending on drug use.

Indications
- Replacement therapy in adrenal cortical insufficiency
- Hypercalcemia associated with cancer
- Short-term inflammatory and allergic disorders, such as rheumatoid arthritis, collagen diseases (SLE), dermatologic diseases (pemphigus), status asthmaticus, and autoimmune disorders
- Hematologic disorders—thrombocytopenic purpura, erythroblastopenia
- Trichinosis with neurologic or myocardial involvement
- Ulcerative colitis, acute exacerbations of multiple sclerosis, and palliation in some leukemias and lymphomas
- *Intra-articular or soft-tissue administration:* Arthritis, psoriatic plaques
- *Retention enema:* For ulcerative colitis, proctitis
- *Dermatologic preparations:* To relieve inflammatory and pruritic manifestations of dermatoses that are steroid responsive
- *Anorectal cream, suppositories:* To relieve discomfort of hemorrhoids and perianal itching or irritation

Contraindications and cautions
- *Systemic administration:* infections, especially tuberculosis, fungal infections, amebiasis, hepatitis B, vaccinia, or varicella, and antibiotic-resistant infections; kidney disease (risk to edema); liver disease, cirrhosis, hypothyroidism; ulcerative colitis with impending perforation; diverticulitis; recent GI surgery; active or latent peptic ulcer; inflammatory bowel disease (risks exacerbations or bowel perforation); hypertension, CHF; thromboembolitic tendencies, thrombophlebitis, osteoporosis, convulsive disorders, metastatic carcinoma, diabetes mellitus; lactation.
- *Retention enemas, intrarectal foam:* systemic fungal infections, recent intestinal surgery, extensive fistulas.
- *Topical dermatologic administration:* fungal, tubercular, herpes simplex skin infections; vaccinia, varicella; ear application when eardrum is perforated; lactation.

Available forms

Tablets—5, 10, 20 mg; oral suspension—10 mg/5 mL, 25, 50 mg/mL; injection—50 mg/mL, 100, 250, 500, 1,000 mg/vial; topical lotion—1%, 2%, 2.5%; topical liquid—1%; topical oil—1%; topical solution—1%; topical spray—1%; cream—0.5%

Dosages
Adults

Individualize dosage, based on severity and response. Give daily dose before 9 AM to minimize adrenal suppression. If long-term therapy is needed, alternate-day therapy should be considered. After long-term therapy, withdraw drug slowly to avoid adrenal insufficiency. For maintenance therapy, reduce initial dose in small increments at intervals until lowest clinically satisfactory dose is reached.

IM, IV (hydrocortisone sodium succinate)

100–500 mg initially and q 2–10 hr, based on condition and response.

• *Acute adrenal insufficiency (hydrocortisone sodium phosphate):* 100 mg IV followed by 100 mg q 8 hr in IV fluids.

Pediatric patients

Individualize dosage based on severity and response rather than on formulae that correct adult doses for age or weight. Carefully observe growth and development in infants and children on prolonged therapy.

Oral (hydrocortisone and cypionate)

20–240 mg/day in single or divided doses.

Adults and pediatric patients
IV, IM or SC (hydrocortisone and hydrocortisone sodium phosphate)

20–240 mg/day usually in divided doses q 12 hr.

IM, IV (hydrocortisone sodium succinate)

Reduce dose, based on condition and response, but give no less than 25 mg/day.

• *Retention enema (hydrocortisone):* 100 mg nightly for 21 days.

Intrarectal foam (hydrocortisone acetate)

1 applicator daily or bid for 2 wk and every second day thereafter.

Intra-articular, intralesional (hydrocortisone acetate)

5–25 mg, depending on joint or soft-tissue injection site.

Topical dermatologic preparations

Apply sparingly to affected area bid–qid.

Pharmacokinetics

Route	Onset	Peak	Duration
Oral	1–2 hr	1–2 hr	1–1.5 days
IM	Rapid	4–8 hr	1–1.5 days
IV	Immediate		1–1.5 days
PR	Slow	3–5 days	4–6 days

Metabolism: Hepatic; $T_{1/2}$: 80–120 min
Distribution: Crosses placenta; enters breast milk
Excretion: Urine

▼IV facts

Preparation: Give directly or dilute in normal saline or D_5W. Administer within 24 hr of diluting

Infusion: Inject slowly, directly or dilute, and infuse hydrocortisone phosphate at a rate of 25 mg/min; hydrocortisone sodium succinate at rate of each 500 mg over 30–60 sec.

Incompatibilities: Do not mix or inject at Y-site with amobarbital, ampicillin, bleomycin, dimenhydrinate, doxapram, doxorubicin, ephedrine, ergotamine, heparin, hydralazine, metaraminol, methicillin, nafcillin, pentobarbital, phenobarbital, phenytoin, prochlorperazine, promethazine, secobarbital, tetracyclines.

Adverse effects
Systemic

• **CNS:** *Vertigo, headache,* paresthesias, insomnia, **convulsions,** psychosis
• **CV:** *Hypotension, shock,* hypertension and CHF secondary to fluid retention, **thromboembolism,** thrombophlebitis, fat embolism, cardiac arrhythmias secondary to electrolyte disturbances
• **Dermatologic:** *Thin, fragile skin; petechiae; ecchymoses;* purpura; striae; subcutaneous fat atrophy
• **EENT:** Cataracts, glaucoma (long-term therapy), increased intraocular pressure

---

Adverse effects in *Italics* are most common; those in **Bold** are life-threatening.

- **Endocrine:** *Amenorrhea, irregular menses,* growth retardation, decreased carbohydrate tolerance and diabetes mellitus, cushingoid state (long-term therapy), hypothalamic-pituitary-adrenal (HPA) suppression systemic with therapy longer than 5 days
- **GI:** *Peptic or esophageal ulcer, pancreatitis,* abdominal distention, nausea, vomiting, increased appetite and weight gain (long-term therapy)
- **Hematologic:** *Na⁺ and fluid retention, hypokalemia,* hypocalcemia, increased blood sugar, increased serum cholesterol, decreased serum T_1 and T_4 levels
- **Hypersensitivity:** Anaphylactoid or hypersensitivity reactions
- **Musculoskeletal:** *Muscle weakness,* steroid myopathy and loss of muscle mass, osteoporosis, spontaneous fractures (long-term therapy)
- **Other:** *Immunosuppression, aggravation or masking of infections, impaired wound healing*

Adverse effects related to specific routes of administration
- **IM repository injections:** Atrophy at injection site
- **Intra-articular:** Osteonecrosis, tendon rupture, infection
- **Intralesional therapy, head and neck:** Blindness (rare)
- **Intraspinal:** Meningitis, adhesive arachnoiditis, conus medullaris syndrome
- **Intrathecal administration:** Arachnoiditis
- **Retention enema:** Local pain, burning; rectal bleeding; systemic absorption and adverse effects (above)
- **Topical dermatologic ointments, creams, sprays:** Local burning, irritation, acneiform lesions, striae, skin atrophy

Interactions
✶ **Drug-drug** • Increased steroid blood levels with hormonal contraceptives, troleandomycin • Decreased steroid blood levels with phenytoin, phenobarbital, rifampin, cholestyramine • Decreased serum level of salicylates • Decreased effectiveness of anticholinesterases (ambenonium, edrophonium, neostigmine, pyridostigmine)

✶ **Drug-lab test** • False-negative nitrobluetetrazolium test for bacterial infection (with systemic absorption) • Suppression of skin test reactions

■ **Nursing considerations**
Assessment
- **History:** Infections; kidney disease; liver disease, hypothyroidism; ulcerative colitis with impending perforation; diverticulitis; recent GI surgery; active or latent peptic ulcer; inflammatory bowel disease; hypertension, CHF; thromboembolitic tendencies, thrombophlebitis, osteoporosis, convulsive disorders, metastatic carcinoma, diabetes mellitus; lactation. *Retention enemas, intrarectal foam:* Systemic fungal infections; recent intestinal surgery, extensive fistulas. *Topical dermatologic administration:* Fungal, tubercular, herpes simplex skin infections; vaccinia, varicella; ear application when eardrum is perforated
- **Physical:** *Systemic administration:* weight, T; reflexes, affect, bilateral grip strength, ophthalmologic exam; BP, P, auscultation, peripheral perfusion, discoloration, pain or prominence of superficial vessels; R, adventitious sounds, chest x-ray; upper GI x-ray (history or symptoms of peptic ulcer), liver palpation; CBC, serum electrolytes, 2-hr postprandial blood glucose, urinalysis, thyroid function tests, serum cholesterol. *Topical, dermatologic preparations:* Affected area, integrity of skin

Interventions
Systemic administration
- Give daily before 9 AM to mimic normal peak diurnal corticosteroid levels and minimize HPA suppression.
- Space multiple doses evenly throughout the day.
- Do not give IM injections if patient has thrombocytopenic purpura.
- Rotate sites of IM repository injections to avoid local atrophy.
- Use minimal doses for minimal duration to minimize adverse effects.
- Taper doses when discontinuing high-dose or long-term therapy.
- Arrange for increased dosage when patient is subject to unusual stress.

- Use alternate-day maintenance therapy with short-acting corticosteroids whenever possible.
- Do not give live virus vaccines with immunosuppressive doses of hydrocortisone.
- Provide antacids between meals to help avoid peptic ulcer.

Topical dermatologic administration

- Use caution with occlusive dressings; tight or plastic diapers over affected area can increase systemic absorption.
- Avoid prolonged use, especially near eyes, in genital and rectal areas, on face, and in skin creases.

Teaching points
Systemic administration

- Take this drug exactly as prescribed. Do not stop taking this drug without notifying your health care provider; slowly taper dosage to avoid problems.
- Take with meals or snacks if GI upset occurs.
- Take single daily or alternate-day doses before 9 AM; mark calendar or use other measures as reminder of treatment days.
- Do not overuse joint after intra-articular injections, even if pain is gone.
- Frequent follow-ups to your health care provider are needed to monitor drug response and adjust dosage.
- These side effects may occur: increase in appetite, weight gain (some of gain may be fluid retention; monitor intake); heartburn, indigestion (small, frequent meals, use of antacids may help); increased susceptibility to infection (avoid crowds during peak cold or flu seasons, and avoid anyone with a known infection); poor wound healing (if injured or wounded, consult health care provider); muscle weakness, fatigue (frequent rest periods may help).
- Wear a medical alert ID (long-term therapy) so that any emergency medical personnel will know that you are taking this drug.
- Report unusual weight gain, swelling of lower extremities, muscle weakness, black or tarry stools, vomiting of blood, epigastric burning, puffing of face, menstrual irregularities, fever, prolonged sore throat, cold or other infection, worsening of symptoms.

- Dosage reductions may create adrenal insufficiency. Report any of these: fatigue, muscle and joint pains, anorexia, nausea, vomiting, diarrhea, weight loss, weakness, dizziness, low blood sugar (if you monitor blood sugar).

Intra-articular, intralesional administration

- Do not overuse the injected joint even if the pain is gone. Adhere to rules of proper rest and exercise.

Topical dermatologic administration

- Apply sparingly, and rub in lightly
- Avoid eye contact.
- Report burning, irritation, or infection of the site, worsening of the condition.
- Avoid prolonged use.

Anorectal preparations

- Maintain normal bowel function with proper diet, adequate fluid intake, and regular exercise.
- Use stool softeners or bulk laxatives if needed.
- Notify your health care provider if symptoms do not improve in 7 days or if bleeding, protrusion, or seepage occurs.

▽ hydroflumethiazide
(hye droe floo me thye' a zide)

Diucardin, Saluron

PREGNANCY CATEGORY C

Drug class
Thiazide diuretic

Therapeutic actions
Inhibits reabsorption of sodium and chloride in distal renal tubule, increasing the excretion of sodium, chloride, and water by the kidney.

Indications
- Adjunctive therapy in edema associated with CHF, cirrhosis, corticosteroid, and estrogen therapy; renal dysfunction
- Hypertension, alone or with other antihypertensives
- Unlabeled uses: calcium nephrolithiasis alone or with amiloride or allopurinal to

prevent recurrences in hypercalciuric or normal calciuric patients, diabetes insipidus, especially nephrogenic diabetes insipidus, osteoporosis

Contraindications and cautions
• Contraindicated with allergy to thiazides, sulfonamides; fluid or electrolyte imbalance; renal disease (azotemia); liver disease (hepatic coma); gout (risk of attack); SLE; glucose tolerance abnormalities, diabetes mellitus; hyperparathyroidism; manic-depressive disorder (aggravated by hypercalcemia); pregnancy; lactation.

Available forms
Tablets—50 mg

Dosages
Adults
• *Edema:* 50 mg daily–bid PO. Maintenance: 25–200 mg daily PO; divide doses if dose exceeds 100 mg/day.
• *Hypertension:* 50 mg PO bid. Maintenance: 50–100 mg/day PO. Do not exceed 200 mg/day.

Pharmacokinetics

Route	Onset	Peak	Duration
Oral	2 hr	4 hr	6–12 hr

Metabolism: Hepatic; $T_{1/2}$: 17 hr
Distribution: Crosses placenta; enters breast milk
Excretion: Urine

Adverse effects
• **CNS:** *Dizziness, vertigo,* paresthesias, weakness, headache, drowsiness, fatigue, leukopenia, thrombocytopenia, agranulocytosis, aplastic anemia, neutropenia
• **CV:** Orthostatic hypotension, venous thrombosis, volume depletion, cardiac arrhythmias, chest pain
• **Dermatologic:** Photosensitivity, rash, purpura, exfoliative dermatitis, hives
• **GI:** *Nausea, anorexia, vomiting, dry mouth,* diarrhea, constipation, jaundice, hepatitis, pancreatitis
• **GU:** *Polyuria, nocturia,* impotence, loss of libido

• **Other:** Muscle cramps and muscle spasms, fever, gouty attacks, flushing, weight loss, rhinorrhea

Interactions
✱ **Drug-drug** • Increased thiazide effects if taken with diazoxide • Decreased absorption with cholestyramine, colestipol • Increased risk of cardiac glycoside toxicity if hypokalemia occurs • Increased risk of lithium toxicity • Decreased effectiveness of antidiabetic agents when taken concurrently with hydrochlorothiazide

✱ **Drug-lab test** • Decreased PBI levels without clinical signs of thyroid disturbance

H

■ Nursing considerations
Assessment
• **History:** Allergy to thiazides, sulfonamides; fluid or electrolyte imbalance; renal or liver disease; gout; SLE; glucose tolerance abnormalities; hyperparathyroidism; manic-depressive disorders; lactation, pregnancy
• **Physical:** Skin color, lesions, edema; orientation, reflexes, muscle strength; pulses, baseline ECG, BP, orthostatic BP, perfusion; R, pattern, adventitious sounds; liver evaluation, bowel sounds, urinary output patterns; CBC, serum electrolytes, blood glucose, liver and renal function tests, serum uric acid, urinalysis

Interventions
• Give with food or milk if GI upset occurs.
• Mark calendars, other reminders for alternate day or 3–5 days/wk therapy for edema.
• Reduce dosage of other antihypertensive drugs by at least 50% if given with thiazides; readjust dosages gradually as BP responds.
• Give early so increased urination will not disturb sleep.
• Measure and record regular body weights to monitor fluid changes.

Teaching points
• Record intermittent therapy on a calendar, or use prepared, dated envelopes. Take the drug early in the day so increased urination will not disturb sleep. Take drug with food or meals if GI upset occurs.
• Weigh yourself on a regular basis, at the same time and in the same clothing, record the weight on your calendar.

- These side effects may occur: increased volume and frequency of urination; dizziness, feeling faint on arising, drowsiness (avoid rapid position changes; hazardous activities, like driving; and alcohol); sensitivity to sunlight (use sunglasses, wear protective clothing, or use a sunscreen); decrease in sexual function; increased thirst (sucking on sugarless lozenges and frequent mouth care may help).
- Report weight change of more than 3 lb in 1 day, swelling in your ankles or fingers, unusual bleeding or bruising, dizziness, trembling, numbness, fatigue, muscle weakness or cramps.

▷ hydromorphone hydrochloride

(bye droe mor' fone)

Dilaudid, Dilaudid-5, Dilaudid-HP, Hydromorph Contin (CAN), PMS-Hydromorphone (CAN)

PREGNANCY CATEGORY C

PREGNANCY CATEGORY D
(LABOR AND DELIVERY)

C-II CONTROLLED SUBSTANCE

Drug class
Narcotic agonist analgesic

Therapeutic actions
Acts as agonist at specific opioid receptors in the CNS to produce analgesia, euphoria, sedation; the receptors mediating these effects are thought to be the same as those mediating the effects of endogenous opioids (enkephalins, endorphins).

Indications
- Relief of moderate to severe pain

Contraindications and cautions
- Contraindicated with hypersensitivity to narcotics, tartrazine (2- and 4-mg tablets, *Dilaudid*; physical dependence on a narcotic analgesic (drug may precipitate withdrawal); lactation.
- Use cautiously with pregnancy (readily crosses placenta; neonatal withdrawal if mothers used drug during pregnancy); labor or delivery (safety to mother and fetus has not been established); bronchial asthma, COPD, respiratory depression, anoxia, increased intracranial pressure, acute MI, ventricular failure, coronary insufficiency, hypertension, biliary tract surgery, renal or hepatic dysfunction.

Available forms
Injection—1, 2, 4, 10 mg/mL; tablets—2, 3, 4, 8 mg; suppositories—3 mg; liquid—5 mg/ 5 mL; powder for injection—250 mg

Dosages
Adults
Oral
Tablet—2–4 mg q 4–6 hr; > 4 mg may be needed for severe pain. Liquid—2.5–10 mg q 4–6 hr.
Parenteral
1–4 mg IM, SC q 4–6 hr as needed. May be given by slow IV injection if no other route is tolerated.
Rectal
3 mg q 6–8 hr.
Pediatric patients
Safety and efficacy not established. Contraindicated in premature infants.
Geriatric patients or impaired adults
Use caution; respiratory depression may occur in elderly, the very ill, those with respiratory problems. Reduced dosage may be necessary.

Pharmacokinetics

Route	Onset	Peak	Duration
Oral	Varies	30–60 min	4–5 hr
IM	15–30 min	30–60 min	4–5 hr

Metabolism: Hepatic; $T_{1/2}$: 2–3 hr
Distribution: Crosses placenta; enters breast milk
Excretion: Urine

▽ IV facts
Preparations: Administer undiluted or diluted in normal saline or D_5W.

Infusion: Inject slowly, each 2 mg over 2–5 min, directly into vein or into tubing of running IV.

Adverse effects

- **CNS:** *Light-headedness, dizziness, sedation,* euphoria, dysphoria, delirium, insomnia, agitation, anxiety, fear, hallucinations, disorientation, drowsiness, lethargy, impaired mental and physical performance, coma, mood changes, weakness, headache, tremor, convulsions, miosis, visual disturbances, suppression of cough reflex
- **CV:** Facial flushing, peripheral circulatory collapse, tachycardia, bradycardia, arrhythmia, palpitations, chest wall rigidity, hypertension, hypotension, orthostatic hypotension, syncope
- **Dermatologic:** Pruritus, urticaria, laryngospasm, bronchospasm, edema
- **GI:** *Nausea, vomiting,* dry mouth, anorexia, constipation, biliary tract spasm; increased colonic motility in patients with chronic ulcerative colitis
- **GU:** Ureteral spasm, spasm of vesical sphincters, urinary retention or hesitancy, oliguria, antidiuretic effect, reduced libido or potency
- **Hypersensitivity:** Anaphylactoid reactions (IV administration)
- **Local:** Phlebitis following IV injection pain at injection site; tissue irritation and induration (SC injection)
- **Major hazards: Respiratory depression, apnea, circulatory depression, respiratory arrest, shock, cardiac arrest**
- **Other:** *Sweating,* physical tolerance and dependence, psychological dependence

Interactions

✳ **Drug-drug** • Potentiation of effects of hydromorphone with barbiturate anesthetics; decrease dose of hydromorphone when coadministering.

✳ **Drug-lab test** • Elevated biliary tract pressure (an effect of narcotics) may cause increases in plasma amylase, lipase; determinations of these levels may be unreliable for 24 hr after administration of narcotics.

■ Nursing considerations
Assessment

- **History:** Hypersensitivity to narcotics, tartrazine; physical dependence on a narcotic analgesic; pregnancy; lactation; COPD, respiratory depression, anoxia, increased intracranial pressure, acute MI, ventricular failure, coronary insufficiency, hypertension, biliary tract surgery, renal or hepatic dysfunction
- **Physical:** Orientation, reflexes, bilateral grip strength, affect; pupil size, vision; P, auscultation, BP; R, adventitious sounds; bowel sounds, normal output; thyroid, liver, kidney function tests

Interventions

- Give to nursing women 4–6 hr before the next scheduled feeding to minimize drug in milk.
- Provide narcotic antagonist, facilities for assisted or controlled respiration on standby during parenteral administration.
- Use caution when injecting SC into chilled body areas or in patients with hypotension or in shock; impaired perfusion may delay absorption. With repeated doses, an excessive amount may be absorbed when circulation is restored.
- Refrigerate rectal suppositories.

Teaching points

- Learn how to administer rectal suppositories; refrigerate suppositories.
- Take drug exactly as prescribed.
- Avoid alcohol, antihistamines, sedatives, tranquilizers, OTC drugs.
- These side effects may occur: nausea, loss of appetite (take drug with food and lie quietly, eat frequent small meals); constipation (laxative may help); dizziness, sedation, drowsiness, impaired visual acuity (avoid driving, performing tasks that require alertness, visual acuity).
- Do not take leftover medication for other disorders, and do not let anyone else take the prescription.
- Report severe nausea, vomiting, constipation, shortness of breath or difficulty breathing.

▷hydroxocobalamin crystalline (vitamin B₁₂ₐ)
*(hye drox oh koe **bal' a** min)*

Acti-B₁₂ (CAN), Hydro-Crysti-12, Hydro-Cobex, LA-12 Injection

PREGNANCY CATEGORY C

Drug class
Vitamin

Therapeutic actions
Essential to growth, cell reproduction, hematopoiesis, and nucleoprotein and myelin synthesis; physiologic function is associated with nucleic acid and protein synthesis; acts the same way as cyanocobalamin.

Indications
- Vitamin B₁₂ deficiency due to malabsorption; GI pathology, dysfunction, or surgery; fish tapeworm; gluten enteropathy, sprue; small bowel bacterial overgrowth; folic acid deficiency
- Increased vitamin B₁₂ requirements—pregnancy, thyrotoxicosis, hemolytic anemia, hemorrhage, malignancy, hepatic and renal disease
- Unlabeled use: prevention and treatment of cyanide toxicity associated with sodium nitroprusside (forms cyanocobalamin with cyanide, thus lowering plasma and RBC cyanide concentrations)

Contraindications and cautions
- Contraindicated with allergy to cobalt, vitamin B₁₂, or their components; Leber's disease.
- Use cautiously with pregnancy (safety not established, but is an essential vitamin required during pregnancy—4 mcg/day); lactation—secreted in breast milk (required nutrient during lactation—4 mcg/day).

Available forms
Injection—1,000 mcg/mL

Dosages
For IM use only; folic acid therapy should be given concurrently if needed.

Adults
30 mcg/day for 5–10 days IM, followed by 100–200 mcg/mo.

Pediatric patients
1–5 mg over 2 or more wk in doses of 100 mcg IM, then 30–50 mcg every 4 wk for maintenance.

Pharmacokinetics

Route	Onset	Peak
IM	Intermediate	60 min

Metabolism: Hepatic; $T_{1/2}$: 24–36 hr
Distribution: Crosses placenta; enters breast milk
Excretion: Urine

Adverse effects
- **CNS:** Severe and swift optic nerve atrophy (patients with early Leber's disease)
- **CV:** Pulmonary edema, CHF, peripheral vascular thrombosis
- **Dermatologic:** *Itching, transitory exanthema,* urticaria
- **GI:** *Mild, transient diarrhea*
- **Hematologic:** Polycythemia vera
- **Hypersensitivity: Anaphylactic shock and death**
- **Local:** *Pain at injection site*
- **Other:** Feeling of total body swelling; hypokalemia

Interactions
※ **Drug-lab test** • Invalid folic acid and vitamin B₁₂ diagnostic blood assays if patient is taking methotrexate, pyrimethamine, most antibiotics

■ Nursing considerations
Assessment
- **History:** Allergy to cobalt, vitamin B₁₂, or any component of these medications; Leber's disease
- **Physical:** Skin color, lesions; ophthalmic exam; P, BP, peripheral perfusion; R, adventitious sounds; CBC, Hct, Hgb, vitamin B₁₂, and folic acid levels

Interventions
- Give in parenteral form for pernicious anemia.

Adverse effects in *Italics* are most common; those in **Bold** are life-threatening.

- Give with folic acid if needed; check serum levels.
- Monitor serum potassium levels, especially during the first few days of treatment; arrange for appropriate treatment of hypokalemia.
- Maintain emergency drugs and life support equipment on standby in case of severe anaphylactic reaction.
- Arrange for periodic checks for stomach cancer with pernicious anemia; risk is three times greater in these patients.

Teaching points
- The IM route is the only one available. Monthly injections needed for life with pernicious anemia. Without it, anemia will return and irreversible neurologic damage will develop.
- These side effects may occur: mild diarrhea (transient); rash, itching; pain at injection site.
- Report swelling of the ankles, leg cramps, fatigue, difficulty breathing, pain at injection site.

▷hydroxychloroquine sulfate

(hye drox ee klor' ob kwin)

Plaquenil

PREGNANCY CATEGORY C

Drug classes
Antimalarial
Antirheumatic agent
4-aminoquinoline

Therapeutic actions
Inhibits protozoal reproduction and protein synthesis, preventing the replication of DNA, the transcription of RNA, and the synthesis of protein. Anti-inflammatory action in rheumatoid arthritis, lupus: mechanism of action is not known but is thought to involve the suppression of the formation of antigens, which cause hypersensitivity reactions and symptoms.

Indications
- Suppression and treatment of acute attacks of malaria caused by susceptible strains of plasmodia; *Note:* Radical cure of vivax malaria requires concomitant primaquine therapy; some strains of *Plasmodium falciparum* are resistant to chloroquine and related drugs
- Treatment of acute or chronic rheumatoid arthritis
- Treatment of chronic discoid and systemic lupus erythematosus

Contraindications and cautions
- Contraindicated with allergy to 4-aminoquinolines, porphyria, psoriasis, retinal disease (irreversible retinal damage may occur); pregnancy.
- Use cautiously with hepatic disease, alcoholism, G-6-PD deficiency.

Available forms
Tablets—200 mg

Dosages
200 mg hydroxychloroquine sulfate is equivalent to 155 mg hydroxychloroquine base.
Adults
- *Suppression of malaria:* 310 mg base/wk PO on the same day each week, beginning 1–2 wk prior to exposure and continuing for 4 wk after leaving the endemic area. If suppressive therapy is not begun prior to exposure, double the initial loading dose (620 mg base), and give in two doses, 6 hr apart.
- *Acute attack of malaria:*

Dose	Time	Dosage (mg Base)
1st dose	Day 1	620 mg
2nd dose	6 hr later	310 mg
3rd dose	Day 2	310 mg
4th dose	Day 3	310 mg

- *Rheumatoid arthritis:* Initial dosage 400–600 mg/day PO taken with meals or a glass of milk. From 5–10 days later, gradually increase dosage to optimum effectiveness. *Maintenance dosage:* When good response is obtained (usually 4–12 wk), reduce dosage to 200–400 mg/day PO.
- *Lupus erythematosus:* 400 mg daily–bid PO continued for several weeks or months; for prolonged use, 200–400 mg/day may be sufficient.
Pediatric patients
- *Suppression of malaria:* 5 mg base/kg weekly PO up to a maximum adult dose (above).

• *Acute attack of malaria:*

Dose	Time	Dosage (mg Base)
1st dose	Day 1	10 mg/kg
2nd dose	6 hr later	5 mg/kg
3rd dose	Day 2	5 mg/kg
4th dose	Day 3	5 mg/kg

Pharmacokinetics

Route	Onset	Peak
Oral	Varies	1–6 hr

Metabolism: Hepatic; $T_{1/2}$: 70–120 hr
Distribution: Crosses placenta; enters breast milk
Excretion: Urine

Adverse effects

• **CNS:** Tinnitus, loss of hearing (ototoxicity), exacerbation of porphyria, muscle weakness, absent or hypoactive deep tendon reflexes, irritability, nervousness, emotional changes, nightmares, psychosis, headache, dizziness, vertigo, nystagmus, convulsions, ataxia
• **Dermatologic:** *Pruritus, bleaching of hair,* alopecia, skin and mucosal pigmentation, skin eruptions, psoriasis, exfoliative dermatitis
• **EENT:** *Retinal changes, corneal changes*—edema, opacities, decreased sensitivity; ciliary body changes—disturbance of accommodation, blurred vision
• **GI:** *Nausea, vomiting, diarrhea,* abdominal cramps, loss of appetite
• **Hematologic:** *Blood dyscrasias,* immunoblastic lymphadenopathy, hemolysis in patients with G-6-PD deficiency

■ Nursing considerations

Assessment

• **History:** Allergy to 4-aminoquinolines, porphyria, psoriasis, retinal disease, hepatic disease, alcoholism, G-6-PD deficiency, pregnancy, lactation
• **Physical:** Skin color, lesions; hair; reflexes, muscle strength, auditory and ophthalmological screening, affect, reflexes; liver palpation, abdominal exam, mucous membranes; CBC, G-6-PD in deficient patients, liver function tests

Interventions

• Administer with meals or milk.
• Adjust long-term therapy to smallest effective dose; incidence of retinopathy increases with larger doses.
• Schedule malaria suppressive doses for weekly same-day therapy on a calendar.
• Double-check pediatric doses; children are very susceptible to overdosage.
• Arrange for administration of ammonium chloride (8 g/day in divided doses for adults) 3–4 days/wk for several months after therapy has been stopped if serious toxic symptoms occur.
• Arrange for ophthalmologic examinations during long-term therapy.

Teaching points

• Take full course of drug as prescribed.
• Take drug with meals or milk.
• Mark your calendar with the drug days for malarial prophylaxis.
• These side effects may occur: stomach pain, loss of appetite, nausea, vomiting or diarrhea; irritability, emotional changes, nightmares, headache (reversible).
• Arrange for regular ophthalmologic exams if long-term use is indicated.
• Report blurring of vision, loss of hearing, ringing in the ears, muscle weakness, skin rash or itching, unusual bleeding or bruising, yellow color of eyes or skin, mood swings or mental changes.

▷ hydroxyprogesterone caproate in oil
*(hye **drox**' ee proe **jess**' te rone)*

Hy/Gestrone (CAN), Hylutin, Prodrox (CAN)

PREGNANCY CATEGORY X

Drug classes
Hormonal agent
Progestin

Therapeutic actions
Progesterone derivative. Endogenous progesterone transforms proliferative endometrium

into secretory endometrium; inhibits the secretion of pituitary gonadotropins, which prevents follicular maturation and ovulation; and inhibits spontaneous uterine contraction. Progestins have varying profiles of estrogenic, antiestrogenic, anabolic, and androgenic activity.

Indications

- Treatment of amenorrhea (primary or secondary); abnormal uterine bleeding due to hormonal imbalance
- Production of secretory endometrium and desquamation

Contraindications and cautions

- Contraindicated with allergy to progestins; thrombophlebitis, thromboembolic disorders, cerebral hemorrhage, or history of these; hepatic disease, carcinoma of the breast or genital organs, undiagnosed vaginal bleeding, missed abortion; pregnancy (fetal abnormalities, including masculinization of the female fetus); lactation.
- Use cautiously with epilepsy, migraine, asthma, cardiac or renal dysfunction.

Available forms

Injection—125, 250 mg/mL

Dosages

Administer IM only.
Adults

- *Amenorrhea; abnormal uterine bleeding:* 375 mg IM at any time. After 4 days of desquamation or if no bleeding occurs in 21 days after hydroxyprogesterone alone, start cyclic therapy (administer 20 mg estradiol valerate on day 1 of each cycle; 2 wk after day 1, administer 250 mg hydroxyprogesterone caproate and 5 mg estradiol valerate; 4 wk after day 1 is day 1 of the next cycle). Repeat every 4 wk, and stop after four cycles. Observe patient for onset of normal cycling for 2 to 3 cycles after cessation of therapy.
- *Production of secretory endometrium and desquamation:* Start cyclic therapy any time (see above); repeat every 4 wk until no longer required. Give 125–250 mg IM given on 10th day of cycle; repeat q 7 days until suppression is no longer necessary.

Pharmacokinetics

Route	Onset	Duration
IM	Slow	9–17 days

Metabolism: Hepatic; $T_{1/2}$: unknown
Distribution: Crosses placenta; enters breast milk
Excretion: Urine

Adverse effects

- **CNS:** Sudden, partial, or complete loss of vision, proptosis, diplopia, migraine, precipitation of acute intermittent porphyria, mental depression, pyrexia, insomnia, somnolence
- **CV:** Thrombophlebitis, cerebrovascular disorders, retinal thrombosis, pulmonary embolism, thromboembolic and thrombotic disease, increased BP
- **Dermatologic:** *Rash with or without pruritus, acne,* melasma or chloasma, alopecia, hirsutism, photosensitivity
- **General:** *Fluid retention, edema, increase or decrease in weight*
- **GI:** Cholestatic jaundice, nausea
- **GU:** *Breakthrough bleeding, spotting, change in menstrual flow, amenorrhea,* changes in cervical erosion and cervical secretions, breast tenderness and secretion
- **Other:** Decreased glucose tolerance

Interactions

✻ Drug-lab test • Inaccurate tests of hepatic and endocrine function

■ Nursing considerations
Assessment

- **History:** Allergy to progestins; thromboembolic disorders, cerebral hemorrhage; hepatic disease, carcinoma of the breast or genital organs, undiagnosed vaginal bleeding, missed abortion; epilepsy, migraine, asthma, cardiac or renal dysfunction, pregnancy, lactation
- **Physical:** Skin color, lesions, turgor; hair; breasts; pelvic exam; orientation, affect; ophthalmologic exam; P, auscultation, peripheral perfusion, edema; R, adventitious sounds; liver evaluation; liver and renal function tests, glucose tolerance, Pap smear

Interventions

- Arrange for pretreatment and periodic (at least annual) history and physical, which

H

should include BP, breasts, abdomen, pelvic organs, and a Pap smear.
- Alert patient before therapy to avoid pregnancy during treatment and to have frequent medical follow-ups.
- Administer IM only.
- Discontinue medication and consult physician if sudden partial or complete loss of vision occurs; if papilledema or retinal vascular lesions are present on exam, discontinue drug.
- Arrange to discontinue medication and consult physician at the first sign of thromboembolic disease (leg pain, swelling, peripheral perfusion changes, shortness of breath).

Teaching points
- Prepare a calendar of drug days to remind you about doses.
- This drug can be given only by IM injection.
- These side effects may occur: sensitivity to light (avoid exposure to the sun; use sunscreen and protective clothing); dizziness, sleeplessness, depression (use caution if driving or performing tasks that require alertness); rash, color changes, loss of hair; fever; nausea.
- Do not take drug during pregnancy; serious fetal abnormalities have occurred.
- Report pain or swelling and warmth in the calves, acute chest pain or shortness of breath, sudden severe headache or vomiting, dizziness or fainting, visual disturbances, numbness or tingling in the arm or leg.

▷hydroxyurea
(bye drox ee yoor ee' a)

Droxia, Hydrea, Mylocel

PREGNANCY CATEGORY D

Drug class
Antineoplastic agent

Therapeutic actions
Cytotoxic: inhibits an enzyme that is crucial for DNA synthesis, but exact mechanism of action is not fully understood.

Indications
- Melanoma
- Resistant chronic myelocytic leukemia
- Recurrent, metastatic, or inoperable ovarian cancer
- Concomitant therapy with irradiation for primary squamous cell carcinoma of the head and neck, excluding the lip
- To reduce the frequency of painful crises and to reduce the need for blood transfusions in adult patients with sickle cell anemia (*Droxia*)
- Unlabeled uses: essential thrombocythemia, psoriasis, HIV treatment with didanosine

Contraindications and cautions
- Allergy to hydroxyurea, irradiation, leukopenia, impaired hepatic and renal function, pregnancy, lactation.

Available forms
Capsules—500 mg; *Droxia* capsules—200, 300, 400 mg; tablets—1,000 mg (*Mylocel*)

Dosages
Adults
Base dosage on ideal or actual body weight, whichever is less. Interrupt therapy if WBC falls below 2,500/mm^3 or platelet count below 100,000/mm^3. Recheck in 3 days and resume therapy when counts approach normal.
- *Solid tumors:* Intermittent therapy: 80 mg/kg PO as a single dose every third day. Continuous therapy: 20–30 mg/kg PO as a single daily dose.
- *Concomitant therapy with irradiation:* 80 mg/kg as a single daily dose every third day. Begin hydroxyurea 7 days before irradiation, and continue during and for a prolonged period after radiotherapy.
- *Resistant chronic myelocytic leukemia:* 20–30 mg/kg as a single daily dose.
- *Reduction of sickle cell anemia crises (Droxia):* 15 mg/kg/day PO as a single dose; may be increased by 5 mg/kg/day every 12 wk until maximum tolerated dose or 35 mg/kg/day is reached.
Pediatric patients
Dosage regimen not established.

Adverse effects in *Italics* are most common; those in **Bold** are life-threatening.

Pharmacokinetics

Route	Onset	Peak	Duration
Oral	Varies	2 hr	18–20 hr

Metabolism: Hepatic; $T_{1/2}$: 3–4 hr
Distribution: Crosses placenta; enters breast milk
Excretion: Urine

Adverse effects

- **CNS:** *Headache, dizziness,* disorientation, hallucinations
- **Dermatologic:** Maculopapular rash, facial erythema
- **GI:** *Stomatitis, anorexia, nausea, vomiting,* diarrhea, constipation, elevated hepatic enzymes
- **GU:** Impaired renal tubular function
- **Hematologic:** *Bone marrow depression*
- **Local:** Mucositis at the site, especially in combination with irradiation
- **Other:** Fever, chills, malaise, **cancer**

Interactions

✳ Drug-lab test • Serum uric acid, BUN, and creatinine levels may increase with hydroxyurea therapy • Drug causes self-limiting abnormalities in erythrocytes that resemble those of pernicious anemia but are not related to vitamin B_{12} or folate deficiency

■ Nursing considerations
Assessment

- **History:** Allergy to hydroxyurea, irradiation, leukopenia, impaired hepatic and renal function, lactation, pregnancy
- **Physical:** Weight; T; skin color, lesions; reflexes, orientation, affect; mucous membranes, abdominal exam; CBC, renal and liver function tests

Interventions

- Give in oral form only. If patient is unable to swallow capsules, empty capsules into a glass of water, and give immediately (inert products may not dissolve).
- Encourage patient to drink 10–12 glasses of fluid each day.
- Check CBC before administration of each dose of drug
- Caution patient to avoid pregnancy while using this drug; use of barrier contraceptives is advised.

Teaching points

- Prepare a calendar for dates to return for diagnostic testing and treatment days. If you are unable to swallow the capsule, empty the capsule into a glass of water, and take immediately (some of the material may not dissolve).
- These side effects may occur: loss of appetite, nausea, vomiting, mouth sores (frequent mouth care, small frequent meals may help; maintain good nutrition; an antiemetic may be ordered); constipation or diarrhea (a bowel program may be established); disorientation, dizziness, headache (take precautions to avoid injury); red face, rash (reversible).
- Avoid pregnancy while on this drug, fetal abnormalities have been reported; use of barrier contraceptives is advised.
- Arrange for regular blood tests to monitor the drug's effects.
- Drink at least 10–12 glasses of fluid each day while on this drug.
- Report fever, chills, sore throat, unusual bleeding or bruising, severe nausea, vomiting, loss of appetite, sores in the mouth or on the lips, pregnancy (it is advisable to use birth control while on this drug).

▽hydroxyzine
(bye drox' i zeen)

hydroxyzine hydrochloride
Oral preparations:
Apo-Hydroxyzine (CAN), Atarax, Novo-Hydroxyzine (CAN), Vistaril
Parenteral preparations: Multipax (CAN), Vistaril

hydroxyzine pamoate
Oral preparations: Vistaril

PREGNANCY CATEGORY C

Drug classes
Antianxiety drug
Antihistamine
Antiemetic

Therapeutic actions
Mechanisms of action not understood; actions may be due to suppression of subcortical ar-

eas of the CNS; has clinically demonstrated antihistaminic, analgesic, antispasmodic, antiemetic, mild antisecretory, and bronchodilator activity

Indications

- Symptomatic relief of anxiety and tension associated with psychoneurosis; adjunct in organic disease states in which anxiety is manifested; alcoholism and asthma; prior to dental procedures
- Management of pruritus due to allergic conditions, such as chronic urticaria, atopic and contact dermatosis, and in histamine-mediated pruritus
- Sedation when used as premedication and following general anesthesia
- Control of nausea and vomiting and as adjunct to analgesia pre- and post-op (parenteral) to allow decreased narcotic dosage
- Management of the acutely disturbed or hysterical patient; the acute or chronic alcoholic with anxiety withdrawal symptoms or delirium tremens; as preoperative and postoperative and prepartum and postpartum adjunctive medication to permit reduction in narcotic dosage, allay anxiety, and control emesis (IM administration)

Contraindications and cautions

- Allergy to hydroxyzine; uncomplicated vomiting in children (may contribute to Reye's syndrome or unfavorably influence its outcome; extrapyramidal effects may obscure diagnosis of Reye's syndrome); pregnancy; lactation.

Available forms

Tablets—10, 25, 50, 100 mg; syrup—10 mg/ 5 mL; capsules—25, 50, 100 mg; oral suspension—25 mg/5 mL; injection—25, 50 mg/mL

Dosages

Start patients on IM therapy when indicated; use oral therapy for maintenance. Adjust dosage to patient's response.
Adults
Oral
- *Symptomatic relief of anxiety:* 50–100 mg qid.
- *Management of pruritus:* 25 mg tid–qid.

- *Sedative (preoperative and postoperative):* 50–100 mg.
IM
- *Psychiatric and emotional emergencies, including alcoholism:* 50–100 mg immediately and q 4–6 hr as needed.
- *Nausea and vomiting:* 25–100 mg.
- *Preoperative and postoperative, prepartum and postpartum:* 25–100 mg.
Pediatric patients
Oral
- *Anxiety, pruritus:*
- *> 6 yr:* 50–100 mg/day in divided doses.
- *< 6 yr:* 50 mg/day in divided doses.
- *Sedative:* 0.6 mg/kg.
IM
- *Nausea, preoperative and postoperative:* 1.1 mg/kg (0.5 mg/lb).

Pharmacokinetics

Route	Onset	Peak	Duration
Oral, IM	15–30 min	3 hr	4–6 hr

Metabolism: Hepatic; $T_{1/2}$: 3 hr
Distribution: Crosses placenta; may enter breast milk
Excretion: Urine

Adverse effects

- **CNS:** *Drowsiness,* involuntary motor activity, including tremor and convulsions
- **GI:** *Dry mouth*
- **Hypersensitivity:** Wheezing, dyspnea, chest tightness

■ Nursing considerations
Assessment

- **History:** Allergy to hydroxyzine, uncomplicated vomiting in children, lactation, pregnancy
- **Physical:** Skin color, lesions, texture; orientation, reflexes, affect; R, adventitious sounds

Interventions

- Determine and treat underlying cause of vomiting. Drug may mask signs and symptoms of serious conditions, such as brain tumor, intestinal obstruction, appendicitis.
- Do not administer parenteral solution SC, IV, or intra-arterially; tissue necrosis has oc-

curred with SC and intra-arterial injection, hemolysis with IV injection.
- Give IM injections deep into a large muscle: *Adults:* upper outer quadrant of buttocks or midlateral thigh; *Children:* midlateral thigh muscles; use deltoid area only if well developed.

Teaching points
- Take this drug as prescribed. Avoid excessive dosage.
- These side effects may occur: dizziness, sedation, drowsiness (use caution if driving or performing tasks that require alertness); avoid alcohol, sedatives, sleep aids (serious overdosage could result); dry mouth (frequent mouth care, sucking sugarless lozenges may help).
- Report difficulty breathing, tremors, loss of coordination, sore muscles, or muscle spasms.

▽hylan G-F 20
See *Less Commonly Used Drugs,* p. 1344.

▽hyoscyamine sulfate (L-hyoscyamine)
(high ab' ska meen)

Anaspaz, Cytospaz, Cytospaz-M, ED-SPAZ, Levsin, Levsin/SL, Levsinex Timecaps, NuLev, Symax-SC

PREGNANCY CATEGORY C

Drug classes
Antispasmodic
Anticholinergic
Antimuscarinic
Parasympatholytic

Therapeutic actions
Direct GI smooth muscle relaxant; competitively blocks the effects of acetylcholine at muscarinic cholinergic receptors that mediate the effects of parasympathetic postganglionic impulses, thus relaxing the GI tract.

Indications
- Adjunctive therapy in irritable bowel syndrome, peptic ulcer, spastic or functional GI disorders, cystitis, neurogenic bladder or bowel disorders, parkinsonism, biliary or renal colic
- Treatment of rhinitis and anticholinesterase poisoning
- Partial heart block associated with vagal activity
- Preoperatively to decrease secretions

Contraindications and cautions
- Contraindicated with glaucoma, adhesions between iris and lens, stenosing peptic ulcer, pyloroduodenal obstruction, paralytic ileus, intestinal atony, severe ulcerative colitis, toxic megacolon, symptomatic prostatic hypertrophy, bladder neck obstruction, bronchial asthma, COPD, myocardial ischemia, myasthenia gravis.
- Use cautiously with high environmental temperatures, fever, diarrhea, hyperthyroidism, cardiovascular disease, hypertension, CHF, arrhythmias, renal disease, hiatal hernia, pregnancy, lactation.

Available forms
Tablets—0.125 mg, 0.15 mg; sublingual tablets—0.125 mg; sustained-release tablets—0.375 mg; extended-release capsules—0.375 mg; solution—0.125 mg/mL; injection—0.5 mg/mL

Dosages
Adults
Oral or sublingual
0.125–0.25 mg 3–4 times per day.
Sustained-release
0.375–0.75 mg PO q 12 hr.
Parenteral
0.25–0.5 mg SC, IM, or IV 2–4 times per day as needed.
Pediatric patients 2 yr–< 12 yr
Give dose based on weight (see following) q 4 hr as needed. Daily dose should not exceed 0.75 mg.

Weight (kg)	Dose (mcg)
10	31.3–33.3
20	62.5
40	93.8
50	125

Pharmacokinetics

Route	Onset	Duration
Oral	1–2 hr	4 hr

Metabolism: Hepatic; $T_{1/2}$: 9–10 hr
Distribution: Crosses placenta; passes into breast milk
Excretion: Urine

Adverse effects

- **CNS:** *Dizziness,* blurred vision, confusion, *drowsiness,* psychosis
- **CV:** *Palpitations,* hypertension, chest pain
- **GI:** *Nausea, dry mouth,* taste loss
- **GU:** *Urinary hesitancy,* impotence
- **Other:** *Decreased sweating*

Interactions

✳ **Drug-drug** • Additive effects with other anticholinergics, amantadine, haloperidol, phenothiazines, MAOIs, TCAs, or antihistamines; monitor patient closely and adjust dosages as needed • Decreased absorption if combined with antacids; space 2–4 hr apart

■ Nursing considerations
Assessment

- **History:** Glaucoma, adhesions between iris and lens, stenosing peptic ulcer, pyloroduodenal obstruction, paralytic ileus, intestinal atony, severe ulcerative colitis, toxic megacolon, symptomatic prostatic hypertrophy, bladder neck obstruction, bronchial asthma, COPD, myocardial ischemia, myasthenia gravis, fever, diarrhea, hyperthyroidism, cardiovascular disease, hypertension, CHF, arrhythmias, renal disease, hiatal hernia, pregnancy, lactation
- **Physical:** Bowel sounds, normal output; normal urinary output, prostate palpation; respiratory rate, adventitious sounds; P, BP; intraocular pressure, vision; bilateral grip strength, reflexes; liver palpation, liver function tests; renal function tests; skin color, lesions, texture

Interventions

- Ensure adequate hydration; provide environmental control (temperature) to prevent hyperpyrexia.

- Encourage patient to void before each dose if urinary retention becomes a problem.
- Monitor lighting to minimize discomfort of photophobia.
- Establish safety precautions (siderails, assistance with ambulation, proper lighting, etc.) if visual effects occur.
- Provide sugarless lozenges, ice chips to suck (if permitted) if dry mouth occurs.
- Provide small, frequent meals if GI upset is severe.

Teaching points

- Take drug exactly as prescribed.
- Avoid hot environments while taking this drug (you will be heat-intolerant and dangerous reactions may occur).
- These side effects may occur: dry mouth (sugarless lozenges, frequent mouth care may help; this effect sometimes lessens over time); blurred vision, sensitivity to light (these effects will go away when you discontinue the drug; avoid tasks that require acute vision and wear sunglasses when in bright light); impotence (this effect will go away when you discontinue the drug; you may wish to discuss it with your nurse or physician); difficulty in urination (it may help to empty the bladder immediately before taking each dose).
- Report skin rash, flushing, eye pain, difficulty breathing, tremors, loss of coordination, irregular heartbeat, palpitations, headache, abdominal distention, hallucinations, difficulty swallowing, difficulty urinating.

▷ **ibritumomab**

See *Less Commonly Used Drugs,* p. 1344.

▷ **ibuprofen**
(eye byoo' proe fen)

Actiprofen (CAN), Advil, Advil Liqui-Gels, Advil Migraine, Alti-Ibuprofen (CAN), Apo-Ibuprofen (CAN), Children's Advil, Children's Motrin, Genpril, Haltran, Infants' Motrin, Junior Strength Advil, Junior Strength Motrin, Menadol, Midol,

Midol Maximum Strength Cramp, Motrin, Motrin IB, Motrin Migraine Pain, Novo-Profen (CAN), Nuprin, PediaCare Fever, Pediatric Advil Drops

PREGNANCY CATEGORY B

Drug classes
Nonsteroidal anti-inflammatory drug (NSAID)
Analgesic (non-narcotic)
Propionic acid derivative

Therapeutic actions
Anti-inflammatory, analgesic, and antipyretic activities largely related to inhibition of prostaglandin synthesis; exact mechanisms of action are not known

Indications
- Relief of signs and symptoms of rheumatoid arthritis and osteoarthritis
- Relief of mild to moderate pain
- Treatment of primary dysmenorrhea
- Fever reduction

Contraindications and cautions
- Contraindicated with allergy to ibuprofen, salicylates, or other NSAIDs (more common in patients with rhinitis, asthma, chronic urticaria, nasal polyps); CV dysfunction, hypertension; peptic ulceration, GI bleeding; pregnancy; lactation.
- Use cautiously with impaired hepatic or renal function.

Available forms
Tablets—100, 200, 400, 600, 800 mg; chewable tablets—50, 100 mg; capsules—200 mg; suspension—100 mg/2.5 mL, 100 mg/5 mL; oral drops—40 mg/mL

Dosages
Adults
Do not exceed 3,200 mg/day.
- *Mild to moderate pain:* 400 mg q 4–6 hr PO.
- *Osteoarthritis or rheumatoid arthritis:* 1,200–3,200 mg/day PO (300 mg qid or 400, 600, 800 mg tid or qid; individualize dosage. Therapeutic response may occur in a few days, but often takes 2 wk).

- *Primary dysmenorrhea:* 400 mg q 4 hr PO.
- *OTC use:* 200–400 mg q 4–6 hr PO while symptoms persist; do not exceed 1,200 mg/day. Do not take for more than 10 days for pain or 3 days for fever, unless so directed by health care provider.

Pediatric patients
- *Juvenile arthritis:* 30–40 mg/kg/day PO in three to four divided doses; 20 mg/kg/day for milder disease.
- *Fever (6 mo–12 yr):* 5–10 mg/kg PO q 6–8 hr; do not exceed 40 mg/kg/day.

Pharmacokinetics

Route	Onset	Peak	Duration
Oral	30 min	1–2 hr	4–6 hr

Metabolism: Hepatic; $T_{1/2}$: 1.8–2.5 hr
Distribution: Crosses placenta; may enter breast milk
Excretion: Urine

Adverse effects
NSAIDs
- **CNS:** *Headache, dizziness, somnolence, insomnia,* fatigue, tiredness, dizziness, tinnitus, ophthalmologic effects
- **Dermatologic:** *Rash,* pruritus, sweating, dry mucous membranes, stomatitis
- **GI:** *Nausea, dyspepsia, GI pain,* diarrhea, vomiting, *constipation,* flatulence, GI bleeding
- **GU:** Dysuria, renal impairment, menorrhagia
- **Hematologic:** Bleeding, platelet inhibition with higher doses, neutropenia, eosinophilia, leukopenia, pancytopenia, thrombocytopenia, agranulocytosis, granulocytopenia, aplastic anemia, decreased Hgb or Hct, bone marrow depression
- **Respiratory:** Dyspnea, hemoptysis, pharyngitis, bronchospasm, rhinitis
- **Other:** Peripheral edema, **anaphylactoid reactions to anaphylactic shock**

Interactions
✳ Drug-drug • Increased toxic effects of lithium with ibuprofen • Decreased diuretic effect with loop diuretics: bumetanide, furosemide, ethacrynic acid • Potential decrease in antihypertensive effect of beta-adrenergic blocking agents

■ Nursing considerations

Assessment

- **History:** Allergy to ibuprofen, salicylates or other NSAIDs; CV dysfunction, hypertension; peptic ulceration, GI bleeding; impaired hepatic or renal function; pregnancy; lactation
- **Physical:** Skin color, lesions; T; orientation, reflexes, ophthalmologic evaluation, audiometric evaluation, peripheral sensation; P, BP, edema; R, adventitious sounds; liver evaluation, bowel sounds; CBC, clotting times, urinalysis, renal and liver function tests, serum electrolytes, stool guaiac

Interventions

- Administer drug with food or after meals if GI upset occurs.
- Arrange for periodic ophthalmologic examination during long-term therapy.
- Discontinue drug if eye changes, symptoms of liver dysfunction, renal impairment occur.
- Institute emergency procedures if overdose occurs: gastric lavage, induction of emesis, supportive therapy.

Teaching points

- Use drug only as suggested; avoid overdose. Take the drug with food or after meals if GI upset occurs. Do not exceed the prescribed dosage.
- These side effects may occur: nausea, GI upset, dyspepsia (take drug with food); diarrhea or constipation; drowsiness, dizziness, vertigo, insomnia (use caution when driving or operating dangerous machinery).
- Avoid OTC drugs. Many of these drugs contain similar medications, and serious overdosage can occur.
- Report sore throat, fever, rash, itching, weight gain, swelling in ankles or fingers, changes in vision, black or tarry stools.

⏷**ibutilide fumarate**
(eye byu' ti lyed)

Corvert

PREGNANCY CATEGORY C

Drug class

Antiarrhythmic

Therapeutic actions

Prolongs cardiac action potential, increases atrial and ventricular refractoriness; produces mild slowing of sinus rate and AV conduction.

Indications

- Rapid conversion of atrial fibrillation or flutter of recent onset to sinus rhythm; most effective in arrhythmias of < 90 days' duration

Contraindications and cautions

- Contraindicated with hypersensitivity to ibutilide; second- or third-degree AV heart block, prolonged QTc intervals; pregnancy, lactation.
- Use cautiously with ventricular arrhythmias.

Available forms

Solution—0.1 mg/mL

Dosages

Adults

≥ 60 *kg (132 lb):* 1 vial (1 mg) infused over 10 min; may be repeated after 10 min if arrhythmia is not terminated.

< 60 *kg:* 0.1 mL/kg (0.01 mg/kg) infused over 10 min; may be repeated after 10 min if arrhythmia is not terminated.

Pediatric patients

Not recommended.

Pharmacokinetics

Route	Onset	Peak
IV	Immediate	10 min

Metabolism: Hepatic; $T_{1/2}$: 6 hr
Distribution: Crosses placenta, may be excreted in breast milk
Excretion: Urine and feces

⏷IV facts

Preparation: May be diluted in 50 mL of diluent, 0.9% sodium chloride, or 5% dextrose injection; one 10-mL vial added to 50 mL of diluent yields a concentration of 0.017 mg/mL; may also be infused undiluted; diluted solu-

---

tion is stable for 24 hr at room temperature or for 48 hr refrigerated.

Infusion: Infuse slowly over 10 min.

Compatibilities: Compatible with 5% dextrose injection, 0.9% sodium chloride injection.

Incompatibilities: Do not mix in solution with any other drugs.

Adverse effects

- **CNS:** Headache, light-headedness, dizziness, tingling in arms, numbness
- **CV: Ventricular arrhythmias,** hypotension, hypertension
- **GI:** *Nausea*

Interactions

✳ **Drug-drug** • Increased risk of serious to life-threatening arrhythmias with disopyramide, quinidine, procainamide, amiodarone, sotalol; do not give together • Increased risk of proarrhythmias with phenothiazines, TCAs, antihistamines

■ Nursing considerations
Assessment

- **History:** Hypersensitivity to ibutilide; second- or third-degree AV heart block, time of onset of atrial arrhythmia; prolonged QTc intervals; pregnancy, lactation; ventricular arrhythmias
- **Physical:** Orientation; BP, P, auscultation, ECG; R, adventitious sounds

Interventions

- Determine time of onset of arrhythmia and potential benefit before beginning therapy. Conversion is more likely in patients with arrhythmias of short (< 90 days) duration.
- Ensure that patient is adequately anticoagulated, generally for at least 2 wk, if atrial fibrillation lasts > 2–3 days.
- Monitor ECG continually during and for at least 4 hr after administration. Be alert for possible arrhythmias, including PVCs, sinus tachycardia, sinus bradycardia, varying degrees of block at time of conversion.
- Maintain emergency equipment on standby during and for at least 4 hr after administration.
- Provide appointments for continued follow-up, including ECG monitoring; tendency to revert to atrial arrhythmia after conversion

increases with length of time patient was in abnormal rhythm.

Teaching points

- This drug can only be given by IV infusion. You will need ECG monitoring during and for 4 hours after administration.
- Arrange for follow-up medical evaluation, including ECG, which is important to monitor the effect of the drug on your heart.
- These side effects may occur: rapid or irregular heartbeat (usually passes shortly), headache.
- Report chest pain, difficulty breathing, numbness or tingling.

▽**idarubicin hydrochloride**
*(eye da **roo'** bi sin)*

Idamycin, Idamycin PFS

PREGNANCY CATEGORY D

Drug classes

Antibiotic (anthracycline)
Antineoplastic

Therapeutic actions

Cytotoxic: binds to DNA and inhibits DNA synthesis in susceptible cells.

Indications

- In combination with other approved antileukemic drugs for the treatment of acute myeloid leukemia (AML) in adults
- Orphan drug uses: acute nonlymphocytic leukemia, acute lymphoblastic leukemia in pediatric patients

Contraindications and cautions

- Contraindicated with allergy to idarubicin, other anthracycline antibiotics; myelosuppression; cardiac disease; pregnancy; lactation.
- Use cautiously with impaired hepatic or renal function.

Available forms

Powder for injection—5, 10, 20 mg; injection—1 mg/mL

Dosages
Adults
- *Induction therapy in adults with AML:* 12 mg/m^2 daily for 3 days by slow IV injections in combination with cytarabine; 100 mg/m^2 daily given by continuous infusion for 7 days or as a 25-mg/m^2 IV bolus of cytarabine followed by cytarabine 200 mg/m^2 daily for 5 days by continuous infusion. A second course may be administered when toxicity has subsided, if needed.

Pediatric patients
Safety and efficacy not established.

Geriatric patients or patients with renal or hepatic impairment
Reduce dosage by 25%. Do not administer if bilirubin level is > 5 mg/dL.

Pharmacokinetics

Route	Onset	Peak
IV	Rapid	Minutes

Metabolism: Hepatic; T$_{1/2}$: 22 hr
Distribution: Crosses placenta; enters breast milk
Excretion: Bile and urine

▼IV facts
Preparation: Reconstitute the 5-, 10-, and 20-mg vials with 5, 10, and 20 mL, respectively, of 0.9% sodium chloride injection to give a final concentration of 1 mg/mL. Do not use bacteriostatic diluents. Use extreme caution when preparing drug. Use of goggles and gloves is recommended as drug can cause severe skin reactions. If skin is accidently exposed to idarubicin, wash with soap and water; use standard irrigation techniques if eyes are contaminated. Vials are under negative pressure; use care when inserting needle to minimize inhalation of any aerosol that is released. Reconstituted solution is stable for 7 days if refrigerated and 72 hr at room temperature.
Infusion: Administer slowly (over 10–15 min) into tubing of a freely running IV infusion of sodium chloride injection or 5% dextrose injection. Attach the tubing to a butterfly needle inserted into a large vein; avoid veins over joints or in extremities with poor perfusion.

Incompatibilities: Do not mix idarubicin with other drugs, especially heparin (a precipitate forms, and the IV solution must not be used) and any alkaline solution.

Adverse effects
- **CV: Cardiac toxicity,** CHF, phlebosclerosis
- **Dermatologic:** *Complete but reversible alopecia,* hyperpigmentation of nailbeds and dermal creases, facial flushing
- **GI:** *Nausea, vomiting, mucositis,* anorexia, diarrhea
- **Hematologic: Myelosuppression,** hyperuricemia due to cell lysis
- **Hypersensitivity:** Fever, chills, urticaria, **anaphylaxis**
- **Local:** Severe local cellulitis, vesication and tissue necrosis if extravasation occurs
- **Other:** Carcinogenesis, infertility

■ Nursing considerations
Assessment
- **History:** Allergy to idarubicin, other anthracycline antibiotics; myelosuppression; cardiac disease; impaired hepatic or renal function; pregnancy; lactation
- **Physical:** T; skin color, lesions; weight; hair; nailbeds; local injection site; cardiac auscultation, peripheral perfusion, pulses, ECG; R, adventitious sounds; liver evaluation, mucous membranes; CBC, liver and renal function tests, uric acid levels

Interventions
- Do not give IM or SC because severe local reaction and tissue necrosis occur. Give IV only.
- Monitor injection site for extravasation: reports of burning or stinging. If extravasation occurs discontinue infusion immediately, and restart in another vein. For local SC extravasation, local infiltration with corticosteroid may be ordered; flood area with normal saline, and apply cold compress to area. If ulceration begins, arrange consultation with plastic surgeon.
- Monitor patient's response to therapy frequently at beginning of therapy: serum uric acid level, CBC, cardiac output (listen for S$_3$). CBC changes may require a decrease in the dose; consult with physician.

- Ensure adequate hydration to prevent hyperuricemia.
- Ensure that patient is not pregnant; explain the importance of avoiding pregnancy.

Teaching points

- Prepare a calendar for days to return for drug therapy. Drug can only be given IV.
- These side effects may occur: rash, skin lesions, loss of hair, changes in nails (obtain a wig before hair loss occurs; skin care may help); loss of appetite, nausea, mouth sores (frequent mouth care, small frequent meals may help; maintain good nutrition; consult a dietitian; an antiemetic may be ordered); red urine (transient).
- This drug should not be used during pregnancy; use of barrier contraceptives is advised.
- Have regular medical follow-up, including blood tests to monitor the drug's effects.
- Report difficulty breathing, sudden weight gain, swelling, burning or pain at injection site, unusual bleeding or bruising.

▽ **ifosfamide**
(eye foss' fa mide)

Ifex

PREGNANCY CATEGORY D

Drug classes
Alkylating agent
Nitrogen mustard
Antineoplastic

Therapeutic actions
Cytotoxic: Exact mechanism of action is not known, although metabolite of ifosfamide alkylates DNA, interferes with the replication of susceptible cells; immunosuppressive: lymphocytes are especially sensitive to drug effects.

Indications

- In combination with other approved neoplastic agents for third-line chemotherapy of germ cell testicular cancer; should be used with an agent for hemorrhagic cystitis
- Orphan drug uses: third-line chemotherapy in the treatment of bone sarcomas, soft-tissue sarcomas

- Unlabeled uses: possible effectiveness in the treatment of lung, breast, ovarian, pancreatic and gastric cancer, sarcomas, acute leukemias, malignant lymphomas

Contraindications and cautions

- Allergy to ifosfamide, hematopoietic depression, impaired hepatic or renal function, pregnancy, lactation.

Available forms
Powder for injection—1, 3 g

Dosages
Adults
Administer IV at a dose of 1.2 g/m^2 per day for 5 consecutive days. Treatment is repeated every 3 wk or after recovery from hematologic toxicity.
Pediatric patients
Safety and efficacy not established.
Geriatric patients or patients with renal or hepatic impairment
Data not available on appropriate dosage. Reduced dosage is advisable.

Pharmacokinetics

Route	Onset
IV	Rapid

Metabolism: Hepatic; T$_{1/2}$: 15 hr
Distribution: Crosses placenta; enters breast milk
Excretion: Urine

▽ IV facts
Preparation: Add sterile water for injection or bacteriostatic water for injection to the vial, and shake gently. Use 20 mL diluent with 1-g vial, giving a final concentration of 50 mg/mL, or use 60-mL diluent with 3-g vial, giving a final concentration of 50 mg/mL. Solutions may be further diluted to achieve concentrations of 0.6–20 mg/mL in 5% dextrose injection, 0.9% sodium chloride injection, lactated Ringer's injection, and sterile water for injection. Solution is stable for at least 1 wk at room temperature or 6 wk if refrigerated. Dilutions not prepared with bacteriostatic water for injection should be refrigerated and used within 6 hr.
Infusion: Administer as a slow IV infusion lasting a minimum of 30 min.

Adverse effects

- **CNS:** *Somnolence, confusion, hallucinations,* coma, depressive psychosis, dizziness, seizures
- **Dermatologic:** *Alopecia,* darkening of skin and fingernails
- **GI:** *Anorexia, nausea, vomiting,* diarrhea, stomatitis
- **GU:** *Hemorrhagic cystitis,* bladder fibrosis, *hematuria* to **potentially fatal hemorrhagic cystitis,** increased urine uric acid levels, gonadal suppression
- **Hematologic:** *Leukopenia,* thrombocytopenia, anemia (rare), increased serum uric acid levels
- **Other:** Immunosuppression, secondary neoplasia

Interactions

✴ **Drug-food** • Decreased metabolism and risk of toxic effects if taken with grapefruit juice; avoid this combination

■ Nursing considerations

Assessment

- **History:** Allergy to ifosfamide, hematopoietic depression, impaired hepatic or renal function, pregnancy, lactation
- **Physical:** Reflexes; affect; skin lesions, hair; urinary output, renal function; renal and hepatic function tests, CBC, Hct

Interventions

- Arrange for blood tests to evaluate hematopoietic function before beginning therapy and weekly during therapy.
- Arrange for extensive hydration consisting of at least 2 L of oral or IV fluid per day to prevent bladder toxicity.
- Arrange to administer a protector, such as mesna, to prevent hemorrhagic cystitis.
- Counsel male patients not to father a child during or immediately after therapy; infant cardiac and limb abnormalities have occurred. Counsel female patients not to become pregnant while on this drug; severe birth defects have occurred.

Teaching points

- This drug can only be given IV.

- Have frequent blood tests to monitor your response to this drug. All appointments for follow-up should be kept.
- These side effects may occur: nausea, vomiting, loss of appetite (take drug with food, have small frequent meals); maintain your fluid intake and nutrition (drink at least 10–12 glasses of fluid each day); darkening of the skin and fingernails, loss of hair (obtain a wig or arrange for some other head covering before hair loss occurs; keep head covered in extremes of temperature).
- Avoid grapefruit juice while on this drug.
- Use birth control while on drug and for a time afterwards (male and female patients); this drug can cause severe birth defects.
- Report unusual bleeding or bruising, fever, chills, sore throat, cough, shortness of breath, blood in the urine, painful urination, unusual lumps or masses, flank, stomach or joint pain, sores in mouth or on lips, yellow discoloration of skin or eyes.

▷ imatinib mesylate
(eh mat' eh nib)

Gleevec

PREGNANCY CATEGORY D

Drug classes

Protein tyrosine kinase inhibitor
Antineoplastic

Therapeutic actions

A protein tyrosine kinase inhibitor that selectively inhibits the Bcr-Abl tyrosine kinase created by the Philadelphia chromosome abnormality in chronic myeloid leukemia; this inhibits proliferation and induces apoptosis in the Bcr-Abl positive cell lines as well as fresh leukemic cells, leading to an inhibition of tumor growth in chronic myeloid leukemia (CML) patients in blast crisis

Indications

- Treatment of patients with CML in blast crisis, accelerated phase or in chronic phase after failure with interferon-alpha therapy

---

- Treatment of patients with Kit (CD117) positive unresectable or metastatic malignant GI stromal tumors (GIST)
- First-line treatment of patients with chronic myeloid leukemia (CML)

Contraindications and cautions
- Contraindicated with allergy to imatinib or any of its components, pregnancy, lactation.
- Use cautiously with hepatic or renal dysfunction.

Available forms
Capsules—100 mg

Dosages
Adults
- *Chronic phase CML:* 400 mg/day PO as a once-a-day dose; increase to 600 mg/day may be considered if response is not satisfactory and patient can tolerate the drug.
- *Accelerated phase or blast crisis CML:* 600 mg/day PO as a single dose; increase to 400 mg PO bid may be considered if response is not satisfactory and patient can tolerate the drug.
- *First-line treatment of CML:* 400 mg/day PO.
- *GIST:* 400–600 mg/day PO.
Pediatric patients
Safety and efficacy not established.

Pharmacokinetics

Route	Onset	Peak
Oral	Slow	2–4 hr

Metabolism: Hepatic; $T_{1/2}$: 18 and 40 hr
Distribution: Crosses placenta; may enter breast milk
Excretion: Feces and urine

Adverse effects
- **CNS:** Malaise, *muscle cramps,* insomnia, *headache*
- **GI:** *Vomiting, nausea, diarrhea,* dyspepsia, anorexia, constipation, hepatotoxicity
- **Hematologic:** *Neutropenia, thrombocytopenia*
- **Respiratory:** Pulmonary edema, pneumonia
- **Other:** Myalgia, cough, fever, *rash, sudden weight gain, fluid retention,* night sweats

Interactions
✳ **Drug-drug** • Risk of increased imatinib effects with ketoconazole, itraconazole, erythromycin, clarithromycin; use caution if this combination is used • Risk of decreased imatinib effects if combined with dexamethasone, phenytoin, carbamazepine, rifampicin, or phenobarbital; use caution if this combination is required • Increased serum levels of simvastatin, cyclosporine, pimozide when combined with imatinib, avoid these combinations if possible • Increased risk of bleeding with warfarin; if anticoagulation is needed, use of a heparin is recommended

✳ **Drug-alternative therapy** • Decreased effectiveness of imatinib if taken with St. John's wort; avoid this combination

■ Nursing considerations
- **History:** Allergy to imatinib or any of its components, pregnancy, lactation, hepatic or renal dysfunction
- **Physical:** Body temperature, body weight, P, BP, R, adventitious sounds, CBC

Interventions
- Administer once a day with a meal and a large glass of water.
- Provide small, frequent meals if GI upset occurs.
- Arrange for nutritional consult if nausea and vomiting are persistent.
- Provide analgesics if headache, muscle pain are a problem.
- Advise women of child-bearing age to use a barrier form of contraception while taking this drug.
- Monitor CBC before and periodically during therapy; arrange for dosage adjustment as indicated if bone marrow suppression occurs.
- Monitor patient for fluid retention and edema; severe cases may require dosage reduction or discontinuation of drug.
- Arrange for appropriate consultation to help patient cope with the high cost of drug.

Teaching points
- This drug should be taken once a day as a single dose, with a meal and a large glass of water.
- This drug has been linked to serious fetal abnormalities; women of child-bearing age

who are taking this drug should use a form of barrier contraceptive.

- Avoid infection while taking this drug; avoid crowded areas or people with known infections.
- These side effects may occur: nausea, vomiting (small frequent meals or sucking on sugarless lozenges or chewing gum may help); headache, muscle cramps, pain (use of an analgesic may help; consult your health care provider); fluid retention and sudden weight gain (monitor daily weights and report sudden increases or difficulty breathing).
- Do not use any alternative therapy, including St. John's wort, while you are in this treatment program; it may decrease the effectiveness of the drug.
- You will need to be followed with blood tests to monitor the effects of this drug on your blood.
- Report fever, chills, unusual bleeding or bruising, difficulty breathing, yellowing of your skin or eyes, any signs of infection, sudden weight gain, severe swelling.

▽ imipramine

*(im **ip'** ra meen)*

imipramine hydrochloride

Apo-Imipramine (CAN), Impril (CAN), Novopramine (CAN), Tofranil

imipramine pamoate

Tofranil-PM

PREGNANCY CATEGORY D

Drug class

Tricyclic antidepressant (TCA) (tertiary amine)

Therapeutic actions

Mechanism of action unknown; the TCAs are structurally related to the phenothiazine antipsychotic drugs (eg, chlorpromazine), but unlike the phenothiazines, TCAs inhibit the presynaptic reuptake of the neurotransmitters norepinephrine and serotonin; anticholinergic at CNS and peripheral receptors; sedative;

the relation of these effects to clinical efficacy is unknown.

Indications

- Relief of symptoms of depression (endogenous depression most responsive); sedative effects of tertiary amine TCAs may be helpful in patients whose depression is associated with anxiety and sleep disturbance
- Enuresis in children 6 yr or older
- Unlabeled use: control of chronic pain (eg, intractable pain of cancer, peripheral neuropathies, postherpetic neuralgia, tic douloureux, central pain syndromes)

Contraindications and cautions

- Contraindicated with hypersensitivity to any tricyclic drug or to tartrazine (in preparations marketed as *Tofranil, Tofranil PM;* patients with aspirin allergy are often allergic to tartrazine); concomitant therapy with an MAO inhibitor; EST with coadministration of TCAs; recent MI; myelography within previous 24 hr or scheduled within 48 hr; pregnancy; lactation.
- Use cautiously with preexisting CV disorders; seizure disorders (TCAs lower the seizure threshold); hyperthyroidism; angle-closure glaucoma, increased intraocular pressure, urinary retention, ureteral or urethral spasm; impaired hepatic, renal function; psychiatric patients (schizophrenic or paranoid patients may exhibit a worsening of psychosis with TCA therapy; manic-depressive patients may shift to hypomanic or manic phase); elective surgery.

Available forms

Tablets (imipramine hydrochloride)—10, 25, 50 mg; capsules (imipramine pamoate)—75, 100, 125, 150 mg

Dosages
Adults

- *Depression:* Hospitalized patients: initially, 100–150 mg/day PO in divided doses. Gradually increase to 200 mg/day as required. If no response after 2 wk, increase to 250–300 mg/day. Total daily dosage may be given hs. Outpatients: initially, 75 mg/day PO, increasing to 150 mg/day. Dosages > 200 mg/

day not recommended. Total daily dosage may be given hs. Maintenance dose is 50–150 mg/day.

- *Chronic pain:* 50–200 mg/day PO.

Adolescent and geriatric patients

- *Depression:* 30–40 mg/day PO; doses > 100 mg/day generally are not needed.

Pediatric patients ≥ 6 yr

- *Childhood enuresis:* Initially, 25 mg/day 1 hr before bedtime. If response is not satisfactory after 1 wk, increase to 50 mg nightly in children < 12 yr, 75 mg nightly in children > 12 yr. Doses > 75 mg/day do not have greater efficacy but are more likely to increase side effects. Do not exceed 2.5 mg/kg per day. Early-night bedwetters may be more effectively treated with earlier and divided dosage (25 mg midafternoon, repeated hs). Institute drug-free period after successful therapy, gradually tapering dosage.

Pharmacokinetics

Route	Onset	Peak
Oral	Varies	2–4 hr

Metabolism: Hepatic; $T_{1/2}$: 8–16 hr
Distribution: Crosses placenta; enters breast milk
Excretion: Urine

Adverse effects
Adult use

- **CNS:** *Sedation and anticholinergic effects,* dry mouth, blurred vision, disturbance of accommodation for near vision, mydriasis, increased intraocular pressure; *confusion, disturbed concentration,* hallucinations, disorientation, decreased memory, feelings of unreality, delusions, anxiety, nervousness, restlessness, agitation, panic, insomnia, nightmares, hypomania, mania, exacerbation of psychosis, drowsiness, weakness, fatigue, headache, numbness, tingling, paresthesias of extremities, incoordination, motor hyperactivity, akathisia, ataxia, tremors, peripheral neuropathy, extrapyramidal symptoms, *seizures,* dysarthria, tinnitus, altered EEG
- **CV:** *Orthostatic hypotension,* hypertension, syncope, tachycardia, palpitations, MI, arrhythmias, heart block, precipitation of CHF, stroke

- **Endocrine:** Elevated or depressed blood sugar, elevated prolactin levels, inappropriate ADH secretion
- **GI:** *Dry mouth, constipation,* paralytic ileus, *nausea,* vomiting, anorexia, epigastric distress, diarrhea, flatulence, dysphagia, peculiar taste, increased salivation, stomatitis, glossitis, parotid swelling, abdominal cramps, black tongue, hepatitis
- **GU:** Urinary retention, delayed micturition, dilation of the urinary tract, gynecomastia, testicular swelling in men; breast enlargement, menstrual irregularity and galactorrhea in women; increased or decreased libido; impotence
- **Hematologic:** Bone marrow depression, including agranulocytosis; eosinophilia, purpura, thrombocytopenia, leukopenia
- **Hypersensitivity:** Rash, pruritus, vasculitis, petechiae, photosensitization, edema (generalized, facial, tongue), drug fever
- **Withdrawal:** Abrupt discontinuation of prolonged therapy: nausea, headache, vertigo, nightmares, malaise
- **Other:** Nasal congestion, excessive appetite, weight gain or loss; sweating (paradoxical effect in a drug with prominent anticholinergic effects), alopecia, lacrimation, hyperthermia, flushing, chills

Pediatric use for enuresis

- **CNS:** *Nervousness, sleep disorders, tiredness,* convulsions, anxiety, emotional instability, syncope, collapse
- **CV:** ECG changes of unknown significance when given in doses of 5 mg/kg/day
- **GI:** Constipation, *mild GI disturbances*
- **Other:** Adverse reactions reported with adult use

Interactions
✱ **Drug-drug** • Increased TCA levels and pharmacologic (especially anticholinergic) effects with cimetidine, fluoxetine, ranitidine • Increased serum levels and risk of bleeding with oral anticoagulants • Altered response, including arrhythmias and hypertension, with sympathomimetics • Risk of severe hypertension with clonidine • Hyperpyretic crises, severe convulsions, hypertensive episodes, and deaths when MAO inhibitors are given with TCAs • Decreased hypotensive activity of guanethidine with imipramine

Note: MAOIs and TCAs have been used successfully in some patients resistant to therapy with single agents; however, the combination can cause serious and potentially fatal adverse effects.

■ Nursing considerations
Assessment
- **History:** Hypersensitivity to any tricyclic drug or to tartrazine; concomitant therapy with an MAO inhibitor; EST with coadministration of TCAs; recent MI; myelography within previous 24 hr or scheduled within 48 hr; preexisting CV disorders; seizure disorders; hyperthyroidism; angle-closure glaucoma, increased intraocular pressure, urinary retention, ureteral or urethral spasm; impaired hepatic, renal function; psychiatric patients; elective surgery; pregnancy; lactation
- **Physical:** Weight; T; skin color, lesions; orientation, affect, reflexes, vision and hearing; P, BP, auscultation, orthostatic BP, perfusion; bowel sounds, normal output, liver evaluation; urine flow, normal output; usual sexual function, frequency of menses, breast and scrotal examination; liver function tests, urinalysis, CBC, ECG

Interventions
- Limit drug access for depressed and potentially suicidal patients.
- Give IM only when oral therapy is impossible. Do not give IV.
- Give major portion of dose hs if drowsiness, severe anticholinergic effects occur (note that elderly may not tolerate single daily dose therapy).
- Reduce dosage if minor side effects develop; discontinue if serious side effects occur.
- Arrange for CBC if patient develops fever, sore throat, or other sign of infection during therapy.

Teaching points
- Take drug exactly as prescribed. Do not stop taking drug abruptly or without consulting your health care provider.
- Avoid prolonged exposure to sunlight or sunlamps; use a sunscreen or protective garments.
- These side effects may occur: headache, dizziness, drowsiness, weakness, blurred vision (reversible; safety measures may need to be taken if severe; avoid driving or performing tasks that require alertness); nausea, vomiting, loss of appetite (small frequent meals, frequent mouth care may help); dry mouth (sucking sugarless candies may help); disorientation, difficulty concentrating, emotional changes; changes in sexual function, impotence, changes in libido.
- Report dry mouth, difficulty in urination, excessive sedation, fever, chills, sore throat, palpitations.

▽**inamrinone lactate**
(*in **am**' ri none*)

Inocor

PREGNANCY CATEGORY C

Drug classes
Cardiotonic drug
Inotropic agent

Therapeutic actions
Increases force of contraction of ventricles (positive inotropic effect); causes vasodilation by a direct relaxant effect on vascular smooth muscle.

Indications
- CHF: short-term management of patients who have not responded to digitalis, diuretics, or vasodilators.

Contraindications and cautions
- Allergy to inamrinone or bisulfites, severe aortic or pulmonic valvular disease, acute MI, decreased fluid volume, lactation

Available forms
Injection—5 mg/mL

Dosages
Adults
- *Initial dose:* 0.75 mg/kg IV bolus, given over 2–3 min. A supplemental IV bolus of 0.75 mg/kg may be given after 30 min if needed.
- *Maintenance infusion:* 5–10 mcg/kg/min. Do not exceed a total of 10 mg/kg/day.

Adverse effects in *Italics* are most common; those in **Bold** are life-threatening.

Pediatric patients
Not recommended.

Pharmacokinetics

Route	Onset	Peak	Duration
IV	Immediate	10 min	2 hr

Metabolism: Hepatic; $T_{1/2}$: 3.6–5.8 hr
Distribution: Crosses placenta; may pass into breast milk
Excretion: Urine (63%) and feces (18%)

▽ IV facts

Preparation: Give as supplied or dilute in normal or one-half normal saline solution to a concentration of 1–3 mg/mL. Use diluted solution within 24 hr. Protect ampules from exposure to light.

Infusion: Administer IV bolus slowly over 2–3 min. Maintenance infusion should not exceed 5—10 mcg/kg/min. Monitor doses; do not exceed a daily dose of 10 mg/kg.

Incompatibilities: Do not mix directly with dextrose-containing solutions; may be injected into a Y-connector or into tubing when a dextose solution is running.

Y-site incompatibilities: Do not mix with furosemide, sodium bicarbonate. Do not inject with furosemide.

Adverse effects

- **CV:** *Arrhythmias,* hypotension
- **GI:** Nausea, vomiting, abdominal pain, anorexia, hepatoxicity
- **Hematologic:** *Thrombocytopenia*
- **Hypersensitivity:** Pericarditis, pleuritis, ascites, vasculitis
- **Other:** Fever, chest pain, burning at injection site

Interactions

❋ **Drug-drug** • Precipitate formation in solution if given in the same IV line with furosemide

■ Nursing considerations

CLINICAL ALERT!
Name confusion had occurred between amiodarone when drug name was amrinone; although inamrinone is a new name, confusion may still occur.

Assessment

- **History:** Allergy to inamrinone or bisulfites, severe aortic or pulmonic valvular disease, acute MI, decreased fluid volume, lactation
- **Physical:** Weight, orientation, P, BP, cardiac auscultation; peripheral pulses, peripheral perfusion; R, adventitious sounds; bowel sounds, liver evaluation; urinary output; serum electrolyte levels, platelet count, liver enzymes

Interventions

- Protect drug vial from light.
- Monitor BP and P, and reduce dose if marked decreases occur.
- Monitor I&O and electrolyte levels; record daily weights.
- Monitor platelet counts if patient is on prolonged therapy. Reduce dose if platelet levels fall to < 150,000 mm³.

Teaching points

- You will need frequent BP and P monitoring.
- You may experience increased voiding while on this drug.
- Report pain at IV injection site; dizziness; weakness, fatigue; numbness or tingling.

▽ indapamide
*(in **dap'** a mide)*

Lozol

PREGNANCY CATEGORY B

Drug class
Thiazide-like diuretic (actually an indoline)

Therapeutic actions
Inhibits reabsorption of sodium and chloride in distal renal tubule, increasing excretion of sodium, chloride, and water by the kidney.

Indications
- Edema associated with CHF
- Hypertension, as sole therapy or in combination with other antihypertensives
- Unlabeled use: diabetes insipidus, especially nephrogenic diabetes insipidus

Contraindications and cautions

- Contraindicated with allergy to thiazides, sulfonamides; fluid or electrolyte imbalance; renal disease (risk of azotemia); liver disease (may precipitate hepatic coma); gout (risk of precipitation of attack); SLE; glucose tolerance abnormalities, diabetes mellitus; hyperparathyroidism; manic-depressive disorder (aggravated by hypercalcemia); pregnancy; lactation.

Available forms

Tablets—1.25, 2.5 mg

Dosages
Adults

- *Edema:* 2.5 mg/day PO as single dose in the morning. May be increased to 5 mg/day if response is not satisfactory after 1 wk.
- *Hypertension:* 1.25 mg/day PO. May be increased up to 2.5 mg/day if response is not satisfactory after 4 wk. May increase to a maximum of 5 mg/day. If combination antihypertensive therapy is needed, reduce the dosage of other agents by 50%, then adjust according to patient's response.

Pharmacokinetics

Route	Onset	Peak	Duration
Oral	1–2 hr	2 hr	36 hr

Metabolism: Hepatic; $T_{1/2}$: 14 hr
Distribution: Crosses placenta; enters breast milk
Excretion: Urine

Adverse effects

- **CNS:** *Dizziness, vertigo,* paresthesias, weakness, headache, drowsiness, fatigue, leukopenia, thrombocytopenia, agranulocytosis, aplastic anemia, neutropenia
- **CV:** Orthostatic hypotension, venous thrombosis, volume depletion, cardiac arrhythmias, chest pain
- **Dermatologic:** Photosensitivity, rash, purpura, exfoliative dermatitis, hives
- **GI:** *Nausea, anorexia, vomiting, dry mouth,* diarrhea, constipation, jaundice, hepatitis, pancreatitis
- **GU:** *Polyuria, nocturia,* impotence, decreased libido

- **Other:** Muscle cramps and muscle spasms, fever, gouty attacks, flushing, weight loss, rhinorrhea

Interactions

✳ **Drug-drug** • Increased thiazide effects if taken with diazoxide • Decreased absorption with cholestyramine, colestipol • Increased risk of cardiac glycoside toxicity if hypokalemia occurs • Increased risk of lithium toxicity • Decreased effectiveness of antidiabetic agents
✳ **Drug-lab test** • Decreased PBI levels without clinical signs of thyroid disturbance

■ Nursing considerations
Assessment

- **History:** Allergy to thiazides, sulfonamides; fluid or electrolyte imbalance; renal or liver disease; gout; SLE; glucose tolerance abnormalities; diabetes mellitus; hyperparathyroidism; manic-depressive disorders; lactation, pregnancy
- **Physical:** Skin color, lesions, edema; orientation, reflexes, muscle strength; pulses, baseline ECG, BP, orthostatic BP, perfusion; R, pattern, adventitious sounds; liver evaluation, bowel sounds, urinary output patterns; CBC, serum electrolytes, blood glucose, liver and renal function tests, serum uric acid, urinalysis

Interventions

- Give with food or milk if GI upset occurs.
- Mark calendars or provide other reminders for outpatients on alternate-day or 3–5 days/wk therapy.
- Give early in the day so increased urination will not disturb sleep.
- Measure and record regular weight to monitor fluid changes.

Teaching points

- Record intermittent therapy on a calendar, or use prepared, dated envelopes. Take the drug early so increased urination will not disturb sleep. The drug may be taken with food or meals if GI upset occurs.
- Weigh yourself on a regular basis, at the same time of the day and in the same clothing; record the weight on your calendar.

Adverse effects in *Italics* are most common; those in **Bold** are life-threatening.

- These side effects may occur: increased volume and frequency of urination; dizziness, feeling faint on arising, drowsiness (avoid rapid position changes; hazardous activities, like driving a car; and alcohol, which can intensify these problems); sensitivity to sunlight (use sunglasses, wear protective clothing, or use a sunscreen); decrease in sexual function; increased thirst (sucking on sugarless lozenges, frequent mouth care may help).
- Report weight change of more than 3 lb in 1 day, swelling in ankles or fingers, unusual bleeding or bruising, dizziness, trembling, numbness, fatigue, muscle weakness or cramps.

▽ indinavir sulfate
(in **din'** ah ver)

Crixivan

PREGNANCY CATEGORY C

Drug classes
Antiviral
Antiretroviral

Therapeutic actions
Antiviral activity; inhibits HIV protease activity, leading to production of immature, non-infective HIV particles

Indications
- Treatment of HIV infection in adults when antiretroviral therapy is indicated; used in combination with other drugs

Contraindications and cautions
- Contraindicated with allergy to component of indinavir
- Use cautiously with pregnancy, hepatic or renal impairment, lactation

Available forms
Capsules—100, 200, 333, 400 mg

Dosages
Adults
800 mg PO q 8 hr. With delavirdine: 600 mg PO q 8 hr with delavirdine 400 mg tid; with didanosine: administer ≥ 1 hr apart on an empty stomach; with efavirenz: 1,000 mg PO q 8 hr; with itraconazole: 600 mg PO q 8 hr with itraconazole 200 mg bid; with ketoconazole: 600 mg PO q 8 hr; with rifabutin: 1,000 mg PO q 8 hr, reduce rifabutin by 50%.

Pediatric patients
Safety and efficacy not established in children < 12 yr.

Patients with hepatic impairment
600 mg PO q 8 hr with mild to moderate hepatic impairment.

Pharmacokinetics

Route	Onset	Peak
Oral	Rapid	0.8 hr

Metabolism: Hepatic; $T_{1/2}$: 3–4 hr
Distribution: Crosses placenta; passes into breast milk
Excretion: Feces and urine

Adverse effects
- **CNS:** *Headache,* dizziness, insomnia, somnolence
- **CV:** Palpitations
- **Dermatologic:** Acne, dry skin, contact dermatitis, rash, body odor
- **GI:** *Nausea, vomiting, diarrhea,* anorexia, dry mouth, acid regurgitation, *hyperbilirubinemia*
- **GU:** Dysuria, hematuria, nocturia, pyelonephritis, nephrolithiasis
- **Respiratory:** Cough, dyspnea, sinusitis
- **Other:** Hypothermia, chills, back pain, flank pain, flulike illness

Interactions
✳ Drug-drug • Potentially large increase in serum concentration of triazolam, midazolam with indinavir; potential for serious arrhythmias, seizure, and fatal reactions; do not administer indinavir with any of these drugs • Decreased effectiveness with didanosine; give these two drugs 1 hr apart on empty stomach to decrease effects of interaction • Significant decrease in serum levels with nevirapine—avoid this combination; if combination is necessary, increase indinavir to 1,000 mg q 8 hr with nevirapine 200 mg bid; carefully monitor effectiveness of indinavir if starting or stopping nevirapine
✳ Drug-food • Absorption is decreased by presence of food and grapefruit juice; give on empty stomach with full glass of water

✴ Drug-alternative therapy • Decreased effectiveness if combined with St. John's wort

■ Nursing considerations
Assessment
- **History:** Allergy to indinavir, hepatic or renal dysfunction, pregnancy, lactation
- **Physical:** T; orientation, reflexes; BP, P, peripheral perfusion; R, adventitious sounds; bowel sounds; urinary output; skin color, perfusion; liver and renal function tests

Interventions
- Capsules should be protected from moisture; store in container provided and keep desiccant in bottle. Give drug every 8 hr around the clock.
- Give on an empty stomach, 1 hr before or 2 hr after meal with a full glass of water. If GI upset is severe, give with a light meal; avoid grapefruit juice, foods high in calories, fat, or protein.
- Carefully screen drug history to avoid potentially dangerous drug–drug interactions.
- Monitor patient to maintain hydration; if nephrolithiasis occurs, therapy will need to be interrupted or stopped.

Teaching points
- Take this drug on an empty stomach, 1 hr before or 2 hr after a meal, with a full glass of water. If GI upset is severe, take with a light meal; avoid grapefruit juice, foods high in calories, fat, or protein.
- Store the capsules in the original container and leave the desiccant in the bottle. These capsules are very sensitive to moisture.
- Take the full course of therapy as prescribed; do not double up doses if one is missed; do not change dosage without consulting your physician. Take drug every 8 hr around the clock.
- This drug does not cure HIV infection; long-term effects are not yet known; continue to take precautions as the risk of transmission is not reduced by this drug.
- Do not take any other drug, prescription or OTC, without consulting your health care provider; this drug interacts with many other drugs and serious problems can occur.

- These side effects may occur: nausea, vomiting, loss of appetite, diarrhea, abdominal pain, headache, dizziness, insomnia.
- Report severe diarrhea, severe nausea, personality changes, changes in color of urine or stool, flank pain, fever or chills.

▷ indomethacin
(in doe meth' a sin)

indomethacin
Indocid P.D.A. (CAN), Indocin, Indocin-SR, Novo-Methacin (CAN)

indomethacin sodium trihydrate
Apo-Indomethacin (CAN), Indocid (CAN), Indocin I.V., Indotec (CAN), Novomethacin (CAN), Rhodacine (CAN)

PREGNANCY CATEGORY B

PREGNANCY CATEGORY D (THIRD TRIMESTER)

Drug class
Nonsteroidal anti-inflammatory drug (NSAID)

Therapeutic actions
Anti-inflammatory, analgesic, and antipyretic activities largely related to inhibition of prostaglandin synthesis; exact mechanisms of action are not known.

Indications
Oral, topical, suppositories
- Relief of signs and symptoms of moderate to severe rheumatoid arthritis and moderate to severe osteoarthritis, moderate to severe ankylosing spondylitis, acute painful shoulder (bursitis, tendinitis), acute gouty arthritis (*not* sustained-release form)
- Unlabeled uses for oral form: pharmacologic closure of persistent patent ductus arteriosus in premature infants; juvenile rheumatoid arthritis
- Unlabeled use of topical eye drops: cystoid macular edema

Adverse effects in *Italics* are most common; those in **Bold** are life-threatening.

IV preparation
- Closure of hemodynamically significant patent ductus arteriosus in premature infants weighing between 500–1,750 g, if 48 hr of usual medical management is not effective

Contraindications and cautions
- *Oral and rectal preparations:* allergy to indomethacin, salicylates, or other NSAIDs; CV dysfunction, hypertension; peptic ulceration, GI bleeding; history of proctitis or rectal bleeding; impaired hepatic or renal function; pregnancy; labor and delivery; lactation.
- *IV preparations:* proven or suspected infection; bleeding, thrombocytopenia, coagulation defects; necrotizing enterocolitis; renal impairment; local irritation if extravasation occurs.

Available forms
Capsules—25, 50 mg; SR capsules—75 mg; oral suspension—25 mg/5 mL; suppositories—50 mg; powder for injection—1 mg

Dosages
Adults
- *Osteoarthritis or rheumatoid arthritis, ankylosing spondylitis:* 25 mg PO bid or tid. If tolerated, increase dose by 25- or 50-mg increments if needed up to total daily dose of 150–200 mg/day PO.
- *Acute painful shoulder:* 75–150 mg/day PO, in 3–4 divided doses. Discontinue drug after inflammation is controlled, usually 7–14 days.
- *Acute gouty arthritis:* 50 mg PO, tid until pain is tolerable, then rapidly decrease dose until no longer needed, usually within 3–5 days.
Pediatric patients
Safety and efficacy have not been established. When special circumstances warrant use in children older than 2 yr, initial dose is 2 mg/kg/day in divided doses PO. Do not exceed 4 mg/kg/day or 150–200 mg/day, whichever is less.
IV
Three IV doses given at 12- to 24-hr intervals.

Age	1st Dose	2nd Dose	3rd Dose
< 48 hr	0.2 mg/kg	0.1 mg/kg	0.1 mg/kg
2–7 days	0.2 mg/kg	0.2 mg/kg	0.2 mg/kg
> 7 days	0.2 mg/kg	0.25 mg/kg	0.25 mg/kg

If marked anuria or oliguria occurs, do not give additional doses. If ductus reopens, course of therapy may be repeated at 12- to 24-hr intervals.

Pharmacokinetics

Route	Onset	Peak	Duration
Oral	30 min	1–2 hr	4–6 hr
IV	Immediate		15–30 min

Metabolism: Hepatic; $T_{1/2}$: 4.5–6 hr
Distribution: Crosses placenta; enters breast milk
Excretion: Urine

▼ IV facts
Preparation: Reconstitute solution with 1–2 mL of 0.9% sodium chloride injection or water for injection; diluents should be preservative free. If 1 mL of diluent is used, concentration is 0.1 mg/0.1 mL. If 2 mL of diluent is used, concentration is 0.05 mg/0.1 mL. Discard any unused portion of the solution; prepare fresh solution before each dose.
Infusion: Inject reconstituted solution IV over 5–10 sec; further dilution is not recommended.

Adverse effects
NSAIDs: Oral, suppositories
- **CNS:** *Headache, dizziness, somnolence, insomnia,* fatigue, tiredness, dizziness, tinnitus, ophthalmologic effects
- **Dermatologic:** *Rash,* pruritus, sweating, dry mucous membranes, stomatitis
- **GI:** *Nausea, dyspepsia, GI pain,* diarrhea, vomiting, *constipation,* flatulence
- **GU:** Dysuria, renal impairment
- **Hematologic:** Bleeding, platelet inhibition with higher doses, neutropenia, eosinophilia, leukopenia, pancytopenia, thrombocytopenia, agranulocytosis, granulocytopenia, aplastic anemia, decreased Hgb or Hct, bone marrow depression, mennorhagia
- **Respiratory:** Dyspnea, hemoptysis, pharyngitis, bronchospasm, rhinitis
- **Other:** Peripheral edema, **anaphylactoid reactions to anaphylactic shock**
IV preparation
- **GI:** *GI bleeding, vomiting,* abdominal distention, transient ileus
- **GU:** Renal dysfunction
- **Hematologic:** *Increased bleeding problems,* including intracranial bleed, **dis-**

seminated intravascular coagulopathy, hyponatremia, hyperkalemia, hypoglycemia, fluid retention
- **Respiratory:** *Apnea, exacerbation of pulmonary infection,* **pulmonary hemorrhage**
- **Other:** Retrolental fibroplasia

Interactions
✳ Drug-drug • Increased toxic effects of lithium • Decreased diuretic effect with loop diuretics: bumetanide, furosemide, ethacrynic acid • Potential decrease in antihypertensive effect of beta-adrenergic blocking agents, captopril, lisinopril, enalapril

■ Nursing considerations
Assessment
- **History:** Oral and rectal preparations: allergy to indomethacin, salicylates, or other NSAIDs; CV dysfunction, hypertension; peptic ulceration, GI bleeding; history of proctitis or rectal bleeding; impaired hepatic or renal function; pregnancy; labor and delivery. IV preparations: proven or suspected infection; bleeding, thrombocytopenia, coagulation defects; necrotizing enterocolitis; renal impairment; local irritation if extravasation occurs
- **Physical:** Skin color, lesions; T; orientation, reflexes, ophthalmologic evaluation, audiometric evaluation, peripheral sensation; P, BP, edema; R, adventitious sounds; liver evaluation, bowel sounds; CBC, clotting times, urinalysis, renal and liver function tests, serum electrolytes, stool guaiac

Interventions
Oral and rectal preparations
- Give drug with food or after meals if GI upset occurs.
- Do not give sustained-release tablets for gouty arthritis.
- Arrange for periodic ophthalmologic examination during long-term therapy.
- Discontinue drug if eye changes, symptoms of liver or renal dysfunction occur.
- Institute emergency procedures if overdose occurs: gastric lavage, induction of emesis, support.

- Test renal function between doses. If severe renal impairment is noted, do not give the next dose.

Teaching points
- Use the drug only as suggested; avoid overdose. Take the drug with food or after meals if GI upset occurs. Do not exceed the prescribed dosage.
- These side effects may occur: nausea, GI upset, dyspepsia (take drug with food); diarrhea or constipation; drowsiness, dizziness, vertigo, insomnia (use caution if driving or operating dangerous machinery).
- Report sore throat, fever, rash, itching, weight gain, swelling in ankles or fingers, changes in vision, black tarry stools.
- Parents of infants receiving IV therapy for PDA will need support and encouragement and an explanation of the drug's action; this is best incorporated into the teaching about the disease.

▽ infliximab
See *Less Commonly Used Drugs,* p. 1344.

▽ insulin
(in' su lin)

Insulin injection: Humulin R, Humulin R Regular U-500 (concentrated), Novolin R, Novolin R PenFill, Novolin ge Toronto (CAN), Regular Iletin II, Velosulin Human BR

Insulin lispro: Humalog

Isophane insulin suspension (NPH): Humulin N, Novolin N, Novolin N PenFill, Novolin ge (CAN), NPH Iletin II

Insulin zinc suspension (Lente): Humulin-L, Lente Iletin II, Lente L, Novolin ge lente (CAN), Novolin L

Protamine zinc suspension (PZI): Iletin PZI (CAN)

Insulin zinc suspension, extended (Ultralente): Humulin U

(CAN), Humulin U Ultralente
Insulin injection concentrated:
Novolin ge Ultralente (CAN), Regular (concentrated) Iletin II
Insulin Aspart: Novolog
Insulin Glargine: Lantus
Combination insulins: Humalog 75/25, Humalog 50/50, Humulin 70/30, Humulin 50/50, Novolin 70/30

PREGNANCY CATEGORY B

Drug classes
Antidiabetic agent
Hormone

Therapeutic actions
Insulin is a hormone that, by receptor-mediated effects, promotes the storage of the body's fuels, facilitating the transport of metabolites and ions (potassium) through cell membranes and stimulating the synthesis of glycogen from glucose, of fats from lipids, and proteins from amino acids.

Indications
- Treatment of diabetes mellitus type 1
- Treatment of diabetes mellitus type 2 that cannot be controlled by diet or oral agents
- Treatment of severe ketoacidosis or diabetic coma (regular insulin injection)
- Treatment of hyperkalemia with infusion of glucose to produce a shift of potassium into the cells
- Highly purified and human insulins promoted for short courses of therapy (surgery, intercurrent disease), newly diagnosed patients, patients with poor metabolic control, and patients with gestational diabetes
- Insulin injection concentrated indicated for treatment of diabetic patients with marked insulin resistance (requirements of > 200 units/day)

Contraindications and cautions
- Allergy to pork products (varies with preparations; use of human insulin removes this caution); pregnancy (keep patients under close supervision; rigid control is desired; following delivery, requirements may drop for 24–72 hr, rising to normal levels during next 6 wk); lactation (monitor mother carefully; insulin requirements may decrease during lactation).

Available forms
Injection—100 units/mL, 500 units/mL (concentrated); pre-filled cartridges—100 units/mL

Dosages
Adults and pediatric patients
General guidelines: 0.5–1 unit/kg/day. The number and size of daily doses, times of administration, and type of insulin preparation are determined after close medical scrutiny of the patient's blood and urine glucose, diet, exercise, and intercurrent infections and other stresses. Usually given SC. Regular insulin may be given IV or IM in diabetic coma or ketoacidosis. Insulin injection concentrated may be given SC or IM, but do not administer IV.

Pharmacokinetics

Type	Onset	Peak	Duration
Regular	30–60 min	2–3 hr	6–8 hr
Semilente	1–1.5 hr	5–10 hr	12–16 hr
NPH	1–1.5 hr	4–12 hr	24 hr
Lente	1–2.5 hr	7–15 hr	24 hr
PZI	4–8 hr	14–24 hr	36 hr
Ultralente	4–8 hr	10–30 hr	> 36 hr
Lispro	< 15 min	30–90 min	6–8 hr
Aspart	10–20 min	1–3 hr	3–5 hr
Glargine	60 min	None	24 hr
Combination Insulins	30–60 min, then 1–2 hr	2–4 hr, then 6–12 hr	6–8 hr, then 18–24 hr

Metabolism: Cellular; $T_{1/2}$: varies with preparation
Distribution: Crosses placenta; does not enter breast milk

▼IV facts
Preparation: May be mixed with standard IV solutions; use of plastic tubing or bag will change the amount of insulin delivered.
Infusion: Use of a monitored delivery system is suggested. Rate should be determined by patient response and glucose levels.
Incompatibilities: Do not add to aminophylline, amobarbital, chlorothiazide, cytarabine, dobutamine, methylprednisolone, pentobarbital, phenobarbital, phenytoin, secobarbital, sodium bicarbonate, thiopental.

Adverse effects

- **Hypersensitivity:** Rash, **anaphylaxis or angioedema**
- **Local:** Allergy—local reactions at injection site—redness, swelling, itching; usually resolves in a few days to a few weeks; a change in type or species source of insulin may be tried
- **Metabolic:** Hypoglycemia; ketoacidosis

Interactions

✳ **Drug-drug** • Increased hypoglycemic effects of insulin with monoamine oxidase inhibitors, beta-blockers, salicylates, alcohol • Delayed recovery from hypoglycemic episodes and masked signs and symptoms of hypoglycemia if taken with beta-adrenergic blocking agents

✳ **Drug-alternative therapy** • Increased risk of hypoglycemia if taken with juniper berries, ginseng, garlic, fenugreek, coriander, dandelion root, celery

■ Nursing considerations

CLINICAL ALERT!
Name confusion may occur between Lantus and Lente insulin; use *extreme* caution.

Assessment

- **History:** Allergy to pork products; pregnancy; lactation
- **Physical:** Skin color, lesions; eyeball turgor; orientation, reflexes, peripheral sensation; P, BP, adventitious sounds; R, adventitious sounds; urinalysis, blood glucose

Interventions

- Ensure uniform dispersion of insulin suspensions by rolling the vial gently between hands; avoid vigorous shaking.
- Give maintenance doses SC, rotating injection sites regularly to decrease incidence of lipodystrophy; give regular insulin IV or IM in severe ketoacidosis or diabetic coma.
- Monitor patients receiving insulin IV carefully; plastic IV infusion sets have been reported to remove 20%–80% of the insulin; dosage delivered to the patient will vary.

- Do not give insulin injection concentrated IV; severe anaphylactic reactions can occur.
- Use caution when mixing two types of insulin; always draw the regular insulin into the syringe first; if mixing with insulin lispro, draw the lispro first; use mixtures of regular and NPH or regular and Lente insulins within 5–15 min of combining them; *Lantus* insulin (insulin glargine) cannot be mixed in solution with any other drug, including other insulins.
- Double-check, or have a colleague check, the dosage drawn up for pediatric patients, for patients receiving concentrated insulin injection, or patients receiving very small doses; even small errors in dosage can cause serious problems.
- Monitor patients being switched from one type of insulin to another carefully; dosage adjustments are often needed. Human insulins often require smaller doses than beef or pork insulin; monitor cautiously if patients are switched; lispro insulin is given 15 min before a meal.
- Store insulin in a cool place away from direct sunlight. Refrigeration is preferred. Do not freeze insulin. Insulin prefilled in glass or plastic syringes is stable for 1 wk refrigerated; this is a safe way of ensuring proper dosage for patients with limited vision or who have problems with drawing up insulin.
- Monitor urine or serum glucose levels frequently to determine effectiveness of drug and dosage. Patients can learn to adjust insulin dosage on a sliding scale based on test results.
- Monitor insulin needs during times of trauma or severe stress; dosage adjustments may be needed.
- Maintain life support equipment, glucose on standby to deal with ketoacidosis or hypoglycemic reactions.

Teaching points

- Use the same type and brand of syringe; use the same type and brand of insulin to avoid dosage errors.
- Do not change the order of mixing insulins. Rotate injection sites regularly (keep a chart) to prevent breakdown at injection sites.

Adverse effects in *Italics* are most common; those in **Bold** are life-threatening.

- Dosage may vary with activities, stress, diet. Monitor blood or urine glucose levels, and consult physician if problems arise.
- Store drug in the refrigerator or in a cool place out of direct sunlight; do not freeze insulin.
- Monitor your urine or blood for glucose and ketones as prescribed.
- Wear a medical alert tag stating that you are a diabetic taking insulin so that emergency medical personnel will take proper care of you.
- Avoid alcohol; serious reactions can occur.
- Report fever, sore throat, vomiting, hypoglycemic or hyperglycemic reactions, rash.

▽interferon alfa-2a (IFLrA, rIFN-A)
(in ter feer' on)

Roferon-A

PREGNANCY CATEGORY C

Drug classes
Antineoplastic
Interferon

Therapeutic actions
Inhibits growth of tumor cells: mechanism of action is not clearly understood; prevents tumor cells from multiplying and modulates host immune response. Interferons are produced by human leukocytes in response to viral infections and other stimuli. Interferon alfa-2a is produced by recombinant DNA technology using *Escherichia coli*.

Indications
- Treatment of hepatitis C in select patients ≥ 18 yr
- Hairy cell leukemia in selected patients ≥ 18 yr
- AIDS-related Kaposi's sarcoma in selected patients ≥ 18 yr
- Treatment of chronic myelogenous leukemia in chronic phase in Philadelphia chromosome–positive patient
- Orphan drug uses: treatment of advanced colorectal cancer, esophageal carcinoma, metastatic malignant melanoma, renal cell carcinoma

- Unlabeled uses: treatment of several malignant and viral conditions, phase I AIDS, ARC

Contraindications and cautions
- Contraindicated with allergy to interferon alfa or any components of the product; pregnancy, lactation.
- Use cautiously with pancreatitis, hepatic or renal disease, seizure disorders, compromised CNS function, cardiac disease or history of cardiac disease, bone marrow depression, suicidal tendencies, neuropsychiatric disorders, autoimmune diseases.

Available forms
Injection solution—3 million IU/mL, 6 million IU/mL, 9 million IU/0.9 mL, 36 million IU/mL; prefilled syringes 6 million, 9 million IU/0.5 mL

Dosages
Adults
- *Chronic hepatitis C:* 3 million IU IM or SC 3 times/wk for 12 mo.
- *Hairy cell leukemia:* Induction dose: 3 million IU/day SC or IM for 16–24 wk. Maintenance dose: 3 million IU/day 3 times/wk. Treat patient for approximately 6 mo, then evaluate response before continuing therapy. Treatment for up to 20 mo has been reported. Dosage may need to be adjusted downward based on adverse reactions.
- *AIDS-related Kaposi's sarcoma:* 36 million IU daily for 10–12 wk IM or SC. Maintenance: 36 million IU 3 times/wk. Reduce dose by one-half or withhold individual doses when severe adverse reactions occur. Continue treatment until tumor disappears or until discontinuation is required.
- *CML:* Induction dose: 9 million IU daily IM or SC. Continue therapy until disease progresses or adverse effects are severe.

Pediatric patients
Safety and efficacy not established in patients < 18 yr.

Pharmacokinetics

Route	Onset	Peak
IM	Rapid	3.8 hr
SC	Slow	7.3 hr

Metabolism: Hepatic and renal; $T_{1/2}$: 3.7–8.5 hr

Distribution: Crosses placenta; may enter breast milk

Excretion: Urine

Adverse effects

- **CNS:** *Dizziness, confusion,* paresthesias, numbness, lethargy, decreased mental status, depression, **suicidal ideation,** visual disturbances, sleep disturbances, nervousness
- **CV:** Hypotension, edema, hypertension, chest pain, arrhythmias, palpitations
- **Dermatologic:** Rash, dryness, or inflammation of the oropharynx; dry skin; pruritus; partial alopecia
- **GI:** *Anorexia, nausea,* diarrhea, vomiting, change in taste
- **GU:** Impairment of fertility in women, transient impotence in men
- **Hematologic:** Leukopenia, neutropenia, thrombocytopenia, anemia, decreased Hgb; increased levels of AST, LDH, alkaline phosphatase, bilirubin, uric acid, serum creatinine, BUN, blood sugar, serum phosphorus, neutralizing antibodies; hypocalcemia
- **Other:** *Flulike syndrome,* weight loss, diaphoresis, arthralgia

■ Nursing considerations
Assessment

- **History:** Allergy to interferon alfa or any product components, pancreatitis, hepatic or renal disease, seizure disorders, compromised CNS function, cardiac disease or history of cardiac disease, bone marrow depression, pregnancy, lactation
- **Physical:** Weight; T; skin color, lesions; orientation, reflexes; P, BP, edema, ECG; liver evaluation; CBC, blood glucose, liver and renal function tests, urinalysis

Interventions

- Obtain laboratory tests (CBC, differential, granulocytes and hairy cells, bone marrow hairy cells, and liver function tests) before therapy and monthly during therapy.
- Monitor for severe reactions; notify physician immediately; dosage reduction or discontinuation may be necessary.
- Refrigerate solution; do not shake.

- Ensure that patient is well hydrated, especially during initiation of treatment.
- Provide small, frequent meals if GI problems occur.
- Counsel female patients to use some form of birth control. Drug is contraindicated in pregnancy.
- Assure patient that all steps possible are taken to ensure that there is little risk of hepatitis and AIDS from use of human blood products.

Teaching points

- Prepare a calendar to check off as drug is given. You and a significant other should learn the proper technique for SC or IM injection for outpatient use. Do not change brands of interferon without consulting with physician.
- Refrigerate solution; do not shake.
- These side effects may occur: loss of appetite, nausea, vomiting (frequent mouth care, small frequent meals may help; maintain good nutrition; a dietitian may be able to help; an antiemetic also may be ordered); fatigue, confusion, dizziness, numbness, visual disturbances, depression (transient; avoid injury; avoid driving or using dangerous machinery); impotence (transient); fetal deformities or death (use birth control); depression, suicidal ideation (advise health care provider immediately if these occur).
- Arrange for regular blood tests to monitor the drug's effects.
- Report fever, chills, sore throat, unusual bleeding or bruising, chest pain, palpitations, dizziness, changes in mental status, depression, suicidal ideation.

▷interferon alfa-2b
(IFN-α2, rIFN-a2,
a-2-interferon)
(in ter feer' on)

Intron-A

PREGNANCY CATEGORY C

Drug classes
Antineoplastic
Interferon

Adverse effects in *Italics* are most common; those in **Bold** are life-threatening.

Therapeutic actions

Inhibits growth of tumor cells; mechanism of action is not clearly understood; prevents the replication of tumor cells and enhances host immune response. Interferons are produced by human leukocytes in response to viral infections and other stimuli. Interferon alfa-2b is produced by recombinant DNA technology using *Escherichia coli.*

Indications

- Hairy cell leukemia in patients ≥ 18 yr
- Intralesional treatment of condylomata acuminata in patients ≥ 18 yr
- AIDS-related Kaposi's sarcoma in patients ≥ 18 yr
- Treatment of malignant melanoma in patients > 18 yr
- Treatment of chronic hepatitis C in patients ≥ 18 yr
- Treatment of chronic hepatitis B in patients ≥ 18 yr
- Orphan drug uses: chronic myelogenous leukemia, metastatic renal cell carcinoma, ovarian carcinoma, invasive carcinoma of cervix, primary malignant brain tumors, laryngeal papillomatosis, carcinoma in situ of urinary bladder, chronic delta hepatitis, acute hepatitis B
- Unlabeled uses: treatment of several malignant and viral conditions

Contraindications and cautions

- Contraindicated with allergy to interferon-alfa or any components of the product; lactation.
- Use cautiously with cardiac disease, pulmonary disease, diabetes mellitus prone to ketoacidosis, coagulation disorders, bone marrow depression, pregnancy, neuropsychiatric disorders, autoimmune diseases.

Available forms

Powder for injection—3, 5, 10, 18, 25, 50 million IU/vial; solution for injection—3, 5, 10, 18, 25 million IU

Dosages
Adults

- *Hairy cell leukemia:* 2 million IU/m^2 SC or IM 3 times/wk. Continue for several months, depending on clinical and hematologic response.

- *Condylomata acuminata:* 1 million IU/lesion 3 times/wk for 3 wk intralesionally. Maximum response occurs 4–8 wk after initiation of therapy.
- *Chronic hepatitis C:* 3 million IU SC or IM, 3 times/wk for 18–24 mo.
- *AIDS-related Kaposi's sarcoma:* 30 million IU/m^2 3 times/wk SC or IM. Maintain dosage until disease progresses rapidly or severe intolerance occurs.
- *Chronic hepatitis B:* 30–35 million IU/wk SC or IM either as 5 million IU daily or 10 million IU 3 times/wk for 16 wk.
- *Malignant melanoma:* 20 million IU/m^2 IV on 5 consecutive days/wk for 4 wk; maintenance: 10 million IU/m^2 IV 3 times/wk for 48 wk.

Pediatric patients

Safety and efficacy not established in patients < 18 yr.

Pharmacokinetics

Route	Onset	Peak
IM, SC	Rapid	3–12 hr
IV	Rapid	End of infusion

Metabolism: Renal; T$_{1/2}$: 2–3 hr
Distribution: Crosses placenta; may enter breast milk
Excretion: Unknown

▼IV facts

Preparation: Inject diluent (bacteriostatic water for injection) into vial using chart provided by manufacturer; agitate gently, withdraw with sterile syringe, inject into 100 mL of normal saline.
Infusion: Administer each dose slowly over 20 min.

Adverse effects

- **CNS:** *Dizziness, confusion,* paresthesias, numbness, lethargy, decreased mental status, depression, visual disturbances, sleep disturbances, nervousness
- **CV:** Hypotension, edema, hypertension, chest pain, arrhythmias, palpitations
- **Dermatologic:** *Rash,* dryness or inflammation of the oropharynx, *dry skin, pruritus,* partial alopecia
- **GI:** *Anorexia, nausea,* diarrhea, vomiting, change in taste

- **GU:** Impaired fertility in women, transient impotence
- **Hematologic:** Leukopenia, neutropenia, thrombocytopenia, anemia, decreased Hgb; increased levels of AST, LDH, alkaline phosphatase, bilirubin, uric acid, serum creatinine, BUN, blood sugar, serum phosphorus, neutralizing antibodies; hypocalcemia
- **Other:** *Flulike syndrome,* weight loss, diaphoresis, arthralgia

■ Nursing considerations
Assessment

- **History:** Allergy to interferon-alfa or product components, cardiac or pulmonary disease, diabetes mellitus prone to ketoacidosis, coagulation disorders, bone marrow depression, pregnancy, lactation
- **Physical:** Weight; T; skin color, lesions; orientation, reflexes; P, BP, edema, ECG; liver evaluation; CBC, blood glucose, liver and renal function tests, urinalysis

Interventions

- Obtain laboratory tests (CBC, differential, granulocytes and hairy cells, bone marrow and hairy cells) before therapy and monthly during therapy.
- Prepare solution as follows:

Vial Strength In Million IU	Amount of Diluent in mL	Final Concentration in Million IU/mL
3	1	3
5	1	5
10	2	5
25	5	5
10	1	10
50	1	50

- Use bacteriostatic water for injection as diluent. Agitate gently. After reconstitution, stable for 1 mo if refrigerated.
- Administer IM or SC.
- Monitor for severe reactions, including hypersensitivity reactions; notify physician immediately; dosage reduction or discontinuation may be necessary.
- Ensure that patient is well hydrated, especially during initiation of treatment.

Teaching points

- Prepare a calendar to check off as drug is given. You and a significant other should learn the proper technique for SC or IM injection for outpatient use. Do not change brands of interferon without consulting your health care provider.
- These side effects may occur: loss of appetite, nausea, vomiting (frequent mouth care, small frequent meals may help; maintain good nutrition; a dietitian may be able to help; an antiemetic also may be ordered); fatigue, confusion, dizziness, numbness, visual disturbances, depression (use special precautions to avoid injury; avoid driving or using dangerous machinery); flulike syndrome (take drug at bedtime; ensure rest periods for yourself; a medication may be ordered for fever).
- Arrange for regular blood tests to monitor the drug's effects.
- Report fever, chills, sore throat, unusual bleeding or bruising, chest pain, palpitations, dizziness, changes in mental status.

▽interferon alfa-n3

See *Less Commonly Used Drugs,* p. 1344.

▽interferon alfacon-1
(in ter feer' on)

Infergen

PREGNANCY CATEGORY C

Drug class
Interferon

Therapeutic actions

Interferons are produced by human leukocytes in response to viral infections and other stimuli; interferon alfacon-1 blocks replication of viruses and stimulates the host immunoregulatory activities; type 1 interferons exhibit antiviral, natural killer cell activation, cytokine induction activity; produced by recombinant DNA technology with *E. coli* bacteria.

Adverse effects in *Italics* are most common; those in **Bold** are life-threatening.

Indications
- Treatment of chronic hepatitis C infection in patients > 18 yr of age with compensated liver disease who have HCV antibodies
- Unlabeled uses: treatment of hairy cell leukemia in combination with G-CSF therapy

Contraindications and cautions
- Contraindicated with allergy to alfa interferons or product derived from *E. coli*, pregnancy, lactation.
- Use cautiously with a history of psychotic events, cardiac disease, hepatic dysfunction.

Available forms
Injection—9, 15 mcg

Dosages
Adults
9 mcg SC as a single injection, 3 times/wk for 24 wk; at least 48 hr must elapse between doses.
Pediatric patients
Safety and efficacy not established in patients < 18 yr.

Pharmacokinetics

Route	Onset	Peak
SC	Slow	24–36 hr

Metabolism: Hepatic and renal; $T_{1/2}$: unknown
Distribution: Crosses placenta; may pass into breast milk
Excretion: Urine

Adverse effects
- **CNS:** *Dizziness, insomnia,* paresthesias, amnesia, hypoesthesia, **psychotic episodes,** depression, anxiety, *nervousness*
- **CV:** Hypertension, chest pain, palpitations
- **Dermatologic:** *Alopecia, pruritus,* rash, erythema, dry skin
- **GI:** *Anorexia, nausea, diarrhea,* vomiting, change in taste, *abdominal pain*
- **GU:** Impairment of fertility in women, transient impotence
- **Hematologic:** *Granulocytosis, thrombocytopenia,* leukopenia
- **Respiratory:** *Pharyngitis, upper respiratory infection, cough, sinusitis,* rhinitis, congestion, dyspnea
- **Other:** *Flulike syndrome,* weight loss, diaphoresis, arthralgia, *injection site reaction*

■ Nursing considerations
Assessment
- **History:** Allergy to alfa interferon or *E. coli*–produced products, mental disorders, cardiac or hepatic disease, pregnancy, lactation
- **Physical:** Weight; T; skin color, lesions; orientation, reflexes; P, BP, edema; R, adventitious sounds; liver evaluation; CBC

Interventions
- Arrange for laboratory tests (CBC, differential, HCV antibodies) before beginning therapy.
- Monitor for severe reactions of any kind; notify prescriber immediately. Dosage reduction or discontinuation of drug may be necessary.
- Refrigerate vials; avoid vigorous shaking; discard any unused portions.
- Ensure that patient is well hydrated, especially during initiation of treatment.
- Arrange for supportive treatment if flulike syndrome occurs: rest, acetaminophen for fever and headache, environmental control.
- Monitor patients with any history of mental disorders or suicidal tendencies carefully for any evidence of psychotic reaction, which can be severe.
- Consult with physician for antiemetic for severe nausea and vomiting.
- Counsel female patients to use some form of birth control while on this drug. Drug is contraindicated in pregnancy.

Teaching points
- Store vial in refrigerator; do not shake. Inject SC into arms, abdomen, hips, thighs. Vial is for single use only. Discard any unused portions.
- Keep a chart of injection sites to prevent overuse of one area.
- These side effects may occur: loss of appetite, nausea, vomiting (use frequent mouth care; eat small, frequent meals; an antiemetic may also be ordered); fatigue, confusion, dizziness, numbness, visual disturbances, depression (use special precautions to avoid

injury; avoid driving or using dangerous machinery).
- Arrange for regular follow-up; this drug will be given for 24 wk.
- Avoid pregnancy while on this drug; use of barrier contraceptives is advised.
- Report fever, chills, sore throat, unusual bleeding or bruising, chest pain, palpitations, dizziness, changes in mental status.

▽interferon beta-1a
(in ter feer' on)

Avonex, Rebif

PREGNANCY CATEGORY C

Drug class
Interferon

Therapeutic actions
Interferons are produced by human leukocytes in response to viral infections and other stimuli; interferon beta-1a blocks replication of viruses and stimulates the host immunoregulatory activities. It is produced by Chinese hamster ovary cells.

Indications
- Multiple sclerosis—treatment of relapsing forms of MS to slow accumulation of physical disability and decrease frequency of clinical exacerbations
- Unlabeled uses: treatment of AIDS, AIDS-related Kaposi's sarcoma, metastatic renal-cell carcinoma, malignant melanoma, cutaneous T-cell lymphoma, acute non-A non-B hepatitis

Contraindications and cautions
- Contraindicated with allergy to beta interferon or any components of product, pregnancy, lactation
- Use cautiously with chronic progressive MS, suicidal tendencies or mental disorders, cardiac disease, seizures

Available forms
Powder for injection—33 mcg (*Avonex*); 22, 44 mcg (*Rebif*)

Dosages
Adults
30 mcg IM once/wk (*Avonex*); 44 mcg SC 3 times/wk (*Rebif*)—start with 8.8 mcg 3 times/wk and titrate up over 5 wk.
Pediatric patients
Safety and efficacy not established in patients < 18 yr.

Pharmacokinetics

Route	Onset	Peak	Duration
IM	12 hr	48 hr	4 days

Metabolism: Hepatic and renal; $T_{1/2}$: 10 hr
Distribution: Crosses placenta; may pass into breast milk
Excretion: Urine

Adverse effects
- **CNS:** *Dizziness, confusion,* paresthesias, numbness, lethargy, decreased mental status, depression, visual disturbances, sleep disturbances, nervousness
- **CV:** Hypotension, edema, hypertension, chest pain, arrhythmias, palpitations
- **Dermatologic:** *Photosensitivity,* rash, alopecia, sweating
- **GI:** *Anorexia, nausea,* diarrhea, vomiting, change in taste
- **GU:** Impairment of fertility in women, transient impotence
- **Hematologic:** Leukopenia, neutropenia, thrombocytopenia, anemia, decreased Hgb; increased levels of AST, LDH, alkaline phosphatase, bilirubin, uric acid, serum creatinine, BUN, blood sugar, serum phosphorus, neutralizing antibodies; hypocalcemia
- **Other:** *Flulike syndrome,* weight loss, diaphoresis, arthralgia, injection site reaction

■ Nursing considerations
Assessment
- **History:** Allergy to beta interferon or any component of product, mental disorders, suicidal tendencies, cardiac disease, seizures, depression, pregnancy, lactation
- **Physical:** Weight; T; skin color, lesions; orientation, reflexes; P, BP, edema, ECG; liver evaluation; CBC, blood glucose, liver and renal function tests, urinalysis

Interventions

- Arrange for laboratory tests—CBC, differential, granulocytes and hairy cells and bone marrow hairy cells, and liver function tests—before and monthly during therapy.
- Reconstitute with 1.1 mL of diluent and swirl gently to dissolve; use within 6 hr (*Avonex*).
- Ensure that patient is well hydrated, especially during initiation of treatment.
- Ensure regular follow-up and treatment of MS; this drug is not a cure.
- Arrange for supportive treatment if flulike syndrome occurs: rest, acetaminophen for fever and headache, environmental control.
- Carefully monitor patients with any history of mental disorders or suicidal tendencies.
- Counsel female patients to use birth control while on this drug. Drug is contraindicated in pregnancy.

Teaching points

- *Avonex* needs to be given weekly. If you or significant other can give an IM injection: store vial in refrigerator, reconstitute with 1.1 mL of diluent and swirl gently, use within 6 hr. Do not give in the same site each week.
- *Rebif* needs to be given 3 times per wk subcutaneously, preferably at the same time of day and on the same days of the week. Store in refrigerator, reconstitute with solution provided, discard any solution remaining in the syringe. Rotate injection sites.
- Keep a chart of injection sites to prevent overuse of one area.
- These side effects may occur: loss of appetite, nausea, vomiting (use frequent mouth care; eat small, frequent meals; maintain good nutrition if possible—dietitian may be able to help; antiemetics may be ordered); fatigue, confusion, dizziness, numbness, visual disturbances, depression (use caution to avoid injury; avoid driving or using dangerous machinery); impotence (usually transient); sensitivity to sunlight (use a sunscreen, wear protective clothing if exposure to sun cannot be prevented).
- Arrange for regular treatment and follow-up of MS; this drug is not a cure.
- Report fever, chills, sore throat, unusual bleeding or bruising, chest pain, palpitations, dizziness, changes in mental status.

▽interferon beta-1b (rIFN-B)

(in ter feer' on)

Betaseron

PREGNANCY CATEGORY C

Drug class
Interferon

Therapeutic actions
Interferons are produced by human leukocytes in response to viral infections and other stimuli; interferon beta-1b block replication of viruses and stimulate the host immunoregulatory activities. Interferon beta-1b are produced by recombinant DNA technology using *E. coli.*

Indications
- Reduce the frequency of clinical exacerbations in relapsing, remitting multiple sclerosis (MS)
- Unlabeled uses: treatment of AIDS, AIDS-related Kaposi's sarcoma, metastatic renal cell carcinoma, malignant melanoma, cutaneous T-cell lymphoma, acute non-A, non-B hepatitis

Contraindications and cautions
- Contraindicated with allergy to beta interferon, human albumin, or product components; pregnancy, lactation.
- Use cautiously with chronic progressive MS, suicidal tendencies, or mental disorders.

Available forms
Powder for injection—0.3 mg

Dosages
Adults
0.25 mg SC every other day; discontinue use if disease is unremitting > 6 mo.
Pediatric patients
Safety and efficacy not established in patients < 18 yr.

Pharmacokinetics

Route	Onset	Peak
SC	Slow	1–8 hr

Metabolism: Hepatic and renal; $T_{1/2}$: 8 min–4.3 hr
Distribution: Crosses placenta; may enter breast milk
Excretion: Urine

Adverse effects

- **CNS:** *Dizziness, confusion,* paresthesias, numbness, lethargy, decreased mental status, depression, visual disturbances, sleep disturbances, nervousness
- **CV:** Hypotension, edema, hypertension, chest pain, arrhythmias, palpitations
- **Dermatologic:** *Photosensitivity,* rash, alopecia, sweating
- **GI:** *Anorexia, nausea,* diarrhea, vomiting, change in taste
- **GU:** Impairment of fertility in women, transient impotence
- **Hematologic:** Leukopenia, neutropenia, thrombocytopenia, anemia, decreased Hgb; increased levels of AST, LDH, alkaline phosphatase, bilirubin, uric acid, serum creatinine, BUN, blood sugar, serum phosphorus, neutralizing antibodies; hypocalcemia
- **Other:** *Flulike syndrome,* weight loss, diaphoresis, arthralgia, injection site reaction

■ Nursing considerations
Assessment

- **History:** Allergy to interferon beta or any components of the product, mental disorders, suicidal tendencies, pregnancy, lactation
- **Physical:** Weight; T; skin color, lesions; orientation, reflexes; P, BP, edema, ECG; liver evaluation; CBC, blood glucose, liver and renal function tests, urinalysis

Interventions

- Obtain laboratory tests (CBC, differential, granulocytes and hairy cells, bone marrow hairy cells, and liver function tests) before therapy and monthly during therapy.
- Monitor for severe reactions; notify physician immediately; dosage reduction or discontinuation may be necessary.
- Reconstitute by using a sterile syringe and needle to inject 1.2 mL supplied diluent into vial; gently swirl vial to dissolve drug completely; do not shake. Discard if any partic-

ulate matter or discoloration has occurred. After reconstitution, vial contains 0.25 mg/mL solution. Withdraw 1 mL of reconstituted solution with a sterile syringe fitted with a 27-gauge needle. Inject SC into arms, abdomen, hips, thighs. Vial is for single use only. Discard any unused portions. Refrigerate. Use reconstituted solution within 3 hr.
- Ensure that patient is well hydrated, especially during initiation of treatment.
- Ensure regular follow-up and treatment of MS; this drug is not a cure.
- Monitor patients with any mental disorders or suicidal tendencies carefully.
- Counsel female patients to use birth control. Drug is contraindicated in pregnancy.

Teaching points

- Reconstitute by using a sterile syringe and needle to inject 1.2 mL supplied diluent into vial; gently swirl the vial to dissolve the drug completely; do not shake. Discard if any particulate matter or discoloration has occurred. After reconstitution, vial contains 0.25 mg/mL solution. Withdraw 1 mL of reconstituted solution with a sterile syringe fitted with a 27-gauge needle. Inject SC into arms, abdomen, hips, thighs. Vial is for single use only. Discard any unused portions. Refrigerate. Use reconstituted solution within 3 hr.
- Keep a chart of injection sites to prevent overuse of one area.
- These side effects may occur: loss of appetite, nausea, vomiting (frequent mouth care, small frequent meals may help; maintain good nutrition; a dietitian may be able to help; an antiemetic also may be ordered); fatigue, confusion, dizziness, numbness, visual disturbances, depression (use special precautions to avoid injury; avoid driving or using dangerous machinery); impotence (transient and reversible); sensitivity to the sun (use sunscreen and wear protective clothing if exposed to sun).
- Arrange for regular treatment and follow-up of MS; this drug is not a cure.
- Report fever, chills, sore throat, unusual bleeding or bruising, chest pain, palpitations, dizziness, changes in mental status.

▽interferon gamma-1b
(in ter feer' on)

Actimmune

PREGNANCY CATEGORY C

Drug class
Interferon

Therapeutic actions
Interferons are produced by human leukocytes in response to viral infections and other stimuli; interferon gamma-1b block has potent phagocyte-activating effects; acts as an interleukin; produced by *E. coli* bacteria.

Indications
- For reducing the frequency and severity of serious infections associated with chronic granulomatous disease
- For delaying time to disease progression in patients with severe, malignant osteopetrosis
- Orphan drug use: renal cell carcinoma

Contraindications and cautions
- Contraindicated with allergy to interferon gamma, *E. coli,* or product components; pregnancy, lactation.
- Use cautiously with seizure disorders, compromised CNS function, cardiac disease, myelosuppression.

Available forms
Injection—100 mcg

Dosages
Adults
50 mcg/m^2 (1 million IU/m^2) SC 3 times/wk in patients with body surface area > 0.5 m^2; 1.5 mcg/kg per dose in patients with body surface area < 0.5 m^2.
Pediatric patients
Safety and efficacy not established in patients < 18 yr.

Pharmacokinetics

Route	Onset	Peak
SC	Slow	7 hr

Metabolism: Hepatic and renal; $T_{1/2}$: 2.9–5.9 hr

Distribution: Crosses placenta; may enter breast milk
Excretion: Urine

Adverse effects
- **CNS:** *Dizziness, confusion,* paresthesias, numbness, lethargy, decreased mental status, depression, visual disturbances, sleep disturbances, nervousness
- **CV:** Hypotension, edema, hypertension, chest pain, arrhythmias, palpitations
- **GI:** *Anorexia, nausea,* diarrhea, vomiting, change in taste, pancreatitis
- **Other:** *Flulike syndrome,* weight loss, diaphoresis, arthralgia, injection site reaction

■ Nursing considerations
Assessment
- **History:** Allergy to interferon gamma, *E. coli,* or product components; pregnancy, lactation, seizure disorders, compromised CNS function, cardiac disease, myelosuppression
- **Physical:** Weight; T; skin color, lesions; orientation, reflexes; P, BP, edema, ECG; liver evaluation; CBC, blood glucose, liver and renal function tests, urinalysis

Interventions
- Obtain laboratory tests (CBC, differential, granulocytes and hairy cells, bone marrow and hairy cells, and liver function tests) before therapy and monthly during therapy.
- Monitor for severe reactions; notify physician immediately; dosage reduction or discontinuation may be necessary.
- Store in refrigerator; each vial is for one use only, discard after that time. Discard any vial that has been unrefrigerated for 12 hr.
- Give drug hs if flulike symptoms become a problem.

Teaching points
- Store in refrigerator; each vial is for one use only; discard after that time. Discard vial that has been unrefrigerated for 12 hr. You and a significant other should learn the proper technique for SC injections.
- Keep a chart of injection sites to prevent overuse of one area.
- These side effects may occur: loss of appetite, nausea, vomiting (frequent mouth care, small frequent meals may help; maintain good nutrition; a dietitian may be able to

help; an antiemetic also may be ordered); fatigue, confusion, dizziness, numbness, visual disturbances, depression (use special precautions to avoid injury; avoid driving or using dangerous machinery); flulike symptoms (eg, fever, chills, aches, pains; rest, acetaminophen for fever and headache; take drug at bedtime).

- Report fever, chills, sore throat, unusual bleeding or bruising, chest pain, palpitations, dizziness, changes in mental status.

▽ iodine thyroid products
(eye' oh dine)

Lugol's Solution, Strong Iodine Solution, Thyro-Block

PREGNANCY CATEGORY D

Drug class
Thyroid suppressant

Therapeutic actions
Inhibits synthesis of the active thyroid hormones T_3 and T_4 and inhibits the release of these hormones into circulation.

Indications
- Hyperthyroidism: adjunctive therapy with antithyroid drugs in preparation for thyroidectomy, treatment of thyrotoxic crisis, or neonatal thyrotoxicosis
- Thyroid blocking in a radiation emergency
- Unlabeled uses: potassium iodide has been effective with Sweet's syndrome, treatment of lymphocutaneous sporotrichosis

Contraindications and cautions
- Allergy to iodides; pulmonary edema, pulmonary tuberculosis (sodium iodide); pregnancy; lactation.

Available forms
Solution—5% iodine, 10% potassium iodide; tablets—130 mg potassium iodide

Dosages
Adults
- *RDA:* 150 mcg PO.
- *Preparation for thyroidectomy:* 2–6 drops strong iodine solution tid PO for 10 days prior to surgery.
- *Thyroid blocking in a radiation emergency used as directed by state or local health authorities:* 1 tablet (130 mg potassium iodide) PO or 6 drops (21 mg potassium iodide/drop) added to half glass of liquid per day for 10 days.

Pediatric patients
- *Thyroid blocking in a radiation emergency:* > 1 yr: Adult dose. < 1 yr: one-half of a crushed tablet or 3 drops in a small amount of liquid per day for 10 days. *Note:* Potassium iodide tablets and drops are available only to state and federal agencies.

Pharmacokinetics

Route	Onset	Peak	Duration
Oral	24 hr	10–15 days	6 wk

Metabolism: Hepatic; $T_{1/2}$: unknown
Distribution: Crosses placenta; may enter breast milk
Excretion: Urine

Adverse effects
- **Dermatologic:** *Rash*
- **Endocrine:** Hypothyroidism, hyperthyroidism, goiter
- **GI:** *Swelling of the salivary glands, iodism* (metallic taste, burning mouth and throat, sore teeth and gums, head cold symptoms, stomach upset, diarrhea)
- **Hypersensitivity:** Allergic reactions— fever, joint pains, swelling of the face or body, shortness of breath

Interactions
✷ **Drug-drug** • Increased risk of hypothyroidism if taken concurrently with lithium

■ Nursing considerations

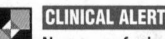 **CLINICAL ALERT!**
Name confusion has occurred between iodine and Lodine (etodolac); use caution.

Assessment

- **History:** Allergy to iodides, pulmonary edema, pulmonary tuberculosis, lactation
- **Physical:** Skin color, lesions, edema; R, adventitious sounds; gums, mucous membranes; T_3 and T_4

Interventions

- Test skin for idiosyncrasy to iodine before giving parenteral doses.
- Dilute strong iodine solution with fruit juice or water to improve taste.
- Crush tablets for small children.
- Discontinue drug if symptoms of acute iodine toxicity occur: vomiting, abdominal pain, diarrhea, circulatory collapse.

Teaching points

- Drops may be diluted in fruit juice or water. Tablets may be crushed.
- Discontinue use and report fever, rash, swelling of the throat, metallic taste, sore teeth and gums, head cold symptoms, severe GI distress, enlargement of the thyroid gland.

▽ **iodoquinol**
(diiodohydroxyquinoline)

(eye oh doe kwin' ole)

Diodoquin (CAN), Yodoquinal (CAN), Yodoxin

PREGNANCY CATEGORY C

Drug class

Amebicide

Therapeutic actions

Directly amebicidal by an unknown mechanism; is poorly absorbed in the GI tract and is able to exert its amebicidal action directly in the large intestine.

Indications

- Acute or chronic intestinal amebiasis

Contraindications and cautions

- Contraindicated with hepatic failure, allergy to iodine preparations or 8-hydroxyquinolines.

- Use cautiously with thyroid disease, pregnancy, lactation.

Available forms

Tablets—210, 650 mg

Dosages

Adults

650 mg tid PO after meals for 20 days.

Pediatric patients

40 mg/kg/day PO, in 3 divided doses for 20 days. Maximum dose: 650 mg/dose. Do not exceed 1.95 g in 24 hr for 20 days.

Pharmacokinetics

Route	Onset
Oral	Slow

Very poorly absorbed; exerts effects locally in the intestine.

Adverse effects

- **CNS:** Blurring of vision, weakness, fatigue, numbness, headache
- **Dermatologic:** *Rash, pruritus*
- **GI:** *Nausea, vomiting, diarrhea,* anorexia
- **Other:** Thyroid enlargement, fever, chills

Interactions

✱ **Drug-lab test** • Interferes with many tests of thyroid function; interference may last up to 6 mo after drug is discontinued

■ Nursing considerations

Assessment

- **History:** Hepatic failure, allergy to iodine preparations or 8-hydroxyquinolines, thyroid disease, lactation, pregnancy
- **Physical:** Skin rashes, lesions; check reflexes, ophthalmologic exam; BP, P, R; liver and thyroid function tests (PBI, T_3 and T_4)

Interventions

- Administer drug after meals.
- Administer for full course of therapy.
- Maintain patient's nutrition.

Teaching points

- Take drug after meals.

- These side effects often occur: GI upset, nausea, vomiting, diarrhea (small frequent meals, frequent mouth care often help).
- Report severe GI upset, rash, blurring of vision, unusual fatigue, fever.

▽ipecac syrup
(ip' e kak)

PMS-Ipecac (CAN)

PREGNANCY CATEGORY C

Drug class
Emetic agent

Therapeutic actions
Produces vomiting by a local GI mucosa irritant effect and a central medullary effect (CTZ stimulation).

Indications
- Treatment of drug overdose and certain poisonings

Contraindications and cautions
- Contraindicated with unconscious, semiconscious, convulsing states; poisoning with corrosives, such as alkalies, strong acids, petroleum distillates.
- Use cautiously with pregnancy.

Available forms
Syrup—1.5%–1.75% alcohol in 15 and 30 mL, 2% alcohol in 15 and 30 mL

Dosages
Repeat dosage if vomiting does not occur within 20–30 min. If vomiting does not occur within 30–45 min of second dose, perform gastric lavage.
Adults
15–30 mL PO followed by 3–4 glasses of water.
Pediatric patients
< 1 yr: 5–10 mL PO followed by one-half to 1 glass of water.
> 1–12 yr: 15 mL PO followed by 2–3 glasses of water.

Pharmacokinetics

Route	Onset	Peak
Oral	Varies	20–30 min

Minimal systemic absorption occurs if taken correctly.

Adverse effects
- **CNS:** *Mild CNS depression*
- **CV:** Heart conduction disturbances, atrial fibrillation, fatal myocarditis if drug is not vomited
- **GI:** *Diarrhea, mild GI upset*

■ Nursing considerations
Assessment
- **History:** Unconscious, semiconscious, convulsing states; poisoning with corrosives; lactation, pregnancy
- **Physical:** Orientation, affect; P, baseline ECG, auscultation; stools, bowel sounds

Interventions
- Give to conscious patients only.
- Give as soon after poisoning as possible.
- Ipecac syrup differs from ipecac fluid extract, which is 14 times stronger and has caused some deaths.
- Consult with a Poison Control Center if in doubt and if vomiting does not occur within 20 min of second dose.
- Give with adequate amounts of water.
- Maintain life support equipment on standby for poisoning and overdose; cardiac support will be needed if vomiting of ipecac does not occur.
- Use activated charcoal if vomiting of ipecac does not occur or if overdose of ipecac occurs.

Teaching points
- Drug is available in premeasured doses for emergency home use.
- Call physician, Poison Control Center, or emergency room in cases of accidental ingestion.
- Give drug with adequate amounts of water. Do not exceed recommended dose.
- These side effects may occur: diarrhea, GI upset, drowsiness and lethargy.

Adverse effects in *Italics* are most common; those in **Bold** are life-threatening.

▽ipratropium bromide
*(i pra **roe'** pee um)*

Alti-Ipratropium (CAN), Apo-Ipravent (CAN), Atrovent, Novo-Ipramide (CAN)

PREGNANCY CATEGORY B

Drug classes
Anticholinergic
Antimuscarinic agent
Parasympatholytic

Therapeutic actions
Anticholinergic, chemically related to atropine, which blocks vagally mediated reflexes by antagonizing the action of acetylcholine.

Indications
- Bronchodilator for maintenance treatment of bronchospasm associated with COPD (solution, aerosol)
- Symptomatic relief of rhinorrhea associated with perennial rhinitis, common cold (nasal spray)

Contraindications and cautions
- Contraindicated with hypersensitivity to atropine or its derivatives, acute episodes of bronchospasm.
- Use cautiously with narrow-angle glaucoma, prostatic hypertrophy, bladder neck obstruction, pregnancy, lactation.

Available forms
Aerosol—18 mcg/actuation; solution for inhalation—0.02%; nasal spray—0.03% (21 mcg/spray), 0.06% (42 mcg/spray)

Dosages
Adults
Inhalation
The usual dosage is 2 inhalations (36 mcg) qid. Patients may take additional inhalations as required. Do not exceed 12 inhalations/24 hr. Solution for inhalation: 500 mcg, tid to qid with doses 6–8 hr apart.
Nasal spray
2 sprays 0.03% per nostril bid to tid or 2 sprays 0.06% per nostril tid to qid for relief with common cold.

Pediatric patients
Safety and efficacy not established for children < 12 yr.

Pharmacokinetics

Route	Onset	Peak	Duration
Inhalation	15 min	1–2 hr	3–4 hr

Adverse effects
- **CNS:** *Nervousness, dizziness, headache,* fatigue, insomnia, *blurred vision*
- **GI:** *Nausea,* GI distress, dry mouth
- **Respiratory:** *Cough,* exacerbation of symptoms, hoarseness
- **Other:** Palpitations, rash

■ Nursing considerations
Assessment
- **History:** Hypersensitivity to atropine; acute bronchospasm, narrow-angle glaucoma, prostatic hypertrophy, bladder neck obstruction, pregnancy, lactation
- **Physical:** Skin color, lesions, texture; T; orientation, reflexes, bilateral grip strength; affect; ophthalmic exam; P, BP; R, adventitious sounds; bowel sounds, normal output; normal urinary output, prostate palpation

Interventions
- Protect solution for inhalation from light. Store unused vials in foil pouch.
- Ensure adequate hydration, provide environmental control (temperature) to prevent hyperpyrexia.
- Have patient void before taking medication to avoid urinary retention.
- Teach patient proper use of inhalator.

Teaching points
- Use this drug as an inhalation product. Review the proper use of inhalator; for nasal spray, initiation of pump requires 7 actuations; if not used for 24 hr, 2 actuations will be needed before use. Protect from light; do not freeze.
- These side effects may occur: dizziness, headache, blurred vision (avoid driving or performing hazardous tasks); nausea, vomiting, GI upset (proper nutrition is important; consult with your dietitian to maintain nutrition); cough.

- Report rash, eye pain, difficulty voiding, palpitations, vision changes.

▽irbesartan
(er bah sar' tan)

Avapro

PREGNANCY CATEGORY D
(SECOND AND THIRD TRIMESTERS)

PREGNANCY CATEGORY C
(FIRST TRIMESTER)

Drug classes
Angiotensin II receptor antagonist (ARB)
Antihypertensive

Therapeutic actions
Selectively blocks the binding of angiotensin II to specific tissue receptors found in the vascular smooth muscle and adrenal gland; this action blocks the vasoconstriction effect of the renin-angiotensin system as well as the release of aldosterone, leading to decreased blood pressure.

Indications
- Treatment of hypertension as monotherapy or in combination with other antihypertensives
- Slowing of the progression of kidney disease in patients with hypertension and type 2 diabetes

Contraindications and cautions
- Contraindicated with hypersensitivity to irbesartan, pregnancy (use during the second or third trimester can cause injury or even death to the fetus), lactation.
- Use cautiously with hepatic or renal dysfunction, hypovolemia.

Available forms
Tablets—75, 150, 300 mg

Dosages
Adults
- *Diabetic neuropathy:* 300 mg/day PO as a single dose.

- *Hypertension:* 150 mg PO daily as one dose; adjust slowly to determine effective dose; maximum daily dose—300 mg.

Pediatric patients
< 6 yr: Not recommended.
6–12 yr: 75 mg/day PO, titrate to a maximum of 150 mg/day.
13–16 yr: 150 mg/day PO; maximum dose 300 mg.

Patients who are volume or salt depleted
75 mg/day PO.

Pharmacokinetics

Route	Onset	Peak
Oral	Varies	1–3 hr

Metabolism: Hepatic; $T_{1/2}$: 11–15 hr
Distribution: Crosses placenta; passes into breast milk
Excretion: Feces and urine

Adverse effects
- **CNS:** *Headache, dizziness,* syncope, muscle weakness
- **CV:** Hypotension, orthostatic hypotension
- **Dermatologic:** Rash, inflammation, urticaria, pruritus, alopecia, dry skin
- **GI:** *Diarrhea, abdominal pain, nausea,* constipation, dry mouth, dental pain
- **Respiratory:** *URI symptoms, cough,* sinus disorders
- **Other:** Cancer in preclinical studies, back pain, fever, gout, *fatigue*

■ Nursing considerations
Assessment
- **History:** Hypersensitivity to irbesartan, pregnancy, lactation, hepatic or renal dysfunction, hypovolemia
- **Physical:** Skin lesions, turgor; T; reflexes, affect; BP; R, respiratory auscultation; liver and kidney function tests

Interventions
- Administer without regard to meals.
- Ensure that patient is not pregnant before beginning therapy; suggest the use of barrier birth control while using irbesartan; fetal injury and deaths have been reported.

Adverse effects in *Italics* are most common; those in **Bold** are life-threatening.

- Find an alternative method of feeding the baby if giving drug to a nursing mother. Depression of the renin-angiotensin system in infants is potentially very dangerous.
- Alert surgeon and mark patient's chart with notice that irbesartan is being taken. The blockage of the renin-angiotensin system following surgery can produce problems. Hypotension may be reversed with volume expansion.
- Monitor patient closely in any situation that may lead to a decrease in blood pressure secondary to reduction in fluid volume (excessive perspiration, dehydration, vomiting, diarrhea); excessive hypotension can occur.

Teaching points

- Take this drug without regard to meals. Do not stop taking this drug without consulting your health care provider.
- Use a barrier method of birth control while on this drug; if you become pregnant or desire to become pregnant, consult with your physician.
- These side effects may occur: dizziness (more likely to occur in any situation where you may be fluid depleted [extreme heat, exertion, etc.]; avoid driving or performing hazardous tasks); headache (medications may be available to help); nausea, vomiting, diarrhea (proper nutrition is important; consult with your dietitian); symptoms of upper respiratory tract infection, cough (do not self-medicate; consult with your nurse or physician if this becomes uncomfortable).
- Report fever, chills, dizziness, pregnancy.

▽**irinotecan hydrochloride**

(eh rin ob' te kan)

Camptosar

PREGNANCY CATEGORY D

Drug class
Antineoplastic

Therapeutic actions
Cytotoxic: causes death of cells during cell division by causing damage to the DNA strand during DNA synthesis; specific to cells using topoisomerase I, DNA and irinotecan complexes

Indications

- First-line therapy in combination with 5-FU and leucovorin for patients with metastatic colon or rectal carcinomas
- Treatment of patients with metastatic colon or rectal cancer whose disease has recurred or progressed following 5-FU therapy

Contraindications and cautions

- Contraindicated with allergy to irinotecan, pregnancy
- Use cautiously with bone marrow depression, severe diarrhea, lactation

Available forms
Injection—20 mg/mL

Dosages
Adults

- *Single-agent use:* 125 mg/m² IV over 90 min once weekly for 4 wk, then a 2-wk rest; repeat 6-wk regimen or 350 mg/m² IV over 90 min once every 3 wks.
- *Combination agents:* 125 mg/m² IV over 90 min, days 1, 8, 15, 22 with leucovorin 20 mg/m² IV bolus days 1, 8, 15, and 22 and 5-FU, 500 mg/m² IV days 1, 8, 15, and 22. Restart cycle on day 43. *Or* 180 mg/m² IV over 90 min days 1, 15, 29 with leucovorin—200 mg/m² IV over 2 hr day 1, 2, 15, 16, 29, and 30 and 5-FU—400 mg/m² as IV bolus days 1, 2, 15, 16, 29, and 30 followed by 5-FU 600 mg/m² IV infusion over 22 hr. Restart cycle on day 43.

Pediatric patients
Not recommended.

Pharmacokinetics

Route	Onset	Peak
IV	Immediate	1–2 hr

Metabolism: Hepatic; $T_{1/2}$: 6 hr
Distribution: Crosses placenta; may pass into breast milk
Excretion: Urine and bile

▽IV facts

Preparation: Dilute in 5% dextrose injection or 0.9% sodium chloride injection to final concentration of 0.12–1.1 mg/mL. Store diluted drug protected from light; use within 24 hr if refrigerated or within 6 hr if at room temperature. Store vials at room temperature, protected from light.

Infusion: Infuse total dose over 90 min.

Adverse effects

- **CNS:** Insomnia, dizziness, asthenia
- **Dermatologic:** *Alopecia,* sweating, flushing, rashes
- **GI:** *Nausea, vomiting, diarrhea,* constipation, stomatitis, flatulence, dyspepsia
- **Hematologic: Neutropenia, leukopenia, anemia**
- **Respiratory:** *Dyspnea,* cough, rhinitis
- **Other:** Fatigue, malaise, pain, infections, fever, cramping

■ Nursing considerations

Assessment

- **History:** Allergy to irinotecan, diarrhea, pregnancy, lactation, bone marrow depression
- **Physical:** T; skin lesions, color, turgor; orientation, affect, reflexes; R; abdominal exam, bowel sounds; CBC with differential

Interventions

- Obtain CBC before each infusion; do not give to patients with a baseline neutrophil count of < 1,500 cells/mm^2; consult with physician for reduction in dose or withholding of drug if bone marrow depression becomes evident.
- Ensure that patient is not pregnant before beginning therapy; advise the use of barrier contraceptives.
- Monitor infusion site; if extravasation occurs, flush with sterile water and apply ice.
- Monitor for diarrhea; assess hydration and arrange to decrease dose if 4–6 stools/day; omit a dose if 7–9 stools/day; if 10 or more stools/day, consult with physician. Early diarrhea may be prevented or ameliorated by atropine 0.25–1 mg IV or SC; treat late diarrhea > 24 hr with loperamide.
- Protect patient from any exposure to infection.
- Arrange for wig or other appropriate head covering when alopecia occurs.

Teaching points

- This drug can only be given by IV infusion, which will run over 90 min. Mark calendar with days to return for infusion. A blood test will be required before each dose.
- These side effects may occur: increased susceptibility to infection (avoid crowded areas or people with known infections; report any injury); nausea, vomiting (eat small, frequent meals; medication may be ordered); headache; loss of hair (arrange for a wig or other head covering; it is important to protect the head from extremes of temperature); diarrhea.
- This drug cannot be used during pregnancy; use of barrier contraceptives is suggested.
- Report pain at injection site, any injury or illness, fatigue, severe nausea or vomiting, increased, severe, or bloody diarrhea.

▽iron dextran

DexFerrum, InFeD, Infufer (CAN)

PREGNANCY CATEGORY B

Drug class

Iron preparation

Therapeutic actions

Elevates the serum iron concentration and is then converted to Hgb or trapped in the reticuloendothelial cells for storage and eventual conversion to usable form of iron.

Indications

- Treatment of iron deficiency anemia only when oral administration of iron is unsatisfactory or impossible
- Unlabeled use: may be required for patients receiving epoetin therapy

Contraindications and cautions

- Contraindicated with allergy to iron dextran, anemias other than iron deficiency anemia, pregnancy.
- Use cautiously with impaired liver function, rheumatoid arthritis, allergies, asthma, lactation.

Available forms
Injection—50 mg/mL

Dosages
Adults and pediatric patients
- *Iron deficiency anemia:* Administer a 0.5 mL IM or IV test dose before therapy. Base dosage on hematologic response with frequent Hgb determinations.

For patients weighing > 15 kg (33 lb), use the following formula:

Dose (mL) = 0.0442 (desired Hgb − observed Hgb) × LBW + (0.26 × LBW), where Hgb = Hgb in g/dL and LBW = lean body weight. Determine LBW as follows:

For males: LBW = 50 kg + 2.3 kg for each inch of patient's height over 5 feet.

For females: LBW = 45.5 kg + 2.3 kg for each inch of patients' height over 5 feet.

For children 5–15 kg (11–33 lb) and > 4 mo, use the following formula:

Dose (mL) = 0.0442 (desired Hgb − observed Hgb) × W (0.26 × W), where W = actual weight in kg.

- *Iron replacement for blood loss:* Determine dosage by the following formula: replacement iron (in mg) = blood loss (in mL) × Hct

IM
Inject only into the upper outer quadrant of the buttocks. Give test dose of 0.5 mL IM. If tolerated, do not exceed 0.5 mL (25 mg) for infants < 5 kg; 1 mL for < 10 kg; 2 mL for all others.

Pharmacokinetics

Route	Onset	Peak
IM	Slow	1–2 wk

Metabolism: $T_{1/2}$: 6 hr
Distribution: Crosses placenta; enters breast milk
Excretion: Blood loss

▽IV facts
Preparation: Intermittent IV: Calculate dose from formula. Give individual doses of 2 mL or less per day. Use single dose ampules without preservatives. IV infusion: dilute needed dose in 200–250 mL of normal saline.
Infusion: Intermittent IV: give undiluted and slowly—1 mL or less/min. IV infusion (not approved by the FDA): infuse over 1–2 hr after a test dose of 25 mL.

Adverse effects
- **CNS:** Headache, backache, dizziness, malaise, transitory paresthesias
- **CV:** Hypotension, chest pain, shock, tachycardia
- **GI:** *Nausea, vomiting*
- **Hypersensitivity:** Hypersensitivity reactions including **anaphylaxis;** dyspnea, urticaria, rash and itching, arthralgia and myalgia, fever, sweating, purpura
- **Local:** *Pain, inflammation and sterile abscesses at injection site, brown skin discoloration* (IM use); *lymphadenopathy, local phlebitis, peripheral vascular flushing* (IV administration)
- **Other:** *Arthritic reactivation,* fever, shivering, **cancer**

Interactions
✳ **Drug-drug** • Delayed response to iron dextran therapy in patients taking chloramphenicol.
✳ **Drug-lab test** • Use caution when interpreting serum iron levels when done within 1–2 wk of iron dextran injection • Serum may be discolored to a brownish color following IV injection • Bone scans using Tc-99m diphosphonate may have abnormal areas following IM injection

■ Nursing considerations
Assessment
- **History:** Allergy to iron dextran, anemias other than iron deficiency anemia, impaired liver function, rheumatoid arthritis, allergies or asthma, lactation
- **Physical:** Skin lesions, color; T; injection site exam; range of motion, joints; R, adventitious sounds; liver evaluation; CBC, Hgb, Hct, serum ferritin assays, liver function tests

Interventions
- Ensure that patient does have iron deficiency anemia before treatment.
- Arrange treatment of underlying cause of iron deficiency anemia.
- Give IM injections using the Z-track technique (displace skin laterally before injection) to avoid injection into the tissue and tissue staining. Use a large-gauge needle; if standing, have patient support self on leg not receiving the injection. If lying, have the injection site uppermost.

- Monitor patient for hypersensitivity reactions; test dose is highly recommended. Maintain epinephrine on standby in case severe hypersensitivity reaction occurs.
- Monitor serum ferritin levels periodically; these correlate well with iron stores. Do not give with oral iron preparations.
- Caution patients with rheumatoid arthritis that acute exacerbation of joint pain and swelling may occur; provide appropriate comfort measures.

Teaching points
- Treatment will end if anemia is corrected.
- Have periodic blood tests during therapy to assess drug response and determine appropriate dosage.
- Do not take oral iron products or vitamins with iron added while on this drug.
- These side effects may occur: pain at injection site, headache, joint and muscle aches, GI upset.
- Report difficulty breathing, pain at injection site, rash, itching.

▽ iron sucrose

See *Less Commonly Used Drugs*, p. 1344.

▽ isocarboxazid

See *Less Commonly Used Drugs*, p. 1346.

▽ isoetharine hydrochloride
*(eye soe **eth'** a reen)*

PREGNANCY CATEGORY C

Drug classes
Sympathomimetic
Beta₂-selective adrenergic agonist
Bronchodilator
Antiasthmatic agent

Therapeutic actions
In low doses, acts relatively selectively at beta₂-adrenergic receptors to cause bronchodilation; at higher doses, beta₂-selectivity is lost, and the drug acts at beta₂-receptors to cause typical sympathomimetic cardiac effects.

Indications
- Prophylaxis and treatment of bronchial asthma and reversible bronchospasm that may occur with bronchitis and emphysema

Contraindications and cautions
- Contraindicated with hypersensitivity to isoetharine; allergy to sulfites; tachyarrhythmias, tachycardia caused by digitalis intoxication; general anesthesia with halogenated hydrocarbons or cyclopropane (sensitize the myocardium to catecholamines); unstable vasomotor system disorders.
- Use cautiously with hypertension, coronary insufficiency, CAD, history of stroke, COPD patients with degenerative heart disease, hyperthyroidism, history of seizure disorders, psychoneurotic individuals, labor and delivery (may inhibit labor; parenteral use of beta₂-adrenergic agonists can accelerate fetal heart beat, cause hypoglycemia, hypokalemia, and pulmonary edema in the mother and hypoglycemia in the neonate); lactation.

Available forms
Solution for inhalation—1%

Dosages
Adults
- *Hand bulb nebulizer:* 4 inhalations or 3–7 inhalations of 1:3 dilution (one part isoetharine, 3 parts normal saline).
- *Oxygen aerosolization:* 1–2 mL of 1:3 dilution with O₂ flow at 4–6 L/min over 15–20 min; usual dose of 0.5 mL.
- *IPPB:* 1–4 mL of 1:3 dilution; usual dose of 0.5 mL.

Pediatric patients
Dosage not established.

Geriatric patients
Patients > 60 yr are more likely to develop adverse effects; use with extreme caution.

Pharmacokinetics

Route	Onset	Duration
Inhalation	5 min	1–3 hr

Adverse effects in *Italics* are most common; those in **Bold** are life-threatening.

Metabolism: Tissue
Distribution: Crosses placenta; may enter breast milk
Excretion: Urine

Adverse effects

- **CNS:** *Restlessness, apprehension, anxiety, fear,* CNS stimulation, hyperkinesia, insomnia, tremor, drowsiness, irritability, weakness, vertigo, headache
- **CV:** *Cardiac arrhythmias, tachycardia, palpitations,* PVCs, anginal pain
- **GI:** *Nausea,* vomiting, heartburn, unusual or bad taste
- **Respiratory:** *Respiratory difficulties, pulmonary edema, coughing,* bronchospasm, paradoxical airway resistance with repeated, excessive use of inhalation preparations
- **Other:** Sweating, pallor, flushing

Interactions

✳ **Drug-drug •** Increased likelihood of cardiac arrhythmias with halogenated hydrocarbon anesthetics (halothane), cyclopropane

■ Nursing considerations
Assessment

- **History:** Hypersensitivity to isoetharine, allergy to sulfites, tachyarrhythmias, general anesthesia with halogenated hydrocarbons or cyclopropane, unstable vasomotor system disorders, hypertension, coronary insufficiency, history of stroke, COPD patients who have developed degenerative heart disease, hyperthyroidism, history of seizure disorders, psychoneuroses
- **Physical:** Weight; skin color, temperature, turgor; orientation, reflexes; P, BP; R, adventitious sounds; blood and urine glucose, serum electrolytes, thyroid function tests, ECG

Interventions

- Use minimal doses for minimal periods of time; drug tolerance can occur with prolonged use.
- Maintain a beta-adrenergic blocker (a cardioselective beta-blocker, such as atenolol, should be used in patients with respiratory distress) on standby in case cardiac arrhythmias occur.
- Do not exceed recommended dosage; give aerosol during second half of inspiration,

because the airways are open wider, and the aerosol distribution is more extensive.

Teaching points

- Do not exceed recommended dosage; adverse effects or loss of effectiveness may result. Read the instructions that come with the aerosol product, and ask your health care provider or pharmacist if you have any questions.
- These side effects may occur: dizziness, drowsiness, fatigue, apprehension (use caution if driving or performing tasks that require alertness); nausea, heartburn, unusual taste (small, frequent meals may help); fast heart rate, anxiety, changes in breathing.
- Report chest pain, dizziness, insomnia, weakness, tremor or irregular heart beat, difficulty breathing, productive cough, failure to respond to usual dosage.

▽**isoniazid
(isonicotinic acid
hydrazide, INH)**
*(eye soe **nye'** a zid)*

Isotamine (CAN), Nydrazid, PMS
Isoniazid (CAN)

PREGNANCY CATEGORY C

Drug class
Antituberculous agent

Therapeutic actions
Bactericidal: interferes with lipid and nucleic acid biosynthesis in actively growing tubercle bacilli.

Indications
- Tuberculosis, all forms in which organisms are susceptible
- Prophylaxis in specific patients who are tuberculin reactors or household members of recently diagnosed tuberculars or who are considered to be high risk (patients with HIV, IV drug users, etc.)
- Unlabeled use of 300–400 mg/day, increased over 2 wk to 20 mg/kg/day for improvement of severe tremor in patients with multiple sclerosis

Contraindications and cautions

- Contraindicated with allergy to isoniazid, isoniazid-associated hepatic injury or other severe adverse reactions to isoniazid, acute hepatic disease, pregnancy.
- Use cautiously with renal dysfunction, lactation.

Available forms

Tablets—100, 300 mg; syrup—50 mg/5 mL; injection—100 mg/mL

Dosages
Adults

- *Treatment of active TB:* 5 mg/kg/day (up to 300 mg) PO in a single dose, with other effective agents or 15 mg/kg (up to 900 mg) PO 2–3 times/wk. "First-line treatment" is considered to be 300 mg INH plus 600 mg rifampin, each given in a single daily oral dose. Consult manufacturer's guidelines for other possible combinations.
- *Prophylaxis for TB:* 300 mg/day PO in a single dose. Concomitant administration of 6–50 mg/day of pyridoxine is recommended for those who are malnourished or predisposed to neuropathy (alcoholics, diabetics).

Pediatric patients

- *Treatment of active TB:* 10–15 mg/kg/day (up to 300 mg) PO in a single dose, with other effective agents or 20–40 mg/kg (up to 400 mg/day) 2–3 times/wk.
- *Prophylaxis for TB:* 10 mg/kg/day (up to 300 mg) PO in a single dose.

Pharmacokinetics

Route	Onset	Peak	Duration
Oral	Varies	1–2 hr	24 hr

Metabolism: Hepatic; $T_{1/2}$: 1–4 hr
Distribution: Crosses placenta; enters breast milk
Excretion: Urine

Adverse effects

- **CNS:** *Peripheral neuropathy,* convulsions, toxic encephalopathy, optic neuritis and atrophy, memory impairment, toxic psychosis

- **GI:** *Nausea, vomiting, epigastric distress,* bilirubinemia, bilirubinuria, *elevated AST, ALT levels,* jaundice, **hepatitis**
- **Hematologic:** Agranulocytosis, hemolytic or aplastic anemia, thrombocytopenia, eosinophilia, pyridoxine deficiency, pellagra, hyperglycemia, metabolic acidosis, hypocalcemia, hypophosphatemia due to altered vitamin D metabolism
- **Hypersensitivity:** Fever, skin eruptions, lymphadenopathy, vasculitis
- **Local:** *Local irritation at IM injection site*
- **Other:** Gynecomastia, rheumatic syndrome, systemic lupus erythematosus syndrome

Interactions

✹ **Drug-drug** • Increased incidence of isoniazid-related hepatitis with alcohol and possibly if taken in high doses with rifampin • Increased serum levels of phenytoin • Increased effectiveness and risk of toxicity of carbamazepine • Risk of high output renal failure in fast INH acetylators with enflurane

✹ **Drug-food** • Risk of sympathetic-type reactions with tyramine-containing foods and exaggerated response (headache, palpitations, sweating, hypotension, flushing, diarrhea, itching) to histamine-containing food (fish [skipjack, tuna] sauerkraut juice, yeast extracts)

■ Nursing considerations
Assessment

- **History:** Allergy to isoniazid, isoniazid-associated adverse reactions; acute hepatic disease; renal dysfunction; lactation
- **Physical:** Skin color, lesions; T; orientation, reflexes, peripheral sensitivity, bilateral grip strength; ophthalmologic examination; R, adventitious sounds; liver evaluation; CBC, liver and kidney function tests, blood glucose

Interventions

- Give on an empty stomach, 1 hr before or 2 hr after meals; may be given with food if GI upset occurs.
- Give in a single daily dose. Reserve parenteral dose for patients unable to take oral medications.
- Decrease tyramine-containing and histamine-containing food in diet.

Adverse effects in *Italics* are most common; those in **Bold** are life-threatening.

- Consult with physician and arrange for daily pyridoxine in diabetic, alcoholic, or malnourished patients; also for patients who develop peripheral neuritis.
- Discontinue drug, and consult with physician if signs of hypersensitivity occur.

Teaching points
- Take this drug in a single daily dose. Take on an empty stomach, 1 hr before or 2 hr after meals. If GI distress occurs, may be taken with food.
- Take this drug regularly; avoid missing doses; do not discontinue without first consulting with your prescriber.
- Do not drink alcohol, or drink as little as possible. There is an increased risk of hepatitis if these two drugs are combined.
- Avoid tyramine-containing foods; consult a dietitian to obtain a list of tyramine-containing and histamine-containing foods.
- These side effects may occur: nausea, vomiting, epigastric distress (take drug with meals); skin rashes or lesions; numbness, tingling, loss of sensation (use caution to prevent injury or burns).
- Have periodic medical check-ups, including an eye examination and blood tests to evaluate the drug effects.
- Report weakness, fatigue, loss of appetite, nausea, vomiting, yellowing of skin or eyes, darkening of the urine, numbness or tingling in hands or feet.

▽**isoproterenol**
*(eye soe proe **ter' e** nole)*

isoproterenol hydrochloride
Isuprel, Isuprel Mistometer

isoproterenol sulfate
Medihaler-Iso

PREGNANCY CATEGORY C

Drug classes
Sympathomimetic
Beta$_1$- and beta$_2$-adrenergic agonist
Bronchodilator
Antiasthmatic agent
Drug used in shock

Therapeutic actions
Effects are mediated by beta$_1$- and beta$_2$-adrenergic receptors; acts on beta$_1$-receptors in the heart to produce positive chronotropic and positive inotropic effects and to increase automaticity; acts on beta$_2$-receptors in the bronchi to cause bronchodilation; acts on beta$_2$-receptors in smooth muscle in the walls of blood vessels in skeletal muscle and splanchnic beds to cause dilation (cardiac stimulation, vasodilation may be adverse effects when drug is used as bronchodilator).

Indications
- Inhalation: treatment of bronchospasm associated with acute and chronic bronchial asthma, pulmonary emphysema, bronchitis, bronchiectasis
- Injection: management of bronchospasm during anesthesia; a vasopressor in shock
- Adjunct in the management of shock (hypoperfusion syndrome) and in the treatment of cardiac standstill or arrest; carotid sinus hypersensitivity; heart block; Stokes-Adams syndrome; ventricular tachycardia and ventricular arrhythmias that require increased inotropic activity for therapy
- Sublingual: management of patients with bronchopulmonary disease; Stokes-Adams syndrome and AV heart block
- Rectal: Stokes-Adams syndrome and AV heart block

Contraindications and cautions
- Contraindicated with hypersensitivity to isoproterenol; tachyarrhythmias, tachycardia caused by digitalis intoxication; general anesthesia with halogenated hydrocarbons or cyclopropane (sensitize the myocardium to catecholamines); labor and delivery (may delay second stage of labor; can accelerate fetal heart beat; may cause hypoglycemia, hypokalemia, pulmonary edema in the mother, and hypoglycemia in the neonate); lactation.
- Use cautiously with unstable vasomotor system disorders, hypertension, coronary insufficiency, history of stroke, COPD patients with degenerative heart disease, diabetes mellitus, hyperthyroidism, history of seizure disorders, psychoneuroses.

Available forms
Solution for inhalation—0.5%, 1%; aerosol—103 mcg/mist, 80 mcg/dose; injection—0.02, 0.2 mg/mL

Dosages
Adults
Injection
- *Bronchospasm during anesthesia:* 0.01–0.02 mg (0.5–1 mL of diluted solution) IV; repeat when necessary.
- *Shock:* Dilute to 2 mcg/mL and infuse IV at a rate adjusted on the basis of HR, central venous pressure, systemic BP, and urine flow.
- *Cardiac standstill and arrhythmias:* IV injection: 0.02–0.06 mg using diluted solution. IV infusion: 5 mcg/min using diluted solution. IM, SC: 0.2 mg of undiluted 1:5,000 solution. Intracardiac: 0.02 mg of undiluted 1:5,000 solution.

Inhalation
- *Acute bronchial asthma: Hand bulb nebulizer:* Administer the 1:200 solution in a dosage of 5–15 deep inhalations. If desired, administer the 1:100 solution in 3–7 deep inhalations. If no relief after 5–10 min, repeat doses once more. If acute attack recurs, may repeat treatment up to five times per day. *Metered-dose inhaler:* Start with one inhalation; if no relief after 2–5 min, repeat. *Daily maintenance:* 1–2 inhalations 4–6 times/day. Do not take more than 2 inhalations at a time. Do not take more than 6 inhalations per hour.
- *Bronchospasm in COPD: Hand bulb nebulizer:* 5–15 inhalations using the 1:200 solution. Patients with severe attacks may require 3–7 inhalations using the 1:100 solution. Do not use at less than 3- to 4-hr intervals. *Nebulization by compressed air or O₂, IPPB:* 0.5 mL of a 1:200 solution is diluted to 2–2.5 mL with appropriate diluent for a concentration of 1:800 to 1:1,000 and delivered over 10–20 min. May repeat up to 5 times/day. *Metered-dose inhaler:* 1 or 2 inhalations; repeat at no less than 3- to 4-hr intervals.

Pediatric patients
- *Nebulization (bronchospasm):* Administration is similar to that of adults; children's smaller ventilatory exchange capacity provides smaller aerosol intake. Use the 1:200 solution for an acute attack; do not use more than 0.25 mL of the 1:200 solution for each 10- to 15-min programmed treatment.

Geriatric patients
Patients > 60 yr are more likely to experience adverse effects; use with extreme caution.

Pharmacokinetics

Route	Onset	Duration
Inhalation	Rapid	50–60 min
IV	Immediate	1–2 min
PR	Slow	2–4 hr

Metabolism: Tissue; $T_{1/2}$: unknown
Distribution: Crosses placenta; enters breast milk
Excretion: Urine

▼IV facts
Preparation: Dilute the 1:5,000 solutions for IV injection or infusion with 5% dextrose injection; a convenient dilution is 1 mg isoproterenol (5 mL) in 500 mL diluent (final concentration 1:500,000 or 2 mcg/mL).
Infusion: Dosage of 5 mcg/min is provided by infusing 2.5 mL/min; adjust dosage to keep heart rate < 110.
Incompatibilities: Do not combine with aminophylline, barbiturates, lidocaine, sodium bicarbonate.

Adverse effects
- **CNS:** *Restlessness, apprehension, anxiety, fear,* CNS stimulation, hyperkinesia, insomnia, tremor, drowsiness, irritability, weakness, vertigo, headache
- **CV:** *Cardiac arrhythmias, tachycardia, palpitations,* anginal pain, changes in BP, paradoxical precipitation of Stokes-Adams seizures during normal sinus rhythm or transient heart block
- **GI:** *Nausea, vomiting, heartburn,* unusual or bad taste, swelling of the parotid glands
- **Respiratory:** *Respiratory difficulties,* **pulmonary edema,** *coughing, bronchospasm, paradoxical airway resistance with repeated, excessive use*
- **Other:** *Sweating, pallor,* flushing, muscle cramps

Adverse effects in *Italics* are most common; those in **Bold** are life-threatening.

Interactions

* Drug-drug • Increased peripheral vaso-constriction if given with ergot alkaloids. If this combination is used, monitor blood pressure and perfusion carefully **•** Increased blood pressure response may occur if combined with tricyclic antidepressants, halogenated hydrocarbon anesthetics, bretylium. Monitor patient closely and adjust dosage as needed

■ Nursing considerations
Assessment

- **History:** Hypersensitivity to isoproterenol; tachyarrhythmias; general anesthesia with halogenated hydrocarbons or cyclopropane; unstable vasomotor system disorders; hypertension; coronary artery disease; history of stroke; COPD patients with degenerative heart disease; diabetes mellitus; hyperthyroidism; history of seizure disorders; psychoneurotic individuals; labor and delivery; lactation
- **Physical:** Weight; skin color, temperature, turgor; orientation, reflexes; P, BP; R, adventitious sounds; blood and urine glucose, serum electrolytes, thyroid function tests, ECG

Interventions

- Use minimal doses for minimum periods; drug tolerance can occur with prolonged use.
- Maintain a beta-adrenergic blocker (a cardioselective beta-blocker, such as atenolol, should be used in patients with respiratory distress) on standby in case cardiac arrhythmias occur.
- Do not exceed recommended dosage of inhalation products; administer pressurized inhalation drug forms during second half of inspiration, because the airways are open wider and the aerosol distribution is more extensive. If a second inhalation is needed, give at peak effect of previous dose, 3–5 min.

Teaching points

- Do not exceed recommended dosage; adverse effects or loss of effectiveness may result. Read product instructions (respiratory inhalant products), and ask your health care provider or pharmacist if you have any questions. Use inhalator correctly for best results and avoiding adverse effects.

- These side effects may occur: drowsiness, dizziness, inability to sleep (use caution if driving or performing tasks that require alertness); nausea, vomiting (small, frequent meals may help); anxiety; rapid heart rate.
- Report chest pain, dizziness, insomnia, weakness, tremor or irregular heart beat, failure to respond to usual dosage.

▽isosorbide
*(eye soe **sor'** bide)*

Ismotic

PREGNANCY CATEGORY B

Drug class
Osmotic diuretic

Therapeutic actions
Elevates the osmolarity of the glomerular filtrate, hindering the reabsorption of water and leading to a loss of water, sodium, and chloride; creates an osmotic gradient in the eye between plasma and ocular fluids, reducing intraocular pressure.

Indications

- Glaucoma: to interrupt acute attacks; poses less risk of nausea and vomiting than other oral osmotic agents
- Short-term reduction of intraocular pressure prior to and after ocular surgery

Contraindications and cautions

- Allergy to isosorbide, anuria due to severe renal disease, severe dehydration, pulmonary edema, CHF, diseases associated with salt retention.

Available forms
Solution—100 g/220 mL

Dosages
Adults
PO use only. 1.5 g/kg (range 1–3 mg/kg) bid–qid as needed.

Pharmacokinetics

Route	Onset	Peak	Duration
Oral	10–30 min	60–90 min	5–6 hr

Metabolism: $T_{1/2}$: 5–9.5 hr
Distribution: Crosses placenta
Excretion: Urine

Adverse effects

- **CNS:** *Headache, confusion, disorientation, dizziness,* light-headedness, syncope, vertigo, irritability
- **GI:** Nausea, vomiting, GI discomfort, thirst, hiccoughs
- **Hematologic:** Hypernatremia, hyperosmolarity
- **Other:** Rash

■ Nursing considerations
Assessment

- **History:** Allergy to isosorbide, anuria due to severe renal disease, severe dehydration, pulmonary edema, CHF, diseases associated with salt retention
- **Physical:** Skin color, edema; orientation, reflexes, muscle strength, pupillary reflexes; pulses, BP, perfusion; R, pattern, adventitious sounds; urinary output patterns; serum electrolytes, urinalysis

Interventions

- Administer by oral route only; not for injection.
- Pour over cracked ice, and have patient sip drug to improve palatability.
- Monitor urinary output carefully.
- Monitor BP regularly and carefully.

Teaching points

- Pour the drug over cracked ice to make it easier to take.
- These side effects may occur: increased urination; GI upset (small, frequent meals may help); dry mouth (sucking sugarless lozenges may help); headache, blurred vision, feelings of irritability (use caution when moving around; ask for assistance).
- Report severe headache, confusion, dizziness.

▽**isosorbide nitrates**
(eye soe sor' bide)

isosorbide dinitrate
Apo-ISDN (CAN), Cedocard SR (CAN), Dilatrate SR, Isordil, Isordil Tembids, Isordil Titradose, Sorbitrate

isosorbide mononitrate
ISMO, Imdur, Isotrate ER, Monoket

PREGNANCY CATEGORY C

Drug classes

Antianginal agent
Nitrate

Therapeutic actions

Relaxes vascular smooth muscle with a resultant decrease in venous return and decrease in arterial BP, which reduces left ventricular workload and decreases myocardial oxygen consumption.

Indications

- Treatment and prevention of angina pectoris (dinitrate)
- Prevention of angina pectoris (mononitrate)

Contraindications and cautions

- Allergy to nitrates, severe anemia, head trauma, cerebral hemorrhage, hypertrophic cardiomyopathy, pregnancy, lactation.

Available forms

Dinitrate: tablets—5, 10, 20, 30, 40 mg; SR tablets—40 mg; SR capsules—40 mg; SL tablets—2.5, 5, 10 mg; chewable tablets—5, 10 mg *Mononitrate:* tablets —10, 20 mg; ER tablets —30, 60, 120 mg

Dosages
Adults
Isosorbide dinitrate

- *Angina pectoris:* Starting dose: 2.5–5 mg sublingual, 5-mg chewable tablets, 5- to 20-mg oral tablets. Maintenance: 10–40 mg q 6 hr oral tablets or capsules; sustained release, initially 40 mg, then 40–80 mg PO q 8–12 hr.

- *Acute prophylaxis:* Initial dosage: 5–10 mg sublingual or chewable tablets q 2–3 hr.

Isosorbide mononitrate

- Prevention of angina 20 mg PO bid given at least 7 hr apart; ER tablets—30–60 mg/day PO may be increased to 120 mg/day if needed.

Pediatric patients

Safety and efficacy not established.

Pharmacokinetics

Route	Onset	Duration
Oral	15–45 min	4 hr
SL	2–5 min	1–2 hr

Metabolism: Hepatic; $T_{1/2}$: 5 min, then 2–5 hr
Distribution: May cross placenta; may enter breast milk
Excretion: Urine

Adverse effects

- **CNS:** *Headache, apprehension, restlessness, weakness,* vertigo, dizziness, faintness
- **CV:** *Tachycardia, retrosternal discomfort, palpitations, hypotension,* **syncope,** *collapse, orthostatic hypotension, angina*
- **Dermatologic:** Rash, exfoliative dermatitis, cutaneous vasodilation with flushing
- **GI:** *Nausea,* vomiting, incontinence of urine and feces, abdominal pain
- **Other:** Muscle twitching, pallor, perspiration, cold sweat

Interactions

✳ **Drug-drug** • Increased systolic BP and decreased antianginal effect if taken concurrently with ergot alkaloids
✳ **Drug-lab test** • False report of decreased serum cholesterol if done by the Zlatkis-Zak color reaction

■ Nursing considerations

CLINICAL ALERT!
Name confusion has occurred between Isordil (isosorbide) and Plendil (felodipine); use caution.

Assessment

- **History:** Allergy to nitrates, severe anemia, GI hypermobility, head trauma, cerebral hemorrhage, hypertrophic cardiomyopathy, pregnancy, lactation
- **Physical:** Skin color, temperature, lesions; orientation, reflexes, affect; P, BP, orthostatic BP, baseline ECG, peripheral perfusion; R, adventitious sounds; liver evaluation, normal output; CBC, Hgb

Interventions

- Give sublingual preparations under the tongue or in the buccal pouch; encourage the patient not to swallow.
- Give chewable tablets slowly, only 5 mg initially because severe hypotension can occur; ensure that patient does not chew or crush sustained-release preparations.
- Give oral preparations on an empty stomach, 1 hr before or 2 hr after meals; take with meals if severe, uncontrolled headache occurs.
- Maintain life support equipment on standby if overdose occurs or cardiac condition worsens.
- Gradually reduce dose if anginal treatment is being terminated; rapid discontinuation can lead to problems of withdrawal.

Teaching points

- Place sublingual tablets under your tongue or in your cheek; do not chew or swallow the tablet. Take the isosorbide before chest pain begins, when activities or situation may precipitate an attack. Take oral isosorbide dinitrate on an empty stomach, 1 hr before or 2 hr after meals; do not chew or crush sustained-release preparations.
- These side effects may occur: dizziness, lightheadedness (may be transient; use care to change positions slowly); headache (lie down in a cool environment, rest; OTC preparations may not help; take drug with meals); flushing of the neck or face (reversible).
- Report blurred vision, persistent or severe headache, rash, more frequent or more severe angina attacks, fainting.

isotretinoin (13-*cis*-retinoic acid, vitamin A metabolite)

(eye so tret' i noyn)

Accutane, Amnesteem, Isotrex (CAN)

PREGNANCY CATEGORY X

Drug classes
Vitamin metabolite
Acne product

Therapeutic actions
Decreases sebaceous gland size and inhibits sebaceous gland differentiation, resulting in a reduction in sebum secretion; inhibits follicular keratinization; exact mechanism of action is not known.

Indications
- Treatment of severe recalcitrant nodular acne unresponsive to conventional treatments
- Unlabeled uses: treatment of cutaneous disorders of keratinization; cutaneous T-cell lymphoma and leukoplakia, psoriasis

Contraindications and cautions
- Contraindicated with allergy to isotretinoin, parabens, or product component; pregnancy (has caused severe fetal malformations and spontaneous abortions); lactation; history of severe depression, suicidal ideation.
- Use cautiously with diabetes mellitus, pediatric patients with genetic predisposition to age-related osteoporosis, a history of childhood osteoporosis, osteomalacia, other diseases of bone metabolism.

Available forms
Capsules—10, 20, 40 mg

Dosages
Individualize dosage based on side effects and disease response. Initial dose: 0.5–1 mg/kg/day PO; usual dosage range is 0.5–2 mg/kg/day divided into 2 doses for 15–20 wk. Maximum daily dose: 2 mg/kg. If a second course of therapy is needed, allow a rest period of at least 8 wk between courses.

Pharmacokinetics

Route	Onset	Peak	Duration
Oral	Varies	2.9–3.2 hr	6–20 hr

Metabolism: Hepatic; $T_{1/2}$: 10–20 hr
Distribution: Crosses placenta; may enter breast milk
Excretion: Urine

Adverse effects
- **CNS:** *Lethargy, insomnia, fatigue, headache,* pseudotumor cerebri (papilledema, headache, nausea, vomiting, visual disturbances); depression, psychoses, **suicide**, aggressive or violent behavior
- **Dermatologic:** *Skin fragility, dry skin, pruritus, rash,* thinning of hair, peeling of palms and soles, skin infections, photosensitivity, nail brittleness, petechiae
- **EENT:** *Cheilitis, eye irritation, conjunctivitis,* corneal opacities
- **GI:** *Nausea, vomiting, abdominal pain,* anorexia, inflammatory bowel disease
- **GU:** *White cells in the urine, proteinuria, hematuria*
- **Hematologic:** *Elevated sedimentation rate, hypertriglyceridemia,* abnormal liver function tests, increased fasting serum glucose
- **Musculoskeletal:** Skeletal hyperostosis, arthralgia, bone and joint pain and stiffness
- **Respiratory:** *Epistaxis, dry nose, dry mouth*

Interactions
✳ **Drug-drug** • Increased toxicity when taken with vitamin A; avoid this combination
• Risk of increased adverse effects if combined with systemic corticosteroids, phenytoin; use caution if these combinations are used

■ Nursing considerations
Assessment
- **History:** Allergy to isotretinoin, parabens, or product component; diabetes mellitus; pregnancy; lactation; history of depression
- **Physical:** Skin color, lesions, turgor, texture; joints—range of motion; orientation, reflexes, affect, ophthalmologic exam; mucous membranes, bowel sounds; serum

triglycerides, HDL, sedimentation rate, CBC and differential, urinalysis, pregnancy test

Interventions

- Ensure that patient is not pregnant before therapy; test for pregnancy within 2 wk of beginning therapy. Advise patient to use two forms of contraception starting 1 mo before therapy, during treatment and for 1 mo after treatment is discontinued. Patient must sign consent acknowledging this information; form should be kept in patient's medical record.
- Do not give a second course of therapy within 8 wk of first course.
- Give drug with meals; do not crush capsules.
- Do not give vitamin supplements that contain vitamin A.
- Discontinue drug if signs of papilledema occur; consult with a neurologist for further care.
- Discontinue drug at any indication of severe depression; psychoses. Patient must sign informed consent concerning risk of suicide; form should be kept in patient's medical record.
- Discontinue drug if visual disturbances occur; arrange for an ophthalmologic exam.
- Discontinue drug if abdominal pain, rectal bleeding, or severe diarrhea occurs; consult with physician.
- Monitor triglycerides during therapy; if elevation occurs, institute measures to lower serum triglycerides: reduce weight, reduce dietary fat, exercise, increase intake of insoluble fiber, decrease alcohol consumption.
- Monitor diabetic patients with frequent blood glucose determinations.
- Do not allow blood donation from patients taking isotretinoin due to the teratogenic effects of the drug.

Teaching points

- Only 1 month's prescription can be given at a time.
- Take drug with meals; do not crush capsules.
- Transient flare-ups of acne may occur at the beginning of therapy.
- There is a risk of injury in pediatric patients who participate in sports that involve repetitive impact; parents should monitor activity and alert coaches.

- Use two forms of contraception 1 mo prior to, during treatment, and for 1 mo after treatment is discontinued. This drug has been associated with severe birth defects and miscarriages; it is contraindicated in pregnant women. If you think that you are pregnant, consult your physician immediately. You must sign a consent stating your understanding of the need for contraception.
- Do not donate blood while on this drug because of its potential effects on the fetus of a blood recipient.
- These side effects may occur: dizziness, lethargy, headache, visual changes (avoid driving or performing tasks that require alertness); sensitivity to the sun (avoid sunlamps, exposure to the sun; use sunscreens, protective clothing); diarrhea, abdominal pain, loss of appetite (take drug with meals); dry mouth (sucking sugarless lozenges may help); eye irritation and redness, inability to wear contact lenses; dry skin, itching, redness.
- Avoid vitamin supplements containing vitamin A; serious toxic effects may occur. Limit your consumption of alcohol. You also may need to limit your intake of fats and increase exercise to limit drug effects on blood triglyceride levels.
- Report headache with nausea and vomiting, severe diarrhea or rectal bleeding, visual difficulties, depression, suicidal ideation, violent or aggressive behavior.

▽isradipine
*(eyes **rad'** i peen)*

DynaCirc, DynaCirc CR

PREGNANCY CATEGORY C

Drug classes
Calcium channel-blocker
Antihypertensive

Therapeutic actions
Inhibits the movement of calcium ions across the membranes of cardiac and arterial muscle cells; calcium is involved in the generation of the action potential in specialized automatic and conducting cells in the heart and in arterial smooth muscle and excitation-contraction coupling in cardiac muscle cells; inhibition of

transmembrane calcium flow results in the depression of impulse formation in specialized cardiac pacemaker cells, slowing of the velocity of conduction of the cardiac impulse, the depression of myocardial contractility, and the dilation of coronary arteries and arterioles and peripheral arterioles. These effects lead to decreased cardiac work, cardiac energy consumption, and blood pressure.

Indications

- Management of hypertension alone or in combination with thiazide-type diuretics

Contraindications and cautions

- Contraindicated with allergy to isradipine; sick sinus syndrome, except with ventricular pacemaker; heart block (second or third degree); IHSS; cardiogenic shock, severe CHF; pregnancy; lactation.
- Use cautiously with hypotension, impaired hepatic or renal function (repeated doses may accumulate).

Available forms

Capsules—2.5, 5 mg; CR tablets—5, 10 mg

Dosages
Adults

Initial dose of 2.5 mg PO bid. An antihypertensive effect is usually seen within 2–3 hr; maximal response may require 2–4 wk. Dosage may be increased in increments of 5 mg/day at 2- to 4-wk intervals. Maximum dose: 20 mg/day. CR: 5–10 mg PO daily as monotherapy or combined with thiazide diuretic.

Pharmacokinetics

Route	Onset	Peak
Oral	40 min	90 min

Metabolism: Hepatic; $T_{1/2}$: 8 hr
Distribution: Crosses placenta; enters breast milk
Excretion: Urine

Adverse effects

- **CNS:** *Dizziness,* vertigo, emotional depression, sleepiness, *headache*
- **CV:** *Peripheral edema, hypotension,* arrhythmias, bradycardia, **AV heart block, angina, MI, stroke** (increased risk with isradipine than with other calcium channel-blockers)
- **GI:** *Nausea,* constipation
- **Other:** Muscle fatigue, diaphoresis

Interactions

✷ **Drug-drug** • Increased cardiac depression with beta-adrenergic blocking agents • Increased serum levels of digoxin, carbamazepine, prazosin, quinidine • Increased respiratory depression with atracurium, gallamine, pancuronium, tubocurarine, vecuronium • Decreased effects with calcium, rifampin

■ Nursing considerations
Assessment

- **History:** Allergy to isradipine; sick sinus syndrome, heart block; IHSS; cardiogenic shock, severe CHF; hypotension; impaired hepatic or renal function; pregnancy; lactation
- **Physical:** Skin color, edema; orientation, reflexes; P, BP, baseline ECG, peripheral perfusion, auscultation; R, adventitious sounds; liver evaluation, normal output; liver and renal function tests, urinalysis

Interventions

- Consider increased risk of angina, MI, stroke with use of this drug; select patients carefully.
- Monitor patient carefully (BP, cardiac rhythm, and output) while drug is being adjusted to therapeutic dose.
- Monitor BP very carefully with concurrent doses of other antihypertensive drugs.
- Monitor cardiac rhythm regularly during stabilization of dosage and periodically during long-term therapy.
- Monitor patients with renal or hepatic impairment carefully for drug accumulation and adverse reactions.

Teaching points

- These side effects may occur: nausea, vomiting (small, frequent meals may help); headache (monitor lighting, noise, and temperature; medication may be ordered if severe); dizziness, sleepiness (avoid driving or operating dangerous equipment); emotional depression (should pass when the drug is

stopped); constipation (measures may be taken to alleviate this problem).
- Report irregular heart beat, shortness of breath, swelling of the hands or feet, pronounced dizziness, constipation.

▽ **itraconazole**

*(eye tra **kon'** a zole)*

Sporanox

PREGNANCY CATEGORY C

Drug class
Antifungal

Therapeutic actions
Binds to sterols in the fungal cell membrane, changing membrane permeability; fungicidal or fungistatic depending on concentration and organism.

Indications
- Treatment of blastomycosis, histoplasmosis in immunocompromised and nonimmunocompromised patients (parenteral and oral)
- Treatment of aspergillosis in patients intolerant to amphotericin B (parenteral)
- Treatment of onychomycosis due to dermatophytes
- Treatment of fungal infections of the esophagus or mouth (oral solution)
- Unlabeled uses: treatment of superficial and systemic mycoses, fungal keratitis, cutaneous leishmaniasis

Contraindications and cautions
- Contraindicated with hypersensitivity to itraconazole or other azoles, lactation, congestive heart failure, history of prolonged QTc interval.
- Use cautiously with hepatic impairment.

Available forms
Capsules—100 mg; oral solution—10 mg/mL; injection—10 mg/mL

Dosages
Adults
- *Oropharyngeal and esophageal candidiasis:* 100 mg/day PO for 1–2 wk; continue for 4 wk with esophageal candidiasis.
- *Blastomycosis or chronic histoplasmosis:* 200 mg/day PO for a minimum of 3 mo, may increase to a maximum of 400 mg/day.
- *Other systemic mycoses:* 100–200 mg/day for 3–6 mo.
- *Dermatocytoses:* 100–200 mg/day to bid for 7–28 days, determined by specific infection.
- *Fingernail onychomycosis:* 200 mg bid PO for 1 wk, followed by 3-wk rest period; repeat.
- *Toenail onychomycosis:* 200 mg/day PO for 12 wk.
- *Blastomycosis, histoplasmosis, aspergillosis:* 200 mg IV bid for a total of 4 doses, followed by 200 mg/day.

Oral solution
100–200 mg (10–20 mL), rinse and hold, swallow solution daily for 1–3 wk.

Pediatric patients
Safety and efficacy not established.

Patients with renal impairment
Do not give to patients if creatine clearance < 30 mL/min.

Pharmacokinetics

Route	Onset	Peak	Duration
Oral	Slow	4.6 hr	4–6 days
IV	Rapid	–	End of infusion

Metabolism: Hepatic; $T_{1/2}$: 21 hr, then 64 hr
Distribution: Crosses placenta; may enter breast milk
Excretion: Urine

▽ **IV facts**
Preparation: Add full contents of provided ampule to 50 mL of 0.9% sodium chloride injection, mix gently.
Infusion: Use a flow control device to infuse over 60 min. Flush line with normal saline, dispose of infusion line.
Incompatibilities: Do not mix with D_5W or lactated Ringer's. Do not infuse with any other medications.

Adverse effects
- **CNS:** *Headache,* dizziness
- **GI:** *Nausea, vomiting, diarrhea, abdominal pain,* anorexia
- **Other:** *Rash, edema,* fever, malaise

Interactions

✳ Drug-drug • Increased serum levels and therefore therapeutic and toxic effects of cyclosporine, digoxin, oral hypoglycemics, warfarin anticoagulants, phenytoin, buspirone • Decreased serum levels with H_2 antagonists, antacids, proton pump inhibitors, isoniazid, phenytoin, rifampin • Potential for serious CV events, including ventricular tachycardia and death, with lovastatin, simvastatin, cisapride, triazolam, midazolam, pimozide, dofetilide; avoid these combinations • Potential for prolonged sedation if combined with benzodiazepines

■ Nursing considerations
Assessment

• **History:** Hypersensitivity to itraconazole, hepatic impairment, lactation, CHF, prolonged QTc interval
• **Physical:** Skin color, lesions; T; orientation, reflexes, affect; bowel sounds, BP, P, auscultation; hepatic function tests; culture of area involved, ECG

Interventions

• Culture of infection before beginning therapy; begin treatment before laboratory results are returned.
• Screen medications to prevent serious drug–drug interactions.
• Decrease dosage in cases of hepatic failure.
• Do not administer to patients with evidence of cardiac dysfuntion, CHF.
• Give oral capsules with meals to facilitate absorption.
• Monitor hepatic function tests regularly in patients with a history of hepatic dysfunction; discontinue or decrease dosage at signs of increased renal toxicity.
• Discontinue drug at any sign of active liver disease—elevated enzymes, hepatitis; or signs of CHF.

Teaching points

• Take the full course of drug therapy that has been prescribed. Therapy may need to be long term.
• Take capsules with food; take oral solution without food.

• Adopt hygiene measures to prevent reinfection or spread of infection.
• Have frequent follow-up while you are on this drug. Keep all appointments, which may include blood tests.
• Women of child-bearing age should use contraceptives during therapy and for 1 mo after therapy is stopped.
• These side effects may occur: nausea, vomiting, diarrhea (small frequent meals may help); headache (analgesics may be ordered); rash, itching (appropriate medication may help).
• Report unusual fatigue, anorexia, vomiting, jaundice, dark urine, pale stool, edema, difficulty breathing.

▽ivermectin

See *Less Commonly Used Drugs,* p. 1346.

▽kanamycin sulfate
(kan a mye' sin)

Kantrex

PREGNANCY CATEGORY C

Drug class
Aminoglycoside antibiotic

Therapeutic actions
Bactericidal: inhibits protein synthesis in strains of gram-negative bacteria; functional integrity of cell membrane appears to be disrupted, causing cell death.

Indications

• Infections caused by susceptible strains of *E. coli, Proteus, Enterobacter aerogenes, Klebsiella pneumoniae, Serratia marcescens, Acinetobacter*
• Treatment of severe infections due to susceptible strains of staphylococci in patients allergic to other antibiotics
• Suppression of GI bacterial flora (oral, adjunctive therapy)
• Hepatic coma, to reduce ammonia-forming bacteria in the GI tract (oral)

- As part of a multidrug therapy for *Mycobacterium avium* complex (an infection in AIDS patients)

Contraindications and cautions
- Contraindicated with allergy to aminoglycosides; intestinal obstruction, pregnancy, lactation.
- Use cautiously with elderly or any patient with diminished hearing, decreased renal function, dehydration, neuromuscular disorders.

Available forms
Injection—500 mg, 1 g; pediatric injection—75 mg; capsules—500 mg

Dosages
Adults or pediatric patients
Do not exceed 1.5 g/day.
IM
7.5 mg/kg q 12 hr or 15 mg/kg/day in equally divided doses q 6–8 hr. Usual duration is 7–10 days. If no effect in 3–5 days, discontinue therapy.
IV
15 mg/kg/day divided into 2 to 3 equal doses, administered over 30–60 min.
Intraperitoneal
500 mg diluted in 20 mL sterile water instilled into the wound closure.
Aerosol
250 mg bid–qid, nebulized.
Oral
- *Suppression of intestinal bacteria:* 1 g every hour for 4 hr followed by 1 g q 6 hr for 36–72 hr.
- *Hepatic coma:* 8–12 g/day in divided doses PO.
Geriatric patients or patients with renal failure
Reduce dosage, and carefully monitor serum drug levels and renal function tests. When not possible, reduce frequency of administration. Calculate dosing interval from the following: dosage interval in hr = serum creatinine (mg/dL) $\times$ 9.

Pharmacokinetics

Route	Onset	Peak
IM, IV	Rapid	30–120 min
Oral	Slow; not absorbed systemically	

Metabolism: $T_{1/2}$: 2–3 hr
Distribution: Crosses placenta; enters breast milk
Excretion: Urine

▽ IV facts
Preparation: Do not mix with other antibacterial agents; administer separately; dilute contents of 500-mg vial with 100–200 mL of normal saline or 5% dextrose in water; dilute 1 g-vial with 200–400 mL of diluent; vials may darken during storage, does not affect potency.
Infusion: Administer dose slowly over 30–60 min (especially important in children).
Incompatibilities: Do not combine with amphotericin B, cephalothin, cephapirin, chlorpheniramine, colistimethate, heparin, methohexital, or other antibacterials.

Adverse effects
Although oral kanamycin is only negligibly absorbed from the intact GI mucosa, there is a risk of absorption from ulcerated areas or when used as an irrigant or aerosol.
- **CNS:** *Ototoxicity–tinnitus, dizziness, vertigo, deafness* (partially reversible to irreversible), confusion, disorientation, depression, lethargy, nystagmus, visual disturbances, headache, fever, tremor, paresthesias, muscle twitching, convulsions, muscular weakness, neuromuscular blockade, apnea
- **CV:** Palpitations, hypotension, hypertension
- **GI:** *Nausea, vomiting, anorexia, diarrhea,* weight loss, increased salivation, malabsorption syndrome
- **GU:** *Nephrotoxicity* (may be irreversible)
- **Hematologic:** Leukemoid reaction, agranulocytosis, granulocytosis, leukopenia, leukocytosis, thrombocytopenia, eosinophilia, anemia, hemolytic anemia, increased or decreased reticulocyte count
- **Hepatic:** Hepatic toxicity; hepatomegaly
- **Hypersensitivity:** Purpura, rash, urticaria, exfoliative dermatitis
- **Other:** *Superinfections, pain and irritation at IM injection sites*

Interactions
✳ **Drug-drug** • Increased ototoxic and nephrotoxic effects with potent diuretics and other ototoxic and nephrotoxic drugs (cephalosporins, penicillins) • Increased likelihood of neuromuscular blockade if given shortly af-

ter general anesthetics, depolarizing and non-depolarizing neuromuscular junction blockers, succinylcholine • Decreased absorption and therapeutic levels of digoxin with kanamycin and methotrexate • Increased effect of warfarin with oral kanamycin due to decreased absorption of vitamin K

■ Nursing considerations
Assessment
- **History:** Allergy to aminoglycosides; intestinal obstruction, lactation, diminished hearing, decreased renal function, dehydration, neuromuscular disorders; pregnancy
- **Physical:** Site of infection, skin color, lesions; orientation, reflexes, eighth cranial nerve function; P, BP; R, bowel sounds; urinalysis, BUN, serum creatinine, serum electrolytes, liver function tests, CBC

Interventions
- Arrange culture and sensitivity tests on infection before beginning therapy.
- Therapeutic serum levels are peaks of 15–40 mcg/mL and troughs of < 10 mcg/mL. Monitor with fourth dose, then weekly thereafter.
- Monitor length of treatment: usual duration 7–10 days. If clinical response does not occur within 3–5 days, stop therapy. Prolonged treatment risks increased toxicity. If drug is used longer than 10 days, monitor auditory and renal function daily.
- Give IM dosage by deep IM injection in upper outer quadrant of the gluteal muscle.
- Ensure that patient is well hydrated before and during therapy.
- Monitor patients receiving a total dose of > 15 g for signs of 8th cranial nerve damage.

Teaching points
- Complete the full course of drug therapy.
- These side effects may occur: ringing in the ears, headache, dizziness (reversible; use safety); nausea, vomiting, loss of appetite (small frequent meals, frequent mouth care may help).
- Report severe headache, dizziness, loss of hearing, severe diarrhea, increased urine output.

▽ketoconazole
*(kee toe **koe'** na zole)*

Nizoral

PREGNANCY CATEGORY C

Drug class
Antifungal

Therapeutic actions
Impairs the synthesis of ergosterol, the main sterol of fungal cell membranes, allowing increased permeability and leakage of cellular components and causing cell death.

Indications
- Treatment of systemic fungal infections: candidiasis, chronic mucocutaneous candidiasis, oral thrush, candiduria, blastomycosis, coccidioidomycosis, histoplasmosis, chromomycosis, paracoccidioidomycosis
- Treatment of dermatophytosis (recalcitrant infections not responding to topical or griseofulvin therapy)
- Topical treatment of tinea corporis and tinea cruris caused by *Trichophyton rubrum, Trichophyton mentagrophytes,* and *Epidermophyton floccosun* and the treatment of tinea versicolor caused by *Malassezia furfur* (topical administration)
- Reduction of scaling due to dandruff (shampoo)
- Orphan drug use: with cyclosporine to diminish cyclosporine-induced nephrotoxicity in organ transplant
- Unlabeled uses: treatment of onychomycosis, pityriasis versicolor, vaginal candidiasis; CNS fungal infections at high doses (800–1,200 mg/day); treatment of advanced prostate cancer at doses of 400 mg q 8 hr; treatment of Cushing's syndrome (800–1,200 mg/day).

Contraindications and cautions
- Contraindicated with allergy to ketoconazole; fungal meningitis; pregnancy; lactation.
- Use cautiously with hepatic failure (increased risk of hepatocellular necrosis).

Adverse effects in *Italics* are most common; those in **Bold** are life-threatening.

Available forms
Tablets—200 mg; topical cream—2%; shampoo—2%

Dosages
Adults
200 mg PO daily. Up to 400 mg/day in severe infections. Treatment period must be long enough to prevent recurrence, 3 wk–6 mo, depending on infecting organism and site.
Pediatric patients
< 2 yr: Safety and efficacy not established.
> 2 yr: 3.3–6.6 mg/kg/day PO as a single dose.
Topical cream
Apply once daily to affected area and immediate surrounding area. Severe cases may be treated twice daily. Continue treatment for at least 2 wk.
Shampoo
Moisten hair and scalp thoroughly with water; apply sufficient shampoo to produce a lather; gently massage for 1 min; rinse hair with warm water; repeat, leaving on hair for 3 min. Shampoo twice a week for 4 wk with at least 3 days between shampooing.

Pharmacokinetics

Route	Onset	Peak
Oral	Varies	1–4 hr
Topical	Slow; not appreciably systemically absorbed	

Metabolism: Hepatic; $T_{1/2}$: 8 hr
Distribution: Crosses placenta; enters breast milk
Excretion: Bile

Adverse effects
- **CNS:** Headache, dizziness, somnolence, photophobia
- **GI:** Hepatotoxicity, *nausea, vomiting,* abdominal pain
- **GU:** Impotence, oligospermia (with very high doses)
- **Hematologic:** Thrombocytopenia, leukopenia, hemolytic anemia
- **Hypersensitivity:** Urticaria to **anaphylaxis**
- **Local:** Severe irritation, *pruritus, stinging* with topical application
- **Other:** *Pruritus,* fever, chills, gynecomastia

Interactions
✳ **Drug-drug** • Decreased blood levels of ketoconazole with rifampin • Increased blood levels of cyclosporine and risk of toxicity • Increased duration of adrenal suppression with corticosteroids • Decreased absorption if taken with antacids, H_2 blockers, proton pump inhibitors; space these at least 2 hr apart • Potent inhibitor of cytochrome P450 3A4 enzyme system. Use with drugs metabolized via this system may lead to increased plasma levels and toxicity (eg, tacrolimus, warfarin)

■ Nursing considerations
Assessment
- **History:** Allergy to ketoconazole, fungal meningitis, hepatic failure, pregnancy, lactation
- **Physical:** Skin color, lesions; orientation, reflexes, affect; bowel sounds; liver function tests; CBC and differential; culture of area involved

Interventions
- Culture fungus prior to therapy; begin treatment before return of laboratory results.
- Maintain epinephrine on standby in case of severe anaphylaxis after first dose.
- Administer oral drug with food to decrease GI upset.
- Do not administer with antacids, H_2 blockers, proton pump inhibitors; ketoconazole requires an acid environment for absorption; if antacids are required, administer at least 2 hr apart.
- Continue administration for long-term therapy until infection is eradicated: candidiasis, 1–2 wk; other systemic mycoses, 6 mo; chronic mucocutaneous candidiasis, often requires maintainance therapy; tineaversicolor, 2 wk of topical application.
- Stop treatment, and consult physician about diagnosis if no improvement is seen within 2 wk of topical application.
- Discontinue topical applications if sensitivity or chemical reaction occurs.
- Administer shampoo as follows: moisten hair and scalp thoroughly with water; apply sufficient shampoo to produce a lather; gently massage for 1 min; rinse hair with warm water; repeat, leaving on hair for 3 min.

- Arrange to monitor hepatic function tests before therapy and monthly or more frequently throughout treatment.

Teaching points
- Take the full course of drug therapy. Long-term use of the drug will be needed; beneficial effects may not be seen for several weeks.
- Take oral drug with meals to decrease GI upset.
- Apply topical drug to affected area and surrounding area. Avoid contact with eyes.
- If using shampoo, moisten hair and scalp thoroughly with water; apply sufficient shampoo to produce a lather; gently massage for 1 min; rinse hair with warm water; repeat, leaving on hair for 3 min. Shampoo twice a week for 4 wk with at least 3 days between shampooing.
- Use appropriate hygiene measures to prevent reinfection or spread of infection.
- These side effects may occur: nausea, vomiting, diarrhea (take drug with food); sedation, dizziness, confusion (avoid driving or performing tasks that require alertness); stinging, irritation (local application).
- Do not take antacids, H₂ blockers, proton pump inhibitors with this drug; if they are needed, take this drug at least 2 hr after their administration.
- Report rash, severe nausea, vomiting, diarrhea, fever, sore throat, unusual bleeding or bruising, yellow skin or eyes, dark urine or pale stools, severe irritation (local application).

▽ketoprofen
(kee toe proe' fen)

Nu-Ketoprofen (CAN), Orafen (CAN), Orudis KT, Oruvail, Rhodis (CAN), Rhovail (CAN)

PREGNANCY CATEGORY B

Drug classes
NSAID
Non-opioid analgesic

Therapeutic actions
Anti-inflammatory and analgesic activity; inhibits prostaglandin and leukotriene synthesis and has antibradykinin and lysosomal membrane-stabilizing actions.

Indications
- Acute and long-term treatment of rheumatoid arthritis and osteoarthritis (capsules or sustained release—*Oruvail*)
- Relief of mild to moderate pain
- Treatment of dysmenorrhea
- Reduction of fever
- OTC use: temporary relief of minor aches and pains

Contraindications and cautions
- Contraindicated with significant renal impairment, pregnancy, lactation.
- Use cautiously with impaired hearing, allergies, hepatic, CV, and GI conditions.

Available forms
Tablets—12.5 mg; capsules—25, 50, 75 mg; ER capsules—100, 150, 200 mg

Dosages
Adults
Do not exceed 300 mg/day, or 200 mg/day ER.
- *Rheumatoid arthritis, osteoarthritis:* Starting dose: 75 mg tid or 50 mg qid PO. Maintenance dose: 150–300 mg PO in 3 to 4 divided doses. Extended release: 200 mg PO daily.
- *Mild to moderate pain, primary dysmenorrhea:* 25–50 mg PO q 6–8 hr as needed. Do not use *Oruvail.*
- *OTC:* 12.5 mg PO q 4–6 hr; do not exceed 25 mg in 4–6 hr or 75 mg in 24 hr.
Pediatric patients
Safety and efficacy not established.
Geriatric patients or patients with hepatic or renal impairment
Reduce starting dose by one-half or one-third. Do not use *Oruvail.*

Pharmacokinetics
Route	Onset	Peak
Oral	30–60 min	0.5–2 hr, 6–7 hr for ER

Adverse effects in *Italics* are most common; those in **Bold** are life-threatening.

Metabolism: Hepatic; $T_{1/2}$: 2–4 hr, 5–6 hr for ER

Distribution: Crosses placenta; enters breast milk

Excretion: Urine

Adverse effects
NSAIDs

- **CNS:** *Headache, dizziness,* somnolence, *insomnia,* fatigue, tiredness, tinnitus, ophthalmologic effects
- **Dermatologic:** *Rash,* pruritus, sweating, dry mucous membranes
- **GI:** *Nausea, dyspepsia, GI pain,* diarrhea, vomiting, *constipation,* flatulence, **gastric or duodenal ulcer**
- **GU:** Dysuria, **renal impairment**
- **Hematologic:** Bleeding, platelet inhibition with higher doses, neutropenia, eosinophilia, leukopenia, thrombocytopenia, agranulocytosis, aplastic anemia, menorrhagia
- **Respiratory:** Dyspnea, hemoptysis, pharyngitis, bronchospasm, rhinitis
- **Other:** Peripheral edema, **anaphylactoid reactions to anaphylactic shock**

Interactions
✱ Drug-drug • Increased risk of nephrotoxicity with other nephrotoxins (aminoglycosides, cyclosporine) • Increased risk of bleeding with anticoagulants (warfarin)

■ Nursing considerations
Assessment

- **History:** Renal impairment, impaired hearing, allergies, hepatic, CV, and GI conditions, lactation, pregnancy
- **Physical:** Skin color and lesions; orientation, reflexes, ophthalmologic and audiometric evaluation, peripheral sensation; P, edema; R, adventitious sounds; liver evaluation; CBC, clotting times, renal and liver function tests; serum electrolytes, stool guaiac

Interventions

- Administer drug with food or after meals if GI upset occurs.
- Arrange for periodic ophthalmologic examination during long-term therapy.

- Institute emergency procedures if overdose occurs: gastric lavage, induction of emesis, supportive therapy.

Teaching points

- Take drug with food or meals if GI upset occurs; take only the prescribed dosage.
- Use during pregnancy is not advised; if an analgesic is needed, consult your health care provider.
- Dizziness, drowsiness can occur (avoid driving or the use of dangerous machinery).
- For OTC use—do not take for > 3 days for fever and > 10 days for pain. If symptoms persist, contact your health care provider.
- Report sore throat, fever, rash, itching, weight gain, swelling in ankles or fingers; changes in vision; black, tarry stools, easy bruising.

K

▷ketorolac tromethamine
(kee' toe role ak)

Acular (ophthalmic), Toradol

PREGNANCY CATEGORY B

Drug classes
NSAID
Non-opioid analgesic

Therapeutic actions
Anti-inflammatory and analgesic activity; inhibits prostaglandins and leukotriene synthesis.

Indications

- Short-term management of pain (up to 5 days)
- Relief of ocular itching due to seasonal conjunctivitis (ophthalmic)

Contraindications and cautions

- Contraindicated with significant renal impairment, pregnancy, lactation; patients wearing soft contact lenses (ophthalmic).
- Use cautiously with impaired hearing; allergies; hepatic, CV and GI conditions.

Available forms
Ophthalmic solution—0.5%; tablets—10 mg; injection—15, 30 mg/mL

Dosages
For short-term use only (up to 5 days). Potent NSAID with many adverse effects.
Adults
- *Single-dose treatment:* 60 mg IM or 30 mg IV.
- *Multiple-dose treatment:* 30 mg IM or IV q 6 hr to a maximum 120 mg/day.
- *Transfer to oral:* 20 mg PO as a first dose for patients who received 60 mg IM or 30 mg IV as a single dose or 30-mg multiple dose, followed by 10 mg q 4–6 hr; do not exceed 40 mg/24 hr.
- *Ophthalmic:* 1 drop (0.25 mg) qid.
Pediatric patients
Safety and efficacy not established.
Geriatric patients ≥ 65 yr, patients with renal impairment, and patients < 50 kg
- *Single-dose treatment:* 30 mg IM or 15 mg IV.
- *Multiple-dose treatment:* 15 mg IM or IV q 6 hr to a maximum of 60 mg/day.
- *Transfer to oral:* 10 mg PO as first dose for patients who received 30 mg IM or 15 mg IV single dose or 15 mg IM or IV multiple dose, then 10 mg PO q 4–6 hr; do not exceed 40 mg/24 hr.

Pharmacokinetics

Route	Onset	Peak	Duration
Oral	Varies	30–60 min	6 hr
IM, IV	30 min	1–2 hr	6 hr

Metabolism: Hepatic; $T_{1/2}$: 2.4–8.6 hr
Distribution: Crosses placenta; enters breast milk
Excretion: Urine

▼IV facts
Preparation: No further preparation is required.
Infusion: Infuse slowly as a bolus over no less than 15 sec.
Incompatibilities: Do not mix with morphine, sulfate, meperidine, promethazine, or hydroxyzine; a precipitate will form. Protect injection from light.

Adverse effects
- **CNS:** *Headache, dizziness, somnolence, insomnia,* fatigue, dizziness, tinnitus, ophthalmologic effects
- **Dermatologic:** *Rash,* pruritus, sweating, dry mucous membranes
- **GI:** *Nausea, dyspepsia, GI pain,* diarrhea, vomiting, *constipation,* flatulence, **gastric or duodenal ulcers**
- **GU:** Dysuria, **renal impairment**
- **Hematologic:** Bleeding, platelet inhibition with higher doses, neutropenia, eosinophilia, leukopenia, pancytopenia, thrombocytopenia, agranulocytosis, granulocytopenia, aplastic anemia, decreased Hgb or Hct, bone marrow depression, menorrhagia
- **Respiratory:** Dyspnea, hemoptysis, pharyngitis, bronchospasm, rhinitis
- **Other:** Peripheral edema; **anaphylactoid reactions to anaphylactic shock;** *local burning, stinging* (ophthalmic)

Interactions
✳ Drug-drug • Increased risk of nephrotoxicity with other nephrotoxins (aminoglycosides, cyclosporine) • Increased risk of bleeding with anticoagulants (warfarin)

■ Nursing considerations

 CLINICAL ALERT!
Name confusion has occurred between Fovadil (formoterol) and Toradol (ketorolac) and between tramadol and Toradol (ketorolac); use caution.

Assessment
- **History:** Renal impairment; impaired hearing; allergies; hepatic, CV, and GI conditions; lactation
- **Physical:** Skin color and lesions; orientation, reflexes, ophthalmologic and audiometric evaluation, peripheral sensation; P, edema; R, adventitious sounds; liver evaluation; CBC, clotting times, renal and liver function tests; serum electrolytes, stool guaiac

Interventions

- Maintain emergency equipment on standby at time of initial dose, in case of severe hypersensitivity reaction.
- Protect drug vials from light.
- Administer every 6 hr to maintain serum levels and control pain.

Teaching points

- Every effort will be made to administer the drug on time to control pain; dizziness, drowsiness can occur (avoid driving or using dangerous machinery); burning and stinging on application (ophthalmic).
- Report sore throat, fever, rash, itching, weight gain, swelling in ankles or fingers; changes in vision; black, tarry stools, easy bruising.

▽labetalol hydrochloride

*(la **bet**' a lol)*

Normodyne, Trandate

PREGNANCY CATEGORY C

Drug classes

Alpha- and beta-adrenergic blocker
Antihypertensive

Therapeutic actions

Competitively blocks alpha$_1$- and beta$_1$- and beta$_2$-adrenergic receptors, and has some sympathomimetic activity at beta$_2$-receptors. Alpha- and beta-blocking actions contribute to the BP-lowering effect; beta blockade prevents the reflex tachycardia seen with most alpha-blocking drugs and decreases plasma renin activity.

Indications

- Hypertension, alone or with other oral drugs, especially diuretics
- Severe hypertension (parenteral preparations)
- Unlabeled uses: control of BP in pheochromocytoma; clonidine withdrawal hypertension

Contraindications and cautions

- Contraindicated with sinus bradycardia, second or third-degree heart block, cardio-

genic shock, CHF, asthma, pregnancy, lactation.
- Use cautiously with diabetes or hypoglycemia (can mask cardiac signs of hypoglycemia), nonallergic bronchospasm (oral drug—IV is absolutely contraindicated), pheochromocytoma (paradoxical increases in BP have occurred).

Available forms

Tablets—100, 200, 300 mg; injection—5 mg/mL

Dosages

Adults

Oral

Initial dose 100 mg bid. After 2–3 days, using standing BP as indicator, adjust dosage in increments of 100 mg bid q 2–3 days. *Maintenance:* 200 to 400 mg bid. Up to 2,400 mg/day may be required; to improve tolerance, divide total daily dose and give tid.

Parenteral

- *Severe hypertension: Repeated IV injection:* 20 mg (0.25 mg/kg) slowly over 2 min. Individualize dosage using supine BP; additional doses of 40 or 80 mg can be given at 10-min intervals until desired BP is achieved or until a 300-mg dose has been injected. *Continuous IV infusion:* Dilute ampule (below), infuse at the rate of 2 mg/min, adjust according to BP response up to 300 mg total dose. Transfer to oral therapy as soon as possible.

Pediatric patients

Safety and efficacy not established.

Geriatric patients

Generally require lower maintenance doses.

Pharmacokinetics

Route	Onset	Peak	Duration
Oral	Varies	1–2 hr	8–12 hr
IV	Immediate	5 min	5.5 hr

Metabolism: Hepatic; $T_{1/2}$: 6–8 hr
Distribution: Crosses placenta; enters breast milk
Excretion: Urine

▽IV facts

Preparation: Add 200 mg to 160 mL of a compatible IV fluid to make a 1 mg/mL solution; infuse at 2 mL/min, or add 200 mg (2 ampules) to 250 mg of IV fluid to make a 2 mg/ 3 mL solution, infuse at 3 mL/min. Compatible IV fluids include Ringer's, lactated Ringer's, 0.9% sodium chloride, 2.5% dextrose and 0.45% sodium chloride, 5% dextrose, 5% dextrose and Ringer's, 5% dextrose and 5% lactated Ringer's, and 5% dextrose and 0.2%, 0.33%, or 0.9% sodium chloride. Stable for 24 hr in these solutions at concentrations between 1.25 and 3.75 mg/mL.

Infusion: Administer infusion at 2–3 mL/ min; inject slowly over 2 min.

Incompatibilities: Do not dilute drug in 5% sodium bicarbonate injection or other alkaline solutions, including furosemide.

Y-site incompatibilities: Do not give with cefoperazone, nafcillin.

Adverse effects

- **CNS:** *Dizziness, vertigo, fatigue,* depression, paresthesias, sleep disturbances, hallucinations, disorientation, memory loss, slurred speech
- **CV:** CHF, cardiac arrhythmias, peripheral vascular insufficiency, claudication, cerebrovascular accident, pulmonary edema, hypotension
- **Dermatologic:** Rash, pruritus, sweating, dry skin
- **EENT:** Eye irritation, dry eyes, conjunctivitis, blurred vision
- **GI:** *Gastric pain, flatulence, constipation, diarrhea, nausea, vomiting,* anorexia, ischemic colitis, renal and mesenterial arterial thrombosis, retroperitoneal fibrosis, hepatomegaly, acute pancreatitis
- **GU:** *Impotence, decreased libido,* Peyronie's disease, dysuria, nocturia, polyuria, priapism, urinary retention
- **Respiratory:** *Bronchospasm, dyspnea, cough,* bronchial obstruction, nasal stuffiness, rhinitis, pharyngitis
- **Other:** *Decreased exercise tolerance,* development of antinuclear antibodies, hyperglycemia or hypoglycemia, elevated liver enzymes

Interactions

✳ **Drug-drug** • Risk of excessive hypotension with enflurane, halothane, or isoflurane
• Potential for added anithypertensive effects

with nitroglycerin • Additive A-V block with calcium channel-blockers

✳ **Drug-lab test** • Possible falsely elevated urinary catecholamines in lab tests using a trihydroxyindole reaction

■ Nursing considerations
Assessment

- **History:** Sinus bradycardia, second- or third-degree heart block, cardiogenic shock, CHF, asthma, pregnancy, lactation, diabetes or hypoglycemia, nonallergic bronchospasm, pheochromocytoma
- **Physical:** Weight, skin condition, neurologic status, P, BP, ECG, respiratory status, kidney and thyroid function, blood and urine glucose

Interventions

- Do not discontinue drug abruptly after long-term therapy. (Hypersensitivity to catecholamines may have developed, causing exacerbation of angina, MI and ventricular arrhythmias; taper drug gradually over 2 wk with monitoring.)
- Consult with physician about withdrawing the drug if the patient is to undergo surgery (withdrawal is controversial).
- Keep patient supine during parenteral therapy, and assist initial ambulation.
- Position to decrease effects of edema.
- Provide support and encouragement to deal with drug effects and disease.

Teaching points

- Take drug with meals.
- Do not stop taking unless instructed to do so by a health care provider.
- These side effects may occur: dizziness, lightheadedness, loss of appetite, nightmares, depression, sexual impotence.
- Report difficulty breathing, night cough, swelling of extremities, slow pulse, confusion, depression, rash, fever, sore throat.
- Diabetic patients: this drug may mask usual symptoms of hypoglycemia; monitor blood glucose carefully.

Adverse effects in *Italics* are most common; those in **Bold** are life-threatening.

▽lactulose
(lak' tyoo lose)

Laxative: Chronulac, Constilac, Constulose, Duphalac, Lactulax (CAN), Laxilose (CAN)

Ammonia-reducing agent: Acilac (CAN), Cephulac, Cholac, Enulose

PREGNANCY CATEGORY B

Drug classes
Laxative
Ammonia reduction agent

Therapeutic actions
The drug passes unchanged into the colon where bacteria break it down to organic acids that increase the osmotic pressure in the colon and slightly acidify the colonic contents, resulting in an increase in stool water content, stool softening, laxative action. This also results in migration of blood ammonia into the colon contents with subsequent trapping and expulsion in the feces.

Indications
- Treatment of constipation
- Prevention and treatment of portal-systemic encephalopathy

Contraindications and cautions
- Contraindicated with allergy to lactulose, low-galactose diet.
- Use cautiously with diabetes and lactation.

Available forms
Syrup, solution—10 g/15 mL

Dosages
Adults
- *Laxative:* 15–30 mL/day PO; may be increased to 60 mL/day as needed.
- *Portal-systemic encephalopathy:*
Oral
30–45 mL tid or qid. Adjust dosage every day or two to produce 2–3 soft stools/day. 30–45 mL/hr may be used if necessary. Return to standard dose as soon as possible.

Rectal
300 mL lactulose mixed with 700 mL water or physiologic saline as a retention enema, retained for 30–60 min. May be repeated q 4–6 hr. Start oral drug as soon as feasible and before stopping enemas.
Pediatric patients
- *Laxative:* Safety and efficacy not established.
- *Portal-systemic encephalopathy:*
Oral
Standards not clearly established. Initial dose of 2.5–10 mL/day in divided dose for small children or 40–90 mL/day for older children is suggested. Attempt to produce 2–3 soft stools daily.

Pharmacokinetics

Route	Onset	Peak	Duration
Oral	Varies	20 hr	24–48 hr

Very minimally absorbed systemically

Adverse effects
- **GI:** *Transient flatulence, distension, intestinal cramps, belching,* diarrhea, nausea
- **Other:** Acid–base imbalances

■ Nursing considerations
Assessment
- **History:** Allergy to lactulose, low-galactose diet, diabetes, lactation, pregnancy
- **Physical:** Abdominal exam, bowel sounds, serum electrolytes, serum ammonia levels

Interventions
- Do not freeze laxative form. Extremely dark or cloudy syrup may be unsafe; do not use.
- Give laxative syrup orally with fruit juice, water, or milk to increase palatability.
- Administer retention enema using a rectal balloon catheter. Do not use cleansing enemas containing soap suds or other alkaline agents that counteract the effects of lactulose.
- Do not administer other laxatives while using lactulose.
- Monitor serum ammonia levels.
- Monitor with long-term therapy for potential electrolyte and acid–base imbalances.
- Monitor blood glucose levels carefully in diabetic patients.

Teaching points

- Do not use other laxatives. The drug may be mixed in water, juice, or milk to make it more tolerable.
- For laxative use: do not use continuously for > 1 wk unless directed by a physician.
- These side effects may occur: abdominal fullness, flatulence, belching.
- Ensure ready access to bathroom; bowel movements will be increased to 2–3 per day.
- Report diarrhea, severe belching, abdominal fullness.

▷lamivudine (3TC)

*(lam ah **vew**' den)*

Epivir, Epivir-HBV

PREGNANCY CATEGORY C

Drug classes

Antiviral
Reverse transcriptase inhibitor

Therapeutic actions

Nucleoside analogue inhibitor of HIV reverse transcriptase via DNA viral chain termination.

Indications

- Treatment of HIV infection in combination with other antiretroviral drugs
- Treatment of chronic hepatitis B (*Epivir-HBV*) with active liver inflammation

Contraindications and cautions

- Contraindicated with life-threatening allergy to any component; pregnancy, lactation.
- Use cautiously with compromised bone marrow function, impaired renal function, liver dysfunction, obesity.

Available forms

Tablets—100 (*Epivir–HBV*), 150 mg; oral solution—5 (*Epivir–HBV*), 10 mg/mL

Dosages
Adults

- *Hepatitis B:* 100 mg PO daily.

Adults and patients ≥ 16 yr

- *HIV infection:* 150 mg PO bid or 300 mg/day PO as a single dose in combination with other antiretroviral drugs.

Pediatric patients

- *HIV infection: 3 mo–16 yr:* 4 mg/kg PO bid; up to a maximum of 150 mg bid.
- *Hepatitis B: 2–17 yr:* 3 mg/kg PO daily up to a maximum of 100 mg daily.

Patients with impaired renal function

- *HIV infection:*

Creatinine Clearance (mL/min)	Dosage
≥ 50	150 mg PO bid
30–49	150 mg PO daily
15–29	150 mg PO first dose, then 100 mg PO daily
5–14	150 mg PO first dose, then 50 mg PO daily
< 5	50 mg PO first dose, then 25 mg PO daily

- *Hepatitis B:*

Creatinine Clearance (mL/min)	Dosage
≥ 50	100 mg PO daily
30–49	100 mg first dose, then 50 mg daily
15–29	100 mg first dose, then 25 mg daily
5–14	35 mg first dose, then 15 mg daily
< 5	35 mg first dose, then 10 mg daily

Pharmacokinetics

Route	Onset	Peak
Oral	Slow	2–4 hr

Metabolism: Unknown; $T_{1/2}$: 5–7 hr
Distribution: Crosses placenta; passes into breast milk
Excretion: Urine

Adverse effects

- **CNS:** *Headache,* insomnia, myalgia, *asthenia,* malaise, dizziness, paresthesias, somnolence
- **GI:** *Nausea, GI pain, diarrhea,* anorexia, vomiting, dyspepsia, **pancreatitis** (chil-

---

Adverse effects in *Italics* are most common; those in **Bold** are life-threatening.

dren), **hepatomegaly with lactic acidosis, steatosis**
- **Hematologic:** *Agranulocytosis*
- **Respiratory:** *Nasal signs and symptoms, cough*
- **Other:** *Fever, rash,* taste perversion

Interactions
⁕ Drug-drug • Increased levels of lamivudine taken concurrently with trimethoprim-sulfamethoxazole • Lamivudine and zalcitabine inhibit the effects of each other; avoid concurrent use

■ Nursing considerations
Assessment
- **History:** Life-threatening allergy to any component, compromised bone marrow function, impaired renal function, pregnancy, lactation, liver dysfunction, obesity
- **Physical:** Skin rashes, lesions, texture; T; affect, reflexes, peripheral sensation; bowel sounds, liver evaluation; renal function tests, CBC and differential

Interventions
- Arrange to monitor hematologic indices and liver function every 2 wk during therapy.
- Monitor children for any sign of pancreatitis and discontinue immediately if it occurs.
- Monitor patient for signs of opportunistic infections that will need to be treated appropriately.
- Administer the drug concurrently with other antiretroviral agents for HIV infection.
- Offer support and encouragement to the patient to deal with the diagnosis as well as the effects of drug therapy and the high expense of treatment.

Teaching points
- Take drug as prescribed; take concurrently with other agents prescribed for HIV treatment.
- These drugs are not a cure for AIDS or ARC or hepatitis B; opportunistic infections may occur and regular medical care should be sought to deal with the disease.
- Arrange for frequent blood tests, needed during the course of treatment; results of blood counts may indicate a need for decreased dosage or discontinuation of the drug for a period of time.

- These side effects may occur: nausea, loss of appetite, change in taste (small, frequent meals may help); dizziness, loss of feeling (take appropriate precautions); headache, fever, muscle aches (an analgesic may help, consult with your health care provider).
- Lamivudine does not reduce the risk of transmission of HIV or hepatitis B to others by sexual contact or blood contamination—use appropriate precautions.
- Avoid pregnancy while on this drug; use of barrier contraceptives is urged.
- Report extreme fatigue, lethargy, severe headache, severe nausea, vomiting, difficulty breathing, rash.

▽ lamotrigine
(la mo' tri geen)

Lamictal, Lamictal Chewable Dispersible Tablets

PREGNANCY CATEGORY C

Drug class
Antiepileptic agent

Therapeutic actions
Mechanism not well understood; may inhibit voltage-sensitive sodium channels, stabilizing the neuronal membrane and modulating calcium-dependent presynaptic release of excitatory amino acids.

Indications
- Adjuvant therapy in the treatment of partial seizures in adults with epilepsy
- Adjunctive therapy for the treatment of Lennox-Gastaut syndrome in infants, children, and adults
- Monotherapy in adults with partial seizures
- Unlabeled use: generalized tonic-clonic, absence, and myoclonic seizures (adults), bipolar disorder

Contraindications and cautions
- Contraindicated with allergy to drug, lactation, pregnancy.
- Use cautiously with impaired hepatic, renal, or cardiac function; patients < 16 yr

Available forms

Tablets—25, 100, 150, 200 mg; chewable tablets—2, 5, 25 mg

Dosages

Adults

- Patients taking enzyme-inducing antiepiletic drugs: 50 mg PO daily for 2 wk; then 100 mg PO daily in 2 divided doses for 2 wk; may increase by 100 mg/day every wk up to a maintenance dose of 300–700 mg/day in 2 divided doses. If valproic acid is also being taken: 25 mg PO every other day for 2 wk; then 25 mg PO daily for 2 wk, then may increase by 25–50 mg every 1–2 wk up to a maintenance dose of 100–200 mg/day PO in 2 divided doses.
- Conversion of patients to lamotrigine monotherapy: titrate as above to a target dose of 500 mg/day in 2 divided doses, then attempt to decrease other antiepileptic by 20% weekly.

Pediatric patients

- 2–12 yr: Patients taking enzyme-inducing antiepileptic drugs—0.15 mg/kg/day in 1–2 divided doses for 2 wk. If calculated dose is 2.5–5 mg, take 5 mg on alternate days for 2 wk, then 0.3 mg/kg/day in 1–2 divided doses, rounded down to nearest 5 mg for 2 wk. Maintenance: 1–5 mg/kg/day in 1–2 divided doses, to a maximum of 200 mg/day. Without valproic acid: 0.6 mg/kg/day in 2 divided doses for 2 wk, then 1.2 mg/kg/day in 2 divided doses for 2 wk. Maintenance: 5–15 mg/kg/day in 2 divided doses, to a maximum of 400 mg/day.
- > 12 yr: Patients taking enzyme-inducing antiepileptic drugs—25 mg PO every other day for 2 wk, then 25 mg PO daily for 2 wk. Maintenance: 100–400 mg/day in 1–2 divided doses. With valproic acid: 50 mg/day PO for 2 wk, then 100 mg/day in 2 divided doses for 2 wk. Maintenance: 300–500 mg/day in 1–2 divided doses.

Pharmacokinetics

Route	Onset	Peak
Oral	Rapid	2–5 hr

Metabolism: Hepatic; $T_{1/2}$: 25–33 hr

Distribution: Crosses placenta; may pass into breast milk
Excretion: Urine

Adverse effects

- **CNS:** *Dizziness,* insomnia, headache, somnolence, *ataxia,* diplopia, blurred vision
- **Dermatologic: Rash, Stevens-Johnson syndrome, toxic epidermal necrosis with multiorgan failure**
- **GI:** *Nausea,* vomiting

Interactions

✴ **Drug-drug** • 40%–50% decrease in lamotrigine levels with enzyme-inducing antiepiletic agents: carbamazepine, phenytoin, phenobarbital, primidone • Decreased clearance of lamotrigine, requiring a lower dose, if taken with valproic acid

■ Nursing considerations

 CLINICAL ALERT!
Name confusion has occurred between Lamictal (lamotrigine) and Lamisel (terbinafine); use extreme caution.

Assessment

- **History:** Lactation; impaired hepatic, renal or cardiac function; pregnancy
- **Physical:** Weight; T; skin color, lesions; orientation, affect, reflexes; P, BP, perfusion; bowel sounds, normal output; liver and renal function tests

Interventions

- Monitor renal and hepatic function before and periodically during therapy; if abnormal, reevaluate therapy.
- Monitor drug doses carefully when starting therapy and with each increase in dose; special care will be needed when changing the dose or frequency of any other antiepiletic.
- Monitor patient for any sign of rash; discontinue lamotrigine immediately if rash appears and be prepared with appropriate life support if needed.
- Administer only whole dispersable tablets.
- Administer chewable, dispersible tablets with a small amount of water or fruit juice if chewed; to disperse, add tablet to 1 tsp wa-

ter, wait 1 min, swirl and administer immediately.
- Taper drug slowly over a 2-wk period when discontinuing.

Teaching points
- Take this drug exactly as prescribed.
- Do not discontinue this drug abruptly or change dosage, except on the advice of your health care provider.
- These side effects may occur: dizziness, drowsiness (avoid driving or performing tasks requiring alertness or visual acuity); GI upset (take drug with food or milk, frequent small meals may help); headache (medication can be ordered).
- Wear a medical ID tag to alert emergency medical personnel that you are an epileptic taking antiepileptic medication.
- Notify health care provider immediately if rash occurs.
- Report yellowing of skin, abdominal pain, changes in color of urine or stools, fever, sore throat, mouth sores, unusual bleeding or bruising, rash.

▽**lansoprazole**
(lanz ab' pray zol)

Prevacid

PREGNANCY CATEGORY B

Drug classes
Antisecretory agent
Proton pump inhibitor

Therapeutic actions
Gastric acid-pump inhibitor: suppresses gastric acid secretion by specific inhibition of the hydrogen–potassium ATPase enzyme system at the secretory surface of the gastric parietal cells; blocks the final step of acid production.

Indications
- Short-term treatment of active duodenal ulcer (≤ 4 wk)
- Short-term treatment of gastroesophageal reflux disease: severe erosive esophagitis; poorly responsive symptomatic gastroesophageal reflux disease (≤ 8 wk)

- Treatment of pathological hypersecretory conditions (eg, Zollinger-Ellison syndrome, multiple adenomas, systemic mastocytosis)—long-term therapy
- Maintenance therapy for healing of erosive esophagitis, duodenal ulcers
- Eradication of *Helicobacter pylori* infection in patients with active or recurrent duodenal ulcers in combination with clarithromycin and amoxicillin
- Short-term treatment of symptomatic gastroesophageal reflux disease and erosive esophagitis in children 1–11 yr

Contraindications and cautions
- Contraindicated with hypersensitivity to lansoprazole or any of its components.
- Use cautiously with pregnancy, lactation.

Available forms
DR capsules—15, 30 mg; DR granules for oral suspension—15, 30 mg

Dosages
Adults
- *Active duodenal ulcer:* 15 mg PO daily before eating for 4 wk. Maintenance: 15 mg PO daily.
- *Gastric ulcer:* 30 mg/day PO for ≤ 8 wk.
- *Risk reduction of gastric ulcer with NSAIDS:* 15 mg/day PO for ≤ 12 wk.
- *Duodenal ulcers associated with H. pylori:* 30 mg lansoprazole, 500 mg clarithromycin, 1 g amoxicillin, all give PO bid for 10–14 days; or 30 mg lansoprazole and 1 g amoxicillin PO tid for 14 days.
- *Erosive esophagitis or poorly responsive gastroesophageal reflux disease:* 30 mg PO daily before eating for up to 8 wk. An additional 8-wk course may be helpful for patients who do not heal with 8-wk therapy.
- *Maintenance of healing of erosive esophagitis:* 15 mg/day PO.
- *Pathological hypersecretory conditions:* Individualize dosage. Initial dose is 60 mg PO daily. Doses up to 90 mg bid have been used. Administer daily doses of > 120 mg in divided doses.
Pediatric patients 1–11 yr
< 30 kg: 15 mg/day PO; > 30 kg: 30 mg/day PO. Give as oral suspension, or capsules may be opened and the granules sprinkled on soft food. Do not cut, crush, or chew granules.

Patients with hepatic dysfunction
Consider lowering dose and monitoring patient response.

Pharmacokinetics

Route	Onset	Peak
Oral	Varies	1.7 hr

Metabolism: Hepatic; $T_{1/2}$: 2 hr
Distribution: Crosses placenta; may pass into breast milk
Excretion: Bile

Adverse effects

- **CNS:** *Headache,* dizziness, asthenia, vertigo, insomnia, anxiety, paresthesias, dream abnormalities
- **Dermatologic:** Rash, inflammation, urticaria, pruritus, alopecia, dry skin, acne
- **GI:** *Diarrhea, abdominal pain, nausea, vomiting,* constipation, dry mouth
- **Respiratory:** *URI symptoms,* cough, epistaxis
- **Other:** Gastric cancer in preclinical studies, back pain, fever

Interactions

✳ Drug-drug ● Decreased serum levels if taken concurrently with sucralfate ● Decreased serum levels of ketoconazole, theophylline when taken with lansoprazole

■ Nursing considerations
Assessment

- **History:** Hypersensitivity to lansoprazole or any of its components; pregnancy; lactation
- **Physical:** Skin lesions; body temperature; reflexes, affect; urinary output, abdominal exam; respiratory auscultation

Interventions

- Administer before meals. Caution patient to swallow capsules whole, not to open, chew, or crush. If patient has difficulty swallowing, open capsule and sprinkle granules on apple sauce, *Ensure,* yogurt, cottage cheese, or strained pears; for NG tube, mix granules from capsule with 40 mL apple juice and inject through tube, flush tube with additional apple juice; or granules for oral suspension can be added to 30 mL water, stir well, and have patient drink immediately.
- Arrange for further evaluation of patient after 4 wk of therapy for acute gastroreflux disorders if symptomatic improvement does not rule out gastric cancer, which did occur in preclinical studies.

Teaching points

- Take the drug before meals. Swallow the capsules whole—do not chew, open, or crush. If you are unable to swallow capsule, open and sprinkle granules on apple sauce, or use granules, which can be added to 30 mL water, stirred, and drunk immediately.
- Arrange to have regular medical follow-up while you are on this drug.
- These side effects may occur: dizziness (avoid driving a car or performing hazardous tasks); headache (medications may be available to help); nausea, vomiting, diarrhea (proper nutrition is important, consult with your dietitian to maintain nutrition); symptoms of upper respiratory tract infection, cough (reversible; do not self-medicate, consult with your health care provider if this becomes uncomfortable).
- Report severe headache, worsening of symptoms, fever, chills.

▷ leflunomide
(leh flew' no mide)

Arava

PREGNANCY CATEGORY X

Drug classes
Antiarthritis drug
Pyrimidine synthesis inhibitor

Therapeutic actions
Reversibly inhibits the enzyme DHODH, which is active in the autoimmune process that leads to rheumatoid arthritis; blocking this enzyme relieves the signs and symptoms of inflammation and blocks the structural damage caused by the inflammatory response to the autoimmune process.

Indications

- Treatment of active rheumatoid arthritis; to relieve symptoms and slow progression of the disease

Contraindications and cautions

- Contraindicated with allergy to leflunomide, lactation, pregnancy, or child-bearing age when not using a reliable method of contraception, significant hepatic impairment, hepatitis B or C.
- Use cautiously with renal or hepatic disorders.

Available forms

Tablets—10, 20, 100 mg

Dosages
Adults

Loading dose: 100 mg PO daily for 3 days; maintenance dose: 20 mg PO daily. If not well tolerated or if ALT elevates to more than 2 times upper level of normal, may reduce to 10 mg PO daily.
Pediatric patients

Safety and efficacy not established.
Patients with hepatic impairment

Do not use with serious hepatic impairment. Decrease dosage and monitor patient closely with mild to moderate hepatic impairment.

Pharmacokinetics

Route	Onset	Peak
Oral	Varies	6–12 hr

Metabolism: Hepatic; $T_{1/2}$: 14 days
Distribution: Crosses placenta; passes into breast milk
Excretion: Urine

Adverse effects

- **CNS:** *Headache,* drowsiness, blurred vision, fatigue, dizziness, paresthesias
- **Dermatologic:** *Erythematous rashes,* pruritus, urticaria, *transient alopecia*
- **GI:** Nausea, vomiting, *diarrhea,* **hepatic toxicity**
- **Other: Serious birth defects**

Interactions

✳ **Drug-drug** • Possible severe liver dysfunction if combined with other hepatotoxic drugs; use with caution • Decreased absorption and effectiveness if combined with charcoal, cholestyramine • Increased risk of toxicity if combined with rifampin; monitor patient closely if this combination is used

■ Nursing considerations
Assessment

- **History:** Allergy to leflunomide, childbearing age, pregnancy, lactation, hepatitis B or C, severe hepatic impairment
- **Physical:** Weight; skin lesions, color; hair; orientation, liver evaluation, abdominal exam; liver function tests

Interventions

- Monitor liver function tests prior to and periodically during therapy. Discontinue drug if hepatic impairment occurs.
- Advise patient that this drug does not cure the disease and appropriate therapies for rheumatoid arthritis should be used.
- Arrange for patient to obtain a wig or some other suitable head covering if alopecia occurs; ensure that head is covered at extremes of temperature; loss of hair is usually reversible.
- Provide appropriate skin care; arrange for treatment of skin lesions as needed.
- Advise women of childbearing age of the risks associated with becoming pregnant while on this drug. Arrange for counseling for appropriate contraceptive measures while this drug is being used. If patient decides to become pregnant, a withdrawal program to rid the body of leflunomide is recommended. Cholestyramine may be used to rapidly decrease serum levels if unplanned pregnancy occurs.

Teaching points

- Take this drug exactly as prescribed. Note that this drug does not cure rheumatoid arthritis, and appropriate therapies to deal with the disease should be followed.
- These side effects may occur: nausea, vomiting, diarrhea (medication may be ordered to help; small frequent meals may also help); dizziness, drowsiness (these are all effects of the drug; consult with your nurse or physician if these occur; dosage adjustment may be needed; it is advisable to avoid driving or operating dangerous machinery if these occur); loss of hair (you may wish to obtain a

wig or other suitable head covering; it is important to keep the head covered at extremes of temperature); rash (avoid exposure to the sun, use a sunscreen and protective clothing if exposed to sun—lotion may be recommended).
- Be aware that this drug may cause birth defects or miscarriages. It is advisable to use birth control while on this drug and for 8 wk thereafter. Consult with your health care provider if you decide to become pregnant; a withdrawal program is available.
- Arrange for frequent, regular medical follow-up, including frequent blood tests to follow the effects of the drug on your body.
- Report black, tarry stools; fever, chills, sore throat; unusual bleeding or bruising; cough or shortness of breath; darkened or bloody urine; abdominal, flank, or joint pain; yellow color to the skin or eyes; mouth sores.

▷ lepirudin

See *Less Commonly Used Drugs,* p. 1346.

▷ letrozole
(le' tro zol)

Femara

PREGNANCY CATEGORY D

Drug classes
Antiestrogen
Aromatase inhibitor

Therapeutic actions
Inhibits the conversion of androgens to estrogens by the aromatase enzyme system (in postmenopausal women, the aromatase system is the main source of estrogens); reduces estrogen levels in all tissues, including tumors.

Indications
- Treatment of advanced breast cancer in postmenopausal women as a first-line treatment and with disease progression following traditional antiestrogen therapy

Contraindications and cautions
- Contraindicated with allergy to letrozole, pregnancy.
- Use cautiously with hepatic impairment, lactation.

Available forms
Tablets—2.5 mg

Dosages
Adults
2.5 mg PO daily; continue until tumor progression is evident.

Pharmacokinetics

Route	Onset	Peak
Oral	Varies	2–6 wk

Metabolism: Hepatic; $T_{1/2}$: 2 days
Distribution: Crosses placenta; may pass into breast milk
Excretion: Urine

Adverse effects
- **CNS:** Depression, *headache,* fatigue
- **Dermatologic:** Alopecia, *hot flashes,* rash
- **GI:** *Nausea, GI upset,* elevated liver enzymes
- **Other:** Peripheral edema; arthralgia

■ Nursing considerations
Assessment
- **History:** Allergy to letrozole, hepatic impairment, pregnancy, lactation
- **Physical:** Skin lesions, color, turgor; orientation, affect, reflexes; peripheral pulses, edema; liver function tests, estrogen receptor evaluation of tumor cells

Interventions
- Counsel patient about the need to use contraceptive measures to avoid pregnancy while taking this drug; inform patient that serious fetal harm could occur.
- Provide comfort measures to help patient deal with drug effects: hot flashes (environmental temperature control); headache, depression (monitoring of light and noise); vaginal bleeding (hygiene measures).
- Discontinue drug at signs that tumor is progressing.

Adverse effects in *Italics* are most common; those in **Bold** are life-threatening.

Teaching points

- These side effects may occur: hot flashes (stay in cool temperatures); nausea, GI upset (eat small, frequent meals); headache, light-headedness (use caution if driving or performing tasks that require alertness).
- This drug can cause serious fetal harm and must not be taken during pregnancy. Contraceptive measures should be used while you are taking this drug. If you become pregnant or decide that you would like to become pregnant, consult with your physician or nurse immediately.
- Report changes in color of urine or stool, increased fatigue, rash, fever, chills, severe depression.

▷ leucovorin calcium (citrovorum factor, folinic acid)

(loo koe vor' in)

Wellcovorin

PREGNANCY CATEGORY C

Drug class
Folic acid derivative

Therapeutic actions
Active reduced form of folic acid; required for nucleoprotein synthesis and maintenance of normal hematopoiesis.

Indications
- "Leucovorin rescue"—after high-dose methotrexate therapy for various cancers
- Treatment of megaloblastic anemias due to sprue, nutritional deficiency, pregnancy, and infancy when oral folic acid therapy is not feasible—parenteral form
- With 5-fluorouracil for palliative treatment of metastatic colorectal cancer (IV)
- To decrease toxicity of methotrexate due to decreased elimination or for inadvertent overdose of folic acid antagonists such as trimethoprim

Contraindications and cautions
- Allergy to leucovorin on previous exposure, pernicious anemia or other megaloblastic anemias in which vitamin B_{12} is deficient, lactation, pregnancy

Available forms
Tablets—5, 15, 25 mg; injection—3 mg/mL; powder for injection—50, 100, 350 mg/vial

Dosages
Adults

- *Rescue after methotrexate therapy:* Begin therapy within 48 hr of methotrexate dose. 10 mg/m^2 PO q 6 hr for 72 hr or until methotrexate level is < 0.05 micromolar. If at 24 hr following methotrexate administration, the serum creatinine is 50% greater than the pretreatment level, or based on methotrexate levels, increase the leucovorin dose to 100 mg/m^2 q 3 hr until the serum methotrexate level is < 0.05 micromolar. For drugs with less affinity for mammalian dihydrofolate reductase (eg, trimethoprim), 5 to 15 mg/day has been used.
- *Megaloblastic anemia:* Up to 1 mg/day IM may be used. Do not exceed 1 mg/day.
- *Metastatic colon cancer:* Give 200 mg/m^2 by slow IV injection over ≥ 3 min, followed by 5-FU 370 mg/m^2 IV *or* 20 mg/m^2 IV, followed by 5-FU 425 mg/m^2 IV. Repeat daily for 5 days; may be repeated at 4-wk intervals.

Pharmacokinetics

Route	Onset	Peak	Duration
Oral	30 min	2.4 hr	3–6 hr
IM	Rapid	52 min	3–6 hr
IV	Immediate	10 min	3–6 hr

Metabolism: Hepatic; $T_{1/2}$: unknown
Distribution: Crosses placenta; enters breast milk
Excretion: Urine and feces

▽ IV facts
Preparation: Prepare solution by diluting a 50-mg vial of powder with 5 mL bacteriostatic water for injection that contains benzyl alcohol and use within 7 days, or reconstitute with water for injection, and use immediately. Protect from light.
Infusion: Infuse slowly over 3–5 min; not more than 160 mg/min.
Incompatibilities: Do not mix with floxuridine.

Y-site incompatibilities: Do not inject with droperidol.

Adverse effects
- **Hypersensitivity:** Allergic reactions
- **Local:** *Pain and discomfort at injection site*

Interactions
✱ **Drug-drug** • Leucovorin increases the efficacy and potential side effects of 5-FU; avoid this combination.

■ Nursing considerations

 CLINICAL ALERT!
Name confusion has occurred between leucovorin and Leukeran (chlorambucil) and between folinic acid (leucovorin) and folic acid; use extreme caution.

Assessment
- **History:** Allergy to leucovorin on previous exposure, pernicious anemia or other megaloblastic anemias, lactation, pregnancy
- **Physical:** Skin lesions, color; R, adventitious sounds; CBC, Hgb, Hct, serum folate levels, serum methotrexate levels

Interventions
- Do not use benzyl alcohol solutions when giving leucovorin to premature infants; a fatal gasping syndrome has occurred.
- Begin leucovorin rescue within 48 hr of methotrexate administration. Arrange for fluid loading and urine alkalinization during this procedure to decrease methotrexate toxicity.
- Give drug orally unless intolerance to oral route develops due to nausea and vomiting from chemotherapy or clinical condition. Switch to oral drug when feasible. Doses > 25 mg should be divided or given IV.
- Monitor patient for hypersensitivity reactions, especially if drug has been used previously. Maintain supportive equipment and emergency drugs on standby in case of serious allergic response.

Teaching points
- Leucovorin "rescues" normal cells from the effects of methotrexate and allows them to survive.
- Leucovorin used to treat anemias or colorectal cancer must be given IV. Mark calendars with treatment days.
- Report rash, difficulty breathing, pain, or discomfort at injection site.

▷ leuprolide acetate
*(loo **proe'** lide)*

Lupron, Lupron Depot, Lupron Depot-Ped, Lupron Depot—3 Month, Lupron Depot—4 Month, Viadur

PREGNANCY CATEGORY X

Drug class
Gonadotropin-releasing hormone analog

Therapeutic actions
An LH-RH agonist that occupies pituitary gonadotropin-releasing hormone receptors and desensitizes them; inhibits gonoadotropin secretion when given continuously, leading to an initial increase, then profound decrease in LH and FSH levels.

Indications
- Advanced prostatic cancer—palliation, alternative to orchiectomy or estrogen therapy
- Endometriosis (depot only)
- Central precocious puberty
- Uterine leiomyomata (depot only)
- Unlabeled uses: treatment of breast, ovarian, and endometrial cancer; infertility; prostatic hypertrophy

Pharmacokinetics

Route	Onset	Peak	Duration
IM depot	4 hr	Variable	1, 3, or 4 mo

Metabolism: Unknown; $T_{1/2}$: 3 hr (SC injection)

Contraindications and cautions
- Allergy to leuprolide; pregnancy

Available forms

Injection—5 mg/mL; *Depot*—3.75, 7.5 mg/mL; *Depot-ped*—7.5, 11.25, 15 mg; 3-mo *Depot*—11.25, 22.5 mg; 4-mo *Depot*—30 mg; 12 mo implant (*Viadur*)—72 mg

Dosages
Adults

- *Advanced prostate cancer:* 1 mg/day SC; use only the syringes that come with the drug.

Depot: 7.5 mg IM monthly (q 28–33 days). Do not use needles smaller than 22 gauge.

3-mo depot: 22.5 mg IM every 3 mo (84 days).

4-mo depot: 30 mg IM every 4 mo.

12-mo implant (Viadur): 72 mg IM every 12 mo.

- *Endometriosis:* 3.75 mg as a single monthly IM injection or 11.25 mg IM q 3 mo. Continue for 6 mo.
- *Uterine leiomyomata:* 3.75 mg as a single monthly injection for 3 mo *or* 11.25 mg IM once.

Pediatric patients

- *Central precocious puberty:* 50 mcg/kg/day SC; may be titrated up by 10 mcg/kg/day increments.

Depot: 0.3 mg/kg IM monthly every 4 wk. Round to nearest depot size.

Adverse effects

- **CNS:** *Dizziness, headache, pain,* paresthesia, blurred vision, lethargy, fatigue, insomnia, memory disorder
- **CV:** *Peripheral edema,* cardiac arrhythmias, thrombophlebitis, CHF, **MI**
- **Dermatologic:** Rash, alopecia, itching, erythema
- **GI:** GI bleeding, *nausea, vomiting, anorexia,* sour taste, *constipation*
- **GU:** *Frequency, hematuria,* decrease in size of testes, increased BUN and creatinine, impotence, decreased libido, gynecomastia
- **Local:** Ecchymosis at injection site
- **Respiratory:** Difficulty breathing, pleural rub, worsening of pulmonary fibrosis
- **Other:** *Hot flashes, sweats,* bone pain

■ Nursing considerations
Assessment

- **History:** Allergy to leuprolide; pregnancy
- **Physical:** Skin lesions, color, turgor; testes; injection sites; orientation, affect, reflexes, peripheral sensation; peripheral pulses, edema, P; R, adventitious sounds; serum testosterone and serum PSA levels

Interventions

- Administer only with the syringes provided with the drug.
- Administer SC; monitor injection sites for bruising and rash; rotate injection sites to decrease local reaction.
- Give depot injection deep into muscle. Prepare a calendar of monthly (28–33 days every 3 or 4 mo) return visits for new injection.
- Refrigerate the vials until dispensed; must be stored below 30° C if unrefrigerated.
- Arrange for periodic serum testosterone and PSA determinations.
- Consider stopping therapy for central precocious puberty before 11 yr in females, 12 yr in males. Monitor patient with GnRH stimulation test, sex steroids, and Tanner staging.
- Advise the use of barrier contraceptives; serious fetal harm can occur.
- Teach patient and significant other the technique for SC injection, and observe administration before home administration.

Teaching points

- Administer SC only, using the syringes that come with the drug. If depot route is used, prepare calendar for return dates, stressing the importance of receiving each injection.
- Do not stop taking this drug without first consulting the health care provider.
- These side effects may occur: bone pain, difficulty urinating (usually transient); hot flashes (staying in cool temperatures may help); nausea, vomiting (small, frequent meals may help); dizziness, headache, lightheadedness (use caution when driving or performing tasks that require alertness); decreased libido, impotence.
- This drug cannot be taken during pregnancy; use of barrier contraceptives is advised.
- Report injection site pain, burning, itching, swelling, numbness, tingling, severe GI upset, pronounced hot flashes.

▽ levalbuterol
*(lev al **byoo'** ter ole)*

Xopenex

PREGNANCY CATEGORY C

Drug classes
Sympathomimetic drug
Beta$_2$-selective adrenergic agonist
Bronchodilator
Antiasthmatic drug

Therapeutic actions
In low doses, acts relatively selectively at beta$_2$-adrenergic receptors to cause bronchodilation and vasodilation; at higher doses, beta$_2$-selectivity is lost and the drug also acts at beta$_1$ receptors to cause typical sympathomimetic cardiac effects.

Indications
• Treatment and prevention of bronchospasm in adults and children ≥ 6 yr with reversible obstructive pulmonary disease

Contraindications and cautions
• Contraindicated with hypersensitivity to albuterol or levalbuterol; tachyarrhythmias, tachycardia caused by digitalis intoxication; general anesthesia with halogenated hydrocarbons or cyclopropane (these sensitize the myocardium to catecholamines); unstable vasomotor system disorders; hypertension; coronary insufficiency, coronary artery disease; history of stroke; COPD in patients who have developed degenerative heart disease.
• Use cautiously with hyperthyroidism; history of seizure disorders; psychoneurotic individuals; pregnancy and lactation.

Available forms
Solution for inhalation—0.31 mg/3 mL, 0.63 mg/3 mL, 1.25 mg/3 mL

Dosages
Adults and patients ≥ 12 yr
0.63 mg tid, every 6–8 hr by nebulization; if patient does not respond, the dose may be increased to up to 1.25 mg tid by nebulization.
Pediatric patients
6–11 yr: 0.31 mg tid by nebulization; do not exceed 0.63 mg tid.
< *6 yr:* Safety and efficacy not established.

Pharmacokinetics

Route	Onset	Peak	Duration
Inhalation	5 min	1 hr	6–8 hr

Metabolism: Hepatic; T$_{1/2}$: 4–6 hr
Distribution: Crosses placenta; passes into breast milk
Excretion: Urine

Adverse effects
• **CNS:** *Apprehension, anxiety, fear, CNS stimulation,* hyperkinesia, insomnia, tremor, dizziness, irritability, weakness, vertigo, headache
• **CV:** Cardiac arrhythmias, tachycardia, palpitations, PVCs (rare), anginal pain (less likely with bronchodilator doses of this drug than with bronchodilator doses of a nonselective beta-agonist, eg, isoproterenol), changes in BP (increases or decreases)
• **Dermatologic:** Sweating, pallor, flushing
• **GI:** *Nausea,* vomiting, heartburn, unusual or bad taste
• **Respiratory:** Respiratory difficulties, pulmonary edema, coughing, bronchospasm

Interactions
✳ **Drug-drug** • Risk of increased sympathomimetic effects when given with other sympathomimetic drugs • Risk of increased toxicity, especially cardiac, when used in combination with theophylline, aminophylline, oxtriphylline • Possible decreased bronchodilating effects when given with beta-adrenergic blockers (propranolol, etc.)

■ Nursing considerations
Assessment
• **History:** Hypersensitivity to levalbuterol or albuterol; tachyarrhythmias, tachycardia caused by digitalis intoxication; general anesthesia with halogenated hydrocarbons or cyclopropane; unstable vasomotor system disorders; hypertension; coronary artery dis-

---

Adverse effects in *Italics* are most common; those in **Bold** are life-threatening.

ease; history of stroke; COPD in patients who have developed degenerative heart disease; diabetes mellitus; hyperthyroidism; history of seizure disorders; history of psychiatric illness; pregnancy, lactation
- **Physical:** Weight, skin color, T, turgor; orientation, reflexes, affect; P, BP; R, adventitious sounds; blood and urine glucose, serum electrolytes, thyroid function tests, ECG

Interventions
- Keep unopened drug in foil pouch until ready to use; protect from heat and light. Once foil pouch is open, use the vial within 2 wk, protected from light and heat. Once a vial is removed from foil pouch, use immediately. If not used, protect from light and use within 1 wk. Discard vial if solution is not colorless.
- Continue use to control recurrent bouts of bronchospasm; most effective with regular use.
- Do not exceed recommended dosage; administer inhalation drug forms during second half of inspiration, because the airways are open wider and the aerosol distribution is more extensive.
- Monitor patient response; if usual effective dosage regimen does not provide relief, this usually indicates a serious worsening of the asthma and indicates need for reassessment of drug regimen.
- Establish safety precautions if CNS changes occur.
- Reassure patients with acute respiratory distress; provide appropriate supportive measures.
- Monitor environmental temperature if flushing, sweating occur.

Teaching points
- Do not exceed recommended dosage—adverse effects or loss of effectiveness may result; read the instructions for use that come with the product for proper administration of nebulized drug.
- Keep unopened drug in foil pouch until ready to use; protect from heat and light. Once foil pouch is open, use the vial within 2 wk, protected from light and heat. Once a vial is removed from foil pouch, use immediately. If not used, protect from light and use within 1 wk. Discard vial if solution is not colorless.

- These side effects may occur: dizziness, fatigue, headache (use caution if driving or performing tasks that require alertness if these effects occur); nausea, vomiting, change in taste (small, frequent meals may help, consult your nurse or physician if this is prolonged); rapid heart rate, anxiety, sweating, flushing.
- Report chest pain, dizziness, insomnia, weakness, tremors or irregular heartbeat, difficulty breathing, productive cough, failure to respond to usual dosage.

▽levamisole hydrochloride

See *Less Commonly Used Drugs,* p. 1346.

▽levetiracetam
*(lev ah ty **ray'** ca tam)*

Keppra

PREGNANCY CATEGORY C

Drug class
Antiepileptic

Therapeutic actions
Mechanism of action not well understood; antiepileptic activity may be related to its ability to inhibit polysynaptic responses and block post-tetanic potentiation.

Indications
- Adjunctive therapy in the treatment of partial onset seizures in adults with epilepsy, when used in combination with other epilepsy medication

Contraindications and cautions
- Hypersensitivity to levetiracetam; lactation, pregnancy, renal dysfunction.

Available forms
Tablets—250, 500, 750 mg

Dosages
Adults
1,000 mg/day given as 500 mg PO bid; may be increased in 1,000 mg/day increments every 2 wk; maximum dose: 3,000 mg/day.

Pediatric patients
Safety and efficacy not established.
Patients with renal impairment
For creatinine clearance > 80 mL/min: 500–1,500 mg q 12 hr; creatinine clearance 50–80 mL/min: 500–1,000 mg q 12 hr; creatinine clearance 30–50 mL/min: 250–750 mg q 12 hr; creatinine clearance < 30 mL/min: 250–500 mg q 12 hr. For patients on dialysis: 500–1,000 mg q 12 hr.

Pharmacokinetics

Route	Onset	Peak	Duration
Oral	Rapid	1 hr	N/A

Metabolism: $T_{1/2}$: 6–8 hr
Distribution: Crosses placenta; may pass into breast milk
Excretion: Unchanged in the urine

Adverse effects
- **CNS:** *Dizziness, headache,* vertigo, nervousness, fatigue, *somnolence, ataxia,* diplopia
- **Dermatologic:** Pruritus
- **GI:** Dyspepsia, vomiting, nausea, constipation, anorexia
- **Respiratory:** Rhinitis, pharyngitis
- **Other:** Weight gain, facial edema, impotence

■ Nursing considerations
Assessment
- **History:** Hypersensitivity to levetiracetam; lactation, renal impairment, pregnancy
- **Physical:** Body weight; body temperature; skin color, lesions; orientation, affect, reflexes; P, R, adventitious sounds; bowel sounds, normal output, renal function tests

Interventions
- Give drug with food to prevent GI upset.
- Establish safety precautions if CNS, vision, coordination changes occur (siderails, accompany patient when ambulating, etc.).
- Advise the use of barrier contraceptives while this drug is being used.
- Offer support and encouragement for dealing with epilepsy and adverse drug effects; arrange for consultation with support groups for epileptics as needed.

Teaching points
- Take this drug exactly as prescribed.
- Do not discontinue this drug abruptly or change dosage, except on the advice of your physician.
- Do not take this drug if you are pregnant or plan to become pregnant, serious fetal effects can occur, use of barrier contraceptives is recommended.
- These side effects may occur: dizziness, blurred vision (avoid driving a car or performing other tasks requiring alertness or visual acuity if this occurs); GI upset (taking the drug with food or milk and eating frequent small meals may help); headache, nervousness (if these become severe, consult with your health care provider); fatigue (periodic rest periods may be helpful).
- Wear a medical alert tag at all times so that any emergency medical personnel taking care of you will know that you are an epileptic patient taking antiepileptic medication.
- Report severe headache, sleepwalking, rash, severe vomiting, chills, fever, difficulty breathing.

▽ levodopa
*(lee voe **doe' pa**)*

Dopar, Larodopa

PREGNANCY CATEGORY C

Drug class
Antiparkinsonian agent

Therapeutic actions
Biochemical precursor of the neurotransmitter dopamine, which is deficient in the basal ganglia of parkinsonism patients; unlike dopamine, levodopa penetrates the blood–brain barrier. It is transformed in the brain to dopamine; thus, levodopa is a form of replacement therapy. It is efficacious for 2–5 yr in relieving the symptoms of parkinsonism but not drug-induced extrapyramidal disorders.

Indications
- Treatment of parkinsonism (postencephalitic, arteriosclerotic, and idiopathic types)

Adverse effects in *Italics* are most common; those in **Bold** are life-threatening.

and symptomatic parkinsonism, following injury to the nervous system by carbon monoxide or manganese intoxication
- Given with carbidopa (*Lodosyn*; fixed combinations, *Sinemet*), an enzyme inhibitor that decreases the activity of dopa decarboxylase in the periphery, thus reducing blood levels of levodopa and decreasing the intensity and incidence of many of the adverse effects of levodopa
- Unlabeled use: relief of herpes zoster (shingles) pain; restless leg syndrome

Contraindications and cautions
- Contraindicated with hypersensitivity to levodopa; allergy to tartrazine (marketed as *Dopar*); glaucoma, especially angle-closure glaucoma; history of melanoma; suspicious or undiagnosed skin lesions; lactation.
- Use cautiously with severe CV or pulmonary disease; occlusive cerebrovascular disease; history of MI with residual arrhythmias; bronchial asthma; renal, hepatic, endocrine disease; history of peptic ulcer; psychiatric patients, especially the depressed or psychotic; pregnancy.

Available forms
Tablets—100, 250, 500 mg; capsules—100, 250, 500 mg

Dosages
Adults
Individualize dosage. Increase dosage gradually to minimize side effects; titrate dosage carefully to optimize benefits and minimize side effects. Initially, 0.5–1 g PO daily divided into 2 or more doses given with food. Increase gradually in increments not exceeding 0.75 g/day q 3–7 days as tolerated. Do not exceed 8 g/day, except for exceptional patients. A significant therapeutic response may not be obtained for 6 mo.
Pediatric patients
Safety for use in children < 12 yr not established.

Pharmacokinetics

Route	Onset	Peak
Oral	Varies	0.5–2 hr

Metabolism: Hepatic; $T_{1/2}$: 1–3 hr

Distribution: Crosses placenta; enters breast milk
Excretion: Urine

Adverse effects
- **CNS:** *Adventitious movement (eg, dystonic movements), ataxia, increased hand tremor, headache, dizziness, numbness, weakness and faintness,* bruxism, confusion, insomnia, nightmares, hallucinations and delusions, *agitation and anxiety, malaise, fatigue, euphoria,* mental changes (including paranoid ideation), psychotic episodes, depression with or without suicidal tendencies, dementia, bradykinesia ("on-off" phenomenon), muscle twitching and blepharospasm, diplopia, blurred vision, dilated pupils
- **CV:** Cardiac irregularities, palpitations, orthostatic hypotension
- **Dermatologic:** Flushing, hot flashes, increased sweating, rash
- **GI:** *Anorexia, nausea, vomiting, abdominal pain or distress, dry mouth, dysphagia, dysgeusia,* bitter taste, sialorrhea, trismus, burning sensation of the tongue, diarrhea, constipation, flatulence, weight change, upper GI hemorrhage in patients with history of peptic ulcer
- **GU:** Urinary retention, urinary incontinence
- **Hematologic:** Leukopenia, anemia, elevated BUN, AST, ALT, LDH, bilirubin, alkaline phosphatase, protein-bound iodine
- **Respiratory:** Bizarre breathing patterns

Interactions
✳ Drug-drug • Increased therapeutic effects and possible hypertensive crisis with MAOIs; withdraw MAOIs at least 14 days before starting levodopa therapy • Decreased efficacy with pyridoxine (vitamin B_6), phenytoin, papaverine, TCAs

✳ Drug-lab test • May interfere with urine tests for sugar or ketones • False Coombs' test results • False elevations of uric acid when using colorimetric method

■ Nursing considerations
Assessment
- **History:** Hypersensitivity to levodopa, tartrazine; glaucoma; history of melanoma; suspicious or undiagnosed skin lesions; severe CV or pulmonary disease; occlusive cere-

brovascular disease; history of MI with residual arrhythmias; bronchial asthma; renal,
hepatic, endocrine disease; history of peptic
ulcer; psychiatric disorders; lactation, pregnancy
- **Physical:** Weight; T; skin color, lesions; orientation, affect, reflexes, bilateral grip
strength, vision exam; P, BP, orthostatic BP;
auscultation; R, depth, adventitious sounds;
bowel sounds, normal output, liver evaluation; voiding pattern, normal output, prostate
palpation; liver and kidney function tests;
CBC with differential

Interventions
- Arrange to decrease dosage if therapy is in-
terrupted; observe for the development of sui-
cidal tendencies.
- Give with meals if GI upset occurs.
- Ensure that patient voids before receiving
dose if urinary retention is a problem.
- Monitor hepatic, renal, hematopoietic, and
CV function.
- For patients who take multivitamins provide
Larobec, a preparation without pyridoxine.

Teaching points
- Take this drug exactly as prescribed.
- Do not take multivitamin preparations with
pyridoxine. These may prevent any therapeutic effect of levodopa. Notify your health
care provider if you need vitamins.
- These side effects may occur: drowsiness,
dizziness, confusion, blurred vision (avoid
driving or engaging in activities that require
alertness and visual acuity); nausea (take
with meals, frequent small meals); dry mouth
(sucking sugarless lozenges or ice chips may
help); painful or difficult urination (empty
bladder before each dose); constipation
(maintain adequate fluid intake and exercise regularly, request correctives); dark sweat
or urine (not harmful); dizziness or faintness when you get up (change position slowly and use caution when climbing stairs).
- Report fainting, light-headedness, dizziness;
uncontrollable movements of the face, eyelids, mouth, tongue, neck, arms, hands, or
legs; mental changes; irregular heartbeat or
palpitations; difficult urination; severe or
persistent nausea or vomiting.

▽levofloxacin
(lee voe flox' a sin)

Levaquin

PREGNANCY CATEGORY C

Drug classes
Antibiotic
Fluoroquinolone

Therapeutic actions
Bactericidal: interferes with DNA by inhibiting
DNA synase replication in susceptible gram-
negative and gram-positive bacteria, preventing cell reproduction.

Indications
- Treatment of adults with community-
acquired pneumonia, acute maxillary sinusitis caused by susceptible bacteria
- Treatment of acute exacerbation of chronic
bronchitis caused by susceptible bacteria
- Treatment of complicated and uncomplicated skin and skin structure infections
caused by susceptible bacteria
- Treatment of complicated and uncomplicated UTIs and acute pyelonephritis caused
by susceptible bacteria
- Treatment of nosocomial pneumonia due
to methicillin-sensitive *Staphylococcus aureus, Pseudomonas* strains, *Serratia, Escherichia coli, Klebsiella, Haemophilus influenzae, Streptococcus pneumoniae*

Contraindications and cautions
- Contraindicated with allergy to fluoroquinolones, pregnancy, lactation.
- Use cautiously with renal dysfunction,
seizures.

Available forms
Tablets—250, 500, 750 mg; injection—500,
750 mg; premixed injection—250, 500, 750 mg

Dosages
Adults
- *Pneumonia:* 500 mg daily PO or IV for
7–14 days.
- *Sinusitis:* 500 mg daily PO or IV for
10–14 days.

- *Chronic bronchitis:* 500 mg daily PO or IV for 7 days.
- *Skin infection:* 500–750 mg daily PO or IV for 7–10 days.
- *UTIs:* 250 mg daily PO or IV for 3–10 days.
- *Pyelonephritis:* 250 mg daily PO or IV for 10 days.
- *Nosocomial pneumonia:* 750 mg daily PO or IV for 7–14 days.

Pediatric patients
Not recommended in patients < 18 yr.

Patients with renal impairment

Creatinine Clearance (mL/min)	Dose
50–80	No adjustment
20–49	500 mg initially, then 250 mg daily
10–19	500 mg initially, then 250 mg q 48 hr

Pharmacokinetics

Route	Onset	Peak	Duration
Oral	Varies	1–2 hr	3–5 hr
IV	Rapid	End of infusion	3–5 hr

Metabolism: Hepatic; $T_{1/2}$: 4–7 hr
Distribution: Crosses placenta; passes into breast milk
Excretion: Urine

▼ IV facts
Preparation: No further preparation is needed if using the premixed solution; dilute single-use vials in 50–100 mL D₅W.
Infusion: Administer slowly over at least 60 min. Do not administer IM or SC.
Compatibilities: Can be further diluted in 0.9% sodium chloride injection, 5% dextrose injection, 5% dextrose/0.9% sodium chloride, 5% dextrose in lactated Ringer's, *Plasma-Lyte 56 and 5% Dextrose* injection, 9% dextrose/0.45% sodium chloride, 0.15% potassium chloride, sodium lactate injection.

Adverse effects
- **CNS:** *Headache*, dizziness, *insomnia,* fatigue, somnolence, blurred vision
- **GI:** *Nausea,* vomiting, dry mouth, *diarrhea,* abdominal pain (occur less with this drug than with ofloxacin), constipation, flatulence

- **Hematologic:** Elevated BUN, AST, ALT, serum creatinine, and alkaline phosphatase; neutropenia, anemia
- **Other:** Fever, rash, **photosensitivity,** *muscle and joint tenderness*

Interactions
✳ Drug-drug • Decreased therapeutic effect with iron salts, sulcrafate, antacids, zinc, magnesium (separate by at least 2 hr) • Increased risk of seizures with NSAIDs; avoid this combination

✳ Drug-alternative therapy • Increased risk of severe photosensitivity reactions if combined with St. John's wort therapy

■ Nursing considerations
Assessment
- **History:** Allergy to fluoroquinolones, renal dysfunction, seizures, lactation, pregnancy
- **Physical:** Skin color, lesions; T; orientation, reflexes, affect; mucous membranes, bowel sounds; renal and liver function tests

Interventions
- Arrange for culture and sensitivity tests before beginning therapy.
- Continue therapy as indicated for condition being treated.
- Administer oral drug 1 hr before or 2 hr after meals with a glass of water; separate oral drug from other cation administration, including antacids, by at least 2 hr.
- Ensure that patient is well hydrated during course of therapy.
- Discontinue drug at any sign of hypersensitivity (rash, photophobia) or at complaint of tendon pain, inflammation, or rupture.
- Monitor clinical response; if no improvement is seen or a relapse occurs, repeat culture and sensitivity test.

Teaching points
- Take oral drug on an empty stomach, 1 hr before or 2 hr after meals. If an antacid is needed, do not take it within 2 hr of levofloxacin dose.
- Drink plenty of fluids while you are on this drug.
- These side effects may occur: nausea, vomiting, abdominal pain (eat small, frequent meals); diarrhea or constipation (consult nurse or physician); drowsiness, blurred vi-

sion, dizziness (use caution if driving or operating dangerous equipment); sensitivity to sunlight (avoid exposure, use a sunscreen if necessary).
• Report rash, visual changes, severe GI problems, weakness, tremors.

▽ levomethadyl acetate hydrochloride
*(lev oh **meth**' a dil)*

Orlaam

PREGNANCY CATEGORY C

C-II CONTROLLED SUBSTANCE

Drug class
Opioid agonist analgesic

Therapeutic actions
Acts at specific opioid receptors, causing analgesia, respiratory depression, physical dependence, euphoria.

Indications
• Management of opiate dependence in those patients who do not respond to other therapies
• Orphan drug use: treatment of heroin addicts suitable for maintenance on opiate agonists

Contraindications and cautions
• Contraindicated with hypersensitivity to opioids, diarrhea caused by poisoning, acute bronchial asthma, upper airway obstruction, history of prolonged QTc interval or patients at risk of QT prolongation (CHF, hypokalemia, diuretic use, bradycardia).
• Not recommended during pregnancy. If patient becomes pregnant, switch to methadone.
• Use cautiously with bradycardia, history of seizures, lactation.

Available forms
Solution—10 mg/mL

Dosages
Must be given in an opiate withdrawal clinic that maintains control over drug delivery.

Adults
• *Usual induction dose:* 20–40 mg PO, increase in increments of 5–10 mg every 48–72 hr as tolerated.
• *Maintenance:* 60–90 mg PO 3 times a wk. Maximum dose recommended is 140 mg 3 times/wk or 130 mg/130 mg/180 mg on a 3 times/wk schedule.
• *Transfer from methadone:* Higher initial doses may be needed.
• *Transfer from levomethadyl to methadone:* Start methadone at 80% of the usual dose, giving the initial methadone dose no sooner than 48 hr after the last levomethadyl dose.

Pediatric patients
Safety and efficacy not established.

Pharmacokinetics

Route	Onset	Duration
Oral	Varies	Up to 72 hr

Metabolism: Plasma; $T_{1/2}$: 15–40 hr
Distribution: Crosses placenta; enters breast milk

Adverse effects
• **CNS:** *Sedation, clamminess, sweating, headache, vertigo, floating feeling, dizziness, lethargy, confusion, light-headedness,* nervousness, unusual dreams, agitation, euphoria, hallucinations, delirium, insomnia, anxiety, fear, disorientation, impaired mental and physical performance, coma, mood changes, weakness, headache, tremor, convulsions
• **CV:** Palpitations, increase or decrease in BP, circulatory depression, **cardiac arrest, shock,** arrhythmia
• **Dermatologic:** Rash, hives, pruritus, flushing, warmth, sensitivity to cold
• **EENT:** Diplopia, blurred vision
• **GI:** *Nausea, vomiting,* dry mouth, anorexia, *constipation,* biliary tract spasm
• **Respiratory:** Slow, shallow respiration; apnea; suppression of cough reflex; laryngospasm; bronchospasm
• **Other:** Physical tolerance and dependence, psychological dependence

Adverse effects in *Italics* are most common; those in **Bold** are life-threatening.

Interactions

✳ Drug-drug • Potentiation of CNS effects with ethanol, barbiturates, antihistamines, or another sedating drug • Risk of serious to fatal arrhythmia if combined with other drugs known to prolong the QTc interval • Levomethadyl is metabolized by the cytochrome P450 3A4 enzyme system. Use caution when administering drugs that inhibit (fluconazole, diltiazem) or induce (rifampin, phenytoin, phenobarbital) those enzymes

✳ Drug-lab test • Elevated biliary tract pressure may cause increases in plasma amylase and lipase; determinations of these levels may be unreliable for 24 hr after administration of opioids

■ Nursing considerations
Assessment

- **History:** Hypersensitivity to opioids, physical dependence on an opioid analgesic, pregnancy, lactation, bronchial asthma, COPD, respiratory depression, anoxia, increased intracranial pressure, acute MI, ventricular failure, prolonged QTc interval; coronary insufficiency, hypertension, biliary tract surgery, and renal or hepatic dysfunction
- **Physical:** Orientation, reflexes, bilateral grip strength, affect; pupil size, vision; P, auscultation, BP; R, adventitious sounds; bowel sounds, normal output; liver and kidney function tests; baseline ECG

Interventions

- Reserve use for patients who do not respond to other therapies because of risk of cardiac arrhythmia.
- Give to lactating women 4–6 hr before the next feeding to minimize amount in milk.
- Provide opioid antagonist, and have facilities for assisted or controlled respiration on standby during parenteral administration.
- Caution patient that clinic visits must be kept; use of street drugs can cause serious complications and even death.
- To be assessed for prolonged QT, patients must have a baseline ECG, then additional ECGs 10–14 days after initiation and periodically thereafter.

Teaching points

- Return to the clinic for scheduled dosing; skipping doses can cause serious side effects.

Use of street drugs can cause serious complications.
- These side effects may occur: dizziness, sedation, drowsiness, impaired visual acuity (ask for assistance to move); nausea, loss of appetite (lying quietly, frequent small meals may help); constipation (request laxative).
- Report severe nausea, vomiting, palpitations, shortness of breath, or difficulty breathing.

▷ levorphanol tartrate
(lee vor' fa nole)

Levo-Dromoran

PREGNANCY CATEGORY C

C-II CONTROLLED SUBSTANCE

Drug class
Narcotic agonist analgesic

Therapeutic actions
Acts as agonist at specific opioid receptors in the CNS to produce analgesia, euphoria, sedation; the receptors are thought to be the same as those mediating the effects of endogenous opioids (enkephalins, endorphins).

Indications
- Relief of moderate to severe acute and chronic pain
- Preoperative medication to allay apprehension, provide prolonged analgesia, reduce thiopental requirements, and shorten recovery time

Contraindications and cautions
- Contraindicated with hypersensitivity to narcotics, diarrhea caused by poisoning (before toxins are eliminated), pregnancy (neonatal withdrawal), labor or delivery (respiratory depression of neonate—premature infants are especially at risk; may prolong labor), bronchial asthma, acute alcoholism, increased intracranial pressure, respiratory depression, anoxia.
- Use cautiously with COPD, cor pulmonale, acute abdominal conditions, CV disease, supraventricular tachycardias, myxedema, convulsive disorders, delirium tremens, cerebral arteriosclerosis, ulcerative colitis, kyphoscoliosis, Addison's disease, prostatic hy-

pertrophy, urethral stricture, recent GI or GU surgery, toxic psychosis, and renal or hepatic dysfunction.

Available forms

Tablets—2 mg

Dosages

Adults

Starting dose is 2 mg PO repeated q 6–8 hr. Increase to 3 mg if necessary. Higher doses may be needed in narcotic-tolerant patients or patients with severe pain.

Geriatric patients or impaired adults

Use caution—respiratory depression may occur in the elderly, the very ill, and those with respiratory problems. Reduced dosage may be necessary.

Pharmacokinetics

Route	Onset	Peak	Duration
Oral	30–90 min	0.5–1 hr	6–8 hr

Metabolism: Hepatic; $T_{1/2}$: 12–16 hr
Distribution: Crosses placenta; enters breast milk
Excretion: Urine

Adverse effects

- **CNS:** *Light-headedness, dizziness, sedation,* euphoria, dysphoria, delirium, insomnia, agitation, anxiety, fear, hallucinations, disorientation, drowsiness, lethargy, impaired mental and physical performance, coma, mood changes, weakness, headache, tremor, convulsions, miosis, visual disturbances, suppression of cough reflex
- **CV:** Facial flushing, peripheral circulatory collapse, tachycardia, bradycardia, arrhythmia, palpitations, chest wall rigidity, hypertension, hypotension, orthostatic hypotension, syncope
- **Dermatologic:** Pruritus, urticaria, laryngospasm, bronchospasm, edema, hemorrhagic urticaria (rare)
- **GI:** *Nausea, vomiting,* dry mouth, anorexia, *constipation,* biliary tract spasm; increased colonic motility in patients with chronic ulcerative colitis

- **GU:** Ureteral spasm, spasm of vesicle sphincters, urinary retention or hesitancy, oliguria, antidiuretic effect, reduced libido or potency
- **Major hazards:** Respiratory depression, apnea, circulatory depression, **respiratory arrest, shock, cardiac arrest**
- **Other:** *Sweating* (more common in ambulatory patients and those without severe pain), physical tolerance and dependence, psychological dependence

Interactions

✳ **Drug-drug** • Potentiation of effects of levorphanol when given with barbiturate anesthetics; decrease dose of levorphanol when coadministering • Increased risk of CNS effects with ethanol, barbiturates, antihistamines, and other sedating drugs

✳ **Drug-lab test** • Elevated biliary tract pressure may cause increases in plasma amylase and lipase; determinations of these levels may be unreliable for 24 hr after administration of narcotics

■ Nursing considerations

Assessment

- **History:** Hypersensitivity to narcotics, diarrhea caused by poisoning, labor or delivery, bronchial asthma, acute alcoholism, increased intracranial pressure, respiratory depression, cor pulmonale, acute abdominal conditions, CV disease, myxedema, convulsive disorders, delirium tremens, cerebral arteriosclerosis, ulcerative colitis, fever, kyphoscoliosis, Addison's disease, prostatic hypertrophy, urethral stricture, recent GI or GU surgery, toxic psychosis, renal or hepatic dysfunction
- **Physical:** T; skin color, texture, lesions; orientation, reflexes, pupil size, bilateral grip strength, affect; P, auscultation, BP, orthostatic BP, perfusion; R, adventitious sounds; bowel sounds, normal output; frequency and pattern of voiding, normal output; ECG; EEG; thyroid, liver, kidney function tests

Interventions

- Give to lactating women 4–6 hr before the next feeding to minimize the amount in milk.
- Reassure about addiction liability; most patients who receive opiates for medical rea-

sons do not develop psychological dependency.

Teaching points
- Take drug exactly as prescribed.
- These side effects may occur: nausea, loss of appetite (take with food, lie quietly, eat frequent small meals); constipation (laxative may help); dizziness, sedation, drowsiness, impaired visual acuity (avoid driving, performing other tasks that require alertness, visual acuity).
- Do not take leftover medication for other disorders, do not let anyone else take your prescription.
- Report severe nausea, vomiting, constipation, shortness of breath, or difficulty breathing.

▽levothyroxine sodium (L-thyroxine, T$_4$)
(lee voe thye rox' een)

Eltroxin, Levo-T, Levothroid, Levoxine, Levoxyl, Synthroid, Unithroid

PREGNANCY CATEGORY A

Drug class
Thyroid hormone

Therapeutic actions
Increases the metabolic rate of body tissues, thereby increasing oxygen consumption; respiration and heart rate; rate of fat, protein, and carbohydrate metabolism; and growth and maturation.

Indications
- Replacement therapy in hypothyroidism
- Pituitary TSH suppression in the treatment and prevention of euthyroid goiters and in the management of thyroid cancer
- Thyrotoxicosis in conjunction with antithyroid drugs and to prevent goitrogenesis, hypothyroidism, and thyrotoxicosis during pregnancy
- Treatment of myxedema coma

Contraindications and cautions
- Contraindicated with allergy to active or extraneous constituents of drug, thyrotoxico-

sis, and acute MI uncomplicated by hypothyroidism.
- Use cautiously with Addison's disease (treat hypoadrenalism with corticosteroids before thyroid therapy), lactation, patients with coronary artery disease or angina.

Available forms
Tablets—0.025, 0.05, 0.075, 0.088, 0.1, 0.112, 0.125, 0.137, 0.15, 0.175, 0.2, 0.3 mg; powder for injection—200, 500 mcg/vial

Dosages
0.05–0.06 mg equals approximately 60 mg (1 grain) thyroid.
Adults
- *Hypothyroidism:* Initial dose: 0.05 mg PO, with increasing increments of 0.025 mg PO q 2–4 wk; maintenance of up to 0.2 mg/day. IV or IM injection can be substituted for the oral dosage form when oral ingestion is not possible. Usual IV dose is 50% of oral dose. Start at ≤ 0.025 mg/day in patients with long-standing hypothyroidism or known cardiac disease.
- *Myxedema coma without severe heart disease:* 0.4 mg IV as initial dose, then 0.1 to 0.2 mg IV daily; daily maintenance of 0.05 to 0.1 mg once a euthyroid state is established. Switch to PO once patient is able.
- *TSH suppression in thyroid cancer, nodules, and euthyroid goiters:* Larger amounts than used for normal suppression.
- *Thyroid suppression therapy:* 2.6 mcg/kg/day PO for 7–10 days.
Pediatric patients
- *Congenital hypothyroidism:* Infants require replacement therapy from birth.
0–1 yr: 8–10 mcg/kg/day.
1–5 yr: 4–6 mcg/kg/day.
> 5 yr: 3–4 mcg/kg/day.

Pharmacokinetics

Route	Onset	Peak
Oral	Slow	1–3 wk
IV	6–8 hr	24–48 hr

Metabolism: Hepatic; T$_{1/2}$: 6–7 days
Distribution: Crosses placenta; enters breast milk
Excretion: Bile

▽IV facts

Preparation: Add 5 mL 0.9% sodium chloride injection, USP or bacteriostatic sodium chloride injection, USP with benzyl alcohol. Shake the vial to ensure complete mixing. Use immediately after reconstitution. Discard any unused portion.

Infusion: Inject directly, each 100 mcg over 1 min.

Incompatibilities: Do not mix with any other IV fluids.

Adverse effects

- **CNS:** Tremors, headache, nervousness, insomnia
- **CV:** Palpitations, tachycardia, angina, **cardiac arrest**
- **Dermatologic:** Allergic skin reactions, partial loss of hair in first few months of therapy in children
- **GI:** Diarrhea, nausea, vomiting

Interactions

✳ Drug-drug ● Decreased absorption of oral thyroid preparation with cholestyramine ● Increased risk of bleeding with warfarin, anisindione—reduce dosage of anticoagulant when T_4 is begun ● Decreased effectiveness of digitalis glycosides if taken with thyroid replacement ● Decreased theophylline clearance when patient is in hypothyroid state; monitor levels and patient response as euthyroid state is achieved

■ Nursing considerations
Assessment

- **History:** Allergy to active or extraneous constituents of drug, thyrotoxicosis, acute MI uncomplicated by hypothyroidism, Addison's disease, lactation
- **Physical:** Skin lesions, color, temperature, texture; T; muscle tone, orientation, reflexes; P, auscultation, baseline ECG, BP; R, adventitious sounds; thyroid function tests

Interventions

- Monitor response carefully at start of therapy, adjust dosage. Full therapeutic effect may not be seen for several days.
- Do not change brands of T_4 products, due to possible bioequivalence problems.

- Do not add IV doses to other IV fluids.
- Use caution in patients with CV disease.
- Administer oral drug as a single daily dose before breakfast.
- Arrange for regular, periodic blood tests of thyroid function.
- For children and other patients who cannot swallow tablets, crush and suspend in a small amount of water or formula, or sprinkle over soft food. Take immediately.
- Most CV and CNS adverse effects indicate a too high dose. Stop medication for several days and reinstitute at a lower dose.

Teaching points

- Take as a single dose before breakfast.
- This drug replaces an important hormone and will need to be taken for life. Do not discontinue without consulting your health care provider; serious problems can occur.
- Wear a medical ID tag to alert emergency medical personnel that you are on this drug.
- Arrange to have periodic blood tests and medical evaluations. Keep your scheduled appointments.
- Report headache, chest pain, palpitations, fever, weight loss, sleeplessness, nervousness, irritability, unusual sweating, intolerance to heat, diarrhea.

▷L-hyoscyamine sulfate

See *Less Commonly Used Drugs,* p. 1346.

▷lidocaine hydrochloride
(lye' doe kane)

lidocaine HCl in 5% dextrose

lidocaine HCl without preservatives

Antiarrhythmic preparations: LidoPen AutoInjector, Xylocaine HCl IV for Cardiac Arrhythmias

Local anesthetic preparations: Dilocaine, Lidoject, Octocaine,

---

Nervocaine, Xylocaine HCl (injectable)

Topical for mucous membranes: Anestacon, Burn-O-Jel, DermaFlex, Dentipatch, ELA-Max, Xylocaine, Zilactin-L

Topical dermatologic: Lidoderm, Numby Stuff, Xylocaine

PREGNANCY CATEGORY B

Drug classes
Antiarrhythmic
Local anesthetic

Therapeutic actions
Type 1 antiarrhythmic: decreases diastolic depolarization, decreasing automaticity of ventricular cells; increases ventricular fibrillation threshold.
Local anesthetic: blocks the generation and conduction of action potentials in sensory nerves by reducing sodium permeability, reducing height and rate of rise of the action potential, increasing excitation threshold, and slowing conduction velocity.

Indications
- As antiarrhythmic: Management of acute ventricular arrhythmias during cardiac surgery and MI (IV use). Use IM when IV administration is not possible or when ECG monitoring is not available and the danger of ventricular arrhythmias is great (single-dose IM use, for example, by paramedics in a mobile coronary care unit)
- As anesthetic: Infiltration anesthesia, peripheral and sympathetic nerve blocks, central nerve blocks, spinal and caudal anesthesia, retrobulbar and transtracheal injection; topical anesthetic for skin disorders and accessible mucous membranes

Contraindications and cautions
- Contraindicated with allergy to lidocaine or amide-type local anesthetics, CHF, cardiogenic shock, second- or third-degree heart block (if no artificial pacemaker), Wolff-Parkinson-White syndrome, Stokes-Adams syndrome.
- Use cautiously with hepatic or renal disease, inflammation or sepsis in the region of injection (local anesthetic), labor and delivery (epidural anesthesia may prolong the second stage of labor; monitor for fetal and neonatal CV and CNS toxicity), and lactation.

Available forms
IM injection (*LidoPen Autoinjection*)—300 mg/3 mL; direct injection—10, 20 mg/mL; IV injection (admixture) 40, 100, 200 mg/mL; IV infusion—2, 4, 8 mg/mL; topical liquid—2.5%, 5%; topical ointment—2.5%, 5%; topical cream—0.5%; topical gel—0.5%, 2.5%; topical spray—0.5%, 10%; topical solution—2%, 4%; topical jelly—2%; injection—0.5%, 1%, 1.5%, 2%, 4%, 5%; patch (varies)

Dosages
Adults
IM
Use only the 10% solution for IM injection. 300 mg in deltoid or thigh muscle. Switch to IV lidocaine or oral antiarrhythmic as soon as possible.
IV bolus
Use only lidocaine injection labeled for IV use and without preservatives or catecholamines. Monitor ECG constantly. Give 50 to 100 mg at rate of 20–50 mg/min. One-third to one-half the initial dose may be given after 5 min if needed. Do not exceed 200–300 mg in 1 hr.
IV
- *Continuous infusion:* Give 1–4 mg/min (or 20–50 mcg/kg/min). Titrate the dose down as soon as the cardiac rhythm stabilizes. Use lower doses in patients with CHF, liver disease, and in patients > 70 yr.
Pediatric patients
Safety and efficacy have not been established. American Heart Association recommends bolus of 0.5–1 mg/kg IV, followed by 30 mcg/kg/min with caution. The IM auto-injector device is not recommended.
- *As local anesthetic:* Preparations containing preservatives should not be used for spinal or epidural anesthesia. Drug concentration and diluent should be appropriate to particular local anesthetic use: 5% solution with glucose is used for spinal anesthesia, 1.5% solution with dextrose for low spinal or "saddle block"; anesthesia. Dosage varies with the area to be anesthetized and the reason for the anesthesia; use the lowest dose possible to achieve results. Caution: Use lower

concentrations in debilitated, elderly, and pediatric patients.

Pharmacokinetics

Route	Onset	Peak	Duration
IM	5–10 min	5–15 min	2 hr
IV	Immediate	Immediate	10–20 min
Topical	Minimally absorbed systemically		

Metabolism: Hepatic; $T_{1/2}$: 10 min, then 1.5 to 3 hr
Distribution: Crosses placenta; enters breast milk
Excretion: Urine

▼IV facts

Preparation: Prepare solution for IV infusion as follows: 1–2 g lidocaine to 1 L 5% dextrose in water = 0.1%–0.2% solution; 1–2 mg lidocaine/mL. Stable for 24 hr after dilution.
Infusion: IV bolus: give 50–100 mg at rate of 20–50 mg/min. An infusion rate of 1–4 mL/min will provide 1–4 mg lidocaine/min. Use only preparations of lidocaine specifically labeled for IV infusion.

Adverse effects

Antiarrhythmic with systemic administration

- **CNS:** *Dizziness or light-headedness, fatigue, drowsiness,* unconsciousness, tremors, twitching, vision changes; may progress to **seizures**
- **CV:** *Cardiac arrhythmias,* **cardiac arrest,** vasodilation, *hypotension*
- **GI:** *Nausea,* vomiting
- **Hypersensitivity:** Rash, **anaphylactoid reactions**
- **Respiratory:** Respiratory depression and **arrest**
- **Other:** Malignant hyperthermia, fever, local injection-site reaction

Injectable local anesthetic for epidural or caudal anesthesia

- **CNS:** *Headache, backache,* septic meningitis, persistent sensory, motor, or autonomic deficit of lower spinal segments, sometimes with incomplete recovery
- **CV:** *Hypotension* due to sympathetic block
- **Dermatologic:** Urticaria, pruritus, erythema, edema

- **GU:** *Urinary retention, urinary or fecal incontinence*

Topical local anesthetic

- **Dermatologic:** Contact dermatitis, urticaria, cutaneous lesions
- **Hypersensitivity:** Anaphylactoid reactions
- **Local:** *Burning, stinging, tenderness, swelling, tissue irritation,* tissue sloughing and necrosis
- **Other:** Methemoglobinemia, **seizures** (children)

Interactions

✳ **Drug-drug** • Increased lidocaine levels with beta-blockers (propranolol, metoprolol, nadolol, pindolol, atenolol), cimetidine, ranitidine • Prolonged apnea with succinylcholine
✳ **Drug-lab test** • Increased CPK if given IM

■ Nursing considerations
Assessment

- **History:** Allergy to lidocaine or amide-type local anesthetics, CHF, cardiogenic shock, second- or third-degree heart block, Wolff-Parkinson-White syndrome, Stokes-Adams syndrome, hepatic or renal disease, inflammation or sepsis in region of injection, lactation
- **Physical:** T; skin color, rashes, lesions; orientation, speech, reflexes, sensation and movement (local anesthetic); P, BP, auscultation, continuous ECG monitoring during use as antiarrhythmic; edema; R, adventitious sounds; bowel sounds, liver evaluation; urine output; serum electrolytes, liver and renal function tests

Interventions

- Check drug concentration carefully; many concentrations are available.
- Reduce dosage with hepatic or renal failure.
- Continuously monitor response when used as antiarrhythmic or injected as local anesthetic.
- Maintain life-support equipment, and have vasopressors on standby if severe adverse reaction (CNS, CV, or respiratory) occurs when lidocaine is injected.
- Establish safety precautions if CNS changes occur; have IV diazepam or short-acting bar-

biturate (thiopental, thiamylal) on standby in case of convulsions.
- Monitor for malignant hyperthermia (jaw muscle spasm, rigidity); have life-support equipment and IV dantrolene on standby.
- Titrate dose to minimum needed for cardiac stability, when using lidocaine as antiarrhythmic.
- Reduce dosage when treating arrhythmias in CHF, digitalis toxicity with AV block, and geriatric patients.
- Monitor fluid load carefully; more concentrated solutions can be used to treat arrhythmias in patients on fluid restrictions.
- Have patients who have received lidocaine as a spinal anesthetic remain lying flat for 6–12 hr afterward, and ensure that they are adequately hydrated to minimize risk of headache.
- Check lidocaine preparation carefully; epinephrine is added to solutions of lidocaine to retard the absorption of the local anesthetic from the injection site. Be sure that such solutions are used *only* to produce local anesthesia. These solutions should be injected cautiously in body areas supplied by end arteries and used cautiously in patients with peripheral vascular disease, hypertension, thyrotoxicosis, or diabetes.
- Use caution to prevent choking. Patient may have difficulty swallowing following use of oral topical anesthetic. Do not give food or drink for 1 hr after use of oral anesthetic.
- Treat methemoglobinemia with 1% methylene blue, 0.1 mg/kg, IV over 10 min.
- Apply lidocaine ointments or creams to a gauze or bandage before applying to the skin.
- Monitor for safe and effective serum drug concentrations (antiarrhythmic use: 1–5 mcg/mL). Doses > 6–10 mcg/mL are usually toxic.

Teaching points
- Dosage is changed frequently in response to cardiac rhythm on monitor.
- These side effects may occur: drowsiness, dizziness, numbness, double vision; nausea, vomiting; stinging, burning, local irritation (local anesthetic).
- Oral lidocaine can cause numbness of the tongue, cheeks, and throat. Do not eat or drink for 1 hr after using oral lidocaine to prevent biting cheeks or tongue and choking.

- Report difficulty speaking, thick tongue, numbness, tingling, difficulty breathing, pain or numbness at IV site, swelling, or pain at site of local anesthetic use.

▷ **lincomycin hydrochloride**
(lin koe mye' sin)

Lincocin, Lincorex

PREGNANCY CATEGORY B

Drug class
Lincosamide antibiotic

Therapeutic actions
Inhibits protein synthesis in susceptible bacteria, causing cell death.

Indications
- Treatment of serious infections caused by staphylococcal, streptococcal, and pneumococcal infections resistant to other antibiotics in penicillin-allergic patients or when penicillin is inappropriate. Less toxic antibiotics (erythromycin or clindamycin) should be considered. Use in conjunction with other antibiotics when indicated.

Contraindications and cautions
- Contraindicated with allergy to lincomycin, history of asthma or other allergies, and lactation.
- Use cautiously with hepatic or renal dysfunction, pregnancy.

Available forms
Capsules—500 mg; injection—300 mg/mL

Dosages
Adults
Oral
500 mg q 6–8 hr, depending on severity of infection.
IM
600 mg q 12–24 hr, depending on severity of infection.
IV
600 mg–1 g q 8–12 hr, up to 8 g/day in severe infections.

Pediatric patients > 1 mo
Oral
30–60 mg/kg/day in 3–4 equally divided doses.
IM
10 mg/kg q 12–24 hr, depending on severity of infection.
IV
10–20 mg/kg/day in divided doses, depending on severity of infection.
Newborns
Not indicated for use in newborns.
Geriatric patients or patients with renal failure
Reduce dose to 25% to 30% of that normally recommended.

Pharmacokinetics

Route	Onset	Peak	Duration
Oral	Varies	2–4 hr	6–8 hr
IM	20–30 min	0.5 hr	24 hr
IV	Immediate	Immediate	14 hr

Metabolism: Hepatic; $T_{1/2}$: 5 hr
Distribution: Crosses placenta; enters breast milk
Excretion: Urine and feces

▼IV facts
Preparation: Dilute to a concentration of 1 g/100 mL minimum. Severe cardiopulmonary reactions have occurred when given at greater than recommended concentrations and rate. IV administration in 250–500 mL of 5% dextrose in water or normal saline produces no local irritation or phlebitis. Use with 5% dextrose in water or in saline.
Infusion: Do not inject as a bolus, infuse over 1–4 hr depending on dose.
Incompatibilities: Lincomycin is not compatible in solution with novobiocin, kanamycin, or phenytoin sodium.

Adverse effects
- **CNS:** Tinnitus, vertigo
- **CV:** Hypotension, **cardiopulmonary arrest** (infusion rate related)
- **Dermatologic:** Rashes, urticaria to anaphylactoid reactions, angioneurotic edema
- **GI:** Severe colitis, including **pseudomembranous colitis,** *nausea, vomit-ing, diarrhea, stomatitis, glossitis, pruritus ani,* jaundice, liver function changes
- **GU:** Vaginitis, kidney function changes
- **Hematologic:** Neutropenia, leukopenia, agranulocytosis, thrombocytopenia, aplastic anemia
- **Local:** *Pain following injection*
- **Other:** Serum sickness

Interactions
✻ **Drug-drug** • Increased neuromuscular blockade with neuromuscular blocking agents • Decreased GI absorption with kaolin, aluminum salts, magaldrate

■ Nursing considerations
Assessment
- **History:** Allergy to lincomycin, history of asthma or other allergies, hepatic or renal dysfunction, lactation
- **Physical:** Site of infection, skin color, lesions; orientation, reflexes, auditory function; BP; R, adventitious sounds; bowel sounds, output, liver evaluation; CBC, renal and liver function tests

Interventions
- Administer oral drug on an empty stomach, 1 hr before or 2–3 hr after meals. Give with a full glass of water.
- Culture infection site before therapy.
- Do not use for minor bacterial or viral infections.
- Monitor renal function tests with prolonged therapy.
- Arrange for metronidazole or vancomycin and corticosteroids to be available for serious colitis.

Teaching points
- Take drug on an empty stomach, 1 hr before or 2–3 hr after meals. Take the drug with a full glass of water.
- Take prescribed course. Do not stop taking without notifying your health care provider.
- These side effects may occur: nausea, vomiting (small frequent meals may help); superinfections in the mouth, vagina (use frequent hygiene measures, request treatment if severe); rash, flulike sickness (report if severe).

Adverse effects in *Italics* are most common; those in **Bold** are life-threatening.

- Report severe or watery diarrhea, inflamed mouth or vagina, skin rash or lesions.

▽ linezolid
*(lah **nez'** oh lid)*

Zyvox

PREGNANCY CATEGORY C

Drug class
Oxazolidinone antibiotic

Therapeutic actions
Bacteriostatic and bacteriocidal: interferes with protein synthesis on the bacterial ribosome; effective in vancomycin-resistant *Enterococcus* (VRE), *Staphylococcus,* and methicillin-resistant *S. aureus* (MRSA) and penicillin-resistant pneumococci and *S. aureus;* is a reversible, nonselective MAO inhibitor.

Indications
- Treatment of infections due to vancomycin-resistant *Enterococcus faecium*
- Treatment of nosocomial and community-acquired pneumonia due to *S. aureus* and penicillin-susceptible *Streptococcus pneumoniae*
- Treatment of skin and skin structure infections including those caused by methicillin-resistant *S. aureus*

Contraindications and cautions
- Contraindicated with allergy to linezolid; pregnancy, lactation; phenylketonuria (oral form).
- Use cautiously with bone marrow suppression, hepatic dysfunction, hypertension, hyperthyroidism, pheochromocytoma, carcinoid syndrome.

Available forms
Tablets—400, 600 mg; powder for oral suspension—100 mg/5 mL; injection—2 mg/mL

Dosages
No dosage adjustment is needed if switching between oral and IV forms.
Adults
- *VRE, MRSA, pneumonia, complicated skin and skin structure infections:* 600 mg IV or PO q 12 hr for 10–28 days, depending on infection.
- *Uncomplicated skin and skin structure infections:* 400 mg PO q 12 hr for 10–14 days.
Pediatric patients
Safety and efficacy not established.

Pharmacokinetics

Route	Onset	Peak
Oral	Rapid	1–2 hr

Metabolism: Hepatic; $T_{1/2}$: 5 hr
Distribution: Crosses placenta; passes into breast milk
Excretion: Urine

▼ IV facts
Preparation: Use premixed solution—available in 100, 200, and 300 mL forms; store at room temperature, protect from light, leave overwrap in place until ready to use.
Infusion: Infuse over 30–120 min, switch to oral form as soon as appropriate. May be infused into line using 5% dextrose injection, 0.9% NaCL, or lactated Ringer's.
Incompatibilities: Do not introduce additives into this solution; do not mix in solution or at Y-connection with any other drugs. If other drugs are being given through the same line, the line should be flushed before and after linezolid administration.

Adverse effects
- **CNS:** *Headache,* dizziness, *insomnia,* fatigue, somnolence, depression, nervousness
- **GI:** *Nausea,* vomiting, dry mouth, *diarrhea,* anorexia, gastritis, **pseudomembranous colitis**
- **Hematologic:** Altered prothrombin time, **thrombocytopenia**
- **Other:** Fever, rash, sweating, photosensitivity, tendinitis

Interactions
✳ **Drug-drug** • Risk of hypertension and related adverse effects if combined with drugs containing pseudoephedrine, SSRIs, MAOIs; use caution and monitor patient carefully if any of these combinations are used • Increased risk of bleeding and thrombocytopenia if combined with antiplatelet drugs (aspirin, dipyridamole, NSAIDs); monitor platelet counts carefully

⁕ Drug-food • Risk of severe hypertension if combined with large amounts of food containing tyramine (see *Appendix O* for tyramine food lists); patient should be cautioned to avoid large amounts of these foods

■ Nursing considerations

 CLINICAL ALERT!
Name confusion has occurred between Zyvox (linezolid) and Vioxx (rofecoxib); use caution.

Assessment

- **History:** Allergy to linezolid; hepatic dysfunction, bone marrow depression, hypertension, phenylketonuria, hyperthyroidism, carcinoid syndrome, pheochromocytoma, pregnancy, lactation
- **Physical:** Culture site; skin—color, lesions; body temperature; orientation, reflexes, affect; P, BP; mucous membranes, bowel sounds; liver function tests, CBC, and differential

Interventions

- Arrange for culture and sensitivity tests before beginning therapy.
- Reserve use of this drug for cases of well-documented bacteria-sensitive infections.
- Continue therapy as indicated for condition being treated.
- Monitor platelet counts regularly if drug is used for ≥ 2 weeks.
- Monitor blood pressure before and periodically during therapy if patient is on antidepressants or drugs containing sympathomimetics.
- Advise patient to avoid foods high in tyramine to avoid risk of severe hypertension.
- Advise patient of high cost of drug and refer for financial support as needed.
- Monitor clinical response—if no improvement is seen or a relapse occurs, repeat culture and sensitivity.

Teaching points

- Take drug q 12 hr as prescribed; take the full course of the drug; drug may be taken with or without food.

- Avoid foods high in tyramine (a list will be provided) while you are on this drug.
- These side effects may occur: nausea, vomiting, abdominal pain (small, frequent meals may help, taking the drug with food may also help); diarrhea (consult nurse or physician if this occurs).
- Report rash, severe GI problems, weakness, tremors, anxiety, increased bleeding.

▽liothyronine sodium (T₃, triiodithyronine)
(lye' oh thye' roe neen)

Cytomel, Triostat

PREGNANCY CATEGORY A

Drug class
Thyroid hormone

Therapeutic actions
Increases the metabolic rate of body tissues, thereby increasing oxygen consumption; respiratory and heart rate; rate of fat, protein, and carbohydrate metabolism; and growth and maturation.

Indications

- Replacement therapy in hypothyroidism
- Pituitary TSH suppression in the treatment and prevention of euthyroid goiters and in the management of thyroid cancer
- Thyrotoxicosis in conjunction with antithyroid drugs and to prevent goitrogenesis, hypothyroidism, and thyrotoxicosis during pregnancy
- Synthetic hormone used with patients allergic to desiccated thyroid or thyroid extract derived from pork or beef
- Diagnostic use: T₃ suppression test to differentiate suspected hyperthyroidism from euthyroidism
- Treatment of myxedema coma and precoma

Contraindications and cautions

- Contraindicated with allergy to active or extraneous constituents of drug, thyrotoxicosis, and acute MI uncomplicated by hypothyroidism.

Adverse effects in *Italics* are most common; those in **Bold** are life-threatening.

- Use cautiously with Addison's disease (treat hypoadrenalism with corticosteroids before thyroid therapy), lactation, patients with coronary artery disease or angina.

Available forms
Tablets—5, 25, 50 mcg; injection—10 mcg/mL

Dosages
15–37.5 mcg equals approximately 60 mg (1 grain) thyroid.
Adults
- *Hypothyroidism:* Initial dosage: 25 mcg/day PO. May be increased every 1–2 wk in 12.5- to 25-mcg increments. Maintenance: 25–75 mcg/day.
- *Myxedema:* Initial dosage: 5 mcg/day PO. Increase in 5- to 10-mcg increments every 1–2 wk. Maintenance: 50–100 mcg/day.
- *Myxedema coma and precoma:* 25–50 mcg IV q 4–12 hr; do not give IM or SC. In patients with cardiac disease, start at 10–20 mcg IV.
- *Simple goiter:* Initial dosage: 5 mcg/day PO. May be increased by 5- to 10-mcg increments every 1–2 wk. Maintenance: 75 mcg/day.
- *T₃ suppression test:* 75–100 mcg/day PO for 7 days, then repeat I-131 uptake test. I-131 uptake will be unaffected in the hyperthyroid patient but will be decreased by 50% or more in the euthyroid patient.
Pediatric patients
- *Congenital hypothyroidism:* Infants require replacement therapy from birth. Starting dose is 5 mcg/day PO with 5-mcg increments q 3–4 days until the desired dosage is reached. Usual maintenance dosage: 20 mcg/day PO up to 1 yr of age; 50 mcg/day for 1–3 yr of age. Adult dosage after 3 yr.
Geriatric patients
Start therapy with 5 mcg/day PO. Increase by only 5-mcg increments, and monitor patient response.

Pharmacokinetics

Route	Onset	Peak	Duration
Oral	Varies	2–3 days	3–4 days
IV	Rapid	End of infusion	

Metabolism: Hepatic; $T_{1/2}$: 1–2 days
Distribution: Does not cross placenta; enters breast milk
Excretion: Urine

▼IV facts
Preparation: No further preparation is needed; refrigerate vials before use; discard unused portions.
Infusion: Infuse slowly, each 10 mcg over 1 min. Switch to oral form as soon as possible.

Adverse effects
- **Dermatologic:** Allergic skin reactions, partial loss of hair in first few months of therapy in children
- **Endocrine:** Mainly symptoms of hyperthyroidism: *palpitations, elevated pulse pressure, tachycardia, arrhythmias,* angina pectoris, **cardiac arrest;** tremors, *headache, nervousness, insomnia; nausea,* diarrhea, changes in appetite; weight loss, menstrual irregularities, sweating, heat intolerance, fever

Interactions
✳ Drug-drug • Decreased absorption of oral thyroid preparation with cholestyramine • Increased risk of bleeding with warfarin—reduce dosage of anticoagulant when thyroid hormone is begun • Decreased effectiveness of cardiac glycosides with thyroid replacement • Decreased clearance of theophyllines if patient is in hypothyroid state; monitor response and adjust dosage as patient approaches euthyroid state

■ Nursing considerations
Assessment
- **History:** Allergy to active or extraneous constituents of drug, thyrotoxicosis, acute MI uncomplicated by hypothyroidism, Addison's disease, lactation
- **Physical:** Skin lesions, color, temperature, texture; T; muscle tone, orientation, reflexes; P, auscultation, baseline ECG, BP; R, adventitious sounds; thyroid function tests

Interventions
- Monitor patient response carefully at start of therapy, adjust dosage.
- Monitor exchange from one form of thyroid replacement to T₃. Discontinue the other medication, then begin this drug at a low dose with gradual increases based on the patient's response.
- Most CV and CNS adverse effects indicate a too high dose. Stop medication for several days and reinstitute at a lower dose.

- Administer as a single daily dose before breakfast.
- Arrange for regular, periodic blood tests of thyroid function.
- Monitor cardiac response.

Teaching points

- Take as a single dose before breakfast.
- This drug replaces an important hormone and will need to be taken for life. Do not discontinue for any reason without consulting your health care provider; serious problems can occur.
- Wear a medical ID tag to alert emergency medical personnel that you are on this drug.
- Nausea and diarrhea may occur (dividing the dose may help).
- Have periodic blood tests and medical evaluations.
- Report headache, chest pain, palpitations, fever, weight loss, sleeplessness, nervousness, irritability, unusual sweating, intolerance to heat, diarrhea.

▽ liotrix
(lye' oh trix)

Thyrolar

PREGNANCY CATEGORY A

Drug class

Thyroid hormone (contains synthetic T_3 and T_4 in a ratio of 1 to 4 by weight)

Therapeutic actions

Increases the metabolic rate of body tissues, thereby increasing oxygen consumption; respiratory and heart rate; rate of fat, protein, and carbohydrate metabolism; and growth and maturation.

Indications

- Replacement therapy in hypothyroidism
- Congenital hypothyroidism
- Pituitary TSH suppression in the treatment and prevention of euthyroid goiters and in the management of thyroid cancer
- Thyrotoxicosis in conjunction with antithyroid drugs and to prevent goitrogenesis, hypothyroidism, and thyrotoxicosis during pregnancy

Contraindications and cautions

- Contraindicated with allergy to active or extraneous constituents of drug, thyrotoxicosis, and acute MI uncomplicated by hypothyroidism.
- Use cautiously with Addison's disease (hypoadrenalism; treat with corticosteroids before thyroid therapy), lactation, coronary artery disease, or angina.

Available forms

Tablets—1/4, 1/2, 1, 2, 3 grains

Dosages

60 mg equals 65 mg (1 grain) thyroid; administered only PO.

Adults

- *Hypothyroidism:* Initial dosage: 30 mg/day PO. Increase gradually every 1–2 wk in 15-mg increments (2 wk in children). In patients with cardiac disease, start with 15 mg/day.
- *Maintenance dose:* 60 to 120 mg/day PO.
- *Thyroid cancer:* Use larger doses than required for replacement surgery.

Pediatric patients

0–6 mo: 25–50 mcg/day (8–10 mcg/kg/day PO).

6–12 mo: 50–75 mcg/day (6–8 mcg/kg/day PO).

1–5 yr: 75–100 mcg/day (5–6 mcg/kg/day PO).

6–12 yr: 100–150 mcg/day (4–5 mcg/kg/day PO).

> 12 yr: > 150 mcg/day (2–3 mcg/kg/day PO).

Pharmacokinetics

Route	Onset	Peak	Duration
Oral	Varies	2–3 days	3 days

Metabolism: Hepatic; $T_{1/2}$: 1–6 days
Distribution: Does not cross placenta; enters breast milk
Excretion: Urine

Adverse effects in *Italics* are most common; those in **Bold** are life-threatening.

Adverse effects
- **Dermatologic:** Allergic skin reactions, partial hair loss in first few months of therapy in children
- **Endocrine:** Mainly symptoms of hyperthyroidism: *palpitations, elevated pulse pressure, tachycardia, arrhythmias,* angina pectoris, **cardiac arrest;** tremors, *headache, nervousness, insomnia; nausea,* diarrhea, changes in appetite; weight loss, menstrual irregularities, sweating, heat intolerance, fever

Interactions
✻ **Drug-drug •** Decreased absorption of oral thyroid preparation with cholestyramine • Increased risk of bleeding with warfarin—reduce dosage of anticoagulant when T_4 is begun • Decreased effectiveness of cardiac glycosides if taken with thyroid replacement • Decreased clearance of theophyllines in hypothyroid state; monitor response and adjust dosage as patient approaches euthyroid state

■ Nursing considerations
Assessment
- **History:** Allergy to active or extraneous constituents of drug, thyrotoxicosis, acute MI uncomplicated by hypothyroidism, Addison's disease, lactation
- **Physical:** Skin lesions, color, temperature, texture; T; muscle tone, orientation, reflexes; P, auscultation, baseline ECG, BP; R, adventitious sounds; thyroid function tests

Interventions
- Monitor response carefully at start of therapy, and adjust dosage.
- Most CV and CNS adverse effects indicate a too high dose. Stop medication for several days and reinstitute at a lower dose.
- Administer as a single daily dose before breakfast.
- Arrange for regular, periodic blood tests of thyroid function.
- Monitor cardiac response.

Teaching points
- Take as a single dose before breakfast.
- This drug replaces an important hormone and will need to be taken for life. Do not discontinue without consulting your health care provider; serious problems can occur.

- Wear a medical ID tag to alert emergency medical personnel that you take this drug.
- Nausea and diarrhea may occur (divide the dose).
- Have periodic blood tests and medical evaluations.
- Report headache, chest pain, palpitations, fever, weight loss, sleeplessness, nervousness, irritability, unusual sweating, intolerance to heat, diarrhea.

▷ lisinopril
*(lyse **in'** oh pril)*

Apo-Lisinopril (CAN), Privinil, Zestril

PREGNANCY CATEGORY C
(FIRST TRIMESTER)

PREGNANCY CATEGORY D
(SECOND AND THIRD TRIMESTERS)

Drug classes
Antihypertensive
Angiotensin-converting enzyme inhibitor (ACE inhibitor)

Therapeutic actions
Renin, synthesized by the kidneys, is released into the circulation where it acts on a plasma precursor to produce angiotensin I, which is converted by angiotensin-converting enzyme to angiotensin II, a potent vasoconstrictor that also causes release of aldosterone from the adrenals. Lisinopril blocks the conversion of angiotensin I to angiotensin II, leading to decreased BP, decreased aldosterone secretion, a small increase in serum potassium levels, and sodium and fluid loss.

Indications
- Treatment of hypertension alone or in combination with thiazide-type diuretics
- Adjunctive therapy in CHF for patients unresponsive to diuretics and digitalis alone
- Treatment of stable patients within 24 hr of acute MI to improve survival with beta blocker, aspirin, or thrombolytics

Contraindications and cautions
- Contraindicated with allergy to lisinopril or enalapril.

- Use cautiously with impaired renal function, CHF, salt or volume depletion, and lactation, pregnancy.

Available forms
Tablets—2.5, 5, 10, 20, 40 mg

Dosages
Adults not taking diuretics
Initial dose: 10 mg/day PO. Adjust dosage based on response. Usual range is 20–40 mg/day as a single dose.
Adults taking diuretics
Discontinue diuretic for 2–3 days. If it is not possible to discontinue, give initial dose of 5 mg, and monitor for excessive hypotension.
- *CHF:* 5 mg PO daily with diuretics and digitalis. Effective range: 5 to 20 mg/day.
- *Acute MI:* Start within 24 hr of MI with 5 mg PO followed in 24 hr by 5 mg PO; 10 mg PO after 48 hr, then 10 mg PO daily for 6 wk.
Pediatric patients
Safety and efficacy not established.
Geriatric patients and patients with renal impairment
Excretion is reduced in renal failure. Use smaller initial dose, and adjust upward to a maximum of 40 mg/day PO.

Creatinine Clearance (mL/min)	Initial Dose
> 30	10 mg/day
10–30	5 mg/day (2.5 mg for CHF)
< 10	2.5 mg/day
Dialysis	2.5 mg on dialysis day

Pharmacokinetics

Route	Onset	Peak	Duration
Oral	1 hr	7 hr	24 hr

Metabolism: Hepatic; $T_{1/2}$: 12 hr
Distribution: Crosses placenta; enters breast milk
Excretion: Urine

Adverse effects
- **CNS:** *Headache, dizziness, insomnia, fatigue,* paresthesias
- **CV:** *Orthostatic hypotension,* tachycardia, angina pectoris, MI, Raynaud's syndrome, CHF, severe hypotension in salt or volume depleted patients
- **GI:** *Gastric irritation, nausea, diarrhea,* peptic ulcers, dysgeusia, cholestatic jaundice, hepatocellular injury, anorexia, constipation
- **GU:** Proteinuria, renal insufficiency, renal failure, polyuria, oliguria, frequency
- **Hematologic:** Neutropenia, agranulocytosis, thrombocytopenia, hemolytic anemia, **pancytopenia**
- **Other:** *Angioedema* (particularly of the face, extremities, lips, tongue, larynx; death has been reported with **airway obstruction**; *cough,* muscle cramps, impotence, rash, pruritis

Interactions
✳ **Drug-drug** • Decreased antihypertensive effects if taken with indomethacin • Exacerbation of cough if combined with capsaicin

■ Nursing considerations

CLINICAL ALERT!
Name confusion has occurred between lisinopril and fosinopril; use caution.

Assessment
- **History:** Allergy to lisinopril or enalapril, impaired renal function, CHF, salt or volume depletion, lactation, pregnancy
- **Physical:** Skin color, lesions, turgor; T; P, BP, peripheral perfusion; mucous membranes, bowel sounds, liver evaluation; urinalysis, renal and liver function tests, CBC and differential

Interventions
- Begin drug within 24 hr of acute MI; ensure that patient is also receiving standard treatment (thrombolytics, aspirin, beta-blockers, etc.).
- Maintain epinephrine on standby in case of angioedema of the face or neck region; if breathing difficulty occurs, consult physician, and administer epinephrine.
- Alert surgeon, and mark patient's chart with notice that lisinopril is being taken. The angiotensin II formation subsequent to compensatory renin release during surgery will

be blocked. Hypotension may be reversed with volume expansion.

- Monitor patients on diuretic therapy for excessive hypotension following the first few doses of lisinopril.
- Monitor patients closely in any situation that may lead to a decrease in BP secondary to reduction in fluid volume, excessive perspiration and dehydration, vomiting, diarrhea because excessive hypotension may occur.
- Arrange for reduced dosage in patients with impaired renal function.

Teaching points

- Take this drug once a day. It may be taken with meals. Do not stop taking without consulting your prescriber.
- These side effects may occur: GI upset, loss of appetite, change in taste perception (may be transient; take with meals); rash; fast heart rate; dizziness, light-headedness (transient; change position slowly, and limit activities to those that do not require alertness and precision); headache, fatigue, sleeplessness.
- Be careful in situations that may lead to a drop in BP—diarrhea, sweating, vomiting, dehydration. If light-headedness or dizziness occurs, consult your health care provider.
- Report mouth sores; sore throat; fever; chills; swelling of the hands or feet; irregular heartbeat; chest pains; swelling of the face, eyes, lips, or tongue; and difficulty breathing.

▽ lithium
(lith' ee um)

lithium carbonate
Carbolith (CAN), Duralith (CAN), Eskalith, Eskalith CR, Lithizine (CAN), Lithobid, Lithonate, Lithotabs, PMS-Lithium Carbonate (CAN)

lithium citrate
Cibalith-S (CAN)

PREGNANCY CATEGORY D

Drug class
Antimanic agent

Therapeutic actions
Mechanism is not known; alters sodium transport in nerve and muscle cells; inhibits release of norepinephrine and dopamine, but not serotonin, from stimulated neurons; slightly increases intraneuronal stores of catecholamines; decreases intraneuronal content of second messengers and may thereby selectively modulate the responsiveness of hyperactive neurons that might contribute to the manic state.

Indications
- Treatment of manic episodes of manic-depressive illness; maintenance therapy to prevent or diminish frequency and intensity of subsequent manic episodes
- Unlabeled use: improvement of neutrophil counts in patients with cancer chemotherapy–induced neutropenia and in children with chronic neutropenia and HIV patients on zidovudine therapy (doses of 300–1,000 mg/day, serum levels of 0.5 and 1 mEq/L); prophylaxis of cluster headache and cyclic migraine headache, treatment of SIADH, hypothyroidism (doses of 600–900 mg/day)

Contraindications and cautions
- Contraindicated with hypersensitivity to tartrazine; significant renal or CV disease; severe debilitation, dehydration; sodium depletion, patients on diuretics (lithium decreases sodium reabsorption, and hyponatremia increases lithium retention); pregnancy; lactation.
- Use cautiously with protracted sweating and diarrhea; suicidal or impulsive patients; infection with fever.

Available forms
Capsules—150, 300, 600 mg; tablets—300 mg; SR tablets—300 mg; CR tablets—450 mg; syrup—300 mg/5 mL

Dosages
Individualize dosage according to serum levels and clinical response.
Adults
- *Acute mania:* 600 mg PO tid or 900 mg slow-release form PO bid to produce effective serum levels between 1 and 1.5 mEq/L. Serum levels should be determined twice per

wk in samples drawn immediately before a dose (at least 8–12 hr after previous dose).
- *Long-term use:* 300 mg PO tid to qid to produce a serum level of 0.6 to 1.2 mEq/L. Serum levels should be determined at least every 2 mo in samples drawn immediately before a dose (at least 8–12 hr after previous dose).
- *Conversion from conventional to slow-release dosage forms:* Give the same total daily dose divided into 2 or 3 doses.

Pediatric patients
Safety and efficacy for children < 12 yr not established.

Geriatric patients and patients with renal impairment
Reduced dosage may be necessary. Elderly patients often respond to reduced dosage and may exhibit signs of toxicity at serum levels tolerated by other patients. Plasma half-life is prolonged in renal impairment.

Pharmacokinetics

Route	Onset	Peak
Oral	5–7 days	10–21 days

Metabolism: Hepatic; $T_{1/2}$: 17–36 hr
Distribution: Crosses placenta; enters breast milk
Excretion: Urine

Adverse effects
Reactions are related to serum lithium levels (toxic lithium levels are close to therapeutic levels: therapeutic levels in acute mania range between 1 and 1.5 mEq/L; therapeutic levels for maintenance are 0.6 to 1.2 mEq/L).

< 1.5 mEq/L
- **CNS:** *Lethargy, slurred speech, muscle weakness, fine hand tremor*
- **GI:** *Nausea, vomiting, diarrhea, thirst*
- **GU:** *Polyuria*

1.5–2 mEq/L (mild to moderate toxic reactions)
- **CNS:** Coarse hand tremor, mental confusion, hyperirritability of muscles, drowsiness, incoordination
- **CV:** ECG changes
- **GI:** Persistent GI upset, gastritis, salivary gland swelling, abdominal pain, excessive salivation, flatulence, indigestion

2–2.5 mEq/L (moderate to severe toxic reactions)
- **CNS:** Ataxia, giddiness, fasciculations, tinnitus, blurred vision, clonic movements, seizures, stupor, coma
- **CV:** Serious ECG changes, severe hypotension with **cardiac arrythmias**
- **GU:** Large output of dilute urine
- **Respiratory:** Fatalities secondary to **pulmonary complications**

> 2.5 mEq/L (life-threatening toxicity)
- **General:** Complex involvement of multiple organ systems, including seizures, arrythmias, CV collapse, stupor, coma

Reactions unrelated to serum levels
- **CNS:** Headache, worsening of organic brain syndromes, fever, reversible short-term memory impairment, dyspraxia
- **CV:** ECG changes; hyperkalemia associated with ECG changes; syncope; tachycardia-bradycardia syndrome; rarely, arrhythmias, CHF, diffuse myocarditis, **death**
- **Dermatologic:** Pruritus with or without rash; maculopapular, acneiform, and follicular eruptions; cutaneous ulcers; edema of ankles or wrists
- **Endocrine:** Diffuse nontoxic goiter; hypothyroidism; hypercalcemia associated with hyperparathyroidism; transient hyperglycemia; irreversible nephrogenic diabetes insipidus, which improves with diuretic therapy; impotence or sexual dysfunction
- **GI:** Dysgeusia (taste distortion), salty taste; swollen lips; dental caries
- **Other:** Weight gain (5–10 kg); chest tightness; swollen or painful joints, eye irritation, worsening of cataracts, disturbance of visual accommodation, leukocytosis

Interactions
✽ **Drug-drug** • Increased risk of toxicity with thiazide diuretics due to decreased renal clearance of lithium—reduced lithium dosage may be necessary • Increased plasma lithium levels with indomethacin and some other NSAIDs—phenylbutazone, piroxicam, ibuprofen, as well as fluoxetine and methyldopa • Increased CNS toxicity with carbamazepine • Encephalopathic syndrome (weakness, lethargy, fever, tremulousness, confusion, extrapyrami-

Adverse effects in *Italics* are most common; those in **Bold** are life-threatening.

dal symptoms, leukocytosis, elevated serum enzymes) with irreversible brain damage when taken with haloperidol • Greater risk of hypothyroidism with iodide salts • Decreased effectiveness due to increased excretion of lithium with urinary alkalinizers, including antacids, tromethamine

✳ Drug-alternative therapy • Increased effects and toxicity with juniper, dandelion

■ Nursing considerations
Assessment
- **History:** Hypersensitivity to tartrazine; significant renal or CV disease; severe debilitation, dehydration; sodium depletion, patients on diuretics; protracted sweating, diarrhea; suicidal or impulsive patients; infection with fever; pregnancy; lactation
- **Physical:** Weight and T; skin color, lesions; orientation, affect, reflexes; ophthalmic exam; P, BP, R, adventitious sounds; bowel sounds, normal output; normal fluid intake, normal output, voiding pattern; thyroid, renal glomerular and tubular function tests, urinalysis, CBC and differential, baseline ECG

Interventions
- Give with caution and daily monitoring of serum lithium levels to patients with renal or CV disease, debilitation, or dehydration or life-threatening psychiatric disorders.
- Give drug with food or milk or after meals.
- Monitor clinical status closely, especially during initial stages of therapy; monitor for therapeutic serum levels of 0.6–1.2 mEq/L.
- Individuals vary in their reponse to this drug; some patients may exhibit toxic signs at serum lithium levels considered within the therapeutic range.
- Advise patient that this drug may cause serious fetal harm and cannot be used during pregnancy; urge use of barrier contraceptives.
- Decrease dosage after the acute manic episode is controlled; lithium tolerance is greater during the acute manic phase and decreases when manic symptoms subside.
- Ensure that patient maintains adequate intake of salt and adequate intake of fluid (2,500–3,000 mL/day).

Teaching points
- Take this drug exactly as prescribed, after meals or with food or milk.
- Eat a normal diet with normal salt intake; maintain adequate fluid intake (at least 2.5 quarts/day).
- Arrange for frequent checkups, including blood tests. Keep all appointments for checkups to receive maximum benefits and minimum risks of toxicity.
- These side effects may occur: drowsiness, dizziness (avoid driving or performing tasks that require alertness); GI upset (frequent small meals may help); mild thirst, greater than usual urine volume, fine hand tremor (may persist throughout therapy; notify heath care provider if severe).
- Use contraception to avoid pregnancy. If you wish to become pregnant or believe that you have become pregnant, consult your care provider.
- Discontinue drug, and notify care provider if toxicity occurs: diarrhea, vomiting, ataxia, tremor, drowsiness, lack of coordination or muscular weakness.
- Report diarrhea or fever.

▷lomefloxacin hydrochloride
*(low ma **flox'** a sin)*

Maxaquin

PREGNANCY CATEGORY C

Drug classes
Antibiotic
Fluoroquinolone

Therapeutic actions
Bactericidal: interferes with DNA replication by inhibiting DNA synase in susceptible gram-negative and gram-positive bacteria, preventing cell reproduction and causing cell death.

Indications
- For the treatment of infections in adults caused by susceptible organisms: lower respiratory tract infections caused by *Haemophilus influenzae, Moraxella catarrhalis*
- Treatment of acute exacerbations of chronic bronchitis caused by *H. influenzae* or *M. catarrhalis*
- Treatment of urinary tract infections due to *Escherichia coli, Klebsiella pneumoniae,*

Proteus mirabilis, Staphylococcus epidermidis, Enterobacter cloacae, Citrobacter diversus, Pseudomonas aeruginosa

- Prophylaxis: preoperatively to reduce the incidence of urinary tract infections in early postoperative period in patients undergoing transurethral procedures
- Preoperative prevention of infection in transrectal prostate biopsy
- Treatment of uncomplicated gonococcal infections

Contraindications and cautions
- Contraindicated with allergy to lomefloxacin, or any fluoroquinolone; syphilis; pregnancy, lactation.
- Use cautiously with renal dysfunction and seizures.

Available forms
Tablets—400 mg

Dosages
Adults
- *Lower respiratory tract infection:* 400 mg daily PO for 10 days.
- *Uncomplicated UTIs:* 400 mg daily PO for 3–10 days.
- *Complicated UTIs:* 400 mg daily PO for 14 days.
- *Prophylaxis:* Single dose of 400 mg PO 2–6 hr prior to surgery when oral preoperative medication is appropriate.
- *Uncomplicated gonococcal infections:* 400 mg PO as a single dose.
Pediatric patients
Not recommended for patients < 18 yr; produced lesions of joint cartilage in immature experimental animals.
Patients with impaired renal function
Creatinine clearance > 10 to < 40 mL/min: initial dose of 400 mg followed by 200 mg daily for the rest of the course.

Pharmacokinetics

Route	Onset	Peak	Duration
Oral	Varies	1–1.5 hr	8–10 hr

Metabolism: Hepatic; T$_{1/2}$: 8 hr

Distribution: Crosses placenta; enters breast milk
Excretion: Urine and feces

Adverse effects
- **CNS:** *Headache, dizziness,* insomnia, fatigue, somnolence, depression, blurred vision
- **GI:** *Nausea, vomiting,* dry mouth, diarrhea, abdominal pain
- **Hematologic:** Elevated BUN, AST, ALT, serum creatinine, and alkaline phosphatase; neutropenia, anemia
- **Other:** Fever, rash, *photosensitivity*

Interactions
✳ **Drug-drug** • Decreased therapeutic effect with iron salts • Decreased absorption with antacids • Increased serum levels and toxic effects of theophyllines

✳ **Drug-alternative therapy** • Increased risk of severe photosensitivity reactions if combined with St. John's wort therapy

■ Nursing considerations
Assessment
- **History:** Allergy to any fluoroquinolone; renal dysfunction; seizures; lactation, pregnancy
- **Physical:** Skin color, lesions; T; orientation, reflexes, affect; mucous membranes, bowel sounds; renal and liver function tests

Interventions
- Arrange for culture and sensitivity tests before beginning therapy.
- Continue therapy for full prescription, even if the signs and symptoms of infection have disappeared.
- Give oral drug without regard to meals.
- Ensure that patient is well hydrated.
- Give antacids at least 2 hr after dosing.
- Monitor clinical response; if no improvement is seen or a relapse occurs, repeat culture and sensitivity.

Teaching points
- Take oral drug without regard to meals. If an antacid is needed, do not take it within 2 hr of lomefloxacin dose.
- Drink plenty of fluids.
- These side effects may occur: nausea, vomiting, abdominal pain (small, frequent meals

may help); drowsiness, blurred vision, dizziness (observe caution if driving or using dangerous equipment), increased sensitivity to sun and ultraviolet light (use sunscreen and wear protective clothing).
• Report rash, visual changes, severe GI problems, weakness, tremors.

▽lomustine (CCNU)
(loe us' teen)

CeeNu

PREGNANCY CATEGORY D

Drug classes
Alkylating agent, nitrosourea
Antineoplastic

Therapeutic actions
Cytotoxic: exact mechanism of action not known, but it involves alkylation of DNA, thus inhibiting DNA, RNA, and protein synthesis; cell-cycle nonspecific.

Indications
• Treatment with other agents for primary and metastatic brain tumors and Hodgkin's disease

Contraindications and cautions
• Contraindicated with allergy to lomustine, myelosuppression, pregnancy (teratogenic and embryotoxic in preclinical studies), and lactation.
• Use cautiously with impaired renal or hepatic function.

Available forms
Capsules—10, 40, 100 mg

Dosages
Adults and pediatric patients
130 mg/m² PO as a single dose every 6 wk. Adjustments must be made with bone marrow suppression; initially reduce the dose to 100 mg/m² PO every 6 wk; do not give a repeat dose until platelets are > 100,000/mm³ and leukocytes are > 4,000/mm³; adjust dosage after initial dose based on hematologic response as follows:

Minimum (nadir) count after prior dose:

Leukocytes	Platelets	Percentage of Prior Dose to Give
> 4,000	> 100,000	100
3,000–3,999	75,000–99,999	100
2,000–2,999	25,000–74,999	70
< 2,000	< 25,000	50

Pharmacokinetics

Route	Onset	Peak	Duration
Oral	10 min	3 hr	48 hr

Metabolism: Hepatic; $T_{1/2}$: 16 to 72 hr
Distribution: Crosses placenta; enters breast milk
Excretion: Urine

Adverse effects
• **CNS:** Ataxia, lethargy
• **Dermatologic:** Alopecia
• **GI:** *Nausea, vomiting,* stomatitis, hepatotoxicity
• **GU:** Renal toxicity
• **Hematologic:** *Leukopenia; thrombocytopenia; anemia,* delayed for 4 to 6 wk; immunosuppression
• **Respiratory:** Pulmonary fibrosis
• **Other:** Secondary malignancies

■ Nursing considerations
Assessment
• **History:** Allergy to lomustine, radiation therapy, chemotherapy, hematopoietic depression, impaired renal or hepatic function, pregnancy, lactation
• **Physical:** T; weight; mucous membranes, liver evaluation; CBC, differential; urinalysis, liver and renal function tests

Interventions
• Arrange for blood tests to evaluate hematopoietic function before therapy and weekly for at least 6 wk thereafter.
• Do not give full dosage within 2–3 wk after a full course of radiation therapy or chemotherapy due to risk of severe bone marrow depression; reduced dosage may be needed.
• Advise patient that drug cannot be taken during pregnancy; suggest use of barrier contraceptives.

- Reduce dosage in patients with depressed bone marrow function.
- Administer tablets on an empty stomach to decrease GI upset; antiemetics may be needed for nausea and vomiting.

Teaching points
- Take this drug on an empty stomach.
- These side effects may occur: nausea, vomiting, loss of appetite (take on an empty stomach, an antiemetic may be ordered; small frequent meals may help), hair loss.
- Maintain your fluid intake and nutrition.
- Use birth control; this drug can cause severe birth defects.
- Report unusual bleeding or bruising, fever, chills, sore throat, stomach or flank pain, sores on your mouth or lips, unusual tiredness, confusion, difficulty breathing.

▷**loperamide hydrochloride**
(loe **per'** a mide)

Prescription: Apo-Loperamide (CAN), Imodium, Novo-Loperamide (CAN)

OTC: Diar-Aid Caplets, Diarr-Eze (CAN), Imodium A-D, Kaopectate II, Maalox Anti-Diarrheal Caplets, Neo-Diaral, Pepto Diarrhea Control

PREGNANCY CATEGORY B

Drug class
Antidiarrheal agent

Therapeutic actions
Slows intestinal motility and affects water and electrolyte movement through the bowel by inhibiting peristalsis through direct effects on the circular and longitudinal muscles of the intestinal wall.

Indications
- Control and symptomatic relief of acute nonspecific diarrhea and chronic diarrhea associated with inflammatory bowel disease
- Reduction of volume of discharge from ileostomies

- OTC use: control of diarrhea, including traveler's diarrhea

Contraindications and cautions
- Contraindicated with allergy to loperamide, patients who must avoid constipation, diarrhea associated with organisms that penetrate the intestinal mucosa (*Escherichia coli, Salmonella, Shigella, Clostridium difficile*).
- Use cautiously with hepatic dysfunction, acute ulcerative colitis, pregnancy, and lactation.

Available forms
Tablets—2 mg; capsules—2 mg; liquid—1 mg/5 mL; 1 mg/mL

Dosages
Adults
- *Acute diarrhea:* Initial dose of 4 mg PO followed by 2 mg after each unformed stool. Do not exceed 16 mg/day unless directed by a physician. Clinical improvement is usually seen within 48 hr.
- *Chronic diarrhea:* Initial dose of 4 mg PO followed by 2 mg after each unformed stool until diarrhea is controlled. Individualize dose based on patient response. Optimal daily dose is 4–8 mg. If no clinical improvement is seen with dosage of 16 mg/day for 10 days, further treatment will probably not be effective.
- *Traveler's diarrhea (OTC):* 4 mg PO after first loose stool, followed by 2 mg after each subsequent stool; do not exceed 8 mg/day for > 2 days.

Pediatric patients
Avoid use in children < 2 yr, and use extreme caution in younger children. Do not use OTC product with children.
- *Acute diarrhea:* First-day dosage schedule:

Age	Weight	Dose Form	Dosage
2–5 yr	13–20 kg	Liquid	1 mg tid
5–8 yr	20–30 kg	Liquid or capsule	2 mg bid
8–12 yr	> 30 kg	Liquid or capsule	2 mg tid

Subsequent doses: Administer 1 mg/10 kg PO only after a loose stool. Daily dosage should not exceed recommended first-day dosage.

Adverse effects in *Italics* are most common; those in **Bold** are life-threatening.

- *Chronic diarrhea:* Dosage schedule has not been established.
- *Traveler's diarrhea (OTC):*

9–11 yr: 2 mg PO after first loose stool followed by 1 mg after each subsequent stool

6–8 yr: 1 mg PO after first loose stool, followed by 1 mg after each subsequent loose stool—do not exceed 4 mg/day

< 6 yr: Consult with physician; not recommended.

Pharmacokinetics

Route	Onset	Peak
Oral	Varies	5 hr

Metabolism: Hepatic; $T_{1/2}$: 10.8 hr
Distribution: May cross placenta and enter breast milk
Excretion: Urine and feces

Adverse effects

- **CNS:** Tiredness, drowsiness, or dizziness
- **GI: Toxic megacolon** (in patients with ulcerative colitis), *abdominal pain, distention or discomfort, constipation, dry mouth, nausea,* vomiting
- **Hypersensitivity:** Rash

■ Nursing considerations
Assessment

- **History:** Allergy to loperamide, patients who must avoid constipation, diarrhea associated with organisms that penetrate the intestinal mucosa (*E. coli, Salmonella, Shigella*); hepatic dysfunction, acute ulcerative colitis, lactation
- **Physical:** Skin color, lesions; orientation, reflexes; abdominal exam, bowel sounds, liver evaluation; serum electrolytes (with extended use)

Interventions

- Monitor for response. If improvement is not seen within 48 hr, discontinue treatment and notify health care provider.
- Give drug after each unformed stool. Keep track of amount given to avoid exceeding the recommended daily dosage unless directed by a physician.
- Have the narcotic antagonist naloxone on standby in case of overdose and CNS depression.

Teaching points

- Take drug as prescribed. Do not exceed prescribed dosage or recommended daily dosage.
- These side effects may occur: abdominal fullness, nausea, vomiting; dry mouth (suck on sugarless lozenges); dizziness.
- Report abdominal pain or distention, fever, and diarrhea that does not stop after a few days.

▷**lopinavir
(lopinavir and ritonavir)**
*(low **pin'** ah ver)*

Kaletra

PREGNANCY CATEGORY C

Drug classes
Antiviral drug
Protease inhibitor combination

Therapeutic action
Lopinavir in this combination exhibits antiviral activity; inhibits HIV protease activity, leading to the decrease in production of HIV particles; ritonavir in this preparation blocks the excretion of lopinavir, allowing for increased plasma levels of lopinavir.

Indications
- Treatment of HIV infection in combination with other antiretroviral agents

Contraindications and cautions
- Contraindicated with allergy to lopinavir, ritonavir.
- Use cautiously with pregnancy, hepatic impairment, pancreatitis, lactation.

Available forms
Gel caps—133.3 mg lopinavir/33.3 mg ritonavir; oral solution—80 mg lopinavir/20 mg ritonavir/mL

Dosages
Adults
400 mg lopinavir and 100 mg ritonavir PO bid, taken with food (3 capsules or 5 mL)
Taken with efavirenz or nevirapine: 533 mg lopinavir and 133 mg ritonavir PO bid (4 capsules or 6.5 mL)

Pediatric patients

< 6 mo: Not recommended. 7–15 kg: 12 mg/kg PO bid; 15–40 kg: 10 mg/kg PO bid; > 40 kg: Use adult dose.
- *Taken with efavirenz or nevirapine:* 7–15 kg: 13 mg/kg PO bid; 15–50 kg: 11 mg/kg PO bid; > 50 kg: adult dose.

Pharmacokinetics

Route	Onset	Peak
Oral	Varies	3–4 hr

Metabolism: Hepatic; $T_{1/2}$: 5–6 hr
Distribution: Crosses placenta; may pass into breast milk
Excretion: Feces and urine

Adverse effects

- **CNS:** *Asthenia, peripheral and circumoral paresthesias,* anxiety, dreams, *headache,* dizziness, hallucinations, personality changes
- **CV:** DVTs, hypotension, syncope, tachycardia, chest pain
- **Dermatologic:** Rash, acne, alopecia, dry skin, exfoliative dermatitis
- **Endocrine:** *Increased triglycerides and cholesterol,* hyperglycemia, hyperuricemia, gynecomastia, hypothyroidism, hypogonadism
- **GI:** *Nausea, vomiting, diarrhea, anorexia, abdominal pain,* pancreatitis, *taste perversion,* dry mouth, hepatitis, liver dysfunction, dehydration
- **Hematologic:** Leukopenia, anemia
- **Other:** Hypothermia, chills, back pain, edema, cachexia

Interactions

✳ **Drug-drug** • Potentially large increase in the serum concentration of drugs metabolized by cytochrome P450 3A4 (due to ritonavir). These include amiodarone, bepridil, buproprion, cloxapine, encainide, flecainide, meperidine, piroxicam, propafenone, propoxyphene, quinidine, and rifabutin, when taken with lopinavir. Potential for serious arrhythmias, seizures, and fatal reactions. **Do not administer lopinavir with any of these drugs** • May decrease the effectiveness of hormonal contraceptives; use of barrier contraceptives is advised • Potentially large increases in the serum concentration of these sedatives and hypnotics: alprazolam, clorazepam, diazepam, estazolam, flurazepam, midazolam, triazolam, zolpidem. Extreme sedation and respiratory depression could occur. **Do not administer lopinavir with any of these drugs**

✳ **Drug-food** • Absorption of lopinavir is increased by the presence of food; taking the drug with food is strongly recommended

✳ **Drug-alternative therapy** • Potential for reduced effectiveness if combined with St. John's wort; avoid this combination

■ Nursing considerations
Assessment

- **History:** Allergy to lopinavir, ritonavir, hepatic dysfunction, pancreatitis, pregnancy, lactation
- **Physical:** T; orientation, reflexes; BP, P, peripheral perfusion; R, adventitious sounds; bowel sounds; skin color, perfusion; liver function tests, serum amylase levels, triglycerides, cholesterol, electrolytes

Interventions

- Capsules and solution should be stored in the refrigerator; may be left at room temperature, but should be used within 60 days; protect from light and extreme heat. Be aware that oral solution contains 42% alcohol.
- Obtain baseline triglycerides, cholesterol levels, electrolytes and glucose levels. Monitor periodically during therapy.
- Screen medication history before administration to avoid potentially serious drug–drug interactions.
- Administer with meals or food to increase absorption.
- Administer didanosine 1 hr before or 2 hr after lopinavir.

Teaching points

- Take this drug with meals or food; store the capsules or solution in the refrigerator. The taste of the solution may be improved if mixed with chocolate milk, *Ensure,* or *Advera* 1 hour before taking.
- Take the full course of therapy as prescribed; do not double up doses if one is missed; do

---

Adverse effects in *Italics* are most common; those in **Bold** are life-threatening.

not change dosage without consulting your health care provider. Take this drug with your other HIV medications.
- This drug does not cure HIV infection; long-term effects are not yet known; continue to take precautions as the risk of transmission is not reduced by this drug.
- This drug may cause hormonal contraceptives to be ineffective; use of barrier contraceptives is advised.
- Do not take any other drug, prescription or over-the-counter, or use any herbal therapies without consulting with your health care provider; this drug interacts with many other drugs and serious problems can occur.
- These side effects may occur: nausea, vomiting, loss of appetite, diarrhea, abdominal pain; headache, dizziness, numbness, and tingling.
- Report severe diarrhea, severe nausea, personality changes, changes in the color of urine or stool, fever or chills, severe abdominal pain.

▽ loracarbef
*(lor ah **kar' bef**)*

Lorabid

PREGNANCY CATEGORY B

Drug classes
Antibiotic
Cephalosporin (second generation)

Therapeutic actions
Bactericidal: inhibits synthesis of bacterial cell wall, causing cell death.

Indications
- Pharyngitis and tonsillitis caused by *Streptococcus pyogenes*
- Secondary bacterial infection of acute bronchitis and exacerbation of chronic bronchitis caused by *S. pneumoniae, H. influenzae, M. catarrhalis*
- Pneumonia caused by *S. pneumoniae, H. influenzae*
- Uncomplicated skin and skin structure infections caused by *Staphylococcus aureus, S. pyogenes*

- Uncomplicated urinary tract infections caused by *E. coli, Staphylococcus saprophyticus*
- Uncomplicated pyelonephritis caused by *E. coli*
- Otitis media caused by *S. pneumoniae, H. influenzae, M. catarrhalis, S. pyogenes*

Contraindications and cautions
- Allergy to cephalosporins or penicillins, renal failure, lactation.

Available forms
Capsules—200, 400 mg; powder for suspension—100, 200 mg/5 mL

Dosages
Adults
200 to 400 mg PO q 12 hr. Continue treatment for 7 to 14 days, depending on the severity of the infection.
Pediatric patients
15 to 30 mg/kg/day in divided doses q 12 hr PO. Continue treatment for 7 to 10 days.
Geriatric patients or patients with renal impairment
Creatinine clearance > 50 mL/min: Use standard dose. Creatinine clearance 10–49 mL/min: Use 50% of standard dose.

Pharmacokinetics
Route	Peak
Oral	90 min

Metabolism: Hepatic; $T_{1/2}$: 60 min
Distribution: Crosses the placenta, enters breast milk
Excretion: Renal, unchanged

Adverse effects
- **CNS:** Headache, dizziness, lethargy, paresthesias
- **GI:** *Nausea, vomiting, diarrhea, anorexia, abdominal pain, flatulence,* **pseudomembranous colitis,** liver toxicity
- **GU:** Nephrotoxicity
- **Hematologic:** Bone marrow depression
- **Hypersensitivity:** *Ranges from rash to fever* to **anaphylaxis;** serum sickness reaction
- **Other:** *Superinfections*

Interactions

❋ Drug-drug • Increased nephrotoxicity with aminoglycosides • Increased bleeding effects if taken with oral anticoagulants; decreased dose of anticoagulant may be needed • Disulfiram-like reaction if alcohol is taken within 72 hr after loracarbef administration **❋ Drug-lab test •** Possibility of false results on tests of urine glucose using Benedict's solution, Fehling's solution, *Clinitest* tablets, urinary 17-ketosteroids, direct Coombs' test

■ Nursing considerations
Assessment
- **History:** Penicillin or cephalosporin allergy, pregnancy or lactation
- **Physical:** Kidney function, respiratory status, skin status; culture and sensitivity tests of infected area

Interventions
- Culture infection before drug therapy.
- Give drug on an empty stomach, 1 hr before or 2 hr after meals.
- Reconstitute solution by adding 30–60 mL water in two portions to the dry mixture in the 50- or 100-mL bottle, respectively.
- Keep suspension at room temperature after reconstitution, discard after 14 days.
- Stop drug if hypersensitivity reaction occurs.
- Arrange for oral vancomycin or metronidazole for serious colitis that fails to respond to discontinuation.
- Reculture infected area if infection fails to respond.

Teaching points
- Take this drug on an empty stomach, 1 hr before or 2 hr after meals. Store suspension at room temperature, and discard any unused portions after 14 days.
- Complete the full course of this drug, even if you feel better before the treatment is over.
- This drug is prescribed for this infection; do not self-treat other infections.
- These side effects may occur: stomach upset, loss of appetite, nausea (take with food); diarrhea, headache, dizziness.
- Report severe diarrhea with blood, pus, or mucus; rash or hives; difficulty breathing; unusual tiredness or fatigue; unusual bleeding or bruising.

▽loratadine
*(lor **at**' a deen)*

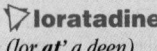

Alavert, Claritin, Claritin Reditabs

PREGNANCY CATEGORY B

Drug class
Antihistamine (nonsedating type)

Therapeutic actions
Competitively blocks the effects of histamine at peripheral H_1 receptor sites; has anticholinergic (atropine-like) and antipruritic effects.

Indications
- Symptomatic relief of perennial and seasonal allergic rhinitis, vasomotor rhinitis, allergic conjunctivitis, and mild, uncomplicated urticaria and angioedema
- Treatment of rhinitis and chronic urticaria in children ≥ 2 yr

Contraindications and cautions
- Allergy to any antihistamines; narrow-angle glaucoma, stenosing peptic ulcer, symptomatic prostatic hypertrophy, asthma, bladder neck obstruction, pyloroduodenal obstruction (avoid use or use with caution, condition may be exacerbated by drug); lactation, pregnancy.

Available forms
Tablets—10 mg; syrup—1 mg/mL; rapidly disintegrating tablets (*Reditabs*)—10 mg

Dosages
Place rapid dissolving tablets on tongue. Swallow with or without water.
Adults and patients ≥ 6 yr
10 mg daily PO on an empty stomach.
Pediatric patients 2–5 yr
5 mg PO daily (syrup).

Geriatric patients or patients with hepatic impairment
10 mg PO every other day.

Pharmacokinetics

Route	Onset	Peak	Duration
Oral	1–3 hr	8–12 hr	24 hr

Metabolism: Hepatic; $T_{1/2}$: 8.4 hr
Distribution: Crosses placenta; enters breast milk
Excretion: Urine and feces

Adverse effects

- **CNS:** *Headache, nervousness, dizziness,* depression, drowsiness
- **CV:** Palpitations, edema
- **GI:** *Appetite increase,* nausea, diarrhea, abdominal pain
- **Respiratory:** Bronchospasm, pharyngitis
- **Other:** Fever, photosensitivity, rash, myalgia, arthralgia, angioedema, *weight gain*

Interactions

✴ **Drug-drug** • Additive CNS depressant effects with alcohol or other CNS depressants
• Increased and prolonged anticholinergic (drying) effects with MAO inhibitors; avoid this combination
✴ **Drug-lab test** • False skin testing procedures if done while patient is on antihistamines

■ Nursing considerations
Assessment
- **History:** Allergy to any antihistamines; narrow-angle glaucoma, stenosing peptic ulcer, symptomatic prostatic hypertrophy, asthma, bladder neck obstruction, pyloroduodenal obstruction; lactation, pregnancy
- **Physical:** Skin color, lesions, texture; orientation, reflexes, affect; vision exams; R, adventitious sounds; prostate palpation; serum transaminase levels

Interventions
- Administer on an empty stomach 1 hr before or 2 hr after meals.

Teaching points
- Take this drug on an empty stomach 1 hr before or 2 hr after meals or food.

- If using rapid dissolving tablets, place on tongue, tablet will dissolve within seconds, swallow with or without water.
- These side effects may occur: dizziness, sedation, drowsiness (use caution if driving or performing tasks that require alertness); headache; thickening of bronchial secretions, dryness of nasal mucosa (use a humidifier).
- Avoid the use of alcohol; serious sedation could occur.
- Report difficulty breathing, hallucinations, tremors, loss of coordination, irregular heartbeat.

▽ lorazepam
(lor a' ze pam)

Apo-Lorazepam (CAN), Ativan, Novo-Lorazem (CAN), Nu-Loraz (CAN)

PREGNANCY CATEGORY D

C-IV CONTROLLED SUBSTANCE

Drug classes
Benzodiazepine
Antianxiety agent
Sedative and hypnotic

Therapeutic actions
Exact mechanisms are not understood; acts mainly at subcortical levels of the CNS, leaving the cortex relatively unaffected. Main sites of action may be the limbic system and reticular formation; benzodiazepines potentiate the effects of GABA, an inhibitory neurotransmitter; anxiolytic effects occur at doses well below those necessary to cause sedation and ataxia.

Indications
- Management of anxiety disorders or for short-term relief of symptoms of anxiety or anxiety associated with depression (oral)
- Preanesthetic medication in adults to produce sedation, relieve anxiety, and decrease recall of events related to surgery (parenteral)
- Unlabeled parenteral use: management of status epilepticus, chemotherapy-induced nausea and vomiting, acute alcohol withdrawal

Contraindications and cautions

- Contraindicated with hypersensitivity to benzodiazepines, propylene glycol, polyethylene glycol or benzyl alcohol (parenteral lorazepam); psychoses; acute narrow-angle glaucoma; shock; coma; acute alcoholic intoxication with depression of vital signs; pregnancy (crosses placenta; risk of congenital malformations and neonatal withdrawal syndrome); labor and delivery ("floppy infant" syndrome); and lactation.
- Use cautiously with impaired liver or kidney function.

Available forms

Injection—2, 4 mg/mL; oral solution—2 mg/mL; tablets—0.5, 1, 2 mg

Dosages

Adults

Oral

Usual dose is 2–6 mg/day; range 1–10 mg/day given in divided doses with largest dose hs.
- *Insomnia due to transient stress:* 2–4 mg given hs.

IM

0.05 mg/kg up to a maximum of 4 mg administered at least 2 hr before operative procedure.

IV

Initial dose is 2 mg total or 0.044 mg/kg, whichever is smaller. Do not exceed this dose in patients older than 50 yr. Doses as high as 0.05 mg/kg up to a total of 4 mg may be given 15 to 20 min before the procedure to those benefited by a greater lack of recall. Continuous infusion 0.5–1 mg/hr titrated, based on patient response.

Pediatric patients

Drug should not be used in children < 12 yr.

Geriatric patients or patients with hepatic disease

Initially, 1 to 2 mg/day in divided doses. Adjust as needed and tolerated.

Pharmacokinetics

Route	Onset	Peak	Duration
Oral	Intermed	1–6 hr	12–24 hr
IM	15–30 min	60–90 min	12–24 hr
IV	1–5 min	10–15 min	12–24 hr

Metabolism: Hepatic; $T_{1/2}$: 10–20 hr
Distribution: Crosses placenta; enters breast milk
Excretion: Urine

▼ IV facts

Preparation: Dilute lorazepam immediately prior to IV use. For direct IV injection or injection into IV line, dilute with an equal volume of compatible solution (sterile water for injection, sodium chloride injection, or 5% dextrose injection); do not use if solution is discolored or contains a precipitate. Protect from light.

Infusion: Direct inject slowly, or infuse at maximum rate of 2 mg/min.

Y-site incompatibilities: Do not mix with foscarnet, ondansetron.

Adverse effects

- **CNS:** *Transient, mild drowsiness initially; sedation, depression, lethargy, apathy, fatigue, light-headedness, disorientation, anger, hostility,* episodes of mania and hypomania, *restlessness, confusion,* crying, delirium, *headache,* slurred speech, dysarthria, stupor, rigidity, tremor, dystonia, vertigo, euphoria, nervousness, difficulty concentrating, vivid dreams, psychomotor retardation, extrapyramidal symptoms; *mild paradoxical excitatory reactions during first 2 wk of treatment*
- **CV:** Bradycardia, tachycardia, **CV collapse**, hypertension and hypotension, palpitations, edema
- **Dermatologic:** Urticaria, pruritus, rash, dermatitis
- **EENT:** Visual and auditory disturbances, diplopia, nystagmus, depressed hearing, nasal congestion
- **GI:** Constipation, diarrhea, *dry mouth,* salivation, *nausea,* anorexia, vomiting, difficulty in swallowing, gastric disorders, hepatic dysfunction
- **GU:** Incontinence, urinary retention, changes in libido, menstrual irregularities
- **Hematologic:** Elevations of blood enzymes: LDH, alkaline phosphatase, AST, ALT; blood dyscrasias: agranulocytosis, leukopenia

---

Adverse effects in *Italics* are most common; those in **Bold** are life-threatening.

- **Other:** Hiccups, fever, diaphoresis, paresthesias, muscular disturbances, gynecomastia. *Drug dependence with withdrawal syndrome when drug is discontinued; more common with abrupt discontinuation of higher dosage used for > 4 mo*

Interactions

✻ **Drug-drug** • Increased CNS depression with alcohol and other sedating medications, such as barbiturates and opioids • Decreased effectiveness with theophyllines

✻ **Drug-herb** • Kava kava increases the sedative effects of benzodiazepines; coma has been reported with concurrent use

■ Nursing considerations

 CLINICAL ALERT!
Name confusion has occurred between lorazepam and alprazolam; use caution.

Assessment

- **History:** Hypersensitivity to benzodiazepines, propylene glycol, polyethylene glycol or benzyl alcohol; psychoses; acute narrow-angle glaucoma; shock; coma; acute alcoholic intoxication with depression of vital signs; pregnancy; lactation; impaired liver or kidney function, debilitation
- **Physical:** Skin color, lesions; T; orientation, reflexes, affect, ophthalmologic exam; P, BP; R, adventitious sounds; liver evaluation, abdominal exam, bowel sounds, normal output; CBC, liver and renal function tests

Interventions

- Be aware that SL administration has more rapid absorption than PO, and bioavailability compares to IM use.
- Do not administer intra-arterially; arteriospasm, gangrene may result.
- Give IM injections of undiluted drug deep into muscle mass, monitor injection sites.
- Do not use solutions that are discolored or contain a precipitate. Protect drug from light, and refrigerate oral solution.
- Keep equipment to maintain a patent airway on standby when drug is given IV.
- Reduce dose of opioid analgesics by at least half in patients who have received parenteral lorazepam.

- Keep patients who have received parenteral doses under close observation, preferably in bed, up to 3 hr. Do not permit ambulatory patients to drive following an injection.
- Taper dosage gradually after long-term therapy, especially in epileptic patients.

Teaching points

- Take drug exactly as prescribed; do not stop taking drug (long-term therapy) without consulting health care provider.
- These side effects may occur: drowsiness, dizziness (may be transient; avoid driving or engaging in dangerous activities); GI upset (take drug with food); nocturnal sleep disturbances for several nights after discontinuing the drug if used as a sedative and hypnotic; depression, dreams, emotional upset, crying.
- Report severe dizziness, weakness, drowsiness that persists, rash or skin lesions, palpitations, edema of the extremities; visual changes; difficulty voiding.

▽losartan potassium
*(low **sar'** tan)*

Cozaar

PREGNANCY CATEGORY C
(FIRST TRIMESTER)

PREGNANCY CATEGORY D
(SECOND AND THIRD TRIMESTERS)

Drug classes

Angiotensin II receptor blocker (ARB)
Antihypertensive

Therapeutic actions

Selectively blocks the binding of angiotensin II to specific tissue receptors found in the vascular smooth muscle and adrenal gland; this action blocks the vasoconstriction effect of the renin-angiotensin system as well as the release of aldosterone leading to decreased blood pressure.

Indications

- Treatment of hypertension, alone or in combination with other antihypertensive agents
- Treatment of diabetic neuropathy with an elevated serum creatinine and proteinuria

in patients with type 2 diabetes and a history of hypertension

Contraindications and cautions
- Contraindicated with hypersensitivity to losartan, pregnancy (use during the second or third trimester can cause injury or even death to the fetus), lactation.
- Use cautiously with hepatic or renal dysfunction, hypovolemia.

Available forms
Tablets—25, 50, 100 mg

Dosages
Adults
- *Hypertension:* Starting dose of 50 mg PO daily. Patients on diuretics or hypovolemic patients may only require 25 mg daily. Dosage ranges from 25–100 mg PO given once or twice a day have been used.
- *Diabetic neuropathy:* 50 mg/day PO once daily; may be increased to 100 mg/day once daily based on blood pressure response.

Pediatric patients
Safety and efficacy not established.

Pharmacokinetics

Route	Onset	Peak
Oral	Varies	1–3 hr

Metabolism: Hepatic; $T_{1/2}$: 2 hr, then 6–9 hr
Distribution: Crosses placenta; passes into breast milk
Excretion: Feces and urine

Adverse effects
- **CNS:** Headache, *dizziness,* syncope, insomnia
- **CV:** Hypotension
- **Dermatologic:** Rash, urticaria, pruritus, alopecia, dry skin
- **GI:** *Diarrhea, abdominal pain, nausea,* constipation, dry mouth
- **Respiratory:** *URI symptoms, cough,* sinus disorders
- **Other:** Back pain, fever, gout, muscle weakness

Interactions
✱ **Drug-drug** • Decreased serum levels and effectiveness if taken concurrently with phenobarbital • Losartan is converted to an active metabolite by cytochrome P450 3A4. Drugs that inhibit 3A4 (ketoconazole, fluconazole, diltiazem) may decrease the antihypertensive effects of losartan

■ Nursing considerations
Assessment
- **History:** Hypersensitivity to losartan, pregnancy, lactation, hepatic or renal dysfunction, hypovolemia
- **Physical:** Skin lesions, turgor; T; reflexes, affect; BP; R, respiratory auscultation; liver and kidney function tests

Interventions
- Administer without regard to meals.
- Ensure that patient is not pregnant before beginning therapy, suggest the use of barrier birth control while using losartan; fetal injury and deaths have been reported.
- Find an alternative method of feeding the baby if given to a nursing mother. Depression of the renin-angiotensin system in infants is potentially very dangerous.
- Alert surgeon and mark patient's chart with notice that losartan is being taken. The blockage of the renin-angiotensin system following surgery can produce problems. Hypotension may be reversed with volume expansion.
- Monitor patient closely in any situation that may lead to a decrease in blood pressure secondary to reduction in fluid volume—excessive perspiration, dehydration, vomiting, diarrhea—excessive hypotension can occur.

Teaching points
- Take drug without regard to meals. Do not stop taking this drug without consulting your health care provider.
- Use a barrier method of birth control while on this drug; if you become pregnant or desire to become pregnant, consult with your health care provider.
- These side effects may occur: dizziness (avoid driving a car or performing hazardous tasks);

Adverse effects in *Italics* are most common; those in **Bold** are life-threatening.

2004 Quick-Access Photoguide to Pills and Capsules

This photoguide presents nearly 400 pills and capsules, representing the most commonly prescribed generic and trade drugs. These drugs, organized alphabetically by generic name, are shown in actual size and color, with cross-references to drug information. Each product is labeled with its trade name and its strength.

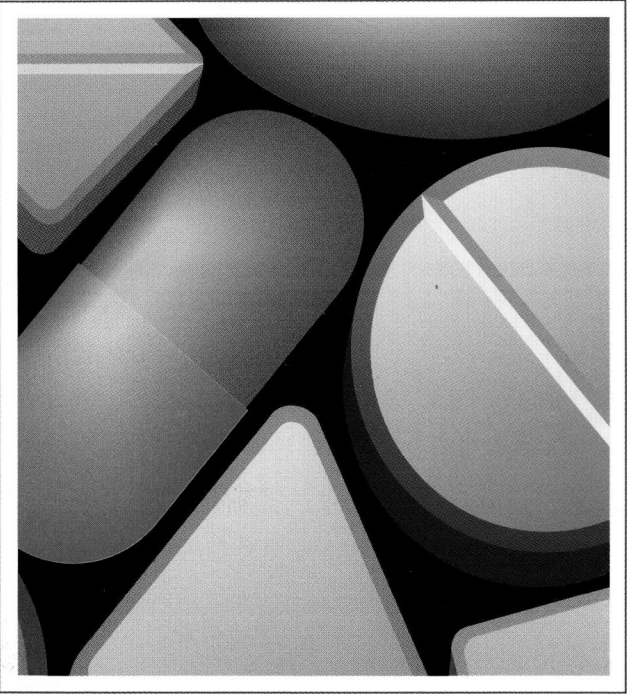

Adapted from Facts and Comparisons, St. Louis, Missouri

ACETAMINOPHEN AND CODEINE

Tylenol and Codeine #3
(page 1278)

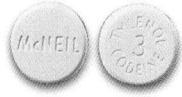

300/30 mg

ACYCLOVIR

Zovirax
(page 74)

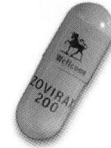
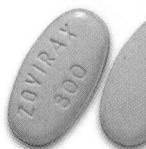

200 mg   400 mg   800 mg

ALENDRONATE SODIUM

Fosamax
(page 86)

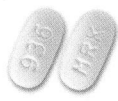

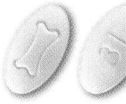

10 mg   40 mg   70 mg

ALOSETRON HYDROCHLORIDE

Lotronex
(page 90)

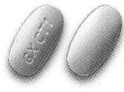

1 mg

ALPRAZOLAM

Xanax
(page 91)

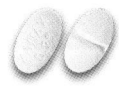
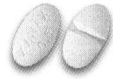
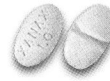

0.25 mg   0.5 mg   1 mg

AMIODARONE HYDROCHLORIDE

Cordarone
(page 113)

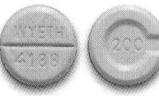

200 mg

MITRIPTYLINE HYDROCHLORIDE

lavil
age 115)

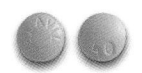

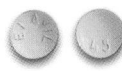

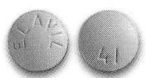

10 mg   25 mg   50 mg

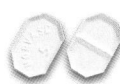

75 mg   100 mg   150 mg

MLODIPINE BESYLATE

orvasc
age 117)

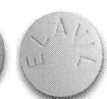

2.5 mg   5 mg

MOXICILLIN AND CLAVULANIC ACID

ugmentin
age 1281)

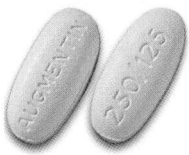

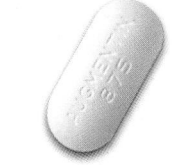

250 mg   500 mg   875 mg

ugmentin Chewable
age 1281)

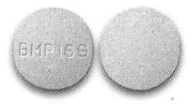

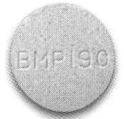

125 mg   250 mg

MOXICILLIN TRIHYDRATE

moxil
age 123)

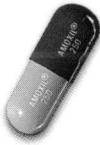

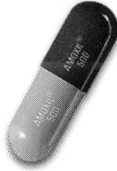

250 mg   500 mg

ARIPIPRAZOLE

Abilify

(page 140)

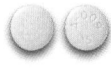

15 mg

ATENOLOL

Tenormin

(page 146)

25 mg   50 mg   100 mg

ATOMOXETINE HYDROCHLORIDE

Strattera

(page 147)

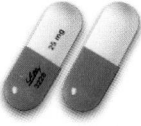 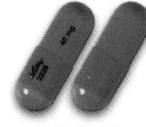

25 mg   40 mg

ATORVASTATIN CALCIUM

Lipitor

(page 149)

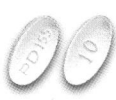 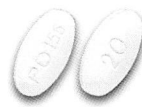

10 mg   20 mg

AZITHROMYCIN

Zithromax

(page 160)

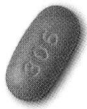

250 mg

BENAZEPRIL HYDROCHLORIDE

Lotensin

(page 168)

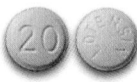

20 mg   40 mg

BUMETANIDE

Bumex
(page 199)

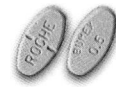 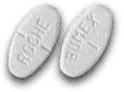 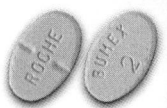

0.5 mg   1 mg   2 mg

BUPROPION HYDROCHLORIDE

Wellbutrin
(page 203)

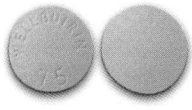 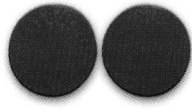

75 mg   100 mg

Wellbutrin SR
(page 203)

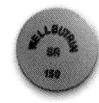

150 mg

Zyban
(page 203)

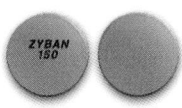

150 mg

BUSPIRONE HYDROCHLORIDE

BuSpar
(page 204)

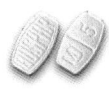 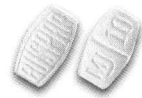

5 mg   10 mg

CAPTOPRIL

Capoten
(page 221)

12.5 mg   25 mg

CARISOPRODOL

Soma
(page 229)

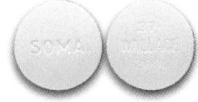

350 mg

CARVEDILOL

Coreg
(page 233)

3.125 mg

6.25 mg

12.5 mg

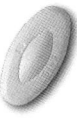

25 mg

CEFADROXIL

Duricef
(page 236)

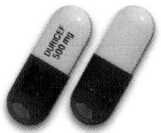

500 mg

1,000 mg

CEFPROZIL

Cefzil
(page 255)

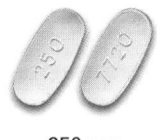

250 mg

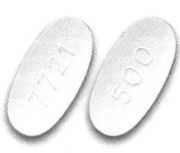

500 mg

CEFUROXIME AXETIL

Ceftin
(page 262)

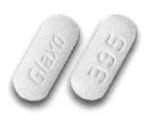

125 mg

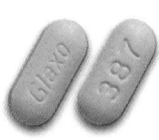

250 mg

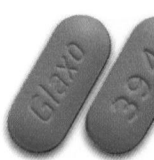

500 mg

CELECOXIB

Celebrex
(page 264)

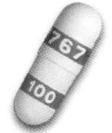 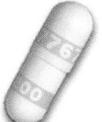

100 mg 200 mg

CETIRIZINE HYDROCHLORIDE

Zyrtec
(page 271)

5 mg 10 mg

CILOSTAZOL

Pletal
(page 298)

50 mg 100 mg

CIMETIDINE

Tagamet
(page 299)

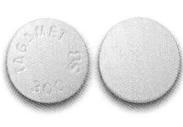 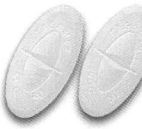 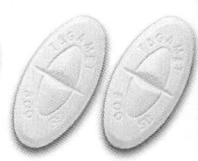

300 mg 400 mg 800 mg

CIPROFLOXACIN

Cipro
(page 301)

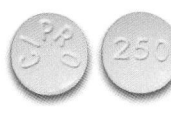 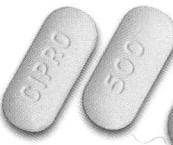  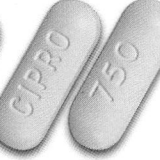

250 mg 500 mg 750 mg

CITALOPRAM HYDROBROMIDE

Celexa
(page 305)

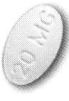

20 mg 40 mg

CLARITHROMYCIN

Biaxin
(page 307)

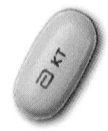 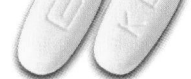

250 mg   500 mg

Biaxin XL
(page 307)

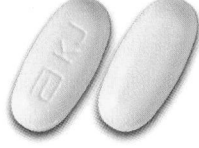

500 mg

CLONAZEPAM

Klonopin
(page 317)

0.5 mg   1 mg   2 mg

CO-TRIMOXAZOLE

Bactrim DS
(page 1282)

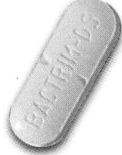

160/800 mg

DESLORATADINE

Clarinex
(page 369)

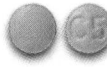

5 mg

DIAZEPAM

Valium
(page 385)

2 mg   5 mg   10 mg

DIGOXIN

Lanoxicaps
(page 396)

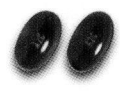 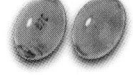

0.05 mg   0.1 mg   0.2 mg

Lanoxin
(page 396)

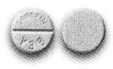 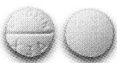

0.125 mg   0.25 mg

DILTIAZEM HYDROCHLORIDE

Cardizem
(page 401)

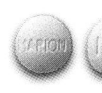 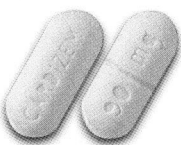

30 mg   90 mg

Cardizem CD
(page 401)

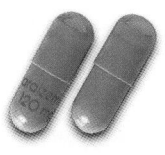 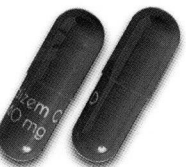

120 mg   240 mg

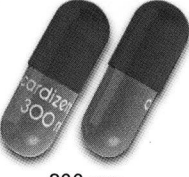

300 mg

Cardizem SR
(page 401)

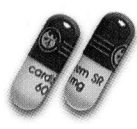 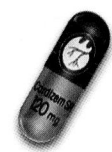

60 mg   120 mg

DOXAZOSIN MESYLATE

Cardura
(page 424)

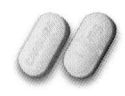

1 mg

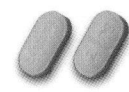

2 mg

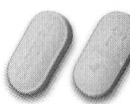

4 mg

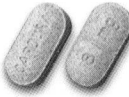

8 mg

ENALAPRIL MALEATE

Vasotec
(page 442)

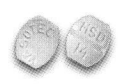

2.5 mg

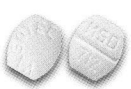

5 mg

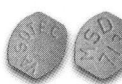

10 mg

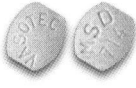

20 mg

ERYTHROMYCIN BASE

E-Mycin
(page 464)

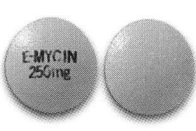

250 mg   333 mg

Eryc
(page 464)

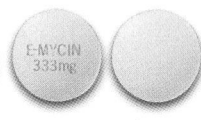

250 mg

Ery-Tab
(page 464)

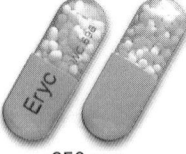

333 mg

ESCITALOPRAM OXALATE

Lexapro
(page 468)

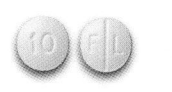 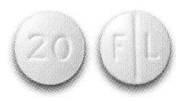

10 mg   20 mg

ESTRADIOL

Estrace
(page 473)

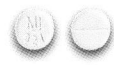   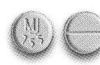   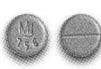

0.5 mg   1 mg   2 mg

ESTROGENS, CONJUGATED

Premarin
(page 477)

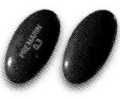   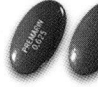   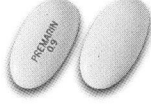

0.3 mg   0.625 mg   0.9 mg

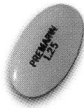   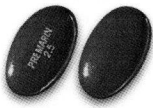

1.25 mg   2.5 mg

ETHINYL ESTRADIOL AND ETHYNODIOL DIACETATE

Demulen
(page 1299)

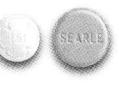   

1/35-28   1/50-28

ETHINYL ESTRADIOL AND NORETHINDRONE

Ovcon-35
(page 1299)

0.4/35-28

EZETIMIBE

Zetia
(page 500)

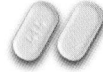

10 mg

FAMOTIDINE

Pepcid
(page 504)

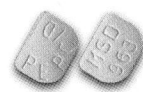   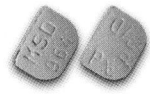

20 mg   40 mg

FEXOFENADINE HYDROCHLORIDE

Allegra
(page 513)

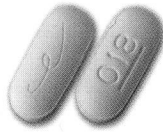

180 mg

FLUCONAZOLE

Diflucan
(page 521)

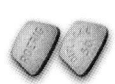   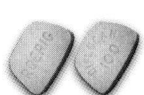   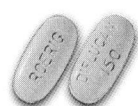

50 mg   100 mg   150 mg

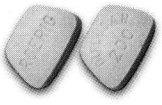

200 mg

FLUOXETINE HYDROCHLORIDE

Prozac
(page 530)

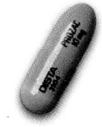

10 mg

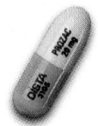

20 mg

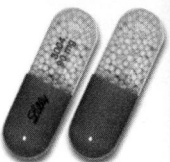

90 mg

Sarafem
(page 530)

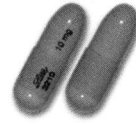

10 mg

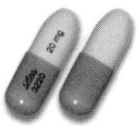

20 mg

FLUVASTATIN SODIUM

Lescol
(page 540)

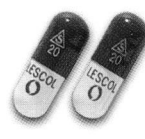

20 mg

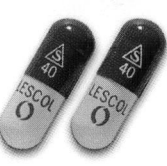

40 mg

FOSINOPRIL SODIUM

Monopril
(page 549)

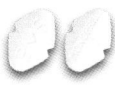

10 mg

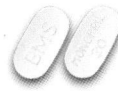

20 mg

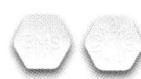

40 mg

FROVATRIPTAN SUCCINATE

Frova
(page 552)

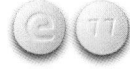

2.5 mg

FUROSEMIDE

Lasix
(page 554)

20 mg

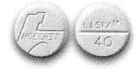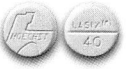

40 mg

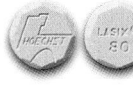

80 mg

GABAPENTIN

Neurontin
(page 556)

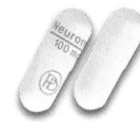 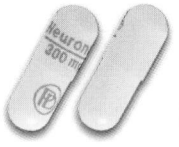 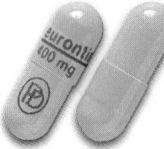

100 mg 300 mg 400 mg

GEMFIBROZIL

Lopid
(page 564)

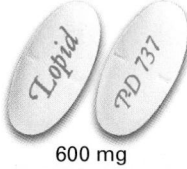

600 mg

GLIPIZIDE

Glucotrol
(page 570)

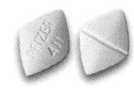 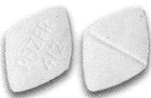

5 mg 10 mg

Glucotrol XL
(page 570)

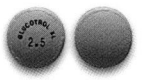 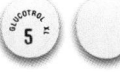 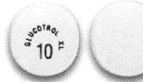

2.5 mg 5 mg 10 mg

GLYBURIDE

DiaBeta
(page 574)

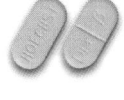 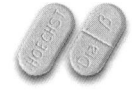 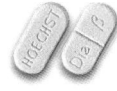

1.25 mg 2.5 mg 5 mg

Micronase
(page 574)

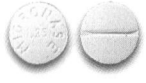   

1.25 mg 2.5 mg 5 mg

HYDROCHLOROTHIAZIDE

HydroDIURIL
(page 597)

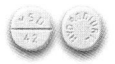 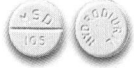

25 mg   50 mg

HYDROCODONE BITARTRATE AND ACETAMINOPHEN

Lortab
(page 1279)

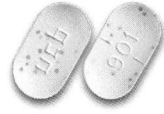 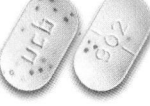 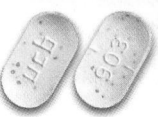

2.5/500 mg   5/500 mg   7.5/500 mg

Vicodin
(page 1279)

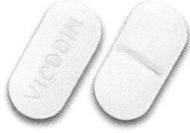

5/500 mg

Vicodin ES
(page 1279)

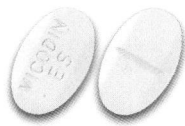

7.5/750 mg

IBUPROFEN

Motrin
(page 614)

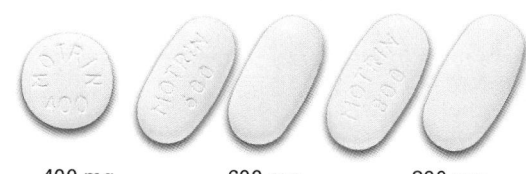

400 mg   600 mg   800 mg

IMATINIB MESYLATE

Gleevec
(page 620)

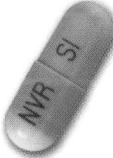

100 mg

INDINAVIR SULFATE

Crixivan
(page 627)

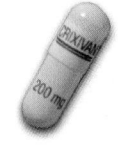 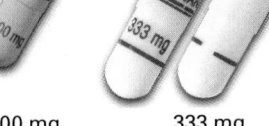 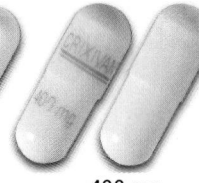

200 mg   333 mg   400 mg

LAMIVUDINE AND ZIDOVUDINE

Combivir
(page 1294)

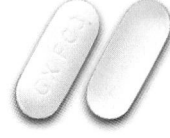

150/300 mg

LANSOPRAZOLE

Prevacid
(page 675)

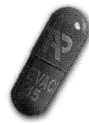 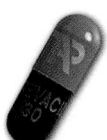

15 mg   30 mg

LEVODOPA AND CARBIDOPA

Sinemet
(page 1292)

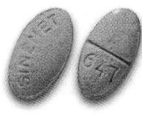 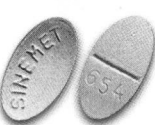

10/100 mg   25/250 mg

Sinemet CR
(page 1292)

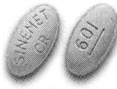

25/100 mg

LEVOFLOXACIN

Levaquin
(page 686)

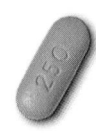 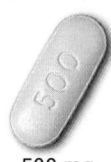

250 mg   500 mg

LEVOTHYROXINE SODIUM

Levoxyl
(page 691)

 25 mcg

 50 mcg

 75 mcg

 88 mcg

 100 mcg

 112 mcg

 125 mcg

 137 mcg

 150 mcg

 175 mcg

 200 mcg

 300 mcg

Synthroid
(page 691)

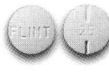 0.025 mg

 0.05 mg

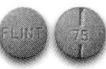 0.075 mg

 0.088 mg

  0.1 mg

  0.112 mg

  0.125 mg

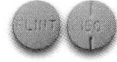 0.15 mg

 0.175 mg

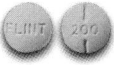 0.2 mg

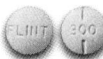 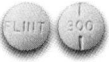  0.3 mg

LISINOPRIL

Prinivil
(page 701)

2.5 mg

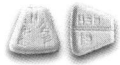
5 mg

10 mg

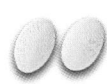
20 mg

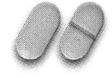
40 mg

Zestril
(page 701)

2.5 mg

5 mg

10 mg

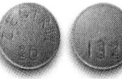
20 mg

40 mg

LOPINAVIR AND RITONAVIR

Kaletra
(page 709)

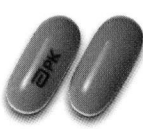
133.3/33.3 mg

LORATADINE

Claritin
(page 712)

10 mg

Claritin Reditabs
(page 712)

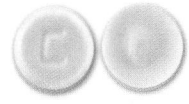

10 mg

LOSARTAN POTASSIUM

Cozaar
(page 715)

25 mg   50 mg

LOVASTATIN

Mevacor
(page 717)

   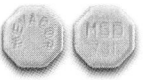

10 mg   20 mg   40 mg

MEDROXYPROGESTERONE ACETATE

Provera
(page 734)

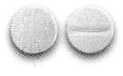   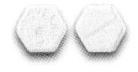   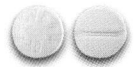

2.5 mg   5 mg   10 mg

MEPERIDINE HYDROCHLORIDE

Demerol
(page 743)

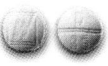

50 mg   100 mg

METFORMIN HYDROCHLORIDE

Glucophage
(page 760)

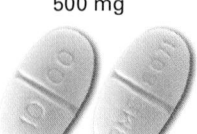

500 mg   850 mg

1,000 mg

Glucophage XR
(page 760)

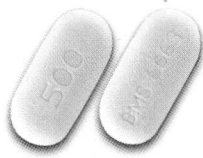

500 mg

METHYLPHENIDATE HYDROCHLORIDE

Concerta
(page 780)

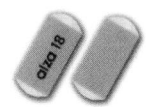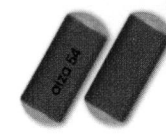

18 mg   36 mg   54 mg

Ritalin
(page 780)

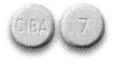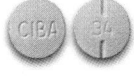

5 mg   10 mg   20 mg

Ritalin SR
(page 780)

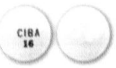

20 mg

METHYLPREDNISOLONE

Medrol
(page 782)

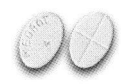 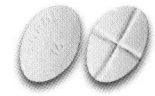

4 mg   16 mg

METOPROLOL SUCCINATE

Toprol-XL
(page 787)

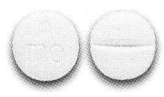 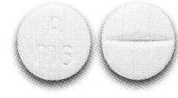 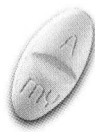

50 mg   100 mg   200 mg

MONTELUKAST SODIUM

Singulair
(page 814)

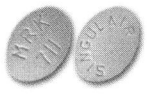

4 mg   5 mg   10 mg

NABUMETONE

Relafen
(page 824)

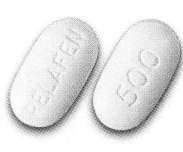 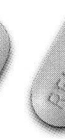 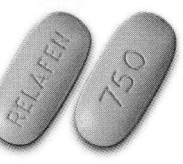

500 mg   750 mg

NAPROXEN

Naprosyn
(page 837)

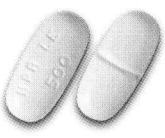

500 mg

NEFAZODONE HYDROCHLORIDE

Serzone
(page 843)

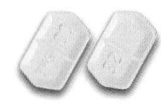

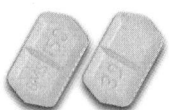

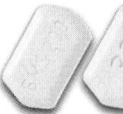

100 mg   150 mg   200 mg

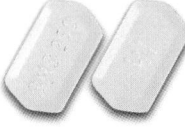

250 mg

NIFEDIPINE

Procardia
(page 859)

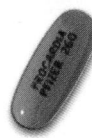

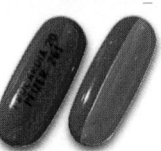

10 mg   20 mg

Procardia XL
(page 859)

30 mg   60 mg   90 mg

NITROFURANTOIN MACROCRYSTALS

Macrobid
(page 863)

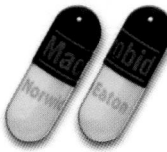

100 mg

NITROGLYCERIN

Nitrostat
(page 865)

0.4 mg

NORTRIPTYLINE HYDROCHLORIDE

Pamelor
(page 876)

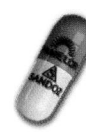

10 mg

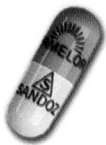

25 mg

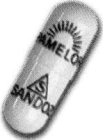

50 mg

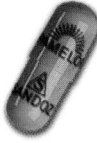

75 mg

OFLOXACIN

Floxin
(page 881)

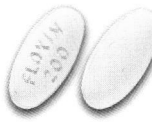

200 mg

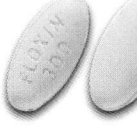

300 mg

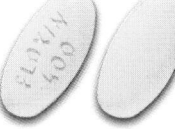

400 mg

OLMESARTAN MEDOXOMIL

Benicar
(page 885)

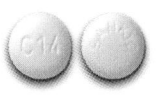

20 mg

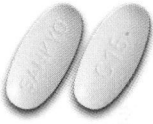

40 mg

OMEPRAZOLE

Prilosec
(page 887)

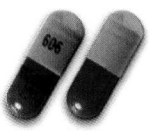

10 mg

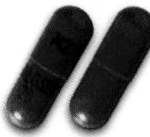

20 mg

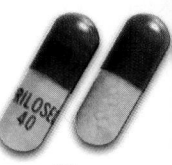

40 mg

OXYCODONE HYDROCHLORIDE

OxyContin
(page 903)

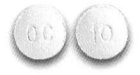  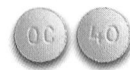

10 mg   20 mg   40 mg

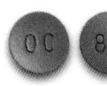

80 mg

PAROXETINE HYDROCHLORIDE

Paxil
(page 922)

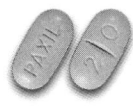 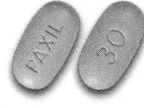

20 mg   30 mg

PENICILLIN V

Pen Vee K
(page 936)

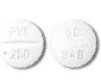 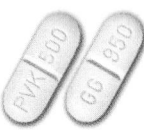

250 mg   500 mg

PENTOXIFYLLINE

Trental
(page 944)

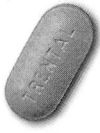

400 mg

PHENYTOIN

Dilantin Infatab
(page 961)

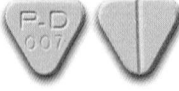

50 mg

PHENYTOIN SODIUM

Dilantin Kapseals
(page 961)

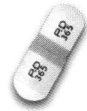 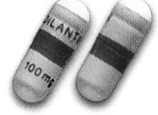

30 mg   100 mg

POTASSIUM CHLORIDE

K-Dur 20
(page 977)

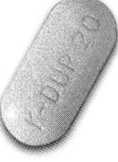

20 mEq

PRAVASTATIN SODIUM

Pravachol
(page 982)

     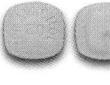   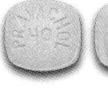 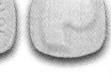

10 mg   20 mg   40 mg

PREDNISONE

Deltasone
(page 987)

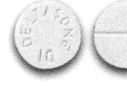   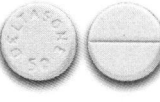

10 mg   50 mg

PROCHLORPERAZINE

Compazine
(page 994)

5 mg   10 mg

PROMETHAZINE HYDROCHLORIDE

Phenergan
(page 1001)

    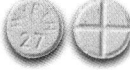   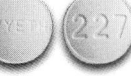

12.5 mg   25 mg   50 mg

PROPRANOLOL HYDROCHLORIDE

Inderal
(page 1007)

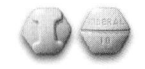

10 mg

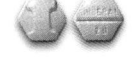

20 mg

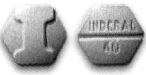

40 mg

60 mg

80 mg

Inderal LA
(page 1007)

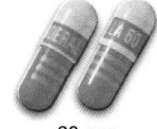

60 mg

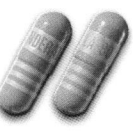

80 mg

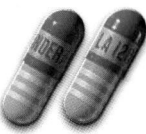

120 mg

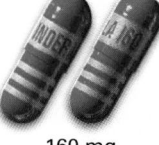

160 mg

QUINAPRIL HYDROCHLORIDE

Accupril
(page 1022)

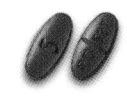

5 mg

10 mg

20 mg

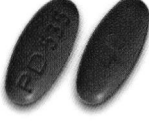

40 mg

RALOXIFENE HYDROCHLORIDE

Evista
(page 1026)

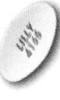

60 mg

RANITIDINE HYDROCHLORIDE

Zantac
(page 1029)

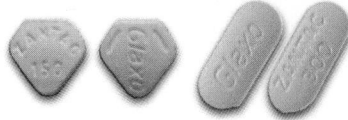

150 mg   300 mg

RISEDRONATE SODIUM

Actonel
(page 1039)

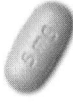

5 mg

RISPERIDONE

Risperdal
(page 1040)

                    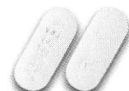

0.25 mg   0.5 mg   1 mg

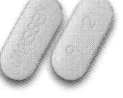   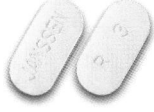   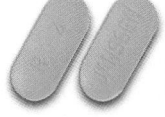

2 mg   3 mg   4 mg

ROFECOXIB

Vioxx
(page 1045)

                    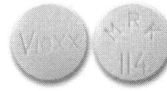

12.5 mg   25 mg   50 mg

ROSIGLITAZONE MALEATE

Avandia
(page 1048)

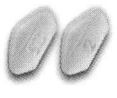   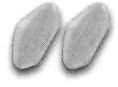   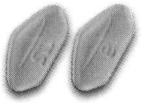

2 mg   4 mg   8 mg

SERTRALINE HYDROCHLORIDE

Zoloft
(page 1060)

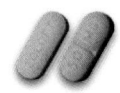

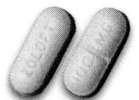

50 mg   100 mg

SILDENAFIL CITRATE

Viagra
(page 1062)

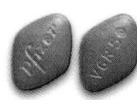

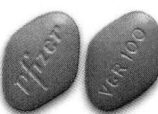

50 mg   100 mg

SIMVASTATIN

Zocor
(page 1065)

5 mg   10 mg   20 mg

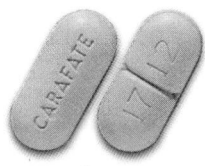

40 mg

SUCRALFATE

Carafate
(page 1089)

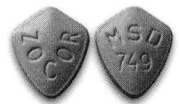

1 g

SUMATRIPTAN SUCCINATE

Imitrex
(page 1098)

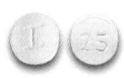

25 mg   50 mg

TAMOXIFEN CITRATE

Nolvadex
(page 1103)

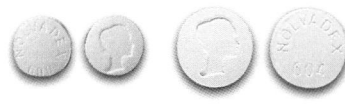

10 mg 20 mg

TEMAZEPAM

Restoril
(page 1108)

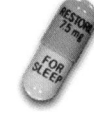 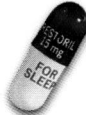 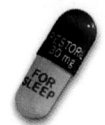

7.5 mg 15 mg 30 mg

TENOFOVIR DISOPROXIL FUMARATE

Viread
(page 1113)

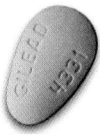

300 mg

TERAZOSIN HYDROCHLORIDE

Hytrin
(page 1114)

1 mg 2 mg 5 mg

10 mg

TICLOPIDINE HYDROCHLORIDE

Ticlid
(page 1142)

250 mg

TOLTERODINE TARTRATE

Detrol
(page 1158)

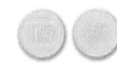 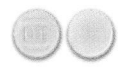

1 mg   2 mg

TRAMADOL HYDROCHLORIDE AND ACETAMINOPHEN

Ultracet
(page 1280)

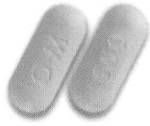

37.5/325 mg

TRAZODONE HYDROCHLORIDE

Desyrel
(page 1169)

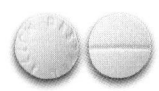 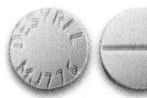

50 mg   100 mg

VALDECOXIB

Bextra
(page 1204)

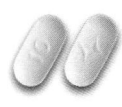 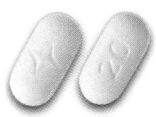

10 mg   20 mg

VALPROIC ACID

Depakote
(page 1207)

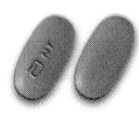 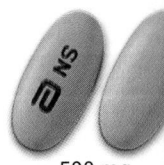

125 mg   250 mg   500 mg

Depakote Sprinkle
(page 1207)

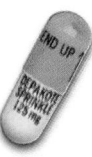

125 mg

VENLAFAXINE HYDROCHLORIDE

Effexor
(page 1213)

25 mg

37.5 mg

50 mg

75 mg

100 mg

Effexor XR
(page 1213)

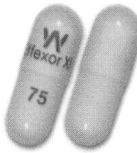

75 mg

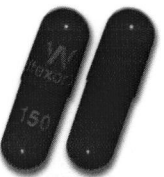

150 mg

VERAPAMIL HYDROCHLORIDE

Calan
(page 1214)

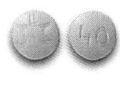

40 mg

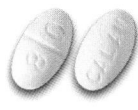

80 mg

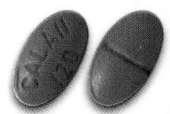

120 mg

Isoptin SR
(page 1214)

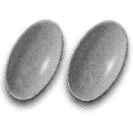

120 mg

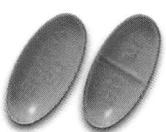

180 mg

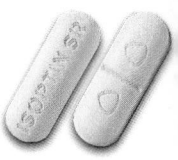

240 mg

Verelan
(page 1214)

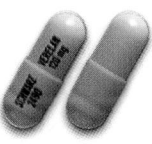

120 mg

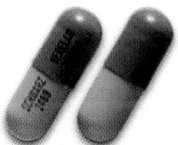

180 mg

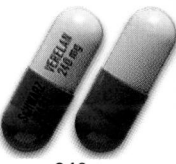

240 mg

WARFARIN SODIUM

Coumadin
(page 1223)

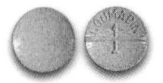 1 mg

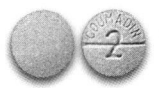 2 mg

 2.5 mg

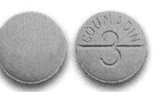 3 mg

 4 mg

 5 mg

 6 mg

 7.5 mg

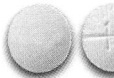 10 mg

ZALEPLON

Sonata
(page 1229)

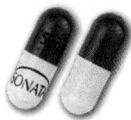 5 mg

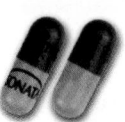 10 mg

ZIDOVUDINE

Retrovir
(page 1231)

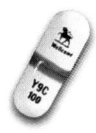 100 mg

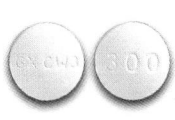 300 mg

ZOLPIDEM TARTRATE

Ambien
(page 1238)

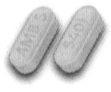 5 mg

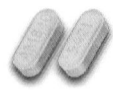 10 mg

headache (request medications); nausea, vomiting, diarrhea (proper nutrition is important, consult with your dietitian to maintain nutrition); symptoms of upper respiratory tract infection, cough (do not self-medicate; consult your health care provider if uncomfortable).

• Report fever, chills, dizziness, pregnancy.

▽lovastatin (mevinolin)
*(loe va **sta'** tin)*

Altocor, Apo-Lovastatin (CAN), Mevacor

PREGNANCY CATEGORY X

Drug classes
Antihyperlipidemic
HMG-CoA reductase inhibitor

Therapeutic actions
Inhibits the enzyme that catalyzes the rate-limiting step in the cholesterol synthesis pathway, resulting in a decrease in serum cholesterol, serum LDLs (the lipids associated with the development of coronary artery disease), and either an increase or no change in serum HDLs (the lipids associated with decreased risk of CAD).

Indications
• Treatment of familial hypercholesterolemia
• Adjunctive treatment of type II hyperlipidemia
• To slow the progression of atherosclerosis in patients with CAD
• Primary prevention of coronary heart disease in patients without symptomatic disease; average to moderately elevated total cholesterol and LDL cholesterol, and low HDLs
• As adjunct to diet to reduce total cholesterol, LDLs, apoliprotein B levels in adolescent boys and girls who are at least 1 yr post-menarche who have heterozygous familial hypercholesterolemia

Contraindications and cautions
• Contraindicated with allergy to lovastatin, pregnancy.

• Use cautiously with impaired hepatic function, cataracts, and lactation.

Available forms
Tablets—10, 20, 40 mg; ER tablets—10, 20, 40, 60 mg

Dosages
Adults
Initially 20 mg/day PO given in the evening. Maintenance dose range: 20–80 mg/day PO. Do not exceed 80 mg/day; or 10–60 mg/day PO ER tablets, taken in the evening. Adjust at intervals of 4 wk or more. Patients receiving cyclosporine should start at 10 mg daily and not exceed 20 mg daily. May be combined with bile acid sequestrants. If combined with fibrates or niacin, do not exceed 20 mg daily.
Pediatric patients
Adolescents at least 1 yr post-menarche: 20 mg/day PO; may increase to a maximum of 80 mg/day.
Patients with renal impairment
Creatinine clearance < 30 mL/min, use doses > 20 mg/day with caution.

Pharmacokinetics

Route	Onset	Peak
Oral	2 wk	4–6 wk

Metabolism: Hepatic; $T_{1/2}$: 3–4 hr
Distribution: Crosses placenta; enters breast milk
Excretion: Bile and feces

Adverse effects
• **CNS:** *Headache,* blurred vision, dizziness, insomnia, fatigue, muscle cramps, cataracts
• **GI:** *Flatulence, abdominal pain, cramps, constipation, nausea,* dyspepsia, heartburn, elevations of alkaline phosphatase, transaminases
• **Other:** Myalgia, rhabdomyolysis, rash, photosensitivity

Interactions
✳ **Drug-drug** • Possibility of severe myopathy or rhabdomyolysis with cyclosporine or gemfibrozil or other HMG-CoA inhibitors; avoid these combinations • Increased serum levels and risk of myopathy if combined with drugs that inhibit cytochrome P450 3A4 (eg, itraconazole, ketoconazole). Reduce lovastatin

dose or interrupt treatment if these drugs are needed

✱ Drug-food • Decreased metabolism and increased risk of toxic effects if taken with grapefruit juice; avoid this combination

■ Nursing considerations
Assessment
- **History:** Allergy to lovastatin, impaired hepatic function, cataracts, pregnancy, lactation
- **Physical:** Orientation, affect, ophthalmologic exam; liver evaluation; lipid studies, liver function tests

Interventions
- Give in the evening; highest rates of cholesterol synthesis are between midnight and 5 AM.
- Arrange for regular check-ups.
- Advise patient that this drug cannot be taken during pregnancy; urge the use of barrier contraceptives
- Arrange for periodic ophthalmologic exams to check for cataract development, and liver function studies q 4–6 wk during first 15 mo and then periodically.
- Adminster only when diet restricted in cholesterol and saturated fats fails to lower cholesterol and lipids adequately.

Teaching points
- Take drug in the evening. Continue following a cholesterol-lowering diet while on this medication. Avoid drinking grapefruit juice while on this drug.
- Do not cut, crush, or chew extended-release tablets.
- Use a barrier contraceptive while you are on this drug; if you feel you are pregnant or wish to become pregnant, consult with your health care provider.
- These side effects may occur: nausea (small frequent meals may help), headache, muscle and joint aches and pains (may lessen).
- Have periodic ophthalmic exams.
- Report severe GI upset, changes in vision, unusual bleeding or bruising, dark urine, or light-colored stools, severe muscle pain, soreness.

▽**loxapine**
(*lox' a peen*)

loxapine hydrochloride

loxapine succinate
Oral capsules: Loxapac (CAN), Loxitane, PMS-Loxapine (CAN)
Oral concentrate: Loxitane C
IM injection: Loxitane IM

PREGNANCY CATEGORY C

Drug classes
Dopaminergic blocking agent
Antipsychotic

Therapeutic actions
Mechanism of action is not fully understood: antipsychotic drugs block postsynaptic dopamine receptors in the brain, but this may not be necessary and sufficient for antipsychotic activity.

Indications
- Management of manifestations of psychotic disorders

Contraindications and cautions
- Contraindicated with coma or severe CNS depression; bone marrow depression; blood dyscrasia; circulatory collapse; subcortical brain damage; Parkinson's disease; liver disease; cerebral arteriosclerosis; coronary disease; severe hypotension or hypertension.
- Use cautiously with respiratory disorders ("silent pneumonia"); glaucoma, prostatic hypertrophy; epilepsy or history of epilepsy; breast cancer (elevations in prolactin may stimulate a prolactin-dependent tumor); thyrotoxicosis; peptic ulcer, decreased renal function; exposure to heat or phosphorus insecticides; pregnancy; and lactation.

Available forms
Capsules—5, 10, 25, 50 mg; concentrate—25 mg/mL; injection—50 mg/mL

Adverse effects in *Italics* are most common; those in **Bold** are life-threatening.

Dosages
Adults
Oral
Individualize dosage, and administer in divided doses bid to qid, initially 10 mg bid. Severely disturbed patients may need up to 50 mg/day. Increase dosage fairly rapidly over the first 7–10 days until symptoms are controlled. Usual dosage range is 60–100 mg/day; dosage greater than 250 mg/day is not recommended. Maintenance: reduce to minimum effective dose. Usual range is 20–60 mg/day.
IM
For prompt control of symptoms in acutely agitated patients, 12.5 to 50 mg q 4–6 hr or longer, depending on response. Once symptoms are controlled (about 5 days), change to oral medication.
Pediatric patients
Not recommended for patients < 16 yr.
Geriatric patients
Use lower doses, and increase dosage more gradually than in younger patients.

Pharmacokinetics

Route	Onset	Peak	Duration
Oral	30 min	1.5–3 hr	12 hr
IM	Rapid		

Metabolism: Hepatic; $T_{1/2}$: 19 hr
Distribution: Not known
Excretion: Urine

Adverse effects
- **Autonomic:** Dry mouth, salivation, nasal congestion, nausea, vomiting, anorexia, fever, pallor, facial flushing, sweating, constipation, paralytic ileus, urinary retention, incontinence, polyuria, enuresis, priapism, ejaculation dysfunction, male impotence
- **CNS:** *Drowsiness,* insomnia, vertigo, headache, weakness, tremor, ataxia, slurring, cerebral edema, seizures, exacerbation of psychotic symptoms, extrapyramidal syndromes—*pseudoparkinsonism; dystonias; akathisia,* tardive dyskinesias, potentially irreversible, **neuroleptic malignant syndrome**
- **CV:** Hypotension, orthostatic hypotension, hypertension, tachycardia, bradycardia, cardiac arrest, CHF, cardiomegaly, **refractory arrhythmias,** pulmonary edema
- **Endocrine:** Lactation, breast engorgement, galactorrhea; syndrome of inappropriate ADH secretion; amenorrhea, menstrual irregularities; gynecomastia; changes in libido; hyperglycemia or hypoglycemia; glycosuria; hyponatremia; pituitary tumor with hyperprolactinemia; inhibition of ovulation, infertility, pseudopregnancy; reduced urinary levels of gonadotropins, estrogens, progestins
- **Hematologic:** Eosinophilia, leukopenia, leukocytosis, anemia; aplastic anemia; hemolytic anemia; thrombocytopenic or nonthrombocytopenic purpura; pancytopenia
- **Hypersensitivity:** Jaundice, urticaria, angioneurotic edema, laryngeal edema, photosensitivity, eczema, asthma, anaphylactoid reactions, exfoliative dermatitis
- **Respiratory:** Bronchospasm, laryngospasm, dyspnea; suppression of cough reflex and potential for aspiration

■ Nursing considerations
Assessment
- **History:** Coma or severe CNS depression; blood dyscrasia; circulatory collapse; subcortical brain damage; Parkinson's disease; liver damage; cerebral arteriosclerosis; coronary disease; severe hypotension or hypertension; respiratory disorders; glaucoma; prostatic hypertrophy; epilepsy; breast cancer; thyrotoxicosis; peptic ulcer, decreased renal function; myelography within previous 24 hr or myelography scheduled within 48 hr; exposure to heat or phosphorus insecticides; pregnancy
- **Physical:** Weight, T; reflexes, orientation, intraocular pressure; P, BP, orthostatic BP; R, adventitious sounds; bowel sounds and normal output, liver evaluation; urinary output, prostate size; CBC, urinalysis, thyroid, liver, and kidney function tests

Interventions
- Mix the oral concentrate with orange or grapefruit juice shortly before administration.
- Do not give *Loxitane IM* intravenously.
- Arrange for discontinuation if serum creatinine or BUN become abnormal or if WBC count is depressed.
- Monitor elderly patients for dehydration, and institute remedial measures promptly; sedation and decreased sensation of thirst due to CNS effects can lead to severe dehydration.

- Consult physician regarding appropriate warning of patient or patient's guardian about tardive dyskinesias.
- Consult physician about dosage reduction and use of anticholinergic antiparkinsonian drugs (controversial) if extrapyramidal effects occur.

Teaching points

- Take drug exactly as prescribed.
- Avoid driving or engaging in dangerous activities if CNS or vision changes occur.
- Avoid prolonged exposure to sun or use a sunscreen or covering garments.
- Maintain fluid intake, and use precautions against heat stroke in hot weather.
- Report sore throat, fever, unusual bleeding or bruising, rash, weakness, tremors, impaired vision, dark urine, pale stools, and yellowing of the skin or eyes.

▽ magaldrate (hydroxymagnesium aluminate)

(mag' al drate)

Iosopan, Riopan

PREGNANCY CATEGORY C

Drug class

Antacid

Therapeutic actions

Neutralizes or reduces gastric acidity, resulting in an increase in the pH of the stomach and duodenal bulb and inhibiting the proteolytic activity of pepsin; the combination of magnesium (causes diarrhea when administered alone) and aluminum (constipating when administered alone) salts usually minimizes adverse GI effects.

Indications

- Symptomatic relief of upset stomach associated with hyperacidity
- Hyperacidity associated with peptic ulcer, gastritis, peptic esophagitis, gastric hyperacidity, and hiatal hernia

Contraindications and cautions

- Contraindicated with allergy to magnesium or aluminum products.
- Use cautiously with renal insufficiency, gastric outlet obstruction (aluminum salt may inhibit gastric emptying).

Available forms

Suspension—540 mg/5 mL; liquid—540 mg/ 5 mL

Dosages

Adults

480–1,080 mg (5–10 mL) PO between meals and hs.

Pharmacokinetics

Route	Onset	Peak
Oral	30 min	30–60 min

Generally no systemic absorption.

Adverse effects

- **GI:** *Rebound hyperacidity*
- **Metabolic:** Decreased absorption of fluoride and accumulation of aluminum in serum, bone, CNS (aluminum may be neurotoxic, especially in patients with renal failure); *alkalosis;* hypermagnesemia and toxicity in patients with renal failure

Interactions

✳ **Drug-drug** • Do not administer other oral drugs within 1–2 hr of antacid administration; change in gastric pH may interfere with absorption of oral drugs • Decreased pharmacologic effect of tetracyclines, penicillamine, nitrofurantoin, fluoroquinolones, ketoconazole • Decreased absorption and therapeutic effects of clindamycin and lincomycin

■ Nursing considerations
Assessment

- **History:** Allergy to magnesium or aluminum products, renal insufficiency, gastric outlet obstruction
- **Physical:** Bone and muscle strength; abdominal exam, bowel sounds; renal function tests, serum magnesium as appropriate

Interventions

- Do not administer oral drugs within 1–2 hr of antacid administration.
- Give between meals and hs.
- Monitor patients on long-term therapy for signs of aluminum accumulation: bone pain, muscle weakness, malaise. Discontinue drug as needed.

Teaching points

- Take between meals and at bedtime.
- Do not take with any other oral medications; absorption of those medications can be inhibited. Take other oral medications at least 1–2 hr after aluminum salt.
- Report bone pain, muscle weakness, coffee-ground vomitus, black tarry stools, no relief from symptoms being treated.

▽**magnesium salts**
(*mag nee' zhum*)

magnesium citrate
Citro-Mag (CAN)

magnesium hydroxide
Milk of Magnesia

magnesia

magnesium oxide
Mag-Ox 400, Maox 420, Uro-Mag

PREGNANCY CATEGORY C

Drug classes
Antacid
Laxative

Therapeutic actions

Antacid (magnesium hydroxide, magnesium oxide): neutralizes or reduces gastric acidity, resulting in an increase in the pH of the stomach and duodenal bulb and inhibition of the proteolytic activity of pepsin. Laxative (magnesium citrate, magnesium hydroxide): attracts and retains water in intestinal lumen and distends bowel; causes the duodenal secretion of cholecystokinin, which stimulates fluid secretion and intestinal motility.

Indications

- Symptomatic relief of upset stomach associated with hyperacidity
- Hyperacidity associated with peptic ulcer, gastritis, peptic esophagitis, gastric hyperacidity, and hiatal hernia
- Prophylaxis of GI bleeding, stress ulcers, aspiration pneumonia
- Short-term relief of constipation; evacuation of the colon for rectal and bowel examination

Contraindications and cautions

- Contraindicated with allergy to magnesium products.
- Use cautiously with renal insufficiency.

Available forms

Tablets—311 (chewable), 400, 420, 500 mg; capsules—140 mg; liquid—various

Dosages
Adults
Magnesium citrate
1 glassful (240 mL) PO as needed.
Magnesium hydroxide
- *Antacid:* 5–15 mL liquid or 622–1,244 mg tablets PO qid (adult and children older than 12 yr).
- *Laxative:* 15–60 mL PO taken with liquid.

Magnesium oxide
Capsules: 140 mg PO tid–qid. Tablets: 400–800 mg/day PO.
Pediatric patients
Magnesium citrate
Half the adult dose; repeat as needed.
Magnesium hydroxide
- *Laxative:*
6–11 yr: 15–30 mL PO.
2–5 yr: 5–15 mL PO.
< 2 yr: Do not administer unless directed by a physician.

Pharmacokinetics

Route	Onset
Oral	3–6 hr

Minimal systemic absorption.
Excretion: Renal

Adverse effects

- **CNS:** Dizziness, fainting, sweating
- **GI:** *Diarrhea, nausea, perianal irritation*

M

- **Metabolic:** Hypermagnesemia and toxicity in patients with renal failure

Interactions
✳ **Drug-drug** • Do not give other oral drugs within 1–2 hr of antacid administration; change in gastric pH may interfere with absorption • Decreased pharmacologic effect of tetracyclines, penicillamine, nitrofurantoin, fluoroquinolones, ketoconazole

■ Nursing considerations
Assessment
- **History:** Allergy to magnesium products; renal insufficiency
- **Physical:** Abdominal exam, bowel sounds; renal function tests, serum magnesium

Interventions
- Do not administer oral drugs within 1–2 hr of antacid administration.
- Have patient chew antacid tablets thoroughly before swallowing; follow with a glass of water.
- Give antacid between meals and hs.

Teaching points
- Take antacid between meals and at bedtime. If tablets are being used, chew thoroughly before swallowing, and follow with a glass of water.
- Do not use laxatives with abdominal pain, nausea, or vomiting.
- Refrigerate magnesium citrate solutions to retain potency and increase palatability.
- Do not take with any other oral medications; absorption of those medications can be inhibited. Take other oral medications at least 1–2 hr after aluminum salt.
- Diarrhea may occur with antacid therapy.
- These side effects may occur as a result of laxative therapy: excessive bowel activity, gripping, diarrhea, nausea, dizziness (exercise precaution not to fall).
- Do not use laxatives long-term. Prolonged or excessive use can lead to serious problems. You should increase your intake of water (6–8 glasses/day) and fiber, and exercise regularly.
- Report: Antacid use—diarrhea; coffee-ground vomitus; black, tarry stools; no re-

lief from symptoms being treated. Laxative use—rectal bleeding, muscle cramps or pain, weakness, dizziness (not related to abdominal cramps and bowel movement), unrelieved constipation.

▽ magnesium sulfate (epsom salt)
*(mag **nee'** zee-um)*

PREGNANCY CATEGORY A

Drug classes
Electrolyte
Anticonvulsant
Laxative

Therapeutic actions
Cofactor of many enzyme systems involved in neurochemical transmission and muscular excitability; prevents or controls convulsions by blocking neuromuscular transmission; attracts and retains water in the intestinal lumen and distends the bowel to promote mass movement and relieve constipation.

Indications
- Acute nephritis (children), to control hypertension
- Hypomagnesemia, replacement therapy (IV)
- Preeclampsia/eclampsia (IV, IM)
- Short-term treatment of constipation (PO)
- Evacuation of the colon for rectal and bowel examinations (PO)
- To correct or prevent hypomagnesemia in patients on parenteral nutrition
- Treatment of atypical ventricular arrhythmias (Torsades de pointes) (IV)
- Adjunctive therapy for the treatment of acute MI (IV)
- Unlabeled uses: inhibition of premature labor (parenteral), adjunct treatment of exacerbations of acute asthma

Contraindications and cautions
- Contraindicated with allergy to magnesium products; heart block, myocardial damage; abdominal pain, nausea, vomiting or other symptoms of appendicitis; acute surgical abdomen, fecal impaction, intestinal and

biliary tract obstruction, hepatitis. Do not give during 2 hr preceding delivery because of risk of magnesium toxicity in the neonate.
• Use cautiously with renal insufficiency.

Available forms

Granules—40 mEq/5 g; injection—0.8, 1, 4 mEq/mL

Dosages
Adults
• *Parenteral nutrition:* 8–24 mEq/day IV.
• *Mild magnesium deficiency:* 1 g IM or IV q 6 hr for four doses (32.5 mEq/24 hr).
• *Severe hypomagnesemia:* Up to 2 mEq/kg IM within 4 hr or 5 g (40 mEq)/1,000 mL D$_5$W IV infused over 3 hr.
• *Toxemia, eclampsia, nephritis:*
IM
4–5 g of a 50% solution q 4 hr as necessary.
IV
1–4 g of a 10%–20% solution. Do not exceed 1.5 mL/min of a 10% solution.
IV infusion
4–5 g in 250 mL of 5% dextrose. Do not exceed 3 mL/min.
• *Arrhythmias:* 1–6 g IV over several min; then 3–20 mg/min continuous infusion for 5–48 hr.
• *Acute MI:* 2 g IV over 5–15 min followed by 18 g IV over 24 hr.
• *Laxative:* 10–15 g PO epsom salt in glass of water.
Pediatric patients
• *Parenteral nutrition (infants):* 2–10 mEq/day IV.
• *Anticonvulsant:* 20–40 mg/kg in a 20% solution, IM. Repeat as necessary.
• *Laxative:* 5–10 g PO epsom salt in glass of water.

Pharmacokinetics

Route	Onset	Duration
IV	Immediate	30 min
IM	60 min	3–4 hr
Oral	1–2 hr	3–4 hr

Metabolism: T$_{1/2}$: unknown
Distribution: Crosses placenta, enters breast milk
Excretion: Urine

▼ IV facts
Preparation: Dilute IV infusion to a concentration of 20% or less prior to IV administration; dilute 4–5 g in 250 mL D$_5$W or sodium chloride solution.
Infusion: Do not exceed 1.5 mL of a 10% solution per minute IV or 3 mL/min IV infusion.
Incompatibilities: Do not mix with calcium gluceptate, dobutamine, polymyxin, procaine hydrochloride, sodium bicarbonate, tobramycin.

Adverse effects
• **CNS:** *Weakness, dizziness,* fainting, sweating (PO)
• **CV:** Palpitations
• **GI:** *Excessive bowel activity, perianal irritation* (PO)
• **Metabolic:** *Magnesium intoxication* (flushing, sweating, hypotension, depressed reflexes, flaccid paralysis, hypothermia, circulatory collapse, cardiac and CNS depression—parenteral); hypocalcemia with tetany (secondary to treatment of eclampsia—parenteral)

Interactions
✳ **Drug-drug •** Potentiation of neuromuscular blockade produced by nondepolarizing neuromuscular relaxants (tubocurarine, atracurium, gallamine, pancuronium, vecuronium)

■ Nursing considerations
Assessment
• **History:** Allergy to magnesium products; renal insufficiency; heart block, myocardial damage; symptoms of appendicitis; acute surgical abdomen, fecal impaction, intestinal and biliary tract obstruction, hepatitis
• **Physical:** Skin color, texture; muscle tone; T; orientation, affect, reflexes, peripheral sensation; P, auscultation, BP, rhythm strip; abdominal exam, bowel sounds; renal function tests, serum magnesium and calcium, liver function tests (oral use)

Interventions
• Reserve IV use in eclampsia for immediate life-threatening situations.
• Give IM route by deep IM injection of the undiluted (50%) solution for adults; dilute to a 20% solution for children.

M

- Monitor serum magnesium levels during parenteral therapy. Arrange to discontinue administration as soon as levels are within normal limits (1.5–3 mEq/L) and desired clinical response is obtained.
- Monitor knee-jerk reflex before repeated parenteral administration. If knee-jerk reflexes are suppressed, do not administer magnesium because respiratory center failure may occur.
- Give oral magnesium sulfate as a laxative only as a temporary measure. Arrange for dietary measures (fiber, fluids) and exercise, environmental control to return to normal bowel activity.
- Do not give oral magnesium sulfate with abdominal pain, nausea, vomiting.
- Monitor bowel function; if diarrhea and cramping occur, discontinue oral drug.
- Maintain urine output at a level of 100 mL q 4 hr during parenteral administration.

Teaching points

- Use only as a temporary measure to relieve constipation. Do not take if abdominal pain, nausea, or vomiting occur.
- These side effect may occur: diarrhea (discontinue drug, consult care provider—oral use).
- Report sweating, flushing, muscle tremors or twitching, inability to move extremities.

▽ mannitol
(man' i tole)

Osmitrol, Resectisol

PREGNANCY CATEGORY C

Drug classes
Osmotic diuretic
Diagnostic agent
Urinary irrigant

Therapeutic actions
Elevates the osmolarity of the glomerular filtrate, thereby hindering the reabsorption of water and leading to a loss of water, sodium, chloride (used for diagnosis of glomerular filtration rate); creates an osmotic gradient in the eye between plasma and ocular fluids, thereby reducing intraocular pressure; creates an osmotic effect, leading to decreased swelling in post-transurethral prostatic resection.

Indications

- Prevention and treatment of the oliguric phase of renal failure
- Reduction of intracranial pressure and treatment of cerebral edema; of elevated intraocular pressure when the pressure cannot be lowered by other means
- Promotion of the urinary excretion of toxic substances
- Measurement of glomerular filtration rate (diagnostic use)
- Irrigant in transurethral prostatic resection or other transurethral procedures

Contraindications and cautions

- Anuria due to severe renal disease, pulmonary congestion, active intracranial bleeding (except during craniotomy), dehydration, renal disease, CHF.

Available forms
Injection—5%, 10%, 15%, 20%, 25%; solution—5 g/100 mL

Dosages
Adults
IV infusion only; individualize concentration and rate of administration. Dosage is 50–200 g/day. Adjust dosage to maintain urine flow of 30–50 mL/hr.

- *Prevention of oliguria:* 50–100 g IV as a 5%–25% solution.
- *Treatment of oliguria:* 50–100 g IV of a 15%–25% solution.
- *Reduction of intracranial pressure and cerebral edema:* 1.5–2 g/kg IV as a 15%–25% solution over 30–60 min. Evidence of reduced pressure should be seen in 15 min.
- *Reduction of intraocular pressure:* Infuse 1.5–2 g/kg IV as a 25% solution, 20% solution, or 15% solution over 30 min. If used preoperatively, use 60–90 min before surgery.
- *Adjunctive therapy to promote diuresis in intoxications:* Maximum of 200 g IV of mannitol with other fluids and electrolytes.

Adverse effects in *Italics* are most common; those in **Bold** are life-threatening.

- *Measurement of glomerular filtration rate:* Dilute 100 mL of a 20% solution with 180 mL of sodium chloride injection. Infuse this 280 mL of 7.2% solution IV at a rate of 20 mL/min. Collect urine with a catheter for the specified time for measurement of mannitol excreted in mg/min. Draw blood at the start and at the end of the time for measurement of mannitol in mg/mL plasma.
- *Test dose of mannitol for patients with inadequate renal function:* 0.2 g/kg IV (about 60 mL of a 25% solution, 75 mL of a 20% solution, or 100 mL of a 15% solution) in 3–5 min to produce a urine flow of 30–50 mL/hr. If urine flow does not increase, repeat dose. If no response to second dose, reevaluate patient situation.
- *Urologic irrigation:* Use prepared 5 g/100 mL distilled water solution; irrigate as needed.

Pediatric patients
Dosage for children < 12 yr not established.

Pharmacokinetics

Route	Onset	Peak	Duration
IV	30–60 min	1 hr	6–8 hr
Irrigant	Rapid	Rapid	Short

Metabolism: $T_{1/2}$: 15–100 min
Distribution: Crosses placenta; may enter breast milk
Excretion: Urine

▽ **IV facts**
Preparation: Mannitol may crystallize at lower temperatures, especially solutions of > 15%. If crystals are observed, warm solution to dissolve.
Infusion: Infuse at rates listed (above).
Incompatibilities: Do not add to blood products.

Adverse effects

- **CNS:** *Dizziness,* headache, blurred vision, **seizures**
- **CV:** Hypotension, hypertension, edema, thrombophlebitis, tachycardia, chest pain
- **Dermatologic:** Uriticaria, skin necrosis with infiltration
- **GI:** *Nausea, anorexia, dry mouth, thirst*
- **GU:** *Diuresis,* urinary retention

- **Hematologic:** Fluid and electrolyte imbalances, hyponatremia
- **Respiratory:** Pulmonary congestion, rhinitis

■ Nursing considerations
Assessment

- **History:** Pulmonary congestion, active intracranial bleeding, dehydration, renal disease, CHF
- **Physical:** Skin color, lesions, edema, hydration; orientation, reflexes, muscle strength, pupils; pulses, BP, perfusion; R, pattern, adventitious sounds; urinary output patterns; serum electrolytes, urinalysis, renal function tests

Interventions

- Do not give electrolyte-free mannitol with blood. If blood must be given, add at least 20 mEq of sodium chloride to each liter of mannitol solution.
- Do not expose solutions to low temperatures; crystallization may occur. If crystals are seen, warm the bottle in a hot water bath, then cool to body temperature before administering.
- Make sure the infusion set contains a filter if giving concentrated mannitol.
- Monitor serum electrolytes periodically with prolonged therapy.

Teaching points

- These side effects may occur: increased urination; GI upset (small, frequent meals may help); dry mouth (sugarless lozenges to suck may help); headache, blurred vision (use caution when moving, ask for assistance).
- Report difficulty breathing, pain at the IV site, chest pain.

▽ **maprotiline hydrochloride**
(*ma **proe'** ti leen*)

Novo-Maprotiline (CAN)

PREGNANCY CATEGORY B

Drug class
Antidepressant

Therapeutic actions

Mechanism of action unknown; appears to act similarly to TCAs; the TCAs act to inhibit the presynaptic reuptake of the neurotransmitters norepinephrine (primarily) and serotonin; anticholinergic at CNS and peripheral receptors; sedating; the relation of these effects to clinical efficacy is unknown.

Indications

- Treatment of depressive illness in patients with depressive neurosis (dysthymic disorder)
- Treatment of depression in patients with manic-depressive illness (depressed type)
- Unlabeled use: Treatment of anxiety associated with depression

Contraindications and cautions

- Contraindicated with hypersensitivity to any tricyclic drug, concomitant therapy with an MAO inhibitor, recent MI, myelography within previous 24 hr or scheduled within 48 hr, pregnancy (limb reduction abnormalities reported), lactation.
- Use cautiously with EST; preexisting CV disorders (increased risk of serious CVS toxicity); angle-closure glaucoma, increased intraocular pressure, urinary retention, ureteral or urethral spasm; seizure disorders (lower seizure threshold); hyperthyroidism (predisposes to CVS toxicity, including cardiac arrhythmias); impaired hepatic, renal function; psychiatric patients (schizophrenic or paranoid patients may worsen); manic-depressives (may shift to hypomanic or manic phase); elective surgery (discontinue as long as possible before surgery).

Available forms

Tablets—25, 50, 75 mg

Dosages
Adults

- *Mild to moderate depression:* Initially, 75 mg/day PO in outpatients. Maintain initial dosage for 2 wk due to long drug half-life. Dosage may then be increased gradually in 25-mg increments. Most patients respond to 150 mg/day, but some may require up to 225 mg/day.

- *More severe depression:* Initially, 100–150 mg/day PO in hospitalized patients. If needed, may gradually increase to 300 mg/day.
- *Maintenance:* Reduce dosage to lowest effective level, usually 75–150 mg/day PO.

Pediatric patients
Not recommended in patients < 18 yr.

Geriatric patients
Give lower doses to patients > 60 yr; begin at 25 mg PO daily and gradually increase to 50–75 mg/day PO for maintenance.

Pharmacokinetics

Route	Onset	Peak	Duration
Oral	Slow	12 hr	2–4 wk

Metabolism: Hepatic; $T_{1/2}$: 27–58 hr
Distribution: Crosses placenta; enters breast milk
Excretion: Urine and feces

Adverse effects

- **CNS:** *Sedation and anticholinergic (atropine-like) effects; confusion* (especially in elderly), *disturbed concentration,* hallucinations, disorientation, decreased memory, feelings of unreality, delusions, anxiety, nervousness, restlessness, agitation, panic, insomnia, nightmares, hypomania, mania, exacerbation of psychosis, drowsiness, weakness, fatigue, headache, numbness, tingling, paresthesia of extremities, incoordination, motor hyperactivity, akathisia, ataxia, tremors, peripheral neuropathy, extrapyramidal symptoms, **seizures,** speech blockage, dysarthria, tinnitus, altered EEG
- **CV:** *Orthostatic hypotension,* hypertension, syncope, tachycardia, palpitations, MI, arrhythmias, heart block, precipitation of CHF, stroke
- **Endocrine:** Elevated or depressed blood sugar, elevated prolactin levels, inappropriate ADH secretion
- **GI:** *Dry mouth, constipation,* paralytic ileus, *nausea,* vomiting, anorexia, epigastric distress, diarrhea, flatulence, dysphagia, peculiar taste, increased salivation, stomatitis, glossitis, parotid swelling, abdominal cramps, black tongue, hepatitis, jaundice

Adverse effects in *Italics* are most common; those in **Bold** are life-threatening.

(rare), elevated transaminases, altered alkaline phosphatase
- **GU:** Urinary retention, delayed micturition, dilation of the urinary tract, gynecomastia, testicular swelling; breast enlargement, menstrual irregularity and galactorrhea; increased or decreased libido; impotence
- **Hematologic:** Bone marrow depression, eosinophilia, thrombocytopenia, leukopenia
- **Hypersensitivity:** Rash, pruritus, vasculitis, petechiae, photosensitization, edema
- **Withdrawal:** Symptoms with abrupt discontinuation of prolonged therapy: nausea, headache, vertigo, nightmares, malaise
- **Other:** Nasal congestion, excessive appetite, weight gain or loss; sweating (paradoxical effect in a drug with prominent anticholinergic effects), alopecia, lacrimation, hyperthermia, flushing, chills

Interactions
✷ Drug-drug • Risk of seizures if taken with benzodiazepines (or if benzodiazepines are rapidly tapered during maprotiline therapy), phenothiazines • Additive atropine-like effects if combined with anticholinergics, sympathomimetics; monitor patient closely and adjust dosages as needed • Increased risk of cardiotoxicity if taken with thyroid medications

■ Nursing considerations

CLINICAL ALERT!
Name confusion has occurred with Ludiomil (maprotiline) and Lomotil (diphenoxylate/atropine); use caution.

Assessment
- **History:** Hypersensitivity to any tricyclic drug; concomitant therapy with an MAO inhibitor; recent MI; myelography within previous 24 hr or scheduled within 48 hr; lactation; EST; preexisting CV disorders; angle-closure glaucoma, increased intraocular pressure, urinary retention, ureteral or urethral spasm; seizure disorders; hyperthyroidism; impaired hepatic, renal function; psychiatric problems; manic-depressive patients; elective surgery
- **Physical:** Weight; T; skin color, lesions; orientation, affect, reflexes, vision and hearing; P, BP, orthostatic BP, perfusion; bowel

sounds, normal output, liver evaluation; urine flow, normal output; usual sexual function, frequency of menses, breast and scrotal examination; liver function tests, urinalysis, CBC, ECG

Interventions
- Limit drug access to depressed and potentially suicidal patients.
- Expect clinical response in 3–7 days or up to 2–3 wk (the latter is more usual).
- Give major portion of dose hs if drowsiness, severe anticholinergic effects occur.
- Reduce dosage with minor side effects; discontinue drug if serious side effects occur.
- Arrange for CBC if patient develops fever, sore throat, or signs of infection.

Teaching points
- Take drug exactly as prescribed, and do not stop taking this drug without consulting your health care provider.
- Avoid pregnancy while on this drug, fetal abnormalities have been reported; barrier contraceptive use is advised.
- Avoid alcohol, sleep-inducing drugs, OTC drugs.
- Avoid prolonged exposure to sunlight or sunlamps, use sunscreen or protective garments if exposure is unavoidable.
- These side effects may occur: headache, dizziness, drowsiness, weakness, blurred vision (reversible; use caution if severe, avoid driving or performing tasks that require alertness); nausea, vomiting, loss of appetite, dry mouth (small frequent meals, frequent mouth care, sucking sugarless candies may help); nightmares, inability to concentrate, confusion; changes in sexual function.
- Report dry mouth, difficulty in urination, excessive sedation, chest pain.

▽ mebendazole
*(me **ben'** da zole)*

Vermox

PREGNANCY CATEGORY C

Drug class
Anthelmintic

Therapeutic actions

Irreversibly blocks glucose uptake by susceptible helminths, depleting glycogen stores needed for survival and reproduction of the helminths, causing death.

Indications

- Treatment of *Trichuris trichiura* (whipworm), *Enterobius vermicularis* (pinworm), *Ascaris lumbricoides* (roundworm), *Ancylostoma duodenale* (common hookworm), *Necator americanus* (American hookworm)

Contraindications and cautions

- Contraindicated with allergy to mebendazole, pregnancy (embryotoxic and teratogenic; avoid use, especially during first trimester).
- Use cautiously with lactation.

Available forms

Chewable tablets—100 mg

Dosages

Adults and patients ≥ 2 yr

- *Trichuriasis, ascariasis, hookworm infections:* 1 tablet PO morning and evening on 3 consecutive days.
- *Enterobiasis:* 1 tablet PO once. If not cured 3 wk after treatment, a second treatment course is advised.

Pediatric patients

Safety and efficacy for use in children < 2 yr not established.

Pharmacokinetics

Route	Onset	Peak
Oral	Slow	2–4 hr

Metabolism: Hepatic; $T_{1/2}$: 2.5–9 hr
Distribution: Crosses placenta; may enter breast milk
Excretion: Feces

Adverse effects

- **GI:** *Transient abdominal pain, diarrhea*
- **Other:** Fever

■ Nursing considerations

Assessment

- **History:** Allergy to mebendazole, pregnancy, lactation
- **Physical:** T; bowel sounds, output

Interventions

- Culture for ova and parasites.
- Administer drug with food; tablets may be chewed, swallowed whole, or crushed and mixed with food.
- Arrange for second course of treatment if patient is not cured 3 wk after treatment.
- Treat all family members for pinworm infestation.
- Disinfect toilet facilities after patient use (pinworms).
- Arrange for daily laundry of bed linens, towels, nightclothes, and undergarments (pinworms).

Teaching points

- Chew or swallow whole or crushed and mixed with food.
- Pinworms are easily transmitted; all family members should be treated for complete eradication.
- Use strict handwashing and hygiene measures. Launder undergarments, bedlinens, nightclothes daily. Disinfect toilet facilities daily and bathroom floors periodically (pinworms).
- These side effects may occur: nausea, abdominal pain, diarrhea (small, frequent meals may help).
- Report fever, return of symptoms, severe diarrhea.

▽**mecamylamine hydrochloride**
(mek a mill' a meen)

Inversine

PREGNANCY CATEGORY C

Drug classes

Antihypertensive
Ganglionic blocker

Adverse effects in *Italics* are most common; those in **Bold** are life-threatening.

Therapeutic actions

Occupies cholinergic receptors of autonomic postganglionic neurons, blocking the effects of acetylcholine released from preganglionic nerve terminals, decreasing the effects of the sympathetic (and parasympathetic) nervous systems on effector organs; reduces sympathetic tone on the vasculature, causing vasodilation and decreased BP; decreases sympathetic impulses to the heart; and decreases the release of catecholamines from the adrenal medulla.

Indications

- Moderately severe to severe hypertension
- Uncomplicated malignant hypertension

Contraindications and cautions

- Contraindicated with hypersensitivity to mecamylamine; coronary insufficiency, recent MI; uncooperative patients; uremia; chronic pyelonephritis when patient is receiving antibiotics and sulfonamides; glaucoma; organic pyloric stenosis; lactation.
- Use cautiously with prostatic hypertrophy, bladder neck obstruction, urethral stricture (urinary retention, may be more serious with these disorders); cerebral or renal insufficiency; high ambient temperature, fever, infection, hemorrhage, surgery, vigorous exercise; salt depletion resulting from diminished intake or increased excretion due to diarrhea, vomiting, sweating, or diuretics; pregnancy.

Available forms

Tablets—2.5 mg

Dosages
Adults

Initially 2.5 mg PO bid. Adjust dosage in increments of 2.5 mg in intervals of at least 2 days until desired BP response occurs (dosage below that causing signs of mild orthostatic hypotension). Average total daily dosage is 25 mg, usually in three divided doses. Partial tolerance may develop, necessitating increased dosage. With other antihypertensives, reduce both the dosage of the other agents and mecamylamine; exception: give thiazides at usual dosage while decreasing mecamylamine by at least 50%.

Pharmacokinetics

Route	Onset	Peak	Duration
Oral	30 min–2 hr	3–5 hr	6–12 hr

Metabolism: $T_{1/2}$: 4–6 hr
Distribution: Crosses placenta; enters breast milk
Excretion: Urine

Adverse effects

- **CNS:** Syncope, paresthesia, *weakness, fatigue, sedation,* dilated pupils and blurred vision, tremor, choreiform movements, mental aberrations, convulsions
- **CV:** *Orthostatic hypotension* and dizziness
- **GI:** *Anorexia, dry mouth, glossitis, nausea,* vomiting, constipation and paralytic ileus
- **GU:** *Decreased libido, impotence, urinary retention*
- **Respiratory:** Interstitial pulmonary edema and fibrosis

■ Nursing considerations

 CLINICAL ALERT!
Name confusion has occurred between Inversine (mecamylamine) and Invirase (saquinavir); use caution.

M

Assessment

- **History:** Hypersensitivity to mecamylamine; coronary insufficiency, recent MI; uremia; chronic pyelonephritis; glaucoma; organic pyloric stenosis; prostatic hypertrophy, bladder neck obstruction, urethral stricture; cerebral or renal insufficiency; high ambient temperature, fever, infection, hemorrhage, surgery, vigorous exercise, salt depletion, vomiting, sweating, or diuretics; lactation
- **Physical:** T; orientation, affect, reflexes; ophthalmic exam, including tonometry; P, BP, orthostatic BP, supine BP, perfusion, edema, auscultation; bowel sounds, normal output; normal urinary output, voiding pattern, prostate palpation; renal, hepatic function tests

Interventions

- Give after meals for more gradual absorption and smoother control of BP; timing of doses with regard to meals should be consistent.

- Consider giving larger doses at noontime and in the evening rather than in the morning; the response is greater in the morning. The morning dose should be relatively small or omitted, based on BP response, and symptoms of faintness, light-headedness.
- Determine the initial and maintenance dosage by BP readings in the erect position at the time of maximal drug effect and by other signs and symptoms of orthostatic hypotension.
- Discontinue drug gradually; concurrently replace with another antihypertensive drug. Abrupt discontinuation in patients with malignant hypertension may cause return of hypertension and fatal CVAs or acute CHF.
- Decrease dosage with fever, infection, salt depletion, which decrease drug requirements.
- Monitor patient for orthostatic hypotension: most marked in the morning, accentuated by hot weather, alcohol, exercise.
- Ensure adequate salt intake; use caution where increased sodium loss exists.
- Monitor bowel function carefully; paralytic ileus has occurred. Prevent constipation by giving pilocarpine or neostigmine with each dose. Treat constipation with *Milk of Magnesia* or similar laxative; do not use bulk laxatives.
- Discontinue drug immediately, and arrange for remedial steps at the first signs of paralytic ileus: frequent loose bowel movements with abdominal distention and decreased borborygmi.

Teaching points

- Take after meals and in a consistent relation to meals. Do not stop taking without consulting your health care provider.
- Learn, alone or with a significant other, to monitor your BP frequently to ensure safe, effective therapy (may be given instructions to reduce or omit a dose if readings fall below a designated level or if faintness or light-headedness occurs).
- Ensure an adequate intake of salt, especially in hot weather, during exercise, or if sweating excessively.
- These side effects may occur: dizziness, weakness (most likely on changing position, in the early morning, after exercise, in hot weather, and with alcohol consumption; some tolerance to drug may occur; avoid driving or engaging in tasks that require alertness, and change position slowly; use caution in climbing stairs); blurred vision, dilated pupils, sensitivity to bright light (revised eyeglass prescription, wearing sunglasses may help); constipation (request a laxative or GI stimulant); dry mouth (sucking sugarless lozenges, ice chips may help); GI upset (frequent, small meals may help); impotence, decreased libido.
- Report tremor, seizure, frequent dizziness or fainting, severe or persistent constipation, or frequent loose stools with abdominal distention.

▽ mechlorethamine hydrochloride (HN₂, nitrogen mustard)

*(me klor **eth' a** meen)*

Mustargen

PREGNANCY CATEGORY D

Drug classes

Alkylating agent
Nitrogen mustard
Antineoplastic

Therapeutic actions

Cytotoxic: reacts chemically with DNA, RNA, other proteins to prevent replication and function of susceptible cells, causing cell death; cell cycle nonspecific.

Indications

- Treatment of Hodgkin's disease, lymphosarcoma, chronic myelocytic or chronic lymphocytic leukemia, polycythemia vera, cutaneous T-cell lymphoma, lung carcinoma (IV use)
- Treatment of effusion secondary to metastatic carcinoma (intrapleural, intraperitoneal, intrapericardial use)
- Unlabeled use: topical treatment of cutaneous T-cell lymphoma

---

Adverse effects in *Italics* are most common; those in **Bold** are life-threatening.

Contraindications and cautions

- Contraindicated with allergy to mechlorethamine, active infection, pregnancy, lactation.
- Use cautiously with amyloidosis, hematopoietic depression, chronic lymphocytic leukemia, concomitant steroid therapy.

Available forms

Powder for injection—10 mg

Dosages

Individualize dosage based on hematologic profile and response.

Adults

- *Usual dose:* total of 0.4 mg/kg IV for each course of therapy as a single dose *or* in 2 to 4 divided doses of 0.1–0.2 mg/kg/day. Give at night in case sedation is required for side effects. Interval between courses of therapy is usually 3–6 wk.
- *Intracavitary administration:* Dose and preparation vary considerably with cavity and disease being treated: consult manufacturer's label.

Pharmacokinetics

Route	Onset	Peak	Duration
IV	Immediate	Seconds	Minutes

Metabolism: $T_{1/2}$: minutes
Distribution: Crosses placenta; may enter breast milk
Excretion: Urine

▽ IV facts

Preparations: Reconstitute vial with 10 mL of sterile water for injection or sodium chloride injection; resultant solution contains 1 mg/mL of mechlorethamine HCl. Prepare solution immediately before use; decomposes on standing.
Infusion: Inject into tubing of a flowing IV infusion slowly over 3–5 min.

Adverse effects

- **CNS:** *Weakness,* vertigo, tinnitus, diminished hearing
- **Dermatologic:** Maculopapular rash, alopecia
- **GI:** *Nausea, vomiting, anorexia,* diarrhea, jaundice
- **GU:** *Impaired fertility*
- **Hematologic:** *Bone marrow depression,* immunosuppression, hyperuricemia
- **Local:** *Vesicant thrombosis, thrombophlebitis,* tissue necrosis if extravasation occurs

■ Nursing considerations
Assessment

- **History:** Allergy to mechlorethamine, active infection, amyloidosis, hematopoietic depression, chronic lymphocytic leukemia, concomitant steroid therapy, pregnancy, lactation
- **Physical:** T; weight; skin color, lesions; injection site; orientation, reflexes, hearing evaluation; CBC, differential, uric acid

Interventions

- Arrange for blood tests to evaluate hematopoietic function before and during therapy.
- Use caution when preparing drug for administration; use chemo-safe nonpermeable gloves for handling drug; drug is highly toxic and a vesicant. Avoid inhalation of dust or vapors and contact with skin or mucous membranes (especially the eyes). If eye contact occurs, immediately irrigate with copious amount of ophthalmic irrigating solution, and obtain an ophthalmologic consultation. If skin contact occurs, irrigate with copious amount of water for 15 min, followed by application of 2% sodium thiosulfate.
- Use caution when determining correct amount of drug for injection. The margin of safety is very small; double check dosage before administration.
- Monitor injection site for any sign of extravasation. Painful inflammation and induration or sloughing of skin may occur. If leakage is noted, promptly infiltrate with sterile isotonic sodium thiosulfate (1/6 molar), and apply an ice compress for 6–12 hr. Notify physician.
- Consult physician for premedication with antiemetics or sedatives to prevent severe nausea and vomiting. Giving at night may help alleviate the problem.
- Ensure that patient is well hydrated before treatment.
- Caution patient to avoid pregnancy while on this drug; advise use of barrier contraceptives.

- Monitor uric acid levels; ensure adequate fluid intake, and prepare for appropriate treatment if hyperuricemia occurs.

Teaching points
- This drug must be given IV or directly into a body cavity.
- These side effects may occur: nausea, vomiting, loss of appetite (use antiemetic or sedative at night; maintain fluid intake and nutrition); weakness, dizziness, ringing in the ears or loss of hearing (use special precautions to avoid injury); infertility, from irregular menses to complete amenorrhea; men may stop producing sperm (may be irreversible).
- Use birth control. This drug cannot be taken during pregnancy; serious fetal effects can occur. If you think you are pregnant or wish to become pregnant, consult your prescriber.
- Report pain, burning at IV site, severe GI distress, sore throat, rash, joint pain, fever.

▷meclizine hydrochloride
(mek' li zeen)

Bonamine (CAN), Bonine, D-Vert (CAN)

Oral prescription tablets:
Antivert, Antrizine, Dramamine Less Drowsy Formula, Meni-D

PREGNANCY CATEGORY B

Drug classes
Antiemetic
Anti-motion sickness agent
Antihistamine
Anticholinergic

Therapeutic actions
Reduces sensitivity of the labyrinthine apparatus; probably acts at least partly by blocking cholinergic synapses in the vomiting center, which receives input from the chemoreceptor trigger zone and from peripheral nerve pathways; peripheral anticholinergic effects may contribute to efficacy.

Indications
- Prevention and treatment of nausea, vomiting, motion sickness
- Possibly effective for the management of vertigo associated with diseases affecting the vestibular system

Contraindications and cautions
- Contraindicated with allergy to meclizine or cyclizine, pregnancy.
- Use cautiously with lactation, narrow-angle glaucoma, stenosing peptic ulcer, symptomatic prostatic hypertrophy, bronchial asthma, bladder neck obstruction, pyloroduodenal obstruction, cardiac arrhythmias, postoperative state (hypotensive effects may be confusing and dangerous).

Available forms
Tablets—12.5, 25, 50 mg; chewable tablets—25 mg; capsules—25, 30 mg

Dosages
Adults
- *Motion sickness:* 25–50 mg PO 1 hr prior to travel. May repeat dose every 24 hr for the duration of the journey.
- *Vertigo:* 25–100 mg PO daily in divided doses.
Pediatric patients
Not recommended for use in children < 12 yr.
Geriatric patients
More likely to cause dizziness, sedation, syncope, toxic confusional states, and hypotension in elderly patients; use with caution.

Pharmacokinetics

Route	Onset	Peak	Duration
Oral	1 hr	1–2 hr	12–24 hr

Metabolism: $T_{1/2}$: 6 hr
Distribution: Crosses placenta; may enter breast milk
Excretion: Feces

Adverse effects
- **CNS:** *Drowsiness, confusion,* euphoria, nervousness, restlessness, insomnia and excitement, seizures, vertigo, tinnitus, blurred vision, diplopia, auditory and visual hallucinations

Adverse effects in *Italics* are most common; those in **Bold** are life-threatening.

- **CV:** Hypotension, palpitations, tachycardia
- **Dermatologic:** Urticaria, rash
- **GI:** *Dry mouth, anorexia, nausea,* vomiting, diarrhea or constipation
- **GU:** *Urinary frequency, difficult urination,* urinary retention
- **Respiratory: Respiratory depression, death** (due to overdose, especially in young children), dry nose and throat

Interactions
✳ Drug-drug • Increased sedation with alcohol or other CNS depressants

■ Nursing considerations
Assessment
- **History:** Allergy to meclizine or cyclizine, pregnancy, narrow-angle glaucoma, stenosing peptic ulcer, symptomatic prostatic hypertrophy, bronchial asthma, bladder neck obstruction, pyloroduodenal obstruction, cardiac arrhythmias, postoperative patients, lactation
- **Physical:** Skin color, lesions, texture; orientation, reflexes, affect; ophthalmic exam; P, BP; R, adventitious sounds; bowel sounds, normal output, status of mucous membranes; prostate palpation, urinary output

Interventions
- Monitor I & O, and take appropriate measures with urinary retention.

Teaching points
- Take as prescribed. Avoid excessive dosage. Chew the chewable tablets carefully before swallowing.
- Anti-motion sickness drugs work best if used prophylactically.
- These side effects may occur: dizziness, sedation, drowsiness (use caution driving or performing tasks that require alertness); epigastric distress, diarrhea, or constipation (take with food); dry mouth (frequent mouth care, sucking sugarless lozenges may help); dryness of nasal mucosa (try another motion sickness, antivertigo remedy).
- Avoid alcohol; serious sedation could occur.
- Report difficulty breathing, hallucinations, tremors, loss of coordination, visual disturbances, irregular heartbeat.

▷ **meclofenamate sodium**
*(me kloe fen **am**' ate)*

Meclomen (CAN)

PREGNANCY CATEGORY C

Drug class
Nonsteroidal anti-inflammatory drug (NSAID)

Therapeutic actions
Anti-inflammatory, analgesic, and antipyretic activities related to inhibition of prostaglandin synthesis; exact mechanisms of action are not known.

Indications
- Acute and chronic rheumatoid arthritis and osteoarthritis (not recommended as initial therapy due to adverse GI effects: severe diarrhea)
- Relief of mild to moderate acute pain
- Treatment of idiopathic heavy menstrual blood loss
- Treatment of primary dysmenorrhea

Contraindications and cautions
- Contraindicated with pregnancy and lactation, hypersensitivity to meclofenamate.
- Use cautiously with asthma, renal or liver dysfunction, peptic ulcer disease, GI bleeding, hypertension, CHF.

Available forms
Capsules—50, 100 mg

Dosages
Adults
- *Rheumatoid arthritis:* Usual dosage 200–400 mg/day PO in 3 to 4 equal doses. Initiate therapy with a lower dose, and increase as needed. Do not exceed 400 mg/day. 2–3 wk may be needed to achieve optimum therapeutic effect.
- *Mild to moderate pain:* 50 mg PO q 4–6 hr. Doses of 100 mg may be required for optimal pain relief. Do not exceed 400 mg/day.
- *Excessive menstrual blood loss and primary dysmenorrhea:* 100 mg PO tid for up to 6 days, starting at the onset of menstrual flow.

Pediatric patients
Safety and efficacy in patients < 14 yr not established.

Pharmacokinetics

Route	Onset	Peak
Oral	Varies	30–60 min

Metabolism: Hepatic; $T_{1/2}$: 2–4 hr
Distribution: Crosses placenta; enters breast milk
Excretion: Urine

Adverse effects
NSAIDs
- **CNS:** *Headache, dizziness,* somnolence, *insomnia,* fatigue, tiredness, dizziness, tinnitus, ophthalmologic effects
- **Dermatologic:** *Rash,* pruritus, sweating, dry mucous membranes, stomatitis
- **GI:** *Nausea, dyspepsia, GI pain, diarrhea,* vomiting, constipation, flatulence
- **GU:** Dysuria, renal impairment
- **Hematologic:** Bleeding, platelet inhibition with higher doses, neutropenia, eosinophilia, leukopenia, pancytopenia, thrombocytopenia, agranulocytosis, granulocytopenia, aplastic anemia, decreased hemoglobin or Hct, bone marrow depression, mennorhagia
- **Respiratory:** Dyspnea, hemoptysis, pharyngitis, bronchospasm, rhinitis
- **Other:** Peripheral edema, **anaphylactoid reactions to anaphylaxis shock**

■ Nursing considerations
Assessment
- **History:** Asthma, renal or liver dysfunction, peptic ulcer disease, GI bleeding, hypertension, CHF, pregnancy, lactation
- **Physical:** Skin color and lesions; orientation, reflexes, ophthalmologic and audiometric evaluation, peripheral sensation; P, edema; R, adventitious sounds; liver evaluation; CBC, clotting times, renal and liver function tests; serum electrolytes, stool guaiac

Interventions
- Give with milk or food to decrease GI upset.
- Arrange for periodic ophthalmologic examination during long-term therapy.

- Institute emergency procedures if overdose occurs: gastric lavage, induction of emesis, supportive therapy.

Teaching points
- Take drug with food; take only the prescribed dosage.
- Dizziness, drowsiness can occur (avoid driving or the use of dangerous machinery).
- Report sore throat, fever, rash, itching, weight gain, swelling in ankles or fingers; changes in vision; black, tarry stools; severe diarrhea.

▷ medroxyprogesterone acetate

(me drox' ee proe jess' te rone)

Oral: Alti-MPA (CAN), Amen, Curretab, Cycrin, Gen-Medroxy (CAN), Novo-Medrone (CAN), Provera
Parenteral, antineoplastic: Depo-Provera

PREGNANCY CATEGORY X

Drug classes
Hormone
Progestin
Antineoplastic

Therapeutic actions
Progesterone derivative; endogenous progesterone transforms proliferative endometrium into secretory endometrium; inhibits the secretion of pituitary gonadotropins, which prevents follicular maturation and ovulation; inhibits spontaneous uterine contraction.

Indications
- Reduction of endometrial hyperplasia in postmenopausal women
- Treatment of secondary amenorrhea (oral)
- Abnormal uterine bleeding due to hormonal imbalance in the absence of organic pathology (oral)
- Adjunctive therapy and palliation of inoperable, recurrent, and metastatic endometrial carcinoma or renal carcinoma (parenteral)

- Unlabeled use for depot form: long-acting contraceptive, treatment of breast cancer

Contraindications and cautions
- Contraindicated with allergy to progestins; thrombophlebitis, thromboembolic disorders, cerebral hemorrhage or history of these conditions; hepatic disease, carcinoma of the breast, ovaries, or endometrium, undiagnosed vaginal bleeding, missed abortion; pregnancy (fetal abnormalities, including masculinization of the female fetus have been reported); lactation.
- Use cautiously with epilepsy, migraine, asthma, cardiac or renal dysfunction.

Available forms
Tablets—2.5, 5, 10 mg; with estradiol—25 mg medroxyprogesterone and 5 mg estradiol cypionate per 0.5 mL; injection—150, 400 mg/mL

Dosages
Adults
- *Contraception monotherapy:* 150 mg IM q 3 mo.
- *Secondary amenorrhea:* 5–10 mg/day PO for 5–10 days. A dose for inducing an optimum secretory transformation of an endometrium that has been primed with exogenous or endogenous estrogen is 10 mg/day for 10 days. Start therapy at any time; withdrawal bleeding usually occurs 3–7 days after therapy ends.
- *Abnormal uterine bleeding:* 5–10 mg/day PO for 5–10 days, beginning on the 16th or 21st day of the menstrual cycle. To produce an optimum secretory transformation of an endometrium that has been primed with estrogen, give 10 mg/day PO for 10 days, beginning on the 16th day of the cycle. Withdrawal bleeding usually occurs 3–7 days after discontinuing therapy. If bleeding is controlled, administer two subsequent cycles.
- *Endometrial or renal carcinoma:* 400–1,000 mg/wk IM. If improvement occurs within a few weeks or months and the disease appears stabilized, it may be possible to maintain improvement with as little as 400 mg/mo IM.
- *Reduction of endometrial hyperplasia:* 5–10 mg/day PO for 12–14 days/mo.

Pharmacokinetics

Route	Onset	Peak
Oral	Slow	Unknown
IM	Weeks	Months

Metabolism: Hepatic; $T_{1/2}$: unknown
Distribution: Crosses placenta; enters breast milk
Excretion: Unknown

Adverse effects
- **CNS:** Sudden, partial, or complete loss of vision; proptosis, diplopia, migraine, precipitation of acute intermittent porphyria, mental depression, pyrexia, insomnia, somnolence, nervousness, fatigue
- **CV:** Thrombophlebitis, cerebrovascular disorders, retinal thrombosis, pulmonary embolism, thromboembolic and thrombotic disease, increased BP
- **Dermatologic:** *Rash with or without pruritus, acne,* melasma or chloasma, alopecia, hirsutism, photosensitivity, pruritus, urticaria
- **GI:** Cholestatic jaundice, nausea
- **GU:** *Breakthrough bleeding, spotting, change in menstrual flow, amenorrhea,* changes in cervical erosion and cervical secretions, breast tenderness and secretion
- **Other:** *Fluid retention, edema, increase or decrease in weight,* decreased glucose tolerance

Interactions
✳ Drug-lab test • Inaccurate tests of hepatic and endocrine function

■ Nursing considerations
Assessment
- **History:** Allergy to progestins; thrombophlebitis; thromboembolic disorders; cerebral hemorrhage; hepatic disease; carcinoma of the breast, ovaries, or endometrium; undiagnosed vaginal bleeding; missed abortion; epilepsy; migraine; asthma; cardiac or renal dysfunction; pregnancy; lactation
- **Physical:** Skin color, lesions, turgor; hair; breasts; pelvic exam; orientation, affect; ophthalmologic exam; P, auscultation, peripheral perfusion, edema; R, adventitious sounds; liver evaluation; liver and renal function tests, glucose tolerance, Pap smear

Interventions

- Arrange for pretreatment and periodic (at least annual) history and physical, which should include BP, breasts, abdomen, pelvic organs, and a Pap smear.
- Alert patient before therapy to prevent pregnancy and to have frequent medical follow-ups.
- Discontinue medication and consult physician if sudden, partial, or complete loss of vision occurs; if papilledema or retinal vascular lesions are present, discontinue drug.
- Discontinue medication and consult physician at the first sign of thromboembolic disease (leg pain, swelling, peripheral perfusion changes, shortness of breath).

Teaching points

- Prepare a calendar, marking drug days (oral drug).
- These side effects may occur: sensitivity to light (avoid exposure to the sun; use sunscreen and protective clothing); dizziness, sleeplessness, depression (use caution driving or performing tasks that require alertness); skin rash, color changes, loss of hair; fever; nausea.
- This drug should not be taken during pregnancy due to risk of serious fetal abnormalities; use of barrier contraceptives is suggested.
- Report pain or swelling and warmth in the calves, acute chest pain or shortness of breath, sudden severe headache or vomiting, dizziness or fainting, visual disturbances, numbness or tingling in the arm or leg.

▽ mefenamic acid

(me fe nam' ik)

Apo-Mefenamic (CAN), PMS-Mefenamic Acid (CAN), Ponstan (CAN), Ponstel

PREGNANCY CATEGORY C

Drug class

Nonsteroidal anti-inflammatory drug (NSAID)

Therapeutic actions

Anti-inflammatory, analgesic, and antipyretic activities related to inhibition of prostaglandin synthesis; exact mechanisms of action are not known.

Indications

- Relief of moderate pain when therapy will not exceed 1 wk
- Treatment of primary dysmenorrhea

Contraindications and cautions

- Contraindicated with hypersensitivity to mefenamic acid, pregnancy, lactation.
- Use cautiously with asthma, renal or liver dysfunction, peptic ulcer disease, GI bleeding, hypertension, CHF.

Available forms

Capsules—250 mg

Dosages

Adults and patients > 14 yr

- *Acute pain:* Initially 500 mg PO followed by 250 mg q 6 hr as needed. Do not exceed 1 wk of therapy.
- *Primary dysmenorrhea:* Initially 500 mg PO then 250 mg q 6 hr starting with the onset of bleeding. Can be initiated at start of menses and should not be necessary for longer than 2–3 days.

Pediatric patients

Safety and efficacy for patients < 14 yr not established.

Pharmacokinetics

Route	Onset	Peak	Duration
Oral	Varies	2–4 hr	6 hr

Metabolism: Hepatic; $T_{1/2}$: 2–4 hr
Distribution: Crosses placenta; enters breast milk
Excretion: Urine and feces

Adverse effects

- **CNS:** *Headache, dizziness,* somnolence, *insomnia,* fatigue, tiredness, dizziness, tinnitus, ophthalmic effects
- **Dermatologic:** *Rash,* pruritus, sweating, dry mucous membranes, stomatitis

---

*Adverse effects in Italics are most common; those in **Bold** are life-threatening.*

- **GI:** *Nausea, dyspepsia, GI pain, diarrhea,* vomiting, *constipation,* flatulence
- **GU:** Dysuria, **renal impairment**
- **Hematologic:** Bleeding, platelet inhibition with higher doses, neutropenia, eosinophilia, leukopenia, pancytopenia, thrombocytopenia, agranulocytosis, granulocytopenia, aplastic anemia, decreased Hgb or Hct, bone marrow depression, menorrhagia
- **Respiratory:** Dyspnea, hemoptysis, pharyngitis, bronchospasm, rhinitis
- **Other:** Peripheral edema, **anaphylactoid reactions to anaphylactic shock**

Interactions

✴ **Drug-lab test** • False-positive reaction for urinary bile using the diazo tablet test

■ Nursing considerations
Assessment

- **History:** Allergies; renal, hepatic, CV, GI conditions; pregnancy; lactation
- **Physical:** Skin color and lesions; orientation, reflexes, ophthalmologic and audiometric evaluation, peripheral sensation; P, edema; R, adventitious sounds; liver evaluation; CBC, clotting times, renal and liver function tests; serum electrolytes, stool guaiac

Interventions

- Give with milk or food to decrease GI upset.
- Arrange for periodic ophthalmologic examination during long-term therapy.
- Institute emergency procedures if overdose occurs: gastric lavage, induction of emesis, supportive therapy.

Teaching points

- Take drug with food; take only the prescribed dosage; do not take the drug longer than 1 wk.
- Dizziness, drowsiness can occur (avoid driving or the use of dangerous machinery).
- Discontinue drug and consult care provider if rash, diarrhea, or digestive problems occur.
- Report sore throat, fever, rash, itching, weight gain, swelling in ankles or fingers; changes in vision; black, tarry stools; severe diarrhea.

▽ **megestrol acetate**
(*me* **jess'** *trole*)

Apo-Megestrol (CAN), Megace, Megace-OS (CAN)

PREGNANCY CATEGORY X

Drug classes
Hormone
Progestin
Antineoplastic

Therapeutic actions
Synthetic progestational agent; mechanism of antineoplastic activity is unknown but may be due to a pituitary-mediated antileutinizing effect.

Indications
- Palliation of advanced carcinoma of the breast or endometrium and as an adjunct to surgery or radiation
- Orphan drug use: Appetite stimulant in HIV-related cachexia

Contraindications and cautions
- Contraindicated with allergy to progestins; thrombophlebitis, thromboembolic disorders, cerebral hemorrhage or history of these conditions; hepatic disease, undiagnosed vaginal bleeding, missed abortion; pregnancy (masculinization of female fetus); lactation.
- Use cautiously with epilepsy, migraine, asthma, cardiac or renal dysfunction.

Available forms
Tablets—20, 40 mg; suspension—40 mg/mL

Dosages
Adults
- *Breast cancer:* 160 mg/day PO (40 mg qid).
- *Endometrial cancer:* 40–320 mg/day PO in divided doses.
- *Cachexia:* 160–800 mg/day PO.
- *Cachexia with HIV:* Initially 800 mg/day; normal range, 100–800 mg/day.

Pharmacokinetics

Route	Onset	Peak
Oral	Slow	Weeks

M

Metabolism: Hepatic; T$_{1/2}$: unknown
Distribution: Crosses placenta; enters breast milk
Excretion: Urine

Adverse effects

- **CNS:** Sudden, partial, or complete loss of vision; proptosis; diplopia; migraine; precipitation of acute intermittent porphyria; mental depression; pyrexia; insomnia; somnolence, nervousness, fatigue
- **CV:** Thrombophlebitis, cerebrovascular disorders, retinal thrombosis, **pulmonary embolism,** thromboembolic and thrombotic disease, increased BP
- **Dermatologic:** *Rash with or without pruritus, acne,* melasma or chloasma, alopecia, hirsutism, photosensitivity, pruritus, urticaria
- **GI:** Cholestatic jaundice, nausea
- **GU:** *Breakthrough bleeding, spotting, change in menstrual flow, amenorrhea,* changes in cervical erosion and cervical secretions, breast tenderness and secretion
- **Other:** *Fluid retention, edema, increase in weight,* decreased glucose tolerance

Interactions

✳ **Drug-lab test** • Inaccurate tests of hepatic and endocrine function

■ Nursing considerations
Assessment

- **History:** Allergy to progestins; thrombophlebitis, thromboembolic disorders, cerebral hemorrhage; hepatic disease; carcinoma of the breast or genital organs, undiagnosed vaginal bleeding, missed abortion; epilepsy, migraine, asthma, cardiac or renal dysfunction; pregnancy; lactation
- **Physical:** Skin color, lesions, turgor; hair; breasts; pelvic exam; orientation; affect; ophthalmologic exam; P, auscultation, peripheral perfusion, edema; R, adventitious sounds; liver evaluation; liver and renal function tests, glucose tolerance, Pap smear

Interventions

- Discontinue drug and consult physician at signs of thromboembolic disease: leg pain,

swelling, peripheral perfusion changes, shortness of breath.
- Caution patient to avoid use of this drug during pregnancy because of risks to the fetus; advise the use of barrier contraceptives.

Teaching points

- These side effects may occur: sensitivity to light (avoid exposure to the sun; use sunscreen and protective clothing); dizziness, sleeplessness, depression (use caution if driving or performing tasks that require alertness); skin rash, color changes, loss of hair; fever; nausea.
- This drug causes serious fetal abnormalities or fetal death; avoid pregnancy. Use of barrier contraceptives is advised.
- Report pain or swelling and warmth in the calves, acute chest pain or shortness of breath, sudden severe headache or vomiting, dizziness or fainting, numbness or tingling in the arm or leg.

▽ **meloxicam**
(mel ox' i kam)

Mobic

PREGNANCY CATEGORY B

Drug class

NSAID (nonsteroidal anti-inflammatory drug—oxicam derivative)

Therapeutic actions

Anti-inflammatory, analgesic, and antipyretic activities related to inhibition of the enzyme cyclooxygenase (COX), which is required for the synthesis of prostaglandins and thromboxanes. Somewhat more selective for COX-2 sites (found in the brain, kidney, ovary, uterus, cartilage, bone, and at sites of inflammation) than for COX-1 sites, which are found throughout the tissues and are related to protection of the GI mucosa.

Indications

- Treatment of osteoarthritis

Contraindications and cautions

- Contraindicated with pregnancy, lactation, aspirin allergy.
- Use cautiously with allergies; renal, hepatic, cardiovascular, GI conditions; bleeding disorders.

Available forms

Tablets—7.5, 15 mg

Dosages

Adults

Starting dose: 7.5 mg PO daily. Maximum dosage: 15 mg PO daily.

Pediatric patients

Safety and efficacy not established.

Pharmacokinetics

Route	Onset	Peak
Oral	1 hr	4–5 hr

Metabolism: Hepatic; $T_{1/2}$: 15–20 hr
Distribution: Crosses placenta; passes into breast milk
Excretion: Urine and feces

Adverse effects

- **CNS:** *Headache, dizziness,* somnolence, *insomnia,* fatigue, tiredness, dizziness, tinnitus, ophthamologic effects
- **Dermatologic:** *Rash,* pruritus, sweating, dry mucous membranes, stomatitis
- **GI:** *Nausea, dyspepsia, GI pain, diarrhea,* vomiting, constipation, flatulence
- **GU:** Dysuria, renal impairment
- **Hematologic:** Bleeding, platelet inhibition—with higher doses, neutropenia, eosinophilia, leukopenia, pancytopenia, thrombocytopenia, agranulocytosis, granulocytopenia, aplastic anemia, decreased hemoglobin or hematocrit, bone marrow depression, menorrhagia
- **Respiratory:** Dyspnea, hemoptysis, pharyngitis, bronchospasm, rhinitis
- **Other:** Peripheral edema, anaphylactoid reactions to **anaphylactic shock**

Interactions

✳ Drug-drug • Increased serum lithium levels and risk of toxicity if taken concurrently; monitor patient carefully • Possible increased risk of renal failure if combined with ACE inhibitors, diuretics • Increased risk of GI bleeding if combined with aspirin, anticoagulants, oral corticosteroids

■ Nursing considerations
Assessment

- **History:** Allergies, renal, hepatic, cardiovascular, and GI bleeding, history of ulcers, pregnancy, lactation, bleeding disorders
- **Physical:** Skin color and lesions; orientation, reflexes, peripheral sensation; P, edema; R, adventitious sounds; liver evaluation; CBC, clotting times, renal and liver function tests; serum electrolytes, stool guaiac

Interventions

- Administer drug with food or milk if GI upset occurs.
- Establish safety measures if CNS disturbances occur.
- Monitor patient on prolonged therapy for signs of GI bleeding, hepatic toxicity.
- Institute emergency procedures if overdose occurs—gastric lavage, induction of emesis, supportive therapy.
- Provide further comfort measures to reduce pain (positioning, environmental control, etc), and to reduce inflammation (warmth, positioning, rest, etc).

Teaching points

- Take drug with food if GI upset occurs.
- Take only the prescribed dosage.
- Know that dizziness, drowsiness can occur (avoid driving or the use of dangerous machinery while on this drug).
- Report sore throat, fever, rash, itching, weight gain, swelling in ankles or fingers, changes in vision, black, tarry stools.

▷ **melphalan (L-Pam, L-Phenylalanine Mustard, L-Sarcolysin)**
(mel' fa lan)

Alkeran

PREGNANCY CATEGORY D

Drug classes

Alkylating agent
Nitrogen mustard
Antineoplastic

Therapeutic actions

Cytotoxic: alkylates cellular DNA, thus interfering with the replication of susceptible cells, causing cell death; cell-cycle nonspecific.

Indications

- Treatment of multiple myeloma, nonresectable epithelial ovarian carcinoma; use IV only when oral therapy is not possible

Contraindications and cautions

- Allergy to melphalan or chlorambucil, radiation therapy, chemotherapy, pregnancy (potentially mutagenic and teratogenic; avoid use in the first trimester), lactation.

Available forms

Tablets—2 mg; powder for injection—50 mg

Dosages

Individualize dosage based on hematologic profile and response.

Adults

Oral

- *Multiple myeloma:* 6 mg/day PO. After 2–3 wk, stop drug for up to 4 wk, and monitor blood counts. When blood counts are rising, institute maintenance dose of 2 mg/day PO. Response may occur gradually over many months (many alternative regimens, some including prednisone, are used).
- *Epithelial ovarian carcinoma:* 0.2 mg/kg/day PO for 5 days as a single course. Repeat courses every 4–5 wk, depending on hematologic response.

IV

16 mg/m^2 administered as a single infusion over 15–20 min; administered at 2-wk intervals for 4 doses, then at 4-wk intervals.

Pharmacokinetics

Route	Onset	Peak
Oral	Varies	2 hr
IV	Rapid	1 hr

Metabolism: T$_{1/2}$: 90 min
Distribution: Crosses placenta; enters breast milk
Excretion: Urine

▽ IV facts

Preparation: Reconstitute with 10 mL of supplied diluent, and shake vigorously until a clear solution is obtained; this provides 5 mg/mL solution. Immediately dilute in 0.9% sodium chloride injection to a dilution of < 0.45 mg/mL. Complete infusion within 60 min of reconstitution. Protect from light. Dispense in glass containers. Do not refrigerate reconstituted solution.

Infusion: Administer dilute product over a minimum of 15 min; complete within 60 min of reconstitution.

Adverse effects

- **Dermatologic:** Maculopapular rash, urticaria, *alopecia*
- **GI:** *Nausea, vomiting,* oral ulceration
- **Hematologic: Bone marrow depression,** hyperuricemia
- **Respiratory:** Bronchopulmonary dysplasia, **pulmonary fibrosis**
- **Other:** *Amenorrhea,* cancer, acute leukemia

Interactions

✳ **Drug-lab test** ● Increased urinary 5-hydroxyindole acetic acid levels (5-HIAA) due to tumor cell destruction

■ Nursing considerations

Assessment

- **History:** Allergy to melphalan or chlorambucil, radiation therapy, chemotherapy, pregnancy, lactation
- **Physical:** T; weight; skin color, lesions; R, adventitious sounds; liver evaluation; CBC, differential, hemoglobin, uric acid, renal function tests

Interventions

- Arrange for blood tests to evaluate hematopoietic function before therapy and weekly during therapy.
- Do not give full dosage until 4 wk after a full course of radiation therapy or chemotherapy due to risk of severe bone marrow depression.
- Consider dosage reductions in patients with impaired renal function.
- Ensure that patient is well hydrated before treatment.

- Caution patient to avoid pregnancy while on this drug.
- Monitor uric acid levels; ensure adequate fluid intake, and prepare for appropriate treatment if hyperuricemia occurs.
- Divide single daily dose if nausea and vomiting occur with single dose.

Teaching points

- Take drug once a day. If nausea and vomiting occur, consult with care provider about dividing the dose.
- These side effects may occur: nausea, vomiting, loss of appetite (divided dose, small frequent meals may help; maintain fluid intake and nutrition; drink at least 10–12 glasses of fluid each day); skin rash, loss of hair (obtain a wig if hair loss occurs; head should be covered at extremes of temperature).
- This drug causes severe birth defects; use of barrier contraceptives is advised.
- Report unusual bleeding or bruising, fever, chills, sore throat, cough, shortness of breath, black tarry stools, flank or stomach pain, joint pain.

▽ menotropins

*(men oh **troe'** pins)*

Pergonal, Repronex

PREGNANCY CATEGORY C

Drug classes

Hormone
Fertility drug

Therapeutic actions

A purified preparation of human gonadotropins; in women, produces ovarian follicular growth; when followed by administration of human chorionic gonadotropin (HCG), produces ovulation; used with HCG for at least 3 mo to induce spermatogenesis in men with primary or secondary pituitary hypofunction who have previously achieved adequate masculinization with HCG administration.

Indications

- Women: Given with HCG sequentially to induce ovulation and pregnancy in anovulatory infertile patients without primary ovar-

ian failure. Used with HCG to stimulate multiple follicles for in vitro fertilization programs.
- Men: With concomitant HCG therapy to stimulate spermatogenesis in men with primary hypogonadotropic hypogonadism due to a congenital factor or prepubertal hypophysectomy and in men with secondary hypogonadotropic hypogonadism due to hypophysectomy, craniopharyngioma, cerebral aneurysm, or chromophobe adenoma (*Pergonal*).

Contraindications and cautions

- Known sensitivity to menotropins; high gonadotropin levels, indicating primary ovarian failure; overt thyroid or adrenal dysfunction; abnormal bleeding of undetermined origin; ovarian cysts or enlargement not due to polycystic ovary syndrome; intracranial lesion, such as pituitary tumor; pregnancy (women); normal gonadotropin levels, indicating pituitary function; elevated gonadotropin levels, indicating primary testicular failure; infertility disorders other than hypogonadotropin hypogonadism (men).

Available forms

Powder for injection—75 IU FSH/75 IU LH; 150 IU FSH/150 IU LH

Dosages
Women

To achieve ovulation, HCG must be given following menotropins when clinical assessment indicates sufficient follicular maturation as indicated by urinary excretion of estrogens.
Pergonal

Initial dose is 75 IU FSH/75 IU LH/day IM for 7–12 days. Follow administration with 5,000–10,000 units HCG 1 day after the last dose of menotropins. Do not administer for longer than 12 days. Treat until estrogen levels are normal or slightly higher than normal. When urinary estrogen excretion is < 100 mcg/24 hr, and urinary estriol excretion is < 50 mcg/24 hr prior to HCG administration, there is less risk of ovarian overstimulation. Do not administer if urinary excretion exceeds these values. Couple should engage in intercourse daily beginning on the day prior to the HCG administration and until ovulation occurs. If there is evidence of ovulation but pregnancy does not occur, repeat regimen for at least 2 more courses before increasing dose to 150 IU FSH/150 IU LH/day IM for 7–12 days followed by 10,000 units HCG 1 day after the last dose of menotropins. If there is evidence of ovulation but pregnancy does not occur, repeat this regimen twice more. Larger doses are not recommended.

Repronex

Initially 150 IU SC or IM daily for first 5 days; adjust dose as needed after 2 or more days. Do not adjust by more than 150 IU per adjustment and do not exceed maximum daily dose of 450 IU. Do not use > 12 days. If patient response is adequate, give HCG 5,000–10,000 units 1 day following last dose of menotropins.

Men

Pergonal

Pretreat with HCG (5,000 units 3 times/wk) until serum testosterone levels are in normal range and masculinization has occurred. Pretreatment may take 4–6 mo. Then give 1 ampule (75 IU FSH/75 IU LH) menotropins IM 3 times/wk and HCG 2,000 units 2 times/wk. Continue for a minimum of 4 mo. If increased spermatogenesis has not occurred at the end of 4 mo, continue treatment with 1 ampule menotropins 3 times/wk or 2 ampules (dose of 150 IU FSH/150 IU LH) menotropins 3 times/wk with the HCG dose unchanged.

Pharmacokinetics

Route	Onset	Peak	Duration
IM	Slow	Weeks	Months

Metabolism: $T_{1/2}$: Unknown
Distribution: Crosses placenta
Excretion: Urine

Adverse effects

Women

- **CV:** Arterial thromboembolism
- **GU:** *Ovarian enlargement,* hyperstimulation syndrome, hemoperitoneum
- **Hypersensitivity:** Hypersensitivity reactions
- **Other:** *Febrile reactions;* birth defects in resulting pregnancies, *multiple pregnancies*

Men

- **Endocrine:** Gynecomastia

■ Nursing considerations

Assessment

- **History:** Sensitivity to menotropins; high gonadotropin levels; overt thyroid or adrenal dysfunction, abnormal bleeding of undetermined origin, ovarian cysts or enlargement not due to polycystic ovary syndrome, intracranial lesion (women); normal gonadotropin levels; elevated gonadotropin levels; infertility disorders other than hypogonadotropin hypogonadism (men)
- **Physical:** T; masculinization (men); abdominal exam; pelvic exam; testicular exam; serum gonadotropin levels; 24 hr urinary estrogens and estriol excretion (women); serum testosterone levels (men)

Interventions

- Dissolve contents of 1 ampule in 1–2 mL of sterile saline. Administer IM immediately. Discard any unused portion.
- Store ampules at room temperature or in refrigerator; do not freeze.
- Monitor women at least every other day during treatment and for 2 wk after treatment for any sign of ovarian enlargement.
- Discontinue drug at any sign of ovarian overstimulation, and arrange to have patient admitted to the hospital for observation and supportive measures. Do not attempt to remove ascitic fluid because of the risk of injury to the ovaries. Have the patient refrain from intercourse if ovarian enlargement occurs.
- Provide women with calendar of treatment days and explanations about what signs of estrogen and progesterone activity to watch for. Caution patient that 24-hr urine collections will be needed periodically, that HCG also must be given to induce ovulation, and that daily intercourse should begin 1 day prior to HCG administration and until ovulation occurs.
- Alert patient to risks and hazards of multiple births.
- Provide support and encouragement to the male patient, explaining the need for long-term treatment, regular sperm counts, and masculinizing effects of HCG.

Adverse effects in *Italics* are most common; those in **Bold** are life-threatening.

Teaching points

- Prepare a calendar showing the treatment schedule; drug can only be given IM and must be used with HCG to achieve the desired effects.
- Have intercourse daily beginning on the day prior to HCG therapy until ovulation occurs.
- These side effects may occur: breast enlargement (men); ovarian enlargement, abdominal discomfort, fever, multiple births (women).
- Report pain at injection site, severe abdominal or lower back pain, fever, fluid in the abdomen.

▽ meperidine hydrochloride (pethidine)
(me per' i deen)

Demerol

PREGNANCY CATEGORY C

C-II CONTROLLED SUBSTANCE

Drug class
Opioid agonist analgesic

Therapeutic actions
Acts as agonist at specific opioid receptors in the CNS to produce analgesia, euphoria, sedation; the receptors mediating these effects are thought to be the same as those mediating the effects of endogenous opioids (enkephalins, endorphins).

Indications
- Relief of moderate to severe acute pain (oral, parenteral)
- Preoperative medication, support of anesthesia, and obstetric analgesia (parenteral)

Contraindications and cautions
- Contraindicated with hypersensitivity to narcotics, diarrhea caused by poisoning (before toxins are eliminated), bronchial asthma, COPD, cor pulmonale, respiratory depression, anoxia, kyphoscoliosis, acute alcoholism, increased intracranial pressure, pregnancy, seizure disorder, renal dysfunction.

- Use cautiously with acute abdominal conditions, CV disease, supraventricular tachycardias, myxedema, delirium tremens, cerebral arteriosclerosis, ulcerative colitis, fever, Addison's disease, prostatic hypertrophy, urethral stricture, recent GI or GU surgery, toxic psychosis, labor or delivery (narcotics given to the mother can cause respiratory depression of neonate; premature infants are especially at risk), renal or hepatic dysfunction.

Available forms
Tablets—50, 100 mg; syrup—50 mg/mL; injection—10, 25, 50, 75, 100 mg/mL

Dosages
Adults
- *Relief of pain:* Individualize dosage; 50–150 mg IM, SC, or PO q 3–4 hr as necessary. Diluted solution may be given by slow IV injection. IM route is preferred for repeated injections.
- *Preoperative medication:* 50–100 mg IM or SC, 30–90 min before beginning anesthesia.
- *Support of anesthesia:* Dilute to 10 mg/mL, and give repeated doses by slow IV injection, or dilute to 1 mg/mL and infuse continuously. Individualize dosage.
- *Obstetric analgesia:* When pains become regular 50–100 mg IM or SC; repeat q 1–3 hr.

Pediatric patients
Contraindicated in premature infants.
- *Relief of pain:* 1.1–1.75 mg/kg IM, SC, or PO up to adult dose q 3–4 hr as necessary.
- *Preoperative medication:* 1.1–2.2 mg/kg IM or SC, up to adult dose, 30–90 min before beginning anesthesia.

Geriatric patients or impaired adults
Use caution; respiratory depression may occur in elderly, the very ill, those with respiratory problems. Reduced dosage may be necessary.

Pharmacokinetics

Route	Onset	Peak	Duration
Oral	15 min	60 min	2–4 hr
IM, SC	10–15 min	30–60 min	2–4 hr
IV	Immediate	5–7 min	2–4 hr

Metabolism: Hepatic; $T_{1/2}$: 3–8 hr
Distribution: Crosses placenta; enters breast milk
Excretion: Urine

M

▼IV facts

Preparation: Dilute parenteral solution prior to IV injection using 5% dextrose and lactated Ringer's; dextrose-saline combinations; 2.5%, 5%, or 10% dextrose in water, Ringer's, or lactated Ringer's; 0.45% or 0.9% sodium chloride; 1/6 molar sodium lactate.

Infusion: Administer by slow IV injection over 4–5 min or by continuous infusion when diluted to 1 mg/mL.

Incompatibilities: Do *not* mix meperidine solutions with solutions of barbiturates, aminophylline, heparin, morphine sulfate, methicillin, phenytoin, sodium bicarbonate, iodide, sulfadiazine, sulfisoxazole.

Y-site incompatibilities: Do not give with cefoperazone, mezlocillin, minocycline, tetracycline.

Adverse effects

- **CNS:** *Light-headedness, dizziness, sedation,* euphoria, dysphoria, delirium, insomnia, agitation, anxiety, fear, hallucinations, disorientation, drowsiness, lethargy, impaired mental and physical performance, coma, mood changes, weakness, headache, tremor, seizures, miosis, visual disturbances, suppression of cough reflex
- **CV:** Facial flushing, peripheral circulatory collapse, tachycardia, bradycardia, arrhythmia, palpitations, chest wall rigidity, hypertension, hypotension, orthostatic hypotension, syncope
- **Dermatologic:** Pruritus, urticaria, laryngospasm, bronchospasm, edema
- **GI:** *Nausea, vomiting,* dry mouth, anorexia, *constipation,* biliary tract spasm, increased colonic motility in patients with chronic ulcerative colitis
- **GU:** Ureteral spasm, spasm of vesical sphincters, urinary retention or hesitancy, oliguria, antidiuretic effect, reduced libido or potency
- **Local:** Tissue irritation and induration (SC injection)
- **Major hazards: Respiratory depression, apnea, circulatory depression, respiratory arrest, shock, cardiac arrest**
- **Other:** *Sweating,* physical tolerance and dependence, psychological dependence

Interactions

✳ **Drug-drug** • Potentiation of effects with barbiturate anesthetics; decrease dose of meperidine when coadministering • Severe and sometimes fatal reactions (resembling narcotic overdose; characterized by seizures, hypertension, hyperpyrexia) when given to patients receiving or who have recently received MAOIs; do not give meperidine to patients on MAOIs • Increased likelihood of respiratory depression, hypotension, profound sedation, or coma with phenothiazines

✳ **Drug-lab test** • Elevated biliary tract pressure may cause increases in plasma amylase, lipase; determinations of these levels may be unreliable for 24 hr after administration of opioids

■ Nursing considerations
Assessment

- **History:** Hypersensitivity to opioids, diarrhea caused by poisoning, bronchial asthma, COPD, cor pulmonale, respiratory depression, anoxia, kyphoscoliosis, acute alcoholism, increased intracranial pressure; acute abdominal conditions, CV disease, supraventricular tachycardias, myxedema, seizure disorders, delirium tremens, cerebral arteriosclerosis, ulcerative colitis, fever, Addison's disease, prostatic hypertrophy, urethral stricture, recent GI or GU surgery, toxic psychosis, renal or hepatic dysfunction, pregnancy
- **Physical:** T; skin color, texture, lesions; orientation, reflexes, bilateral grip strength, affect, pupil size; P, auscultation, BP, orthostatic BP, perfusion; R, adventitious sounds; bowel sounds, normal output; frequency and pattern of voiding, normal output; ECG; EEG; thyroid, liver, kidney function tests

Interventions

- Administer to lactating women 4–6 hr before the next feeding to minimize the amount in milk.
- Provide narcotic antagonist, facilities for assisted or controlled respiration on standby during parenteral administration.
- Use caution when injecting SC into chilled areas of the body or in patients with hypotension or in shock; impaired perfusion may delay absorption; with repeated doses,

an excessive amount may be absorbed when circulation is restored.

- Reduce dosage of meperidine by 25%–50% in patients receiving phenothiazines or other tranquilizers.
- Give each dose of the oral syrup in half glass of water. If taken undiluted, it may exert a slight local anesthetic effect on mucous membranes.
- Reassure patient about addiction liability; most patients who receive opiates for medical reasons do not develop dependence syndromes.
- Use meperidine with extreme caution in patients with renal dysfunction or those requiring repeated dosing due to accumulation of normeperidine, a toxic metabolite that may cause seizures.

Teaching points

- Take drug exactly as prescribed.
- Avoid alcohol, antihistamines, sedatives, tranquilizers, OTC drugs.
- These side effects may occur: nausea, loss of appetite (take with food and lie quietly, eating frequent small meals may help); constipation (request a laxative); dizziness, sedation, drowsiness, impaired visual acuity (avoid driving, performing other tasks that require alertness, visual acuity).
- Do not take leftover medication for other disorders, and do not let anyone else take this prescription.
- Report severe nausea, vomiting, constipation, shortness of breath, or difficulty breathing.

▽mephentermine sulfate

(me fen' ter meen)

Wyamine Sulfate

PREGNANCY CATEGORY C

Drug class

Sympathomimetic

Therapeutic actions

Sympathomimetic amine that acts directly and indirectly (causes norepinephrine release); increases cardiac output, increases peripheral resistance.

Indications

- Treatment of hypotension secondary to ganglionic blockade, spinal anesthesia
- Emergency maintenance of BP until blood or blood substitute is available

Contraindications and cautions

- Contraindicated with hypotension induced by chlorpromazine (drug interaction will potentiate hypotension); use of MAO inhibitors.
- Use cautiously with CV disease, chronic illness, pregnancy, lactation.

Available forms

Injection—15, 30 mg/mL

Dosages
Adults

- *Prevention of hypotension attendant to spinal anesthesia:* 30–45 mg IM, 10–20 min prior to procedure.
- *Hypotension following spinal anesthesia:* 30–45 mg IV as a single injection. Repeat doses of 30 mg as necessary.
- *Hypotension following spinal anesthesia in obstetric patients:* Initial dose of 15 mg IV; repeat as needed.
- *Treatment of shock following hemorrhage:* Continuous IV infusion of 0.1% solution in 5% dextrose in water just until blood replacement can be achieved.

Pharmacokinetics

Route	Onset	Peak	Duration
IM	10–15 min	30–60 min	1–2 hr
IV	Immediate	Unknown	15–30 min

Metabolism: Hepatic; $T_{1/2}$: 15–20 min
Distribution: Crosses placenta; may enter breast milk
Excretion: Urine

▽IV facts

Preparation: Prepare 0.1% solution by adding 10 or 20 mL mephentermine, 30 mg/mL, to 250 or 500 mL of 5% dextrose in water, respectively.
Infusion: Administer as a single IV injection, each 30 mg over 1 min, or by continuous infusion of 0.1% solution; regulate dose based on BP response.

Adverse effects
- **CNS:** *Anxiety,* fear, hallucinations
- **CV:** *BP changes,* arrhythmias (most likely with heart disease)

Interactions
✳ Drug-drug • Decreased effects of guanethidine with mephentermine • Severe and sometimes fatal reactions (including hypertensive crisis and intracranial hemorrhage) with MAOIs, furazolidone • Increased likelihood of serious arrhythmias with halogenated hydrocarbon anesthetics

■ Nursing considerations
Assessment
- **History:** Hypotension induced by chlorpromazine; use of MAOIs, CV disease, chronic illness, pregnancy, lactation
- **Physical:** T; skin color, texture, lesions; orientation; P, auscultation, BP, orthostatic BP, perfusion; R, adventitious sounds; liver, kidney function tests

Interventions
- Monitor BP continously during and for several hours after administration.
- Arrange for immediate replacement with blood or blood products if used in emergency situation for shock.
- Drug teaching should be incorporated into total teaching plan of patient receiving spinal anesthesia.

Teaching points
- Drug may produce a feeling of anxiety.
- Report difficulty breathing, numbness or tingling, palpitations.

▷ mephenytoin
(me fen' i toyn)

Mesantoin

PREGNANCY CATEGORY C

Drug classes
Antiepileptic agent
Hydantoin

Therapeutic actions
Has antiepileptic activity without causing general CNS depression; stabilizes neuronal membranes and prevents hyperexcitability caused by excessive stimulation; limits the spread of seizure activity from an active focus.

Indications
- Control of grand mal (tonic-clonic), psychomotor, focal, and Jacksonian seizures in patients refractory to less toxic antiepileptic drugs

Contraindications and cautions
- Contraindicated with hypersensitivity to hydantoins; pregnancy; lactation; hepatic abnormalities; hematologic disorders.
- Use cautiously with acute intermittent porphyria; hypotension, severe myocardial insufficiency; diabetes mellitus, hyperglycemia.

Available forms
Tablets—100 mg

Dosages
Adults
Start with 50–100 mg/day PO during the first wk. Thereafter increase the daily dose by 50–100 mg at weekly intervals. No dose should be increased until it has been taken for at least 1 wk. Average dose ranges from 200–600 mg/day PO. Up to 800 mg/day may be needed for full seizure control.
- *Replacement therapy:* 50–100 mg/day PO during the first wk. Gradually increase (above), while decreasing the dose of discontinued drug, over 3–6 wk. If patient is also receiving phenobarbital, continue until the transition is completed, then gradually withdraw phenobarbital.

Pediatric patients
Usual dose is 100–400 mg/day PO.
Geriatric patients and patients with hepatic impairment
Use caution and monitor for early signs of toxicity; mephenytoin is metabolized in the liver.

Pharmacokinetics

Route	Onset	Peak	Duration
Oral	30 min	1–3 hr	24–48 hr

Adverse effects in *Italics* are most common; those in **Bold** are life-threatening.

Metabolism: Hepatic; $T_{1/2}$: 144 hr
Distribution: Crosses placenta; enters breast milk
Excretion: Urine

Adverse effects

- **CNS:** *Nystagmus, ataxia, dysarthria, slurred speech, mental confusion, dizziness, drowsiness, insomnia, transient nervousness, motor twitchings, fatigue, irritability, depression, numbness, tremor, headache,* photophobia, diplopia, conjunctivitis
- **Dermatologic:** Scarlatiniform, morbilliform, maculopapular, urticarial and nonspecific rashes; also serious **dermatologic reactions**—bullous, exfoliative, or purpuric dermatitis, lupus erythematosus, and **Stevens-Johnson syndrome;** toxic epidermal necrolysis, hirsutism, alopecia, coarsening of the facial features, enlargement of the lips, Peyronie's disease
- **GI:** *Nausea,* vomiting, diarrhea, constipation, *gingival hyperplasia,* toxic hepatitis, **liver damage;** hypersensitivity reactions with hepatic involvement, including hepatocellular degeneration and **hepatocellular necrosis**
- **GU:** Nephrosis
- **Hematologic: Hematopoietic complications:** thrombocytopenia, leukopenia, granulocytopenia, agranulocytosis, pancytopenia; macrocytosis and megaloblastic anemia that usually respond to folic acid therapy; eosinophilia, monocytosis, leukocytosis, simple anemia, hemolytic anemia, aplastic anemia, hyperglycemia
- **Respiratory:** Pulmonary fibrosis, acute pneumonitis
- **Other:** Lymph node hyperplasia, sometimes progressing to frank malignant lymphoma; monoclonal gammopathy and multiple myeloma (prolonged therapy); polyarthropathy; osteomalacia; weight gain; chest pain; periarteritis nodosa

Interactions

✻ Drug-drug • Increased effects with: chloramphenicol, cimetidine, disulfiram, isoniazid, phenacemide, phenylbutazone, sulfonamides, trimethoprim • Complex interactions and effects when hydantoins and valproic acid are given together: toxicity with apparently normal serum ethotoin levels; decreased plasma levels of valproic acid; breakthrough seizures when the two drugs are given together • Decreased effects with antineoplastics, diazoxide, folic acid, rifampin, theophyllines • Increased effects and toxicity when primidone, oxyphenbutazone, fluconazole, amiodarone are given with hydantoins • Increased hepatotoxicity with acetaminophen • Decreased effects of the following drugs with hydantoins: corticosteroids, cyclosporine, dicumarol, disopyramide, doxycycline, estrogens, levodopa, methadone, metyrapone, mexiletine, hormonal contraceptives, quinestrol, carbamazepine

✻ Drug-lab test • Interference with the metyrapone and the 1-mg dexamethasone tests; avoid hydantoins for at least 7 days prior to metyrapone testing

■ Nursing considerations
Assessment

- **History:** Hypersensitivity to hydantoins; hepatic abnormalities; hematologic disorders; acute intermittent porphyria; hypotension, severe myocardial insufficiency; diabetes mellitus, hyperglycemia; pregnancy; lactation
- **Physical:** T; skin color, lesions; lymph node palpation; orientation, affect, reflexes, vision exam; P, BP; R, adventitious sounds; bowel sounds, normal output, liver evaluation; periodontal exam; liver function tests, urinalysis, CBC and differential, blood proteins, blood and urine glucose, EEG and ECG

Interventions

- Give with food to enhance absorption and reduce GI upset.
- Reduce dosage, discontinue mephenytoin, or substitute other antiepileptic medication gradually; abrupt discontinuation may precipitate status epilepticus.
- Mephenytoin is ineffective in controlling absence (petit mal) seizures; patients with combined seizures will need other medication for their absence seizures.
- Discontinue drug if rash, depression of blood count, enlarged lymph nodes, hypersensitivity reaction, signs of liver damage, or Peyronie's disease (induration of the corpora cavernosa of the penis) occurs; arrange to institute another antiepileptic drug promptly.

- Monitor CBC and differential before therapy is instituted, at 2 wk, 4 wk, and monthly thereafter for the first year, then every 3 mo. If neutrophils drop to between 2,500 and 1,600/mm^3, counts should be made every 2 wk. If neutrophils drop to < 1,600/mm^3, discontinue drug.
- Monitor hepatic function periodically during long-term therapy.
- Have lymph node enlargement occurring during therapy evaluated carefully, lymphadenopathy simulates Hodgkin's disease; lymph node hyperplasia may progress to lymphoma.
- Arrange dental instruction in oral hygiene techniques for long-term patients to prevent gum hyperplasia.
- Arrange counseling for childbearing-age women who need long-term maintenance therapy with antiepileptic drugs and who wish to become pregnant.

Teaching points
- Take this drug exactly as prescribed, with food to enhance absorption and reduce GI upset. Do not discontinue abruptly or change dosage, except on the advice of your health care provider.
- Be especially careful not to miss a dose if you are on once-a-day therapy.
- Maintain good oral hygiene (regular brushing and flossing) to prevent gum disease; have frequent dental checkups to prevent serious gum disease.
- Have frequent checkups to monitor drug response. Keep all follow-up appointments.
- These side effects may occur: drowsiness, dizziness, confusion, blurred vision (avoid driving or performing other tasks requiring alertness or visual acuity); GI upset (take with food; frequent, small meals may help).
- Wear a medical alert tag so that emergency medical personnel will know that you are an epileptic taking antiepileptic medication.
- This drug is associated with fetal abnormalities; it is advisable to use barrier contraceptives while on this drug; if you wish to become pregnant, consult with your health care provider.
- Report rash, severe nausea or vomiting, drowsiness, slurred speech, impaired coordination (ataxia), swollen glands, bleeding, swollen or tender gums, yellowish discoloration of the skin or eyes, joint pain, unexplained fever, sore throat, unusual bleeding or bruising, persistent headache, malaise, any indication of an infection or bleeding tendency, abnormal erection, pregnancy.

▽ **mephobarbital**
*(me foe **bar**' bi tal)*

Mebaral

PREGNANCY CATEGORY D

C-IV CONTROLLED SUBSTANCE

Drug classes
Barbiturate
Sedative and hypnotic
Antiepileptic agent

Therapeutic actions
General CNS depressant; barbiturates inhibit impulse conduction in the ascending RAS, depress the cerebral cortex, alter cerebellar function, depress motor output, and can produce excitation (especially with subanesthetic doses used with pain), sedation, hypnosis, anesthesia, and deep coma

Indications
- Sedative for the relief of anxiety, tension, and apprehension
- Antiepileptic for the treatment of partial and generalized tonic-clonic and cortical focal seizures

Contraindications and cautions
- Contraindicated with hypersensitivity to barbiturates; manifest or latent porphyria; marked liver impairment; nephritis; severe respiratory distress; previous addiction to sedative or hypnotic drugs; pregnancy.
- Use cautiously with acute or chronic pain (may cause paradoxical excitement or mask important symptoms); seizure disorders (abrupt discontinuation of daily doses can result in status epilepticus); lactation (secreted in breast milk; causes drowsiness in nursing infants); fever, hyperthyroidism, di-

abetes mellitus, severe anemia, pulmonary or cardiac disease, status asthmaticus, shock, uremia; impaired liver or kidney function, debilitation.

Available forms
Tablets—32, 50, 100 mg

Dosages
Adults
- *Daytime sedation:* 32–100 mg PO tid–qid. Optimum dose is 50 mg tid–qid PO.
- *Epilepsy:* Average dose is 400–600 mg/day PO. Start treatment with a low dose and gradually increase over 4–5 days until optimum dosage is reached. Give hs if seizures occur at night, during the day if attacks are diurnal. May be given with phenobarbital or with phenytoin; decrease dose of mephobarbital and phenobarbital to about half that when drug is used alone. Decrease dose of phenytoin, but not mephobarbital, when phenytoin is given with mephobarbital. Satisfactory results have been obtained with an average daily dose of 230 mg phenytoin and 600 mg mephobarbital.

Pediatric patients
Use caution: barbiturates may produce irritability, excitability, inappropriate tearfulness, and aggression. Base dosage on body weight, age (see Appendix K), and response.
- *Sedative:* 16–32 mg PO tid–qid.
- *Epilepsy:*
  < 5 yr: 16–32 mg tid–qid PO.
  > 5 yr: 32–64 mg tid–qid PO.

Geriatric patients or patients with debilitating disease
Reduce dosage and monitor closely; may produce excitement, depression, confusion.

Pharmacokinetics

Route	Onset	Peak	Duration
Oral	30–60 min	3–4 hr	10–16 hr

Metabolism: Hepatic; $T_{1/2}$: 11–67 hr
Distribution: Crosses placenta; enters breast milk
Excretion: Urine

Adverse effects
- **CNS:** *Somnolence,* agitation, confusion, hyperkinesia, ataxia, vertigo, CNS depression, nightmares, lethargy, residual sedation (hangover), paradoxical excitement, nervousness, psychiatric disturbance, hallucinations, insomnia, anxiety, dizziness, thinking abnormality
- **CV:** Bradycardia, hypotension, syncope
- **GI:** *Nausea, vomiting, constipation, diarrhea, epigastric pain*
- **Hypersensitivity:** Rashes, angioneurotic edema, serum sickness, morbiliform rash, urticaria; rarely, exfoliative dermatitis, **Stevens-Johnson syndrome**
- **Respiratory:** Hypoventilation, apnea, respiratory depression, laryngospasm, bronchospasm, **circulatory collapse**
- **Other:** Tolerance, psychological and physical dependence; **withdrawal syndrome**

Interactions
✱ **Drug-drug** • Increased CNS depression with alcohol and other CNS depressants • Increased risk of nephrotoxicity with methoxyflurane • Decreased effects of the following with barbiturates: theophyllines, oral anticoagulants, beta-blockers, doxycycline, griseofulvin, corticosteroids, hormonal contraceptives and estrogens, metronidazole, phenylbutazones, quinidine, carbamazepine

■ Nursing considerations
Assessment
- **History:** Hypersensitivity to barbiturates, manifest or latent porphyria; marked liver impairment, nephritis, severe respiratory distress; previous addiction to sedative-hypnotic drugs, acute or chronic pain, seizure disorders, fever, hyperthyroidism, diabetes mellitus, severe anemia, pulmonary or cardiac disease, shock, uremia, debilitation, pregnancy, lactation
- **Physical:** Weight; T; skin color, lesions; orientation, affect, reflexes; P, BP, orthostatic BP; R, adventitious sounds; bowel sounds, normal output, liver evaluation; liver and kidney function tests, blood and urine glucose, BUN

Interventions
- Monitor patient responses, blood levels when above interacting drugs are given with mephobarbital; suggest alternate contraception to women on hormonal contraceptives.

- Provide resuscitative equipment on standby in case of respiratory depression, hypersensitivity reaction.
- Taper dosage gradually after repeated use, especially in epileptic patients. When changing antiepileptic medications, taper dosage of discontinued drug while replacement drug dosage is increased.

Teaching points

- Take this drug exactly as prescribed; do not reduce the dosage or discontinue this drug (when used for epilepsy) without consulting care provider; the abrupt discontinuation of the drug could result in a serious increase in seizures.
- This drug is habit forming.
- Avoid alcohol, sleep-inducing, or OTC drugs because these could cause dangerous effects.
- Change birth control method from oral contraception to barrier contraceptives while on mephobarbital; avoid becoming pregnant.
- These side effects may occur: drowsiness, dizziness, hangover, impaired thinking (may be transient; avoid driving or engaging in dangerous activities); GI upset (taking the drug with food may help); dreams, nightmares, difficulty concentrating, fatigue, nervousness (reversible).
- Wear a medical ID tag to alert emergency medical personnel that you are an epileptic taking this medication.
- Report severe dizziness, weakness, drowsiness that persists, rash or skin lesions, fever, sore throat, mouth sores, easy bruising or bleeding, nosebleed, petechiae, pregnancy.

▽meprobamate
*(me proe **ba'** mate)*

Apo-Meprobamate (CAN), Equanil, Miltown, Novomepro (CAN)

PREGNANCY CATEGORY D

C-IV CONTROLLED SUBSTANCE

Drug class
Antianxiety agent

Therapeutic actions
Has effects at many sites in the CNS, including the thalamus and limbic system; inhibits multineuronal spinal reflexes; is mildly tranquilizing; has some anticonvulsant and central skeletal muscle relaxing properties.

Indications
- Management of anxiety disorders for the short-term relief of the symptoms of anxiety (anxiety or tension associated with the stress of everyday life usually does not require treatment with anxiolytic drugs); effectiveness for longer than 4 mo not established.

Contraindications and cautions
- Contraindicated with hypersensitivity to meprobamate or to related drugs, such as carisoprodol; acute intermittent porphyria; hepatic or renal impairment; pregnancy; lactation.
- Use cautiously with epilepsy (drug may precipitate seizures).

Available forms
Tablets—200, 400 mg

Dosages
Adults
1,200–1,600 mg/day PO in 3 to 4 divided doses. Do not exceed 2,400 mg/day.
Pediatric patients
6–12 yr: 100–200 mg PO bid–tid.
< 6 yr: Safety and efficacy not established.
Geriatric patients
Use lowest effective dose to avoid oversedation.

Pharmacokinetics

Route	Onset	Peak
Oral	Varies	1–3 hr

Metabolism: Hepatic; $T_{1/2}$: 6–17 hr
Distribution: Crosses placenta; enters breast milk
Excretion: Urine

Adverse effects
- **CNS:** *Drowsiness, ataxia, dizziness, slurred speech, headache, vertigo, weakness, impairment of visual accommodation,* eu-

---

Adverse effects in *Italics* are most common; those in **Bold** are life-threatening.

phoria, overstimulation, paradoxical excitement, paresthesias
- **CV:** *Palpitations, tachycardia,* various arrhythmias, syncope, **hypotensive crisis**
- **GI:** *Nausea, vomiting, diarrhea*
- **Hematologic:** Agranulocytosis, aplastic anemia; thrombocytopenic purpura; exacerbation of porphyric symptoms
- **Hypersensitivity:** Allergic or idiosyncratic reactions (usually seen between first and fourth doses in patients without previous drug exposure): *itchy, urticarial or erythematous maculopapular rash;* leukopenia, acute nonthrombocytopenic purpura, petechiae, ecchymoses, eosinophilia, peripheral edema, adenopathy, fever, fixed drug eruption; hyperpyrexia, chills, angioneurotic edema, bronchospasm, oliguria, anuria, anaphylaxis, erythema multiforme, exfoliative dermatitis, stomatitis, proctitis; **Stevens-Johnson syndrome,** bullous dermatitis
- **Other:** Physical, psychological dependence; withdrawal reaction

Interactions
✳ **Drug-drug** • Additive CNS depression with alcohol, narcotics, barbiturates, and other CNS depressants

■ Nursing considerations
Assessment
- **History:** Hypersensitivity to meprobamate or to related drugs; acute intermittent porphyria; hepatic or renal impairment; epilepsy; pregnancy; lactation
- **Physical:** T; skin color, lesions; orientation, affect, reflexes, vision exam; P, BP; R, adventitious sounds; bowel sounds, normal output, liver evaluation; liver and kidney function tests, CBC and differential, EEG and ECG

Interventions
- Supervise dose and amount for patients who are addiction prone or alcoholic.
- Dispense least amount of drug feasible to patients who are depressed or suicidal.
- Withdraw gradually over 2 wk if patient has been maintained on high doses for weeks or months.
- Withdraw drug if allergic or idiosyncratic reactions occur.

- Caution patient about the need to avoid pregnancy while on this drug.
- Provide epinephrine, antihistamines, corticosteroids, life support equipment on standby in case allergic or idiosyncratic reaction occurs.

Teaching points
- Take this drug exactly as prescribed. This drug may not be effective after several months of therapy; continue to see your health care provider.
- Avoid alcohol, sleep-inducing, or OTC drugs; these could cause dangerous effects.
- These side effects may occur: drowsiness, dizziness, light-headedness, blurred vision (avoid driving or performing other tasks requiring alertness or visual acuity); GI upset (frequent, small meals may help).
- Use barrier method of birth control while on this drug; do not take this drug during pregnancy. Consult your physician immediately if you decide to become pregnant or find that you are pregnant.
- Report rash, sore throat, fever, easy bruising, bleeding.

M

▽ mercaptopurine (6-mercaptopurine, 6-MP)
*(mer kap toe **pyoor' een**)*

Purinethol

PREGNANCY CATEGORY D

Drug classes
Antimetabolite
Antineoplastic

Therapeutic actions
Tumor-inhibiting properties, probably due to interference with purine nucleotide synthesis and hence with RNA and DNA synthesis, leading to cell death; cell-cycle specific.

Indications
- Remission induction, remission consolidation, and maintenance therapy of acute leukemia (lymphocytic, myelogenous)

Contraindications and cautions

- Contraindicated with allergy to mercaptopurine, prior resistance to mercaptopurine (cross-resistance with thioguanine is frequent), hematopoietic depression, pregnancy, lactation.
- Use cautiously with impaired renal function (slower elimination and greater accumulation; reduce dosage).

Available forms

Tablets—50 mg

Dosages

Adults and pediatric patients

- *Induction therapy:* Usual initial dose is 2.5 mg/kg/day PO (about 100–200 mg in adults, 50 mg in the average 5-year-old). Continue daily for several weeks. After 4 wk, if no clinical improvement or toxicity, increase to 5 mg/kg/day.
- *Maintenance therapy after complete hematologic remission:* 1.5–2.5 mg/kg/day PO as a single daily dose. Often effective in children with acute lymphatic leukemia, especially in combination with methotrexate.

Patients with renal impairment

Reduce dosage and monitor patient closely.

Pharmacokinetics

Route	Onset	Peak
Oral	Varies	2 hr

Metabolism: Hepatic; $T_{1/2}$ 20–50 min
Distribution: Crosses placenta; enters breast milk
Excretion: Urine

Adverse effects

- **GI:** Hepatotoxicity; oral lesions—resemble thrush; nausea; vomiting; anorexia, pancreatitis
- **Hematologic:** *Bone marrow depression, immunosuppression, hyperuricemia* as consequence of antineoplastic effect and cell lysis
- **Other:** Drug fever, **cancer,** chromosomal aberrations, rash, hyperpigmentation

Interactions

✳ **Drug-drug** • Increased risk of severe toxicity with allopurinol; reduce mercaptopurine to one-third to one-fourth the usual dose • Decreased or reversed actions of nondepolarizing neuromuscular relaxants (atracurium, gallamine, pancuronium, tubocurarine, vecuronium)

■ Nursing considerations

Assessment

- **History:** Allergy to mercaptopurine; prior resistance to mercaptopurine; hematopoietic depression; impaired renal function; pregnancy; lactation
- **Physical:** T; mucous membranes, liver evaluation, abdominal exam; CBC, differential, Hgb, platelet counts; renal and liver function tests; urinalysis; serum uric acid

Interventions

- Evaluate hematopoietic status before and frequently during therapy.
- Round dose to nearest 25 mg (tablets are scored).
- Ensure that patient is well hydrated before and during therapy to minimize adverse effects of hyperuricemia.
- Caution patient about the risk of serious fetal harm while on this drug; advise the use of barrier contraceptives.
- Administer as a single daily dose.

Teaching points

- Drink adequate fluids; drink at least 8–10 glasses of fluid each day.
- These side effects may occur: mouth sores (frequent mouth care will be needed); miscarriages (use barrier contraceptive method of birth control); nausea, vomiting.
- Have frequent, regular medical follow-ups, including blood tests to follow the drug effects.
- Report fever, chills, sore throat, unusual bleeding or bruising, yellow discoloration of the skin or eyes, abdominal pain, flank pain, joint pain, fever, weakness, diarrhea.

Adverse effects in *Italics* are most common; those in **Bold** are life-threatening.

▽ **meropenem**

*(mare ob **pen**' ehm)*

Merrem IV

PREGNANCY CATEGORY B

Drug class
Antibiotic (carbapenem)

Therapeutic actions
Bactericidal: inhibits synthesis of bacterial cell wall and causes cell death in susceptible cells.

Indications
- Susceptible intra-abdominal infections caused by viridans group streptococci, *E. coli, K. pneumoniae, P. aeruginosa, B. fragilis, B. thetaiotaomicron,* and Peptostreptococcus
- Bacterial meningitis caused by *S. pneumoniae, H. influenzae, N. meningitidis* in pediatric patients ≥ 3 mo only

Contraindications and cautions
- Contraindicated with allergy to cephalosporins, penicillins, beta-lactams; renal failure; lactation.
- Use cautiously with CNS disorders, seizures, renal or hepatic impairment, pregnancy.

Available forms
Powder for injection—500 mg, 1 g

Dosages
Adults
1 g IV q 8 hr.
Pediatric patients
< 3 mo: Not recommended.
> 3 mo:
- *Intra-abdominal infections:* < 50 kg: 20 mg/kg IV q 8 hr. > 50 kg: 1 g IV q 8 hr.
- *Meningitis:* < 50 kg: 40 mg/kg IV q 8 hr. > 50 kg: 2 g IV q 8 hr.
Geriatric patients or patients with impaired renal function

Creatinine Clearance (mL/min)	Dose
26–50	1 g IV q 12 hr
10–25	500 mg IV q 12 hr
< 10	500 mg IV q 24 hr

Pharmacokinetics

Route	Onset	Peak	Duration
IV	Immediate	5 min	10–12 min

Metabolism: $T_{1/2}$: 0.8–1.1 hr
Distribution: Crosses placenta; passes into breast milk
Excretion: Renal—unchanged

▽ IV facts
Preparation: Dilute in 0.9% sodium chloride injection; 5% or 10% dextrose injection; dextrose in sodium chloride, potassium chloride, sodium bicarbonate, Normosol-M, Ringer's lactate; mannitol injection; Ringer's injection; Ringer's lactate injection; sodium lactate injection 1/6N; sodium bicarbonate or sterile water for injection. Store at room temperature; stability in each solution varies—consult manufacturer's instructions if not used immediately.
Infusion: Infuse over 15–30 min or give by direct IV injection over 3–5 min.
Incompatibilities: Do not mix in solution with other drugs.

Adverse effects
- **CNS:** *Headache,* dizziness, lethargy, paresthesias, **seizures,** insomnia
- **GI:** *Nausea, vomiting, diarrhea, anorexia, abdominal pain, flatulence,* **pseudomembranous colitis,** liver toxicity
- **Other:** *Superinfections,* abscess (redness, tenderness, heat, tissue sloughing), inflammation at injection site, *phlebitis, rash,* urticaria, pruritus

Interactions
✷ **Drug-drug •** Possible toxic levels if combined with probenecid; avoid this combination

■ Nursing considerations
Assessment
- **History:** Allergy to cephalosporins, penicillins, beta lactams; renal failure; CNS disorders, seizures, renal or hepatic impairment; pregnancy, lactation
- **Physical:** Orientation; affect; skin color, lesions; culture site of infection; R, adventitious sounds; bowel sounds, abdominal exam; renal and liver function tests

M

Interventions

- Culture infected area and arrange for sensitivity tests before beginning therapy.
- Monitor for occurrence of superinfections and arrange treatment as appropriate.
- Discontinue drug at any sign of colitis and arrange for appropriate supportive treatment.

Teaching points

- This drug can only be given IV.
- These side effects may occur: stomach upset, loss of appetite, nausea (take drug with food); diarrhea (stay near bathroom); headache, dizziness.
- Report severe diarrhea, difficulty breathing, unusual tiredness, pain at injection site.

▽mesalamine (5-aminosalicylic acid, 5-ASA)

(me sal' a meen)

Asacol, Mesasal (CAN), Pentasa, Quintasa (CAN), Rowasa, Salofalk (CAN)

PREGNANCY CATEGORY B

Drug class

Anti-inflammatory agent

Therapeutic actions

Mechanism of action is unknown; thought to be a direct, local anti-inflammatory effect in the colon where mesalamine blocks cyclooxygenase and inhibits prostaglandin production in the colon.

Indications

- Treatment of active mild to moderate distal ulcerative colitis (oral)
- Treatment of active, ulcerative proctitis or proctosigmoiditis (suppository)

Contraindications and cautions

- Contraindicated with hypersensitivity to mesalamine, salicylates, any component of the formulation.
- Use cautiously with renal impairment, pregnancy, lactation.

Available forms

DR tablets—400 mg; CR capsules—250 mg; suppositories—500 mg; rectal suspension—4 g/60 mL

Dosages
Adults
Rectal

- *Suspension enema:* 60 mL units in one rectal instillation (4 g) once a day, preferably hs, and retained for approximately 8 hr. Usual course of therapy is 3–6 wk. Effects may be seen within 3–21 days.
- *Rectal suppository:* 500 mg (1 suppository) bid. Retain suppository for 1–3 hr or more. Usual course is 3–6 wk.

Oral

Tablets—800 mg PO tid for 6 wk; capsules—1 g PO qid for up to 8 wk.

Pediatric patients

Safety and efficacy not established.

Pharmacokinetics

Route	Onset	Peak
Oral	Varies	3–6 hr
Rectal	Slow	3–6 hr

Metabolism: $T_{1/2}$: 5–10 hr
Distribution: Unknown
Excretion: Feces

Adverse effects

- **CNS:** *Headache, fatigue, malaise,* dizziness, asthenia, insomnia
- **GI:** *Abdominal pain, cramps, discomfort; gas; flatulence; nausea;* diarrhea, bloating, hemmorhoids, rectal pain, constipation
- **GU:** UTI, urinary burning
- **Other:** *Flulike symptoms, fever, cold,* rash, back pain, hair loss, peripheral edema, pruritus

■ Nursing considerations
Assessment

- **History:** Hypersensitivity to mesalamine, salicylates, any component of the formulation; renal impairment; lactation
- **Physical:** T, hair status; reflexes, affect; abdominal exam, rectal exam; urinary output; renal function tests

Interventions

- Administer enemas as follows: Shake bottle well to ensure suspension is homogeneous. Remove protective applicator sheath; hold bottle at the neck to ensure that none of the dose is lost. Have patient lie on the left side (to facilitate migration of drug into the sigmoid colon) with the lower leg extended and the upper leg flexed forward. Knee-chest position can be used if more acceptable to the patient. Gently insert the application tip into the rectum pointing toward the umbilicus; steadily squeeze the bottle to discharge the medication. Patient must retain medication for approximately 8 hr.
- Administer rectal suppository as follows: remove the foil wrapper; avoid excessive handling (suppository will melt at body temperature); insert completely into the rectum with pointed end first; have patient retain for 3 hr or more.
- Caution patient not to chew tablet; swallow whole. Notify physician if intact tablets are found in the stool.
- Monitor patients with renal impairment for possible adverse effects.

Teaching points

- This drug may be given as a suspension enema, so the medication must be retained for approximately 8 hr; it is best given hs to facilitate the retention; the effects of the drug are usually seen within 3–21 days, but a full course of therapy is about 6 wk. (Review administration with patient and significant other.)
- Administer rectal suppository as follows: remove the foil wrapper; avoid excessive handling (suppository will melt at body temperature); insert completely into the rectum with pointed end first; retain for 3 hr or more; staining of clothing may occur, use of a protective pad is suggested.
- Do not chew oral tablets; swallow whole. If intact tablets are seen in the stool, notify physician.
- These side effects may occur: abdominal cramping, discomfort, pain, gas (relax; maintain the position used for insertion to relieve pressure on the abdomen); headache, fatigue, fever, flulike symptoms (request medication); hair loss (usually mild and transient).
- Report difficulty breathing, rash, severe abdominal pain, fever, headache.

▷ mesna

See *Less Commonly Used Drugs*, p. 1346.

▷ mesoridazine besylate

*(mez oh **rid'** a zeen)*

Serentil

PREGNANCY CATEGORY C

Drug classes

Phenothiazine (piperidine)
Dopaminergic blocking agent
Antipsychotic
Antianxiety agent

Therapeutic actions

Mechanism not fully understood: antipsychotic drugs block postsynaptic dopamine receptors in the brain, depressing the RAS, including the parts of the brain involved with wakefulness and emesis; anticholinergic, antihistaminic (H_1), and alpha-adrenergic blocking activity also may contribute to some of its therapeutic (and adverse) actions.

Indications

- Treatment of refractory schizophrenia

Contraindications and cautions

- Contraindicated with coma or severe CNS depression; bone marrow depression; blood dyscrasia; circulatory collapse; subcortical brain damage; Parkinson's disease; liver damage; cerebral arteriosclerosis; coronary disease; severe hypotension or hypertension; history of prolonged QTc intervals.
- Use cautiously with respiratory disorder ("silent pneumonia"); glaucoma, prostatic hypertrophy, epilepsy or history of epilepsy, breast cancer, thyrotoxicosis, peptic ulcer, decreased renal function, myelography within previous 24 hr or scheduled within 48 hr, exposure to heat or phosphorous insecticides; pregnancy; lactation; children < 12 yr, especially those with chickenpox, CNS infections (children are especially sus-

ceptible to dystonias that may confound the diagnosis of Reye's syndrome).

Available forms

Tablets—10, 25, 50, 100 mg; concentrate—25 mg/mL; injection—25 mg/mL

Dosages

Full clinical effects may require 6 wk–6 mo of therapy.

Adults

Initial dosage 50 mg PO tid (optimal total dosage range 100–400 mg/day).

IM

Initial dose 25 mg; may repeat in 30–60 min if necessary (optimum dosage range 25–200 mg/day).

Pediatric patients

Generally not recommended for children < 12 yr.

Geriatric patients

Use lower doses, and increase dosage more gradually than in younger patients.

Pharmacokinetics

Route	Onset	Peak	Duration
Oral	Varies	2–4 hr	4–6 hr
IM	Rapid	30 min	6–8 hr

Metabolism: Hepatic; $T_{1/2}$: 24–48 hr
Distribution: Crosses placenta; enters breast milk
Excretion: Urine and feces

Adverse effects

- **Autonomic:** *Dry mouth,* salivation, nasal congestion, nausea, vomiting, anorexia, fever, pallor, flushed facies, sweating, constipation, paralytic ileus, urinary retention, incontinence, polyuria, enuresis, priapism, ejaculation inhibition, male impotence
- **CNS:** *Drowsiness,* insomnia, vertigo, headache, weakness, tremor, ataxia, slurring, cerebral edema, **seizures,** exacerbation of psychotic symptoms, extrapyramidal syndromes—*pseudoparkinsonism; dystonias; akathisia,* tardive dyskinesias, potentially irreversible (no known treatment), neuroleptic malignant syndrome (NMS)
- **CV:** Hypotension, *orthostatic hypotension,* hypertension, tachycardia, bradycardia, cardiac arrest, CHF, cardiomegaly, **refractory arrhythmias, QTc interval prolongation** (which has been associated with arrhythmias and sudden death), pulmonary edema
- **Endocrine:** Lactation, breast engorgement in females, galactorrhea; SIADH; amenorrhea, menstrual irregularities; gynecomastia; changes in libido; hyperglycemia or hypoglycemia; glycosuria; hyponatremia; pituitary tumor with hyperprolactinemia; inhibition of ovulation; infertility; pseudopregnancy; reduced urinary levels of gonadotropins, estrogens, progestins
- **Hematologic:** Eosinophilia, leukopenia, leukocytosis, anemia; aplastic anemia; hemolytic anemia; thrombocytopenic or nonthrombocytopenic purpura; pancytopenia
- **Hypersensitivity:** Jaundice, urticaria, angioneurotic edema, laryngeal edema, photosensitivity, eczema, asthma, anaphylactoid reactions, exfoliative dermatitis
- **Respiratory:** Bronchospasm, laryngospasm, dyspnea, suppression of cough reflex and potential for aspiration

Interactions

✱ Drug-drug • Additive CNS depression with alcohol and other CNS depressants • Additive anticholinergic effects and possibly decreased antipsychotic efficacy with anticholinergic drugs • Increased likelihood of seizures with metrizamide (contrast agent used in myelography) • Decreased antihypertensive effect of guanethidine with antipsychotic drugs • Risk of serious to fatal cardiac arrhythmias if combined with drugs that prolong the QTc interval, including disopyramide, procainamide, quinidine, fluoxetine, and paroxetine; avoid these combinations

✱ Drug-lab test • False-positive pregnancy tests (less likely if serum test is used) • Increase in PBI, not attributable to an increase in thyroxine

■ Nursing considerations
Assessment

- **History:** Coma or severe CNS depression, bone marrow depression, circulatory collapse, subcortical brain damage, Parkinson's disease, liver damage, cerebral arteriosclerosis, coronary disease, history of prolonged QTc interval, severe hypotension or hypertension, respiratory disorders, glaucoma, prostatic hypertrophy, epilepsy, breast cancer, thyrotoxicosis, peptic ulcer, decreased renal function, myelography within previous 24 hr or scheduled within 48 hr, exposure to heat or phosphorous insecticides, lactation, children < 12 yr

- **Physical:** Weight, T; reflexes, orientation, intraocular pressure; P, BP, orthostatic BP; R, adventitious sounds; bowel sounds and normal output, liver evaluation; urinary output, prostate size; baseline ECG; serum K^+ levels, CBC, urinalysis, thyroid, liver and kidney function tests

Interventions

- Obtain baseline and periodic ECG and serum K^+ levels; ensure that serum K^+ is maintained within normal limits. If QTc interval becomes prolonged, over 450 msec, discontinue drug and monitor patient carefully.
- Do not change dosage in long-term therapy more often than weekly; drug requires 4–7 days to achieve steady state plasma levels.
- Avoid skin contact with oral solution; contact dermatitis has occurred.
- Discontinue drug if serum creatinine, BUN become abnormal or if WBC count is depressed.
- Monitor elderly patients for dehydration, and institute remedial measures promptly; sedation and decreased sensation related to CNS effects of drug can lead to severe dehydration.
- Consult physician regarding appropriate warning of patient or patient's guardian about tardive dyskinesias.
- Consult physician about dosage reduction; use of anticholinergic antiparkinsonian drugs (controversial) if extrapyramidal effects occur.

Teaching points

- Take drug exactly as prescribed.
- Avoid skin contact with drug solutions.
- Avoid driving or engaging in other dangerous activities if CNS, vision changes occur.
- Avoid prolonged exposure to sun or use a sunscreen or covering garments.
- Maintain fluid intake and use precautions against heatstroke in hot weather.

- Report sore throat, fever, unusual bleeding or bruising, rash, weakness, tremors, impaired vision, dark colored urine (pink or reddish brown urine), pale stools, yellowing of the skin or eyes.

▽ metaproterenol sulfate

(met a proe ter' e nole)

Alupent, Orcipren (CAN), Tanta Orciprenaline (CAN)

PREGNANCY CATEGORY C

Drug classes

Sympathomimetic
Beta$_2$-selective adrenergic agonist
Bronchodilator
Antiasthmatic agent

Therapeutic actions

In low doses, acts relatively selectively at beta$_2$-adrenergic receptors to cause bronchodilation; at higher doses, beta$_2$ selectivity is lost and the drug also acts at beta$_1$ receptors to cause typical sympathomimetic cardiac effects.

Indications

- Prophylaxis and treatment of bronchial asthma and reversible bronchospasm that may occur with bronchitis and emphysema
- Treatment of acute asthmatic attacks in children ≥ 6 yr (5% solution for inhalation only)

Contraindications and cautions

- Contraindicated with hypersensitivity to metaproterenol; tachyarrhythmias, tachycardia caused by digitalis intoxication; general anesthesia with halogenated hydrocarbons or cyclopropane, which sensitize the myocardium to catecholamines.
- Use cautiously with unstable vasomotor system disorders; hypertension; CAD; history of stroke; COPD patients who have developed degenerative heart disease; hyperthyroidism; history of seizure disorders; psychoneurotic individuals; pregnancy; labor and delivery (may inhibit labor; parenteral use of beta$_2$-adrenergic agonists can accelerate fetal heartbeat, cause hypoglycemia, hypokalemia, and pulmonary edema in the mother

M

and hypoglycemia in the neonate); lactation.

Available forms
Aerosol solution for inhalation—0.4%, 0.6%, 5%; canister—0.65 mg/actuation

Dosages
Adults
Inhalation
- *Metered-dose inhaler:* 2–3 inhalations q 3–4 hr. Do not exceed 12 inhalations/day.
- *Inhalant solutions:* Administer tid–qid from hand bulb nebulizer or using an IPPB device, following manufacturer's instructions.
Pediatric patients
Inhalation
> *12 yr:* Same as adult.
< *12 yr:* Not recommended.
Nebulizer
6–*12 yr:* 0.1–0.2 mL in saline to a total volume of 3 mL.
Geriatric patients
Patients > 60 yr are more likely to develop adverse effects, use extreme caution.

Pharmacokinetics

Route	Onset	Peak	Duration
Inhalation	1–4 min	1 hr	3–4 hr

Metabolism: Liver and tissue; $T_{1/2}$: unknown
Excretion: Bile and feces

Adverse effects
- **CNS:** *Restlessness, apprehension, anxiety, fear, CNS stimulation,* hyperkinesia, insomnia, tremor, drowsiness, irritability, weakness, vertigo, headache
- **CV:** Cardiac arrhythmias, *tachycardia,* palpitations, PVCs (rare), anginal pain—less likely with bronchodilator doses of this drug than with bronchodilator doses of a nonselective beta-agonist (isoproterenol), changes in BP
- **GI:** *Nausea, vomiting, heartburn,* unusual or bad taste
- **Respiratory:** Respiratory difficulties, pulmonary edema, coughing, bronchospasm, paradoxical airway resistance with repeated, excessive use of inhalation preparations
- **Other:** *Sweating, pallor, flushing*

■ Nursing considerations
Assessment
- **History:** Hypersensitivity to metaproterenol; tachyarrhythmias; general anesthesia with halogenated hydrocarbons or cyclopropane; unstable vasomotor system disorders; hypertension; CAD; stroke; COPD patients who have developed degenerative heart disease; hyperthyroidism; seizure disorders; psychoneuroses; pregnancy; labor; lactation.
- **Physical:** Weight; skin color, temperature, turgor; orientation, reflexes; P, BP; R, adventitious sounds; blood and urine glucose, serum electrolytes, thyroid function tests, ECG

Interventions
- Use minimal doses for minimal periods of time—drug tolerance can occur with prolonged use.
- Maintain a beta-adrenergic blocker (a cardioselective beta-blocker such as atenolol should be used in patients with respiratory distress) on standby in case cardiac arrhythmias occur.
- Do not exceed recommended dosage. Administer aerosol during second half of inspiration, when airways are wider and distribution is more extensive.
- Consult manufacturer's instructions for use of aerosal delivery equipment; specifics of administration vary with each product.

Teaching points
- Do not exceed recommended dosage; adverse effects or loss of effectiveness may result. Read product instructions and ask your health care provider or pharmacist if you have any questions.
- These side effects may occur: nausea, vomiting, change in taste (small, frequent meals may help); dizziness, drowsiness, fatigue, weakness (use caution if driving or performing tasks that require alertness); irritability, apprehension, sweating, flushing.
- Report chest pain, dizziness, insomnia, weakness, tremor or irregular heartbeat, difficulty breathing, productive cough, failure to respond to usual dosage.

Adverse effects in *Italics* are most common; those in **Bold** are life-threatening.

▽metaxalone
*(me **tax**' ah lone)*

Skelaxin

PREGNANCY CATEGORY C

Drug class
Centrally acting skeletal muscle relaxant

Therapeutic actions
Precise mechanism of action not known, but may be due to general CNS depression; does not directly relax tense skeletal muscles or directly affect the motor endplate or motor nerves.

Indications
- Adjunct to rest, physical therapy, and other measures for the relief of discomfort associated with acute, painful musculoskeletal disorders

Contraindications and cautions
- Contraindicated with hypersensitivity to metaxalone; tendency for hemolytic or other anemias; severe renal or hepatic dysfunction, lactation.
- Use cautiously with mild liver dysfunction, pregnancy.

Available forms
Tablets—400 mg

Dosages
Adults and patients > 12 yr
800 mg PO tid–qid.
Pediatric patients < 12 yr
Not recommended.

Pharmacokinetics

Route	Onset	Peak	Duration
Oral	60 min	2 hr	4–6 hr

Metabolism: Hepatic; $T_{1/2}$: 2–3 hr
Distribution: Crosses placenta; may pass into breast milk
Excretion: Urine

Adverse effects
- **CNS:** *Lightheadedness, dizziness, drowsiness,* headache, fever, blurred vision
- **Dermatologic:** Urticaria, pruritus, rash
- **GI:** *Nausea,* vomiting, GI upset, liver dysfunction
- **Other: Hemolytic anemia, leukopenia**

Interactions
✳ **Drug-drug** • Increased risk of sedation with other CNS depressants and alcohol
✳ **Drug-lab test** • False-positive Benedict's test; use of a more specific glucose test is advised

■ Nursing considerations
Assessment
- **History:** Hypersensitivity to metaxalone; tendency for hemolytic or other anemias; severe renal or hepatic dysfunction; lactation, pregnancy
- **Physical:** Body temperature; skin—color, lesions; orientation, affect, vision exam, reflexes; bowel sounds, normal output; CBC, renal and hepatic function tests

Interventions
- Establish safety precautions if dizziness, drowsiness, blurred vision occur (siderails, accompany patient when ambulating, etc.).
- Arrange for analgesics if headache occurs (and possibly as adjunct for relief of discomfort of muscle spasm).
- Provide positioning, massage, warm soaks as appropriate for relief of pain of muscle spasm.
- Provide support and encouragement to deal with discomfort of underlying condition, drug effects.

Teaching points
- Take this drug exactly as prescribed. Do not take a higher dosage than that prescribed.
- Continue the use of rest, physical therapy, and other measures to relieve the discomfort.
- Avoid the use of alcohol, sleep-inducing or over-the-counter drugs while you are on this drug. These could cause dangerous effects. If you feel that you need one of these preparations, consult your health care provider.
- These side effects may occur: drowsiness, dizziness (avoid driving a car or engaging in activities that require alertness if these occur); nausea (taking drug with food and eating frequent small meals may help).

M

- Report rash, itching, yellow discoloration of the skin or eyes.

▽ metformin hydrochloride

(met fore' min)

Glucophage, Glucophage XR

PREGNANCY CATEGORY B

Drug class
Antidiabetic agent

Therapeutic actions
Exact mechanism is not understood; possibly increases peripheral utilization of glucose, increases production of insulin, decreases hepatic glucose production and alters intestinal absorption of glucose.

Indications
- Adjunct to diet to lower blood glucose with non–insulin-dependent diabetes mellitus (type 2) in patients ≥ 10 yr; extended release in patients ≥ 17 yr.
- As part of combination therapy with a sulfonylurea or insulin when either drug alone cannot control glucose levels in patients with non–insulin-dependent diabetes mellitus

Contraindications and cautions
- Allergy to metformin; CHF; diabetes complicated by fever, severe infections, severe trauma, major surgery, ketosis, acidosis, coma (use insulin); type 1 or juvenile diabetes, serious hepatic impairment, serious renal impairment, uremia, thyroid or endocrine impairment, glycosuria, hyperglycemia associated with primary renal disease; labor and delivery—if metformin is used during pregnancy, discontinue drug at least 1 mo before delivery; lactation, safety not established.

Available forms
Tablets—500, 850, 1,000 mg; extended-release tablets—500 mg

Dosages
Adults
500–850 mg/day PO in divided doses to a maximum of 2,550 mg/day. Dose should be adjusted based on response and blood glucose level. *ER tablet:* Initially 500 mg/day PO with the evening meal; may be increased by 500 mg each wk to a maximum of 2,550 mg once daily.
Pediatric patients 10–16 yr
500 mg/day PO in divided doses with meals; may be increased by 500 mg each wk to a maximum of 2,000 mg/day. *ER tablet:* Not recommended.
Geriatric patients and patients with renal impairment
Smaller doses may be necessary; monitor closely and adjust slowly

Pharmacokinetics

Route	Peak	Duration
Oral	2–2.5 hr	10–16 hr

Metabolism: Hepatic; $T_{1/2}$: 6.2 and 17.6 hr
Distribution: Crosses placenta; passes into breast milk
Excretion: Urine

Adverse effects
- **Endocrine:** *Hypoglycemia,* **lactic acidosis**
- **GI:** *Anorexia, nausea,* vomiting, *epigastric discomfort, heartburn, diarrhea*
- **Hypersensitivity:** *Allergic skin reactions, eczema, pruritus, erythema, urticaria*

Interactions
✳ **Drug-drug** • Increased risk of hypoglycemia with cimetidine, furosemide, cationic drugs such as digoxin, amiloride, vancomycin • Increased risk of lactic acidosis with glucocorticoids or ethanol • Increased risk of acute renal failure and lactic acidosis with iodinated contrast material used in radiologic studies; stop metformin for 48 hr before and after such studies

✳ **Drug-alternative therapy** • Increased risk of hypoglycemia if taken with juniper berries, ginseng, garlic, fenugreek, coriander, dandelion root, celery

Adverse effects in *Italics* are most common; those in **Bold** are life-threatening.

■ Nursing considerations

Assessment

- **History:** Allergy to metformin; diabetes complicated by fever, severe infections, severe trauma, major surgery, ketosis, acidosis, coma; type 1 or juvenile diabetes, serious hepatic or renal impairment, uremia, thyroid or endocrine impairment, glycosuria, hyperglycemia associated with primary renal disease, CHF
- **Physical:** Skin color, lesions; T, orientation, reflexes, peripheral sensation; R, adventitious sounds; liver evaluation, bowel sounds; urinalysis, BUN, serum creatinine, liver function tests, blood glucose, CBC

Interventions

- Monitor urine or serum glucose levels frequently to determine effectiveness of drug and dosage.
- Arrange for transfer to insulin therapy during periods of high stress (infections, surgery, trauma).
- Use IV glucose if severe hypoglycemia occurs as a result of overdose.

Teaching points

- Do not discontinue this medication without consulting your health care provider.
- Monitor urine or blood for glucose and ketones as prescribed.
- Do not use this drug during pregnancy.
- Avoid the use of alcohol while on this drug.
- Report fever, sore throat, unusual bleeding or bruising, rash, dark urine, light-colored stools, hypo- or hyperglycemic reactions.

▽ methadone hydrochloride

(meth' a done)

Dolophine, Methadone HCl Diskets, Methadone HCl Intensol, Methadose

PREGNANCY CATEGORY C

C-II CONTROLLED SUBSTANCE

Drug class

Narcotic agonist analgesic

Therapeutic actions

Acts as agonist at specific opioid receptors in the CNS to produce analgesia, euphoria, sedation; the receptors mediating these effects are thought to be the same as those mediating the effects of endogenous opioids (enkephalins, endorphins); when used in approved methadone maintenance programs, can substitute for heroin, other illicit narcotics in patients who want to terminate a drug use.

Indications

- Relief of severe pain
- Detoxification and temporary maintenance treatment of narcotic addiction (ineffective for relief of general anxiety)

Contraindications and cautions

- Contraindicated with hypersensitivity to narcotics, diarrhea caused by poisoning (before toxins are eliminated), bronchial asthma, COPD, cor pulmonale, respiratory depression, anoxia, kyphoscoliosis, acute alcoholism, increased intracranial pressure.
- Use cautiously with acute abdominal conditions, CV disease, supraventricular tachycardias, myxedema, convulsive disorders, delirium tremens, cerebral arteriosclerosis, ulcerative colitis, fever, Addison's disease, prostatic hypertrophy, urethral stricture, recent GI or GU surgery, toxic psychosis, pregnancy prior to labor (crosses placenta; neonatal withdrawal observed in infants born to drug-using mothers; safety for use in pregnancy before labor not established), labor or delivery (administration of narcotics to mother can cause respiratory depression of neonate—risk greatest for prematures), renal or hepatic dysfunction, lactation.

Available forms

Tablets—5, 10 mg; oral solution—5 mg/5 mL, 10 mg/5 mL; oral concentrate—10 mg/mL; injection—10 mg/mL; dispersible tablets—40 mg

Dosages

Oral methadone is approximately one-half as potent as parenteral methadone.

Adults

- *Relief of pain:* 2.5–10 mg IM, SC, or PO q 3–4 hr as necessary. IM route is preferred to SC for repeated doses (SC may cause local irritation). Individualize dosage: patients with excessively severe pain and those who have become tolerant to the analgesic effect of narcotics may need higher dosage.

- *Detoxification:* Initially, 15–20 mg PO or parenteral–PO preferred. Increase dose to suppress withdrawal signs. 40 mg/day in single or divided doses is usually an adequate stabilizing dose for those physically dependent on high doses. Continue stabilizing doses for 2–3 days, then gradually decrease dosage every day or every 2 days. A daily reduction of 20% of the total dose may be tolerated. Provide sufficient dosage to keep withdrawal symptoms at tolerable level. Treatment should not exceed 21 days and may not be repeated earlier than 4 wk after completion of previous course. Detoxification treatment continued longer than 21 days becomes maintenance treatment, which may be undertaken only by approved programs (addicts hospitalized for other medical conditions may receive methadone maintenance treatment).
- *Maintenance treatment:* For patients who are heavy heroin users up until hospital admission, initial dose of 20 mg 4–8 hr after heroin is stopped or 40 mg in a single dose PO. For patients with little or no narcotic tolerance, half this dose may suffice. Dosage should suppress withdrawal symptoms but not produce acute narcotic effects of sedation, respiratory depression. Give additional 10 mg doses if needed to suppress withdrawal syndrome. Adjust dosage, up to 120 mg/day.

Pediatric patients

Not recommended for relief of pain in children due to insufficient documentation.

Geriatric patients or impaired adults

Use caution—respiratory depression may occur in the elderly, the very ill, those with respiratory problems. Reduced dosage may be necessary.

Pharmacokinetics

Route	Onset	Peak	Duration
PO	30–60 min	1.5–2 hr	4–12 hr
IM	10–20 min	1–2 hr	4–6 hr
SC	10–20 min	1–2 hr	4–6 hr

Metabolism: Liver; $T_{1/2}$: 25 hr
Distribution: Crosses placenta and enters breast milk
Excretion: Bile and feces

Adverse effects

- **CNS:** *Light-headedness, dizziness, sedation,* euphoria, dysphoria, delirium, insomnia, agitation, anxiety, fear, hallucinations, disorientation, drowsiness, lethargy, impaired mental and physical performance, coma, mood changes, weakness, headache, tremor, convulsions, miosis, visual disturbances, suppression of cough reflex
- **CV:** Facial flushing, peripheral circulatory collapse, arrhythmia, palpitations, chest wall rigidity, hypertension, hypotension, orthostatic hypotension, syncope
- **Dermatologic:** Pruritus, urticaria, laryngospasm, bronchospasm, edema, hemorrhagic urticaria (rare)
- **GI:** *Nausea, vomiting,* dry mouth, anorexia, constipation, biliary tract spasm; increased colonic motility in patients with chronic ulcerative colitis
- **GU:** Ureteral spasm, spasm of vesical sphincters, urinary retention or hesitancy, oliguria, antidiuretic effect, reduced libido or potency
- **Local:** Tissue irritation and induration (SC injection)
- **Major hazards: Respiratory depression, apnea, circulatory depression, respiratory arrest, shock, cardiac arrest**
- **Other:** Sweating (more common in ambulatory patients and those without severe pain), physical tolerance and dependence, psychological dependence

Interactions

✳ Drug-drug • Potentiation of effects of methadone with barbiturate anesthetics—decrease dose of meperidine when coadministering • Decreased effectiveness of methadone with hydantoins, rifampin, urinary acidifiers (ammonium chloride, potassium acid phosphate, sodium acid phosphate) • Increased effects and toxicity of methadone with cimetidine, ranitidine

✳ Drug-lab test • Elevated biliary tract pressure (narcotic effect) may cause increases in

---

Adverse effects in *Italics* are most common; those in **Bold** are life-threatening.

plasma amylase, lipase; determinations of these levels may be unreliable for 24 hr after administration of narcotics

■ Nursing considerations
Assessment
- **History:** Hypersensitivity to narcotics, diarrhea caused by poisoning, bronchial asthma, COPD, cor pulmonale, respiratory depression, kyphoscoliosis, acute alcoholism, increased intracranial pressure; acute abdominal conditions, CV disease, supraventricular tachycardias, myxedema, convulsive disorders, delirium tremens, cerebral arteriosclerosis, ulcerative colitis, fever, Addison's disease, prostatic hypertrophy, urethral stricture, recent GI or GU surgery, toxic psychosis; pregnancy; labor; lactation
- **Physical:** T; skin color, texture, lesions; orientation, reflexes, bilateral grip strength, affect, pupil size; pulse, auscultation, BP, orthostatic BP, perfusion; R, adventitious sounds; bowel sounds, normal output; frequency and pattern of voiding, normal output; ECG; EEG; thyroid, liver, kidney function tests

Interventions
- Give to lactating women 4–6 hr before the next feeding to minimize the amount in milk.
- Provide narcotic antagonist, equipment for assisted or controlled respiration on standby during parenteral administration.
- Use caution when injecting SC into chilled areas of the body or in patients with hypotension or in shock—impaired perfusion may delay absorption; with repeated doses, an excessive amount may be absorbed when circulation is restored.

Teaching points
- Take drug exactly as prescribed.
- Avoid alcohol—serious adverse effects may occur.
- These side effects may occur: nausea, loss of appetite (take with food, lie quietly, eat frequent small meals); constipation (laxative may help); dizziness, sedation, drowsiness, impaired visual acuity (avoid driving, performing other tasks that require alertness, visual acuity).

- Do not take leftover medication for other disorders; do not let anyone else take the prescription.
- Avoid pregnancy while on this drug; use of barrier contraceptives is advised.
- Report severe nausea, vomiting, constipation, shortness of breath, or difficulty breathing.

▷ methazolamide
(meth a zoe' la mide)

GlaucTabs

PREGNANCY CATEGORY C

Drug classes
Carbonic anhydrase inhibitor
Antiglaucoma agent
Sulfonamide, nonbacteriostatic

Therapeutic actions
Inhibits the enzyme carbonic anhydrase, thereby decreasing aqueous humor formation and hence decreasing intraocular pressure; decreasing hydrogen ion secretion by renal tubule cells and hence increasing sodium, potassium, bicarbonate, and water excretion by the kidney.

Indications
- Adjunctive treatment of chronic open-angle glaucoma, secondary glaucoma
- Preoperative use in acute angle-closure glaucoma where delay of surgery is desired to lower intraocular pressure
- Unlabeled uses: treatment of hyperkalemia and hypokalemia periodic paralysis

Contraindications and cautions
- Contraindicated with allergy to dichlorphenamide, sulfonamides.
- Use cautiously with renal or liver disease; adrenocortical insufficiency; respiratory acidosis; COPD; chronic noncongestive angle-closure glaucoma; decreased sodium, potassium; hyperchloremic acidosis; pregnancy; lactation.

Available forms
Tablets—25, 50 mg

Dosages
Adults
50–100 mg PO bid or tid. Most effective if taken with other miotics.

Pharmacokinetics

Route	Onset	Peak	Duration
Oral	2–4 hr	6–8 hr	10–18 hr

Metabolism: Liver; $T_{1/2}$: 14 hr
Distribution: Crosses placenta and enters breast milk
Excretion: Urine

Adverse effects
- **CNS:** *Photophobia,* weakness, fatigue, nervousness, sedation, drowsiness, dizziness, depression, tremor, ataxia, headache, paresthesias, convulsions, flaccid paralysis, transient myopia
- **Dermatologic:** Urticaria, pruritis, rash, *photosensitivity,* erythema multiforme
- **GI:** *Anorexia, nausea, vomiting, constipation,* melena, hepatic insufficiency
- **GU:** Hematuria, glycosuria, urinary frequency, renal colic, renal calculi, crystalluria, polyuria
- **Hematologic:** Bone marrow depression
- **Other:** Weight loss, fever, acidosis

Interactions
✳ **Drug-drug** • Increased risk of salicylate toxicity, due to metabolic acidosis with salicylates
✳ **Drug-lab test** • False-positive results on tests for urinary protein

■ Nursing considerations
Assessment
- **History:** Allergy to dichlorphenamide, sulfonamides; renal or liver disease; adrenocortical insufficiency; respiratory acidosis; COPD; chronic noncongestive angle-closure glaucoma; pregnancy; lactation
- **Physical:** Skin color and lesions; T; weight; orientation, reflexes, muscle strength, ocular pressure; R, pattern, adventitious sounds; liver evaluation and bowel sounds; CBC, serum electrolytes, liver and renal function tests, urinalysis

Interventions
- Administer with food if GI upset occurs; provide small, frequent meals.

Teaching points
- Take this drug with food if GI upset is a problem.
- Have periodic checks of intraocular pressure.
- Sensitivity to sun: use sunscreen or wear protective clothing.
- Report loss or gain of more than 3 lb/day, unusual bleeding or bruising, dizziness, muscle cramps or weakness, rash.

▽ **methenamine**
*(meth **en' a** meen)*

methenamine
Dehydral (CAN), Urasal (CAN)

methenamine hippurate
Hiprex, Hip-Rex (CAN), Urex

methenamine mandelate
Mandelamine

PREGNANCY CATEGORY C

Drug classes
Urinary tract anti-infective
Antibacterial

Therapeutic actions
Hydrolyzed in acid urine to ammonia and formaldehyde, which is bactericidal; the hippurate and mandelate salts help to maintain an acid urine.

Indications
- Suppression or elimination of bacteriuria associated with pyelonephritis, cystitis, chronic UTIs, residual urine (accompanying some neurologic disorders), and in anatomic abnormalities of the urinary tract

Contraindications and cautions
- Contraindicated with allergy to methenamine, tartrazine (in methenamine hippurate marketed as *Hiprex*), aspirin (associ-

ated with tartrazine allergy), pregnancy, lactation.
- Use cautiously with hepatic or renal dysfunction; gout (causes urate crystals to precipitate in urine).

Available forms

Tablets—0.5, 1 g; suspension—0.5 g/5 mL

Dosages
Adults
Methenamine
1 g qid PO.
Methenamine hippurate
1 g bid PO.
Methenamine mandelate
1 g qid PO after meals and at hs.
Pediatric patients
Methenamine
< 6 yr: 50 mg/kg/day PO divided into 3 doses.
6–12 yr: 500 mg qid PO.
Methenamine hippurate
6–12 yr: 0.5–1 g bid PO.
> 12 yr: 1 g bid PO.
Methenamine mandelate
< 6 yr: 0.25 g/14 kg qid PO.
6–12 yr: 0.5 g qid PO.

Pharmacokinetics

Route	Onset	Peak
Oral	Rapid	2–3 hr

Metabolism: Hepatic; $T_{1/2}$: 3–6 hr
Distribution: Crosses placenta; enters breast milk
Excretion: Urine

Adverse effects

- **Dermatologic:** Pruritus, urticaria, erythematous eruptions
- **GI:** *Nausea, abdominal cramps, vomiting, diarrhea,* anorexia, stomatitis
- **GU:** *Bladder irritation, dysuria,* proteinuria, hematuria, frequency, urgency, crystalluria
- **Other:** Headache, dyspnea, generalized edema, elevated serum transaminase (with hippurate salt)

Interactions

✴ Drug-lab test ● False increase in 17-hydroxycorticosteroids, catecholamines ● False decrease in 5-hydroxyindoleacetic acid ● In-

accurate measurement of urine estriol levels by acid hydrolysis procedures during pregnancy

■ Nursing considerations
Assessment

- **History:** Allergy to methenamine, tartrazine, aspirin; renal or hepatic dysfunction; dehydration; gout; pregnancy, lactation
- **Physical:** Skin color, lesions; hydration; ear lobes—tophi; joints; liver evaluation; urinalysis, liver function tests; serum uric acid

Interventions

- Arrange for culture and sensitivity tests before and during therapy.
- Administer drug with food to prevent GI upset; give drug around the clock for best effects.
- Ensure avoidance of foods or medications that alkalinize the urine.
- Ensure adequate hydration for patient.
- Monitor clinical response; if no improvement is seen or a relapse occurs, repeat urine culture and sensitivity tests.
- Monitor liver function tests with methenamine hippurate.

Teaching points

- Take drug with food. Complete the full course of therapy to resolve the infection.
- Take this drug at regular intervals around the clock; develop a schedule with the help of your health care provider.
- Avoid alkalinizing foods: citrus fruits, milk products; or alkalinizing medications (sodium bicarbonate).
- Review other medications with your care provider.
- Drink plenty of fluids.
- These side effects may occur: nausea, vomiting, abdominal pain (small, frequent meals may help); diarrhea; painful urination, frequency, blood in urine (drink plenty of fluids).
- Report rash, painful urination, severe GI upset.

M

▷ **methimazole**
*(meth **im**' a zole)*

Tapazole

PREGNANCY CATEGORY D

Drug class
Antithyroid agent

Therapeutic actions
Inhibits the synthesis of thyroid hormones.

Indications
• Hyperthyroidism

Contraindications and cautions
• Allergy to antithyroid products, pregnancy (use only if absolutely necessary and when mother has been informed about potential harm to the fetus; if an antithyroid agent is required, propylthiouracil is the drug of choice), lactation.

Available forms
Tablets—5, 10 mg, usually in three equal doses q 8 hr.

Dosages
Adults
Initial dose: 15 mg/day PO up to 30–60 mg/day in severe cases. *Maintenance dose:* 5–15 mg/day PO.
Pediatric patients
Initially, give 0.4 mg/kg/day PO, followed by maintenance dose of approximately one-half the initial dose; actual dose is determined by the patient's response. Alternatively, give initial dose of 0.5–0.7 mg/kg/day or 15–20 mg/m^2/day PO in three divided doses, followed by maintenance dose of one-third to two-thirds of initial dose, starting when patient becomes euthyroid. Maximum dose is 30 mg/24 hr.

Pharmacokinetics

Route	Onset	Peak	Duration
Oral	30–40 min	60 min	2–4 hr

Metabolism: $T_{1/2}$: 6–13 hr

Distribution: Crosses placenta; enters breast milk
Excretion: Urine

Adverse effects
• **CNS:** *Paresthesias, neuritis,* vertigo, drowsiness, neuropathies, depression, headache
• **Dermatologic:** *Rash,* urticaria, pruritus, skin pigmentation, exfoliative dermatitis, lupuslike syndrome, loss of hair
• **GI:** Nausea, vomiting, epigastric distress, loss of taste, sialadenopathy, jaundice, hepatitis
• **GU:** Nephritis
• **Hematologic:** *Agranulocytosis, granulocytopenia, thrombocytopenia, hypoprothrombinemia, bleeding,* vasculitis, periarteritis
• **Other:** Arthralgia, myalgia, edema, lymphadenopathy, drug fever

Interactions
✳ **Drug-drug** • Increased theophylline clearance and decreased effectiveness if given to hyperthyroid patients; clearance will change as patient approaches euthyroid state • Altered effects of oral anticoagulants with methimazole • Increased therapeutic effects and toxicity of digitalis glycosides, metroprolol, propranolol when hyperthyroid patients become euthyroid

■ **Nursing considerations**
Assessment
• **History:** Allergy to antithyroid products; pregnancy, lactation
• **Physical:** Skin color, lesions, pigmentation; orientation, reflexes, affect; liver evaluation; CBC, differential, prothrombin time, liver and renal function tests

Interventions
• Give drug in three equally divided doses at 8-hr intervals; try to schedule to allow patient to sleep at his or her regular time.
• Obtain regular, periodic blood tests to monitor bone marrow depression and bleeding tendencies.
• Advise medical and surgical personnel that patient is taking this drug, thereby increasing the risk of bleeding problems.

Adverse effects in *Italics* are most common; those in **Bold** are life-threatening.

- Ensure patient is not pregnant before giving this drug; advise the use of barrier contraceptives.

Teaching points

- Take this drug around the clock at 8-hr intervals. Establish a schedule that fits your routine, with the aid of your health care provider.
- This drug will need to be taken for a prolonged period to achieve the desired effects.
- These side effects may occur: dizziness, weakness, vertigo, drowsiness (use caution driving or operating dangerous machinery); nausea, vomiting, loss of appetite (small, frequent meals may help); rash, itching.
- Use of barrier contraceptives is advised while on this drug; serious fetal abnormalities may occur.
- Report fever, sore throat, unusual bleeding or bruising, headache, general malaise.

▽ **methocarbamol**

(meth oh kar' ba mole)

Robaxin, Robaxin-750

PREGNANCY CATEGORY C

Drug class

Skeletal muscle relaxant, centrally acting

Therapeutic actions

Precise mechanism of action not known but may be due to general CNS depression; does not directly relax tense skeletal muscles or directly affect the motor end plate or motor nerves.

Indications

- Relief of discomfort associated with acute, painful musculoskeletal conditions, as an adjunct to rest, physical therapy, and other measures
- May have a beneficial role in the control of neuromuscular manifestations of tetanus

Contraindications and cautions

- Contraindicated with hypersensitivity to methocarbamol; known or suspected renal pathology (parenteral methocarbamol is contraindicated because of presence of polyethylene glycol 300 in vehicle).

- Use cautiously in patients with epilepsy, pregnancy, lactation.

Available forms

Tablets—500, 750 mg; injection—100 mg/mL

Dosages
Adults
Parenteral

IV and IM use only. Do not use SC. Do not exceed total dosage of 3 g/days for more than 3 consecutive days, except in the treatment of tetanus. Repeat treatment after a lapse of 48 hr if condition persists. Injection need not be repeated, because tablets will sustain the relief.

IV

Administer undiluted at a maximum rate of 3 mL/min.

- *Tetanus:* Give 1–2 g directly IV and add 1–2 g to IV infusion bottle so that initial dose is 3 g. Repeat q 6 hr until conditions allow for insertion of nasogastric tube and administration of crushed tablets suspended in water or saline. Total daily oral doses up to 24 g may be required.

IM

Do not give more than 5 mL at any gluteal injection site. Repeat q 8 hr if needed.

Oral

- *Initially:* 1.5 g qid PO. For the first 48–72 hr, 6 g/day or up to 8 g/day is recommended.
- *Maintenance:* 1 g qid or 750 mg q 4 hr PO or 1.5 g bid–tid for total dosage of 4–4.5 g/day.

Pediatric patients

- *Tetanus:* A minimum initial dose of 15 mg/kg IV by direct IV injection or IV infusion. Repeat q 6 hr as needed.

Pharmacokinetics

Route	Onset	Peak
Oral	30 min	2 hr
IM, IV	Rapid	Unknown

Metabolism: Hepatic; $T_{1/2}$: 1–2 hr
Distribution: Crosses placenta; may enter breast milk
Excretion: Urine and feces

▽ IV facts

Preparation: Administer undiluted. May be added to IV drip of sodium chloride injection or 5% dextrose injection; do not dilute one vial

M

given as a single dose to more than 250 mL for IV infusion.

Infusion: Inject directly 1 or 2 g into IV tubing at maximum rate of 3 mL/min; may add 1–2 g to infusion for a total of 3 g.

Adverse effects
Parenteral
- **CNS:** *Syncope, dizziness, light-headedness, vertigo, headache, mild muscular incoordination,* convulsions during IV administration, blurred vision
- **CV:** *Hypotension*
- **Dermatologic:** *Urticaria,* pruritus, rash, flushing
- **GI:** GI upset, metallic taste
- **Local:** Sloughing or pain at injection site
- **Other:** Nasal congestion
Oral
- **CNS:** *Light-headedness, dizziness, drowsiness,* headache, fever, blurred vision
- **Dermatologic:** *Urticaria,* pruritus, rash
- **GI:** *Nausea*
- **Other:** Conjunctivitis with nasal congestion

Interactions
✳ **Drug-lab test** • May cause interference with color reactions in tests for 5-HIAA and vanillylmandelic acid (VMA)

■ Nursing considerations
Assessment
- **History:** Hypersensitivity to methocarbamol; known or suspected renal pathology, epilepsy (use caution with parenteral administration)
- **Physical:** T; skin color, lesions; nasal mucous membranes, conjunctival exam; orientation, affect, vision exam, reflexes; P, BP; bowel sounds, normal output; urinalysis, renal function tests

Interventions
- Ensure patient is not pregnant before use; use in pregnancy only if benefits clearly outweigh risk to the fetus.
- Ensure patient is recumbent during IV injection and for at least 15 min thereafter.
- Administer IV slowly to minimize risk of CVS reactions, seizures.

- Monitor IV injection sites carefully to prevent extravasation; solution is hypertonic; can cause sloughing of tissue.
- Ensure that patients receiving methocarbamol for tetanus receive other appropriate care—debridement of wound, penicillin, tetanus antitoxin, tracheotomy, attention to fluid/electrolyte balance.
- Provide epinephrine, injectable steroids, or injectable antihistamines on standby in case syncope, hypotension occur with IV administration.
- Patient's urine may darken on standing.

Teaching points
- Take this drug exactly as prescribed. Do not take a higher dosage than prescribed, and do not take it longer than prescribed.
- Avoid alcohol, sleep-inducing, or OTC drugs; these could cause dangerous effects.
- Your urine may darken to a brown, black, or green color on standing.
- These side effects may occur: drowsiness, dizziness, blurred vision (avoid driving or engaging in activities that require alertness); nausea (take with food, eat frequent, small meals).
- Report rash, itching, fever, or nasal congestion.

▽ methotrexate (methopterin, MTX)
(meth oh trex' ate)
Rheumatrex, Rheumatrex Dose Pak, Trexall

PREGNANCY CATEGORY X

Drug classes
Antimetabolite
Antineoplastic
Antipsoriatic
Antirheumatic

Therapeutic actions
Inhibits folic acid reductase, leading to inhibition of DNA synthesis and inhibition of cellular replication; selectively affects the most rapidly dividing cells (neoplastic and psoriatic cells).

Indications

- Treatment of gestational choriocarcinoma, chorioadenoma destruens, hydatidiform mole
- Treatment and prophylaxis of meningeal leukemia
- Symptomatic control of severe, recalcitrant, disabling psoriasis
- Management of severe, active, classical, or definite rheumatoid arthritis
- Unlabeled uses: high-dose regimen followed by leucovorin rescue for adjuvant therapy of nonmetastatic osteosarcoma (orphan drug designation); to reduce corticosteroid requirements in patients with severe corticosteroid-dependent asthma
- Orphan drug use: treatment of juvenile rheumatoid arthritis

Contraindications and cautions

- Use cautiously with hematopoietic depression; leukopenia, thrombocytopenia, anemia, severe hepatic or renal disease, infection, peptic ulcer, ulcerative colitis, debility.

Available forms

Tablets—2.5, 5, 7.5, 10, 15 mg; powder for injection—20 mg, 50 mg, 1 g per vial; injection—25 mg/mL, 2.5 mg/mL; preservative-free injection—25 mg/mL

Dosages
Adults

- *Choriocarcinoma and other trophoblastic diseases:* 15–30 mg PO or IM daily for a 5-day course. Repeat courses 3–5 times with rest periods of 1 wk or more between courses until toxic symptoms subside. Continue 1–2 courses of methotrexate after chorionic gonadotropin hormone levels are normal.
- *Leukemia:* Induction: 3.3 mg/m² of methotrexate PO or IM with 60 mg/m² of prednisone daily for 4–6 wk. Maintenance: 30 mg/m² methotrexate PO or IM twice weekly or 2.5 mg/m² IV every 14 days. If relapse occurs, return to induction doses.
- *Meningeal leukemia:* Give methotrexate intrathecally in cases of lymphocytic leukemia as prophylaxis. 12 mg/m² intrathecally at intervals of 2–5 days and repeat until cell count of CSF is normal.
- *Lymphomas:* Burkitt's tumor, stages I and II: 10–25 mg/day PO for 4–8 days. In stage

III, combine with other neoplastic drugs. All usually require several courses of therapy with 7- to 10-day rest periods between doses.
- *Mycosis fungoides:* 2.5–10 mg/day PO for weeks or months or 50 mg IM once weekly or 25 mg IM twice weekly.
- *Osteosarcoma:* Starting dose is 12 g/m² or up to 15 g/m² PO, IM, or IV to give a peak serum concentration of 1,000 micromol. Must be used as part of a cytotoxic regimen with leucovorin rescue.
- *Severe psoriasis:* 10–25 mg/wk PO, IM, or IV as a single weekly dose. Do not exceed 50 mg/wk or 2.5 mg PO at 12-hr intervals for 3 doses or at 8-hr intervals for 4 doses each wk. Do not exceed 30 mg/wk. Alternatively, 2.5 mg/day PO for 5 days followed by at least 2 days rest. Do not exceed 6.25 mg/day. After optimal clinical response is achieved, reduce dosage to lowest possible with longest rest periods and consider return to conventional, topical therapy.
- *Severe rheumatoid arthritis:* Starting dose: single doses of 7.5 mg/wk PO or divided dosage of 2.5 mg PO at 12-hr intervals for 3 doses given as a course once weekly. Dosage may be gradually increased, based on response. Do not exceed 20 mg/wk. Therapeutic response usually begins within 3–6 wk, and improvement may continue for another 12 wk. Improvement may be maintained for up to 2 yr with continued therapy.

Pharmacokinetics

Route	Onset	Peak
Oral	Varies	1–4 hr
IM, IV	Rapid	0.5–2 hr

Metabolism: $T_{1/2}$: 2–4 hr
Distribution: Crosses placenta; enters breast milk
Excretion: Urine

▼IV facts

Preparation: Reconstitute 20- and 50-mg vials with an appropriate sterile preservative-free medium, 5% dextrose solution or sodium chloride injection to a concentration no greater than 25 mg/mL; reconstitute 1-g vial with 19.4 mL to a concentration of 50 mg/mL.
Infusion: Administer diluted drug by direct IV injection at a rate of not more than 10 mg/min.

Incompatibilities: Do not combine with bleomycin, fluorouracil, prednisolone.
Y-site incompatibility: Do not give with droperidol.

Adverse effects

- **CNS:** Headache, drowsiness, blurred vision, aphasia, hemiparesis, paresis, seizures, *fatigue, malaise, dizziness*
- **Dermatologic:** *Erythematous rashes,* pruritus, urticaria, photosensitivity, depigmentation, *alopecia,* ecchymosis, telangiectasia, acne, furunculosis
- **GI:** *Ulcerative stomatitis,* gingivitis, pharyngitis, anorexia, *nausea,* vomiting, diarrhea, hematemesis, melena, GI ulceration and bleeding, enteritis, **hepatic toxicity**
- **GU:** Renal failure, *effects on fertility* (defective oogenesis, defective spermatogenesis, transient oligospermia, menstrual dysfunction, infertility, abortion, fetal defects)
- **Hematologic: Severe bone marrow depression,** *increased susceptibility to infection*
- **Hypersensitivity: Anaphylaxis, sudden death**
- **Respiratory: Interstitial pneumonitis,** chronic interstitial obstructive pulmonary disease
- **Other:** *Chills and fever,* metabolic changes (diabetes, osteoporosis), cancer

Interactions

✱ **Drug-drug** • Increased risk of toxicity with salicylates, phenytoin, probenecid, sulfonamides • Decreased serum levels and therapeutic effects of digoxin • Potentially serious to fatal reactions when given with NSAIDs; use extreme caution if this combination is used • Risk of toxicity if combined with alcohol; avoid this combination

■ Nursing considerations

Assessment

- **History:** Allergy to methotrexate, hematopoietic depression, severe hepatic or renal disease, infection, peptic ulcer, ulcerative colitis, debility, psoriasis, pregnancy, lactation
- **Physical:** Weight; T; skin lesions, color; hair; vision, speech, orientation, reflexes, sensation; R, adventitious sounds; mucous membranes, liver evaluation, abdominal exam; CBC, differential; renal and liver function tests; urinalysis, blood and urine glucose, glucose tolerance test, chest x-ray

Interventions

- Arrange for tests to evaluate CBC, urinalysis, renal and liver function tests, chest x-ray before therapy, during therapy, and for several weeks after therapy.
- Ensure that patient is not pregnant before administering this drug; counsel patient about the severe risks of fetal abnormalities associated with this drug.
- Reduce dosage or discontinue if renal failure occurs.
- Reconstitute powder for intrathecal use with preservative-free sterile sodium chloride injection; intended for one dose only; discard remainder. The solution for injection contains benzyl alcohol and should *not* be given intrathecally.
- Arrange to have leucovorin readily available as antidote for methotrexate overdose or when large doses are used. In general, doses of leucovorin (calcium leucovorin) should be equal or higher than doses of methotrexate and should be given within the first hour. Up to 75 mg IV within 12 hr, followed by 12 mg IM q 6 hr for 4 doses. For average doses of methotrexate that cause adverse effects, give 6–12 mg leucovorin IM, q 6 hr for 4 doses or 10 mg/m^2 PO followed by 10 mg/m^2 q 6 hr for 72 hr.
- Arrange for an antiemetic if nausea and vomiting are severe.
- Arrange for adequate hydration during therapy to reduce the risk of hyperuricemia.
- Do not administer any other medications containing alcohol.

Teaching points

- Prepare a calendar of treatment days.
- These side effects may occur: nausea, vomiting (request medication; small, frequent meals may help); numbness, tingling, dizziness, drowsiness, blurred vision, difficulty speaking (drug effects; seek dosage adjustment; avoid driving or operating dangerous machinery): mouth sores (frequent mouth care is needed); infertility; loss of hair (ob-

tain a wig or other suitable head covering; keep the head covered at extremes of temperature); rash, sensitivity to sun and ultraviolet light (avoid sun; use a sunscreen and protective clothing).

- This drug may cause birth defects or miscarriages. Use birth control while on this drug and for 8 wk thereafter. Males using this drug should also use barrier contraceptives.
- Avoid alcohol; serious side effects may occur.
- Arrange for frequent, regular medical follow-up, including blood tests to follow the drug's effects.
- Report black, tarry stools; fever; chills; sore throat; unusual bleeding or bruising; cough or shortness of breath; darkened or bloody urine; abdominal, flank, or joint pain; yellow color to the skin or eyes; mouth sores.

▷methotrimeprazine hydrochloride

*(meth oh trye **mep'** ra zeen)*

Levoprome, Novo-Meprazine (CAN), Nozinan (CAN)

PREGNANCY CATEGORY C

Drug classes
Analgesic (non-narcotic)
Phenothiazine

Therapeutic actions
CNS depressant; suppresses sensory impulses; reduces motor activity; produces sedation and tranquilization; raises pain threshold; produces amnesia. Also has antihistaminic, anticholinergic, antiadrenergic activity.

Indications
- Relief of moderate to marked pain in nonambulatory patients
- Obstetric analgesia and sedation where respiratory depression is to be avoided
- Preanesthetic for producing sedation, somnolence, relief of apprehension and anxiety

Contraindications and cautions
- Contraindicated with hypersensitivity to phenothiazines, sulfites; coma; severe myocardial, hepatic, or renal disease; hypotension.

- Use cautiously with heart disease, pregnancy prior to labor, lactation.

Available forms
Injection—20 mg/mL

Dosages
For IM use only. Do not give SC or IV. Do not administer for longer than 30 days, unless narcotic analgesics are contraindicated or patient has terminal illness.
Adults
- *Analgesia:* 10–20 mg IM q 4–6 hr as required (range, 5–40 mg q 1–24 hr).
- *Obstetric analgesia:* During labor, an initial dose of 15–20 mg PO. May be repeated or adjusted as needed.
- *Preanesthetic medication:* 2–20 mg IM 45 min–3 hr before surgery; 10 mg is often satisfactory. 15–20 mg IM may be given for more sedation. Atropine sulfate or scopolamine HBr may be used concurrently in lower than usual doses.
- *Postoperative analgesia:* 2.5–7.5 mg IM in the immediate postoperative period. Supplement q 4–6 hr as needed.
Pediatric patients
Not recommended in children < 12 yr.
Geriatric patients
Initial dose of 5–10 mg IM; gradually increase subsequent doses if needed and tolerated.

Pharmacokinetics

Route	Onset	Peak	Duration
IM	20 min	30–90 min	4 hr

Metabolism: Hepatic; $T_{1/2}$: 15–30 hr
Distribution: Crosses placenta; enters breast milk
Excretion: Urine

Adverse effects
- **CNS:** *Weakness,* disorientation, dizziness, excessive sedation, slurring of speech
- **CV:** *Orthostatic hypotension, fainting, syncope*
- **GI:** Abdominal discomfort, nausea, vomiting, *dry mouth,* jaundice
- **GU:** Difficult urination, uterine inertia
- **Local:** Local inflammation, swelling, pain at injection site
- **Other:** Nasal congestion, agranulocytosis, chills

Interactions

* Drug-drug • Additive anticholinergic effects and possibly decreased antipsychotic efficacy with anticholinergic drugs • Increased likelihood of seizures with metrizamide (contrast agent used in myelography)

* Drug-lab test • False-positive pregnancy tests (less likely if serum test is used) • Increase in PBI, not attributable to an increase in thyroxine

■ Nursing considerations
Assessment

- **History:** Hypersensitivity to phenothiazines, sulfites; coma; severe myocardial, hepatic, renal, or heart disease; hypotension; lactation, pregnancy
- **Physical:** Weight, T; reflexes, orientation, intraocular pressure; P, BP, orthostatic BP; R, adventitious sounds; bowel sounds and normal output, liver evaluation; urinary output, prostate size; CBC, urinalysis, thyroid, liver, and kidney function tests

Interventions

- Do not mix drugs other than atropine or scopolamine in the same syringe with methotrimeprazine.
- Rotate IM injection sites.
- Keep patient supine for about 6–12 hr after injection to prevent severe hypotension, syncope; tolerance to hypotensive effects usually occurs with repeated administration but may be lost if dosage is interrupted for several days.
- Provide methoxamine, phenylephrine on standby in case severe hypotension occurs. Do not give epinephrine; paradoxical hypotension may occur.

Teaching points

- These side effects may occur: dizziness, sedation, drowsiness (remain supine for 12 hr after the injection; request assistance if you need to sit or stand); nausea, vomiting (frequent, small meals may help).
- Report severe nausea, vomiting, urinary difficulty, yellowing of the skin or eyes, pain at injection site.

▽ methoxsalen

See *Less Commonly Used Drugs,* p. 1346.

▽ methscopolamine bromide

*(meth skoe **pol'** a meen)*

Pamine

PREGNANCY CATEGORY C

Drug classes
Anticholinergic
Antimuscarinic agent
Parasympatholytic
Antispasmodic

Therapeutic actions
Competitively blocks the effects of acetylcholine at muscarinic cholinergic receptors that mediate the effects of parasympathetic postganglionic impulses, relaxing the GI tract and inhibiting gastric acid secretion.

Indications
- Adjunctive therapy in the treatment of peptic ulcer

Contraindications and cautions
- Contraindicated with glaucoma; adhesions between iris and lens, stenosing peptic ulcer, pyloroduodenal obstruction, paralytic ileus, intestinal atony, severe ulcerative colitis, toxic megacolon, symptomatic prostatic hypertrophy, bladder neck obstruction, bronchial asthma, COPD, cardiac arrhythmias, myocardial ischemia; sensitivity to anticholinergic drugs; bromides, tartrazine (tartrazine sensitivity is more common with allergy to aspirin); impaired metabolic, liver, or kidney function; myasthenia gravis.
- Use cautiously with Down syndrome, brain damage, spasticity, hypertension, hyperthyroidism, pregnancy, lactation.

Available forms
Tablets—2.5 mg

Adverse effects in *Italics* are most common; those in **Bold** are life-threatening.

Dosages
Adults
2.5 mg PO 30 min before meals and 2.5–5 mg hs.
Pediatric patients
Safety and efficacy not established.

Pharmacokinetics

Route	Onset	Duration
Oral	1 hr	4–6 hr

Metabolism: Hepatic; T$_{1/2}$: 2–3 hr
Distribution: Crosses placenta; may enter breast milk
Excretion: Urine and bile

Adverse effects
- **CNS:** *Blurred vision,* mydriasis, cycloplegia, photophobia, increased intraocular pressure
- **CV:** Palpitations, tachycardia
- **GI:** *Dry mouth, altered taste perception, nausea, vomiting, dysphagia,* heartburn, constipation, bloated feeling, paralytic ileus, gastroesophageal reflux
- **GU:** *Urinary hesitancy and retention;* impotence
- **Local:** *Irritation at site of IM injection*
- **Other:** Decreased sweating and predisposition to heat prostration, suppression of lactation, nasal congestion

Interactions
✻ Drug-drug • Decreased antipsychotic effectiveness of haloperidol with anticholinergic drugs

■ Nursing considerations
Assessment
- **History:** Glaucoma, adhesions between iris and lens, stenosing peptic ulcer, pyloroduodenal obstruction, paralytic ileus, intestinal atony, severe ulcerative colitis, toxic megacolon, symptomatic prostatic hypertrophy, bladder neck obstruction, bronchial asthma, COPD, cardiac arrhythmias, myocardial ischemia; sensitivity to anticholinergic drugs; bromides, tartrazine, impaired metabolic, liver, or kidney function; myasthenia gravis, Down syndrome, brain damage, spasticity, hypertension, hyperthyroidism, pregnancy, lactation
- **Physical:** Bowel sounds, normal output; urinary output, prostate palpation; R; adventitious sounds; P, BP; intraocular pressure, vision; bilateral grip strength, reflexes; liver palpation, liver and renal function tests; skin color, lesions, texture

Interventions
- Ensure adequate hydration; provide environmental control (temperature) to prevent hyperpyrexia.
- Encourage patient to void before each dose of medication if urinary retention becomes a problem.

Teaching points
- Take drug exactly as prescribed.
- Avoid hot environments (you will be heat intolerant, and dangerous reactions may occur).
- These side effects may occur: constipation (ensure adequate fluid intake, proper diet); dry mouth (sugarless lozenges, frequent mouth care may help); blurred vision, sensitivity to light (avoid tasks that require acute vision; wear sunglasses when in bright light); impotence (reversible); difficulty in urination (empty bladder immediately before taking dose).
- Report rash, flushing, eye pain, difficulty breathing, tremors, loss of coordination, irregular heartbeat, palpitations, headache, abdominal distention, hallucinations, severe or persistent dry mouth, difficulty swallowing, difficulty in urination, severe constipation, sensitivity to light.

▽ methsuximide
(meth sux' i mide)

Celontin Kapseals

PREGNANCY CATEGORY C

Drug classes
Antiepileptic agent
Succinimide

Therapeutic actions
Suppresses the paroxysmal three-cycle-per-second spike-and-wave EEG pattern associated with lapses of consciousness in absence (petit mal) seizures; reduces frequency of attacks; mechanism of action not understood.

Indications

- Control of absence (petit mal) seizures when refractory to other drugs

Contraindications and cautions

- Contraindicated with hypersensitivity to succinimides.
- Use cautiously with hepatic, renal abnormalities; pregnancy (there is an association between antiepileptic drugs in epileptic women and elevated risk of birth defects in their children; therapy for major seizures should continue; the effect of seizures on fetus is unknown); lactation.

Available forms

Capsules—150, 300 mg

Dosages

Determine optimal dosage by trial.

Adults

Suggested schedule is 300 mg/day PO for the first week. If required, increase at weekly intervals by increments of 300 mg/day for 3 wk, up to a dosage of 1.2 g/day. Individualize therapy according to response. May be given with other antiepileptic drugs when other forms of epilepsy coexist with absence (petit mal) seizures.

Pediatric patients

150-mg half-strength capsules aid pediatric administration; determine dosage by trial.

Pharmacokinetics

Route	Onset	Peak
Oral	Rapid	1–4 hr

Metabolism: Hepatic; $T_{1/2}$: 2.6–4 hr
Distribution: Crosses placenta; may enter breast milk
Excretion: Urine

Adverse effects

- **CNS:** *Drowsiness, ataxia, dizziness,* irritability, nervousness, headache, blurred vision, myopia, photophobia, hiccups, euphoria, dreamlike state, lethargy, hyperactivity, fatigue, insomnia, confusion, instability, mental slowness, depression, hypochondriacal behavior, sleep disturbances
- **Dermatologic: Stevens-Johnson syndrome,** pruritus, urticaria, pruritic erythematous rashes, skin eruptions, erythema multiforme, systemic lupus erythematosus, alopecia, hirsutism
- **GI:** *Nausea, vomiting, vague gastric upset, epigastric and abdominal pain,* cramps, anorexia, diarrhea, constipation, weight loss, swelling of tongue, gum hypertrophy
- **Hematologic:** Eosinophilia, granulocytopenia, leukopenia, agranulocytosis, aplastic anemia, monocytosis, **pancytopenia**
- **Other:** Periorbital edema, hyperemia, muscle weakness, abnormal liver and kidney function tests, vaginal bleeding

Interactions

✳ **Drug-drug** • Decreased serum levels and therapeutic effects of primidone

■ Nursing considerations
Assessment

- **History:** Hypersensitivity to succinimides; hepatic, renal abnormalities; pregnancy; lactation
- **Physical:** Skin color, lesions; orientation, affect, reflexes, bilateral grip strength, vision exam; bowel sounds, normal output, liver evaluation; liver and kidney function tests, urinalysis, CBC with differential, EEG

Interventions

- Reduce dosage, discontinue, or substitute other antiepileptic medication gradually; abrupt discontinuation may precipitate absence (petit mal) seizures.
- Monitor CBC and differential before therapy and frequently during therapy.
- Discontinue drug if rash, depression of blood count, or unusual depression, aggressiveness, or behavioral alterations occur.

Teaching points

- Take this drug exactly as prescribed; do not discontinue abruptly or change dosage, except on the advice of your health care provider.
- Avoid alcohol, sleep-inducing, or OTC drugs. These could cause dangerous effects. If you need one of these preparations, consult your health care provider.
- Have frequent check-ups to monitor drug response.

Adverse effects in *Italics* are most common; those in **Bold** are life-threatening.

- These side effects may occur: drowsiness, dizziness, confusion, blurred vision (avoid driving a car or performing other tasks requiring alertness or visual acuity); GI upset (take with food or milk, eat frequent, small meals).
- Wear a medical ID tag to alert emergency medical personnel that you are an epileptic taking antiepileptic medication.
- Report rash, joint pain, unexplained fever, sore throat, unusual bleeding or bruising, drowsiness, dizziness, blurred vision, pregnancy.

▽methyclothiazide
*(meth i kloe **thye'** a zide)*

Aquatensen, Duretic (CAN), Enduron

PREGNANCY CATEGORY C

Drug class
Thiazide diuretic

Therapeutic actions
Inhibits reabsorption of sodium and chloride in distal renal tubule, thereby increasing excretion of sodium, chloride, and water by the kidney.

Indications
- Adjunctive therapy in edema associated with CHF, cirrhosis, corticosteroid and estrogen therapy, renal dysfunction
- Hypertension, as sole therapy or in combination with other antihypertensives
- Unlabeled use: diabetes insipidus, especially nephrogenic diabetes insipidus

Contraindications and cautions
- Contraindicated with hypersensitivity to thiazides, pregnancy.
- Use cautiously with fluid or electrolyte imbalances, renal or liver disease, gout, SLE, glucose tolerance abnormalities, hyperparathyroidism, manic-depressive disorders, lactation.

Available forms
Tablets—2.5, 5 mg

Dosages
Adults
- *Edema:* 2.5–10 mg daily PO. Maximum single dose is 10 mg.
- *Hypertension:* 2.5–5 mg daily PO. If BP is not controlled by 5 mg daily within 8–12 wk, another antihypertensive may be needed.

Pharmacokinetics

Route	Onset	Peak	Duration
Oral	2 hr	6 hr	24 hr

Metabolism: $T_{1/2}$: unknown
Distribution: Crosses placenta; enters breast milk
Excretion: Urine

Adverse effects
- **CNS:** *Dizziness, vertigo,* paresthesias, weakness, headache, drowsiness, fatigue, leukopenia, thrombocytopenia, agranulocytosis, aplastic anemia, neutropenia
- **CV:** Orthostatic hypotension, venous thrombosis, volume depletion, cardiac arrhythmias, chest pain
- **Dermatologic:** Photosensitivity, rash, purpura, exfoliative dermatitis, hives
- **GI:** *Nausea, anorexia, vomiting, dry mouth,* diarrhea, constipation, jaundice, hepatitis
- **GU:** *Polyuria, nocturia,* impotence, loss of libido
- **Other:** Muscle cramp

Interactions
✴ Drug-drug • Risk of hyperglycemia with diazoxide • Decreased absorption with cholestyramine, colestipol • Increased risk of digitalis glycoside toxicity if hypokalemia occurs • Increased risk of lithium toxicity when taken with thiazides • Increased fasting blood glucose leading to need to adjust dosage of antidiabetic agents

✴ Drug-lab test • Decreased PBI levels without clinical signs of thyroid disturbances

■ Nursing considerations
Assessment
- **History:** Fluid or electrolyte imbalances, renal or liver disease, gout, SLE, glucose tolerance abnormalities, hyperparathyroidism, manic-depressive disorders, pregnancy, lactation

M

- **Physical:** Skin color and lesions; orientation, reflexes, muscle strength; pulses, BP, orthostatic BP, perfusion, edema, baseline ECG; R, adventitious sounds; liver evaluation, bowel sounds; CBC, serum electrolytes, blood glucose, liver and renal function tests, serum uric acid, urinalysis

Interventions

- Give with food or milk if GI upset occurs.
- Administer early in the day so increased urination will not disturb sleep.
- Measure and record regular body weights to monitor fluid changes.

Teaching points

- Take drug early in day so sleep will not be disturbed by increased urination.
- Weigh yourself daily, and record weight on a calendar.
- Protect skin from exposure to sun or bright lights (sensitivity may occur).
- Increased urination will occur.
- Use caution if dizziness, drowsiness, feeling faint occur.
- Report rapid weight change, swelling in ankles or fingers, unusual bleeding or bruising, muscle cramps.

▷ **methyldopa**
(meth ill doe' pa)

methyldopa
Aldomet, Dopamet (CAN),
Novomedopa (CAN), Nu-Medopa
(CAN)

methyldopate
hydrochloride
Aldomet

PREGNANCY CATEGORY B (ORAL)

PREGNANCY CATEGORY C (IV)

Drug classes
Antihypertensive
Sympatholytic, centrally acting

Therapeutic actions
Mechanism of action not conclusively demonstrated; probably due to drug's metabolism to alpha-methyl norepinephrine, which lowers arterial blood pressure by stimulating central (CNS) alpha$_2$-adrenergic receptors, which in turn decreases sympathetic outflow from the CNS.

Indications
- Hypertension
- Acute hypertensive crisis (IV methyldopa); not drug of choice because of slow onset of action

Contraindications and cautions
- Contraindicated with hypersensitivity to methyldopa, active hepatic disease, previous methyldopa therapy associated with liver disorders.
- Use cautiously with previous liver disease, renal failure, dialysis, bilateral cerebrovascular disease, pregnancy, lactation.

Available forms
Tablets—125, 250, 500 mg; oral suspension—50 mg/mL; injection—50 mg/mL

Dosages
Adults
- *Oral therapy (methyldopa):* Initial therapy: 250 mg bid–tid in the first 48 hr. Adjust dosage at minimum intervals of at least 2 days until response is adequate. Increase dosage in the evening to minimize sedation. Maintenance: 500 mg–3 g/day in 2 to 4 doses. Usually given in 2 doses; some patients may be controlled with a single hs dose.
- *Concomitant therapy:* With antihypertensives other than thiazides, limit initial dosage to 500 mg/day in divided doses. When added to a thiazide, dosage of thiazide need not be changed.
- *IV therapy (methyldopate):* 250–500 mg q 6 hr as required (maximum 1 g q 6 hr). Switch to oral therapy as soon as control is attained; use the dosage schedule used for parenteral therapy.
Pediatric patients
- *Oral therapy (methyldopa):* Individualize dosage; initial dosage is based on 10 mg/kg/

day in 2 to 4 doses. Maximum dosage is 65 mg/kg/day or 3 g/day, whichever is less.
• *IV therapy (methyldopate):* 20–40 mg/kg/day in divided doses q 6 hr. Maximum dosage is 65 mg/kg or 3 g/day, whichever is less.

Geriatric patients or patients with impaired renal function
Reduce dosage. Drug is largely excreted by the kidneys.

Pharmacokinetics

Route	Onset	Peak	Duration
Oral	Varies	2–4 hr	24–48 hr
IV	4–6 hr	Unknown	10–16 hr

Metabolism: Hepatic; $T_{1/2}$: 1.7 hr
Distribution: Crosses placenta; enters breast milk
Excretion: Urine

▼ IV facts

Preparation: Add the dose to 100 mL of 5% dextrose, or give in 5% dextrose in water in a concentration of 10 mg/mL.
Infusion: Administer over 30–60 min.
Incompatibilities: Do not combine with barbiturates or sulfonamides.

Adverse effects

• **CNS:** *Sedation, headache, asthenia, weakness* (usually early and transient), dizziness, light-headedness, symptoms of cerebrovascular insufficiency, paresthesias, parkinsonism, Bell's palsy, decreased mental acuity, involuntary choreoathetotic movements, psychic disturbances
• **CV:** *Bradycardia,* prolonged carotid sinus hypersensitivity, aggravation of angina pectoris, paradoxical pressor response, pericarditis, **myocarditis,** orthostatic hypotension, edema
• **Dermatologic:** Rash seen as eczema or lichenoid eruption, toxic epidermal necrolysis fever, lupuslike syndrome
• **Endocrine:** Breast enlargement, gynecomastia, lactation, hyperprolactinemia, amenorrhea, galactorrhea, impotence, failure to ejaculate, decreased libido
• **GI:** *Nausea, vomiting, distention, constipation,* flatus, diarrhea, colitis, dry mouth, sore or black tongue, pancreatitis, sialadenitis, abnormal liver function tests, jaundice, hepatitis, **hepatic necrosis**
• **Hematologic:** Positive Coombs' test, hemolytic anemia, bone marrow depression, leukopenia, granulocytopenia, thrombocytopenia, positive tests for antinuclear antibody, LE cells, and rheumatoid factor
• **Other:** Nasal stuffiness, mild arthralgia, myalgia, septic shock–like syndrome

Interactions

✱ **Drug-drug** • Potentiation of the pressor effects of sympathomimetic amines • Increased hypotension with levodopa • Risk of hypotension during surgery with central anesthetics; monitor patient carefully

✱ **Drug-lab test** • Methyldopa may interfere with tests for urinary uric acid, serum creatinine, AST, urinary catecholamines

■ Nursing considerations
Assessment

• **History:** Hypersensitivity to methyldopa; hepatic disease; previous methyldopa therapy associated with liver disorders; renal failure; dialysis; bilateral cerebrovascular disease; lactation
• **Physical:** Weight; body temperature; skin color, lesions; mucous membrane color, lesions; orientation, affect, reflexes; P, BP, orthostatic BP, perfusion, edema, auscultation; bowel sounds, normal output, liver evaluation; breast exam; liver and kidney function tests, urinalysis, CBC and differential, direct Coombs' test

Interventions

• Administer IV slowly over 30–60 min; monitor injection site.
• Monitor hepatic function, especially in the first 6–12 wk of therapy or if unexplained fever appears. Discontinue drug if fever, abnormalities in liver function tests, or jaundice occurs. Ensure that methyldopa is not reinstituted in such patients.
• Monitor blood counts periodically to detect hemolytic anemia; a direct Coombs' test before therapy and 6 and 12 mo later may be helpful. Discontinue drug if Coombs'-positive hemolytic anemia occurs. If hemolytic anemia is related to methyldopa, ensure that drug is not reinstituted.
• Discontinue therapy if involuntary choreoathetotic movements occur.

M

- Discontinue if edema progresses or signs of CHF occur.
- Add a thiazide to drug regimen or increase dosage if methyldopa tolerance occurs (second and third mo of therapy).
- Monitor BP carefully when discontinuing methyldopa; drug has short duration of action, and hypertension usually returns within 48 hr.

Teaching points

- Take this drug exactly as prescribed; it is important that you not miss doses.
- These side effects may occur: drowsiness, dizziness, light-headedness, headache, weakness (often transient; avoid driving or engaging in tasks that require alertness); GI upset (frequent, small meals may help); dreams, nightmares, memory impairment (reversible); dizziness, light-headedness when you get up (get up slowly; use caution when climbing stairs); urine that darkens on standing (expected effect); impotence, failure of ejaculation, decreased libido; breast enlargement, sore breasts.
- Report unexplained, prolonged general tiredness; yellowing of the skin or eyes; fever; bruising; rash.

▽ methylene blue
(meth' i leen)

Methblue 65, Urolene Blue

PREGNANCY CATEGORY C

Drug classes
Urinary tract anti-infective
Antidote

Therapeutic actions
Oxidation-reduction agent that converts the ferrous iron of reduced Hgb to the ferric form, producing methemoglobin; weak germicide in lower doses; tissue staining.

Indications
- Treatment of cyanide poisoning and drug-induced methemoglobinemia

- May be useful in the management of patients with oxalate urinary tract calculi
- GU antiseptic for cystitis and urethritis
- Unlabeled uses: delineation of body structures and fistulas through dye effect; neonatal glutaricaciduria II unresponsive to riboflavin

Contraindications and cautions
- Contraindicated with allergy to methylene blue, renal insufficiency, intraspinal injections.
- Use cautiously with G-6-PD deficiency; anemias; CV deficiencies; pregnancy.

Available forms
Tablets—65 mg; injection—10 mg/mL

Dosages
Adults
Oral
65–130 mg tid with a full glass of water.
IV
1–2 mg/kg (0.1–0.2 mL/kg) injected over several minutes.

Pharmacokinetics

Route	Onset	Peak
Oral	Varies	Unknown
IV	Immediate	End of infusion

Metabolism: Tissue; $T_{1/2}$: unknown
Excretion: Urine, bile, and feces

▼ IV facts
Preparation: No preparation required.
Infusion: Inject directly IV or into tubing of actively running IV; inject slowly over several minutes.

Adverse effects
- **CNS:** Dizziness, headache, mental confusion, sweating
- **CV:** Precordial pain
- **GI:** *Nausea,* vomiting, diarrhea, abdominal pain, *blue-green stool*
- **GU:** *Discolored urine* (blue-green); bladder irritation
- **Other:** Necrotic abscess (SC injection); fetal anemia and distress (amniotic injection);

Adverse effects in *Italics* are most common; those in **Bold** are life-threatening.

neural damage, paralysis (intrathecal injection); *skin stained blue*

■ Nursing considerations
Assessment
- **History:** Allergy to methylene blue, renal insufficiency, presence of G6PD deficiency; anemias; CV deficiencies; pregnancy
- **Physical:** Skin color, lesions; urinary output, bladder palpation; abdominal exam, normal output; CBC with differential

Interventions
- Give oral drug after meals with a full glass of water.
- Give IV slowly over several minutes; avoid exceeding recommended dosage.
- Use care to avoid SC injection; monitor intrathecal sites used for diagnostic injection for necrosis and damage.
- Contact with skin will dye the skin blue; stain may be removed by hypochlorite solution.
- Monitor CBC for signs of marked anemia.

Teaching points
- Take drug after meals with a full glass of water.
- Avoid bubble baths, excessive ingestion of citrus juice, and sexual contacts if bladder infection or urethritis is being treated.
- These side effects may occur: urine or stool discolored blue-green; abdominal pain, nausea, vomiting (small frequent meals may help).
- Report difficulty breathing, severe nausea or vomiting, fatigue.

▷ methylergonovine maleate

*(meth ill er goe **noe**' veen)*

Methergine

PREGNANCY CATEGORY C

Drug class
Oxytocic

Therapeutic actions
A partial agonist or antagonist at alpha receptors; as a result, it increases the strength,
duration, and frequency of uterine contractions.

Indications
- Routine management after delivery of the placenta
- Treatment of postpartum atony and hemorrhage; subinvolution of the uterus
- Uterine stimulation during the second stage of labor following the delivery of the anterior shoulder, under strict medical supervision

Contraindications and cautions
- Contraindicated with allergy to methylergonovine, hypertension, toxemia, lactation, pregnancy.
- Use cautiously with sepsis, obliterative vascular disease, hepatic or renal impairment.

Available forms
Tablets—0.2 mg; injection—0.2 mg/mL

Dosages
Adults
IM
0.2 mg after delivery of the placenta, after delivery of the anterior shoulder, during puerperium. May be repeated q 2–4 hr.
IV
Same dosage as IM; infuse slowly over at least 60 sec. Monitor BP very carefully as severe hypertensive reaction can occur.
Oral
0.2 mg PO tid or qid daily in the puerperium for up to 1 wk.

Pharmacokinetics

Route	Onset	Peak	Duration
Oral	5–10 min	30–60 min	3 hr
IM	2–5 min	30 min	3 hr
IV	Immediate	2–3 min	1–3 hr

Metabolism: Hepatic; $T_{1/2}$: 30 min
Distribution: Crosses placenta; enters breast milk
Excretion: Urine

▼ IV facts
Preparation: No additional preparation required.
Infusion: Inject directly IV or into tubing of running IV; inject very slowly, over no less than

60 sec; rapid infusion can result in sudden hypertension or cerebral events.

Adverse effects
- **CNS:** *Dizziness, headache,* tinnitus, diaphoresis
- **CV:** *Transient hypertension,* palpitations, chest pain, dyspnea
- **GI:** *Nausea,* vomiting

■ Nursing considerations
Assessment
- **History:** Allergy to methylergonovine, hypertension, toxemia, sepsis, obliterative vascular disease, hepatic or renal impairment, lactation, pregnancy
- **Physical:** Uterine tone, vaginal bleeding; orientation, reflexes, affect; P, BP, edema; CBC, renal and liver function tests; fetal monitoring when used during labor

Interventions
- Administer by IM injection or orally unless emergency requires IV use. Complications are more frequent with IV use.
- Monitor postpartum women for BP changes and amount and character of vaginal bleeding.
- Discontinue if signs of toxicity occur.
- Avoid prolonged use of the drug.
- The patient receiving a parenteral oxytocic is usually receiving it as part of an immediate medical situation, and the drug teaching should be incorporated into the teaching about delivery. The patient needs to know the name of the drug and what she can expect after it is administered.

Teaching points
- This drug should not be needed for longer than 1 wk.
- These side effects may occur: nausea, vomiting, dizziness, headache, ringing in the ears (short time use may make it tolerable).
- Report difficulty breathing, headache, numb or cold extremities, severe abdominal cramping.

▽ methylphenidate hydrochloride
*(meth ill **fen**' i date)*

Concerta, Metadate CD, Metadate ER, Methylin, Methylin ER, PMS-Methylphenidate (CAN), Riphenidate (CAN), Ritalin, Ritalin LA, Ritalin SR

PREGNANCY CATEGORY C

C-II CONTROLLED SUBSTANCE

Drug class
Central nervous system stimulant

Therapeutic actions
Mild cortical stimulant with CNS actions similar to those of the amphetamines; efficacy in hyperkinetic syndrome, attention-deficit disorders in children appears paradoxical and is not understood

Indications
- Narcolepsy (*Ritalin, Ritalin SR, Metadate ER*)
- Attention-deficit disorders, hyperkinetic syndrome, minimal brain dysfunction in children or adults with a behavioral syndrome characterized by the following symptoms: moderate to severe distractibility, short attention span, hyperactivity, emotional lability, and impulsivity, not secondary to environmental factors or psychiatric disorders
- Unlabeled use: treatment of depression in the elderly, cancer and stroke patients; alleviation of neurobehavioral symptoms after traumatic brain injury; improvement in pain control and sedation in patients receiving opiates

Contraindications and cautions
- Contraindicated with hypersensitivity to methylphenidate; marked anxiety, tension, and agitation; glaucoma; motor tics, family history or diagnosis of Tourette's syndrome; severe depression of endogenous or exogenous origin; normal fatigue states, pregnancy.

- Use cautiously with seizure disorders; hypertension; drug dependence, alcoholism; emotional instability; lactation.

Available forms

Tablets—5, 10, 20 mg; SR tablets—20 mg; ER tablets—10, 18, 20, 27, 36, 54 mg; ER capsules—20 mg (*Metadate CD*); 20, 30, 40 mg (*Ritalin*); and 20, 30, 40 mg (*Ritalin LA*)

Dosages
Adults

Individualize dosage. Give orally in divided doses bid–tid, preferably 30–45 min before meals; dosage ranges from 10–60 mg/day PO. If insomnia is a problem, drug should be taken before 6 PM. Timed-release tablets have a duration of 8 hr and may be used when timing and dosage are adjusted to the 8-hr daily regimen. ER tablets (*Concerta*): 18 mg PO daily in the morning; may be increased by 18 mg/day at 1-wk intervals to a maximum of 54 mg/day.

Pediatric patients

Start with small oral doses (5 mg PO before breakfast and lunch with gradual increments of 5–10 mg weekly). Daily dosage > 60 mg not recommended. Discontinue use after 1 mo if no improvement. Discontinue periodically to assess condition; usually discontinued after puberty.

$\geq 6\ yr$: Use adult dose of *Concerta*.

$< 6\ yr$: Not recommended.

Pharmacokinetics

Route	Onset	Peak	Duration
Oral	Varies	1–3 hr	4–6 hr

Metabolism: Hepatic; $T_{1/2}$: 1–3 hr
Distribution: Crosses placenta; enters breast milk
Excretion: Urine

Adverse effects

- **CNS:** *Nervousness, insomnia,* dizziness, headache, dyskinesia, chorea, drowsiness, Tourette syndrome, toxic psychosis, blurred vision, accommodation difficulties
- **CV:** *Increased or decreased pulse and BP; tachycardia,* angina, cardiac arrhythmias, palpitations
- **Dermatologic:** Rash, urticaria, fever, arthralgia, exfoliative dermatitis, erythema multiforme with necrotizing vasculitis and thrombocytopenic purpura, loss of scalp hair
- **GI:** *Anorexia, nausea, abdominal pain,* weight loss
- **Hematologic:** Leukopenia, anemia
- **Other:** Tolerance, psychological dependence, abnormal behavior with abuse

Interactions

✳ **Drug-drug** • Decreased effects of guanethidine; avoid this combination • Increased effects and toxicity of methylphenidate with MAOIs • Increased serum levels of phenytoin, TCAs, oral anticoagulants, SSRIs with methylphenidate; monitor for toxicity

✳ **Drug-lab test** • Methylphenidate may increase the urinary excretion of epinephrine

■ Nursing considerations
Assessment

- **History:** Hypersensitivity to methylphenidate; marked anxiety, tension, and agitation; glaucoma; motor tics, Tourette syndrome; severe depression; normal fatigue state; seizure disorders; hypertension; drug dependence, alcoholism, emotional instability; pregnancy, lactation
- **Physical:** Weight; T; skin color, lesions; orientation, affect, ophthalmologic exam (tonometry); P, BP, auscultation; R, adventitious sounds; bowel sounds, normal output; CBC with differential, platelet count, baseline ECG

Interventions

- Ensure proper diagnosis before administering to children for behavioral syndromes; drug should not be used until other causes/concomitants of abnormal behavior (learning disability, EEG abnormalities, neurologic deficits) are ruled out.
- Interrupt drug dosage periodically in children to determine if symptoms warrant continued drug therapy.
- Monitor growth of children on long-term methylphenidate therapy.
- Ensure that all timed-release tablets and capsules are swallowed whole, not chewed or crushed.
- Dispense the least feasible dose to minimize risk of overdose.
- Give before 6 PM to prevent insomnia.

- Monitor CBC, platelet counts periodically in patients on long-term therapy.
- Monitor BP frequently early in treatment.

Teaching points

- Take this drug exactly as prescribed. Timed-release tablets and capsules must be swallowed whole, not chewed or crushed. *Metadate CD* capsules may be opened and entire contents sprinkled on soft food—do not chew or crush granules.
- Take drug before 6 PM to avoid night-time sleep disturbance.
- Avoid alcohol and OTC drugs, including nose drops, cold remedies; some OTC drugs could cause dangerous effects.
- These side effects may occur: nervousness, restlessness, dizziness, insomnia, impaired thinking (may lessen; avoid driving or engaging in activities that require alertness); headache, loss of appetite, dry mouth.
- Report nervousness, insomnia, palpitations, vomiting, rash, fever.

▽methylprednisolone
*(meth ill pred **niss'** oh lone)*

methylprednisolone
Oral: Medrol, Meprolone (CAN)

methylprednisolone sodium succinate
IV, IM injection: A-Methapred, Solu-Medrol

PREGNANCY CATEGORY C

Drug classes
Corticosteroid
Glucocorticoid
Hormone

Therapeutic actions
Enters target cells and binds to intracellular corticosteroid receptors, initiating many complex reactions that are responsible for its anti-inflammatory and immunosuppressive effects.

Indications
- Hypercalcemia associated with cancer

- Short-term management of various inflammatory and allergic disorders, such as rheumatoid arthritis, collagen diseases (eg, SLE), dermatologic diseases (eg, pemphigus), status asthmaticus, and autoimmune disorders
- Hematologic disorders: thrombocytopenia purpura, erythroblastopenia
- Ulcerative colitis, acute exacerbations of multiple sclerosis, and palliation in some leukemias and lymphomas
- Trichinosis with neurologic or myocardial involvement
- Unlabeled use: septic shock

Contraindications and cautions
- Contraindicated with infections, especially tuberculosis, fungal infections, amebiasis, vaccinia and varicella, and antibiotic-resistant infections; lactation; allergy to tartrazine or aspirin in products labeled *Medrol*.
- Use cautiously with kidney or liver disease, hypothyroidism, ulcerative colitis with impending perforation, diverticulitis, active or latent peptic ulcer, inflammatory bowel disease, CHF, hypertension, thromboembolic disorders, osteoporosis, convulsive disorders, diabetes mellitus.

Available forms
Tablets—2, 4, 8, 16, 24, 32 mg; powder for injection—40, 125, 500 mg/mL, 1, 2 g/vial

Dosages
Adults
Individualize dosage, depending on severity and response. Give daily dose before 9 AM to minimize adrenal suppression. For maintenance, reduce initial dose in small increments at intervals until the lowest satisfactory clinical dose is reached. If long-term therapy is needed, consider alternate-day therapy with a short-acting corticosteroid. After long-term therapy, withdraw drug slowly to prevent adrenal insufficiency.
Oral
4–48 mg/day. Alternate-day therapy: twice the usual dose every other morning.
IV, IM
10–40 mg IV administered over 1 to several min. Give subsequent doses IV or IM. Caution:

Adverse effects in *Italics* are most common; those in **Bold** are life-threatening.

Rapid IV administration of large doses (more than 0.5–1 g in less than 10–120 min) has caused serious cardiac complications.

Pediatric patients

Individualize dosage on the basis of severity and response rather than by formulae that correct doses for age or weight. Carefully observe growth and development in infants and children on prolonged therapy. Minimum dose of methylprednisolone is 0.5 mg/kg per 24 hr.

• *High-dose therapy:* 30 mg/kg IV infused over 10–20 min; may repeat q 4–6 hr, but not beyond 48–72 hr.

Pharmacokinetics

Route	Onset	Peak	Duration
Oral	Varies	1–2 hr	1.2–1.5 days
IV	Rapid	Rapid	Unknown
IM	Rapid	4–8 days	1–5 wk

Metabolism: Hepatic; $T_{1/2}$: 78–188 min
Distribution: Crosses placenta; enters breast milk
Excretion: Urine

▽ IV facts

Preparation: No additional preparation is required.

Infusion: Inject directly into vein or into tubing of running IV; administer slowly, over 1–20 min to reduce cardiac effects.

Incompatibilities: Do not combine with calcium gluconate, glycopyrrolate, insulin, nafcillin, penicillin G sodium, tetracycline.

Adverse effects

Effects depend on dose, route, and duration of therapy.

• **CNS:** *Vertigo, headache,* paresthesias, insomnia, convulsions, psychosis, cataracts, increased intraocular pressure, glaucoma

• **CV:** Hypotension, **shock**, hypertension and CHF secondary to fluid retention, thromboembolism, thrombophlebitis, fat embolism, cardiac arrhythmias

• **Electrolyte imbalance:** *Na+ and fluid retention,* hypokalemia, hypocalcemia

• **Endocrine:** Amenorrhea, irregular menses, growth retardation, decreased carbohydrate tolerance, diabetes mellitus, cushingoid state (long-term effect), increased blood sugar, increased serum cholesterol, decreased T_3

and T_4 levels, hypothalamic-pituitary-adrenal (HPA) suppression with systemic therapy longer than 5 days

• **GI:** Peptic or esophageal ulcer, pancreatitis, abdominal distention, nausea, vomiting, *increased appetite, weight gain*

• **Hypersensitivity:** Anaphylactoid reactions

• **Musculoskeletal:** Muscle weakness, steroid myopathy, loss of muscle mass, osteoporosis, spontaneous fractures

• **Other:** *Immunosuppression; aggravation or masking of infections; impaired wound healing;* thin, fragile skin; petechiae, ecchymoses, purpura, striae; subcutaneous fat atrophy

Interactions

✷ **Drug-drug** • Increased therapeutic and toxic effects with erythromycin, ketoconazole, troleandomycin • Risk of severe deterioration of muscle strength when given to myasthenia gravis patients who are receiving ambenonium, edrophonium, neostigmine, pyridostigmine • Decreased steroid blood levels with barbiturates, phenytoin, rifampin • Decreased effectiveness of salicylates

✷ **Drug-lab test** • False-negative nitroblue-tetrazolium test for bacterial infection • Suppression of skin test reactions

■ Nursing considerations
Assessment

• **History:** Infections; kidney or liver disease, hypothyroidism, ulcerative colitis, diverticulitis, active or latent peptic ulcer, inflammatory bowel disease, CHF, hypertension, thromboembolic disorders, osteoporosis, convulsive disorders, diabetes mellitus; pregnancy; lactation

• **Physical:** Weight, T, reflexes and grip strength, affect and orientation, P, BP, peripheral perfusion prominence of superficial veins, R and adventitious sounds, serum electrolytes, blood glucose

Interventions

• Use caution with the 24-mg tablets marketed as *Medrol;* these contain tartrazine, which may cause allergic reactions, especially in people who are allergic to aspirin.

• Give daily dose before 9 AM to mimic normal peak corticosteroid blood levels.

- Increase dosage when patient is subject to stress.
- Taper doses when discontinuing high-dose or long-term therapy.
- Do not give live virus vaccines with immunosuppressive doses of corticosteroids.

Teaching points

- Do not to stop taking the oral drug without consulting your health care provider.
- Avoid exposure to infections.
- Report unusual weight gain, swelling of the extremities, muscle weakness, black or tarry stools, fever, prolonged sore throat, colds or other infections, worsening of disorder.

▷ metoclopramide
*(met oh kloe **pra'** mide)*

Apo-Metoclop (CAN), Maxeran (CAN), Maxolon, Nu-Metoclopramide (CAN), Octamide PFS, Reglan

PREGNANCY CATEGORY B

Drug classes
GI stimulant
Antiemetic
Dopaminergic blocking agent

Therapeutic actions
Stimulates motility of upper GI tract without stimulating gastric, biliary, or pancreatic secretions; appears to sensitize tissues to action of acetylcholine; relaxes pyloric sphincter, which, when combined with effects on motility, accelerates gastric emptying and intestinal transit; little effect on gallbladder or colon motility; increases lower esophageal sphincter pressure; has sedative properties; induces release of prolactin.

Indications
- Relief of symptoms of acute and recurrent diabetic gastroparesis
- Short-term therapy (4–12 wk) for adults with symptomatic gastroesophageal reflux who fail to respond to conventional therapy

- Prevention of nausea and vomiting associated with emetogenic cancer chemotherapy (parenteral)
- Prophylaxis of postoperative nausea and vomiting when nasogastric suction is undesirable
- Facilitation of small-bowel intubation when tube does not pass the pylorus with conventional maneuvers (single-dose parenteral use)
- Stimulation of gastric emptying and intestinal transit of barium when delayed emptying interferes with radiologic exam of the stomach or small intestine (single-dose parenteral use)
- Unlabeled uses: improvement of lactation (doses of 30–45 mg/day); treatment of nausea and vomiting of a variety of etiologies: emesis during pregnancy and labor, gastric ulcer, anorexia nervosa

Contraindications and cautions
- Contraindicated with allergy to metoclopramide; GI hemorrhage, mechanical obstruction or perforation; pheochromocytoma (may cause hypertensive crisis); epilepsy.
- Use cautiously with previously detected breast cancer (one third of such tumors are prolactin dependent); lactation.

Available forms
Tablets—5, 10 mg; syrup—5 mg/5 mL; concentrated solution—10 mg/mL; injection—5 mg/mL

Dosages
Adults
- *Relief of symptoms of gastroparesis:* 10 mg PO 30 min before each meal and hs for 2–8 wk. If symptoms are severe, initiate therapy with IM or IV administration for up to 10 days until symptoms subside.
- *Symptomatic gastroesophageal reflux:* 10–15 mg PO up to 4 times/day 30 min before meals and hs. If symptoms occur only at certain times or in relation to specific stimuli, single doses of 20 mg may be preferable; guide therapy by endoscopic results. Do not use longer than 12 wk.

Adverse effects in *Italics* are most common; those in **Bold** are life-threatening.

- *Prevention of postoperative nausea and vomiting:* 10–20 mg IM at the end of surgery.
- *Prevention of chemotherapy-induced emesis:* Dilute and give by IV infusion over not less than 15 min. Give first dose 30 min before chemotherapy; repeat q 2 hr for 2 doses, then q 3 hr for 3 doses. The initial 2 doses should be 2 mg/kg for highly emetogenic drugs (cisplatin, dacarbazine); 1 mg/kg may suffice for other chemotherapeutic agents.
- *Facilitation of small bowel intubation, gastric emptying:* 10 mg (2 mL) by direct IV injection over 1–2 min.

Pediatric patients
- *Facilitation of intubation, gastric emptying:*

6–14 yr: 2.5–5 mg by direct IV injection over 1–2 min.

< 6 yr: 0.1 mg/kg by direct IV injection over 1–2 min.

Pharmacokinetics

Route	Onset	Peak	Duration
Oral	30–60 min	60–90 min	1–2 hr
IM	10–15 min	60–90 min	1–2 hr
IV	1–3 min	60–90 min	1–2 hr

Metabolism: Hepatic; $T_{1/2}$: 5–6 hr
Distribution: Crosses placenta; enters breast milk
Excretion: Urine

▼IV facts
Preparation: Dilute dose in 50 mL of a parenteral solution (dextrose 5% in water, sodium chloride injection, dextrose 5% in 0.45% sodium chloride, Ringer's injection, or lactated Ringer's injection). May be stored for up to 48 hr if protected from light or up to 24 hr under normal light.
Infusion: Give direct IV doses slowly (over 1–2 min); give infusions over at least 15 min.
Incompatibilities: Do not mix with solutions containing chloramphenicol, sodium bicarbonate, cisplatin, erythromycin.
Y-site incompatibility: Do not give with furosemide.

Adverse effects
- **CNS:** *Restlessness, drowsiness, fatigue, lassitude,* insomnia, *extrapyramidal reac-*

tions, parkinsonism-like reactions, akathisia, dystonia, myoclonus, dizziness, anxiety
- **CV:** Transient hypertension
- **GI:** *Nausea, diarrhea*

Interactions
✳ Drug-drug • Decreased absorption of digoxin from the stomach • Increased toxic and immunosuppressive effects of cyclosporine

■ Nursing considerations
Assessment
- **History:** Allergy to metoclopramide, GI hemorrhage, mechanical obstruction or perforation, pheochromocytoma, epilepsy, lactation, previously detected breast cancer
- **Physical:** Orientation, reflexes, affect; P, BP; bowel sounds, normal output; EEG

Interventions
- Monitor BP carefully during IV administration.
- Monitor for extrapyramidal reactions, and consult physician if they occur.
- Monitor diabetic patients, arrange for alteration in insulin dose or timing if diabetic control is compromised by alterations in timing of food absorption.
- Provide diphenhydramine injection on standby in case extrapyramidal reactions occur (50 mg IM).
- Provide phentolamine on standby in case of hypertensive crisis (most likely to occur with undiagnosed pheochromocytoma).

Teaching points
- Take this drug exactly as prescribed.
- Do not use alcohol, sleep remedies, sedatives; serious sedation could occur.
- These side effects may occur: drowsiness, dizziness (do not drive or perform other tasks that require alertness); restlessness, anxiety, depression, headache, insomnia (reversible); nausea, diarrhea.
- Report involuntary movement of the face, eyes, or limbs, severe depression, severe diarrhea.

▽metolazone
(*me tole' a zone*)

Mykrox, Zaroxolyn

PREGNANCY CATEGORY B

Drug class
Thiazide-like diuretic

Therapeutic actions
Inhibits reabsorption of sodium and chloride in distal renal tubule, increasing excretion of sodium, chloride, and water by the kidney.

Indications
- Adjunctive therapy in edema associated with CHF, cirrhosis, corticosteroid and estrogen therapy, renal dysfunction
- Hypertension, as monotherapy or in combination with other antihypertensives
- Unlabeled uses: calcium nephrolithiasis alone or with amiloride or allopurinol to prevent recurrences in hypercalciuric or normal calciuric patients; diabetes insipidus, especially nephrogenic diabetes insipidus

Contraindications and cautions
- Contraindicated with hypersensitivity to thiazides, hepatic coma, fluid or electrolyte imbalances, renal or liver disease.
- Use cautiously with gout, SLE, glucose tolerance abnormalities, hyperparathyroidism, manic-depressive disorders, lactation.

Available forms
Tablets: *Zaroxolyn*—2.5, 5, 10 mg; *Mykrox*—0.5 mg

Dosages
Adults
Zaroxolyn
- *Hypertension:* 2.5–5 mg daily PO.
- *Edema of renal disease:* 5–20 mg daily PO.
- *Edema of CHF:* 5–10 mg daily PO.
- *Calcium nephrolithiasis:* 2.5–10 mg/day PO.

Mykrox
- *Mild to moderate hypertension:* 0.5 mg daily PO taken as a single dose early in the morning. May be increased to 1 mg daily; do not exceed 1 mg/day. If switching from *Zaroxolyn* to *Mykrox,* determine the dose by adjustment starting at 0.5 mg daily and increasing to 1 mg daily. If absolutely need to change brands from *Zaroxolyn* to *Mykrox,* start at *Mykrox* 0.5 mg PO daily and increase to 1 mg PO daily if needed.

Pediatric patients
Not recommended.

Pharmacokinetics

Brand	Onset	Peak	Duration
Mykrox	20–30 min	2–4 hr	12–24 hr
Zaroxolyn	1 hr	2 hr	12–24 hr

Metabolism: Hepatic; $T_{1/2}$: 14 hr (*Mykrox*), unknown (*Zaroxolyn*)
Distribution: Crosses placenta; enters breast milk
Excretion: Urine

Adverse effects
- **CNS:** *Dizziness, vertigo,* paresthesias, weakness, *headache,* drowsiness, *fatigue*
- **CV:** Orthostatic hypotension, venous thrombosis, volume depletion, cardiac arrhythmias, chest pain
- **Dermatologic:** Photosensitivity, rash, purpura, exfoliative dermatitis
- **GI:** *Nausea, anorexia, vomiting, dry mouth, diarrhea, constipation,* jaundice, hepatitis, pancreatitis
- **GU:** *Polyuria, nocturia, impotence,* decreased libido
- **Hematologic:** Leukopenia, thrombocytopenia, agranulocytosis, aplastic anemia, neutropenia, fluid and electrolyte imbalances
- **Other:** Muscle cramps and muscle spasms, fever, hives, gouty attacks, flushing

Interactions
✳ **Drug-drug** • Increased thiazide effects and chance of acute hyperglycemia with diazoxide • Decreased absorption with cholestyramine, colestipol • Increased risk of cardiac glycoside toxicity if hypokalemia occurs • Increased risk of lithium toxicity • Increased dosage of antidiabetic agents may be needed

• Increased risk of hyperglycemia if taken with diazoxide

✻ Drug-lab test • Decreased PBI levels without clinical signs of thyroid disturbances

■ Nursing considerations
Assessment
• **History:** Fluid or electrolyte imbalances, renal or liver disease, gout, SLE, glucose tolerance abnormalities, hyperparathyroidism, manic-depressive disorders, hepatic coma or precoma, lactation
• **Physical:** Skin color and lesions; orientation, reflexes, muscle strength; pulses, BP, orthostatic BP, perfusion, edema, baseline ECG; R, adventitious sounds; liver evaluation, bowel sounds; CBC, serum electrolytes, blood glucose, liver and function tests, serum uric acid, urinalysis

Interventions
• Note that metolazone formulations (*Mykrox, Zaroxolyn*) are not therapeutically equivalent. Do not interchange brands.
• Withdraw drug 2–3 days before elective surgery; if emergency surgery is indicated, reduce dosage of preanesthetic or anesthetic agents.
• Administer with food or milk if GI upset occurs.
• Measure and record body weights to monitor fluid changes.

Teaching points
• Take drug early in the day so sleep will not be disturbed by increased urination.
• Weigh yourself daily, and record weights.
• Protect skin from exposure to the sun or bright lights.
• These side effects may occur: increased urination; dizziness, drowsiness, feeling faint (use caution; avoid driving or operating dangerous machinery); headache.
• Report rapid weight change, swelling in ankles or fingers, unusual bleeding or bruising, muscle cramps.

▽ **metoprolol**
*(me **toe'** proe lole)*

Apo-Metoprolol (CAN), Betaloc (CAN), Lopresor (CAN), Lopressor, Novometoprol (CAN), Nu-Metop (CAN), Toprol-XL

PREGNANCY CATEGORY C

Drug classes
Beta$_1$-selective adrenergic blocker
Antihypertensive

Therapeutic actions
Competitively blocks beta-adrenergic receptors in the heart and juxtaglomerular apparatus, decreasing the influence of the sympathetic nervous system on these tissues and the excitability of the heart, decreasing cardiac output and the release of renin, and lowering BP; acts in the CNS to reduce sympathetic outflow and vasoconstrictor tone.

Indications
• Hypertension, alone or with other drugs, especially diuretics
• Prevention of reinfarction in MI patients who are hemodynamically stable or within 3–10 days of the acute MI (immediate-release tablets and injection)
• Treatment of angina pectoris
• Treatment of stable, symptomatic CHF of ischemic, hypertensive, or cardiomyopathic origin (*Toprol-XL* only)

Contraindications and cautions
• Contraindicated with sinus bradycardia (HR < 45 beats/min), second- or third-degree heart block (PR interval > 0.24 sec), cardiogenic shock, CHF, systolic BP < 100 mm Hg; lactation.
• Use cautiously with diabetes or thyrotoxicosis; asthma or COPD; pregnancy.

Available forms
Tablets—50, 100 mg; ER tablets—25, 50, 100, 200 mg; injection—1 mg/mL

Dosages
Adults
• *Hypertension:* Initially 100 mg/day PO in single or divided doses; gradually increase

M

dosage at weekly intervals. Usual maintenance dose is 100–450 mg/day.
- *Angina pectoris:* Initially 100 mg/day PO
in 2 divided doses; may be increased gradually, effective range 100–400 mg/day.
- *MI, early treatment:* Three IV bolus doses
of 5 mg each at 2-min intervals with careful monitoring. If these are tolerated, give
50 mg PO 15 min after the last IV dose and
q 6 hr for 48 hr. Thereafter, give a maintenance dosage of 100 mg PO bid. Reduce initial PO doses to 25 mg, or discontinue in patients who do not tolerate the IV doses.
- *MI, late treatment:* 100 mg PO bid as soon
as possible after infarct, continuing for at
least 3 mo and possibly for 1–3 yr.

Extended-release tablets
- *Hypertension:* 50–100 mg/day PO as one
dose.
- *Angina:* 100 mg/day PO as one dose.
- *CHF:* 12.5–25 mg/day *Toprol-XL* for 2 wk;
may then be increased by 25 mg every 2 wk
to a maximum of 200 mg.

Pediatric patients
Safety and efficacy not established.

Pharmacokinetics

Route	Onset	Peak	Duration
Oral	15 min	90 min	15–19 hr
IV	Immediate	60–90 min	15–19 hr

Metabolism: Hepatic; $T_{1/2}$: 3–4 hr
Distribution: Crosses placenta; enters breast
milk
Excretion: Urine

▽IV facts
Preparation: No additional preparation is
required.
Infusion: Inject directly into vein or into tubing of running IV over 1 min. Inject as a bolus; monitor carefully; wait 2 min between doses; do not give if bradycardia of < 45 beats/min,
heart block, systolic pressure < 100 mm Hg.
Incompatibilities: Do not mix with amino
acids, aztreonam, dopamine.

Adverse effects
- **Allergic:** Pharyngitis, erythematous rash,
fever, sore throat, laryngospasm

- **CNS:** Dizziness, vertigo, tinnitus, fatigue,
emotional depression, paresthesias, sleep disturbances, hallucinations, disorientation,
memory loss, slurred speech
- **CV:** *CHF, cardiac arrhythmias,* peripheral vascular insufficiency, claudication, CVA,
pulmonary edema, hypotension
- **Dermatologic:** Rash, pruritus, sweating,
dry skin
- **EENT:** Eye irritation, dry eyes, conjunctivitis, blurred vision
- **GI:** *Gastric pain, flatulence, constipation,
diarrhea, nausea, vomiting,* anorexia, ischemic colitis, renal and mesenteric arterial thrombosis, retroperitoneal fibrosis, hepatomegaly, acute pancreatitis
- **GU:** *Impotence, decreased libido,* Peyronie's
disease, dysuria, nocturia, frequent urination
- **Musculoskeletal:** Joint pain, arthralgia,
muscle cramp
- **Respiratory:** Bronchospasm, dyspnea,
cough, bronchial obstruction, nasal stuffiness, rhinitis, pharyngitis
- **Other:** *Decreased exercise tolerance, development of antinuclear antibodies (ANA),*
hyperglycemia or hypoglycemia, elevated
serum transaminase, alkaline phosphatase

Interactions
✱ Drug-drug • Increased effects of metoprolol with verapamil, cimetidine, methimazole, propylthiouracil • Increased effects of
both drugs if metoprolol is taken with hydralazine • Increased serum levels and toxicity of IV lidocaine, if given concurrently • Increased risk of orthostatic hypotension with
prazosin • Decreased antihypertensive effects
if taken with NSAIDs, clonidine, rifampin • Decreased therapeutic effects with barbiturates
• Hypertension followed by severe bradycardia
if given concurrently with epinephrine
✱ Drug-lab test • Possible false results with
glucose or insulin tolerance tests (oral)

■ Nursing considerations
Assessment
- **History:** Sinus bradycardia (HR < 45 beats/
min), second- or third-degree heart block
(PR interval > 0.24 sec), cardiogenic shock,
CHF, systolic BP < 100 mm Hg; diabetes or
thyrotoxicosis; asthma or COPD; lactation

- **Physical:** Weight, skin condition, neurologic status, P, BP, ECG, respiratory status, kidney and thyroid function, blood and urine glucose

Interventions

- Do not discontinue drug abruptly after long-term therapy (hypersensitivity to catecholamines may have developed, causing exacerbation of angina, MI, and ventricular arrhythmias). Taper drug gradually over 2 wk with monitoring.
- Ensure that patient swallows the ER tablets whole; do not cut, crush, or chew.
- Consult physician about withdrawing drug if patient is to undergo surgery (controversial).
- Give oral drug with food to facilitate absorption.
- Provide continual cardiac monitoring for patients receiving IV metoprolol.

Teaching points

- Do not stop taking this drug unless instructed to do so by a health care provider.
- Swallow the ER tablets whole; do not cut, crush, or chew.
- These side effects may occur: dizziness, drowsiness, light-headedness, blurred vision (avoid driving or dangerous activities); nausea, loss of appetite (small, frequent meals may help); nightmares, depression (discuss change of medication); sexual impotence.
- Report difficulty breathing, night cough, swelling of extremities, slow pulse, confusion, depression, rash, fever, sore throat.

▽ **metronidazole**
*(me troe **ni'** da zole)*

Apo-Metronidazole (CAN), Flagyl, Flagyl 375, Flagyl ER, Flagyl IV, Flagyl IV RTU, MetroCream (CAN), MetroGel, Metro I.V., Neo-Tric (CAN), NidaGel (CAN), Noritate, Novonidazol (CAN), PMS-Metronidazole (CAN), Protostat, Trikacide (CAN)

PREGNANCY CATEGORY B

Drug classes
Antibiotic
Antibacterial
Amebicide
Antiprotozoal

Therapeutic actions
Bactericidal: inhibits DNA synthesis in specific (obligate) anaerobes, causing cell death; antiprotozoal-trichomonacidal, amebicidal: biochemical mechanism of action is not known.

Indications
- Acute infection with susceptible anaerobic bacteria
- Acute intestinal amebiasis
- Amebic liver abscess
- Trichomoniasis (acute and partners of patients with acute infection)
- Preoperative, intraoperative, postoperative prophylaxis for patients undergoing colorectal surgery
- Topical application in the treatment of inflammatory papules, pustules, and erythema of rosacea
- Unlabeled uses: prophylaxis for patients undergoing gynecologic, abdominal surgery; hepatic encephalopathy; Crohn's disease; antibiotic-associated pseudomembranous colitis; treatment of *Gardnerella vaginalis,* giardiasis (use recommended by the CDC)

Contraindications and cautions
- Contraindicated with hypersensitivity to metronidazole; pregnancy (do not use for trichomoniasis in first trimester).
- Use cautiously with CNS diseases, hepatic disease, candidiasis (moniliasis), blood dyscrasias, lactation.

Available forms
Tablets—250, 500 mg; ER tablets—750 mg; capsules—375 mg; powder for injection—500 mg; injection—500 mg/100 mL

Dosages
Adults
- *Anaerobic bacterial infection:* 15 mg/kg IV infused over 1 hr; then 7.5 mg/kg infused over 1 hr q 6 hr for 7–10 days, not to exceed 4 g/day.
- *Amebiasis:* 750 mg/tid PO for 5–10 days. (In amebic dysentery, combine with iodoquinol 650 mg PO tid for 20 days.)

- *Trichomoniasis:* 2 g PO in 1 day (1-day treatment) *or* 250 mg tid PO for 7 days.
- *Prophylaxis:* 15 mg/kg infused IV over 30–60 min and completed about 1 hr before surgery. Then 7.5 mg/kg infused over 30–60 min at 6- to 12-hr intervals after initial dose during the day of surgery only.
- *Gardnerella vaginalis:* 500 mg bid PO for 7 days.
- *Giardiasis:* 250 mg tid PO for 7 days.
- *Antibiotic-associated pseudomembranous colitis:* 1–2 g/day PO for 7– 10 days.
- *Treatment of inflammatory papules, pustules, and erythema of rosacea* (Metro-Gel)*:* Apply and rub in a thin film twice daily, morning and evening, to entire affected areas after washing; results should be seen within 3 wk; treatment through 9 wk has been effective.

Pediatric patients

- *Anaerobic bacterial infection:* Not recommended.
- *Amebiasis:* 35–50 mg/kg/day PO in three doses for 10 days.

Pharmacokinetics

Route	Onset	Peak
Oral	Varies	1–2 hr
IV	Rapid	1–2 hr
Topical	Generally no systemic absorption	

Metabolism: Hepatic; $T_{1/2}$: 6–8 hr
Distribution: Crosses placenta; enters breast milk
Excretion: Urine and feces

▼▼IV facts

Preparation: Reconstitute by adding 4.4 mL of sterile water for injection, bacteriostatic water for injection, 0.9% sodium chloride injection, bacteriostatic 0.9% sodium chloride injection to the vial and mix thoroughly. Resultant volume is 5 mL with a concentration of 100 mg/mL. Solution should be clear to pale yellow to yellow-green; do not use if cloudy or if containing precipitates; use within 24 hr; protect from light. Add reconstituted solution to glass or plastic container containing 0.9% sodium chloride injection, 5% dextrose injection or lactated Ringer's; discontinue other solutions while running metronidazole.
Infusion: Prior to administration, add 5 mEq sodium bicarbonate injection for each 500 mg used (if not using premixed bags); mix thoroughly. Do not refrigerate neutralized solution. Do not administer solution that has not been neutralized. Infuse over 1 hr.

Adverse effects

- **CNS:** *Headache, dizziness, ataxia,* vertigo, incoordination, insomnia, seizures, peripheral neuropathy, fatigue
- **GI:** *Unpleasant metallic taste, anorexia, nausea, vomiting, diarrhea,* GI upset, cramps
- **GU:** Dysuria, incontinence, *darkening of the urine*
- **Local:** Thrombophlebitis (IV); *redness, burning, dryness, and skin irritation* (topical)
- **Other:** Severe, disulfiram-like interaction with alcohol, candidiasis (superinfection)

Interactions

✱ **Drug-drug** ● Decreased effectiveness with barbiturates ● Disulfiram-like reaction (flushing, tachycardia, nausea, vomiting) with alcohol ● Psychosis if taken with disulfiram ● Increased bleeding tendencies with oral anticoagulants

✱ **Drug-lab test** ● Falsely low (or zero) values in AST, ALT, LDH, triglycerides, hexokinase glucose tests

■ Nursing considerations
Assessment

- **History:** CNS or hepatic disease; candidiasis (moniliasis); blood dyscrasias; pregnancy; lactation
- **Physical:** Reflexes; affect; skin lesions, color (with topical application); abdominal exam, liver palpation; urinalysis, CBC, liver function tests

Interventions

- Avoid use unless necessary. Metronidazole is carcinogenic in some rodents.
- Administer oral doses with food.
- Apply topically (*MetroGel, MetroCream*) after cleansing the area. Advise patient that

cosmetics may be used over the area after application.
- Reduce dosage in hepatic disease.

Teaching points
- Take full course of drug therapy; take the drug with food if GI upset occurs.
- These side effects may occur: dry mouth with strange metallic taste (frequent mouth care, sucking sugarless candies may help); nausea, vomiting, diarrhea (small, frequent meals may help).
- Do not drink alcohol (beverages or preparations containing alcohol, cough syrups); severe reactions may occur.
- Be aware that your urine may appear dark; this is expected.
- Refrain from sexual intercourse unless partner wears a condom during treatment for trichomoniasis.
- Report severe GI upset, dizziness, unusual fatigue or weakness, fever, chills.

Topical application
- Apply the topical preparation by cleansing the area and then rubbing a thin film into the affected area. Avoid contact with the eyes. Cosmetics may be applied to the area after application.

▽ metyrosine

See *Less Commonly Used Drugs*, p. 1346.

▽ mexiletine hydrochloride
(mex ill' i teen)

Mexitil, Novo-Mexiletine (CAN)

PREGNANCY CATEGORY C

Drug class
Antiarrhythmic

Therapeutic actions
Type 1 antiarrhythmic: decreases automaticity of ventricular cells by membrane stabilization.

Indications
- Treatment of documented life-threatening ventricular arrhythmias (use with lesser arrhythmias is not recommended)
- Unlabeled uses: prophylactic use to decrease arrhythmias in acute phase of acute MI (mortality may not be affected); reduction of pain, dysesthesia, and paresthesia associated with diabetic neuropathy

Contraindications and cautions
- Contraindicated with allergy to mexiletine, CHF, cardiogenic shock, hypotension, second- or third-degree heart block (without artificial pacemaker), lactation.
- Use cautiously with hepatic disease, seizure disorders, pregnancy.

Available forms
Capsules—150, 200, 250 mg

Dosages
Adults
200 mg q 8 hr PO. Increase in 50- to 100-mg increments every 2–3 days until desired antiarrhythmic effect is obtained. Maximum dose: 1,200 mg/day PO. Rapid control: 400 mg loading dose, then 200 mg q 8 hr PO.
- *Transferring from other antiarrhythmics: Lidocaine.* Stop the lidocaine with the first dose of mexiletine; leave IV line open until adequate arrhythmia suppression is ensured. *Quinidine sulfate.* Initial dose of 200 mg 6–12 hr PO after the last dose of quinidine. *Procainamid.* Initial dose of 200 mg 3–6 hr PO after the last dose of procainamide. *Disopyramid.* 200 mg 6–12 hr PO after the last dose of disopyramide. *Tocainide.* 200 mg 8–12 hr PO after the last dose of tocainide.

Pediatric patients
Safety and efficacy not established.

Pharmacokinetics

Route	Onset	Peak
Oral	Varies	2–3 hr

Metabolism: Hepatic; $T_{1/2}$: 10–12 hr
Distribution: Crosses placenta; enters breast milk
Excretion: Urine

Adverse effects

- **CNS:** *Dizziness/light-headedness, head-ache,* fatigue, drowsiness, *tremors, coordination difficulties, visual disturbances,* numbness, nervousness, *sleep difficulties*
- **CV:** *Cardiac arrhythmias, chest pain*
- **GI:** *Nausea, vomiting, heartburn,* abdominal pain, diarrhea, liver injury
- **Hematologic:** Positive ANA, thrombocytopenia, leukopenia
- **Respiratory:** *Dyspnea*
- **Other:** *Rash*

Interactions

✳ Drug-drug • Decreased mexiletine levels with hydantoins • Increased theophylline levels and toxicity with mexiletine

■ Nursing considerations
Assessment

- **History:** Allergy to mexiletine, CHF, cardiogenic shock, hypotension, second- or third-degree heart block, hepatic disease, seizure disorders, lactation, pregnancy
- **Physical:** Weight; orientation, reflexes; P, BP, auscultation; ECG, edema; R, adventitious sounds; bowel sounds, liver evaluation; urinalysis, urine pH, CBC, electrolytes, liver and renal function tests

Interventions

- Monitor patient response carefully, especially when beginning therapy.
- Reduce dosage with hepatic failure.
- Monitor for safe and effective serum levels (0.5–2 mcg/mL).

Teaching points

- Take with food to reduce GI problems.
- Frequent monitoring of cardiac rhythm is necessary.
- These side effects may occur: drowsiness, dizziness, numbness, visual disturbances (avoid driving or working with dangerous machinery); nausea, vomiting, heartburn (small, frequent meals may help); diarrhea; headache; sleep disturbances.
- Do not stop taking this drug without checking with your health care provider.
- Return for regular follow-ups to check your heart rhythm; and have blood tests.

- Do not change your diet. Maintain acidity level in urine. Discuss dietary change with your health care provider.
- Report fever, chills, sore throat, excessive GI discomfort, chest pain, excessive tremors, numbness, lack of coordination, headache, sleep disturbances.

▽ miconazole nitrate
(mi **kon'** *a zole)*

Topical: Absorbine Antifungal Foot Powder, Breeze Mist Antifungal, Fungoid Tincture, Lotrimin AF, Maximum Strength Desenex Antifungal, Ony Clear, Tetterine, Zeasorb-AF

Vaginal suppositories, topical: Micatin, Micozole (CAN), Monazole 7 (CAN), Monistat 3, Monistat 7, Monistat-Derm, Monistat Dual Pak

PREGNANCY CATEGORY B

Drug class
Antifungal

Therapeutic actions
Fungicidal: alters fungal cell membrane permeability, causing cell death; also may alter fungal cell DNA and RNA metabolism or cause accumulation of toxic peroxides intracellularly.

Indications

- Local treatment of vulvovaginal candidiasis (moniliasis; vaginal suppositories)
- Tinea pedis, tinea cruris, tinea corporis caused by *Trichophyton rubrum, Trichophyton mentagrophytes, Epidermophyton floccosum;* cutaneous candidiasis (moniliasis), tinea versicolor (topical administration)

Contraindications and cautions

- Contraindicated with allergy to miconazole or components used in preparation.
- Use cautiously with pregnancy, lactation.

Adverse effects in *Italics* are most common; those in **Bold** are life-threatening.

Available forms

Vaginal suppositories—100, 200, 1,200 mg; topical cream—2%; vaginal cream—2%; topical powder—2%; topical spray—2%; topical ointment—2%; spray powder or liquid—2%; solution—2%

Dosages
Adults

• *Vaginal suppositories: Monistat 3.* Insert 1 suppository intravaginally once daily hs for 3 days. *Monistat 7.* One applicator cream or 1 suppository in the vagina daily hs for 7 days. Repeat course if necessary. Alternatively, one 1,200-mg suppository at hs for one dose.
• *Topical:* Cream and lotion. Cover affected areas bid, morning and evening. Powder. Spray or sprinkle powder liberally over affected area in the morning and evening.
Pediatric patients
• *Topical:* Not recommended for children < 2 yr.

Pharmacokinetics

Route	Onset	Peak
Topical	Rapid	Unknown

Metabolism: Hepatic; $T_{1/2}$: 21–24 hr
Distribution: Crosses placenta; may enter breast milk
Excretion: Urine and feces

Adverse effects
Vaginal suppositories
• **Local:** *Irritation,* sensitization or vulvovaginal burning, pelvic cramps
• **Other:** Rash, headache
Topical application
• **Local:** *Irritation, burning, maceration,* allergic contact dermatitis

■ Nursing considerations
Assessment
• **History:** Allergy to miconazole or components used in preparation; lactation
• **Physical:** Skin color, lesions, area around lesions; T; orientation, affect; culture of area involved

Interventions
• Culture fungus involved before therapy.

• Insert vaginal suppositories high into the vagina; have patient remain recumbent for 10–15 min after insertion; provide sanitary napkin to protect clothing from stains.
• Monitor response; if none is noted, arrange for further cultures to determine causative organism.
• Apply lotion to intertriginous areas if topical application is required; if cream is used, apply sparingly to avoid maceration of the area.
• Ensure patient receives the full course of therapy to eradicate the fungus and to prevent recurrence.
• Discontinue topical or vaginal administration if rash or sensitivity occurs.

Teaching points
• Take the full course of drug therapy even if symptoms improve. Continue during menstrual period even if vaginal route is being used. Long-term use will be needed; beneficial effects may not be seen for several weeks.
• Insert vaginal suppositories high into the vagina.
• Use hygiene measures to prevent reinfection or spread of infection.
• This drug is for the fungus being treated; do not self-medicate other problems with this drug.
• Refrain from sexual intercourse, or advise partner to use a condom to avoid reinfection; use a sanitary napkin to prevent staining of clothing (vaginal use).
• These side effects may occur: irritation, burning, stinging.
• Report local irritation, burning (topical application); rash, irritation, pelvic pain (vaginal use).

▽midodrine hydrochloride
(mid' oh dryn)

Amatine (CAN), ProAmatine

PREGNANCY CATEGORY C

Drug classes
Antihypotensive
Alpha agonist

Therapeutic actions

Activates alpha receptors in the arteriolar and venous vasculature, producing an increase in vascular tone and elevation of BP.

Indications

- Treatment of symptomatic orthostatic hypotension in patients whose lives are considerably impaired by the disorder and who do not respond to other therapy
- Unlabeled use: management of urinary incontinence at doses of 2.5–5 mg bid–tid

Contraindications and cautions

- Contraindicated with severe CAD, acute renal disease; urinary retention; pheochromocytoma; thyrotoxicosis; persistent or excessive supine hypertension
- Use cautiously with renal or hepatic impairment, lactation, pregnancy, visual problems

Available forms

Tablets—2.5, 5 mg

Dosages
Adults

10 mg PO tid during daytime hours when upright.
Pediatric patients
Safety and efficacy not established.
Patients with renal impairment
Starting dose of 2.5 mg PO tid.

Pharmacokinetics

Route	Onset	Peak
Oral	Rapid	30 min

Metabolism: Hepatic and tissue; $T_{1/2}$: 25 min
Distribution: Crosses placenta; may pass into breast milk
Excretion: Urine

Adverse effects

- **CNS:** Headache, *paresthesias, pain,* dizziness, vertigo, visual field changes
- **CV:** *Supine hypertension, bradycardia*
- **Dermatologic:** *Piloerection, pruritus,* rash
- **Other:** *Dysuria, chills*

Interactions

✳ **Drug-drug** • Increased effects and toxicity of cardiac glycosides, beta-blockers, alpha-adrenergic agents, steroids (fludrocortisone) with midodrine; monitor patient carefully and adjust dosage as needed

■ Nursing considerations
Assessment

- **History:** Severe CAD, acute renal disease; urinary retention; pheochromocytoma; thyrotoxicosis; persistent or excessive supine hypertension; renal or hepatic impairment, lactation, pregnancy; visual problems
- **Physical:** T; orientation, visual field checks; skin color, lesions, temperature; BP—sitting, standing, supine, P; renal and hepatic function tests

Interventions

- Establish baseline hepatic and renal function and evaluate periodically during therapy.
- Monitor BP carefully, especially if used with any agent that causes vasoconstriction; give only to patients who are up and about—do not give to bedridden patients or before bed.
- Monitor heart rate when beginning therapy. Bradycardia is common as therapy begins; persistent bradycardia should be evaluated and drug discontinued.
- Monitor patients with known visual problems or who are taking fludrocortisone for any change in visual fields. Discontinue drug and consult physician if changes occur.
- Encourage patient to take drug after voiding if urinary retention is a problem.

Teaching points

- Take this drug during the day when you will be up and around. Do not take it before bed or lying down.
- Empty your bladder before taking this drug if urinary retention has been a problem.
- Return for regular medical evaluation of your BP and response to this drug.
- These side effects may occur: numbness or tingling in the extremities (avoid injury); slow heart rate; rash, goose bumps.

- Report changes in vision, pounding in the head when lying down, very slow heart rate, difficulty urinating.

▽mifepristone (RU-486)

*(miff eh **prist**' own)*

Mifeprex

PREGNANCY CATEGORY X

Drug class
Abortifacient

Therapeutic actions
Acts as an antagonist of progesterone sites in the endometrium, allowing prostaglandins to stimulate uterine contractions, causing implanted trophoblast to separate from the placental wall; may also decrease placental viability and accelerate degenerative changes resulting in sloughing of the endometrium.

Indications
- Termination of pregnancy through 49 days gestational age; most effective when combined with a prostaglandin
- Unlabeled uses: postcoital contraception, endometriosis, unresectable meningioma, fetal death or nonviable early pregnancy

Contraindications and cautions
- Contraindicated with allergy to prostaglandin preparations; acute PID; active cardiac, hepatic, pulmonary, renal disease
- Use cautiously with history of asthma; anemia; jaundice; diabetes; epilepsy; scarred uterus; cervicitis, infected endocervical lesions, acute vaginitis

Available forms
Tablets—200 mg

Dosages
Adults
- *Day 1:* 600 mg (3 tablets) PO taken as a single dose.
- *Day 3:* If termination of pregnancy cannot be confirmed, 400 mcg (2 tablets) misoprostol (*Cytotec*).

- *Day 14:* Evaluation for termination of pregnancy; if unsuccessful, surgical intervention is suggested at this time.

Pharmacokinetics

Route	Onset	Peak
Oral	Rapid	1–3 hr

Metabolism: Tissue; $T_{1/2}$: 20–54 hr
Distribution: Crosses placenta; passes into breast milk
Excretion: Urine

Adverse effects
- **CNS:** *Headache*
- **GI:** *Vomiting, diarrhea, nausea, abdominal pain*
- **GU:** Heavy uterine bleeding, endometritis, uterine or vaginal pain

■ Nursing considerations

 CLINICAL ALERT!
Name confusion has occurred between mifepristone and misoprostol; use extreme caution.

M

Assessment
- **History:** Allergy to prostaglandin preparations; acute PID; active cardiac, hepatic, pulmonary, renal disease; history of asthma; hypotension; hypertension; CV, adrenal, renal, or hepatic disease; anemia; jaundice; diabetes; epilepsy; scarred uterus; cervicitis, infected endocervical lesions, acute vaginitis
- **Physical:** T; BP, P, auscultation; bowel sounds, liver evaluation; vaginal discharge, pelvic exam, uterine tone; liver and renal function tests, WBC, urinalysis, CBC

Interventions
- Provide appropriate referrals and counseling for abortion.
- Alert patient that menses usually begins within 5 days of treatment and lasts for 1–2 wk.
- Arrange to follow drug within 48 hr with a prostaglandin (*Cytotec*) as appropriate.
- Ensure that abortion is complete or that other measures are used to complete the abortion if drug effects are not sufficient.

- Prepare for D & C if heavy bleeding does not resolve.
- Provide analgesic and antiemetic agents as needed to increase comfort.

Teaching points
Teaching about mifepristone should be incorporated into the total teaching plan for the patient undergoing an abortion; specific information that should be included follows:

- Menses begin within 5 days of treatment and will last 1–2 wk.
- These side effects may occur: nausea, vomiting, diarrhea (medication may be ordered); uterine or vaginal pain, headache (an analgesic may be ordered).
- Report severe pain; persistent, heavy bleeding; extreme fatigue, dizziness on arising.

▽ **miglitol**
(*mig' lah tall*)

Glyset

PREGNANCY CATEGORY B

Drug class
Antidiabetic agent

Therapeutic actions
An alpha-glucosidase inhibitor that delays the digestion of ingested carbohydrates, leading to a smaller rise in blood glucose following meals and a decrease in glycosylated hemoglobin; does not enhance insulin secretion and so its effects are additive to those of the sulfonylureas in controlling blood glucose.

Indications
- Adjunct to diet to lower blood glucose in patients with non–insulin-dependent diabetes mellitus (type 2) whose hyperglycemia cannot be managed by diet alone
- Combination therapy with a sulfonylurea to enhance glycemic control in those patients who do not receive adequate control with diet and either drug

Contraindications and cautions
- Contraindicated with hypersensitivity to the drug; diabetic ketoacidosis; cirrhosis; inflammatory bowel disease; intestinal obstruction or predisposition to intestinal obstruction; type 1 diabetes; conditions that would deteriorate with increased gas in the bowel.
- Use cautiously with renal impairment, pregnancy, lactation.

Available forms
Tablets—25, 50, 100 mg

Dosages
Adults
- *Initial dose:* 25 mg PO tid at the first bite of each meal; may start at 25 mg PO daily if severe GI effects are seen. *Maintenance:* 50 mg PO tid at first bite of each meal. *Maximum dose:* 100 mg PO tid.
- *Combination with a sulfonylurea:* Blood glucose may be much lower; monitor closely and adjust dosages of each drug accordingly.

Pediatric patients
Safety and efficacy not established.

Pharmacokinetics

Route	Onset	Peak
Oral	Rapid	2–3 hr

Metabolism: Not metabolized; $T_{1/2}$: 2 hr
Distribution: Very little
Excretion: Urine

Adverse effects
- **Dermatologic:** Rash
- **Endocrine:** *Hypoglycemia* (taken in combination with other antidiabetic drugs)
- **GI:** *Abdominal pain, flatulence, diarrhea,* anorexia, nausea, vomiting

Interactions
✱ Drug-drug • Decreased bioavailability and effectiveness of propranolol, ranitidine • Reduced effectiveness of miglitol if taken with digestive enzymes or charcoal; avoid these combinations
✱ Drug-alternative therapy • Increased risk of hypoglycemia if taken with juniper

---

berries, ginseng, garlic, fenugreek, coriander, dandelion root, celery

■ Nursing considerations

Assessment
- **History:** Hypersensitivity to the drug; diabetic ketoacidosis; cirrhosis; inflammatory bowel disease; intestinal obstruction or predisposition to intestinal obstruction; type 1 diabetes; conditions that would deteriorate with increased gas in the bowel; renal impairment; pregnancy; lactation
- **Physical:** Skin color, lesions; T; orientation, reflexes, peripheral sensation; R, adventitious sounds; liver evaluation, bowel sounds; urinalysis, BUN, blood glucose

Interventions
- Administer drug tid with the first bite of each meal.
- Monitor urine and serum glucose levels frequently to determine effectiveness of drug and dosage being used.
- Inform patient of likelihood of abdominal pain and flatulence.
- Arrange for consult with dietitian to establish weight loss program and dietary control as appropriate.
- Arrange for thorough diabetic teaching program to include disease, dietary control, exercise, signs and symptoms of hypo- and hyperglycemia, avoidance of infection, hygiene.

Teaching points
- Do not discontinue this medication without consulting your health care provider.
- Take this drug three times a day with the first bite of each meal.
- Monitor urine or blood for glucose and ketones as prescribed.
- Continue diet and exercise program established for control of diabetes.
- These side effects may occur: abdominal pain, flatulence, bloating.
- Report fever, sore throat, unusual bleeding or bruising, severe abdominal pain.

▷milrinone lactate
(*mill' ri none*)

Primacor

PREGNANCY CATEGORY C

Drug class
Cardiotonic agent

Therapeutic actions
Increases force of contraction of ventricles (positive inotropic effect); causes vasodilation by a direct relaxant effect on vascular smooth muscle.

Indications
- CHF: short-term IV management of those patients who are receiving digitalis and diuretics

Contraindications and cautions
- Contraindicated with allergy to milrinone or bisulfites; severe aortic or pulmonic valvular disease.
- Use cautiously with the elderly, pregnancy.

Available forms
Injection—1 mg/mL; premixed injection—200 mcg/mL

Dosages
Adults
- *Loading dose:* 50 mcg/kg IV bolus, given over 10 min. *Maintenance infusion:* 0.375–0.75 mcg/kg/min. Do not exceed a total of 1.13 mg/kg/day.

Pediatric patients
Not recommended.

Geriatric patients or patients with renal impairment
Do not exceed 1.13 mg/kg/day. For patients with renal impairment, refer to the following table:

Creatinine Clearance (mL/min)	Infusion Rate (mcg/kg/min)
5	0.2
10	0.23
20	0.28
30	0.3
40	0.38
50	0.43

Pharmacokinetics

Route	Onset	Peak	Duration
IV	Immediate	5–15 min	8 hr

Metabolism: Hepatic; $T_{1/2}$: 2.3–2.5 hr
Distribution: Crosses placenta; may enter breast milk
Excretion: Urine

▼IV facts

Preparation: Add diluent of 0.45% or 0.9% sodium chloride injection, USP or 5% dextrose injection, USP. Add 180 mL per 20-mg vial to prepare solution of 100 mcg/mL^2; 113 mL per 20-mg vial to prepare a solution of 150 mcg/mL^2; add 80 mL diluent to 20-mg vial to prepare solution of 200 mcg/mL^2.

Infusion: Administer while carefully monitoring patient's hemodynamic and clinical response; see manufacturer's insert for detailed guidelines.

Incompatibilities: Do not mix directly with furosemide.

Adverse effects

- **CV:** *Ventricular arrhythmias,* hypotension, supraventricular arrhythmias, chest pain, angina, **death**
- **Hematologic:** Thrombocytopenia, hypokalemia

Interactions

✳ **Drug-drug** • Precipitate formation in solution if given in the same IV line with furosemide; avoid this combination

■ Nursing considerations

Assessment

- **History:** Allergy to milrinone or bisulfites, severe aortic or pulmonic valvular disease, lactation, pregnancy
- **Physical:** Weight, orientation, P, BP, cardiac auscultation, peripheral pulses and perfusion, R, adventitious sounds, serum electrolyte levels, platelet count, ECG

Interventions

- Monitor cardiac rhythm continually.
- Monitor BP and P and reduce dose if marked decreases occur.
- Monitor intake and output and electrolyte levels.

Teaching points

- You will need frequent BP and P and heart activity monitoring during therapy.
- You may experience increased voiding; appropriate bathroom arrangements will be made.
- Report pain at IV injection site, numbness or tingling, shortness of breath, chest pain.

▷ minocycline hydrochloride
(mi noe sye' kleen)

Alti-Minocycline (CAN), Arestin, Dynacin, Gen-Minocycline (CAN), Minocin IV, Novo-Minocycline (CAN), Vectrin

PREGNANCY CATEGORY D

Drug classes
Antibiotic
Tetracycline

Therapeutic actions
Bacteriostatic: inhibits protein synthesis of susceptible bacteria, causing cell death.

Indications

- Infections caused by rickettsiae; *Mycoplasma pneumoniae;* agents of psittacosis, ornithosis, lymphogranuloma venereum and granuloma inguinale; *Borrelia recurrentis; Hemophilus ducreyi; Pasteurella pestis; Pasteurella tularensis; Bartonella bacilliformis; Bacteroides; Vibrio comma; Vibrio fetus; Brucella; E. coli; Enterobacter aerogenes; Shigella; Acinetobacter calcoaceticus; H. influenzae; Klebsiella; Diplococcus pneumoniae; S. aureus*
- When penicillin is contraindicated, infections caused by *N. gonorrhoeae, Treponema pallidum, Treponema pertenue, Listeria monocytogenes, Clostridium, Bacillus anthracis.* As an adjunct to amebicides in acute intestinal amebiasis

---

Adverse effects in *Italics* are most common; those in **Bold** are life-threatening.

- Oral tetracyclines are indicated for treatment of acne, uncomplicated urethral, endocervical, or rectal infections in adults caused by *Chlamydia trachomatis*
- Oral minocycline is indicated in treatment of asymptomatic carriers of *Neisseria meningitidis* (not useful for treating the infection); infections caused by *Mycobacterium marinum;* uncomplicated urethral, endocervical, or rectal infections caused by *Ureaplasma urealyticum;* uncomplicated gonococcal urethritis in men in due to *N. gonorrhoeae*
- Adjunct to scaling and root planing to reduce pocket depth in patients with adult periodontitis (*Arestin*)
- Unlabeled use: alternative to sulfonamides in the treatment of nocardiosis

Contraindications and cautions
- Contraindicated with allergy to tetracyclines.
- Use cautiously with renal or hepatic dysfunction, pregnancy, lactation.

Available forms
Capsules—50, 100 mg; pellet filled capsules—50, 100 mg; powder for injection—100 mg

Dosages
Adults
200 mg followed by 100 mg q 12 hr IV. Do not exceed 400 mg/day. Or 200 mg initially, followed by 100 mg q 12 hr PO. May be given as 100–200 mg initially and then 50 mg qid PO.
- *Syphilis:* Usual PO dose for 10–15 days.
- *Urethral, endocervical, rectal infections:* 100 mg bid PO for 7 days.
- *Gonococcal urethritis in men:* 100 mg bid PO for 5 days.
- *Gonorrhea:* 200 mg PO followed by 100 mg q 12 hr for 4 days; get post-therapy cultures within 2–3 days.
- *Meningococcal carrier state:* 100 mg q 12 hr PO for 5 days.
- *Adult peridontitis:* Unit dose cartridge discharged in subgingival area.
Pediatric patients > 8 yr
4 mg/kg IV followed by 2 mg/kg q 12 hr IV or PO.
Geriatric patients or patients with renal failure
IV doses of minocycline are not as toxic as other tetracyclines in these patients.

Pharmacokinetics

Route	Onset	Peak
Oral	Rapid	2–3 hr
IV	Immediate	End of infusion

Metabolism: Hepatic; $T_{1/2}$: 11–26 hr
Distribution: Crosses placenta; enters breast milk
Excretion: Urine and feces

▽ IV facts
Preparation: Dissolve powder and then further dilute to 500–1,000 mL with sodium chloride injection, dextrose injection, dextrose and sodium chloride injection, Ringer's injection, or lactated Ringer's injection; administer immediately.
Infusion: Infuse slowly over 6 hr; discard any diluted solution not used within 24 hr.
Incompatibilities: Avoid solutions with calcium; a precipitate may form.
Y-site incompatibilities: Do not inject with hydromorphone, meperidine, morphine.

Adverse effects
- **Dental:** *Discoloring and inadequate calcification of primary teeth of fetus if used by pregnant women; discoloring and inadequate calcification of permanent teeth if used during period of dental development*
- **Dermatologic:** *Phototoxic reactions, rash,* exfoliative dermatitis (more frequent, more severe with this tetracycline than with any others)
- **GI:** Fatty liver, liver failure, *anorexia, nausea, vomiting, diarrhea, glossitis,* dysphagia, enterocolitis, esophageal ulcer
- **Hematologic:** Hemolytic anemia, thrombocytopenia, neutropenia, eosinophilia, leukocytosis, leukopenia
- **Local:** Local irritation at injection site
- **Other:** Superinfections, nephrogenic diabetes insipidus syndrome

Interactions
✳ **Drug-drug** • Decreased absorption of minocycline with antacids, iron, alkali • Increased digoxin toxicity • Increased nephrotoxicity with methoxyflurane • Decreased activity of penicillin
✳ **Drug-food** • Decreased absorption of minocycline if taken with food, dairy products

■ Nursing considerations
Assessment
- **History:** Allergy to tetracyclines, renal or hepatic dysfunction, pregnancy, lactation
- **Physical:** Skin status, orientation and reflexes, R and sounds, GI function and liver evaluation, urinalysis and BUN, liver and renal function tests; culture infected area

Interventions
- Administer oral medication without regard to food or meals; if GI upset occurs, give with meals.

Teaching points
- Take drug throughout the day for best results.
- Take with meals if GI upset occurs.
- These side effects may occur: sensitivity to sunlight (wear protective clothing, use sunscreen); diarrhea, nausea (take with meals; small, frequent meals may help).
- Report rash, itching; difficulty breathing; dark urine or light-colored stools; severe cramps, watery diarrhea.

▽ minoxidil
(mi nox' i dill)

Oral: Loniten, Minox (CAN)
Topical: Minoxigaine(CAN), Rogaine, Rogaine Extra Strength

PREGNANCY CATEGORY C

Drug classes
Antihypertensive
Vasodilator

Therapeutic actions
Acts directly on vascular smooth muscle to cause vasodilation, reducing elevated systolic and diastolic BP; does not interfere with CV reflexes; does not usually cause orthostatic hypotension but does cause reflex tachycardia and renin release, leading to sodium and water retention; mechanism in stimulating hair growth is not known, possibly related to arterial dilation.

Indications
- Severe hypertension that is symptomatic or associated with target organ damage and is not manageable with maximum therapeutic doses of a diuretic plus two other antihypertensive drugs; use in milder hypertension not recommended
- Alopecia areata and male pattern alopecia—topical use when compounded as a 1%–5% lotion or 1% ointment

Contraindications and cautions
- Contraindicated with hypersensitivity to minoxidil or any component of the topical preparation (topical); pheochromocytoma (may stimulate release of catecholamines from tumor); acute MI; dissecting aortic aneurysm; lactation.
- Use cautiously with malignant hypertension; CHF (use diuretic); angina pectoris (use a beta-blocker); pregnancy.

Available forms
Tablets—2.5, 10 mg; topical 2%, 5%

Dosages
Adults and patients ≥ 12 yr
Oral
Initial dosage is 2.5–5 mg/day PO as a single dose. Daily dosage can be increased to 10, 20, then 40 mg in single or divided doses. Effective range is usually 10–40 mg/day PO. Maximum dosage is 100 mg/day. If supine diastolic BP has been reduced less than 30 mm Hg, administer the drug only once a day. If reduced more than 30 mm Hg, divide the daily dose into two equal parts. Dosage adjustment should normally be at least at 3-day intervals; in emergencies, q 6 hr with careful monitoring is possible.
- *Concomitant therapy:*
Diuretics: Use minoxidil with a diuretic in patients relying on renal function for maintaining salt and water balance; the following diuretic dosages have been used when starting minoxidil therapy: hydrochlorothiazide, 50 mg bid; chlorthalidone, 50–100 mg daily; furosemide, 40 mg bid. If excessive salt and water retention result in weight gain > 5 lb, change diuretic therapy to furosemide; if patient already takes furosemide, increase dosage. *Beta-*

Adverse effects in *Italics* are most common; those in **Bold** are life-threatening.

adrenergic blockers or other sympatholytics: The following dosages are recommended when starting minoxidil therapy: propranolol, 80–160 mg/day; other beta-blockers, dosage equivalent to the above; methyldopa 250–750 mg bid (start methyldopa at least 24 hr before minoxidil); clonidine, 0.1–0.2 mg bid.

Topical
Apply 1 mL to the total affected areas of the scalp twice daily. The total daily dosage should not exceed 2 mL. Twice daily application for > 4 mo may be required before evidence of hair regrowth is observed. Once hair growth is realized, twice daily application is necessary for continued and additional hair regrowth. Balding process reported to return to untreated state 3–4 mo after cessation of the drug.

Pediatric patients < 12 yr
Experience is limited, particularly in infants; use recommendations as a guide; careful adjustment is necessary. Initial dosage is 0.2 mg/kg/day PO as a single dose. May increase by 50%–100% increments until optimum BP control is achieved. Effective range is usually 0.25–1 mg/kg/day; maximum dose is 50 mg daily. Experience in children is limited; monitor carefully.

Geriatric patients or patients with impaired renal function
Smaller doses may be required; closely supervise to prevent cardiac failure or exacerbation of renal failure.

Pharmacokinetics

Route	Onset	Peak	Duration
Oral	30 min	2–3 hr	75 hr
Topical	Generally no systemic absorption		

Metabolism: Hepatic; $T_{1/2}$: 4.2 hr
Distribution: Crosses placenta; enters breast milk
Excretion: Urine

Adverse effects
- **CNS:** Fatigue, headache
- **CV:** Tachycardia (unless given with beta-adrenergic blocker or other sympatholytic drug), pericardial effusion and tamponade; *changes in direction and magnitude of T-waves;* cardiac necrotic lesions (reported in patients with known ischemic heart dis-

ease, but risk of minoxidil-associated cardiac damage cannot be excluded)
- **Dermatologic:** *Temporary edema, hypertrichosis* (elongation, thickening, and enhanced pigmentation of fine body hair occurring within 3–6 wk of starting therapy; usually first noticed on temples, between eyebrows and extending to other parts of face, back, arms, legs, scalp); rashes including bullous eruptions; **Stevens-Johnson syndrome;** darkening of the skin
- **GI:** Nausea, vomiting
- **Hematologic:** Initial decrease in Hct, Hgb, RBC count
- **Local:** *Irritant dermatitis, allergic contact dermatitis, eczema, pruritus, dry skin/scalp, flaking, alopecia* (topical use)
- **Respiratory:** *Bronchitis, upper respiratory infection, sinusitis* (topical use)

Interactions
✴ Drug-drug • Risk of profound orthostatic hypotension if given with guanethidine. Stop guanethidine; if not possible, hospitalize patient

■ Nursing considerations
Assessment
- **History:** Hypersensitivity to minoxidil or any component of the topical preparation; pheochromocytoma; acute MI, dissecting aortic aneurysm; malignant hypertension; CHF; angina pectoris; lactation, pregnancy
- **Physical:** Skin color, lesions, hair, scalp; P, BP, orthostatic BP, supine BP, perfusion, edema, auscultation; bowel sounds, normal output; CBC with differential, kidney function tests, urinalysis, ECG

Interventions
- Apply topical preparation to affected area; if fingers are used to facilitate drug application, wash hands thoroughly afterward.
- Do not apply other topical agents, including topical corticosteroids, retinoids, and petrolatum or agents known to enhance cutaneous drug absorption.
- Do not apply topical preparation to open lesions or breaks in the skin, which could increase risk of systemic absorption.
- Arrange to withdraw oral drug gradually, especially from children; rapid withdrawal may cause a sudden increase in BP (rebound hy-

pertension has been reported in children, even with gradual withdrawal; use caution and monitor BP closely when withdrawing from children).

• Arrange for echocardiographic evaluation of possible pericardial effusion; more vigorous diuretic therapy, dialysis, other treatment (including minoxidil withdrawal) may be required.

Teaching points
Oral

• Take this drug exactly as prescribed. Take all other medications that have been prescribed. Do not discontinue any drug or reduce the dosage without consulting your health care provider.

• These side effects may occur: enhanced growth and darkening of fine body and face hair (do not discontinue medication without consulting health care provider); GI upset (frequent small meals may help).

• Report increased heart rate of ≥ 20 beats per minute over normal (your normal heart rate is ___ beats per minute); rapid weight gain of more than 5 lb; unusual swelling of the extremities, face, or abdomen; difficulty breathing, especially when lying down; new or aggravated symptoms of angina (chest, arm, or shoulder pain); severe indigestion; dizziness, light-headedness, or fainting.

Topical

• Apply the prescribed amount to affected area twice a day. If using the fingers to facilitate application, wash hands thoroughly after application. It may take 4 mo or longer for any noticeable hair regrowth to appear. Response to this drug is very individual. If no response is seen within 4 mo, consult with your health care provider about efficacy of continued use.

• Do not apply more frequent or larger applications. This will not speed up or increase hair growth but may increase side effects.

• If one or two daily applications are missed, restart twice-daily applications, and return to usual schedule. Do not attempt to make up missed applications.

• Do not apply any other topical medication to the area while you are using this drug.

• Do not apply to any sunburned, broken skin or open lesions; this increases the risk of systemic effects. Do not apply to any part of the body other than the scalp.

• Twice daily use of the drug will be necessary to retain or continue the hair regrowth.

▽ mirtazapine
(mer tab' zah peen)

Remeron, Remeron SolTab

PREGNANCY CATEGORY C

Drug class
Antidepressant (tetracyclic)

Therapeutic actions
Mechanism of action unknown; appears to act similarly to TCAs, which inhibit the presynaptic reuptake of the neurotransmitters norepinephrine and serotonin; anticholinergic at CNS and peripheral receptors; sedating; relation of these effects to clinical efficacy is unknown.

Indications
• Relief of symptoms of depression (endogenous depression most responsive)

Contraindications and cautions
• Contraindicated with hypersensitivity to any tricyclic or tetracyclic drug; comcomitant therapy with an MAOI; recent MI; myelography within previous 24 hr or scheduled within 48 hr; pregnancy (limb reduction abnormalities reported); lactation

• Use cautiously with ECT; preexisting CV disorders, eg, severe coronary heart disease, progressive heart failure, angina pectoris, paroxysmal tachycardia (possible increased risk of serious CVS toxicity with TCAs); angle-closure glaucoma, increased intraocular pressure, urinary retention, ureteral or urethral spasm; seizure disorders (TCAs lower the seizure threshold); hyperthyroidism (predisposes to CVS toxicity, including cardiac arrhythmias); impaired hepatic, renal function; psychiatric patients (schizophrenic or paranoid patients may exhibit a worsening of psychosis with TCAs); manic-depressive patients (may shift to hypomanic or manic phase); elective surgery (TCAs should be discontinued as long as possible before surgery)

Available forms

Tablets—15, 30, 45 mg; orally disintegrating tablet—15, 30, 45 mg

Dosages
Adults

Initial dose: 15 mg PO daily, as a single dose in evening. May be increased up to 45 mg/day as needed. Change dose only at intervals greater than 1–2 wk. Continue treatment for up to 6 mo for acute episodes.

- *Switching from MAOI:* Allow at least 14 days between discontinuation of MAOI and beginning of mirtazapine therapy. Allow 14 days after stopping mirtazapine before starting MAOI.

Pediatric patients

Not recommended in patients < 18 yr.
Geriatric patients and patients with renal or hepatic dysfunction

Give lower doses to patients > 60 yr.

Pharmacokinetics

Route	Onset	Peak	Duration
Oral	Slow	2–4 hr	2–4 wk

Metabolism: Hepatic; $T_{1/2}$: 20–40 hr
Distribution: Crosses placenta; passes into breast milk
Excretion: Urine and feces

Adverse effects

- **CNS:** *Sedation and anticholinergic (atropine-like) effects; confusion* (especially in elderly), *disturbed concentration,* hallucinations, disorientation, decreased memory, feelings of unreality, delusions, anxiety, nervousness, restlessness, agitation, panic, insomnia, nightmares, hypomania, mania, exacerbation of psychosis, drowsiness, weakness, fatigue, headache, numbness, agitation (less likely with this drug than with other antidepressants)
- **CV:** Orthostatic hypotension, hypertension, syncope, tachycardia, palpitations, MI, arrhythmias, **heart block,** precipitation of CHF, stroke
- **Endocrine:** Elevated or depressed blood sugar; elevated prolactin levels; inappropriate ADH secretion

- **GI:** *Dry mouth, constipation,* paralytic ileus, *nausea* (less likely with this drug than with other antidepressants), vomiting, anorexia, epigastric distress, diarrhea, flatulence, dysphagia, peculiar taste, increased salivation, stomatitis, glossitis, parotid swelling, abdominal cramps, black tongue, liver enzyme elevations
- **GU:** Urinary retention, delayed micturition, dilation of urinary tract, gynecomastia, testicular swelling in men; breast enlargement, menstrual irregularity, galactorrhea in women; increased or decreased libido; impotence
- **Hematologic: Agranulocytosis,** *neutropenia*
- **Hypersensitivity:** Rash, pruritus, vasculitis, petechiae, photosensitization, edema

Interactions

✳ **Drug-drug** • Risk of serious, sometimes fatal reactions if combined with MAOIs; do not use this combination or within 14 days of MAOI therapy

■ Nursing considerations
Assessment

- **History:** Hypersensitivity to any antidepressant; concomitant therapy with MAOI; recent MI; myelography within previous 24 hr or scheduled within 48 hr; lactation; ECT; preexisting CV disorders; angle-closure glaucoma; increased intraocular pressure, urinary retention, ureteral or urethral spasm; seizure disorders; hyperthyroidism; impaired hepatic, renal function; psychiatric problems; manic-depressive patients; elective surgery; pregnancy
- **Physical:** Body weight; T; skin color, lesions; orientation, affect, reflexes, vision and hearing; P, BP, orthostatic BP, perfusion; bowel sounds, normal output, liver evaluation; urine flow, normal output; usual sexual function, frequency of menses, breast and scrotal examination; liver function tests, urinalysis, CBC, ECG

Interventions

- Ensure that depressed and potentially suicidal patients have access only to limited quantities of the drug.
- Administer orally disintegrating tablets to patients who have difficulty swallowing: open

blister pack and have patient place tablet on tongue. Do not split tablet.

- Expect clinical response in 3–7 days up to 2–3 wk (latter is more usual).
- Arrange for CBC if patient develops fever, sore throat, or other sign of infection during therapy.
- Establish safety precautions if CNS changes occur (side rails, accompany patient when ambulating, etc).

Teaching points

- Take this drug exactly as prescribed; do not stop taking the drug abruptly or without consulting your health care provider.
- Place orally disintegrating tablet on tongue, can be swallowed without water. Open blister pack with dry hands and use tablet immediately; do not cut or break tablet.
- Avoid using alcohol, other sleep-inducing drugs, OTC drugs while on this drug.
- Avoid prolonged exposure to sunlight or sunlamps; use a sunscreen or protective garments if long exposure to sunlight is unavoidable.
- These side effects may occur: headache, dizziness, drowsiness, weakness, blurred vision (reversible; avoid driving or performing tasks that require alertness); nausea, vomiting, loss of appetite, dry mouth (eat small, frequent meals; frequent mouth care and sucking on sugarless candies may help); nightmares, inability to concentrate, confusion; changes in sexual function.
- Report fever, flulike illness, any infection, dry mouth, difficulty urinating, excessive sedation.

▽ **misoprostol**

*(mye soe **prost'** ole)*

Cytotec

PREGNANCY CATEGORY X

Drug class
Prostaglandin

Therapeutic actions
A synthetic prostaglandin E_1 analog; inhibits gastric acid secretion and increases bicarbonate and mucus production, protecting the lining of the stomach.

Indications

- Prevention of NSAID (including aspirin)-induced gastric ulcers in patients at high risk of complications from a gastric ulcer (the elderly; patients with concomitant debilitating disease, history of ulcers)
- With mifepristone as an abortifacient (see mifepristone)
- Unlabeled use: appears effective in treating duodenal ulcers in those patients unresponsive to H_2 antagonists; cervical ripening and labor induction

Contraindications and cautions

- History of allergy to prostaglandins; pregnancy (abortifacient; advise women of childbearing age in written and oral form of use, have a negative serum pregnancy test within 2 wk prior to therapy, provide contraceptives, and begin therapy on the second or third day of the next normal menstrual period); lactation.

Available forms
Tablets—100, 200 mcg

Dosages
Adults
200 mcg four times daily PO with food. If this dose cannot be tolerated, 100 mcg can be used. Take misoprostol for the duration of the NSAID therapy. Take the last dose of the day hs.
Pediatric patients
Safety and efficacy in patients < 18 yr not established.
Geriatric patients or patients with renal impaired
Adjustment in dosage is usually not necessary, but dosage can be reduced if 200-mcg PO dose cannot be tolerated.

Pharmacokinetics

Route	Onset	Peak
Oral	Rapid	12–15 min

Adverse effects in *Italics* are most common; those in **Bold** are life-threatening.

Metabolism: Hepatic; $T_{1/2}$: 20–40 min
Distribution: Crosses placenta; enters breast milk
Excretion: Urine

Adverse effects

- **GI:** *Nausea, diarrhea, abdominal pain, flatulence,* vomiting, dyspepsia, constipation
- **GU:** *Miscarriage,* excessive bleeding, *spotting, cramping,* hypermenorrhea, menstrual disorders, dysmenorrhea
- **Other:** Headache

■ Nursing considerations

CLINICAL ALERT!
Name confusion has occurred between misoprostol and mifepristone; use extreme caution.

Assessment

- **History:** Allergy to prostaglandins; pregnancy, lactation
- **Physical:** Abdominal exam, normal output; urinary output

Interventions

- Give to patients at high risk for developing NSAID-induced gastric ulcers; give for the full term of the NSAID use.
- Arrange for serum pregnancy test for any woman of childbearing age; must have a negative test within 2 wk of beginning therapy.
- Arrange for oral and written explanation of the risks to pregnancy; appropriate contraceptive measures must be taken; begin therapy on the second or third day of a normal menstrual period.

Teaching points

- Take this drug four times a day, with meals and at bedtime. Continue to take your NSAID while on this drug. Take the drug exactly as prescribed. Do not give this drug to anyone else.
- These side effects may occur: abdominal pain, nausea, diarrhea, flatulence (take with meals); menstrual cramping, abnormal menstrual periods, spotting, even in postmenopausal women (request analgesics); headache.

- This drug can cause miscarriage, and is often associated with dangerous bleeding. Do not take if pregnant; do not become pregnant while taking this medication. If pregnancy occurs, discontinue drug, and consult physician immediately.
- Report severe diarrhea, spotting or menstrual pain, severe menstrual bleeding, pregnancy.

▽mitomycin (mitomycin-C, MTC)

*(mye toe **mye'** sin)*

Mutamycin

PREGNANCY CATEGORY D

Drug classes

Antibiotic
Antineoplastic

Therapeutic actions

Cytotoxic: inhibits DNA synthesis and cellular RNA and protein synthesis in susceptible cells, causing cell death.

Indications

- Disseminated adenocarcinoma of the stomach or pancreas; part of combination therapy or as palliative measure when other modalities fail
- Unlabeled use: superficial bladder cancer (intravesical route)

Contraindications and cautions

- Allergy to mitomycin; thrombocytopenia, coagulation disorders, or increase in bleeding tendencies, impaired renal function (creatinine > 1.7 mg/dL); myelosuppression; pregnancy; lactation.

Available forms

Powder for injection—5, 20, 40 mg

Dosages
Adults

After hematologic recovery from previous chemotherapy, use either of the following schedules at 6- to 8-wk intervals: 20 mg/m²/day IV as a single dose or 2 mg/m²/day IV for 5 days followed by a drug-free interval of 2 days and then 2 mg/m²/day for 5 days (total of 20 mg/m² for 10 days). Reevaluate patient for hematologic response between courses of therapy; adjust dose accordingly:

Leukocytes	Platelets	% of Prior Dose to Be Given
> 4,000	> 100,000	100
3,000–3,999	75,000–99,999	100
2,000–2,999	25,000–74,999	70
< 2,000	< 25,000	50

Do not repeat dosage until leukocyte count has returned to 3,000/mm^3 and platelet count to 75,000/mm^3.

Pharmacokinetics

Route	Onset	Peak
IV	Slow	Unknown

Metabolism: Hepatic; T$_{1/2}$: 17 min
Distribution: Crosses placenta; enters breast milk
Excretion: Urine

▼IV facts

Preparation: Reconstitute 5- to 20-mg vial with 10 or 40 mL of sterile water for injection, respectively; reconstitute 40-mg vial with 80 mL sterile water. If product does not dissolve immediately, allow to stand at room temperature until solution is obtained. This solution is stable for 14 days if refrigerated, 7 days at room temperature; further dilution in various IV fluids reduces stability—check manufacturer's insert.
Infusion: Infuse slowly over 5–10 min; monitor injection site to avoid local reaction.
Incompatibilities: Do not mix with bleomycin.

Adverse effects

- **CNS:** Headache, blurred vision, confusion, drowsiness, syncope, fatigue
- **GI:** *Anorexia, nausea, vomiting,* diarrhea, hematemesis, stomatitis
- **GU:** Renal toxicity
- **Hematologic: Bone marrow toxicity,** microangiopathic hemolytic anemia (a syndrome of anemia, thrombocytopenia, renal failure, hypertension)
- **Respiratory: Pulmonary toxicity**

- **Other:** *Fever,* cancer in preclinical studies, *cellulitis at injection site, alopecia*

■ Nursing considerations

Assessment

- **History:** Allergy to mitomycin; thrombocytopenia, coagulation disorders or increase in bleeding tendencies, impaired renal function; myelosuppression; pregnancy; lactation
- **Physical:** T; skin color, lesions; weight; hair; local injection site; orientation, reflexes; R, adventitious sounds; mucous membranes; CBC, clotting tests, renal function tests

Interventions

- Do not give IM or SC due to severe local reaction and tissue necrosis.
- Monitor injection site for extravasation: reports of burning or stinging; discontinue infusion immediately and restart in another vein.
- Monitor response frequently at beginning of therapy (CBC, renal function tests, pulmonary exam); adverse effects may require a decreased dose or discontinuation of drug; consult with physician.

Teaching points

- Prepare a calendar with return dates for drug therapy; this drug can only be given IV.
- These side effects may occur: rash, skin lesions, loss of hair (obtain a wig; skin care may help); loss of appetite, nausea, mouth sores (frequent mouth care, small frequent meals may help; maintain good nutrition; consult a dietician; request an antiemetic); drowsiness, dizziness, syncope, headache (use caution driving or operating dangerous machinery; take special precautions to prevent injuries).
- Take precautions to avoid pregnancy while on this drug; use of barrier contraceptives is advised.
- Have regular medical follow-ups, including blood tests to monitor drug's effects.
- Report difficulty breathing, sudden weight gain, swelling, burning or pain at injection site, unusual bleeding or bruising.

Adverse effects in *Italics* are most common; those in **Bold** are life-threatening.

▽mitotane (o, p'-DDD)
(mye' toe tane)

Lysodren

PREGNANCY CATEGORY C

Drug classes
Antineoplastic
Adrenal cytotoxic drug

Therapeutic actions
Acts by unknown mechanism to reduce plasma and urinary levels of adrenocorticosteroids; selectively cytotoxic to normal and neoplastic adrenal cortical cells.

Indications
- Treatment of inoperable adrenal cortical carcinoma, functional (hormone-secreting) and nonfunctional
- Treatment of Cushing's syndrome

Contraindications and cautions
- Contraindicated with allergy to mitotane, lactation.
- Use cautiously with impaired liver function, pregnancy.

Available forms
Tablets—500 mg

Dosages
Adults
Institute therapy in a hospital. Start at 2–6 g/day PO in divided doses tid or qid. Increase dose incrementally to 9–10 g/day. If severe side effects occur, reduce to maximum tolerated dose (2–16 g/day), usually 9–10 g/day. Continue therapy as long as benefits are observed. If no clinical benefits are seen after 3 mo, consider the case a clinical failure.
- *Cushing's syndrome:* 1–12 g/day PO in 3–4 divided doses, usual dose is 3–6 g/day.

Pharmacokinetics

Route	Onset	Peak	Duration
Oral	Slow	Varies	10 wk

Metabolism: Hepatic; $T_{1/2}$: 18–159 days
Distribution: Crosses placenta; may enter breast milk
Excretion: Urine and bile

Adverse effects
- **CNS:** *Depression, sedation, lethargy, vertigo, dizziness,* visual blurring, diplopia, lens opacity, toxic retinopathy, brain damage and possible behavioral and neurologic changes (therapy longer than 2 yr)
- **CV:** Hypertension, orthostatic hypotension, flushing
- **Endocrine:** *Adrenal insufficiency*
- **GI:** *Nausea, vomiting, diarrhea, anorexia*
- **GU:** Hematuria, hemorrhagic cystitis, proteinuria
- **Other:** *Rash,* fever, generalized aching

Interactions
✷ Drug-lab test • Decreased levels of PBI, urinary 17-hydroxycorticosteroids

■ Nursing considerations
Assessment
- **History:** Allergy to mitotane; impaired liver function; lactation, pregnancy
- **Physical:** Weight, skin integrity; orientation, affect, vestibular nerve function, ophthalmologic exam; BP, P, orthostatic BP; bowel sounds, output; liver and renal function tests, urinalysis, plasma cortisol, serum electrolytes

Interventions
- Large metastatic tumor masses are usually removed surgically before therapy to minimize risk of tumor infarction and hemorrhage.
- Administer cautiously with impaired liver function; drug metabolism may be impaired, and drug may accumulate to toxic levels if usual dosage is continued.
- Discontinue temporarily following shock or severe trauma; administration of adrenal steriods may also be necessary to help patient deal with stress.
- Monitor for adrenal insufficiency; adrenal steroid replacement therapy may be necessary.

Teaching points
- Have frequent follow-ups and monitoring.
- Use contraceptives during therapy; this drug can cause birth defects or fetal death.
- These side effects may occur: dizziness, drowsiness, tiredness (avoid driving or performing hazardous tasks); nausea, vomit-

M

ing, diarrhea (small, frequent meals, proper nutrition may help); aching muscles, fever (request medication).

• Report severe nausea, vomiting, loss of appetite, diarrhea, aching muscles, muscle twitching, fever, flushing, emotional depression, rash or darkening of skin.

▽mitoxantrone hydrochloride

*(mye toe **zan**' trone)*

Novantrone

PREGNANCY CATEGORY D

Drug classes

Antineoplastic
Multiple sclerosis drug

Therapeutic actions

Cytotoxic; cell cycle nonspecific, appears to be DNA reactive, causing the death of both proliferating and nonproliferating cells.

Indications

• As part of combination therapy in the treatment of acute nonlymphocytic leukemia (ANLL) in adults, including myelogenous, promyelocytic, monocytic, and erythroid acute leukemias
• Treatment of bone pain in patients with advanced prostatic cancer, in combination with steroids
• Treatment of chronic progressive, progressive relapsing, or worsening relapsing-remitting multiple sclerosis
• Unlabeled uses: treatment of breast cancer, refractory lymphomas

Contraindications and cautions

• Contraindicated with hypersensitivity to mitoxantrone, pregnancy
• Use cautiously with bone marrow suppression, CHF, lactation

Available forms

Injection—2 mg/mL

Dosages
Adults

• *Combination therapy:* For induction, 12 mg/m^2 IV per day on days 1–3, with 100 mg/m^2 of cytosine arabinoside for 7 days given as a continuous infusion on days 1–7. If remission does not occur, a second series can be used, with mitoxantrone given for 2 days and cytosine arabinoside for 5 days.
• *Consolidation therapy:* Mitoxantrone 12 mg/m^2 IV for days 1 and 2, and cytosine arabinoside 100 mg/m^2 given as a continuous 24-hr infusion on days 1–5; given 6 wk after induction therapy if needed. Severe myelosuppression may occur.
• *Multiple sclerosis:* 12 mg/m^2 IV over 5–15 min every 3 mo; do not exceed cumulative lifetime dose of $\geq$ 140 mg/m^2.

Pediatric patients

Safety and efficacy not established.

Pharmacokinetics

Route	Onset	Duration
IV	Rapid	2–3 days

Metabolism: Hepatic; T$_{1/2}$: 5.8 days
Distribution: Crosses placenta; may enter breast milk
Excretion: Bile and urine

▽IV facts

Preparation: Dilute solution to at least 50 mL in either 0.9% sodium chloride injection or 5% dextrose injection; may be further diluted in dextrose 5% in water, normal saline, or dextrose 5% in normal saline if needed. Inject this solution into tubing of a freely running IV of 0.9% sodium chloride injection or 5% dextrose injection over period of at least 3 min. Use immediately after dilution and discard any leftover solution immediately. Wear gloves and goggles and avoid any contact with skin or mucous membranes.
Infusion: Inject slowly over at least 3 min.
Incompatibilities: Do not mix in solution with heparin; a precipitate may form. Do not mix in solution with any other drug; studies are not yet available regarding the safety of such mixtures.

Adverse effects in *Italics* are most common; those in **Bold** are life-threatening.

Adverse effects
- **CNS:** Headache, seizures
- **CV: CHF,** potentially fatal; arrhythmias; chest pain
- **GI:** *Nausea, vomiting, diarrhea,* abdominal pain, mucositis, GI bleeding, jaundice
- **Hematologic: Bone marrow depression,** *infections of all kinds, hyperuricemia*
- **Pulmonary:** *Cough,* dyspnea
- **Other:** *Fever, alopecia, cancer in laboratory animals*

■ Nursing considerations
Assessment
- **History:** Hypersensitivity to mitoxantrone, bone marrow depression; CHF; pregnancy, lactation
- **Physical:** Neurologic status, T; P, BP, auscultation, peripheral perfusion; R, adventitious sounds; abdominal exam, mucous membranes; liver function tests, CBC with differential

Interventions
- Follow CBC and liver function tests carefully before and frequently during therapy; dose adjustment may be needed if myelosuppression becomes severe.
- Monitor patient for hyperuricemia, which frequently occurs as a result of rapid tumor lysis; monitor serum uric acid levels and arrange for appropriate treatment as needed.
- Handle drug with great care; the use of gloves, gowns, and goggles is recommended; if drug comes in contact with skin, wash immediately with warm water; clean spills with calcium hypochlorite solution.
- Monitor IV site for signs of extravasation; if extravasation occurs, stop administration and restart at another site immediately.
- Monitor BP, P, cardiac output regularly during administration; supportive care for CHF should be started at the first sign of failure.
- Protect patient from exposure to infection; monitor occurrence of infection at any site and arrange for appropriate treatment.

Teaching points
- This drug will need to be given IV for 3 days in conjunction with cytosine therapy; mark calendar with days of treatment. Regular blood tests will be needed to evaluate the effects of this treatment (antineoplastic).
- This drug will be given IV every 3 mo when being used to treat MS.
- Use of barrier contraceptives is advised; fetal harm may occur if pregnant while taking this drug.
- These side effects may occur: nausea, vomiting (may be severe; antiemetics may be helpful; eat small, frequent meals); increased susceptibility to infection (avoid crowds and exposure to disease); loss of hair (obtain a wig; it is important to keep the head covered in extremes of temperature); blue-green color of the urine (may last for 24 hr after treatment is finished; the whites of the eyes may also be tinted blue for a time; this is expected and will pass).
- Report severe nausea and vomiting; fever, chills, sore throat; unusual bleeding or bruising; fluid retention or swelling; severe joint pain.

▽ modafinil
*(moe **daff**' in ill)*

Provigil

PREGNANCY CATEGORY C

C-IV CONTROLLED SUBSTANCE

Drug classes
CNS stimulant
Narcolepsy agent

Therapeutic actions
A central nervous system stimulant that helps to improve vigilance and decrease excessive daytime sleepiness associated with narcolepsy and other sleep disorders; may act through dopaminergic mechanisms; exact mechanism of action is not known. Not associated with the cardiac and other systemic stimulatory effects of amphetamines.

Indications
- Treatment of narcolepsy with excessive daytime sleepiness

Contraindications and cautions
- Contraindicated with hypersensitivity to modafinil, left ventricular hypertrophy, ischemic EKG changes, mitral valve prolapse.

- Use cautiously with impaired renal function, epilepsy, emotional instability, pregnancy, lactation.

Available forms
Tablets—100, 200 mg

Dosages
Adults
200 mg PO daily given as a single dose. Up to 400 mg/day as a single dose may be used.
Pediatric patients
Safety and efficacy not established.
Patients with hepatic impairment
With severe hepatic impairment, reduce dose to 50%.
Geriatric patients
Elimination may be reduced; monitor response and consider use of lower dose.

Pharmacokinetics

Route	Onset	Peak
Oral	Gradual	2–3 hr

Metabolism: Hepatic; $T_{1/2}$: 8–10 hours
Distribution: Crosses placenta; may pass into breast milk
Excretion: Urine

Adverse effects
- **CNS:** *Insomnia, headache, nervousness, anxiety,* fatigue
- **Dermatologic:** Rashes
- **GI:** Dry mouth, choking

Interactions
✷ Drug-drug • Possible decreased effectiveness of hormonal contraceptives; suggest the use of barrier contraceptives • Risk of increased levels and effects of warfarin, phenytoin, and TCAs; monitor patient and decrease dose as appropriate

■ Nursing considerations
Assessment
- **History:** Hypersensitivity to modafinil; left ventricular hypertrophy, mitral valve prolapse, ischemic EKG changes; epilepsy; pregnancy, lactation, drug dependence, emotional instability

- **Physical:** Body weight; T; skin color, lesions; orientation, affect, reflexes; P, BP, auscultation; R, adventitious sounds; bowel sounds, normal output; liver and kidney function tests, baseline ECG

Interventions
- Ensure proper diagnosis before administering to rule out underlying medical problems.
- Arrange to dispense the least feasible amount of drug at any one time to minimize risk of overdose.
- Administer drug once a day in the morning.
- Arrange to monitor liver function tests periodically in patients on long-term therapy.
- Establish safety precautions if CNS changes occur—use siderails, accompany patient when ambulating, etc.

Teaching points
- Take this drug exactly as prescribed.
- These side effects may occur: insomnia, nervousness, restlessness, dizziness, impaired thinking (these effects may become less pronounced after a few days; avoid driving a car or engaging in activities that require alertness if these effects occur, notify your health care provider if they are pronounced or bothersome), headache.
- Avoid pregnancy while on this drug; use of barrier contraceptives is advised.
- Report insomnia, abnormal body movements, rash, severe diarrhea, pale-colored stools, yellowing of the skin or eyes.

▽ moexipril
(mo ex' ah pril)

Univasc

PREGNANCY CATEGORY C
(FIRST TRIMESTER)

PREGNANCY CATEGORY D
(SECOND AND THIRD TRIMESTERS)

Drug classes
Antihypertensive
Angiotensin-converting enzyme inhibitor (ACE inhibitor)

Adverse effects in *Italics* are most common; those in **Bold** are life-threatening.

Therapeutic actions

Renin, synthesized by the kidneys, is released into the circulation where it acts on a plasma precursor to produce angiotensin I, which is converted by angiotensin converting enzyme to angiotensin II, a potent vasoconstrictor that also causes release of aldosterone from the adrenals. Both of these actions increase BP; moexipril blocks the conversion of angiotensin I to angiotensin II, leading to decreased BP, decreased aldosterone secretion, a small increase in serum potassium levels, and sodium and fluid loss; increased prostaglandin synthesis may also be involved in the antihypertensive action.

Indications

- Treatment of hypertension, alone or in combination with thiazide-type diuretics

Contraindications and cautions

- Contraindicated with allergy to ACE inhibitors; impaired renal function; CHF; salt or volume depletion; lactation, pregnancy.

Available forms

Tablets—7.5, 15 mg

Dosages
Adults

Not receiving diuretics: initially, 7.5 mg PO daily, given 1 hr before a meal; maintenance—7.5–30 mg PO daily or in 1–2 divided doses given 1 hr before meals. *Receiving diuretics:* discontinue diuretic for 2–3 days before beginning moexipril; follow dosage listed above, if BP is not controlled, diuretic therapy may be added. If diuretic cannot be stopped, start moexipril therapy with 3.75 mg and monitor for symptomatic hypotension.
Pediatric patients

Safety and efficacy not established.
Geriatric patients and patients with renal impairment

Excretion is reduced in renal failure; use with caution; if cretinine clearance ≤ 40 mL/min, start with 3.75 mg PO daily, adjust up to a maximum of 15 mg/day.

Pharmacokinetics

Route	Onset	Peak	Duration
Oral	1 hr	3–4 hr	24 hr

Metabolism: $T_{1/2}$: 2–9 hr
Distribution: Crosses placenta; passes into breast milk
Excretion: Urine

Adverse effects

- **CV:** *Tachycardia,* angina pectoris, **myocardial infarction,** Raynaud's syndrome, CHF, hypotension in salt- or volume-depleted patients
- **GI:** *Gastric irritation, aphthous ulcers, peptic ulcers, diarrhea, dysgeusia,* cholestatic jaundice, hepatocellular injury, anorexia, constipation
- **GU:** *Proteinuria,* renal insufficiency, renal failure, polyuria, oliguria, urinary frequency
- **Hematologic:** Neutropenia, agranulocytosis, thrombocytopenia, hemolytic anemia, **pancytopenia**
- **Skin:** *Rash, pruritus, flushing,* scalded mouth sensation, exfoliative dermatitis, photosensitivity, alopecia
- **Other:** *Cough,* malaise, dry mouth, lymphadenopathy, *flulike syndrome, dizziness*

Interactions

✻ Drug-drug • Increased risk of hyperkalemia with K^+ supplements, K^+-sparing diuretics, salt substitutes • Risk of excessive hypotension with diuretics • Risk of abnormal response with lithium

✻ Drug-lab test • False-positive test for urine acetone

■ Nursing considerations
Assessment

- **History:** Allergy to ACE inhibitors; impaired renal function; CHF; salt or volume depletion; pregnancy; lactation
- **Physical:** Skin color, lesions, turgor; T; P; BP, peripheral perfusion; mucous membranes, bowel sounds, liver evaluation; urinalysis, renal and liver function tests, CBC and differential

Interventions

- Alert surgeon and mark patient's chart with notice that moexipril is being taken; the angiotensin II formation subsequent to compensatory renin release during surgery will be blocked; hypotension may be reversed with volume expansion.

M

- Monitor patient closely for a fall in BP secondary to reduction in fluid volume from excessive perspiration and dehydration, vomiting, or diarrhea; excessive hypotension may occur. Monitor K+ levels carefully in patients receiving K+ supplements, using K+-sparing diuretics or salt substitutes.
- Reduce dosage in patients with impaired renal function.
- Monitor for excessive hypotension with any diuretic therapy.

Teaching points

- Do not stop taking this drug without consulting your health care provider.
- These side effects may occur: GI upset, diarrhea, loss of appetite, change in taste perception; mouth sores (frequent mouth care may help); rash; fast heart rate; dizziness, light-headedness (transient; change position slowly and limit activities to those that do not require alertness and precision).
- This drug is associated with fetal defects; use of barrier contraceptives is advised to prevent pregnancy.
- Be careful in any situation that may lead to a drop in blood pressure (diarrhea, sweating, vomiting, dehydration); if light-headedness or dizziness occurs, consult your health care provider.
- Report mouth sores; sore throat, fever, chills; swelling of the hands or feet; irregular heartbeat, chest pains; swelling of the face, eyes, lips, tongue; difficulty breathing; leg cramps.

▽ molindone hydrochloride

(moe lin' done)

Moban

PREGNANCY CATEGORY C

Drug classes

Dopaminergic blocking agent
Antipsychotic

Therapeutic actions

Mechanism of action not fully understood: antipsychotic drugs block postsynaptic dopamine receptors in the brain, but this may not be necessary and sufficient for antipsychotic activity; clinically resembles the piperazine phenothiazines (fluphenazine).

Indications

- Management of manifestations of psychotic disorders

Contraindications and cautions

- Contraindicated with coma or severe CNS depression, bone marrow depression, blood dyscrasia, circulatory collapse, subcortical brain damage, Parkinson's disease, liver damage, cerebral arteriosclerosis, coronary disease, severe hypotension or hypertension.
- Use cautiously with respiratory disorders ("silent pneumonia"); glaucoma, prostatic hypertrophy; epilepsy or history of epilepsy (drug lowers seizure threshold); breast cancer (elevations in prolactin may stimulate a prolactin-dependent tumor); thyrotoxicosis; peptic ulcer, decreased renal function; exposure to heat or phosphorous insecticides; pregnancy; lactation; children < 12 yr, especially those with chickenpox, CNS infections (children are especially susceptible to dystonias that may confound the diagnosis of Reye's syndrome).

Available forms

Tablets—5, 10, 25, 50, 100 mg; oral concentrate—20 mg/mL

Dosages
Adults

Initially 50–75 mg/day PO increased to 100 mg/day in 3–4 divided doses. Individualize dosage; severe symptoms may require up to 225 mg/day. Maintenance: mild symptoms, 5–15 mg PO tid–qid; moderate symptoms, 10–25 mg PO tid–qid; severe symptoms, 225 mg/day.
Pediatric patients

Not recommended for children < 12 yr.
Geriatric patients

Use lower doses and increase dosage more gradually than in younger patients.

Adverse effects in *Italics* are most common; those in **Bold** are life-threatening.

Pharmacokinetics

Route	Onset	Peak	Duration
Oral	Varies	90 min	24–36 hr

Metabolism: Hepatic; $T_{1/2}$: 1.5 hr
Distribution: Crosses placenta; enters breast milk
Excretion: Urine and feces

Adverse effects

- **Autonomic:** Dry mouth, salivation, nasal congestion, nausea, vomiting, anorexia, fever, pallor, flushed facies, sweating, constipation, paralytic ileus, urinary retention, incontinence, polyuria, enuresis, priapism, ejaculation inhibition, male impotence
- **CNS:** *Drowsiness,* insomnia, vertigo, headache, weakness, tremor, ataxia, slurring, cerebral edema, seizures, exacerbation of psychotic symptoms, extrapyramidal syndromes—*pseudoparkinsonism; dystonias; akathisia,* tardive dyskinesias, potentially irreversible (no known treatment), **NMS**—extrapyramidal symptoms, hyperthermia, autonomic disturbances (rare, but 20% fatal)
- **CV:** Hypotension, orthostatic hypotension, hypertension, tachycardia, bradycardia, cardiac arrest, CHF, cardiomegaly, **refractory arrhythmias,** pulmonary edema
- **Endocrine:** Lactation, breast engorgement, galactorrhea; SIADH; amenorrhea, menstrual irregularities; gynecomastia; changes in libido; hyperglycemia or hypoglycemia; glycosuria; hyponatremia; pituitary tumor with hyperprolactinemia; inhibition of ovulation; infertility, pseudopregnancy; reduced urinary levels of gonadotropins, estrogens, progestins
- **Hematologic:** Eosinophilia, leukopenia, leukocytosis, anemia; aplastic anemia; hemolytic anemia; thrombocytopenic or nonthrombocytopenic purpura
- **Hypersensitivity:** Jaundice, urticaria, angioneurotic edema, laryngeal edema, eczema, asthma, anaphylactoid reactions, exfoliative dermatitis
- **Respiratory:** Bronchospasm, laryngospasm, dyspnea; suppression of cough reflex and potential for aspiration (sudden death related to **asphyxia** or **cardiac arrest**)

Interactions

✴ **Drug-drug** • Decreased absorption of oral phenytoin, tetracycline
✴ **Drug-lab test** • False-positive pregnancy tests (less likely if serum test is used) • Increase in PBI, not attributable to an increase in thyroxine

■ Nursing considerations
Assessment

- **History:** Coma or severe CNS depression; bone marrow depression; circulatory collapse; subcortical brain damage; Parkinson's disease; liver damage; cerebral arteriosclerosis; coronary disease; severe hypotension or hypertension; respiratory disorders; glaucoma, prostatic hypertrophy; epilepsy; breast cancer; thyrotoxicosis; peptic ulcer, decreased renal function; exposure to heat or phosphorous insecticides; pregnancy; lactation; children < 12 yr
- **Physical:** Weight; T; reflexes, orientation, intraocular pressure; P, BP, orthostatic BP; R, adventitious sounds; bowel sounds and normal output, liver evaluation; urinary output, prostate size; CBC, urinalysis, thyroid, liver and kidney function tests

Interventions

- Discontinue drug if serum creatinine, BUN become abnormal or if WBC count is depressed.
- Monitor elderly for dehydration, and institute remedial measures promptly; sedation and decreased sensation of thirst related to CNS effects can lead to severe dehydration.
- Consult physician regarding appropriate warning of patient or patient's guardian about tardive dyskinesias.
- Consult physician about dosage reduction, use of anticholinergic antiparkinsonian drugs (controversial) if extrapyramidal effects occur.

Teaching points

- Take drug exactly as prescribed.
- Avoid driving or engaging in other dangerous activities if CNS, vision changes occur.
- Maintain fluid intake, and use precautions against heat stroke in hot weather.
- Report sore throat, fever, unusual bleeding or bruising, rash, weakness, tremors, impaired vision, dark urine (pink or reddish

brown urine is to be expected), pale stools, yellowing of the skin or eyes.

▷ monoctanoin

See *Less Commonly Used Drugs,* p. 1346.

▷ montelukast sodium
(mon tell oo' kast)

Singulair

PREGNANCY CATEGORY B

Drug classes
Antiasthmatic drug
Leukotriene receptor antagonist

Therapeutic actions
Selectively and competitively blocks the receptor that inhibits leukotriene formation, thus blocking many of the signs and symptoms of asthma—neutrophil and eosinophil migration, neutrophil and monocyte aggregation, leukocyte adhesion, increased capillary permeability, and smooth muscle contraction. These actions contribute to inflammation, edema, mucus secretion, and bronchoconstriction associated with the signs and symptoms of asthma.

Indications
- Prophylaxis and chronic treatment of asthma in adults and children > 12 mo
- Relief of symptoms of seasonal allergic rhinitis in adults and children > 2 yr

Contraindications and cautions
- Contraindicated with hypersensitivity to montelukast or any of its components; acute asthma attacks; status asthmaticus.
- Use cautiously with pregnancy and lactation.

Available forms
Tablets—10 mg; chewable tablets—4, 5 mg; granules—4 mg/packet

Dosages
Adults and patients > 15 yr
One 10 mg tablet PO daily, taken in the evening.
Pediatric patients
6–14 yr: One 5-mg chewable tablet PO daily, taken in the evening.
2–5 yr: One 4-mg chewable tablet PO daily, taken in the evening.
12–23 mo (asthma only): 4 mg granules PO daily, taken in the evening.

Pharmacokinetics

Route	Onset	Peak
Oral	Rapid	2–4 hr

Metabolism: Hepatic; $T_{1/2}$: 2.7–5.5 hr
Distribution: Crosses placenta and enters breast milk
Excretion: Feces, urine

Adverse effects
- **CNS:** Headache, dizziness
- **GI:** Nausea, diarrhea, abdominal pain, dental pain
- **Respiratory:** Influenza, cold, nasal congestion
- **Other:** Generalized pain, fever, rash, fatigue

Interactions
✳ Drug-drug • Decreased effects and bioavailability if taken with phenobarbital, rifampin; monitor patient and adjust dosage as needed

■ Nursing considerations
Assessment
- **History:** Hypersensitivity to montelukast or any of its components; acute asthma attacks; status asthmaticus, pregnancy and lactation
- **Physical:** T; orientation, reflexes; R, adventitious sounds; GI evaluation

Interventions
- Administer in the evening without regard to food.
- Ensure that drug is taken continually for optimal effect.

Adverse effects in *Italics* are most common; those in **Bold** are life-threatening.

- Do not administer for acute asthma attack or acute bronchospasm.
- Avoid the use of aspirin or NSAIDs in patients with known sensitivities while they are on this drug.
- Ensure that patient has a readily available rescue medication for acute asthma attacks or situations when a short-acting inhaled agent is needed.

Teaching points

- Take this drug regularly as prescribed; do not stop taking this drug during symptom-free periods; do not stop taking this drug without consulting your health care provider. Continue taking any other antiasthma drugs that have been prescribed for you. Notify your health care provider if your asthma becomes worse.
- Do not take this drug for an acute asthma attack or acute bronchospasm; this drug is not a bronchodilator, and routine emergency procedures should be followed during acute attacks.
- These side effects may occur: dizziness (use caution when driving or performing activities that require alertness if these effects occur); nausea, vomiting (small, frequent meals may help, taking the drug with food may also help); headache (analgesics may be helpful).
- Avoid the use of aspirin or NSAIDs if you have a known sensitivity to these drugs. Montelukast will not prevent reactions.
- Report fever, acute asthma attacks, flulike symptoms, lethargy.

▽moricizine hydrochloride

(mor i' siz een)

Ethmozine

PREGNANCY CATEGORY B

Drug class
Antiarrhythmic

Therapeutic actions
Type I antiarrhythmic with potent local anesthetic activity; decreases diastolic depolarization, decreasing automaticity of ventricular cells; increases ventricular fibrillation threshold.

Indications
- Treatment of documented ventricular arrhythmias, such as sustained ventricular tachycardias, that are deemed to be life threatening; because of proarrhythmic effects, reserve use for patients in whom the benefit outweighs the risk

Contraindications and cautions
- Contraindicated with hypersensitivity to moricizine; preexisting second- or third-degree AV block; right bundle branch block when associated with left hemiblock (unless a pacemaker is present), cardiogenic shock, CHF; pregnancy; lactation.
- Use cautiously with sick sinus syndrome, hepatic or renal impairment.

Available forms
Tablets—200, 250, 300 mg

Dosages
Adults
600–900 mg/day PO, given q 8 hr in three equally divided doses. Adjust dosage within this range in increments of 150 mg/day at 3-day intervals until the desired effect is seen. Patients with good response may be retained on the same dosage at q 12 hr intervals instead of q 8 hr if this is more convenient. Patients with malignant arrhythmias who respond well may be maintained on long-term therapy.

- *Transfer from another antiarrhythmic:* Withdraw previous antiarrhythmic for 1–2 half-lives before starting moricizine therapy. Hospitalize patients in whom withdrawal may precipitate serious arrhythmias. Transferring from quinidine, disopyramide, start moricizine 6–12 hr after last dose; procainamide, start moricizine 3–6 hr after last dose; encainide, propafenone, tocainide, mexiletine, start moricizine 8–12 hr after last dose.

Pediatric patients
Safety and efficacy not established for patients < 18 yr.

M

Geriatric patients or patients with hepatic impairment

Start < 600 mg/day, and monitor closely, including measurement of ECG intervals, before adjusting dosage.

Pharmacokinetics

Route	Onset	Peak	Duration
Oral	2 hr	0.5–2 hr	10–24 hr

Metabolism: Hepatic; $T_{1/2}$: 1.5–3.5 hr
Distribution: Crosses placenta; enters breast milk
Excretion: Urine

Adverse effects

- **CNS:** *Headache, dizziness, fatigue, hypoesthesias, asthenia, nervousness, sleep disorders,* tremor, anxiety, depression, euphoria, confusion, seizure, nystagmus, ataxia, loss of memory
- **CV:** *Arrhythmias, palpitations, ventricular tachycardia, CHF,* **death** (up to 5% occurrence), *conduction defects, heart block, hypotension,* **cardiac arrest,** *MI*
- **GI:** *Nausea, vomiting, diarrhea, abdominal pain, dyspepsia,* flatulence, anorexia, bitter taste, paralytic ileus
- **GU:** Urinary retention, dysuria, urinary incontinence, kidney pain, impotence
- **Respiratory:** *Dyspnea,* hyperventilation, apnea, asthma, pharyngitis, cough, sinusitis
- **Other:** Sweating, muscle pain, dry mouth, blurred vision, fever

Interactions

* Drug-drug • Increased serum levels of moricizine with cimetidine • Increased risk of heart block with digoxin, propranolol • Decreased serum levels and therapeutic effects of theophylline

■ Nursing considerations
Assessment

- **History:** Hypersensitivity to moricizine; preexisting second- or third-degree AV block; right bundle branch block associated with left hemiblock; cardiogenic shock, CHF; sick sinus syndrome; hepatic or renal impairment; lactation
- **Physical:** T; reflexes, affect; BP, P, ECG including interval monitoring, exercise testing; R, auscultation; abdominal exam, normal output; urinary output; liver and renal function tests, serum electrolytes

Interventions

- Administer only to patients with life-threatening arrhythmias who do not respond to conventional therapy and in whom the benefits outweigh the risks.
- Correct electrolyte disturbances (hypokalemia, hyperkalemia, hypomagnesemia), which may alter the effects of class I antiarrhythmics, before therapy.
- Patient should be hospitalized and monitored continually during start of therapy.
- Reduce dosage for patients with hepatic failure.
- Maintain life support equipment and vasopressor agents on standby in case of severe reactions or generation of arrhythmias.
- Administer with food if severe GI upset occurs; food delays but does not change peak serum levels.
- Frequently monitor heart rhythm, including ECG intervals, during long-term therapy.

Teaching points

- Take drug exactly as prescribed. Arrange schedule to decrease interruptions in your day.
- Frequent monitoring will be necessary to determine the drug effects on your heart and to determine the dosage needed. Keep appointments for these tests, which may include Holter monitoring, stress tests.
- These side effects may occur: arrhythmias or abnormal heart rhythm (hospitalization is required to start drug therapy and to monitor drug response until dosage is determined and stabilized); dizziness, headache, fatigue, nervousness (avoid driving or performing hazardous tasks); nausea, vomiting, diarrhea (eat small, frequent meals; maintain proper nutrition); cough, difficulty breathing, sweating.
- Report palpitations, lethargy, vomiting, difficulty breathing, edema of the extremities, chest pain.

Adverse effects in *Italics* are most common; those in **Bold** are life-threatening.

▽morphine sulfate
(mor' feen)

Immediate-release tablets: MSIR

Timed-release: Kadian, M-Eslon (CAN), MS Contin, Oramorph SR, Roxanol SR

Oral solution: MSIR, Rescudose, Roxanol, Roxanol T

Rectal suppositories: RMS

Injection: Astramorph PF, Duramorph, Epimorph (CAN)

Preservative-free concentrate for microinfusion devices for intraspinal use: Infumorph

PREGNANCY CATEGORY C

C-II CONTROLLED SUBSTANCE

Drug class
Narcotic agonist analgesic

Therapeutic actions
Principal opium alkaloid; acts as agonist at specific opioid receptors in the CNS to produce analgesia, euphoria, sedation; the receptors mediating these effects are thought to be the same as those mediating the effects of endogenous opioids (enkephalins, endorphins).

Indications
- Relief of moderate to severe acute and chronic pain
- Preoperative medication to sedate and allay apprehension, facilitate induction of anesthesia, and reduce anesthetic dosage
- Analgesic adjunct during anesthesia
- Component of most preparations that are referred to as Brompton's cocktail or mixture, an oral alcoholic solution that is used for chronic severe pain, especially in terminal cancer patients
- Intraspinal use with microinfusion devices for the relief of intractable pain
- Unlabeled use: dyspnea associated with acute left ventricular failure and pulmonary edema

Contraindications and cautions
- Contraindicated with hypersensitivity to narcotics; diarrhea caused by poisoning until toxins are eliminated; during labor or delivery of a premature infant (may cross immature blood–brain barrier more readily); after biliary tract surgery or following surgical anastomosis; pregnancy; labor (respiratory depression in neonate; may prolong labor).
- Use cautiously with head injury and increased intracranial pressure; acute asthma, COPD, cor pulmonale, preexisting respiratory depression, hypoxia, hypercapnia (may decrease respiratory drive and increase airway resistance); lactation (wait 4–6 hr after administration to nurse the baby); acute abdominal conditions, CV disease, supraventricular tachycardias, myxedema, convulsive disorders, acute alcoholism, delirium tremens, cerebral arteriosclerosis, ulcerative colitis, fever, kyphoscoliosis, Addison's disease, prostatic hypertrophy, urethral stricture, recent GI or GU surgery, toxic psychosis, renal or hepatic dysfunction.

Available forms
Injection—0.5, 1, 2, 4, 5, 8, 10, 15, 25, 50 mg/mL; tablets—15, 30 mg; CR tablets—15, 60, 100, 200 mg; ER tablets—30, 60, 100 mg; soluble tablets—10, 15, 30 mg; oral solution—10, 20, 100 mg/5 mL; concentrated oral solution—20 mg/mL, 100 mg/5 mL; suppositories—5, 10, 20, 30 mg; capsules—15, 30 mg; SR capsules—20, 30, 50, 60, 100 mg

Dosages
Adults
Oral
One-third to one-sixth as effective as parenteral administration because of first-pass metabolism; 10–30 mg q 4 hr PO. *Controlled-release:* 30 mg q 8–12 hr PO or as directed by physician; *Kadian:* 20–100 mg PO daily–24-hr release system; *MS Contin:* 200 mg PO q 12 hr.
SC and IM
10 mg (range, 5–20 mg)/70 kg q 4 hr or as directed by physician.
IV
2.5–15 mg/70 kg of body weight in 4–5 mL water for injection administered over 4–5 min, or as directed by physician. *Continuous IV infusion:* 0.1–1 mg/mL in 5% dextrose in water by controlled infusion device.

Rectal
10–30 mg q 4 hr or as directed by physician.

Epidural
Initial injection of 5 mg in the lumbar region may provide pain relief for up to 24 hr. If adequate pain relief is not achieved within 1 hr, incremental doses of 1–2 mg may be given at intervals sufficient to assess effectiveness, up to 10 mg/24 hr. For continuous infusion, initial dose of 2–4 mg/24 hr is recommended. Further doses of 1–2 mg may be given if pain relief is not achieved initially.

Intrathecal
Dosage is usually one-tenth that of epidural dosage; a single injection of 0.2–1 mg may provide satisfactory pain relief for up to 24 hr. Do not inject > 2 mL of the 5 mg/10 mL ampule or > 1 mL of the 10 mg/10 mL ampule. Use only in the lumbar area. Repeated intrathecal injections are not recommended; use other routes if pain recurs. For epidural or intrathecal dosing, use preservative-free morphine preparations only.

Pediatric patients
Do not use in premature infants.

SC or IM
0.05–0.2 mg/kg (up to 15 mg per dose) q 4 hr or as directed by physician.

Geriatric patients or impaired adults
Use caution. Respiratory depression may occur in the elderly, the very ill, those with respiratory problems. Reduced dosage may be necessary.

Epidural
Use extreme caution; injection of < 5 mg in the lumbar region may provide adequate pain relief for up to 24 hr.

Intrathecal
Use lower dosages than recommended for adults above.

Pharmacokinetics

Route	Onset	Peak	Duration
Oral	Varies	60 min	5–7 hr
TPR	Rapid	20–60 min	5–7 hr
SC	Rapid	50–90 min	5–7 hr
IM	Rapid	30–60 min	5–6 hr
IV	Immediate	20 min	5–6 hr

Metabolism: Hepatic; $T_{1/2}$: 1.5–2 hr
Distribution: Crosses placenta; enters breast milk
Excretion: Urine and bile

▼IV facts
Preparation: No further preparation needed for direct injection; prepare infusion by adding 0.1–1 mg/mL to 5% dextrose in water.
Infusion: Inject slowly directly IV or into tubing of running IV, each 15 mg over 4–5 min; monitor by controlled infusion device to maintain pain control.
Incompatibilities: Do not mix with aminophylline, amobarbital, chlorothiazide, heparin, meperidine, phenobarbital, phenytoin, sodium bicarbonate, sodium iodide, thiopental.
Y-site incompatibilities: Do not give with minocycline, tetracycline.

Adverse effects
- **CNS:** *Light-headedness, dizziness, sedation,* euphoria, dysphoria, delirium, insomnia, agitation, anxiety, fear, hallucinations, disorientation, drowsiness, lethargy, impaired mental and physical performance, coma, mood changes, weakness, headache, tremor, convulsions, miosis, visual disturbances, suppression of cough reflex
- **CV:** Facial flushing, peripheral circulatory collapse, tachycardia, bradycardia, arrhythmia, palpitations, chest wall rigidity, hypertension, hypotension, orthostatic hypotension, syncope
- **Dermatologic:** Pruritus, urticaria, laryngospasm, bronchospasm, edema
- **GI:** *Nausea, vomiting,* dry mouth, anorexia, constipation, biliary tract spasm; increased colonic motility in patients with chronic ulcerative colitis
- **GU:** Ureteral spasm, spasm of vesical sphincters, urinary retention or hesitancy, oliguria, antidiuretic effect, reduced libido or potency
- **Local:** Tissue irritation and induration (SC injection)
- **Major hazards: Respiratory depression, apnea, circulatory depression, respiratory arrest, shock, cardiac arrest**

Adverse effects in *Italics* are most common; those in **Bold** are life-threatening.

- **Other:** *Sweating,* physical tolerance and dependence, psychological dependence

Interactions

✳ **Drug-drug** • Increased likelihood of respiratory depression, hypotension, profound sedation or coma in patients receiving barbiturate general anesthetics

✳ **Drug-lab test** • Elevated biliary tract pressure (an effect of narcotics) may cause increases in plasma amylase, lipase; determinations of these levels may be unreliable for 24 hr

■ Nursing considerations
Assessment

- **History:** Hypersensitivity to narcotics; diarrhea caused by poisoning; labor or delivery of a premature infant; biliary tract surgery or surgical anastomosis; head injury and increased intracranial pressure; acute asthma, COPD, cor pulmonale, preexisting respiratory depression; acute abdominal conditions, CV disease, supraventricular tachycardias, myxedema, convulsive disorders, acute alcoholism, delirium tremens, cerebral arteriosclerosis, ulcerative colitis, fever, kyphoscoliosis, Addison's disease, prostatic hypertrophy, urethral stricture, recent GI or GU surgery, toxic psychosis, renal or hepatic dysfunction; pregnancy; lactation
- **Physical:** T; skin color, texture, lesions; orientation, reflexes, bilateral grip strength, affect; P, auscultation, BP, orthostatic BP, perfusion; R, adventitious sounds; bowel sounds, normal output; urinary frequency, voiding pattern, normal output; ECG; EEG; thyroid, liver, kidney function tests

Interventions

- Caution patient not to chew or crush controlled-release preparations.
- Dilute and administer slowly IV to minimize likelihood of adverse effects.
- Direct patient to lie down during IV administration.
- Provide narcotic antagonist, facilities for assisted or controlled respiration on standby during IV administration.
- Use caution when injecting SC or IM into chilled areas or in patients with hypotension or in shock; impaired perfusion may delay absorption; with repeated doses, an excessive amount may be absorbed when circulation is restored.
- Reassure patient about addiction liability; most patients who receive opiates for medical reasons do not develop dependence syndromes.

Teaching points

- Take this drug exactly as prescribed. Avoid alcohol, antihistamines, sedatives, tranquilizers, OTC drugs.
- Swallow controlled-release preparation (*MS Contin, Oramorph SR*) whole; do not cut, crush, or chew.
- These side effects may occur: nausea, loss of appetite (take with food, lie quietly); constipation (use laxative); dizziness, sedation, drowsiness, impaired visual acuity (avoid driving or performing tasks that require alertness and visual acuity).
- Do not take leftover medication for other disorders, and do not let anyone else take your prescription.
- Report severe nausea, vomiting, constipation, shortness of breath or difficulty breathing, rash.

▷ **moxifloxacin hydrochloride**
(mocks ah flox' a sin)

Avelox, Avelox IV

PREGNANCY CATEGORY C

Drug classes
Antibiotic
Fluoroquinolone

Therapeutic actions
Bactericidal; interferes with DNA replication, repair, transcription, and recombination in susceptible gram-negative and gram-positive bacteria, preventing cell reproduction and leading to cell death.

Indications

- Treatment of adults with community-acquired pneumonia caused by susceptible strains of *Streptococcus pneumoniae, Haemophilus influenzae, Mycoplasma pneu-*

moniae, Chlamydia pneumoniae, Moraxella catarrhalis
- Treatment of bacterial sinusitis caused by *S. pneumoniae, H. influenzae, M. catarrhalis*
- Treatment of acute bacterial exacerbation of chronic bronchitis caused by *S. pneumoniae, H. influenzae, H. parainfluenzae, Klebsiella pneumoniae, Staphylococcus aureus, M. catarrhalis*
- Treatment of uncomplicated skin and skin structure infections

Contraindications and cautions
- Contraindicated with allergy to fluoroquinolones, pregnancy, lactation; presence of prolonged QT interval, hypokalemia.
- Use cautiously with hepatic dysfunction, seizures.

Available forms
Tablets—400 mg; injection—400 mg in 250 mL

Dosages
Adults
- *Pneumonia:* 400 mg PO or IV daily for 10 days.
- *Sinusitis:* 400 mg PO or IV daily for 10 days.
- *Acute exacerbation of chronic bronchitis:* 400 mg PO or IV daily for 5 days.
- *Uncomplicated skin and skin structure infections:* 400 mg PO daily for 7 days.
Pediatric patients
Not recommended in patients < 18 yr.

▽ IV facts
Preparation: Supplied in premixed 250-mL bags; do not refrigerate; single use only, discard any excess.
Infusion: Infuse over 60 min by direct infusion or into Y-site of running IV.
Compatibilities: Compatible with 0.9% sodium chloride injection, 1M sodium chloride injection, 5% or 10% dextrose injection, sterile water for injection, lactated Ringer's for injection.

Pharmacokinetics

Route	Onset	Peak
Oral	Varies	1–3 hr
IV	Rapid	Minutes

Metabolism: Hepatic; $T_{1/2}$: 12–13.5 hr
Distribution: Crosses placenta; passes into breast milk
Excretion: Urine and feces

Adverse effects
- **CNS:** *Headache,* dizziness, *insomnia,* fatigue, somnolence, depression, nervousness, anxiety, paresthesia
- **CV:** Palpitations, tachycardia, hypertension, hypotension, **prolonged QT interval**
- **GI:** *Nausea,* vomiting, dry mouth, *diarrhea,* anorexia, gastritis, stomatitis
- **Hematologic:** Altered prothrombin time, thrombocytopenia, eosinophilia
- **Respiratory:** Asthma, cough, dyspnea, pharyngitis, rhinitis
- **Other:** Fever, rash, sweating, photosensitivity, tendonitis

Interactions
✳ Drug-drug • Decreased absorption and therapeutic effectiveness of moxifloxacin if taken with sucralfate, metal medications (antacids), multivitamins, didanosine chewable; moxifloxacin should be taken 4 hr before or at least 8 hr after any of these drugs • Risk of severe cardiac arrhythmias if combined with any other drug known to prolong the QTc interval (quinidine, procainamide, amiodarone, sotalol); avoid these combinations • Increased risk of seizures if fluoroquinolones are combined with NSAIDs; monitor patient closely

■ Nursing considerations
Assessment
- **History:** Allergy to fluoroquinolones; prolonged QTc interval, hypokalemia, hepatic dysfunction; seizures; lactation; pregnancy
- **Physical:** Skin color, lesions; T; orientation, reflexes, affect; R, adventitious sounds; P, BP; mucous membranes, bowel sounds; liver function tests, ECG, CBC

Interventions
- Arrange for culture and sensitivity tests before beginning therapy.
- Continue therapy as indicated for condition being treated.

Adverse effects in *Italics* are most common; those in **Bold** are life-threatening.

- Administer oral drug 4 hr before or at least 8 hr after antacids or other anion-containing drugs.
- Do not change dosage when switching from IV to oral dose.
- Discontinue drug at any sign of hypersensitivity (rash, photophobia) or with severe diarrhea.
- Discontinue drug and monitor ECG if palpitations, dizziness occur.
- Monitor clinical response—if no improvement is seen or a relapse occurs, repeat culture and sensitivity.

Teaching points

- Take oral drug once a day for the period prescribed. If antacids are being taken, take drug 4 hr before or at least 8 hr after the antacid.
- These side effects may occur: nausea, vomiting, abdominal pain (small, frequent meals may help); diarrhea or constipation (consult nurse or physician if this occurs); drowsiness, blurring of vision, dizziness (observe caution if driving or using dangerous equipment); sensitivity to the sun (avoid exposure, use a sunscreen if needed).
- Report rash, visual changes, severe GI problems, weakness, tremors, palpitations, sensitivity to light.

▽ muromonab-CD3

(mew ro' mon ab)

Orthoclone OKT3

PREGNANCY CATEGORY C

Drug classes

Immunosuppressant
Monoclonal antibody

Therapeutic actions

A murine monoclonal antibody to the antigen of human T cells; functions as an immunosuppressant by enabling T cells.

Indications

- Acute allograft rejection in renal transplant patients

- Treatment of steroid-resistant acute allograft rejection in cardiac and hepatic transplant patients

Contraindications and cautions

- Contraindicated with allergy to muromonab or any murine product, fluid overload as evidenced by chest x-ray, or > 3% weight gain in 1 wk.
- Use cautiously with fever (use antipyretics to decrease fever before therapy); previous administration of muromonab-CD3 (antibodies frequently develop, risks serious reactions on repeat administration); pregnancy.

Available forms

Injection—5 mg/5 mL

Dosages

Give only as an IV bolus in < 1 min. Do not infuse or give by any other route.

Adults

5 mg/day for 10–14 days. Begin treatment once acute renal rejection is diagnosed. It is strongly recommended that methylprednisolone sodium succinate 1 mg/kg IV be given prior to muromonab-CD3 and IV hydrocortisone sodium succinate 100 mg be given 30 min after muromonab-CD3 administration.

Pediatric patients

Safety and efficacy not established.

Pharmacokinetics

Route	Onset	Peak	Duration
IV	Minutes	2–7 days	7 days

Metabolism: Tissue; $T_{1/2}$: 47–100 hr
Distribution: Crosses placenta

▽ IV facts

Preparation: Draw solution into a syringe through a low protein-binding 0.2- or 0.22-μm filter. Discard filter and attach needle for IV bolus injection. Solution may develop fine translucent particles that do not affect its potency. Refrigerate solution; do not freeze or shake.

Infusion: Administer as an IV bolus over < 1 min. Do not give as an IV infusion or with other drug solutions.

M

Incompatibilities: Do not mix with any other drug solution; do not infuse simultaneously with any other drug.

Adverse effects
- **CNS:** Malaise, *tremors*
- **GI:** *Vomiting, nausea, diarrhea*
- **Respiratory: Acute pulmonary edema,** *dyspnea, chest pain,* wheezing
- **Other:** Lymphomas, *increased susceptibility to infection, fever, chills,* **cytokine-release syndrome** ("flu" to shock)

Interactions
✳ **Drug-drug** • Reduce dosage of other immunosuppressive agents; severe immunosuppression can lead to increased susceptibility to infection and increased risk of lymphomas; other immunosuppressives can be restarted about 3 days prior to cessation of muromonab
• Risk of encephalopathy and CNS effects with indomethacin

■ Nursing considerations
Assessment
- **History:** Allergy to muromonab or any murine product; fluid overload; fever; previous administration of muromonab-CD3; pregnancy; lactation
- **Physical:** T, weight; P, BP; R, adventitious sounds; chest x-ray, CBC

Interventions
- Obtain chest x-ray within 24 hr of therapy to ensure chest is clear.
- Arrange for antipyretics (acetaminophen) if patient is febrile before therapy.
- Monitor WBC levels and circulating T cells periodically during therapy.
- Monitor patient very closely after first dose; acetaminophen prn should be ordered to cover febrile reactions; cooling blanket may be needed in severe cases. Equipment for intubation and respiratory support should be on standby for severe pulmonary reactions.

Teaching points
- There is often a severe reaction to the first dose, including high fever and chills, difficulty breathing, and chest congestion (you will be closely watched, and comfort measures will be given).
- Avoid infection; people may wear masks and rubber gloves when caring for you; visitors may be limited.
- Report chest pain, difficulty breathing, nausea, chills.

▷ mycophenolate mofetil
(my coe fin' oh late)

CellCept

PREGNANCY CATEGORY C

Drug class
Immunosuppressant

Therapeutic actions
Immunosuppressant; inhibits T-lymphocyte activation; exact mechanism of action unknown, but binds to intracellular protein, which may prevent the generation of nuclear factor of activated T cells, and suppresses the immune activation and response of T cells; inhibits proliferative responses of T and B cells.

Indications
- Prophylaxis of organ rejection in patients receiving allogeneic renal, hepatic, and heart transplants; intended to be used concomitantly with corticosteroids and cyclosporine
- Unlabeled use: refractory uveitis as 2 g/day alone or in combination therapy

Contraindications and cautions
- Contraindicated with allergy to mycophenolate, pregnancy, lactation.
- Use cautiously with impaired renal function.

Available forms
Capsules—250 mg; tablets—500 mg; powder for oral suspension: 200 mg/mL; powder for injection—500 mg

Dosages
Adults
- *Renal transplantation:* 1 g bid PO or IV (administered over ≥ 2 hr) starting within 24 hr of transplant.
- *Cardiac transplantation:* 1.5 g bid PO or IV (IV over ≥ 2 hr).
- *Hepatic transplantation:* 1 g bid IV or 1.5 g PO bid (over ≥ 2 hr).

Pediatric patients
Safety and efficacy not established.
Patients with severe renal impairment
Avoid doses > 1 g/day. Monitor patient carefully for adverse response.

Pharmacokinetics

Route	Onset	Peak
Oral	Varies	45–60 min

Metabolism: Hepatic; $T_{1/2}$: 17.9 hr
Distribution: Crosses placenta; enters breast milk
Excretion: Urine

▽ IV facts
Preparation: Reconstitute and dilute to 6 mg/mL with 5% dextrose injection. Reconstitute each vial with 14 mL 5% dextrose injection. Gently shake. Solution should be slightly yellow without precipitates. For a large dose, dilute contents of two reconstituted vials into 140 mL of D_5W; for a 1.5 g dose, dilute contents of three reconstituted vials into 210 mL of D_5W. Use caution to avoid contact with solution. If contact occurs, wash with soap and water.
Infusion: Infuse over ≥ 2 hr. Begin ≤ 24 hr of transplant and continue for ≤ 14 days.
Incompatibilities: Do not mix with any other drugs or infusion admixtures.

Adverse effects
- **CNS:** *Tremor, headache, insomnia,* paresthesias
- **CV:** Chest pain, hypertension, peripheral edema
- **GI: Hepatotoxicity,** *constipation, diarrhea, nausea, vomiting,* anorexia
- **GU:** *Renal dysfunction,* nephrotoxicity, *UTI,* oliguria
- **Hematologic:** Leukopenia, *anemia,* hyperkalemia, hypokalemia, hyperglycemia
- **Other:** Abdominal pain, fever, asthenia, back pain, ascites, neoplasms, *infection*

Interactions
✳ **Drug-drug** • Decreased levels and effectiveness with cholestyramine • Decreased levels and effectiveness of theophylline, phenytoin

■ Nursing considerations
Assessment
- **History:** Allergy to mycophenolate; pregnancy, lactation; renal function
- **Physical:** T; skin color, lesions; BP, peripheral perfusion; liver evaluation, bowel sounds, gum evaluation; renal and liver function tests, CBC

Interventions
- Monitor renal and liver function before and periodically during therapy; marked decreases in function may require dosage change or discontinuation of therapy.
- Prepare oral suspension by tapping closed bottle several times, adding 47 mL water to bottle, and shaking closed bottle for 1 min. Add another 47 mL water; shake for 1 min.
- Protect patient from exposure to infections and maintain sterile technique for invasive procedures.

Teaching points
- Avoid infection while on this drug; avoid crowds or people with infections. Notify your physician immediately if you injure yourself.
- These side effects may occur: nausea, vomiting (take drug with food); diarrhea; headache (request analgesics).
- This drug should not be taken during pregnancy. If you think you are pregnant or you want to become pregnant, discuss this with your physician.
- Have periodic blood tests to monitor your response to the drug and its effects.
- Do not discontinue this drug without your physician's advice.
- Report unusual bleeding or bruising, fever, sore throat, mouth sores, tiredness.

▽ nabumetone

(nah bye' meh tone)

Relafen

PREGNANCY CATEGORY C
(FIRST AND SECOND TRIMESTERS)

PREGNANCY CATEGORY D
(THIRD TRIMESTER)

Drug classes
Nonsteroidal anti-inflammatory drug (NSAID)
Analgesic (non-narcotic)

Therapeutic actions
Analgesic, anti-inflammatory, and antipyretic activities largely related to inhibition of prostaglandin synthesis; exact mechanisms of action are not known.

Indications
• Acute and long-term treatment of signs and symptoms of rheumatoid arthritis and osteoarthritis

Contraindications and cautions
• Contraindicated with significant renal impairment, pregnancy, lactation.
• Use cautiously with impaired hearing; allergies; hepatic, CV, and GI conditions.

Available forms
Tablets—500, 750 mg

Dosages
Adults
1,000 mg PO as a single dose with or without food. 1,500–2,000 mg/day have been used. May be given in divided doses.
Pediatric patients
Safety and efficacy have not been established.

Pharmacokinetics

Route	Onset	Peak
Oral	30 min	30–60 min

Metabolism: Hepatic; $T_{1/2}$: 22.5–30 hr
Distribution: Crosses placenta; enters breast milk
Excretion: Urine

Adverse effects
• **CNS:** *Headache, dizziness, somnolence, insomnia,* fatigue, tiredness, dizziness, tinnitus, ophthalmic effects
• **Dermatologic:** *Rash,* pruritus, sweating, dry mucous membranes, stomatitis
• **GI:** *Nausea, dyspepsia, GI pain,* diarrhea, vomiting, *constipation,* flatulence
• **GU:** Dysuria, **renal impairment**
• **Hematologic:** Bleeding, platelet inhibition with higher doses, neutropenia, eosinophilia, leukopenia, pancytopenia, thrombocytopenia, agranulocytosis, granulocytopenia, aplastic anemia, decreased Hgb or Hct, bone marrow depression, menorrhagia
• **Respiratory:** Dyspnea, hemoptysis, pharyngitis, bronchospasm, rhinitis
• **Other:** Peripheral edema, **anaphylactoid reactions to fatal anaphylactic shock**

■ Nursing considerations
Assessment
• **History:** Renal impairment; impaired hearing; allergies; hepatic, CV, and GI conditions; lactation
• **Physical:** Skin color and lesions; orientation, reflexes, ophthalmic and audiometric evaluation, peripheral sensation; P, edema; R, adventitious sounds; liver evaluation; CBC, clotting times, renal and liver function tests; serum electrolytes, stool guaiac

Interventions
• Administer drug with food or after meals if GI upset occurs.
• Arrange for periodic ophthalmologic examination during long-term therapy.
• Institute emergency procedures if overdose occurs: gastric lavage, induction of emesis, supportive therapy.

Teaching points
• Take drug with food or meals if GI upset occurs; take only the prescribed dosage.
• Dizziness, drowsiness can occur (avoid driving or the use of dangerous machinery).
• Report sore throat, fever, rash, itching, weight gain, swelling in ankles or fingers; changes in vision; black, tarry stools.

Adverse effects in *Italics* are most common; those in **Bold** are life-threatening.

▽ nadolol
(nay doe' lol)

Alti-Nadolol (CAN), Apo-Nadolol (CAN), Corgard, Novo-Nadolol (CAN)

PREGNANCY CATEGORY C

Drug classes
Beta-adrenergic blocker (nonselective)
Antianginal agent
Antihypertensive

Therapeutic actions
Competitively blocks beta-adrenergic receptors in the heart and juxtaglomerular apparatus, decreasing the influence of the sympathetic nervous system on these tissues and decreasing the excitability of the heart, cardiac output, oxygen consumption, and the release of renin, and lowering BP.

Indications
- Hypertension alone or with other drugs, especially diuretics
- Long-term management of angina pectoris
- Unlabeled uses: treatment of ventricular arrhythmias, migraines, lithium-induced tremors, essential tremors

Contraindications and cautions
- Contraindicated with sinus bradycardia (HR < 45 beats/min), second- or third-degree heart block (PR interval > 0.24 sec), cardiogenic shock, CHF, asthma, COPD, pregnancy, lactation.
- Use cautiously with diabetes or thyrotoxicosis.

Available forms
Tablets—20, 40, 80, 120, 160 mg

Dosages
Adults
- **Hypertension:** Initially 40 mg PO daily; gradually increase dosage in 40- to 80-mg increments until optimum response is achieved. Usual maintenance dose is 40–80 mg/day; up to 320 mg daily may be needed.
- **Angina:** Initially 40 mg PO daily; gradually increase dosage in 40- to 80-mg increments at 3- to 7-day intervals until optimum

response is achieved or heart rate markedly decreases. Usual maintenance dose is 40–80 mg daily; up to 240 mg/day may be needed. Safety and efficacy of larger doses not established. To discontinue, reduce dosage gradually over 1- to 2-wk period.

Pediatric patients
Safety and efficacy not established.

Geriatric patients or patients with renal failure

Creatinine Clearance (mL/min)	Dosage Intervals (hr)
> 50	24
31–50	24–36
10–30	24–48
< 10	40–60

Pharmacokinetics

Route	Onset	Peak	Duration
Oral	Varies	2–4 hr	17–24 hr

Metabolism: $T_{1/2}$: 20–24 hr
Distribution: Crosses placenta; enters breast milk
Excretion: Urine

Adverse effects
- **Allergic reactions:** Pharyngitis, erythematous rash, fever, sore throat, laryngospasm, respiratory distress
- **CNS:** Dizziness, vertigo, tinnitus, fatigue, emotional depression, paresthesias, sleep disturbances, hallucinations, disorientation, memory loss, slurred speech
- **CV:** *CHF, cardiac arrhythmias,* peripheral vascular insufficiency, claudication, CVA, **pulmonary edema,** hypotension
- **Dermatologic:** Rash, pruritus, sweating, dry skin
- **EENT:** Eye irritation, dry eyes, conjunctivitis, blurred vision
- **GI:** *Gastric pain, flatulence, constipation, diarrhea, nausea, vomiting,* anorexia, ischemic colitis, renal and mesenteric arterial thrombosis, retroperitoneal fibrosis, hepatomegaly, acute pancreatitis
- **GU:** *Impotence, decreased libido,* Peyronie's disease, dysuria, nocturia, urinary frequency
- **Musculoskeletal:** Joint pain, arthralgia, muscle cramp
- **Respiratory:** Bronchospasm, dyspnea, cough, bronchial obstruction, nasal stuffi-

N

ness, rhinitis, pharyngitis (less likely than with propranolol)
• **Other:** *Decreased exercise tolerance, development of antinuclear antibodies,* hyperglycemia or hypoglycemia, elevated serum transaminase

Interactions
✴ **Drug-drug** • Increased effects with verapamil • Increased serum levels and toxicity of IV lidocaine, aminophylline • Increased risk of orthostatic hypotension with prazosin • Increased risk of peripheral ischemia with ergotamine, methysergide, dihydroergotamine • Decreased antihypertensive effects with NSAIDs, clonidine • Hypertension followed by severe bradycardia with epinephrine
✴ **Drug-lab test** • Possible false results with glucose or insulin tolerance tests

■ Nursing considerations
Assessment
• **History:** Sinus bradycardia, second- or third-degree heart block, cardiogenic shock, CHF, asthma, COPD; diabetes or thyrotoxicosis; pregnancy; lactation
• **Physical:** Weight, skin condition, neurologic status, P, BP, ECG, respiratory status, kidney and thyroid function, blood and urine glucose

Interventions
• Do not discontinue drug abruptly after long-term therapy (hypersensitivity to catecholamines may have developed, causing exacerbation of angina, MI, and ventricular arrhythmias). Taper drug gradually over 2 wk with monitoring.
• Consult with physician about withdrawing drug if patient is to undergo surgery (controversial).

Teaching points
• Do not stop taking unless instructed to do so by a health care provider; drug must be gradually stopped to prevent serious adverse effects.
• Avoid driving or dangerous activities if CNS effects occur.

• Report difficulty breathing, night cough, swelling of extremities, slow pulse, confusion, depression, rash, fever, sore throat.

▷ nafarelin acetate
(naf' a re lin)

Synarel

PREGNANCY CATEGORY X

Drug class
GnRH (gonadotropin-releasing hormone)

Therapeutic actions
A potent agonistic analog of gonadotropin-releasing hormone (GnRH), which is released from the hypothalamus to stimulate LH and FSH release from the pituitary; these hormones are responsible for regulating reproductive status. Repeated dosing abolishes the stimulatory effect on the pituitary gland, leading to decreased secretion of gonadal steroids by about 4 wk; consequently, tissues and functions that depend on gonadal steroids for their maintenance become quiescent.

Indications
• Treatment of endometriosis, including pain relief and reduction of endometriotic lesions
• Treatment of central precocious puberty in children of both sexes

Contraindications and cautions
• Known sensitivity to GnRH, GnRH-agonist analogs, excipients in the product; undiagnosed abnormal genital bleeding; pregnancy; lactation (potential androgenic effects on the fetus).

Available forms
Nasal solution—2 mg/mL

Dosages
Adults
• *Endometriosis:* 400 mcg/day. One spray (200 mcg) into one nostril in the morning and one spray into the other nostril in the evening. Start treatment between days 2 and 4 of the menstrual cycle. 800-mcg dose may

---

Adverse effects in *Italics* are most common; those in **Bold** are life-threatening.

be administered as one spray into each nostril in the morning (a total of two sprays) and again in the evening for patients with persistent regular menstruation after months of treatment. Treatment for 6 mo is recommended. Retreatment is not recommended because safety has not been established.

Pediatric patients

- *Central precocious puberty:* 1,600 mcg/day. Two sprays (400 mcg) in each nostril in the morning and two sprays in each nostril in the evening; may be increased to 1,800 mcg/day. If 1,800 mcg are needed, give 3 sprays into alternating nostrils 3 times/day. Continue until resumption of puberty is desired.

Pharmacokinetics

Route	Onset	Peak
Nasal	Rapid	4 wk

Metabolism: $T_{1/2}$: 2–4 hr
Distribution: Crosses placenta; enters breast milk
Excretion: Urine

Adverse effects

- **CNS:** Dizziness, headache, sleep disorders, fatigue, tremor
- **Endocrine:** *Androgenic effects* (acne, edema, mild hirsutism, decrease in breast size, deepening of the voice, oily skin or hair, weight gain, clitoral hypertrophy or testicular atrophy), *hypoestrogenic effects* (flushing, sweating, vaginitis, nervousness, emotional lability)
- **GI:** Hepatic dysfunction
- **GU:** Fluid retention
- **Local:** *Nasal irritation*
- **Other:** With prolonged therapy, bone density loss has been noted

■ Nursing considerations
Assessment

- **History:** Sensitivity to GnRH, GnRH-agonist analogs, excipients in the product; undiagnosed abnormal genital bleeding; pregnancy; lactation
- **Physical:** Weight; hair distribution pattern; skin color, texture, lesions; breast exam; nasal mucosa; orientation, affect, reflexes; P, auscultation, BP, peripheral edema; liver evaluation; bone density studies in long-term therapy

Interventions

- Ensure that patient is not pregnant before therapy; begin therapy for endometriosis during menstrual period, days 2–4; advise the use of barrier contraceptives.
- Store drug upright; protect from exposure to light.
- Arrange for bone density studies before therapy if retreatment is suggested because of return of endometriosis.
- Ensure patient has enough of the drug to prevent interruption of therapy.
- Caution patient that androgenic effects may not be reversible when the drug is withdrawn.
- Monitor nasal mucosa for signs of erosion during course of therapy.
- Provide topical decongestant to be used at least 2 hr after dosing with nafarelin.

Teaching points

- Use this drug without interruption; be sure that you have enough on hand to prevent interruption. Store the drug upright. Protect the bottle from exposure to light.
- Regular menstruation should cease within 4–6 wk of therapy. Breakthrough bleeding or ovulation may still occur.
- These side effects may occur: masculinizing effects (acne, hair growth, deepening of voice, oily skin or hair; may not be reversible); low estrogen effects (flushing, sweating, vaginal irritation, nervousness); nasal irritation.
- Consult with your nurse or physician if you need a topical nasal decongestant; a decongestant should be used at least 2 hr after nafarelin use.
- This drug is contraindicated during pregnancy; use a nonhormonal form of birth control during therapy. If you become pregnant, discontinue the drug and consult with your physician immediately.
- Report abnormal growth of facial hair, deepening of the voice, unusual bleeding or bruising, fever, chills, sore throat, vaginal itching or irritation; nasal irritation, burning.

N

▽nafcillin sodium
(naf sill' in)

PREGNANCY CATEGORY B

Drug classes
Antibiotic
Penicillinase-resistant penicillin

Therapeutic actions
Bactericidal: inhibits cell wall synthesis of sensitive organisms, causing cell death.

Indications
- Infections due to penicillinase-producing staphylococci; may be used to initiate therapy when such infection is suspected
- Treatment of streptococcal pharyngitis

Contraindications and cautions
- Contraindicated with allergies to penicillins, cephalosporins, or other allergens.
- Use cautiously with renal disorders, pregnancy, lactation (may cause diarrhea or candidiasis in infant).

Available forms
Capsules—250 mg; powder for injection—500 mg; 1, 2 g

Dosages
Adults
IV
500–1,000 mg q 4 hr for short-term (24–48 hr) therapy only, especially in the elderly.
IM
500 mg q 6 hr (q 4 hr in severe infections).
PO
250–500 mg q 4–6 hr, up to 1 g q 4–6 hr in severe infections.
Pediatric patients
IM
25 mg/kg bid.
- *Newborns:* 10 mg/kg bid.
PO
- *Staphylococcal infections:* 50 mg/kg/day in four divided doses; newborns: *10* mg/kg tid–qid.
- *Scarlet fever, pneumonia:* 25 mg/kg/day in four divided doses.

- *Streptococcal pharyngitis:* 250 mg tid (penicillin G is preferred).

Pharmacokinetics

Route	Onset	Peak	Duration
Oral	Varies	60 min	4 hr
IM	Rapid	3–90 min	4–6 hr
IV	Immediate	15 min	4 hr

Metabolism: Hepatic; $T_{1/2}$: 1 hr
Distribution: Crosses placenta; enters breast milk
Excretion: Urine and bile

▽IV facts
Preparation: Dilute solution for IV use in 15–30 mL sodium chloride injection or sterile water for injection; dilute reconstituted solution with compatible IV solution: 0.9% sodium chloride injection, sterile water for injection, 5% dextrose in water or in 0.4% sodium chloride solution, M/6 sodium lactate solution, or Ringer's solution. Solutions at concentrations of 2–40 mg/mL are stable for 24 hr at room temperature or 4 days refrigerated; discard solution after this time.
Infusion: Infuse slowly, each 500 mg over 5–10 min.
Incompatibilities: Do not mix in the same IV solution as other antibiotics.

Adverse effects
- **CNS:** Lethargy, hallucinations, seizures
- **GI:** *Glossitis, stomatitis, gastritis, sore mouth,* furry tongue, black "hairy" tongue, *nausea, vomiting, diarrhea,* abdominal pain, bloody diarrhea, enterocolitis, pseudomembranous colitis, nonspecific hepatitis
- **GU:** Nephritis—oliguria, proteinuria, hematuria, casts, azotemia, pyuria
- **Hematologic:** Anemia, thrombocytopenia, leukopenia, neutropenia, prolonged bleeding time (more common than with other penicillinase-resistant penicillins)
- **Hypersensitivity:** *Rash, fever, wheezing,* **anaphylaxis**
- **Local:** *Pain, phlebitis,* thrombosis at injection site
- **Other:** Superinfections—oral and rectal moniliasis, vaginitis

Adverse effects in *Italics* are most common; those in **Bold** are life-threatening.

Interactions
* **Drug-drug** • Decreased effectiveness with tetracyclines • Inactivation of parenteral aminoglycosides: amikacin, gentamicin, kanamycin, neomycin, metilmicin, streptomycin, tobramycin
* **Drug-lab test** • False-positive Coombs' test with IV use

■ Nursing considerations
Assessment
* **History:** Allergies to penicillins, cephalosporins, or other allergens; renal disorders; pregnancy; lactation
* **Physical:** Culture the infection; skin color, lesions; R, adventitious sounds; bowel sounds; CBC, liver and renal function tests, serum electrolytes, Hct, urinalysis

Interventions
* Culture the infection before treatment; reculture if response is not as expected.
* Continue therapy for at least 2 days after signs of infection have disappeared, usually 7–10 days.
* Reconstitute powder for IM use with sterile or bacteriostatic water for injection or sodium chloride injection. Administer by deep intragluteal injection. Reconstituted solution is stable for 7 days if refrigerated or 3 days at room temperature.
* Do not give IM injections repeatedly in the same site; atrophy can occur; monitor injection sites.
* Administer oral drug on an empty stomach, 1 hr before or 2 hr after meals, with a full glass of water. Do not administer with fruit juices or soft drinks.

Teaching points
* Take oral drug on an empty stomach with a full glass of water; take the full course of drug therapy.
* Avoid self-treating other infections with this antibiotic because it is specific to the infection being treated.
* Nausea, vomiting, diarrhea, mouth sores, pain at injection sites may occur.
* Report difficulty breathing, rashes, severe diarrhea, severe pain at injection site, mouth sores, unusual bleeding or bruising.

▽**nalbuphine hydrochloride**
(*nal' byoo feen*)

Nubain

PREGNANCY CATEGORY C

Drug class
Narcotic agonist-antagonist analgesic

Therapeutic actions
Nalbuphine acts as an agonist at specific opioid receptors in the CNS to produce analgesia, sedation but also acts to cause hallucinations and is an antagonist at mu receptors.

Indications
* Relief of moderate to severe pain
* Preoperative analgesia, as a supplement to surgical anesthesia, and for obstetric analgesia during labor and delivery

Contraindications and cautions
* Contraindicated with hypersensitivity to nalbuphine, sulfites; lactation.
* Use cautiously with emotionally unstable patients or those with a history of narcotic abuse; pregnancy prior to labor (neonatal withdrawal may occur if mothers used drug during pregnancy), labor or delivery (use with caution during delivery of premature infants, who are especially sensitive to respiratory depressant effects of narcotics), bronchial asthma, COPD, respiratory depression, anoxia, increased intracranial pressure, acute MI when nausea and vomiting are present, biliary tract surgery (may cause spasm of the sphincter of Oddi).

Available forms
Injection—10 mg/mL, 20 mg/mL

Dosages
Adults
Usual dose is 10 mg/70 kg of body weight, SC, IM, or IV q 3–6 hr as necessary. Individualize dosage. In nontolerant patients, the recommended single maximum dose is 20 mg, with a maximum total daily dose of 160 mg. Patients dependent on narcotics may experience withdrawal symptoms with administration of nalbuphine; control by small increments of

morphine by slow IV administration until relief occurs. If the previous narcotic was morphine, meperidine, codeine, or another narcotic with similar duration of activity, administer one-fourth the anticipated nalbuphine dose initially, and observe for signs of withdrawal. If no untoward symptoms occur, progressively increase doses until analgesia is obtained.

Pediatric patients < 18 yr
Not recommended.

Geriatric patients or patients with renal or hepatic impairment
Reduce dosage.

Pharmacokinetics

Route	Onset	Peak	Duration
IV	2–3 min	15–20 min	3–6 hr
SC/IM	< 15 min	30–60 min	3–6 hr

Metabolism: Hepatic; $T_{1/2}$: 5 hr
Distribution: Crosses placenta; enters breast milk
Excretion: Urine

▽IV facts

Preparation: No additional preparation is required.
Infusion: Administer by direct injection or into the tubing of a running IV.
Y-site incompatibilities: Do not give with nafcillin.

Adverse effects

- **CNS:** *Sedation, clamminess, sweating, headache,* nervousness, restlessness, depression, crying, confusion, faintness, hostility, unusual dreams, hallucinations, euphoria, dysphoria, unreality, *dizziness, vertigo,* floating feeling, feeling of heaviness, numbness, tingling, flushing, warmth, blurred vision
- **CV:** Hypotension, hypertension, bradycardia, tachycardia
- **Dermatologic:** Itching, burning, urticaria
- **GI:** Nausea, vomiting, cramps, dyspepsia, bitter taste, *dry mouth*
- **GU:** Urinary urgency
- **Respiratory:** Respiratory depression, dyspnea, asthma

Interactions

✳ **Drug-drug** • Potentiation of effects with barbiturate anesthetics

■ Nursing considerations
Assessment

- **History:** Hypersensitivity to nalbuphine, sulfites; lactation; emotional instability or history of narcotic abuse; pregnancy; bronchial asthma, COPD, respiratory depression, anoxia, increased intracranial pressure, MI, biliary tract surgery
- **Physical:** Orientation, reflexes, bilateral grip strength, affect; pupil size, vision; pulse, auscultation, BP; R, adventitious sounds; bowel sounds, normal output; urine output; liver, kidney function tests

Interventions

- Taper dosage when discontinuing after prolonged use to avoid withdrawal symptoms.
- Provide narcotic antagonist, facilities for assisted or controlled respiration on standby in case of respiratory depression.
- Reassure patient about addiction liability; most patients who receive opiates for medical reasons do not develop dependence syndromes.

Teaching points

- These side effects may occur: dizziness, sedation, drowsiness, impaired visual acuity (avoid driving, performing tasks that require alertness); nausea, loss of appetite (lying quietly, eating frequent small meals may help).
- Report severe nausea, vomiting, palpitations, shortness of breath, or difficulty breathing.

▽nalidixic acid
*(nal i **dix'** ik)*

NegGram

PREGNANCY CATEGORY B

Drug classes
Urinary tract anti-infective
Antibacterial

Adverse effects in *Italics* are most common; those in **Bold** are life-threatening.

Therapeutic actions
Bactericidal; interferes with DNA and RNA synthesis in susceptible gram-negative bacteria, causing cell death.

Indications
- Urinary tract infections caused by susceptible gram-negative bacteria, including *Proteus* strains, *Klebsiella* species, Enterobacter species, *Escherichia coli*

Contraindications and cautions
- Contraindicated with allergy to nalidixic acid, seizures, epilepsy, pregnancy, lactation.
- Use cautiously with G6PD deficiency, renal or liver dysfunction, cerebral arteriosclerosis.

Available forms
Caplets—250, 500 mg, 1 g; suspension—250 mg/5 mL

Dosages
Adults
Initial therapy, 1 g PO qid for 1–2 wk. For prolonged therapy, total dose may be reduced to 2 g/day.
Pediatric patients
< 3 mo: Not recommended.

3 mo–< 12 yr: Exact dosage is based on weight; total daily dose for initial therapy, 55 mg/kg/day PO divided into four equal doses. For prolonged therapy, may be reduced to 33 mg/kg/day.

Pharmacokinetics

Route	Onset	Peak
Oral	Varies	1–2 hr

Metabolism: Hepatic; $T_{1/2}$: 1–2.5 hr
Distribution: Crosses placenta; enters breast milk
Excretion: Urine

Adverse effects
- **CNS:** *Drowsiness, weakness, headache, dizziness, vertigo,* visual disturbances
- **Dermatologic:** Photosensitivity reactions
- **GI:** *Abdominal pain, nausea, vomiting, diarrhea*
- **Hematologic:** Thrombocytopenia, leukopenia, hemolytic anemia
- **Hypersensitivity:** Rash, pruritus, urticaria, angioedema, eosinophilia, arthralgia

Interactions
✳ **Drug-drug** • Increased risk of bleeding if given with oral anticoagulants
✳ **Drug-lab test** • False-positive urinary glucose results when using Benedict's reagent, Fehling's reagent, *Clinitest* tablets • False elevations of urinary 17-keto and ketogenic steroids when assay uses m-dinitrobenzene

■ Nursing considerations
Assessment
- **History:** Allergy to nalidixic acid, seizures, epilepsy, G6PD deficiency, renal or liver dysfunction, cerebral arteriosclerosis, pregnancy, lactation
- **Physical:** Skin color, lesions; joints; orientation, reflexes; CBC, liver and renal function tests

Interventions
- Arrange for culture and sensitivity tests.
- Give with food if GI upset occurs.
- Obtain periodic blood counts, renal and liver function tests during prolonged therapy.
- Encourage patient to implement nondrug measures to help fight UTIs— avoid bubble baths, void after intercourse, avoid alkaline ash foods, use proper hygiene, increase fluid intake.
- Monitor clinical response; if no improvement is seen or a relapse occurs, send urine for repeat culture and sensitivity.

Teaching points
- Take drug with food. Complete the full course of therapy to ensure resolution of the infection.
- These side effects may occur: nausea, vomiting, abdominal pain (small, frequent meals may help); diarrhea; sensitivity to sunlight (wear protective clothing, and use sunscreen); drowsiness, blurring of vision, dizziness (observe caution if driving or using dangerous equipment).

- Report severe rash, visual changes, weakness, tremors, severe headaches, seizures, changes in behavior.

▽nalmefene hydrochloride

(nal' me feen)

Revex

PREGNANCY CATEGORY B

Drug class
Narcotic antagonist

Therapeutic actions
Pure opiate antagonist; prevents or blocks the effects of opioids, including respiratory depression, sedation, and hypotension.

Indications
- Complete or partial reversal of opioid drug effects, including respiratory depression, induced by either natural or synthetic opioids
- Management of known or suspected opioid overdose

Contraindications and cautions
- Contraindicated with allergy to narcotic antagonists, pregnancy.
- Use cautiously with narcotic addiction (may produce withdrawal), liver or renal impairment, lactation.

Available forms
Injection—100 mcg/mL (blue label), 1 mg/mL (green label)

Dosages
Adults
Titrate dose to reverse the undesired effects of opioids; once reversal has been achieved, no further administration is required.

- *Postoperative use:* Use 100 mcg/mL strength (blue label) 0.25 mcg/kg IV, repeat at 2- to 5-min intervals until reversal is achieved, then stop administration:

Body Weight (kg)	Nalmefene (mL of 100 mcg/mL solution)
50	0.125
60	0.15
70	0.175
80	0.2
90	0.225
100	0.25

- *Management of known or suspected overdose:* Use 1 mg/mL strength (green label); initial dose of 0.5 mg/70 kg of body weight IV; if needed, a second dose of 1 mg/70 kg of body weight IV is given 2–5 min later; maximum effective dose is 1.5 mg/70 kg.
- *Suspected opioid dependency:* Challenge dose of 0.1 mg/70 kg of body weight IV; if no evidence of withdrawal within 2 min, proceed as above.
- *Loss of IV access:* Single 1-mg dose IM or SC should be effective within 5–15 min.

Pediatric patients
Safety has not been established in patients < 18 years.

Geriatric patients or patients with renal impairment
Slowly administer incremental doses over 60 sec to minimize side effects.

Pharmacokinetics

Route	Onset	Peak
IV	Immediate	15 min
SC, IM	5–15 min	1–3 hr

Metabolism: Hepatic; $T_{1/2}$: 10.8 hr
Distribution: Crosses placenta; enters breast milk
Excretion: Urine

▽IV facts
Preparation: No further preparation is required; ensure that correct concentration is being used for indication: blue label—postoperative reversal; green label—overdose.
Infusion: Inject initial dose directly into line of running IV over 15–30 sec or directly into vein in emergency situations; titrate subsequent doses based on patient response.

Adverse effects in *Italics* are most common; those in **Bold** are life-threatening.

Adverse effects
- **CNS:** *Difficulty sleeping, anxiety, nervousness, headache, low energy,* increased energy, irritability, dizziness
- **CV:** Hypertension, hypotension, arrhythmias
- **GI:** Hepatocellular injury, *abdominal pain or cramps, nausea, vomiting,* loss of appetite, diarrhea, constipation
- **Other:** *Chills,* fever, pharyngitis, pruritus

■ Nursing considerations
Assessment
- **History:** Allergy to narcotic antagonists, pregnancy, narcotic addiction, liver or renal impairment, lactation
- **Physical:** Sweating; skin lesions, color; reflexes, affect, orientation, muscle strength; P, BP, edema, baseline ECG, renal and liver function tests

Interventions
- Administer challenge test in situations of suspected or known opioid dependency.
- Check vial carefully to ensure use of correct concentration for indication: blue label—postoperative reversal of effects; green label—overdose.
- Monitor patient carefully during treatment; discontinue drug as soon as reversal is achieved.
- The effects of the drug may continue for several days because of the long half-life of nalmefene.
- Do not use opioid drugs for analgesia, cough and cold; do not use opioid antidiarrheal preparations; patient will not have a response to these drugs for an extended period of time—use a nonopioid preparation if possible.

Teaching points
- This drug blocks the effects of narcotics and other opiates.
- These side effects may occur for several days: drowsiness, dizziness, blurred vision, anxiety (avoid driving or operating dangerous machinery); nausea, vomiting; headache.
- Report unusual bleeding or bruising; dark, tarry stools; yellowing of eyes or skin; dizziness; headache; palpitations.

▽ **naloxone hydrochloride**
*(nal **ox'** one)*

Narcan

PREGNANCY CATEGORY B

Drug classes
Narcotic antagonist
Diagnostic agent

Therapeutic actions
Pure narcotic antagonist; reverses the effects of opioids, including respiratory depression, sedation, hypotension; can reverse the psychotomimetic and dysphoric effects of narcotic agonist-antagonists, such as pentazocine.

Indications
- Complete or partial reversal of narcotic depression, including respiratory depression induced by opioids, including natural and synthetic narcotics, propoxyphene, methadone, nalbuphine, butorphanol, pentazocine
- Diagnosis of suspected acute opioid overdose
- Unlabeled uses: improvement of circulation in refractory shock, reversal of alcoholic coma, dementia of Alzheimer or schizophrenic type

Contraindications and cautions
- Contraindicated with allergy to narcotic antagonists.
- Use cautiously with narcotic addiction, CV disorders, pregnancy, lactation.

Available forms
Injection—0.4, 1 mg/mL, neonatal injection—0.02 mg/mL

Dosages
IV administration is recommended in emergencies when rapid onset of action is required.
Adults
- *Narcotic overdose:* Initial dose of 0.4–2 mg, IV. Additional doses may be repeated at 2- to 3-min intervals. If no response after 10 mg, question the diagnosis. IM or SC routes may be used if IV route is unavailable.
- *Postoperative narcotic depression:* Titrate dose to patient's response. Initial dose of 0.1–0.2 mg IV at 2- to 3-min intervals un-

N

til desired degree of reversal. Repeat doses may be needed within 1- to 2-hr intervals, depending on amount and type of narcotic. Supplemental IM doses produce a longer-lasting effect.

Pediatric patients

- *Narcotic overdose:* Initial dose is 0.01 mg/kg IV. Subsequent dose of 0.1 mg/kg may be administered if needed. May be given IM or SC in divided doses.
- *Postoperative narcotic depression:* For the initial reversal of respiratory depression, inject in increments of 0.005–0.01 mg IV at 2- to 3-min intervals to the desired degree of reversal.

Neonates

- *Narcotic-induced depression:* Initial dose of 0.01 mg/kg IV, SC, IM. May be repeated as indicated in the adult guidelines.

Pharmacokinetics

Route	Onset	Duration
IV	2 min	4–6 hr
IM, SC	3–5 min	4–6 hr

Metabolism: Hepatic; $T_{1/2}$: 30–81 min
Distribution: Crosses placenta; enters breast milk
Excretion: Urine

▼ IV facts

Preparation: Dilute in normal saline or 5% dextrose solutions for IV infusions. The addition of 2 mg in 500 mL of solution provides a concentration of 0.004 mg/mL; titrate rate by response. Use diluted mixture within 24 hr. After that time, discard any remaining solution.
Infusion: Inject directly, or titrate rate of infusion based on response.
Incompatibilities: Do not mix naloxone with preparations containing bisulfite, metabisulfite, high molecular weight anions, alkaline pH solutions.

Adverse effects

- **Acute narcotic abstinence syndrome:** *Nausea, vomiting, sweating, tachycardia, increased BP, tremulousness*
- **CNS:** Reversal of analgesia and excitement (postoperative use)
- **CV:** *Hypotension, hypertension,* ventricular tachycardia and **fibrillation, pulmonary edema** (postoperative use)

■ Nursing considerations
Assessment

- **History:** Allergy to narcotic antagonists; narcotic addiction; CV disorders; lactation
- **Physical:** Sweating; reflexes, pupil size; P, BP; R, adventitious sounds

Interventions

- Monitor patient continuously after use of naloxone; repeat doses may be necessary, depending on duration of narcotic and time of last dose.
- Maintain open airway and provide artificial ventilation, cardiac massage, vasopressor agents if needed to counteract acute narcotic overdose.

Teaching points

- Report sweating, feelings of tremulousness.

naltrexone hydrochloride
*(nal **trex**' one)*

Depade, ReVia, Trexan (CAN)

PREGNANCY CATEGORY C

Drug class
Narcotic antagonist

Therapeutic actions
Pure opiate antagonist; markedly attenuates or completely, reversibly blocks the subjective effects of IV opioids, including those with mixed narcotic agonist-antagonist properties.

Indications

- Adjunct to treatment of alcohol or narcotic dependence as part of a comprehensive treatment program
- Unlabeled uses: treatment of postconcussional syndrome unresponsive to other treatments; eating disorders

---

Adverse effects in *Italics* are most common; those in **Bold** are life-threatening.

Contraindications and cautions

- Contraindicated with allergy to narcotic antagonists, pregnancy, acute hepatitis, liver failure.
- Use cautiously with narcotic addiction (may produce withdrawal symptoms; do not administer unless patient has been opioid free for 7–10 days); opioid withdrawal; lactation; depression, suicidal tendencies.

Available forms

Tablets—50 mg

Dosages
Adults

Give naloxone challenge before use except in patients showing clinical signs of opioid withdrawal.

IV

Draw 2 ampules of naloxone, 2 mL (0.8 mg) into a syringe. Inject 0.5 mL (0.2 mg). Leave needle in vein, and observe for 30 sec. If no signs of withdrawal occur, inject remaining 1.5 mL (0.6 mg), and observe for 20 min for signs and symptoms of withdrawal (stuffiness or running nose, tearing, yawning, sweating, tremor, vomiting, piloerection, feeling of temperature change, joint or bone and muscle pain, abdominal cramps, skin crawling).

SC

Administer 2 mL (0.8 mg), and observe for signs and symptoms of withdrawal for 45 min. If any of the signs and symptoms of withdrawal occur or if there is any doubt that the patient is opioid free, do not administer naltrexone. Confirmatory rechallenge can be done within 24 hr. Inject 4 mL IV, and observe for signs and symptoms of withdrawal. Repeat until no signs and symptoms are seen and patient is no longer at risk.

- *Naltrexone maintenance (alcoholism):* 50 mg/day PO.
- *Narcotic dependence:* Initial dose of 25 mg PO. Observe for 1 hr; if no signs or symptoms are seen, complete dose with 25 mg. Usual maintenance dose is 50 mg/24 hr PO. Flexible dosing schedule can be used with 100 mg every other day or 150 mg every third day, and so forth.

Pediatric patients

Safety has not been established in patients < 18 yr.

Pharmacokinetics

Route	Onset	Peak	Duration
Oral	15–30 min	60 min	24–72 hr

Metabolism: Hepatic; $T_{1/2}$: 3.9–12.9 hr
Distribution: Crosses placenta; enters breast milk
Excretion: Urine

Adverse effects

- **CNS:** *Difficulty sleeping, anxiety, nervousness, headache, low energy,* increased energy, irritability, dizziness, blurred vision, burning, light sensitivity
- **CV:** Phlebitis, edema, increased BP, nonspecific ECG changes
- **Dermatologic:** *Rash,* itching, oily skin, pruritus, acne
- **GI: Hepatocellular injury,** *abdominal pain/cramps, nausea, vomiting,* loss of appetite, diarrhea, constipation
- **GU:** *Delayed ejaculation, decreased potency,* increased frequency of or discomfort with voiding
- **Respiratory:** Nasal congestion, rhinorrhea, sneezing, sore throat, excess mucus or phlegm, sinus trouble, epistaxis
- **Other:** *Chills, increased thirst,* increased appetite, weight change, yawning, swollen glands, *joint and muscle pain*

Interactions

＊ Drug-drug • Decreased effectiveness of opioid analgesics or other opioid-containing preparations

■ Nursing considerations
Assessment

- **History:** Allergy to narcotic antagonists; narcotic addiction; opioid withdrawal; acute hepatitis, liver failure; lactation; depression, suicidal tendencies
- **Physical:** Sweating; skin lesions, color; reflexes, affect, orientation, muscle strength; P, BP, edema, baseline ECG; R, adventitious sounds; liver evaluation; urine screen for opioids, liver function tests

Interventions

- Do not use until patient has been opioid free for 7–10 days; check urine opioid levels.
- Do not administer until patient has passed a naloxone challenge.

N

- Initiate treatment slowly, and monitor until patient has been given naltrexone in the full daily dose with no signs and symptoms of withdrawal.
- Obtain periodic liver function tests during therapy; discontinue therapy at sign of increasing liver dysfunction.
- Do not use opioid drugs for analgesia, cough, and cold; do not use opioid antidiarrheal preparations; patient will not respond; use a nonopioid preparation.
- Ensure that patient is actively participating in a comprehensive treatment program.

Teaching points

- This drug will help facilitate abstinence from alcohol.
- This drug blocks the effects of narcotics and other opiates.
- Wear a medical ID tag to alert emergency medical personnel that you are taking this drug.
- Small doses of heroin or other opiate drugs will not have an effect. Self-administration of large doses of heroin or other narcotics can overcome the blockade effect but may cause death, serious injury, or coma.
- These side effects may occur: drowsiness, dizziness, blurred vision, anxiety (avoid driving or operating dangerous machinery); diarrhea, nausea, vomiting; decreased sexual function.
- Report unusual bleeding or bruising; dark, tarry stools; yellowing of eyes or skin; running nose; tearing; sweating; chills; joint or muscle pain.

▽nandrolone decanoate

(*nan' droe lone*)

Deca-Durabolin, Kabolin (CAN)

PREGNANCY CATEGORY X

C-III CONTROLLED SUBSTANCE

Drug classes

Anabolic steroid
Hormone

Therapeutic actions

Testosterone analogue; promotes body tissue–building processes and reverses catabolic or tissue-depleting processes; increases Hgb and red cell mass.

Indications

- Management of anemia related to renal insufficiency

Contraindications and cautions

- Known sensitivity to nandrolone or anabolic steroids; prostate or breast cancer in males; benign prostatic hypertrophy; breast cancer (females); pituitary insufficiency; MI (contraindicated because of effects on cholesterol); nephrosis; liver disease; hypercalcemia; pregnancy; lactation.

Available forms

Injection—100, 200 mg/mL

Dosages

Administer by deep IM injection; therapy should be intermittent.
Adults
Women: 50–100 mg/wk IM.
Men: 100–200 mg/wk IM.
Pediatric patients 2–13 yr
25–50 mg IM every 3–4 wk.

Pharmacokinetics

Route	Onset	Peak
IM	Slow	Unknown

Metabolism: Hepatic; $T_{1/2}$: unknown
Distribution: Crosses placenta; enters breast milk
Excretion: Unknown

Adverse effects

- **CNS:** *Excitation, insomnia,* chills, toxic confusion
- **Endocrine:** *Virilization; in prepubertal males,* phallic enlargement, hirsutism, increased skin pigmentation; *in postpubertal males,* inhibition of testicular function, gynecomastia, testicular atrophy, priapism, baldness, epididymitis, change in libido; *in females,* hirsutism, hoarseness, deepening of the voice, clitoral enlargement, menstru-

---

Adverse effects in *Italics* are most common; those in **Bold** are life-threatening.

al irregularities, baldness; decreased glucose tolerance
- **GI:** Hepatotoxicity, peliosis, hepatitis with life-threatening **liver failure** or **intra-abdominal hemorrhage; liver cell tumors,** sometimes malignant, *nausea, vomiting, diarrhea, abdominal fullness, loss of appetite, burning of tongue*
- **GU:** Increased risk of prostatic hypertrophy, carcinoma in geriatric patients
- **Hematologic:** *Blood lipid changes* (increased risk of atherosclerosis); iron-deficiency anemia, hypercalcemia, altered serum cholesterol levels; *retention of sodium, chloride, water,* potassium, phosphates, and calcium
- **Other:** *Acne,* premature closure of the epiphyses

Interactions

✱ **Drug-drug** • Potentiation of oral anticoagulants with anabolic steroids • Decreased need for insulin, oral hypoglycemia agents with anabolic steroids

✱ **Drug-lab test** • Altered glucose tolerance tests • Decrease in thyroid function tests, which may persist for 2–3 wk after stopping therapy • Increased creatinine, creatinine clearance, which may last for 2 wk after therapy

■ Nursing considerations
Assessment

- **History:** Sensitivity to nandrolone or anabolic steroids; prostate or breast cancer in males; benign prostatic hypertrophy; breast cancer in females; pituitary insufficiency; MI; nephrosis; liver disease; hypercalcemia; pregnancy; lactation
- **Physical:** Skin color, texture; hair distribution pattern; affect, orientation; abdominal exam, liver evaluation; serum electrolytes, serum cholesterol levels, glucose tolerance tests, thyroid function tests, long-bone x-ray (in children)

Interventions

- Ensure that patient is not pregnant before administering; advise the use of barrier contraceptives during therapy.
- Inject nandrolone deeply into gluteal muscle.
- Intermittent administration decreases adverse effects.

- Monitor effect on children with long-bone x-rays every 3–6 mo; discontinue drug well before the bone age reaches the norm for the patient's chronologic age.
- Monitor patient for edema; arrange for diuretic therapy.
- Monitor liver function, serum electrolytes, and consult with physician for appropriate corrective measures.
- Measure cholesterol levels periodically in patients with high risk for CAD.
- Monitor diabetic patients closely because glucose tolerance may change; adjustments may be needed in insulin, oral hypoglycemic dosage, and diet.

Teaching points

- This drug can only be given IM; mark calendar indicating days to return for injection.
- These side effects may occur: nausea, vomiting, diarrhea, burning of the tongue (small, frequent meals); body hair growth, baldness, deepening of the voice, decrease in libido, impotence (most effects are reversible); excitation, confusion, insomnia (avoid driving, performing tasks that require alertness); swelling of the ankles, fingers (request medication).
- This drug is associated with severe fetal effects; do not use drug during pregnancy; use of barrier contraceptives is advised.
- Diabetic patients—monitor urine sugar closely because glucose tolerance may change. Report any abnormalities to physician, so corrective action can be taken.
- Report ankle swelling, skin color changes, severe nausea, vomiting, hoarseness, body hair growth, deepening of the voice, acne, menstrual irregularities (women).

▽**naproxen**
*(na **prox'** en)*

naproxen
Apo-Naproxen (CAN), EC-Naprosyn, Naprelan, Naprosyn, Naxen (CAN), Novo-Naprox (CAN)

naproxen sodium
Aleve, Anaprox, Anaprox DS, Apo-Napro-Na (CAN), Synflex (CAN)

PREGNANCY CATEGORY B
(FIRST AND SECOND TRIMESTERS)

PREGNANCY CATEGORY D
(THIRD TRIMESTER)

Drug classes
Nonsteroidal anti-inflammatory drug (NSAID)
Analgesic (non-narcotic)

Therapeutic actions
Analgesic, anti-inflammatory, and antipyretic activities largely related to inhibition of
prostaglandin synthesis; exact mechanisms of
action are not known.

Indications
- Mild to moderate pain
- Treatment of primary dysmenorrhea, rheumatoid arthritis, osteoarthritis, ankylosing
  spondylitis, tendinitis, bursitis, acute gout
- OTC use: temporary relief of minor aches
  and pains associated with the common cold,
  headache, toothache, muscular aches, backache, minor pain of arthritis, pain of menstrual cramps, reduction of fever
- Treatment of juvenile arthritis (naproxen
  only)

Contraindications and cautions
- Contraindicated with allergy to naproxen,
  salicylates, other NSAIDs; pregnancy; lactation.
- Use cautiously with asthma, chronic urticaria, CV dysfunction; hypertension; GI
  bleeding; peptic ulcer; impaired hepatic or
  renal function.

Available forms
Tablets—250, 375, 500 mg; 220, 275, 500 mg
(as naproxen sodium); DR tablets—375,
500 mg; CR tablets—375, 500 mg; suspension—125 mg/5 mL

Dosages
Do not exceed 1,250 mg/day (1,375 mg/day
naproxen sodium).
Adults
- *Rheumatoid arthritis or osteoarthritis,
  ankylosing spondylitis:*

Delayed-release (EC-Naprosyn)
375–500 mg PO bid.
Controlled-release (Naprelan)
750–1,000 mg PO daily.
Naproxen sodium
275–550 mg bid PO. May increase to 1.65 g/day
for a limited period.
- *Acute gout:*
Controlled-release (Naprelan)
1,000–1,500 mg PO daily.
Naproxen sodium
825 mg PO followed by 275 mg q 8 hr until
the attack subsides.
- *Mild to moderate pain:*
Controlled-release (Naprelan)
1,000 mg PO daily.
Naproxen sodium
550 mg PO followed by 275 mg q 6–8 hr.
OTC
200 mg PO q 8–12 hr with a full glass of liq-
uid while symptoms persist. Do not exceed
600 mg in 24 hr.
Pediatric patients
- *Juvenile arthritis:*
Naproxen sodium
Safety and efficacy not established.
OTC
Do not give to children < 12 yr unless under
advice of physician.
Geriatric patients
Do not take > 200 mg q 12 hr PO.

Pharmacokinetics

Drug	Onset	Peak	Duration
Naproxen	1 hr	2–4 hr	≤ 7 hr
Naproxen sodium	1 hr	1–2 hr	≤ 7 hr

Metabolism: Hepatic; $T_{1/2}$: 12–15 hr
Distribution: Crosses placenta; enters breast
milk
Excretion: Urine

Adverse effects
- **CNS:** *Headache, dizziness, somnolence,
  insomnia,* fatigue, tiredness, dizziness, tinnitus, ophthalmic effects
- **Dermatologic:** *Rash,* pruritus, sweating,
  dry mucous membranes, stomatitis
- **GI:** *Nausea, dyspepsia, GI pain,* diarrhea,
  vomiting, *constipation,* flatulence

Adverse effects in *Italics* are most common; those in **Bold** are life-threatening.

- **GU:** Dysuria, renal impairment, including renal failure, interstitial nephritis, hematuria
- **Hematologic:** Bleeding, platelet inhibition with higher doses, neutropenia, eosinophilia, leukopenia, pancytopenia, thrombocytopenia, agranulocytosis, granulocytopenia, aplastic anemia, decreased Hgb or Hct, bone marrow depression, menorrhagia
- **Respiratory:** Dyspnea, hemoptysis, pharyngitis, bronchospasm, rhinitis
- **Other:** Peripheral edema, **anaphylactoid reactions to anaphylactic shock**

Interactions
✻ Drug-drug • Increased serum lithium levels and risk of toxicity with naproxen
✻ Drug-lab test • Falsely increased values for urinary 17-ketogenic steroids; discontinue naproxen therapy for 72 hr before adrenal function tests • Inaccurate measurement of urinary 5-hydroxyindoleacetic acid

■ Nursing considerations
Assessment
- **History:** Allergy to naproxen, salicylates, other NSAIDs; asthma, chronic urticaria, CV dysfunction; hypertension; GI bleeding; peptic ulcer; impaired hepatic or renal function; pregnancy; lactation
- **Physical:** Skin color and lesions; orientation, reflexes, ophthalmologic and audiometric evaluation, peripheral sensation; P, edema; R, adventitious sounds; liver evaluation; CBC, clotting times, renal and liver function tests; serum electrolytes; stool guaiac

Interventions
- Give with food or after meals if GI upset occurs.
- Arrange for periodic ophthalmologic examination during long-term therapy.
- Institute emergency procedures if overdose occurs: gastric lavage, induction of emesis, supportive therapy.

Teaching points
- Take drug with food or meals if GI upset occurs; take only the prescribed dosage.
- Dizziness, drowsiness can occur (avoid driving or the use of dangerous machinery).

- Report sore throat; fever; rash; itching; weight gain; swelling in ankles or fingers; changes in vision; black, tarry stools.

> ## ▽ naratriptan
> *(nar ah **trip'** tan)*
>
> Amerge
>
> **PREGNANCY CATEGORY C**

Drug classes
Antimigraine agent (triptan)
Serotonin selective agonist

Therapeutic actions
Binds to serotonin receptors to cause vascular constrictive effects on cranial blood vessels, causing the relief of migraine in selective patients; migraine is believed to be caused by vasodilation of cranial blood vessels in these patients.

Indications
- Treatment of acute migraine attacks with or without aura

Contraindications and cautions
- Contraindicated with allergy to any triptan, active coronary artery disease, uncontrolled hypertension, cardiovascular or peripheral vascular syndromes, severe renal or hepatic impairment, pregnancy.
- Use cautiously with the elderly; lactation.

Available forms
Tablets—1, 2.5 mg

Dosages
Adults

Single dose of 1 mg PO or 2.5 mg PO; may be repeated in 4 hr if needed. Do not exceed 5 mg/24 hr. Take drug with fluid.
Pediatric patients
Safety and efficacy not established.
Patients with renal or hepatic impairment

Contraindicated with severe renal or hepatic impairment. Start with lowest dose and do not exceed 2.5 mg/24 hr with moderate to mild impairment.

Pharmacokinetics

Route	Onset	Peak
Oral	Slow	2–3 hr

Metabolism: Hepatic; $T_{1/2}$: 6 hr
Distribution: Crosses placenta; passes into breast milk
Excretion: Urine

Adverse effects

- **CNS:** *Dizziness,* headache, anxiety, fatigue, drowsiness, paresthesias, corneal defects
- **CV:** Blood pressure alterations, tightness or pressure in chest
- **Other:** *Neck, throat, or jaw discomfort;* generalized pain

Interactions

✳ **Drug-drug** • Prolonged vasoactive reactions when taken concurrently with ergot-containing drugs • Increased blood levels and prolonged effects if combined with hormonal contraceptives; monitor patient and adjust dosage as appropriate

■ Nursing considerations
Assessment

- **History:** Allergy to any triptan, active coronary artery disease, uncontrolled hypertension, severe renal or hepatic impairment, pregnancy, lactation
- **Physical:** Orientation, reflexes, peripheral sensation; P, BP; renal and liver function tests

Interventions

- Administer to relieve acute migraine, not as a prophylactic measure; administer with food.
- Establish safety measures if CNS, visual disturbances occur.
- Provide appropriate analgesics as needed for pains related to therapy.
- Recommend the use of barrier contraceptives to women of child-bearing age; serious birth defects could occur.
- Provide environmental control as appropriate to help relieve migraine (lighting, temperature, etc).
- Monitor BP of patients with possible coronary artery disease; discontinue naratriptan

at any sign of angina, prolonged high blood pressure, etc.

Teaching points

- Take this drug to relieve migraine; do not use as a means of prevention. Take drug with food.
- Dosage may be repeated in 4 hr if headache returns or has not been relieved. Do not take more than 5 mg in one 24-hr period.
- Be aware that this drug should not be taken during pregnancy; if you suspect that you are pregnant, contact physician and refrain from using drug.
- These side effects may occur: dizziness, drowsiness (avoid driving or the use of dangerous machinery while on this drug); numbness, tingling, feelings of tightness or pressure.
- Maintain any procedures you usually use during a migraine—controlled lighting, noise, etc.
- Contact health care provider immediately if you experience chest pain or pressure that is severe or does not go away.
- Report severe pain or discomfort, visual changes, palpitations, unrelieved headache.

▷ nateglinide
*(nah **teg'** lah nyde)*

Starlix

PREGNANCY CATEGORY C

Drug class
Antidiabetic agent

Therapeutic actions

Closes potassium channels in the beta cells of the pancreas, which causes the opening of calcium channels and a resultant increase in insulin release; highly selective for pancreatic potassium channels with little effect on the vasculature. Glucose-lowering abilities depend on the existence of functioning beta cells in the pancreas.

Indications
- Adjunct to diet and exercise to lower blood glucose in patients with non–insulin-dependent diabetes mellitus (type 2) whose hyperglycemia cannot be managed by diet and exercise alone
- Combination therapy with metformin for glycemic control in those patients who do not receive adequate control with diet and either drug

Contraindications and cautions
- Contraindicated with hypersensitivity to the drug; diabetic ketoacidosis; type 1 diabetes.
- Use cautiously with renal or hepatic impairment, pregnancy, lactation.

Available forms
Tablets—60, 120 mg

Dosages
Adults
120 mg PO tid taken 1–30 min before meals; 60 mg PO tid may be tried if patient is near HbA$_{1c}$ goal.
Pediatric patients
Safety and efficacy not established.

Pharmacokinetics

Route	Onset	Peak	Duration
Oral	Rapid	1 hr	4 hr

Metabolism: Hepatic; T$_{1/2}$: 1.5 hr
Distribution: Crosses placenta and may enter breast milk
Excretion: Feces, urine

Adverse effects
- **CNS:** *Headache,* paresthesias, dizziness
- **Endocrine:** Hypoglycemia (low risk)
- **GI:** Nausea, diarrhea, constipation, vomiting, dyspepsia
- **Respiratory:** *URI,* sinusitis, rhinitis, bronchitis

Interactions
✱ Drug-drug • Increased risk of hypoglycemia if taken with alcohol, salicylates, NSAIDS, beta blockers, MAO inhibitors; monitor patient closely

■ Nursing considerations
Assessment
- **History:** Hypersensitivity to the drug; diabetic ketoacidosis; type 1 diabetes; renal or hepatic impairment; pregnancy; lactation
- **Physical:** Skin color, lesions; T; orientation, reflexes, peripheral sensation; R, adventitious sounds; liver evaluation, bowel sounds; blood glucose, liver and renal function tests

Interventions
- Administer drug three times a day before meals; if a patient skips or adds a meal, the dosage should be skipped or added appropriately.
- Monitor urine or serum glucose levels and HbA$_{1c}$ levels frequently to determine effectiveness of drug and dosage being used.
- Arrange for consult with dietitian to establish weight loss program and dietary control as appropriate.
- Arrange for thorough diabetic teaching program to include disease, dietary control, exercise, signs and symptoms of hypoglycemia and hyperglycemia, avoidance of infection, hygiene.

Teaching points
- Do not discontinue this medication without consulting health care provider.
- Take this drug before meals (3 times a day); if you skip a meal, skip the dosage; if you add a meal, take your dosage before that meal also.
- Monitor urine or blood for glucose and ketones as prescribed.
- Return for regular follow up and monitoring of your response to the drug and possible need for dosage adjustment.
- Continue diet and exercise program established for control of diabetes.
- Know the signs and symptoms of hypoglycemia and hyperglycemia and appropriate treatment as indicated; report the incidence of either to your health care provider.
- You may experience headache, increased upper respiratory infections, nausea with this drug.
- Report fever, sore throat, unusual bleeding or bruising; severe abdominal pain.

▽nedocromil sodium
*(nee **doc'** ro mill)*
Alocril, Mireze (CAN), Tilade

PREGNANCY CATEGORY B

Drug classes
Antiasthmatic agent
Antiallergic agent

Therapeutic actions
Inhibits the mediators of a variety of inflammatory cells, including eosinophils, neutrophils, macrophages, mast cells; decreases the release of histamine and blocks the overall inflammatory reaction.

Indications
- Maintenance therapy in the management of patients with mild to moderate bronchial asthma (aerosol)
- Treatment of itching associated with allergic conjunctivitis (ophthalmic)

Contraindications and cautions
- Allergy to nedocromil or any other ingredients in the preparation; pregnancy; lactation.

Available forms
Aerosol—1.75 mg/actuation; ophthalmic solution—2%

Dosages
Adults and patients > 12 yr
- *Asthma:* 2 inhalations qid at regular intervals to provide 14 mg/day; to lower dose, first reduce to tid inhalations (10.5 mg/day), then after several weeks to bid (7 mg/day).
- *Allergic conjunctivitis:* 1–2 drops in each eye bid.

Pharmacokinetics

Route	Onset	Peak	Duration
Inhalation	Rapid	28 min	10–12 hr

Metabolism: Hepatic; $T_{1/2}$: 3.3 hr
Distribution: Crosses placenta; may enter breast milk
Excretion: Urine

Adverse effects
- **CNS:** Dizziness, *headache,* fatigue, lacrimation
- **GI:** *Nausea,* vomiting, dyspepsia, diarrhea, *unpleasant taste*
- **Respiratory:** *Cough, pharyngitis, rhinitis, URI,* increased sputum, dyspnea, bronchitis

■ Nursing considerations
Assessment
- **History:** Allergy to nedocromil, lactation
- **Physical:** Skin color, lesions; orientation; R, auscultation, patency of nasal passages; abdominal exam, normal output; kidney and liver function tests, urinalysis

Interventions
- Do not use during acute bronchospasm; begin therapy when acute episode has subsided and patient can inhale adequately.
- Continue treatment; nedocromil must be taken continuously, even during periods with no asthmatic attacks; use ophthalmic preparation continually during pollen season.
- Use caution if cough or bronchospasm occurs after inhalation; this may (rarely) preclude continuation of treatment.
- Administer with corticosteroids.

Teaching points
- Take drug at regular intervals, even during periods with no asthmatic attacks. Do not use during acute bronchospasm; use ophthalmic solution continually during pollen season.
- Take the drug according to guidelines in manufacturer's insert; the effect of the drug depends on contact with the lungs; therefore you must follow the manufacturer's directions.
- Do not discontinue drug abruptly except on advice of your health care provider.
- These side effects may occur: dizziness, drowsiness, fatigue (avoid driving or operating dangerous machinery); headache (if severe, request analgesics); coughing, running nose.
- Report coughing, wheezing, dizziness.

Adverse effects in *Italics* are most common; those in **Bold** are life-threatening.

▽ nefazodone hydrochloride
(ne faz' oh don)

Serzone

PREGNANCY CATEGORY C

Drug classes
Antidepressant
Reuptake inhibitor

Therapeutic actions
Acts as an antidepressant by inhibiting CNS neuronal uptake of serotonin and norepinephrine; also thought to antagonize alpha$_1$-adrenergic receptors.

Indications
- Treatment of depression

Contraindications and cautions
- Contraindicated with pregnancy, allergy to nefazodone, active liver disease.
- Use cautiously with CV or cerebrovascular disorders, dehydration, hypovolemia, mania, hypomania, suicidal patients, hepatic cirrhosis, EST, debilitation, lactation.

Available forms
Tablets—50, 100, 150, 200, 250 mg

Dosages
Adults

200 mg/day PO in 2 divided doses; increase at 1-wk intervals in increments of 100–200 mg/day; usual range is 300–600 mg/day. *Switching to or from an MAO inhibitor:* Allow 14 days to elapse between stopping the MAOI and starting nefazodone. Wait at least 7 days after stopping nefazodone before starting MAOI.
Pediatric patients

Not recommended in patients < 18 yr.
Geriatric patients or debilitated patients

Initially 100 mg/day PO in 2 divided doses.

Pharmacokinetics

Route	Onset	Peak
Oral	Slow	1 hr

Metabolism: Hepatic; T$_{1/2}$: 2–4 hr

Distribution: Crosses placenta; passes into breast milk
Excretion: Urine and feces

Adverse effects
- **CNS:** *Headache, nervousness, insomnia, drowsiness, anxiety, tremor, dizziness, light-headedness,* agitation, sedation, abnormal gait, confusion
- **CV:** *Orthostatic hypotension*
- **Dermatologic:** *Sweating, rash, pruritus,* acne, alopecia, contact dermatitis
- **GI:** *Nausea, vomiting, diarrhea, dry mouth, anorexia, dyspepsia, constipation, taste changes,* flatulence, gastroenteritis, dysphagia, gingivitis

Interactions
✳ Drug-drug • Increased risk of severe toxic effects with MAOIs, carbamazepine; avoid these combinations • Risk of serious effects if combined with triazolam, alprazolam; decrease dose of triazolam or alprazolam by 75%; avoid this combination with the elderly • Risk of prolonged QTc interval and potential for serious arrhythmias if combined with cisapride, pimozide; avoid this combination • Risk of increased depression with general anesthetics • Risk of serotonin syndrome with sibutramine, trazodone; avoid combining these drugs

✳ Drug-alternative therapy • Increased sedative-hypnotic effects may occur with St. John's wort

■ Nursing considerations
Assessment
- **History:** Pregnancy, CV or cerebrovascular disorders, dehydration, hypovolemia, mania, hypomania, suicidal patients, hepatic cirrhosis, EST, debilitation, lactation, pregnancy
- **Physical:** Weight, T, skin rash, lesions; reflexes, affect; bowel sounds, liver evaluation; P, BP, peripheral perfusion; urinary output, renal function; renal and liver function tests

Interventions
- Give lower doses or less frequently in the elderly or debilitated.
- Monitor patient closely for signs of liver dysfunction; discontinue drug and consult prescriber.

N

- Establish suicide precautions for severely depressed patients. Limit number of capsules dispensed.
- Ensure that patient is well hydrated while on this therapy; monitor for orthostatic hypotension.
- Recommend the use of barrier contraceptives while patient is on this drug.
- Ensure at least 14 days elapse between discontinuing MAO inhibitor and starting nefazodone; at least 7 days between stopping nefazodone and starting MAO inhibitor.

Teaching points

- Take this drug exactly as prescribed; do not increase dosage or combine with other drugs without consulting prescriber; several weeks may be needed to see full effects.
- These side effects may occur: dizziness, drowsiness, nervousness, insomnia (avoid driving or performing hazardous tasks, change positions slowly, take care in conditions of extremes of temperature); nausea, vomiting, weight loss (small, frequent meals; if weight loss becomes marked, consult with your health care provider).
- Avoid pregnancy while on this drug; use of barrier contraceptives is advised.
- Report changes in stool or urine; chest pain, dizziness, vision changes, malaise, anorexia, yellowing of skin or eyes, GI complaints.

▽nelfinavir mesylate
(nell fin' a veer)

Viracept

PREGNANCY CATEGORY B

Drug class
Antiviral

Therapeutic actions
Inhibitor of the HIV-1 protease; prevents viral cleavage resulting in the production of immature, non-infectious virus. Though no controlled trials of the effectiveness of nelfinavir exist, studies may indicate effectiveness in combination with nucleoside analogs.

Indications
- Treatment of HIV infection when antiretroviral therapy is warranted in combination with nucleoside analogs or other antiretroviral agents

Contraindications and cautions
- Contraindicated with life-threatening allergy to any component.
- Use cautiously with renal and hepatic impairment, hemophilia, pregnancy, lactation.

Available forms
Tablets—250 mg; powder—50 mg/g

Dosages
Adults and patients > 13 yr
750 mg PO tid or 1,250 mg PO bid in combination with nucleoside analogs.
Pediatric patients ≤ 13 yr
2–13 yr: 20–30 mg/kg/dose PO tid.
< 2 yr: Not recommended.

Pharmacokinetics

Route	Onset	Peak
Oral	Slow	2–4 hr

Metabolism: Hepatic; T$_{1/2}$: 3.5–5 hr
Distribution: May cross placenta; may pass into breast milk
Excretion: Feces

Adverse effects
- **CNS:** Anxiety, depression, insomnia, myalgia, dizziness, paresthesias, **seizures,** suicide ideation
- **Dermatologic:** Dermatitis, folliculitis, fungal dermatitis, rash, sweating, urticaria
- **GI:** *Diarrhea, nausea, GI pain,* anorexia, vomiting, dyspepsia, liver enzyme elevations
- **Respiratory:** Dyspnea, pharyngitis, rhinitis, sinusitis
- **Other:** Eye disorders, sexual dysfunction

Interactions
✳ Drug-drug • Decreased effectiveness with rifabutin, phenobarbital, phenytoin, dexamethasone, carbamazepine • Risk of severe toxic effects and life-threatening arrhythmias with rifampin, triazolam, midazolam; avoid these combinations • Possible loss of effectiveness

---

Adverse effects in *Italics* are most common; those in **Bold** are life-threatening.

of hormonal contraceptives with nelfinavir; recommend use of barrier contraceptives

✻ **Drug–food** • Decreased metabolism and risk of toxic effects if combined with grapefruit juice; avoid this combination

✻ **Drug-alternative therapy** • Decreased effectiveness of nelfinavir if combined with St. John's wort

■ Nursing considerations

CLINICAL ALERT!
Name confusion has occurred between Viracept (nelfinavir) and Viramune (nevirapine); use caution.

Assessment

- **History:** Life-threatening allergy to any component, impaired hepatic or renal function, pregnancy, lactation, hemophilia
- **Physical:** T; affect, reflexes, peripheral sensation; R, adventitious sounds; bowel sounds, liver evaluation; liver and renal function tests

Interventions

- Administer with meals or a light snack; powder may be mixed with a small amount of non-acidic food or beverage; use within 6 hr of mixing.
- Monitor patient for signs of opportunistic infections that will need to be treated appropriately.
- Administer the drug concurrently with nucleoside analogs.
- Arrange for loperamide to control diarrhea if it occurs.
- Recommend the use of barrier contraceptives while on this drug.

Teaching points

- Take drug exactly as prescribed; take missed doses as soon as possible and return to normal schedule; do not double up skipped doses.
- Take with meals or a light snack; do not drink grapefruit juice while on this drug.
- Powder may be mixed with water, milk, or formula; use within 6 hr of mixing; take in combination with nucleoside analogs.
- These drugs are not a cure for AIDS or ARC; opportunistic infections may occur and reg-

ular medical care should be sought to deal with the disease.

- The long-term effects of this drug are not yet known.
- These side effects may occur: nausea, loss of appetite, diarrhea (eat small, frequent meals; medication is available to control diarrhea); dizziness, loss of feeling (take appropriate precautions).
- This drug combination does not reduce the risk of transmission of HIV to others by sexual contact or blood contamination; use appropriate precautions.
- Use barrier contraceptives; this drug may block the effectiveness of hormonal contraceptives.
- Report extreme fatigue, lethargy, severe headache, severe nausea, vomiting, difficulty breathing, rash, changes in color of urine or stool.

▽neomycin sulfate
*(nee o **mye'** sin)*

Systemic: Mycifradin, Neo-fradin, Neo-Tabs

Topical dermatologic preparations: Mycifradin (CAN), Myciguent

PREGNANCY CATEGORY D

Drug class
Aminoglycoside

Therapeutic actions
Bactericidal: inhibits protein synthesis in susceptible strains of gram-negative bacteria; functional integrity of bacterial cell membrane appears to be disrupted, causing cell death. Due to poor PO absorption, oral neomycin is used to suppress GI bacterial flora.

Indications
- Preoperative suppression of GI bacterial flora (oral)
- Hepatic coma to reduce ammonia-forming bacteria in the GI tract (oral)
- Infection prophylaxis in minor skin wounds and treatment of superficial skin infections due to susceptible organisms (topical dermatologic preparations)

Contraindications and cautions

- Contraindicated with allergy to aminoglycosides, intestinal obstruction, pregnancy, lactation.
- Use cautiously with the elderly or with any patient with diminished hearing, decreased renal function, dehydration, neuromuscular disorders (myasthenia gravis, parkinsonism, infant botulism).

Available forms

Tablets—500 mg; oral solution—125 mg/5 mL; ointment, cream—0.5% (0.35% neomycin)

Dosages
Adults
Oral
Preoperative preparation for elective colorectal surgery: see manufacturer's recommendations for a complex 3-day regimen that includes oral erythromycin, magnesium sulfate, enemas, and dietary restrictions.

- *Hepatic coma:* 4–12 g/day in divided doses for 5–6 days, as adjunct to protein-free diet and supportive therapy, including transfusions, as needed.

Topical dermatologic
Apply to affected area one to five times daily, except burns affecting more than 20% of the body surface should be treated once daily.

Pediatric patients
Oral
- *Hepatic coma:* 50–100 mg/kg/day in divided doses for 5–6 days, as adjunct to protein-free diet and supportive therapy including transfusions, as needed.

Geriatric patients or patients with renal failure
Reduce dosage and carefully monitor serum drug levels and renal function tests throughout treatment. If this is not possible, reduce frequency of administration.

Pharmacokinetics

Route	Onset	Peak
Oral	Varies	1–4 hr
Topical	Generally no systemic absorption	

Metabolism: $T_{1/2}$: 3 hr

Distribution: Crosses placenta; enters breast milk
Excretion: Feces and urine

Adverse effects

While limited absorption occurs across the intact GI mucosa, the risk of absorption from ulcerated area requires consideration of all side effects with oral and parenteral therapy. These side effects also should be considered with dermatologic applications to ulcerated, burned skin or large skin areas where absorption is possible.

- **CNS:** Ototoxicity—*tinnitus, dizziness,* vertigo, deafness (partially reversible to irreversible), vestibular paralysis, confusion, disorientation, depression, lethargy, nystagmus, visual disturbances, headache, *numbness, tingling,* tremor, paresthesias, muscle twitching, **seizures**
- **CV:** Palpitations, hypotension, hypertension
- **GI:** Hepatic toxicity, *nausea, vomiting, anorexia,* weight loss, stomatitis, increased salivation
- **GU: Nephrotoxicity**
- **Hematologic:** *Leukemoid reaction,* agranulocytosis, granulocytosis, leukopenia, leukocytosis, thrombocytopenia, eosinophilia, pancytopenia, anemia, hemolytic anemia, increased or decreased reticulocyte count, electrolyte disturbances
- **Hypersensitivity:** Hypersensitivity reactions: *purpura, rash,* urticaria, exfoliative dermatitis, itching
- **Local:** *Pain, irritation*
- **Other:** Fever, apnea, splenomegaly, joint pain, *superinfection*

Interactions

✴ **Drug-drug** • Increased ototoxic, nephrotoxic, neurotoxic effects with other aminoglycosides, potent diuretics • Increased neuromuscular blockade and muscular paralysis with anesthetics, nondepolarizing neuromuscular blocking drugs, succinylcholine, citrate-anticoagulated blood • Potential inactivation of both drugs if mixed with beta-lactam–type antibiotics • Increased bactericidal effect with penicillins, cephalosporins, carbenicillin, ticarcillin • Decreased absorption and therapeutic effects of digoxin

---

Adverse effects in *Italics* are most common; those in **Bold** are life-threatening.

✳ **Drug-lab test** • Falsely low serum aminoglycoside levels with penicillin or cephalosporin therapy; these antibiotics can inactivate aminoglycosides after the blood sample is drawn

■ **Nursing considerations**
Assessment
- **History:** Allergy to aminoglycosides; intestinal obstruction, diminished hearing, decreased renal function, dehydration, neuromuscular disorders; pregnancy, lactation
- **Physical:** Renal function, eighth cranial nerve function, state of hydration, CBC, skin color and lesions, orientation and affect, reflexes, bilateral grip strength, body weight, bowel sounds

Interventions
- Ensure that the patient is well hydrated.

Teaching points
- Report hearing changes, dizziness, severe diarrhea.

▷**neostigmine methylsulfate**
(nee oh stig' meen)

PMS-Neostigmine Methylsulfate (CAN), Prostigmin

PREGNANCY CATEGORY C

Drug classes
Cholinesterase inhibitors
Parasympathomimetic
Urinary tract agent
Antimyasthenic agent
Antidote

Therapeutic actions
Increases the concentration of acetylcholine at the sites of cholinergic transmission, and prolongs and exaggerates the effects of acetylcholine by reversibly inhibiting the enzyme acetylcholinesterase, causing parasympathomimetic effects and facilitating transmission at the skeletal neuromuscular junction; also has direct cholinomimetic activity on skeletal muscle; may have direct cholinomimetic activity on neurons in autonomic ganglia and the CNS.

Indications
- Prevention and treatment of postoperative distention and urinary retention
- Symptomatic control of myasthenia gravis
- Diagnosis of myasthenia gravis (edrophonium preferred)
- Antidote for nondepolarizing neuromuscular junction blockers (tubocurarine) after surgery

Contraindications and cautions
- Contraindicated with hypersensitivity to anticholinesterases; adverse reactions to bromides (neostigmine bromide); intestinal or urogenital tract obstruction, peritonitis; pregnancy (may stimulate uterus and induce premature labor); lactation.
- Use cautiously with asthma, peptic ulcer, bradycardia, cardiac arrhythmias, recent coronary occlusion, vagotonia, hyperthyroidism, epilepsy.

Available forms
Tablets—15 mg; injection—1:1,000 (1 mg/mL), 1:2,000 (0.5 mg/mL), 1:4,000 (0.25 mg/mL)

Dosages
Adults
- *Prevention of postoperative distention and urinary retention:* 1 mL of the 1:4,000 solution (0.25 mg) neostigmine methylsulfate SC or IM as soon as possible after operation. Repeat q 4–6 hr for 2–3 days.
- *Treatment of postoperative distention:* 1 mL of the 1:2,000 solution (0.5 mg) neostigmine methylsulfate SC or IM, as required.
- *Treatment of urinary retention:* 1 mL of the 1:2,000 solution (0.5 mg) neostigmine methylsulfate SC or IM. If urination does not occur within 1 hr, catheterize the patient. After the bladder is emptied, continue 0.5 mg injections q 3 hr for at least 5 injections.
- *Symptomatic control of myasthenia gravis:* 1 mL of the 1:2,000 solution (0.5 mg) SC or IM. Individualize subsequent doses.
- *Diagnosis of myasthenia gravis:* 0.022 mg/kg IM.
- *Antidote for nondepolarizing neuromuscular blockers:* Give atropine sulfate 0.6–1.2 mg IV several min before slow IV injection of neostigmine 0.5–2 mg. Repeat as re-

quired. Total dose should usually not exceed 5 mg.

Pediatric patients

- *Prevention, treatment of postoperative distention and urinary retention:* Safety and efficacy not established.
- *Symptomatic control of myasthenia gravis:* 0.01–0.04 mg/kg per dose IM, IV, or SC q 2–3 hr as needed.
- *Diagnosis of myasthenia gravis:* 0.04 mg/kg IM.
- *As antidote for nondepolarizing neuromuscular blocker:* Give 0.008–0.025 mg/kg atropine sulfate IV several min before slow IV injection of neostigmine 0.025–0.08 mg/kg.

Pharmacokinetics

Route	Onset	Peak	Duration
SC, IM	20–30 min	20–30 min	2.5–4 hr
IV	10–30 min	20–30 min	2.5–4 hr

Metabolism: Hepatic; $T_{1/2}$: 47–60 min
Distribution: May cross placenta or enter breast milk
Excretion: Urine

▽ IV facts

Preparation: No further preparation is required.
Infusion: Inject slowly directly into vein or into tubing of running IV, each 0.5 mg over 1 min.

Adverse effects

- **CNS:** Convulsions, dysarthria, dysphonia, drowsiness, dizziness, headache, loss of consciousness
- **CV:** *Cardiac arrhythmias,* **cardiac arrest,** decreased cardiac output leading to hypotension, syncope
- **Dermatologic:** Diaphoresis, flushing, rash, urticaria, anaphylaxis
- **EENT:** *Lacrimation, miosis,* spasm of accommodation, diplopia, conjunctival hyperemia
- **GI:** *Salivation, dysphagia, nausea, vomiting, increased peristalsis, abdominal cramps,* flatulence, diarrhea
- **GU:** *Urinary frequency and incontinence,* urinary urgency
- **Local:** Thrombophlebitis after IV use

- **Peripheral:** Skeletal muscle weakness, fasciculations, muscle cramps, arthralgia
- **Respiratory:** *Increased pharyngeal and tracheobronchial secretions,* laryngospasm, bronchospasm, bronchiolar constriction, dyspnea, respiratory muscle paralysis, central respiratory paralysis

Interactions

✱ **Drug-drug** • Decreased neuromuscular blockade of succinylcholine • Decreased effects and possible muscular depression with corticosteroids

■ Nursing considerations

Assessment

- **History:** Hypersensitivity to anticholinesterases; adverse reactions to bromides; intestinal or urogenital tract obstruction, peritonitis; asthma, peptic ulcer, cardiac arrhythmias, recent coronary occlusion, vagotonia, hyperthyroidism, epilepsy; lactation, pregnancy
- **Physical:** Skin color, texture, lesions; reflexes, bilateral grip strength; P, auscultation, BP; R, adventitious sounds; salivation, bowel sounds, normal output; frequency, voiding pattern, normal output; EEG, thyroid tests

Interventions

- Administer IV slowly.
- Overdose with anticholinesterase drugs can cause muscle weakness (cholinergic crisis) that is difficult to differentiate from myasthenic weakness. The administration of atropine may mask the parasympathetic effects of anticholinesterase overdose and further confound the diagnosis.
- Maintain atropine sulfate on standby as an antidote and antagonist in case of cholinergic crisis or hypersensitivity reaction.
- Discontinue drug, and consult physician if excessive salivation, emesis, frequent urination, or diarrhea occurs.
- Decrease dosage if excessive sweating, nausea occur.

Teaching points

- Take this drug exactly as prescribed; patient and a significant other should receive extensive teaching about the effects of the drug,

---

Adverse effects in *Italics* are most common; those in **Bold** are life-threatening.

the signs and symptoms of myasthenia gravis, the fact that muscle weakness may be related both to drug overdose and to exacerbation of the disease, and that it is important to report muscle weakness promptly to the nurse or physician so that proper evaluation can be made.

- These side effects may occur: blurred vision, difficulty with far vision, difficulty with dark adaptation (use caution while driving, especially at night, or performing hazardous tasks in reduced light); increased urinary frequency, abdominal cramps; sweating (avoid hot or excessively humid environments).
- Report muscle weakness, nausea, vomiting, diarrhea, severe abdominal pain, excessive sweating, excessive salivation, frequent urination, urinary urgency, irregular heartbeat, difficulty breathing.

▽nesiritide (hBNP)
(neb sir' ah tide)

Natrecor

PREGNANCY CATEGORY C

Drug classes
Human B-type natriuretic peptide
Vasodilator

Therapeutic actions
A form of the natural peptide produced in human ventricles—human natriuretic peptide—produced by recombinant DNA technology. Binds to vascular smooth muscle and endothelial cells causing smooth muscle relaxation and dilation of veins and arteries. This dilation results in a decrease in pulmonary capillary wedge pressure (PCWP), decrease in systemic arterial pressure, and a diuretic effect.

Indications
- Intravenous treatment of patients with acutely decompensated congestive heart failure who have dyspnea at rest or with minimal activity

Contraindications and cautions
- Contraindicated with allergy to any components of the drug, with low cardiac filling pressure, and as a primary therapy for cardiogenic shock.
- Use cautiously with restrictive or obstructive cardiomyopathy, constrictive pericarditis, pericardial tamponade, renal dysfunction, hypotension, pregnancy, and lactation.

Available forms
Injection—1.58 mg, single-use vials

Dosages
Adults
IV bolus of 2 mcg/kg followed by a continuous infusion at a rate of 0.01 mcg/kg/min; use for longer than 48 hr has not been studied.
Pediatric patients
Safety and efficacy not established.

Pharmacokinetics

Route	Onset	Peak
IV	Immediate	15 min

Metabolism: Tissue; $T_{1/2}$: 18 min
Distribution: May cross placenta; may enter breast milk
Excretion: Urine

▽IV facts
Preparation: Reconstitute one vial by adding 5 mL of diluent removed from a pre-filled 250-mL plastic IV bag containing 5% dextrose injection, 0.9% sodium chloride injection, 5% dextrose, and 0.45% sodium chloride, or 5% dextrose and 0.2% sodium chloride injection; do not shake vial, but rock gently to ensure complete reconstitution. Use only a clear, colorless solution. Withdraw reconstituted solution and add to 250-mL bag, giving a concentration of 6 mcg/mL. Invert bag several times to mix. Use within 24 hr.
Infusion: Prime IV tubing with 25 mL prior to connecting to patient. Withdraw bolus volume from the infusion bag and infuse over 60 sec. Immediately follow with constant infusion at a flow rate of 0.1 mL/kg/hr, which will deliver a dose of 0.01 mcg/kg/min.
Incompatibilities: Do not mix with any other drug solution. Always administer via a separate line. Physically incompatible with heparin, insulin, ethacrynate sodium, bumetanide, enalaprilat, hydralazine, furosemide.

Adverse effects
- **CNS:** *Headache,* dizziness, insomnia, anxiety
- **CV:** *Hypotension,* ventricular tachycardia, angina, bradycardia
- **GI:** *Nausea,* vomiting
- **Other:** *Abdominal pain, back pain*

Interactions
✳ Drug-drug • Increased risk of hypotension if given with other drugs that decrease blood pressure (ACE inhibitors, possibly nitrate vasodilators)

■ Nursing considerations
Assessment
- **History:** Presence of allergy to known components of the drug; cardiovascular disorders; renal dysfunction, pregnancy, lactation
- **Physical:** P, BP, R, ECG, skin color, perfusion, PCW pressure, urinary output, renal function tests

Interventions
- Monitor ECG, blood pressure, PAW pressure continually during administration and for several hours after finishing infusion.
- Monitor urinary output and assess patient for hydration status.
- Arrange to discontinue drug if serious hypotension occurs; if drug is to be restarted, omit the bolus dose and start drug at 30% dose and slowly titrate.
- Ensure that reconstituted solution is replaced every 24 hr.
- Provide small, frequent meals if GI upset occurs.
- Arrange for nutritional consult if nausea and vomiting are persistent.

Teaching points
- This drug must be given by continuous IV infusion; you will be closely monitored during the infusion and for several hours afterward.
- These side effects may occur: headache (an analgesic may be ordered for you); nausea, vomiting (small, frequent meals may help); low blood pressure (this will be closely monitored).

- Report chest pain, changes in vision, dizziness, palpitations.

▷ netilmicin sulfate
*(ne til **mye'** sin)*

Netromycin

PREGNANCY CATEGORY D

Drug classes
Aminoglycoside
Antibiotic

Therapeutic actions
Bactericidal: inhibits protein synthesis in strains of gram-negative bacteria; mechanism of lethal action not fully understood, but functional integrity of cell membrane appears to be disrupted, leading to cell death.

Indications
- Short-term treatment of serious infections caused by susceptible strains of *E. coli, Klebsiella pneumoniae, Pseudomonas aeruginosa, Enterobacter* species, *Proteus mirabilis,* indole-positive *Proteus* species, *Serratia, Citrobacter* species, *Staphylococcus aureus*
- Treatment of staphylococcal infections when other antibiotics are ineffective or contraindicated
- Treatment of staphylococcal infections or infections of which the cause is unknown, before antibiotic susceptibility studies can be completed (often given in conjunction with a penicillin or cephalosporin)

Contraindications and cautions
- Contraindicated with allergy to aminoglycosides, intestinal obstruction (oral), lactation.
- Use cautiously with the elderly or any patient with diminished hearing, decreased renal function, dehydration, neuromuscular disorders (myasthenia gravis, parkinsonism, infant botulism); pregnancy.

Available forms
Injection—100 mg/mL IM or IV

Adverse effects in *Italics* are most common; those in **Bold** are life-threatening.

Dosages
IV and IM dosages are the same.
Adults
- *Complicated UTIs:* 1.5–2 mg/kg q 12 hr.
- *Systemic infections:* 1.3–2.2 mg/kg q 8 hr or 2–3.25 mg/kg q 12 hr.
Pediatric patients
Neonates: 2–3.25 mg/kg q 12 hr.
6 wk–12 yr: 1.8–2.7 mg/kg q 8 hr or 2.7–4 mg/kg q 12 hr.
Geriatric patients or patients with renal failure
Reduce dosage, and carefully monitor serum drug levels and renal function tests throughout treatment. Manufacturer suggests three ways to adjust dosage based on serum creatinine or creatinine clearance; see package insert.

Pharmacokinetics

Route	Onset	Peak
IM	Rapid	30–60 min
IV	Immediate	End of infusion

Metabolism: Hepatic; $T_{1/2}$: 2–2.5 hr
Distribution: Crosses placenta; enters breast milk
Excretion: Urine

▼IV facts
Preparation: Dilute with 50–200 mL of solution. Stable when stored in glass in concentrations of 2.1–3 mg/mL for up to 72 hr at room temperature or refrigerated. Discard after that time.
Infusion: Infuse over 30 min–2 hr.
Compatibilities: Compatible with sterile water for injection; 0.9% sodium chloride injection alone or with 5% dextrose; 5% or 10% dextrose injection in water; 5% dextrose with electrolyte 48 or 75; Ringer's and lactated Ringer's; lactated Ringer's and 5% dextrose injection; *Plasma-Lyte 56 or 148* injection with 5% dextrose; 10% *Travert with Electrolyte 2 or 3* injection; *Isolyte E, M, or P* with 5% dextrose injection; *10% Dextran 40* or *6% Dextran 75 in 5% Dextrose* injection; *Plasma-Lyte M* injection with 5% dextrose; *Ionosol B in D_5W; Normosol-R; Plasma-Lyte 148* injection; 10% fructose injection; *Electrolyte 3* with 10% invert sugar injection; *Normosol-M or R in D_5W, Isolyte H or S* with 5% dextrose;

Isolyte S; Plasma-Lyte 148 injection in water; *Normosol-R pH 7.4.*
Incompatibilities: Do not mix in solution with other drugs.
Y-site incompatibilities: Do not give with furosemide, heparin.

Adverse effects
- **CNS:** Ototoxicity—*tinnitus, dizziness,* vertigo, deafness (partially reversible to irreversible), vestibular paralysis, confusion, disorientation, depression, lethargy, nystagmus, visual disturbances, headache, *numbness, tingling,* tremor, paresthesias, muscle twitching, convulsions, muscular weakness, neuromuscular blockade
- **CV:** Palpitations, hypotension, hypertension
- **GI:** Hepatic toxicity, *nausea, vomiting, anorexia,* weight loss, stomatitis
- **GU:** *Nephrotoxicity*
- **Hematologic:** *Leukemoid reaction,* agranulocytosis, granulocytosis, leukopenia, leukocytosis, thrombocytopenia, eosinophilia, pancytopenia, anemia, hemolytic anemia, changed reticulocyte count, electrolyte disturbances
- **Hypersensitivity:** *Purpura, rash,* urticaria, exfoliative dermatitis, itching
- **Local:** *Pain, irritation, arachnoiditis at IM injection sites*
- **Other:** Fever, apnea, splenomegaly, joint pain, *superinfections*

Interactions
✷ Drug-drug • Increased ototoxic, nephrotoxic, neurotoxic effects with other aminoglycosides, potent diuretics • Increased neuromuscular blockade and muscular paralysis with anesthetics, nondepolarizing neuromuscular blocking drugs, succinylcholine, citrate-anticoagulated blood • Potential inactivation of both drugs if mixed with beta-lactam–type antibiotics. Increased bactericidal effect with penicillins, cephalopsorins, carbenicillin, ticarcillin

■ Nursing considerations
Assessment
- **History:** Allergy to aminoglycosides; intestinal obstruction (oral); pregnancy; lactation; diminished hearing; decreased renal function, dehydration, neuromuscular disorders

- **Physical:** Weight, renal function, eighth cranial nerve function, state of hydration, hepatic function, CBC, skin color and lesions, orientation and affect, reflexes, bilateral grip strength, bowel sounds

Interventions
- Arrange culture and sensitivity tests of infection before beginning therapy.
- Limit duration of treatment to short term to reduce the risk of toxicity; usual duration of treatment is 7–14 days.
- Give IM dose by deep IM injection.
- Ensure that patient is well hydrated before and during therapy.

Teaching points
- These side effects may occur: nausea, loss of appetite (small, frequent meals may help); diarrhea; superinfections in mouth, vagina (request treatment).
- Report any hearing changes, dizziness, lesions in mouth, vaginal itching.

▽ **nevirapine**
(neh veer' ah pine)

Viramune

PREGNANCY CATEGORY C

Drug class
Antiviral

Therapeutic actions
Antiretroviral activity; binds directly to HIV-1 reverse transcriptase and blocks the replication of HIV by changing the structure of the HIV enzyme.

Indications
- Treatment of HIV-1–infected patients who have experienced clinical or immunologic deterioration; used in combination with nucleoside analogues

Contraindications and cautions
- Contraindicated with allergy to nevirapine; pregnancy, lactation.

- Use cautiously with renal or hepatic impairment, rash.

Available forms
Tablets—200 mg; oral suspension—50 mg/5 mL

Dosages
Adults
200 mg PO daily for 14 days; if no rash appears, then 200 mg PO bid.
Pediatric patients
2 mo–8 yr: 4 mg/kg PO daily for 14 days, then 7 mg/kg PO bid.
≥ 8 yr: 4 mg/kg PO daily for 14 days, then 4 mg/kg PO bid.

Pharmacokinetics

Route	Onset	Peak
Oral	Rapid	4 hr

Metabolism: Hepatic; $T_{1/2}$: 45 hr, then 25–30 hr
Distribution: Crosses placenta; passes into breast milk
Excretion: Urine

Adverse effects
- **CNS:** *Headache*
- **Dermatologic: Rash**
- **GI:** *Nausea, vomiting, diarrhea,* dry mouth, **liver dysfunction**
- **Other:** Infection, chills, fever

Interactions
✳ **Drug-drug** • Avoid concurrent use with protease inhibitors, hormonal contraceptives (metabolism is increased and effectiveness decreased) • Decreased ketoconazole levels and effects; avoid this combination
✳ **Drug-alternative therapy** • Decreased effectiveness if combined with St. John's wort

■ Nursing considerations

 CLINICAL ALERT!
Name confusion has occurred between Viramune (nevirapine) and Viracept (nelfinavir); use caution.

Assessment

- **History:** Allergy to nevirapine; renal or hepatic dysfunction, pregnancy, lactation, rash
- **Physical:** T; orientation, reflexes; peripheral perfusion; urinary output; skin color, perfusion, hydration; hepatic and renal function tests

Interventions

- Monitor renal and hepatic function tests before and during treatment. Discontinue drug at any sign of hepatic dysfunction.
- Do not administer if severe rash occurs, especially accompanied by fever, blistering, lesion, swelling, general malaise; discontinue if rash recurs on rechallenge.
- Shake suspension gently before use. Rinse oral dosing cup and administer rinse to patient.

Teaching points

- Take this drug exactly as prescribed; do not double up missed doses.
- Use some method of barrier birth control (not hormonal contraceptives) while on this medication. Severe birth defects can occur, and this drug causes loss of effectiveness of hormonal contraceptives.
- This drug does not cure HIV infection. Follow routine preventive measures and continue any other medication that has been prescribed.
- These side effects may occur: nausea, vomiting, loss of appetite, diarrhea, headache, fever.
- Report rash, any lesions or blistering, changes in color of stool or urine, fever, muscle or joint pain.

▽**niacin**

(nye' ah sin)

Niacor, Niaspan

PREGNANCY CATEGORY C

Drug classes

Antihyperlipidemic
Vitamin

Therapeutic actions

May partially inhibit the release of free fatty acids from adipose tissue and increase lipoprotein activity, which could increase the rate of triglyceride removal from plasma; these actions reduce the total LDL and triglycerides and increase HDL. Niacin also decreases serum levels of apo B and lipoprotein A.

Indications

- Adjunct to diet for treatment of adults with very high serum triglyceride levels (types IV and V hyperlipidemia) who present a risk of pancreatitis and who do not respond adequately to dietary control

Contraindications and cautions

- Contraindicated with hepatic dysfunction, active peptic ulcer disease, arterial bleeding, lactation.
- Use cautiously with history of jaundice, hepatobiliary disease, peptic ulcer, high alcohol consumption, renal dysfunction, unstable angina, gout, recent surgery, pregnancy.

Available forms

ER tablets—500, 750, 1,000 mg; tablet—500 mg

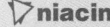

Dosages
Adults and patients > 16 yr
ER tablets

500 mg PO q hs for 1–4 wk, then 1,000 mg PO q hs during weeks 5–8. If response is not adequate, may continue to adjust by increasing 500 mg each 4 wk to a maximum 2,000 mg/day.
Tablets
Start at 250 mg PO at the evening meal, may increase at 4- to 7-day intervals to a dose of 1.5–2 g/day PO in divided doses; do not exceed 6 g/day.
Pediatric patients < 16 yr
Safety and efficacy not established.

Pharmacokinetics

Route	Onset	Peak
Oral	Rapid	45 min

Metabolism: Hepatic; $T_{1/2}$: unknown
Distribution: Crosses placenta, enters breast milk
Excretion: Urine

Adverse effects
- **CNS:** *Headache,* anxiety
- **CV:** Arrhythmias, hypotension
- **Dermatologic:** *Flushing,* acanthosis nigricans, dry skin
- **GI:** *GI upset,* peptic ulcer, abnormal liver function tests
- **Hematologic:** Hyperuricemia
- **Other:** Glucose intolerance

Interactions
✳ Drug-drug• Increased risk of rhabdomyolysis with HMG-CoA inhibitors • Increased effectiveness of antihypertensives, vasoactive drugs • Increased risk of bleeding with anticoagulants; monitor PT and platelet counts and adjust dose accordingly • Decreased absorption with bile acid sequestrants; separate doses by at least 4–6 hr

■ Nursing considerations
Assessment
- **History:** Hepatic dysfunction, active peptic ulcer disease, arterial bleeding, lactation, hepatobiliary disease, peptic ulcer; high alcohol consumption, renal dysfunction, unstable angina, gout, recent surgery, pregnancy
- **Physical:** Skin lesions, color, temperature; orientation, affect, reflexes; P, auscultation, baseline ECG, BP; liver evaluation; lipid studies, liver function tests

Interventions
- Administer drug at bedtime to minimize effects of flushing if using ER forms; give *Niacor* with meals.
- Administer bile sequestrants at least 4–6 hr apart from niacin.
- Consult with dietitian regarding low-cholesterol diets.
- Arrange for regular follow-up during long-term therapy.

Teaching points
- Take drug at bedtime (ER) or with meals (*Niacor*). The dose will change each week until the desired response is achieved.
- Take your bile acid sequestrant (if appropriate) 4–6 hr apart from niacin; avoid alcohol while on this drug.

- These side effects may occur: nausea, heartburn, loss of appetite (eat small, frequent meals); headache (may lessen over time; if bothersome, consult with your nurse or physician); rash, flushing (take drug at bedtime).
- Report unusual bleeding or bruising, palpitations, fainting, rash, fever.

▷ nicardipine hydrochloride
*(nye **kar**' de peen)*

Cardene, Cardene IV, Cardene SR

PREGNANCY CATEGORY C

Drug classes
Calcium channel-blocker
Antianginal agent
Antihypertensive

Therapeutic actions
Inhibits the movement of calcium ions across the membranes of cardiac and arterial muscle cells; calcium is involved in the generation of the action potential in specialized automatic and conducting cells in the heart, in arterial smooth muscle, and in excitation-contraction coupling in cardiac muscle cells. Inhibition of calcium flow results in the depression of impulse formation in specialized cardiac pacemaker cells, in slowing of the velocity of conduction of the cardiac impulse, in the depression of myocardial contractility, and in the dilation of coronary arteries and arterioles and peripheral arterioles; these effects lead to decreased cardiac work, decreased cardiac energy consumption, and increased delivery of oxygen to myocardial cells.

Indications
- Chronic stable (effort-associated) angina. Use alone or with beta-blockers (immediate release only)
- Management of essential hypertension alone or with other antihypertensives (immediate release and sustained release)
- Short-term treatment of hypertension when oral use is not feasible (IV)

Adverse effects in *Italics* are most common; those in **Bold** are life-threatening.

Contraindications and cautions

- Contraindicated with allergy to nicardipine, pregnancy, lactation.
- Use cautiously with impaired hepatic or renal function, sick sinus syndrome, heart block (second- or third-degree).

Available forms

Capsules—20, 30 mg; SR capsules—30, 45, 60 mg; injection—2.5 mg/mL

Dosages
Adults

- *Angina:* Immediate release only. Individualize dosage. Usual initial dose is 20 mg tid PO. Range 20–40 mg tid PO. Allow at least 3 days before increasing dosage to ensure steady-state plasma levels.
- *Hypertension:* Immediate release. *Initial dose:* 20 mg tid PO. Range 20–40 mg tid. The maximum BP-lowering effect occurs in 1–2 hr. Adjust dosage based on BP response, allow at least 3 days before increasing dosage. *IV:* 0.5–2.2 mg/hr; regulate by patient response; switch to oral drug as soon as possible. *Sustained-release:* Initial dose is 30 mg bid PO. *Range:* 30–60 mg bid.

Pediatric patients
Safety and efficacy not established.

Geriatric patients or patients with renal or hepatic impairment

- *Renal impairment:* Adjust dose beginning with 20 mg tid PO (immediate release) or 30 mg bid PO (sustained release).
- *Hepatic impairment:* Starting dose 20 mg bid PO (immediate-release) with individual adjustment.

Pharmacokinetics

Route	Onset	Peak
Oral	20 min	0.5–2 hr

Metabolism: Hepatic; $T_{1/2}$: 2–4 hr
Distribution: Crosses placenta; enters breast milk
Excretion: Urine

▼ IV facts

Preparation: Dilute each ampule with 240 mL of solution; store at room temperature; protect from light; stable for 24 hr.
Infusion: Slow IV infusion, 0.5–2.2 mg/hr based on patient response.

Compatibilities: Compatible with dextrose 5% injection, dextrose 5% and sodium chloride 0.45% or 0.9% injection; dextrose 5% with potassium; 0.45% or 0.9% sodium chloride.
Incompatibilities: Do not mix with 5% sodium bicarbonate or lactated Ringer's.

Adverse effects

- **CNS:** *Dizziness, light-headedness, headache, asthenia,* fatigue
- **CV:** *Peripheral edema, angina,* hypotension, arrhythmias, *bradycardia, AV block,* asystole
- **Dermatologic:** *Flushing,* rash
- **GI:** *Nausea,* hepatic injury

Interactions

✳ Drug-drug • Increased serum levels and toxicity of cyclosporine

■ Nursing considerations
Assessment

- **History:** Allergy to nicardipine, impaired hepatic or renal function, sick sinus syndrome, heart block (second or third degree), pregnancy, lactation
- **Physical:** Skin lesions, color, edema; P, BP, baseline ECG, peripheral perfusion, auscultation; R, adventitious sounds; liver evaluation, normal GI output; liver and renal function tests, urinalysis

Interventions

- Monitor patient carefully (BP, cardiac rhythm, and output) while drug is being titrated to therapeutic dose; dosage may be increased more rapidly in hospitalized patients under close supervision.
- Monitor BP very carefully with concurrent doses of nitrates.
- Monitor cardiac rhythm regularly during stabilization of dosage and long-term therapy.
- Provide small, frequent meals if GI upset occurs.

Teaching points

- These side effects may occur: nausea, vomiting (small, frequent meals may help); headache (monitor lighting, noise, and temperature; request medication if severe).
- Report irregular heart beat, shortness of breath, swelling of the hands or feet, pronounced dizziness, constipation.

▽nicotine
(*nik' oh teen*)

Habitrol, Nicoderm, Nicoderm CQ, Nicotrol, Nicotrol NS

PREGNANCY CATEGORY X

Drug class
Smoking deterrent

Therapeutic actions
Nicotine acts at nicotinic receptors in the peripheral and CNS; produces behavioral stimulation and depression, cardiac acceleration, peripheral vasoconstriction, and elevated BP.

Indications
- Temporary aid to the cigarette smoker seeking to give up smoking while in a behavioral modification program under medical supervision
- Unlabeled use: improvement of symptoms of Tourette's syndrome

Contraindications and cautions
- Contraindicated with allergy to nicotine; nonsmokers; post-MI period; arrhythmias; angina pectoris; pregnancy; lactation.
- Use cautiously with hyperthyroidism, pheochromocytoma, type 2 diabetes (releases catecholamines from the adrenal medulla); hypertension, peptic ulcer disease.

Available forms
Transdermal system—7, 14, 21 mg/day (*Habitrol*); 15 mg/16 hr (*Nicotrol*); nasal spray— 0.5 mg/actuation

Dosages
Adults
Topical
Apply system, 5–21 mg, once every 24 hr. Dosage is based on response and stage of withdrawal. *Habitrol, Nicoderm:* 21 mg/day for first 6 wk; 14 mg/day for next 2 wk; 7 mg/day for next 2 wk. *Nicotrol:* 15 mg/day for 6 wk.
Nasal spray
1 spray in each nostril as needed—one to two doses each hour, up to 40 doses/day.

Pediatric patients
Safety and efficacy in children and adolescents who smoke have not been established.

Pharmacokinetics

Route	Onset	Peak	Duration
Dermal	1–2 hr	4–6 min	4–24 hr
Nasal	Rapid	15 min	NA

Metabolism: Hepatic; $T_{1/2}$: 1–4 hr
Distribution: Crosses placenta; enters breast milk
Excretion: Urine

Adverse effects
- **CNS:** *Headache, insomnia,* abnormal dreams, dizziness, light-headedness, sweating
- **GI:** Diarrhea, constipation, nausea, dyspepsia, abdominal pain, dry mouth
- **Local:** *Erythema, burning, pruritus* at site of patch; local edema
- **Respiratory:** Cough, pharyngitis, sinusitis
- **Other:** Backache, chest pain, asthenia, dysmenorrhea

Interactions
✳ **Drug-drug** • Increased circulating levels of cortisol, catecholamines with nicotine use; smoking dosage of adrenergic agonists, adrenergic blockers may need to be adjusted according to nicotine, smoking status of patient • Smoking increases metabolism and lowers blood levels of caffeine, theophylline, imipramine, pentazocine; decreases effects of furosemide, propranolol • Cessation of smoking may decrease absorption of glutethimide, decrease metabolism of propoxyphene

■ Nursing considerations
Assessment
- **History:** Allergy to nicotine; nonsmoker; post-MI period; arrhythmias; angina pectoris; hyperthyroidism, pheochromocytoma, type II diabetes; hypertension, peptic ulcer disease; pregnancy; lactation
- **Physical:** Orientation, affect; P, auscultation, BP; oral mucous membranes, abdominal exam; thyroid function tests

---

Adverse effects in *Italics* are most common; those in **Bold** are life-threatening.

Interventions

- Protect systems from heat; slight discoloration of system is not significant.
- Apply system to nonhairy, clean, dry skin site on upper body or upper outer arm; use only when the pouch is intact; use immediately after removal from pouch; use each system only once.
- Wash hands thoroughly after application; do not touch eyes.
- Wrap used system in foil pouch of newly applied system; fold over and dispose of immediately to prevent access by pets or children.
- Apply new system after 24 hr; do not reuse same site for at least 1 wk. *Nicotrol:* Apply a new system each day after waking, and remove at bedtime.
- Handle nasal spray carefully; if it comes in contact with skin, flush immediately; dispose of bottle with cap in place.
- Ensure that patient has stopped smoking; if the patient is unable to stop smoking within the first 4 wk of therapy, drug therapy should be stopped.
- Encourage patients who have been unsuccessful at any dose to take a "therapy holiday" before trying again; counseling should explore factors contributing to their failure and other means of success.

Teaching points

- Protect systems from heat; slight discoloration of system is not significant.
- Apply system to nonhairy, clean, dry skin site on upper body or upper outer arm; use only when the pouch is intact; use immediately after removal from pouch; use each system only once.
- Wash hands thoroughly after application; do not touch eyes. Wrap used system in foil pouch of newly applied system; fold over and dispose of immediately to prevent access by pets or children.
- Apply new system after 24 hr; do not reuse same site for at least 1 wk. *Nicotrol:* Apply a new system each day after waking, and remove at bedtime.
- Tilt head back to administer spray; do not sniff, swallow, or inhale while spray is administered. If spray comes in contact with skin, flush immediately; discard bottle with cap in place.

- Abstain from smoking.
- These side effects may occur: dizziness, headache, light-headedness (use caution driving or performing tasks that require alertness); nausea, vomiting, constipation or diarrhea (small, frequent meals, regular mouth care may help); skin redness, swelling at application site (good skin care, switching sites daily may help).
- Report nausea and vomiting, diarrhea, cold sweat, chest pain, palpitations, burning or swelling at application site.

▷nicotine polacrilex (nicotine resin complex)
(nik' oh teen)

Nicorette, Nicorette DS, Nicorette Gum, Nicotrol Inhaler

PREGNANCY CATEGORY X

Drug class
Smoking deterrent

Therapeutic actions
Acts as an agonist at nicotinic receptors in the peripheral and CNS; produces behavioral stimulation and depression, cardiac acceleration, peripheral vasoconstriction, and elevated BP.

Indications
- Temporary aid to the cigarette smoker seeking to give up smoking while in a behavioral modification program under medical supervision

Contraindications and cautions
- Contraindicated with allergy to nicotine or resin used; nonsmoker; post-MI period; arrhythmias; angina pectoris; active TMJ disease; pregnancy; lactation.
- Use cautiously with hyperthyroidism, pheochromocytoma, type 2 diabetes (releases catecholamines from the adrenal medulla); hypertension, peptic ulcer disease.

Available forms
Chewing gum—2 or 4 mg/square; inhaler— 4 mg/actuation

Dosages
Adults
Chewing gum
Have patient chew one piece of gum whenever the urge to smoke occurs. Chew each piece slowly and intermittently for about 30 min to promote even, slow, buccal absorption of nicotine. Patients often require 10 pieces/day during the first month. Do not exceed 24 pieces/day. Therapy may be effective for up to 3 mo; 4–6 mo for complete cessation has been used. Should not be used for longer than 4 mo.
Nasal spray inhaler
1 spray in each nostril, 1–2 doses/hr to a maximum of 5 doses/hr or 40 doses/day. Dosage is individualized; in studies, best results were achieved by continuous frequent puffing over 20 min. Do not use > 6 mo. Patients are treated for 12 wk, then are weaned off the daily dose over next 6–12 wk.
Pediatric patients
Safety and efficacy in children and adolescents who smoke have not been established.

Pharmacokinetics

Route	Onset	Peak
Oral	Slow	15–30 min
Nasal	Immediate	5–10 min

Metabolism: Hepatic; $T_{1/2}$: 30–120 min
Distribution: Crosses placenta; enters breast milk
Excretion: Urine

Adverse effects
- **CNS:** Dizziness, light-headedness
- **GI:** *Mouth or throat soreness; hiccoughs, nausea, vomiting,* nonspecific GI distress, excessive salivation
- **Local:** Mechanical effects of chewing gum—traumatic injury to oral mucosa or teeth, *jaw ache,* eructation secondary to air swallowing

Interactions
* Drug-drug • Increased circulating levels of cortisol, catecholamines with nicotine use, smoking—dosage of adrenergic agonists, adrenergic blockers may need to be adjusted according to nicotine, smoking status of patient • Smoking increases metabolism and lowers blood levels of caffeine, theophylline, imipramine, pentazocine; decreases effects of furosemide, propranolol • Cessation of smoking may decrease absorption of glutethimide, decrease metabolism of propoxyphene

■ Nursing considerations
Assessment
- **History:** Allergy to nicotine or resin used; nonsmoker; post-MI period; arrhythmias; angina pectoris; active TMJ disease; hyperthyroidism, pheochromocytoma, type 2 diabetes; hypertension, peptic ulcer disease; pregnancy; lactation
- **Physical:** Jaw strength, symmetry; orientation, affect; P, auscultation, BP; oral mucous membranes, abdominal exam; thyroid function tests

Interventions
- Review mechanics of chewing gum with patient; patient must chew the gum slowly and intermittently to promote even, slow absorption of nicotine; discard chewed gum in wrapper to prevent access by children or pets.
- Arrange to withdraw or taper use of gum in abstainers at 3 mo; effectiveness after that time has not been established, and patients may be using gum as substitute source for nicotine dependence.

Teaching points
- Chew one piece of gum every time you have the desire to smoke. Chew slowly and intermittently for about 30 min; do not chew more than 24 pieces of gum each day. Discard chewed gum in wrapper to prevent access by children or pets.
- Store reusable mouthpiece for inhaler in plastic case; wash with soap and water. Throw inhaler cartridge away out of reach of children and pets.
- Do not consume liquids within 15 min before or while chewing gum—may interfere with nicotine absorption.
- Abstain from smoking.
- These side effects may occur: dizziness, headache, light-headedness (use caution driving or performing tasks that require alertness); nausea, vomiting, increased burping; jaw muscle ache (modify chewing technique).

- Report nausea and vomiting, increased salivation, diarrhea, cold sweat, headache, disturbances in hearing or vision, chest pain, palpitations.
- Do not offer to nonsmokers; serious reactions can occur if used by nonsmokers.

▽**nifedipine**
(nye fed' i peen)

Adalat, Adalat CC, Adalat XL (CAN), Apo-Nifed (CAN), Gen-Nifedipine (CAN), Nifedical XL, Novo-Nifedin (CAN), Procardia, Procardia XL

PREGNANCY CATEGORY C

Drug classes
Calcium channel-blocker
Antianginal agent
Antihypertensive

Therapeutic actions
Inhibits the movement of calcium ions across the membranes of cardiac and arterial muscle cells; inhibition of transmembrane calcium flow results in the depression of impulse formation in specialized cardiac pacemaker cells, in slowing of the velocity of conduction of the cardiac impulse, in the depression of myocardial contractility, and in the dilation of coronary arteries and arterioles and peripheral arterioles; these effects lead to decreased cardiac work, decreased cardiac energy consumption, and increased delivery of oxygen to myocardial cells.

Indications
- Angina pectoris due to coronary artery spasm (Prinzmetal's variant angina)
- Chronic stable angina (effort-associated angina)
- Treatment of hypertension (sustained-release preparation only)
- Orphan drug use: treatment of interstitial cystitis

Contraindications and cautions
- Contraindicated with allergy to nifedipine; pregnancy.
- Use cautiously with lactation.

Available forms
ER tablets—30, 60, 90 mg; capsules—10, 20 mg

Dosages
Adults
10 mg tid PO initial dose. Maintenance range: 10–20 mg tid. Higher doses (20–30 mg tid–qid) may be required, depending on patient response. Adjust over 7–14 days. More than 180 mg/day is not recommended.
Sustained-release
30–60 mg PO once daily. Adjust over 7–14 days. Usual maximum dose is 90–120 mg/day.

Pharmacokinetics

Route	Onset	Peak
Oral	20 min	30 min
SR	20 min	2.5–6 hr

Metabolism: Hepatic; $T_{1/2}$: 2–5 hr
Distribution: Crosses placenta; enters breast milk
Excretion: Urine and feces

Adverse effects
- **CNS:** *Dizziness, light-headedness, headache, asthenia, fatigue, nervousness,* sleep disturbances, blurred vision
- **CV:** *Peripheral edema, angina,* hypotension, arrhythmias, *AV block,* asystole
- **Dermatologic:** *Flushing, rash,* dermatitis, pruritus, urticaria
- **GI:** *Nausea, diarrhea, constipation,* cramps, flatulence, hepatic injury
- **Other:** *Nasal congestion, cough,* fever, chills, shortness of breath, muscle cramps, joint stiffness, sexual difficulties

Interactions
✳ **Drug-drug** • Increased effects with cimetidine

■ Nursing considerations
Assessment
- **History:** Allergy to nifedipine; pregnancy; lactation
- **Physical:** Skin lesions, color, edema; orientation, reflexes; P, BP, baseline ECG, peripheral perfusion, auscultation; R, adventitious sounds; liver evaluation, normal GI output; liver function tests

N

Interventions

- Monitor patient carefully (BP, cardiac rhythm, and output) while drug is being adjusted to therapeutic dose; the dosage may be increased more rapidly in hospitalized patients under close supervision. Do not exceed 30 mg/dose increases.
- Ensure that patients do not chew or divide sustained-release tablets.
- Taper dosage of beta-blockers before nifedipine therapy.
- Protect drug from light and moisture.

Teaching points

- Do not chew, cut, or crush sustained-release tablets. Swallow whole.
- These side effects may occur: nausea, vomiting (small, frequent meals may help); dizziness, light-headedness, vertigo (avoid driving, operating dangerous machinery; take special precautions to avoid falling); muscle cramps, joint stiffness, sweating, sexual difficulties (reversible).
- Report irregular heartbeat, shortness of breath, swelling of the hands or feet, pronounced dizziness, constipation.

▽nilutamide
*(nah **loo'** ta mide)*

Anandron (CAN), Nilandron

PREGNANCY CATEGORY C

Drug class
Antiandrogen

Therapeutic actions
Nonsteroidal agent; exerts potent antiandrogenic activity by inhibiting androgen uptake or inhibiting nuclear binding of androgen in target tissues.

Indications

- Treatment of metastatic prostatic carcinoma (stage D2) in combination with surgical castration

Contraindications and cautions

- Contraindicated with hypersensitivity to nilutamide or any component of preparation; severe hepatic impairment; severe respiratory insufficiency.
- Use cautiously in patients with impaired liver function; Asian patients (adverse effects more pronounced); pregnancy, lactation.

Available forms
Tablets—50, 150 mg; tablets (CAN)— 50, 100 mg

Dosages
Adults
300 mg PO daily for 30 days beginning day of or day following surgery then 150 mg PO daily thereafter.
Pediatric patients
Safety and efficacy not established.

Pharmacokinetics

Route	Onset	Peak	Duration
Oral	Rapid	Days	Weeks

Metabolism: Hepatic and tissue; $T_{1/2}$: days
Distribution: Crosses placenta; may pass into breast milk
Excretion: Urine

Adverse effects

- **CNS:** Dizziness, headache, insomnia, asthenia, *impaired adaptation to dark or light,* abnormal vision, hyperesthesia
- **CV:** Hypertension, peripheral edema
- **Endocrine:** *Gynecomastia, hot flashes*
- **GI:** *GI upset,* constipation, anorexia
- **GU:** *Impotence, decreased libido,* UTIs, liver failure
- **Hematologic:** Elevated AST, ALT
- **Respiratory: Interstitial pneumonia,** dyspnea
- **Other:** *Flulike syndrome,* pain

Interactions
✳ **Drug-drug** • Antabuse-type reaction with alcohol; avoid this combination • Increased serum levels and risk of toxicity with anticoagulants, phenytoin, theophylline; monitor patient and reduce dosage as needed

---

Adverse effects in *Italics* are most common; those in **Bold** are life-threatening.

■ Nursing considerations
Assessment

- **History:** Hypersensitivity to nilutamide or any component of preparation; severe hepatic impairment, severe respiratory insufficiency; pregnancy, lactation; date of surgical castration
- **Physical:** Skin color, lesions; reflexes, affect, vision exam; urinary output; bowel sounds, liver evaluation; R, adventitious sounds; CBC, Hct, electrolytes, liver function tests, chest x-ray

Interventions

- Arrange for baseline and periodic monitoring of liver function tests during therapy; discontinue drug and notify physician if transaminases exceed 2–3 times normal.
- Monitor for baseline respiratory function, including chest x-ray; discontinue if any sign of interstitial pneumonia occurs.
- Begin drug on the day of or the day after surgical castration; do not interrupt therapy.
- Offer support and encouragement to deal with diagnosis, change in self-concept, and alteration in sexual functioning.

Teaching points

- Take this drug exactly as prescribed. Do not interrupt dosing or stop taking the medication without consulting your health care provider. Note that the dosage will be changed after 30 days of treatment.
- Periodic blood tests will need to be done to monitor the drug effects. It is important that you keep these appointments.
- These side effects may occur: dizziness, drowsiness (avoid driving or performing hazardous tasks); loss of ability to accommodate to light and dark (avoid night driving and take special care in low-light or changing-light situations); impotence, loss of libido (drug effects; consult with your nurse or physician if bothersome or if you desire to talk about them); alcohol intolerance (do not drink alcohol while on this drug; serious reactions could occur).
- Report change in stool or urine color, yellow skin, difficult or painful breathing, cough, chest pain, difficulty voiding.

▽ nimodipine
*(nye **moe'** di peen)*

Nimotop

PREGNANCY CATEGORY C

Drug class
Calcium channel-blocker

Therapeutic actions
Inhibits the movement of calcium ions across the membranes of cardiac and arterial muscle cells; inhibition of transmembrane calcium flow results in the depression of impulse formation in specialized cardiac pacemaker cells, in slowing of the velocity of conduction of the cardiac impulse, in the depression of myocardial contractility, and in the dilation of coronary arteries and arterioles and peripheral arterioles.

Indications

- Improvement of neurologic deficits due to spasm following subarachnoid hemorrhage (SAH) from ruptured congenital intracranial aneurysms in patients who are in good neurologic condition postictus (Hunt and Hess Grades I–III)
- Unlabeled uses: treatment of common and classic migraines and chronic cluster headaches

Contraindications and cautions

- Allergy to nimodipine, impaired hepatic function, pregnancy (teratogenic), lactation.

Available forms
Capsules, liquid—30 mg

Dosages
Adults
Begin therapy within 96 hr of the SAH. 60 mg q 4 hr PO for 21 consecutive days.
Pediatric patients
- *Hepatic impairment:* 30 mg q 4 hr with close monitoring of BP and pulse.

Pharmacokinetics

Route	Onset	Peak
Oral	Unknown	> 60 min

Metabolism: Hepatic; $T_{1/2}$: 1–2 hr
Distribution: Crosses placenta; may enter breast milk
Excretion: Urine, feces

Adverse effects
- **CNS:** Dizziness, light-headedness, *headache*, asthenia, fatigue
- **CV:** Peripheral edema, angina, *hypotension*, **arrhythmias,** bradycardia, AV block, **asystole**
- **Dermatologic:** Flushing, *rash*
- **GI:** *Diarrhea,* nausea, hepatic injury

Interactions
✳ **Drug–food** • Decreased metabolism and increased risk of toxic effects if combined with grapefruit juice; avoid this combination

■ Nursing considerations
Assessment
- **History:** Allergy to nimodipine; impaired hepatic function; pregnancy, lactation
- **Physical:** Skin lesions, color, edema; reflexes, affect, complete neurologic exam; P, BP, baseline ECG, peripheral perfusion, auscultation; R, adventitious sounds; liver evaluation, normal output; liver function tests, urinalysis

Interventions
- Begin therapy within 96 hr of subarachnoid hemorrhage.
- Administer PO. If patient is unable to swallow capsule, make a hole in both ends of the capsule with an 18-gauge needle, and extract the contents into a syringe. Empty the contents into the patient's in-situ nasogastric tube, and wash down the tube with 30 mL of normal saline.
- Monitor neurologic effects closely to determine progress and patient response.

Teaching points
- Take drug for 21 consecutive days.
- Do not drink grapefruit juice while on this drug.
- These side effects may occur: nausea, diarrhea (small, frequent meals may help); headache (monitor lighting, noise, and temperature; request medication if severe).

- Report irregular heart beat, shortness of breath, swelling of the hands or feet, pronounced dizziness, constipation.

▽**nisoldipine**
*(nye **sole'** di peen)*

Sular

PREGNANCY CATEGORY C

Drug classes
Calcium channel-blocker
Antihypertensive

Therapeutic actions
Inhibits the movement of calcium ions across the membranes of cardiac and arterial muscle cells; inhibits transmembrane calcium flow, which results in the depression of impulse formation in specialized cardiac pacemaker cells, slowing of the velocity of conduction of the cardiac impulse, depression of myocardial contractility, and dilation of coronary arteries and arterioles and peripheral arterioles; these effects in turn lead to decreased cardiac work, decreased cardiac energy consumption.

Indications
- Essential hypertension, alone or in combination with other antihypertensives

Contraindications and cautions
- Contraindicated with allergy to nisoldipine, impaired hepatic function, sick sinus syndrome, CHF, heart block (second- or third-degree).
- Use cautiously with MI or severe CAD (increased severity of disease has occurred), lactation.

Available forms
ER tablets—10, 20, 30, 40 mg

Dosages
Adults
Initial dose of 20 mg PO daily; increase in weekly increments of 10 mg/wk until BP control is achieved. Usual maintenance dose is 20–40 mg PO daily. Maximum dose 60 mg/day.

Adverse effects in *Italics* are most common; those in **Bold** are life-threatening.

Pediatric patients
Safety and efficacy not established.
Geriatric patients or patients with hepatic impairment
Monitor BP very carefully. Lower starting doses and lower maintenance doses are recommended.

Pharmacokinetics

Route	Onset	Peak	Duration
Oral	Slow	6–12 hr	24 hr

Metabolism: Hepatic; $T_{1/2}$: 7–12 hr
Distribution: Crosses placenta; may enter breast milk
Excretion: Urine

Adverse effects
- **CNS:** *Dizziness, light-headedness, headache,* asthenia, *fatigue, lethargy*
- **CV:** *Peripheral edema,* arrhythmias, **MI, increased angina**
- **Dermatologic:** *Flushing,* rash
- **GI:** *Nausea,* abdominal discomfort

Interactions
✳ **Drug-drug** • Possible increased serum levels and toxicity of cyclosporine • Possible increased serum levels and toxicity with cimetidine • Increased risk of toxic cardiac effects with quinidine
✳ **Drug-food** • Decreased metabolism and increased risk of toxic effects if combined with grapefruit juice; avoid this combination

■ Nursing considerations
Assessment
- **History:** Allergy to nisoldipine, impaired hepatic function, sick sinus syndrome, heart block (second- or third-degree), lactation, CHF, CAD
- **Physical:** Skin lesions, color, edema; P, BP; baseline ECG, peripheral perfusion, auscultation, R, adventitious sounds; liver evaluation, GI normal output; liver function tests, renal function tests, urinalysis

Interventions
- Monitor patient carefully (BP, cardiac rhythm and output) while drug is being adjusted to therapeutic dose; dosage may be increased

more rapidly in hospitalized patients under close supervision.
- Monitor BP very carefully if patient is on concurrent doses of nitrates or other antihypertensives.
- Monitor cardiac rhythm regularly during stabilization of dosage and periodically during long-term therapy.
- Administer drug without regard to meals.

Teaching points
- Take this drug with meals if upset stomach occurs; do not take with high-fat meals or grapefruit juice. Do not drink grapefruit juice while on this drug.
- Swallow tablet whole; do not chew, cut, or crush.
- These side effects may occur: nausea, vomiting (small, frequent meals may help); headache (monitor lighting, noise, and temperature; request medication if severe).
- Report irregular heart beat, shortness of breath, swelling of the hands or feet, pronounced dizziness, constipation, chest pain.

▽ nitazoxanide
See *Less Commonly Used Drugs,* p. 1348.

▽ nitisinone
See *Less Commonly Used Drugs,* p. 1348.

▽ nitrofurantoin
*(nye troe fyoor **an'** toyn)*

nitrofurantoin
Apo-Nitrofurantoin (CAN),
Furadantin, Novo-Furantoin (CAN)

nitrofurantoin macrocrystals
Macrobid, Macrodantin

PREGNANCY CATEGORY B

Drug classes
Urinary tract anti-infective
Antibacterial

Therapeutic actions

Bacteriostatic in low concentrations, possibly by interfering with bacterial carbohydrate metabolism; bactericidal in high concentrations, possibly by disrupting bacterial cell wall formation, causing cell death.

Indications

- Treatment of UTIs caused by susceptible strains of *E. coli, S. aureus, Klebsiella, Enterobacter, Proteus*
- Prophylaxis or long-term suppression of UTIs

Contraindications and cautions

- Contraindicated with allergy to nitrofurantoin; renal dysfunction; pregnancy, lactation.
- Use cautiously in patients with G6PD deficiency, anemia, diabetes.

Available forms

Capsules—25, 50, 100 mg; ER capsules—100 mg; oral suspension—25 mg/5 mL

Dosages
Adults
50–100 mg PO qid for 10–14 days or 100 mg bid for 7 days (ER capsules). Do not exceed 400 mg/day.
- *Long-term suppressive therapy:* 50–100 mg PO at bedtime.
Pediatric patients
5–7 mg/kg/day in 4 divided doses PO. Not recommended in children < 1 mo.
- *Long-term suppressive therapy:* As low as 1 mg/kg/day PO in 1 to 2 doses.

Pharmacokinetics

Route	Onset	Peak
Oral	Rapid	30 min

Metabolism: Hepatic; $T_{1/2}$: 20–60 min
Distribution: Crosses placenta; enters breast milk
Excretion: Urine

Adverse effects

- **CNS:** Peripheral neuropathy, headache, dizziness, nystagmus, drowsiness, vertigo

- **Dermatologic:** Exfoliative dermatitis, **Stevens-Johnson syndrome,** alopecia, pruritus, urticartia, angioedema
- **GI:** *Nausea, abdominal cramps, vomiting, diarrhea, anorexia,* parotitis, pancreatitis, **hepatotoxicity**
- **Hematologic:** Hemolytic anemia in G6PD deficiency; granulocytopenia, agranulocytosis, leukopenia, thrombocytopenia, eosinophilia, megaloblastic anemia
- **Respiratory: Pulmonary hypersensitivity**
- **Other:** Superinfections of the GU tract; hypotension; muscular aches; *brown-rust urine*

Interactions

✳ **Drug-drug** • Delayed or decreased absorption with magnesium trisilicate, magaldrate

✳ **Drug-lab test** • False elevations of urine glucose, bilirubin, alkaline phosphatase, BUN, urinary creatinine • False-positive urine glucose when using Benedict's or Fehling's reagent

■ Nursing considerations
Assessment

- **History:** Allergy to nitrofurantoin, renal dysfunction, G6PD deficiency, anemia, diabetes, pregnancy, lactation
- **Physical:** Skin color, lesions; orientation, reflexes; R, adventitious sounds; liver evaluation; CBC; liver and kidney function tests; serum electrolytes; blood, urine glucose, urinalysis

Interventions

- Arrange for culture and sensitivity tests before and during therapy.
- Give with food or milk to prevent GI upset.
- Continue drug for at least 3 days after a sterile urine specimen is obtained.
- Monitor clinical response; if no improvement is seen or a relapse occurs, send urine for repeat culture and sensitivity.
- Monitor pulmonary function carefully; reactions can occur within hours or weeks of nitrofurantoin therapy.
- Arrange for periodic CBC and liver function tests during long-term therapy.

Adverse effects in *Italics* are most common; those in **Bold** are life-threatening.

Teaching points

- Take drug with food or milk. Complete the full course of drug therapy to ensure a resolution of the infection. Take this drug at regular intervals around the clock; consult your nurse or pharmacist to set up a convenient schedule.
- These side effects may occur: nausea, vomiting, abdominal pain (small, frequent meals may help); diarrhea; drowsiness, blurring of vision, dizziness (observe caution driving or using dangerous equipment); brown or yellow-rust urine (expected effect).
- Report fever, chills, cough, chest pain, difficulty breathing, rash, numbness or tingling of the fingers or toes.

▽nitroglycerin
(nye troe gli' ser in)

Intravenous: Nitro-Bid IV, Nitroject (CAN), Tridil
Spray: Nitrolingual Pumpspray
Sublingual: NitroQuick, Nitrostat
Sustained-release: Nitroglyn E-R, Nitrong, Nitro-Time
Topical: Nitrobid, Nitrol, Nitrong
Transdermal: Deponit, Minitran, Nitrek, Nitro-Derm, Nitro-Dur, Nitrodisc, Transderm-Nitro
Translingual: Nitrolingual
Transmucosal: Nitrogard

PREGNANCY CATEGORY C

Drug classes
Antianginal agent
Nitrate

Therapeutic actions
Relaxes vascular smooth muscle with a resultant decrease in venous return and decrease in arterial BP, which reduces left ventricular workload and decreases myocardial oxygen consumption.

Indications
- Acute angina: sublingual, translingual preparations
- Prophylaxis of angina: oral sustained release, sublingual, topical, transdermal, translingual, transmucosal preparations
- Angina unresponsive to recommended doses of organic nitrates or beta-blockers (IV preparations)
- Perioperative hypertension (IV preparations)
- CHF associated with acute MI (IV preparations)
- To produce controlled hypertension during surgery (IV preparations)
- Unlabeled uses: reduction of cardiac workload in acute MI and in CHF (sublingual, topical); adjunctive treatment of Raynaud's disease (topical)

Contraindications and cautions
- Contraindicated with allergy to nitrates, severe anemia, early MI, head trauma, cerebral hemorrhage, hypertrophic cardiomyopathy, pregnancy, lactation.
- Use cautiously with hepatic or renal disease, hypotension or hypovolemia, increased intracranial pressure, constrictive pericarditis, pericardial tamponade, low ventricular filling pressure or low PCWP.

Available forms
Injection—0.5, 5 mg/mL; injection solution—25, 50, 100, 200 mg; sublingual tablets—0.3, 0.4, 0.6 mg; translingual spray—0.4 mg/spray; transmucosal tablets—1, 2, 3 mg; transmucosal SR tablets—1, 2, 2.5, 3, 5 mg; oral SR capsules—2.5, 6.5, 9 mg; transdermal—0.1, 0.2, 0.3, 0.4, 0.6, 0.8 mg/hr; topical ointment—2%

Dosages
Adults
IV
- *Initial dose:* 5 mcg/min delivered through an infusion pump. Increase by 5-mcg/min increments every 3–5 min as needed. If no response at 20 mcg/min, increase increments to 10–20 mcg/min. Once a partial BP response is obtained, reduce dose and lengthen dosage intervals; continually monitor response and titrate carefully.
Sublingual
- *Acute attack:* Dissolve 1 tablet under tongue or in buccal pouch at first sign of anginal attack; repeat every 5 min until relief is obtained. Do not take more than 3 tablets/

15 min. If pain continues or increases, patient should call physician or go to hospital.
- *Prophylaxis:* Use 5–10 min before activities that might precipitate an attack.

Sustained-release (oral)
- *Initial dose:* 2.5–9 mg q 12 hr. Increase to q 8 hr as needed and tolerated. Doses as high as 26 mg given qid have been used.

Topical
- *Initial dose:* One-half inch q 8 hr. Increase by one-half inch to achieve desired results. Usual dose is 1–2 inches q 8 hr; up to 4–5 inches q 4 hr have been used. 1 inch = 15 mg nitroglycerin.

Transdermal
Apply one patch each day. Adjust to higher doses by using patches that deliver more drug or by applying more than one patch. Apply patch to arm; remove at bedtime.

Translingual
Spray preparation delivers 0.4 mg/metered dose. At onset of attack, spray 1–2 metered doses into oral mucosa; no more than 3 doses/15 min should be used. If pain persists, seek medical attention. May be used prophylactically 5–10 min prior to activity that might precipitate an attack.

Transmucosal
1 mg q 3–5 hr during waking hours. Place tablet between lip and gum above incisors, or between cheek and gum.

Pediatric patients
Safety and efficacy not established.

Pharmacokinetics

Route	Onset	Duration
IV	1–2 min	3–5 min
Sublingual	1–3 min	30–60 min
Translingual spray	2 min	30–60 min
Transmucosal tablet	1–2 min	3–5 min
Oral, sustained-release	20–45 min	8–12 hr
Topical ointment	30–60 min	4–8 hr
Transdermal	30–60 min	24 hr

Metabolism: Hepatic; $T_{1/2}$: 1–4 min
Distribution: Crosses placenta; enters breast milk
Excretion: Urine

▼IV facts
Preparations: Dilute in 5% dextrose injection or 0.9% sodium chloride injection. Do not mix with other drugs; check the manufacturer's instructions carefully because products vary considerably in concentration and volume per vial. Use only with glass IV bottles and the administration sets provided. Protect from light and extremes of temperature.
Infusion: Do not give by IV push; regulate rate based on patient response.
Incompatibilities: Do not mix in solution with other drugs.

Adverse effects
- **CNS:** Headache, apprehension, restlessness, weakness, vertigo, dizziness, faintness
- **CV:** Tachycardia, retrosternal discomfort, palpitations, **hypotension,** syncope, collapse, orthostatic hypotension, angina
- **Dermatologic:** Rash, exfoliative dermatitis, cutaneous vasodilation with flushing, pallor, perspiration, cold sweat, contact dermatitis—transdermal preparations, topical allergic reactions—topical nitroglycerin ointment
- **GI:** Nausea, vomiting, incontinence of urine and feces, abdominal pain
- **Local:** Local burning sensation at the point of dissolution (sublingual)
- **Other:** Ethanol intoxication with high-dose IV use (alcohol in diluent)

Interactions
✳ **Drug-drug** • Increased risk of hypertension and decreased antianginal effect with ergot alkaloids • Decreased pharmacologic effects of heparin
✳ **Drug-lab test** • False report of decreased serum cholesterol if done by the Zlatkis-Zak color reaction

■ Nursing considerations
Assessment
- **History:** Allergy to nitrates, severe anemia, early MI, head trauma, cerebral hemorrhage, hypertrophic cardiomyopathy, hepatic or renal disease, hypotension or hypovolemia, increased intracranial pressure, constrictive pericarditis, pericardial tamponade, low ven-

tricular filling pressure or low PCWP, pregnancy, lactation

• **Physical:** Skin color, temperature, lesions; orientation, reflexes, affect; P, BP, orthostatic BP, baseline ECG, peripheral perfusion; R, adventitious sounds; liver evaluation, normal output; liver and renal function tests (IV); CBC, Hgb

Interventions

• Give sublingual preparations under the tongue or in the buccal pouch. Encourage patient not to swallow. Ask patient if the tablet "fizzles" or burns. Always check the expiration date on the bottle; store at room temperature, protected from light. Discard unused drug 6 mo after bottle is opened (conventional tablets); stabilized tablets (*Nitrostat*) are less subject to loss of potency.

• Give sustained-release preparations with water; warn the patient not to chew the tablets or capsules; do not crush these preparations.

• Administer topical ointment by applying the ointment over a 6 x 6 inch area in a thin, uniform layer using the applicator. Cover area with plastic wrap held in place by adhesive tape. Rotate sites of application to decrease the chance of inflammation and sensitization; close tube tightly when finished.

• Administer transdermal systems to skin site free of hair and not subject to much movement. Shave areas that have a lot of hair. Do not apply to distal extremities. Change sites slightly to decrease the chance of local irritation and sensitization. Remove transdermal system before attempting defibrillation or cardioversion.

• Administer transmucosal tablets by placing them between the lip and gum above the incisors or between the cheek and gum. Encourage patient not to swallow and not to chew the tablet.

• Administer the translingual spray directly onto the oral mucosa; preparation is not to be inhaled.

• Arrange to withdraw drug gradually; 4–6 wk is the recommended withdrawal period for the transdermal preparations.

Teaching points

• Place sublingual tablets under your tongue or in your cheek; do not chew or swallow the tablet; the tablet should burn or "fizzle" un-der the tongue. Take the nitroglycerin before chest pain begins, when you anticipate that your activities or situation may precipitate an attack. Do not buy large quantities; this drug does not store well. Keep the drug in a dark, dry place, in a dark-colored glass bottle with a tight lid; do not combine with other drugs. You may repeat your dose every 5 min for a total of 3 tablets. If the pain is still not relieved, go to an emergency room.

• Do not chew or crush the timed-release preparations; take on an empty stomach.

• Spread a thin layer of topical ointment on the skin using the applicator. Do not rub or massage the area. Cover with plastic wrap held in place with adhesive tape. Wash your hands after application. Keep the tube tightly closed. Rotate the sites frequently to prevent local irritation.

• To use transdermal systems, you may need to shave an area for application. Apply to a slightly different area each day. Use care if changing brands; each system has a different concentration.

• Place transmucosal tablets between the lip and gum or between the gum and cheek. Do not chew; try not to swallow.

• Spray translingual spray directly onto oral mucous membranes; do not inhale. Use 5–10 min before activities that you anticipate will precipitate an attack.

• These side effects may occur: dizziness, lightheadedness (may be transient; change positions slowly); headache (lie down in a cool environment and rest; OTC preparations may not help); flushing of the neck or face (transient).

• Report blurred vision, persistent or severe headache, rash, more frequent or more severe angina attacks, fainting.

▽**nitroprusside sodium**
*(nye troe **pruss'** ide)*

Nipride (CAN), Nitropress

PREGNANCY CATEGORY C

Drug classes

Antihypertensive
Vasodilator

Therapeutic actions

Acts directly on vascular smooth muscle to cause vasodilation (arterial and venous) and reduce BP. Mechanism involves interference with calcium influx and intracellular activation of calcium. CV reflexes are not inhibited and reflex tachycardia, increased renin release occur.

Indications

- Hypertensive crises for immediate reduction of BP
- Controlled hypotension during anesthesia to reduce bleeding in surgical procedures
- Acute CHF
- Unlabeled uses: acute MI, with dopamine; left ventricular failure, with O_2, morphine, loop diuretic

Contraindications and cautions

- Contraindicated with treatment of compensatory hypertension; to produce controlled hypotension during surgery with known inadequate cerebral circulation; emergency use in moribund patients.
- Use cautiously with hepatic, renal insufficiency (drug decomposes to cyanide, which is metabolized by the liver and kidneys to thiocyanate ion); hypothyroidism (thiocyanate inhibits the uptake and binding of iodine); pregnancy; lactation.

Available forms

Powder for injection—50 mg/vial

Dosages

Administer only by continuous IV infusion with sterile 5% dextrose in water.

Adults and pediatric patients

In patients not receiving antihypertensive medication, the average dose is 3 mcg/kg/min (range 0.5–10 mcg/kg/min). At this rate, diastolic BP is usually lowered by 30%–40% below pretreatment diastolic levels. Use smaller doses in patients on antihypertensive medication. Do not exceed infusion rate of 10 mcg/kg/min. If this rate of infusion does not reduce BP within 10 min, discontinue administration.

Geriatric patients or patients with renal impairment

Use with caution and in initial low dosage. The elderly may be more sensitive to the hypotensive effects.

Pharmacokinetics

Route	Onset	Duration
IV	1–2 min	1–10 min

Metabolism: Hepatic; $T_{1/2}$: 2 min
Distribution Crosses placenta; may enter breast milk
Excretion: Urine

▽ IV facts

Preparation: Dissolve the contents of the 50-mg vial in 2–3 mL of 5% dextrose in water. Dilute the prepared stock solution in 250–1,000 mL of 5% dextrose in water, and promptly wrap container in aluminum foil or other opaque material to protect from light; the administration set tubing does not need to be covered. Observe solution for color changes. The freshly prepared solution has a faint brown tint; discard it if it is highly colored (blue, green, or dark red). If properly protected from light, reconstituted solution is stable for 24 hr. Do not use the infusion fluid for administration of any other drugs.
Infusion: Infuse slowly to reduce likelihood of adverse effects; use an infusion pump, microdrip regulator, or similar device to allow precise control of flow rate; carefully monitor BP and regulate dose based on response.
Incompatibilities: Do not mix in solution with any other drugs.

Adverse effects

- **CNS:** *Apprehension, headache, restlessness, muscle twitching,* dizziness
- **CV:** *Restrosternal pressure, palpitations,* bradycardia, tachycardia, ECG changes
- **Cyanide toxicity:** Increasing tolerance to drug and metabolic acidosis are early signs, followed by dyspnea, headache, vomiting, dizziness, ataxia, loss of consciousness, imperceptible pulse, absent reflexes, widely dilated pupils, pink skin color, distant heart sounds, shallow breathing (seen in overdose)

Adverse effects in *Italics* are most common; those in **Bold** are life-threatening.

- **Dermatologic:** *Diaphoresis,* flushing
- **Endocrine:** Hypothyroidism
- **GI:** *Nausea, vomiting, abdominal pain*
- **Hematologic:** Methemoglobinemia, antiplatelet effects
- **Local:** Irritation at injection site

■ Nursing considerations
Assessment
- **History:** Hepatic or renal insufficiency, hypothyroidism, pregnancy, lactation
- **Physical:** Reflexes, affect, orientation, pupil size; BP, P, orthostatic BP, supine BP, perfusion, edema, auscultation; R, adventitious sounds; renal, liver, and thyroid function tests, blood acid–base balance

Interventions
- Monitor injection site carefully to prevent extravasation.
- Do not allow BP to drop too rapidly; do not lower systolic BP below 60 mm Hg.
- Provide amyl nitrate inhalation, materials to make 3% sodium nitrite solution, sodium thiosulfate on standby in case overdose of nitroprusside, depletion of patient's body stores of sulfur occur, leading to cyanide toxicity.
- Monitor blood acid–base balance (metabolic acidosis is early sign of cyanide toxicity), serum thiocyanate levels daily during prolonged therapy, especially in patients with renal impairment.

Teaching points
- Anticipate frequent monitoring of BP, blood tests, checks of IV dosage and rate.
- Report pain at injection site, chest pain.

▽nizatidine
(ni za' ti deen)
Apo-Nizatidine (CAN), Axid, Axid AR

PREGNANCY CATEGORY B

Drug class
Histamine$_2$ (H$_2$) antagonist

Therapeutic actions
Inhibits the action of histamine at the histamine H$_2$ receptors of the parietal cells of the stomach, inhibiting basal gastric acid secretion and gastric acid secretion that is stimulated by food, caffeine, insulin, histamine, cholinergic agonists, gastrin, and pentagastrin. Total pepsin output also is reduced.

Indications
- Short-term and maintenance treatment of duodenal ulcer
- Short-term treatment of benign gastric ulcer
- Gastroesophageal reflux disease
- Prevention of heartburn, acid indigestion, and sour stomach brought on by eating (OTC)

Contraindications and cautions
- Contraindicated with allergy to nizatidine, lactation.
- Use cautiously with impaired renal or hepatic function, pregnancy.

Available forms
Capsules—150, 300 mg; OTC tablets—75 mg

Dosages
Adults
- *Active duodenal ulcer:* 300 mg PO daily hs. 150 mg PO bid may be used.
- *Maintenance of healed duodenal ulcer:* 150 mg PO daily hs.
- *GERD:* 150 mg PO bid.
- *Benign gastric ulcer:* 150 mg PO bid or 300 mg daily.
- *Prevention of heartburn, acid indigestion:* 75 mg PO 30–60 min before food or beverages that cause the problem, taken with water.

Pediatric patients
Safety and efficacy not established.

Geriatric patients or patients with renal impairment
Creatinine clearance 20–50 mL/min: 150 mg/day PO for active ulcer; 150 mg every other day for maintenance. Creatinine clearance < 20 mL/min: 150 mg PO every other day for active ulcer; 150 mg PO every 3 days for maintenance.

Pharmacokinetics

Route	Onset	Peak
Oral	Varies	0.5–3 hr

Metabolism: Hepatic; $T_{1/2}$: 1–2 hr
Distribution: Crosses placenta; enters breast milk
Excretion: Urine

Adverse effects

- **CNS:** *Dizziness, somnolence, headache, confusion, hallucinations,* peripheral neuropathy; symptoms of brainstem dysfunction (dysarthria, ataxia, diplopia)
- **CV:** Cardiac arrhythmias, **cardiac arrest**
- **GI:** *Diarrhea,* hepatitis, pancreatitis, hepatic fibrosis
- **Hematologic:** Neutropenia, agranulocytosis, increases in plasma creatinine, serum transaminase
- **Other:** *Impotence,* gynecomastia, rash, arthralgia, myalgia

Interactions

✳ **Drug-drug** • Increased serum salicylate levels with aspirin

✳ **Drug-lab test** • False-positive tests for urobilinogen

■ Nursing considerations
Assessment

- **History:** Allergy to nizatidine, impaired renal or hepatic function, pregnancy, lactation
- **Physical:** Skin lesions; orientation, affect; P, baseline ECG; liver evaluation, abdominal exam, normal output; CBC, liver and renal function tests

Interventions

- Administer drug at bedtime.
- Decrease doses in renal and liver dysfunction.
- Prepare liquid by mixing 150 or 300 mg in apple juice, *Gatorade,* cranberry juice; stable for 48 hr refrigerated or at room temperature.
- Arrange for regular follow-up, including blood tests to evaluate effects.

Teaching points

- Prepare liquid by mixing 150 or 300 mg in apple juice, *Gatorade,* cranberry juice; stable for 48 hr refrigerated or at room temperature.

- Take OTC drug 30–60 min before the food or beverage that causes the problem; take with water.
- Take drug at bedtime. Therapy may continue for 4–6 wk or longer.
- Take antacids exactly as prescribed, being careful of the times of administration. Do not take OTC drugs, and avoid alcohol. Many OTC drugs contain ingredients that might interfere with this drug's effectiveness.
- Tell all physicians, nurses, or dentists that you are taking this drug. Dosage and timing of all your medications must be coordinated. If anything changes the drugs that you are taking, consult with your nurse or physician.
- Have regular medical follow-ups to evaluate drug response.
- Report sore throat, fever, unusual bruising or bleeding, tarry stools, confusion, hallucinations, dizziness, muscle or joint pain.

▽**norepinephrine bitartrate (levarterenol)**
*(nor ep i **nef'** rin)*

Levophed

PREGNANCY CATEGORY C

Drug classes

Sympathomimetic
Alpha-adrenergic agonist
Beta$_1$-adrenergic agonist
Cardiac stimulant
Vasopressor

Therapeutic actions

Vasopressor and cardiac stimulant; effects are mediated by alpha$_1$- or beta$_1$-adrenergic receptors in target organs; potent vasoconstrictor (alpha effect) acting in arterial and venous beds; potent positive inotropic agent (beta$_1$ effect), increasing the force of myocardial contraction and increasing coronary blood flow.

Indications

- Restoration of BP in controlling certain acute hypotensive states (pheochromocytomectomy, sympathectomy, poliomyelitis, spinal

---

Adverse effects in *Italics* are most common; those in **Bold** are life-threatening.

anesthesia, MI, septicemia, blood transfusion, and drug reactions)
- Adjunct in the treatment of cardiac arrest and profound hypotension

Contraindications and cautions
- Hypovolemia (not a substitute for restoration of fluids, plasma, electrolytes, and should not be used when there are blood volume deficits except as an emergency measure to maintain coronary and cerebral perfusion until blood volume replacement can be effected; if administered continuously to maintain BP when there is hypovolemia, perfusion of vital organs may be severely compromised and tissue hypoxia may result); general anesthesia with halogenated hydrocarbons or cyclopropane; profound hypoxia or hypercarbia; mesenteric or peripheral vascular thrombosis (risk of extending the infarct); pregnancy.

Available forms
Injection—1 mg/mL

Dosages
Individualize infusion rate based on response. Norepinephrine bitartrate 2 mg = 1 mg norepinephrine base.
Adults
- *Restoration of BP in acute hypotensive states:* Add 4 mL of the solution (1 mg/mL) to 1,000 mL of 5% dextrose solution for a concentration of 4 mcg base/mL. Initially give 8–12 mcg base per min. Adjust dose gradually to maintain desired BP (usually 80–100 mm Hg systolic). Average maintenance dose is 2–4 mcg base per min. Occasionally enormous daily doses are necessary (68 mg base/day). Continue the infusion until adequate BP and tissue perfusion are maintained without therapy. Treatment may be required up to 6 days (vascular collapse due to acute MI). Reduce infusion gradually.
- *Adjunct in cardiac arrest:* Administer IV during cardiac resuscitation to restore and maintain BP after effective heartbeat and ventilation established.

Pharmacokinetics

Route	Onset	Duration
IV	Rapid	1–2 min

Metabolism: Neural; $T_{1/2}$: unknown
Distribution: Crosses placenta
Excretion: Urine

▼ IV facts
Preparation: Dilute drug in 5% dextrose solution in distilled water or 5% dextrose in saline solution; these dextrose solutions protect against oxidation. Do not administer in saline solution alone.
Infusion: Infusion rate is determined by response with constant BP monitoring; check manufacturer's insert for detailed guidelines.
Incompatibilities: Do not mix with blood products, aminophylline, amobarbital, cephapirin, lidocaine, pentobarbital, phenobarbital, phenytoin, secobarbital, sodium bicarbonate, thiopental.

Adverse effects
- **CNS:** *Headache*
- **CV:** *Bradycardia,* hypertension

Interactions
✳ **Drug-drug** • Increased hypertensive effects with TCAs (imipramine), guanethidine or reserpine, furazolidone, methyldopa • Decreased vasopressor effects with phenothiazines

■ Nursing considerations
Assessment
- **History:** Hypovolemia, general anesthesia with halogenated hydrocarbons or cyclopropane, profound hypoxia or hypercarbia, mesenteric or peripheral vascular thrombosis, lactation
- **Physical:** Weight; skin color, temperature, turgor; P, BP; R, adventitious sounds; urine output; serum electrolytes, ECG

Interventions
- Give whole blood or plasma separately, if indicated.
- Administer IV infusions into a large vein, preferably the antecubital fossa, to prevent extravasation.
- Do not infuse into femoral vein in elderly patients or those suffering from occlusive vascular disease (atherosclerosis, arteriosclerosis, diabetic endarteritis, Buerger's disease); occlusive vascular disease is more likely to occur in lower extremity.

- Avoid catheter tie-in technique, if possible, because stasis around tubing may lead to high local concentrations of drug.
- Monitor BP every 2 min from the start of infusion until desired BP is achieved, then monitor every 5 min if infusion is continued.
- Monitor infusion site for extravasation.
- Provide phentolamine on standby in case extravasation occurs (5–10 mg phentolamine in 10–15 mL saline should be used to infiltrate the affected area).
- Do not use drug solutions that are pink or brown; drug solutions should be clear and colorless.

Teaching points

Because norepinephrine is used only in acute emergency situations, patient teaching will depend on patient's awareness and will relate mainly to patient's status and to monitoring being done, rather than specifically to therapy with norepinephrine.

▽norethindrone acetate

(nor eth in' drone)

Aygestin, Norlutate (CAN)

PREGNANCY CATEGORY X

Drug classes

Hormone
Progestin

Therapeutic actions

Progesterone derivative. Progesterone transforms proliferative endometrium into secretory endometrium; inhibits the secretion of pituitary gonadotropins, which prevents follicular maturation and ovulation; and inhibits spontaneous uterine contraction. Progestins have varying profiles of estrogenic, antiestrogenic, anabolic, and androgenic activity.

Indications

- Treatment of amenorrhea; abnormal uterine bleeding due to hormonal imbalance
- Treatment of endometriosis

- Component of some hormonal contraceptive preparations (base)

Contraindications and cautions

- Contraindicated with allergy to progestins; thrombophlebitis, thromboembolic disorders, cerebral hemorrhage or history of these conditions; hepatic disease, carcinoma of the breast or genital organs, undiagnosed vaginal bleeding, missed abortion; pregnancy; lactation.
- Use cautiously with epilepsy, migraine, asthma, cardiac or renal dysfunction.

Available forms

Tablets—5 mg

Dosages

Administer PO only.
Adults
- *Amenorrhea; abnormal uterine bleeding:* 2.5–10 mg PO starting with day 5 of the menstrual cycle and ending on day 25.
- *Endometriosis:* 5 mg/day PO for 2 wk. Increase in increments of 2.5 mg/day every 2 wk until 15 mg/day is reached. May be maintained for 6–9 mo or until breakthrough bleeding demands temporary termination.

Pharmacokinetics

Route	Onset
Oral	Varies

Metabolism: Hepatic; $T_{1/2}$: unknown
Distribution: Crosses placenta; enters breast milk
Excretion: Urine and feces

Adverse effects

- **CNS:** Sudden, partial, or complete loss of vision; proptosis; diplopia; migraine; precipitation of acute intermittent porphyria; mental depression; pyrexia; insomnia; somnolence
- **CV:** Thrombophlebitis, cerebrovascular disorders, retinal thrombosis, pulmonary embolism, thromboembolic and thrombotic disease, increased blood pressure

---

Adverse effects in *Italics* are most common; those in **Bold** are life-threatening.

- **Dermatologic:** *Rash with or without pruritus, acne,* melasma or chloasma, alopecia, hirsutism, photosensitivity
- **GI:** Cholestatic jaundice, nausea
- **GU:** *Breakthrough bleeding, spotting, change in menstrual flow, amenorrhea,* changes in cervical erosion and cervical secretions, breast tenderness and secretion
- **Other:** Decreased glucose tolerance, *fluid retention, edema, increase in weight*

Interactions
✳ **Drug-lab test** • Inaccurate tests of hepatic and endocrine function

■ Nursing considerations
Assessment
- **History:** Allergy to progestins; thrombophlebitis, thromboembolic disorders, cerebral hemorrhage; hepatic disease, carcinoma of the breast or genital organs, undiagnosed vaginal bleeding, missed abortion; pregnancy; lactation; epilepsy, migraine, asthma, cardiac or renal dysfunction
- **Physical:** Skin color, lesions, turgor; hair; breasts; pelvic exam; orientation, affect; ophthalmologic exam; P, auscultation, peripheral perfusion, edema; R, adventitious sounds; liver evaluation; liver and renal function tests, glucose tolerance, Pap smear

Interventions
- Arrange for pretreatment and periodic (at least annual) history and physical, including BP, breasts, abdomen, pelvic organs, and a Pap smear.
- Warn patient prior to therapy to prevent pregnancy and to obtain frequent medical follow-ups.
- Use caution when administering drug to ensure preparation ordered is the one being used; norethindrone acetate is approximately twice as potent as norethindrone.
- Discontinue medication and consult physician if sudden partial or complete loss of vision occurs; if papilledema or retinal vascular lesions are present, discontinue drug.
- Discontinue medication and consult physician at sign of thromboembolic disease: leg pain, swelling, peripheral perfusion changes, shortness of breath.

Teaching points
- Take drugs in accordance with marked calendar.
- These side effects may occur: sensitivity to light (avoid exposure to the sun; use sunscreen and protective clothing); dizziness, sleeplessness, depression (use caution driving or performing tasks that require alertness); skin rash, color changes, loss of hair; fever; nausea.
- Avoid pregnancy; serious fetal abnormalities or fetal death could occur.
- Report pain or swelling and warmth in the calves, acute chest pain or shortness of breath, sudden severe headache or vomiting, dizziness or fainting, numbness or tingling in the arm or leg.

▽ norfloxacin
(nor flox' a sin)
Noroxin

PREGNANCY CATEGORY C

Drug classes
Urinary tract anti-infective
Antibiotic
Fluoroquinolone

Therapeutic actions
Bactericidal; interferes with DNA replication in susceptible gram-negative bacteria, leading to cell death.

Indications
- For the treatment of adults with UTIs caused by susceptible gram-negative bacteria, including *E. coli, Proteus mirabilis, K. pneumoniae, Enterobacter cloacae, Proteus vulgaris, Providencia rettgeri, Morganella morganii, Proteus aeruginosa, Citrobacter freundii, S. aureus, Staphylococcus epidermidis,* group D streptococci
- Uncomplicated urethral and cervical gonorrhea caused by *Neisseria gonorrhoeae*
- Prostatitis caused by *E. coli*

Contraindications and cautions
- Contraindicated with allergy to norfloxacin, nalidixic acid, or cinoxacin; pregnancy; lactation.

- Use cautiously in patients with renal dysfunction, seizures.

Available forms
Tablets—400 mg

Dosages
Adults
- *Uncomplicated UTIs:* 400 mg q 12 hr PO for 7–10 days. Maximum dose of 800 mg/day.
- *Uncomplicated cystitis due to* E. coli, K. pneumonia *or* P. mirabilis: 400 mg q 12 hr PO for 3 days.
- *Uncomplicated gonorrhea:* 800 mg PO as a single dose.
- *Prostatitis:* 400 mg q 12 hr PO for 28 days.
Pediatric patients
Not recommended; produced lesions of joint cartilage in immature experimental animals.
Geriatric patients or patients with impaired renal function
Creatinine clearance < 30 mL/min: 400 mg/day, PO for 7–10 days.

Pharmacokinetics

Route	Onset	Peak
Oral	Varies	2–3 hr

Metabolism: Hepatic; $T_{1/2}$: 3–4.5 hr
Distribution: Crosses placenta; enters breast milk
Excretion: Urine

Adverse effects
- **CNS:** *Headache,* dizziness, insomnia, fatigue, somnolence, depression, blurred vision
- **GI:** *Nausea,* vomiting, dry mouth, diarrhea, abdominal pain, dyspepsia, flatulence, constipation, heartburn
- **Hematologic:** Elevated BUN, AST, ALT, serum creatinine and alkaline phosphatase; decreased WBC, neutrophil count, Hct
- **Other:** Fever, rash, photosensitivity

Interactions
✳ **Drug-drug** ● Decreased therapeutic effect with iron salts, sucralfate ● Decreased absorption with antacids ● Increased serum levels and toxic effects of theophyllines, cyclosporine

✳ **Drug-alternative therapy** ● Increased risk of severe photosensitivity reactions if combined with St. John's wort therapy

■ Nursing considerations
Assessment
- **History:** Allergy to norfloxacin, nalidixic acid, or cinoxacin; renal dysfunction; **seizures;** pregnancy; lactation
- **Physical:** Skin color, lesions; T; orientation, reflexes, affect; mucous membranes, bowel sounds; renal and liver function tests

Interventions
- Arrange for culture and sensitivity tests before therapy.
- Administer drug 1 hr before or 2 hr after meals with a glass of water.
- Ensure that patient is well hydrated.
- Administer antacids at least 2 hr after dosing.
- Monitor clinical response; if no improvement is seen or a relapse occurs, send urine for repeat culture and sensitivity.

Teaching points
- Take drug on an empty stomach, 1 hr before or 2 hr after meals. If an antacid is needed, do not take it within 2 hr of norfloxacin dose.
- Drink plenty of fluids.
- These side effects may occur: nausea, vomiting, abdominal pain (small, frequent meals may help); diarrhea or constipation; drowsiness, blurring of vision, dizziness (observe caution driving or using dangerous equipment).
- Report rash, visual changes, severe GI problems, weakness, tremors.

▽ **norgestrel**
(nor jess' trel)

Ovrette

PREGNANCY CATEGORY X

Drug classes
Hormone
Progestin
Hormonal contraceptive

Adverse effects in *Italics* are most common; those in **Bold** are life-threatening.

Therapeutic actions

Progestational agent; the endogenous female progestin, progesterone, transforms proliferative endometrium into secretory endometrium; inhibits the secretion of pituitary gonadotropins, which prevents follicular maturation and ovulation; and inhibits spontaneous uterine contractions. The primary mechanism by which norgestrel prevents conception is not known, but progestin-only hormonal contraceptives alter the cervical mucus, exert a progestional effect on the endometrium that interferes with implantation, and in some patients, suppress ovulation.

Indications

- Prevention of pregnancy using hormonal contraceptives; somewhat less efficacious (3 pregnancies per 100 woman years) than the combined estrogen/progestin hormonal contraceptives (about 1 pregnancy per 100 woman years, depending on formulation)

Contraindications and cautions

- Contraindicated with allergy to progestins, tartrazine; thrombophlebitis, thromboembolic disorders, cerebral hemorrhage, or history of these conditions; CAD; hepatic disease, carcinoma of the breast or genital organs, undiagnosed vaginal bleeding, missed abortion; as a diagnostic test for pregnancy; pregnancy (fetal abnormalities: masculinization of the female fetus, congenital heart defects, and limb reduction defects); lactation.
- Use cautiously with epilepsy, migraine, asthma, cardiac or renal dysfunction.

Available forms

Tablets—0.075 mg

Dosages
Adults

Administer daily, starting on the first day of menstruation. Take one tablet, PO, at the same time each day, every day of the year. *Missed dose:* 1 tablet—take as soon as remembered, then take the next tablet at regular time; 2 consecutive tablets—take 1 of the missed tablets, discard the other, and take daily tablet at usual time; 3 consecutive tablets—discontinue

immediately and use additional form of birth control until menses or pregnancy is ruled out.

Pharmacokinetics

Route	Onset
Oral	Varies

Metabolism: Hepatic; $T_{1/2}$: unknown
Distribution: Crosses placenta; enters breast milk
Excretion: Urine

Adverse effects

- **CNS:** Neuro-ocular lesions, mental depression, migraine, *changes in corneal curvature,* contact lens intolerance
- **CV:** *Thrombophlebitis, thrombosis,* **pulmonary embolism,** coronary thrombosis, MI, cerebral thrombosis, Raynaud's disease, arterial thromboembolism, renal artery thrombosis, **cerebral hemorrhage,** hypertension
- **Dermatologic:** Rash with or without pruritus, acne, melasma
- **GI:** Gallbladder disease, liver tumors, hepatic lesions, *nausea, vomiting,* abdominal cramps, bloating, cholestatic jaundice
- **GU:** *Breakthrough bleeding, spotting, change in menstrual flow, amenorrhea,* changes in cervical erosion and cervical secretions, endocervical hyperplasia, vaginal candidiasis
- **Other:** *Breast tenderness and secretion, enlargement;* fluid retention, edema, increase or decrease in weight

Interactions

✳ Drug-drug • Decreased effectiveness of hormonal contraceptives with barbiturates, hydantoins, carbamazepine, rifampin, griseofulvin, penicillins, tetracyclines; use alternate form of birth control if these drugs are needed
✳ Drug-alternative therapy • Decreased effectiveness if taken with St. John's wort

■ Nursing considerations
Assessment

- **History:** Allergy to progestins, tartrazine; thrombophlebitis, thromboembolic disorders, cerebral hemorrhage; CAD; hepatic disease, carcinoma of the breast or genital organs, undiagnosed vaginal bleeding, missed abortion; epilepsy, migraine, asthma, car-

N

diac or renal dysfunction; pregnancy; lactation

- **Physical:** Skin color, lesions, turgor; hair; breasts; pelvic exam; orientation, affect; ophthalmologic exam; P, auscultation, peripheral perfusion, edema; R, adventitious sounds; liver evaluation; liver and renal function tests, glucose tolerance, Pap smear, pregnancy test

Interventions

- Arrange for pretreatment and periodic (at least annual) history and physical, including BP, breasts, abdomen, pelvic organs, and a Pap smear.
- Start no earlier than 4 wk postpartum for postpartum use.
- Discontinue medication and consult physician if sudden partial or complete loss of vision occurs; if papilledema or retinal vascular lesions are present on exam, discontinue.
- Discontinue medication and consult physician at any sign of thromboembolic disease: leg pain, swelling, peripheral perfusion changes, shortness of breath.

Teaching points

- Take exactly as prescribed at intervals not exceeding 24 hr. Take at bedtime or with a meal to establish a routine; medication must be taken daily for prevention of pregnancy; if you miss one tablet, take as soon as remembered, then take the next tablet at regular time. If you miss two consecutive tablets, take 1 of the missed tablets, discard the other, and take daily tablet at usual time. If you miss three consecutive tablets, discontinue immediately, and use another method of birth control until your cycle starts again. It is a good idea to use an additional method of birth control if any tablets are missed.
- Discontinue drug and consult your health care provider if you decide to become pregnant. It may be suggested that you use a nonhormonal form of birth control for a few months before becoming pregnant.
- These side effects may occur: sensitivity to light (avoid exposure to the sun; use sunscreen and protective clothing); dizziness, sleeplessness, depression (use caution driv-

ing or performing tasks that require alertness); rash, skin color changes, loss of hair; fever; nausea; breakthrough bleeding or spotting (transient); intolerance to contact lenses due to corneal changes.

- Do not take this drug during pregnancy; serious fetal abnormalities have been reported. If you think that you are pregnant consult physician immediately.
- Tell your nurse, physician, or dentist that you take this drug. If other medications are prescribed, they may decrease the effectiveness of hormonal contraceptives and an additional method of birth control may be needed.
- Report pain or swelling and warmth in the calves, acute chest pain or shortness of breath, sudden severe headache or vomiting, dizziness or fainting, visual disturbances, numbness or tingling in the arm or leg, breakthrough bleeding or spotting that lasts into the second month of therapy.

▽ nortriptyline hydrochloride
*(nor **trip**' ti leen)*

Aventyl, Norventyl (CAN), Pamelor, PMS-Nortriptyline (CAN)

PREGNANCY CATEGORY C

Drug class

Tricyclic antidepressant (TCA) (secondary amine)

Therapeutic actions

Mechanism of action unknown; the TCAs are structurally related to the phenothiazine antipsychotic drugs (eg, chlorpromazine), but inhibit the presynaptic reuptake of the neurotransmitters norepinephrine and serotonin; anticholinergic at CNS and peripheral receptors; sedating; the relationship of these effects to clinical efficacy is unknown.

Indications

- Relief of symptoms of depression (endogenous depression most responsive)

Adverse effects in *Italics* are most common; those in **Bold** are life-threatening.

- Unlabeled uses: treatment of panic disorders (25–75 mg/day), premenstrual depression (50–125 mg/day), dermatologic disorders (75 mg/day), chronic pain, headache prophylaxis

Contraindications and cautions

- Contraindicated with hypersensitivity to any tricyclic drug; concomitant therapy with an MAO inhibitor; recent MI; myelography within previous 24 hr or scheduled within 48 hr; pregnancy (limb reduction abnormalities); lactation.
- Use cautiously with EST (increased hazard with TCAs); preexisting CV disorders (possibly increased risk of serious CVS toxicity); angle-closure glaucoma, increased intraocular pressure; urinary retention, ureteral or urethral spasm (anticholinergic effects may exacerbate these conditions); seizure disorders; hyperthyroidism (predisposes to CVS toxicity, including cardiac arrhythmias); impaired hepatic, renal function; psychiatric patients (schizophrenic or paranoid patients may exhibit a worsening of psychosis); manic-depressive patients (may shift to hypomanic or manic phase); elective surgery (discontinued as long as possible before surgery).

Available forms

Capsules—10, 25, 50, 75 mg; solution—10 mg/5 mL

Dosages

Adults
25 mg tid–qid PO. Begin with low dosage and gradually increase as required and tolerated. Doses > 150 mg/day are not recommended.
Pediatric patients
≥ *12 yr:* 30–50 mg/day PO in divided doses.
< *12 yr:* Not recommended.
Geriatric patients
30–50 mg/day PO in divided doses.

Pharmacokinetics

Route	Onset	Peak	Duration
Oral	Varies	2–4 hr	2–4 wk

Metabolism: Hepatic; $T_{1/2}$: 18–28 hr
Distribution: Crosses placenta; enters breast milk
Excretion: Urine

Adverse effects

- **CNS:** *Sedation and anticholinergic (atropine-like) effects* (dry mouth, blurred vision, disturbance of accommodation for near vision, mydriasis, increased intraocular pressure), *confusion* (especially in elderly), *disturbed concentration,* hallucinations, disorientation, decreased memory, feelings of unreality, delusions, anxiety, nervousness, restlessness, agitation, panic, insomnia, nightmares, hypomania, mania, exacerbation of psychosis, drowsiness, weakness, fatigue, headache, numbness, tingling, paresthesias of extremities, incoordination, motor hyperactivity, akathisia, ataxia, tremors, peripheral neuropathy, extrapyramidal symptoms, **seizures,** speech blockage, dysarthria
- **CV:** *Orthostatic hypotension,* hypertension, syncope, tachycardia, palpitations, MI, arrhythmias, heart block, precipitation of CHF, stroke
- **Endocrine:** Elevated or depressed blood sugar; elevated prolactin levels; inappropriate ADH secretion
- **GI:** *Dry mouth, constipation,* paralytic ileus, *nausea,* vomiting, anorexia, epigastric distress, diarrhea, flatulence, dysphagia, peculiar taste, increased salivation, stomatitis, glossitis, parotid swelling, abdominal cramps, black tongue, hepatitis; elevated transaminase, altered alkaline phosphatase
- **GU:** Urinary retention, delayed micturition, dilation of the urinary tract, gynecomastia, testicular swelling; breast enlargement, menstrual irregularity and galactorrhea; increased or decreased libido; impotence
- **Hematologic:** Bone marrow depression, including agranulocytosis; eosinophilia; purpura; thrombocytopenia; leukopenia
- **Hypersensitivity:** Rash, pruritus, vasculitis, petechiae, photosensitization, edema (generalized, facial, tongue), drug fever
- **Withdrawal:** Symptoms with abrupt discontinuation of prolonged therapy: nausea, headache, vertigo, nightmares, malaise
- **Other:** Nasal congestion, excessive appetite, weight gain or loss; sweating, alopecia, lacrimation, hyperthermia, flushing, chills

Interactions

✳ Drug-drug • Increased TCA levels and pharmacologic (especially anticholinergic) effects with cimetidine, fluoxetine • Altered response, including arrhythmias and hypertension with sympathomimetics • Risk of severe hypertension with clonidine • Hyperpyretic crises, severe convulsions, hypertensive episodes, and deaths when MAO inhibitors are given with TCAs • Decreased hypotensive activity of guanethidine

Note: MAOIs and tricyclic antidepressants have been used successfully in some patients resistant to therapy with single agents; however, case reports indicate that the combination can cause serious and potentially fatal adverse effects.

■ Nursing considerations
Assessment
- **History:** Hypersensitivity to any tricyclic drug; concomitant therapy with an MAO inhibitor; recent MI; myelography within previous 24 hr or scheduled within 48 hr; pregnancy; lactation; EST; preexisting CV disorders; angle-closure glaucoma, increased intraocular pressure, urinary retention, ureteral or urethral spasm; seizure disorders; hyperthyroidism; impaired hepatic, renal function; psychiatric patients; manic-depressive patients; elective surgery
- **Physical:** Weight; T; skin color, lesions; orientation, affect, reflexes, vision and hearing; P, BP, orthostatic BP, perfusion; bowel sounds, normal output, liver evaluation; urine flow, normal output; usual sexual function, frequency of menses, breast and scrotal examination; liver function tests, urinalysis, CBC, ECG

Interventions
- Limit drug access to depressed and potentially suicidal patients.
- Give major portion of dose hs if drowsiness, severe anticholinergic effects occur.
- Reduce dosage if minor side effects develop; discontinue if serious side effects occur.
- Arrange for CBC if patient develops fever, sore throat, or other sign of infection.

Teaching points
- Take drug exactly as prescribed; do not stop taking this drug abruptly or without consulting your health care provider.

- Avoid alcohol, other sleep-inducing, OTC drugs.
- Avoid prolonged exposure to sunlight or sunlamps; use a sunscreen or protective garments if possible.
- These side effects may occur: headache, dizziness, drowsiness, weakness, blurred vision (reversible; use safety measures if severe; avoid driving or performing tasks that require alertness); nausea, vomiting, loss of appetite, dry mouth (small, frequent meals, frequent mouth care and sucking sugarless candies may help); nightmares, inability to concentrate, confusion; changes in sexual function.
- Report dry mouth, difficulty in urination, excessive sedation.

▽nystatin
(nye stat' in)

Oral, oral suspensions, oral troche: Candistatin (CAN), Mycostatin, Nadostine (CAN), Nilstat, Nystex, PMS Nystatin (CAN)

Vaginal preparations: Mycostatin, Nadostine (CAN), Nilstat (CAN)

Topical application: Mycostatin, Nadostine (CAN), Nilstat, Nystex

PREGNANCY CATEGORY C

Drug class
Antifungal

Therapeutic actions
Fungicidal and fungistatic: binds to sterols in the cell membrane of the fungus with a resultant change in membrane permeability, allowing leakage of intracellular components and causing cell death.

Indications
- Treatment of oropharyngeal candidiasis (oral)
- Treatment of oral candidiasis (oral suspension, troche)
- Local treatment of vaginal candidiasis (moniliasis; vaginal)

Adverse effects in *Italics* are most common; those in **Bold** are life-threatening.

• Treatment of cutaneous or mucocutaneous mycotic infections caused by *Candida albicans* and other *Candida* species (topical applications)

Contraindications and cautions
• Contraindicated with allergy to nystatin or components used in preparation.
• Use cautiously with pregnancy, lactation.

Available forms
Tablets—500,000 units; oral suspension—100,000 units/mL; troche—200,000 units; vaginal tablets—100,000 units; topical cream, ointment, powder—100,000 units/g

Dosages
Adults and pediatric patients except infants
Oral
500,000–1,000,000 units tid. Continue for at least 48 hr after clinical cure.
• *Oral suspension:* 400,000–600,000 units qid (one-half of dose in each side of mouth, retaining the drug as long as possible before swallowing).
• *Troche:* Dissolve 1–2 tablets in mouth 4–5 times/day for up to 14 days.
Infants
Oral suspension
200,000 units qid (100,000 in each side of mouth).
Premature and low-birth-weight infants: 100,000 units qid.
Adults
Vaginal preparations
1 tablet (100,000 units) or 1 applicator of cream (100,000 units) daily–bid for 2 wk.
Topical
• *Vaginal preparations:* Apply to affected area 2–3 times/day until healing is complete.
• *Topical foot powder:* For fungal infections of the feet, dust powder on feet and in shoes and socks.

Pharmacokinetics
No general systemic absorption. Excreted unchanged in the feces after oral use.

Adverse effects
Oral
• **GI:** *Nausea, vomiting, diarrhea, GI distress*

Vaginal
• **Local:** *Irritation, vulvovaginal burning*
Topical
• **Local:** *Local irritation*

■ Nursing considerations
Assessment
• **History:** Allergy to nystatin or components used in preparation, pregnancy, lactation
• **Physical:** Skin color, lesions, area around lesions; bowel sounds; culture of area involved

Interventions
• Culture fungus before therapy.
• Have patient retain oral suspension in mouth as long as possible before swallowing. Paint suspension on each side of the mouth. Continue local treatment for at least 48 hr after clinical improvement is noted.
• Prepare nystatin in the form of frozen flavored popsicles to improve oral retention of the drug for local application.
• Administer nystatin troche orally for the treatment of oral candidiasis; have patient dissolve 1–2 tablets in mouth.
• Insert vaginal suppositories high into the vagina. Have patient remain recumbent for 10–15 min after insertion. Provide sanitary napkin to protect clothing from stains.
• Cleanse affected area before topical application, unless otherwise indicated.
• Monitor response to drug therapy. If no response is noted, arrange for further cultures to determine causative organism.
• Ensure that patient receives the full course of therapy to eradicate the fungus and to prevent recurrence.
• Discontinue topical or vaginal administration if rash or sensitivity occurs.

Teaching points
• Take the full course of drug therapy even if symptoms improve. Continue during menstrual period if vaginal route is being used. Long-term use of the drug may be needed; beneficial effects may not be seen for several weeks. Vaginal suppositories should be inserted high into the vagina.
• Use appropriate hygiene measures to prevent reinfection or spread of infection.

- This drug is for the fungus being treated; do not self-medicate other problems.
- Refrain from sexual intercourse or advise partner to use a condom to avoid reinfection; use a sanitary napkin to prevent staining of clothing with vaginal use.
- These side effects may occur: nausea, vomiting, diarrhea (oral use); irritation, burning, stinging (local use).
- Report worsening of condition; local irritation, burning (topical application); rash, irritation, pelvic pain (vaginal use); nausea, GI distress (oral administration).

▽ octreotide acetate
*(ok **trye' oh tide**)*

Sandostatin, Sandostatin LAR Depot

PREGNANCY CATEGORY B

Drug classes
Hormone
Antidiarrheal

Therapeutic actions
Mimics the natural hormone somatostatin; suppresses secretion of serotonin, gastrin, vasoactive intestinal peptide, insulin, glucagon, secretin, motilin, and pancreatic polypeptide; also suppresses growth hormone and decreases splanchnic blood flow.

Indications
- Symptomatic treatment of patients with metastatic carcinoid tumors to suppress or inhibit the associated severe diarrhea and flushing episodes
- Treatment of the profuse watery diarrhea associated with vasoactive intestinal polypeptide tumors (VIPomas)
- Reduction of growth hormone blood levels in patients with acromegaly not responsive to other treatment
- Unlabeled uses: GI fistula, variceal bleeding, diarrheal states, pancreatic fistulas, irritable bowel syndrome, dumping syndrome

Contraindications and cautions
- Contraindicated with hypersensitivity to octreotide or any of its components.
- Use cautiously with renal impairment, thyroid disease, diabetes mellitus, pregnancy, lactation.

Available forms
Injection—0.05, 0.1, 0.2, 0.5, 1 mg/mL; depot injection—10, 20, 30 mg/vial

Dosages
Adults
SC injection is the route of choice. Initial dose is 50 mcg SC daily or bid; the number of injections is increased based on response, usually bid–tid. IV bolus injections have been used in emergency situations—not recommended. *Depot injection:* Do not administer IV or SC; inject intragluteally at 4-wk intervals. Patients should be stabilized on SC octreotide for at least 2 wk before switching to long-acting depot.
- *Carcinoid tumors:* First 2 wk of therapy: 100–600 mcg/day SC in 2 to 4 divided doses (mean daily dosage, 300 mcg).
- *VIPomas:* 200–300 mcg SC in 2 to 4 divided doses during initial 2 wk of therapy to control symptoms. Range: 150–750 mcg SC; doses above 450 mcg are usually not required. *Depot injection:* 20 mg IM q 4 wk.
- *Acromegaly:* 50 mcg tid SC, adjusted up to 100–500 mcg tid. Withdraw for 4 wk once yearly. *Depot injection:* 20 mg IM intragluteally once every 4 wk; after 2–3 mo, reevaluate patient to adjust dose as needed.

Pediatric patients
Safety and efficacy for depot injection not established.
- *GI tumors:* 1–10 mcg/kg/day SC.

Geriatric patients or patients with renal impairment
Half-life may be prolonged; adjust dose.

Pharmacokinetics

Route	Onset	Peak
SC	Rapid	15 min

Metabolism: Hepatic; $T_{1/2}$: 1.5 hr
Distribution: May cross placenta; may enter breast milk
Excretion: Urine

Adverse effects
- **CNS:** *Headache, dizziness, light-headedness,* fatigue, anxiety, convulsions, depression, drowsiness, vertigo, hyperesthesia, irritability, forgetfulness, malaise, nervousness, visual disturbances
- **CV:** Shortness of breath, hypertension, thrombophlebitis, ischemia, CHF, palpitations, bradycardia
- **Dermatologic:** *Flushing,* edema, hair loss, thinning of skin, skin flaking, bruising, pruritus, rash
- **Endocrine:** *Hyperglycemia, hypoglycemia,* galactorrhea, clinical hypothyroidism
- **GI:** *Nausea, vomiting, diarrhea, abdominal pain, loose stools,* fat malabsorption, constipation, flatulence, hepatitis, rectal spasm, GI bleeding, heartburn, cholelithiasis, dry mouth, burning mouth
- **Local:** *Injection site pain*
- **Musculoskeletal:** Asthenia/weakness, leg cramps, muscle pain
- **Respiratory:** Rhinorrhea

■ Nursing considerations
Assessment
- **History:** Hypersensitivity to octreotide or any of its components; renal impairment; thyroid disease, diabetes mellitus; lactation
- **Physical:** Skin lesions, hair; reflexes, affect; BP, P, orthostatic BP; abdominal exam, liver evaluation, mucous membranes; renal and thyroid function tests, blood glucose, electrolytes

Interventions
- Administer by SC injection; avoid multiple injections in the same site within short periods of time.
- Administer depot injection by deep IM intragluteal injection; avoid deltoid injections.
- Monitor patients with renal function impairment closely; reduced dosage may be necessary.
- Store ampules in the refrigerator; may be at room temperature on day of use. Do not use if particulates or discoloration are observed.
- Monitor patient closely for endocrine reactions: blood glucose alterations, thyroid hormone changes, growth hormone level.
- Arrange for baseline and periodic gall bladder ultrasound to pick up cholelithiasis.

- Monitor blood glucose, especially at start of therapy, to detect hypoglycemia or hyperglycemia. Diabetic patients will require close monitoring.
- Arrange to withdraw the drug for 4 weeks once yearly in treating acromegaly.

Teaching points
- This drug must be injected. You and a significant other can be instructed in the procedure of SC injections. Review technique and process periodically. Do not use the same site for repeated injections; rotate injection sites. Dosage will be adjusted based on your response. Depot injection must be given IM once every 4 wk.
- These side effects may occur: headache, dizziness, light-headedness, fatigue (avoid driving or performing tasks that require alertness); nausea, diarrhea, abdominal pain (small, frequent meals may help; maintain nutrition); flushing, dry skin, flaking of skin (skin care may prevent breakdown); pain at the injection site.
- Arrange for periodic medical exams, including blood tests and gall bladder tests.
- Report sweating, dizziness, severe abdominal pain, fatigue, fever, chills, infection, or severe pain at injection sites.

▷ ofloxacin
(oe flox' a sin)

Floxin, Ocuflox

PREGNANCY CATEGORY C

Drug classes
Antibiotic
Fluoroquinolone

Therapeutic actions
Bactericidal; interferes with DNA replication in susceptible gram-positive and gram-negative bacteria, preventing cell reproduction.

Indications
- Lower respiratory tract infections caused by *Haemophilus influenzae, Streptococcus pneumoniae*
- Acute, uncomplicated urethral and cervical gonorrhea due to *Neisseria gonorrhoeae,*

nongonococcal urethritis, and cervicitis due to *Chlamydia trachomatis,* mixed infections due to both

- Skin and soft tissue infections due to *Staphylococcus aureus, Staphylococcus pyogenes, Proteus mirabilis*
- Urinary tract infections due to *Citrobacter diversus, Enterobacter aerogenes, Escherichia coli, Klebsiella pneumoniae, Pseudomonas aeruginosa*
- Primary treatment of PID (oral)
- Prostatitis due to *E. coli*
- Treatment of ocular infections caused by susceptible organisms (ophthalmic solution)
- Orphan drug use: treatment of bacterial corneal ulcers
- Otic: otitis externa, chronic suppurative otitis media, acute otitis media

Contraindications and cautions

- Contraindicated with allergy to fluoroquinolones, pregnancy, lactation.
- Use cautiously with renal dysfunction, seizures.

Available forms

Ophthalmic solution—3 mg/mL (0.3%); tablets—200, 300, 400 mg; injection—200, 400 mg; otic solution—0.3%

Dosages
Adults

- *Uncomplicated UTIs:* 200 mg q 12 hr PO for 3 days.
- *Complicated UTIs:* 200 mg bid PO or IV for 10 days.
- *Lower respiratory tract infections:* 400 mg q 12 hr PO or IV for 10 days.
- *Mild to moderate skin infections:* 400 mg q 12 hr PO or IV for 10 days.
- *Prostatitis:* 300 mg q 12 hr PO or IV for 6 wk.
- *Acute, uncomplicated gonorrhea:* 400 mg PO or IV as a single dose.
- *Cervicitis, urethritis:* 300 mg q 12 hr PO or IV for 7 days.
- *Ocular infections:* 1–2 drops per eye as indicated.
- *Otic infections:* 10 drops in affected ear tid for 10–14 days.

Pediatric patients < 18 yr
Not recommended; produced lesions of joint cartilage in immature experimental animals.
Geriatric patients or patients with impaired renal function
Creatinine clearance 20–50 mL/min: use a 24-hr interval; creatinine clearance < 20 mL/min: use a 24-hr interval and half the recommended dose.

Pharmacokinetics

Route	Onset	Peak	Duration
Oral	Varies	1–2 hr	9 hr
IV	10 min	30 min	9 hr

Metabolism: Hepatic; $T_{1/2}$: 5–10 hr
Distribution: Crosses placenta; enters breast milk
Excretion: Urine and bile

▼ IV facts
Preparation: Dilute the single-dose vial to a final concentration of 4 mg/mL using 0.9% NaCl injection, 5% dextrose injection, 5% dextrose/0.9% sodium chloride; 5% dextrose in lactated Ringer's; 5% sodium bicarbonate; *Plasma-Lyte 56* in 5% dextrose; 5% dextrose, 0.45% sodium chloride and 0.15% potassium chloride; sodium lactate (M/6); water for injection. Premixed bottles require no further dilution. Discard any unused portion.
Infusion: Administer slowly over 60 min.

Adverse effects

- **CNS:** *Headache,* dizziness, *insomnia,* fatigue, somnolence, depression, blurred vision
- **GI:** *Nausea,* vomiting, dry mouth, *diarrhea,* abdominal pain
- **Hematologic:** Elevated BUN, AST, ALT, serum creatinine and alkaline phosphatase; decreased WBC, neutrophil count, Hct
- **Other:** Fever, rash, *photosensitivity*

Interactions
✻ Drug-drug • Decreased therapeutic effect with iron salts, zinc, sucralfate • Decreased absorption with antacids

✻ Drug-alternative therapy • Increased risk of severe photosensitivity reactions if combined with St. John's wort therapy

---

Adverse effects in *Italics* are most common; those in **Bold** are life-threatening.

■ Nursing considerations
Assessment
- **History:** Allergy to fluoroquinolones, renal dysfunction, seizures, lactation, pregnancy
- **Physical:** Skin color, lesions; T; orientation, reflexes, affect; mucous membranes, bowel sounds; renal and liver function tests

Interventions
- Arrange for culture and sensitivity tests before beginning therapy.
- Continue therapy for 2 days after the signs of infection have disappeared.
- Administer oral drug 1 hr before or 2 hr after meals with a glass of water.
- Ensure that patient is well hydrated.
- Administer antacids at least 2 hr after dosing.
- Monitor clinical response; if no improvement is seen or a relapse occurs, repeat culture and sensitivity.

Teaching points
- Take oral drug on an empty stomach, 1 hr before or 2 hr after meals. If an antacid is needed, do not take it within 2 hr of ofloxacin dose.
- Drink plenty of fluids.
- These side effects may occur: nausea, vomiting, abdominal pain (small, frequent meals may help); diarrhea or constipation; drowsiness, blurring of vision, dizziness (observe caution if driving or using dangerous equipment).
- Report rash, visual changes, severe GI problems, weakness, tremors.

▽ olanzapine
(oh lan' za peen)

Zyprexa, Zyprexa Zydis

PREGNANCY CATEGORY C

Drug classes
Antipsychotic
Dopaminergic blocking agent

Therapeutic actions
Mechanism of action not fully understood; blocks dopamine receptors in the brain, depresses the RAS; blocks serotonin receptor sites; anticholinergic, antihistaminic (H_1), and alpha-adrenergic blocking activity may contribute to some of its therapeutic (and adverse) actions; produces fewer extrapyramidal effects than most antipsychotics.

Indications
- Treatment of schizophrenia
- Treatment of acute manic episodes associated with bipolar 1 disorder
- Unlabeled use: dementia related to Alzheimer's disease

Contraindications and cautions
- Contraindicated with allergy to olanzapine, myeloproliferative disorders, severe CNS depression, comatose states, lactation.
- Use cautiously with CV or cerebrovascular disease, dehydration, seizure disorders, Alzheimer's disease, prostate enlargement, narrow-angle glaucoma, history of paralytic ileus or breast cancer, elderly or debilitated patients, pregnancy.

Available forms
Tablets—2.5, 5, 7.5, 10, 15, 20 mg; orally disintegrating tablets—5, 10, 15, 20 mg

Dosages
Adults
- *Schizophrenia:* Initially, 5–10 mg PO daily, increase to 10 mg PO daily within several days; may be increased by 5 mg/day at 1-wk intervals to achieve desired effect. Do not exceed 20 mg/day.
- *Bipolar mania:* 10–15 mg/day PO; adjust at 5-mg intervals as needed, not less than q 24 hr. Maximum dose, 20 mg/day.

Pediatric patients
Safety and efficacy not established in patients < 18 yr.

Debilitated patients
Start with initial dose of 5 mg.

Pharmacokinetics

Route	Onset	Peak	Duration
Oral	Varies	6 hr	Weeks

Metabolism: Hepatic; $T_{1/2}$: 30 hr
Distribution: Crosses placenta; passes into breast milk
Excretion: Urine and feces

Adverse effects

- **CNS:** *Somnolence, dizziness,* nervousness, headache, akathisia, personality disorders, tardive dyskinesia, **neuroleptic malignant syndrome**
- **CV:** *Orthostatic hypotension,* peripheral edema, tachycardia
- **GI:** *Constipation,* abdominal pain
- **Respiratory:** Cough, pharyngitis
- **Other:** *Fever,* weight gain, joint pain

Interactions

✳ **Drug-drug** • Increased risk of orthostatic hypotension with antihypertensives, alcohol, benzodiazepines; avoid use of alcohol and use caution with antihypertensives • Increased risk of seizures with anticholinergics, CNS drugs • May decrease effectiveness of levodopa, dopamine agonists • Decreased effectiveness with rifampin, omeprazole, carbamazepine, smoking • Increased risk of toxicity with fluvoxamine

■ Nursing considerations

 CLINICAL ALERT!
Name confusion has occurred between Zyprexa (olanzapine) and Zyrtec (cetirizine); use caution.

Assessment

- **History:** Allergy to olanzapine, myeloproliferative disorders, severe CNS depression, comatose states, history of seizure disorders, lactation; CV or cerebrovascular disease, dehydration, Alzheimer's disease, prostate enlargement, narrow-angle glaucoma, history of paralytic ileus or breast cancer, elderly or debilitated patients, pregnancy
- **Physical:** T, weight; reflexes, orientation, intraocular pressure, ophthalmologic exam; P, BP, orthostatic BP, ECG; R, adventitious sounds; bowel sounds, normal output, liver evaluation; prostate palpation, normal urine output; CBC, urinalysis, liver and renal function tests

Interventions

- Do not dispense more than 1-wk supply at a time.

- Peel back foil on blister pack of disintegrating tablets; do not push through foil; use dry hands to remove tablet and place in mouth.
- Monitor for the many possible drug–drug interactions before beginning therapy.
- Monitor elderly patients for dehydration and institute remedial measures promptly; sedation and decreased sensation of thirst related to CNS effects of drug can lead to dehydration.
- Encourage patient to void before taking the drug to help decrease anticholinergic effects of urinary retention.
- Monitor for elevations of temperature and differentiate between infection and neuroleptic malignant syndrome.
- Monitor for orthostatic hypotension and provide appropriate safety measures as needed.

Teaching points

- Take this drug exactly as prescribed; do not change dose without consulting your health care provider.
- Peel back foil on blister pack of disintegrating tablets; do not push through foil; use dry hands to remove tablet, place entire tablet in mouth.
- These side effects may occur: drowsiness, dizziness, sedation, seizures (avoid driving, operating machinery, or performing tasks that require concentration); dizziness, faintness on arising (change positions slowly, use caution); increased salivation (if bothersome, contact your nurse or physician); constipation (consult with your nurse or physician for appropriate relief measures); fast heart rate (rest and take your time if this occurs).
- This drug cannot be taken during pregnancy. If you think you are pregnant or wish to become pregnant, contact your nurse or physician.
- Report lethargy, weakness, fever, sore throat, malaise, mouth ulcers, and flulike symptoms.

Adverse effects in Italics are most common; those in Bold are life-threatening.

▽olmesartan medoxomil
(ol ma sar' tan)

Benicar

PREGNANCY CATEGORY C
(FIRST TRIMESTER)

PREGNANCY CATEGORY D
(SECOND AND THIRD TRIMESTERS)

Drug classes
Angiotensin II receptor antagonist
Antihypertensive

Therapeutic actions
Selectively blocks the binding of angiotensin II to specific tissue receptors found in the vascular smooth muscle and adrenal gland; this action blocks the vasoconstricting effect of the renin–angiotensin system as well as the release of aldosterone leading to decreased blood pressure; may prevent the vessel remodeling associated with the development of atherosclerosis.

Indications
- Treatment of hypertension, alone or in combination with other antihypertensive agents

Contraindications and cautions
- Contraindicated with hypersensitivity to any component of the drug; pregnancy (use during the second or third trimester can cause injury or even death to the fetus), lactation.
- Use cautiously with renal dysfunction, hypovolemia, salt depletion.

Available forms
Tablets—5, 20, 40 mg

Dosages
Adults
20 mg/day PO as a once daily dose; may titrate to 40 mg/day if needed after 2 wk.
Pediatric patients
Safety and efficacy not established.

Pharmacokinetics

Route	Onset	Peak
Oral	Varies	1–2 hr

Metabolism: Hydrolyzed in GI tract; $T_{1/2}$: 13 hr
Distribution: Crosses placenta; passes into breast milk
Excretion: Feces and urine

Adverse effects
- **CNS:** *Headache,* dizziness, syncope, muscle weakness
- **CV:** Hypotension, tachycardia
- **Dermatologic:** Rash, inflammation, urticaria, pruritus, alopecia, dry skin
- **GI:** *Diarrhea, abdominal pain, nausea,* constipation, dry mouth, dental pain
- **Hematologic:** Increased CPK, hyperglycemia, hypertriglyceridemia
- **Respiratory:** *URI symptoms, bronchitis, cough,* sinusitis, rhinitis, pharyngitis
- **Other:** *Back pain, flulike symptoms,* fatigue, hematuria, arthritis, **angioedema**

■ Nursing considerations
Assessment
- **History:** Hypersensitivity to any component of the drug, pregnancy, lactation, hepatic or renal dysfunction, hypovolemia, salt depletion
- **Physical:** Skin lesions, turgor; body temperature; reflexes, affect; BP; R, respiratory auscultation; liver and kidney function tests, serum electrolytes

Interventions
- Administer without regard to meals.
- Ensure that patient is not pregnant before beginning therapy; suggest the use of barrier birth control while using olmesartan; fetal injury and deaths have been reported.
- Find an alternate method of feeding the infant if given to a nursing mother. Depression of the renin–angiotensin system in infants is potentially very dangerous.
- Alert surgeon and mark patient's chart with notice that olmesartan is being taken. The blockage of the renin–angiotensin system following surgery can produce problems. Hypotension may be reversed with volume expansion.
- Monitor patient closely in any situation that may lead to a decrease in blood pressure secondary to reduction in fluid volume—excessive perspiration, dehydration, vomiting,

diarrhea—excessive hypotension can occur.

Teaching points
- Take drug without regard to meals. Do not stop taking this drug without consulting your health care provider.
- Use a barrier method of birth control while on this drug; if you become pregnant or desire to become pregnant, consult with your health care provider.
- Take special precautions to maintain your fluid intake and provide safety precautions in any situation that might cause a loss of fluid volume—excessive perspiration, dehydration, vomiting, diarrhea—excessive hypotension can occur.
- These side effects may occur: dizziness (avoid driving a car or performing hazardous tasks); headache (medications may be available to help); nausea, vomiting, diarrhea (proper nutrition is important, consult with your dietitian to maintain nutrition); symptoms of upper respiratory tract, cough (do not self-medicate, consult with your nurse or physician if this becomes uncomfortable).
- Report fever, chills, dizziness, pregnancy, swelling.

▽olsalazine sodium
*(ole **sal'** a zeen)*

Dipentum

PREGNANCY CATEGORY C

Drug class
Anti-inflammatory agent

Therapeutic actions
Mechanism of action is unknown; thought to be a direct, local anti-inflammatory effect in the colon where olsalazine is converted to mesalamine (5-ASA), which blocks cyclooxygenase and inhibits prostaglandin production in the colon.

Indications
- Maintenance of remission of ulcerative colitis in patients intolerant of sulfasalazine

Contraindications and cautions
- Contraindicated with hypersensitivity to salicylates, pregnancy (fetal abnormalities).
- Use cautiously with lactation.

Available forms
Capsules—250 mg

Dosages
Adults
1 g/day PO in two divided doses.
Pediatric patients
Safety and efficacy not established.

Pharmacokinetics

Route	Onset	Peak
Oral	Varies	60 min

Metabolism: Hepatic; $T_{1/2}$: 0.9 hr
Distribution: Crosses placenta; may enter breast milk
Excretion: Feces and urine

Adverse effects
- **CNS:** *Headache, fatigue, malaise, depression,* dizziness, asthenia, insomnia
- **GI:** *Abdominal pain, cramps, discomfort; gas; flatulence; nausea; diarrhea, dyspepsia,* bloating, hemmorhoids, rectal pain, constipation
- **Other:** *Flulike symptoms, rash,* fever, cold, back pain, hair loss, peripheral edema, *arthralgia*

■ Nursing considerations
Assessment
- **History:** Hypersensitivity to salicylates, pregnancy, lactation
- **Physical:** T, hair status; reflexes, affect; abdominal and rectal exam; urinary output, renal function tests

Interventions
- Administer with meals in evenly divided doses.
- Monitor patients with renal impairment for possible adverse effects.

Teaching points
- Take the drug with meals in evenly divided doses.

Adverse effects in *Italics* are most common; those in **Bold** are life-threatening.

- These side effects may occur: abdominal cramping, discomfort, pain, diarrhea (take with meals); headache, fatigue, fever, flu-like symptoms (request medications); rash, itching (skin care may help).
- Report severe diarrhea, malaise, fatigue, fever, blood in the stool.

▽ omeprazole
(oh me' pray zol)

Losec (CAN), Prilosec

PREGNANCY CATEGORY C

Drug classes
Antisecretory agent
Proton pump inhibitor

Therapeutic actions
Gastric acid-pump inhibitor: suppresses gastric acid secretion by specific inhibition of the hydrogen/potassium ATPase enzyme system at the secretory surface of the gastric parietal cells; blocks the final step of acid production.

Indications
- Short-term treatment of active duodenal ulcer
- First-line therapy in treatment of heartburn or symptoms of gastroesophageal reflux disease (GERD)
- Short-term treatment of active benign gastric ulcer
- GERD, severe erosive esophagitis, poorly responsive symptomatic GERD
- Treatment of pathologic hypersecretory conditions (Zollinger-Ellison syndrome, multiple adenomas, systemic mastocytosis) (long-term therapy)
- Eradication of *H. pylori* with amoxicillin or metronidazole and clarithromycin
- Unlabeled use: posterior laryngitis; enhance efficacy of pancreatin for the treatment of steatorrhea in cystic fibrosis

Contraindications and cautions
- Contraindicated with hypersensitivity to omeprazole or its components.
- Use cautiously with pregnancy, lactation.

Available forms
DR capsules—10, 20, 40 mg

Dosages
Adults
- *Active duodenal ulcer:* 20 mg PO daily for 4–8 wk. Should not be used for maintenance therapy.
- *Active gastric ulcer:* 40 mg PO daily for 4–8 wk.
- *Severe erosive esophagitis or poorly responsive GERD:* 20 mg PO daily for 4–8 wk. Do not use as maintenance therapy. An additional 4–8 wk course can be considered if needed.
- *Pathologic hypersecretory conditions:* Individualize dosage. Initial dose is 60 mg PO daily. Doses up to 120 mg tid have been used. Administer daily doses of > 80 mg in divided doses.

Pediatric patients
Safety and efficacy not established.

Pharmacokinetics

Route	Onset	Peak
Oral	Varies	0.5–3.5 hr

Metabolism: Hepatic; $T_{1/2}$: 0.5–1 hr
Distribution: Crosses placenta; may enter breast milk
Excretion: Urine and bile

Adverse effects
- **CNS:** *Headache, dizziness,* asthenia, vertigo, insomnia, apathy, anxiety, paresthesias, dream abnormalities
- **Dermatologic:** Rash, inflammation, urticaria, pruritus, alopecia, dry skin
- **GI:** *Diarrhea, abdominal pain, nausea, vomiting,* constipation, dry mouth, tongue atrophy
- **Respiratory:** *URI symptoms,* cough, epistaxis
- **Other:** Cancer in preclinical studies, back pain, fever

Interactions
✳ Drug-drug • Increased serum levels and potential increase in toxicity of benzodiazepines, phenytoin, warfarin; if these combinations are used, monitor patient very closely
- Decreased absorption with sucralfate; give these drugs at least 30 min apart

■ Nursing considerations
Assessment
- **History:** Hypersensitivity to omeprazole or any of its components; pregnancy, lactation
- **Physical:** Skin lesions; T; reflexes, affect; urinary output, abdominal exam; respiratory auscultation

Interventions
- Administer before meals. Caution patient to swallow capsules whole—not to open, chew, or crush.
- Arrange for further evaluation of patient after 8 wk of therapy for gastroreflux disorders; not intended for maintenance therapy. Symptomatic improvement does not rule out gastric cancer, which did occur in preclinical studies.
- Administer antacids with omeprazole, if needed.

Teaching points
- Take the drug before meals. Swallow the capsules whole; do not chew, open, or crush. This drug will need to be taken for up to 8 wk (short-term therapy) or for a prolonged period (> 5 yr in some cases).
- Have regular medical follow-ups.
- These side effects may occur: dizziness (avoid driving or performing hazardous tasks); headache (request medications); nausea, vomiting, diarrhea (maintain proper nutrition); symptoms of upper respiratory tract infection, cough (do not self-medicate; consult with your health care provider if uncomfortable).
- Report severe headache, worsening of symptoms, fever, chills.

▽ ondansetron hydrochloride
(on **dan'** sah tron)

Zofran, Zofran ODT

PREGNANCY CATEGORY B

Drug class
Antiemetic

Therapeutic actions
Blocks specific receptor sites (5-HT$_3$), which are associated with nausea and vomiting in the CTZ (chemoreceptor trigger zone) centrally and at specific sites peripherally. It is not known whether its antiemetic actions are from actions at the central, peripheral, or combined sites.

Indications
- Treatment of nausea and vomiting associated with emetogenic cancer chemotherapy (parenteral and oral)
- Treatment of postoperative nausea and vomiting—to prevent further episodes or, when postoperative nausea and vomiting must be avoided (oral), prophylactically (parenteral)
- Treatment of nausea and vomiting associated with radiotherapy
- Unlabeled uses: Treatment of nausea and vomiting associated with acetaminophen poisoning, prostacyclen therapy; treatment of acute levodopa-induced psychosis; reduction of episodes in bulimia nervosa; treatment of spinal or epidural morphine-induced pruritus

Contraindications and cautions
- Contraindicated with allergy to ondansetron.
- Use cautiously with pregnancy, lactation.

Available forms
Tablets—4, 8, 24 mg; orally disintegrating tablets—4, 8 mg; oral solution—4 mg/5 mL; injection—2 mg/mL, 32 mg/50 mL

Dosages
Adults
- *Antiemetic:*
Parenteral
Three 0.15 mg/kg doses IV: first dose is given over 15 min, beginning 30 min before the chemotherapy; subsequent doses are given at 4 and 8 hr, or a single 32-mg dose infused over 15 min beginning 30 min before the start of the chemotherapy.
Oral
8 mg PO tid; administer the first dose 30 min before beginning the chemotherapy and at 4 and 8 hr; continue q 12 hr for 1–2 days after the chemotherapy treatment; for radiotherapy, administer 1–2 hr before radiation.

Adverse effects in *Italics* are most common; those in **Bold** are life-threatening.

- *Prevention of nausea and vomiting associated with cancer chemotherapy:* 8 mg 30 min prior to chemotherapy, then 8 mg 8 hr later; give 8 mg q 12 hr for 1–2 days after completion of chemotherapy.
- *Prevention of postoperative nausea and vomiting:* 4 mg undiluted IV, preferably over 2–5 min, or as a single IM dose immediately prior to induction of anesthesia or 16 mg PO 1 hr before anesthesia.

Pediatric patients
- *Antiemetic:*
< 4 yr: Safety and efficacy not established.
4–12 yr: 4 mg PO 30 min prior to chemotherapy, 4 mg at 4 and 8 hr, then 4 mg PO tid for 1–2 days after completion of chemotherapy.
4–18 yr: IV dose same as adult.
- *Prevention of postoperative nausea and vomiting:* Safety and efficacy not established.
Patients with hepatic impairment
Maximum daily dose of 8 mg IV or PO.

Pharmacokinetics

Route	Onset	Peak
Oral	30–60 min	1.7–2.2 hr
IV	Immediate	Immediate

Metabolism: Hepatic; $T_{1/2}$: 3.5–6 hr
Distribution: Crosses placenta; may enter breast milk
Excretion: Urine

▽IV facts
Preparation: Dilute in 50 mL of 5% dextrose injection or 0.9% sodium chloride injection; stable for 48 hr at room temperature after dilution.
Infusion: Infuse slowly over 15 min diluted or 2–5 min undiluted.
Compatibilities: May be diluted with 0.9% sodium chloride injection, 5% dextrose injection, 5% dextrose and 0.9% sodium chloride injection; 5% dextrose and 0.45% sodium chloride injection; 3% sodium chloride injection.
Incompatibilities: Do not mix with alkaline solutions.

Adverse effects
- **CNS:** *Headache, dizziness,* drowsiness, shivers, malaise, fatigue, weakness, *myalgia*
- **CV:** Chest pain, hypotension
- **Dermatologic:** Pruritus
- **GI:** Abdominal pain, constipation
- **GU:** Urinary retention

- **Local:** Pain at injection site

Interactions
✳ **Drug-food** • Increased extent of absorption if taken orally with food

■ Nursing considerations
Assessment
- **History:** Allergy to ondansetron, pregnancy, lactation, nausea and vomiting
- **Physical:** Skin color and texture; orientation, reflexes, bilateral grip strength, affect; P, BP; abdominal exam; urinary output

Interventions
- Ensure that the timing of drug doses corresponds to that of the chemotherapy or radiation.
- Administer oral drug for 1–2 days following completion of chemotherapy or radiation.

Teaching points
- Take oral drug for 1–2 days following chemotherapy or radiation therapy to maximize prevention of nausea and vomiting. Take the drug every 8 hr around the clock for best results.
- These side effects may occur: weakness, dizziness (change position slowly to avoid injury); dizziness, drowsiness (do not drive or perform tasks that require alertness).
- Report continued nausea and vomiting, pain at injection site, chest pain, palpitations.

▷ **opium preparations**
(ob' pee um)

Camphorated tincture:
Paregoric
Deodorized tincture:
Opium Tincture, Deodorized

PREGNANCY CATEGORY C

C-III CONTROLLED SUBSTANCE
(PAREGORIC)

C-II CONTROLLED SUBSTANCE
(OPIUM TINCTURE, DEODORIZED)

Drug classes
Narcotic agonist analgesic
Antidiarrheal agent

Therapeutic actions

Activity is primarily due to morphine content; acts as agonist at specific opioid receptors in the CNS to produce analgesia, euphoria, sedation; the receptors mediating these effects are thought to be the same as those mediating the effects of endogenous opioids (enkephalins, endorphins); inhibits peristalsis and diarrhea by producing spasm of GI tract smooth muscle.

Indications

- Antidiarrheal
- Disorders requiring the analgesic, sedative or hypnotic, narcotic, or opiate effect
- For relief of severe pain in place of morphine (not a drug of choice)
- Unlabeled uses: neonatal abstinence syndrome, management of short bowel syndrome

Contraindications and cautions

- Contraindicated with hypersensitivity to narcotics, diarrhea caused by poisoning (before toxins are eliminated), pregnancy, labor or delivery (narcotics given to mother can cause respiratory depression of neonate; premature infants are at special risk; may prolong labor), bronchial asthma, COPD, cor pulmonale, respiratory depression, anoxia, kyphoscoliosis, acute alcoholism, increased intracranial pressure.
- Use cautiously with acute abdominal conditions, CV disease, supraventricular tachycardias, myxedema, convulsive disorders, delirium tremens, cerebral arteriosclerosis, ulcerative colitis, fever, Addison's disease, prostatic hypertrophy, urethral stricture, recent GI or GU surgery, toxic psychosis, renal or hepatic dysfunction.

Available forms

Liquid—2 mg morphine equivalent/5 mL (*Paregoric*); 10% (*Opium Tincture, Deodorized*)

Dosages

Caution: *Opium Tincture, Deodorized* contains 25 times more morphine than *Paregoric*. Do not confuse dosage—severe toxicity can occur.

Adults
Paregoric
5–10 mL PO daily–qid (5 mL is equivalent to 2 mg morphine).
Opium Tincture, Deodorized
0.6 mL qid.
Pediatric patients
Contraindicated in premature infants.
Paregoric
0.25–0.5 mL/kg PO daily–qid.
Geriatric patients or impaired adults
Use caution; respiratory depression may occur in the elderly, the very ill, those with respiratory problems. Reduced dosage may be necessary.

Pharmacokinetics

Route	Onset	Peak	Duration
Oral	Varies	0.5–1 hr	3–7 hr

Metabolism: Hepatic; $T_{1/2}$: 1.5–2 hr
Distribution: Crosses placenta; enters breast milk
Excretion: Urine

Adverse effects

- **CNS:** *Light-headedness, dizziness, sedation,* euphoria, dysphoria, delirium, insomnia, agitation, anxiety, fear, hallucinations, disorientation, drowsiness, lethargy, impaired mental and physical performance, coma, mood changes, weakness, headache, tremor, convulsions, miosis, visual disturbances
- **CV:** Facial flushing, peripheral circulatory collapse, tachycardia, bradycardia, arrhythmia, palpitations, chest wall rigidity, hypertension, hypotension, orthostatic hypotension, syncope, circulatory depression, **shock, cardiac arrest**
- **Dermatologic:** Pruritus, urticaria, edema, hemorrhagic urticaria (rare)
- **GI:** *Nausea, vomiting, sweating,* dry mouth, anorexia, constipation, biliary tract spasm; increased colonic motility with chronic ulcerative colitis
- **GU:** Ureteral spasm, spasm of vesical sphincters, urinary retention or hesitancy, oliguria, antidiuretic effect, reduced libido or potency

- **Respiratory:** Suppression of cough reflex, respiratory depression, apnea, **respiratory arrest,** laryngospasm, bronchospasm
- **Other:** Physical tolerance and dependence, psychological dependence

Interactions
✴ Drug-drug • Increased likelihood of respiratory depression, hypotension, profound sedation or coma with barbiturate general anesthetics

✴ Drug-lab test • Elevated biliary tract pressure may cause increases in plasma amylase, lipase determinations 24 hr after administration

■ Nursing considerations
Assessment
- **History:** Hypersensitivity to narcotics, diarrhea caused by poisoning, bronchial asthma, COPD, cor pulmonale, respiratory depression, kyphoscoliosis, acute alcoholism, increased intracranial pressure, acute abdominal conditions, CV disease, supraventricular tachycardias, myxedema, convulsive disorders, delirium tremens, cerebral arteriosclerosis, ulcerative colitis, fever, Addison's disease, prostatic hypertrophy, urethral stricture, recent GI or GU surgery, toxic psychosis, renal or hepatic dysfunction
- **Physical:** T; skin color, texture, lesions; orientation, reflexes, bilateral grip strength, affect, pupil size; P, auscultation, BP, orthostatic BP, perfusion; R, adventitious sounds; bowel sounds, normal output; frequency and pattern of voiding, normal output; thyroid, liver, kidney function tests

Interventions
- Give to lactating women 4–6 hr before the next feeding to minimize the amount in milk.
- Reassure patient about addiction liability; most patients who receive opiates for medical reasons do not develop dependence syndromes.

Teaching points
- Take this drug exactly as prescribed.
- These side effects may occur: nausea, loss of appetite (take with food and lie quietly; eating frequent, small meals may help); con-

stipation (a laxative may help); dizziness, sedation, drowsiness, impaired visual acuity (avoid driving, performing other tasks that require alertness, visual acuity).
- Do not take leftover medication for other disorders, and do not let anyone else take the prescription.
- Report severe nausea, vomiting, constipation, shortness of breath, or difficulty breathing.

▽ **oprelvekin**
See *Less Commonly Used Drugs,* p. 1348.

▽ **orlistat**
(ore' lab stat)

Xenical

PREGNANCY CATEGORY B

Drug classes
Weight loss agent
Lipase inhibitor

Therapeutic actions
Synthetic derivative of lipostatin, a naturally occurring lipase inhibitor or so-called fat blocker. Binds to gastric and pancreatic lipase to prevent the digestion of fats. When taken with fat-containing foods, the fat passes through the intestines unchanged and is not absorbed.

Indications
- Treatment of obesity as part of weight loss program

Contraindications and cautions
- Contraindicated with hypersensitivity to orlistat; pregnancy, lactation.
- Use cautiously with impaired hepatic function, biliary obstruction, pancreatic disease.

Available forms
Capsules—120 mg

Dosages
Adults
120 mg tid PO with meals.

Pediatric patients
Safety and efficacy not established.

Pharmacokinetics
Not absorbed systemically

Adverse effects
- **Dermatologic:** *Rash, dry skin*
- **GI:** *Dry mouth,* nausea, flatulence, *loose stools,* oily stools, fecal incontinence or urgency
- **Other:** Vitamin deficiency of fat-soluble vitamins (A, D, E, K)

Interactions
❋ **Drug-drug** ● Decreased absorption of fat-soluble vitamins ● Additive lipid-lowering effects with pravastatin; monitor patient response ● Increased risk of bleeding related to decreased vitamin K; when taking with oral anticoagulants, monitor patient closely

■ Nursing considerations
Assessment
- **History:** Hypersensitivity to orlistat; impaired hepatic or pancreatic function; pregnancy, biliary obstruction, lactation
- **Physical:** Weight, temperature, skin—rash, lesions; liver evaluation; liver function tests

Interventions
- Ensure that patient is participating in a weight-loss diet and exercise program.
- Administer with meals.
- Arrange for administration of fat-soluble vitamins. Do not administer with orlistat; separate doses.
- Provide sugarless lozenges, frequent mouth care if dry mouth is a problem.
- Ensure ready access to bathroom facilities if diarrhea occurs.
- Counsel patient about the use of barrier contraceptives while on this drug; pregnancy should be avoided because of the possible risk to the fetus.

Teaching points
- Take this drug with meals.
- You may need to take a vitamin supplement while you are on this drug. Take the supplement at least 2 hr before or after orlistat.
- These side effects may occur: dry mouth (sucking sugarless lozenges and frequent mouth care may help); nausea, loose stools, flatulence (ensure ready access to bathroom facilities, this may pass in time).
- Do not take this drug during pregnancy. If you think that you are pregnant, or wish to become pregnant, consult with your health care provider.
- Report rash, glossy tongue, vision changes, bruising, changes in stool or urine color.

▷ orphenadrine citrate
(or fen′ a dreen)

Banflex, Flexoject, Flexon, Norflex, Orfenate (CAN)

PREGNANCY CATEGORY C

Drug classes
Skeletal muscle relaxant, centrally acting

Therapeutic actions
Precise mechanisms not known; acts in the CNS; does not directly relax tense skeletal muscles; does not directly affect the motor endplate or motor nerves.

Indications
- Relief of discomfort associated with acute, painful musculoskeletal conditions; as an adjunct to rest, physical therapy, and other measures
- Unlabeled use: 100 mg hs for the treatment of quinidine-resistant leg cramps

Contraindications and cautions
- Contraindicated with hypersensitivity to orphenadrine; glaucoma; pyloric or duodenal obstruction; stenosing peptic ulcers; achalasia; cardiospasm (megaesophagus); prostatic hypertrophy; obstruction of bladder neck; myasthenia gravis; lactation.
- Use cautiously with cardiac decompensation, coronary insufficiency, cardiac arrhythmias, hepatic or renal dysfunction, pregnancy.

Available forms

SR tablets—100 mg; injection—30 mg/mL

Dosages
Adults
60 mg IV or IM. May repeat q 12 h. Inject IV over 5 min. Alternatively, give 100 mg PO every morning and evening.
Pediatric patients
Safety and efficacy not established; not recommended.
Geriatric patients
Use caution and regulate dosage carefully; patients older than 60 yr frequently develop increased sensitivity to adverse CNS effects of anticholinergic drugs.

Pharmacokinetics

Route	Onset	Peak	Duration
IM, IV	Rapid	2 hr	4–6 hr
Oral	–	2 hr	4–6 hr

Metabolism: Hepatic; $T_{1/2}$: 14 hr
Distribution: Crosses placenta; enters breast milk
Excretion: Urine and feces

▼IV facts
Preparation: No further preparation is required.
Infusion: Administer slowly IV, each 60 mg over 5 min.

Adverse effects
- **CNS:** *Weakness, headache, dizziness, confusion* (especially in elderly), hallucinations, drowsiness, memory loss, psychosis, agitation, nervousness, delusions, delirium, paranoia, euphoria, depression, paresthesia, blurred vision, pupil dilation, increased intraocular tension
- **CV:** *Tachycardia,* palpitation, transient syncope, hypotension, orthostatic hypotension
- **Dermatologic:** Urticaria, other dermatoses
- **GI:** *Dry mouth, gastric irritation, vomiting, nausea, constipation,* dilation of the colon, paralytic ileus
- **GU:** *Urinary hesitancy and retention,* dysuria, difficulty achieving or maintaining an erection

- **Other:** *Flushing, decreased sweating,* elevated temperature, muscle weakness, cramping

Interactions
✻ Drug-drug • Additive anticholinergic effects with other anticholinergic drugs • Additive adverse CNS effects with phenothiazines • Possible masking of the development of persistent extrapyramidal symptoms, tardive dyskinesia in long-term therapy with phenothiazines, halperidol

■ Nursing considerations
Assessment
- **History:** Hypersensitivity to orphenadrine; glaucoma; pyloric or duodenal obstruction; stenosing peptic ulcers; achalasia; cardiospasm; prostatic hypertrophy; obstruction of bladder neck; myasthenia gravis; cardiac, hepatic, or renal dysfunction; lactation, pregnancy
- **Physical:** Weight; T; skin color, lesions; orientation, affect, reflexes, bilateral grip strength, vision exam with tonometry; P, BP, orthostatic BP, auscultation; bowel sounds, normal output, liver evaluation; prostate palpation, normal output, voiding pattern; urinalysis, CBC with differential, liver and renal function tests, ECG

Interventions
- Ensure that patient is supine during IV injection and for at least 15 min thereafter; assist patient from the supine position after treatment.
- Ensure that patients swallow SR tablets whole; do not cut, crush, or chew.
- Decrease or discontinue drug temporarily if dry mouth is so severe that swallowing or speaking becomes difficult.
- Give with caution, reduce dosage in hot weather; drug interferes with sweating and body's ability to thermoregulate in hot environments.
- Arrange for analgesics if headache occurs (adjunct for relief of muscle spasm).

Teaching points
- Swallow SR tablets whole; do not cut, crush, or chew.

- Do not use alcohol while on this drug.
- These side effects may occur: drowsiness, dizziness, blurred vision (avoid driving or engaging in activities that require alertness and visual acuity); dry mouth (sucking on sugarless lozenges or ice chips may help); nausea (frequent, small meals may help); difficulty urinating (be sure that you empty the bladder just before taking the medication); constipation (increase fluid and fiber intake and exercise regularly); headache (request medication).
- Report dry mouth, difficult urination, constipation, headache, or GI upset that persists; rash or itching; rapid heart rate or palpitations; mental confusion; eye pain; fever; sore throat; bruising.

▽ oseltamivir phosphate
*(oz el **tam' ah** ver)*

Tamiflu

PREGNANCY CATEGORY C

Drug classes
Antiviral drug
Neuroaminidase inhibitor

Therapeutic action
Selectively inhibits influenza virus neuroaminidase; by blocking the actions of this enzyme, there is decreased viral release from infected cells, increased formation of viral aggregates, and decreased spread of the virus.

Indications
- Treatment of uncomplicated acute illness due to influenza virus (A or B) in adults and children > 1 yr who have been symptomatic for ≤ 2 days.
- Prevention of naturally occurring influenza A and B in adults and children ≥ 13 yr in close contact with the flu.

Contraindications and cautions
- Contraindicated with allergy to any component of the drug.

- Use cautiously with pregnancy, lactation, asthma, COPD.

Available forms
Capsules—75 mg; powder for oral suspension—12 mg/mL

Dosages
Adults and patients ≥ 13 yr
- *Treatment:* 75 mg PO bid for 5 days, starting within 2 days of the onset of symptoms.
- *Prevention:* 75 mg/day PO for ≥ 7 days; begin treatment within 2 days of exposure.

Pediatric patients 1–12 yr
- *Treatment:* 30–75 mg PO bid for 5 days based on weight—use solution.
- *Prevention:* Not recommended.

Patients with renal impairment
Creatinine clearance < 30 mL/min: 75 mg/day PO for 5 days.

Pharmacokinetics

Route	Onset	Peak
Oral	Varies	2.5–6 hr

Metabolism: Hepatic; $T_{1/2}$: 6–10 hr
Distribution: Crosses placenta; may pass into breast milk
Excretion: Urine

Adverse effects
- **CNS:** *Headache,* dizziness
- **GI:** *Nausea,* vomiting, *diarrhea, anorexia*
- **Respiratory:** Cough, *rhinitis,* bronchitis

■ Nursing considerations
Assessment
- **History:** Allergy to any components of the drug; COPD, asthma, pregnancy, lactation
- **Physical:** T; orientation, reflexes; R, adventitious sounds; bowel sounds

Interventions
- Administer within 2 days of the onset of flu symptoms.
- Encourage patient to complete full 5-day course of therapy; advise patient that treatment does not decrease the risk of transmission of the flu to others.

Adverse effects in *Italics* are most common; those in **Bold** are life-threatening.

- Start dosage for prevention within 2 days of exposure and continue for 7 days.
- Prepare solution by adding 52 mL of water to bottle containing powder; shake well for 15 sec. Shake solution well before each dose.

Teaching points

- Take the full course of therapy as prescribed; be advised that this drug does not decrease the risk of transmitting the virus to others.
- Shake solution well before each use; store in refrigerator.
- These side effects may occur: nausea, vomiting, loss of appetite, diarrhea; headache, dizziness (use caution if driving an automobile or operating dangerous machinery).
- Report severe diarrhea, severe nausea, worsening of respiratory symptoms.

▷oxacillin sodium
*(ox a **sill'** in)*

Bactocill

PREGNANCY CATEGORY B

Drug classes
Antibiotic
Penicillinase-resistant penicillin

Therapeutic actions
Bactericidal: inhibits cell wall synthesis of sensitive organisms, causing cell death.

Indications
- Infections due to penicillinase-producing staphylococci

Contraindications and cautions
- Contraindicated with allergies to penicillins, cephalosporins, or other allergens.
- Use cautiously with renal disorders, pregnancy, lactation (may cause diarrhea or candidiasis in infants).

Available forms
Powder for injection—250, 500 mg; 1, 2, 4, 10 g; capsules—250, 500 mg; powder for oral solution—250 mg/5 mL

Dosages
Maximum recommended dosage is 6 g/day.
Adults
PO
500 mg q 4–6 hr PO for at least 5 days. Follow-up therapy after parenteral oxacillin in severe infections: 1 g q 4–6 hr PO for up to 1–2 wk.
Parenteral
250–500 mg q 4–6 hr IM or IV. Up to 2 g q 4–6 hr in severe infections.
Pediatric patients ≥ 40 kg
Use adult dose.
Pediatric patients < 40 kg
PO
12.5–25 mg/kg/dose q 6 hr.
Parenteral
- *Bacterial meningitis: Neonates < 2 kg:* 25–50 mg/kg/dose IV or IM q 12 hr during first week of life, then 50 mg/kg/dose q 8 hr IV or IM thereafter. *Neonates ≥ 2 kg:* 50 mg/kg/dose q 8 hr IV or IM during first wk of life, then 50 mg/kg/dose q 6 hr IV or IM thereafter.
- *All other infections: Premature infants and neonates:* 6.25 mg q 6 hr IV or IM. *Children < 40 kg:* 12.5–25 mg/kg/dose q 6 hr IV or IM or 16.7 mg/kg q 4 hr. *Children ≥ 40 kg:* Use adult dose.

Pharmacokinetics

Route	Onset	Peak	Duration
Oral	Varies	30–60 min	4 hr
IM	Rapid	30–60 min	4–6 hr
IV	Rapid	15 min	Length of infusion

Metabolism: Hepatic; $T_{1/2}$: 0.5–1 hr
Distribution: Crosses placenta; enters breast milk
Excretion: Urine and bile

▼IV facts
Preparation: Dilute for direct IV administration to a maximum concentration of 1 g/10 mL using sodium chloride injection or sterile water for injection. For IV infusion: reconstituted solution may be diluted with compatible IV solution: 0.9% sodium chloride injection, 5% dextrose in water or in normal saline, 10% D-fructose in water or in normal saline, lactated Ringer's solution, lactated potassic saline injections, 10% invert sugar in

water or in normal saline, 10% invert sugar plus 0.3% potassium chloride in water, *Travert 10% Electrolyte 1, 2, or 3*. 0.5–40 mg/mL solutions are stable for up to 12 hr at room temperature. Discard after that time.

Infusion: Give by direct administration slowly to avoid vein irritation, each 1 g over 10 min; infusion—up to 6 hr.

Incompatibilities: Do not mix in the same IV solution as other antibiotics.

Adverse effects
- **CNS:** Lethargy, hallucinations, **seizures**
- **GI:** *Glossitis, stomatitis, gastritis, sore mouth,* "furry" or black "hairy" tongue, *nausea, vomiting, diarrhea,* abdominal pain, bloody diarrhea, enterocolitis, pseudomembranous colitis, nonspecific hepatitis
- **GU:** Nephritis—oliguria, proteinuria, hematuria, casts, azotemia, pyuria
- **Hematologic:** Anemia, thrombocytopenia, leukopenia, neutropenia, prolonged bleeding time (more common than with other penicillinase-resistant penicillins)
- **Hypersensitivity:** *Rash, fever, wheezing,* **anaphylaxis**
- **Local:** *Pain, phlebitis,* thrombosis at injection site
- **Other:** *Superinfections,* sodium overload leading to CHF

Interactions
✱ **Drug-drug** • Decreased effectiveness with tetracyclines • Inactivation of aminoglycosides in parenteral solutions with oxacillin

✱ **Drug-lab test** • False-positive Coombs' test with IV oxacillin

■ Nursing considerations
Assessment
- **History:** Allergies to penicillins, cephalosporins, or other allergens; renal disorders; pregnancy; lactation
- **Physical:** Culture infection; skin color, lesions; R, adventitious sounds; bowel sounds; CBC, liver and renal function tests, serum electrolytes, Hct, urinalysis

Interventions
- Culture infection before treatment; reculture if response is not as expected.

- Continue therapy for at least 2 days after infection has disappeared, usually 7–10 days.
- Reconstitute for IM use to a dilution of 250 mg/1.5 mL using sterile water for injection or sodium chloride injection. Discard after 3 days at room temperature or after 7 days if refrigerated.
- Maintain epinephrine, IV fluids, vasopressors, bronchodilators, oxygen, and emergency equipment on standby in case of serious hypersensitivity reaction.

Teaching points
- These side effects may occur: upset stomach, nausea, diarrhea (small, frequent meals may help), mouth sores (frequent mouth care may help), pain at the injection site.
- Report difficulty breathing, rashes, severe diarrhea, severe pain at injection site, mouth sores.

▷ **oxaliplatin**

See *Less Commonly Used Drugs*, p. 1348.

▷ **oxandrolone**
*(ox **an'** droh lone)*

Oxandrin

PREGNANCY CATEGORY X

C-III CONTROLLED SUBSTANCE

Drug classes
Anabolic steroid
Hormone

Therapeutic actions
Testosterone analog with androgenic and anabolic activity; promotes body tissue-building processes; reverses catabolic or tissue-depleting processes; increases Hgb and red cell mass.

Indications
- Adjunctive therapy to promote weight gain after weight loss following extensive surgery, chronic infections, trauma
- Offset protein catabolism associated with prolonged use of corticosteroids

---

Adverse effects in *Italics* are most common; those in **Bold** are life-threatening.

- Orphan drug uses: short stature associated with Turner syndrome, HIV wasting syndrome, and HIV-associated muscle weakness
- Unlabeled use: alcoholic hepatitis

Contraindications and cautions

- Known sensitivity to anabolic steroids; prostate, breast cancer; benign prostatic hypertrophy; pituitary insufficiency; MI (contraindicated because of effects on cholesterol); nephrosis; liver disease; hypercalcemia; pregnancy, lactation.

Available forms

Tablets—2.5 mg

Dosages
Adults
2.5 mg PO bid–qid: up to 20 mg has been used to achieve the desired effect; 2–4 wk needed to evaluate response.
Pediatric patients
Total daily dose of < 0.1 mg/kg or < 0.045 mg/lb PO; may be repeated intermittently.

Pharmacokinetics

Route	Onset
Oral	Slow

Metabolism: Hepatic; $T_{1/2}$: 9 hr
Distribution: Crosses placenta; enters breast milk
Excretion: Urine

Adverse effects

- **CNS:** *Excitation, insomnia,* chills, toxic confusion
- **Endocrine:** *Virilization: prepubertal males*—phallic enlargement, hirsutism, increased skin pigmentation; *postpubertal males*—inhibition of testicular function, gynecomastia, testicular atrophy, priapism, baldness, epididymitis, change in libido; *females*—hirsutism, hoarseness, deepening of the voice, clitoral enlargement, menstrual irregularities, baldness; decreased glucose tolerance
- **GI:** Hepatotoxicity, peliosis, **hepatitis** with **liver failure or intra-abdominal hemorrhage; liver cell tumors,** sometimes malignant, *nausea, vomiting, diarrhea, abdominal fullness, loss of appetite, burning of tongue*

- **GU:** Possible increased risk of prostatic hypertrophy, carcinoma in geriatric patients
- **Hematologic:** *Blood lipid changes;* iron deficiency anemia, hypercalcemia, altered serum cholesterol levels; *retention of sodium, chloride, water,* potassium, phosphates and calcium
- **Other:** *Acne,* premature closure of the epiphyses

Interactions

✹ **Drug-drug** • Potentiation of oral anticoagulants with anabolic steroids • Decreased need for insulin, oral hypoglycemia agents with anabolic steroids

✹ **Drug-lab test** • Altered glucose tolerance tests • Decrease in thyroid function tests (may persist for 2–3 wk after stopping therapy) • Increased creatinine, creatinine clearance, which may last for 2 wk after therapy

■ Nursing considerations
Assessment

- **History:** Sensitivity to anabolic steroids; prostate or breast cancer; benign prostatic hypertrophy; pituitary insufficiency; MI; nephrosis; liver disease; hypercalcemia; pregnancy; lactation
- **Physical:** Skin color, texture; hair distribution pattern; affect, orientation; abdominal exam, liver evaluation; serum electrolytes and cholesterol levels, glucose tolerance tests, thyroid function tests, long-bone x-ray (in children)

Interventions

- Administer with food if GI upset or nausea occurs.
- Monitor effect on children with long-bone x-rays every 3–6 mo; discontinue drug well before the bone age reaches the norm for the patient's chronologic age because effects may continue for 6 mo after therapy.
- Ensure that women of childbearing age are not pregnant and understand the need to use contraceptive measures to prevent pregnancy.
- Monitor patient for occurrence of edema; arrange for diuretic therapy.
- Monitor liver function, serum electrolytes periodically and consult with physician for corrective measures.

- Measure cholesterol levels periodically in patients who are at high risk for CAD.
- Monitor diabetic patients closely because glucose tolerance may change. Adjustments may be needed in insulin, oral hypoglycemic dosage, and diet.

Teaching points

- Take drug with food if nausea or GI upset occurs.
- These side effects may occur: nausea, vomiting, diarrhea, burning of the tongue (eat small, frequent meals); body hair growth, baldness, deepening of the voice, decrease in libido, impotence (most reversible); excitation, confusion, insomnia (avoid driving, performing tasks that require alertness); swelling of the ankles, fingers (request medication).
- Diabetic patients need to monitor urine or blood sugar closely because glucose tolerance may change; report any abnormalities to physician for corrective action.
- These drugs do not enhance athletic ability but do have serious effects. They should not be used for increasing muscle strength.
- This drug cannot be taken during pregnancy; serious adverse effects can occur. Use of barrier contraceptives is advised.
- Report ankle swelling, skin color changes, severe nausea, vomiting, hoarseness, body hair growth, deepening of the voice, acne, menstrual irregularities.

▽ oxaprozin
(oks a pro' zin)

Daypro

PREGNANCY CATEGORY C

Drug classes

Analgesic (non-narcotic)
Antipyretic
Nonsteroidal anti-inflammatory drug (NSAID)

Therapeutic actions

Inhibits prostaglandin synthetase to cause antipyretic and anti-inflammatory effects; the exact mechanism of action is not known.

Indications

- Acute or long-term use in the management of signs and symptoms of osteoarthritis and rheumatoid arthritis

Contraindications and cautions

- Contraindicated with significant renal impairment, pregnancy, lactation.
- Use cautiously with impaired hearing, allergies, hepatic, CV, and GI conditions.

Available forms

Tablets—600 mg

Dosages

Adjust to the lowest effective dose to minimize side effects. Maximum daily dose: 1,800 mg or 26 mg/kg, whichever is lower.
Adults
- *Osteoarthritis:* 1,200 mg PO daily; use initial dose of 600 mg with low body weight or milder disease.
- *Rheumatoid arthritis:* 1,200 mg PO daily.
Pediatric patients
Safety and efficacy not established.

Pharmacokinetics

Route	Onset	Peak	Duration
Oral	Varies	3–5 hr	24–36 hr

Metabolism: Hepatic; $T_{1/2}$: 42–50 hr
Distribution: Crosses placenta; enters breast milk
Excretion: Urine and feces

Adverse effects

- **CNS:** Dizziness, somnolence, insomnia, fatigue, tiredness, dizziness, tinnitus, ophthalmic effects
- **Dermatologic:** Rash, pruritus, sweating, dry mucous membranes, stomatitis
- **GI:** *Nausea, dyspepsia,* GI pain, *diarrhea,* vomiting, *constipation,* flatulence
- **GU:** Dysuria, renal impairment
- **Hematologic:** Bleeding, platelet inhibition with higher doses
- **Other:** Peripheral edema, **anaphylactoid reactions to anaphylactic shock**

Adverse effects in *Italics* are most common; those in **Bold** are life-threatening.

■ Nursing considerations
Assessment
- **History:** Renal impairment; impaired hearing; allergies; hepatic, CV, and GI conditions; lactation, pregnancy
- **Physical:** Skin color and lesions; orientation, reflexes, ophthalmologic and audiometric evaluation; peripheral sensation; P, edema; R, adventitious sounds; liver evaluation; CBC, clotting times, renal and liver function tests; serum electrolytes, stool guaiac

Interventions
- Administer drug with food or after meals if GI upset occurs.
- Arrange for periodic ophthalmologic examination during long-term therapy.
- Institute emergency procedures if overdose occurs (gastric lavage, induction of emesis, supportive therapy).

Teaching points
- Take drug with food or meals if GI upset occurs.
- Dizziness, drowsiness can occur (avoid driving or the use of dangerous machinery).
- Report sore throat, fever, rash, itching, weight gain, swelling in ankles or fingers, changes in vision, black tarry stools.

▽oxazepam
(ox a' ze pam)

Apo-Oxazepam (CAN), Novoxapam (CAN), Serax

PREGNANCY CATEGORY D

C-IV CONTROLLED SUBSTANCE

Drug classes
Benzodiazepine
Antianxiety agent

Therapeutic actions
Exact mechanisms not understood; acts mainly at subcortical levels of the CNS, leaving the cortex relatively unaffected; main sites of action may be the limbic system and reticular formation; benzodiazepines potentiate the effects of GABA, an inhibitory eurotransmitter; anxiolytic effects occur at doses well below those necessary to cause sedation, ataxia.

Indications
- Management of anxiety disorders or for short-term relief of symptoms of anxiety; anxiety associated with depression also is responsive
- Management of anxiety, tension, agitation, and irritability in older patients
- Alcoholics with acute tremulousness, inebriation, or anxiety associated with alcohol withdrawal

Contraindications and cautions
- Contraindicated with hypersensitivity to benzodiazepines, tartrazine (in the tablets); psychoses; acute narrow-angle glaucoma; shock; coma; acute alcoholic intoxication with depression of vital signs; pregnancy (risk of congenital malformations, neonatal withdrawal syndrome); labor and delivery ("floppy infant" syndrome); lactation (may cause infants to become lethargic and lose weight).
- Use cautiously with impaired liver or kidney function, debilitation.

Available forms
Capsules—10, 15, 30 mg; tablets—15 mg

Dosages
Increase dosage gradually to avoid adverse effects.
Adults
10–15 mg PO or up to 30 mg PO tid–qid, depending on severity of symptoms of anxiety. The higher dosage range is recommended in alcoholics.
Pediatric patients 6–12 yr
Dosage not established.
Geriatric patients or patients with debilitating disease
Initially 10 mg PO tid. Gradually increase to 15 mg PO tid–qid if needed and tolerated.

Pharmacokinetics

Route	Onset	Peak
Oral	Slow	2–4 hr

Metabolism: Hepatic; $T_{1/2}$: 5–20 hr
Distribution: Crosses placenta; enters breast milk
Excretion: Urine

Adverse effects

- **CNS:** *Transient, mild drowsiness* (initially), *sedation, depression, lethargy, apathy, fatigue, light-headedness, disorientation,* restlessness, confusion, crying, delirium, headache, slurred speech, dysarthria, stupor, rigidity, tremor, dystonia, vertigo, euphoria, nervousness, difficulty in concentration, vivid dreams, psychomotor retardation, extrapyramidal symptoms, mild paradoxical excitatory reactions during first 2 wk of treatment, visual and auditory disturbances, diplopia, nystagmus, depressed hearing
- **CV:** Bradycardia, tachycardia, **CV collapse,** hypertension and hypotension, palpitations, edema
- **Dermatologic:** Urticaria, pruritus, rash, dermatitis
- **GI:** *Constipation, diarrhea, dry mouth,* salivation, nausea, anorexia, vomiting, difficulty in swallowing, gastric disorders
- **GU:** *Incontinence, urinary retention,* changes in libido, menstrual irregularities
- **Hematologic:** Elevations of blood enzymes, hepatic dysfunction, blood dyscrasias: agranulocytosis, leukopenia
- **Other:** *Nasal congestion, hiccups, fever, diaphoresis,* paresthesias, muscular disturbances, gynecomastia, drug dependence with withdrawal syndrome when drug is discontinued: more common with abrupt discontinuation of higher dosage used for longer than 4 mo

Interactions

✳ **Drug-drug** ● Increased CNS depression with alcohol ● Decreased sedation when given to heavy smokers of cigarettes or if taken concurrently with theophyllines

■ Nursing considerations
Assessment

- **History:** Hypersensitivity to benzodiazepines, tartrazine; psychoses; acute narrow-angle glaucoma; shock; coma; acute alcoholic intoxication; pregnancy; labor and delivery; lactation; impaired liver or kidney function, debilitation
- **Physical:** Skin color, lesions; T; orientation, reflexes, affect, ophthalmologic exam; P, BP; R, adventitious sounds; liver evaluation, abdominal exam, bowel sounds, normal output; CBC, liver and renal function tests

Interventions

- Taper dosage gradually after long-term therapy, especially in epileptic patients.

Teaching points

- Take this drug exactly as prescribed; do not stop taking drug (long-term therapy) without consulting health care provider.
- These side effects may occur: drowsiness, dizziness (may lessen; avoid driving or engaging in other dangerous activities); GI upset (take with food); depression, dreams, emotional upset, crying.
- Report severe dizziness, weakness, drowsiness that persists, palpitations, swelling of the extremities, visual changes, difficulty voiding, rash or skin lesion.

▷**oxcarbazepine**
(oks car baz' e peen)

Trileptal

PREGNANCY CATEGORY C

Drug class
Antiepileptic

Therapeutic actions
Mechanism of action not understood; antiepileptic activity may be related to its ability to block voltage-sensitive sodium channels, increase potassium conductance, and affect high-voltage activated calcium channels, leading to enhanced membrane stability.

Indications

- As monotherapy or adjunct therapy in the treatment of partial seizures in adults
- Adjunct therapy in the treatment of partial seizures in children 4–16 yr
- Unlabeled use: atypical panic disorder

Contraindications and cautions
- Contraindicated with hypersensitivity to carbamazepine or oxcarbazepine; pregnancy and lactation.
- Use cautiously with the elderly and with hyponatremia, renal or hepatic dysfunction.

Available forms
Tablets—150, 300, 600 mg

Dosages
Adults
- *Adjunctive therapy:* 300 mg PO bid, may be increased to a total of 1,200 mg PO bid if clinically needed.
- *Conversion to monotherapy:* 300 mg PO bid started while reducing the dose of other antiepileptic drugs; other drugs should be reduced over 3–6 wks while increasing oxcarbazepine to the maximum dose of 2,400 mg/day (in divided doses)
- *Starting as monotherapy:* Start with 300 mg/day and increase by 300 mg/day every third day until the desired dose of 1,200 mg/day is reached. Some patients may benefit from doses as high as 2,400 mg/day, but should be carefully monitored.

Pediatric patients 4–16 yr
- *Adjunctive therapy:* 8–10 mg/kg/day PO given in 2 equally divided doses not to exceed 600 mg/day. Achieve the target dose over 2 wk. Suggested target dosages: 20–29 kg: 900 mg/day; 29.1–39 kg: 1,200 mg/day; > 39 kg: 1,800 mg/day.

Geriatric patients or patients with renal impairment
Use caution, drug may cause confusion, agitation. Creatinine clearance < 30 mL/min; initiate dosage at one-half the usual starting dose for the indication, increase slowly until desired clinical response is seen; monitor patient carefully.

Pharmacokinetics

Route	Onset	Peak
Oral	Slow	4–5 hr

Metabolism: Hepatic; $T_{1/2}$: 2 hr, then 9 hr
Distribution: Crosses placenta; passes into breast milk
Excretion: Urine and feces

Adverse effects
- **CNS:** *Dizziness, drowsiness, unsteadiness,* disturbance of coordination, confusion, headache, fatigue, visual hallucinations, depression with agitation, behavioral changes in children
- **CV:** *Hypotension, hypertension, bradycardia, tachycardia,* atrial fibrillation
- **GI:** *Nausea, vomiting,* gastric distress, abdominal pain, diarrhea, increased liver enzymes
- **GU:** *Impaired fertility,* hematuria, dysuria, priapism, renal calculi
- **Metabolic and nutritional:** Respiratory acidosis, hyperkalemia, *hyponatremia,* thirst
- **Respiratory: Pulmonary edema,** pleural effusion, hypoventilation, *hypoxia,* dyspnea, bronchospasm
- **Other:** Fever, hypovolemia, sweating, rigors, acne, alopecia

Interactions
✳ Drug-drug • Possible decreased oxcarbazepine effectiveness if combined with phenytoin, carbamazepine, phenobarbital, valproic acid, verapamil; if these combinations are used, monitor patient closely • Decreased effectiveness of felodipine if combined with oxcarbazepine • Decreased effectiveness of hormonal contraceptives if combined with oxcarbazepine; suggest the use of barrier contraceptives if this combination is used • Increased serum levels and risk of toxicity of phenytoin, phenobarbital; if this combination is used, monitor patient closely for signs of toxicity and arrange to decrease drug dosage as needed • Possible increased sedation if combined with alcohol; avoid this combination

■ Nursing considerations
Assessment
- **History:** Hypersensitivity to carbamazepine or oxcarbazepine; hyponatremia; renal or hepatic dysfunction; pregnancy, lactation
- **Physical:** T; skin color, lesions; orientation, affect, reflexes; P, BP, perfusion; ECG; R, adventitious sounds; bowel sounds, normal output; normal urinary output, voiding pattern; renal and hepatic function tests; serum sodium

Interventions

- Monitor serum sodium prior to and periodically during therapy with oxcarbazepine; serious hyponatremia can occur. Signs and symptoms of hyponatremia include nausea, malaise, headache, lethargy, confusion, and decreased sensation.
- Investigate if patient has a history of hypersensitivity to carbamazepine. Stop drug if signs or symptoms of hypersensitivity occur.
- Give drug with food or milk to prevent GI upset. Arrange for patient to have small, frequent meals if GI upset occurs.
- Arrange to reduce dosage or discontinue oxcarbazepine, or substitute other antiepileptic medication gradually. Abrupt discontinuation of antiepileptic medication may precipitate status epilepticus.
- Monitor patient carefully when converting to monotherapy from combined therapy or when adding oxcarbazepine to an established regimen.
- Ensure ready access to bathroom facilities if GI effects occur.
- Establish safety precautions if CNS changes occur (use siderails, accompany patient when ambulating).
- Arrange for appropriate counseling for women of childbearing age who wish to become pregnant; the use of a barrier contraceptive is recommended while on this drug.
- Offer support and encouragement for dealing with epilepsy and adverse drug effects; arrange for consultation with support groups for epileptics as needed.

Teaching points

- Take this drug exactly as prescribed.
- Do not discontinue this drug abruptly or change dosage, except on the advice of your physician.
- Avoid the use of alcohol, sleep-inducing, or OTC drugs while you are on this drug; these could cause dangerous effects. If you feel that you need one of these preparations, consult your nurse or physician.
- Use barrier contraceptive techniques at all times; if you wish to become pregnant while you are taking this drug, you should consult your physician. Hormonal contraceptives may be ineffective.

- Blood tests to measure your blood sodium levels will be needed periodically while you are on this drug.
- These side effects may occur: drowsiness, dizziness, blurred vision (avoid driving a car or performing other tasks requiring alertness or visual acuity if this occurs); GI upset (taking the drug with food or milk and eating frequent small meals may help).
- Wear a medical alert tag at all times so that any emergency medical personnel taking care of you will know that you are an epileptic taking antiepileptic medication.
- Report bruising, unusual bleeding, abdominal pain, yellowing of the skin or eyes, pale-colored feces, darkened urine, impotence, severe CNS disturbances, edema, fever, chills, thirst, pregnancy.

▷ **oxybutynin chloride**
*(ox i **byoo'** ti nin)*

Albert Oxybutynin (CAN), Apo-Oxybutynin (CAN), Ditropan, Ditropan XL, Novo-Oxybutynin (CAN)

PREGNANCY CATEGORY B

Drug classes

Anticholinergic
Urinary antispasmodic

Therapeutic actions

Acts directly to relax smooth muscle and inhibits the effects of acetylcholine at muscarinic receptors; reported to be less potent an anticholinergic than atropine but more potent as antispasmodic and devoid of antinicotinic activity at skeletal neuromuscular junctions or autonomic ganglia.

Indications

- Relief of symptoms of bladder instability associated with voiding in patients with uninhibited neurogenic and reflex neurogenic bladder
- Treatment of signs and symptoms of overactive bladder (incontinence, urgency, frequency)—ER tablets

Contraindications and cautions

- Contraindicated with allergy to oxybutynin, pyloric or duodenal obstruction, obstructive intestinal lesions or ileus, intestinal atony, megacolon, colitis, obstructive uropathies, glaucoma, myasthenia gravis, CV instability in acute hemorrhage.
- Use cautiously with hepatic, renal impairment; pregnancy; lactation.

Available forms

Tablets—5 mg; syrup—5 mg/5 mL; ER tablets—5, 10, 15 mg

Dosages

Adults

5 mg PO bid or tid. Maximum dose is 5 mg qid. ER tablets—5 mg PO daily, up to a maximum of 30 mg/day.

Pediatric patients > 5 yr

5 mg PO bid. Maximum dose is 5 mg tid.

Pharmacokinetics

Route	Onset	Peak	Duration
Oral	30–60 min	3–6 hr	6–10 hr

Metabolism: Hepatic; $T_{1/2}$: unknown
Distribution: Crosses placenta; may enter breast milk
Excretion: Urine

Adverse effects

- **CNS:** *Drowsiness, dizziness, blurred vision,* dilatation of the pupil, cycloplegia, increased ocular tension, weakness
- **CV:** Tachycardia, palpitations
- **GI:** *Dry mouth, nausea,* vomiting, constipation, bloated feeling
- **GU:** *Urinary hesitancy,* retention, impotence
- **Hypersensitivity:** Allergic reactions including urticaria, dermal effect
- **Other:** *Decreased sweating,* heat prostration in high environmental temperatures secondary to loss of sweating

Interactions

* **Drug-drug** • Decreased effectiveness of phenothiazines with oxybutynin • Decreased effectiveness of haloperidol and development of tardive dyskinesia • Increased toxicity if combined with amantadine, nitrofurantoin

■ Nursing considerations

Assessment

- **History:** Allergy to oxybutynin, intestinal obstructions or lesions, intestinal atony, obstructive uropathies, glaucoma, myasthenia gravis, CV instability in acute hemorrhage, hepatic or renal impairment, pregnancy
- **Physical:** Skin color, lesions; T; orientation, affect, reflexes; ophthalmologic exam, ocular pressure measurement; P, rhythm, BP; bowel sounds, liver evaluation; renal and liver function tests, cystometry

Interventions

- Arrange for cystometry and other diagnostic tests before and during treatment.
- Arrange for ophthalmologic exam before therapy and periodically during therapy.

Teaching points

- Take this drug as prescribed.
- Periodic bladder exams will be needed during this treatment to evaluate therapeutic response.
- These side effects may occur: dry mouth (sucking on sugarless lozenges and frequent mouth care may help); GI upset; blurred vision; drowsiness (avoid driving or performing tasks that require alertness); decreased sweating (avoid high temperatures; serious complications can occur because you will be heat intolerant).
- Report blurred vision, fever, rash, nausea, vomiting.

▷ **oxycodone hydrochloride**
(ox i koe' done)

Endocodone, M-oxy, OxyContin, OxyFAST, OxyIR, Percolone, Roxicodone, Roxicodone Intensol, Supeudol (CAN)

PREGNANCY CATEGORY C

C-II CONTROLLED SUBSTANCE

Drug class

Narcotic agonist analgesic

Therapeutic actions

Acts as agonist at specific opioid receptors in the CNS to produce analgesia, euphoria, sedation; the receptors mediating these effects are thought to be the same as those mediating the effects of endogenous opioids (enkephalins, endorphins).

Indications

- Relief of moderate to moderately severe pain
- Management of moderate to severe pain when a continuous, around-the-clock analgesic is needed for an extended period of time (CR tablets)

Contraindications and cautions

- Contraindicated with hypersensitivity to narcotics, diarrhea caused by poisoning (before toxins are eliminated); pregnancy (readily crosses placenta; neonatal withdrawal); labor or delivery (narcotics given to the mother can cause respiratory depression in neonate; premature infants are at special risk; may prolong labor); bronchial asthma, COPD, cor pulmonale, respiratory depression, anoxia, kyphoscoliosis, acute alcoholism, increased intracranial pressure, lactation.
- Use cautiously with acute abdominal conditions, CV disease, supraventricular tachycardias, myxedema, convulsive disorders, delirium tremens, cerebral arteriosclerosis, ulcerative colitis, fever, Addison's disease, prostatic hypertrophy, urethral stricture, recent GI or GU surgery, toxic psychosis, renal or hepatic dysfunction.

Available forms

Tablets—5 mg; IR capsules—5 mg; IR tablets—15, 30 mg; CR tablets—10, 20, 40, 80, 160 mg; oral solution—5 mg/5 mL; solution concentrate—20 mg/ml

Dosages

Individualize dosage.
Adults
10–30 mg PO q 4 hr.
OxyIR, OxyFAST
5 mg q 3–6 hr.
Controlled-release (OxyContin)
10–20 mg PO q 12 hr.

Immediate-release (OxyIR)
- *Breakthrough pain:* 5 mg PO q 4 hr.
Pediatric patients
Controlled-release is not recommended for pediatric patients. Regular and IR dosage should be individualized based on patient's age and size.
Geriatric patients or impaired adults
Use caution. Respiratory depression may occur in the elderly, the very ill, those with respiratory problems.

Pharmacokinetics

Route	Onset	Peak	Duration
Oral	15–30 min	1 hr	4–6 hr

Metabolism: Hepatic; $T_{1/2}$: 2–3 hr
Distribution: Crosses placenta; enters breast milk
Excretion: Urine

Adverse effects

- **CNS:** *Light-headedness, dizziness, sedation,* euphoria, dysphoria, delirium, insomnia, agitation, anxiety, fear, hallucinations, disorientation, drowsiness, lethargy, impaired mental and physical performance, coma, mood changes, weakness, headache, tremor, convulsions, miosis, visual disturbances
- **CV:** Facial flushing, peripheral circulatory collapse, tachycardia, bradycardia, arrhythmia, palpitations, chest wall rigidity, hypertension, hypotension, orthostatic hypotension, syncope, circulatory depression, **shock, cardiac arrest**
- **Dermatologic:** Pruritus, urticaria, edema, hemorrhagic urticaria (rare)
- **GI:** *Nausea, vomiting, sweating* (more common in ambulatory patients and those without severe pain), dry mouth, anorexia, constipation, biliary tract spasm; increased colonic motility in patients with chronic ulcerative colitis
- **GU:** Ureteral spasm, spasm of vesical sphincters, urinary retention or hesitancy, oliguria, antidiuretic effect, reduced libido or potency
- **Respiratory:** Suppression of cough reflex, respiratory depression, apnea, **respiratory arrest,** laryngospasm, bronchospasm

Adverse effects in *Italics* are most common; those in **Bold** are life-threatening.

- **Other:** Physical tolerance and dependence, psychological dependence

Interactions
✻ Drug-drug • Increased likelihood of respiratory depression, hypotension, profound sedation or coma in patients receiving barbiturate general anesthetics, protease inhibitors
✻ Drug-lab test • Elevated biliary tract pressure may cause increases in plasma amylase, lipase; determinations for 24 hr after administration

■ Nursing considerations
Assessment
- **History:** Hypersensitivity to narcotics, diarrhea caused by poisoning, pregnancy, labor or delivery, bronchial asthma, COPD, cor pulmonale, respiratory depression, kyphoscoliosis, acute alcoholism, increased intracranial pressure, acute abdominal conditions, CV disease, myxedema, convulsive disorders, cerebral arteriosclerosis, ulcerative colitis, fever, Addison's disease, prostatic hypertrophy, urethral stricture, recent GI or GU surgery, toxic psychosis, renal or hepatic dysfunction
- **Physical:** T; skin color, texture, lesions; orientation, reflexes, bilateral grip strength, affect, pupil size; P, auscultation, BP, orthostatic BP, perfusion; R, adventitious sounds; bowel sounds, normal output; frequency and pattern of voiding, normal output; ECG; EEG; thyroid, liver, kidney function tests

Interventions
- Administer to nursing women 4–6 hr before the next feeding to minimize amount in milk.
- Do not crush or allow patient to chew controlled-release preparations.
- Administer immediate-release preparations to cover breakthrough pain.
- *OxyFAST* and *Roxicodone Intensol* are highly concentrated preparations. Use extreme care with these preparations.
- Provide narcotic antagonist, facilities for assisted or controlled respiration on standby during parenteral administration.
- Reassure patient about addiction liability; most patients who receive opiates for medical reasons do not develop dependence syndromes.

Teaching points
- Take drug exactly as prescribed. Do not crush or chew controlled-release preparations.
- These side effects may occur: nausea, loss of appetite (take with food, lie quietly, eat frequent, small meals); constipation (use a laxative); dizziness, sedation, drowsiness, impaired visual acuity (avoid driving, performing other tasks that require alertness, visual acuity).
- Do not take any leftover medication for other disorders, and do not let anyone else take the prescription.
- Report severe nausea, vomiting, constipation, shortness of breath, or difficulty breathing.

▽ oxymetazoline
(ox i met az' oh leen)

Afrin, Afrin Children's Pump Mist, Afrin Sinus, Dristan 12 Hr Nasal, Duramist Plus, Genasal, Nasal Relief, Neo-Synephrine 12 Hour, Nostrilla, Vicks Sinex 12-Hour, 4-Way Long Lasting Nasal

PREGNANCY CATEGORY C

Drug class
Nasal decongestant

Therapeutic actions
Acts directly on alpha receptors to produce vasoconstriction of arterioles in nasal passages, which produces a decongestant response; no effect on beta receptors.

Indications
- Symptomatic relief of nasal and nasopharyngeal mucosal congestion due to colds, hay fever, or other respiratory allergies (topical)

Contraindications and cautions
- Contraindicated with allergy to oxymetalozine, angle-closure glaucoma, anesthesia with cyclopropane or halothane, thyrotoxicosis, diabetes, hypertension, CV disorders, women in labor whose BP > 130/80.

- Use cautiously with angina, arrhythmias, prostatic hypertrophy, unstable vasomotor syndrome, lactation.

Available forms
Nasal spray—0.05%

Dosages
Adults
2–3 sprays of 0.05% solution in each nostril bid, morning and evening or q 10–12 hr.
Pediatric patients > 6 yr
Use adult dosage.

Pharmacokinetics

Route	Onset	Duration
Nasal	5–10 min	6–10 hr

Metabolism: Hepatic; $T_{1/2}$: unknown
Distribution: Crosses placenta; may enter breast milk
Excretion: Urine

Adverse effects
Systemic effects are less likely with topical administration than with systemic administration, but because systemic absorption can take place, the systemic effects should be considered:
- **CNS:** *Fear, anxiety, tenseness, restlessness, headache, light-headedness, dizziness,* drowsiness, tremor, insomnia, hallucinations, psychological disturbances, convulsions, CNS depression, weakness, blurred vision, ocular irritation, tearing, photophobia, symptoms of paranoid schizophrenia
- **CV:** Arrhythmias, hypertension resulting in intracranial hemorrhage, **CV collapse** with hypotension, palpitations, tachycardia, precordial pain in patients with ischemic heart disease
- **GI:** *Nausea,* vomiting, anorexia
- **GU:** Constriction of renal blood vessels, *dysuria, vesical sphincter spasm* resulting in difficult and painful urination, urinary retention with prostatism
- **Local:** *Rebound congestion* with topical nasal application
- **Other:** *Pallor,* respiratory difficulty, orofacial dystonia, sweating

Interactions
✳ Drug-drug • Severe hypertension with MAO inhibitors, TCAs, furazolidone • Additive effects and increased risk of toxicity if taken with urinary alkalinizers • Decreased vasopressor response with reserpine, methyldopa, urinary acidifiers • Decreased hypotensive action of guanethidine

■ Nursing considerations
Assessment
- **History:** Allergy to oxymetazoline; angle-closure glaucoma; anesthesia with cyclopropane or halothane; thyrotoxicosis, diabetes, hypertension, CV disorders; prostatic hypertrophy, unstable vasomotor syndrome; lactation
- **Physical:** Skin color, temperature; orientation, reflexes, peripheral sensation, vision; P, BP, auscultation, peripheral perfusion; R, adventitious sounds; urinary output pattern, bladder percussion, prostate palpation; nasal mucous membrane evaluation

Interventions
- Monitor CV effects carefully; patients with hypertension may experience changes in BP because of the additional vasoconstriction. If a nasal decongestant is needed, pseudoephedrine is the drug of choice.

Teaching points
- Do not exceed recommended dose. Demonstrate proper administration technique for topical nasal application. Avoid prolonged use because underlying medical problems can be disguised.
- These side effects may occur: dizziness, weakness, restlessness, light-headedness, tremor (avoid driving or operating dangerous equipment); urinary retention (void before taking drug).
- Rebound congestion may occur when this drug is stopped; drink plenty of fluids, use a humidifier, and avoid smoke-filled areas to help decrease problems.
- Report nervousness, palpitations, sleeplessness, sweating.

Adverse effects in *Italics* are most common; those in **Bold** are life-threatening.

oxymetholone
*(ox i **meth**' ob lone)*

Anadrol-50, Anapolon 50 (CAN)

PREGNANCY CATEGORY X

C-III CONTROLLED SUBSTANCE

Drug classes
Anabolic steroid
Hormone

Therapeutic actions
Testosterone analog with androgenic and anabolic activity; promotes body tissue–building processes and reverses catabolic or tissue-depleting processes; increases Hgb and red cell mass.

Indications
- Anemias caused by deficient red cell production
- Acquired or congenital aplastic anemia
- Myelofibrosis and hypoplastic anemias due to myelotoxic drugs

Contraindications and cautions
- Known sensitivity to oxymetholone or anabolic steroids, prostate or breast cancer; benign prostatic hypertrophy, pituitary insufficiency, MI, nephrosis, liver disease, hypercalcemia, pregnancy, lactation.

Available forms
Tablets—50 mg

Dosages
Adults
1–5 mg/kg/day PO. Usual effective dose is 1–2 mg/kg/day. Give for a minimum trial of 3–6 mo. Following remission, patients may be maintained without the drug or on a lower daily dose. Continuous therapy is usually needed in cases of congenital aplastic anemia.
Pediatric patients
Long-term therapy is contraindicated due to risk of serious disruption of growth and development; weigh benefits and risks.

Pharmacokinetics

Route	Onset
Oral	Rapid

Metabolism: Hepatic; $T_{1/2}$: 9 hr
Distribution: Crosses placenta; enters breast milk
Excretion: Urine

Adverse effects
- **CNS:** *Excitation, insomnia,* chills, toxic confusion
- **Endocrine:** *Virilization: prepubertal males*—phallic enlargement, hirsutism, increased skin pigmentation; *postpubertal males*—inhibition of testicular function, gynecomastia, testicular atrophy, priapism, baldness, epididymitis, change in libido; *females*—hirsutism, hoarseness, deepening of the voice, clitoral enlargement, menstrual irregularities, baldness; decreased glucose tolerance
- **GI:** Hepatotoxicity, peliosis, **hepatitis with liver failure or intra-abdominal hemorrhage; liver cell tumors,** sometimes malignant and fatal, *nausea, vomiting, diarrhea, abdominal fullness, loss of appetite, burning of tongue*
- **GU:** Possible increased risk of prostatic hypertrophy, carcinoma in geriatric patients
- **Hematologic:** *Blood lipid changes:* decreased HDL and sometimes increased LDL; iron deficiency anemia, hypercalcemia, altered serum cholesterol levels; *retention of sodium, chloride, water,* potassium, phosphates, and calcium
- **Other:** *Acne,* premature closure of the epiphyses

Interactions
✳ **Drug-drug** • Potentiation of oral anticoagulants with anabolic steroids • Decreased need for insulin, oral hypoglycemia agents
✳ **Drug-lab test** • Altered glucose tolerance tests • Decrease in thyroid function tests, which may persist for 2–3 wk after therapy • Increased creatinine, decreased creatinine clearance, which may last for 2 wk after therapy

■ Nursing considerations
Assessment
- **History:** Known sensitivity to oxymetholone or anabolic steroids; prostate or breast can-

cer; benign prostatic hypertrophy; pituitary insufficiency; MI; nephrosis; liver disease; hypercalcemia; pregnancy; lactation
- **Physical:** Skin color, texture; hair distribution pattern; affect, orientation; abdominal exam, liver evaluation; serum electrolytes and cholesterol levels, glucose tolerance tests, thyroid function tests, long-bone x-ray (in children)

Interventions
- Administer with food if GI upset or nausea occurs.
- Monitor effect on children with long-bone x-rays every 3–6 mo; discontinue drug well before the bone age reaches the norm for the patient's chronologic age because effects may continue for 6 mo after therapy.
- Monitor for occurrence of edema; arrange for diuretic therapy as needed.
- Monitor liver function, serum electrolytes during therapy, and consult with physician for corrective measures.
- Measure cholesterol levels in patients who are at high risk for CAD.
- Caution patients that this drug cannot be used during pregnancy; advise the use of barrier contraceptives.
- Monitor diabetic patients closely because glucose tolerance may change. Adjust insulin, oral hypoglycemic dosage, and diet.

Teaching points
- Take with food if nausea or GI upset occurs.
- These side effects may occur: nausea, vomiting, diarrhea, burning of the tongue (small, frequent meals may help); body hair growth, baldness, deepening of the voice, decrease in libido, impotence (most reversible); excitation, confusion, insomnia (avoid driving, performing tasks that require alertness); swelling of the ankles, fingers (request medication).
- Diabetic patients need to monitor urine sugar closely as glucose tolerance may change; report any abnormalities to physician, so corrective action can be taken.
- This drug cannot be taken during pregnancy; use barrier contraceptives while on this drug.

- These drugs do not enhance athletic ability but do have serious effects and should not be used for increasing muscle strength.
- Report ankle swelling, skin color changes, severe nausea, vomiting, hoarseness, body hair growth, deepening of the voice, acne, menstrual irregularities in women.

▷ oxymorphone hydrochloride
(ox i mor' fone)

Numorphan

PREGNANCY CATEGORY C

C-II CONTROLLED SUBSTANCE

Drug class
Narcotic agonist analgesic

Therapeutic actions
Acts as agonist at specific opioid receptors in the CNS to produce analgesia, euphoria, sedation; the receptors mediating these effects are thought to be the same as those mediating the effects of endogenous opioids (enkephalins, endorphins).

Indications
- Relief of moderate to moderately severe pain
- Parenterally for preoperative medication, support of anesthesia, obstetric analgesia
- For relief of anxiety with dyspnea associated with acute left ventricular failure and pulmonary edema

Contraindications and cautions
- Contraindicated with hypersensitivity to narcotics, diarrhea caused by poisoning (before toxins are eliminated), pregnancy (readily crosses placenta; neonatal withdrawal), labor or delivery (narcotics given to the mother can cause respiratory depression of neonate; premature infants are at special risk; may prolong labor), bronchial asthma, COPD, cor pulmonale, respiratory depression, anoxia, kyphoscoliosis, acute alcoholism, increased intracranial pressure, lactation.
- Use cautiously with acute abdominal conditions, CV disease, supraventricular tachy-

cardias, myxedema, convulsive disorders, delirium tremens, cerebral arteriosclerosis, ulcerative colitis, fever, Addison's disease, prostatic hypertrophy, urethral stricture, recent GI or GU surgery, toxic psychosis, renal or hepatic dysfunction.

Available forms

Injection—1, 1.5 mg/mL; suppositories—5 mg

Dosages

Adults

IV

Initially 0.5 mg.

SC or IM

Initially 1–1.5 mg q 3–6 hr as needed. For analgesia during labor, 0.5–1 mg IM.

Rectal suppositories

5 mg q 4–6 hr. After initial dosage, cautiously increase dose in nondebilitated patients until pain relief is obtained.

Pediatric patients

Safety and efficacy not established for children < 12 yr.

Geriatric patients or impaired adults

Use caution; respiratory depression may occur in elderly, the very ill, those with respiratory problems.

Pharmacokinetics

Route	Onset	Peak	Duration
IV	5–10 min	15–60 min	3–6 hr
IM, SC	10–15 min	30–60 min	3–6 hr
PR	15–30 min	1–2 hr	3–6 hr

Metabolism: Hepatic; $T_{1/2}$: 2.6–4 hr
Distribution: Crosses placenta; enters breast milk
Excretion: Urine

▼ IV facts

Preparation: No further preparation needed.
Infusion: Inject slowly over 5 min directly into vein or into tubing of running IV.

Adverse effects

- **CNS:** *Light-headedness, dizziness, sedation,* euphoria, dysphoria, delirium, insomnia, agitation, anxiety, fear, hallucinations, disorientation, drowsiness, lethargy, impaired mental and physical performance, coma, mood changes, weakness, headache, tremor, convulsions, miosis, visual disturbances
- **CV:** Facial flushing, peripheral circulatory collapse, tachycardia, bradycardia, arrhythmia, palpitations, chest wall rigidity, hypertension, hypotension, orthostatic hypotension, syncope, circulatory depression, **shock, cardiac arrest**
- **Dermatologic:** Pruritus, urticaria, edema, hemorrhagic urticaria (rare)
- **GI:** *Nausea, vomiting, sweating* (more common in ambulatory patients and those without severe pain), dry mouth, anorexia, constipation, biliary tract spasm; increased colonic motility in patients with chronic ulcerative colitis
- **GU:** Ureteral spasm, spasm of vesical sphincters, urinary retention or hesitancy, oliguria, antidiuretic effect, reduced libido or potency
- **Local:** Pain at injection site, tissue irritation and induration (SC injection)
- **Respiratory:** Suppression of cough reflex, respiratory depression, apnea, **respiratory arrest,** laryngospasm, bronchospasm
- **Other:** Physical tolerance and dependence, psychological dependence

Interactions

✳ **Drug-drug** • Increased likelihood of respiratory depression, hypotension, profound sedation or coma in patients receiving barbiturate general anesthetics

✳ **Drug-lab test** • Elevated biliary tract pressure may cause increases in plasma amylase, lipase; determinations for 24 hr after administration of narcotics

■ Nursing considerations

Assessment

- **History:** Hypersensitivity to narcotics, diarrhea caused by poisoning, pregnancy; labor or delivery; bronchial asthma, COPD, cor pulmonale, respiratory depression, kyphoscoliosis, acute alcoholism, increased intracranial pressure, acute abdominal conditions, CV disease, myxedema, convulsive disorders, delirium tremens, cerebral arteriosclerosis, ulcerative colitis, fever, Addison's disease, prostatic hypertrophy, urethral stricture, recent GI or GU surgery, toxic psychosis, renal or hepatic dysfunction
- **Physical:** T; skin color, texture, lesions; orientation, reflexes, bilateral grip strength, af-

fect, pupil size; P, auscultation, BP, ortho-static BP, perfusion; R, adventitious sounds; bowel sounds, normal output; frequency and pattern of voiding, normal output; ECG; EEG; thyroid, liver, kidney function tests

Interventions

- Give to lactating women 4–6 hr before the next feeding to minimize amount in milk.
- Refrigerate rectal suppositories.
- Provide narcotic antagonist, facilities for assisted or controlled respiration on standby during parenteral administration.
- Use caution when injecting SC into chilled areas of the body or in patients with hypotension or in shock; impaired perfusion may delay absorption; with repeated doses, an excessive amount may be absorbed when circulation is restored.
- Reassure patient about addiction liability; most patients who receive opiates for medical reasons do not develop dependence syndromes.

Teaching points

- Take drug exactly as prescribed.
- These side effects may occur: nausea, loss of appetite (take drug with food and lie quietly, eating frequent small meals may help); constipation (use a laxative); dizziness, sedation, drowsiness, impaired visual acuity (avoid driving, performing other tasks that require alertness, visual acuity).
- Do not take leftover medication for other disorders, and do not let anyone else take the prescription.
- Report severe nausea, vomiting, constipation, shortness of breath or difficulty breathing.

▷ oxytetracycline
(ox i tet ra sye' kleen)

Terramycin, Terramycin IM, Uri-Tet

PREGNANCY CATEGORY D

Drug classes
Antibiotic
Tetracycline antibiotic

Therapeutic actions
Bacteriostatic: inhibits protein synthesis of susceptible bacteria

Indications

- Infections caused by rickettsiae; *Mycoplasma pneumoniae;* agents of psittacosis, ornithosis, lymphogranuloma venereum and granuloma inguinale; *Borrelia recurrentis; Hemophilus ducreyi; Pasteurella pestis; Pasteurella tularensis; Bartonella bacilliformis; Bacteroides; Vibrio comma; Vibrio fetus; Brucella; E. coli; E. aerogenes; Shigella; Acinetobacter calcoaceticus; H. influenzae; Klebsiella; Streptococcus pneumoniae; S. aureus*
- When penicillin is contraindicated, infections caused by *N. gonorrhoeae, Treponema pallidum, Treponema pertenue, Listeria monocytogenes, Clostridium, Bacillus anthracis, Fusobacterium fusiforme, Actinomyces, Neisseria meningitidis*
- As an adjunct to amebicides in acute intestinal amebiasis

Contraindications and cautions
- Allergy to tetracylines, allergy to lidocaine (IM), renal or hepatic dysfunction, pregnancy, lactation.

Available forms
Capsules—250 mg; injection—50, 125 mg/mL

Dosages
Adults
IM
250 mg daily or 300 mg in divided doses q 8–12 hr IM. Note: Injection contains 2% lidocaine. Do not exceed 500 mg/day IM.
Oral
250–500 mg PO q 6 hr. Do not exceed 4 g/day PO.
Pediatric patients > 8 yr
IM
15–25 mg/kg/day IM. May be given in single dose of up to 250 mg, or divided into equal doses q 8–12 hr.
Oral
6.25–12.5 mg/kg/dose q 6 hr.

Adverse effects in *Italics* are most common; those in **Bold** are life-threatening.

Geriatric patients or patients with renal failure

IV and IM doses of tetracyclines have been associated with severe hepatic failure and death with renal dysfunction. Lower than normal doses are required, and serum levels should be checked regularly.

Pharmacokinetics

Route	Onset	Peak
Oral	Varies	2–4 hr
IM	Rapid	2–4 hr

Metabolism: Hepatic; $T_{1/2}$: 6–12 hr
Distribution: Crosses placenta; enters breast milk
Excretion: Urine

Adverse effects

- **Dental:** *Discoloring and inadequate calcification of primary teeth of fetus if used by pregnant women; discoloring and inadequate calcification of permanent teeth if used during period of dental development*
- **Dermatologic:** *Phototoxic reactions, rash,* exfoliative dermatitis (more frequent and more severe with this tetracycline)
- **GI:** Fatty liver, liver failure, *anorexia, nausea, vomiting, diarrhea, glossitis,* dysphagia, enterocolitis, esophageal ulcer
- **Hematologic:** Hemolytic anemia, thrombocytopenia, neutropenia, eosinophilia, leukocytosis, leukopenia
- **Local:** Local irritation at injection site
- **Other:** Superinfections, nephrogenic diabetes insipidus syndrome

Interactions

✳ Drug-drug • Decreased absorption with antacids, iron, urine alkalinizers • Increased digoxin toxicity • Increased nephrotoxicity with methoxyflurane • Decreased activity of penicillins
✳ Drug-food • Decreased absorption with alkaline ash food, dairy products

■ Nursing considerations
Assessment

- **History:** Allergy to tetracylines; renal or hepatic dysfunction; pregnancy, lactation
- **Physical:** Skin status; orientation and reflexes; R, sounds; GI function and liver eval-

uation; urinalysis and BUN; liver and renal function tests; culture infection before therapy

Interventions

- Do not take within 1–3 hr of other medications, milk, or other dairy products. If GI upset occurs, this medication can be taken with food. Take with a full glass of water.
- Advise patient that drug should not be used during pregnancy; advise the use of barrier contraceptives.

Teaching points

- Take drug throughout the day.
- Do not take within 1–3 hr of other medications, milk, or other dairy products. If GI upset occurs, this medication can be taken with food. Take with a full glass of water.
- Sensitivity to sunlight may occur (wear protective clothing, and use a sunscreen).
- Do not take this drug during pregnancy; use of barrier contraceptives is advised.
- Report rash, itching; difficulty breathing; dark urine or light-colored stools; severe cramps, watery diarrhea.

▽oxytocin
*(ox i **toe'** sin)*

Pitocin, Syntocinon

PREGNANCY CATEGORY X

Drug classes
Oxytocic
Hormone

Therapeutic actions

Synthetic form of an endogenous hormone produced in the hypothalamus and stored in the posterior pituitary; stimulates the uterus, especially the gravid uterus just before parturition, and causes myoepithelium of the lacteal glands to contract, which results in milk ejection in lactating women.

Indications

- Antepartum: to initiate or improve uterine contractions to achieve early vaginal delivery; stimulation or reinforcement of labor

in selected cases of uterine inertia; management of inevitable or incomplete abortion; second trimester abortion
- Postpartum: to produce uterine contractions during the third stage of labor and to control postpartum bleeding or hemorrhage
- Lactation deficiency
- Unlabeled use: antepartum fetal heart rate testing (oxytocin challenge test), treatment of breast engorgement

Contraindications and cautions

- Significant cephalopelvic disproportion, unfavorable fetal positions or presentations, obstetric emergencies that favor surgical intervention, prolonged use in severe toxemia, uterine inertia, hypertonic uterine patterns, induction or augmentation of labor when vaginal delivery is contraindicated, previous cesarean section, pregnancy (nasal).

Available forms

Injection—10 units/mL; nasal solution—40 units/mL

Dosages

Adjust dosage based on uterine response.
Adults
- *Induction or stimulation of labor:* Initial dose of no more than 1–2 milliunits/min (0.001–0.002 units/min) by IV infusion through an infusion pump. Increase the dose in increments of no more than 1–2 milliunits/min at 15- to 60-min intervals until a contraction pattern similar to normal labor is established. Do not exceed 20 milliunits/min. Discontinue in event of uterine hyperactivity, fetal distress.
- *Control of postpartum uterine bleeding:* **IV drip**
Add 10–40 units to 1,000 mL of a nonhydrating diluent, run at a rate to control uterine atony.
IM
Administer 10 units after delivery of the placenta.
- *Treatment of incomplete or inevitable abortion:* IV infusion of 10 units of oxytocin with 500 mL physiologic saline solution or 5% dextrose in physiologic saline infused at

a rate of 10–20 milliunits (20–40 drops)/min.
Nasal
- *Lactation stimulant:* 1 spray into one or both nostrils 2–3 min before nursing or pumping of breasts.

Pharmacokinetics

Route	Onset	Duration
IV	Immediate	60 min
IM	3–5 min	2–3 hr

Metabolism: Hepatic; $T_{1/2}$: 1–6 min
Distribution: Crosses placenta; enters breast milk
Excretion: Urine

▼IV facts

Preparation: Add 1 mL (10 units) to 1,000 mL of 0.9% aqueous sodium chloride or other IV fluid; the resulting solution will contain 10 milliunits/mL (0.01 units/mL).
Infusion: Infuse via constant infusion pump to ensure accurate control of rate; rate determined by uterine response; begin with 1–2 mL/min and increase at 15- to 60-min intervals.
Compatibilities: Compatible at a concentration of 5 units/L in dextrose–Ringer's combinations; dextrose–lactated Ringer's combinations; dextrose–saline combinations; dextrose 2%, 5%, and 10% in water; fructose 10% in water; Ringer's injection; lactated Ringer's injection; sodium chloride 0.45% and 0.9% injection; and 1/6 M sodium lactate.
Incompatibilities: Do not combine in solution with fibrinolysin or heparin.

Adverse effects

- **CV:** *Cardiac arrhythmias,* PVCs, hypertension, subarachnoid hemorrhage
- **Fetal effects:** *Fetal bradycardia,* neonatal jaundice, low Apgar scores
- **GI:** *Nausea, vomiting*
- **GU:** Postpartum hemorrhage, uterine rupture, pelvic hematoma, *uterine hypertonicity,* spasm, tetanic contraction, rupture of the uterus with excessive dosage or hypersensitivity
- **Hypersensitivity: Anaphylactic reaction**

Adverse effects in *Italics* are most common; those in **Bold** are life-threatening.

- **Other:** Maternal and fetal deaths when used to induce labor or in first or second stages of labor; **afibrinogenemia; severe water intoxication** with convulsions and coma, **maternal death** (associated with slow oxytocin infusion over 24 hr; oxytocin has antidiuretic effects)

■ Nursing considerations
Assessment
- **History:** Significant cephalopelvic disproportion, unfavorable fetal positions or presentations, severe toxemia, uterine inertia, hypertonic uterine patterns, previous cesarean section
- **Physical:** Fetal heart rate (continuous monitoring is recommended); fetal positions; fetal-pelvic proportions; uterine tone; timing and rate of contractions; breast exam; orientation, reflexes; P, BP, edema; R, adventitious sounds; CBC, bleeding studies, urinary output

Interventions
- Ensure fetal position and size and absence of complications that are contraindicated with oxytocin before therapy.
- Ensure continuous observation of patient receiving IV oxytocin for induction or stimulation of labor; fetal monitoring is preferred. A physician should be immediately available to deal with complications if they arise.
- Regulate rate of oxytocin delivery to establish uterine contractions that are similar to normal labor; monitor rate and strength of contractions; discontinue drug and notify physician at any sign of uterine hyperactivity or spasm.
- Monitor maternal BP during oxytocin administration, discontinue drug and notify physician with any sign of hypertensive emergency.
- Monitor neonate for the occurrence of jaundice.

Teaching points
- The patient receiving parenteral oxytocin is usually receiving it as part of an immediate medical situation, and the drug teaching should be incorporated into the teaching about delivery. The patient needs to know the name of the drug and what she can expect after it is administered.

▽ paclitaxel
*(pass leh **tax' ell**)*

Onxol, Taxol

PREGNANCY CATEGORY D

Drug class
Antineoplastic

Therapeutic actions
Inhibits the normal dynamic reorganization of the microtubule network that is essential for dividing cells; leads to cell death in rapidly dividing cells.

Indications
- Treatment of metastatic carcinoma of the ovary after failure of first-line or subsequent therapy (*Onxol* and *Taxol*)
- Treatment of breast cancer after failure of combination therapy (*Onxol* and *Taxol*)
- First-line treatment of non–small-cell lung cancer (*Taxol*)
- Second-line treatment of AIDS-related Kaposi's sarcoma (*Taxol*)
- Unlabeled uses: treatment of advanced head and neck cancer, previously untreated extensive-stage small-cell lung cancer, adenocarcinoma of the upper GI tract, hormone-refractory prostate cancer, leukemias

Contraindications and cautions
- Contraindicated with hypersensitivity to paclitaxel or drug formulated with polyoxyethylated castor oil, bone marrow depression, severe neurologic toxicity, lactation, pregnancy.
- Use cautiously with cardiac conduction defects, severe hepatic impairment.

Available forms
Injection—6 mg/mL

Dosages
Adults
- *Ovarian cancer:* 135 mg/m^2 IV over 24 hr *or* 175 mg/m^2 IV over 3 hr every 3 wk followed by 75 mg/m^2 IV cisplatin (*Taxol* only) in previously untreated patients. 135 mg/m^2 *or* 175 mg/m^2 IV over 3 hr every 3 wk in previously treated patients. Do not repeat until neutrophil count is at least

1,500 cells/mm² and platelet count is at least 100,000 cells/mm².

- *Breast cancer:* 175 mg/m² IV over 3 hr every 3 wk after failure of chemotherapy (*Taxol* only).
- *AIDS-related Kaposi's sarcoma:* 135 mg/m² IV over 3 hr every 3 wk *or* 100 mg/m² IV over 3 hr every 2 wk.
- *Non–small-cell-lung cancer:* 135 mg/m² IV over 24 hr followed by 75 mg/m² cisplatin IV every 3 wk. Reduce dose by 20% if neutrophils < 500/mm³ for a week or more.

Pediatric patients
Safety and efficacy not established.

Pharmacokinetics

Route	Onset	Duration
IV	Rapid	6–12 hr

Metabolism: Hepatic; $T_{1/2}$: 5.3–17.4 hr
Distribution: Crosses placenta; enters breast milk
Excretion: Bile

▼ IV facts

Preparation: Use extreme caution when handling drug; dilute prior to infusion in 0.9% sodium chloride, 5% dextrose injection, 5% dextrose and 0.9% sodium chloride injection, 5% dextrose in Ringer's injection to a concentration of 0.3–1.2 mg/mL; stable at room temperature for 24 hr. Refrigerate unopened vials; avoid use of PVC infusion bags and tubing.

Infusion: Administer over 3 hr or 24 hr through an in-line filter not greater than 0.22 mcg.

Y-site compatibilities: May be given with fluconazole.

Adverse effects

- **CNS:** Peripheral sensory neuropathy, mild to severe
- **CV:** Bradycardia, hypotension, severe CV events
- **GI:** *Nausea, vomiting,* mucositis, anorexia, elevated liver enzymes
- **Hematologic: Bone marrow depression, infection**
- **Other: Hypersensitivity reactions,** *myalgia, arthralgia, alopecia*

Interactions

✳ **Drug-drug** • Increased myelosuppression with cisplatin • Increased paclitaxel effects with ketoconazole, verapamil, diazepam, quinidine, dexamethasone, cyclosporine, teniposide, etoposide, vincristine, testosterone

■ Nursing considerations

 CLINICAL ALERT!
Name confusion has occurred between *Taxol* (paclitaxel) and *Taxotere* (docetaxel). Serious adverse effects can occur; use extreme caution.

Assessment

- **History:** Hypersensitivity to paclitaxel, castor oil; bone marrow depression; cardiac conduction defects; severe hepatic impairment; pregnancy; lactation
- **Physical:** Neurologic status; T; P, BP, peripheral perfusion; skin color, texture, hair distribution; abdominal exam, mucous membranes; kidney and liver function tests, CBC

Interventions

- Do not administer drug unless blood counts are within acceptable parameters.
- Handle drug with great care; gloves are recommended. If drug comes in contact with skin, wash immediately with soap and water.
- Premedicate with one of the following drugs to prevent severe hypersensitivity reactions: oral dexamethasone 20 mg, 12 hr and 6 hr before paclitaxel, 10 mg if AIDS-related Kaposi's sarcoma; diphenhydramine 50 mg IV 30–60 min before paclitaxel; and cimetidine 300 mg IV 30–60 min before paclitaxel.
- Monitor BP and pulse during administration.
- Obtain blood counts before and at least monthly during treatment.
- Monitor patient's neurologic status frequently during treatment.
- Advise patient to avoid pregnancy; serious fetal harm can occur; advise use of barrier contraceptives.

Adverse effects in *Italics* are most common; those in **Bold** are life-threatening.

Teaching points

- This drug will need to be given over a 3-hr or 24-hr period once every 3 wk. Mark a calendar noting drug days.
- Have regular blood tests and neurologic exams while receiving this drug.
- Avoid pregnancy while you are on this drug, serious fetal harm can occur; use of barrier contraceptives is advised.
- These side effects may occur: nausea and vomiting (if severe, request antiemetics; small frequent meals also may help); weakness, lethargy (frequent rest periods will help); increased susceptibility to infection (avoid crowds and exposure to diseases); numbness and tingling in the fingers or toes (avoid injury to these areas; use care with tasks requiring precision); loss of hair (obtain a wig or other head covering; keep the head covered at extremes of temperature).
- Report severe nausea and vomiting; fever, chills, sore throat; unusual bleeding or bruising; numbness or tingling in your fingers or toes; chest pain.

▷ palivizumab

(pa live ah zoo' mab)

Synagis

PREGNANCY CATEGORY C

Drug class

Monoclonal antibody

Therapeutic actions

A murine and human monoclonal antibody produced by recombinant DNA technology specific to an antigenic site of the respiratory syncytial virus (RSV); has neutralizing effects on the RSV.

Indications

- Prevention of serious lower respiratory tract disease caused by RSV in pediatric patients at high risk for RSV disease

Contraindications and cautions

- Contraindicated with allergy to palivizumab or any murine product.
- Use cautiously with fever (antipyretics should be used to decrease fever before beginning

therapy); previous administration of palivizumab (antibodies frequently develop causing a risk of serious reactions on repeat administration); pregnancy.

Available forms

Injection—50, 100 mg

Dosages

Administer IM only.
Pediatric patients
15 mg/kg IM as a single injection, once a month during the RSV season with the first dose given before the start of the RSV season.

Pharmacokinetics

Route	Onset	Peak
IM	Slow	2–7 days

Metabolism: Tissue; $T_{1/2}$: 18 days
Distribution: Unknown

Adverse effects

- **CNS:** Malaise
- **GI:** Nausea, vomiting, gastroenteritis
- **Respiratory:** Upper respiratory infection, pharyngitis, otitis media
- **Other:** Increased susceptibility to infection; **risk of severe anaphylactoid reaction,** especially with repeated administrations, *fever, chills*

Interactions

❋ **Drug-drug** • Reduce dosage of other immunosuppressive agents; severe immunosuppression can lead to increased susceptibility to infection and increased risk of lymphomas

■ Nursing considerations

Assessment

- **History:** Allergy to palivizumab or any murine product; previous administration of palivizumab
- **Physical:** T, body weights; P, BP; R, adventitious sounds; CBC

Interventions

- Prepare by slowly adding 1 mL of sterile water for injection to the 100-mg vial; gently swirl for 30 sec to avoid foaming; do not shake vial. Allow to stand at room temperature for 20 min until the solution clears.

Use within 6 hr of reconstituting. Discard any leftover medication.
- Monitor WBC levels and circulating T cells periodically during therapy.
- Monitor for any sign of RSV infection; do not use during acute RSV infection, only used for prophylaxis.
- Protect patient from exposure to infections and maintain sterile technique for invasive procedures.
- Arrange for nutritional consult if nausea and vomiting are persistent.

Teaching points
- Protect your child from exposure to infection while you are on this drug; people may wear masks and rubber gloves when caring for your child; visitors may have to be limited.
- Report fever, fussiness, other infections; difficulty breathing.

▽ pamidronate disodium
(pah mih' dro nate)

Aredia

PREGNANCY CATEGORY D

Drug classes
Calcium regulator
Bisphosphonate

Therapeutic actions
Slows normal and abnormal bone resorption without inhibiting bone formation and mineralization.

Indications
- Treatment of hypercalcemia of malignancy
- Treatment of moderate to severe Paget's disease
- Treatment of osteolytic lesions in breast cancer patients receiving chemotherapy and hormonal therapy
- Treatment of osteolytic bone lesions of multiple myeloma
- Unlabeled uses: postmenopausal osteoporosis, hyperparathyroidism, prostatic carcinoma, multiple myeloma, immobilization-related hypercalcemia to prevent fractures and bone pain

Contraindications and cautions
- Contraindicated with allergy to pamidronate disodium or bisphosphonates.
- Use cautiously with renal failure, enterocolitis, pregnancy, lactation.

Available forms
Powder for injection—30, 60, 90 mg

Dosages
Adults
- *Hypercalcemia:* 60–90 mg IV given over 2–24 hr as a single dose.
- *Paget's disease:* 30 mg/day IV as a 4-hr infusion on 3 consecutive days for a total dose of 90 mg.
- *Osteolytic bone lesions:* 90 mg IV as a 4-hr infusion every 3–4 wk.
Patients with renal impairment
Do not exceed single dose of 90 mg.
Pediatric patients
Safety and efficacy not established.

Pharmacokinetics

Route	Onset	Duration
IV	Rapid	72 hr

Metabolism: Hepatic; $T_{1/2}$: 1.6 hr, then 27.3 hr
Distribution: Crosses placenta; may enter breast milk
Excretion: Urine

▽IV facts
Preparation: Reconstitute by adding 10 mL sterile water for injection to each vial; allow drug to dissolve. May be further diluted in 1,000 mL sterile 0.45% or 0.9% sodium chloride or 5% dextrose injection; stable for 24 hr at room temperature.
Infusion: Infuse over 2–24 hr (90-mg dose); over 4 hr (30–60-mg dose).
Incompatibilities: Do not mix with calcium-containing infusions, such as Ringer's; give in a single IV infusion and keep line separate from all other drugs.

Adverse effects in Italics *are most common; those in* **Bold** *are life-threatening.*

Adverse effects
- **GI:** *Nausea, diarrhea*
- **Musculoskeletal:** *Increased or recurrent bone pain* at pagetic sites, focal osteomalacia

■ Nursing considerations
Assessment
- **History:** Allergy to pamidronate disodium or any bisphosphonates, renal failure, enterocolitis, lactation
- **Physical:** Skin lesions, color, T; muscle tone, bone pain; bowel sounds; urinalysis, serum calcium

Interventions
- Provide saline hydration before administration.
- Monitor serum calcium levels before, during, and after therapy. Consider retreatment if hypercalcemia recurs, but allow at least 7 days between treatments.
- Do not give foods high in calcium, vitamins with mineral supplements, or antacids high in metals within 2 hr of dosing.
- Maintain adequate nutrition, particularly intake of calcium and vitamin D.
- Monitor patients with renal impairment carefully; arrange for reduction of dosage if glomerular filtration rate is reduced.
- Maintain calcium on standby in case hypocalcemic tetany develops.

Teaching points
- Do not take foods high in calcium, antacids, or vitamins with minerals within 2 hr of receiving this drug.
- These side effects may occur: nausea, diarrhea, recurrent bone pain.
- Report twitching, muscle spasms, dark urine, severe diarrhea.

▽pancreatic enzymes
(pan kre at' ik)

pancrelipase
Prescription products: Cotazym Capsules; Cotazym-S; Creon (CAN); Creon 10, 20, 25 Capsules; Ilozyme; Kutrase; Ku-Zyme; Pancrease Capsules; Pancrease MT 4, 10, 16,

and 20; Protilase, Ultrase MT 12, 18, and 20; Viokase; Zymase

pancreatin
Creon Capsules, Digepepsin Tablets, Hi-Vegi-Lip Tablets
OTC products: Pancrezyme 4X, 4X and 8X Pancreatin

PREGNANCY CATEGORY C

Drug class
Digestive enzyme

Therapeutic actions
Replacement of pancreatic enzymes: helps to digest and absorb fat, proteins, and carbohydrates.

Indications
- Replacement therapy in patients with deficient exocrine pancreatic secretions, cystic fibrosis, chronic pancreatitis, postpancreatectomy, ductal obstructions, pancreatic insufficiency, steatorrhea or malabsorption syndrome, and postgastrectomy
- Presumptive test for pancreatic function
- Treatment of steatorrhea due to exocrine pancreatic enzyme deficiency in cystic fibrosis and chronic pancreatitis (*Cotazym*)

Contraindications and cautions
- Contraindicated with allergy to any component, pork products.
- Use cautiously with pregnancy, lactation.

Available forms
Pancrelipase capsules—4,000, 5,000, 8,000, 12,000, 16,000, 20,000, 24,000, 25,000 units; powder—16,800 units; *Pancreatin* tablets—250; 300; 500; 2,400; 7,200 mg

Dosages
Adults
Pancrelipase
Capsules and tablets: 4,000–48,000 units PO with each meal and with snacks, usually 1–3 capsules or tablets before or with meals and snacks. May be increased to 8 tablets in severe cases. Patients with pancreatectomy or obstruction, 8,000–16,000 units PO lipase at

P

2-hr intervals, may be increased to 64,000–88,000 units.

Powder: 0.7 g PO with meals.

Pancreatin

Capsules and tablets: 1–2 PO with meals or snacks.

Pediatric patients

6 mo–1 yr: 2,000 units lipase PO per meal.

1–6 yr: 4,000–8,000 units PO lipase with each meal and 4,000 units with snacks.

7–12 yr: 4,000–12,000 units PO lipase with each meal and with snacks.

Pharmacokinetics

Generally no systemic absorption.

Adverse effects

- **GI:** *Nausea, abdominal cramps, diarrhea*
- **GU:** Hyperuricosuria, hyperuricemia with extremely high doses
- **Hypersensitivity:** Asthma with inhalation of fine-powder concentrates in sensitized individuals

■ Nursing considerations

Assessment

- **History:** Allergy to any component, pork products; pregnancy; lactation
- **Physical:** R, adventitious sounds; abdominal exam, bowel sounds; pancreatic function tests

Interventions

- Administer before or with meals and snacks.
- Avoid inhaling or spilling powder on hands because it may irritate skin or mucous membranes.
- Do not crush or let patient chew the enteric-coated capsules; drug will not survive acid environment of the stomach.

Teaching points

- Take drug before or with meals and snacks.
- Do not crush or chew the enteric-coated capsules; swallow whole.
- Do not inhale powder dosage forms; severe reaction can occur.
- These side effects may occur: abdominal discomfort, diarrhea.

- Report joint pain, swelling, soreness; difficulty breathing; GI upset.

▽ pantoprazole

(pan toe' pray zol)

Protonix, Protonix IV, Pantoloc (CAN)

PREGNANCY CATEGORY B

Drug classes

Antisecretory agent
Proton pump inhibitor

Therapeutic actions

Gastric acid-pump inhibitor: suppresses gastric acid secretion by specific inhibition of the hydrogen/potassium ATPase enzyme system at the secretory surface of the gastric parietal cells; blocks the final step of acid production.

Indications

- Short-term (≤ 8 wk) and long-term treatment of GERD (gastric esophageal reflux disease) (oral)
- Short-term (7–10 days) treatment of GERD in patients unable to continue oral therapy (IV)
- Treatment of pathological hypersecretory conditions associated with Zollinger-Ellison syndrome and other neoplastic conditions
- Unlabeled uses: treatment of peptic ulcer

Contraindications and cautions

- Contraindicated with hypersensitivity to any proton pump inhibitor or any drug components.
- Use cautiously with pregnancy, lactation.

Available forms

DR tablet—40 mg; powder for injection—40 mg/vial

Dosages

Adults

40 mg PO daily to bid for ≤ 8 wk; 40 mg/day IV for 7–10 days.

Pediatric patients < 18 yr

Safety and efficacy not established.

Adverse effects in *Italics* are most common; those in **Bold** are life-threatening.

Patients with hepatic impairment
Use caution and monitor patient closely.

Pharmacokinetics

Route	Onset	Peak
Oral	1 hr	3–5 hr
IV	Rapid	3–5 hr

Metabolism: Hepatic; $T_{1/2}$: 1.5 hr
Distribution: Crosses placenta; may pass into breast milk
Excretion: Urine and bile

▽IV facts

Preparation: Reconstitute with 10 mL 0.9% sodium chloride; may then be further diluted with 100 mL 5% dextrose injection, 0.9% sodium chloride injection or lactated Ringer's, final concentration 0.4 mg/mL; reconstituted solution can be stored 2 hr, dilution up to 12 hr at room temperature.
Infusion: Infuse over at least 15 min using in-line filter.
Incompatibilities: Do not mix with or administer through the same line as other IV solutions.

Adverse effects

- **CNS:** *Headache, dizziness,* asthenia, vertigo, insomnia, apathy, anxiety, paresthesias, dream abnormalities
- **Dermatologic:** Rash, inflammation, urticaria, pruritus, alopecia, dry skin
- **GI:** *Diarrhea, abdominal pain, nausea, vomiting,* constipation, dry mouth, tongue atrophy
- **Respiratory:** *URI symptoms,* cough, epistaxis
- **Other:** Cancer in preclinical studies, back pain, fever

Interactions

✳ **Drug-drug** • Fewer drug interactions reported than with other proton pump inhibitors

■ Nursing considerations
Assessment

- **History:** Hypersensitivity to any proton pump inhibitor or any drug components; pregnancy; lactation
- **Physical:** Skin lesions; T; reflexes, affect; urinary output, abdominal exam; respiratory auscultation

Interventions

- Administer once or twice a day. Caution patient to swallow tablets whole; not to cut, chew, or crush.
- Arrange for further evaluation of patient after 4 wk of therapy for gastroreflux disorders. Symptomatic improvement does not rule out gastric cancer, which did occur in preclinical studies.
- Maintain supportive treatment as appropriate for underlying problem.
- Switch patients on IV therapy to oral dosage as soon as possible.
- Provide additional comfort measures to alleviate discomfort from GI effects, headache, etc.

Teaching points

- Take the drug once or twice a day. Swallow the tablets whole—do not chew, cut, or crush.
- Arrange to have regular medical follow-up while you are on this drug.
- These side effects may occur: dizziness (avoid driving a car or performing hazardous tasks); headache (consult with your nurse if these become bothersome, medications may be available to help); nausea, vomiting, diarrhea (proper nutrition is important, consult with your dietitian to maintain nutrition; ensure ready access to bathroom facilities); symptoms of URI, cough (it may help to know that this is a drug effect, do not self-medicate, consult with your nurse or physician if this becomes uncomfortable).
- Report severe headache, worsening of symptoms, fever, chills, blurred vision, periorbital pain.
- Maintain all of the usual activities and restrictions that apply to your condition. If this becomes difficult, consult with your nurse or physician.

▽ **paraldehyde**
*(par **al**' de byde)*

Paral

PREGNANCY CATEGORY C

C-IV CONTROLLED SUBSTANCE

Drug class
Sedative or hypnotic (nonbarbiturate)

Therapeutic actions
Hypnotic that produces nonspecific, reversible depression of the CNS.

Indications
- Oral, rectal: sedative and hypnotic; quiets the patient and produces sleep in delirium tremens and other psychiatric states characterized by excitement

Contraindications and cautions
- Contraindicated with hypersensitivity to paraldehyde, gastroenteritis.
- Use cautiously with bronchopulmonary disease, hepatic insufficiency, pregnancy, lactation.

Available forms
Liquid—1 g/mL

Dosages
All doses expressed in volume refer to the 1 g/mL solution of paraldehyde that is commercially available.
Adults
Oral
4–8 mL in milk or iced fruit juice to mask the taste and odor.
- *Hypnosis:* 10–30 mL.
- *Sedation:* 5–10 mL.
- *Delirium tremens:* 10–35 mL.
Rectal
Dissolve in oil as a retention enema; mix 10–20 mL, as appropriate, with 1 or 2 parts of olive oil or isotonic sodium chloride solution
- *Hypnosis:* 10–30 mL of the 1 g/mL solution diluted as described above.
- *Sedation:* 5–10 mL of the 1 g/mL solution.
Pediatric patients
- *Hypnosis:* Give 0.3 mL/kg of the 1-g/mL solution PO or rectally.
- *Sedation:* Give 0.15 mL/kg or 6 mL/m^2 PO or rectally.

Pharmacokinetics

Route	Onset	Peak	Duration
Oral	10–15 min	30–60 min	8–12 hr
PR	Slow	2.5 hr	8–12 hr

Metabolism: Hepatic; T$_{1/2}$: 3.4–9.8 hr

Distribution: Crosses placenta; may enter breast milk
Excretion: Lungs and bile

Adverse effects
- **CV:** Unusually slow heart beat, right heart edema, dilation, and failure
- **Dermatologic:** Rash, redness
- **GI:** *GI upset, irritation of the mucous membranes,* esophagitis, gastritis, proctitis, hepatitis, *strong, unpleasant breath for up to 24 hr after ingestion*
- **Hematologic:** *Metabolic acidosis,* particularly with high dosage or addiction
- **Local:** Swelling or pain at injection site (thrombophlebitis), severe and permanent nerve damage, including paralysis, particularly of the sciatic nerve, when injected too close to a nerve trunk
- **Respiratory:** Shortness of breath, troubled breathing, coughing
- **Other:** *Addiction resembling alcoholism,* with withdrawal syndrome characterized by delirium tremens, hallucinations (prolonged use)

■ Nursing considerations
Assessment
- **History:** Hypersensitivity to paraldehyde, bronchopulmonary disease, hepatic insufficiency, gastroenteritis, lactation, pregnancy
- **Physical:** Skin injection site; orientation, reflexes; P, BP, perfusion; R, depth, adventitious sounds; bowel sounds, liver evaluation; liver function tests

Interventions
- Dilute before oral or rectal use, as described in dosage section.
- Give with food or mix with milk or iced fruit juice to improve taste and reduce GI upset when administering drug orally.
- Do not let paraldehyde contact plastic surfaces (eg, syringes, glasses, spoons); paraldehyde reacts with plastic.
- Discard unused paraldehyde after opening bottle; paraldehyde decomposes to acetaldehyde if exposed to light and air.
- Do not use drug solutions that are brownish or have a sharp odor of acetic acid (vinegar).

- Keep away from heat, open flame, or sparks.
- Liquefy drug solution that has solidified due to exposure to temperatures less than 12° C or 54° F.
- Do not store in direct sunlight or expose to temperatures < 25° C (77° F).
- Taper drug to withdraw after long-term use.

Teaching points

- Take this drug exactly as directed, diluted in iced fruit juice or milk.
- Do not let this drug contact plastic; avoid plastic glasses, spoons, and so forth.
- Do not use if liquid is brownish or has a strong odor of vinegar.
- Discard any unused drug.
- These side effects may occur: drowsiness (use caution and avoid driving or performing other tasks that require alertness); GI upset (take drug with food or with milk or iced juices); strong, unpleasant-smelling breath for up to 24 hr after you have taken this drug (you may be unaware of this).
- Report yellowing of the skin or eyes, pale stools, bloody stools.

▷ **paricalcitol**

See *Less Commonly Used Drugs,* p. 1348.

▷ **paromomycin sulfate**
*(par oh moe **mye'** sin)*

Humatin

PREGNANCY CATEGORY C

Drug classes

Amebicide
Antibiotic and antibacterial
Cesticide

Therapeutic actions

Bactericidal: inhibits bacterial protein synthesis, effective against *Shigella* and *Salmonella,* amebicidal, cesticidal.

Indications

- Acute or chronic intestinal amebiasis (not indicated in extraintestinal amebiasis because it is poorly absorbed)

- Adjunctive use in hepatic coma (reduces population of ammonia-forming intestinal bacteria)
- Unlabeled uses: tapeworm (cestode) infestations and *Dientamoeba fragilis* infections

Contraindications and cautions

- Contraindicated with allergy to paromomycin, intestinal obstruction.
- Use cautiously with pregnancy, lactation.

Available forms

Capsules—250 mg

Dosages

Absorption is very poor; nearly 100% is excreted unchanged in the stool.

Adults

- *Intestinal amebiasis:* 25–35 mg/kg/day PO in 3 divided doses for 5–10 days.
- *Hepatic coma:* 4 g/day PO in divided doses for 5–6 days.
- *Fish, beef, pork, dog tapeworm:* 1 g q 15 min PO for four doses.
- *Dwarf tapeworm:* 45 mg/kg/day PO in one dose for 5–7 days.
- *Dientamoeba fragilis:* 25–30 mg/kg/day PO in three doses for 7 days.

Pediatric patients

- *Intestinal amebiasis:* 25–35 mg/kg/day PO, in 3 divided doses for 5–10 days.
- *Fish, beef, pork, dog tapeworm:* 11 mg/kg PO q 15 min for four doses.
- *Dwarf tapeworm:* 45 mg/kg/day PO in one dose for 5–7 days.

Pharmacokinetics

Not generally absorbed systemically.

Adverse effects

- **CNS:** Vertigo, headache, change in hearing, ringing in the ears
- **GI:** *Nausea, abdominal cramps, diarrhea,* heartburn, vomiting
- **GU:** BUN increase, decrease in urinary output, hematuria
- **Other:** *Superinfections*

Interactions

✳ **Drug-drug** • Increased or decreased bioavailability of digoxin • Increased neuromuscular blockade with succinylcholine; delay administration of paromomycin as long as possible after recovery of spontaneous respirations after use of succinylcholine

■ Nursing considerations
Assessment
- **History:** Allergy to paromomycin, renal failure, intestinal obstruction, lactation, pregnancy
- **Physical:** Reflexes, eighth cranial nerve function; bowel sounds; BUN, urinalysis

Interventions
- Administer drug with meals.

Teaching points
- Take drug three times a day with meals; small, frequent meals will help if stomach upset occurs.
- These side effects may occur: nausea, vomiting, diarrhea.
- Report ringing in the ears, dizziness, rash, fever, severe GI upset.

▽ paroxetine hydrochloride
(pah rox' a teen)

Paxil, Paxil CR

PREGNANCY CATEGORY C

Drug class
Antidepressant

Therapeutic actions
Potentiates serotonergic activity in the CNS, resulting in antidepressant effect.

Indications
- Treatment of major depressive disorder
- Treatment of obsessive-compulsive disorders
- Treatment of panic disorders
- Treatment of social anxiety disorder (social phobia)
- Treatment of generalized anxiety disorder
- Treatment of posttraumatic stress disorder
- Unlabeled uses: treatment of diabetic neuropathy, headaches, premature ejaculation

Contraindications and cautions
- Contraindicated with MAO inhibitor use.
- Use cautiously with renal or hepatic impairment, the elderly, pregnancy, lactation, suicidal patients.

Available forms
Tablets—10, 20, 30, 40 mg; CR tablets, 12.5, 25, 37.5 mg; suspension—10 mg/5 mL

Dosages
Adults
- *Depression:* 20 mg/day PO as a single daily dose. Range: 20–50 mg/day. Or 25–62.5 mg/day CR tablet.
- *Obsessive-compulsive disorder:* 20 mg/day PO as a single dose, may increase in 10-mg/day increments; do not exceed 60 mg/day.
- *Panic disorder:* 10 mg/day, increase in increments of 10 mg/wk; usual range: 10–60 mg/day. Or 12.5–75 mg/day CR tablet; do not exceed 75 mg/day.
- *Social anxiety disorder:* 20 mg/day PO as a single dose in the morning. May increase up to 60 mg/day.
- *Generalized anxiety disorder:* 20 mg/day PO as a single daily dose. Range: 20–50 mg/day.
- *Posttraumatic stress disorder:* 20 mg/day as a single dose. Range: 20–50 mg/day PO.
- *Switching to or from an MAO inhibitor:* At least 14 days should elapse between discontinuation of MAO inhibitor and initiation of paroxetine therapy; similarly, allow 14 days between discontinuing paroxetine and beginning MAO inhibitor.

Pediatric patients
Safety and efficacy not established.

Geriatric patients or patients with renal or hepatic impairment
10 mg/day PO. Do not exceed 40 mg/day. 12.5 mg/day PO of CR tablets. Do not exceed 50 mg/day.

Pharmacokinetics

Route	Onset
Oral	Slow

Metabolism: Hepatic; $T_{1/2}$: 24 hr

Adverse effects in *Italics* are most common; those in **Bold** are life-threatening.

Distribution: Crosses placenta; enters breast milk
Excretion: Urine

Adverse effects

- **CNS:** *Somnolence, dizziness, insomnia, tremor, nervousness, headache,* anxiety, paresthesia, blurred vision
- **CV:** Palpitations, vasodilation, orthostatic hypotension, hypertension
- **Dermatologic:** *Sweating,* rash, redness
- **GI:** *Nausea, dry mouth, constipation, diarrhea,* anorexia, flatulence, vomiting
- **GU:** *Ejaculatory disorders, male genital disorders,* urinary frequency
- **Respiratory:** Yawns, pharyngitis, cough
- **Other:** *Headache, asthenia*

Interactions

✳ **Drug-drug** • Increased paroxetine levels and toxicity with cimetidine, MAOIs • Decreased therapeutic effects of phenytoin, digoxin • Decreased effectiveness of paroxetine with phenobarbital, phenytoin • Increased serum levels and possible toxicity of procyclidine, tryptophane, warfarin • Risk of serotonin syndrome (hypertension, hyperthermia, mental status changes) if used with SSRIs

✳ **Drug-alternative therapy** • Increased sedative-hypnotic effects with St. John's wort

■ Nursing considerations
Assessment

- **History:** Hypersensitivity to paroxetine, lactation, renal or hepatic impairment, seizure disorder; pregnancy, lactation
- **Physical:** Orientation, reflexes; P, BP, perfusion; R, adventitious sounds; bowel sounds, normal output; urinary output; liver evaluation; liver and renal function tests

Interventions

- Administer once a day in the morning.
- Shake suspension well before using.
- Ensure that patient swallows CR tablets whole; do not cut, crush, or chew.
- Limit amount of drug given to potentially suicidal patients.
- Advise patient to avoid use if pregnant or lactating.

Teaching points

- Take this drug exactly as directed and as long as directed. Shake suspension well before using. Swallow CR tablets whole; do not cut, crush, or chew.
- Abrupt discontinuation may result in discontinuation symptoms (agitation, palpitations); consider tapering.
- These side effects may occur: drowsiness, dizziness, tremor (use caution and avoid driving or performing other tasks that require alertness); GI upset (small, frequent meals, frequent mouth care may help); alterations in sexual function.
- This drug should not be taken during pregnancy or when nursing a baby; use of barrier contraceptives is advised.
- Report severe nausea, vomiting; palpitations; blurred vision; excessive sweating.

▽ pegaspargase

See *Less Commonly Used Drugs,* p. 1348.

▽ pegfilgrastim (G-CSF conjugate)
*(peg fill **grass'** stim)*

Neulasta

PREGNANCY CATEGORY C

Drug class
Colony-stimulating factor

Therapeutic actions
Covalent conjugate of the human granulocyte colony-stimulating factor (filgrastim) produced by recombinant DNA technology; increases the production of neutrophils within the bone marrow with little effect on the production of other hematopoietic cells.

Indications

- To decrease the incidence of infection in patients with nonmyeloid malignancies receiving myelosuppressive anticancer drugs associated with a significant incidence of severe febrile neutropenia

Contraindications and cautions

- Contraindicated with hypersensitivity to *Escherichia coli* products, filgrastim.
- Use cautiously with sickle cell disease, pregnancy, lactation.

Available forms

Injection—6 mg/0.6 mL in prefilled syringes

Dosages

Adults

6 mg SC as a single dose once per chemotherapy cycle. Do not administer in the period 14 days before and 24 hr after administration of cytotoxic chemotherapy.

Pediatric patients

Safety and efficacy not established.

Pharmacokinetics

Route	Peak	Duration
SC	8 hr	Varies

Metabolism: Unknown; $T_{1/2}$: 15–80 hr
Distribution: Crosses placenta; may enter breast milk

Adverse effects

- **CNS:** *Headache, generalized weakness, fatigue, dizziness, insomnia*
- **Dermatologic:** *Alopecia, rash, mucositis*
- **GI:** *Nausea, vomiting, stomatitis, anorexia, diarrhea, constipation, taste perversion, dyspepsia, abdominal pain*
- **Respiratory: ARDS**
- **Other: Splenic rupture,** aggravation of sickle cell disease, *fever, arthralgia, peripheral edema, myalgia, bone pain, granulocytopenic allergic reactions* (anaphylaxis, rash, urticaria), *increased LDH, alkaline phosphatase, uric acid*

Interactions

✳ **Drug-drug** • Risk of increased effects if combined with lithium; if this combination is used, monitor neutrophil counts frequently

■ Nursing considerations
Assessment

- **History:** Hypersensitivity to *E. coli* products, filgrastim, sickle cell disease, pregnancy, lactation

- **Physical:** Skin color, lesions, hair; T; orientation, affect; abdominal exam, status of mucous membranes; CBC, platelets.

Interventions

- Obtain CBC and platelet count prior to and twice weekly during therapy.
- Administer no earlier than 24 hr after cytotoxic chemotherapy and not in the period of 14 days before the administration of chemotherapy.
- Give one injection with each course of chemotherapy.
- Store in refrigerator; allow to warm to room temperature before use; if syringe is at room temperature for ≥ 48 hr, discard. Use each syringe for one dose.
- Do not shake syringe before use. Make sure the syringe is free of particulate matter and that the solution is not discolored before using.
- Monitor patient for any sign of infection and arrange for appropriate treatment.
- Protect patient from exposure to infection.
- Provide appropriate comfort and supportive measures for headache, bone pain, GI discomfort.
- Arrange for patient to obtain wig or other head covering if alopecia occurs; cover head at extremes of temperature.
- Arrange for small, frequent meals if nausea and vomiting are a problem.
- Offer support and encouragement to deal with pain, discomfort, and hair loss.

Teaching points

- This drug will be given by subcutaneous injection once with each cycle of your chemotherapy.
- Avoid exposure to infection while you are receiving this drug (eg, avoid crowds).
- These side effects may occur: bone pain (analgesia may be ordered), nausea and vomiting (eat small, frequent meals), loss of hair (you may want to arrange for appropriate head covering; it is very important to cover head in extreme temperatures).
- Keep appointments for frequent blood tests to evaluate effects of drug on your blood count.

- Report fever, chills, severe bone pain, sore throat, weakness, pain or swelling at injection site.

▽ peginterferon alfa-2a
(peg in ter feer' on)

Pegasys

PREGNANCY CATEGORY C

Drug class
Interferon

Therapeutic actions
Interferons are produced by human leukocytes in response to viral infections and other stimuli. Binds to specific cell receptor sites and causes many biological effects including the inhibition of viral replication in infected cells, inhibition of cell proliferation and immune modulation. Peginterferon alfa-2a is produced by recombinant DNA technology using *Escherichia coli.*

Indications
- Treatment of adults with hepatitis C who have compensated liver disease and who have not been previously treated with interferon alfa.

Contraindications and cautions
- Contraindicated with allergy to peginterferon alfa-2a or any components of the product, autoimmune hepatitis, decompensated hepatic disease.
- Use cautiously with history of depression or suicidal ideation, bone marrow suppression with neutrophil count < 1,500 cells/mm³, platelet counts < 90,000 cells/mm³ or baseline hemoglobin < 10 g/dL; preexisting cardiac disease; thyroid disease; diabetes mellitus; autoimmune disorders; pulmonary disease; preexisting ophthalmologic disorders; impaired renal function, pregnancy, lactation.

Available forms
Single dose vial—180 mcg/mL

Dosages
Adults
180 mcg SC once each week for 48 weeks.
- *Neutrophil count > 500 and < 750 cell/mm³:* 135 mcg SC each week; if neutrophil count falls below 500, suspend treatment and restart at 90 mcg SC each week when neutrophil count returns to > 1,000.
- *Platelet count < 50,000 cells/mm³:* 90 mcg SC each week; stop therapy if platelet count falls below 25,000.
- *End-stage renal disease requiring dialysis:* 135 mcg SC each week with close monitoring.
- *Liver disease:* 90 mcg SC each week if ALT is above baseline levels; discontinue drug if ALT continues to rise or is accompanied by increased bilirubin or hepatic decompensation.

Pediatric patients < 18 yr
Safety and efficacy not established.

Pharmacokinetics

Route	Onset	Peak
SC	Gradual	72–96 hr

Metabolism: Renal; $T_{1/2}$: 80 hr
Distribution: May cross placenta; may enter breast milk
Excretion: Unknown

Adverse effects
- **CNS:** *Headache, dizziness, insomnia,* memory impairment, concentration impairment, **depression,** *irritability,* anxiety, depressed mood, **suicidal ideation, cerebral hemorrhage**
- **CV: Arrhythmia, endocarditis**
- **Dermatologic:** *Alopecia, pruritus,* increased sweating, dermatitis, rash
- **GI:** *Nausea, diarrhea, abdominal* pain, vomiting, dry mouth, *anorexia,* **hepatic decompensation, GI bleeding, pancreatitis, colitis**
- **Hematologic:** Leukopenia, *neutropenia,* thrombocytopenia
- **Pulmonary: Interstitial pneumonitis, pulmonary embolism,** pneumonia
- **Other:** *Fatigue, fever, rigors, injection-site reaction, pain,* asthenia, *myalgia, arthralgia,* corneal ulcer, **retinopathy, autoimmune phenomena, diabetes**

mellitus, hypersensitivity reactions, back pain.

■ Nursing considerations
Assessment

- **History:** Allergy to peginterferon alfa-2a or any components of the product, autoimmune hepatitis, decompensated hepatic disease, lactation, pregnancy, history of depression or suicidal ideation, bone marrow suppression; preexisting cardiac disease; thyroid disease; diabetes mellitus; autoimmune disorders; pulmonary disease; preexisting ophthalmologic disorders; impaired renal function
- **Physical:** T; skin color, lesions; orientation, reflexes; P; R, adventitious sounds, liver function tests, renal function tests, CBC, TSH, T_4, blood glucose

Interventions

- Arrange for laboratory tests: CBC, differential, TSH, T_4, liver and renal function tests prior to and periodically during therapy.
- Examine solution for particulate matter or discoloring before using. If particulate matter is seen or discoloration has occurred, do not use the vial.
- Store vials in the refrigerator; protect from light; do not shake vial.
- Use each vial only once; discard any leftover solution.
- Inject drug subcutaneously into the abdomen or thigh.
- Monitor for severe reactions of any kind, including hypersensitivity reactions, bone marrow suppression, liver impairment, pulmonary dysfunction, suicidal ideation; notify prescriber immediately, dosage reduction or discontinuation of drug may be necessary.
- Arrange for supportive treatment if flulike syndrome occurs—rest, acetaminophen for treatment of fever and headache, environmental control, bedtime dosage may also help.
- Provide small, frequent meals if GI problems occur.
- Arrange for dietary consult if weight loss or loss of appetite become a problem.
- Establish safety precautions if CNS effects occur.

- Protect patient from exposure to infections.
- Provide skin care as appropriate for dermatologic reactions.
- Advise women of child bearing age to use contraceptives during drug therapy; if a woman is nursing, another method of feeding the baby should be used.

Teaching points

- Prepare a calendar to check off as drug is given. You and a significant other should learn the proper technique for subcutaneous injection. The drug is given once each week by injection into the abdomen or thigh.
- Store the vials in the refrigerator; protect from light. Examine the vial for any particulate matter or discoloration before use. If particulate matter appears or the solution appears discolored, return it to the pharmacy. Do not shake the vial. Dispose of the needles and syringes in the appropriate container as directed.
- These side effects may occur: loss of appetite, nausea, diarrhea (frequent mouth care, small frequent meals may help); fatigue, confusion, dizziness, numbness, visual disturbances, depression (it may help to know that these are drug effects; use special precautions to avoid injury if these occur; avoid driving a car or using dangerous machinery if these effects occur); flulike syndrome (taking the drug at bedtime may help, ensure rest periods for yourself, a medication may be ordered for fever); depression, mental changes (alert your health care provider if you begin to feel depressed or anxious).
- Arrange for regular follow-up, including blood tests, to monitor the drug's effects on your body.
- Use of barrier contraceptives is advised if you are a woman of child-bearing age.
- Avoid crowded areas or people with known infections while on this drug, you may be more susceptible to infection.
- Report fever, chills, sore throat, unusual bleeding or bruising, chest pain, palpitations, dizziness, changes in mental status.

▽ peginterferon alfa-2b

See *Less Commonly Used Drugs*, p. 1348.

▽ pemoline
(pem' oh leen)

Cylert, PemADD, PemADD CT

PREGNANCY CATEGORY B

C-IV CONTROLLED SUBSTANCE

Drug class
Central nervous system stimulant

Therapeutic actions
CNS actions similar to those of the amphetamines and methylphenidate but has minimal sympathomimetic effects; may act through dopaminergic mechanisms; efficacy in hyperkinetic syndrome, attention-deficit disorders in children appears paradoxical and is not understood.

Indications
- Attention-deficit disorders, hyperkinetic syndrome, minimal brain dysfunction in children with behavioral syndrome characterized by the following symptoms: moderate to severe distractibility, short attention span, hyperactivity, emotional lability and impulsivity not secondary to environmental factors or psychiatric disorders (part of treatment program)
- Unlabeled use: narcolepsy and excessive daytime sleepiness at doses of 50–200 mg/day

Contraindications and cautions
- Contraindicated with hypersensitivity to pemoline, impaired hepatic function.
- Use cautiously with impaired renal function, psychosis in children, epilepsy, drug dependence, alcoholism, emotional instability, lactation.

Available forms
Tablets—18.75, 37.5, 75 mg; chewable tablets—37.5 mg

Dosages
Adults and patients > 6 yr
Administer as a single oral dose each morning. Recommended starting dose is 37.5 mg/day PO. Gradually increase at 1-wk intervals using increments of 18.75 mg until desired response is obtained. Mean effective dose range is 56.25–75 mg/day. Do not exceed 112.5 mg/day.
Pediatric patients
Not recommended in children < 6 yr.

Pharmacokinetics

Route	Onset	Peak
Oral	Gradual	2–4 hr

Metabolism: Hepatic; $T_{1/2}$: 12 hr
Distribution: Crosses placenta; may enter breast milk
Excretion: Urine

Adverse effects
- **CNS:** *Insomnia, anorexia with weight loss* (most common), dyskinetic movements of tongue, lips, face, and extremities; Tourette's syndrome; nystagmus; oculogyric crisis; convulsive seizures; increased irritability; mild depression; dizziness; headache; drowsiness; hallucinations
- **Dermatologic:** Rashes
- **GI:** *Stomach ache,* nausea, hepatitis; elevations of AST, ALT, LDH; jaundice
- **Other:** Aplastic anemia; tolerance, psychological or physical dependence

■ Nursing considerations
Assessment
- **History:** Hypersensitivity to pemoline; impaired hepatic or renal function, psychosis in children, epilepsy; drug dependence, alcoholism, emotional instability; lactation
- **Physical:** Body weight; T; skin color, lesions; orientation, affect, reflexes; P, BP, auscultation; R, adventitious sounds; bowel sounds, normal output; CBC with differential, liver and kidney function tests, baseline ECG

Interventions
- Ensure proper diagnosis before administering to children for behavioral syndromes: drug should not be used until other causes or concomitants of abnormal behavior

(learning disability, EEG abnormalities, neurologic deficits) are ruled out.
- Interrupt drug dosage periodically in children to determine if symptoms warrant continued drug therapy.
- Monitor growth of children on long-term pemoline therapy.
- Dispense the smallest feasible amount of drug to minimize risk of overdose.
- Give drug in the morning to prevent insomnia.
- Monitor liver function tests every 2 wk during long-term therapy.

Teaching points
- Take this drug exactly as prescribed.
- These side effects may occur: insomnia, nervousness, restlessness, dizziness, impaired thinking (may lessen after a few days; avoid driving or engaging in activities that require alertness); diarrhea; headache, loss of appetite, weight loss.
- Report insomnia, abnormal body movements, rash, severe diarrhea, pale stools, yellowing of the skin or eyes.

▷penbutolol sulfate
(pen byoo' toe lole)

Levatol

PREGNANCY CATEGORY C

Drug classes
Beta-adrenergic blocker
Antihypertensive

Therapeutic actions
Competitively blocks beta adrenergic receptors in the heart and juxtaglomerular apparatus, reducing the influence of the sympathetic nervous system on these tissues; decreasing the excitability of the heart, cardiac output, and release of renin; and lowering BP.

Indications
- Treatment of mild to moderate hypertension, alone or as part of combination therapy

Contraindications and cautions
- Contraindicated with sinus bradycardia, second- or third-degree heart block, cardiogenic shock, CHF, pregnancy, lactation.
- Use cautiously with renal failure, diabetes or thyrotoxicosis, asthma, COPD, impaired hepatic function.

Available forms
Tablets—20 mg

Dosages
Adults
Usual starting dose, maintenance dose, and dose used in combination with other antihypertensives: 20 mg PO daily. Doses of 40–80 mg daily have been used but with no additional antihypertensive effect.
Pediatric patients
Safety and efficacy not established.

Pharmacokinetics

Route	Onset	Peak	Duration
Oral	Varies	2–3 hr	20 hr

Metabolism: Hepatic; $T_{1/2}$: 5 hr
Distribution: Crosses placenta; enters breast milk
Excretion: Urine

Adverse effects
- **Allergic reactions:** Pharyngitis, erythematous rash, fever, sore throat, laryngospasm, respiratory distress
- **CNS:** Dizziness, vertigo, tinnitus, fatigue, emotional depression, paresthesias, sleep disturbances, hallucinations, disorientation, memory loss, slurred speech
- **CV:** *Bradycardia, CHF, cardiac arrhythmias, sinoatrial or AV nodal block, tachycardia,* peripheral vascular insufficiency, claudication, **CVA, pulmonary edema,** hypotension
- **Dermatologic:** Rash, pruritus, sweating, dry skin
- **EENT:** Eye irritation, dry eyes, conjunctivitis, blurred vision
- **GI:** *Gastric pain, flatulence, constipation, diarrhea, nausea, vomiting,* anorexia, ischemic colitis, mesenteric arterial throm-

Adverse effects in *Italics* are most common; those in **Bold** are life-threatening.

bosis, retroperitoneal fibrosis, hepatomegaly, acute pancreatitis
- **GU:** *Impotence, decreased libido,* Peyronie's disease, dysuria, nocturia, frequent urination, renal arterial thrombosis
- **Musculoskeletal:** Joint pain, arthralgia, muscle cramp
- **Respiratory:** Bronchospasm, dyspnea, cough, bronchial obstruction, nasal stuffiness, rhinitis, pharyngitis (less likely than with propranolol)
- **Other:** *Decreased exercise tolerance, development of antinuclear antibodies (ANA),* hyperglycemia or hypoglycemia, elevated serum transaminase, alkaline phosphatase, and LDH

Interactions
✻ Drug-drug • Increased effects with verapamil • Decreased effects with epinephrine • Increased risk of peripheral ischemia, even gangrene, with ergot alkaloids (dihydroergotamine, methysergide, ergotamine) • Prolonged hypoglycemic effects of insulin • Increased first-dose response to prazosin • Paradoxical hypertension when clonidine is given with beta-blockers; increased rebound hypertension when clonidine is discontinued in patients on beta-blockers • Decreased hypertensive effect if given with NSAIDs (piroxicam, indomethacin, ibuprofen) • Decreased bronchodilator effects of theophylline and decreased bronchial and cardiac effects of sympathomimetics with penbutolol
✻ Drug-lab test • Possible false results with glucose or insulin tolerance tests

■ Nursing considerations
Assessment
- **History:** Sinus bradycardia, heart block, cardiogenic shock, CHF, renal failure, diabetes or thyrotoxicosis, asthma or COPD, impaired hepatic function, lactation, pregnancy
- **Physical:** Weight, skin condition, neurologic status, P, BP, ECG, respiratory status, kidney and thyroid function, blood and urine glucose

Interventions
- Give drug once a day. Monitor response and maintain at lowest possible dose.
- Do not discontinue drug abruptly after long-term therapy (hypersensitivity to catechol-

amines may have developed, causing exacerbation of angina, MI, and ventricular arrhythmias; taper drug gradually over 2 wk with monitoring).
- Consult with physician about withdrawing drug if patient is to undergo surgery (withdrawal is controversial).

Teaching points
- Do not stop taking this drug unless instructed to do so by a health care provider.
- Avoid driving or dangerous activities if dizziness, drowsiness occur.
- Report difficulty breathing, night cough, swelling of extremities, slow pulse, confusion, depression, rash, fever, sore throat.

▽ penicillamine
(pen i sill' a meen)

Cuprimine, Depen

PREGNANCY CATEGORY C

Drug classes
Chelating agent
Antirheumatic

Therapeutic actions
Chelating agent that removes excessive copper in Wilson's disease; exact mechanism of action as antirheumatoid agent is not known, but penicillamine lowers IgM rheumatoid factor; reduces excessive cystine excretion by disulfide interchange with cystine, resulting in a substance more soluble than cystine that is readily excreted.

Indications
- Rheumatoid arthritis: severe active disease in patients in whom other therapies have failed
- Wilson's disease
- Cystinuria when conventional measures are inadequate to control stone formation
- Unlabeled uses: primary biliary cirrhosis, scleroderma

Contraindications and cautions
- Contraindicated with allergy to penicillamine, penicillin; history of penicillamine-

related aplastic anemia or agranulocytosis; renal insufficiency; pregnancy (teratogenic).
- Use cautiously with lactation.

Available forms

Capsules—125, 250 mg; titratable tablets—250 mg

Dosages

Warning: interruptions of daily therapy of Wilson's disease or cystinuria for even a few days have been followed by sensitivity reactions when the drug is reinstituted.

Adults

- *Wilson's disease:* Base dosage on urinary copper excretion. Suggested initial dosage is 1 g/day PO given in divided doses qid. Up to 2 g/day may be needed.
- *Rheumatoid arthritis (2–3 mo may be required for a clinical response):* Initial therapy: A single daily dose of 125–250 mg PO. Thereafter increase dose at 1- to 3-mo intervals by 125 or 250 mg/day based on patient response, tolerance, and toxicity. Continue increases at 2- to 3-mo intervals. Doses of 1,000–1,500 mg/day for 3–4 mo with no improvement indicate that patient will not respond. Maintenance: Many patients respond to 500–750 mg/day PO. Dosage above 1 g/day is unusual.
- *Exacerbations:* Some patients experience exacerbation of disease activity that can subside in 12 wk. Treatment with NSAIDs is usually sufficient for control. Increase maintenance dose only if flare fails to subside within the 12-wk time period. *Duration of therapy:* After 6 mo of remission, attempt a gradual, stepwise dosage reduction in decrements of 125–250 mg/day at 3-mo intervals.
- *Cystinuria:* Usual dosage is 2 g/day (range 1–4 g/day) PO in divided doses qid, with the last dose hs. Initiate dosage with 250 mg/day and increase gradually. Individualize dosage to limit cystine excretion to 100–200 mg/day in those with no history of stones, and to < 100 mg/day in those with a history of stones.

Pediatric patients

- *Wilson's disease:* Base dosage on urinary copper excretion. Suggested intial dosage is 1 g/d PO given in divided doses qid. Up to 2 g/day may be needed.
- *Rheumatoid arthritis:* Efficacy in juvenile rheumatoid arthritis has not been established.
- *Cystinuria:* 30 mg/kg/day PO in divided doses qid with the last dose hs. Consider patient's age, size, and rate of growth in determining dosage.

Pharmacokinetics

Route	Onset	Peak
Oral	Varies	1–3 hr

Metabolism: Hepatic; $T_{1/2}$: 1.7–3.2 hr
Distribution: Crosses placenta; enters breast milk
Excretion: Urine

Adverse effects

- **CNS:** Tinnitus, reversible optic neuritis, **myasthenic syndrome**
- **GI:** *Anorexia, epigastric pain, nausea, vomiting, diarrhea, altered taste perception,* intrahepatic cholestasis and toxic hepatitis, *oral ulcerations,* cheilosis, glossitis, colitis
- **GU:** *Proteinuria,* hematuria, which may progress to nephrotic syndrome
- **Hematologic:** *Bone marrow depression*—leukopenia, thrombocytopenia, thrombocytic thrombocytopenic purpura, hemolytic anemia, red cell aplasia, monocytosis, leukocytosis, eosinophilia—fatalities from **thrombocytopenia, agranulocytosis, aplastic anemia**
- **Hypersensitivity:** Allergic reactions: *generalized pruritus,* lupus erythematosus-like syndrome, pemphigoid-type reactions, drug eruptions, urticaria and exfoliative dermatitis, migratory polyarthralgia, **polymyositis,** Goodpasture's syndrome, alveolitis, obliterative bronchiolitis

Interactions

✳ Drug-drug • Decreased absorption with iron salts, antacids • Decreased serum levels of digoxin
✳ Drug-food • Decreased absorption if taken with food

Adverse effects in *Italics* are most common; those in **Bold** are life-threatening.

■ Nursing considerations

Assessment

- **History:** Allergy to penicillamine, penicillin; history of penicillamine-related aplastic anemia or agranulocytosis; renal insufficiency; pregnancy; lactation
- **Physical:** Skin color, lesions; T; orientation, reflexes, ophthalmologic evaluation, audiometric evaluation, peripheral sensation; R, adventitious sounds; liver evaluation, bowel sounds, mucous membranes; CBC, clotting times, urinalysis, renal and liver function tests, x-ray for renal stones

Interventions

- Use caution when administering this drug due to potential serious side effects.
- Arrange for monitoring of urinalysis, CBC before and every 2 wk during the first 6 mo of therapy and monthly thereafter; also monitor liver function tests and x-ray for renal stones before and periodically during therapy.
- Discontinue therapy if drug fever occurs—briefly in Wilson's disease and cystinuria, permanently in rheumatoid arthritis—and switch to another therapy.
- Consult physician about the advisability of decreasing dosage to 250 mg/day when surgery is contemplated; wound healing may be delayed by the effects on collagen and elastin.
- Administer drug on an empty stomach, 1 hr before or 2 hr after meals and at least 1 hr apart from any other drug, food, or milk.
- Administer drug for Wilson's disease on an empty stomach, 30–60 min before meals and hs, at least 2 hr after the evening meal.
- Administer drug for cystinuria in four equal doses; if this is not possible, give the larger dose hs; the bedtime dose is of utmost importance.
- Ensure that patient with cystinuria drinks 1 pint of fluid hs and another pint once during night; the greater the fluid intake, the lower the dose of penicillamine required.
- Arrange for nutritional consultation; pyridoxine supplements may be needed; ensure that multivitamin preparations do not contain copper for patients with Wilson's disease; iron deficiency may occur; if iron supplements are used, ensure that they are given with at least a 2-hr interval between iron and

penicillamine; hypogeusia (loss of taste) may lead to anorexia or inappropriate eating habits.

Teaching points

- Take drug on an empty stomach 1 hr before or 2 hr after meals and at least 1 hr apart from any other drug, food, or milk.
- Wilson's disease: take 30–60 min before meals and at bedtime. Cystinuria: be sure to take the bedtime dose; drink one pint of fluid at bedtime and one pint during the night; drink copious amounts of fluid during the day.
- These side effects may occur: nausea, GI upset, vomiting (take drug with food); diarrhea; rash, delays in healing (use good skin care; avoid injury); mouth sores, loss of taste perception (frequent mouth care will help; taste perception usually returns within 2–3 mo).
- This drug is not to be used during pregnancy; if you become pregnant or want to become pregnant, consult your physician.
- Report rash, unusual bruising or bleeding, sore throat, difficulty breathing, cough or wheezing, fever, chills.
- Keep this drug and all medications out of the reach of children; this drug can be very dangerous for children.

P

▽ penicillin G benzathine

(pen i sill' in)

Megacillin (CAN)

PREGNANCY CATEGORY B

Drug classes

Antibiotic
Penicillin antibiotic

Therapeutic actions

Bactericidal: inhibits synthesis of cell wall of sensitive organisms, causing cell death.

Indications

- Severe infections caused by sensitive organisms (streptococci)
- Upper respiratory infection caused by sensitive streptococci

- Treatment of syphilis, neurosyphilis, congenital syphilis, yaws, uncomplicated erysipeloid infection
- Prophylaxis of rheumatic fever and chorea

Contraindications and cautions

- Contraindicated with allergies to penicillins, cephalosporins, or other allergens.
- Use cautiously with renal disorders, pregnancy, lactation (may cause diarrhea or candidiasis in the infant).

Available forms

Injection—600,000; 1,200,000; 2,400,000; 3,000,000 units/dose

Dosages
Adults

- *Streptococcal infections (including otitis media, URIs of mild to moderate severity):* 1.2 million units IM as a single dose.
- *Early syphilis:* 2.4 million units IM as a single dose.
- *Syphilis lasting > 1 yr:* 7.2 million units given as 2.4 million units IM weekly for 3 wk.
- *Yaws:* 1.2 million units IM as a single dose.
- *Erysipeloid:* 1.2 million units IM as a single dose.
- *Prophylaxis of rheumatic fever or chorea:* 1.2 million units IM q month.

Pediatric patients

- *Streptococcal infections (including otitis media, URIs of mild to moderate severity):* Older children: 900,000–1.2 million units IM as a single injection.
Children < 60 lb: 300,000–600,000 units IM as a single injection.
Neonates: 50,000 units/kg IM as a single injection (congenital syphilis).

Pharmacokinetics

Route	Onset	Peak	Duration
IM	Slow	12–24 hr	Days

Metabolism: Hepatic; $T_{1/2}$: 30–60 min
Distribution: Crosses placenta; enters breast milk
Excretion: Urine

Adverse effects

- **CNS:** Lethargy, hallucinations, seizures

- **GI:** *Glossitis, stomatitis, gastritis, sore mouth,* furry tongue, black "hairy" tongue, *nausea, vomiting, diarrhea,* abdominal pain, bloody diarrhea, enterocolitis, pseudomembranous colitis, nonspecific hepatitis
- **GU:** Nephritis
- **Hematologic:** Anemia, thrombocytopenia, leukopenia, neutropenia, prolonged bleeding time (more common than with other penicillinase-resistant penicillins)
- **Hypersensitivity:** *Rash, fever, wheezing,* **anaphylaxis**
- **Local:** *Pain, phlebitis,* thrombosis at injection site, Jarisch-Herxheimer reaction when used to treat syphilis
- **Other:** *Superinfections,* sodium overload, leading to CHF

Interactions

✳ Drug-drug • Decreased effectiveness of penicillin G benzathine with tetracyclines • Inactivation of parenteral aminoglycosides (amikacin, gentamicin, kanamycin, neomycin, metilmicin, tobramycin); separate administration times

■ Nursing considerations
Assessment

- **History:** Allergies to penicillins, cephalosporins, other allergens; renal disorders; pregnancy, lactation
- **Physical:** Culture infection; skin color, lesions; R, adventitious sounds; bowel sounds: CBC, liver and renal function tests, serum electrolytes, Hct, urinalysis

Interventions

- Culture infection before beginning treatment; reculture if response is not as expected.
- Give by IM route only.
- Continue therapy for at least 2 days after infection has disappeared, usually 7–10 days.
- Give IM injection in upper outer quadrant of the buttock. In infants and small children, the midlateral aspect of the thigh may be preferred.

Teaching points

- You will need to receive a full course of drug therapy.

*Adverse effects in Italics are most common; those in **Bold** are life-threatening.*

- These side effects may occur: nausea, vomiting, diarrhea, mouth sores, pain at injection sites.
- Report difficulty breathing, rashes, severe diarrhea, severe pain at injection site, mouth sores, unusual bleeding or bruising.

▷penicillin G
(pen i sill' in)

penicillin G potassium (aqueous)
Falapen (CAN), Novo-Pen G (CAN), Pentids (CAN), Pfizerpen

penicillin G sodium
Crystapen (CAN)

PREGNANCY CATEGORY B

Drug classes
Antibiotic
Penicillin antibiotic

Therapeutic actions
Bactericidal: inhibits synthesis of cell wall of sensitive organisms, causing cell death.

Indications
- Treatment of severe infections caused by sensitive organisms—streptococci, pneumococci, staphylococci, *Neisseria gonorrhoeae*, *Treponema pallidum*, meningococci, *Actinomyces israelii*, *Clostridium perfringens* and *tetani*, *Leptotrichia buccalis* (Vincent's disease), *Spirillum minus* or *Streptobacillus moniliformis*, *Listeria monocytogenes*, *Pasteurella multocida*, *Erysipelothrix insidiosa*, *Escherichia coli*, *Enterobacter aerogenes*, *Alcaligenes faecalis*, *Salmonella*, *Shigella*, *Proteus mirabilis*, *Corynebacterium diphtheriae*, *Bacillus anthracis*
- Treatment of syphilis, gonococcal infections
- Unlabeled use: treatment of Lyme disease

Contraindications and cautions
- Contraindicated with allergy to penicillins, cephalosporins, other allergens.
- Use cautiously with renal disease, pregnancy, lactation (may cause diarrhea or candidiasis in the infant).

Available forms
Injection—1, 2, 3 million units/50 mL; powder for injection—1, 5, 10, 20 million units/vial; oral solution—400,000 units/5 mL; tablets—200,000, 250,000, 400,000, 800,000 units

Dosages
Adults
- *Meningococcal meningitis:* 1–2 million units q 2 hr IM or by continuous IV infusion of 20–30 million units/day.
- *Actinomycosis:* 1–6 million units/day IM or IV for cervicofacial cases; 10–20 million units/day IM or IV for thoracic and abdominal diseases.
- *Clostridial infections:* 20 million units/day IM or IV with antitoxin therapy.
- *Fusospirochetal infections (Vincent's disease):* 5–10 million units/day IM or IV or 200,000–500,000 units q 6–8 hr PO for milder infections.
- *Rat-bite fever:* 12–15 million units/day IM or IV for 3–4 wk.
- *Listeria infections:* 15–20 million units/day IM or IV for 2 or 4 wk (meningitis or endocarditis, respectively).
- *Pasteurella infections:* 4–6 million units/day IM or IV for 2 wk.
- *Erysipeloid endocarditis:* 12–20 million units/day IM or IV for 4–6 wk.
- *Gram-negative bacillary bacteremia:* 20–30 million units/day IM or IV.
- *Diphtheria (adjunctive therapy with antitoxin to prevent carrier state):* 2–3 million units/day IM or IV in divided doses for 10–12 days.
- *Anthrax:* Minimum of 5 million units/day IM or IV in divided doses.
- *Pneumococcal infections:* 5–24 million units/day in divided doses.
- *Syphilis:* 18–24 million units/day IV for 10 days followed by benzathine penicillin G 2.4 million units IM weekly for 3 wk.
- *Gonorrhea:* 10 million units/day IV until improvement occurs, followed by amoxicillin or ampicillin 500 mg qid PO for 7 days.
Pediatric patients
- *Meningitis:* 250,000 units/kg/day IM or IV in divided doses q 4 hr for 7–14 days.
- *Streptococcal infections:* 150,000 units/kg/day IV or IM q 4–6 hr.

P

Infants > 7 days: 75,000 units/kg/day IV in divided doses q 8 hr.
• *Meningitis:* 200,000–300,000 units/kg/day IV.
Infants < 7 days: 50,000 units/kg/day IV in divided doses q 12 hr.
• *Group B streptococcus:* 100,000 units/kg/day IV.
• *Meningitis:* 100,000–150,000 units/kg/day IV.

Pharmacokinetics

Route	Onset	Peak
IM, IV	Rapid	15–30 min

Metabolism: Hepatic; $T_{1/2}$: 30–60 min
Distribution: Crosses placenta; enters breast milk
Excretion: Urine

▼IV facts

Preparation: Prepare solution using sterile water for injection, isotonic sodium chloride injection, or dextrose injection. Do not use with carbohydrate solutions at alkaline pH; do not refrigerate powder; sterile solution is stable for 1 wk refrigerated. IV solutions are stable at 24 hr at room temperature. Discard solution after 24 hr.
Infusion: Administer doses of 10–20 million units by slow infusion.
Incompatibilities: Do not mix with amphotericin B, bleomycin, chlorpromazine, cytarabine, hydroxyzine, methylprednisolone, aminoglycosides.

Adverse effects

• **CNS:** Lethargy, hallucinations, seizures
• **GI:** *Glossitis, stomatitis, gastritis, sore mouth,* furry tongue, black "hairy" tongue, *nausea, vomiting, diarrhea,* abdominal pain, bloody diarrhea, enterocolitis, pseudomembranous colitis, nonspecific hepatitis
• **GU:** Nephritis—oliguria, proteinuria, hematuria, casts, azotemia, pyuria
• **Hematologic:** Anemia, thrombocytopenia, leukopenia, neutropenia, prolonged bleeding time
• **Hypersensitivity reactions:** *Rash, fever, wheezing,* anaphylaxis

• **Local:** *Pain, phlebitis,* thrombosis at injection site, Jarisch-Herxheimer reaction when used to treat syphilis
• **Other:** *Superinfections,* sodium overload, leading to CHF

Interactions

❋ **Drug-drug** • Decreased effectiveness of penicillin G with tetracyclines • Inactivation of parenteral aminoglycosides (amikacin, gentamicin, kanamycin, neomycin, metilmicin, streptomycin, tobramycin)
❋ **Drug-lab test** • False-positive Coombs' test (IV)

■ Nursing considerations
Assessment

• **History:** Allergy to penicillins, cephalosporins, other allergens, renal disease, lactation, pregnancy
• **Physical:** Culture infection; skin rashes, lesions; R, adventitious sounds; bowel sounds, normal output; CBC, liver and renal function tests, serum electrolytes, Hct, urinalysis; skin test with benzylpenicylloyl-polylysine if hypersensitivity reactions to penicillin have occurred

Interventions

• Culture infection before beginning treatment; reculture if response is not as expected.
• Use the smallest dose possible for IM injection to avoid pain and discomfort.
• Continue treatment for 48–72 hr beyond time that the patient is asymptomatic.
• Monitor serum electrolytes and cardiac status if penicillin G is given by IV infusion. Sodium or potassium preparations have been associated with severe electrolyte imbalances.
• Explain the reason for parenteral administration; offer support and encouragement to deal with therapy.
• Maintain epinephrine, IV fluids, vasopressors, bronchodilators, oxygen, and emergency equipment on standby in case of serious hypersensitivity reaction.
• Arrange for the use of corticosteroids, antihistamines for skin reactions.

Adverse effects in *Italics* are most common; those in **Bold** are life-threatening.

Teaching points

- This drug must be given by injection for severe infections.
- These side effects may occur: upset stomach, nausea, vomiting (small, frequent meals may help); sore mouth (frequent mouth care may help); diarrhea; pain or discomfort at the injection site.
- Report unusual bleeding, sore throat, rash, hives, fever, severe diarrhea, difficulty breathing.

▽**penicillin G procaine
(penicillin G procaine,
aqueous, APPG)**
*(pen i **sill**' in)*

Ayercillin (CAN), Crysticillin-AS
(CAN), Wycillin

PREGNANCY CATEGORY B

Drug classes

Antibiotic
Penicillin, long-acting, parenteral

Therapeutic actions

Bactericidal: inhibits cell wall synthesis of sensitive organisms, causing cell death.

Indications

- Treatment of moderately severe infections caused by sensitive organisms—streptococci, pneumococci, staphylococci, meningococci, *A. israelii*, *C. perfringens* and *tetani*, *L. buccalis* (Vincent's disease), *S. minus* or *S. moniliformis*, *L. monocytogenes*, *P. multocida*, *E. insidiosa*, *E. coli*, *E. aerogenes*, *A. faecalis*, *Salmonella*, *Shigella*, *P. mirabilis*, *C. diphtheriae*, *B. anthracis*
- Treatment of specific sexually transmitted diseases

Contraindications and cautions

- Contraindicated with allergies to penicillins, cephalosporins, procaine, or other allergens.
- Use cautiously with renal disorders, pregnancy, lactation (may cause diarrhea or candidiasis in the infant).

Available forms

600,000, 1,200,000, 2,400,000, 3,000,000 units/dose

Dosages

Adults

- *Moderately severe infections caused by sensitive strains of streptococci, pneumococci, staphylococci:* Minimum of 600,000–1.2 million units/day IM.
- *Bacterial endocarditis (group A streptococci):* 600,000–1.2 million units/day IM.
- *Fusospirochetal infections:* 600,000–1.2 million units/day IM.
- *Rat-bite fever:* 600,000–1 million units/day IM.
- *Erysipeloid:* 600,000–1 million units/day IM.
- *Diphtheria:* 300,000–600,000 units/day IM with antitoxin.
- *Diphtheria carrier state:* 300,000 units/day IM for 10 days.
- *Anthrax:* 600,000–1.2 million units/day IM.
- *Syphilis (negative spinal fluid):* 600,000 units/day IM for 8 days.
- *Late syphilis:* 600,000 units/day for 10–15 days.
- *Neurosyphilis:* 2.4 million units/day IM with 500 mg probenecid PO qid for 10–14 days, followed by 2.4 million units IM benzathine penicillin G following completion of treatment regimen.
- *Uncomplicated gonococcal infections:* 4.8 million units IM in divided doses at two sites together with 1 g probenecid.

Pediatric patients

- *Congenital syphilis in patients weighing < 70 lb:* 50,000 units/kg per day IM for 10–14 days.
- *Neurosyphilis in infants:* 50,000 units/kg/ day IM for at least 10 days.

Pharmacokinetics

Route	Onset	Peak	Duration
IM	Varies	4 hr	15–20 hr

Metabolism: Hepatic; $T_{1/2}$: 30–60 min
Distribution: Crosses placenta; enters breast milk
Excretion: Urine

Adverse effects

- **CNS:** Lethargy, hallucinations, seizures

- **GI:** *Glossitis, stomatitis, gastritis, sore mouth,* furry tongue, black "hairy" tongue, *nausea, vomiting, diarrhea,* abdominal pain, bloody diarrhea, enterocolitis, pseudomembranous colitis, nonspecific hepatitis
- **GU:** Nephritis—oliguria, proteinuria, hematuria, casts, azotemia, pyuria
- **Hematologic:** Anemia, thrombocytopenia, leukopenia, neutropenia, prolonged bleeding time
- **Hypersensitivity:** *Rash, fever, wheezing,* **anaphylaxis**
- **Local:** *Pain, phlebitis,* thrombosis at injection site, Jarisch-Herxheimer reaction when used to treat syphilis
- **Other:** *Superinfections,* sodium overload, leading to CHF

Interactions
* Drug-drug • Decreased effectiveness of penicillin G procaine with tetracyclines • Inactivation of parenteral aminoglycosides (amikacin, gentamicin, kanamycin, neomycin, metilmicin, streptomycin, tobramycin)

■ Nursing considerations
Assessment
- **History:** Allergies to penicillins, cephalosporins, procaine, other allergens, renal disorders, pregnancy, lactation
- **Physical:** Culture infection; skin color, lesions; R, adventitious sounds; bowel sounds: CBC, liver and renal function tests, serum electrolytes, Hct, urinalysis

Interventions
- Culture infection before beginning treatment; reculture if response is not as expected.
- Administer by IM route only.
- Continue therapy for at least 2 days after infection has disappeared, usually 7–10 days.
- Administer IM injection in upper outer quadrant of the buttock. In infants and small children, the midlateral aspect of the thigh may be preferred.

Teaching points
- This drug can be given only by IM injection.
- These side effects may occur: nausea, vomiting, diarrhea, mouth sores, pain at injection sites.

- Report difficulty breathing, rashes, severe diarrhea, severe pain at injection site, mouth sores, unusual bleeding or bruising.

▷penicillin V (penicillin V potassium)
(pen i sill' in)

Beepen VK, Nadopen-V (CAN), Novo-Pen VK (CAN), Pen-Vee-K, Veetids

PREGNANCY CATEGORY B

Drug classes
Antibiotic
Penicillin (acid stable)

Therapeutic actions
Bactericidal: inhibits cell wall synthesis of sensitive organisms, causing cell death.

Indications
- Mild to moderately severe infections caused by sensitive organisms—streptococci, pneumococci, staphylococci, fusospirochetes
- Prophylaxis against bacterial endocarditis in patients with valvular heart disease undergoing dental or upper respiratory tract surgery
- Unlabeled uses: prophylactic treatment of children with sickle cell anemia, mild to moderate anaerobic infections, Lyme disease

Contraindications and cautions
- Contraindicated with allergies to penicillins, cephalosporins, or other allergens.
- Use cautiously with renal disorders, pregnancy, lactation (may cause diarrhea or candidiasis in the infant).

Available forms
Tablets—250, 500 mg; powder for oral solution—125, 250 mg/5 mL

Dosages
Adults
- *Fusospirochetal infections:* 250 mg q 6–8 hr PO.
- *Streptococcal infections (including otitis media, URIs of mild to moderate severi-*

Adverse effects in *Italics* are most common; those in **Bold** are life-threatening.

ty, scarlet fever, erysipelas): 125–250 mg q 6–8 hr PO for 10 days.

- *Pneumococcal infections:* 250 mg q 6 hr PO until afebrile for 48 hr.
- *Staphylococcal infections of skin and soft tissues:* 250 mg q 6–8 hr PO.
- *Prophylaxis against bacterial endocarditis, dental or upper respiratory procedures:* 2 g PO 30 min–1 hr before the procedure, then 500 mg q 6 hr for eight doses.
- *Alternate prophylaxis:* 1 million units penicillin G IM mixed with 600,000 units procaine penicillin G 30 min–1 hr before the procedure, then 500 mg penicillin V PO q 6 hr for 8-hr doses.
- *Lyme disease:* 250–500 mg PO qid for 10–20 days.

Pediatric patients < 12 yr
15–62.5 mg/kg/day PO given q 6–8 hr. Calculate doses according to weight.

- *Prophylaxis against bacterial endocarditis, dental or upper respiratory procedures: Children > 60 lb:* 2 g PO 30 min–1 hr before the procedure, then 500 mg q 6 hr for eight doses. *Children < 60 lb:* 1 g PO 30 min–1 hr before the procedure, then 250 mg q 6 hr for eight doses.
- *Alternate prophylaxis: < 30 kg:* 30,000 units penicillin G/kg IM mixed with 600,000 units procaine penicillin G 30 min–1 hr before the procedure and then 250 mg penicillin V PO q 6 hr for eight doses.
- *Sickle cell anemia as prophylaxis of S. pneumoniae septicemia:* 125 mg PO bid.
- *Lyme disease:* 50 mg/kg/day PO in four divided doses for 10–20 days for children < 2 yr.

Pharmacokinetics

Route	Onset	Peak
Oral	Varies	60 min

Metabolism: Hepatic; $T_{1/2}$: 30–60 min
Distribution: Crosses placenta; enters breast milk
Excretion: Urine

Adverse effects

- **CNS:** Lethargy, hallucinations, seizures
- **GI:** *Glossitis, stomatitis, gastritis, sore mouth,* furry tongue, black "hairy" tongue, *nausea, vomiting, diarrhea,* abdominal pain, bloody diarrhea, enterocolitis, pseudomembranous colitis, nonspecific hepatitis
- **GU:** Nephritis—oliguria, proteinuria, hematuria, casts, azotemia, pyuria
- **Hematologic:** Anemia, thrombocytopenia, leukopenia, neutropenia, prolonged bleeding time
- **Hypersensitivity reactions:** *Rash, fever, wheezing,* **anaphylaxis** (sometimes fatal)
- **Other:** *Superinfections,* sodium overload leading to CHF; potassium poisoning—hyperreflexia, coma, cardiac arrhythmias, **cardiac arrest** (potassium preparations)

Interactions

✱ **Drug-drug** • Decreased effectiveness with tetracyclines

■ Nursing considerations
Assessment

- **History:** Allergies to penicillins, cephalosporins, or other allergens; renal disorders; pregnancy; lactation
- **Physical:** Culture infection; skin color, lesions; R, adventitious sounds; bowel sounds: CBC, liver and renal function tests, serum electrolytes, Hct, urinalysis

Interventions

- Culture infection before beginning treatment; reculture if response is not as expected.
- Continue therapy for at least 2 days after infection has disappeared, usually 7–10 days.
- Do not administer oral drug with milk, fruit juices, or soft drinks; a full glass of water is preferred; this oral penicillin is less affected by food than other penicillins.

Teaching points

- Avoid self-treating other infections with this antibiotic because it is specific for the infection being treated.
- These side effects may occur: nausea, vomiting, diarrhea, mouth sores.
- Report difficulty breathing, rashes, severe diarrhea, mouth sores, unusual bleeding or bruising.

▷ pentamidine isethionate

(pen ta' ma deen)

Parenteral: Pentacarinat, Pentam 300
Inhalation: NebuPent

PREGNANCY CATEGORY C

Drug class
Antiprotozoal

Therapeutic actions
Antiprotozoal activity in susceptible *Pneumocystis carinii* infections; mechanism of action is not fully understood, but the drug interferes with nuclear metabolism and inhibits the synthesis of DNA, RNA, phospholipids, and proteins, which lead to cell death.

Indications
- Treatment of *P. carini* pneumonia, especially in patients unresponsive to therapy with the less toxic trimethoprim/sulfamethoxazole combination (injection)
- Prevention of *P. carinii* pneumonia in high-risk, HIV-infected patients (inhalation)
- Unlabeled use (injection): treatment of trypanosomiasis, visceral leishmaniasis

Contraindications and cautions
If the diagnosis of *P. carinii* pneumonia has been confirmed, there are no absolute contraindications to the use of this drug.
- Contraindicated with history of anaphylactic reaction to inhaled or parenteral pentamidine isethionate (inhalation therapy); pregnancy; lactation.
- Use cautiously with hypotension, hypertension, hypoglycemia, hyperglycemia, hypocalcemia, leukopenia, thrombocytopenia, anemia, hepatic or renal dysfunction.

Available forms
Injection—300 mg/vial; powder for injection—300 mg; aerosol—300 mg

Dosages
Adults and pediatric patients
Parenteral
4 mg/kg once a day for 14–21 days by deep IM injection or IV infusion over 60 min.
Inhalation
300 mg once every 4 wk administered through the *Respirgard II* nebulizer.

Pharmacokinetics

Route	Onset
IM	Slow
Inhalation	Rapid

Metabolism: $T_{1/2}$: 6.4–9.4 hr
Distribution: Crosses placenta; enters breast milk
Excretion: Urine

▼ IV facts
Preparation: Prepare solution by dissolving contents of 1 vial in 3–5 mL of sterile water for injection or 5% dextrose injection; do not use saline for reconstitution. Dilute the calculated dose further in 50–250 mL of 5% dextrose solution; solutions of 1 and 2.5 mg/mL in 5% dextrose are stable at room temperature for up to 24 hr. Protect from light.
Infusion: Infuse the diluted solution over 60 min.
Y-site incompatibilities: Do not mix with foscarnet.

Adverse effects
Parenteral
- **CV:** *Hypotension,* tachycardia
- **GI:** *Nausea, anorexia*
- **GU:** *Elevated serum creatinine,* **acute renal failure**
- **Hematologic:** *Leukopenia, hypoglycemia,* thrombocytopenia, hypocalcemia, elevated liver function tests
- **Local:** *Pain, abscess at injection site*
- **Other:** Stevens-Johnson syndrome, *fever, rash,* **severe hypotension,** hypoglycemia, and cardiac arrhythmias
Inhalation
- **CNS:** *Fatigue, dizziness,* headache, tremors, confusion, anxiety, memory loss, seizure, insomnia, drowsiness

Adverse effects in *Italics* are most common; those in **Bold** are life-threatening.

- **CV:** Tachycardia, hypotension, hypertension, palpitations, syncope, vasodilatation
- **GI:** *Metallic taste to mouth, anorexia, nausea, vomiting,* gingivitis, dyspepsia, oral ulcer, gastritis, hypersalivation, dry mouth, melena, colitis, abdominal pain
- **Respiratory:** *Shortness of breath, cough, pharyngitis, congestion, bronchospasm,* rhinitis, laryngitis, laryngospasm, hyperventilation, pneumothorax
- **Other:** *Rash, night sweats, chills*

■ Nursing considerations
Assessment
- **History:** History of anaphylactic reaction to inhaled or parenteral pentamidine isethionate, hypotension, hypertension, hypoglycemia, hyperglycemia, hypocalcemia, leukopenia, thrombocytopenia, anemia, hepatic or renal dysfunction, pregnancy, lactation
- **Physical:** Skin lesions, color; T; reflexes, affect (inhalation); BP, P, baseline ECG; BUN, serum creatinine, blood glucose, CBC, platelet count, liver function tests, serum calcium

Interventions
- Monitor patient closely during administration; fatalities have been reported.
- Arrange for the following tests to be performed before, during, and after therapy: daily BUN, daily serum creatinine, daily blood glucose; regular CBC, platelet counts, liver function tests, serum calcium; periodic ECG.
- Position patient in supine position before parenteral administration to protect patient if BP changes occur.
- Reconstitute for inhalation: Dissolve contents of 1 vial in 6 mL of sterile water for injection. Use only sterile water. Saline cannot be used, precipitates will form. Place entire solution in nebulizer reservoir. Solution is stable for 48 hr in original vial at room temperature if protected from light. Do not mix with other drugs.
- Administer inhalation using the *Respirgard II* nebulizer. Deliver the dose until the chamber is empty (30–45 min).
- For IM use: Prepare IM solution by dissolving contents of 1-g vial in 3 mL of sterile water for injection; protect from light. Discard any unused portions. Inject deeply into large muscle group. Inspect injection site regularly; rotate injection sites.

- Instruct patient and significant other in the reconstitution of inhalation solutions and administration for outpatient use.

Teaching points
- Parenteral drug can be given only IV or IM and must be given every day. Inhalation drug must be given using the *Respirgard II* nebulizer. Prepare the solution as instructed by your health care provider, using only sterile water for injection. Protect the medication from exposure to light. Use freshly reconstituted solution. The drug must be used once every 4 wk. Prepare a calendar with drug days marked as a reminder. Do not mix any other drugs in the nebulizer.
- Have frequent blood tests and BP checks because this drug may cause many changes in your body.
- You may feel weak and dizzy with sudden position changes; take care to change position slowly.
- If using the inhalation, metallic taste and GI upset may occur. Small, frequent meals and mouth care may help.
- Report pain at injection site, confusion, hallucinations, unusual bleeding or bruising, weakness, fatigue.

▽ pentazocine
(pen taz' oh seen)

pentazocine lactate
Parenteral: Talwin

pentazocine hydrochloride with naloxone hydrochloride, 0.5 mg
Oral: Talwin NX

PREGNANCY CATEGORY C

C-IV CONTROLLED SUBSTANCE

Drug class
Narcotic agonist-antagonist analgesic

Therapeutic actions
Pentazocine acts as an agonist at specific (kappa) opioid receptors in the CNS to produce analgesia, sedation; acts as an agonist at sig-

ma opioid receptors to cause dysphoria, hallucinations; acts at mu opioid receptors to antagonize the analgesic and euphoric activities of some other narcotic analgesics. Has lower abuse potential than morphine, other pure narcotic agonists; the oral preparation contains the opioid antagonist naloxone, which has poor bioavailability when given orally and does not interfere with the analgesic effects of pentazocine but serves as a deterrent to the unintended IV injection of solutions made from the oral tablets.

Indications

- Relief of moderate to severe pain (oral and parenteral)
- Preanesthetic medication and as supplement to surgical anesthesia (parenteral)

Contraindications and cautions

- Contraindicated with hypersensitivity to narcotics, to naloxone (oral form); pregnancy (neonatal withdrawal); labor or delivery (narcotics given to the mother can cause neonatal respiratory depression; premature infants are especially at risk; may prolong labor); lactation.
- Use cautiously with physical dependence on a narcotic analgesic (can precipitate a withdrawal syndrome); bronchial asthma, COPD, cor pulmonale, respiratory depression, anoxia, increased intracranial pressure; acute MI with hypertension, left ventricular failure or nausea and vomiting; renal or hepatic dysfunction.

Available forms

Injection—30 mg/mL; tablets—50 mg

Dosages

Adults

Oral

Initially, 50 mg q 3–4 hr. Increase to 100 mg if necessary. Do not exceed a total dose of 600 mg/24 hr.

Parenteral

30 mg IM, SC, or IV. May repeat q 3–4 hr. Doses > 30 mg IV or 60 mg IM or SC are not recommended. Do not exceed 360 mg/24 hr. Give SC only when necessary; repeat injections should be given IM.

- *Patients in labor:* A single 30-mg IM dose is most common. A 20-mg IV dose given 2–3 times at 2- to 3-hr intervals relieves pain when contractions become regular.

Pediatric patients < 12 yr

Not recommended.

Geriatric patients or impaired adults

Use caution; respiratory depression may occur in elderly, very ill, those with respiratory problems. Reduced dosage may be necessary.

Pharmacokinetics

Route	Onset	Peak	Duration
Oral, IM, SC	15–30 min	1–3 hr	3 hr
IV	2–3 min	15 min	3 hr

Metabolism: Hepatic; $T_{1/2}$: 2–3 hr
Distribution: Crosses placenta; enters breast milk
Excretion: Urine and feces

▼IV facts

Preparation: No further preparation is required.
Infusion: Inject directly into vein or into tubing of actively running IV; infuse slowly, each 5 mg over 1 min.
Incompatibilities: Do not mix in same syringe as barbiturates; precipitate will form.

Adverse effects

- **CNS:** *Light-headedness, dizziness, sedation, euphoria,* dysphoria, delirium, insomnia, agitation, anxiety, fear, hallucinations, disorientation, drowsiness, lethargy, impaired mental and physical performance, coma, mood changes, weakness, headache, tremor, convulsions, miosis, visual disturbances
- **CV:** Facial flushing, peripheral circulatory collapse, tachycardia, bradycardia, arrhythmia, palpitations, chest wall rigidity, hypertension, hypotension, orthostatic hypotension, syncope, circulatory depression, **shock, cardiac arrest**
- **Dermatologic:** Pruritus, urticaria, edema
- **GI:** *Nausea, vomiting, sweating* (more common in ambulatory patients and those without severe pain), dry mouth, anorexia,

constipation, biliary tract spasm; increased colonic motility in patients with chronic ulcerative colitis
- **GU:** Ureteral spasm, spasm of vesical sphincters, urinary retention or hesitancy, oliguria, antidiuretic effect, reduced libido or potency
- **Local:** Pain at injection site, tissue irritation and induration (SC injection)
- **Respiratory:** Suppression of cough reflex, respiratory depression, apnea, respiratory arrest, laryngospasm, bronchospasm
- **Other:** Physical tolerance and dependence, psychological dependence (**the oral form has been especially abused in combination with tripelennamine—"Ts and Blues"—with serious and fatal consequences;** the addition of naloxone to the oral formulation may decrease this abuse)

Interactions
✷ **Drug-drug** • Increased likelihood of respiratory depression, hypotension, profound sedation, or coma with barbiturate general anesthetics • Precipitation of withdrawal syndrome in patients previously given other narcotic analgesics, including morphine, methadone (note that this applies to the parenteral preparation without naloxone and to the oral preparation that includes naloxone)

■ Nursing considerations
Assessment
- **History:** Hypersensitivity to narcotics, to naloxone (oral form); physical dependence on a narcotic analgesic; pregnancy; labor or delivery; lactation; respiratory disease; anoxia; increased intracranial pressure; acute MI; renal or hepatic dysfunction
- **Physical:** T; skin color, texture, lesions; orientation, reflexes, bilateral grip strength, affect, pupil size; P, auscultation, BP, orthostatic BP, perfusion; R, adventitious sounds; bowel sounds, normal output; frequency and pattern of voiding, normal output; liver, kidney function tests, CBC with differential

Interventions
- Do not mix parenteral pentazocine in same syringe as barbiturates; precipitate will form.

- Provide narcotic antagonist, equipment for assisted or controlled respiration on standby during parenteral administration.
- Use caution when injecting SC into chilled areas of the body or in patients with hypotension or in shock; impaired perfusion may delay absorption; with repeated doses, an excessive amount may be absorbed when circulation is restored.
- Withdraw drug gradually if it has been given for 4–5 days, especially to emotionally unstable patients or those with a history of drug abuse; a withdrawal syndrome sometimes occurs in these circumstances.
- Reassure patient about addiction liability; most patients who receive opiates for medical reasons do not develop dependence syndromes.

Teaching points
- Take drug exactly as prescribed.
- Avoid alcohol, antihistamines, sedatives, tranquilizers, OTC drugs while taking this drug.
- These side effects may occur: nausea, loss of appetite (take drug with food, lie quietly, eat frequent small meals); constipation (a laxative may help); dizziness, sedation, drowsiness, impaired visual acuity (avoid driving or performing other tasks that require alertness, visual acuity).
- Do not take any leftover medication for other disorders, and do not let anyone else take the prescription.
- Report severe nausea, vomiting, constipation, shortness of breath or difficulty breathing.

▷**pentobarbital
(pentobarbital sodium)**
*(pen toe **bar**' bi tal)*

Nembutal, Nembutal Sodium, Novopentobarb (CAN), Nova Rectal (CAN)

PREGNANCY CATEGORY D

C-II CONTROLLED SUBSTANCE

Drug classes
Barbiturate
Sedative or hypnotic

Hypnotic
Anticonvulsant

Therapeutic actions

General CNS depressant; barbiturates inhibit impulse conduction in the ascending RAS, depress the cerebral cortex, alter cerebellar function, depress motor output, and can produce excitation, sedation, hypnosis, anesthesia, and deep coma; at anesthetic doses, has anticonvulsant activity.

Indications

- Sedative or hypnotic for short-term treatment of insomnia (appears to lose effectiveness for sleep induction and maintenance after 2 wk; oral)
- Preanesthetic medication (oral)
- Sedation when oral or parenteral administration may be undesirable (rectal)
- Hypnotic for short-term treatment of insomnia (rectal)
- Sedative (parenteral)
- Anticonvulsant, in anesthetic doses, for emergency control of certain acute convulsive episodes (eg, status epilepticus, eclampsia, meningitis, tetanus, toxic reactions to strychnine or local anesthetics; parenteral)

Contraindications and cautions

- Contraindicated with hypersensitivity to barbiturates, manifest or latent porphyria, marked liver impairment, nephritis, severe respiratory distress, previous addiction to sedative–hypnotic drugs, pregnancy (fetal damage, neonatal withdrawal syndrome), lactation.
- Use cautiously with acute or chronic pain (paradoxical excitement or masking of important symptoms); seizure disorders (abrupt discontinuation of daily doses can result in status epilepticus); fever, hyperthyroidism, diabetes mellitus, severe anemia, pulmonary or cardiac disease, status asthmaticus, shock, uremia.

Available forms

Capsules—50, 100 mg; elixir—20 mg/5 mL; suppositories—30, 60, 120, 200 mg; injection—50 mg/mL

Dosages

Adults

Oral

- *Daytime sedation:* 20 mg tid–qid.
- *Hypnotic:* 100 mg hs.

Rectal

120–200 mg hs.

Parenteral

Use only when other routes are not feasible or prompt action is imperative.

- *IV:* Give by slow IV injection, 50 mg/min. Initial dose is 100 mg in a 70-kg adult. Wait at least 1 min for full effect. Base dosage on response. Additional small increments may be given up to a total of 200–500 mg. Minimize dosage in convulsive states to avoid compounding the depression that may follow convulsions.
- *IM:* Inject deeply into a muscle mass. Usual adult dose is 150–200 mg. Do not exceed a volume of 5 mL at any site due to tissue irritation.

Pediatric patients

Use caution: barbiturates may produce irritability, aggression, inappropriate tearfulness.

Oral

- *Preoperative sedation:* 2–6 mg/kg/day (maximum: 100 mg), depending on age, weight, degree of sedation desired.
- *Hypnotic:* Base dosage on age and weight.

Rectal

Do not divide suppositories.
12–14 yr (80–110 lb): 60 or 120 mg.
5–12 yr (40–80 lb): 60 mg.
1–4 yr (20–40 lb): 30 or 60 mg.
2 mo–1 yr (10–20 lb): 30 mg.

Parenteral

- *IV:* Reduce initial adult dosage on basis of age, weight, and patient's condition.
- *IM:* Dosage frequently ranges from 25 to 80 mg or 2–6 mg/kg.

Geriatric patients or those with debilitating disease

Reduce dosage and monitor closely. May produce excitement, depression, confusion.

Pharmacokinetics

Route	Onset	Duration
Oral	10–15 min	3–4 hr
IM, IV	Rapid	2–3 hr

Adverse effects in *Italics* are most common; those in **Bold** are life-threatening.

Metabolism: Hepatic; $T_{1/2}$: 15–20 hr
Distribution: Crosses placenta; enters breast milk
Excretion: Urine

▼ IV facts

Preparation: No further preparation is required.
Infusion: Infuse slowly, each 50 mg over 1 min; monitor patient response to dosage.
Incompatibilities: Do not combine with chlorpheniramine, codeine, ephedrine, erythromycin, hydrocortisone, insulin, norepinephrine, penicillin G, potassium, phenytoin, promazine, vancomycin.

Adverse effects

- **CNS:** *Somnolence, agitation, confusion, hyperkinesia, ataxia, vertigo, CNS depression, nightmares, lethargy, residual sedation (hangover), paradoxical excitement, nervousness, psychiatric disturbance, hallucinations, insomnia, anxiety, dizziness, thinking abnormality*
- **CV:** *Bradycardia, hypotension, syncope*
- **GI:** *Nausea, vomiting, constipation, diarrhea, epigastric pain*
- **Hypersensitivity:** Rashes, angioneurotic edema, serum sickness, morbiliform rash, urticaria; rarely, exfoliative dermatitis, **Stevens-Johnson syndrome**
- **Local:** *Pain, tissue necrosis at injection site,* gangrene; arterial spasm with inadvertent intra-arterial injection; thrombophlebitis; permanent neurologic deficit if injected near a nerve
- **Respiratory:** *Hypoventilation, apnea, respiratory depression,* laryngospasm, bronchospasm, **circulatory collapse**
- **Other:** Tolerance, psychological and physical dependence; **withdrawal syndrome**

Interactions

✳ Drug-drug • Increased CNS depression with alcohol • Increased nephrotoxicity with methoxyflurane • Decreased effects of the following drugs: oral anticoagulants, corticosteroids, hormonal contraceptives and estrogens, beta-adrenergic blockers (especially propranolol, metoprolol), theophylline, metronidazole, doxycycline, griseofulvin, phenylbutazones, quinidine

■ Nursing considerations
Assessment

- **History:** Hypersensitivity to barbiturates, manifest or latent porphyria, marked liver impairment, nephritis, severe respiratory distress, previous addiction to sedative-hypnotic drugs, acute or chronic pain, seizure disorders, pregnancy, lactation, fever, hyperthyroidism, diabetes mellitus, severe anemia, pulmonary or cardiac disease, shock, uremia
- **Physical:** Weight; T; skin color, lesions, injection site; orientation, affect, reflexes; P, BP, orthostatic BP; R, adventitious sounds; bowel sounds, normal output, liver evaluation; liver and kidney function tests, blood and urine glucose, BUN

Interventions

- Do not administer intra-arterially; may produce arteriospasm, thrombosis, gangrene.
- Administer IV doses slowly.
- Administer IM doses deep in a muscle mass.
- Do not use parenteral form if solution is discolored or contains a precipitate.
- Monitor injection sites carefully for irritation, extravasation (IV use); solutions are alkaline and very irritating to the tissues.
- Monitor P, BP, respiration carefully during IV administration.
- Taper dosage gradually after repeated use, especially in epileptic patients.

Teaching points

- This drug will make you drowsy and less anxious.
- Do not try to get up after you have received this drug (request assistance to sit up or move about).

Outpatients

- Take this drug exactly as prescribed. This drug is habit-forming; its effectiveness in facilitating sleep disappears after a short time. Do not take this drug longer than 2 wk (for insomnia) and do not increase the dosage without consulting your physician. If the drug appears to be ineffective, consult your health care provider.
- Avoid alcohol, sleep-inducing, or OTC drugs. These could cause dangerous effects.
- Avoid becoming pregnant while you are taking this drug. Use other methods of contraception in place of hormonal contraceptives,

P

which may lose their effectiveness with this drug.

- These side effects may occur: drowsiness, dizziness, hangover, impaired thinking (may lessen after a few days; avoid driving or engaging in activities that require alertness); GI upset (take drug with food); dreams, nightmares, difficulty concentrating, fatigue, nervousness (reversible).
- Report severe dizziness, weakness, drowsiness that persists, rash or skin lesions, pregnancy.

▷ pentosan polysulfate sodium

See *Less Commonly Used Drugs,* p. 1348.

▷ pentostatin

See *Less Commonly Used Drugs,* p. 1348.

▷ pentoxifylline

(pen tox i' fi leen)

Trental

PREGNANCY CATEGORY C

Drug classes

Hemorheologic agent
Xanthine

Therapeutic actions

Reduces RBC aggregation and local hyperviscosity, decreases platelet aggregation, decreases fibrinogen concentration in the blood; precise mechanism of action is not known.

Indications

- Intermittent claudication, to improve function and symptoms
- Unlabeled use: cerebrovascular insufficiency to improve psychopathologic symptoms, diabetic vascular disease

Contraindications and cautions

- Contraindicated with allergy to pentoxifylline or methylxanthines (eg, caffeine, theophyl-

line; drug is a dimethylxanthine derivative), lactation.
- Use cautiously with pregnancy.

Available forms

ER tablets—400 mg

Dosages
Adults

400 mg tid PO with meals. Decrease to 400 mg bid if adverse side effects occur. Continue for at least 8 wk.

Pediatric patients

Safety and efficacy not established.

Pharmacokinetics

Route	Onset	Peak
Oral	Varies	60 min

Metabolism: Hepatic; $T_{1/2}$: 0.4–1.6 hr
Distribution: Crosses placenta; enters breast milk
Excretion: Urine

Adverse effects

- **CNS:** *Dizziness, headache,* tremor, anxiety, confusion
- **CV:** Angina, chest pain, arrhythmia, hypotension, dyspnea
- **Dermatologic:** Brittle fingernails, pruritus, rash, urticaria
- **GI:** *Dyspepsia, nausea,* vomiting
- **Hematologic:** Pancytopenia, purpura, thrombocytopenia

Interactions

✳ **Drug-drug** • Increased therapeutic and toxic effects of theophylline when combined; monitor closely and adjust dosage as needed

■ Nursing considerations
Assessment

- **History:** Allergy to pentoxifylline or methylxanthines, pregnancy, lactation
- **Physical:** Skin color, T; orientation, reflexes; P, BP, peripheral perfusion; CBC

Interventions

- Monitor patient for angina, arrhythmias.
- Administer drug with meals.

Adverse effects in *Italics* are most common; those in **Bold** are life-threatening.

- Caution patient to swallow CR tablets whole—do not cut, crush, or chew.

Teaching points
- Take drug with meals. Swallow CR tablets whole; do not cut, crush, or chew.
- This drug helps the signs and symptoms of claudication, but additional therapy is needed.
- Dizziness may occur as a result of therapy; avoid driving and operating dangerous machinery; take precautions to prevent injury.
- Report chest pain, flushing, loss of consciousness, twitching, numbness and tingling.

▽pergolide mesylate
(per' go lide)

Permax

PREGNANCY CATEGORY B

Drug class
Antiparkinsonian agent

Therapeutic actions
Potent dopamine receptor agonist; inhibits the secretion of prolactin, causes a transient rise in growth hormone and decrease in luteinizing hormone; directly stimulates postsynaptic dopamine receptors in the nigrostriatal system.

Indications
- Adjunctive treatment to levodopa-carbidopa in the management of the signs and symptoms of Parkinson's disease

Contraindications and cautions
- Contraindicated with hypersensitivity to pergolide or ergot derivatives, lactation (suppression of prolactin may inhibit nursing).
- Use cautiously with cardiac arrhythmias, hallucinations, confusion, dyskinesias, pregnancy.

Available forms
Tablets—0.05, 0.25, 1 mg

Dosages
Adults
Initiate with a daily dose of 0.05 mg PO for the first 2 days. Gradually increase dosage by 0.1 or 0.15 mg/day every third day over the next 12 days of therapy. May then be increased by 0.25 mg/day every third day until an optimal therapeutic dosage is achieved. *Usual dose:* 3 mg given in three equally divided doses per day. Maximum 5 mg/day.
Pediatric patients
Safety and efficacy not established.

Pharmacokinetics

Route	Onset	Peak
Oral	Varies	2 hr

Metabolism: Hepatic; $T_{1/2}$: 8–12 hr
Distribution: May cross placenta; may enter breast milk
Excretion: Urine and lungs

Adverse effects
- **CNS:** *Dyskinesias, dizziness, hallucinations, dystonias, confusion, somnolence, insomnia, anxiety, tremor,* fatigue, anxiety, convulsions, depression, drowsiness, vertigo, hyperesthesia, irritability, nervousness, visual disturbances
- **CV:** *Postural hypotension, vasodilation,* palpitation, hypotension, syncope, hypertension, arrhythmia
- **Dermatologic:** Rash, sweating
- **GI:** *Nausea, constipation, diarrhea, dyspepsia,* anorexia, dry mouth, vomiting
- **GU:** Urinary frequency, urinary tract infection, hematuria
- **Respiratory:** *Rhinitis, dyspnea,* epistaxis, hiccups
- **Other:** *Pain, abdominal pain, headache, asthenia,* chest pain, neck pain, chills, *peripheral edema,* edema, weight gain, anemia

■ Nursing considerations
Assessment
- **History:** Hypersensitivity to pergolide or ergot derivatives, cardiac arrhythmias, hallucinations, confusion, dyskinesias, lactation
- **Physical:** Reflexes; affect; BP, P, peripheral perfusion; abdominal exam, normal output; auscultation; R; urinary output

Interventions
- Administer with extreme caution to patients with a history of cardiac arrhythmias, hallucinations, confusion, or dyskinesias.

- Monitor patient while adjusting drug to establish therapeutic dosage. Dosage of levodopa/carbidopa may require adjustment to balance therapeutic effects.

Teaching points

- Take this drug with your levodopa and carbidopa. The dosage will need to be adjusted carefully over the next few weeks to get the best effect for you. Keep appointments to have this dosage evaluated. Instruct a family member or significant other about this medication, because confusion and hallucinations are common effects; you may not be able to remember or follow instructions.
- These side effects may occur: dizziness, confusion, shaking (avoid driving or performing hazardous tasks; change position slowly; use caution when climbing stairs); nausea, diarrhea, constipation (proper nutrition is important); pain, swelling (generalized pain and discomfort may occur); running nose (common problem; do not self-medicate).
- Report hallucinations, palpitations, tingling in the arms or legs, chest pain.

▽ **perindopril erbumine**
(pur in' doh pril)

Aceon

PREGNANCY CATEGORY C
(FIRST TRIMESTER)

PREGNANCY CATEGORY D
(SECOND AND THIRD TRIMESTERS)

Drug classes

Antihypertensive
Angiotensin-converting enzyme inhibitor (ACE inhibitor)

Therapeutic actions

Renin, synthesized by the kidneys, is released into the circulation where it acts on a plasma precursor to produce angiotensin I, which is converted by angiotensin-converting enzyme (ACE) to angiotensin II—a potent vasoconstrictor that also causes release of aldosterone from the adrenals. Perindopril blocks the conversion of angiotensin I to angiotensin II, leading to decreased blood pressure, decreased aldosterone secretion, a small increase in serum potassium levels, and sodium and fluid loss.

Indications

- Treatment of hypertension, alone or in combination with other antihypertensive medication

Contraindications and cautions

- Contraindicated with allergy to any ACE inhibitor, pregnancy.
- Use cautiously with impaired renal function, CHF, salt or volume depletion, lactation.

Available forms

Tablets—2, 4, 8 mg

Dosages

Adults

4 mg PO daily; may be titrated to a maximum of 16 mg/day.

Pediatric patients

Safety and efficacy not established.

Geriatric patients

Maximum daily dosage should not exceed 8 mg/day.

Patients with renal impairment

For creatinine clearance > 30 mL/min, give an initial dose of 2 mg/day PO. Maximum dose: 8 mg/day. For creatinine clearance ≤ 30 mL/min, do not administer drug.

Pharmacokinetics

Route	Onset	Peak
Oral	1 hr	3–7 hr

Metabolism: Hepatic; $T_{1/2}$: 30–120 hr
Distribution: Crosses placenta; passes into breast milk
Excretion: Urine

Adverse effects

- **CNS:** *Headache, dizziness, insomnia, fatigue,* paresthesias
- **CV:** *Orthostatic hypotension,* tachycardia, angina pectoris, myocardial infarction, Raynaud's syndrome, CHF (severe hypotension in salt- or volume-depleted patients)

Adverse effects in *Italics* are most common; those in **Bold** are life-threatening.

- **GI:** *Gastric irritation, nausea, diarrhea,* aphthous ulcers, peptic ulcers, dysgeusia, cholestatic jaundice, hepatocellular injury, anorexia, constipation
- **GU:** *Proteinuria,* renal insufficiency, renal failure, polyuria, oliguria, frequency of urination
- **Hematologic:** Neutropenia, agranulocytosis, thrombocytopenia, hemolytic anemia, **pancytopenia**
- **Other:** *Angioedema* (particularly of the face, extremities, lips, tongue, larynx; death has been reported with **airway obstruction**—greater risk in black patients; *cough,* muscle cramps, impotence

Interactions
✳ **Drug-drug** • Decreased antihypertensive effects if taken with indomethacin

■ Nursing considerations
Assessment
- **History:** Allergy to any ACE inhibitor; impaired renal function; CHF; salt or volume depletion; pregnancy, lactation
- **Physical:** Skin color, lesions, turgor; T; P, BP, peripheral perfusion; mucous membranes; bowel sounds, liver evaluation; urinalysis, renal and liver function tests, CBC and differential

Interventions
- Maintain epinephrine on standby in case of angioedema of the face or neck region; if difficulty breathing occurs, consult with physician and administer epinephrine as appropriate.
- Alert surgeon and mark patient's chart with notice that perindopril is being taken. The angiotensin II formation subsequent to compensatory renin release during surgery will be blocked. Hypotension may be reversed with volume expansion.
- Monitor patients on diuretic therapy for excessive hypotension; the diuretic should be stopped 2–3 days before beginning therapy with perindopril and introduced slowly, monitoring patient response.
- Monitor patient closely in any situation that may lead to a fall in blood pressure secondary to reduction in fluid volume—excessive perspiration and dehydration, vomiting, di-

arrhea—as excessive hypotension may occur.
- Arrange for reduced dosage in patients with impaired renal function.
- Caution patient that this drug can cause serious fetal injury; advise the use of barrier contraceptives.

Teaching points
- Take this drug once a day; it may be taken with meals. Do not stop taking the medication without consulting your physician.
- These side effects may occur: GI upset, loss of appetite, change in taste perception (these may be limited effects which will pass with time; taking the drug with meals may help); mouth sores (frequent mouth care may help); rash; fast heart rate; dizziness, lightheadedness (this usually passes after the first few days of therapy; if it occurs, change position slowly and limit your activities to ones that do not require alertness and precision); headache, fatigue, sleeplessness.
- Be careful with any condition that may lead to a drop in blood pressure—diarrhea, sweating, vomiting, dehydration. If lightheadedness or dizziness should occur, consult your nurse or physician.
- Avoid the use of OTC medications while you are on this drug—especially cough, cold, or allergy medications that may contain ingredients that will interact with this drug. If you feel that you need one of these preparations, consult your nurse or physician.
- Avoid pregnancy while on this drug, serious fetal injury could occur. Use of barrier contraceptives is advised.
- Report mouth sores, sore throat, fever, chills, swelling of the hands, feet, irregular heartbeat, chest pains, swelling of the face, eyes, lips, tongue, difficulty breathing.

▽ perphenazine
(per fen' a zeen)

Apo-Perphenazine (CAN), Phenazine (CAN), Trilafon

PREGNANCY CATEGORY C

Drug classes
Phenothiazine (piperazine)

Dopaminergic blocking agent
Antipsychotic
Antiemetic

Therapeutic actions

Mechanism of action not fully understood: antipsychotic drugs block postsynaptic dopamine receptors in the brain, but this may not be necessary and sufficient for antipsychotic activity; depresses the RAS, including the parts of the brain involved with wakefulness and emesis; anticholinergic, antihistaminic (H_1), and alpha-adrenergic blocking activity also may contribute to some of its therapeutic (and adverse) actions.

Indications

- Management of manifestations of psychotic disorders
- Control of severe nausea and vomiting, intractable hiccups

Contraindications and cautions

- Contraindicated with coma or severe CNS depression, bone marrow depression, blood dyscrasia, circulatory collapse, subcortical brain damage, Parkinson's disease, liver damage, cerebral arteriosclerosis, coronary disease, severe hypotension or hypertension.
- Use cautiously with respiratory disorders ("silent pneumonia" may develop); glaucoma, prostatic hypertrophy; epilepsy or history of epilepsy; breast cancer; thyrotoxicosis; peptic ulcer, decreased renal function; myelography within previous 24 hr or scheduled within 48 hr; exposure to heat or phosphorous insecticides; pregnancy; lactation; children younger than 12 yr, especially those with chickenpox, CNS infections (children are especially susceptible to dystonias that may confound the diagnosis of Reye's syndrome).

Available forms

Tablets—2, 4, 8, 16 mg; concentrate—16 mg/5 mL; injection—5 mg/mL

Dosages

Adults

Full clinical antipsychotic effects may require 6 wk–6 mo of therapy.

- *Moderately disturbed nonhospitalized patients:* 4–8 mg PO tid; reduce as soon as possible to minimum effective dosage.
- *Hospitalized patients:* 8–16 mg PO bid–qid. Avoid dosages > 64 mg/day.

IM

Initial dose 5–10 mg q 6 hr. Total dosage should not exceed 15 mg/day in ambulatory, 30 mg/day in hospitalized patients. Switch to oral dosage as soon as possible.

- *Antiemetic:* 8–16 mg/day PO in divided doses (occasionally 24 mg may be needed); 5–10 mg IM for rapid control of vomiting; 5 mg IV in divided doses by slow infusion of dilute solutions. Give IV only when necessary to control severe vomiting.

Pediatric patients

< 12 yr: Not recommended
> 12 yr: Use lowest adult dosage.

Geriatric patients or debilitated patients

Use lower doses (one-third to one-half adult dose), and increase dosage more gradually than in younger patients.

Pharmacokinetics

Route	Onset	Peak	Duration
Oral	Varies	Unknown	
IM, IV	5–10 min	1–2 hr	6 hr

Metabolism: Hepatic; $T_{1/2}$: unknown
Distribution: Crosses placenta; enters breast milk
Excretion: Urine

▼IV facts

Preparation: Dilute drug to 0.5 mg/mL.
Infusion: Give by either fractional injection or slow drip infusion. When giving as divided doses, give no more than 1 mg/injection at not less than 1- to 2-min intervals. Do not exceed 5 mg total dose; hypotensive and extrapyramidal effects may occur.
Y-site incompatibilities: Do not give with cefoperazone.

Adverse effects

- **Autonomic:** Dry mouth, salivation, nasal congestion, nausea, vomiting, anorexia, fever, pallor, flushed facies, sweating, constipation, paralytic ileus, urinary retention,

incontinence, polyuria, enuresis, priapism, ejaculation inhibition, male impotence
- **CNS:** *Drowsiness,* insomnia, vertigo, headache, weakness, tremor, ataxia, slurring, cerebral edema, seizures, exacerbation of psychotic symptoms, extrapyramidal syndromes—*pseudoparkinsonism; dystonias; akathisia,* tardive dyskinesias, potentially irreversible (no known treatment), **neuroleptic malignant syndrome**
- **CV:** Hypotension, orthostatic hypotension, hypertension, tachycardia, bradycardia, cardiac arrest, CHF, cardiomegaly, **refractory arrhythmias,** pulmonary edema
- **EENT:** Glaucoma, *photophobia, blurred vision,* miosis, mydriasis, deposits in the cornea and lens (opacities), pigmentary retinopathy
- **Endocrine:** Lactation, breast engorgement, galactorrhea; syndrome of inappropriate ADH secretion (SIADH); amenorrhea, menstrual irregularities; gynecomastia; changes in libido; hyperglycemia or hypoglycemia; glycosuria; hyponatremia; pituitary tumor with hyperprolactinemia; inhibition of ovulation, infertility, pseudopregnancy; reduced urinary levels of gonadotropins, estrogens, progestins
- **Hematologic:** Eosinophilia, leukopenia, leukocytosis, anemia; aplastic anemia; hemolytic anemia; thrombocytopenic or nonthrombocytopenic purpura; pancytopenia
- **Hypersensitivity:** Jaundice, urticaria, angioneurotic edema, laryngeal edema, photosensitivity, eczema, asthma, anaphylactoid reactions, exfoliative dermatitis
- **Respiratory:** Bronchospasm, laryngospasm, dyspnea; suppression of cough reflex and potential for aspiration (**sudden death related to asphyxia or cardiac arrest** has been reported)
- **Other:** *Urine discolored pink to red-brown*

Interactions

✳ Drug-drug • Additive CNS depression with alcohol • Additive anticholinergic effects and possibly decreased antipsychotic efficacy with anticholinergic drugs • Increased likelihood of seizures with metrizamide (contrast agent used in myelography) • Increased chance of severe neuromuscular excitation and hypotension with barbiturate anesthetics (methohexital, thiamylal, phenobarbital, thiopental) • Decreased antihypertensive effect of guanethidine when taken with antipsychotics

✳ Drug-lab test • False-positive pregnancy tests (less likely if serum test is used) • Increase in protein-bound iodine, not attributable to an increase in thyroxine

■ Nursing considerations
Assessment

- **History:** Coma or severe CNS depression; bone marrow depression; circulatory collapse; subcortical brain damage; Parkinson's disease; liver damage; cerebral arteriosclerosis; coronary disease; severe hypotension or hypertension; respiratory disorders; glaucoma, prostatic hypertrophy; epilepsy; breast cancer; thyrotoxicosis; peptic ulcer, decreased renal function; myelography within previous 24 hr or myelography scheduled within 48 hr; exposure to heat or phosphorus insecticides; pregnancy; children younger than 12 yr
- **Physical:** Weight, T; reflexes, orientation, intraocular pressure; P, BP, orthostatic BP; R, adventitious sounds; bowel sounds and normal output, liver evaluation; urinary output, prostate size; CBC, urinalysis, thyroid, liver, and kidney function tests

Interventions

- Dilute oral concentrate only with water, saline, *7-Up*, homogenized milk, carbonated orange drink, and pineapple, apricot, prune, orange, *V-8*, tomato, and grapefruit juices; use 60 mL of diluent for each 16 mg (5 mL) of concentrate.
- Do not mix with beverages that contain caffeine (coffee, cola), tannics (tea), or pectinates (apple juice); physical incompatibility may result.
- Give IM injections only to seated or recumbent patients, and observe for adverse effects for a brief period afterward.
- Monitor pulse and BP continuously during IV administration.
- Do not change dosage in long-term therapy more often than weekly; drug requires 4–7 days to achieve steady-state plasma levels.
- Avoid skin contact with oral solution; contact dermatitis has occurred.
- Discontine drug if serum creatinine, BUN become abnormal or if WBC count is depressed.
- Monitor elderly patients for dehydration, and institute remedial measures promptly; se-

dation and decreased sensation of thirst related to CNS effects of drug can lead to severe dehydration.
• Consult physician regarding appropriate warning of patient or patient's guardian about tardive dyskinesias.
• Consult physician about dosage reduction, use of anticholinergic antiparkinsonian drugs (controversial) if extrapyramidal effects occur.

Teaching points
• Take drug exactly as prescribed.
• Avoid skin contact with drug solutions.
• Avoid driving or engaging in other dangerous activities if CNS, vision changes occur.
• Avoid prolonged exposure to sun; use a sunscreen or covering garments.
• Maintain fluid intake, and use precautions against heat stroke in hot weather.
• Report sore throat, fever, unusual bleeding or bruising, rash, weakness, tremors, impaired vision, dark urine (pink or reddish-brown urine is expected), pale stools, yellowing of the skin or eyes.

▽**phenazopyridine hydrochloride (phenylazo-diaminopyridine hydrochloride)**

(fen az oh peer' i deen)

Azo-Standard, Baridium, Geridium, Phenazo (CAN), Prodium, Pyridiate, Pyridium, Pyridium Plus, Urodine, Urogesic, UTI Relief

PREGNANCY CATEGORY B

Drug class
Urinary analgesic

Therapeutic actions
An azo dye that is excreted in the urine and exerts a direct topical analgesic effect on urinary tract mucosa; exact mechanism of action is not understood.

Indications
• Symptomatic relief of pain, urgency, burning, frequency, and discomfort related to irritation of the lower urinary tract mucosa caused by infection, trauma, surgery, endoscopic procedures, passage of sounds or catheters

Contraindications and cautions
• Contraindicated with allergy to phenazopyridine, renal insufficiency.
• Use cautiously with pregnancy, lactation.

Available forms
Tablets—95, 97.2, 100, 200 mg

Dosages
Adults
200 mg PO tid after meals. Do not exceed 2 days if used with antibacterial agent.
Pediatric patients 6–12 yr
12 mg/kg/day or 350 mg/m²/day divided into 3 doses PO.

Pharmacokinetics

Route	Onset
Oral	Rapid

Metabolism: Hepatic; $T_{1/2}$: unknown
Distribution: Crosses placenta; may enter breast milk
Excretion: Urine

Adverse effects
• **CNS:** *Headache*
• **Dermatologic:** *Rash,* yellowish tinge to skin or sclera
• **GI:** *GI disturbances*
• **Hematologic:** Methemoglobinemia, hemolytic anemia
• **Other:** Renal and hepatic toxicity, cancer, *yellow-orange discoloration of urine*

Interactions
✳ **Drug-lab test** • Interference with colorimetric laboratory test procedures

■ Nursing considerations
Assessment
• **History:** Allergy to phenazopyridine, renal insufficiency, pregnancy

Adverse effects in *Italics* are most common; those in **Bold** are life-threatening.

- **Physical:** Skin color, lesions; urinary output; normal GI output, bowel sounds, liver palpation; urinalysis, renal and liver function tests, CBC

Interventions

- Give after meals to avoid GI upset.
- Do not give longer than 2 days if being given with antibacterial agent for treatment of UTI.
- Alert patient that urine may be reddish-orange and may stain fabric.
- Discontinue drug if skin or sclera become yellowish, a sign of drug accumulation.

Teaching points

- Take drug after meals to avoid GI upset.
- Urine may be reddish-orange (normal effect; urine may stain fabric).
- Report yellowish stain to skin or eyes, headache, unusual bleeding or bruising, fever, sore throat.

▽ phenelzine sulfate
(fen' el zeen)

Nardil

PREGNANCY CATEGORY C

Drug classes

Antidepressant
Monoamine oxidase inhibitor (MAO inhibitor)

Therapeutic actions

Irreversibly inhibits MAO, an enzyme that breaks down biogenic amines, such as epinephrine, norepinephrine, and serotonin, thus allowing these biogenic amines to accumulate in neuronal storage sites. According to the biogenic amine hypothesis, this accumulation of amines is responsible for the clinical efficacy of MAOIs as antidepressants.

Indications

- Treatment of patients with depression characterized as atypical, nonendogenous, or neurotic; patients who are unresponsive to other antidepressive therapy; and patients in whom other antidepressive therapy is contraindicated

Contraindications and cautions

- Contraindicated with hypersensitivity to any MAOI, pheochromocytoma, CHF, history of liver disease or abnormal liver function tests, severe renal impairment, confirmed or suspected cerebrovascular defect, CV disease, hypertension, history of headache, myelography within previous 24 hr or scheduled within 48 hr.
- Use cautiously with seizure disorders; hyperthyroidism; impaired Hepatic; renal function; psychiatric patients (agitated or schizophrenic patients may show excessive stimulation; manic-depressive patients may shift to hypomanic or manic phase); patients scheduled for elective surgery; pregnancy; lactation.

Available forms

Tablets—15 mg

Dosages
Adults

Initially, 15 mg PO tid. Increase dosage to at least 60 mg/day at a fairly rapid pace consistent with patient tolerance. Many patients require therapy at 60 mg/day for at least 4 wk before response. Some patients may require 90 mg/day. After maximum benefit is achieved, reduce dosage slowly over several weeks. Maintenance may be 15 mg/day or every other day.
Pediatric patients

Not recommended for patients < 16 yr.
Geriatric patients

Patients > 60 yr are more prone to develop adverse effects; adjust dosage accordingly.

Pharmacokinetics

Route	Onset	Duration
Oral	Slow	48–96 hr

Metabolism: Hepatic; $T_{1/2}$: unknown
Distribution: Crosses placenta; enters breast milk
Excretion: Urine

Adverse effects

- **CNS:** *Dizziness, vertigo, headache, overactivity, hyperreflexia, tremors, muscle twitching, mania, hypomania, jitteriness, confusion, memory impairment, insomnia, weakness, fatigue, drowsiness, restlessness, overstimulation, increased anx-*

iety, agitation, blurred vision, sweating, akathisia, ataxia, coma, euphoria, neuritis, repetitious babbling, chills, glaucoma, nystagmus

- **CV: Hypertensive crises** (sometimes fatal, sometimes with intracranial bleeding, usually attributable to ingestion of contraindicated food or drink containing tyramine; see drug-food interactions below; symptoms include some or all of the following: occipital headache, which may radiate frontally; palpitations; neck stiffness or soreness; nausea; vomiting; sweating; dilated pupils; photophobia; tachycardia or bradycardia; chest pain); *orthostatic hypotension, sometimes associated with falling; disturbed cardiac rate and rhythm,* palpitations, tachycardia
- **Dermatologic:** Minor skin reactions, spider telangiectases, photosensitivity
- **GI:** *Constipation, diarrhea, nausea, abdominal pain, edema, dry mouth, anorexia, weight changes*
- **GU:** Dysuria, incontinence, urinary retention, sexual disturbances
- **Other:** Hematologic changes, black tongue, hypernatremia

Interactions

❋ **Drug-drug** • Increased sympathomimetic effects (hypertensive crisis) with sympathomimetic drugs (norepinephrine, epinephrine, dopamine, dobutamine, levodopa, ephedrine), amphetamines, other anorexiants, local anesthetic solutions containing sympathomimetics • Hypertensive crisis, coma, severe convulsions with TCAs (eg, imipramine, desipramine). Note: MAOIs and TCAs have been used successfully in some patients resistant to therapy with single agents; however, case reports indicate that the combination can cause serious and potentially fatal adverse effects. • Additive hypoglycemic effect with insulin, oral sulfonylureas • Increased risk of adverse interaction with meperidine • Risk of serotonin syndrome if combined with SSRIs

❋ **Drug food** • Tyramine (and other pressor amines) contained in foods are normally broken down by MAO enzymes in the GI tract; in the presence of MAOIs, these vasopressors may be absorbed in high concentrations; in addi-

tion, tyramine releases accumulated norepinephrine from nerve terminals; thus, hypertensive crisis may occur when the following foods that contain tyramine or other vasopressors are ingested by a patient on an MAOI: dairy products (blue, camembert, cheddar, mozzarella, parmesan, romano, roquefort, Stilton cheeses; sour cream; yogurt); meats, fish (liver, pickled herring, fermented sausages—bologna, pepperoni, salami; caviar; dried fish; other fermented or spoiled meat or fish); undistilled beverages (imported beer, ale; red wine, especially Chianti; sherry; coffee, tea, colas containing caffeine; chocolate drinks); fruit/vegetables (avocado, fava beans, figs, raisins, bananas); yeast extracts, soy sauce, chocolate

❋ **Drug-alternative therapy** • May cause headaches, manic episodes if combined with ginseng therapy

■ Nursing considerations
Assessment

- **History:** Hypersensitivity to any MAOI; pheochromocytoma, CHF; abnormal liver function tests; severe renal impairment; cerebrovascular defect; CV disease, hypertension; history of headache; myelography within previous 24 hr or scheduled within 48 hr; seizure disorders; hyperthyroidism; impaired hepatic, renal function; psychiatric patients; elective surgery; pregnancy, lactation
- **Physical:** Weight; T; skin color, lesions; orientation, affect, reflexes, vision; P, BP, orthostatic BP, auscultation, perfusion; bowel sounds, normal output, liver evaluation; urine flow, normal output; thyroid palpation; liver, kidney, and thyroid function tests, urinalysis, CBC, ECG, EEG

Interventions

- Limit amount of drug that is available to suicidal patients.
- Monitor BP and orthostatic BP carefully; arrange for more gradual increase in dosage in patients who show tendency for hypotension.
- Have periodic liver function tests during therapy; discontinue drug at first sign of hepatic dysfunction or jaundice.
- Discontinue drug and monitor BP carefully if patient reports unusual or severe headache.

Adverse effects in *Italics* are most common; those in **Bold** are life-threatening.

- Provide phentolamine or another alpha-adrenergic blocking drug on standby in case hypertensive crisis occurs.
- Provide diet that is low in tyramine-containing foods.

Teaching points

- Take drug exactly as prescribed. Do not stop taking this drug abruptly or without consulting your health care provider.
- Avoid ingestion of tyramine-containing foods while you are taking this drug and for 2 wk afterward (patient and significant other should receive a list of such foods).
- Avoid alcohol; other sleep-inducing drugs; all OTC drugs, including nose drops, cold and hay fever remedies; and appetite suppressants. Many of these contain substances that could cause serious or even life-threatening problems.
- These side effects may occur: dizziness, weakness or fainting when arising from a horizontal or sitting position (transient; change position slowly); drowsiness, blurred vision (reversible; if severe, avoid driving or performing tasks that require alertness); nausea, vomiting, loss of appetite (small, frequent meals, frequent mouth care may help); memory changes, irritability, emotional changes, nervousness (reversible).
- Report headache, rash, darkening of the urine, pale stools, yellowing of the eyes or skin, fever, chills, sore throat, any other unusual symptoms.

▽phenobarbital
(fee noe bar' bi tal)

phenobarbital
Oral preparations: Barbilixir (CAN), Barbita (CAN), Bellatal, Solfoton

phenobarbital sodium
Parenteral: Luminal Sodium

PREGNANCY CATEGORY D

C-IV CONTROLLED SUBSTANCE

Drug classes
Barbiturate (long acting)

Sedative
Hypnotic
Anticonvulsant
Antiepileptic agent

Therapeutic actions
General CNS depressant; barbiturates inhibit impulse conduction in the ascending RAS, depress the cerebral cortex, alter cerebellar function, depress motor output, and can produce excitation, sedation, hypnosis, anesthesia, and deep coma; at subhypnotic doses, has anticonvulsant activity, making it suitable for long-term use as an antiepileptic.

Indications
- Sedative (oral or parenteral)
- Hypnotic, short-term (up to 2 wk) treatment of insomnia (oral or parenteral)
- Long-term treatment of generalized tonic-clonic and cortical focal seizures (oral)
- Emergency control of certain acute convulsive episodes (eg, those associated with status epilepticus, eclampsia, meningitis, tetanus, and toxic reactions to strychnine or local anesthetics; parenteral)
- Preanesthetic (parenteral)
- Anticonvulsant treatment of generalized tonic-clonic and cortical focal seizures (parenteral)
- Emergency control of acute convulsions (tetanus, eclampsia, epilepticus; parenteral)

Contraindications and cautions
- Contraindicated with hypersensitivity to barbiturates, manifest or latent porphyria; marked liver impairment; nephritis; severe respiratory distress; previous addiction to sedative-hypnotic drugs (may be ineffective and may contribute to further addiction); pregnancy (fetal damage, neonatal withdrawal syndrome); lactation.
- Use cautiously with acute or chronic pain (drug may cause paradoxical excitement or mask important symptoms); seizure disorders (abrupt discontinuation of daily doses can result in status epilepticus); lactation (secreted in breast milk; drowsiness in nursing infants); fever, hyperthyroidism, diabetes mellitus, severe anemia, pulmonary or cardiac disease, status asthmaticus, shock, uremia; impaired liver or kidney function, debilitation.

Available forms
Tablets—8, 15, 16, 30, 60, 90, 100 mg; capsules—15 mg; elixir—20 mg/5 mL; injection—30, 60, 65, 130 mg/mL

Dosages
Adults
Oral
- *Sedation:* 30–120 mg/day in two to three divided doses.
- *Hypnotic:* 100–200 mg hs.
- *Anticonvulsant:* 60–100 mg/day.

IM or IV
- *Sedation:* 30–120 mg/day IM or IV in two to three divided doses.
- *Preoperative sedation:* 100–200 mg IM, 60–90 min before surgery.
- *Hypnotic:* 100–320 mg IM or IV.
- *Acute convulsions:* 200–320 mg IM or IV repeated in 6 hr if necessary.

Pediatric patients
Oral
- *Sedation:* 2 mg/kg/dose PO tid.
- *Hypnotic:* Determine dosage using age and weight charts.
- *Anticonvulsant:* 3–5 mg/kg/day.

IM or IV
- *Preoperative sedation:* 1–3 mg/kg IM or IV 60–90 min before surgery.
- *Anticonvulsant:* 4–6 mg/kg/day for 7–10 days to a blood level of 10–15 mcg/mL or 10–15 mg/kg/day IV or IM.
- *Status epilepticus:* 15–20 mg/kg IV over 10–15 min.

Geriatric patients or patients with debilitating disease or renal or hepatic impairment
Reduce dosage and monitor closely—may produce excitement, depression, confusion.

Pharmacokinetics

Route	Onset	Duration
Oral	30–60 min	10–16 hr
IM, SC	10–30 min	4–6 hr
IV	5 min	4–6 hr

Metabolism: Hepatic; $T_{1/2}$: 79 hr
Distribution: Crosses placenta; enters breast milk
Excretion: Urine

▼IV facts
Preparation: No further preparation is needed.

Infusion: Infuse very slowly, each 60 mg over 1 min, directly IV or into tubing or running IV; inject partial dose and observe for response before continuing.

Incompatibilities: Do not combine with chlorpromazine, codeine, ephedrine, hydralazine, hydrocortisone, insulin, meperidine, methadone, procaine, promazine, vancomycin.

Adverse effects
- **CNS:** *Somnolence, agitation, confusion, hyperkinesia, ataxia, vertigo, CNS depression, nightmares, lethargy, residual sedation (hangover), paradoxical excitement, nervousness, psychiatric disturbance, hallucinations, insomnia, anxiety, dizziness, thinking abnormality*
- **CV:** *Bradycardia, hypotension, syncope*
- **GI:** *Nausea, vomiting, constipation, diarrhea, epigastric pain*
- **Hypersensitivity:** Rashes, angioneurotic edema, serum sickness, morbiliform rash, urticaria; rarely, exfoliative dermatitis, **Stevens-Johnson syndrome**
- **Local:** *Pain, tissue necrosis at injection site,* gangrene; arterial spasm with inadvertent intra-arterial injection; thrombophlebitis; permanent neurologic deficit if injected near a nerve
- **Respiratory:** *Hypoventilation, apnea, respiratory depression,* laryngospasm, bronchospasm, circulatory collapse
- **Other:** Tolerance, psychological and physical dependence, **withdrawal syndrome**

Interactions
✳ Drug-drug • Increased serum levels and therapeutic and toxic effects with valproic acid • Increased CNS depression with alcohol • Increased risk of nephrotoxicity with methoxyflurane • Increased risk of neuromuscular excitation and hypotension with barbiturate anesthetics • Decreased effects of the following drugs: theophyllines, oral anticoagulants, beta-blockers, doxycycline, griseofulvin, corticosteroids, hormonal contraceptives and estrogens, metronidazole, phenylbutazones, quinidine

■ Nursing considerations
Assessment

- **History:** Hypersensitivity to barbiturates, manifest or latent porphyria; marked liver impairment; nephritis; severe respiratory distress; previous addiction to sedative-hypnotic drugs; pregnancy; acute or chronic pain; seizure disorders; lactation; fever; hyperthyroidism; diabetes mellitus; severe anemia; cardiac disease; shock; uremia; impaired liver or kidney function; debilitation
- **Physical:** Weight; T; skin color, lesions; orientation, affect, reflexes; P, BP, orthostatic BP; R, adventitious sounds; bowel sounds, normal output, liver evaluation; liver and kidney function tests, blood and urine glucose, BUN

Interventions

- Monitor patient responses, blood levels (as appropriate) if any of the above interacting drugs are given with phenobarbital; suggest alternative means of contraception to women using hormonal contraceptives.
- Do not administer intra-arterially; may produce arteriospasm, thrombosis, gangrene.
- Administer IV doses slowly.
- Administer IM doses deep in a large muscle mass (gluteus maximus, vastus lateralis) or other areas where there is little risk of encountering a nerve trunk or major artery.
- Monitor injection sites carefully for irritation, extravasation (IV use). Solutions are alkaline and very irritating to the tissues.
- Monitor P, BP, respiration carefully during IV administration.
- Arrange for periodic laboratory tests of hematopoietic, renal, and hepatic systems during long-term therapy.
- Taper dosage gradually after repeated use, especially in epileptic patients. When changing from one antiepileptic drug to another, taper dosage of the drug being discontinued while increasing the dosage of the replacement drug.

Teaching points

- This drug will make you drowsy and less anxious; do not try to get up after you have received this drug (request assistance to sit up or move around).

- Take this drug exactly as prescribed; this drug is habit forming; its effectiveness in facilitating sleep disappears after a short time.
- Do not take this drug longer than 2 wk (for insomnia), and do not increase the dosage without consulting the prescriber.
- Do not reduce the dosage or discontinue this drug (when used for epilepsy); abrupt discontinuation could result in a serious increase in seizures.
- These side effects may occur: drowsiness, dizziness, hangover, impaired thinking (may lessen after a few days; avoid driving or engaging in dangerous activities); GI upset (take drug with food); dreams, nightmares, difficulty concentrating, fatigue, nervousness (reversible).
- Wear a medical alert tag so that emergency medical personnel will know you are an epileptic taking this medication.
- Avoid pregnancy while taking this drug; use a means of contraception other than hormonal contraceptives.
- Report severe dizziness, weakness, drowsiness that persists, rash or skin lesions, fever, sore throat, mouth sores, easy bruising or bleeding, nosebleed, petechiae, pregnancy.

▷ phensuximide
(fen sux' i mide)

Milontin Kapseals

PREGNANCY CATEGORY C

Drug classes
Antiepileptic agent
Succinimide

Therapeutic actions
Suppresses the paroxysmal three cycle per second spike and wave EEG pattern associated with lapses of consciousness in absence (petit mal) seizures; reduces frequency of attacks; mechanism of action not understood, but may act in inhibitory neuronal systems that are important in the generation of the three per second rhythm.

Indications
- Control of absence (petit mal) seizures when refractory to other drugs

Contraindications and cautions

- Contraindicated with hypersensitivity to succinimides.
- Use cautiously with hepatic, renal abnormalities, acute intermittent porphyria, pregnancy (association between use of antiepileptic drugs by women with epilepsy and an elevated incidence of birth defects in children born to these women; however, antiepileptic therapy should not be discontinued in pregnant women who are receiving such therapy to prevent major seizures; the effect of even minor seizures on the developing fetus is unknown, and this should be considered when deciding whether to continue antiepileptic therapy in pregnant women), lactation.

Available forms

Capsules—500 mg

Dosages
Adults and pediatric patients

Administer 500–1,000 mg PO bid–tid. The total dosage may vary between 1 and 3 g/day (average, 1.5 g/day). May be administered with other antiepileptic drugs when other forms of epilepsy coexist with absence (petit mal) seizures.

Pharmacokinetics

Route	Onset	Peak
Oral	Varies	1–4 hr

Metabolism: Hepatic; $T_{1/2}$: 4 hr
Distribution: Crosses placenta; enters breast milk
Excretion: Urine and bile

Adverse effects
Succinimides

- **CNS:** *Drowsiness, ataxia, dizziness,* irritability, nervousness, headache, blurred vision, myopia, photophobia, hiccups, euphoria, dreamlike state, lethargy, hyperactivity, fatigue, insomnia, increased frequency of grand mal seizures may occur when used alone; in some patients with mixed types of epilepsy, confusion, instability, mental slowness, depression, hypochondriacal be-

havior, sleep disturbances, night terrors, aggressiveness, inability to concentrate
- **Dermatologic:** Pruritus, urticaria, Stevens-Johnson syndrome, pruritic erythematous rashes, skin eruptions, erythema multiforme, systemic lupus erythematosus, alopecia, hirsutism
- **GI:** *Nausea, vomiting, vague gastric upset, epigastric and abdominal pain,* cramps, anorexia, diarrhea, constipation, weight loss, swelling of tongue, gum hypertrophy
- **Hematologic:** Eosinophilia, granulocytopenia, leukopenia, agranulocytosis, aplastic anemia, monocytosis, **pancytopenia**
- **Other:** Periorbital edema, hyperemia, muscle weakness, abnormal liver and kidney function tests, vaginal bleeding, *discoloration of urine* (pink, red, or brown; not harmful)

Interactions
✳ **Drug-drug** • Decreased serum levels and therapeutic effects of primidone

■ Nursing considerations
Assessment

- **History:** Hypersensitivity to succinimides; hepatic, renal abnormalities; acute intermittent porphyria; pregnancy; lactation
- **Physical:** Skin color, lesions; orientation, affect, reflexes, bilateral grip strength, vision exam; bowel sounds, normal output, liver evaluation; liver and kidney function tests, urinalysis, CBC with differential, EEG

Interventions

- Reduce dosage, discontinue phensuximide, or substitute other antiepileptic medication gradually; abrupt discontinuation may precipitate absence (petit mal) status.
- Monitor CBC and differential before and frequently during therapy.
- Discontinue drug if rash, depression of blood count, or unusual depression, aggressiveness, or behavioral alterations occurs.

Teaching points

- Take this drug exactly as prescribed; do not discontinue this drug abruptly or change

---

Adverse effects in *Italics* are most common; those in **Bold** are life-threatening.

dosage, except on the advice of your prescriber.
- Arrange for frequent checkups to monitor your response to this drug.
- These side effects may occur: drowsiness, dizziness, confusion, blurred vision (avoid driving or performing other tasks requiring alertness or visual acuity); GI upset (take drug with food or milk; eat frequent, small meals).
- Wear a medical alert tag at all times so that emergency medical personnel will know that you are an epileptic taking antiepileptic medication.
- Report rash, joint pain, unexplained fever, sore throat, unusual bleeding or bruising, drowsiness, dizziness, blurred vision, pregnancy.

▽phentolamine mesylate
*(fen **tole'** a meen)*

Regitine, Rogitine (CAN)

PREGNANCY CATEGORY C

Drug classes
Alpha-adrenergic blocker
Diagnostic agent

Therapeutic actions
Competitively blocks postsynaptic alpha$_1$-adrenergic receptors, decreasing sympathetic tone on the vasculature, dilating blood vessels, and lowering arterial BP (no longer used to treat essential hypertension because it also blocks presynaptic alpha$_2$-adrenergic receptors that are believed to mediate a feedback inhibition of further norepinephrine release; this accentuates the reflex tachycardia caused by the lowering of BP); use of phentolamine injection as a test for pheochromocytoma depends on the premise that a greater BP reduction will occur with pheochromocytoma than with other etiologies of hypertension.

Indications
- Pheochromocytoma—prevention or control of hypertensive episodes that may result from stress or manipulation during preoperative preparation and surgical excision

- Pharmacologic test for pheochromocytoma (urinary assays of catecholamines, other biochemical tests have largely supplanted the phentolamine test)
- Prevention and treatment of dermal necrosis and sloughing following IV administration or extravasation of norepinephrine or dopamine
- Unlabeled use: treatment of hypertensive crises secondary to MAOI/sympathomimetic amine interactions, or secondary to rebound hypertension on withdrawal of clonidine, propranolol, or other antihypertensive drugs

Contraindications and cautions
- Contraindicated with hypersensitivity to phentolamine or related drugs, evidence of CAD.
- Use cautiously with pregnancy, lactation.

Available forms
Injection—5 mg/vial; powder for injection—5 mg

Dosages
Adults
- *Prevention or control of hypertensive episodes in pheochromocytoma:* For use in preoperative reduction of elevated BP, inject 5 mg IV or IM 1–2 hr before surgery. Repeat if necessary. Administer 5 mg IV during surgery as indicated to control paroxysms of hypertension, tachycardia, respiratory depression, convulsions.
- *Prevention and treatment of dermal necrosis following IV administration or extravasation of norepinephrine:* For prevention, add 10 mg to each liter of solution containing norepinephrine. The pressor effect of norepinephrine is not affected. For treatment, inject 5–10 mg in 10 mL saline into the area of extravasation within 12 hr.
- *Diagnosis of pheochromocytoma:* See manufacturer's recommendations. This test should be used only to confirm evidence and after the risks have been carefully considered.

Pediatric patients
- *Prevention or control of hypertensive episodes in pheochromocytoma:* For use in preoperative reduction of elevated BP, inject 1 mg IV or IM 1–2 hr before surgery. Repeat

P

if necessary. Administer 1 mg IV during surgery as indicated to control paroxysms of hypertension, tachycardia, respiratory depression, convulsions.

Pharmacokinetics

Route	Onset	Peak	Duration
IM	Rapid	20 min	30–45 min
IV	Immediate	2 min	15–30 min

Metabolism: Unknown
Distribution: Unknown
Excretion: Kidneys

▼IV facts

Preparation: Reconstitute by adding 1 mL of sterile water for injection to the vial, producing a solution of 5 mg/mL.
Infusion: Inject slowly directly into vein or into tubing of actively running IV, each 5 mg over 1 min.

Adverse effects

- **CNS:** *Weakness, dizziness*
- **CV:** *Acute and prolonged hypotensive episodes,* orthostatic hypotension, **MI,** cerebrovascular spasm, cerebrovascular occlusion, *tachycardia, arrhythmias*
- **GI:** *Nausea,* vomiting, diarrhea
- **Other:** Flushing, nasal stuffiness

Interactions

✳ Drug-drug • Decreased vasoconstrictor and hypertensive effects of epinephrine, ephedrine

■ Nursing considerations
Assessment

- **History:** Hypersensitivity to phentolamine or related drugs, evidence of CAD, pregnancy
- **Physical:** Orientation, affect, reflexes; ophthalmologic exam; P, BP, orthostatic BP, supine BP, perfusion, edema, auscultation; bowel sounds, normal output

Interventions

- Change positions slowly.
- Monitor BP response, heart rate carefully.

Teaching points

- Report dizziness, palpitations.

▷ **phenylephrine hydrochloride**
(fen ill ef' rin)

Parenteral: Neo-Synephrine
Oral: AH-Chew D
Topical OTC nasal decongestants: Afrin Children's Pump Mist, Coricidin, Dionephrine (CAN), Little Noses Gentle Formula, Neo-Synephrine, Rhinall, Vicks Sinex Ultra Fine Mist
Ophthalmic preparations (0.12% solutions are OTC): AK-Dilate, AK-Nefrin, Mydfrin, Neo-Synephrine, Ocu-Phrin (CAN), Phenoptic, Preferin Liquifilm, Relief

PREGNANCY CATEGORY C

Drug classes

Sympathomimetic amine
Alpha-adrenergic agonist
Vasopressor
Nasal decongestant
Ophthalmic vasoconstrictor or mydriatic

Therapeutic actions

Powerful postsynaptic alpha-adrenergic receptor stimulant that causes vasoconstriction and increased systolic and diastolic BP with little effect on the beta receptors of the heart. Topical application causes vasoconstriction of the mucous membranes, which in turn relieves pressure and promotes drainage of the nasal passages. Topical ophthalmic application causes contraction of the dilator muscles of the pupil (mydriasis), vasoconstriction, and increased outflow of aqueous humor.

Indications

- Treatment of vascular failure in shock, shocklike states, drug-induced hypotension, or hypersensitivity (parenteral)
- To overcome paroxysmal supraventricular tachycardia (parenteral)
- To prolong spinal anesthesia (parenteral)
- Vasoconstrictor in regional anesthesia (parenteral)

Adverse effects in *Italics* are most common; those in **Bold** are life-threatening.

- To maintain an adequate level of BP during spinal and inhalation anesthesia (parenteral)
- Symptomatic relief of nasal and nasopharyngeal mucosal congestion due to the common cold, hay fever, or other respiratory allergies (topical)
- Adjunctive therapy of middle ear infections by decreasing congestion around the eustachian ostia (topical)
- 10% solution: decongestant and vasoconstrictor and for pupil dilation in uveitis, wide-angle glaucoma and surgery (ophthalmic solution)
- 2.5% solution: decongestant and vasoconstrictor and for pupil dilation in uveitis, open-angle glaucoma in conjunction with miotics, refraction, ophthalmoscopic examination, diagnostic procedures, and before intraocular surgery (ophthalmic solution)
- 0.12% solution: decongestant to provide temporary relief of minor eye irritations caused by hay fever, colds, dust, wind, smog, or hard contact lenses (ophthalmic solution)

Contraindications and cautions
- Contraindicated with hypersensitivity to phenylephrine; severe hypertension, ventricular tachycardia; narrow-angle glaucoma; pregnancy.
- Use cautiously with thyrotoxicosis, diabetes, hypertension, CV disorders; prostatic hypertrophy, unstable vasomotor syndrome; lactation.

Available forms
Chewable tablets—10 mg; nasal solution—0.125%, 0.16%, 0.25%, 0.5%, 1%; ophthalmic solution—0.12%, 2.5%, 10%; injection—10 mg/mL

Dosages
Parenteral preparations may be given IM, SC, by slow IV injection, or as a continuous IV infusion of dilute solutions; for supraventricular tachycardia and emergency use, give by direct IV injection.
Adults
- *Mild to moderate hypotension (adjust dosage on basis of BP response):* 1–10 mg SC or IM; do not exceed an initial dose of 5 mg. A 5-mg IM dose should raise BP for 1–2 hr.

IV
0.1–0.5 mg. Initial dose should not exceed 0.5 mg. Do not repeat more often than q 10–15 min. 0.5 mg IV should raise the pressure for 15 min.
- *Severe hypotension and shock:* Continuous infusion: add 10 mg to 500 mL of dextrose injection or sodium chloride injection. Start infusion at 100–180 mcg/min (based on a drop factor of 20 drops/mL; this would be 100–180 drops/min). When BP is stabilized, maintain at 40–60 mcg/min. If prompt vasopressor response is not obtained, add 10-mg increments to infusion bottle.
- *Spinal anesthesia:* 2–3 mg SC or IM 3–4 min before injection of spinal anesthetic.
- *Hypotensive emergencies during anesthesia:* Give 0.2 mg IV. Do not exceed 0.5 mg/dose.
- *Prolongation of spinal anesthesia:* Addition of 2–5 mg to the anesthetic solution increases the duration of motor block by as much as 50%.
- *Vasoconstrictor for regional anesthesia:* 1:20,000 concentration (add 1 mg of phenylephrine to every 20 mL of local anesthetic solution).
- *Paroxysmal supraventricular tachycardia:* Rapid IV injection (within 20–30 sec) is recommended. Do not exceed an initial dose of 0.5 mg. Subsequent doses should not exceed the preceding dose by more than 0.1–0.2 mg and should never exceed 1 mg. Use only after other treatments have failed.
- *Nasal decongestant:* 1–2 sprays of the 0.25% solution in each nostril q 3–4 hr. In severe cases, the 0.5% or 1% solution may be needed; 10 mg PO bid–qid.
- *Vasoconstriction and pupil dilation:* 1 drop of 2.5% or 10% solution on the upper limbus. May be repeated in 1 hr. Precede instillation with a local anesthetic to prevent tearing and dilution of the drug solution.
- *Uveitis to prevent posterior synechiae:* 1 drop of the 2.5% or 10% solution on the surface of the cornea with atropine.
- *Glaucoma:* 1 drop of 10% solution on the upper surface of the cornea repeated as often as necessary and in conjunction with miotics in patients with wide-angle glaucoma.
- *Intraocular surgery:* 2.5% or 10% solution may be instilled in the eye 30–60 min before the operation.

- *Refraction:* 1 drop of a cycloplegic drug followed in 5 min by 1 drop of phenylephrine 2.5% solution and in 10 min by another drop of the cycloplegic.
- *Ophthalmoscopic exam:* 1 drop of 2.5% phenylephrine solution in each eye. Mydriasis is produced in 15–30 min and lasts for 1–3 hr.
- *Minor eye irritation:* 1–2 drops of the 0.12% solution in eye bid to qid as needed.

Pediatric patients

- *Hypotension during spinal anesthesia:* 0.5–1 mg/25 lb SC or IM.
- *Nasal decongestion:*
  > 6 yr: 1–2 sprays of the 0.25% solution in each nostril q 3–4 hr.
  2–6 yr: 2–3 drops of 0.125% solution in each nostril q 4 hr, prn.
- *Refraction:* 1 drop of atropine sulfate 1% in each eye. Follow in 10–15 min with 1 drop of phenylephrine 2.5% solution and in 5–10 min with a second drop of atropine. Eyes will be ready for refraction in 1–2 hr.

Geriatric patients

These patients are more likely to experience adverse reactions; use with caution.

Pharmacokinetics

Route	Onset	Duration
IV	Immediate	15–20 min
IM, SC	10–15 min	30–120 min

Topical generally not absorbed systemically.
Metabolism: Hepatic and tissue; $T_{1/2}$: 47–100 hr
Distribution: Crosses placenta; enters breast milk

▼IV facts

Preparation: Inject directly for emergency use; dilute phenylephrine 1 mg/L is compatible with dextrose-Ringer's combinations; dextrose-lactated Ringer's combinations; dextrose-saline combinations; dextrose 2 1/2%, 5%, and 10% in water; Ringer's injection; lactated Ringer's injection; 0.45% and 0.9% sodium chloride injection; 1/6 M sodium lactate injection.
Infusion: Give single dose over 20–30 sec to 1 min. Determine actual rate of continuous infusion using an infusion pump by patient response.

Adverse effects

Adverse effects are less likely with topical administration.

Systemic administration

- **CNS:** *Fear, anxiety, tenseness, restlessness, headache, light-headedness, dizziness,* drowsiness, tremor, insomnia, hallucinations, psychological disturbances, convulsions, CNS depression, weakness, blurred vision, ocular irritation, tearing, photophobia, symptoms of paranoid schizophrenia
- **CV: Cardiac arrhythmias**
- **GI:** *Nausea,* vomiting, anorexia
- **GU:** Constriction of renal blood vessels and *decreased urine formation* (initial parenteral administration), *dysuria, vesical sphincter spasm* resulting in difficult and painful urination, urinary retention in males with prostatism
- **Local:** Necrosis and sloughing if extravasation occurs with IV use
- **Other:** *Pallor,* respiratory difficulty, orofacial dystonia, sweating

Nasal solution

- **EENT:** *Blurred vision,* ocular irritation, tearing, photophobia
- **Local:** *Rebound congestion, local burning and stinging,* sneezing, dryness, contact dermatitis

Ophthalmic solutions

- **CNS:** *Headache, browache, blurred vision,* photophobia, difficulty with night vision, *pigmentary (adrenochrome) deposits in the cornea, conjunctiva,* or lids if applied to damaged cornea
- **Local:** *Transitory stinging on initial instillation*
- **Other:** Rebound miosis, decreased mydriatic response in older patients; significant BP elevation in compromised elderly patients with cardiac problems

Interactions

✳ **Drug-drug** • Severe headache, hypertension, hyperpyrexia, possibly resulting in hypertensive crisis with MAO inhibitors (isocarboxazid, phenelzine, tranylcypromine). Do not administer sympathomimetic amines to patients on MAOIs • Increased sympath-omimetic effects with TCAs (eg, imipramine) • Excessive hypertension with furazolidone • Decreased antihypertensive effect of guanethi-dine, methyldopa • Potential for serious ar-rhythmias with halogenated hydrocarbon anes-thetics

■ **Nursing considerations**
Assessment
• **History:** Hypersensitivity to phenylephrine; severe hypertension, ventricular tachycar-dia; narrow-angle glaucoma; thyrotoxico-sis; diabetes; CV disorders; prostatic hyper-trophy; unstable vasomotor syndrome; pregnancy; lactation
• **Physical:** Skin color, T; orientation, re-flexes, affect, peripheral sensation, vision, pupils; BP, P, auscultation, peripheral per-fusion; R, adventitious sounds; urinary out-put, bladder percussion, prostate palpation; ECG

Interventions
• Protect parenteral solution from light; do not administer unless solution is clear; dis-card unused portion.
• Maintain an alpha-adrenergic blocking agent on standby in case of severe reaction or overdose.
• Infiltrate area of extravasation with phen-tolamine (5–10 mg in 10–15 mL of saline), using a fine hypodermic needle; usually ef-fective if area is infiltrated within 12 hr of extravasation.
• Monitor P, BP continuously during parenteral administration.
• Do not administer ophthalmic solution that has turned brown or contains precipitates; prevent prolonged exposure to air and light.
• Administer ophthalmic solution as follows: have patient lie down or tilt head backward and look at ceiling. Hold dropper above eye; drop medicine inside lower lid while patient is looking up. Do not touch dropper to eye, fingers, or any surface. Have patient keep eye open and avoid blinking for at least 30 sec. Apply gentle pressure with fingers to inside corner of the eye for about 1 min. Caution patient not to close eyes tightly and not to blink more often than usual.
• Do not administer other eye drops for at least 5 min after phenylephrine.

• Do not administer nasal decongestant for longer than 3–5 days.
• Do not administer ophthalmic solution for longer than 72 hr.
• Monitor BP and cardiac response regularly in patients with any CV disorders.
• Use topical anesthetics if ophthalmic prepa-rations are painful and burning.
• Monitor CV effects carefully; patients with hypertension who take this drug may expe-rience changes in BP because of the addi-tional vasoconstriction. If a nasal decon-gestant is needed, pseudoephedrine is the drug of choice.

Teaching points
• Do not exceed recommended dose. Demon-strate proper administration technique for topical nasal and ophthalmic preparations.
• Avoid prolonged use, because underlying medical problems can be disguised. Limit is 3–5 days for nasal decongestant, 72 hr for ophthalmic preparations.
• These side effects may occur: dizziness, drowsiness, fatigue, apprehension (use cau-tion if driving or performing tasks that re-quire alertness); *nasal solution,* burning or stinging when first used (transient); *oph-thalmic solution,* slight stinging when first used (usually transient); blurring of vision.
• Report nervousness, palpitations, sleepless-ness, sweating; *ophthalmic solution,* severe eye pain, vision changes, floating spots, eye redness or sensitivity to light, headache.

▷ **phenytoin (diphenylhydantoin, phenytoin sodium)**
(fen' i toe in)

Dilantin-125, Dilantin Infatab, Dilantin Injection, Dilantin Kapseals, Diphenylan (CAN), Phenytek, Phenytex (CAN)

PREGNANCY CATEGORY D

Drug classes
Antiepileptic agent
Hydantoin

Therapeutic actions

Has antiepileptic activity without causing general CNS depression; stabilizes neuronal membranes and prevents hyperexcitability caused by excessive stimulation; limits the spread of seizure activity from an active focus; also effective in treating cardiac arrhythmias, especially those induced by digitalis; antiarrhythmic properties are very similar to those of lidocaine; both are class IB antiarrhythmics.

Indications

- Control of grand mal (tonic-clonic) and psychomotor seizures
- Prevention and treatment of seizures occurring during or following neurosurgery
- Control of status epilepticus of the grand mal type (parenteral administration)
- Unlabeled uses: antiarrhythmic, particularly in digitalis-induced arrhythmias (IV preparations); treatment of trigeminal neuralgia (tic douloureux)

Contraindications and cautions

- Contraindicated with hypersensitivity to hydantoins, sinus bradycardia, sinoatrial block, Stokes-Adams syndrome, pregnancy (data suggest an association between antiepileptic drug use and an elevated incidence of birth defects; however, do not discontinue antiepileptic therapy in pregnant women who are receiving such therapy to prevent major seizures; this is likely to precipitate status epilepticus, with attendant hypoxia and risk to both mother and fetus), lactation.
- Use cautiously with acute intermittent porphyria, hypotension, severe myocardial insufficiency, diabetes mellitus, hyperglycemia.

Available forms

Chewable tablets—50 mg; oral suspension—125 mg/5 mL; capsules—30, 100 mg; ER capsules—200, 300 mg; injection—50 mg/mL

Dosages
Adults
Phenytoin sodium, parenteral

- *Status epilepticus:* 10–15 mg/kg by slow IV. Maintenance: 100 mg PO or IV q 6–8 hr.

Higher doses may be required. Do not exceed an infusion rate of 50 mg/min. Follow each IV injection with an injection of sterile saline through the same needle or IV catheter to avoid local venous irritation by the alkaline solution. Continuous IV infusion is not recommended.

- *Neurosurgery (prophylaxis):* 100–200 mg IM q 4 hr during surgery and the postoperative period (IM route is not recommended because of erratic absorption, pain and muscle damage at the injection site).
- *IM therapy in a patient previously stabilized on oral dosage:* Increase dosage by 50% over oral dosage. When returning to oral dosage, decrease dose by 50% of the original oral dose for 1 wk to prevent excessive plasma levels due to continued absorption from IM tissue sites. Avoid IM route of administration if possible due to erratic absorption and pain and muscle damage at injection site.

Phenytoin and phenytoin sodium, oral

Individualize dosage. Determine serum levels for optimal dosage adjustments. The clinically effective serum level is usually between 10 and 20 mcg/mL.

- *Loading dose (hospitalized patients without renal or liver disease):* Initially, 1 g of phenytoin capsules (phenytoin sodium, prompt) is divided into 3 doses (400 mg, 300 mg, 300 mg) and given q 2 hr. Normal maintenance dosage is then instituted 24 hr after the loading dose with frequent serum determinations.
- *No previous treatment:* Start with 100 mg tid PO. Satisfactory maintenance dosage is usually 300–400 mg/day. An increase to 600 mg/day may be necessary.
- *Single daily dosage (phenytoin sodium, extended):* If seizure control is established with divided doses of three 100-mg extended phenytoin sodium capsules per day, once-a-day dosage with 300 mg PO may be considered.

Pediatric patients
Phenytoin sodium, parenteral

- *Status epilepticus:* Administer phenytoin IV. Determine dosage according to weight in proportion to dose for a 150 lb (70 kg) adult

---

Adverse effects in *Italics* are most common; those in **Bold** are life-threatening.

(see adult dosage on p. 962; see Appendix R for calculation of pediatric doses). Pediatric dosage may be calculated on the basis of 250 mg/m². Dosage for infants and children also may be calculated on the basis of 10–15 mg/kg, given in divided doses of 5–10 mg/kg. For neonates, 15–20 mg/kg in divided doses of 5–10 mg/kg is recommended.

Phenytoin and phenytoin sodium, oral

Children not previously treated: Initially, 5 mg/kg/day in 2–3 equally divided doses. Subsequent dosage should be individualized to a maximum of 300 mg/day. Daily maintenance dosage is 4–8 mg/kg. Children < 6 yr may require the minimum adult dose of 300 mg/day.

Geriatric patients and patients with hepatic impairment

Use caution and monitor for early signs of toxicity; phenytoin is metabolized in the liver.

Pharmacokinetics

Route	Onset	Peak	Duration
Oral	Slow	2–12 hr	6–12 hr
IV	1–2 hr	Rapid	12–24 hr

Metabolism: Hepatic; $T_{1/2}$: 6–24 hr
Distribution: Crosses placenta; enters breast milk
Excretion: Urine

▼IV facts

Preparation: Administration by IV infusion is not recommended because of low solubility of drug and likelihood of precipitation; however, this may be feasible if proper precautions are observed. Use suitable vehicle of 0.9% sodium chloride or lactated Ringer's injection, appropriate concentration; prepare immediately before administration, and use an in-line filter.

Infusion: Infuse slowly in small increments, each 25–50 mg over 1–5 min; infuse flush immediately after drug to reduce the risk of damage to vein and tissues.

Incompatibilities: Do not combine with other medications in solution.

Y-site incompatibilities: Do not give with potassium chloride.

Adverse effects

Some adverse effects are related to plasma concentrations, as follows:

Plasma Concentration	Adverse Effects
5–10 mcg/mL	Some therapeutic effects
10–20 mcg/mL	Usual therapeutic range
> 20 mcg/mL	Far-lateral nystagmus risk
> 30 mcg/mL	Ataxia is usually seen
> 40 mcg/mL	Significantly diminished mental capacity

- **CNS:** *Nystagmus, ataxia, dysarthria, slurred speech, mental confusion, dizziness, drowsiness, insomnia, transient nervousness, motor twitchings, fatigue, irritability, depression, numbness, tremor, headache,* photophobia, diplopia, conjunctivitis
- **Dermatologic:** Dermatologic reactions, scarlatiniform, morbilliform, maculopapular, urticarial and nonspecific rashes; serious and sometimes fatal dermatologic reactions—**bullous, exfoliative, or purpuric dermatitis, lupus erythematosus, and Stevens-Johnson syndrome,** toxic epidermal necrolysis, hirsutism, alopecia, coarsening of the facial features, enlargement of the lips, Peyronie's disease
- **GI:** *Nausea,* vomiting, diarrhea, constipation, *gingival hyperplasia,* toxic hepatitis, **liver damage,** sometimes fatal; hypersensitivity reactions with hepatic involvement, including hepatocellular degeneration and fatal hepatocellular necrosis
- **GU:** Nephrosis
- **Hematologic: Hematopoietic complications,** sometimes fatal: thrombocytopenia, leukopenia, granulocytopenia, agranulocytosis, pancytopenia; macrocytosis and megaloblastic anemia that usually respond to folic acid therapy; eosinophilia, monocytosis, leukocytosis, simple anemia, hemolytic anemia, aplastic anemia, hyperglycemia
- **IV use complications:** Hypotension, transient hyperkinesia, drowsiness, nystagmus, circumoral tingling, vertigo, nausea, cardiovascular collapse, CNS depression
- **Respiratory:** Pulmonary fibrosis, acute pneumonitis

P

- **Other:** Lymph node hyperplasia, sometimes progressing to frank malignant lymphoma, monoclonal gammopathy and multiple myeloma (prolonged therapy), polyarthropathy, osteomalacia, weight gain, chest pain, periarteritis nodosa

Interactions

✳ Drug-drug • Increased pharmacologic effects with chloramphenicol, cimetidine, disulfiram, isoniazid, phenacemide, phenylbutazone, sulfonamides, trimethoprim • Complex interactions and effects when phenytoin and valproic acid are given together; phenytoin toxicity with apparently normal serum phenytoin levels; decreased plasma levels of valproic acid; breakthrough seizures when the two drugs are given together • Decreased pharmacologic effects with antineoplastics, diazoxide, folic acid, sucralfate, rifampin, theophylline (applies only to oral hydantoins, absorption of which is decreased) • Increased pharmacologic effects and toxicity with primidone, oxyphenbutazone, amiodarone, chloramphenicol, fluconazole, isoniazid • Increased hepatotoxicity with acetaminophen • Decreased pharmacologic effects of the following: corticosteroids, cyclosporine, disopyramide, doxycycline, estrogens, furosemide, levodopa, methadone, metyrapone, mexiletine, hormonal contraceptives, quinidine, atracurium, gallamine triethiodide, pancuronium, tubocurarine, vecuronium, carbamazepine, diazoxide • Severe hypotension and bradycardia when IV phenytoin is given with dopamine

✳ Drug-lab test • Interference with the metyrapone and the 1-mg dexamethasone tests for at least 7 days

■ Nursing considerations
Assessment

- **History:** Hypersensitivity to hydantoins; sinus bradycardia, AV heart block, Stokes-Adams syndrome, acute intermittent porphyria, hypotension, severe myocardial insufficiency, diabetes mellitus, hyperglycemia, pregnancy, lactation
- **Physical:** T; skin color, lesions; lymph node palpation; orientation, affect, reflexes, vision exam; P, BP; R, adventitious sounds; bowel sounds, normal output, liver evalua-

tion; periodontal exam; liver function tests, urinalysis, CBC and differential, blood proteins, blood and urine glucose, EEG and ECG

Interventions

- Use only clear parenteral solutions; a faint yellow color may develop, but this has no effect on potency. If the solution is refrigerated or frozen, a precipitate might form, but this will dissolve if the solution is allowed to stand at room temperature. Do not use solutions that have haziness or a precipitate.
- Administer IV slowly to prevent severe hypotension; the margin of safety between full therapeutic and toxic doses is small. Continually monitor patient's cardiac rhythm and check BP frequently and regularly during IV infusion. Suggest use of fosphenytoin sodium if IV route is needed.
- Monitor injection sites carefully; drug solutions are very alkaline and irritating.
- Monitor for therapeutic serum levels of 10–20 mcg/mL.
- Give oral drug with food to enhance absorption and to reduce GI upset.
- Recommend that the oral phenytoin prescription be filled with the same brand each time; differences in bioavailability have been documented.
- Suggest that adult patients who are controlled with 300-mg extended phenytoin capsules try once-a-day dosage to increase compliance and convenience.
- Reduce dosage, discontinue phenytoin, or substitute other antiepileptic medication gradually; abrupt discontinuation may precipitate status epilepticus.
- Phenytoin is ineffective in controlling absence (petit mal) seizures. Patients with combined seizures will need other medication for their absence seizures.
- Discontinue drug if rash, depression of blood count, enlarged lymph nodes, hypersensitivity reaction, signs of liver damage, or Peyronie's disease (induration of the corpora cavernosa of the penis) occurs. Institute another antiepileptic drug promptly.
- Monitor hepatic function periodically during long-term therapy; monitor blood counts, urinalysis monthly.

- Monitor blood or urine sugar of patients with diabetes mellitus regularly. Adjustment of dosage of hypoglycemic drug may be necessary because antiepileptic drug may inhibit insulin release and induce hyperglycemia.
- Have lymph node enlargement occurring during therapy evaluated carefully. Lymphadenopathy that simulates Hodgkin's disease has occurred. Lymph node hyperplasia may progress to lymphoma.
- Monitor blood proteins to detect early malfunction of the immune system (eg, multiple myeloma).
- Arrange dental instruction in proper oral hygiene technique for long-term patients to prevent development of gum hyperplasia.

Teaching points
- Take this drug exactly as prescribed, with food to enhance absorption and reduce GI upset; be especially careful not to miss a dose if you are on once-a-day therapy.
- Do not discontinue this drug abruptly or change dosage, except on the advice of your prescriber.
- Maintain good oral hygiene (regular brushing and flossing) to prevent gum disease; arrange frequent dental checkups to prevent serious gum disease.
- Arrange for frequent checkups to monitor your response to this drug.
- Monitor your blood or urine sugar regularly, and report any abnormality to your health care provider if you are a diabetic.
- This drug is not recommended for use during pregnancy. It is advisable to use some form of contraception other than birth control pills.
- These side effects may occur: drowsiness, dizziness, confusion, blurred vision (avoid driving or performing other tasks requiring alertness or visual acuity); GI upset (take drug with food, eat frequent, small meals).
- Wear a medical alert tag so that any emergency medical personnel will know that you are an epileptic taking antiepileptic medication.
- Report rash, severe nausea or vomiting, drowsiness, slurred speech, impaired coordination (ataxia), swollen glands, bleeding, swollen or tender gums, yellowish discoloration of the skin or eyes, joint pain, un-

explained fever, sore throat, unusual bleeding or bruising, persistent headache, malaise, any indication of an infection or bleeding tendency, abnormal erection, pregnancy.

▷ pilocarpine hydrochloride

See *Less Commonly Used Drugs,* p. 1348.

▷ pimozide

See *Less Commonly Used Drugs,* p. 1348.

▷ pindolol
(pin' doe lole)

Apo-Pindol (CAN), Novo-Pindol (CAN), Nu-Pindol (CAN), Visken

PREGNANCY CATEGORY B

Drug classes
Beta-adrenergic blocker (nonselective)
Antihypertensive

Therapeutic actions
Competitively blocks beta-adrenergic receptors, but also has some intrinsic sympathomimetic activity; however, the mechanism by which it lowers BP is unclear, because it only slightly decreases resting cardiac output and inconsistently affects plasma renin levels.

Indications
- Management of hypertension, alone or with other drugs, especially diuretics
- Unlabeled uses: treatment of ventricular arrhythmias, antipsychotic-induced akathisia, situational anxiety

Contraindications and cautions
- Contraindicated with sinus bradycardia, second- or third-degree heart block, cardiogenic shock, CHF, pregnancy (embryotoxic in preclinical studies), lactation.
- Use cautiously with diabetes or thyrotoxicosis.

Available forms
Tablets—5, 10 mg

Dosages

Adults

Initially 5 mg PO bid. Adjust dose as necessary in increments of 10 mg/day at 3- to 4-wk intervals to a maximum of 60 mg/day. Usual maintenance dose is 5 mg tid.

Pediatric patients

Safety and efficacy not established.

Pharmacokinetics

Route	Onset
Oral	Varies

Metabolism: Hepatic; $T_{1/2}$: 3–4 hr
Distribution: Crosses placenta; enters breast milk
Excretion: Urine

Adverse effects

- **Allergic reactions:** Pharyngitis, erythematous rash, fever, sore throat, laryngospasm, respiratory distress
- **CNS:** Dizziness, vertigo, tinnitus, fatigue, emotional depression, paresthesias, sleep disturbances, hallucinations, disorientation, memory loss, slurred speech
- **CV:** *Bradycardia, CHF, cardiac arrhythmias, sinoatrial or AV nodal block, tachycardia,* peripheral vascular insufficiency, claudication, **CVA**, pulmonary edema, hypotension
- **Dermatologic:** Rash, pruritus, sweating, dry skin
- **EENT:** Eye irritation, dry eyes, conjunctivitis, blurred vision
- **GI:** *Gastric pain, flatulence, constipation, diarrhea, nausea, vomiting,* anorexia, ischemic colitis, renal and mesenteric arterial thrombosis, retroperitoneal fibrosis, hepatomegaly, acute pancreatitis
- **GU:** *Impotence, decreased libido,* Peyronie's disease, dysuria, nocturia, frequency
- **Musculoskeletal:** Joint pain, arthralgia, muscle cramp
- **Respiratory:** Bronchospasm, dyspnea, cough, bronchial obstruction, nasal stuffiness, rhinitis, pharyngitis (less likely than with propranolol)
- **Other:** *Decreased exercise tolerance, development of ANAs,* hyperglycemia or hypoglycemia, elevated serum transaminase, alkaline phosphatase, and LDH

Interactions

✱ Drug-drug • Increased effects with verapamil • Decreased effects with indomethacin, ibuprofen, piroxicam, sulindac • Prolonged hypoglycemic effects of insulin • Peripheral ischemia possible if pindolol combined with ergot alkaloids • Initial hypertensive episode followed by bradycardia with epinephrine • Increased first-dose response to prazosin • Increased serum levels and toxic effects with lidocaine • Paradoxical hypertension when clonidine is given with beta-blockers; increased rebound hypertension when clonidine is discontinued in patients on beta-blockers • Decreased bronchodilator effects of theophyllines
✱ Drug-lab test • Possible false results with glucose or insulin tolerance tests

■ Nursing considerations

CLINICAL ALERT!
Name confusion has been reported between pindolol and Plendil (felodipine); use caution.

Assessment

- **History:** Sinus bradycardia, second- or third-degree heart block, cardiogenic shock, CHF, pregnancy, lactation, diabetes, thyrotoxicosis
- **Physical:** Weight, skin condition, neurologic status, P, BP, ECG, respiratory status, kidney and thyroid function, blood and urine glucose

Indications

- Do not discontinue drug abruptly after long-term therapy (hypersensitivity to catecholamines may have developed, causing exacerbation of angina, MI, and ventricular arrhythmias). Taper drug gradually over 2 wk with monitoring.
- Consult with physician about withdrawing drug if patient is to undergo surgery (withdrawal is controversial).

Adverse effects in *Italics* are most common; those in **Bold** are life-threatening.

Teaching points

- Do not stop taking this drug unless instructed to do so by a health care provider.
- Avoid driving or dangerous activities if CNS effects occur.
- Report difficulty breathing, night cough, swelling of extremities, slow pulse, confusion, depression, rash, fever, sore throat.

▽**pioglitazone**

(pie oh glit' ah zohn)

Actos

PREGNANCY CATEGORY C

Drug classes
Antidiabetic agent
Thiazolidinedione

Therapeutic actions
Resensitizes tissues to insulin; stimulates insulin receptor sites to lower blood glucose and improve the action of insulin; decreases hepatic gluconeogenesis and increases insulin-dependent muscle glucose uptake.

Indications
- Monotherapy as an adjunct to diet and exercise to improve glucose control in patients with type 2 diabetes
- As part of combination with a sulfonylurea, metformin, or insulin when diet, exercise plus a single agent alone does not result in adequate glycemic control in type 2 diabetes

Contraindications and cautions
- Contraindicated with allergy to any thiazolidinedione; type 1 or juvenile diabetes, ketoacidosis, lactation.
- Use cautiously with advanced heart disease, liver failure, pregnancy.

Available forms
Tablets—15, 30, 45 mg

Dosages
Adults

15–30 mg daily as a single oral dose; if adequate response is not seen, dosage may be increased to a maximum 45 mg daily PO.

- *Combination therapy with sulfonylurea or metformin:* 15–30 mg daily PO added to the established dose of the other agent; if hypoglycemia occurs, reduce the dose of the other agent.
- *Combination therapy with insulin:* Decrease insulin dose by 10%–25% when adding pioglitazone.

Pediatric patients
Safety and efficacy not established.

Patients with hepatic impairment
Use caution and monitor patient closely. Do not administer if AST > 2.5 times the upper level of normal.

Pharmacokinetics

Route	Onset	Peak
Oral	Rapid	2–4 hr

Metabolism: Hepatic; $T_{1/2}$: 3–7 hr
Distribution: Crosses placenta; passes into breast milk
Excretion: Urine, feces

Adverse effects
- **CNS:** *Headache, pain, myalgia*
- **Endocrine: Hypoglycemia, hyperglycemia,** *aggravated diabetes*
- **GI:** Diarrhea, liver injury
- **Respiratory:** Sinusitis, URI, rhinitis
- **Other:** *Infections, fatigue,* tooth disorders

Interactions
✳ **Drug-drug** • Decreased effectiveness of hormonal contraceptives, which may result in ovulation and risk of pregnancy; suggest the use of an alternative method of birth control or consider a higher dose of the contraceptive

✳ **Drug-alternative therapy** • Increased risk of hypoglycemia if taken with juniper berries, ginseng, garlic, fenugreek, coriander, dandelion root, celery

■ Nursing considerations
Assessment
- **History:** Allergy to any thiazolidinedione; type 1 or juvenile diabetes, ketoacidosis, serious hepatic impairment, advanced heart disease, pregnancy, lactation
- **Physical:** T; orientation, reflexes, peripheral sensation; R, adventitious sounds; liver

P

evaluation; liver function tests, blood glucose, CBC

Interventions

- Monitor urine or blood glucose levels frequently to determine effectiveness of drug and dosage being used.
- Monitor baseline liver function tests before beginning therapy and periodically during therapy.
- Administer without regard to meals.
- Arrange for consultation with dietitian to establish weight loss program and dietary control as appropriate.
- Arrange for thorough diabetic teaching program to include disease, dietary control, exercise, signs and symptoms of hypo- and hyperglycemia, avoidance of infection, hygiene.

Teaching points

- Do not discontinue this medication without consulting health care provider; continue with diet and exercise program for diabetes control.
- Take this drug with meals. If dose is missed, it may be taken at the next meal. If dose is missed for an entire day, do not double dose the next day.
- Monitor urine or blood for glucose and ketones as prescribed very closely while adjusting to drug.
- Use barrier contraceptives if currently taking hormonal contraceptives; these drugs may be ineffective if combined with pioglitazone.
- Report fever, sore throat, unusual bleeding or bruising, rash, dark urine, light-colored stools, hypoglycemic or hyperglycemic reactions.

▽piperacillin sodium

*(pi **per'** a sill in)*

Pipracil

PREGNANCY CATEGORY B

Drug classes

Antibiotic
Penicillin with extended spectrum

Therapeutic actions

Bactericidal: inhibits synthesis of cell wall of sensitive organisms, causing cell death.

Indications

- Treatment of mixed infections and presumptive therapy prior to identification of organisms
- Lower respiratory tract infections caused by *Haemophilus influenzae, Klebsiella, Pseudomonas aeruginosa, Serratia, Escherichia coli, Bacteroides, Enterobacter*
- Intra-abdominal infections caused by *E. coli, P. aeruginosa, Clostridium, Bacteroides* species, including *Bacteroides fragilis*
- UTIs caused by *E. coli, Proteus* species, including *Proteus mirabilis, Klebsiella, P. aeruginosa,* enterococci
- Gynecologic infections caused by *Neisseria gonorrhoeae, Bacteroides,* enterococci, anaerobic cocci
- Skin and skin-structure infections caused by *E. coli, P. mirabilis,* indole-positive *Proteus, P. aeruginosa, Klebsiella, Enterobacter, Bacteroides, Serratia, Acinetobacter*
- Bone and joint infections caused by *P. aeruginosa, Bacteroides,* enterococci, anaerobic cocci
- Septicemia caused by *E. coli, Klebsiella, Enterobacter, Serratia, P. mirabilis, Streptococcus pneumoniae, P. aeruginosa, Bacteroides,* enterococci, anaerobic cocci
- Infections caused by *Streptococcus* (narrower spectrum antibiotic usually used)
- Prophylaxis in abdominal surgery

Contraindications and cautions

- Contraindicated with allergies to penicillins, cephalosporins, procaine, or other allergens.
- Use cautiously with pregnancy, lactation (may cause diarrhea or candidiasis in the infant).

Available forms

Powder for injection—2, 3, 4 g

Dosages
Adults

3–4 g q 4–6 hr IV or IM. Do not exceed 24 g/day.

---

*Adverse effects in Italics are most common; those in **Bold** are life-threatening.*

Surgery	First Dose	Second Dose	Third Dose
Intra-abdominal	2 g IV just before surgery	2 g during surgery	2 g q 6 hr, no longer than 24 hr
Vaginal hysterectomy	2 g IV just before surgery	2 g at 6 hr	2 g at 12 hr
Cesarean section	2 g IV after cord is clamped	2 g at 4 hr	2 g at 8 hr
Abdominal hysterectomy	2 g IV just before surgery	2 g in recovery room	2 g after 6 hr

Pediatric patients

200–300 mg/kg/day up to a maximum of 24 g/day. Divide dose every 4–6 hr.
Neonates: 75 mg/kg IV q 8 hr for first wk of life, then q 6 hr.
Premature neonates (< 36 wk gestation): 75 mg/kg IV q 12 hr for first week of life, then q 8 hr.

Geriatric patients or patients with renal insufficiency

Creatinine Clearance (mL/min)	UTIs	Systemic Infection
> 40	Usual dosage	Usual dosage
20–40	3 g q 8 hr	4 g q 8 hr
< 20	3 g q 12 hr	4 g q 12 hr

Pharmacokinetics

Route	Onset	Peak
IV	Rapid	End of infusion
IM	Rapid	30–60 min

Metabolism: Hepatic; $T_{1/2}$: 0.7–1.3 hr
Distribution: Crosses placenta; enters breast milk
Excretion: Urine

▽ IV facts

Preparation: Reconstitute each gram for IV use with 5 mL of bacteriostatic water for injection, bacteriostatic sodium chloride injection, bacteriostatic or sterile water for injection, dextrose 5% in water, 0.9% sodium chloride, dextrose 5% and 0.9% sodium chloride, lactated Ringer's injection, dextran 6% in 0.9% sodium chloride, Ringer's injection; stable for 24 hr at room temperature, up to 7 days if refrigerated.

Infusion: Direct injection: Administer as slowly as possible (3–5 min) to avoid vein irritation. Infusion should be run over 20–30 min.
Incompatibilities: Do not mix in solution with aminoglycoside solution; **do not mix in the same IV solution as other antibiotics.**

Adverse effects

- **CNS:** Lethargy, hallucinations, seizures
- **GI:** *Glossitis, stomatitis, gastritis, sore mouth,* furry tongue, black "hairy" tongue, *nausea, vomiting, diarrhea,* abdominal pain, bloody diarrhea, enterocolitis, pseudomembranous colitis, nonspecific hepatitis
- **GU:** Nephritis
- **Hematologic:** Anemia, thrombocytopenia, leukopenia, neutropenia, prolonged bleeding time
- **Hypersensitivity:** *Rash, fever, wheezing,* **anaphylaxis**
- **Local:** *Pain, phlebitis,* thrombosis at injection site
- **Other:** *Superinfections,* sodium overload—CHF

Interactions

✳ Drug-drug • Decreased effectiveness with tetracyclines • Inactivation of parenteral aminoglycosides (amikacin, gentamicin, kanamycin, streptomycin, tobramycin) when infused at the same time

✳ Drug-lab test • False-positive Coombs' test with IV piperacillin

■ Nursing considerations
Assessment

- **History:** Allergies to penicillins, cephalosporins, procaine, or other allergens; pregnancy; lactation
- **Physical:** Culture infection; skin color, lesions; R, adventitious sounds; bowel sounds: CBC, liver and renal function tests, serum electrolytes, Hct, urinalysis

Interventions

- Culture infection before beginning treatment; reculture if response is not as expected.
- Continue therapy for at least 2 days after signs of infection have disappeared, usually 7–10 days.
- Administer by IM or IV routes only.
- Reconstitute each gram for IM use with 2 mL sterile or bacteriostatic water for injection,

0.5% or 1.0% lidocaine HCl without epinephrine, bacteriostatic sodium chloride injection, sodium chloride injection. Do not exceed 2 g per injection. Inject deep into a large muscle, such as upper outer quadrant of the buttock. Do not inject into lower or mid-third of upper arm.

- Carefully check IV site for signs of thrombosis or drug reaction.
- Do not give IM injections repeatedly in the same site, atrophy can occur; monitor injection sites.
- Maintain epinephrine, IV fluids, vasopressors, bronchodilators, oxygen, and emergency equipment on standby in case of serious hypersensitivity reaction.

Teaching points

- This drug must be given by injection.
- These side effects may occur: upset stomach, nausea, diarrhea (small, frequent meals may help), mouth sores (frequent mouth care may help), pain or discomfort at the injection site.
- Report difficulty breathing, rashes, severe diarrhea, severe pain at injection site, mouth sores.

▷ pirbuterol acetate
(peer byoo' ter ole)

Maxair Inhaler

PREGNANCY CATEGORY C

Drug classes

Sympathomimetic
Beta$_2$-selective adrenergic agonist
Bronchodilator
Antiasthmatic agent

Therapeutic actions

Relatively selective beta-adrenergic stimulator; acts at beta$_2$-adrenergic receptors to cause bronchodilation (and vasodilation); at higher doses, beta$_2$-selectivity is lost, and the drug also acts at beta$_2$ receptors to cause typical sympathomimetic cardiac effects.

Indications

- Prophylaxis and treatment of reversible bronchospasm, including asthma

Contraindications and cautions

- Contraindicated with hypersensitivity to pirbuterol, tachyarrhythmias, general anesthesia with halogenated hydrocarbons or cyclopropane, unstable vasomotor system disorders, hypertension.
- Use cautiously with coronary insufficiency, history of stroke, COPD patients who have developed degenerative heart disease, hyperthyroidism, history of seizure disorders, psychoneurotic individuals, pregnancy, lactation.

Available forms

Aerosol—0.2 mg/actuation

Dosages

Adults

2 inhalations (0.4 mg) repeated q 4–6 hr. One inhalation (0.2 mg) may be sufficient. Do not exceed a total daily dose of 12 inhalations.

Pediatric patients

> 12 yr: Same as adult.
< 12 yr: Safety and efficacy not established.

Pharmacokinetics

Route	Onset	Duration
Inhalation	5 min	5 hr

Metabolism: Hepatic and tissue; T$_{1/2}$: unknown
Distribution: Crosses placenta; may enter breast milk
Excretion: Urine

Adverse effects

- **CNS:** *Restlessness, apprehension,* anxiety, fear, CNS stimulation, hyperkinesia, *insomnia,* tremor, drowsiness, *irritability,* weakness, vertigo, headache
- **CV:** Cardiac arrhythmias, tachycardia, palpitations, PVCs (rare), anginal pain (less likely with this drug than with bronchodilator doses of a nonselective beta-agonist, ie, isoproterenol), changes in BP, sweating, pallor, flushing
- **GI:** *Nausea,* vomiting, heartburn, unusual or bad taste

---

Adverse effects in *Italics* are most common; those in **Bold** are life-threatening.

- **Hypersensitivity:** Immediate hypersensitivity (allergic) reactions
- **Respiratory:** Respiratory difficulties, pulmonary edema, coughing, bronchospasm, paradoxical airway resistance with repeated, excessive use of inhalation preparations

Interactions
✳ **Drug-drug** • Increased sympathomimetic effects when given with other sympathomimetic drugs

■ Nursing considerations
Assessment
- **History:** Hypersensitivity to pirbuterol, tachyarrhythmias, general anesthesia with halogenated hydrocarbons or cyclopropane, unstable vasomotor system disorders, hypertension, coronary insufficiency, history of stroke, COPD, hyperthyroidism, seizure disorders, psychoneurotic individuals, pregnancy, lactation
- **Physical:** Weight, skin color, T, turgor; orientation, reflexes, affect; P, BP; R, adventitious sounds; blood and urine glucose, serum electrolytes, thyroid and liver function tests, ECG, CBC

Interventions
- Use smallest dose for least time; drug tolerance can occur with prolonged use.
- Maintain a beta-adrenergic blocker (a cardioselective beta-blocker, such as atenolol, should be used in patients with respiratory distress) on standby in case cardiac arrhythmias occur.
- Do not exceed recommended dosage; administer during second half of inspiration, as the airways are wider and distribution is more extensive.

Teaching points
- Do not exceed recommended dosage; adverse effects or loss of effectiveness may result. Read product instructions and ask your health care provider or pharmacist if you have any questions.
- These side effects may occur: drowsiness, dizziness, fatigue, apprehension (use caution if driving or performing tasks that require alertness); nausea, heartburn, change in taste (small, frequent meals may help); sweating, flushing, rapid heart rate.

- Report chest pain, dizziness, insomnia, weakness, tremor or irregular heart beat, difficulty breathing, productive cough, failure to respond to usual dosage.

▽ piroxicam
(peer ox' i kam)

Alti-Piroxicam (CAN), Apo-Piroxicam (CAN), Feldene, Novo-Pirocam (CAN), Nu-Pirox (CAN)

PREGNANCY CATEGORY B

Drug class
Nonsteroidal anti-inflammatory drug (NSAID) (oxicam derivative)

Therapeutic actions
Anti-inflammatory, analgesic, and antipyretic activities related to inhibition of prostaglandin synthesis; exact mechanisms of action are not known.

Indications
- Relief of the signs and symptoms of acute and chronic rheumatoid arthritis and osteoarthritis

Contraindications and cautions
- Contraindicated with hypersensitivity to piroxicam or any other NSAID, lactation.
- Use cautiously with renal, hepatic; cardiovascular, GI conditions, pregnancy.

Available forms
Capsules—10, 20 mg

Dosages
Adults
Single daily dose of 20 mg PO. Dose may be divided. Steady-state blood levels are not achieved for 7–12 days. Therapeutic response occurs early but progresses over several weeks; do not evaluate for 2 wk.
Pediatric patients
Safety and efficacy not established.

Pharmacokinetics

Route	Onset	Peak
Oral	1 hr	3–5 hr

Metabolism: Hepatic; $T_{1/2}$: 30–86 hr
Distribution: Crosses placenta; enters breast milk
Excretion: Urine

Adverse effects

- **CNS:** *Headache, dizziness, somnolence, insomnia,* fatigue, tiredness, dizziness, tinnitus, ophthalmologic effects
- **Dermatologic:** *Rash,* pruritus, sweating, dry mucous membranes, stomatitis
- **GI:** *Nausea, dyspepsia, GI pain,* diarrhea, vomiting, *constipation,* flatulence
- **GU:** Dysuria, renal impairment
- **Hematologic:** Bleeding, platelet inhibition with higher doses, neutropenia, eosinophilia, leukopenia, pancytopenia, thrombocytopenia, agranulocytosis, granulocytopenia, aplastic anemia, decreased Hgb or Hct, bone marrow depression, mennorhagia
- **Respiratory:** Dyspnea, hemoptysis, pharyngitis, bronchospasm, rhinitis
- **Other:** Peripheral edema, **anaphylactoid reactions to anaphylactic shock**

Interactions

✴ Drug-drug • Increased serum lithium levels and risk of toxicity • Decreased antihypertensive effects of beta-blockers • Decreased therapeutic effects with cholestyramine

■ Nursing considerations
Assessment

- **History:** Allergies; renal, Hepatic; CV, and GI conditions; history of ulcers; pregnancy; lactation
- **Physical:** Skin color and lesions; orientation, reflexes, ophthalmologic and audiometric evaluation, peripheral sensation; P, edema; R, adventitious sounds; liver evaluation; CBC, clotting times, renal and liver function tests; serum electrolytes, stool guaiac

Interventions

- Give drug with food or milk if GI upset occurs.
- Arrange for periodic ophthalmologic examination during long-term therapy.
- Institute emergency procedures if overdose occurs (gastric lavage, induction of emesis, supportive therapy).

Teaching points

- Take drug with food or meals if GI upset occurs.
- These side effects may occur: dizziness, drowsiness (avoid driving or using dangerous machinery).
- Report sore throat, fever, rash, itching, weight gain, swelling in ankles or fingers, changes in vision, black, tarry stools.

▷ plasma protein fraction

Plasmanate, Plasma-Plex, Plasmatein, Protenate

PREGNANCY CATEGORY C

Drug classes
Blood product
Plasma protein

Therapeutic actions

Maintains plasma colloid osmotic pressure and carries intermediate metabolites in the transport and exchange of tissue products; important in the maintenance of normal blood volume.

Indications

- Supportive treatment of shock due to burns, trauma, surgery, and infections
- Hypoproteinemia—nephrotic syndrome, hepatic cirrhosis, toxemia of pregnancy, postoperative patients, tuberculous patients, premature infants
- Acute liver failure
- Sequestration of protein-rich fluids
- Hyperbilirubinemia and erythroblastosis fetalis as an adjunct to exchange transfusions

Contraindications and cautions

- Contraindicated with allergy to albumin, severe anemia, cardiac failure, normal or increased intravascular volume, current use of cardiopulmonary bypass.
- Use cautiously with hepatic or renal failure, pregnancy.

Adverse effects in *Italics* are most common; those in **Bold** are life-threatening.

Available forms
Injection—5%

Dosages
Administer by IV infusion only. Contains 130–160 mEq sodium/L. Do not give more than 250 g in 48 hr; if it seems that more is required, patient probably needs whole blood or plasma.

Adults
- *Hypovolemic shock:* 250–500 mL as an initial dose. Do not exceed 10 mL/min. Adjust dose based on patient response.
- *Hypoproteinemia:* Daily doses of 1,000–1,500 mL are appropriate. Do not exceed 5–8 mL/min. Adjust infusion rate based on patient response.

Pediatric patients
- *Hypovolemic shock:* Infuse a dose of 20–30 mL/kg at a rate not to exceed 10 mL/min. Dose may be repeated depending on patient's response.

Pharmacokinetics

Route	
IV	Stays in the intravascular space

Metabolism: $T_{1/2}$: unknown
Excretion: Unknown

▼IV facts
Preparation: No further preparation required; discard within 4 hr of entering a bottle; store at room temperature; do not use if there is sediment in the bottle.
Infusion: Regulate based on patient response. Do not exceed 10 mL/min.
Compatibilities: Administer in combination with or through the same administration set as the usual IV solutions of saline or carbohydrates.
Incompatibilities: Do not use with alcohol or protein hydrolysates; precipitates may form.

Adverse effects
- **CV:** *Hypotension,* CHF, **pulmonary edema following rapid infusion**
- **Hypersensitivity:** Fever, chills, changes in BP, flushing, nausea, vomiting, changes in respiration, rashes

■ Nursing considerations
Assessment
- **History:** Allergy to albumin, severe anemia, cardiac failure, normal or increased intravascular volume, current use of cardiopulmonary bypass, renal or hepatic failure, pregnancy
- **Physical:** Skin color, lesions; T; P, BP, peripheral perfusion; R, adventitious sounds; liver and renal function tests, Hct, serum electrolytes

Interventions
- Administer by IV infusion only.
- Administer without regard to blood group or type.
- Consider the need for whole blood based on the patient's clinical condition; this infusion only provides symptomatic relief of the patient's hypoproteinemia.
- Monitor BP during infusion; discontinue if hypotension occurs.
- Stop infusion if headache, flushing, fever, changes in BP occur. Arrange to treat reaction with antihistamines. If a plasma protein is still needed, try material from a different lot number.
- Monitor patient's clinical response and adjust infusion rate accordingly.

Teaching points
- Rate will be adjusted based on your response, so constant monitoring is necessary.
- Report headache, nausea, vomiting, difficulty breathing, back pain.

P

▽ polymyxin B sulfate
*(pol i **mix**' in)*

Parenteral: Aerosporin (CAN)
Ophthalmic: Polymyxin B Sulfate Sterile Ophthalmic

PREGNANCY CATEGORY B

Drug class
Antibiotic

Therapeutic actions
Bactericidal: has surfactant (detergent) activity that allows it to penetrate and disrupt the cell membranes of susceptible gram-negative

bacteria, causing cell death; not effective against *Proteus* species.

Indications

- Acute infections caused by susceptible strains of *P. aeruginosa, H. influenzae, E. coli, E. aerogenes, Klebsiella pneumoniae* when less toxic drugs are ineffective or contraindicated
- Infections of the eye caused by susceptible strains of *P. aeruginosa* (ophthalmic preparations)
- Meningeal infections caused by *P. aeruginosa* (intrathecal)

Contraindications and cautions

- Contraindicated with allergy to polymyxins (polymyxin B, colistin, colistimethate).
- Use cautiously with renal disease, pregnancy, lactation.

Available forms

Injection—500,000 units/vial; ophthalmic solution—500,000 units

Dosages
Adults and pediatric patients
IV

15,000–25,000 units/kg/day may be given q 12 hr. Do not exceed 25,000 units/kg/day.
IM

25,000–30,000 units/kg/day divided and given at 4- to 6-hr intervals.
Intrathecal

50,000 units once daily for 3–4 days; then 50,000 units every other day for at least 2 wk after cultures of CSF are negative, and glucose content is normal.
Ophthalmic

1–2 drops in infected eye bid–q 4 hr or as often as needed.
Infants
IV

Up to 40,000 units/kg/day.
IM

Up to 40,000 units/kg/day; doses as high as 45,000 units/kg/day have been used in cases of sepsis caused by *P. aeruginosa.*
Intrathecal

< *2 yr:* 20,000 units once daily for 3–4 days or 25,000 units once every other day. Contin-

ue with 25,000 units once every other day for at least 2 wk after cultures of CSF are negative and glucose content is normal.
Geriatric patients or patients with renal failure

Reduce dosage from the recommended dose, and follow renal function tests during therapy.

Pharmacokinetics

Route	Onset	Peak
IV	Rapid	Unknown
IM	Gradual	2 hr

Metabolism: $T_{1/2}$: 4.3–6 hr
Distribution: Does not cross placenta
Excretion: Urine

▼ IV facts

Preparation: Dissolve 500,000 units in 300–500 mL of 5% dextrose in water. Dissolve 500,000 units in 2 mL sterile distilled water or sodium chloride injection, or 1% procaine hydrochloride solution; refrigerate and discard any unused portion after 72 hr.
Infusion: Administer by continuous IV drip using an infusion pump.
Incompatibilities: Do not mix with amphotericin B, chloramphenicol, heparin, magnesium sulfate, tetracycline.

Adverse effects

- **CNS:** Neurotoxicity—*facial flushing, dizziness, ataxia, drowsiness,* paresthesias
- **Dermatologic:** Rash, urticaria
- **GU:** *Nephrotoxicity*
- **Local:** Pain at IM injection site; *thrombophlebitis at IV injection sites; irritation, burning, stinging, itching, blurring of vision* (ophthalmic preparations)
- **Respiratory:** Apnea (high dosage)
- **Other:** Drug fever, superinfections

Interactions

✳ Drug-drug ● Increased neuromuscular blockade, apnea, and muscular paralysis when given with nondepolarizing neuromuscular blocking drugs

---

Adverse effects in *Italics* are most common; those in **Bold** are life-threatening.

■ Nursing considerations
Assessment
- **History:** Allergy to polymyxins, renal disease, lactation
- **Physical:** Site of infection, skin color, lesions; orientation, reflexes, speech; R; urinary output; urinalysis, serum creatinine, renal function tests

Interventions
- Store drug solutions in refrigerator, and discard any unused portion after 72 hr.
- For intrathecal use: Dissolve 500,000 units in 10 mL sterile physiologic saline for a concentration of 50,000 units/mL.
- For ophthalmic use: Reconstitute powder with 20–50 mL of diluent.
- Culture infection before beginning therapy.
- Monitor renal function tests during therapy.

Teaching points
- Administer ophthalmic preparation as follows: tilt head back; place medication into eyelid and close eyes; gently hold the inner corner of the eye for 1 min. Do not touch dropper to the eye.
- These side effects may occur: vertigo, dizziness, drowsiness, slurring of speech (avoid driving or using hazardous equipment); numbness, tingling of the tongue, extremities (decrease the dosage); superinfections (frequent hygiene measures will help; request medications); burning, stinging, blurring of vision (ophthalmic; transient).
- Report difficulty breathing, rash or skin lesions, pain at injection site or IV site, change in urinary voiding patterns, fever, flulike symptoms, changes in vision, severe stinging or itching (ophthalmic).

▷polythiazide
*(pol i **thye'** a zide)*

Renese

PREGNANCY CATEGORY C

Drug class
Thiazide diuretic

Therapeutic actions
Inhibits reabsorption of sodium and chloride in distal renal tubule, thereby increasing excretion of sodium, chloride, and water by the kidney.

Indications
- Adjunctive therapy in edema associated with CHF, cirrhosis, corticosteroid and estrogen therapy, renal dysfunction
- Hypertension, as sole therapy or in combination with other antihypertensives
- Unlabeled use: diabetes insipidus, especially nephrogenic diabetes insipidus

Contraindications and cautions
- Contraindicated with fluid or electrolyte imbalances, pregnancy, lactation.
- Use cautiously with renal or liver disease, gout, SLE, glucose tolerance abnormalities, hyperparathyroidism, manic-depressive disorders.

Available forms
Tablets—1, 2, 4 mg

Dosages
Adults
- *Edema:* 1–4 mg daily PO.
- *Hypertension:* 2–4 mg daily PO.

Pediatric patients
Safety and efficacy not established.

Pharmacokinetics
Route	Onset	Peak	Duration
Oral	2 hr	6 hr	24–48 hr

Metabolism: $T_{1/2}$: 25.7 hr
Distribution: Crosses placenta; enters breast milk
Excretion: Urine

Adverse effects
- **CNS:** *Dizziness, vertigo,* paresthesias, weakness, headache, drowsiness, fatigue, leukopenia, thrombocytopenia, agranulocytosis, aplastic anemia, neutropenia
- **CV:** Orthostatic hypotension, venous thrombosis, volume depletion, cardiac arrhythmias, chest pain
- **Dermatologic:** Photosensitivity, rash, purpura, exfoliative dermatitis, hives

- **GI:** *Nausea, anorexia, vomiting, dry mouth,* diarrhea, constipation, jaundice, hepatitis, pancreatitis
- **GU:** *Polyuria, nocturia,* impotence, decreased libido
- **Other:** Muscle cramps and muscle spasms, fever, gouty attacks, flushing, weight loss, rhinorrhea

Interactions
✹ **Drug-drug** • Risk of hyperglycemia with diazoxide • Decreased absorption with cholestyramine, colestipol • Increased risk of cardiac glycoside toxicity if hypokalemia occurs • Increased risk of lithium toxicity with thiazides • Increased fasting blood glucose leading to need to adjust dosage of antidiabetic agents
✹ **Drug-lab test** • Monitor for decreased PBI levels without clinical signs of thyroid disturbances

■ Nursing considerations
Assessment
- **History:** Electrolyte imbalances, renal or liver disease, gout, SLE, glucose tolerance abnormalities, hyperparathyroidism, manic-depressive disorders, pregnancy, lactation
- **Physical:** Skin color, lesions; orientation, reflexes, muscle strength; pulses, BP, orthostatic BP, perfusion, edema, baseline ECG; R, adventitious sounds; liver evaluation, bowel sounds; CBC, serum electrolytes, blood glucose, liver and renal function tests, serum uric acid, urinalysis

Interventions
- Administer with food or milk if GI upset occurs.
- Administer early in the day so increased urination will not disturb sleep.
- Measure and record regular body weights to monitor fluid changes.

Teaching points
- Take drug early in the day so sleep will not be disturbed by increased urination.
- Weigh yourself daily and record weights.
- Protect skin from exposure to sun or bright lights.
- Increased urination will occur.

- Use caution if dizziness, drowsiness, feeling faint occur.
- Report rapid weight gain or loss, swelling in ankles or fingers, unusual bleeding or bruising, muscle cramps.

▷ poractant alfa (DDPC, natural lung surfactant)
*(poor **ak'** tant)*
Curosurf

Drug class
Lung surfactant

Therapeutic actions
A natural porcine compound containing lipids and apoproteins that reduce surface tension and allow expansion of the alveoli; replaces the surfactant missing in the lungs of neonates suffering from respiratory distress syndrome (RDS).

Indications
- Rescue treatment of infants who have developed RDS
- Unlabeled use: prophylaxis for RDS, treatment of adult RDS, treatment of adults following near drowning

Contraindications and cautions
- Because poractant is used as an emergency drug in acute respiratory situations, the benefits usually outweigh any possible risks. Caution should be used with any known family history of allergy to porcine products.

Available forms
Suspension for intratracheal instillation: 1.5, 3 mL

Dosages
Accurate determination of birth weight is essential for determining appropriate dosage. Poractant is instilled into the trachea using a catheter inserted into the endotracheal tube.

Administer entire contents of vial (2.5 mL/kg birth weight) intratracheally, one half dose into each bronchi. Administer the first dose as soon as possible after the diagnosis of RDS is made and when the patient is on the ventilator. Up to two subsequent doses of 1.25 mL/kg birth weight at 12-hr intervals may be needed.

Pharmacokinetics

Route	Onset	Peak
Intratracheal	Immediate	3 hr

Metabolism: Normal surfactant metabolic pathways; $T_{1/2}$: 25 hr
Distribution: Lung tissue

Adverse effects

- **CNS:** Seizures
- **CV: Patent ductus arteriosus, intraventricular hemorrhage,** *hypotension, bradycardia*
- **Hematologic:** *Hyperbilirubinemia, thrombocytopenia*
- **Respiratory: Pneumothorax,** *pulmonary air leak,* pulmonary hemorrhage (more often seen with infants < 700 g), *apnea,* pneumomediastinum, emphysema
- **Other:** *Sepsis, nonpulmonary infections*

■ Nursing considerations

Assessment

- **History:** Time of birth, exact birth weight
- **Physical:** T, color; R, adventitious sounds, oximeter, endotracheal tube position and patency, chest movement; ECG, P, BP, peripheral perfusion, arterial pressure (desirable); oxygen saturation, blood gases, CBC; muscular activity, facial expression, reflexes

Interventions

- Arrange for appropriate assessment and monitoring of critically ill infant.
- Monitor ECG and transcutaneous oxygen saturation continually during administration.
- Ensure that endotracheal tube is in the correct position, with bilateral chest movement and lung sounds.
- Arrange for staff to preview teaching videotape, available from the manufacturer, before regular use to cover all of the technical aspects of administration.
- Suction the infant immediately before administration; but do not suction for 2 hr after administration unless clinically necessary.
- Warm vial to room temperature before using, up to 24 hr. No other warming methods should be used.

- Store drug in refrigerator. Protect from light. Enter drug vial only once. Discard remaining drug after use.
- Insert 5 French catheter into the endotracheal tube; do not instill into the main stream bronchus.
- Instill dose slowly; inject one-quarter dose over 2–3 sec; remove catheter and reattach infant to ventilator for at least 30 sec or until stable; repeat procedure administering one-quarter dose at a time.
- Do not suction infant for 1 hr after completion of full dose; do not flush catheter.
- Continually monitor patient color, lung sounds, ECG, oximeter and blood gas readings during administration and for at least 30 min following administration.
- Maintain appropriate interventions for critically ill infant.
- Offer support and encouragement to parents.

Teaching points

Parents of the critically ill infant will need a comprehensive teaching and support program. Details of drug effects and administration are best incorporated into the comprehensive program.

▽ porfimer sodium

See *Less Commonly Used Drugs,* p. 1350.

P

▽ potassium salts

*(po **tass'** ee um)*

potassium acetate

potassium chloride

Oral: Apo-K (CAN), Cena-K, Effer-K, Gen-K, Kaochlor, Kaon-Cl, Kay Ciel, Kaylixir, K-Dur 10, K-Dur 20, K-Lease, K-Lor, K-Norm, K-Tab, Klor-Con, Klorvess, Klotrix, K-Lyte/Cl, Kolyum, K+ Care ET, Micro-K Extentabs, Potasalan, Roychlor (CAN), Rum-K, Slow-K, Ten K

Injection: Potassium Chloride

potassium gluconate
Kaon, K-G Elixir, Kolyum, Tri-K,
Twin-K

PREGNANCY CATEGORY C

Drug class
Electrolyte

Therapeutic actions
Principal intracellular cation of most body tissues, participates in a number of physiologic processes—maintaining intracellular tonicity, transmission of nerve impulses, contraction of cardiac, skeletal, and smooth muscle, maintenance of normal renal function; also plays a role in carbohydrate metabolism and various enzymatic reactions.

Indications
- Prevention and correction of potassium deficiency; when associated with alkalosis, use potassium chloride; when associated with acidosis, use potassium acetate, bicarbonate, citrate, or gluconate
- Treatment of cardiac arrhythmias due to cardiac glycosides (IV)

Contraindications and cautions
- Contraindicated with allergy to tartrazine, aspirin (tartrazine is found in some preparations marketed as *Kaon-Cl, Klor-Con*); severe renal impairment with oliguria, anuria, azotemia; untreated Addison's disease; hyperkalemia; adynamia episodica hereditaria; acute dehydration; heat cramps; GI disorders that delay passage in the GI tract.
- Use cautiously with cardiac disorders, especially if treated with digitalis, pregnancy, lactation.

Available forms
Liquids—20, 30, 40, 45 mEq/15 mL; powders—15, 20, 25 mEq/packet; effervescent tablets—20, 25, 50 mEq; CR tablets—6, 7, 8, 10, 20 mEq; CR capsules—8, 10 mEq; tablets—500, 595 mg; injection—2, 4, 10, 20, 30, 40, 60, 90 mEq

Dosages
Individualize dosage based on patient response using serial ECG and electrolyte determinations in severe cases.
Adults
- *Prevention of hypokalemia:* 16–24 mEq/day PO.
- *Treatment of potassium depletion:* 40–100 mEq/day PO.
- *IV:* Do not administer undiluted. Dilute in dextrose solution to 40–80 mEq/L. Use the following as a guide to administration:

Serum K+	Maximum Infusion Rate	Maximum Concentration	Maximum 24-hr Dose
> 2.6 mEq/L	10 mEq/hr	40 mEq/L	200 mEq
< 2 mEq/L	40 mEq/hr	80 mEq/L	400 mEq

Pediatric patients
- *Replacement:* 3 mEq/kg/day or 40 mg/m^2/day PO or IV.
Geriatric patients or patients with renal impairment
Carefully monitor serum potassium concentration and reduce dosage appropriately.

Pharmacokinetics

Route	Onset	Peak
Oral	Slow	1–2 hr
IV	Rapid	

Metabolism: Cellular; $T_{1/2}$: unknown
Distribution: Crosses placenta; enters breast milk
Excretion: Urine

▼IV facts
Preparation: Do not administer undiluted potassium IV; dilute in dextrose solution to 40–80 mEq/L; in critical states, potassium chloride can be administered in saline.
Infusion: Adjust dosage based on patient response at a maximum of 10 mEq/L.
Incompatibilities: Do not mix with amphotericin B.
Y-site incompatibilities: Do not give with diazepam, ergotamine, phenytoin.

Adverse effects
- **Dermatologic:** Rash

Adverse effects in *Italics* are most common; those in **Bold** are life-threatening.

- **GI:** *Nausea, vomiting, diarrhea, abdominal discomfort,* GI obstruction, GI bleeding, GI ulceration or perforation
- **Hematologic:** Hyperkalemia—increased serum K^+, ECG changes (peaking of T waves, loss of P waves, depression of ST segment, prolongation of QTc interval)
- **Local:** Tissue sloughing, local necrosis, local phlebitis, and venospasm with injection

Interactions

* Drug-drug • Increased risk of hyperkalemia with potassium-sparing diuretics, salt substitutes using potassium

■ Nursing considerations
Assessment

- **History:** Allergy to tartrazine, aspirin; severe renal impairment; untreated Addison's disease; hyperkalemia; adynamia episodica hereditaria; acute dehydration; heat cramps, GI disorders that cause delay in passage in the GI tract, cardiac disorders, lactation
- **Physical:** Skin color, lesions, turgor; injection sites; P, baseline ECG; bowel sounds, abdominal exam; urinary output; serum electrolytes, serum bicarbonate

Interventions

- Arrange for serial serum potassium levels before and during therapy.
- Administer liquid form to any patient with delayed GI emptying.
- Administer oral drug after meals or with food and a full glass of water to decrease GI upset.
- Caution patient not to chew or crush tablets; have patient swallow tablet whole.
- Mix or dissolve oral liquids, soluble powders, and effervescent tablets completely in 3–8 oz of cold water, juice, or other suitable beverage, and have patient drink it slowly.
- Arrange for further dilution or dose reduction if GI effects are severe.
- Agitate prepared IV solution to prevent "layering" of potassium; do not add potassium to an IV bottle in the hanging position.
- Monitor IV injection sites regularly for necrosis, tissue sloughing, phlebitis.
- Monitor cardiac rhythm carefully during IV administration.
- Caution patient that expended wax matrix capsules will be found in the stool.

- Caution patient not to use salt substitutes.

Teaching points

- Take drug after meals or with food and a full glass of water to decrease GI upset. Do not chew or crush tablets, swallow tablets whole. Mix or dissolve oral liquids, soluble powders, and effervescent tablets completely in 3–8 oz of cold water, juice, or other suitable beverage, and drink it slowly. Take the drug as prescribed; do not take more than prescribed.
- These side effects may occur: nausea, vomiting, diarrhea (taking the drugs with meals, diluting them further may help).
- Do not use salt substitutes.
- You may find wax matrix capsules in the stool. The wax matrix is not absorbed in the GI tract.
- Have periodic blood tests and medical evaluation.
- Report tingling of the hands or feet, unusual tiredness or weakness, feeling of heaviness in the legs, severe nausea, vomiting, abdominal pain, black or tarry stools, pain at IV injection site.

▽ pralidoxime chloride (2-PAM)

*(pra li **dox**' eem)*

Protopam Chloride

PREGNANCY CATEGORY C

P

Drug class
Antidote

Therapeutic actions

Reactivates cholinesterase (mainly outside the CNS) inactivated by phosphorylation due to organophosphate pesticide or related compound.

Indications

- Antidote in poisoning due to organophosphate pesticides and chemicals with anticholinesterase activity
- IM use as an adjunct to atropine in poisoning by nerve agents having anticholinesterase activity (autoinjector)
- Control of overdose by anticholinesterase drugs used to treat myasthenia gravis

Contraindications and cautions
- Contraindicated with allergy to any component of drug.
- Use cautiously with impaired renal function, myasthenia gravis, pregnancy, lactation.

Available forms
Injection—1 g

Dosages
Adults
- *Organophosphate poisoning:* In absence of cyanosis, give atropine 2–4 mg IV. If cyanosis is present, give 2–4 mg atropine IM while improving ventilation; repeat every 5–10 min until signs of atropine toxicity appear. Maintain atropinization for at least 48 hr. *Give pralidoxime concomitantly:* inject an initial dose of 1–2 g pralidoxime IV, preferably as a 15- to 30-min infusion in 100 mL of saline. After 1 hr, give a second dose of 1–2 g IV if muscle weakness is not relieved. Give additional doses cautiously. If IV administration is not feasible or if pulmonary edema is present, give IM or SC.
- *Anticholinesterase overdose (eg, neostigmine, pyridostigmine, ambenonium):* 1–2 g IV followed by increments of 250 mg q 5 min.
- *Exposure to nerve agents:* Administer atropine and pralidoxime as soon as possible after exposure. Use the autoinjectors, giving the atropine first; repeat after 15 min. If symptoms exist after an additional 15 min, repeat injections. If symptoms persist after third set of injections, seek medical help.
Pediatric patients
- *Organophosphate poisoning:* 20–40 mg/kg IV per dose given as above.

Pharmacokinetics

Route	Onset	Peak
IV	Rapid	5–15 min
IM	Rapid	10–20 min

Metabolism: Hepatic; $T_{1/2}$: 0.8–2.7 hr
Distribution: May cross placenta or enter breast milk
Excretion: Urine

▼IV facts
Preparation: Dilute in 1–2 g pralidoxime in 100 mL saline.
Infusion: Administer over 15–30 min.

Adverse effects
- **CNS:** *Dizziness, blurred vision, diplopia,* impaired accommodation, *headache,* drowsiness, nausea
- **CV:** Tachycardia
- **Hematologic:** *Transient AST, ALT, CPK elevations*
- **Local:** *Mild to moderate pain at the injection site* 40–60 min after IM injection
- **Respiratory:** Hyperventilation
- **Other:** Muscular weakness

■ Nursing considerations
Assessment
- **History:** Allergy to any component of drug; impaired renal function; myasthenia gravis; lactation, pregnancy
- **Physical:** Reflexes, orientation, vision exam, muscle strength; P, auscultation, baseline ECG; liver evaluation; renal and liver function tests

Interventions
- Remove secretions, maintain patent airway, and provide artificial ventilation as needed for acute organophosphate poisoning; then begin drug therapy.
- Institute treatment as soon as possible after exposure to the poison.
- Remove clothing; thoroughly wash hair and skin with sodium bicarbonate or alcohol as soon as possible after dermal exposure to organophosphate poisoning.
- Use IV sodium thiopental or diazepam if convulsions interfere with respiration after organophosphate poisoning.
- Administer by slow IV infusion; tachycardia, laryngospasm, muscle rigidity have occurred with rapid injection.

Teaching points
- Discomfort may be experienced at IM injection site. If you receive the autoinjector, you need to understand the indications and proper use of the mechanism, review the signs and symptoms of poisoning.

Adverse effects in *Italics* are most common; those in **Bold** are life-threatening.

• Report blurred or double vision, dizziness, nausea.

▽ pramipexole
*(pram ah **pex**' ole)*

Mirapex

PREGNANCY CATEGORY C

Drug classes
Antiparkinsonian agent
Dopamine receptor agonist

Therapeutic actions
Stimulates dopamine receptors in the striatum, leading to decrease in parkinsonian symptoms thought to be related to low dopamine levels.

Indications
• Treatment of the signs and symptoms of idiopathic Parkinson's disease

Contraindications and cautions
• Contraindicated with hypersensitivity to pramipexole.
• Use cautiously with symptomatic hypotension, impaired renal function, pregnancy, lactation.

Available forms
Tablets—0.125, 0.25, 0.5, 1, 1.5 mg

Dosages
Adults
Increase dosage gradually from a starting dose of 0.125 mg PO tid; wk 2—0.25 mg PO tid; wk 3—0.5 mg PO tid; wk 4—0.75 mg PO tid; wk 5—1 mg PO tid; wk 6—1.25 mg PO tid; wk 7—1.5 mg PO tid. If used in combination with levodopa, consider a reduction of dose.
Pediatric patients
Safety and efficacy not established.
Patients with renal impairment

Creatinine Clearance (mL/min)	Starting Dose	Maximum Dose
> 60	0.125 mg PO tid	1.5 mg PO tid
35–59	0.125 mg PO bid	1.5 mg PO bid
15–34	0.125 mg PO daily	1.5 mg PO daily

Pharmacokinetics

Route	Onset	Peak
Oral	Varies	2 hr

Metabolism: Hepatic; $T_{1/2}$: 8 hr
Distribution: May cross placenta; may pass into breast milk
Excretion: Urine

Adverse effects
• **CNS:** *Headache, dizziness, insomnia,* **somnolence,** hallucinations, confusion, amnesia
• **CV:** Orthostatic hypotension, hypertension, arrhythmia, palpitations, hypotension, tachycardia
• **GI:** *Nausea, constipation,* anorexia, dysphagia
• **Other:** Peripheral edema, decreased weight, *asthenia,* fever

Interactions
✳ **Drug-drug•** Increase in levodopa levels and effects if combined • Increase in levels with cimetidine, ranitidine, diltiazem, triamterene, verapamil, quinidine, quinine • Decreased effectiveness with dopamine antagonists

■ Nursing considerations
Assessment
• **History:** Hypersensitivity to pramipexole, symptomatic hypotension, impaired renal function, pregnancy, lactation
• **Physical:** Reflexes, affect; T, BP, P, peripheral perfusion; abdominal exam, normal output; auscultation, R; urinary output, renal function tests

Interventions
• Administer with extreme caution to patients with a history of hypotension, hallucinations, confusion, or dyskinesias.
• Administer with food if GI upset becomes a problem.
• Do not discontinue abruptly; taper gradually over at least 1 wk.
• Monitor patient while adjusting drug to establish therapeutic dosage. Dosage of levodopa/carbidopa may need to be reduced accordingly to balance therapeutic effects.
• Provide safety precautions as needed if hallucinations occur (more common with elderly).

Teaching points

- Take this drug exactly as prescribed, 3 times per day, with breakfast and lunch. Continue to take your levodopa/carbidopa if prescribed. The dosage of the levodopa may need to be decreased after a few days of therapy. The dosage of pramipexole will be slowly increased over a 7-wk period. Write your dose down and follow this pattern.
- Do not stop taking this drug without consulting your health care provider; serious side effects could occur. The drug should be tapered over at least 1 wk.
- These side effects may occur: dizziness, light-headedness, insomnia (avoid driving or operating dangerous machinery); nausea (take drug with meals); edema; weight loss; low blood pressure (change positions slowly; use caution in extremes of heat or exertion); hallucinations (safety precautions may be necessary); falling asleep while engaged in activities of daily living (use caution to avoid injury).
- Avoid becoming pregnant while on this drug; use of barrier contraceptives is advised. If you think you are pregnant, notify your health care provider.
- Report severe nausea, severe swelling, sweating, hallucinations, dizziness, fainting.

▽pravastatin sodium
*(prah va **sta'** tin)*

Pravachol

PREGNANCY CATEGORY X

Drug classes
Antihyperlipidemic
HMG CoA inhibitor

Therapeutic actions
A fungal metabolite that inhibits the enzyme HMG CoA that catalyzes the first step in the cholesterol synthesis pathway, resulting in a decrease in serum cholesterol, serum LDLs (associated with increased risk of CAD), and either an increase or no change in serum HDLs (associated with decreased risk of CAD).

Indications

- Prevention of first MI and reduction of death from CV disease in patients with hypercholesterolemia at risk of first MI
- Adjunct to diet in the treatment of elevated total cholesterol and LDL cholesterol with primary hypercholesterolemia (types IIa and IIb) in patients unresponsive to dietary restriction of saturated fat and cholesterol and other nonpharmacologic measures
- Slow the progression of coronary atherosclerosis in patients with clinically evident CAD to reduce the risk of acute coronary events in hypercholesterolemia patients
- Reduce the risk of stroke or TIA in patients with history of MI and normal cholesterol levels
- Reduce the risk of recurrent MI and death from heart disease in patients with history of MI and normal cholesterol levels

Contraindications and cautions
- Contraindicated with allergy to pravastatin, fungal byproducts, pregnancy, lactation.
- Use cautiously with impaired hepatic function, cataracts, alcoholism.

Available forms
Tablets—10, 20, 40, 80 mg

Dosages
Adults
Initially, 10–40 mg/day PO given once daily. Adjust dose q 4 wk based on response. Maximum daily dose is 40 mg. Maintenance doses range from 40–80 mg/day in single hs dose.
- *Concomitant immunosuppressive therapy:* 10 mg PO daily hs to a maximum of 20 mg/day.
Pediatric patients
Safety and efficacy not established.
Geriatric patients and patients with renal or hepatic impairment
10 mg PO once daily at bedtime; may increase up to 20 mg/day.

Pharmacokinetics

Route	Onset	Peak
Oral	Slow	60–90 min

Adverse effects in *Italics* are most common; those in **Bold** are life-threatening.

Metabolism: Hepatic; T$_{1/2}$: 1.8 hr
Distribution: Crosses placenta; enters breast milk
Excretion: Urine and feces

Adverse effects
- **CNS:** *Headache, blurred vision,* dizziness, insomnia, fatigue, muscle cramps, cataracts
- **GI:** *Flatulence, abdominal pain, cramps, constipation, nausea, vomiting,* heartburn
- **Hematologic:** Elevations of CPK, alkaline phosphatase, and transaminases

Interactions
* **Drug-drug** • Possible severe myopathy or rhabdomyolysis with cyclosporine, erythromycin, gemfibrozil, niacin • Possible increased digoxin, warfarin levels if combined; monitor patient and decrease dosage as needed • Increased pravastatin levels with itraconazole; avoid this combination • Decreased pravastatin levels if combined with bile acid sequestrants; space at least 4 hr apart
* **Drug-food** • Decreased metabolism and risk of toxic effects if combined with grapefruit juice; avoid this combination

■ Nursing considerations
Assessment
- **History:** Allergy to pravastatin, fungal byproducts; impaired hepatic function; cataracts; pregnancy; lactation
- **Physical:** Orientation, affect, ophthalmologic exam; liver evaluation; lipid studies, liver function tests

Interventions
- Caution patient that this drug cannot be used during pregnancy; advise the use of barrier contraceptives.
- Administer drug hs; highest rates of cholesterol synthesis are between midnight and 5 AM.
- Arrange for periodic ophthalmologic exam to check for cataract development; monitor liver function.

Teaching points
- Take drug at bedtime.
- Do not drink grapefruit juice while on this drug.
- These side effects may occur: nausea (small, frequent meals may help); headache, muscle and joint aches and pains (may lessen); sensitivity to sunlight (use sunblock and wear protective clothing).
- This drug cannot be taken during pregnancy; use of barrier contraceptives is advised.
- Have periodic ophthalmic exams while you are on this drug.
- Report severe GI upset, changes in vision, unusual bleeding or bruising, dark urine or light-colored stools, muscle pain or weakness.

▽ praziquantel
See *Less Commonly Used Drugs,* p. 1350.

▽ prazosin hydrochloride
(pra' zoe sin)

Apo-Prazo (CAN), Minipress, Novo-Prazin (CAN), Nu-Prazo (CAN)

PREGNANCY CATEGORY C

Drug classes
Antihypertensive
Alpha-adrenergic blocker

Therapeutic actions
Selectively blocks postsynaptic alpha$_1$-adrenergic receptors, decreasing sympathetic tone on the vasculature, dilating arterioles and veins, and lowering supine and standing BP; unlike conventional alpha-adrenergic blocking agents (eg, phentolamine), it does not also block alpha$_2$ presynaptic receptors, so it does not cause reflex tachycardia.

Indications
- Treatment of hypertension, alone or in combination with other agents
- Unlabeled uses: refractory CHF, management of Raynaud's vasospasm, treatment of prostatic outflow obstruction

Contraindications and cautions
- Contraindicated with hypersensitivity to prazosin, lactation.
- Use cautiously with CHF, renal failure, pregnancy.

Available forms

Capsules—1, 2, 5 mg

Dosages
Adults

First dose may cause syncope with sudden loss of consciousness. First dose should be limited to 1 mg PO and given hs. Initial dosage is 1 mg PO bid–tid. Increase dosage to a total of 20 mg/day given in divided doses. When increasing dosage, give the first dose of each increment hs. Maintenance dosages most commonly range from 6–15 mg/day given in divided doses.

• *Concomitant therapy:* When adding a diuretic or other antihypertensive drug, reduce dosage to 1–2 mg PO tid and then readjust.

Pediatric patients
0.5–7 mg PO tid.

Pharmacokinetics

Route	Onset	Peak
Oral	Varies	1–3 hr

Metabolism: Hepatic; $T_{1/2}$: 2–3 hr
Distribution: Crosses placenta; may enter breast milk
Excretion: Bile/feces, urine

Adverse effects

• **CNS:** *Dizziness, headache, drowsiness, lack of energy, weakness,* nervousness, vertigo, depression, paresthesia
• **CV:** *Palpitations,* sodium and water retention, increased plasma volume, edema, dyspnea, syncope, tachycardia, orthostatic hypotension
• **Dermatologic:** Rash, pruritus, alopecia, lichen planus
• **EENT:** Blurred vision, reddened sclera, epistaxis, tinnitus, dry mouth, nasal congestion
• **GI:** *Nausea,* vomiting, diarrhea, constipation, abdominal discomfort or pain
• **GU:** Urinary frequency, incontinence, impotence, priapism
• **Other:** Diaphoresis, lupus erythematosus

Interactions

＊**Drug-drug** • Severity and duration of hypotension following first dose of prazosin may be greater in patients receiving beta-adrenergic blocking drugs (eg, propranolol), verapamil; first dose of prazosin should be only 0.5 mg or less

■ Nursing considerations
Assessment

• **History:** Hypersensitivity to prazosin, CHF, renal failure, lactation, pregnancy
• **Physical:** Weight; skin color, lesions; orientation, affect, reflexes; ophthalmologic exam; P, BP, orthostatic BP, supine BP, perfusion, edema, auscultation; R, adventitious sounds; status of nasal mucous membranes; bowel sounds, normal output; voiding pattern, normal output; kidney function tests, urinalysis

Interventions

• Administer, or have patient take, first dose just before bedtime to lessen likelihood of first dose effect (syncope)—believed due to excessive orthostatic hypotension.
• Have patient lie down and treat supportively if syncope occurs; condition is self-limiting.
• Monitor for orthostatic hypotension, which is most marked in the morning and is accentuated by hot weather, alcohol, exercise.
• Monitor edema, weight in patients with incipient cardiac decompensation, and add a thiazide diuretic to the drug regimen if sodium and fluid retention, signs of impending CHF occur.

Teaching points

• Take this drug exactly as prescribed. Take the first dose just before bedtime. Do not drive or operate machinery for 4 hr after the first dose.
• These side effects may occur: dizziness, weakness (more likely when changing position, in the early morning, after exercise, in hot weather, and with alcohol; some tolerance may occur; avoid driving or engaging in tasks that require alertness; change position slowly, and use caution when climbing stairs; lie down for a while if dizziness persists); GI upset (frequent, small meals may help); impotence; dry mouth (sucking on sugarless lozenges, ice chips may help); stuffy nose. Most effects are transient.
• Report frequent dizziness or faintness.

Adverse effects in *Italics* are most common; those in **Bold** are life-threatening.

▽ prednisolone
*(pred **niss'** oh lone)*

prednisolone
Oral: Delta-Cortef, Novo-Prednisolone (CAN), Prelone

prednisolone acetate
IM, ophthalmic solution: Econopred, Key-Pred, Predalone, Predcor-50, Pred-Forte, Pred Mild, and others

prednisolone sodium phosphate IM, intra-articular, prednisolone sodium phosphate
IV, IM, intra-articular injection, ophthalmic solution: AK-Pred, Hydeltrasol, Hydrocortone, Inflamase, Key-Pred, Pediapred

prednisolone tebutate
Intra-articular, intralesional injection: Hydeltrasol, Prednisol TBA

PREGNANCY CATEGORY C

Drug classes
Corticosteroid (intermediate acting)
Glucocorticoid
Hormone

Therapeutic actions
Enters target cells and binds to intracellular corticosteroid receptors, thereby initiating many complex reactions that are responsible for its anti-inflammatory and immunosuppressive effects.

Indications
- Hypercalcemia associated with cancer (systemic)
- Short-term management of various inflammatory and allergic disorders, such as rheumatoid arthritis, collagen diseases (eg, SLE), dermatologic diseases (eg, pemphigus), status asthmaticus, and autoimmune disorders (systemic)
- Hematologic disorders: thrombocytopenia purpura, erythroblastopenia (systemic)
- Ulcerative colitis, acute exacerbations of mutiple sclerosis and palliation in some leukemias and lymphomas (systemic)
- Trichinosis with neurologic or myocardial involvement (systemic)
- Arthritis, psoriatic plaques (intra-articular, soft tissue administration)
- Inflammation of the lid, conjunctiva, cornea, and globe (ophthalmic)
- Prednisolone has weaker mineralocorticoid activity than hydrocortisone and is not used as physiologic replacement therapy (ophthalmic)

Contraindications and cautions
- Contraindicated with infections, especially tuberculosis, fungal infections, amebiasis, vaccinia and varicella, and antibiotic-resistant infections; lactation.
- Use cautiously with kidney or liver disease, hypothyroidism, ulcerative colitis with impending perforation, diverticulitis, active or latent peptic ulcer, inflammatory bowel disease, CHF, hypertension, thromboembolic disorders, osteoporosis, convulsive disorders, diabetes mellitus, pregnancy.

Ophthalmic preparations
- Contraindicated with acute superficial herpes simplex keratitis; fungal infections of ocular structures; vaccinia, varicella, and other viral diseases of the cornea and conjunctiva; ocular tuberculosis.

Available forms
Tablets—5 mg; oral syrup—15 mg/5 mL; injection—20, 25, 50 mg/mL; ophthalmic suspension—0.12%, 0.125%, 1%

Dosages
Adults
Individualize dosage, depending on severity of condition and patient's response. Administer daily dose before 9 AM to minimize adrenal suppression. If long-term therapy is needed, consider alternate-day therapy. After long-term therapy, withdraw drug slowly to avoid adrenal insufficiency. Maintenance therapy: reduce initial dose in small increments at intervals until the lowest dose that maintains satisfactory clinical response is reached.

Oral
Prednisolone: 5–60 mg/day.
- *Acute exacerbations of multiple sclerosis:* 200 mg/day for 1 wk, followed by 80 mg every other day for 1 mo.

IM
Prednisolone acetate: 4–60 mg/day.
- *Acute exacerbations of multiple sclerosis:* 200 mg/day for 1 wk followed by 80 mg every other day for 1 mo.

IM, IV
Prednisolone sodium phosphate:
- *Initial dosage,* 4–60 mg/day. Acute exacerbations of multiple sclerosis: 200 mg/day for 1 wk followed by 80 mg every other day for 1 mo.

Intra-articular, intralesional (dose will vary with joint or soft tissue site to be injected)
Prednisolone acetate: 5–100 mg.
Prednisolone acetate and sodium phosphate: 0.25–0.5 mL.
Prednisolone sodium phosphate: 2–30 mg.
Prednisolone tebutate: 4–30 mg.

Pediatric patients
Individualize dosage depending on severity of condition and patient's response rather than by strict adherence to formulae that correct adult doses for age or weight. Carefully observe growth and development in infants and children on prolonged therapy.

Ophthalmic
Prednisolone acetate suspension; prednisolone sodium phosphate solution
1–2 drops into the conjunctival sac every hour during the day and every 2 hr during the night. After a favorable response, reduce dose to 1 drop q 4 hr and then 1 drop tid or qid.

Pharmacokinetics

Route	Onset	Peak	Duration
Oral	Varies	1–2 hr	1–1.5 days

Metabolism: Hepatic; $T_{1/2}$: 3.5 hr
Distribution: Crosses placenta; enters breast milk
Excretion: Urine

▽IV facts
Preparation: May be given undiluted or added to D_5W or normal saline solution; use within 24 hr if diluted.
Infusion: Infuse slowly, each 10 mg over 1 min—slower if discomfort at the injection site.
Incompatibilities: Do not mix in solution with other drugs.

Adverse effects
Effects depend on dose, route, and duration of therapy. The following are primarily associated with systemic absorption.
- **CNS:** *Vertigo, headache,* paresthesias, insomnia, convulsions, psychosis, cataracts, increased intraocular pressure, glaucoma (long-term therapy)
- **CV:** Hypotension, **shock,** hypertension and CHF secondary to fluid retention, thromboembolism, thrombophlebitis, fat embolism, cardiac arrhythmias
- **Electrolyte imbalance:** *Na+ and fluid retention,* hypokalemia, hypocalcemia
- **Endocrine:** Amenorrhea, irregular menses, growth retardation, decreased carbohydrate tolerance, diabetes mellitus, cushingoid state (long-term effect), increased blood sugar, increased serum cholesterol, decreased T_3 and T_4 levels, hypothalamic-pituitary-adrenal (HPA) suppression with systemic therapy longer than 5 days
- **GI:** Peptic or esophageal ulcer, pancreatitis, abdominal distention, nausea, vomiting, *increased appetite, weight gain* (long-term therapy)
- **Hypersensitivity:** Hypersensitivity or anaphylactoid reactions
- **Musculoskeletal:** Muscle weakness, steroid myopathy, loss of muscle mass, osteoporosis, spontaneous fractures (long-term therapy)
- **Other:** *Immunosuppression, aggravation, or masking of infections; impaired wound healing;* thin, fragile skin; petechiae, ecchymoses, purpura, striae; subcutaneous fat atrophy

The following effects are related to various local routes of steroid administration:

Intra-articular
- **Local:** Osteonecrosis, tendon rupture, infection

Intralesional (face and head)
- **Local:** Blindness (rare)

Ophthalmic solutions, ointments
- **Local:** Infections, especially fungal; glaucoma, cataracts with long-term therapy
- **Other:** Systemic absorption and adverse effects (see above) with prolonged use

Interactions
✳ **Drug-drug** • Increased therapeutic and toxic effects of prednisolone with troleandomycin, ketoconazole • Increased therapeutic and toxic effects of estrogens, including hormonal contraceptives • Risk of severe deterioration of muscle strength in myasthenia gravis patients who also are receiving ambenonium, edrophonium, neostigmine, pyridostigmine • Decreased steroid blood levels with barbiturates, phenytoin, rifampin • Decreased effectiveness of salicylates
✳ **Drug-lab test** • False-negative nitrobluetetrazolium test for bacterial infection • Suppression of skin test reactions

■ Nursing considerations
Assessment
- **History:** Infections; kidney or liver disease; hypothyroidism; ulcerative colitis with impending perforation; diverticulitis; active or latent peptic ulcer; inflammatory bowel disease; CHF; hypertension; thromboembolic disorders; osteoporosis; convulsive disorders; diabetes mellitus; pregnancy; lactation. Ophthalmic: acute superficial herpes simplex keratitis; fungal infections of ocular structures; vaccinia, varicella, and other viral diseases of the cornea and conjunctiva; ocular tuberculosis
- **Physical:** Weight, T, reflexes and grip strength, affect and orientation, P, BP, peripheral perfusion, prominence of superficial veins, R, adventitious sounds, serum electrolytes, blood glucose

Interventions
- Administer once-a-day doses before 9 AM to mimic normal peak corticosteroid blood levels.
- Increase dosage when patient is subject to stress.
- Taper doses when discontinuing high-dose or long-term therapy.
- Do not give live virus vaccines with immunosuppressive doses of corticosteroids.

Teaching points
Systemic
- Do not stop taking the drug without consulting your health care provider.
- Avoid exposure to infections.
- Report unusual weight gain, swelling of the extremities, muscle weakness, black or tarry stools, fever, prolonged sore throat, colds or other infections, worsening of the disorder for which the drug is being taken.

Intra-articular administration
- Do not overuse joint after therapy, even if pain is gone.

Ophthalmic preparations
- Learn the proper administration technique: Lie down or tilt head backward, and look at ceiling. Drop suspension inside lower eyelid while looking up. After instilling eye drops, release lower lid, but do not blink for at least 30 sec; apply gentle pressure to the inside corner of the eye for 1 min. Do not close eyes tightly, and try not to blink more often than usual. Do not touch dropper to eye, fingers, or any surface. Wait at least 5 min before using any other eye preparations.
- Eyes may be sensitive to bright light; sunglasses may help.
- Report worsening of the condition, pain, itching, swelling of the eye, failure of the condition to improve after 1 wk.

▷ prednisone
(pred' ni sone)

Apo-Prednisone (CAN), Deltasone, Liquid Pred, Meticorten, Novo-Prednisone (CAN), Orasone, Panasol-S, Prednicen-M, Prednisone-Intensol, Sterapred DS, Winpred (CAN)

PREGNANCY CATEGORY C

Drug classes
Corticosteroid (intermediate acting)
Glucocorticoid
Hormone

Therapeutic actions

Enters target cells and binds to intracellular corticosteroid receptors, thereby initiating many complex reactions that are responsible for its anti-inflammatory and immunosuppressive effects.

Indications

- Replacement therapy in adrenal cortical insufficiency
- Hypercalcemia associated with cancer
- Short-term management of various inflammatory and allergic disorders, such as rheumatoid arthritis, collagen diseases (eg, SLE), dermatologic diseases (eg, pemphigus), status asthmaticus, and autoimmune disorders
- Hematologic disorders: thrombocytopenia purpura, erythroblastopenia
- Ulcerative colitis, acute exacerbations of multiple sclerosis and palliation in some leukemias and lymphomas
- Trichinosis with neurologic or myocardial involvement

Contraindications and cautions

- Contraindicated with infections, especially tuberculosis, fungal infections, amebiasis, vaccinia and varicella, and antibiotic-resistant infections; lactation.
- Use cautiously with kidney or liver disease, hypothyroidism, ulcerative colitis with impending perforation, diverticulitis, active or latent peptic ulcer, inflammatory bowel disease, CHF, hypertension, thromboembolic disorders, osteoporosis, convulsive disorders, diabetes mellitus; hepatic disease; pregnancy (monitor infants for adrenal insufficiency).

Available forms

Tablets—1, 2.5, 5, 10, 20, 50 mg; oral solution—5 mg/5 mL, 5 mg/mL; syrup—5 mg/ 5 mL

Dosages
Adults

Individualize dosage depending on severity of condition and patient's response. Administer daily dose before 9 AM to minimize adrenal suppression. If long-term therapy is needed, consider alternate-day therapy. After long-term therapy, withdraw drug slowly to avoid adrenal insufficiency. Initial dose: 5–60 mg/day PO. Maintenance therapy: reduce initial dose in small increments at intervals until lowest dose that maintains satisfactory clinical response is reached.

Pediatric patients

- *Physiologic replacement:* 0.05–2 mg/kg/day PO or 4–5 mg/m^2/day PO in equal divided doses q 12 hr.
- *Other indications:* Individualize dosage depending on severity of condition and patient's response rather than by strict adherence to formulae that correct adult doses for age or body weight. Carefully observe growth and development in infants and children on prolonged therapy.

Pharmacokinetics

Route	Onset	Peak	Duration
Oral	Varies	1–2 hr	1–1.5 days

Metabolism: Hepatic; $T_{1/2}$: 3.5 hr
Distribution: Crosses placenta; enters breast milk
Excretion: Urine

Adverse effects

- **CNS:** *Vertigo, headache,* paresthesias, insomnia, convulsions, psychosis, cataracts, increased intraocular pressure, glaucoma (long-term therapy)
- **CV:** Hypotension, **shock,** hypertension and CHF secondary to fluid retention, thromboembolism, thrombophlebitis, fat embolism, cardiac arrhythmias
- **Electrolyte imbalance:** *Na+ and fluid retention,* hypokalemia, hypocalcemia
- **Endocrine:** Amenorrhea, irregular menses, growth retardation, decreased carbohydrate tolerance, diabetes mellitus, cushingoid state (long-term effect), increased blood sugar, increased serum cholesterol, decreased T_3 and T_4 levels, HPA suppression with systemic therapy longer than 5 days
- **GI:** Peptic or esophageal ulcer, pancreatitis, abdominal distention, nausea, vomiting, *increased appetite, weight gain* (long-term therapy)
- **Hypersensitivity:** Hypersensitivity or anaphylactoid reactions

Adverse effects in *Italics* are most common; those in **Bold** are life-threatening.

- **Musculoskeletal:** Muscle weakness, steroid myopathy, loss of muscle mass, osteoporosis, spontaneous fractures (long-term therapy)
- **Other:** *Immunosuppression, aggravation or masking of infections; impaired wound healing;* thin, fragile skin; petechiae, ecchymoses, purpura, striae; subcutaneous fat atrophy

Interactions

✴ Drug-drug ● Increased therapeutic and toxic effects with troleandomycin, ketoconazole ● Increased therapeutic and toxic effects of estrogens, including hormonal contraceptives ● Risk of severe deterioration of muscle strength in myasthenia gravis patients who also are receiving ambenonium, edrophonium, neostigmine, pyridostigmine ● Decreased steroid blood levels with barbiturates, phenytoin, rifampin ● Decreased effectiveness of salicylates

✴ Drug-lab test ● False-negative nitrobluetetrazolium test for bacterial infection ● Suppression of skin test reactions

■ Nursing considerations
Assessment

- **History:** Infections; kidney or liver disease, hypothyroidism, ulcerative colitis with impending perforation, diverticulitis, active or latent peptic ulcer, inflammatory bowel disease, CHF, hypertension, thromboembolic disorders, osteoporosis, convulsive disorders, diabetes mellitus; hepatic disease; lactation
- **Physical:** Weight, T, reflexes and grip strength, affect and orientation, P, BP, peripheral perfusion, prominence of superficial veins, R, adventitious sounds, serum electrolytes, blood glucose

Interventions

- Administer once-a-day doses before 9 AM to mimic normal peak corticosteroid blood levels.
- Increase dosage when patient is subject to stress.
- Taper doses when discontinuing high-dose or long-term therapy.
- Do not give live virus vaccines with immunosuppressive doses of corticosteroids.

Teaching points
- Do not stop taking the drug without consulting your health care provider.
- Avoid exposure to infections.
- Report unusual weight gain, swelling of the extremities, muscle weakness, black or tarry stools, fever, prolonged sore throat, colds or other infections, worsening of the disorder for which the drug is being taken.

▷ primidone
(pri′ mi done)

Apo-Primidone (CAN), Mysoline

PREGNANCY CATEGORY D

Drug class
Antiepileptic agent

Therapeutic actions
Mechanism of action not understood; primidone and its two metabolites, phenobarbital and phenylethylmalonamide, all have antiepileptic activity.

Indications
- Control of grand mal, psychomotor, or focal epileptic seizures, either alone or with other antiepileptics; may control grand mal seizures refractory to other antiepileptics
- Unlabeled use: treatment of benign familial tremor (essential tremor)—750 mg/day

Contraindications and cautions
- Contraindicated with hypersensitivity to phenobarbital, porphyria, lactation (somnolence and drowsiness may occur in nursing newborns).
- Use cautiously with pregnancy (association between use of antiepileptic drugs and an elevated incidence of birth defects; however, do not discontinue antiepileptic therapy in pregnant women who are receiving such therapy to prevent major seizures; discontinuing medication is likely to precipitate status epilepticus, with attendant hypoxia and risk to both mother and fetus; to prevent neonatal hemorrhage, primidone should be given with prophylactic vitamin K_1 therapy for 1 mo prior to and during delivery).

Available forms

Tablets—50, 250 mg; oral suspension—250 mg/5 mL

Dosages

Adults

- *Regimen for patients who have received no previous therapy:* Days 1–3, 100–125 mg PO hs; days 4–6, 100–125 mg bid; days 7–9, 100–125 mg tid; day 10–maintenance, 250 mg tid. The usual maintenance dosage is 250 mg tid–qid. If required, increase dosage to 250 mg five to six times daily, but do not exceed dosage of 500 mg qid (2 g/day).
- *Regimen for patients already receiving other antiepileptic drugs:* Start primidone at 100–125 mg PO hs. Gradually increase to maintenance level as the other drug is gradually decreased. Continue this regimen until satisfactory dosage level is achieved for the combination, or the other medication is completely withdrawn. When use of primidone alone is desired, the transition should not be completed in less than 2 wk.

Pediatric patients

- *Regimen for patients who have received no previous therapy:*

> 8 yr: Days 1–3, 100–125 mg PO hs; days 4–6, 100–125 mg bid; days 7–9, 100–125 mg tid; day 10–maintenance, 250 mg tid. The usual maintenance dosage is 250 mg tid–qid. If required, increase dosage to 250 mg five to six times daily, but do not exceed dosage of 500 mg qid (2 g/day).

< 8 yr: Days 1–3, 50 mg PO at bedtime; days 4–6, 50 mg bid; days 7–9, 100 mg bid; day 10–maintenance, 125–250 mg tid. The usual maintenance dosage is 125–250 mg tid or 10–25 mg/kg/day in divided doses.

Pharmacokinetics

Route	Onset	Peak
Oral	Varies	3–7 hr

Metabolism: Hepatic; $T_{1/2}$: 3–24 hr
Distribution: Crosses placenta; enters breast milk
Excretion: Urine

Adverse effects

- **CNS:** *Ataxia, vertigo, fatigue, hyperirritability,* emotional disturbances, nystagmus, diplopia, drowsiness, personality deterioration with mood changes and paranoia
- **GI:** *Nausea, anorexia,* vomiting
- **GU:** Sexual impotence
- **Hematologic:** Megaloblastic anemia that responds to folic acid therapy
- **Other:** Morbiliform skin eruptions

Interactions

✳ **Drug-drug** • Toxicity with phenytoins • Increased CNS effects, impaired hand-eye coordination, and death may occur with acute alcohol ingestion • Decreased serum concentrations of primidone and increased serum concentrations of carbamazepine if taken concurrently • Decreased serum concentrations with acetazolamide • Increased levels with isoniazid, nicotinamide, succinimides

■ Nursing considerations

Assessment

- **History:** Hypersensitivity to phenobarbital, porphyria, pregnancy, lactation
- **Physical:** Skin color, lesions; orientation, affect, reflexes, vision exam; bowel sounds, normal output; CBC and a sequential multiple analysis-12 (SMA-12), EEG

Interventions

- Reduce dosage, discontinue primidone, or substitute other antiepileptic medication gradually; abrupt discontinuation may precipitate status epilepticus.
- Arrange for patient to have CBC and SMA-12 test every 6 mo during therapy.
- Arrange for folic acid therapy if megaloblastic anemia occurs; primidone does not need to be discontinued.
- Obtain counseling for women of childbearing age who wish to become pregnant.
- Evaluate for therapeutic serum levels: 5–12 mcg/mL for primidone.

Teaching points

- Take this drug exactly as prescribed; do not discontinue this drug abruptly or change dosage, except on the advice of your prescriber.

Adverse effects in *Italics* are most common; those in **Bold** are life-threatening.

- Arrange for frequent checkups, including blood tests, to monitor your response to this drug. Keep all appointments for checkups.
- Use contraception at all times. If you wish to become pregnant while you are taking this drug, you should consult your health care provider.
- These side effects may occur: drowsiness, dizziness, muscular incoordination (transient; avoid driving or performing other tasks requiring alertness); vision changes (avoid performing tasks that require visual acuity); GI upset (take drug with food or milk, eat frequent, small meals).
- Wear a medical alert tag at all times so that emergency medical personnel will know that you are an epileptic taking antiepileptic medication.
- Report rash, joint pain, unexplained fever, pregnancy.

▷ probenecid
(proe **ben'** e sid)

Benemid (CAN), Benuryl (CAN)

PREGNANCY CATEGORY B

Drug classes
Uricosuric agent
Antigout agent

Therapeutic actions
Inhibits the renal tubular reabsorption of urate, increasing the urinary excretion of uric acid, decreasing serum uric acid levels, retarding urate deposition, and promoting resorption of urate deposits; also inhibits the renal tubular reabsorption of most penicillins and cephalosporins.

Indications
- Treatment of hyperuricemia associated with gout and gouty arthritis
- Adjuvant to therapy with penicillins or cephalosporins, for elevation and prolongation of plasma levels of the antibiotic

Contraindications and cautions
- Contraindicated with allergy to probenecid, blood dyscrasias, uric acid kidney stones, acute gouty attack, pregnancy.
- Use cautiously with peptic ulcer, acute intermittent porphyria, G-6-PD deficiency, chronic renal insufficiency, lactation.

Available forms
Tablets—0.5 g

Dosages
Adults
- *Gout:* 0.25 g PO bid for 1 wk; then 0.5 g PO bid. Maintenance: continue dosage that maintains the normal serum uric acid levels. When no attacks occur for 6 mo or more, decrease the daily dosage by 0.5 g every 6 mo.
- *Penicillin or cephalosporin therapy:* 2 g/day PO in divided doses.
- *Gonorrhea treatment:* Single 1-g dose PO 30 min before penicillin administration.
Pediatric patients
- *Penicillin or cephalosporin therapy:*
< 2 yr: Do not use.
2–14 yr: 25 mg/kg PO initial dose, then 40 mg/kg/day divided in four doses.
Children ≥ 50 kg: Use adult dosage.
- *Gonorrhea treatment in children < 45 kg:* 23 mg/kg PO in one single dose 30 min before penicillin administration.
Geriatric patients or patients with renal impairment
1 g/day PO may be adequate. Daily dosage may be increased by 0.5 g every 4 wk. Probenecid may not be effective in chronic renal insufficiency when glomerular filtration rate < 30 mL/min.

Pharmacokinetics
Route	Onset	Peak
Oral	Varies	2–4 hr

Metabolism: Hepatic; $T_{1/2}$: 5–8 hr
Distribution: Crosses placenta; may enter breast milk
Excretion: Urine

Adverse effects
- **CNS:** *Headache*
- **GI:** *Nausea, vomiting, anorexia,* sore gums
- **GU:** *Urinary frequency,* exacerbation of gout and uric acid stones
- **Hematologic:** Anemia, hemolytic anemia
- **Hypersensitivity:** Reactions including **anaphylaxis,** dermatitis, pruritus, fever
- **Other:** Blushing, dizziness

Interactions

✱ Drug-drug • Decreased effectiveness with salicylates • Decreased renal excretion and increased serum levels of methotrexate, dyphylline • Increased pharmacologic effects of thiopental, acyclovir, allopurinol, benzodiazepines, clofibrate, dapsone, NSAIDs, sulfonamides, zidovudine, rifampin

✱ Drug-lab test • False-positive test for urine glucose if using Benedict's test, *Clinitest* (use *Clinistix*) • Falsely high determination of theophylline levels • Inhibited excretion of urinary 17-ketosteroids, phenolsulfonphthalein, sulfobromophthalein

■ Nursing considerations

 CLINICAL ALERT!
Name confusion has been reported between probenecid and Procanbid (procainamide); use extreme caution.

Assessment

• **History:** Allergy to probenecid, blood dyscrasias, uric acid kidney stones, acute gouty attack, peptic ulcer, acute intermittent porphyria, G-6-PD deficiency, chronic renal insufficiency, pregnancy, lactation
• **Physical:** Skin lesions, color; reflexes, gait; liver evaluation, normal output, gums; urinary output; CBC, renal and liver function tests, urinalysis

Interventions

• Administer drug with meals or antacids if GI upset occurs.
• Force fluids—2.5 to 3 L/day—to decrease the risk of renal stone development.
• Check urine alkalinity; urates crystallize in acid urine; sodium bicarbonate or potassium citrate may be ordered to alkalinize urine.
• Arrange for regular medical follow-up and blood tests.
• Double-check any analgesics ordered for pain; salicylates should be avoided.

Teaching points

• Take the drug with meals or antacids if GI upset occurs.

• These side effects may occur: headache (monitor lighting, temperature, noise; consult with nurse or physician if severe); dizziness (change position slowly; avoid driving or operating dangerous machinery); exacerbation of gouty attack or renal stones (drink plenty of fluids—2.5–3 L/day); nausea, vomiting, loss of appetite (take drug with meals or request antacids).
• Report flank pain, dark urine or blood in urine, acute gout attack, unusual fatigue or lethargy, unusual bleeding or bruising.

▽ procainamide hydrochloride
(proe kane a' mide)

Apo-Procainamide (CAN), Procan SR (CAN), Procanbid, Pronestyl, Pronestyl-SR

PREGNANCY CATEGORY C

Drug class
Antiarrhythmic

Therapeutic actions
Type 1A antiarrhythmic: decreases rate of diastolic depolarization (decreases automaticity) in ventricles, decreases the rate of rise and height of the action potential, increases fibrillation threshold.

Indications
• Treatment of documented ventricular arrhythmias that are judged to be life-threatening

Contraindications and cautions
• Contraindicated with allergy to procaine, procainamide, or similar drugs; tartrazine sensitivity (tablets marketed as *Pronestyl* contain tartrazine); second- or third-degree heart block (unless electrical pacemaker operative); SLE; torsades de pointes; pregnancy; lactation.
• Use cautiously with myasthenia gravis, hepatic or renal disease.

Available forms

Tablets—250, 375, 500 mg; capsules—250, 375, 500 mg; SR tablets—250, 500, 750, 1,000 mg; injection—100, 500 mg/mL

Dosages
Adults
Oral

50 mg/kg/day PO in divided doses q 3 hr. Maintenance dose of 50 mg/kg/day (sustained release) in divided doses q 6 hr, starting 2–3 hr after last dose of standard oral preparation.

Body Weight	Standard Preparation	Sustained-Release Preparation
< 55 kg	250 mg q 3 hr	500 mg q 6 hr
55–90 kg	375 mg q 3 hr	750 mg q 6 hr
> 90 kg	500 mg q 3 hr	1,000 mg q 6 hr

IM

0.5–1 g q 4–8 hr until oral therapy can be started.

IV

- Direct IV injection: Dilute in 5% dextrose injection. Give 100 mg q 5 min at a rate not to exceed 25–50 mg/min (maximum dose 1 g).
- IV infusion: 500–600 mg over 25–30 min, then 2–6 mg/min. Monitor very closely.

Pediatric patients
Oral

15–50 mg/kg/day divided every 3–6 hr; maximum, 4 g/day.

IM

20–30 mg/kg/day divided every 4–6 hr; maximum 4 g/day.

IV

Loading dose, 3–6 mg/kg per dose over 5 min; maintenance, 20–80 mcg/kg/min per continuous infusion; maximum, 100 mg/day dose or 2 g/day.

Pharmacokinetics

Route	Onset	Peak	Duration
Oral	30 min	60–90 min	3–4 hr
IV	Immediate	20–60 min	3–4 hr
IM	10–30 min	15–60 min	3–4 hr

Metabolism: Hepatic; $T_{1/2}$: 2.5–4.7 hr
Distribution: Crosses placenta; enters breast milk
Excretion: Urine

▼ IV facts

Preparation: Dilute the 100 or 500 mg/mL dose in 5% dextrose in water.
Infusion: Slowly inject directly into vein or into tubing of actively running IV, 100 mg q 5 min, not faster than 25–50 mg/min; maintenance doses should be given by continual IV infusion with a pump to maintain rate—first 500–600 mg over 25–30 min, then 2–6 mg/min.

Adverse effects

- **CNS:** Mental depression, giddiness, convulsions, confusion, psychosis
- **CV:** *Hypotension,* cardiac conduction disturbances
- **Dermatologic:** *Rash,* pruritus, urticaria
- **GI:** *Anorexia, nausea,* vomiting, bitter taste, diarrhea
- **Hematologic:** Granulocytopenia
- **Other:** Lupus syndrome, fever, chills

Interactions

✻ Drug-drug • Increased levels with cimetidine, trimethoprim, amiodarone; monitor for toxicity

■ Nursing considerations

 CLINICAL ALERT!
Name confusion has been reported between Procanbid and probenecid; use extreme caution. Confusion has also been reported between Procanbid and Procan SR (CAN); use caution, dosage varies.

P

Assessment

- **History:** Allergy to procaine, procainamide, or similar drugs; tartrazine sensitivity; second- or third-degree heart block (unless electrical pacemaker operative); myasthenia gravis; hepatic or renal disease; SLE; torsades de pointes; pregnancy; lactation
- **Physical:** Weight, skin color, lesions; bilateral grip strength; P, BP, auscultation, ECG, edema; bowel sounds, liver evaluation; urinalysis, renal and liver function tests, complete blood count

Interventions

- Monitor patient response carefully, especially when beginning therapy.
- Reduce dosage in patients < 120 lb.

- Reduce dosage in patients with hepatic or renal failure.
- Dosage adjustment may be necessary when procainamide is given with other antiarrhythmics, antihypertensives, cimetidine, or alcohol.
- Check to see that patients with supraventricular tachyarrhythmias have been digitalized before giving procainamide.
- Differentiate the sustained-release (SR) form from the regular preparation.
- Monitor cardiac rhythm and BP frequently if IV route is used.
- Arrange for periodic ECG monitoring and determination of ANA titers when on long-term therapy.
- Arrange for frequent monitoring of blood counts.
- Give dosages at evenly spaced intervals, around the clock; determine a schedule that will minimize sleep interruption.
- Evaluate for safe and effective serum drug levels: 4–8 mcg/mL.

Teaching points

- Take this drug at evenly spaced intervals, around the clock. Do not double up doses; do not skip doses; take exactly as prescribed. You may need an alarm clock to wake you up to take the drug. The best schedule for you will be determined to decrease sleep interruption as much as possible. Do not chew the sustained-release tablets.
- You will require frequent monitoring of cardiac rhythm.
- These side effects may occur: nausea, loss of appetite, vomiting (small, frequent meals may help); small wax cores may be passed in the stool (from sustained-release tablet); rash (use careful skin care).
- Do not stop taking this drug for any reason without checking with your health care provider.
- Return for regular follow-up visits to check your heart rhythm and blood counts.
- Report joint pain, stiffness; sore mouth, throat, gums; fever, chills; cold or flulike syndromes; extensive rash, sensitivity to the sun.

▷ procarbazine hydrochloride

See *Less Commonly Used Drugs,* p. 1350.

▷ prochlorperazine
(proe klor per' a zeen)

prochlorperazine
Rectal suppositories: Compazine, Stemetil Suppositories (CAN)

prochlorperazine edisylate
Oral syrup, injection: Compazine, Nu-Prochlor (CAN), Stemetil (CAN)

prochlorperazine maleate
Oral tablets and sustained-release capsules: Compazine, PMS-Prochlorperazine (CAN), Stemetil (CAN)

PREGNANCY CATEGORY C

Drug classes
Phenothiazine (piperazine)
Dopaminergic blocking agent
Antipsychotic
Antiemetic
Antianxiety agent

Therapeutic actions
Mechanism of action not fully understood: antipsychotic drugs block postsynaptic dopamine receptors in the brain, but this may not be necessary and sufficient for antipsychotic activity; depresses the RAS, including the parts of the brain involved with wakefulness and emesis; anticholinergic, antihistaminic (H_1), and alpha-adrenergic blocking activity also may contribute to some of its therapeutic (and adverse) actions.

Indications
- Management of manifestations of psychotic disorders
- Control of severe nausea and vomiting

- Short-term treatment of nonpsychotic anxiety (not drug of choice)
- Unlabeled use: treatment of acute headache

Contraindications and cautions

- Contraindicated with coma or severe CNS depression, bone marrow depression, blood dyscrasia, circulatory collapse, subcortical brain damage, Parkinson's disease, liver damage, cerebral arteriosclerosis, coronary disease, severe hypotension or hypertension.
- Use cautiously with respiratory disorders, glaucoma, prostatic hypertrophy, epilepsy, breast cancer (elevations in prolactin may stimulate a prolactin-dependent tumor), thyrotoxicosis, peptic ulcer, decreased renal function, myelography within previous 24 hr or scheduled within 48 hr, exposure to heat or phosphorous insecticides, pregnancy, lactation, children younger than 12 yr, especially those with chickenpox, CNS infections (children are especially susceptible to dystonias that may confound the diagnosis of Reye's syndrome).

Available forms

Tablets—5, 10, 25 mg; SR capsules—10, 15 mg; syrup—5 mg/5 mL; injection—5 mg/mL; suppositories—2.5, 5, 25 mg

Dosages
Adults

- *Psychotic disturbances:* Initially, 5–10 mg PO tid or qid. Gradually increase dosage every 2–3 days as necessary up to 50–75 mg/day for mild or moderate disturbances, 100–150 mg/day for more severe disturbances. For immediate control of severely disturbed adults, 10–20 mg IM repeated q 2–4 hr (every hour for resistant cases); switch to oral therapy as soon as possible.
- *Antiemetic:* Control of severe nausea and vomiting: 5–10 mg PO tid–qid; 15 mg (sustained-release) on arising; 10 mg (sustained-release) q 12 hr; 25 mg rectally bid; or 5–10 mg IM initially, repeated q 3–4 hr up to 40 mg/day.
- *Nausea, vomiting related to surgery:* 5–10 mg IM 1–2 hr before anesthesia or during and after surgery (may repeat once in 30 min); 5–10 mg IV 15 min before anesthesia or during and after surgery (may repeat once); or as IV infusion, 20 mg/L of isotonic solution added to infusion 15–30 min before anesthesia.

Pediatric patients

Do not use in pediatric surgery.
< 20 lb (9.1 kg) or < 2 yr: Generally not recommended.
2–12 yr: 2.5 mg PO or rectally bid–tid. Do not give more than 10 mg on first day. Increase dosage according to patient response; total daily dose usually does not exceed 20 mg (2–5 yr) or 25 mg (6–12 yr).
< 12 yr: 0.03 mg/kg by deep IM injection. Switch to oral dosage as soon as possible (usually after one dose).

- *Antiemetic—control of severe nausea and vomiting:*

Oral or rectal
> 20 lb or > 2 yr:
9.1–13.2 kg: 2.5 mg daily–bid, not to exceed 7.5 mg/day.
13.6–17.7 kg: 2.5 mg bid–tid, not to exceed 10 mg/day.
18.2–38.6 kg: 2.5 mg tid or 5 mg bid, not to exceed 15 mg/day.

IM
18.2–38.6 kg: 0.132 mg/kg IM (usually only one dose).

Pharmacokinetics

Route	Onset	Duration
Oral	30–40 min	3–4 hr (10–12 SR)
PR	60–90 min	3–4 hr
IM	10–20 min	3–4 hr
IV	Immediate	3–4 hr

Metabolism: Hepatic; $T_{1/2}$: unknown
Distribution: Crosses placenta; enters breast milk
Excretion: Urine

▼IV facts

Preparation: Dilute 20 mg in not less than 1 L of isotonic solution.
Infusion: Inject 5–10 mg directly IV 15–30 min before induction (may be repeated once), or infuse dilute solution 15–30 min before induction; do not exceed 5 mg/mL/min.

Adverse effects

- **Autonomic:** Dry mouth, salivation, nasal congestion, nausea, vomiting, anorexia, fever, pallor, flushed facies, sweating, constipation, paralytic ileus, urinary retention,

incontinence, polyuria, enuresis, priapism, ejaculation inhibition, male impotence
- **CNS:** *Drowsiness,* insomnia, vertigo, headache, weakness, tremor, ataxia, slurring, cerebral edema, seizures, exacerbation of psychotic symptoms, extrapyramidal syndromes—*pseudoparkinsonism; dystonias; akathisia,* tardive dyskinesias, potentially irreversible; **neuroleptic malignant syndrome**
- **CV:** Hypotension, orthostatic hypotension, hypertension, tachycardia, bradycardia, cardiac arrest, CHF, cardiomegaly, **refractory arrhythmias,** pulmonary edema
- **EENT:** Glaucoma, *photophobia, blurred vision,* miosis, mydriasis, deposits in the cornea and lens (opacities), pigmentary retinopathy
- **Endocrine:** Lactation, breast engorgement, galactorrhea; SIADH; amenorrhea, menstrual irregularities; gynecomastia; changes in libido; hyperglycemia or hypoglycemia; glycosuria; hyponatremia; pituitary tumor with hyperprolactinemia; inhibition of ovulation, infertility, pseudopregnancy; reduced urinary levels of gonadotropins, estrogens, progestins
- **Hematologic:** Eosinophilia, leukopenia, leukocytosis, anemia; aplastic anemia; hemolytic anemia; thrombocytopenic or nonthrombocytopenic purpura; pancytopenia
- **Hypersensitivity:** Jaundice, urticaria, angioneurotic edema, laryngeal edema, photosensitivity, eczema, asthma, anaphylactoid reactions, exfoliative dermatitis
- **Respiratory:** Bronchospasm, laryngospasm, dyspnea; suppression of cough reflex and potential for aspiration
- **Other:** *Urine discolored pink to red-brown*

Interactions

✳ **Drug-drug** • Additive CNS depression with alcohol • Additive anticholinergic effects and possibly decreased antipsychotic efficacy with anticholinergic drugs • Increased likelihood of seizures with metrizamide • Increased chance of severe neuromuscular excitation and hypotension with barbiturate anesthetics (methohexital, thiamylal, phenobarbital, thiopental) • Decreased antihypertensive effect of guanethidine

✳ **Drug-lab test** • False-positive pregnancy tests (less likely if serum test is used) • Increase in PBI, not attributable to an increase in thyroxine

■ Nursing considerations
Assessment

- **History:** Coma or severe CNS depression; bone marrow depression; circulatory collapse; subcortical brain damage; Parkinson's disease; liver damage; cerebral arteriosclerosis; coronary disease; severe hypotension or hypertension; respiratory disorders; glaucoma; prostatic hypertrophy; epilepsy; breast cancer; thyrotoxicosis; peptic ulcer, decreased renal function; myelography within previous 24 hr or scheduled within 48 hr; exposure to heat or phosphorous insecticides; pregnancy; lactation; children younger than 12 yr
- **Physical:** Weight; T; reflexes, orientation, intraocular pressure; P, BP, orthostatic BP; R, adventitious sounds; bowel sounds and normal output; liver evaluation; urinary output, prostate size; CBC; urinalysis; thyroid, liver, and kidney function tests

Interventions

- Do not change brand names of oral preparations; bioavailability differences have been documented.
- Do not allow patient to crush or chew sustained-release capsules.
- Do not administer SC because of local irritation.
- Give IM injections deeply into the upper outer quadrant of the buttock.
- Avoid skin contact with oral solution; contact dermatitis has occurred.
- Discontinue drug if serum creatinine, BUN become abnormal or if WBC count is depressed.
- Monitor elderly patients for dehydration, and institute remedial measures promptly; sedation and decreased sensation of thirst related to CNS effects of drug can lead to severe dehydration.
- Consult physician regarding appropriate warning of patient or patient's guardian about tardive dyskinesias.
- Consult physician about dosage reduction, use of anticholinergic antiparkinsonian

drugs (controversial) if extrapyramidal effects occur.

Teaching points
- Take drug exactly as prescribed.
- Do not crush or chew sustained-release capsules.
- Avoid skin contact with drug solutions.
- Avoid driving or engaging in other dangerous activities if CNS, vision changes occur.
- Avoid prolonged exposure to sun, or use a sunscreen or covering garments.
- Maintain fluid intake, and use precautions against heatstroke in hot weather.
- Report sore throat, fever, unusual bleeding or bruising, rash, weakness, tremors, impaired vision, dark urine (expect pink or reddish-brown urine), pale stools, yellowing of the skin or eyes.

▽ procyclidine
(proe sye' kli deen)

Kemadrin, PMS Procyclidine (CAN), Procyclid (CAN)

PREGNANCY CATEGORY C

Drug class
Antiparkinsonian drug (anticholinergic type)

Therapeutic actions
Has anticholinergic activity in the CNS that is believed to help normalize the hypothesized imbalance of cholinergic/dopaminergic neurotransmission created by the loss of dopaminergic neurons in the basal ganglia of the brain in parkinsonism; reduces severity of rigidity and reduces the akinesia and tremor that characterize parkinsonism; less effective overall than levodopa; peripheral anticholinergic effects suppress secondary symptoms of parkinsonism, such as drooling.

Indications
- Treatment of parkinsonism (postencephalitic, arteriosclerotic, and idiopathic types), alone or with other drugs in more severe cases
- Relief of symptoms of extrapyramidal dysfunction that accompany phenothiazine and reserpine therapy

- Control of sialorrhea resulting from neuroleptic medication

Contraindications and cautions
- Contraindicated with hypersensitivity to procyclidine; glaucoma, especially angle-closure glaucoma; pyloric or duodenal obstruction; stenosing peptic ulcers; achalasia (megaesophagus); prostatic hypertrophy or bladder neck obstructions; myasthenia gravis; lactation.
- Use cautiously with tachycardia, cardiac arrhythmias, hypertension, hypotension, hepatic or renal dysfunction, alcoholism, chronic illness, people who work in hot environments, pregnancy.

Available forms
Tablets—5 mg

Dosages
Adults
- *Parkinsonism not previously treated:* Initially 2.5 mg PO tid after meals. If well tolerated, gradually increase dose to 5 mg tid and as needed before retiring.
- *Transferring from other therapy:* Substitute 2.5 mg PO tid for all or part of the original drug, then increase procyclidine while withdrawing other drug.
- *Drug-induced extrapyramidal symptoms:* Initially 2.5 mg PO tid. Increase by 2.5-mg increments until symptomatic relief is obtained. In most cases, results will be obtained with 10–20 mg/day.
Pediatric patients
Safety and efficacy not established.
Geriatric patients
Strict dosage regulation may be necessary. Patients older than 60 yr often develop increased sensitivity to the CNS effects of anticholinergic drugs.

Pharmacokinetics

Route	Onset	Peak
Oral	Varies	1.1–2 hr

Metabolism: Hepatic; $T_{1/2}$: 11.5–12.6 hr
Distribution: Crosses placenta; enters breast milk
Excretion: Urine

Adverse effects
Peripheral anticholinergic effects
- **CNS:** *Blurred vision, mydriasis,* diplopia, increased intraocular tension, angle-closure glaucoma
- **CV:** Tachycardia, palpitations
- **GI:** *Dry mouth, constipation,* dilation of the colon, paralytic ileus
- **GU:** *Urinary retention,* urinary hesitancy, dysuria, difficulty achieving or maintaining an erection
- **Other:** *Flushing, decreased sweating,* elevated temperature

Other effects
- **CNS (some of these are characteristic of centrally acting anticholinergic drugs):** *Disorientation, confusion,* memory loss, hallucinations, psychoses, agitation, nervousness, delusions, delirium, paranoia, euphoria, excitement, *light-headedness, dizziness,* depression, drowsiness, weakness, giddiness, paresthesia, heaviness of the limbs, numbness of fingers
- **CV:** Hypotension, orthostatic hypotension
- **Dermatologic:** Rash, urticaria, other dermatoses
- **GI:** Acute suppurative parotitis, nausea, vomiting, epigastric distress
- **Other:** Muscular weakness, muscular cramping

Interactions
✴ **Drug-drug** ● Paralytic ileus, sometimes fatal, with phenothiazines ● Additive adverse CNS effects, toxic psychosis, with other drugs that have central (CNS) anticholinergic properties, phenothiazines ● Possible masking of the development of persistent extrapyramidal symptoms, tardive dyskinesia, in long-term therapy with phenothiazines, haloperidol ● Decreased therapeutic efficacy of phenothiazines and haloperidol, possibly due to central antagonism

■ Nursing considerations
Assessment
- **History:** Hypersensitivity to procyclidine; glaucoma; pyloric or duodenal obstruction; stenosing peptic ulcers; achalasia; prostatic hypertrophy or bladder neck obstructions; myasthenia gravis; cardiac arrhythmias; hypertension, hypotension; hepatic or renal dysfunction; alcoholism; chronic illness; people who work in hot environments; pregnancy; lactation
- **Physical:** Weight; T; skin color, lesions; orientation, affect, reflexes, bilateral grip strength; visual exam including tonometry; P, BP, orthostatic BP, auscultation; bowel sounds, normal output, liver evaluation; urinary output, voiding pattern, prostate palpation; liver and kidney function tests

Interventions
- Decrease dosage or discontinue drug temporarily if dry mouth is so severe that swallowing or speaking becomes difficult.
- Give with caution, and reduce dosage in hot weather; drug interferes with sweating and ability of body to maintain body heat equilibrium; anhidrosis and fatal hyperthermia have occurred.
- Give with meals if GI upset occurs; give before meals to patients bothered by dry mouth; give after meals if drooling is a problem or if drug causes nausea.
- Have patient void before receiving each dose if urinary retention is a problem.

Teaching points
- Take this drug exactly as prescribed.
- These side effects may occur: drowsiness, dizziness, confusion, blurred vision (avoid driving or engaging in activities that require alertness and visual acuity); nausea (eat frequent, small meals); dry mouth (suck sugarless lozenges or ice chips); painful or difficult urination (empty the bladder immediately before each dose); constipation (if maintaining adequate fluid intake, exercising regularly do not help, consult your nurse or physician); use caution in hot weather (you are more susceptible to heat prostration).
- Report difficult or painful urination, constipation, rapid or pounding heartbeat, confusion, eye pain, or rash.

▽progesterone

(proe jess' ter own)

progesterone in oil (parenteral):
Progestilin (CAN)

progesterone aqueous

progesterone powder

progesterone, micronized:
Prometrium

PREGNANCY CATEGORY X

Drug classes

Hormone
Progestin

Therapeutic actions

Endogenous female progestational substance; transforms proliferative endometrium into secretory endometrium; inhibits the secretion of pituitary gonadotropins, which prevents follicular maturation and ovulation; inhibits spontaneous uterine contractions; may have some estrogenic, anabolic, or androgenic activity.

Indications

- Treatment of primary and secondary amenorrhea
- Treatment of functional uterine bleeding
- Contraception in parous and nulliparous women (intrauterine system)
- Infertility, as part of assisted reproductive technology for infertile women (gel)
- Unlabeled uses: treatment of premenstrual syndrome, prevention of premature labor and habitual abortion in the first trimester, treatment of menorrhagia (intrauterine system)

Contraindications and cautions

- Contraindicated with allergy to progestins, thrombophlebitis, thromboembolic disorders, cerebral hemorrhage or history of these conditions, hepatic disease, carcinoma of the breast or genital organs, undiagnosed vaginal bleeding, missed abortion, diagnostic test for pregnancy, pregnancy (fetal abnormalities, including masculinization of the female fetus have occurred), lactation; PID, venereal disease, postpartum endometritis,

pelvic surgery, uterine or cervical carcinoma (intrauterine system).
- Use cautiously with epilepsy, migraine, asthma, cardiac or renal dysfunction.

Available forms

Injection—50 mg/mL; powder—1, 10, 25, 100, 1,000 g; vaginal gel—45 mg (4%), 90 mg (8%); capsules—100 mg

Dosages

Administer parenteral preparation by IM route only.

Adults

- *Amenorrhea:* 5–10 mg/day IM for 6–8 consecutive days. Expect withdrawal bleeding 48–72 hr after the last injection. Or use 400 mg PO in the evening for 10 days. Spontaneous normal cycles may follow.
- *Functional uterine bleeding:* 5–10 mg/day IM for six doses. Bleeding should cease within 6 days. If estrogen is being given, begin progesterone after 2 wk of estrogen therapy. Discontinue injections when menstrual flow begins.
- *Contraception:* Insert a single intrauterine system into the uterine cavity. Contraceptive effectiveness is retained for 1 yr. The system must be replaced 1 yr after insertion.
- *Infertility:* 90 mg vaginally daily in women requiring progesterone supplementation; 90 mg vaginally bid for replacement—continue for 10–12 wk into pregnancy if it occurs.

Pharmacokinetics

Route	Onset	Peak	Duration
Oral	Varies	3 hr	Unknown
IM	Varies	Unknown	Unknown
Vaginal gel	Slow	Unknown	25–50 hr

Metabolism: Hepatic; $T_{1/2}$: 5 min
Distribution: Crosses placenta; enters breast milk
Excretion: Urine

Adverse effects
Parenteral and oral

- **CNS:** Sudden, partial, or complete loss of vision, proptosis, diplopia, migraine, precipitation of acute intermittent porphyria, mental depression, pyrexia, insomnia, somnolence, *dizziness*

- **CV:** Thrombophlebitis, cerebrovascular disorders, retinal thrombosis, **pulmonary embolism**
- **Dermatologic:** Rash with or without pruritus, acne, melasma or chloasma, alopecia, hirsutism, *photosensitivity*
- **GI:** Cholestatic jaundice, nausea
- **GU:** *Breakthrough bleeding, spotting, change in menstrual flow, amenorrhea, changes in cervical erosion and cervical secretions, breast tenderness* and secretion, transient increase in sodium and chloride excretion
- **Other:** Fluid retention, edema, *change in weight,* effects similar to those seen with oral contraceptives

Oral contraceptives
- **CV:** Increased BP, **thromboembolic and thrombotic disease**
- **Endocrine:** Decreased glucose tolerance
- **GI:** Hepatic adenoma

Intrauterine system
- **CV:** Bradycardia and syncope related to insertional pain
- **GU:** Endometritis, spontaneous abortion, septic abortion, septicemia, perforation of the uterus and cervix, pelvic infection, cervical erosion, vaginitis, leukorrhea, amenorrhea, uterine embedment, *complete or partial expulsion of the device*

Vaginal gel
- **CNS:** *Somnolence, headache,* nervousness, depression
- **GI:** *Constipation,* nausea, diarrhea
- **Other:** *Breast enlargement,* nocturia, perineal pain

Interactions

✳ **Drug-lab test** ● Inaccurate tests of hepatic and endocrine function

✳ **Drug-food** ● Decreased metabolism and risk of toxic effects if combined with grapefruit juice; avoid this combination

■ Nursing considerations
Assessment

- **History:** Allergy to progestins, thrombophlebitis, thromboembolic disorders, cerebral hemorrhage, hepatic disease, carcinoma of the breast or genital organs, undiagnosed vaginal bleeding, missed abortion, epilepsy, migraine, asthma, cardiac or renal dysfunction, PID, venereal disease, postpartum endometritis, pelvic surgery, uterine or cervical carcinoma, pregnancy, lactation
- **Physical:** Skin color, lesions, turgor; hair; breasts; pelvic exam; orientation, affect; ophthalmologic exam; P, auscultation, peripheral perfusion, edema; R, adventitious sounds; liver evaluation; liver and renal function tests, glucose tolerance; Pap smear

Interventions

- Arrange for pretreatment and periodic (at least annual) history and physical, including BP, breasts, abdomen, pelvic organs, and a Pap smear.
- Arrange for insertion of intrauterine system during or immediately after menstrual period to ensure that the patient is not pregnant; arrange to have patient reexamined after first month menses to ensure that system has not been expelled.
- Caution patient before therapy of the need to prevent pregnancy during treatment and to obtain frequent medical follow-up.
- Administer parenteral preparations by IM injection only.
- Discontinue medication and consult physician if sudden partial or complete loss of vision occurs; discontinue if papilledema or retinal vascular lesions are present on exam.
- Discontinue medication and consult physician at the first sign of thromboembolic disease: leg pain, swelling, peripheral perfusion changes, shortness of breath.

Teaching points

- This drug can be given IM; it will be given daily for the specified number of days, or inserted vaginally and can remain for 1 yr (as appropriate), or inserted vaginally using the applicator system 1 to 2 times per day; or given orally for 10 days.
- If used for fertility program, continue vaginal gel 10–12 wk into pregnancy until placental autonomy is achieved.
- Do not drink grapefruit juice while on this drug.
- These side effects may occur: sensitivity to light (avoid exposure to the sun; use sunscreen and protective clothing); dizziness,

sleeplessness, depression (use caution if driving or performing tasks that require alertness); rash, skin color changes, loss of hair; fever; nausea.

- This drug should not be taken during pregnancy (except vaginal gel); serious fetal abnormalities have been reported. If you may be pregnant, consult physician immediately.
- Perform a monthly breast self-exam while on this drug.
- Report pain or swelling and warmth in the calves, acute chest pain or shortness of breath, sudden severe headache or vomiting, dizziness or fainting, visual disturbances, numbness or tingling in the arm or leg.

Intrauterine system
- Report excessive bleeding, severe cramping, abnormal vaginal discharge, fever or flulike symptoms.

Vaginal gel
- Report severe headache, abnormal vaginal bleeding or discharge, acute calf or chest pain, fever.

▽ promethazine hydrochloride
(proe **meth'** a zeen)

Anergan, Phenergan, PMS-Promethazine (CAN)

PREGNANCY CATEGORY C

Drug classes
Phenothiazine
Dopaminergic blocking agent
Antihistamine
Antiemetic
Anti-motion sickness agent
Sedative or hypnotic

Therapeutic actions
Selectively blocks H_1 receptors, diminishing the effects of histamine on cells of the upper respiratory tract and eyes and decreasing the sneezing, mucus production, itching, and tearing that accompany allergic reactions in sensitized people exposed to antigens; blocks cholinergic receptors in the vomiting center that are believed to mediate the nausea and vomiting caused by gastric irritation, by input

from the vestibular apparatus (motion sickness, nausea associated with vestibular neuritis), and by input from the chemoreceptor trigger zone (drug- and radiation-induced emesis); depresses the RAS, including the parts of the brain involved with wakefulness.

Indications
- Symptomatic relief of perennial and seasonal allergic rhinitis, vasomotor rhinitis, allergic conjunctivitis; mild, uncomplicated urticaria and angioedema; amelioration of allergic reactions to blood or plasma; dermatographism, adjunctive therapy (with epinephrine and other measures) in anaphylactic reactions
- Treatment and prevention of motion sickness; prevention and control of nausea and vomiting associated with anesthesia and surgery
- Preoperative, postoperative, or obstetric sedation
- Adjunct to analgesics to control postoperative pain
- Adjunctive IV therapy with reduced amounts of meperidine or other narcotic analgesics in special surgical situations, such as repeated bronchoscopy, ophthalmic surgery, or in poor-risk patients

Contraindications and cautions
- Contraindicated with hypersensitivity to antihistamines or phenothiazines, coma or severe CNS depression, bone marrow depression, vomiting of unknown cause, concomitant therapy with MAOIs, lactation (lactation may be inhibited).
- Use cautiously with lower respiratory tract disorders (may cause thickening of secretions and impair expectoration), glaucoma, prostatic hypertrophy, CV disease or hypertension, breast cancer, thyrotoxicosis, pregnancy (jaundice and extrapyramidal effects in infants; drug may inhibit platelet aggregation in neonate if taken by mother within 2 wk of delivery), children (antihistamine overdose may cause hallucinations, convulsions, and death), a child with a history of sleep apnea, a family history of SIDS, or Reye's syndrome (may mask the symptoms of Reye's syndrome and contribute to its development), the elderly (more likely to cause dizziness, sedation, syncope, toxic confu-

sional states, hypotension, and extrapyramidal effects).

Available forms
Tablets—12.5, 25, 50 mg; syrup—6.25, 25 mg/5 mL; suppositories—12.5, 25, 50 mg; injection—25, 50 mg/mL

Dosages
Adults
- *Allergy:* Average dose is 25 mg PO or by rectal suppository, preferably hs. If necessary, 12.5 mg PO before meals and hs; 25 mg IM or IV for serious reactions. May repeat within 2 hr if necessary.
- *Motion sickness:* 25 mg PO bid. Initial dose should be scheduled 30–60 min before travel; repeat in 8–12 hr if necessary. Thereafter, give 25 mg on arising and before evening meal.
- *Nausea and vomiting:* 25 mg PO; repeat doses of 12.5–25 mg as needed, q 4–6 hr. Give rectally or parenterally if oral dosage is not tolerated. 12.5–25 mg IM or IV, not to be repeated more frequently than q 4–6 hr.
- *Sedation:* 25–50 mg PO, IM, or IV.
- *Preoperative use:* 50 mg PO the night before, or 50 mg with an equal dose of meperidine and the required amount of belladonna alkaloid.
- *Postoperative sedation and adjunctive use with analgesics:* 25–50 mg PO, IM, or IV.
- *Labor:* 50 mg IM or IV in early stages. When labor is established, 25–75 mg with a reduced dose of narcotic. May repeat once or twice at 4-hr intervals. Maximum dose within 24 hr is 100 mg.

Pediatric patients > 2 yr
- *Allergy:* 25 mg PO hs or 6.25–12.5 mg tid.
- *Motion sickness:* 12.5–25 mg PO or rectally bid.
- *Nausea and vomiting:* 1 mg/kg IM q 4–6 hr as needed.
- *Sedation:* 12.5–25 mg PO; 0.25–0.5 mg/kg rectally q 4–6 hr.
- *Preoperative use:* 1 mg/kg PO in combination with an equal dose of meperidine and the required amount of an atropine-like drug.
- *Postoperative sedation and adjunctive use with analgesics:* 1 mg/kg PO, IM, IV or rectally.

Pharmacokinetics

Route	Onset	Duration
Oral	20 min	12 hr
IM	20 min	12 hr
IV	3–5 min	12 hr

Metabolism: Hepatic; $T_{1/2}$: unknown
Distribution: Crosses placenta; enters breast milk
Excretion: Urine

▼IV facts
Preparation: Dilute to a concentration no greater than 25 mg/mL.
Infusion: Infuse no faster than 25 mg/min.
Incompatibilities: Do not combine with aminophylline, chloramphenicol, heparin, hydrocortisone, methicillin, pentobarbital, thiopental.
Y-site incompatibilities: Do not give with cefoperazone, foscarnet, heparin, hydrocortisone, potassium chloride.

Adverse effects
- **CNS:** *Dizziness, drowsiness, poor coordination, confusion, restlessness, excitation,* convulsions, tremors, headache, blurred vision, diplopia, vertigo, tinnitus
- **CV:** Hypotension, palpitations, bradycardia, tachycardia, extrasystoles
- **Dermatologic:** Urticaria, rash, photosensitivity, chills
- **GI:** *Epigastric distress,* nausea, vomiting, diarrhea, constipation
- **GU:** *Urinary frequency, dysuria,* urinary retention, decreased libido, impotence
- **Hematologic:** Hemolytic anemia, hypoplastic anemia, thrombocytopenia, leukopenia, **agranulocytosis, pancytopenia**
- **Respiratory:** *Thickening of bronchial secretions;* chest tightness; dry mouth, nose, and throat; respiratory depression; suppression of cough reflex, potential for aspiration
- **Other:** Tingling, heaviness and wetness of the hands

Interactions
- Additive anticholinergic effects with anticholinergic drugs ● Increased frequency and severity of neuromuscular excitation and hypotension with methohexital, thiamylal,

phenobarbital anesthetic, thiopental • Enhanced CNS depression with alcohol

■ Nursing considerations
Assessment
- **History:** Hypersensitivity to antihistamines or phenothiazines, severe CNS depression, bone marrow depression, vomiting of unknown cause, concomitant therapy with MAO inhibitors, lactation, lower respiratory tract disorders, glaucoma, prostatic hypertrophy, CV disease or hypertension, breast cancer, thyrotoxicosis, pregnancy, history of sleep apnea or a family history of SIDS, child with Reye's syndrome
- **Physical:** Weight; T; reflexes, orientation, intraocular pressure; P, BP, orthostatic BP; R, adventitious sounds; bowel sounds and normal output, liver evaluation; urinary output, prostate size; CBC; urinalysis; thyroid, liver, and kidney function tests

Interventions
- Do not give tablets, rectal suppositories to children < 2 yr.
- Give IM injections deep into muscle.
- Do not administer SC; tissue necrosis may occur.
- Do not administer intra-arterially; arteriospasm and gangrene of the limb may result.
- Reduce dosage of barbiturates given concurrently with promethazine by at least half; arrange for dosage reduction of narcotic analgesics given concomitantly by one-fourth to one-half.

Teaching points
- Take drug exactly as prescribed.
- Avoid using alcohol.
- Avoid driving or engaging in other dangerous activities if CNS, vision changes occur.
- Avoid prolonged exposure to sun, or use a sunscreen or covering garments.
- Maintain fluid intake, and use precautions against heat stroke in hot weather.
- Report sore throat, fever, unusual bleeding or bruising, rash, weakness, tremors, impaired vision, dark urine, pale stools, yellowing of the skin or eyes.

▽propafenone hydrochloride
(proe paf' a non)

Rythmol

PREGNANCY CATEGORY C

Drug class
Antiarrhythmic

Therapeutic actions
Class 1C antiarrhythmic: local anesthetic effects with a direct membrane stabilizing action on the myocardial membranes; refractory period is prolonged with a reduction of spontaneous automaticity and depressed trigger activity.

Indications
- Treatment of documented life-threatening ventricular arrhythmias; reserve use for those patients in whom the benefits outweigh the risks
- Unlabeled uses: treatment of supraventricular tachycardias, including atrial fibrillation associated with Wolff-Parkinson-White syndrome

Contraindications and cautions
- Contraindicated with hypersensitivity to propafenone, uncontrolled CHF, cardiogenic shock, cardiac conduction disturbances in the absence of an artificial pacemaker, bradycardia, marked hypotension, bronchospastic disorders, manifest electrolyte imbalance, pregnancy (teratogenic in preclinical studies), lactation.
- Use cautiously with hepatic, renal dysfunction.

Available forms
Tablets—150, 225, 300 mg

Dosages
Adults
Adjust on the basis of response and tolerance. Initiate with 150 mg PO q 8 hr (450 mg/day). Dosage may be increased at a minimum of 3- to 4-day intervals to 225 mg PO q 8 hr (675 mg/day) and if necessary, to 300 mg PO q 8 hr (900 mg/day). Do not exceed 900 mg/day.

Decrease dosage with significant widening of the QRS complex or with AV block.

Pediatric patients
Safety and efficacy not established.

Geriatric patients
Use with caution; increase dose more gradually during the initial phase of treatment.

Pharmacokinetics

Route	onset	Peak
Oral	Varies	3.5 hr

Metabolism: Hepatic; $T_{1/2}$: 2–10 hr
Distribution: Crosses placenta; enters breast milk
Excretion: Urine

Adverse effects

- **CNS:** *Dizziness, headache, weakness, blurred vision,* abnormal dreams, speech or vision disturbances, coma, confusion, depression, memory loss, numbness, paresthesias, psychosis/mania, seizures, tinnitus, vertigo
- **CV:** *First-degree AV block, intraventricular conduction disturbances,* CHF, atrial flutter, AV dissociation, **cardiac arrest,** sick sinus syndrome, sinus pause, sinus arrest, supraventricular tachycardia
- **Dermatologic:** Alopecia, pruritus
- **GI:** *Unusual taste, nausea, vomiting, constipation,* dyspepsia, cholestasis, gastroenteritis, hepatitis
- **Hematologic:** Agranulocytosis, anemia, granulocytopenia, leukopenia, purpura, thrombocytopenia, positive ANA
- **Musculoskeletal:** Muscle weakness, leg cramps, muscle pain

Interactions

✴ Drug-drug • Increased serum levels of propafenone and risk of increased toxicity with quinidine, cimetidine, beta-blockers • Increased serum levels of digoxin, warfarin

■ Nursing considerations
Assessment

- **History:** Hypersensitivity to propafenone, uncontrolled CHF, cardiogenic shock, cardiac conduction disturbances in the absence of an artificial pacemaker, bradycardia, marked hypotension, bronchospastic disorders, manifest electrolyte imbalance, hepatic or renal dysfunction, pregnancy, lactation
- **Physical:** Reflexes; affect; BP, P, ECG, peripheral perfusion, auscultation; abdomen, normal function; renal and liver function tests; CBC, Hct, electrolytes; ANA

Interventions

- Monitor patient response carefully, especially when beginning therapy. Increase dosage at minimum of 3- to 4-day intervals only.
- Reduce dosage with renal or liver dysfunction and with marked previous myocardial damage.
- Increase dosage slowly in patients with renal, liver, or myocardial dysfunction.
- Arrange for periodic ECG monitoring to monitor effects on cardiac conduction.

Teaching points

- Take the drug every 8 hr around the clock; determine with nurse a schedule that will interrupt sleep the least.
- Frequent monitoring of ECG will be necessary to adjust dosage or determine effects of drug on cardiac conduction.
- These side effects may occur: dizziness, headache (avoid driving or performing hazardous tasks); headache, weakness (request medications; rest periods may help); nausea, vomiting, unusual taste (maintain proper nutrition; take drug with meals); constipation.
- Do not stop taking this drug for any reason without checking with your health care provider.
- Avoid pregnancy while on this drug; use of barrier contraceptives is advised.
- Report swelling of the extremities, difficulty breathing, fainting, palpitations, vision changes, chest pain.

▽ propantheline bromide

*(proe **pan'** the leen)*

Pro-Banthine, Propanthel (CAN)

PREGNANCY CATEGORY C

Adverse effects in *Italics* are most common; those in **Bold** are life-threatening.

Drug classes
Anticholinergic
Antimuscarinic agent
Parasympatholytic
Antispasmodic

Therapeutic actions
Competitively blocks the effects of acetylcholine at muscarinic cholinergic receptors that mediate the effects of parasympathetic postganglionic impulses, relaxing the GI tract and inhibiting gastric acid secretion.

Indications
- Adjunctive therapy in the treatment of peptic ulcer
- Unlabeled uses: antisecretory and antispasmodic

Contraindications and cautions
- Contraindicated with glaucoma, adhesions between iris and lens, stenosing peptic ulcer, pyloroduodenal obstruction, paralytic ileus, intestinal atony, severe ulcerative colitis, toxic megacolon, symptomatic prostatic hypertrophy, bladder neck obstruction, bronchial asthma, COPD, cardiac arrhythmias, tachycardia, myocardial ischemia, sensitivity to anticholinergic drugs or bromides, impaired metabolic, liver or kidney function, myasthenia gravis, lactation.
- Use cautiously with pregnancy, Down syndrome, brain damage, spasticity, hypertension, hyperthyroidism.

Available forms
Tablets—7.5, 15 mg

Dosages
Adults
15 mg PO 30 min before meals and hs.
- *Mild symptoms or person of small stature:* 7.5 mg PO tid.
Pediatric patients
- *Peptic ulcer:* Safety and efficacy not established.
- *Antisecretory:* 1.5 mg/kg/day PO divided into doses tid–qid.
- *Antispasmodic:* 2–3 mg/kg/day PO in divided doses q 4–6 hr and hs.
Geriatric patients
7.5 mg PO tid.

Pharmacokinetics

Route	Onset	Peak	Duration
Oral	30–60 min	2–6 hr	6 hr

Metabolism: Hepatic; $T_{1/2}$: 3–4 hr
Distribution: Crosses placenta; enters breast milk
Excretion: Urine

Adverse effects
- **CNS:** *Blurred vision,* mydriasis, cycloplegia, photophobia, increased intraocular pressure
- **CV:** Palpitations, tachycardia
- **GI:** *Dry mouth, altered taste perception, nausea, vomiting, dysphagia,* heartburn, constipation, bloated feeling, paralytic ileus, gastroesophageal reflux
- **GU:** *Urinary hesitancy and retention;* impotence
- **Local:** *Irritation at site of IM injection*
- **Other:** Decreased sweating and predisposition to heat prostration, suppression of lactation, nasal congestion

Interactions
✳ **Drug-drug** • Decreased antipsychotic effectiveness of haloperidol • Decreased pharmacologic/therapeutic effects of phenothiazines

■ Nursing considerations
Assessment
- **History:** Adhesions between iris and lens, stenosing peptic ulcer, pyloroduodenal obstruction, intestinal atony, severe ulcerative colitis, symptomatic prostatic hypertrophy, bladder neck obstruction, bronchial asthma, COPD, cardiac arrhythmias, myocardial ischemia, sensitivity to anticholinergic drugs; bromides, impaired metabolic, liver or kidney function, myasthenia gravis, lactation, Down syndrome, brain damage, spasticity, hypertension, hyperthyroidism, pregnancy, lactation
- **Physical:** Bowel sounds, normal output; urinary output, prostate palpation; R, adventitious sounds; pulse, BP; intraocular pressure, vision exam; bilateral grip strength, reflexes; liver palpation, liver and renal function tests

Interventions

- Ensure adequate hydration; provide environmental control (temperature) to prevent hyperpyrexia.
- Have patient void before each dose of medication if urinary retention becomes a problem.

Teaching points

- Take drug exactly as prescribed.
- Avoid hot environments (you will be heat intolerant, and dangerous reactions may occur).
- These side effects may occur: constipation (ensure adequate fluid intake, proper diet); dry mouth (sugarless lozenges, frequent mouth care may help; may lessen); blurred vision, sensitivity to light (reversible; avoid tasks that require acute vision; wear sunglasses when in bright light); impotence (reversible); difficulty urinating (empty the bladder immediately before taking drug).
- Report skin rash, flushing, eye pain, difficulty breathing, tremors, loss of coordination, irregular heartbeat, palpitations, headache, abdominal distention, hallucinations, severe or persistent dry mouth, difficulty swallowing, difficulty in urination, severe constipation, sensitivity to light.

▽ **propoxyphene**

(proe **pox***' i feen)*

propoxyphene hydrochloride (dextropropoxyphene)
Darvon, Novo-Propoxyn (CAN)

propoxyphene napsylate
Darvocet-N, Darvon-N

PREGNANCY CATEGORY C

C-IV CONTROLLED SUBSTANCE

Drug class

Narcotic agonist analgesic

Therapeutic actions

Acts as agonist at specific opioid receptors in the CNS to produce analgesia, euphoria, sedation; the receptors mediating these effects are thought to be the same as those mediating the effects of endogenous opioids (enkephalins, endorphins).

Indications

- Relief of mild to moderate pain

Contraindications and cautions

- Contraindicated with hypersensitivity to narcotics, pregnancy (neonatal withdrawal has occurred; neonatal safety not established), labor or delivery (especially when delivery of a premature infant is expected; narcotics given to mother can cause respiratory depression of neonate; may prolong labor), lactation.
- Use cautiously with renal or hepatic dysfunction, emotional depression.

Available forms

Capsules—65 mg; tablets—100 mg

Dosages
Adults
propoxyphene hydrochloride
65 mg PO q 4 hr as needed. Do not exceed 390 mg/day.
propoxyphene napsylate
100 mg PO q 4 hr as needed. Do not exceed 600 mg/day.
Pediatric patients
Not recommended.
Geriatric patients or impaired adults
Use caution; reduced dosage may be necessary.

Pharmacokinetics

Route	Onset	Peak
Oral	Varies	2–2.5 hr

Metabolism: Hepatic; $T_{1/2}$: 6–12 hr
Distribution: Crosses placenta; enters breast milk
Excretion: Urine

Adverse effects
- **CNS:** *Dizziness, sedation,* light-headedness, headache, weakness, euphoria, dysphoria, minor visual disturbances
- **Dermatologic:** Rashes
- **GI:** *Nausea, vomiting,* constipation, abdominal pain, liver dysfunction
- **Other:** Tolerance and dependence, psychological dependence

Interactions
✱ **Drug-drug** • Increased likelihood of respiratory depression, hypotension, profound sedation, or coma with barbiturate general anesthetics • Increased serum levels and toxicity of carbamazepine • Decreased absorption and serum levels with charcoal

■ Nursing considerations
Assessment
- **History:** Hypersensitivity to narcotics, pregnancy, lactation, renal or hepatic dysfunction, emotional depression
- **Physical:** Skin color, texture, lesions; orientation, reflexes, affect; bowel sounds, normal output; liver, kidney function tests

Interventions
- Administer to lactating women 4–6 hr before the next feeding to minimize the amount in milk.
- Limit amount of drug dispensed to depressed, emotionally labile, or potentially suicidal patients; propoxyphene intake alone or with other CNS depressants has been associated with deaths.
- Provide narcotic antagonist, facilities for assisted or controlled respiration on standby in case respiratory depression occurs.
- Give drug with milk or food if GI upset occurs.
- Reassure patient about addiction liability; most patients who receive opiates for medical reasons do not develop dependence syndromes.

Teaching points
- Take drug exactly as prescribed.
- These side effects may occur: nausea, loss of appetite (take drug with food, eat frequent, small meals); constipation (request laxative); dizziness, sedation, drowsiness, impaired visual acuity (avoid driving or performing other tasks that require alertness, visual acuity).
- Do not take leftover medication for other disorders, and do not let anyone else take the prescription.
- Report severe nausea, vomiting, constipation, shortness of breath or difficulty breathing.

▷ propranolol hydrochloride
*(proe **pran'** oh lole)*

Apo-Propranolol (CAN), Inderal, Inderal LA, Novopranol (CAN), PMS-Propranolol (CAN)

PREGNANCY CATEGORY C

Drug classes
Beta-adrenergic blocker (nonselective)
Antianginal agent
Antiarrhythmic
Antihypertensive

Therapeutic actions
Competitively blocks beta-adrenergic receptors in the heart and juxtaglomerular apparatus, decreasing the influence of the sympathetic nervous system on these tissues, the excitability of the heart, cardiac workload and oxygen consumption, and the release of renin and lowering BP; has membrane-stabilizing (local anesthetic) effects that contribute to its antiarrhythmic action; acts in the CNS to reduce sympathetic outflow and vasoconstrictor tone. The mechanism by which it prevents migraine headaches is unknown.

Indications
- Hypertension alone or with other drugs, especially diuretics
- Angina pectoris caused by coronary atherosclerosis
- IHSS to manage associated stress-induced angina, palpitations, and syncope
- Cardiac arrhythmias, especially supraventricular tachycardia, and ventricular tachycardias induced by digitalis or catecholamines

- Prevention of reinfarction in clinically stable patients 1–4 wk after MI
- Pheochromocytoma, an adjunctive therapy after treatment with an alpha-adrenergic blocker to manage tachycardia before or during surgery or if the pheochromocytoma is inoperable
- Prophylaxis for migraine headache
- Management of acute situational stress reaction (stage fright)
- Treatment of essential tremor, familial or hereditary
- Unlabeled uses: recurrent GI bleeding in cirrhotic patients, schizophrenia, tardive dyskinesia, acute panic symptoms, vaginal contraceptive

Contraindications and cautions

- Contraindicated with allergy to beta-blocking agents, sinus bradycardia, second- or third-degree heart block, cardiogenic shock, CHF, bronchial asthma, bronchospasm, COPD, pregnancy (neonatal bradycardia, hypoglycemia, and apnea, and low birth weight with long-term use during pregnancy), lactation.
- Use cautiously with hypoglycemia and diabetes, thyrotoxicosis, hepatic dysfunction.

Available forms

ER capsules—60, 80, 120, 160 mg; tablets—10, 20, 40, 60, 80, 90 mg; SR capsules—60, 80, 120, 160 mg; injection—1 mg/mL; oral solution—4, 8 mg/mL; concentrated oral solution—80 mg/mL

Dosages
Adults
Oral

- *Hypertension:* 40 mg regular propranolol bid or 80 mg sustained-release (SR) daily initially; usual maintenance dose, 120–240 mg/day given bid or tid or 120–160 mg SR daily (maximum dose, 640 mg/day).
- *Angina:* 10–20 mg tid or qid or 80 mg SR daily initially; gradually increase dosage at 3- to 7-day intervals; usual maintenance dose, 160 mg/day (maximum dose, 320 mg/day).
- *IHSS:* 20–40 mg tid or qid or 80–160 mg SR daily.
- *Arrhythmias:* 10–30 mg tid or qid.

- *MI:* 180–240 mg/day given tid or qid (maximum dose, 240 mg/day).
- *Pheochromocytoma:* Preoperatively, 60 mg/day for 3 days in divided doses; inoperable tumor, 30 mg/day in divided doses.
- *Migraine:* 80 mg/day daily (SR) or in divided doses; usual maintenance dose, 160–240 mg/day.
- *Essential tremor:* 40 mg bid; usual maintenance dose, 120 mg/day.
- *Situational anxiety:* 40 mg, timing based on the usual onset of action.

Parenteral

- *Life-threatening arrhythmias:* 1–3 mg IV with careful monitoring, not to exceed 1 mg/min; may give second dose in 2 min, but then do not repeat for 4 hr. (Note: IV dose is markedly less than oral because of first-pass effect with oral propranolol).

Pediatric patients

Safety and efficacy not established.

Pharmacokinetics

Route	Onset	Peak	Duration
Oral	20–30 min	60–90 min	6–12 hr
IV	Immediate	1 min	4–6 hr

Metabolism: Hepatic; $T_{1/2}$: 3–5 hr
Distribution: Crosses placenta; enters breast milk
Excretion: Urine

▼ IV facts

Preparation: No further preparation is needed.
Infusion: Inject directly IV or into tubing of running IV; do not exceed 1 mg/min.

Adverse effects

- **Allergic reactions:** Pharyngitis, erythematous rash, fever, sore throat, laryngospasm, respiratory distress
- **CNS:** Dizziness, vertigo, tinnitus, *fatigue*, emotional depression, paresthesias, sleep disturbances, hallucinations, disorientation, memory loss, slurred speech
- **CV:** *Bradycardia, CHF, cardiac arrhythmias, sinoatrial or AV nodal block,* peripheral vascular insufficiency, claudication, **CVA, pulmonary edema,** hypotension

---

Adverse effects in *Italics* are most common; those in **Bold** are life-threatening.

- **Dermatologic:** Rash, pruritus, sweating, dry skin
- **EENT:** Eye irritation, dry eyes, conjunctivitis, blurred vision
- **GI:** *Gastric pain, flatulence, constipation, diarrhea, nausea, vomiting,* anorexia, ischemic colitis, renal and mesenteric arterial thrombosis, retroperitoneal fibrosis, hepatomegaly, acute pancreatitis
- **GU:** *Impotence, decreased libido,* Peyronie's disease, dysuria, nocturia, frequency
- **Musculoskeletal:** Joint pain, arthralgia, muscle cramp
- **Respiratory:** Bronchospasm, dyspnea, cough, bronchial obstruction, nasal stuffiness, rhinitis, pharyngitis
- **Other:** *Decreased exercise tolerance, development of ANAs,* hyperglycemia or hypoglycemia, elevated serum transaminase, alkaline phosphatase, and LDH

Interactions

✳ **Drug-drug** • Increased effects with verapamil • Decreased effects with indomethacin, ibuprofen, piroxicam, sulindac, barbiturates • Prolonged hypoglycemic effects of insulin • Initial hypertensive episode followed by bradycardia with epinephrine • Increased first-dose response to prazosin • Increased serum levels and toxic effects with lidocaine, cimetidine • Increased serum levels of propranolol and phenothiazines, hydralazine if the two drugs are taken concurrently • Paradoxical hypertension when clonidine is given with beta-blockers; increased rebound hypertension when clonidine is discontinued in patients on beta-blockers • Decreased serum levels and therapeutic effects with methimazole, propylthiouracil • Decreased bronchodilator effects of theophyllines • Decreased antihypertensive effects with NSAIDs (ie, ibuprofen, indomethacin, piroxicam, sulindac), rifampin

✳ **Drug-lab test** • Interference with glucose or insulin tolerance tests, glaucoma screening tests

■ Nursing considerations
Assessment

- **History:** Allergy to beta-blocking agents, sinus bradycardia, second- or third-degree heart block, cardiogenic shock, CHF, bronchial asthma, bronchospasm, COPD, hypo- glycemia and diabetes, thyrotoxicosis, hepatic dysfunction, pregnancy, lactation
- **Physical:** Weight, skin color, lesions, edema, T; reflexes, affect, vision, hearing, orientation; BP, P, ECG, peripheral perfusion; R, auscultation; bowel sounds, normal output, liver evaluation; bladder palpation; liver and thyroid function tests; blood and urine glucose

Interventions

- Do not discontinue drug abruptly after long-term therapy (hypersensitivity to catecholamines may have developed, causing exacerbation of angina, MI, and ventricular arrhythmias). Taper drug gradually over 2 wk with monitoring.
- Ensure that alpha-adrenergic blocker has been given before giving propranolol when treating patients with pheochromocytoma; endogenous catecholamines secreted by the tumor can cause severe hypertension if vascular beta receptors are blocked without concomitant alpha blockade.
- Consult with physician about withdrawing drug if patient is to undergo surgery (withdrawal is controversial).
- Provide continuous cardiac and regular BP monitoring with IV form.
- Give oral drug with food to facilitate absorption.

Teaching points

- Take this drug with meals. Do not discontinue the medication abruptly; abrupt discontinuation can cause a worsening of your disorder.
- These side effects may occur: dizziness, drowsiness, light-headedness, blurred vision (avoid driving or performing hazardous tasks); nausea, loss of appetite (frequent, small meals may help); nightmares, depression (request change of your medication); sexual impotence.
- Report difficulty breathing, night cough, swelling of extremities, slow pulse, confusion, depression, rash, fever, sore throat.
- For diabetic patients: The normal signs of hypoglycemia (sweating, tachycardia) may be blocked by this drug; monitor your blood/urine glucose carefully; eat regular meals and take your diabetic medication regularly.

P

▷ propylthiouracil (PTU)

*(proe pill thye oh **yoor'** a sill)*

Propyl-Thyracil (CAN)

PREGNANCY CATEGORY D

Drug class
Antithyroid agent

Therapeutic actions
Inhibits the synthesis of thyroid hormones; partially inhibits the peripheral conversion of T_4 to T_3, the more potent form of thyroid hormone.

Indications
• Hyperthyroidism

Contraindications and cautions
• Contraindicated with allergy to antithyroid products, pregnancy (can induce hypothyroidism or cretinism in the fetus; use only if absolutely necessary and when mother has been informed about potential harm to the fetus; if antithyroid drug is needed, this is the drug of choice).
• Use cautiously with lactation (if antithyroid drug is needed, this is the drug of choice).

Available forms
Tablets—50 mg

Dosages
Administered usually in three equal doses q 8 hr.
Adults
• Initial: 300 mg/day PO, up to 400–900 mg/day in severe cases. Maintenance: 100–150 mg/day.
Pediatric patients
6–10 yr: Initial: 50–150 mg/day PO.
> 10 yr: Initial: 150–300 mg/day PO. Maintenance is determined by the needs of the patient.

Pharmacokinetics

Route	Onset
Oral	Varies

Metabolism: Hepatic; $T_{1/2}$: 1–2 hr
Distribution: Crosses placenta; enters breast milk
Excretion: Urine

Adverse effects
• **CNS:** *Paresthesias, neuritis, vertigo, drowsiness,* neuropathies, depression, headache
• **CV:** Vasculitis, periarteritis
• **Dermatologic:** *Skin rash, urticaria,* pruritus, skin pigmentation, exfoliative dermatitis, lupus-like syndrome, loss of hair
• **GI:** *Nausea, vomiting, epigastric distress,* loss of taste, jaundice, hepatitis
• **GU:** Nephritis
• **Hematologic:** Agranulocytosis, granulocytopenia, thrombocytopenia, hypoprothrombinemia, bleeding
• **Other:** Arthralgia, myalgia, edema, lymphadenopathy, drug fever

Interactions
✳ **Drug-drug** • Increased risk of bleeding with oral anticoagulants • Alterations in theophylline, metoprolol, propranolol, digitalis glycoside clearance, serum levels and effects as patient moves from hyperthyroid state to euthyroid state

■ Nursing considerations
Assessment
• **History:** Allergy to antithyroid products, pregnancy, lactation
• **Physical:** Skin color, lesions, pigmentation; orientation, reflexes, affect; liver evaluation; CBC, differential, PT time; liver and renal function tests

Interventions
• Administer drug in 3 equally divided doses at 8-hr intervals; schedule to maintain patient's sleep pattern.
• Arrange for regular, periodic blood tests to monitor bone marrow depression and bleeding tendencies.
• Advise medical personnel doing surgical procedures that this patient is using this drug and is at greater risk for bleeding problems.

Adverse effects in *Italics* are most common; those in **Bold** are life-threatening.

Teaching points

- Take around the clock at 8-hr intervals.
- This drug must be taken for a prolonged period to achieve the desired effects.
- These side effects may occur: dizziness, weakness, vertigo, drowsiness (use caution if operating a car or dangerous machinery); nausea, vomiting, loss of appetite (small, frequent meals may help); rash, itching.
- Report fever, sore throat, unusual bleeding or bruising, headache, general malaise.

▽protamine sulfate
(proe' ta meen)

PREGNANCY CATEGORY C

Drug class
Heparin antagonist

Therapeutic actions
Strongly basic proteins found in salmon sperm; protamines form stable salts with heparin, which results in the immediate loss of anticoagulant activity; administered when heparin has not been given; protamine has anticoagulant activity.

Indications
- Treatment of heparin overdose

Contraindications and cautions
- Allergy to protamine sulfate or fish products, pregnancy, lactation.

Available forms
Injection—10 mg/mL

Dosages
Dosage is determined by the amount of heparin in the body and the time that has elapsed since the heparin was given; the longer the interval, the smaller the dose required.
Adults and pediatric patients
1 mg IV neutralizes 90 USP units of heparin derived from lung tissue or 115 USP units of heparin derived from intestinal mucosa.

Pharmacokinetics

Route	Onset	Duration
IV	5 min	2 hr

Metabolism: Degraded in body; $T_{1/2}$: unknown
Distribution: Crosses placenta; may enter breast milk

▽IV facts
Preparation: Administer injection undiluted; if dilution is necessary, use 5% dextrose in water or saline; refrigerate any diluted solution. Do not store diluted solution; no preservatives are added. Reconstitute powder for injection with 5 mL bacteriostatic water for injection with benzyl alcohol added to the 50-mg vial (25 mL to the 250-mg vial); stable at room temperature for 72 hr.
Infusion: Administer very slowly IV over at least 10 min; do not exceed 50 mg in any 10-min period; do not give more than 100 mg over a short period of time.
Incompatibilities: Do not mix in lines with incompatible antibiotics, including many penicillins and cephalosporins.

Adverse effects
- **CV:** *Hypotension*
- **GI:** *Nausea/vomiting*
- **Hypersensitivity:** Anaphylactoid reactions—dyspnea, flushing, hypotension, bradycardia, **anaphylaxis**

■ Nursing considerations
Assessment
- **History:** Allergy to protamine sulfate or fish products, pregnancy, lactation
- **Physical:** Skin color,T; orientation, reflexes; P, BP, auscultation, peripheral perfusion; R, adventitious sounds; plasma thrombin time

Interventions
- Maintain emergency equipment for resuscitation and treatment of shock on standby in case of anaphylactoid reaction.
- Monitor coagulation studies to adjust dosage, and screen for heparin rebound and response to drug.

Teaching points
- Report shortness of breath, difficulty breathing, flushing, feeling of warmth, dizziness, lack of orientation, numbness, tingling.

protriptyline hydrochloride
*proe **trip**' ti leen)*

Triptil (CAN), Vivactil

PREGNANCY CATEGORY C

Drug class
Tricyclic antidepressant (TCA) (secondary amine)

Therapeutic actions
Mechanism of action unknown; the TCAs are structurally related to the phenothiazine antipsychotic drugs (eg, chlorpromazine), but in contrast to the phenothiazines, TCAs inhibit the presynaptic reuptake of the neurotransmitters norepinephrine and serotonin; anticholinergic at CNS and peripheral receptors; the relation of these effects to clinical efficacy is unknown.

Indications
- Relief of symptoms of depression (endogenous depression most responsive; unlike other TCAs, protriptyline is "activating" and may be useful in withdrawn and anergic patients)
- Unlabeled use: treatment of obstructive sleep apnea

Contraindications and cautions
- Contraindicated with hypersensitivity to any tricyclic drug, concomitant therapy with an MAOI, recent MI, myelography within previous 24 hr or scheduled within 48 hr, pregnancy (limb reduction abnormalities), lactation.
- Use cautiously with EST; preexisting CV disorders (eg, severe coronary heart disease, progressive heart failure, angina pectoris, paroxysmal tachycardia); angle-closure glaucoma, increased intraocular pressure, urinary retention, ureteral or urethral spasm; seizure disorders (TCAs lower the seizure threshold); hyperthyroidism (predisposes to CVS toxicity, including cardiac arrhythmias); impaired hepatic, renal function; psychiatric patients (schizophrenic or paranoid patients may exhibit a worsening of psychosis); manic-depressive patients (may shift to hy-

pomanic or manic phase); elective surgery (TCAs should be discontinued as long as possible before surgery).

Available forms
Tablets—5, 10 mg

Dosages
Adults
5–40 mg/day PO in 3–4 divided doses initially. May gradually increase to 60 mg/day if necessary. Do not exceed 60 mg/day. Make increases in dosage in the morning dose.
Pediatric patients
Not recommended.
Geriatric patients and adolescents
Initially 5 mg tid PO. Increase gradually if necessary. Monitor CV system closely if dose exceeds 20 mg/day.

Pharmacokinetics

Route	Onset	peak
Oral	Slow	24–30 hr

Metabolism: Hepatic; $T_{1/2}$: 67–89 hr
Distribution: Crosses placenta; enters breast milk
Excretion: Urine

Adverse effects
- **CNS:** *Sedation and anticholinergic (atropine-like) effects*—dry mouth, blurred vision, disturbance of accommodation for near vision, mydriasis, increased intraocular pressure, *confusion* (especially in elderly), *disturbed concentration,* hallucinations, disorientation, decreased memory, feelings of unreality, delusions, anxiety, nervousness, restlessness, agitation, panic, insomnia, nightmares, hypomania, mania, exacerbation of psychosis, drowsiness, weakness, fatigue, headache, numbness, tingling, paresthesias of extremities, uncoordination, motor hyperactivity, akathisia, ataxia, tremors, peripheral neuropathy, extrapyramidal symptoms, *seizures,* speech blockage, dysarthria, tinnitus, altered EEG
- **CV:** *Orthostatic hypotension,* hypertension, syncope, tachycardia, palpitations, **MI,** arrhythmias, heart block, precipitation of CHF, **stroke**

Adverse effects in *Italics* are most common; those in **Bold** are life-threatening.

- **Endocrine:** Elevated or depressed blood sugar; elevated prolactin levels; inappropriate ADH secretion
- **GI:** *Dry mouth, constipation,* paralytic ileus, *nausea,* vomiting, anorexia, epigastric distress, diarrhea, flatulence, dysphagia, peculiar taste, increased salivation, stomatitis, glossitis, parotid swelling, abdominal cramps, black tongue
- **GU:** Urinary retention, delayed micturition, dilation of the urinary tract, gynecomastia, testicular swelling; breast enlargement, menstrual irregularity and galactorrhea; increased or decreased libido; impotence
- **Hematologic:** Bone marrow depression, including agranulocytosis; eosinophilia; purpura; thrombocytopenia; leukopenia
- **Hypersensitivity:** Skin rash, pruritus, vasculitis, petechiae, photosensitization, edema (generalized or of face and tongue), drug fever
- **Withdrawal:** Symptoms with abrupt discontinuation of prolonged therapy: nausea, headache, vertigo, nightmares, malaise
- **Other:** Nasal congestion, excessive appetite, weight change, sweating, alopecia, lacrimation, hyperthermia, flushing, chills

Interactions
✳ Drug-drug • Increased TCA levels and pharmacologic effects with cimetidine, fluoxetine, ranitidine • Altered response, including arrhythmias and hypertension with sympathomimetics • Risk of severe hypertension with clonidine • Hyperpyretic crises, severe convulsions, hypertensive episodes, and deaths with MAO inhibitors • Decreased hypotensive activity of guanethidine

■ Nursing considerations
Assessment
- **History:** Hypersensitivity to any tricyclic drug; concomitant therapy with an MAOI; recent MI; myelography within previous 24 hr or scheduled within 48 hr; pregnancy; lactation; EST; preexisting CV disorders; angle-closure glaucoma, increased intraocular pressure, urinary retention, ureteral or urethral spasm; seizure disorders; hyperthyroidism; impaired hepatic, renal function; psychiatric patients; manic-depressive patients; elective surgery

- **Physical:** Weight; T; skin color, lesions; orientation, affect, reflexes, vision and hearing; P, BP, orthostatic BP, perfusion; bowel sounds, normal output, liver evaluation; urine flow, normal output; usual sexual function, frequency of menses, breast and scrotal examination; liver function tests, urinalysis, CBC, ECG

Interventions
- Limit drug access for depressed and potentially suicidal patients.
- Reduce dosage if minor side effects develop; discontinue if serious side effects occur.
- Arrange for CBC if patient develops fever, sore throat, or other sign of infection.

Teaching points
- Take drug exactly as prescribed; do not stop taking this drug abruptly or without consulting the physician or nurse.
- Avoid alcohol, other sleep-inducing drugs, OTC drugs.
- Avoid prolonged exposure to sunlight or sunlamps; use a sunscreen or protective garments.
- These side effects may occur: headache, dizziness, drowsiness, weakness, blurred vision (reversible; take safety measures if severe; avoid driving or performing tasks that require alertness); nausea, vomiting, loss of appetite, dry mouth (small, frequent meals, frequent mouth care, and sucking sugarless candies may help); nightmares, inability to concentrate, confusion; changes in sexual function; fetal abnormalities (avoid pregnancy, use contraceptive measures).
- Report dry mouth, difficulty in urination, excessive sedation.

▽pseudoephedrine
(soo dow e fed' rin)

pseudoephedrine hydrochloride (d-isoephedrine hydrochloride)
Cenafed, Decofed, Efidac/24, Eltor (CAN), Sinustop Pro, Sudafed, Sudodrin, Triaminic Allergy Congestion

pseudoephedrine sulfate
Afrin, Drixoral Non-Drowsy Formula

PREGNANCY CATEGORY C

Drug classes
Nasal decongestant
Sympathomimetic amine

Therapeutic actions
Effects are mediated by alpha-adrenergic receptors; causes vasoconstriction in mucous membranes of nasal passages, resulting in their shrinkage, which promotes drainage and improves ventilation.

Indications
- Temporary relief of nasal congestion caused by the common cold, hay fever, other respiratory allergies
- Nasal congestion associated with sinusitis
- Promotes nasal or sinus drainage
- Relief of eustachian tube congestion

Contraindications and cautions
- Contraindicated with allergy or idiosyncrasy to sympathomimetic amines, severe hypertension and coronary artery disease, lactation, pregnancy.
- Use cautiously with hyperthyroidism, diabetes mellitus, arteriosclerosis, ischemic heart disease, increased intraocular pressure, prostatic hypertrophy.

Available forms
Tablets—30, 60 mg; CR tablets—240 mg; ER tablets—120 mg; chewable tablets—15 mg; capsules—30, 60 mg; liquid—15, 30 mg/5 mL; drops—7.5 mg/0.8 mL

Dosages
Adults
60 mg q 4–6 hr PO (sustained-release, 120 mg PO q 12 hr); do not exceed 240 mg in 24 hr.
Pediatric patients
6–12 yr: 30 mg q 4–6 hr PO; do not exceed 120 mg in 24 hr.
2–5 yr: 15 mg as syrup q 4–6 hr PO; do not exceed 60 mg in 24 hr.

1–2 yr: 7 drops (0.02 mL/kg) q 4–6 hr PO; up to four doses per day.
3–12 mo: 3 drops/kg q 4–6 hr PO, up to four doses per day.
Geriatric patients
These patients are more likely to experience adverse reactions; use with caution.

Pharmacokinetics
Route	Onset	Duration
Oral	30 min	4–6 hr

Metabolism: Hepatic; $T_{1/2}$: 7 hr
Distribution: Crosses placenta; enters breast milk
Excretion: Urine

Adverse effects
- **CNS:** *Fear, anxiety, tenseness, restlessness, headache, light-headedness, dizziness, drowsiness, tremors,* insomnia, hallucinations, psychological disturbances, prolonged psychosis, **seizures,** CNS depression, weakness, blurred vision, ocular irritation, tearing, photophobia, orofacial dystonia
- **CV:** *Hypertension, arrhythmias,* CV collapse with hypotension, palpitations, tachycardia, precordial pain
- **Dermatologic:** *Pallor,* sweating
- **GI:** *Nausea/vomiting,* anorexia
- **GU:** Dysuria
- **Respiratory:** Respiratory difficulty

Interactions
✳ **Drug-drug** • Increased hypertension with MAOIs, guanethidine, furazoladine • Increased duration of action with urinary alkalinizers (potassium citrate, sodium citrate, sodium lactate, tromethamine, sodium acetate, sodium bicarbonate) • Decreased therapeutic effects and increased elimination of pseudoephedrine with urinary acidifiers (ammonium chloride, sodium acid phosphate, potassium phosphate) • Decreased antihypertensive effects of methyldopa

■ Nursing considerations
Assessment
- **History:** Allergy or idiosyncrasy to sympathomimetic amines, severe hypertension and

CAD, hyperthyroidism, diabetes mellitus, arteriosclerosis, increased intraocular pressure, prostatic hypertrophy, pregnancy, lactation
- **Physical:** Skin color, T; reflexes, affect, orientation, peripheral sensation, vision; BP, P, auscultation; R, adventitious sounds; urinary output, bladder percussion, prostate palpation

Interventions

- Administer cautiously to patients with CV disease, diabetes mellitus, hyperthyroidism, increased intraocular pressure, hypertension, and to patients > 60 yr who may have increased sensitivity to sympathomimetic amines.
- Avoid prolonged use; underlying medical problems may be causing the congestion.
- Monitor CV effect carefully; hypertensive patients who take this drug may experience changes in BP because of the additional vasoconstriction. However, if a nasal decongestant is needed, pseudoephedrine is the drug of choice.

Teaching points

- Do not exceed the recommended daily dose; serious overdose can occur. Use caution when using more than one OTC preparation because many of these drugs contain pseudoephedrine, and unintentional overdose may occur.
- Avoid prolonged use because underlying medical problems can be disguised.
- These side effects may occur: dizziness, weakness, restlessness, light-headedness, tremors (avoid driving or performing hazardous tasks).
- Report palpitations, nervousness, sleeplessness, sweating.

▷pyrantel pamoate
(pi ran' tel)

Antiminth, Combantrin (CAN), Pin-Rid, Pin-X, Reese's Pinworm

PREGNANCY CATEGORY C

Drug class
Anthelmintic

Therapeutic actions
A depolarizing neuromuscular blocking agent that causes spastic paralysis of *Enterobius vermicularis* and *Ascaris lumbricoides*.

Indications
- Treatment of enterobiasis (pinworm infection)
- Treatment of ascariasis (roundworm infection)

Contraindications and cautions
- Allergy to pyrantel pamoate, pregnancy, lactation, hepatic disease.

Available forms
Capsules—180 mg; oral suspension—50 mg/mL; liquid—50 mg/mL

Dosages
Adults
11 mg/kg (5 mg/lb) PO as a single oral dose. Maximum total dose of 1 g.
Pediatric patients
Safety and efficacy not established for children < 2 yr.

Pharmacokinetics

Route	Onset	Peak
Oral	Slow	1–3 hr

Metabolism: Hepatic; $T_{1/2}$: 47–100 hr
Distribution: Crosses placenta; may enter breast milk
Excretion: Feces and urine

Adverse effects
- **CNS:** Headache, dizziness, drowsiness, insomnia
- **Dermatologic:** Rash
- **GI:** *Anorexia, nausea, vomiting, abdominal cramps, diarrhea,* gastralgia, tenesmus, transient elevation of AST

Interactions
✴ Drug-drug • Pyrantel and piperazine are antagonistic in *Ascaris;* avoid concomitant use

■ Nursing considerations
Assessment
- **History:** Allergy to pyrantel pamoate, pregnancy, lactation

P

- **Physical:** Skin color, lesions; orientation, affect; bowel sounds; AST levels

Interventions

- Culture for ova and parasites.
- Administer drug with fruit juice or milk; ensure that entire dose is taken at once.
- Treat all family members (pinworm infestations).
- Disinfect toilet facilities after patient use (pinworms).
- Launder bed linens, towels, nightclothes, and undergarments (pinworms) daily.

Teaching points

- Take the entire dose at once. Drug may be taken with fruit juice or milk.
- Pinworms are easily transmitted; all family members should be treated for complete eradication.
- Strict handwashing and hygiene measures are important. Launder undergarments, bed linens, nightclothes daily; disinfect toilet facilities daily and bathroom floors periodically (pinworm).
- These side effects may occur: nausea, abdominal pain, diarrhea (small, frequent meals may help); drowsiness, dizziness, insomnia (avoid driving and using dangerous machinery).
- Report rash, joint pain, severe GI upset, severe headache, dizziness.

▽pyrazinamide

*(peer a **zin**' a mide)*

pms-Pyrazinamide (CAN), Tebrazid (CAN)

PREGNANCY CATEGORY C

Drug class

Antituberculous drug

Therapeutic actions

Bacteriostatic or bacteriocidal against *Mycobacterium tuberculosis;* mechanism of action is unknown.

Indications

- Initial treatment of active TB in adults and children when combined with other antituberculous agents
- Treatment of active TB after treatment failure with primary drugs

Contraindications and cautions

- Contraindicated with allergy to pyrazinamide, acute hepatic disease, pregnancy, lactation.
- Use cautiously with gout, diabetes mellitus, acute intermittent porphyria.

Available forms

Tablets—500 mg

Dosages
Adults and pediatric patients

15–30 mg/kg/day PO, given once a day; do not exceed 2 g/day. Always use with up to 4 other antituberculous agents; administer for the first 2 mo of a 6-mo treatment program. 50–70 mg/kg PO twice weekly may increase compliance and is being studied as an alternative dosing schedule. Patients with HIV infection may require a longer course of therapy.

Pharmacokinetics

Route	Onset	Peak
Oral	Rapid	2 hr

Metabolism: Hepatic; $T_{1/2}$: 9–10 hr
Distribution: Crosses placenta; enters breast milk
Excretion: Urine

Adverse effects

- **Dermatologic:** Rashes, photosensitivity
- **GI:** *Hepatotoxicity, nausea, vomiting,* diarrhea
- **Hematologic:** Sideroblastic anemia, adverse effects on clotting mechanism or vascular integrity
- **Other:** Active gout

Interactions

✻ **Drug-lab test** • False readings on *Acetest, Ketostix* urine tests

---

Adverse effects in *Italics* are most common; those in **Bold** are life-threatening.

■ Nursing considerations

Assessment

- **History:** Allergy to pyrazinamide, acute hepatic disease, gout, diabetes mellitus, acute intermittent porphyria, pregnancy, lactation
- **Physical:** Skin color, lesions; joint status; T; liver evaluation; liver function tests, serum and urine uric acid levels, blood and urine glucose, CBC

Interventions

- Administer only in conjunction with other antituberculous agents.
- Administer once a day.
- Arrange for follow-up of liver function tests (AST, ALT) prior to and every 2–4 wk during therapy.
- Discontinue drug if liver damage or hyperuricemia in conjunction with acute gouty arthritis occurs.

Teaching points

- Take this drug once a day; it will need to be taken with your other TB drugs.
- Take this drug regularly; avoid missing doses. Do not discontinue this drug without first consulting your prescriber.
- These side effects may occur: loss of appetite, nausea, vomiting (take drug with food); rash, sensitivity to sunlight (avoid exposure to the sun).
- Have regular, periodic medical checkups, including blood tests to evaluate the drug effects.
- Report fever, malaise, loss of appetite, nausea, vomiting, darkened urine, yellowing of skin and eyes, severe pain in great toe, instep, ankle, heel, knee, or wrist.

▽**pyridostigmine bromide**

*(peer id oh **stig' meen**)*

Mestinon, Regonol

PREGNANCY CATEGORY C

Drug classes

Cholinesterase inhibitor
Antimyasthenic agent
Antidote

Therapeutic actions

Increases the concentration of acetylcholine at the sites of cholinergic transmission and prolongs and exaggerates the effects of acetylcholine by reversibly inhibiting the enzyme acetylcholinesterase, thus facilitating transmission at the skeletal neuromuscular junction.

Indications

- Treatment of myasthenia gravis
- Antidote for nondepolarizing neuromuscular junction blockers (eg, tubocurarine) after surgery (parenteral)

Contraindications and cautions

- Contraindicated with hypersensitivity to anticholinesterases; adverse reactions to bromides; intestinal or urogenital tract obstruction, peritonitis, lactation.
- Use cautiously with asthma, peptic ulcer, bradycardia, cardiac arrhythmias, recent coronary occlusion, vagotonia, hyperthyroidism, epilepsy, pregnancy (given IV near term, drug may stimulate uterus and induce premature labor).

Available forms

Tablets—60 mg; SR tablets—180 mg; syrup—60 mg/5 mL; injection—5 mg/mL

Dosages

Adults

Oral

- *Symptomatic control of myasthenia gravis:* Average dose is 600 mg given over 24 hr; range, 60–1,500 mg, spaced to provide maximum relief. Sustained-release tablets, average dose is 180–540 mg daily or bid. Individualize dosage, allowing at least 6 hr between doses. Optimum control may require supplementation with the more rapidly acting syrup or regular tablets.
- *To supplement oral dosage preoperatively and postoperatively, during labor, during myasthenic crisis, etc:*

Parenteral

Give 1/30 the oral dose IM or very slowly IV. May be given 1 hr before second stage of labor is complete (enables patient to have adequate strength and protects neonate in immediate postnatal period).

- *Antidote for nondepolarizing neuromuscular blockers:* Give atropine sulfate 0.6–1.2 mg IV immediately before slow IV injection of pyridostigmine 0.1–0.25 mg/kg. 10–20 mg pyridostigmine usually suffices. Full recovery usually occurs within 15 min but may take 30 min.

Pediatric patients
Oral
- *Symptomatic control of myasthenia gravis:* 7 mg/kg/day divided into five or six doses.
- *Neonates who have myasthenic mothers and who have difficulty swallowing, sucking, breathing:*

Parenteral
0.05–0.15 mg/kg IM. Change to syrup as soon as possible.

Pharmacokinetics

Route	Onset	Duration
Oral	35–45 min	3–6 hr
IM	15 min	3–6 hr
IV	5 min	3–6 hr

Metabolism: Hepatic and tissue; $T_{1/2}$: 1.9–3.7 hr

Distribution: Crosses placenta; enters breast milk

Excretion: Urine

▼IV facts
Preparation: No further preparation is required.

Infusion: Infuse very slowly, each 0.5 mg over 1 min for myasthenia gravis, each 5 mg over 1 min as a muscle relaxant agonist, directly into vein or into tubing of actively running IV of D_5W, 0.9% sodium chloride, lactated Ringer's, or D_5W and lactated Ringer's.

Adverse effects
Parasympathomimetic effects
- **CV:** *Bradycardia, cardiac arrhythmias,* AV block and nodal rhythm, **cardiac arrest,** decreased cardiac output leading to hypotension, syncope
- **Dermatologic:** Diaphoresis, flushing
- **EENT:** *Lacrimation, miosis,* spasm of accommodation, diplopia, conjunctival hyperemia

- **GI:** *Salivation, dysphagia, nausea, vomiting, increased peristalsis, abdominal cramps,* flatulence, diarrhea
- **GU:** *Urinary frequency and incontinence,* urinary urgency
- **Respiratory:** *Increased pharyngeal and tracheobronchial secretions,* laryngospasm, bronchospasm, bronchiolar constriction, dyspnea

Other effects
- **CNS:** Convulsions, dysarthria, dysphonia, drowsiness, dizziness, headache, loss of consciousness
- **Dermatologic:** Skin rash, urticaria, **anaphylaxis**
- **Local:** Thrombophlebitis after IV use
- **Peripheral:** Skeletal muscle weakness, fasciculations, muscle cramps, arthralgia
- **Respiratory:** Respiratory muscle paralysis, central respiratory paralysis

Interactions
✳ **Drug-drug** • Decreased effectiveness with profound muscular depression with corticosteroids • Increased and prolonged neuromuscular blockade with succinylcholine

■ Nursing considerations
Assessment
- **History:** Hypersensitivity to anticholinesterases; adverse reactions to bromides; intestinal or urogenital tract obstruction, peritonitis, lactation, asthma, peptic ulcer, cardiac arrhythmias, recent coronary occlusion, vagotonia, hyperthyroidism, epilepsy, pregnancy
- **Physical:** Bowel sounds, normal output; urinary frequency, voiding pattern, normal output; R, adventitious sounds; P, auscultation, BP; reflexes, bilateral grip strength, ECG; thyroid function tests; skin color, texture, lesions

Interventions
- Administer IV slowly.
- Overdose with anticholinesterase drugs can cause muscle weakness (cholinergic crisis) that is difficult to differentiate from myasthenic weakness; administration of atropine may mask the parasympathetic effects of anticholinesterase overdose and further confound the diagnosis.

Adverse effects in *Italics* are most common; those in **Bold** are life-threatening.

- Maintain atropine sulfate on standby as an antidote and antagonist to pyridostigmine in case of cholinergic crisis or unusual sensitivity to pyridostigmine.
- Discontinue drug and consult physician if excessive salivation, emesis, frequent urination, or diarrhea occurs.
- Decrease dosage of drug if excessive sweating, nausea occur.

Teaching points
- Take drug exactly as prescribed (patient and significant other should be taught about drug effects, signs and symptoms of myasthenia gravis, the fact that muscle weakness may be related both to drug overdose and to exacerbation of the disease, and the importance of reporting muscle weakness promptly to the nurse or physician for proper evaluation).
- These side effects may occur: blurred vision, difficulty with far vision, difficulty with dark adaptation (use caution while driving, especially at night, or performing hazardous tasks in reduced light); increased urinary frequency, abdominal cramps; sweating (avoid hot or excessively humid environments).
- Report muscle weakness, nausea, vomiting, diarrhea, severe abdominal pain, excessive sweating, excessive salivation, frequent urination, urinary urgency, irregular heartbeat, difficulty breathing.

▽ **quazepam**
(kwa' ze pam)

Doral

PREGNANCY CATEGORY X

C-IV CONTROLLED SUBSTANCE

Drug classes
Benzodiazepine
Sedative and hypnotic

Therapeutic actions
Exact mechanisms of action not understood; acts mainly at subcortical levels of the CNS, leaving the cortex relatively unaffected; main sites of action may be the limbic system and mesencephalic reticular formation; benzodi-azepines potentiate the effects of GABA, an inhibitory neurotransmitter.

Indications
- Insomnia characterized by difficulty in falling asleep, frequent nocturnal awakenings, or early morning awakening
- Recurring insomnia or poor sleeping habits
- Acute or chronic medical situations requiring restful sleep

Contraindications and cautions
- Contraindicated with hypersensitivity to benzodiazepines, established or suspected sleep apnea, psychoses, acute narrow-angle glaucoma, shock, coma, acute alcoholic intoxication with depression of vital signs, pregnancy (congenital malformations, neonatal withdrawal syndrome), labor and delivery ("floppy infant" syndrome), lactation (infants become lethargic and lose weight).
- Use cautiously with impaired liver or kidney function, debilitation, depression, suicidal tendencies.

Available forms
Tablets—7.5, 15 mg

Dosages
Adults
Initially 15 mg PO until desired response is seen. May reduce to 7.5 mg in some patients.
Pediatric patients
Not for use in patients < 18 yr.
Geriatric patients or those with debilitating disease
Attempt to reduce nightly dosage after the first one or two nights of therapy.

Pharmacokinetics

Route	Onset	Peak
Oral	Varies	2 hr

Metabolism: Hepatic; $T_{1/2}$: 39 hr
Distribution: Crosses placenta; enters breast milk
Excretion: Urine

Adverse effects
- **CNS:** *Transient, mild drowsiness initially; sedation; depression; lethargy; apathy; fatigue; light-headedness; disorientation; restlessness; confusion;* crying; delirium;

headache; slurred speech; dysarthria; stupor; rigidity; tremor; dystonia; vertigo; euphoria; nervousness; difficulty in concentration; vivid dreams; psychomotor retardation; extrapyramidal symptoms; *mild paradoxical excitatory reactions during first 2 wk of treatment* (especially in psychiatric patients, aggressive children, and with high dosage); visual and auditory disturbances; diplopia; nystagmus; depressed hearing; nasal congestion

- **CV:** *Bradycardia, tachycardia,* CV collapse, hypertension and hypotension, palpitations, edema
- **Dependence:** *Drug dependence with withdrawal syndrome* when drug is discontinued (more common with abrupt discontinuation of higher dosage used for longer than 4 mo)
- **Dermatologic:** Urticaria, pruritus, skin rash, dermatitis
- **GI:** *Constipation, diarrhea,* dry mouth, salivation, nausea, anorexia, vomiting, difficulty in swallowing, gastric disorders, elevations of blood enzymes, hepatic dysfunction, jaundice
- **GU:** *Incontinence, urinary retention, changes in libido,* menstrual irregularities
- **Hematologic:** Decreased Hct (primarily with long-term therapy), blood dyscrasias (agranulocytosis, leukopenia, neutropenia)
- **Other:** Hiccups, fever, diaphoresis, paresthesias, muscular disturbances, gynecomastia

Interactions
✳ Drug-drug • Increased CNS depression with alcohol, omeprazole • Increased pharmacologic effects with cimetidine, disulfiram, hormonal contraceptives • Decreased sedative effects with theophylline, aminophylline, dyphylline, oxitriphylline

■ Nursing considerations
Assessment
- **History:** Hypersensitivity to benzodiazepines, psychoses, acute narrow-angle glaucoma, shock, coma, acute alcoholic intoxication, pregnancy, labor and delivery, lactation, impaired liver or kidney function, debilitation, depression, suicidal tendencies

- **Physical:** Skin color, lesions; T; orientation, reflexes, affect, ophthalmologic exam; P, BP; R, adventitious sounds; liver evaluation, abdominal exam, bowel sounds, normal output; CBC, liver and renal function tests

Interventions
- Ensure that patient is not pregnant before use; recommend the use of barrier contraceptives.
- Monitor liver and kidney function, CBC during long-term therapy.
- Taper dosage gradually after long-term therapy, especially in epileptics.

Teaching points
- Take drug exactly as prescribed.
- Do not stop taking this drug (long-term therapy) without consulting your health care provider.
- This drug should not be used during pregnancy; use of barrier contraceptives is advised.
- These side effects may occur: drowsiness, dizziness (may lessen; avoid driving or engaging in other dangerous activities); GI upset (take with water); depression, dreams, emotional upset, crying; nocturnal sleep may be disturbed for several nights after discontinuing the drug.
- Report severe dizziness, weakness, drowsiness that persists, rash or skin lesions, palpitations, swelling of the extremities, visual changes, difficulty voiding.

▽ quetiapine fumarate
*(kwe **tie'** ah peen)*

Seroquel

PREGNANCY CATEGORY C

Drug classes
Dibenzothiazepine
Antipsychotic

Therapeutic actions
Mechanism of action not fully understood: blocks dopamine and serotonin receptors in

Adverse effects in *Italics* are most common; those in **Bold** are life-threatening.

the brain; also acts as a receptor antagonist at histamine and adrenergic receptor sites (which may contribute to the adverse effects of orthostatic hypotension and somnolence).

Indications
• Treatment of schizophrenia in patients > 18 yr

Contraindications and cautions
• Contraindicated with coma or severe CNS depression, allergy to quetiapine, lactation, pregnancy.
• Use cautiously with cardiovascular disease, hypotension, hepatic dysfunction, seizures, exposure to extreme heat, autonomic instability, tardive dyskinesia, dehydration, thyroid disease, suicidal tendencies.

Available forms
Tablets—25, 100, 200, 300 mg

Dosages
Adults
25 mg PO bid. Increase in increments of 25–50 mg bid–tid on the 2nd and 3rd days; dosage range by day 4: 300–400 mg/day in 2–3 divided doses. Further increases can be made at 2-day intervals. Maximum dose: 800 mg/day.
Pediatric patients
Not recommended for patients < 18 yr old.
Geriatric or debilitated patients or patients with hepatic impairment
Use lower doses and increase dosage more gradually than in other patients.

Pharmacokinetics

Route	Onset	Peak	Duration
Oral	Slow	2–4 hr	8–10 hr

Metabolism: Hepatic; $T_{1/2}$: 6 hr
Distribution: Crosses placenta; enters breast milk
Excretion: Urine

Adverse effects
• **Autonomic:** Dry mouth, salivation, nasal congestion, nausea, vomiting, anorexia, fever, pallor, flushed facies, sweating, constipation

• **CNS:** *Drowsiness,* insomnia, vertigo, *headache,* weakness, tremor, tardive dyskinesias, **NMS**
• **CV:** Hypotension, *orthostatic hypotension,* syncope
• **Hematologic:** Increased ALT, total cholesterol and triglycerides

Interactions
＊ **Drug-drug** • CNS effects potentiated by alcohol, CNS depressants • Effects decreased with phenytoin, thioridazine, carbamazepine, phenobarbital, rifampin, glucocorticoids; monitor patient closely and adjust dosages appropriately when these drugs are added to or discontinued from regimen • Increased effects of antihypertensives, lorazepam • Decreased effects of levodopa, dopamine antagonists • Potential for heat stroke and intolerance with drugs that affect temperature regulation (anticholinergics); use extreme caution and monitor patient closely

■ Nursing considerations
Assessment
• **History:** Coma or severe CNS depression; allergy to quetiapine, lactation, pregnancy, cardiovascular disease, hypotension, hepatic dysfunction, seizures, exposure to extreme heat, autonomic instability, tardive dyskinesia, dehydration, thyroid disease, suicidal tendencies
• **Physical:** Body weight, T; reflexes, orientation, intraocular pressure; P, BP, orthostatic BP; R, adventitious sounds; CBC, urinalysis, thyroid, liver, and kidney function tests

Interventions
• Administer small quantity to any patient with suicidal ideation.
• Monitor elderly patients for dehydration and institute remedial measures promptly; sedation and decreased sensation of thirst related to CNS effects of drug can lead to severe dehydration.
• Monitor patient closely in any setting that would promote overheating.
• Consult physician about dosage reduction and use of anticholinergic antiparkinsonian drugs (controversial) if extrapyramidal effects occur.

Teaching points

- Take this drug exactly as prescribed.
- These side effects may occur: dizziness, drowsiness, syncope (avoid driving or engaging in other dangerous activities); dry mouth, nausea, loss of appetite (frequent mouth care, small, frequent meals, and increased fluid intake may help).
- This drug should not be used during pregnancy; use of barrier contraceptives is advised.
- Maintain fluid intake and use precautions against heat stroke in hot weather.
- Report sore throat, fever, unusual bleeding or bruising, rash, weakness, tremors, dark-colored urine, pale stools, yellowing of the skin or eyes.

▷**quinapril hydrochloride**

(**kwin' ah pril**)

Accupril

PREGNANCY CATEGORY C
(FIRST TRIMESTER)

PREGNANCY CATEGORY D
(SECOND AND THIRD TRIMESTERS)

Drug classes

Antihypertensive
Angiotensin converting enzyme inhibitor (ACE inhibitor)

Therapeutic actions

Quinapril blocks ACE from converting angiotensin I to angiotensin II, a powerful vasoconstrictor, leading to decreased BP, decreased aldosterone secretion, a small increase in serum potassium levels, and sodium and fluid loss; increased prostaglandin synthesis also may be involved in the antihypertensive action.

Indications

- Treatment of hypertension alone or in combination with thiazide-type diuretics
- Adjunctive therapy in the management of CHF when added to regimen of digitalis and diuretics

Contraindications and cautions

- Contraindicated with allergy to quinapril or other ACE inhibitors, pregnancy.
- Use cautiously with impaired renal function, CHF, salt/volume depletion, lactation.

Available forms

Tablets—5, 10, 20, 40 mg

Dosages

Adults

- *Hypertension:* Initial dose 10 mg PO daily. Maintenance dose, 20–80 mg/day PO as a single dose or two divided doses. Patients on diuretics should discontinue the diuretic 2–3 days before beginning benazepril therapy. If BP is not controlled, add diuretic slowly. If diuretic cannot be discontinued, begin quinapril therapy with 5 mg and monitor carefully for hypotension.
- *CHF:* Initial dose 5 mg PO bid. Dose may be increased as needed to relieve symptoms, 10–20 mg PO bid usual range.

Pediatric patients

Safety and efficacy not established.

Geriatric patients or patients with renal impairment

Initial dose: 10 mg if creatinine clearance > 60 mL/min, 5 mg if creatinine clearance 30–60 mL/min, 2.5 mg if creatinine clearance 10–30 mL/min.

Pharmacokinetics

Route	Onset	Peak	Duration
Oral	1 hr	1 hr	24 hr

Metabolism: Hepatic; $T_{1/2}$: 2 hr
Distribution: Crosses placenta; enters breast milk
Excretion: Urine and feces

Adverse effects

- **CV:** Angina pectoris, orthostatic hypotension in salt/volume depleted patients, palpitations
- **Dermatologic:** Rash, pruritus, diaphoresis, flushing, photosensitivity
- **GI:** *Nausea,* abdominal pain, vomiting, diarrhea
- **Respiratory:** *Cough,* asthma, bronchitis, dyspnea, sinusitis

Adverse effects in *Italics* are most common; those in **Bold** are life-threatening.

- **Other: Angioedema,** asthenia, myalgia, arthralgia

Interactions
✷ **Drug-drug** • Possible increased digoxin levels, monitor patient and decrease dosage as needed • Decreased tetracycline absorption. Separate drugs by 1–2 hr.

■ Nursing considerations
Assessment
- **History:** Allergy to quinapril, other ACE inhibitors; impaired renal function; CHF; salt/volume depletion; lactation, pregnancy
- **Physical:** Skin color, lesions, turgor; T; P, BP, peripheral perfusion; mucous membranes, bowel sounds, liver evaluation; urinalysis, renal and liver function tests, CBC and differential

Interventions
- Alert surgeon and mark patient's chart with notice that quinapril is being taken; the angiotensin II formation subsequent to compensatory renin release during surgery will be blocked; hypotension may be reversed with volume expansion.
- Caution patient that this drug should not be used during pregnancy; advise the use of barrier contraceptives.
- Monitor patient closely in any situation that may lead to a fall in BP secondary to reduction in fluid volume (excessive perspiration and dehydration, vomiting, diarrhea) because excessive hypotension may occur.

Teaching points
- Do not stop taking the medication without consulting your health care provider.
- These side effects may occur: GI upset, loss of appetite (transient); light-headedness (usually transient; change position slowly and limit activities to those that do not require alertness and precision); dry cough (not harmful).
- Be careful in any situation that may lead to a drop in BP (diarrhea, sweating, vomiting, dehydration); if light-headedness or dizziness should occur, consult your health care provider.
- This drug should not be used during pregnancy; barrier contraceptives are advised.

- Report mouth sores; sore throat, fever, chills; swelling of the hands, feet; irregular heartbeat, chest pains; swelling of the face, eyes, lips, tongue; difficulty breathing; persistent cough.

▽ quinidine
(qwin' i deen)

quinidine gluconate
Quinaglute Dura-Tabs, Quinate (CAN)

quinidine sulfate
Apo-Quinidine (CAN), Quinidex Extentabs, Quinora

PREGNANCY CATEGORY C

Drug class
Antiarrhythmic

Therapeutic actions
Type 1A antiarrhythmic: decreases automaticity in ventricles, decreases height and rate of rise of action potential, decreases conduction velocity, increases fibrillation threshold.

Indications
- Treatment of atrial arrhythmias, paroxysmal or chronic ventricular tachycardia without heart block
- Maintenance therapy after electrocardioversion of atrial fibrillation or atrial flutter
- Treatment of life-threatening *P. falciperum* infections when IV therapy (quinidine gluconate) is indicated

Contraindications and cautions
- Contraindicated with allergy or idiosyncrasy to quinidine, second- or third-degree heart block, myasthenia gravis, pregnancy (neonatal thrombocytopenia), lactation.
- Use cautiously with renal disease, especially renal tubular acidosis, CHF, hepatic insufficiency.

Available forms
Tablets—200, 300 mg; SR tablets—300, 324 mg; injection—80 mg/mL

Dosages

Quinidine gluconate contains 62% anhydrous quinidine alkaloid. Quinidine sulfate contains 83% anhydrous quinidine alkaloid.

Adults

Administer a test dose of one tablet PO or 200 mg IM to test for idiosyncratic reaction. 200–300 mg tid or qid PO or 300–600 mg q 8 hr or q 12 hr if sustained-release form is used.

PO

- *Paroxysmal supraventricular arrhythmias:* 400–600 mg PO q 2–3 hr until paroxysm is terminated.

IM

- *Acute tachycardia:* 600 mg IM quinidine gluconate, followed by 400 mg every 2 hr until rhythm is stable.

IV

330 mg quinidine gluconate injected slowly IV at rate of 1 mL/min of diluted solution (10 mL of quinidine gluconate injection diluted to 50 mL with 5% glucose).

Pediatric patients

Safety and efficacy not established.

Pharmacokinetics

Route	Onset	Duration
Oral	1–3 hr	6–8 hr
IM	30–90 min	6–8 hr
IV	Rapid	6–8 hr

Metabolism: Hepatic; $T_{1/2}$: 6–7 hr
Distribution: Crosses placenta; enters breast milk
Excretion: Urine and feces

▽ IV facts

Preparation: Dilute 800 mg quinidine gluconate in 50 mL 5% dextrose injection.
Infusion: Inject slowly at rate of 1 mL/min.
Y-site incompatibility: Do not inject with furosemide.

Adverse effects

- **CNS:** Vision changes (photophobia, blurring, loss of night vision, diplopia)
- **CV: Cardiac arrhythmias,** cardiac conduction disturbances, including heart block, hypotension
- **GI:** *Nausea, vomiting, diarrhea,* liver toxicity

- **Hematologic:** Hemolytic anemia, hypoprothrombinemia, thrombocytopenic purpura, agranulocytosis, lupus erythematosus (resolves after withdrawal)
- **Hypersensitivity:** Rash, flushing, urticaria, angioedema, respiratory arrest
- **Other:** *Cinchonism* (tinnitus, headache, nausea, dizziness, fever, tremor, visual disturbances)

Interactions

✴ Drug-drug • Increased effects and increased risk of toxicity with cimetidine, amiodarone, verapamil • Increased cardiac depressant effects with sodium bicarbonate, antacids • Decreased levels with phenobarbital, hydantoins, rifampin • Increased neuromuscular blocking effects of depolarizing and nondepolarizing neuromuscular blocking agents, succinylcholine • Increased digoxin levels and toxicity • Increased effect of oral anticoagulants and bleeding

✴ Drug-food • Decreased metabolism and increased risk of toxic effects if combined with grapefruit juice; avoid this combination

✴ Drug-lab test • Quinidine serum levels are inaccurate if the patient is also taking triamterene

■ Nursing considerations

Assessment

- **History:** Allergy or idiosyncrasy to quinidine, second- or third-degree heart block, myasthenia gravis, renal disease, CHF, hepatic insufficiency, pregnancy, lactation
- **Physical:** Skin color, lesions; orientation, cranial nerves, reflexes, bilateral grip strength; P, BP, auscultation, ECG, edema; bowel sounds, liver evaluation; urinalysis, renal and liver function tests; CBC

Interventions

- Monitor response carefully, especially when beginning therapy.
- Reduce dosage in patients with hepatic or renal failure.
- Reduced dosage with digoxin; adjust dosage if phenobarbital, hydantoin, or rifampin is added or discontinued.

Adverse effects in *Italics* are most common; those in **Bold** are life-threatening.

rabeprazole sodium

- Check to see that patients with atrial flutter or fibrillation have been digitalized before starting quinidine.
- Differentiate the sustained-release form from the regular form.
- Monitor cardiac rhythm carefully, and frequently monitor BP if given IV or IM.
- Arrange for periodic ECG monitoring when on long-term therapy.
- Monitor blood counts, liver function tests frequently during long-term therapy.
- Evaluate for safe and effective serum drug levels: 2–6 mcg/mL.

Teaching points

- Take this drug exactly as prescribed. Do not chew the sustained-release tablets. If GI upset occurs, take drug with food. Do not drink grapefruit juice while on this drug.
- Frequent monitoring of cardiac rhythm, blood tests will be needed.
- These side effects may occur: nausea, loss of appetite, vomiting (eat small, frequent meals); dizziness, light-headedness, vision changes (do not drive or operate dangerous machinery); rash (use skin care).
- Wear a medical alert tag stating that you are on this drug.
- Return for regular follow-ups to check your heart rhythm and blood counts.
- Report sore mouth, throat, or gums, fever, chills, cold or flulike syndromes, ringing in the ears, severe vision disturbances, headache, unusual bleeding or bruising.

▽rabeprazole sodium
*(rah **beb'** pray zol)*

Aciphex

PREGNANCY CATEGORY B

Drug classes
Antisecretory agent
Proton pump inhibitor

Therapeutic actions
Gastric acid-pump inhibitor: suppresses gastric acid secretion by specific inhibition of the hydrogen and potassium ATPase enzyme system at the secretory surface of the gastric pari-etal cells; blocks the final step of acid production.

Indications

- Healing and maintenance of erosive or ulcerative gastric esophageal reflux disease (GERD) [4–8 wk therapy; may use additional 8 wk as necessary]
- Treatment of daytime and nighttime heartburn and other symptoms of GERD
- Maintenance of healing of erosive or ulcerative GERD and reduction of relapse rates
- Healing of duodenal ulcers as short-term treatment < 4 wk
- Treatment of pathological hypersecretory conditions (eg, Zollinger-Ellison syndrome, multiple adenomas, systemic mastocytosis)
- Eradication of *Helicobacter pylori* infection when used in combination with amoxicillin and clarithromycin

Contraindications and cautions

- Contraindicated with hypersensitivity to any proton pump inhibitor or any drug components.
- Use cautiously with pregnancy, lactation.

Available forms
DR tablet—20 mg

Dosages
Adults
- *Healing of GERD:* 20 mg PO daily for 4 wk.
- *Maintenance of GERD:* 20 mg daily PO.
- *Healing of duodenal ulcer:* 20 mg PO daily for up to 4 wk.
- *Pathological hypersecretory conditions:* 60 mg PO daily to bid for as long as clinically indicated.
- *Eradication of* H. pylori *infection:* Rabeprazole 20 mg PO bid for 7 days with amoxicillin 1,000 mg PO bid for 7 days and clarithromycin 500 mg PO bid for 7 days; take all three drugs twice a day, with the morning and evening meals.
Pediatric patients < 18 yr
Safety and efficacy not established.
Patients with hepatic impairment
Use extreme caution with severe hepatic dysfunction.

Pharmacokinetics

Route	Onset	Peak
Oral	1 hr	3–5 hr

Metabolism: Hepatic; $T_{1/2}$: 1.5 hr
Distribution: Crosses placenta; may pass into breast milk
Excretion: Urine and bile

Adverse effects

- **CNS:** *Headache, dizziness,* asthenia, vertigo, insomnia, apathy, anxiety, paresthesias, dream abnormalities
- **Dermatologic:** Rash, inflammation, urticaria, pruritus, alopecia, dry skin
- **GI:** *Diarrhea, abdominal pain, nausea, vomiting,* constipation, dry mouth, tongue atrophy
- **Respiratory:** *URI symptoms,* cough, epistaxis
- **Other:** Cancer in preclinical studies, back pain, fever

Interactions

✳ **Drug-drug** • Increased serum levels and potential increase in toxicity of benzodiazepines when taken concurrently

■ Nursing considerations
Assessment

- **History:** Hypersensitivity to any proton pump inhibitor or any drug components; pregnancy; lactation
- **Physical:** Skin lesions; body temperature; reflexes, affect; urinary output, abdominal exam; respiratory auscultation

Interventions

- Administer once a day. Caution patient to swallow tablets whole, not to cut, chew, or crush.
- Symptomatic improvement does not rule out gastric cancer, which did occur in preclinical studies.
- If administering antacids, they may be administered concomitantly with rabeprazole.
- Maintain supportive treatment as appropriate for underlying problem.
- Provide additional comfort measures to alleviate discomfort from GI effects, headache, etc.

Teaching points

- Take the drug once a day. Swallow the tablets whole—do not chew, cut, or crush. This drug will need to be taken for up to 4 wk (short-term therapy) or for a prolonged period depending on the condition being treated.
- Arrange to have regular medical follow-up while you are on this drug.
- These side effects may occur: dizziness (avoid driving a car or performing hazardous tasks); headache (consult with your nurse if these become bothersome; medications may be available to help); nausea, vomiting, diarrhea (proper nutrition is important, consult with your dietitian to maintain nutrition; ensure ready access to bathroom facilities); symptoms of upper respiratory tract infection, cough (it may help to know that this is a drug effect, do not self-medicate, consult with your health care provider if this becomes uncomfortable).
- Report severe headache, worsening of symptoms, fever, chills.
- Maintain all of the usual activities and restrictions that apply to your condition. If this becomes difficult, consult with your nurse or physician.

▽ raloxifene hydrochloride
(rah lox' i feen)

Evista

PREGNANCY CATEGORY X

Drug class
Estrogen receptor modulator

Therapeutic actions
Increases bone mineral density without stimulating endometrium in women; modulates effects of endogenous estrogen at specific receptor sites.

Indications
- Prevention and treatment of osteoporosis in postmenopausal women

Contraindications and cautions

- Contraindicated with allergy to raloxifene, pregnancy, lactation, active or history of deep venous thrombosis (DVT), pulmonary embolism, or retinal vein thrombosis.
- Use cautiously with history of smoking, venous thrombosis.

Available forms

Tablets—60 mg

Dosages

Adults

60 mg PO daily.

Pharmacokinetics

Route	Onset	Peak
Oral	Varies	4–7 hr

Metabolism: Hepatic; $T_{1/2}$: 27.7 hr
Distribution: Crosses placenta; passes into breast milk
Excretion: Feces

Adverse effects

- **CNS:** Depression, light-headedness, dizziness, headache, corneal opacity, decreased visual acuity, retinopathy
- **CV: Venous thromboembolism**
- **Dermatologic:** *Hot flashes, skin rash*
- **GI:** *Nausea, vomiting,* food distaste
- **GU:** Vaginal bleeding, vaginal discharge, pruritus vulvae
- **Other:** Peripheral edema

Interactions

✳ **Drug-drug** • Increased risk of bleeding with oral anticoagulants; monitor PT or INR closely • Decreased raloxifene absorption if taken with cholestyramine; avoid this combination

■ Nursing considerations

Assessment

- **History:** Allergy to raloxifene, pregnancy, lactation, smoking, history of venous thrombosis
- **Physical:** Skin lesions, color, turgor; pelvic exam; orientation, affect, reflexes; peripheral pulses, edema; liver function tests, CBC and differential, bone density

Interventions

- Administer daily without regard to food.
- Arrange for periodic blood counts during therapy.
- Monitor patient for possible long-term effects, including cancers, thromboses associated with other drugs in this class.
- Counsel patient about the need to use contraceptive measures to avoid pregnancy while taking this drug; inform patient that serious fetal harm could occur.
- Provide comfort measures to help patient deal with drug effects: hot flashes (environmental temperature control); headache, depression (monitoring of light and noise); vaginal bleeding (hygiene measures).

Teaching points

- Take this drug as prescribed.
- These side effects may occur: bone pain; hot flashes (staying in cool temperatures may help); nausea, vomiting (eat small, frequent meals); weight gain; dizziness, headache, light-headedness (use caution if driving or performing tasks that require alertness).
- This drug can cause serious fetal harm and must not be taken during pregnancy. Contraceptive measures should be used while you are taking this drug. If you become pregnant or would like to become pregnant, consult with your physician immediately.
- Report marked weakness, sleepiness, mental confusion, pain or swelling of the legs, shortness of breath, blurred vision.

R

▽ ramipril

*(ra **mi'** pril)*

Altace

PREGNANCY CATEGORY C
(FIRST TRIMESTER)

PREGNANCY CATEGORY D
(SECOND AND THIRD TRIMESTERS)

Drug classes

Antihypertensive
Angiotensin-converting enzyme (ACE) inhibitor

Therapeutic actions

Ramipril blocks ACE from converting angiotensin I to angiotensin II, a powerful vasoconstrictor, leading to decreased BP, decreased aldosterone secretion, a small increase in serum potassium levels, and sodium and fluid loss; increased prostaglandin synthesis also may be involved in the antihypertensive action.

Indications

- Treatment of hypertension alone or in combination with thiazide-type diuretics
- Treatment of CHF in stable patients in the first few days after MI
- To decrease the risk of cardiovascular disease in patients at risk for developing CAD

Contraindications and cautions

- Contraindicated with allergy to ramipril, pregnancy (embryocidal in preclinical studies).
- Use cautiously with impaired renal function, CHF, salt/volume depletion, lactation.

Available forms

Capsules—1.25, 2.5, 5, 10 mg

Dosages
Adults

- *Hypertension:* Initial dose 2.5 mg PO daily. Adjust dose according to BP response, usually 2.5–20 mg/day as a single dose or in 2 equally divided doses. Discontinue diuretic 2–3 days before beginning therapy; if not possible, administer initial dose of 1.25 mg.
- *CHF:* Initial dose 2.5 mg PO bid; if patient becomes hypotensive, 1.25 mg PO bid may be used while adjusting up to target dose of 5 mg PO bid.
- *Decrease risk of CAD:* Initial dose 2.5 mg PO once daily for 1 wk, then 5 mg PO once daily for next 3 wk, maintenance 10 mg PO daily.

Pediatric patients

Safety and efficacy not established.

Geriatric patients and patients with renal impairment

Excretion is reduced in renal failure; use smaller initial dose, 1.25 mg PO daily in patients with creatinine clearance < 40 mL/min; dosage

may be titrated upward until pressure is controlled or a maximum of 5 mg/day.

Pharmacokinetics

Route	Onset	Peak	Duration
Oral	1–2 hr	1–4 hr	24 hr

Metabolism: Hepatic; $T_{1/2}$: 13–17 hr
Distribution: Crosses placenta; enters breast milk
Excretion: Urine and feces

Adverse effects

- **CV:** *Tachycardia,* angina pectoris, MI, Raynaud's syndrome, CHF, hypotension in salt/volume depleted patients
- **Dermatologic:** *Rash, pruritus,* alopecia pemphigoid-like reaction, scalded mouth sensation, exfoliative dermatitis, photosensitivity
- **GI:** *Gastric irritation, aphthous ulcers, peptic ulcers, dysgeusia,* cholestatic jaundice, hepatocellular injury, anorexia, constipation
- **GU:** *Proteinuria,* renal insufficiency, renal failure, polyuria, oliguria, urinary frequency
- **Hematologic:** Neutropenia, agranulocytosis, thrombocytopenia, hemolytic anemia, **pancytopenia**
- **Other:** *Cough,* malaise, dry mouth, lymphadenopathy, **angioedema**

Interactions

✳ Drug-drug • Exacerbation of cough if taken with capsaicin • Increased serum levels and increased toxicity with lithium; monitor patient closely
✳ Drug-food • Decreased absorption may occur with food
✳ Drug-lab test • False-positive test for urine acetone

■ Nursing considerations
Assessment

- **History:** Allergy to ramipril, impaired renal function, CHF, salt or volume depletion, pregnancy, lactation
- **Physical:** Skin color, lesions, turgor; T; P, BP, peripheral perfusion; mucous membranes, bowel sounds, liver evaluation; uri-

nalysis, renal and liver function tests, CBC and differential

Interventions

- Administer 1 hr before or 2 hr after meals.
- Discontinue diuretic for 2–3 days before beginning therapy, if possible, to avoid severe hypotensive effect.
- Open capsules and sprinkle contents over a small amount of applesauce or mix in applesauce or water if patient has difficulty swallowing capsules. Mixture is stable for 24 hr at room temperature and 48 hr if refrigerated.
- Alert surgeon and mark chart that ramipril is being used; the angiotensin II formation subsequent to compensatory renin release during surgery will be blocked; hypotension may be reversed with volume expansion.
- Monitor patient closely for falling BP secondary to reduction in fluid volume (excessive perspiration and dehydration, vomiting, diarrhea) because excessive hypotension may occur.
- Reduce dosage in patients with impaired renal function.

Teaching points

- Take drug 1 hr before meals. Do not stop taking drug without consulting your prescriber.
- These side effects may occur: GI upset, loss of appetite, change in taste perception (transient) mouth sores (frequent mouth care may help); rash; fast heart rate; dizziness, light-headedness (transient; change position slowly, and limit your activities to those that do not require alertness and precision).
- Be careful in any situation that may lead to a drop in BP (diarrhea, sweating, vomiting, dehydration); if light-headedness or dizziness should occur, consult your health care provider.
- Report mouth sores; sore throat, fever, chills; swelling of the hands, feet; irregular heartbeat, chest pains; swelling of the face, eyes, lips, tongue, difficulty breathing.

▽**ranitidine hydrochloride**

(ra nye' te deen)

Alti-Ranitidine, (CAN), Novo-Ranidine, (CAN), Nu-Ranit (CAN), Zantac, Zantac EFFERdose, Zantac GELdose, Zantac 75

PREGNANCY CATEGORY B

Drug class

Histamine$_2$ (H$_2$) antagonist

Therapeutic actions

Competitively inhibits the action of histamine at the histamine$_2$ (H$_2$) receptors of the parietal cells of the stomach, inhibiting basal gastric acid secretion and gastric acid secretion that is stimulated by food, insulin, histamine, cholinergic agonists, gastrin, and pentagastrin.

Indications

- Short-term treatment of active duodenal ulcer
- Maintenance therapy for duodenal ulcer at reduced dosage
- Short-term treatment of active, benign gastric ulcer
- Short-term treatment of gastroesophageal reflux disease
- Pathologic hypersecretory conditions (eg, Zollinger-Ellison syndrome)
- Treatment of erosive esophagitis
- Treatment of heartburn, acid indigestion, sour stomach

Contraindications and cautions

- Contraindicated with allergy to ranitidine, lactation.
- Use cautiously with impaired renal or hepatic function.

Available forms

Tablets—75, 150, 300 mg; effervescent tablets and granules—150 mg; capsules—150, 300 mg; syrup—15 mg/mL; injection—1, 25 mg/mL

R

Dosages
Adults
- *Active duodenal ulcer:* 150 mg bid PO for 4–8 wk. Alternatively, 300 mg PO once daily hs or 50 mg IM or IV q 6–8 hr *or* by intermittent IV infusion, diluted to 100 mL and infused over 15–20 min. Do not exceed 400 mg/day.
- *Maintenance therapy, duodenal ulcer:* 150 mg PO hs.
- *Active gastric ulcer:* 150 mg bid PO *or* 50 mg IM or IV q 6–8 hr.
- *Pathologic hypersecretory syndrome:* 150 mg bid PO. Individualize dose with patient's response. Do not exceed 6 g/day.
- *Gastroesophageal reflux disease, esophagitis, benign gastric ulcer:* 150 mg bid PO.
- *Treatment of heartburn, acid indigestion:* 75 mg PO as needed.

Pediatric patients
Safety and efficacy not established.

Geriatric patients or patients with impaired renal function
Creatinine clearance < 50 mL/min, accumulation may occur; use lowest dose possible, 150 mg q 24 hr PO or 50 mg IM or IV q 18–24 hr. Dosing may be increased to q 12 hr if patient tolerates it and blood levels are monitored.

Pharmacokinetics

Route	Onset	Peak	Duration
Oral	Varies	1–3 hr	8–12 hr
IM	Rapid	15 min	8–12 hr
IV	Immediate	5–10 min	8–12 hr

Metabolism: Hepatic; $T_{1/2}$: 2–3 hr
Distribution: Crosses placenta; enters breast milk
Excretion: Urine

▼IV facts
Preparation: For IV injection, dilute 50 mg in 0.9% sodium chloride injection, 5% or 10% dextrose injection, lactated Ringer's solution, 5% sodium bicarbonate injection to a volume of 20 mL; solution is stable for 48 hr at room temperature. For intermittent IV, use as follows: dilute 50 mg in 100 mL of 5% dextrose injection or other compatible solution

Infusion: Inject over 5 min or more; for intermittent infusion, infuse over 15–20 min; continuous infusion, 6.25 mg/hr
Incompatibilities: Do not mix with amphotericin B, clindamycin

Adverse effects
- **CNS:** *Headache,* malaise, dizziness, somnolence, insomnia, vertigo
- **CV:** Tachycardia, bradycardia, PVCs (rapid IV administration)
- **Dermatologic:** *Rash,* alopecia
- **GI:** *Constipation, diarrhea, nausea, vomiting, abdominal pain,* hepatitis, increased ALT levels
- **GU:** Gynecomastia, impotence or decreased libido
- **Hematologic:** Leukopenia, granulocytopenia, thrombocytopenia, pancytopenia
- **Local:** *Pain at IM site, local burning or itching at IV site*
- **Other:** Arthralgias

Interactions
✻ **Drug-drug** • Increased effects of warfarin, TCAs • Decreased effectiveness of diazepam • Decreased clearance and possible increased toxicity of lidocaine, nifedipine

■ Nursing considerations
Assessment
- **History:** Allergy to ranitidine, impaired renal or hepatic function, lactation
- **Physical:** Skin lesions; orientation, affect; pulse, baseline ECG; liver evaluation, abdominal exam, normal output; CBC, liver and renal function tests

Interventions
- Administer oral drug with meals and at bedtime.
- Decrease doses in renal and liver failure.
- Provide concurrent antacid therapy to relieve pain.
- Administer IM dose undiluted, deep into large muscle group.
- Arrange for regular follow-up, including blood tests, to evaluate effects.

Teaching points

- Take drug with meals and at bedtime. Therapy may continue for 4–6 wk or longer.
- If you also are on an antacid, take it exactly as prescribed, being careful of the times of administration.
- Have regular medical follow-up to evaluate your response.
- These side effects may occur: constipation or diarrhea (request aid from your health care provider); nausea, vomiting (take drug with meals); enlargement of breasts, impotence or decreased libido (reversible); headache (monitor lights, temperature, noise levels).
- Report sore throat, fever, unusual bruising or bleeding, tarry stools, confusion, hallucinations, dizziness, severe headache, muscle or joint pain.

▽rasburicase

See *Less Commonly Used Drugs,* p. 1350.

▽repaglinide
*(re **pag**' lah nyd)*

Prandin

PREGNANCY CATEGORY C

Drug class
Antidiabetic agent

Therapeutic actions
Closes potassium channels in the beta cells of the pancreas, which causes the opening of calcium channels and a resultant increase in insulin release; highly selective for beta cells in the pancreas. Glucose-lowering abilities depend on the existence of functioning beta cells in the pancreas.

Indications
- Adjunct to diet and exercise to lower blood glucose in patients with non–insulin-dependent diabetes mellitus (type 2) whose hyperglycemia cannot be managed by diet and exercise alone
- Combination therapy with metformin or thiazolidinediones to lower blood glucose in patients whose hyperglycemia cannot be controlled by diet and exercise plus monotherapy with any of the following agents alone: metformin, sulfonylureas, repaglinide, or thiazolidinediones.

Contraindications and cautions
- Contraindicated with hypersensitivity to the drug; diabetic ketoacidosis; type 1 diabetes.
- Use cautiously with renal or hepatic impairment, pregnancy, lactation.

Available forms
Tablets—0.5, 1, 2 mg

Dosages
Adults
0.5–4 mg PO taken before meals; determine dosage based on patient response; maximum dose is 16 mg/day. Monitor patient regularly and adjust dosage as needed.
Pediatric patients
Safety and efficacy not established.
Patients with renal or hepatic impairment
For severe renal impairment, use starting dose of 0.5 mg PO and titrate carefully. Use cautiously with hepatic impairment; monitor closely.

Pharmacokinetics

Route	Onset	Peak
Oral	Rapid	1 hr

Metabolism: Hepatic; $T_{1/2}$: 1 hr
Distribution: Crosses placenta and may enter breast milk
Excretion: Feces, urine

Adverse effects
- **CNS:** *Headache,* paresthesias
- **Endocrine:** *Hypoglycemia, hyperglycemia*
- **GI:** Nausea, diarrhea, constipation, vomiting, dyspepsia
- **Respiratory:** *URI,* sinusitis, rhinitis, bronchitis

Interactions
✳ **Drug-alternative therapy** • Increased risk of hypoglycemia if taken with juniper berries, ginseng, garlic, fenugreek, coriander, dandelion root, celery

■ Nursing considerations
Assessment
- **History:** Hypersensitivity to the drug; diabetic ketoacidosis; type 1 diabetes; renal or hepatic impairment; pregnancy; lactation
- **Physical:** Skin color, lesions; T; orientation, reflexes, peripheral sensation; R, adventitious sounds; liver evaluation, bowel sounds; blood glucose, liver and renal function tests

Interventions
- Administer drug three to four times per day before meals; if a patient skips or adds a meal, the dosage should be skipped or added appropriately.
- Monitor urine or serum glucose levels frequently to determine effectiveness of drug and dosage being used.
- Arrange for consult with dietitian to establish weight loss program and dietary control as appropriate.
- Arrange for thorough diabetic teaching program to include disease, dietary control, exercise, signs and symptoms of hypo- and hyperglycemia, avoidance of infection, hygiene.

Teaching points
- Do not discontinue this medication without consulting health care provider.
- Take this drug before meals (3–4 times a day); if you skip a meal, skip the dose; if you add a meal, take your dose before that meal also.
- Monitor urine or blood for glucose and ketones as prescribed.
- Return for regular follow-up and monitoring of your response to the drug and possible need for dosage adjustment.
- Continue diet and exercise program established for control of diabetes.
- Know the signs and symptoms of hypoglycemia and hyperglycemia and appropriate treatment as indicated; report the incidence of either to your health care provider.
- You may experience headache, increased upper respiratory infections, nausea with this drug.
- Report fever, sore throat, unusual bleeding or bruising; severe abdominal pain.

▽ reteplase (r-PA)
(ret' ah place)

Retavase

PREGNANCY CATEGORY C

Drug class
Thrombolytic enzyme

Therapeutic actions
Human tissue enzyme produced by recombinant DNA techniques; converts plasminogen to the enzyme plasmin (fibrinolysin), which degrades fibrin clots; lyses thrombi and emboli; is most active at site of clot and causes little systemic fibrinolysis.

Indications
- Management of acute MI to improve ventricular function, reduce the incidence of CHF and MI mortality

Contraindications and cautions
- Contraindicated with allergy to r-PA or T-PA (alteplase); active internal bleeding; recent (within 2 mo) CVA; intracranial or intraspinal surgery or neoplasm; recent major surgery, obstetrical delivery, organ biopsy, or rupture of noncompressible blood vessel; recent serious GI bleed; recent serious trauma, including CPR; SBE; hemostatic defects; cerebrovascular disease; early-onset, insulin-dependent diabetes; septic thrombosis; severe uncontrolled hypertension, arteriovenous malformation, or aneurysm.
- Use cautiously with liver disease, age > 75 yr (risk of bleeding may be increased).

Available forms
Powder for injection—10.8 units

Dosages
Adults
- *Acute MI:* 10 units plus 10 units double-bolus IV injection, each over 2 min; second bolus is given 30 min after start of first.

Pharmacokinetics

Route	Onset	Peak
IV	Immediate	End of infusion

Metabolism: None; $T_{1/2}$: 13–16 min
Distribution: Crosses placenta
Excretion: Cleared by liver and kidneys

▼ IV facts

Preparation: Reconstitute with sterile water for injection (no preservatives) for immediate use; stable or 4 hr after reconstitution. Slight foaming may occur with reconstitition; allowing vial to stand undisturbed for several minutes will allow bubbles to dissipate. Protect from light. Do not shake.

Infusion: Infuse each bolus over 2 min into a running IV line in which no other medications are running.

Incompatibilities: Do not mix in the same line with heparin. If heparin has run through the line being used, flush with normal saline or 5% dextrose solution before and after reteplase infusion; do not add any other medications to the solution.

Adverse effects

- **CV:** Cardiac arrhythmias with coronary reperfusion, hypotension
- **Hematologic: Bleeding**—especially at venous or arterial access sites, GI bleeding, intracranial hemorrhage
- **Other:** Urticaria, nausea, vomiting, fever

Interactions

✳ Drug-drug • Increased risk of hemorrhage with heparin or oral anticoagulants, aspirin, dipyridamole, abciximab

■ Nursing considerations
Assessment

- **History:** Allergy to r-PA or T-PA, active internal bleeding, recent (within 2 mo) obstetrical delivery, organ biopsy, or rupture of noncompressible blood vessel, recent serious GI bleed, recent serious trauma (including CPR), SBE, hemostatic defects, cerebrovascular disease, early-onset insulin-dependent diabetes, septic thrombosis, severe uncontrolled hypertension, liver disease
- **Physical:** Skin color, temperature, lesions; orientation, reflexes; P, BP, peripheral perfusion, baseline ECG; R, adventitious sounds; liver evaluation, Hct, platelet count, thrombin time, APTT, PT

Interventions

- Discontinue concurrent heparin and reteplase if serious bleeding occurs.
- Arrange for regular monitoring of coagulation studies.
- Apply pressure and/or pressure dressings to control superficial bleeding (at invaded or disturbed areas).
- Avoid any arterial invasive procedures during therapy.
- Arrange for typing and cross-matching of blood in case serious blood loss occurs and whole blood transfusions are required.
- Institute treatment within 6 hr of onset of symptoms for evolving MI.

Teaching points

- This drug can only be given IV; you will need to be closely monitored during treatment.
- Report difficulty breathing, dizziness, disorientation, headache, numbness, tingling.

▽ ribavirin
(rye ba vye' rin)

Rebetol, Virazole

PREGNANCY CATEGORY X

Drug class
Antiviral

Therapeutic actions
Antiviral activity against respiratory syncytial virus (RSV), influenza virus, and herpes simplex virus; mechanism of action is not known.

Indications

- Treatment of carefully selected hospitalized infants and children with RSV infection of lower respiratory tract
- Treatment of chronic hepatitis C in combination with interferon alfa-2b in patients with compensated liver disease untreated with or refractory to alfa interferon therapy (oral)
- Orphan drug use: treatment of hemorrhagic fever with renal syndrome

- Unlabeled use for aerosol: treatment of some influenza A and B infections
- Unlabeled uses of oral preparation: treatment of some viral diseases, including herpes genitalis, measles, Lassa fever, hemorrhagic fever with renal syndrome

Contraindications and cautions

- Allergy to drug product, COPD, pregnancy or male whose female partner is pregnant (causes fetal damage), lactation.

Available forms

Powder for aerosol reconstitution—6 g/100 mL vial; capsules—200 mg

Dosages
Adults
< 75 kg: Two 200 mg capsules PO in the AM, three 200 mg capsules PO in the PM with *Intron A,* 3 million IU SC 3 times per week.
> 75 kg: Three 200 mg capsules PO in AM, three 200 mg capsules PO in PM with 3 million IU *Intron A,* SC 3 times per week.
Patients with renal impairment or cardiac disease
Use caution if creatinine clearance < 50 mL/min and with cardiac disease.
Pediatric patients
For use only with small-particle aerosol generator. Check operating instructions carefully. Dilute aerosol powder to 20 mg/mL and deliver for 12–18 hr/day for at least 3 but not more than 7 days.

Pharmacokinetics

Route	Onset	Peak
Aerosol	Slow	60–90 min

Metabolism: Cellular; $T_{1/2}$: 9.5 hr
Distribution: Crosses placenta; enters breast milk
Excretion: Urine and feces

Adverse effects

- **CNS:** Depression, suicidal behavior, nervousness
- **CV: Cardiac arrest,** hypotension
- **Dermatologic:** Rash
- **Hematologic:** Anemia

- **Respiratory:** *Deteriorating respiratory function,* pneumothorax, apnea, bacterial pneumonia
- **Other:** Conjunctivitis, testicular lesions in rodents

Interactions

✳ **Drug-drug** • Increased likelihood of digitalis toxicity

■ Nursing considerations
Assessment

- **History:** Allergy to drug product, COPD, pregnancy, lactation
- **Physical:** Skin rashes, lesions; P, BP, auscultation; R, adventitious sounds; Hct

Interventions

- Ensure proper use of small-particle aerosol generator; check operating instructions carefully.
- Ensure that water used as diluent contains no other substance.
- Replace solution in the unit every 24 hr.
- Store reconstituted solution at room temperature.
- Patients on mechanical ventilators should have tubing cleaned and checked to prevent accumulation of drug and malfunction of the machine.
- Monitor respiratory status frequently; pulmonary deterioration, and death have occurred during or shortly after treatment.
- Adults taking oral ribavirin (*Rebetol*) will receive it as part of a combination called *Rebetron* which contains ribavirin capsules and *Intron-A* for injection.
- Caution women to avoid pregnancy while on this drug; use of barrier contraceptives is advised; male partners of pregnant women should not take this drug.
- Use extreme caution in adults with history of depression or psychiatric disorders.
- Monitor BP, P frequently.

Teaching points

- Explain the use of small-particle aerosol generator to patient or family.
- Report any of the following: dizziness, confusion, shortness of breath (pediatric).

Adverse effects in *Italics* are most common; those in **Bold** are life-threatening.

- Take capsules in morning and evening (*Rebetol*), mark calendar with days to inject *Intron-A*.
- Avoid pregnancy while taking this drug; use of barrier contraceptives is advised; male partners of pregnant women should avoid intercourse.
- Report depression, suicidal ideation, difficulty breathing, muscle pain.

▽ rifabutin

See *Less Commonly Used Drugs,* p. 1350.

▽ rifampin
(rif' am pin)

Rifadin, Rimactane, Rofact (CAN)

PREGNANCY CATEGORY C

Drug classes
Antituberculous drug (first-line)
Antibiotic

Therapeutic actions
Inhibits DNA-dependent RNA polymerase activity in susceptible bacterial cells.

Indications
- Treatment of pulmonary TB in conjunction with at least one other effective antituberculous drug
- *Neisseria meningitidis* carriers, for asymptomatic carriers to eliminate meningococci from nasopharynx; not for treatment of meningitis
- Unlabeled uses: infections caused by *Staphylococcus aureus* and *Staphylococcus epidermis,* usually in combination therapy; gram-negative bacteremia in infancy; Legionella (*Legionella pneumophilia*), not responsive to erythromycin; leprosy (in combination with dapsone); prophylaxis of meningitis due to *Haemophilus influenzae*

Contraindications and cautions
- Contraindicated with allergy to any rifamycin, acute hepatic disease, lactation.
- Use cautiously with pregnancy (teratogenic effects have been reported in preclinical stud-

ies; safest antituberculous regimen for use in pregnancy is considered to be rifampin, isoniazid, and ethambutol).

Available forms
Capsules—150, 300 mg; powder for injection—600 mg

Dosages
Adults
- *Pulmonary TB:* 600 mg in a single daily dose PO or IV (used in conjunction with other antituberculous drugs). Continue therapy until bacterial conversion and maximal improvement occur.
- *Meningococcal carriers:* 600 mg PO or IV once daily for 4 consecutive days.
Pediatric patients > 5 yr
- *Pulmonary TB:* 10–20 mg/kg/day PO or IV not to exceed 600 mg/day.
- *Meningococcal carriers: > 1 mo:* 10 mg/kg PO or IV q 12 hr for 2 days, do not exceed 600 mg/dose; *< 1 mo:* 5 mg/kg PO or IV q 12 hr for 2 days.

Pharmacokinetics

Route	Onset	Peak
Oral	Varies	1–4 hr
IV	Rapid	End of infusion

Metabolism: Hepatic; $T_{1/2}$: 3–5.1 hr
Distribution: Crosses placenta; enters breast milk
Excretion: Feces and urine

▽ IV facts
Preparation: Reconstitute by transferring 10 mL sterile water for injection to vial containing 600 mg rifampin; swirl gently. Resultant fluid contains 60 mg/mL; stable at room temperature. Further mix with 500–1,000 mL of dextrose 5% or sterile saline.
Infusion: Infuse over 30–180 min, depending on volume.

Adverse effects
- **CNS:** *Headache, drowsiness, fatigue, dizziness,* inability to concentrate, mental confusion, generalized numbness, ataxia, muscle weakness, visual disturbances, exudative conjunctivitis
- **Dermatologic:** *Rash,* pruritus, urticaria, pemphigoid reaction, flushing, reddish-

orange discoloration of body fluids—tears, saliva, urine, sweat, sputum
- **GI:** *Heartburn, epigastric distress,* anorexia, nausea, vomiting, gas, cramps, diarrhea, pseudomembranous colitis, pancreatitis, *elevations of liver enzymes,* hepatitis
- **GU:** Hemoglobinuria, hematuria, renal insufficiency, **acute renal failure,** menstrual disturbances
- **Hematologic:** *Eosinophilia, thrombocytopenia, transient leukopenia,* hemolytic anemia, decreased Hgb, hemolysis
- **Other:** Pain in extremities, osteomalacia, myopathy, fever, *flulike syndrome*

Interactions
✳ Drug-drug • Increased incidence of rifampin-related hepatitis with isoniazid • Decreased effectiveness of rifampin with p-aminosalicyclic acid, ketoconazole; give the drugs at least 8–12 hr apart • Decreased effectiveness of metoprolol, propranolol, quinidine, corticosteroids, hormonal contraceptives, methadone, oral anticoagulants, oral sulfonylureas, theophyllines, phenytoin, cyclosporine, ketoconazole, verapamil
✳ Drug-lab test • Rifampin inhibits the standard assays for serum folate and vitamin B_{12}

■ Nursing considerations
Assessment
- **History:** Allergy to any rifamycin, acute hepatic disease, pregnancy, lactation
- **Physical:** Skin color, lesions; T; gait, muscle strength; orientation, reflexes, ophthalmologic examination; liver evaluation; CBC, liver and renal function tests, urinalysis

Interventions
- Administer on an empty stomach, 1 hr before or 2 hr after meals.
- Administer in a single daily dose.
- Consult pharmacist for rifampin suspension for patients unable to swallow capsules.
- Prepare patient for the reddish-orange coloring of body fluids (urine, sweat, sputum, tears, feces, saliva); soft contact lenses may be permanently stained; advise patients not to wear them during therapy.

- Arrange for follow-up of liver and renal function tests, CBC, ophthalmologic examinations.

Teaching points
- Take drug in a single daily dose. Take on an empty stomach, 1 hr before or 2 hr after meals.
- Take this drug regularly; avoid missing any doses; do not discontinue this drug without first consulting your health care provider.
- These side effects may occur: reddish-orange coloring of body fluids (tears, sweat, saliva, urine, feces, sputum; stain will wash out of clothing, but soft contact lenses may be permanently stained; do not wear them); nausea, vomiting, epigastric distress; skin rashes or lesions; numbness, tingling, drowsiness, fatigue (use caution if driving or operating dangerous machinery; use precautions to avoid injury).
- Have periodic medical checkups, including an eye examination and blood tests, to evaluate the drug effects.
- Report fever, chills, muscle and bone pain, excessive tiredness or weakness, loss of appetite, nausea, vomiting, yellowing of skin or eyes, unusual bleeding or bruising, skin rash or itching.

▽ rifapentine
*(rif ah **pin'** ten)*

Priftin

PREGNANCY CATEGORY C

Drug classes
Antituberculous drug
Antibiotic

Therapeutic actions
Inhibits DNA-dependent RNA polymerase activity in susceptible strains of *Mycobacterium tuberculosis,* causing cell death.

Indications
- Treatment of pulmonary tuberculosis in conjunction with at least one other effective antituberculous drug

---

Adverse effects in *Italics* are most common; those in **Bold** are life-threatening.

- Orphan drug use: prophylaxis and treatment of *Mycobacterium avium* complex (MAC) in patients with AIDS

Contraindications and cautions
- Contraindicated with allergy to any rifamycin, acute hepatic disease.
- Use cautiously with pregnancy (teratogenic effects have been reported in preclinical studies); lactation, hepatic impairment.

Available forms
Tablets—150 mg

Dosages
Adults
- *TB, intensive phase:* 600 mg PO twice weekly with an interval of at least 72 hr between doses; continue for 2 mo. Always give rifapentine in combination with other antituberculosis drugs.
- *Continuation phase:* 600 mg PO once a week for 4 mo in combination with other agents to which the organism is susceptible.
Pediatric patients
Safety and efficacy not established.

Pharmacokinetics

Route	Onset	Peak
Oral	Slow	5–6 hr

Metabolism: Hepatic; $T_{1/2}$: 13.9 hr
Distribution: Crosses placenta; passes into breast milk
Excretion: Urine and feces

Adverse effects
- **CNS:** *Headache, dizziness*
- **Dermatologic:** Pruritis, acne
- **GI:** Nausea, vomiting, diarrhea, cramps
- **GU:** *Pyuria, proteinuria, hematuria*
- **Hematologic:** *Hyperuricemia,* liver enzyme elevations
- **Other:** Pain, arthralgia, *reddish discoloration of body fluids*

Interactions
✳ **Drug-drug** • Decreased effectiveness of protease inhibitors; use extreme caution if this combination is needed; try to avoid this combination • Decreased effectiveness of rifampin if taken with p-aminosalicylic acid, ketoconazole—give the drugs at least 8–12 hr apart • Decreased effectiveness of metoprolol, propranolol, quinidine, corticosteroids, hormonal contraceptives, methadone, oral anticoagulants, oral sulfonylureas, theophyllines, phenytoin, cyclosporine, ketoconazole, verapamil if taken concurrently with rifapentine. Monitor patient carefully and adjust dosage as needed; suggest the use of barrier contraceptives while using this drug

✳ **Drug-lab test** • Rifapentine inhibits the standard assays for serum folate and vitamin B_{12}

■ Nursing considerations
Assessment
- **History:** Allergy to any rifamycin, acute hepatic disease, pregnancy, lactation
- **Physical:** Skin color, lesions; temperature; gait, muscle strength; orientation, reflexes, CBC, liver function tests, renal function tests, urinalysis

Interventions
- Administer on an empty stomach, 1 hr before 2 hr after meals; if GI upset is severe, drug may be taken with food.
- Always use in combination with other antituberculous drugs.
- Prepare patient for the reddish-orange coloring of body fluids (urine, sweat, sputum, tears, feces, saliva); soft contact lenses may be permanently stained, patients should be advised not to wear them during drug therapy.
- Recommend the use of barrier contraceptives while on this drug; hormonal contraceptives may be ineffective.
- Provide small, frequent meals if GI upset occurs.
- Provide skin care if dermatologic effects occur.

Teaching points
- Take drug along with any other prescribed antituberculous drugs. Take on an empty stomach—1 hr before or 2 hr after meals. If your stomach is very upset by the drug, it may be taken with food.
- Take this drug regularly, avoid missing any doses; do not discontinue this drug without first consulting your health care provider. Make sure doses are at least 72 hr apart.

R

- These side effects may occur: reddish-orange coloring of body fluids (tears, sweat, saliva, urine, feces, sputum; this is an expected occurrence and is not dangerous, do not be alarmed—stain will wash out of clothing but soft contact lenses may be permanently stained, do not wear them when on this drug); nausea, vomiting, epigastric distress (consult your nurse or physician if any of these becomes too uncomfortable); skin rashes or lesions (consult your nurse or physician for appropriate skin care).
- Avoid pregnancy while taking this drug, use of barrier contraceptives is advised.
- Arrange to have periodic medical check-ups, which will include blood tests to evaluate the drug effects.
- Report fever, chills, muscle and bone pain, excessive tiredness or weakness, loss of appetite, yellowing of skin or eyes, unusual bleeding or bruising, skin rash or itching.

▽ riluzole

See *Less Commonly Used Drugs,* p. 1350.

▽ rimantadine hydrochloride
(ri man' ta deen)

Flumadine

PREGNANCY CATEGORY C

Drug class
Antiviral

Therapeutic actions
Synthetic antiviral agent that inhibits viral replication, possibly by preventing the uncoating of the virus.

Indications
- Prophylaxis and treatment of illness caused by influenza A virus in adults
- Prophylaxis against influenza A virus in children

Contraindications and cautions
- Allergy to amantadine, rimantadine; lactation.
- Use cautiously with seizures, liver or renal disease, pregnancy.

Available forms
Tablets—100 mg; syrup—50 mg/5 mL

Dosages
Adults and patients ≥ 10 yr
- *Prophylaxis:* 100 mg/day PO bid.
- *Treatment:* Same dose as above; start treatment as soon after exposure as possible, continuing for 7 days.

Pediatric patients < 10 yr
- *Prophylaxis:* 5 mg/kg PO daily; do not exceed 150 mg/day.

Patients with severe renal disease
Dose of 100 mg PO daily is recommended.

Pharmacokinetics

Route	Onset	Peak
Oral	Slow	6 hr

Metabolism: $T_{1/2}$: 25.4 hr
Distribution: Crosses placenta; enters breast milk
Excretion: Unchanged in the urine

Adverse effects
- **CNS:** *Light-headedness, dizziness, insomnia,* confusion, irritability, ataxia, psychosis, depression, hallucinations
- **CV:** CHF, orthostatic hypotension, dyspnea
- **GI:** *Nausea,* anorexia, constipation, dry mouth
- **GU:** Urinary retention

Interactions
✷ **Drug-drug** • Decreased effectiveness with acetaminophen, aspirin • Increased serum levels and effects with cimetidine

■ Nursing considerations
Assessment
- **History:** Allergy to amantadine, rimantidine; seizures; liver or renal disease; lactation
- **Physical:** Orientation, vision, speech, reflexes; BP, orthostatic BP, P, auscultation,

---

Adverse effects in *Italics* are most common; those in **Bold** are life-threatening.

perfusion, edema; R, adventitious sounds; urinary output; BUN, creatinine clearance

Interventions

- Administer full course of drug to achieve the beneficial antiviral effects. Initiate therapy for treatment within 48 hr of onset of symptoms and continue for 7 days.

Teaching points

- These side effects may occur: drowsiness, blurred vision (use caution in driving or using dangerous equipment); dizziness, lightheadedness (avoid sudden position changes); irritability or mood changes (common; if severe, request a drug change).
- Report swelling of the fingers or ankles, shortness of breath, difficulty urinating, tremors, slurred speech, difficulty walking.

▽ risedronate sodium
*(rah **sed'** dro nate)*

Actonel

PREGNANCY CATEGORY C

Drug class
Bisphosphonate

Therapeutic actions
Affects osteoclast activity by reducing the enzymatic and transport processes that lead to resorption of the bone and by inhibiting the osteoclast protein pump, leading to a rate of bone turnover near normal in patients with Paget's disease.

Indications

- Treatment of Paget's disease of bone in patients with alkaline phosphatase at least 2 times the upper limit of normal, those who are symptomatic, those at risk for future complications
- Treatment and prevention of osteoporosis in postmenopausal women
- Treatment and prevention of glucocorticoid-induced osteoporosis

Contraindications and cautions

- Contraindicated with allergy to biphosphonates; severe renal disease, pregnancy, hypo-

calcemia, inability to stand or sit upright for at least 30 min.
- Use cautiously with renal dysfunction, lactation.

Available forms
Tablets—5, 30, 35 mg

Dosages
Adults

- *Treatment and prevention of osteoporosis:* 5 mg PO once daily taken in an upright position with 6–8 oz of water at least 30 min before or after any other beverage or food. Postmenopausal osteoporosis: may switch to 35 mg tablet taken PO once per wk.
- *Paget's disease:* 30 mg PO once daily for 2 mo taken in an upright position with 6–8 oz of plain water at least 30 min before or after any other beverage or food; may retreat after at least a 2-mo posttreatment period if indicated.

Pediatric patients
Safety and efficacy not established.

Patients with renal impairment
Not recommended with creatinine clearance < 30 mL/min; no dosage adjustment is necessary if creatinine clearance > 30 mL/min.

Pharmacokinetics

Route	Onset	Peak
Oral	Rapid	1 hr

Metabolism: Not metabolized; $T_{1/2}$: 220 hr
Distribution: Crosses placenta; may pass into breast milk
Excretion: Urine

Adverse effects

- **CNS:** *Headache,* paresthesia, *dizziness*
- **CV:** Chest pain, edema, hypertension
- **EENT:** Glaucoma, conjunctivitis, cataract
- **GI:** *Nausea, diarrhea, dyspepsia,* abdominal pain, *anorexia*
- **Skeletal:** *Increased or recurrent bone pain*
- **Other:** *Arthralgia,* bone pain, leg cramps, *rash*

Interactions

＊ **Drug-drug** • Absorption of risedronate decreased by calcium, aspirin, aluminum, magnesium; avoid these drugs for 2 hr before to 2 hr after taking risedronate

■ Nursing considerations
Assessment
- **History:** Allergy to biphosphonates, renal failure, hypocalcemia, pregnancy, lactation
- **Physical:** Muscle tone, bone pain; bowel sounds; eye exam; urinalysis, serum calcium; orientation, affect

Interventions
- Administer with a full glass of plain (not mineral) water, at least 30 min before or after any other beverage, food, or medication; have patient remain in an upright position for at least 30 min to decrease the incidence of GI effects. Patients taking weekly dose should mark calendar as a reminder.
- Monitor serum calcium levels before, during, and after therapy.
- Ensure at least a 2-mo rest period after 2-mo course of treatment if retreatment is required for Paget's disease.
- Ensure adequate vitamin D and calcium intake.
- Provide comfort measures if bone pain returns.

Teaching points
- Take this drug with a full glass of water (plain water, not mineral water), at least 30 min before or after any other beverage, food or medication; remain in an upright position for at least 30 min to decrease the GI side effects of the drug. If taking a once weekly dose, mark calendar as a reminder.
- Maintain adequate vitamin D and calcium intake while you are on this drug.
- These side effects may occur: nausea, diarrhea; bone pain, headache (analgesics may be available to help); rash (appropriate skin care will be suggested).
- Report twitching, muscle spasms, dark-colored urine, edema, bone pain, rash.

▽risperidone
*(ris **peer**' i dohn)*

Risperdal

PREGNANCY CATEGORY C

Drug classes
Antipsychotic
Benzisoxazole

Therapeutic actions
Mechanism of action not fully understood: blocks dopamine and serotonin receptors in the brain, depresses the RAS; anticholinergic, antihistaminic, and alpha-adrenergic blocking activity may contribute to some of its therapeutic and adverse actions.

Indications
- Treatment of schizophrenia
- Delaying relapse in long-term treatment of schizophrenia
- Unlabeled uses: bipolar disorder; treatment of patients with dementia-related psychotic symptoms

Contraindications and cautions
- Contraindicated with hypersensitivity to risperidone, lactation.
- Use cautiously with cardiovascular disease, pregnancy, renal or hepatic impairment, hypotension.

Available forms
Tablets—0.25, 0.5, 1, 2, 3, 4 mg; oral solution—1 mg/mL

Dosages
Adults
Initially: 1 mg PO bid; then gradually increase with daily dosage increments of 1 mg bid on the second and third days to a target dose of 3 mg PO bid by the third day. *Reinitiation of treatment:* Follow initial dosage guidelines, using extreme care due to increased risk of severe adverse effects with reexposure. Switching from other antipsychotics: minimize the overlap period and discontinue other antipsychotic before beginning risperidone therapy.

Adverse effects in *Italics* are most common; those in **Bold** are life-threatening.

Delaying relapse time in long-term treatment: 3 mg PO bid.
Pediatric patients
Safety and efficacy not established.
Geriatric patients or patients with renal or hepatic impairment
Initial dose of 0.5 mg PO bid; monitor patient for adverse effects and response.

Pharmacokinetics

Route	Onset	Peak	Duration
Oral	Varies	3–17 hr	Weeks

Metabolism: Hepatic; $T_{1/2}$: 20 hr
Distribution: Crosses placenta; enters breast milk
Excretion: Urine and feces

Adverse effects

- **CNS:** *Insomnia, anxiety, agitation, headache,* somnolence, aggression, dizziness, tardive dyskinesias
- **CV:** Orthostatic hypotension, **arrhythmias**
- **Dermatologic:** Rash, dry skin, seborrhea, photosensitivity
- **GI:** *Nausea, vomiting, constipation,* abdominal discomfort, dry mouth, increased saliva
- **Respiratory:** Rhinitis, coughing, sinusitis, pharyngitis, dyspnea
- **Other:** Chest pain, arthralgia, back pain, fever, **neuroleptic malignant syndrome**

Interactions

✻ Drug-drug • Increased therapeutic and toxic effects with clozapine • Decreased therapeutic effect with carbamazepine • Decreased effectiveness of levodopa

■ Nursing considerations
Assessment

- **History:** Allergy to risperidone, lactation, CV disease, pregnancy, renal or hepatic impairment, hypotension
- **Physical:** T, weight; reflexes, orientation; P, BP, orthostatic BP; R, adventitious sounds; bowel sounds, normal output, liver evaluation; CBC, urinalysis, liver and kidney function tests

Interventions

- Maintain seizure precautions, especially when initiating therapy and increasing dosage.

- Mix oral solution with 3–4 oz of water, coffee, orange juice, or low-fat milk. Do *not* mix with cola or tea.
- Monitor T. If fever occurs, rule out underlying infection, and consult physician for appropriate comfort measures.
- Advise patient to use contraception during drug therapy.
- Follow guidelines for discontinuation or reinstitution of the drug carefully.

Teaching points

- Dosage will be increased gradually to achieve most effective dose. Do not take more than your prescribed dosage. Do not make up missed doses; contact your health care provider if this occurs. Do not stop taking this drug suddenly; gradual reduction of dosage is needed to prevent side effects.
- Mix oral solution in 3–4 oz of water, coffee, orange juice, or low-fat milk. Do not mix with cola or tea.
- These side effects may occur: drowsiness, dizziness, sedation, seizures (avoid driving, operating machinery, or performing tasks that require concentration); dizziness, faintness on arising (change positions slowly; use caution); increased salivation (reversible); constipation; sensitivity to the sun (use a sunscreen or protective clothing).
- This drug cannot be taken during pregnancy. If you think you are pregnant or wish to become pregnant, contact your health care provider.
- Report lethargy, weakness, fever, sore throat, malaise, mouth ulcers, palpitations.

▽ ritodrine hydrochloride

See *Less Commonly Used Drugs,* p. 1350.

▽ ritonavir
*(ri **ton'** ah ver)*

Norvir

PREGNANCY CATEGORY B

Drug class
Antiretroviral

Therapeutic actions

Antiviral activity; inhibits HIV protease activity, leading to decrease in production of HIV particles.

Indications

- Treatment of HIV infection in combination with other antiretrovirals

Contraindications and cautions

- Contraindicated with allergy to ritonavir.
- Use cautiously with pregnancy, hepatic impairment, lactation.

Available forms

Capsules—100 mg; oral solution—80 mg/mL

Dosages

Adults
600 mg PO bid with food.
Pediatric patients
400 mg/m^2 PO bid; do not exceed 600 mg bid. Use in combination with other antiretrovirals.

Pharmacokinetics

Route	Onset	Peak
Oral	Rapid	2–4 hr

Metabolism: Hepatic; T$_{1/2}$: 6–8 hr
Distribution: Crosses placenta; may pass into breast milk
Excretion: Feces and urine

Adverse effects

- **CNS:** *Asthenia, peripheral and circumoral paresthesias,* anxiety, dreams, headache, dizziness, hallucinations, personality changes
- **CV:** Hemorrhage, hypotension, syncope, tachycardia
- **Dermatologic:** Acne, dry skin, contact dermatitis, rash
- **GI:** *Nausea, vomiting, diarrhea, anorexia, abdominal pain, taste perversion,* dry mouth, hepatitis, liver dysfunction, dehydration
- **GU:** Dysuria, hematuria, nocturia, pyelonephritis
- **Respiratory:** Apnea, dyspnea, cough, rhinitis
- **Other:** Hypothermia, chills, back pain, chest pain, edema, cachexia

Interactions

✳ **Drug-drug** • Potentially large increase in serum concentration of amiodarone, bepridil, bupropion, cisapride, cloxapine, ergotamine, flecainide, meperidine, piroxicam, propafenone, propoxyphene, quinidine, rifabutin; potential for serious arrhythmias, seizure, and fatal reactions; do not administer ritonavir with any of these drugs • Potentially large increases in serum concentration of these sedatives and hypnotics: alprazolam, clorazepam, diazepam, estazolam, flurazepam, midazolam, triazolam, zolpidem; extreme sedation and respiratory depression could occur; do not administer ritonavir with any of these drugs
✳ **Drug-food** • Absorption increased by presence of food; taking drug with food is strongly recommended • Decreased metabolism and risk of toxic effects if combined with grapefruit juice; avoid this combination
✳ **Drug-alternative therapy** • Decreased effectiveness if taken with St. John's wort

■ Nursing considerations

 CLINICAL ALERT!
Name confusion has been reported between Retrovir (zidovudine) and ritonavir; use caution.

Assessment

- **History:** Allergy to ritonavir, hepatic dysfunction, pregnancy, lactation
- **Physical:** T; orientation, reflexes; BP, P, peripheral perfusion; R, adventitious sounds; bowel sounds; skin color, perfusion; liver function tests

Interventions

- Capsules and oral solution should be stored in refrigerator; solution may be refrigerated or left at room temperature if used within 30 days; protect from light and extreme heat.
- Administer with meals or food to increase absorption.
- Carefully screen drug history to avoid potentially dangerous drug–drug interactions.

Teaching points

- Take this drug with meals or food; store capsules in refrigerator. Taste of solution may be improved if mixed with chocolate milk, *Ensure,* or *Advera* 1 hr before taking. Do not drink grapefruit juice while on this drug.
- Take the full course of therapy as prescribed; do not double up doses if one is missed; do not change dosage without consulting your physician. Always take in combination with your other HIV drugs.
- This drug does not cure HIV infection; long-term effects are not yet known; continue to take precautions as the risk of transmission is not reduced by this drug.
- Do not take any other drugs, prescription or OTC, without consulting your health care provider; this drug interacts with many other drugs and serious problems can occur.
- These side effects may occur: nausea, vomiting, loss of appetite, diarrhea, abdominal pain, headache, dizziness, numbness, tingling.
- Report severe diarrhea, severe nausea, personality changes, changes in color of urine or stool, fever, chills.

▽**rituximab**

See *Less Commonly Used Drugs,* p. 1350.

▽**rivastigmine tartrate**
*(riv ah **stig**' meen)*

Exelon, Exelon Oral Solution

PREGNANCY CATEGORY B

Drug classes
Cholinesterase inhibitor
Alzheimer's drug

Therapeutic actions
Centrally acting, selective, long-acting reversible cholinesterase inhibitor; causes elevated acetylcholine levels in the cortex, which slows the neuronal degradation that occurs in Alzheimer's disease.

Indications
- Treatment of mild to moderate dementia of the Alzheimer's type

- Unlabeled use: treatment of behavioral effects of Lewy-body dementia

Contraindications and cautions
- Contraindicated with hypersensitivity to rivastigmine; pregnancy, lactation.
- Use cautiously with sick sinus syndrome; GI bleeding; seizures; asthma; COPD.

Available forms
Capsules—1.5, 3, 4.5, 6 mg; oral solution with dosing syringe—2 mg/mL

Dosages
Adults
Initial dosage: 1.5 mg PO bid with food. If tolerated, may adjust to higher doses at 1.5-mg intervals every 2 wks. Usual range: 6–12 mg/day; should not exceed 12 mg/day. If dose is not tolerated, stop drug for several doses and then restart at the same or a lower level.
Pediatric patients
Safety and efficacy not established.

Pharmacokinetics

Route	Onset	Peak	Duration
Oral	Varies	6 hr	12 hr

Metabolism: Hepatic; $T_{1/2}$: 1 hr
Distribution: Crosses placenta; may pass into breast milk
Excretion: Renal

Adverse effects
- **CNS:** *Insomnia, fatigue,* dizziness, confusion, ataxia, insomnia, somnolence, tremor, agitation, depression, anxiety, abnormal thinking, syncope
- **Dermatologic:** *Rash,* flushing, purpura
- **GI:** *Nausea, vomiting, diarrhea, dyspepsia, anorexia, abdominal pain,* flatulence, constipation

Interactions
✴ **Drug-drug** • Increased effects and risk of toxicity if theophylline, cholinesterase inhibitors taken concurrently • Decreased effects of anticholinergics taken concurrently • Increased risk of GI bleeding if taken with NSAIDs

R

■ Nursing considerations
Assessment
- **History:** Allergy to rivastigmine; pregnancy, lactation; sick sinus syndrome; GI bleeding; seizures; asthma; COPD
- **Physical:** Orientation, affect, reflexes; BP, P; abdominal exam; renal and liver function tests

Interventions
- Establish baseline functional profile to follow evaluation of drug effectiveness.
- Administer with food in the morning and evening to decrease GI discomfort.
- Mix solution with water, fruit juice, or soda to improve compliance. Dosage of capsules and solution are interchangeable.
- Monitor for weight loss, diarrhea, arrhythmias prior to use and periodically with prolonged use.
- Provide small, frequent meals if GI upset is severe.
- Provide patient safety measures if CNS effects occur.
- Notify surgeons that patient is on rivastigmine, exaggerated muscle relaxation may occur if succinylcholine-type drugs are used.

Teaching points
- Take drug exactly as prescribed, take with food to decrease GI upset. Solution may be swallowed directly from the syringe or mixed in a small glass of water, cold fruit juice, or soda.
- Be aware that this drug does not cure the disease, but is thought to slow down the degeneration associated with the disease.
- Be aware that dosage changes may be needed to achieve the best drug levels.
- These side effects may occur: nausea, vomiting (small, frequent meals may help) insomnia, fatigue, confusion (use caution if driving or performing tasks that require alertness).
- Report severe nausea, vomiting, changes in stool or urine color, diarrhea, changes in neurologic functioning, palpitations.

▽**rizatriptan**
*(rib zab **trip' tan)***

Maxalt, Maxalt-MLT

PREGNANCY CATEGORY C

Drug classes
Antimigraine agent
Serotonin selective agonist

Therapeutic actions
Binds to serotonin receptors to cause vascular constrictive effects on cranial blood vessels, causing the relief of migraine in selected patients whose migraines are caused by vasodilation.

Indications
- Treatment of acute migraine attacks with or without aura

Contraindications and cautions
- Contraindicated with allergy to rizatriptan, active coronary artery disease, Printzmetal's angina, uncontrolled hypertension.
- Use cautiously with hepatic dysfunction, dialysis, pregnancy, lactation.

Available forms
Tablets—5, 10 mg; orally disintegrating tablets—5, 10 mg

Dosages
Adults
5 or 10 mg at onset of headache; may repeat in 2 hr if needed. *Maximum dose:* 30 mg/day.
Pediatric patients ≤18 yr
Safety and efficacy not established.
Patients with hepatic or renal impairment
Use lowest possible dose, monitor patient closely.

Pharmacokinetics

Route	Onset	Peak
Oral	Rapid	1 hr

Metabolism: Hepatic; $T_{1/2}$: 2 hr
Distribution: Crosses placenta; may pass into breast milk
Excretion: Urine

Adverse effects

- **CNS:** *Dizziness, vertigo, weakness, somnolence, paresthesias*
- **CV:** Blood pressure alteration
- **GI:** Dry mouth, nausea
- **Other:** *Chest/jaw/throat pressure*

Interactions

✳ Drug-drug ● Prolonged vasoactive reactions when taken concurrently with ergot-containing drugs; do not use within 24 hr of each other ● Risk of severe effects if taken with or ≤ 2 wk of discontinuation of an MAO inhibitor ● Risk of increased serum levels and toxic effects with propanolol

■ Nursing considerations
Assessment

- **History:** Allergy to rizatriptan, active coronary artery disease, Printzmetal's angina, uncontrolled hypertension, hepatic dysfunction, dialysis, pregnancy, lactation
- **Physical:** Skin color and lesions; orientation, reflexes, peripheral sensation; P, BP; renal and liver function tests

Interventions

- Administer to relieve acute migraine, not as a prophylactic measure.
- Have patient place orally disintegrating tablet on tongue and swallow with or without water.
- Establish safety measures if CNS, visual disturbances occur.
- Provide environmental control as appropriate to help relieve migraine (lighting, temperature, etc).
- Monitor BP of patients with possible coronary artery disease; discontinue at any sign of angina, prolonged high blood pressure, etc.

Teaching points

- Take drug exactly as prescribed, at the onset of headache or aura; dosage may be repeated in 2 hr if needed. Place orally disintegrating tablet on tongue and swallow with or without water.
- Be aware that this drug should not be taken during pregnancy; if you suspect that you are pregnant, contact physician and refrain from using drug.
- These side effects may occur: dizziness, drowsiness (avoid driving or the use of dangerous machinery while on this drug); numbness, tingling, feelings of tightness or pressure.
- Maintain any procedures you usually use during a migraine—controlled lighting, noise, etc.
- Contact physician immediately if you experience chest pain or pressure that is severe or does not go away.
- Report feelings of heat, flushing, tiredness, feelings of sickness, chest pain.

▽ rofecoxib
*(rob fah **cox**' bib)*

Vioxx

PREGNANCY CATEGORY C

Drug classes

NSAID (nonsteroidal anti-inflammatory drug)
Analgesic
Selective COX-2 enzyme blocker

Therapeutic actions

Analgesic and anti-inflammatory activities related to inhibition of COX-2 enzyme, which is activated in inflammation to cause the signs and symptoms associated with inflammation; does not effect the COX-1 enzyme, which protects the lining of the GI tract and has blood clotting and renal functions.

Indications

- Relief of signs and symptoms of osteoarthritis and rheumatoid arthritis
- Management of acute pain in adults
- Treatment of primary dysmenorrhea

Contraindications and cautions

- Contraindicated with allergy to celecoxib, salicylates or other NSAIDs (more common in patients with rhinitis, asthma, chronic urticaria, nasal polyps), or any component of the drug; renal impairment, pregnancy, lactation.
- Use cautiously with impaired hepatic or cardiovascular function.

Available forms

Tablets—12.5, 25, 50 mg; suspension—12.5 mg/5 mL, 25 mg/5 mL

Dosages

Adults

- *Osteoarthritis:* 12.5 mg PO daily; do not exceed 25 mg/day.
- *Rheumatoid arthritis:* 25 mg PO daily.
- *Primary dysmenorrhea and acute pain:* 50 mg PO daily. Do not use > 5 days.

Pediatric patients

Safety and efficacy not established.

Pharmacokinetics

Route	Onset	Peak
Oral	45 min	2–3 hr

Metabolism: Hepatic; $T_{1/2}$: 17 hr
Distribution: Crosses placenta; may pass into breast milk
Excretion: Urine

Adverse effects

- **CNS:** *Headache, dizziness, somnolence, insomnia,* fatigue, tiredness, dizziness, tinnitus, ophthamological effects
- **Dermatologic:** *Rash,* pruritus, sweating, dry mucous membranes, stomatitis
- **Hematologic:** Bleeding, leukopenia, pancytopenia, thrombocytopenia, agranulocytosis, granulocytopenia, decreased hemoglobin or hematocrit, bone marrow depression, menorrhagia
- **Respiratory:** Dyspnea, hemoptysis, pharyngitis, bronchospasm, rhinitis
- **Other:** Peripheral edema, **anaphylactoid reactions to fatal anaphylactic shock**

Interactions

✳ **Drug-drug** • Increased risk of bleeding with warfarin, monitor patient closely • Possible increased risk of lithium toxicity, monitor serum levels and adjust dosage appropriately

■ Nursing considerations

CLINICAL ALERT!
Name confusion has occurred between Vioxx (rofecoxib) and Zyvox (linezolid); use caution.

Assessment

- **History:** Allergy to celecoxib, salicylates or other NSAIDs, or any component of the drug; renal impairment, pregnancy, lactation, impaired hepatic or cardiovascular function
- **Physical:** Skin color, lesions;T; orientation, reflexes, audiometric evaluation, peripheral sensation; P, BP, edema; R, adventitious sounds; liver evaluation, CBC, clotting times, liver function tests

Interventions

- Administer drug with food or after meals if GI upset occurs.
- Establish safety measures if CNS, visual disturbances occur.
- Arrange for periodic ophthalmologic examination during long-term therapy.
- Institute emergency procedures if overdose occurs—gastric lavage, induction of emesis, supportive therapy.
- Provide further comfort measures to reduce pain (positioning, environmental control, etc) and inflammation (warmth, positioning, rest, etc).

Teaching points

- Take the drug with food or after meals if GI upset occurs.
- Do not exceed the prescribed dosage.
- These side effects may occur: drowsiness, dizziness, vertigo, insomnia (use caution when driving or operating dangerous machinery if these occur).
- Report sore throat, fever, rash, itching, weight gain, swelling in ankles or fingers, changes in vision.

▽**ropinirole hydrochloride**

*(row **pin'** ah roll)*

Requip

PREGNANCY CATEGORY C

Drug classes

Antiparkinsonian agent
Dopamine receptor agonist

Adverse effects in *Italics* are most common; those in **Bold** are life-threatening.

Therapeutic actions

Acts as a non-ergot dopamine agonist acting directly on postsynaptic dopamine receptors of neurons in the brain, mimicking the effects of the neurotransmitter dopamine, which is thought to be deficient in parkinsonism.

Indications

- Treatment of idiopathic Parkinson's disease in the early stages as well as in the late stages when used in combination with levodopa

Contraindications and cautions

- Contraindicated with hypersensitivity to ropinirole, severe ischemic heart disease or peripheral vascular disease, pregnancy, lactation.
- Use cautiously with dyskinesia, orthostatic hypotension, hepatic or renal impairment.

Available forms

Tablets—0.25, 0.5, 1, 2, 5 mg

Dosages
Adults

Initially 0.25 mg PO tid for 1st wk; 0.5 mg PO tid for 2nd wk; 0.75 mg PO tid for 3rd wk; 1 mg PO tid for 4th wk. May increase by 1.5 mg/day at 1-wk intervals to 9 mg/day, then by up to 3 mg/day at 1-wk intervals to a maximum dose of 24 mg/day.

Pediatric patients

Safety and efficacy not established.

Geriatric patients

Elderly are at higher risk for development of hallucinations; monitor closely and adjust dosage more slowly.

Pharmacokinetics

Route	Onset	Peak	Duration
Oral	Varies	1–2 hr	8 hr

Metabolism: Hepatic; $T_{1/2}$: 6 hr
Distribution: Crosses placenta; enters breast milk
Excretion: Urine

Adverse effects

- **CNS:** *Dizziness, somnolence, insomnia, hypo- or hyperkinesia,* syncope, asthenia, confusion, hallucinations (more common in the elderly), abnormal vision, tremor, anxiety, paresthesias, aggravated parkinsonism
- **CV:** *Orthostatic hypotension*, edema
- **GI:** *Nausea, constipation*
- **Other:** Fatigue, infections, sweating, pharyngitis, pain, arthralgia

Interactions

✳ **Drug-drug** • Increased effects of levodopa; consider decreasing levodopa dose • Increased CNS depression with alcohol, CNS depressants • Monitor and adjust ropinirole dose if estrogen is added to or discontinued from regimen • Increased effects with ciprofloxacin

■ Nursing considerations
Assessment

- **History:** Hypersensitivity to ropinirole, severe ischemic heart disease or peripheral vascular disease, pregnancy, lactation, dyskinesia, orthostatic hypotension, hepatic or renal impairment
- **Physical:** Skin temperature, color, lesions; orientation, affect, reflexes, bilateral grip strength; vision exam including visual fields; P, BP, orthostatic BP, auscultation; liver evaluation; liver and kidney function tests

Interventions

- Administer drug with food if GI upset becomes a problem.
- Monitor patient for orthostatic hypotension and establish safety precautions if necessary (siderails, accompanying patient, etc).
- Withdraw gradually over 1 wk to avoid serious adverse effects.
- Monitor patient carefully and adjust dose more slowly if patient has hypotension or dyskinesias.
- Monitor elderly patients for the development of hallucinations; provide appropriate safety measures as needed.
- Start adjustment of drug over again if drug has been discontinued and is being restarted.
- Monitor hepatic and renal function periodically during therapy.

Teaching points

- Take this drug exactly as prescribed; take with food if GI upset occurs. Dosage will change gradually over several weeks.

R

- Do not discontinue this drug without first consulting with your health care provider; drug must be stopped gradually to prevent serious adverse effects.
- These side effects may occur: drowsiness, dizziness, confusion (avoid driving or engaging in activities that require alertness); nausea (take drug with meals; eat small, frequent meals); dizziness or faintness when you get up (change position slowly, exercise caution when climbing stairs); headache, nasal stuffiness (inform your nurse or physician; it may be possible to have a medication for these).
- Report fainting, light-headedness, dizziness; black, tarry stools; hallucinations.

▽rosiglitazone maleate
*(roh zee **glit**' ah zohn)*

Avandia

PREGNANCY CATEGORY C

Drug classes
Antidiabetic agent
Thiazolidinedione

Therapeutic actions
Resensitizes tissues to insulin; stimulates insulin receptor sites to lower blood glucose and improve the action of insulin; decreases hepatic gluconeogenesis and increases insulin-dependent muscle glucose uptake.

Indications
- Monotherapy as an adjunct to diet and exercise to improve glucose control in patients with type 2 diabetes
- As part of combination with metformin or a sulfonylurea when diet, exercise, and either agent alone does not result in adequate glycemic control in type 2 diabetes, not to be combined with insulin

Contraindications and cautions
- Contraindicated with allergy to any thiazolidinedione; type 1 or juvenile diabetes, ketoacidosis, lactation.

- Use cautiously with advanced heart disease, liver failure, pregnancy.

Available forms
Tablets—2, 4, 8 mg

Dosages
Adults
4 mg as a single oral dose or divided into two doses; if adequate response is not seen in 8–12 wk, may be increased to 8 mg daily PO.
- *Combination therapy with metformin:* 4 mg daily PO added to the established dose of metformin; may be increased after 12 wk to 8 mg daily PO. Do not give in combination with insulin.
Pediatric patients
Safety and efficacy not established.
Patients with hepatic impairment
Use caution and monitor patient closely. Do not administer if AST > 2.5 times the upper level of normal.

Pharmacokinetics

Route	Onset	Peak
Oral	Rapid	1.3–3.5 hr

Metabolism: Hepatic; $T_{1/2}$: 3–4 hr
Distribution: Crosses placenta; passes into breast milk
Excretion: Urine, feces

Adverse effects
- **CNS:** *Headache, pain*
- **Endocrine: Hypoglycemia, hyperglycemia**
- **GI:** Diarrhea, **liver injury**
- **Respiratory:** Sinusitis, URI, rhinitis
- **Other:** *Infections, fatigue, accidental injury*

Interactions
✳ **Drug-drug** • Decreased effectiveness of hormonal contraceptives, which may result in ovulation and risk of pregnancy. Suggest the use of an alternative method of birth control or consider a higher dose of contraceptive
- Increased risk of hypoglycemia and severe reactions with insulin; avoid this combination

Adverse effects in *Italics* are most common; those in **Bold** are life-threatening.

■ Nursing considerations
Assessment
- **History:** Allergy to any thiazolidinedione; type 1 or juvenile diabetes, ketoacidosis, serious hepatic impairment, advanced heart disease, pregnancy, lactation
- **Physical:** T; orientation, reflexes, peripheral sensation; R, adventitious sounds; liver evaluation; liver function tests, blood glucose, CBC

Interventions
- Monitor urine or serum glucose levels frequently to determine effectiveness of drug and dosage being used.
- Monitor baseline liver function tests before beginning therapy and periodically during therapy.
- Administer without regard to meals.
- Arrange for consult with dietitian to establish weight loss program and dietary control as appropriate.
- Arrange for thorough diabetic teaching program to include disease, dietary control, exercise, signs and symptoms of hypo- and hyperglycemia, avoidance of infection, hygiene.

Teaching points
- Do not discontinue this medication without consulting health care provider; continue with diet and exercise program for diabetes control.
- Take this drug with meals if desired. If dose is missed, it may be taken at the next meal. If dose is missed for an entire day, do not double dose the next day.
- Monitor urine or blood for glucose and ketones as prescribed; watch very closely while adjusting to drug.
- Use barrier contraceptives if currently using hormonal contraceptives; these drugs may be ineffective if combined with rosiglitazone.
- Report fever, sore throat, unusual bleeding or bruising, rash, dark urine, light-colored stools, hypo- or hyperglycemic reactions.

▽ sacrosidase

See *Less Commonly Used Drugs*, p. 1350.

▽ saliva substitute
(*sa lie' vah*)

Entertainer's Secret, Moi-Stir, Moi-Stir Swabsticks, MouthKote, Optimoist, Salivart, Salix

PREGNANCY CATEGORY UNKNOWN

Drug class
Saliva substitute

Therapeutic actions
Contains electrolytes and carboxymethylcellulose as a thickening agent to serve as a substitute for saliva in dry mouth syndromes.

Indications
- Management of dry mouth and throat in xerostomia and hyposalivation caused by stroke, medications, radiation therapy, chemotherapy, other illnesses

Contraindications and cautions
- Contraindicated with hypersensitivity to carboxymethylcellulose, parabens, components of the preparation.
- Use cautiously with renal failure, CHF, hypertension.

Available forms
Solution; lozenges; swab sticks

Dosages
Adults
Spray or apply to oral mucosa.
Pediatric patients
Safety and efficacy not established.

Pharmacokinetics
No general systemic absorption. Electrolytes may be absorbed and dealt with in normal electrolyte pathways.

Adverse effects
Other: Excessive absorption of electrolytes (elevated magnesium, sodium, potassium)

■ Nursing considerations
Assessment
- **History:** Allergy to carboxymethylcellulose, parabens, CHF, hypertension, renal failure

- **Physical:** BP, P, auscultation, edema; renal function tests; mucosa evaluation

Interventions
- Give for dry mouth and throat.
- Have patient try to swish saliva substitute around mouth following application.
- Monitor patient while eating; swallowing may be impaired and additional therapy required.

Teaching points
- Apply the drug as instructed; swish it around in your mouth after application.
- Use as needed for dry mouth and throat.
- Take care when eating because swallowing may be difficult; additional therapy may be needed.
- Report swelling, headache, irregular heart beat, leg cramps, failure to relieve discomfort of dry mouth and throat.

▷ salmeterol
(sal mee' ter ol)

Serevent, Serevent Diskus

PREGNANCY CATEGORY C

Drug classes
Beta₂-selective adrenergic agonist
Antasthmatic agent

Therapeutic actions
Long-acting agonist that binds to beta₂ receptors in the lungs, causing bronchodilation; also inhibits the release of inflammatory mediators in the lung, blocking swelling and inflammation.

Indications
- Prevention of and maintenance therapy for bronchospasm in select patients with asthma, chronic obstructive pulmonary disease, and exercise-induced asthma

Contraindications and cautions
- Contraindicated with hypersensitivity to salmeterol, acute asthma attack, worsening or

deteriorating asthma (life-threatening), acute airway obstruction.
- Use cautiously with pregnancy, lactation.

Available forms
Aerosol—mcg/actuation; inhalation powder—50 mcg (*Serevent Diskus*)

Dosages
Adults and patients ≥ 12 yr
- *Asthma or bronchospasm:* Aerosol: 2 inhalations (42 mcg) bid 12 hr apart; inhalation powder: 1 inhalation (50 mcg) bid.
- *Exercise-induced asthma:* Aerosol: 2 inhalations 30–60 min before exertion; inhalation powder: 1 inhalation 30–60 min before exertion.
- *COPD:* Aerosol: 2 inhalations bid 12 hr apart; inhalation powder: 1 inhalation bid.
Pediatric patients 4–12 yr
- *Serevent Diskus:* 1 inhalation bid, 12 hr apart; if used to prevent exercise-induced asthma, 1 inhalation ≥ 30 min before exercising.

Pharmacokinetics
Route	Onset	Peak	Duration
Inhalation	13–20 min	3–4 hr	7.5–17 hr

Metabolism: Hepatic; $T_{1/2}$: unknown
Distribution: Crosses placenta; may enter breast milk
Excretion: Feces

Adverse effects
- **CNS:** *Headache, tremor*
- **CV:** *Tachycardia, palpitations,* hypertension
- **Respiratory:** Worsening of asthma, difficulty breathing, bronchospasm

Interactions
✳ **Drug-drug** ● Risk of severe bronchospasm if combined with beta-blockers; use a cardioselective beta-blocker and monitor patient closely if this combination is used ● Potential for worsened hypokalemia and ECG abnormalities if combined with diuretics; monitor patient very closely ● Administer with extreme caution to patients being treated with MAOIs or TCAs, or within 2 wk of discontinuation of

Adverse effects in *Italics* are most common; those in **Bold** are life-threatening.

such agents because the action of salmeterol may be potentiated by these agents

■ Nursing considerations
Assessment
- **History:** Allergy to salmeterol; pregnancy, acute asthma attack, worsening asthma, lactation
- **Physical:** R, adventitious sounds; P, BP, EKG; orientation, reflexes; liver function tests

Interventions
- Ensure that drug is not used to treat acute asthma or with worsening or deteriorating asthma (risk of death).
- Use aerosol for adults and children ≥ 12 yr; use powder for inhalation (*Serevent Diskus*) for children 4–12 yr.
- Instruct in the proper use of metered inhaler.
- Monitor use of inhaler; use of more than 4 puffs/day may worsen asthma; obtain evaluation by physician.
- Have patients who experience exercise-induced asthma use it 30–60 min before activity.
- Arrange for periodic evaluation of respiratory condition.

Teaching points
- Use the pressurized metered-dose inhaler as instructed. Shake well before using. Use only twice a day. If drug is to be used periodically for exercise-induced asthma, use 30–60 min before activity.
- To gain full therapeutic benefit in the treatment of reversible airway obstruction, administer twice a day (morning and evening).
- Obtain periodic evaluations of your respiratory problem.
- These side effects may occur: headache (request analgesics); tremors (use care in performing dangerous tasks); fast heart, palpitations (monitor activity; rest frequently).
- Report severe headache, irregular heartbeat, worsening of asthma, difficulty breathing.

▽ salsalate (salicylsalicylic acid)
(sal' sa late)

Amigesic, Argesic-SA, Artha-G, Disalcid, Marthritic, Mono-Gesic, Persistin, Salflex, Salsitab

PREGNANCY CATEGORY C

Drug classes
Antipyretic
Analgesic (non-narcotic)
Anti-inflammatory agent
Antirheumatic
Salicylate
Nonsteroidal anti-inflammatory drug (NSAID)

Therapeutic actions
Analgesic and antirheumatic effects are attributable to the ability to inhibit the synthesis of prostaglandins, important mediators of inflammation; antipyretic effects are not fully understood, but salicylates probably act in the thermoregulatory center of the hypothalamus to block the effects of endogenous pyrogen by inhibiting the synthesis of the prostaglandin intermediary; after absorption, this drug is hydrolyzed into two molecules of salicylic acid; insoluble in gastric secretions, it is not absorbed in the stomach, but in the small intestine; reported to cause fewer GI adverse effects than aspirin.

Indications
- Relief of mild to moderate pain
- Reduction of fever
- Relief of symptoms of various inflammatory conditions—rheumatic fever, rheumatoid arthritis, osteoarthritis

Contraindications and cautions
- Allergy to salicylates or NSAIDs, bleeding disorders, impaired hepatic or renal function, GI ulceration (less of a problem than with other anti-inflammatories), lactation, pregnancy.
- Use of salicylates in children and teenagers with influenza or chickenpox may be associated with the development of Reye's syndrome. This acute, life-threatening condition, characterized by vomiting, lethargy, and belligerence, may progress to delirium

S

and coma and has a mortality rate of 20%–30%.

Available forms

Capsules—500 mg; tablets—500, 750 mg

Dosages
Adults
3,000 mg/day PO given in divided doses.
Pediatric patients
Safety and efficacy not established.

Pharmacokinetics

Route	Onset	Peak	Duration
Oral	10–30 min	1–3 hr	3–6 hr

Metabolism: Hepatic; $T_{1/2}$: 2–3 hr (15–30 hr with large doses over extended periods)
Distribution: Crosses placenta; enters breast milk
Excretion: Urine

Adverse effects

- **Acute salicylate toxicity:** Respiratory alkalosis, hyperpnea, tachypnea, hemorrhage, excitement, confusion, asterixis, pulmonary edema, convulsions, tetany, metabolic acidosis, fever, coma, **CV collapse, renal and respiratory failure**
- **CNS:** *Headache, dizziness, somnolence, insomnia,* fatigue, tiredness, dizziness, tinnitus, ophthalmologic effects
- **Dermatologic:** *Rash,* pruritus, sweating, dry mucous membranes, stomatitis
- **GI:** *Nausea, dyspepsia, GI pain,* diarrhea, vomiting, *constipation,* flatulence
- **GU:** Dysuria, renal impairment
- **Hematologic:** Bleeding, platelet inhibition with higher doses, neutropenia, eosinophilia, leukopenia, pancytopenia, thrombocytopenia, agranulocytosis, granulocytopenia, aplastic anemia, decreased Hgb or Hct, bone marrow depression, menorrhagia
- **Respiratory:** Dyspnea, hemoptysis, pharyngitis, bronchospasm, rhinitis
- **Salicylism:** Dizziness, tinnitus, difficulty hearing, nausea, vomiting, diarrhea, mental confusion, lassitude (dose related)
- **Other:** Peripheral edema, **anaphylactoid reactions to anaphylactic shock**

Interactions

✴ **Drug-drug** • Increased risk of GI ulceration with corticosteroids and alcohol • Increased risk of salicylate toxicity with carbonic anhydrase inhibitors • Increased toxicity of carbonic anhydrase inhibitors, valproic acid • Decreased serum salicylate levels with corticosteroids, antacids, urine alkalinizers (sodium acetate, sodium bicarbonate, sodium citrate, sodium lactate, tromethamine) • Increased methotrexate levels and toxicity • Greater glucose-lowering effect of sulfonylureas, insulin with large doses of salicylates • Decreased uricosuric effect of probenecid, sulfinpyrazone • Decreased diuretic effect of spironolactone

✴ **Drug-lab test** • Salicylate competes with thyroid hormone for binding to plasma proteins, which may be reflected in a depressed plasma T_4 value • False-negative readings for urine glucose by glucose oxidase method and copper reduction method • Interference with urine 5-HIAA determinations by fluorescent methods but not by nitrosonaphthol colorimetric method • Interference with urinary ketone determination by ferric chloride method • Falsely elevated urine VMA levels with most tests; false decrease in VMA using the Pisano method • Serum uric acid levels are elevated by salicylate levels < 10 mg/dL and decreased by levels > 10 mg/dL

■ Nursing considerations
Assessment

- **History:** Allergy to salicylates or NSAIDs; bleeding disorders, impaired hepatic or renal function, GI ulceration, lactation, pregnancy
- **Physical:** Skin color and lesions; eighth cranial nerve function, orientation, reflexes, affect; P, BP, perfusion; R, adventitious sounds; liver evaluation and bowel sounds; CBC, urinalysis, stool guiaiac, renal and liver function tests

Interventions

- Administer drug with food or after meals if GI upset occurs.
- Administer drug with a full glass of water to reduce risk of tablet or capsule lodging in the esophagus.

Adverse effects in *Italics* are most common; those in **Bold** are life-threatening.

- Institute emergency procedures if overdose occurs: gastric lavage, induction of emesis, activated charcoal, supportive therapy.
- Provide further comfort measures to reduce pain, fever, and inflammation.

Teaching points
- Take the drug with food or after meals if GI upset occurs.
- Report ringing in the ears, dizziness, confusion, abdominal pain, rapid or difficult breathing, nausea, vomiting.

▽ saquinavir
(sa kwen' a veer)

saquinavir
Fortovase

saquinavir mesylate
Invirase

PREGNANCY CATEGORY B

Drug class
Antiviral

Therapeutic actions
Protease inhibitor which in combination with nucleoside analogues is effective in HIV infections with changes in surrogate markers.

Indications
- Treatment of HIV infection in combination with other antiretroviral agents

Contraindications and cautions
- Contraindicated with life-threatening allergy to any component.
- Use cautiously with hepatic impairment, pregnancy, lactation, hemophilia.

Available forms
Capsules—200 mg (mesylate); soft gel capsules—200 mg

Dosages
Adults and patients > 16 yr
Fortovase: Six 200 mg capsules tid within 2 hr after a meal and in combination with a nucleoside analog. *Invirase (mesylate):* Three 200-mg capsules tid within 2 hr after a meal and in combination with a nucleoside analog.
Pediatric patients < 16 yr
Safety and efficacy not established.
Patients with hepatic impairment
Reduce dose and monitor hepatic function tests.

Pharmacokinetics

Route	Onset	Peak
Oral	Slow	Unknown

Metabolism: Hepatic; $T_{1/2}$: unknown
Distribution: May cross placenta; may pass into breast milk
Excretion: Feces

Adverse effects
- **CNS:** *Headache,* insomnia, myalgia, *asthenia,* malaise, dizziness, paresthesia, fatigue
- **GI:** *Nausea, GI pain, diarrhea,* anorexia, vomiting, dyspepsia
- **Other:** *Asthenia, elevated CPK*

Interactions
✳ **Drug-drug** • Decreased effectiveness with rifampin, rifabutin, phenobarbital, phenytoin, dexamethasone, carbamazepine, nevirapine • Increased saquinavir plasma concentrations with clarithromycin, indinavir, ritonavir, nelfinavir, delavirdine, ketoconazole • Increased sildenafil concentrations when coadministered with saquinavir • Potential for serious to life-threatening reactions with cisapride, ergot derivatives, midazolam, triazolam • Risk of serious hepatic toxicity if combined with HMG-CoA inhibitors (statins); avoid this combination and, if use is required, monitor liver function tests regularly
✳ **Drug-food** • Decreased metabolism and risk of toxic effects if combined with grapefruit juice; avoid this combination
✳ **Drug-alternative therapy** • Decreased effectiveness if combined with St. John's wort

■ Nursing considerations

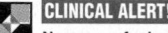 **CLINICAL ALERT!**
Name confusion has occurred between Invirase (saquinavir) and Inversine (mecamylamine); use caution.

S

Assessment

- **History:** Life-threatening allergy to any component; impaired hepatic function, pregnancy, lactation
- **Physical:** T; affect, reflexes, peripheral sensation; bowel sounds, liver evaluation; liver function tests, CPK levels

Interventions

- Administer within 2 hours after a full meal.
- Monitor patient for signs of opportunistic infections that will need to be treated appropriately.
- Administer the drug concurrently with a nucleoside analog.
- Check drug carefully; mesylate capsules and soft-gel capsules are not interchangeable.
- Offer support and encouragement to the patient to deal with the diagnosis as well as the effects of drug therapy and the high expense of treatment.

Teaching points

- Take drug as prescribed; take within 2 hours of a full meal; take concurrently with other prescribed medication. Do not drink grapefruit juice while on this drug.
- Store drug in refrigerator; use by expiration date.
- These drugs are not a cure for AIDS or ARC; opportunistic infections may occur and regular medical care should be sought to deal with the disease.
- The long-term effects of this drug are not yet known.
- These side effects may occur: nausea, loss of appetite, change in taste (small, frequent meals may help); dizziness, loss of feeling (take appropriate precautions).
- This drug combination does not reduce the risk of transmission of HIV to others by sexual contact or blood contamination—use appropriate precautions.
- Report extreme fatigue, lethargy, severe headache, severe nausea, vomiting, difficulty breathing, rash, changes in color of urine or stool.

▽**sargramostim (granulocyte macrophage colony–stimulating factor, GM-CSF)**
*(sar **gram'** ob stim)*

Leukine

PREGNANCY CATEGORY C

Drug class
Colony-stimulating factor

Therapeutic actions
Human GM-CSF produced by recombinant DNA technology; increases the proliferation and differentiation of hematopoietic progenitor cells; can activate mature granulocytes and macrophages.

Indications

- Myeloid reconstitution after autologous bone marrow transplantation
- Treatment of neutropenia associated with bone marrow transplantation failure or engraftment delay
- Induction chemotherapy in AML to shorten neutrophil recovery time
- Acceleration of myeloid recovery in patients with non-Hodgkin's lymphoma, acute lymphoblastic leukemia, and Hodgkin's disease undergoing autologous bone marrow transplantation
- Mobilization of hematopoetic progenitor cells for collection by leukapheresis and to accelerate myeloid reconstitution following PBPC transplantation
- Unlabeled uses: treatment of myelodysplastic syndrome, decreases nadir of leukopenia related to myelosuppression of chemotherapy, corrects neutropenia in aplastic anemia patients, decreases transplant-associated organ system damage, promotes early grafting

Contraindications and cautions

- Contraindicated with hypersensitivity to yeast products, excessive leukemic myeloid blasts in bone marrow or peripheral blood, pregnancy.

- Use cautiously with renal or hepatic failure, lactation; concomitant use with chemotherapy and radiotherapy or within 24 hours preceding or following chemotherapy or radiotherapy.

- Benzyl alcohol is a constituent of leukine liquid and bacteriostatic water for injection diluent and should not be administered to neonates because of association with fatal "gasping syndrome."

Available forms

Powder for injection—250 mcg; liquid—500 mcg/mL

Dosages
Adults

- *Myeloid reconstitution after autologous bone marrow transplantation:* 250 mcg/m²/day for 21 days as a 2-hr IV infusion beginning 2–4 hr after the autologous bone marrow infusion and not less than 24 hr after the last dose of chemotherapy and 12 hr after last dose of radiotherapy.

- *Bone marrow transplantation failure or engraftment delay:* 250 mcg/m²/day for 14 days as a 2-hr IV infusion; the dose can be repeated after 7 days off therapy if engraftment has not occurred.

- *Neutrophil recovery following chemotherapy in AML:* 250 mcg/m²/day IV over 4 hr starting on day 11 or 4 days after chemotherapy induction.

- *Mobilization of PBPC:* 250 mcg/m²/day IV over 24 hr or SC daily; continue throughout harvesting.

- *Post-PBPC transplant:* 250 mcg/m²/day IV over 24 hr or SC daily beginning immediately after infusion of progenitor cells.

Pediatric patients

Safety and efficacy not established.

Pharmacokinetics

Route	Peak	Duration
IV	2 hr	6 hr
SC	1–3 hr	12 hr

Metabolism: Unknown; $T_{1/2}$ (IV): 11 min, then 1.6 hr; $T_{1/2}$ (SC): 2.6 hr

Distribution: Crosses placenta; may enter breast milk

▼ IV facts

Preparation: Reconstitute with 1 mL sterile water for injection; gently swirl contents to avoid foaming; do not shake, and avoid excessive agitation. Resulting solution should be clear, colorless, and isotonic. Do not reenter vial; discard any unused portion. Dilute in 0.9% sodium chloride injection; administer within 6 hr; refrigerate until ready to use.

Infusion: Infuse over 2 hr; do not use an in-line membrane filter; do not mix with any other medication or in any other diluent.

Incompatibilities: Do not mix with any solution other than 0.9% sodium chloride. Do not add to any other medications.

Adverse effects

- **CNS:** Headache, *fever*, generalized weakness, fatigue, *malaise, asthenia*
- **CV:** Edema
- **Dermatologic:** *Alopecia*, rash, mucositis
- **GI:** *Nausea, vomiting*, stomatitis, anorexia, *diarrhea*, constipation
- **Other:** *Bone pain*, generalized pain, sore throat, cough

Interactions

✱ **Drug-drug** • Drugs that may potentiate the myeloproliferative effects of sargramostim, such as lithium and corticosteroids, should be used with caution

■ Nursing considerations
Assessment

- **History:** Hypersensitivity to yeast products; pregnancy, lactation, excessive leukemic myeloid blasts in bone marrow or peripheral blood, renal or hepatic failure
- **Physical:** Skin color, lesions, hair; T; abdominal exam, status of mucous membranes; CBC, platelets, body weight and hydration status

Interventions

- Obtain CBC and platelet count prior to and twice weekly during therapy.
- Administer no less than 24 hr after cytotoxic chemotherapy and within 2–4 hr of bone marrow infusion.
- Administer daily as a 2-hr infusion.
- Store in refrigerator; allow to warm to room temperature before use; if vial is at room temperature for > 6 hr, discard. Use each

vial for one dose; do not reenter the vial; discard any unused drug.
- Do not shake vial before use.

Teaching points
- This drug must be given for as long as needed.
- Avoid exposure to infection (avoid crowds, visitors with infections).
- These side effects may occur: nausea and vomiting (eat small, frequent meals); loss of hair (obtain appropriate head covering; cover head in temperature extremes); fever (request medication).
- This drug should not be taken during pregnancy; use of barrier contraceptives is advised.
- Frequent blood tests will be needed to evaluate drug effects.
- Report fever, chills, sore throat, weakness, pain or swelling at injection site, difficulty breathing, chills.

▷ scopolamine hydrobromide (hyoscine HBr)
*(skoe **pol**' a meen)*

Oral, Parenteral: Scopace, Scopolamine HBr
Transdermal system: Transderm-Scop
Ophthalmic solution: Isopto Hyoscine Ophthalmic

PREGNANCY CATEGORY C

Drug classes
Anticholinergic
Antiemetic
Antimuscarinic agent
Antiparkonsonian agent
Antispasmodic
Parasympatholytic
Anti-motion sickness agent
Belladonna alkaloid

Therapeutic actions
Mechanism of action as antimotion sickness drug not understood; antiemetic action may be mediated by interference with cholinergic impulses to the vomiting center (CTZ); has sedative and amnesia-inducing properties; blocks the effects of acetylcholine at muscarinic cholinergic receptors that mediate the effects of parasympathetic postganglionic impulses, thus depressing salivary and bronchial secretions, inhibiting vagal influences on the heart, relaxing the GI and GU tracts, inhibiting gastric acid secretion, relaxing the pupil of the eye (mydriatic effect), and preventing accommodation for near vision (cycloplegic effect).

Indications
- Prevention and control of nausea and vomiting due to motion sickness and recovery from surgery (transdermal system)
- Adjunctive therapy with antacids and H_2 antihistamines in peptic ulcer supportive treatment of functional GI disorders (diarrhea, pylorospasm, hypermotility, irritable bowel syndrome, spastic colon, acute enterocolitis, pancreatitis, infant colic)
- Treatment of biliary colic with narcotic analgesic
- Relief of urinary frequency and urgency, nocturnal enuresis, and ureteral colic (in conjunction with a narcotic analgesic)
- Suppression of vagally mediated bradycardia
- Preanesthetic medication to control bronchial, nasal, pharyngeal, and salivary secretions; prevent bronchospasm and laryngospasm; block cardiac vagal inhibitory reflexes during induction of anesthesia and intubation; produce sedation
- Induction of obstetric amnesia with analgesics calming delirium
- Treatment of postencephalitic parkinsonism and paralysis agitans; relief of symptoms in spastic states
Ophthalmic solution
- Diagnostically to produce mydriasis and cycloplegia
- Preoperative and postoperative states in the treatment of iridocyclitis

Contraindications and cautions
- Contraindicated with hypersensitivity to anticholinergic drugs; glaucoma; adhesions between iris and lens; stenosing peptic ul-

cer, pyloroduodenal obstruction, paralytic ileus, intestinal atony, severe ulcerative colitis, toxic megacolon, symptomatic prostatic hypertrophy, bladder neck obstruction, bronchial asthma, COPD, cardiac arrhythmias, tachycardia, myocardial ischemia; impaired metabolic, liver, or kidney function (increased likelihood of adverse CNS effects); myasthenia gravis, pregnancy (causes respiratory depression in neonates, contributes to neonatal hemorrhage); lactation.

- Use cautiously with Down syndrome, brain damage, spasticity, hypertension, hyperthyroidism; glaucoma or tendency to glaucoma (ophthalmic solution).

Available forms

Tablets—0.4 mg; injection—0.3, 0.4, 0.86, 1 mg/mL; transdermal system—1.5 mg; ophthalmic solution—0.25%

Dosages
Adults
Oral
0.4–0.8 mg PO daily; may be increased with caution.
Transdermal
- *Motion sickness:* Apply one transdermal system to the postauricular skin at least 4 hr before antiemetic effect is required. Scopolamine 1 mg will be delivered over 3 days. If continued effect is needed, replace system every 3 days.
Parenteral
0.32–0.65 mg SC or IM. May give IV after dilution in sterile water for injection. May repeat if necessary up to 3–4 times daily.
Ophthalmic solution
- *Refraction:* Instill 1–2 drops into the eye(s) 1 hr before refracting.
- *Uveitis:* Instill 1–2 drops into the eye(s) up to qid.
Pediatric patients
Do not use oral scopolamine in children < 6 yr unless directed by physician. Do not use transdermal system in children.
- *Parenteral:* 0.006 mg/kg SC, IM, or IV; maximum dose is 0.3 mg.
Geriatric patients
More likely to cause serious adverse reactions, especially CNS reactions.

Pharmacokinetics

Route	Onset	Peak	Duration
Oral	Unknown	1 hr	8–10 hr
IM, SC	30 min	60 min	4–6 hr
IV	10 min	60 min	2–4 hr
Transdermal	4–5 hr	24 hr	72 hr
Ophthalmic	10–20 min	30–45 min	Days

Metabolism: Hepatic; $T_{1/2}$: 8 hr
Distribution: Crosses placenta; enters breast milk
Excretion: Urine

▼ IV facts
Preparation: Dilute in sterile water for injection.
Infusion: Inject directly into vein or into tubing of actively running IV; inject slowly over 5–10 min.

Adverse effects
- **CNS:** *Pupil dilation, photophobia, blurred vision, headache, drowsiness,* dizziness, mental confusion, excitement, restlessness, hallucinations, delirium in the presence of pain
- **CV:** Palpitations, tachycardia
- **GI:** *Dry mouth, constipation,* paralytic ileus, altered taste perception, nausea, vomiting, dysphagia, heartburn
- **GU:** *Urinary hesitancy and retention,* impotence
- **Hypersensitivity: Anaphylaxis,** urticaria, other dermatologic effects
- **Other:** Suppression of lactation, flushing, fever, *nasal congestion, decreased sweating*

Interactions
✳ Drug-drug • Decreased antipsychotic effectiveness of haloperidol • Decreased effectiveness of phenothiazines, but increased incidence of paralytic ileus • Increased CNS depression with alcohol

■ Nursing considerations
Assessment
- **History:** Hypersensitivity to anticholinergic drugs; glaucoma; adhesions between iris and lens; stenosing peptic ulcer, pyloroduodenal obstruction, intestinal atony, severe ulcerative colitis, symptomatic prostatic hypertrophy, bladder neck obstruction,

S

bronchial asthma, COPD, cardiac arrhythmias, myocardial ischemia; impaired metabolic, liver, or kidney function; myasthenia gravis; Down syndrome, brain damage, spasticity; hypertension, hyperthyroidism; pregnancy; lactation

- **Physical:** Skin color, lesions, texture; T; orientation, reflexes, bilateral grip strength; affect; ophthalmic exam; P, BP; R, adventitious sounds; bowel sounds, normal output; urinary output, prostate palpation; liver and kidney function tests, ECG

Interventions

- Ensure adequate hydration; provide environmental control (temperature) to prevent hyperpyrexia.

Teaching points

- Take as prescribed, 30–60 min before meals. Avoid excessive dosage.
- Avoid hot environments. You will be heat intolerant, and dangerous reactions may occur.
- These side effects may occur: dizziness, sedation, drowsiness (use caution driving or performing tasks that require alertness); constipation (ensure adequate fluid intake, proper diet); dry mouth (sugarless lozenges, frequent mouth care may help; may lessen); blurred vision, sensitivity to light (reversible, avoid tasks that require acute vision; wear sunglasses); impotence (reversible); difficulty urinating (empty bladder before taking drug).
- Avoid alcohol; serious sedation could occur.
- When using transdermal system, take care to wash hands thoroughly after handling patch and dispose of patch properly to avoid contact with children and pets.
- Report rash, flushing, eye pain, difficulty breathing, tremors, loss of coordination, irregular heartbeat, abdominal distention, hallucinations, severe or persistent dry mouth, difficulty urinating, constipation, sensitivity to light.

▽**secobarbital sodium**
*(see koe **bar**' bi tal)*

Novosecobarb (CAN), Seconal Sodium

PREGNANCY CATEGORY D

C-II CONTROLLED SUBSTANCE

Drug classes
Barbiturate (short-acting)
Sedative or hypnotic
Anticonvulsant

Therapeutic actions
General CNS depressant; barbiturates inhibit impulse conduction in the ascending RAS, depress the cerebral cortex, alter cerebellar function, depress motor output, and can produce excitation (especially with subanesthetic doses with pain), sedation, hypnosis, anesthesia, and deep coma; at anesthetic doses, has anticonvulsant activity.

Indications
- Intermittent use as a sedative, hypnotic, or preanesthetic medication

Contraindications and cautions
- Contraindicated with hypersensitivity to barbiturates; manifest or latent porphyria; marked liver impairment; nephritis; severe respiratory distress, respiratory disease with dyspnea, obstruction, or cor pulmonale; previous addiction to sedative-hypnotic drugs (drug may be ineffective, and use may contribute to further addiction); pregnancy (readily crosses placenta and has caused fetal damage, neonatal withdrawal syndrome).
- Use cautiously with acute or chronic pain (drug may cause paradoxical excitement or mask important symptoms); seizure disorders (abrupt discontinuation of daily doses can result in status epilepticus); lactation (has caused drowsiness in nursing infants); fever, hyperthyroidism, diabetes mellitus, severe anemia, pulmonary or cardiac disease, status asthmaticus, shock, uremia; impaired liver or kidney function, debilitation.

Available forms
Capsules—100 mg

Dosages
Adults
Adjust dosage on basis of age, weight, condition.
- *Preoperative sedation*: 200–300 mg PO 1–2 hr before surgery.
- *Bedtime hypnotic:* 100 mg PO hs; do not use > 2 wk.

Pediatric patients
Use caution: barbiturates may produce irritability, excitability, inappropriate tearfulness, and aggression.
- *Preoperative sedation:* 2–6 mg/kg PO 1–2 hours before surgery; maximum dose—100 mg.

Geriatric patients or patients with debilitating disease
Reduce dosage and monitor closely. May produce excitement, depression, confusion.

Patients with hepatic or renal impairment
Reduce dosage.

Pharmacokinetics

Route	Onset	Duration
Oral	10–15 min	3–4 hr

Metabolism: Hepatic; $T_{1/2}$: 15–40 hr
Distribution: Crosses placenta; enters breast milk
Excretion: Urine

Adverse effects
- **CNS:** *Somnolence, agitation, confusion, hyperkinesia, ataxia, vertigo, CNS depression, nightmares, lethargy, residual sedation (hangover), paradoxical excitement, nervousness, psychiatric disturbance, hallucinations, insomnia, anxiety, dizziness, thinking abnormality*
- **CV:** *Bradycardia, hypotension, syncope*
- **GI:** *Nausea, vomiting, constipation, diarrhea, epigastric pain*
- **Hypersensitivity:** Rashes, angioneurotic edema, serum sickness, morbiliform rash, urticaria; rarely, exfoliative dermatitis, **Stevens-Johnson syndrome**
- **Respiratory:** *Hypoventilation, apnea, respiratory depression,* laryngospasm, bronchospasm, circulatory collapse
- **Other:** Tolerance, psychological and physical dependence; **withdrawal syndrome**

Interactions
✳ **Drug-drug** • Increased CNS depression with alcohol • Increased renal toxicity with methoxyflurane • Decreased effects of oral anticoagulants, corticosteroids, hormonal contraceptives and estrogens, metronidazole, metoprolol, propranolol, doxycycline, oxyphenbutazone, phenylbutazone, quinidine with barbiturates • Decreased theophylline serum levels and effectiveness secondary to increased clearance • Decreased bioavailability of verapamil

■ Nursing considerations
Assessment
- **History:** Hypersensitivity to barbiturates; manifest or latent porphyria; nephritis; severe respiratory distress; previous addiction to sedative-hypnotic drugs; pregnancy; acute or chronic pain; seizure disorders; lactation; fever, hyperthyroidism, diabetes mellitus, severe anemia, pulmonary or cardiac disease, shock, uremia; impaired liver or kidney function, debilitation
- **Physical:** Weight; T; skin color, lesions; orientation, affect, reflexes; P, BP, orthostatic BP; R, adventitious sounds; bowel sounds, normal output, liver evaluation; liver and kidney function tests, blood and urine glucose, BUN

Interventions
- Monitor patient responses, blood levels with the above interacting drugs; suggest alternatives to hormonal contraceptives.
- Do not use as a bedtime hypnotic for > 2 wk.
- Stay with children who have received preoperative sedation.
- Taper dosage gradually after repeated use, especially in epileptics.

Teaching points
- This drug will make you drowsy (or induce sleep) and less anxious.
- Do not use this drug during pregnancy, use of barrier contraceptives is recommended.
- Try not to get up after you have received this drug (request assistance if you must sit up or move about).

▷ secretin

See *Less Commonly Used Drugs*, p. 1350.

▷ sermorelin acetate

See *Less Commonly Used Drugs*, p. 1350.

▷ sertraline hydrochloride

(sir' trah leen)

Zoloft

PREGNANCY CATEGORY C

Drug classes
Antidepressant
Selective serotonin reuptake inhibitor (SSRI)

Therapeutic actions
Acts as an antidepressant by inhibiting CNS neuronal uptake of serotonin; blocks uptake of serotonin with little effect on norepinephrine, muscarinic, histaminergic, and alpha₁-adrenergic or dopaminergic receptors.

Indications
- Treatment of major depressive disorder
- Treatment of obsessive-compulsive disorders (OCD)
- Treatment of panic disorder with or without agoraphobia
- Treatment of posttraumatic stress disorder; long-term use to prevent relapse and sustain symptom improvement
- Treatment of premenstrual dysphoric disorder (PMDD)
- Unlabeled use: generalized social phobia

Contraindications and cautions
- Contraindicated with hypersensitivity to sertraline; pregnancy.
- Use cautiously with impaired hepatic or renal function, lactation.

Available forms
Tablets—25, 50, 100 mg; oral concentrate—20 mg/mL

Dosages
Adults
- *Major depressive disorder and OCD:* Administer once a day, morning or evening. 50 mg PO daily; may be increased to up to 200 mg/day; dosage increases should not occur at intervals < 1 wk.
- *Panic disorder and posttraumatic stress disorder:* 25 mg PO daily. After 1 wk increase to 50 mg once daily.
- *PMDD:* 50 mg/day PO daily or just during luteal phase of menstrual cycle.

Pediatric patients
- *6–12 yr:* OCD: 25 mg PO once daily. May be increased slowly as needed.
- *13–17 yr:* OCD: 50 mg PO once daily. May be increased slowly as needed.

Geriatric patients or patients with hepatic impairment
Give a lower or less frequent dose. Use response as dosage guide.

Pharmacokinetics

Route	Onset	Peak
Oral	Slow	4.5–8.4 hr

Metabolism: Hepatic; $T_{1/2}$: 26 hr
Distribution: Crosses placenta; may enter breast milk
Excretion: Urine and feces

Adverse effects
- **CNS:** *Headache, nervousness, drowsiness, anxiety, tremor, dizziness, insomnia,* lightheadedness, agitation, *sedation,* abnormal gait, convulsions, *vision changes, fatigue*
- **CV:** Hot flashes, palpitations, chest pain
- **Dermatologic:** *Sweating,* rash, pruritus, acne, contact dermatitis
- **GI:** *Nausea,* vomiting, *diarrhea, dry mouth,* anorexia, dyspepsia, constipation, taste changes, flatulence, gastroenteritis, dysphagia, gingivitis
- **GU:** *Painful menstruation,* sexual dysfunction, frequency, cystitis, impotence, urgency, vaginitis
- **Respiratory:** Upper respiratory infections, pharyngitis, cough, dyspnea, bronchitis, *rhinitis*
- **Other:** Hot flashes, fever, back pain, thirst

Adverse effects in *Italics* are most common; those in **Bold** are life-threatening.

Interactions

✳ Drug-drug • Serious, sometimes fatal, reactions with MAO inhibitors; allow at least 14 days to elapse between MAOI and sertraline use • Increased serum levels of sertraline with cimetidine • Possible risk of increased QTc interval if combined with pimozide; do not use together

✳ Drug-food • Increased rate of absorption with food

✳ Drug-alternative therapy • Increased risk of severe reaction if combined with St. John's wort therapy

■ Nursing considerations
Assessment

- **History:** Hypersensitivity to sertraline; impaired hepatic or renal function; lactation, pregnancy
- **Physical:** Weight; T; skin rash, lesions; reflexes, affect; bowel sounds, liver evaluation; P, peripheral perfusion; urinary output, renal and liver function tests

Interventions

- Use lower dose in elderly patients and with hepatic or renal impairment.
- Dilute oral concentrate in 4 oz water, gingerale, lemon-lime soda, lemonade, or orange juice only; administer immediately after diluting.
- Establish suicide precautions for severely depressed patients. Limit number of tablets given at any time.
- Give drug once a day, morning or evening.
- Increase dosage at intervals of not less than 1 wk.
- Counsel patient to use nonhormonal contraceptives; pregnancy should be avoided due to risk to fetus.

Teaching points

- Take this drug once a day, at the same time, morning or evening; do not exceed the prescribed dose.
- Dilute concentrate immediately before use in 4 oz water, gingerale, lemon-lime soda, lemonade, or orange juice only.
- These side effects may occur: dizziness, drowsiness, nervousness, insomnia (avoid driving or performing hazardous tasks); nausea, vomiting (eat small frequent meals); dry mouth (sucking sugarless lozenges and frequent mouth care may help); excessive sweating (monitor temperature; avoid overheating).
- Do not take this drug during pregnancy. If you think that you are pregnant or wish to become pregnant, consult with your physician.
- Report rash, mania, seizures, edema, difficulty breathing.

▷ sevelamer hydrochloride

See *Less Commonly Used Drugs,* p. 1352.

▷ sibutramine hydrochloride
*(sih **bu'** trah meen)*

Meridia

PREGNANCY CATEGORY C

C-IV CONTROLLED SUBSTANCE

Drug classes
Anorexiant
Reuptake inhibitor
Weight loss agent

Therapeutic actions
Inhibits the reuptake of norepinephrine, 5-HT, and dopamine; these effects act to suppress the appetite and decrease depression; is nonsedating, nonanticholinergic and has no central depressant effects.

Indications
- Management of obesity, including weight loss, in conjunction with a reduced-calorie diet

Contraindications and cautions
- Contraindicated with hypersensitivity to sibutramine; pregnancy; anorexia nervosa, patients receiving MAOIs or centrally acting appetite suppressant drugs
- Use cautiously with impaired renal or hepatic function, hypertension, arrhythmias.

Available forms
Capsules—5, 10, 15 mg

Dosages
Adults
Initial dose 10 mg PO daily; may increase to up to 15 mg PO daily as tolerated.
Pediatric patients
Safety and efficacy not established in patients < 16 years of age.

Pharmacokinetics

Route	Onset	Peak
Oral	Slow	3–4 hr

Metabolism: Hepatic; $T_{1/2}$: 1.1 hr for parent drug; 14–16 hr
Distribution: Crosses placenta; may enter breast milk
Excretion: Urine and feces

Adverse effects
- **CNS:** *Headache, nervousness, sleep difficulties*
- **CV:** Hypertension, tachycardia, arrhythmias
- **Dermatologic:** *Rash, dry skin*
- **GI:** *Dry mouth,* nausea, anorexia, *constipation*

Interactions
✳ **Drug-drug** • Serious and potentially fatal reactions if taken with MAO inhibitors; avoid this combination • Risk of increased CNS effects if taken with alcohol, CNS stimulants • Risk of serotonin syndrome if combined with other serotogenic agents • Agents that may raise BP or increase heart rate

■ Nursing considerations
Assessment
- **History:** Hypersensitivity to sibutramine; impaired hepatic or renal function; lactation; pregnancy; hypertension; arrhythmias
- **Physical:** Weight, T; skin rash, lesions; reflexes, affect; liver evaluation; P, BP, ECG, peripheral perfusion; renal and liver function test

Interventions
- Ensure that patient is participating in a weight loss diet and exercise program.
- Establish suicide precautions for severely depressed patients. Dispense only a small number of capsules at a time to these patients.

- Administer drug once a day, in the morning or in the evening.
- Increase dosage after 4 wk if adequate response is not achieved.
- Provide sugarless lozenges, frequent mouth care if dry mouth is a problem.
- Counsel patient about the use of nonhormonal contraceptives while on this drug; pregnancy should be avoided because of the possible risk to the fetus.

Teaching points
- Take this drug once a day, at the same time each day, in the morning or in the evening; do not exceed the prescribed dose.
- These side effects may occur: dizziness, drowsiness, nervousness, insomnia (avoid driving or performing hazardous tasks); dry mouth (sucking sugarless lozenges and frequent mouth care may help); dry skin, rash (provide skin care as recommended).
- Do not take this drug during pregnancy. If you think that you are pregnant or wish to become pregnant, consult with your physician.
- Avoid excessive alcohol while on this drug.
- Report rash, mania, seizures, edema, difficulty breathing, palpitations.

▽ sildenafil citrate
(sill den' ah fill)

Viagra

PREGNANCY CATEGORY B

Drug class
Impotence agent

Therapeutic actions
Selectively inhibits cGMP-specific phosphodiesterase type 5. The mechanism of penile erection involves the release of nitric oxide into the corpus cavernosum of the penis during sexual stimulation. Nitrous oxide activates cGMP, which causes smooth muscle relaxation, allowing the flow of blood into the corpus cavernosum. Sildenafil prevents the breakdown of cGMP by phosphodiesterase, leading to increased cGMP levels and prolonged smooth

muscle relaxation, promoting the flow of blood into the corpus cavernosum.

Indications
- Treatment of erectile dysfunction in the presence of sexual stimulation

Contraindications and cautions
- Contraindicated with allergy to any component of the tablet, contraindicated for women or children; concomitant use of nitrates.
- Use cautiously with hepatic or renal dysfunction; with anatomical deformation of the penis; with known cardiac disease (effects of sexual activity need to be evaluated).

Available forms
Tablets—25, 50, 100 mg

Dosages
Adults
50 mg PO taken 1 hr before anticipated sexual activity; range 25–100 mg PO. May be taken 30 min–4 hr before sexual activity. Limit use to once per day.
Pediatric patients
Not intended for use in children.
Geriatric patients
For patients > 65 yr, start dose at 25 mg PO.
Patients with renal or hepatic impairment
Patients with hepatic impairment or creatinine clearance < 30 mL/min may have increased serum levels; start dose at 25 mg PO.

Pharmacokinetics

Route	Onset	Peak
Oral	Rapid	30–120 min

Metabolism: Hepatic; $T_{1/2}$: 4 hr
Distribution: Not intended for use in women, no clear studies on crossing the placenta or entering breast milk
Excretion: Feces and urine

Adverse effects
- **CNS:** *Headache,* abnormal vision, dizziness, nasal congestion
- **CV:** *Flushing*
- **GI:** *Dyspepsia,* diarrhea
- **Other:** Urinary tract infection, rash

Interactions
❋ **Drug-drug** • Possible severe hypotension and serious cardiac events if combined with nitrates; this combination must be avoided
• Possible increased sildenafil levels and effects if taken with cimetidine, amlodipine, erythromycin, protease inhibitors; monitor patient and reduce dosage as needed
❋ **Drug-food** • Decreased rate of absorption and onset of action if taken with a high-fat meal • Decreased metabolism and risk of toxic effects if combined with grapefruit juice; avoid this combination

■ Nursing considerations
Assessment
- **History:** Allergy to any component of the tablet; hepatic or renal dysfunction; with anatomical deformation of the penis, known cardiac disease; concomitant use of nitrates
- **Physical:** Orientation, affect; skin color, lesions; P, BP, ECG, renal and hepatic function tests

Interventions
- Ensure diagnosis of erectile dysfunction and determine underlying causes and other appropriate treatment.
- Advise patient that drug does not work in the absence of sexual stimulation. Limit use to once per day.
- Remind patient that drug does not protect against sexually transmitted diseases and appropriate measures should be taken.
- Advise patient to never take this drug with nitrates; serious and even fatal complications can occur.
- Advise patients receiving HIV medications that there is an increased risk of sidenafil-associated ADRs, including hypotension, visual changes, and priapism. Do not exceed 25 mg of sildenafil in 48 hr.

Teaching points
- Take this drug 30 min to 4 hr before anticipated sexual activity. The usual timing is 1 hr. The drug will have no effect in the absence of sexual stimulation.
- Onset of drug effects will be slowed if taken with a high-fat meal; plan accordingly. Avoid drinking grapefruit juice if using this drug.

S

- This drug will not protect you from sexually transmitted diseases; use appropriate precautions.
- Do not take this drug if you are taking any nitrates; serious side effects and even death can occur.
- These side effects may occur: headache, dizziness, rash, flushing.
- Report difficult or painful urination, rash, dizziness, palpitations.

▽ simethicone
*(sigh **meth' ** ih kohn)*

Degas, Flatulex, Gas-X, Genasyme Drops, Maalox Anti-Gas, Mylanta Gas, Mylicon, Oval (CAN), Phazyme, Phazyme 95, Phazyme 125

PREGNANCY CATEGORY UNKNOWN

Drug class
Antiflatulent

Therapeutic actions
Defoaming action disperses and prevents the formation of mucus surrounded gas pockets in the GI tract; changes the surface tension of gas bubbles in the stomach and small intestine, enabling the bubbles to coalesce, allowing gas to be more easily freed by belching or flatus.

Indications
- Relief of symptoms and pressure of excess gas in the digestive tract; postoperative gaseous distention and pain, use in endoscopic examination; air swallowing; functional dyspepsia; spastic or irritable colon; diverticulosis
- Unlabeled use: treatment of colic in infants

Contraindications and cautions
- Allergy to components of the product.

Available forms
Chewable tablets—40, 80, 125 mg; tablets—60, 95 mg; capsules—125 mg; drops—40 mg/0.6 mL

Dosages
Adults
Oral
Capsules: 125 mg PO qid, after each meal and hs.
Tablets: 40–125 mg PO qid, after each meal and hs.
Drops: 40–80 mg PO qid up to 500 mg/day, after each meal and hs.
Pediatric patients
< 2 yr: 20 mg PO qid after each meal and hs; up to 240 mg/day.
2–12 yr: 40 mg PO qid after each meal and hs.

Pharmacokinetics
Not absorbed systemically; excreted unchanged in the feces.

Adverse effects
- **GI:** Nausea, vomiting, *diarrhea,* constipation, belching, passing of flatus

■ Nursing considerations
Assessment
- **History:** Hypersensitivity to simethicone
- **Physical:** Bowel sounds, normal output

Interventions
- Give after each meal and hs.
- Shake drops thoroughly before each use.
- Add drops to 30 mL cool water, infant formula, or other liquid to ease administration to infants.
- Ensure chewable tablets are chewed thoroughly before swallowing.

Teaching points
- Take this drug after each meal and at bedtime; chew chewable tablets thoroughly before swallowing; shake drops bottle thoroughly before administration. Parents may want to add drops to 30 mL cool water, infant formula, or other liquid to ease administration.
- You may experience increased belching and passing of flatus as gas disperses.
- Report extreme abdominal pain, worsening of condition being treated, vomiting.

Adverse effects in *Italics* are most common; those in **Bold** are life-threatening.

▽ simvastatin
(sim va stah' tin)

Zocor

PREGNANCY CATEGORY X

Drug classes
Antihyperlipidemic
HMG CoA inhibitor

Therapeutic actions
Inhibits HMG co-enzyme A, the enzyme that catalyzes the first step in the cholesterol synthesis pathway, resulting in a decrease in serum cholesterol, serum LDLs, and either an increase or no change in serum HDLs.

Indications
- Adjunct to diet in the treatment of elevated total cholestrol and LDL cholesterol with primary hypercholesterolemia (types IIa and IIb) in those unresponsive to dietary restriction of saturated fat and cholesterol and other nonpharmacologic measures
- To reduce the risk of stroke, TIA, MI in patients with coronary heart disease and hypercholesterolemia
- Treatment of patients with isolated hypertriglyceridemia
- Treatment of type III hyperlipoproteinemia

Contraindications and cautions
- Contraindicated with allergy to simvastatin, fungal byproducts, pregnancy, lactation.
- Use cautiously with impaired hepatic and renal function, cataracts.

Available forms
Tablets—5, 10, 20, 40, 80 mg

Dosages
Adults
Initially, 20 mg PO up to 80 mg PO daily in the evening. Usual range 5–80 mg/day. Maximum dose, 80 mg/day. Adjust at 4-wk intervals.
- *Familial hypercholesterolemia:* 40 mg/day PO in the evening, or 80 mg/day divided into doses of 20 mg, 20 mg, and 40 mg in the evening.
- *Combination therapy:* Do not combine with other statins; if used with fibrates or niacin, do not exceed 10 mg/day; regular dose if combined with bile acid sequestrants. Combined with cyclosporine, start with 5 mg/day; do not exceed 10 mg/day.
Pediatric patients
Safety and efficacy not established.
Geriatric patients and patients with renal impairment
Starting dose, 5 mg/day PO; increase dose slowly, monitoring response.

Pharmacokinetics

Route	Onset	Peak
Oral	Slow	1.3–2.4 hr

Metabolism: Hepatic; $T_{1/2}$: 3 hr
Distribution: Crosses placenta; enters breast milk
Excretion: Urine and feces

Adverse effects
- **CNS:** *Headache,* asthenia, sleep disturbances
- **GI:** *Flatulence, diarrhea, abdominal pain, cramps, constipation, nausea,* dyspepsia, heartburn, **liver failure**
- **Respiratory:** Sinusitis, pharyngitis
- **Other:** **Rhabdomyolysis, acute renal failure,** arthralgia, myalgia

Interactions
✳ **Drug-drug** • Increased risk of myopathy and rhabdomyolysis with amiodarone, verapamil; do not exceed 20 mg simvastatin daily • Increased risk of myopathy and rhabdomyolysis with clarithromycin, erythromycin, HIV protease inhibitors, itraconazole, ketoconazole, nefazodone; avoid concomitant use, or suspend therapy during treatment with clarithromycin, erythromycin, itraconazole, and ketoconazole • Increased risk of myopathy and rhabdomyolysis with cyclosporine, fibrates, niacin; monitor patient closely if use together cannot be avoided. Do not exceed 10 mg simvastatin daily • Digoxin levels may increase slightly; closely monitor plasma digoxin levels at the start of simvastatin therapy • Increased risk for hepatotoxicity with hepatotoxic drugs; avoid concurrent use • Simvastatin may slightly enhance the anticoagulant effect of warfarin; monitor PT and INR at the start of therapy and during dose adjustment
✳ **Drug-food** • Decreased metabolism and risk of toxic effects if combined with grapefruit juice; avoid this combination

■ Nursing considerations

Assessment

- **History:** Allergy to simvastatin, fungal byproducts; impaired hepatic function; pregnancy; lactation
- **Physical:** Orientation, affect; liver evaluation, abdominal exam; lipid studies, liver function tests

Interventions

- Ensure that patient has tried a cholesterol-lowering diet regimen for 3–6 mo before beginning therapy.
- Give in the evening; highest rates of cholesterol synthesis are between midnight and 5 AM.
- Advise patient that this drug cannot be taken during pregnancy; advise the use of barrier contraceptives.
- Arrange for regular follow-up during long-term therapy. Consider reducing dose if cholesterol falls below target.

Teaching points

- Take drug in the evening. Do not drink grapefruit juice while on this drug.
- These side effects may occur: nausea (eating small, frequent meals may help); headache, muscle and joint aches and pains (may lessen); sensitivity to light (use a sunscreen and wear protective clothing).
- Have periodic blood tests.
- This drug cannot be taken during pregnancy; use of barrier contraceptives is recommended.
- Report severe GI upset, changes in vision, unusual bleeding or bruising, dark urine or light-colored stools, fever, muscle pain, or soreness.

▽ **sirolimus**
(*sere ob' lim us*)

Rapamune

PREGNANCY CATEGORY C

Drug class

Immunosuppressant

Therapeutic actions

Immunosuppressant; inhibits T-lymphocyte activation and proliferation; exact mechanism of action not known, but binds to intracellular protein that may prevent the generation of nuclear factor of activated T cells and suppresses the immune activation and response of T cells.

Indications

- Prophylaxis for organ rejection in renal transplants in conjunction with adrenal corticosteroids and cyclosporine
- Unlabeled use: treatment of psoriasis

Contraindications and cautions

- Contraindicated with allergy to sirolimus, pregnancy, lactation.
- Use cautiously with hepatic impairment.

Available forms

Oral solution—1 mg/mL; tablet—1 mg

Dosages

Adults and patients ≥ 13 yr
≥ 40 kg: Loading dose: 6 mg PO as soon after transplant as possible; daily dose 2 mg PO given in combination with cyclosporine and corticosteroids.
< 40 kg: Loading dose of 3 mg/m^2 then 1 mg/m^2/day based on body surface area.
Patients with hepatic impairment
Reduce maintenance dose by one-third.

Pharmacokinetics

Route	Onset	Peak
Oral	Rapid	1 hr

Metabolism: Hepatic; T$_{1/2}$: 62 hr
Distribution: Crosses placenta; passes into breast milk
Excretion: Feces and urine

Adverse effects

- **CNS:** *Tremor,* headache, *insomnia,* paresthesias
- **GI: Hepatotoxicity,** *constipation, diarrhea, nausea, vomiting,* anorexia
- **GU:** Renal dysfunction, nephrotoxicity, UTI, oliguria

Adverse effects in *Italics* are most common; those in **Bold** are life-threatening.

- **Hematologic:** Leukopenia, anemia, hyperkalemia, hypokalemia, hyperglycemia
- **Respiratory:** Dyspnea, pharyngitis, URI
- **Other:** Abdominal pain, fever, asthenia, back pain, ascites, neoplasias, acne

Interactions

✳ **Drug-drug** • Increased risk of toxicity if given with diltiazem, cyclosporine, ketoconazole • Decreased effectiveness if combined with rifampin • Decreased effectiveness of vaccines if combined with sirolimus; avoid the use of live vaccines

✳ **Drug-food** • Decreased metabolism of sirolimus with grapefruit juice

■ Nursing considerations
Assessment

- **History:** Allergy to sirolimus; impaired renal function; pregnancy, lactation
- **Physical:** T; skin color, lesions; R, adventitious sounds, liver evaluation, bowel sounds; renal and liver function tests, CBC with differential

Interventions

- Monitor renal and liver function tests before and periodically during therapy, marked decreases in function could require changes in dosage or discontinuation of the drug.
- Monitor hematologic tests to determine adjustment of dosage as appropriate.
- Administer with cyclosporine and corticosteroids.
- Protect solution from exposure to light; refrigerate. Use solution within 1 mo of opening the bottle.
- Protect patient from exposure to infections and maintain sterile technique for invasive procedures.
- Ensure ready access to bathroom facilities if diarrhea occurs.
- Provide analgesics as appropriate for headache, pain, fever.
- Provide small, frequent meals if GI upset occurs.
- Arrange for nutritional consult if nausea and vomiting are persistent.

Teaching points

- Protect solution from exposure to light; refrigerate. Use solution within 1 mo of opening the bottle.

- Consistently take drug either with food or without food to minimize variability of exposure.
- Take sirolimus 4 hr after cyclosporine.
- Avoid grapefruit juice.
- Avoid infection while you are on this drug— avoid crowds or people who have infections. Notify your health care provider at once if you injure yourself.
- These side effects may occur: nausea, vomiting (taking the drug with food may help); diarrhea (ensure ready access to bathroom facilities if this occurs); headache (analgesics may be ordered).
- This drug should not be taken during pregnancy and you should not become pregnant for 12 weeks after discontinuing the drug. The use of barrier contraceptives is suggested. If you think that you are pregnant or you want to become pregnant, discuss this with your health care provider.
- Arrange to have periodic blood tests to monitor your response to this drug and its effects on your body.
- Do not discontinue this medication without your physician's advice.
- Report unusual bleeding or bruising, fever, sore throat, mouth sores, tiredness.

▷ **sodium bicarbonate**

Parenteral: Neut
Prescription and OTC preparations: Bell/ans

PREGNANCY CATEGORY C

S

Drug classes
Electrolyte
Systemic alkalinizer
Urinary alkalinizer
Antacid

Therapeutic actions
Increases plasma bicarbonate; buffers excess hydrogen ion concentration; raises blood pH; reverses the clinical manifestations of acidosis; increases the excretion of free base in the urine, effectively raising the urinary pH; neutralizes or reduces gastric acidity, resulting in an increase in the gastric pH, which inhibits the proteolytic activity of pepsin.

Indications

- Treatment of metabolic acidosis, with measures to control the cause of the acidosis
- Adjunctive treatment in severe diarrhea with accompanying loss of bicarbonate
- Treatment of certain drug intoxications, hemolytic reactions that require alkalinization of the urine; prevention of methotrexate nephrotoxicity by alkalinization of the urine
- Minimization of uric acid crystalluria in gout, with uricosuric agents
- Minimization of sulfonamide crystalluria
- Symptomatic relief of upset stomach from hyperacidity associated with peptic ulcer, gastritis, peptic esophagitis, gastric hyperacidity, hiatal hernia (oral)
- Prophylaxis of GI bleeding, stress ulcers, aspiration pneumonia (oral)
- To reduce the incidence of chemical phlebitis and patient discomfort due to vein irritation at or near the infusion site by raising the pH of IV acid solutions.

Contraindications and cautions

- Contraindicated with allergy to components of preparations; low serum chloride (secondary to vomiting, continuous GI suction, diuretics associated with hypochloremic alkalosis); metabolic and respiratory alkalosis; hypocalcemia (alkalosis may precipitate tetany).
- Use cautiously with impaired renal function, CHF, edematous or sodium-retaining states, oliguria or anuria, potassium depletion (may predispose to metabolic alkalosis), pregnancy, lactation.

Available forms

Injection—0.5, 0.6, 0.9, 1.0 mEq/mL; neutralizing additive solution—0.48, 0.5 mEq/mL; tablets—325, 520, 650 mg; powder

Dosages
Adults

- *Urinary alkalinization:* 4 g PO initially, then 1–2 g q 4 hr. May need dose of 2.5–4 g q 4 hr, up to 16 g daily.
- *Antacid:* 300 mg–2 g daily to qid PO, usually 1 and 3 hr after meals and hs.
- *Adjunct to advanced cardiovascular life support during CPR:* Although no longer routinely recommended, inject either 300–500 mL of a 5% solution or 200–300 mEq of a 7.5% or 8.4% solution as rapidly as possible. Base further doses on subsequent blood gas values. Alternatively for adults, 1 mEq/kg dose, then repeat 0.5 mEq/kg q 10 min.
- *Severe metabolic acidosis:* Dose depends on blood CO_2 content, pH, and patient's clinical condition. Generally, administer 90–180 mEq/LIV during first hr, then adjust prn.

Adults and adolescents

- *Less urgent metabolic acidosis:* 2–5 mEq/kg as a 4–8 hr IV infusion. May be added to IV fluids, with rate and dosage determined by arterial blood gases and estimation of base deficit.

Pediatric patients

- *Adjunct to advanced cardiovascular life support during CPR in infants ≤ 2 yr:* 1 mEq/kg IV or intraosseous injection of a 4.2% solution. Administer slowly. Do not exceed 8 mEq/kg.
- *Metabolic acidosis:*
Older children: Follow adult recommendation.
Younger children: Use caution, and base dosage on blood gases and calculation of base deficit.
- *Urinary alkalinization:* 84–840 mg/kg PO daily.

Geriatric patients or patients with renal impairment

Reduce dosage and carefully monitor base deficit and clinical response.

Pharmacokinetics

Route	Onset	Peak	Duration
Oral	Rapid	30 min	1–3 hr
IV	Immediate	Rapid	Unknown

Metabolism: $T_{1/2}$: unknown
Distribution: Crosses placenta; enters breast milk
Excretion: Urine

▼IV facts

Preparation: Direct IV push requires no further preparation; continuous infusion may be diluted in saline, dextrose, and dextrose/saline solutions.

Infusion: Administer by IV direct injection slowly; continuous infusion should be regulated with close monitoring of electrolytes and response, 2–5 mEq/kg over 4–8 hr.

Incompatibilities: Avoid solutions containing calcium; precipitation may occur.

Y-site incompatibilities: Do not give with inamrinone, verapamil, calcium. Norepinephrine and dobutamine are also incompatible.

Adverse effects
- **GI:** Gastric rupture following ingestion
- **Hematologic:** *Systemic alkalosis* (headache, nausea, irritability, weakness, tetany, confusion), hypokalemia secondary to intracellular shifting of potassium
- **Local:** Chemical cellulitis, tissue necrosis, ulceration and sloughing at the site of infiltration (parenteral)

Interactions
✳ **Drug-drug** • Increased pharmacologic effects of anorexiants, flecainide, mecamylamine, quinidine, sympathomimetics with oral sodium bicarbonate • Increased half-lives and duration of effects of amphetamines, ephedrine, pseudoephedrine due to alkalinization of urine • Decreased pharmacologic effects of lithium, salicylates, sulfonylureas, methotrexate, demeclocycline, doxycycline, methacycline, and other tetracyclines

■ Nursing considerations
Assessment
- **History:** Allergy to components of preparations; low serum chloride; metabolic and respiratory alkalosis; hypocalcemia; impaired renal function; CHF, edematous, or sodium-retaining states; oliguria or anuria; potassium depletion; pregnancy
- **Physical:** Skin color, turgor; injection sites; P, rhythm, peripheral edema; bowel sounds, abdominal exam; urinary output; serum electrolytes, serum bicarbonate, arterial blood gases, urinalysis, renal function tests

Interventions
- Monitor arterial blood gases, and calculate base deficit when administering parenteral sodium bicarbonate. Adjust dosage based on

response. Administer slowly, and do not attempt complete correction within the first 24 hr; risk of systemic alkalosis is increased.
- Give parenteral preparations by IV route.
- Check serum potassium levels before IV administration; risk of metabolic acidosis is increased in states of hypokalemia, requiring reduction of sodium bicarbonate. Monitor IV injection sites carefully; if infiltration occurs, promptly elevate the site, apply warm soaks, and if needed, arrange for the local injection of lidocaine or hyaluronidase to prevent sloughing.
- Have patient chew oral tablets thoroughly before swallowing, and follow them with a full glass of water.
- Do not give oral sodium bicarbonate within 1–2 hr of other oral drugs to reduce risk of drug-drug interactions.
- Monitor cardiac rhythm carefully during IV administration.

Teaching points
- Chew oral tablets thoroughly, and follow with a full glass of water. Do not take within 1–2 hr of any other drugs to decrease risk of drug interactions.
- Have periodic blood tests and medical evaluations.
- Report irritability, headache, tremors, confusion, swelling of extremities, difficulty breathing, black or tarry stools, pain at IV injection site (parenteral form).

▷ sodium chloride
(klor' ide)

Parenteral: Sodium Chloride Injection (various)
Prescription and OTC oral preparations: Minims Sodium Chloride (CAN), Saline from Otrivin (CAN), Salinex (CAN), Sodium Chloride Tablets

PREGNANCY CATEGORY C

Drug class
Electrolyte

Therapeutic actions

Sodium chloride is the principal salt involved in the maintenance of plasma tonicity; important for maintaining plasma volume, promoting membrane stability and electrolyte balance.

Indications

- Treatment of hyponatremia
- Dilution and reconstitution of parenteral drugs
- Hydration and replacement of fluid loss
- Dilution of bronchodilator solutions for inhalation via nebulization and for tracheal lavage and irrigation
- Urologic irrigation

Contraindications and cautions

- Contraindicated with hypernatremia, fluid retention, pregnancy, any condition when increased sodium or chloride could be detrimental. Bacteriostatic sodium chloride is contraindicated in newborns because of associated toxicity.
- Use cautiously with impaired renal function, CHF, edematous or sodium-retaining states, lactation, surgical patients.

Available forms

Tablets—650 mg; 1, 2.25 g; SR tablets—600 mg; bronchodilator diluent solutions—0.45%, 0.9%; IV infusion for admixture—0.45%, 0.9%, 3%, 5%; concentrated injection—14.6%, 23.4%

Dosages
Adults
Oral

1–2 g PO tid.

IV

Isotonic (replacement) 1 L administered over 1 hr; hypotonic (0.45%; hydration) 1–2 L over 1–2 hr; hypertonic (3%–5%; treatment of hyponatremia) 100 mL over 1 hr.

Pediatric patients

Safety and efficacy not determined; replacement must be monitored closely and based on clinical response.

Geriatric patients and patients with renal impairment

Reduce dosage, and carefully monitor base deficit and clinical response.

Pharmacokinetics

Route	Onset	Peak
Oral	Unknown	Unknown
IV	Immediate	End of infusion

Metabolism: $T_{1/2}$: unknown
Distribution: Crosses placenta; enters breast milk
Excretion: Urine

▼IV facts

Preparation: Concentrated sodium chloride must be further diluted before use; other preparations may be given as provided; change infusion q 24 hr; use only if solution is clear.
Infusion: Administer by IV direct injection slowly; continuous infusion should be regulated with close monitoring of electrolytes and response.
Incompatibilities: Do not mix with amphotericin B, mannitol.

Adverse effects

- **GI:** Anorexia, nausea, abdominal distention
- **Hematologic:** Hypernatremia, fluid overload
- **Local:** Chemical cellulitis, tissue necrosis, ulceration and sloughing at the site of infiltration, pain at site of injection (parenteral)

■ Nursing considerations
Assessment

- **History:** Hypernatremia, fluid retention, pregnancy, impaired renal function, CHF, edematous or sodium-retaining states, lactation, surgical patients
- **Physical:** Skin color, turgor; injection sites; P, rhythm, peripheral edema; bowel sounds, abdominal exam; urinary output; serum electrolytes, urinalysis, renal function tests

Interventions

- Monitor serum electrolytes carefully before and during administration. Administer slowly. Rapid infusion can result in pain and irritation at injection site.

- Give parenteral preparations by IV route.
- Monitor IV injection sites carefully; if infiltration occurs, promptly elevate the site, apply warm soaks, and if needed, arrange for the local injection of lidocaine or hyaluronidase to prevent sloughing.
- Monitor surgical patients for postoperative salt intolerance (weakness, dehydration, disorientation, nausea, distention, oliguria); if this occurs, discontinue infusion and provide supportive measures.
- Assess patients taking oral tablets for actual salt loss; excessive use of these tablets can cause hypernatremia.

Teaching points
- Take these tablets only as prescribed.
- Have periodic blood tests and medical evaluations.
- Report irritability, confusion, tremors, swelling of extremities, difficulty breathing, black or tarry stools.
- Wash hands prior to using ophthalmic preparations.

▷ sodium ferric gluconate complex

See *Less Commonly Used Drugs,* p. 1352.

▷ sodium fluoride
(flor' ide)

AcT, Fluor-A-Day (CAN), Fluoritab, Fluotic (CAN), Flura, Flura-Drops, Flura-Loz, Gel Kam, Gel-Tin, Karidium, Karigel, Karigel-N, Luride Lozi-Tabs, MouthKote F/R, PDF (CAN), Pediaflor, Pedi-Dent (CAN), Pharmaflur, Pharmaflur df, Pharmaflur 1.1, Phos-Flur, PreviDent 5000 Plus, STOP

PREGNANCY CATEGORY C

Drug classes
Mineral
Trace element

Therapeutic actions
Acts systemically before tooth eruption and topically after tooth eruption to increase tooth resistance to acid dissolution and promote remineralization of teeth and inhibit caries formation by microbes.

Indications
- Prevention of dental caries
- Unlabeled use: prevention of osteoporosis

Contraindications and cautions
- Contraindicated in areas where fluoride content of drinking water exceeds 0.7 ppm, with low sodium or sodium-free diets, hypersensitivity to fluoride. Do not use in children < 3 yr of age when the fluoride content of drinking water is ≥ 0.3 ppm. Do not use 1 mg/5 mL (as a supplement) in children < 6 years old.
- Use cautiously with pregnancy, lactation.

Available forms
Chewable tablets—0.25, 0.5, 1 mg; tablets—1 mg; drops—0.125, 0.25, 0.5 mg/mL; lozenges—1 mg; solution—0.2 mg/mL; rinse—0.02%, 0.04%, 0.09%, 0.2%; gel—0.1%, 0.5%, 1.2%, 1.23%

Dosages
Adults
- *Oral tablets:* Up to 60 mg/day PO with calcium supplements, estrogen, vitamin D to prevent osteoporosis.
- *Rinse:* 10 mL; swish around teeth and spit out.
- *Gel or cream:* Apply thin ribbon to toothbrush, brush, rinse, and spit out.

Pediatric patients
Dosage refers to daily dose.
- *Fluoride content of drinking water < 0.3 ppm:* 6 mo–2 yr: 0.25 mg PO daily; 3–5 yr: 0.5 mg PO daily; 6–16 yr: 1 mg PO daily.
- *Fluoride content of drinking water 0.3–0.6 ppm:* 6 mo–2 yr: None; 3–5 yr: 0.25 mg PO daily; 6–16 yr: 0.5 mg PO daily.
- *Fluoride content of drinking water > 0.6 ppm:* none
- *Topical rinse:* 6–16 yr: 5–10 mL/day; ≥ 12 yr: 10 mL; swish around teeth for 1 min and spit out.

S

- *Gel or cream:* Apply thin ribbon to tooth-brush or rub directly on teeth for 2 min, rinse, and spit out.

Pharmacokinetics

Route	Onset
Oral	Unknown

Metabolism: $T_{1/2}$: unknown
Distribution: Crosses placenta; enters breast milk
Excretion: Urine, sweat glands, feces

Adverse effects

- **Dermatologic:** Eczema, atopic dermatitis, urticaria, rash
- **Other:** Gastric distress, headache, weakness, staining of teeth (with stannous fluoride rinse)

Interactions

✸ Drug-food ● Milk, dairy products may decrease absorption; avoid simultaneous use

■ Nursing considerations

Assessment

- **History:** Fluoride content of drinking water; low sodium or sodium-free diets; hypersensitivity to fluoride; pregnancy, lactation
- **Physical:** Skin color, turgor; state of teeth and gums

Interventions

- Do not give with milk or dairy products.
- Tablets may be chewed, swallowed whole, added to drinking water or juice.
- Give drops undiluted, or with fluids, food.
- Ensure that patient has brushed and flossed teeth before the use of rinse and that patient expectorates fluid; it should not be swallowed.
- Ensure that patients using cream or gel rinse thoroughly and spit out fluid.
- Monitor teeth, and arrange for dental consultation if mottling of teeth occurs.
- Monitor patient for signs of overdose (salivation, nausea, abdominal pain, vomiting, diarrhea, irritability, convulsions, respiratory arrest); forced diuresis, gastric lavage, supportive measures may be required.

Teaching points

- Take this drug as prescribed; chew tablets, swallow whole, or add to drinking water or fruit juice.
- Dilute drops in fluids, food, or take undiluted.
- Brush and floss before use of rinse; swish around mouth and spit out liquid; do not eat, drink, or rinse out mouth for 30 min after use. If using cream or gel, apply thin ribbon to toothbrush, brush, rinse thoroughly and spit.
- Avoid simultaneous use of milk or diary products and this drug.
- Arrange to have regular dental exams.
- Report increased salivation, nausea, abdominal pain, diarrhea, irritability, mottling of teeth.

▽ sodium hyaluronate

See *Less Commonly Used Drugs,* p. 1352.

▽ sodium oxybate
(ox' ah bate)

Xyrem

PREGNANCY CATEGORY B

C-III CONTROLLED SUBSTANCE

Drug classes
Central nervous system depressant
Anticataplectic

Therapeutic actions
CNS depressant, its mechanism of action in affecting cataplexy is not understood.

Indications
- Treatment of cataplexy in patients with narcolepsy.

Contraindications and cautions
- Contraindicated with hypersensitivity to any component of the drug; succinic semialdehyde dehydrogenase deficiency, concomitant treatment with sedative-hypnotic agents.

- Use cautiously with respiratory dysfunction, depression, pregnancy, lactation.

Available forms
Solution—500 mg/mL

Dosages
Adults
4.5 g/day PO divided into 2 equal doses of 2.25 g. Administer drug at bedtime and again 2.5–4 hr later. Doses may be increased no more than every 2 wk to a maximum of 9 g/day in increments of 1.5 g/day (0.75 g/dose).
Pediatric patients
Safety and efficacy have not been established.
Patients with hepatic impairment
Reduce initial dose by half and increase in increments of one-half the normal. Monitor patients closely.

Pharmacokinetics

Route	Onset	Peak
Oral	Varies	0.5–1.25 hr

Metabolism: Hepatic; $T_{1/2}$: 0.5–1 hr
Distribution: Crosses placenta; may enter breast milk
Excretion: Converted to CO_2 and excreted by expiration, minimally in urine

Adverse effects
- **CNS:** *Headache, dizziness, somnolence,* sleepwalking, nervousness, confusion, depression, abnormal dreams, asthenia, muscle weakness, loss of consciousness, insomnia
- **GI:** *Diarrhea, nausea,* vomiting, abdominal pain, dyspepsia
- **GU:** Urinary incontinence
- **Respiratory:** *URI symptoms, pharyngitis,* sinusitis, rhinitis, **respiratory depression**
- **Other:** *Flulike symptoms,* accidental injury, back pain, infections

Interactions
✳ **Drug-drug** • Risk for serious CNS depression if combined with any sedative-hypnotic drug, including alcohol; avoid this combination.

■ Nursing considerations
Assessment
- **History:** Hypersensitivity to any component of the drug; succinic semialdehyde dehydrogenase deficiency, concomitant treatment with sedative-hypnotic agents, respiratory dysfunction, depression, pregnancy, lactation
- **Physical:** T; reflexes, affect, orientation; R, respiratory auscultation; liver function tests

Interventions
- Counsel patient that this drug is also known as GHB, a drug known for abuse. The patient will be asked to view an educational program, agree to the safety measures to ensure that only the patient has access to the drug, and agree to return for follow-up at least every 3 mo.
- Dilute each dose with 60 mL water in the child-resistant dosing cups. Prepare both the bedtime dose and the repeat dose at the same time.
- Encourage patient to refrain from eating for at least 2 hr before going to bed and taking the drug.
- Administer first dose of the day when the patient is in bed. Patient should stay in bed after taking the dose. The second dose should be given 2.5–4 hours later, with the patient sitting up in bed. After taking the second dose, the patient should lie in bed.
- Encourage patient to avoid driving or performing tasks that require alertness for at least 6 hr after taking the drug.
- Do not administer any sedative or hypnotic drugs to a patient who is taking sodium oxybate.
- Provide safety precautions for storage and dispensing of the drug.

Teaching points
- Prepare two doses of the drug in the evening before going to bed. Add 60 mL (4 measuring tablespoons) water to the dose of the drug. Place the doses in the child-resistant dosing cups provided with the drug. Take the first dose when you first go to bed. Place the second dose in easy reach from your bed, but out of the reach of children or pets. Set your alarm to take the second dose 2.5–4 hr later. Sit up in bed and take the dose. Lie back down and go back to sleep.

S

- Avoid eating for at least 2 hr before going to bed. Food will interfere with the actions of this drug.
- Take special precautions to ensure the safety of this drug. It is a controlled substance and cannot be shared with or given to any other person. The drug should be locked up and secured from other people and from children. Keep the drug in the original bottle. When the bottle is empty, remove the label, wash out the bottle and throw the bottle away.
- These side effects may occur: dizziness (avoid driving a car or performing hazardous tasks for at least 6 hr after taking the drug); headache (medications may be available to help); nausea, vomiting, diarrhea (proper nutrition is important, consult with your dietitian to maintain nutrition); symptoms of upper respiratory tract infection, cough (do not self-medicate, consult with your nurse or physician if this becomes uncomfortable); urinary incontinence or bed-wetting (consult with your health care provider if this occurs).
- Report fever, difficulty breathing, bed-wetting, confusion, depression, pregnancy.

▽ sodium polystyrene sulfonate

(pol ee stye' reen)

Kayexalate, K-Exit (CAN), Kionex, SPS

PREGNANCY CATEGORY C

Drug class
Potassium-removing resin

Therapeutic actions
An ion exchange resin that releases sodium ions in exchange for potassium ions as it passes along the intestine after oral administration or is retained in the colon after enema, thus reducing elevated serum potassium levels; action is limited and unpredictable.

Indications
- Treatment of hyperkalemia

Contraindications and cautions
- Severe hypertension, severe CHF, marked edema (risk of sodium overload).

Available forms
Suspension—15 g/60 mL; powder 4.1 mEq/g

Dosages
Adults
Oral
15–60 g/day, best given as 15 g daily to qid. May be given as suspension with water or syrup (20–100 mL). Often given with sorbitol to combat constipation. May be introduced into stomach via nasogastric tube.
Enema
30–50 g q 6 hr given in appropriate vehicle and retained for 30–60 min.
Pediatric patients
Give lower doses, using the exchange ratio of 1 mEq potassium/g resin as the basis for calculation; a dose of approximately 1 g/kg q 6 hr has been recommended.

Pharmacokinetics

Route	Onset
Oral	2–12 hr
Rectal	Very long

Excretion: Through the feces or expelled as enema

Adverse effects
- **GI:** *Constipation,* fecal impaction, *gastric irritation, anorexia, nausea, vomiting*
- **Hematologic:** *Hypokalemia,* electrolyte abnormalities (particularly decrease in calcium and magnesium)

Interactions
✳ **Drug-drug** • Risk of metabolic alkalosis with nonabsorbable cation-donating antacids (eg, magnesium hydroxide, aluminum carbonate)

■ Nursing considerations
Assessment
- **History:** Severe hypertension; severe CHF; marked edema
- **Physical:** Orientation, reflexes; P, auscultation, BP, baseline ECG, peripheral edema;

Adverse effects in *Italics* are most common; those in **Bold** are life-threatening.

bowel sounds, abdominal exam; serum electrolytes

Interventions

- Administer resin through plastic stomach tube, or mixed with a diet appropriate for renal failure.
- Give powder form of resin in an oral suspension with a syrup base to increase palatability.
- Administer as an enema after first giving a cleansing enema; insert a soft, large rubber tube into the rectum for a distance of about 20 cm; with the tip well into the sigmoid colon, tape into place. Suspend the resin in 100 mL sorbitol or 20% dextrose in water at body temperature, introduce by gravity, keeping the particles in suspension by stirring. Flush with 50–100 mL fluid and clamp the tube, leaving it in place. If back leakage occurs, elevate hips or have patient assume the knee-chest position. Retain suspension for at least 30–60 min, several hours is preferable, then irrigate the colon with a non–sodium-containing solution at body temperature; 2 qt of solution may be necessary to remove the resin. Drain the return constantly through a Y-tube connection.
- Prepare fresh suspensions for each dose. Do not store beyond 24 hr. Do not heat suspensions; this may alter the exchange properties.
- Monitor patient and consider use of other measures (IV calcium, sodium bicarbonate, or glucose and insulin) in cases of severe hyperkalemia, with rapid tissue breakdown: burns, renal failure.
- Monitor serum electrolytes (potassium, sodium, calcium, magnesium) regularly, and arrange to counteract disturbances.
- Arrange for treatment of constipation with 10–20 mL of 70% sorbitol q 2 hr or as needed to produce two watery stools per day. Establish a bowel training program.

Teaching points

- This drug is often used in emergencies. Drug instruction should be incorporated within general emergency instructions.
- These side effects may occur: GI upset, constipation.
- Frequent blood tests will be necessary to monitor drug effect.

- Report confusion, irregular heartbeats, constipation, severe GI upset.

▷ sodium thiosalicylate
(theye o sall i' sill ayte)

Rexolate

PREGNANCY CATEGORY C

Drug classes

Antipyretic
Analgesic (non-narcotic)
Antigout agent
Anti-inflammatory agent
Antirheumatic
Salicylate
Nonsteroidal anti-inflammatory drug (NSAID)

Therapeutic actions

Analgesic and antirheumatic effects are attributable to the ability to inhibit the synthesis of prostaglandins, important mediators of inflammation; antipyretic effects are not fully understood, but salicylates probably act in the thermoregulatory center of the hypothalamus to block the effects of endogenous pyrogen by inhibiting the synthesis of the prostaglandin intermediary.

Indications

- Acute gout
- Muscular pain and musculoskeletal disturbances
- Rheumatic fever

Contraindications and cautions

- Contraindicated with chickenpox or viral infection in children.
- Use cautiously with allergy to salicylates or NSAIDs, bleeding disorders, impaired hepatic or renal function, GI ulceration (less of a problem with this salicylate than with some others); pregnancy, lactation.

Available forms

Injection—50 mg/mL

Dosages
Adults

- *Acute gout:* 100 mg q 3–4 hr IM for 2 days, then 100 mg/day IM until asymptomatic.

- *Muscular pain and musculoskeletal disturbances:* 50–100 mg/day or on alternate days IM.
- *Rheumatic fever:* 100–150 mg q 4–8 hr IM for 3 days, then reduce to 100 mg bid. Continue until patient is asymptomatic.

Pediatric patients
Dosage schedule not established.

Pharmacokinetics

Route	Onset	Peak
IM	Immediate	15–100 min

Metabolism: Hepatic; $T_{1/2}$: 2–18 hr
Distribution: Crosses placenta; enters breast milk
Excretion: Urine

Adverse effects

- **CNS:** *Headache, dizziness, somnolence, insomnia,* fatigue, tiredness, dizziness, tinnitus, ophthalmologic effects
- **Dermatologic:** *Rash,* pruritus, sweating, dry mucous membranes, stomatitis
- **GI:** *Nausea, dyspepsia, GI pain,* diarrhea, vomiting, *constipation,* flatulence
- **GU:** Dysuria, renal impairment
- **Hematologic:** Bleeding, platelet inhibition with higher doses, neutropenia, eosinophilia, leukopenia, pancytopenia, thrombocytopenia, agranulocytosis, granulocytopenia, aplastic anemia, decreased Hgb or Hct, bone marrow depression, menorrhagia
- **Respiratory:** Dyspnea, hemoptysis, pharyngitis, bronchospasm, rhinitis
- **Other:** Peripheral edema, **anaphylactoid reactions to anaphylactic shock;** salicylism: dizziness, tinnitus, difficulty hearing, nausea, vomiting, diarrhea, mental confusion, lassitude (dose related); acute salicylate toxicity (respiratory alkalosis, hyperpnea, tachypnea, hemmorhage, excitement, confusion, asterixis, pulmonary edema, convulsions, tetany, metabolic acidosis, fever, coma, **CV collapse, renal and respiratory failure** (dose related: 20–25 g in adults)

Interactions

✳ **Drug-drug** • Increased risk of GI ulceration with corticosteroids and alcohol • Increased risk of salicylate toxicity with carbonic anhydrase inhibitors • Increased toxicity of carbonic anhydrase inhibitors, valproic acid • Decreased serum salicylate levels with corticosteroids, antacids, urine alkalinizers (sodium acetate, sodium bicarbonate, sodium citrate, sodium lactate, tromethamine) • Increased methotrexate levels and toxicity • Greater glucose-lowering effect of sulfonylureas, insulin with large doses of salicylates • Decreased uricosuric effect of probenecid, sulfinpyrazone • Decreased diuretic effect of spironolactone

✳ **Drug-lab test** • Decreased serum PBI • False-negative readings for urine glucose by glucose oxidase method and copper reduction method • Interference with urine 5-HIAA determinations by fluorescent methods but not by nitrosonaphthol colorimetric method • Interference with urinary ketone determination by ferric chloride method • Falsely elevated urine VMA levels with most tests; false decrease in VMA using the Pisano method • Serum uric acid levels are elevated by salicylate levels < 10 mg/dL and decreased by levels > 10 mg/dL

■ Nursing considerations

Assessment

- **History:** Allergy to salicylates or NSAIDs; bleeding disorders; impaired hepatic or renal function; GI ulceration; lactation; pregnancy; chickenpox or viral infection
- **Physical:** Skin color and lesions; eighth cranial nerve function, orientation, reflexes, affect; P, BP, perfusion; R, adventitious sounds; liver evaluation and bowel sounds; CBC, urinalysis, stool guaiac; renal and liver function tests

Interventions

- Administer by IM injection.
- Avoid use with sodium restrictions.

Teaching points

- Report ringing in the ears, dizziness, confusion, abdominal pain, rapid or difficult breathing, nausea, vomiting.

Adverse effects in *Italics* are most common; those in **Bold** are life-threatening.

somatrem
(soe' ma trem)

Protropin

PREGNANCY CATEGORY C

Drug class
Hormone

Therapeutic actions
Artificial hormone with identical amino acid sequence of pituitary-derived human growth hormone plus one additional amino acid; therapeutically equivalent to endogenous growth hormone; stimulates skeletal (linear) growth, growth of internal organs, protein synthesis, many other metabolic processes required for normal growth.

Indications
- Long-term treatment of children with growth failure due to lack of adequate endogenous growth hormone secretion
- Orphan drug use: treatment of short stature associated with Turner's syndrome

Contraindications and cautions
- Known sensitivity to somatrem, benzyl alcohol, closed epiphyses, underlying cranial lesions, active neoplasia.

Available forms
Powder for injection—5, 10 mg/vial

Dosages
Adults and pediatric patients
Individualize dosage based on response. A weekly dosage of 0.30 mg/kg (about 0.90 IU/kg) of body weight administered by daily IM or SC injection is recommended. Do not exceed weekly dosage of 0.3 mg/kg.

Pharmacokinetics

Route	Onset	Peak
IM	Varies	Days to weeks

Metabolism: Hepatic; $T_{1/2}$: 20–30 min
Excretion: Urine

Adverse effects
- **Dermatologic:** Rare increased growth of preexisting nevi
- **Endocrine:** Hypothyroidism, insulin resistance, rare gynecomastia, rare pancreatitis
- **Hematologic:** *Development of antibodies to growth hormone*
- **Metabolic:** Infrequent, mild, and transient peripheral edema
- **Musculoskeletal:** Rare carpal tunnel syndrome
- **Local:** Injection site pain

■ Nursing considerations
Assessment
- **History:** Sensitivity to somatrem, benzyl alcohol; closed epiphyses; underlying cranial lesions
- **Physical:** Height; weight; thyroid function tests, glucose tolerance tests, growth hormone levels

Interventions
- Reconstitute each 5-mg or 10-mg vial for administration to adults or older children with 1–5 mL or 1–10 mL respectively of bacteriostatic water for injection (benzyl alcohol preserved) only.
- Reconstitute drug for use in newborns with plain water for injection without benzyl alcohol. Benzyl alcohol has been associated with severe toxicity in newborns. Use only one dose per vial and discard the unused portion.
- Prepare the solution by injecting the diluent into the vial, aiming the stream of liquid against the glass wall. Swirl the product vial with a gentle rotary motion until the contents are completely dissolved. Do not shake. After reconstitution, contents should be clear without particulate matter. Use a needle that is long enough (at least 1 in) to ensure injection deep into the muscle layer.
- Refrigerate vials; reconstituted vials should be used within 14 days; do not freeze drug.
- Arrange for periodic testing of glucose tolerance, thyroid function, and growth hormone antibodies. Arrange for treatment indicated by test results.

Teaching points
- This drug must be given IM or SC.
- You may experience sudden growth; increase in appetite; a decrease in thyroid function (request replacement hormone).

- Report lack of growth, increased hunger, thirst, increased and frequent voiding, fatigue, dry skin, intolerance to cold.

▷ somatropin
*(soe ma **troe'** pin)*

Genotropin, Genotropin Miniquick, Humatrope, Norditropin, Nutropin, Nutropin AQ, Nutropin Depot, Saizen, Serostim

PREGNANCY CATEGORY C

Drug class
Hormone

Therapeutic actions
Hormone of recombinant DNA origin; contains the identical amino acid sequence of pituitary-derived human growth hormone; therapeutically equivalent to endogenous growth hormone; stimulates skeletal (linear) growth, growth of internal organs, protein synthesis, many other metabolic processes required for normal growth.

Indications
- Long-term treatment of children with growth failure due to lack of adequate endogenous growth hormone secretion (all except *Serostim*)
- Treatment of children with growth failure associated with chronic renal failure, chronic renal insufficiency, up to the time of renal transplantation (*Nutropin* and *Nutropin AQ*)
- Treatment of girls suffering from Turner's syndrome (*Nutropin, Nutropin AQ,* and *Humatrope*)
- Treatment of AIDS wasting and cachexia (*Serostim*)
- Long-term treatment of children with growth failure due to Prader-Willi syndrome (*Genotropin*)
- Growth hormone deficiency in adults (*Genotropin, Nutropin, Nutropin AQ, Humatrope*)

- Long-term treatment of growth failure in children of small gestational age who do not catch up by 2 yr (*Genotropin*)

Contraindications and cautions
- Known sensitivity to somatropin, benzyl alcohol, glycerin (*Humatrope*), closed epiphyses, underlying cranial lesions.

Available forms
Powder for injection—varies for each brand name

Dosages
Individualize dosage based on response.
Adults
Genotropin: 0.04–0.08 mg/kg/wk SC divided into 6–7 injections.
Serostim: > 55 kg: 6 mg SC daily; 45–55 kg: 5 mg SC daily; 35–45 kg: 4 mg SC daily; < 35 kg: 0.1 mg/kg SC daily hs.
Humatrope: ≤ 0.006 mg/kg/day SC; may increase to 0.0125 mg/kg/day.
Nutropin/Nutropin AQ: ≤ 0.006 mg/kg/day SC up to 0.025 mg/kg/day in patients < 35 yr and 0.0125 mg/kg/day in patients > 35 yr.
Nutropin Depot: Once-monthly injection: 1.5 mg/kg SC on the same day each month. Patients weighing > 15 kg will require > 1 injection per dose. *Twice-monthly injections:* 0.75 mg/kg SC twice each month on the same days. Patients > 30 kg will require > 1 injection per dose.
Pediatric patients
Humatrope: 0.18–0.3 mg/kg/wk SC or IM divided into doses given 3 times/wk or 6 times/wk.
Nutropin/Nutropin AQ: GH deficiency: 0.3 mg/kg/wk SC or depot injection 1–2 times/mo; chronic renal insufficiency: 0.35 mg/kg/wk SC divided into daily doses; Turner syndrome: ≤ 0.375 mg/kg/wk SC divided into 3–7 injections (also *Humatrope*).
Saizen: 0.06 mg/kg SC or IM 3 times/wk.
Norditropin: 0.024–0.034 mg/kg SC, 6–7 times/wk.
Genotropin: 0.24 mg/kg/wk SC for PWS divided into 6–7 doses; 0.16–0.24 mg/kg/wk SC for GHD divided into 6–7 doses.

Adverse effects in *Italics* are most common; those in **Bold** are life-threatening.

Pharmacokinetics

Route	Onset	Peak
IM, SC	Varies	3–7.5 hr

Metabolism: Hepatic; $T_{1/2}$: 15–50 min
Distribution: Crosses placenta; enters breast milk
Excretion: Urine and feces

Adverse effects

- **Endocrine:** Hypothyroidism, insulin resistance
- **Hematologic:** *Development of antibodies to growth hormone* (not as likely as with somatrem)
- **Other:** Swelling, joint pain, muscle pain, carpal tunnel syndrome, increased growth of preexisting nevi, headache, injection site pain

■ Nursing considerations
Assessment

- **History:** Known sensitivity to somatropin; closed epiphyses; underlying cranial lesions
- **Physical:** Height; weight; thyroid function tests, glucose tolerance tests, growth hormone levels

Interventions

- Administer drug IM or SC.
- Divide total dose into smaller increments given 6–7 times/wk for smaller patients unable to tolerate injections.
- Reconstitute drug carefully following manufacturer's instructions; do not shake; do not inject if solution is cloudy or contains particulate matter.
- Refrigerate vials; reconstituted vials should be used within 7 days; do not freeze drug.
- Arrange for periodic testing of glucose tolerance, thyroid function, and growth hormone antibodies. Arrange for treatment indicated by test results.

Teaching points

- This drug must be given IM or SC. Drug can be given in six to seven smaller doses if needed.
- You may experience sudden growth, increase in appetite, decrease in thyroid function (request replacement hormone).
- Report lack of growth, increased hunger, thirst, increased and frequent voiding, fatigue, dry skin, intolerance to cold.

▽ sotalol hydrochloride
(soh' tal lole)

Apo-Sotalol (CAN), Betapace, Betapace AF, Novo-Sotalol (CAN), Rylosol (CAN), Sotacor (CAN)

PREGNANCY CATEGORY B

Drug classes

Beta-adrenergic blocking agent
Antiarrhythmic

Therapeutic actions

Blocks beta-adrenergic receptors of the sympathetic nervous system in the heart and juxtaglomerular apparatus (kidney), thus decreasing the excitability of the heart, decreasing cardiac output and oxygen consumption.

Indications

- Treatment of life-threatening ventricular arrhythmias; because of proarrhythmic effects, use for less than life-threatening arrhythmias, even symptomatic ones, is not recommended
- Maintenance of normal sinus rhythm—to delay the time to recurrence of atrial fibrillation/flutter in patients with symptomatic atrial fibrillation/flutter who are currently in sinus rhythm—*Betapace AF*

Contraindications and cautions

- Contraindicated with sinus bradycardia (HR < 45 beats/min), second, or third-degree heart block (PR interval > 0.24 sec), cardiogenic shock, CHF, asthma, COPD, lactation; congenital or acquired long QT syndromes; hypokalemia and hypomagnesemia.
- Use cautiously with diabetes or thyrotoxicosis, hepatic or renal impairment, sick sinus syndrome, recent MI.

Available forms

Tablets—80, 120, 160, 240 mg

Dosages
Adults

Initial dose, 80 mg PO bid. Adjust gradually, every 3 days, until appropriate response occurs; may require 240–320 mg/day (*Betapace*); up to 120 mg bid (*Betapace AF*).

S

Pediatric patients
Safety and efficacy not established.
Geriatric patients or patients with renal impairment
Betapace
For creatinine clearance < 10 mL/min, individualize dose based on response. See table below for dosing intervals.

Creatinine Clearance (mL/min)	Dosing Intervals
> 60	12 hr
30–59	24 hr
10–29	36–48 hr

Betapace AF
Betapace AF is contraindicated for creatinine clearance < 40 mL/min. See table below for dosing intervals.

Creatinine Clearance (mL/min)	Dosing Intervals
> 60	12 hr
40–59	24 hr

Pharmacokinetics

Route	Onset	Peak
Oral	Varies	3–4 hr

Metabolism: $T_{1/2}$: 12 hr
Distribution: Crosses placenta; enters breast milk
Excretion: Urine

Adverse effects

- **Allergic reactions:** Pharyngitis, erythematous rash, fever, sore throat, **laryngospasm, respiratory distress**
- **CNS:** Dizziness, vertigo, tinnitus, fatigue, emotional depression, paresthesias, sleep disturbances, hallucinations, disorientation, memory loss, slurred speech
- **CV:** *CHF, cardiac arrhythmias, SA or AV nodal block,* peripheral vascular insufficiency, claudication, **CVA, pulmonary edema,** hypotension
- **Dermatologic:** Rash, pruritus, sweating, dry skin
- **EENT:** Eye irritation, dry eyes, conjunctivitis, blurred vision
- **GI:** *Gastric pain, flatulence, constipation, diarrhea, nausea, vomiting,* anorexia
- **GU:** *Impotence, decreased libido,* Peyronie's disease, dysuria, nocturia, frequent urination
- **Musculoskeletal:** Joint pain, arthralgia, muscle cramp
- **Respiratory:** Bronchospasm, dyspnea, cough, bronchial obstruction, nasal stuffiness, rhinitis
- **Other:** *Decreased exercise tolerance, development of antinuclear antibodies,* hyperglycemia or hypoglycemia, elevated serum transaminase

Interactions

✳ **Drug-drug** ● Possible increased effects with verapamil ● Increased risk of orthostatic hypotension with prazosin ● Possible increased BP lowering effects with aspirin, bismuth subsalicylate, magnesium salicylate, sulfinpyrazone, hormonal contraceptives ● Decreased antihypertensive effects with NSAIDs, clonidine ● Possible increased hypoglycemic effect of insulin ● Risk of potentially fatal arrhythmias if combined with drugs that increase QTc interval

✳ **Drug-lab test** ● Possible false results with glucose or insulin tolerance tests (oral)

■ Nursing considerations
Assessment

- **History:** Sinus bradycardia; second- or third-degree heart block; cardiogenic shock, CHF; asthma, COPD; pregnancy, lactation; diabetes or thyrotoxicosis; prolonged QTc interval
- **Physical:** Weight; skin condition; neurologic status; P, BP, ECG; respiratory status, kidney and thyroid function, blood and urine glucose

Interventions

- Take this drug on an empty stomach.
- Do not give for ventricular arrhythmias unless patient is unresponsive to other antiarrhythmics and has a life-threatening ventricular arrhythmia. Monitor patient response carefully; proarrhythmic effect can be pronounced.
- Maintain patient on continuous cardiac monitoring for at least 3 days when initiating therapy.

Adverse effects in *Italics* are most common; those in **Bold** are life-threatening.

- Do not discontinue drug abruptly after long-term therapy. Taper drug gradually over 2 wk with monitoring (abrupt withdrawal may cause serious beta-adrenergic rebound effects).
- Discontinue other antiarrhythmics gradually, allowing for two to three plasma half-lives of the drug before starting sotalol. After discontinuing amiodarone, do not start sotalol until QTc interval is normalized.
- Consult with physician about withdrawing drug if patient is to undergo surgery (withdrawal is controversial).

Teaching points

- Take drug on an empty stomach.
- Do not stop taking unless told to do so by a health care provider.
- Avoid driving or dangerous activities if dizziness, weakness occur.
- These side effects may occur: dizziness, light-headedness, loss of appetite, nightmares, depression, sexual impotence.
- Report difficulty breathing, night cough, swelling of extremities, slow pulse, confusion, depression, rash, fever, sore throat.

▽ **spectinomycin hydrochloride**
(spek ti noe mye' sin)

Trobicin

PREGNANCY CATEGORY B

Drug class
Antibiotic

Therapeutic actions
Bactericidal: inhibits protein synthesis of susceptible strains of *Neisseria gonorrhoeae*, causing cell death.

Indications
- Acute gonococcal urethritis and proctitis in males
- Acute gonococcal cervicitis and proctitis in females

Contraindications and cautions
- Contraindicated with allergy to spectinomycin, lactation.

- Use cautiously with pregnancy (safety not established; yet drug is recommended for penicillin or probenecid allergic pregnant women with gonococcal infections).

Available forms
Powder for injection—400 mg/mL

Dosages
Adults
2 g IM. In geographic areas where antibiotic resistance is prevalent, 4 g IM divided between two gluteal injection sites is preferred.
- *CDC-recommended treatment for gonorrhea:*
Patients who cannot take cephalosporins or fluoroquinolones or for penicillinase-producing N. gonorrhoeae: 2 g IM.
< 45 kg: 40 mg/kg IM. Maximum: 2 g.
- *Gonococcal infections in pregnant patients allergic to cephalosporins:* 2 gm IM.
- *Disseminated gonococcal infections in patients allergic to beta-lactams:* 2 g IM q 12 hr.

Pediatric patients
≥ 45 kg: Adult regimen.
< 45 kg: Single dose of 40 mg/kg IM. Maximum: 2 g.

Pharmacokinetics

Route	Onset	Peak
IM	Varies	1 hr

Metabolism: $T_{1/2}$: 1.5–2.8 hr
Distribution: Crosses placenta; enters breast milk
Excretion: Urine

Adverse effects
- **CNS:** *Dizziness, chills,* fever, insomnia
- **Dermatologic:** Urticaria
- **GU:** *Decreased urine output without documented renal toxicity*
- **Hematologic:** Decreased Hct, Hgb, creatinine clearance, increased alkaline phosphatase, BUN, ALT
- **Local:** *Soreness at injection site*

■ Nursing considerations
Assessment
- **History:** Allergy to spectinomycin, pregnancy, lactation

S

- **Physical:** Site of infection, skin color, lesions; orientation, reflexes; R, adventitious sounds; CBC, liver and renal function tests

Interventions

- Administer only IM; administer deep into upper outer quadrant of the gluteus to decrease discomfort.
- Reconstitute with bacteriostatic water for injection with 0.9 benzyl alcohol: 3.2 mL diluent for 2-g vial, 6.2 mL diluent for 4-g vial. Stable for 24 hr after being reconstituted.
- Culture infection before therapy.
- Monitor for development of resistant strains on prolonged therapy.
- Monitor blood counts, renal and liver function tests on long-term therapy.

Teaching points

- This drug is given only in the IM form.
- Report worsening of infection, dark urine, yellowing of the skin or eyes, rash or itching.

▷ spironolactone

(speer on oh lak' tone)

Aldactone, Novospiroton (CAN)

PREGNANCY CATEGORY D

Drug classes

Potassium-sparing diuretic
Aldosterone antagonist

Therapeutic actions

Competitively blocks the effects of aldosterone in the renal tubule, causing loss of sodium and water and retention of potassium.

Indications

- Primary hyperaldosteronism, diagnosis, maintenance
- Adjunctive therapy in edema associated with CHF, nephrotic syndrome, hepatic cirrhosis when other therapies are inadequate or inappropriate
- Treatment of hypokalemia or prevention of hypokalemia in patients who would be at high risk if hypokalemia occurred: digitalized patients, patients with cardiac arrhythmias

- Essential hypertension, usually in combination with other drugs
- Unlabeled uses: treatment of hirsutism due to its antiandrogenic properties, palliation of symptoms of PMS, treatment of familial male precocious puberty, short-term treatment of acne vulgaris

Contraindications and cautions

- Contraindicated with allergy to spironolactone, hyperkalemia, renal disease, anuria, amiloride or triamterene use.
- Use cautiously with pregnancy, lactation.

Available forms

Tablets—25, 50, 100 mg

Dosages
Adults

- *Edema:* Initially, 100 mg/day (range 25–200 mg/day) when given as the sole agent; continue ≥ 5 days, then adjust dose and/or add another diuretic.
- *Diagnosis of hyperaldosteronism:* 400 mg/day PO for 3–4 wk (long test). Correction of hypokalemia and hypertension are presumptive evidence of primary hyperaldosteronism. 400 mg/day PO for 4 days (short test). If serum K+ increases but decreases when drug is stopped, presumptive diagnosis can be made.
- *Maintenance therapy for hyperaldosteronism:* 100–400 mg/day PO.
- *Essential hypertension:* 50–100 mg/day PO. May be combined with other diuretics.
- *Hypokalemia:* 25–100 mg/day PO.
Pediatric patients

- *Edema:* 3.3 mg/kg/day PO adjusted to patient's response, administered as single or divided dose.
- *Hypertension:* 1–2 mg/kg PO bid.

Pharmacokinetics

Route	Onset	Peak	Duration
Oral	24–48 hr	48–72 hr	48–72 hr

Metabolism: Hepatic; $T_{1/2}$: 20 hr
Distribution: Crosses placenta; enters breast milk
Excretion: Urine

Adverse effects in *Italics* are most common; those in **Bold** are life-threatening.

Adverse effects
- **CNS:** *Dizziness, headache, drowsiness,* fatigue, ataxia, confusion
- **Dermatologic:** *Rash,* urticaria
- **GI:** *Cramping, diarrhea,* dry mouth, thirst, vomiting.
- **GU:** Impotence, irregular menses, amenorrhea, postmenopausal bleeding
- **Hematologic:** Hyperkalemia, hyponatremia, agranulocytosis
- **Other:** Carcinogenic in animals, *deepening of the voice, hirsutism, gynecomastia*

Interactions
✱ **Drug-drug** • Increased hyperkalemia with potassium supplements, ACE inhibitors, diets rich in potassium • Decreased diuretic effect with salicylates • Decreased hypoprothrombinemic effect of anticoagulants

✱ **Drug-food** • Increased absorption when taken with food

✱ **Drug-lab test** • Interference with radioimmunoassay for digoxin; false increase in serum digoxin levels

✱ **Drug-alternative therapy** • Decreased effectiveness if combined with licorice therapy

■ Nursing considerations
Assessment
- **History:** Allergy to spironolactone; hyperkalemia; renal disease; pregnancy, lactation
- **Physical:** Skin color, lesions, edema; orientation, reflexes, muscle strength; P, baseline ECG, BP; R, pattern, adventitious sounds; liver evaluation, bowel sounds; urinary output patterns, menstrual cycle; CBC, serum electrolytes, renal function tests, urinalysis

Interventions
- Mark calendars of edema outpatients as reminders of alternate day or 3- to 5-day/wk therapy.
- Give daily doses early so that increased urination does not interfere with sleep.
- Make suspension as follows: tablets may be pulverized and given in cherry syrup for young children. This suspension is stable for 1 mo if refrigerated.
- Measure and record regular weight to monitor mobilization of edema fluid.
- Avoid giving food rich in potassium.
- Arrange for regular evaluation of serum electrolytes, BUN.

Teaching points
- Record alternate-day therapy on a calendar, or prepare dated envelopes. Take the drug early because of increased urination.
- Weigh yourself on a regular basis, at the same time and in the same clothing, and record the weight on your calendar.
- Avoid foods that are rich in potassium (fruits, *Sanka*).
- These side effects may occur: increased volume and frequency of urination; dizziness, confusion, feeling faint on arising, drowsiness (avoid rapid position changes, hazardous activities: driving, using alcohol); increased thirst (sucking on sugarless lozenges may help; use frequent mouth care); changes in menstrual cycle, deepening of the voice, impotence, enlargement of the breasts can occur (reversible).
- Report weight change of more than 3 lb in one day, swelling in your ankles or fingers, dizziness, trembling, numbness, fatigue, enlargement of breasts, deepening of voice, impotence, muscle weakness or cramps.

▽ **stanozolol**

See *Less Commonly Used Drugs,* p. 1352.

▽ **stavudine (d4T)**
(stay vew' deen)

Zerit

PREGNANCY CATEGORY C

Drug classes
Antiviral
Nucleoside reverse transcriptase inhibitor

Therapeutic actions
Inhibits replication of some retroviruses, including HIV, HTLV III, LAV, ARV

Indications
Treatment of HIV-1 infection in combination with other antiretroviral therapy

Contraindications and cautions
- Contraindicated with life-threatening allergy to any component, pregnancy, lactation.

S

- Use cautiously with compromised bone marrow, impaired renal or hepatic function, or risk factors for liver disease.

Available forms

Powder for oral solution—1 mg/mL; capsules—15, 20, 30, 40 mg

Dosages
Adults
≥ 60 kg: 40 mg q 12 hr PO.
< 60 kg: 30 mg q 12 hr PO.
Pediatric patients:
< 30 kg: 1 mg/kg/dose PO q 12 hr.
≥ 30 kg: Adult dosage based on weight.
Geriatric patients or patients with renal impairment

Creatinine Clearance (mL/min)	≥ 60 kg	< 60 kg
> 50	40 mg q 12 hr	30 mg q 12 hr
26–50	20 mg q 12 hr	15 mg q 12 hr
10–25	20 mg/day	15 mg/day

Pharmacokinetics

Route	Onset	Peak
Oral	Varies	60–90 min

Metabolism: Unknown; $T_{1/2}$: 30–60 min
Distribution: Crosses placenta; may enter breast milk
Excretion: Urine

Adverse effects
- **CNS:** *Headache,* insomnia, myalgia, *asthenia,* malaise, dizziness, paresthesia, somnolence, motor weakness, peripheral neuropathy
- **GI:** *Nausea, GI pain, diarrhea,* anorexia, vomiting, dyspepsia, hepatomegaly with steatosis, **pancreatitis**
- **Hematologic:** *Agranulocytopenia,* severe anemia requiring transfusions
- **Other:** *Fever,* diaphoresis, dyspnea, *rash,* taste perversion, **lactic acidosis,** body fat redistribution

Interactions
✴ **Drug-drug** • Increased risk of fatal or nonfatal pancreatitis if combined with didanosine; monitor closely • Increased risk of lactic acidosis, severe hepatomegaly when taken with other nucleoside analogs

■ Nursing considerations
Assessment
- **History:** Life-threatening allergy to any component; compromised bone marrow; impaired renal or hepatic function; pregnancy, lactation
- **Physical:** Skin rashes, lesions, texture; T; affect, reflexes, peripheral sensation; bowel sounds, liver evaluation; renal and hepatic function tests, CBC and differential

Interventions
- Monitor hematologic indices every 2 wk during therapy.
- Monitor neurologic function. If neuropathy occurs, discontinue. Restart at 50% dose when neuropathy resolves.
- Give every 12 hr, around the clock; schedule dose so it will not interrupt sleep.
- Monitor LPTs.

Teaching points
- Take drug every 12 hr. Do not share this drug; take exactly as prescribed. Reconstitute powder with 202 mL purified water; discard after 30 days.
- Stavudine is not a cure for AIDS; opportunisitc infections may occur; regular medical care should be sought to deal with the disease.
- Frequent blood tests are needed; results may indicate a need to decrease or discontinue drug for a period of time.
- These side effects may occur: nausea, loss of appetite, change in taste (eat small, frequent meals); dizziness, loss of feeling (take precautions); headache, fever, muscle aches.
- Stavudine does not reduce the risk of transmission of HIV to others by sexual contact or blood contamination; use appropriate precautions.
- This drug should be used during pregnancy only if the potential benefit justifies the potential risk; use of barrier contraceptives is advised.
- Report extreme fatigue, lethargy, severe headache, severe nausea, vomiting, difficulty

breathing, rash, numbness or tingling in feet or hands.

▽ **streptokinase**
*(strep toe **kin**' ase)*

Streptase

PREGNANCY CATEGORY C

Drug class
Thrombolytic agent

Therapeutic actions
Enzyme isolated from streptococcal bacteria; converts endogenous plasminogen to the enzyme plasmin (fibrinolysin) which degrades fibrin clots, fibrinogen, and other plasma proteins; lyses thrombi and emboli.

Indications
- Coronary artery thrombosis, IV or intracoronary use within 24 hr of onset of symptoms of coronary occlusion
- Management of acute evolving transmural myocardial infarction
- Pulmonary embolism—for lysis of diagnosed embolus to restore blood flow
- Deep venous thrombosis for lysis of acute extensive thrombi of the deep veins
- Arterial thrombosis and embolism not originating on the left side of the heart
- Occluded AV cannulae

Contraindications and cautions
- Contraindicated with allergy to streptokinase (Note: most patients have been exposed to streptococci and to streptokinase and therefore have developed resistance to the drug; however, allergic reactions are relatively rare); active internal bleeding; recent (within 2 mo) CVA, intracranial, or intraspinal surgery; intracranial neoplasm; severe uncontrolled hypertension.
- Use cautiously with recent major surgery, obstetric delivery, organ biopsy, puncture of noncompressible blood vessel, serious GI bleed, recent serious trauma, including CPR; severe hypertension; SBE; hemostatic defects; cerebrovascular disease; diabetic hemorrhagic retinopathy; septic thrombosis; pregnancy; lactation; age > 75 yr; any other con-

dition in which bleeding constitutes a serious hazard.

Available forms
Powder for injection—250,000, 750,000, 1,500,000 IU/vial

Dosages
Adults
- *Acute evolving transmural myocardial infarction:* Bolus dose of 20,000 IU directly into the coronary artery. Maintenance dose of 2,000 IU/min for 60 min for a total dose of 140,000 IU *or* 1,500,000 IU administered over 60 min in an infusion of the 1,500,000-IU vial diluted to a total volume of 45 mL. Administer as soon as possible after symptom onset; best within 4 hr but benefit up to 24 hr after onset.
- *Deep vein thrombosis, pulmonary or arterial embolism, arterial thrombosis:* Loading dose of 250,000 IU infused into a peripheral vein over 30 min. Maintenance dose, 100,000 IU/hr for 24–72 hr depending on the response and area treated. After treatment with streptokinase, treat with continuous infusion heparin, beginning after thrombin time decreases to less than twice the control value.
- *AV cannula occlusion:* Slowly instill 250,000 IU in 2 mL IV solution into the occluded cannula; clamp the cannula for 2 hr; then aspirate the catheter and flush with saline.
Pediatric patients
Safety and efficacy not established.

Pharmacokinetics

Route	Onset	Peak
IV	Immediate	30–60 min

Metabolism: $T_{1/2}$: 23 min
Distribution: Crosses placenta; may enter breast milk
Excretion: Unknown

▼ **IV facts**
Preparation: Reconstitute vial with 5 mL of sodium chloride injection or 5% dextrose injection; direct diluent at side of the vial, not directly into the streptokinase. Avoid shaking during reconstitution; gently roll or tilt vial to reconstitute. Further dilute the reconstituted solutions slowly to a total of 45 mL. Solution

S

may be filtered through a ≥ 0.8 mcm filter. Do not add other medications to reconstituted solutions. Discard solutions that contain large amounts of flocculation. Refrigerate reconstituted solution; discard reconstituted solution after 24 hr. Reconstitute the contents of 250,000-IU vial with 2 mL sodium chloride or 5% dextrose injection for use in AV cannulae.
Infusion: Administer as indicated for each specific problem being treated (see Dosages section).
Incompatibilities: Do not mix with any other medications.

Adverse effects
- **CNS:** Headache
- **CV:** Angioneurotic edema, arrhythmias (with intracoronary artery infusion), hypotension, **cholesterol embolism,** pulmonary edema
- **Dermatologic:** Skin rash, urticaria, itching, flushing
- **Hematologic: Bleeding** (*minor or surface* to major internal bleeding)
- **Respiratory:** Breathing difficulty, bronchospasm
- **Other:** Musculoskeletal pain, *fever,* **anaphylactic shock** (rare)

Interactions
✱ **Drug-drug** • Increased risk of hemorrhage with heparin or oral anticoagulants, aspirin, indomethacin, phenylbutazone
✱ **Drug-lab test** • Marked decrease in plasminogen, fibrinogen • Increases in thrombin time (TT), activated partial thromboplastin time (APTT), prothrombin time (PT)

■ Nursing considerations
Assessment
- **History:** Allergy to streptokinase; active internal bleeding, recent CVA; intracranial or intraspinal surgery; intracranial neoplasm; recent major surgery; obstetric delivery; organ biopsy; or rupture of a noncompressible blood vessel; recent serious GI bleed; recent serious trauma; severe hypertension; SBE; hemostatic defects; cerebrovascular disease; diabetic hemorrhagic retinopathy; septic thrombosis; pregnancy; lactation

- **Physical:** Skin color, T, lesions; T; orientation, reflexes; P, BP, peripheral perfusion, baseline ECG; R, adventitous sounds; liver evaluation; Hct, platelet count, TT, APTT, PT

Interventions
- Discontinue heparin, unless ordered specifically for coronary artery infusion.
- Arrange for regular monitoring of coagulation studies.
- Apply pressure or pressure dressings to control superficial bleeding (at invaded or disturbed areas).
- Avoid any arterial invasive procedures.
- Arrange for typing and cross-matching of blood if serious blood loss occurs and whole blood transfusions are required.
- Institute treatment within 2–6 hr of onset of symptoms for evolving MI; within 7 days of other thrombotic event.
- Monitor cardiac rhythm continually during coronary artery infusion.

Teaching points
- You will need frequent blood tests and IV injections.
- Report rash, difficulty breathing, dizziness, disorientation, numbness, tingling.

▽ **streptomycin sulfate**
See *Less Commonly Used Drugs,* p. 1352.

▽ **streptozocin**
(strep toe zoe' sin)
Zanosar
PREGNANCY CATEGORY D

Drug classes
Alkylating agent, nitrosourea
Antineoplastic

Therapeutic actions
Cytotoxic: inhibits DNA synthesis, leading to cell death partially through the production of intrastrand cross-links in DNA; cell cycle nonspecific.

Indications
- Metastatic islet cell carcinoma of the pancreas

Contraindications and cautions
- Contraindicated with allergy to streptozocin; hematopoietic depression; pregnancy (teratogenic and embryotoxic); lactation.
- Use cautiously with impaired renal or hepatic function.

Available forms
Powder for injection—100 mg/mL

Dosages
Two dosage schedules have been used.
Adults
Daily schedule: 500 mg/m² of body surface area IV for 5 consecutive days every 6 wk.
Weekly schedule: Initial dose of 1,000 mg/m² of body surface area IV at weekly intervals for the first 2 wk. Increase subsequent doses if response and toxicity do not occur, but do not exceed a single dose of 1,500 mg/m² of body surface area.

Pharmacokinetics

Route	Onset	Duration
IV	Varies	24 hr

Metabolism: Hepatic; $T_{1/2}$: 35 min
Distribution: Crosses placenta; may enter breast milk
Excretion: Urine

▽ IV facts
Preparation: Reconstitute with 9.5 mL of dextrose injection or 0.9% sodium chloride injection. The resultant pale gold solution contains 100 mg/mL streptozocin. Dilute further with diluents listed above, if needed. Refrigerate vials and protect from light; once reconstituted, use within 12 hr.
Infusion: Infuse slowly over 5–15 min.
Incompatibilities: Do not mix with any other medications.

Adverse effects
- **CNS:** Lethargy, confusion, depression
- **GI:** *Nausea, vomiting,* diarrhea, *hepatotoxicity*
- **GU:** *Renal toxicity*
- **Hematologic: Hematologic toxicity** (rare), glucose intolerance
- **Other:** Infertility, cancer, inflammation at injection site

■ Nursing considerations
Assessment
- **History:** Allergy to streptozocin; hematopoietic depression; impaired renal or hepatic function; pregnancy, lactation
- **Physical:** Weight; orientation, affect; liver evaluation; CBC, differential; urinalysis; blood glucose, serum electrolytes, liver and renal function tests

Interventions
- Arrange for blood and urine tests to evaluate renal function before therapy and weekly during therapy. Monitor liver function tests and CBC.
- Reduce dosage or discontinue if renal toxicity occurs—proteinuria, elevated BUN, plasma creatinine, serum electrolytes.
- Use special precautions when handling the streptozocin; contact with the skin poses a carcinogenic hazard to the area exposed. Wear rubber gloves; if powder or solution comes in contact with the skin, wash immediately with soap and water.
- Administer IV only; intra-arterial administration causes more rapid toxic renal effects.
- Arrange for pretherapy medicating with antiemetic, if needed, to decrease the severity of nausea and vomiting.
- Monitor urine output and perform frequent urinalysis for any sign of renal failure.

Teaching points
- This drug can only be given IV. Prepare a calendar with the course of treatment.
- These side effects may occur: nausea, vomiting, loss of appetite (request an antiemetic; eat small frequent meals); confusion, depression, lethargy.
- This drug can cause severe birth defects. Use birth control with this drug.
- Arrange to have regular medical follow-ups, including blood and urine tests to evaluate drug effects and to determine next dose.
- Report unusual bleeding or bruising, fever, chills, sore throat, stomach or flank pain, changes in urinary output, confusion, depression.

▽ succimer
(sux' i mer)

Chemet

PREGNANCY CATEGORY C

Drug classes
Antidote
Chelating agent

Therapeutic actions
Forms water-soluble chelates with lead, leading to increased urinary excretion of lead.

Indications
• Treatment of lead poisoning in children with blood levels > 45 mcg/dL (not for prophylactic use)
• Orphan drug use: prevention of cystine kidney stones in patients with homozygous cystinuria
• Unlabeled uses: treatment of other heavy metal poisonings (mercury, arsenic)

Contraindications and cautions
• Contraindicated with allergy to succimer, pregnancy (teratogenic and embryotoxic), lactation.
• Use cautiously with impaired renal or hepatic function.

Available forms
Capsules—100 mg

Dosages
Pediatric patients
Starting dose of 10 mg/kg or 350 mg/m^2 q 8 hr PO for 5 days; reduce dosage to 10 mg/kg or 350 mg/m^2 q 12 hr PO for 2 wk (therapy runs for 19 days).

Pharmacokinetics

Route	Onset	Peak
Oral	Varies	1–2 hr

Metabolism: Hepatic; $T_{1/2}$: 2 days
Distribution: Crosses placenta; may enter breast milk
Excretion: Feces and urine

Adverse effects
• **CNS:** Drowsiness, dizziness, sleepiness, otitis media, watery eyes
• **Dermatologic:** Papular rash, herpetic rash, mucocutaneous eruptions, pruritus
• **GI:** *Nausea, vomiting,* diarrhea, metallic taste in mouth, loss of appetite
• **GU:** Decreased urination, voiding difficulty
• **Other:** *Back, stomach, flank, head, rib pain,* chills, fever, flulike symptoms

Interactions
✳ **Drug-drug** • High risk of toxicity with other chelating agents (EDTA)
✳ **Drug-lab test** • False-positive tests of urine ketones using *Ketostix* • False decrease in serum uric acid, CPK

■ Nursing considerations
Assessment
• **History:** Allergy to succimer; lactation, pregnancy; renal or hepatic impairment
• **Physical:** Weight; orientation, affect; liver evaluation; urinalysis; liver and renal function tests; serum lead levels

Interventions
• Test serum blood levels before therapy and monitor weekly.
• Monitor serum transaminase level prior to and weekly during treatment.
• Identify the source of lead and facilitate its removal; succimer is not prophylactic to prevent lead poisoning.
• Ensure that patient continues therapy for full 19 days.
• For children unable to swallow capsules: separate capsules and give medicated beads on a small amount of soft food or by spoon followed by fruit drink.

Teaching points
• For children unable to swallow capsules: separate capsules and give medicated beads on a small amount of soft food or by spoon followed by fruit drink.
• Ensure child maintains good fluid intake.
• These side effects may occur: nausea, vomiting, loss of appetite (eat small, frequent meals); abdominal, back, rib, flank pain (request medications).

Adverse effects in *Italics* are most common; those in **Bold** are life-threatening.

- Report rash, difficulty breathing, difficulty walking, tremors.

▽ sucralfate
*(soo **kral'** fate)*

Apo-sucralfate (CAN), Carafate, Novo-Sucralfate (CAN), Sulcrate (CAN)

PREGNANCY CATEGORY B

Drug class
Antipeptic agent

Therapeutic actions
Forms an ulcer-adherent complex at duodenal ulcer sites, protecting the ulcer against acid, pepsin, and bile salts, thereby promoting ulcer healing; also inhibits pepsin activity in gastric juices.

Indications
- Short-term treatment of duodenal ulcers, up to 8 wk
- Maintenance therapy for duodenal ulcer at reduced dosage after healing
- Orphan drug use: treatment of oral and esophageal ulcers due to radiation, chemotherapy, and sclerotherapy
- Unlabeled uses: accelerates healing of gastric ulcers, long-term treatment of gastric ulcers, treatment of reflux and peptic esophagitis, treatment of NSAID or aspirin-induced GI symptoms and GI damage, prevention of stress ulcers in critically ill patients

Contraindications and cautions
- Allergy to sucralfate, chronic renal failure/dialysis (buildup of aluminum may occur with aluminum-containing products), pregnancy, lactation.

Available forms
Tablets—1 g; suspension—1 g/10 mL

Dosages
Adults
- *Active duodenal ulcer:* 1 g PO qid on an empty stomach (1 hr before meals and hs). Continue treatment for 4–8 wk.

- *Maintenance:* 1 g PO bid.
Pediatric patients
Safety and efficacy not established.

Pharmacokinetics

Route	Onset	Duration
Oral	30 min	5 hr

Metabolism: Hepatic; $T_{1/2}$: 6–20 hr
Distribution: Crosses placenta; may enter breast milk
Excretion: Feces

Adverse effects
- **CNS:** Dizziness, sleeplessness, vertigo
- **Dermatologic:** Rash, pruritus
- **GI:** *Constipation,* diarrhea, nausea, indigestion, gastric discomfort, dry mouth
- **Other:** Back pain

Interactions
❋ **Drug-drug** ● Decreased serum levels and effectiveness of phenytoin, ciprofloxacin, norfloxacin, penicillamine; separate administration by 2 hr ● Risk of aluminum toxicity with aluminum-containing antacids

■ Nursing considerations
Assessment
- **History:** Allergy to sucralfate; chronic renal failure/dialysis; pregnancy, lactation
- **Physical:** Skin color, lesions; reflexes, orientation; mucous membranes, normal output

Interventions
- Give drug on an empty stomach, 1 hr before or 2 hr after meals and hs.
- Monitor pain; use antacids to relieve pain.
- Administer antacids between doses of sucralfate, not within 30 min before or after sucralfate doses.

Teaching points
- Take the drug on an empty stomach, 1 hr before or 2 hr after meals and at bedtime.
- If you are also taking antacids for pain relief; do not take antacids 30 min before or after taking sucralfate.
- These side effects may occur: dizziness, vertigo (avoid driving or operating dangerous machinery); indigestion, nausea (eat small, frequent meals); dry mouth (frequent mouth

S

care, sucking on sugarless candies may help); constipation (request aid).
• Report severe gastric pain.

▷ **sufentanil citrate**
*(soo **fen'** ta nil)*

Sufenta

PREGNANCY CATEGORY C

C-II CONTROLLED SUBSTANCE

Drug class
Narcotic agonist analgesic

Therapeutic actions
Acts at specific opioid receptors, causing analgesia, respiratory depression, physical depression, euphoria.

Indications
• Analgesic adjunct to maintain balanced general anesthesia
• Primary anesthetic with 100% oxygen to induce and maintain anesthesia in major surgical procedures
• Epidural analgesia with bupivacaine during labor and delivery

Contraindications and cautions
• Contraindicated with known sensitivity to sufentanil, pregnancy.
• Use cautiously with obesity, hepatic disease, head injury, diabetes, arrhythmias, lactation, severe debilitation, renal or pulmonary disease.

Available forms
Injection—50 mcg/mL

Dosages
Individualize dosage; monitor vital signs routinely.
Adults
• *Adjunct to general anesthesia:* 1–2 mcg/kg IV initially; 10–25 mcg for maintenance; not to exceed 1 mcg/hr of expected surgical time.
• *With oxygen for anesthesia:* 8–30 mcg/kg IV initially; supplement with doses of 0.5–10 mcg IV; not to exceed 30 mcg/kg for the procedure.
• *Epidural analgesia:* 10–15 mcg via epidural administration with 10 mL bupivacaine 0.125%; may repeat twice at ≥ 1-hr intervals (total of 3 doses).
Pediatric patients 2–12 yr
• *With oxygen for anesthesia:* 10–25 mcg/kg IV initially; supplement with doses of 25–50 mcg IV.

Pharmacokinetics

Route	Onset	Duration
IV	Immediate	5 min

Metabolism: Hepatic; $T_{1/2}$: 2.7 hr
Distribution: Crosses placenta; enters breast milk

▽▼ IV facts
Preparation: Protect vials from light.
Infusion: Give slowly over 1–2 min by direct injection or into running IV tubing.

Adverse effects
• **CNS:** *Sedation, clamminess, sweating, headache, vertigo, floating feeling, dizziness, lethargy, confusion, light-headedness,* nervousness, unusual dreams, agitation, euphoria, hallucinations, delirium, insomnia, anxiety, fear, disorientation, impaired mental and physical performance, coma, mood changes, weakness, headache, tremor, convulsions
• **CV:** Palpitations, change in BP, circulatory depression, **cardiac arrest, shock,** tachycardia, bradycardia, arrhythmia
• **Dermatologic:** Rash, hives, pruritus, flushing, warmth, sensitivity to cold
• **EENT:** Diplopia, blurred vision
• **GI:** *Nausea, vomiting,* dry mouth, anorexia, constipation, biliary tract spasm
• **GU:** Ureteral spasm, spasm of vesical sphincters, urinary retention or hesitancy, oliguria, antidiuretic effect, reduced libido or potency
• **Local:** Phlebitis following IV injection, pain at injection site
• **Respiratory:** Slow, shallow respiration, apnea, suppression of cough reflex, laryngospasm, bronchospasm

---

Adverse effects in *Italics* are most common; those in **Bold** are life-threatening.

- **Other:** Physical tolerance and dependence, psychological dependence

Interactions

✷ **Drug-drug** • Potentiation of effects with barbiturate anesthetics • Increased risk of hypotension and bradycardia if given with beta-blockers, calcium channel blockers

✷ **Drug-food** • Decreased metabolism and risk of toxic effects if combined with grapefruit juice; avoid this combination

✷ **Drug-lab test** • Elevated biliary tract pressure may cause increases in plasma amylase, lipase; determinations of these levels may be unreliable for 24 hr after administration of narcotics

■ Nursing considerations

CLINICAL ALERT!
Name confusion has occurred between sufentanil and fentanyl; use extreme caution.

Assessment

- **History:** Hypersensitivity to sufentanil or narcotics; physical dependence on a narcotic analgesic; pregnancy, lactation; COPD; increased intracranial pressure; acute MI, biliary tract surgery; renal or hepatic dysfunction
- **Physical:** Orientation, reflexes, bilateral grip strength, affect; pupil size, vision; pulse, auscultation, BP; R, adventitious sounds; bowel sounds, normal output; liver and kidney function tests

Interventions

- Give to lactating women 4–6 hr before the next feeding to minimize the amount in milk.
- Ensure that patient avoids grapefruit juice while on this drug.
- Provide narcotic antagonist, facilities for assisted or controlled respiration on standby during parenteral administration.

Teaching points

Incorporate teaching about drug into preoperative or postoperative teaching program.

- These side effects may occur: dizziness, sedation, drowsiness, impaired visual acuity (ask for assistance to move); nausea, loss of appetite (lie quietly, eat frequent, small meals); constipation (use a laxative).
- Report severe nausea, vomiting, palpitations, shortness of breath or difficulty breathing.

▷ sulfadiazine
*(sul fa **dye'** a zeen)*

PREGNANCY CATEGORY C

PREGNANCY CATEGORY D
(LABOR AND DELIVERY)

Drug classes
Antibiotic
Sulfonamide

Therapeutic actions

Bacteriostatic: competitively antagonizes para-aminobenzoic acid (PABA), an essential component of folic acid synthesis in gram-negative and gram-positive bacteria; prevents cell replication.

Indications

- Treatment of acute infections caused by susceptible organisms: urinary tract infections, chancroid, inclusion conjunctivitis, trachoma, nocardiosis, toxoplasmosis (with pyrimethamine), malaria (as adjunctive therapy for chloroquine-resistant strains of *P. falciparum*), acute otitis media (due to *H. influenzae* when used with penicillin or erythromycin), *H. influenzae* meningitis (as adjunctive therapy with parenteral streptomycin), meningococcal meningitis, rheumatic fever
- Orphan drug use: with pyrimethamine for treatment of *Toxoplasma gondii* encephalitis in patients with AIDS

Contraindications and cautions

- Contraindicated with allergy to sulfonamides, sulfonylureas, thiazides; pregnancy (teratogenic; may cause kernicterus); lactation (risk of kernicterus, diarrhea, rash).
- Use cautiously with impaired renal or hepatic function, G-6-PD deficiency, porphyria.

Available forms
Tablets—500 mg

S

Dosages
Adults
Loading dose: 2–4 g PO. Maintenance: 2–4 g/day PO in 3 to 6 divided doses.
- *Prevention of recurrent attacks of rheumatic fever (not for initial therapy of streptococcal infections):*
> *30 kg:* 1 g/day PO.
< *30 kg:* 0.5 g/day PO.
Pediatric patients
< *2 mo:* Not recommended except to treat congenital toxoplasmosis.
> *2 mo:* Initial dose: 75 mg/kg PO. Maintenance: 150 mg/kg/day PO in 4–6 divided doses with a maximum dose of 6 g/day.
- *Treatment of toxoplasmosis for 3–4 wk:*
< *2 mo:* 25 mg/kg PO per dose qid.
> *2 mo:* 25–50 mg/kg PO per dose qid.

Pharmacokinetics

Route	Onset	Peak
Oral	Varies	3–6 hr

Metabolism: Hepatic; $T_{1/2}$: unknown
Distribution: Crosses placenta; enters breast milk
Excretion: Urine

Adverse effects
- **CNS:** *Headache,* peripheral neuropathy, mental depression, convulsions, ataxia, hallucinations, tinnitus, vertigo, insomnia, hearing loss, drowsiness, transient lesions of posterior spinal column, transverse myelitis
- **Dermatologic:** *Photosensitivity,* cyanosis, petechiae, alopecia
- **GI:** *Nausea, emesis, abdominal pains,* diarrhea, bloody diarrhea, anorexia, pancreatitis, stomatitis, impaired folic acid absorption, hepatitis, hepatocellular necrosis
- **GU:** *Crystalluria, hematuria,* proteinuria, nephrotic syndrome, toxic nephrosis with oliguria and anuria, oligospermia, infertility
- **Hematologic:** *Agranulocytosis,* aplastic anemia, thrombocytopenia, leukopenia, hemolytic anemia, hypoprothrombinemia, methemoglobinemia, megaloblastic anemia
- **Hypersensitivity: Stevens-Johnson syndrome,** generalized skin eruptions, epidermal necrolysis, urticaria, serum sickness, pruritus, exfoliative dermatitis, anaphylactoid reactions, periorbital edema, conjunctival and scleral redness, photosensitization, arthralgia, allergic myocarditis, transient pulmonary changes with eosinophilia, decreased pulmonary function
- **Other:** Drug fever, chills, periarteritis nodosum

Interactions
✳ Drug-drug • Increased risk of hypoglycemia when tolbutamide, tolazamide, glyburide, glipizide, acetohexamide, chlorpropamide are taken concurrently • Increased risk of phenytoin toxicity with sulfonamides • Risk of hemorrhage when combined with oral anticoagulants • Increased risk of nephrotoxicity with cyclosporine
✳ Drug-lab test • False-positive urinary glucose tests using Benedict's method

■ Nursing considerations
Assessment
- **History:** Allergy to sulfonamides, sulfonylureas, thiazides; pregnancy, lactation; impaired renal or hepatic function; G-6-PD deficiency
- **Physical:** T; skin color, lesions; culture of infected site; orientation, reflexes, affect, peripheral sensation; R, adventitious sounds; mucous membranes, bowel sounds, liver evaluation; liver and renal function tests, CBC and differential, urinalysis

Interventions
- Arrange for culture and sensitivity tests of infection before therapy; repeat cultures if response is not as expected.
- Administer drug on an empty stomach, 1 hr before or 2 hr after meals, with a full glass of water.
- Ensure adequate fluid intake; sulfadiazine is very insoluble and may cause crystalluria if high concentrations occur in the urine; alkalinization of the urine may be necessary.
- Discontinue drug immediately if hypersensitivity reaction occurs.

Adverse effects in *Italics* are most common; those in **Bold** are life-threatening.

Teaching points

- Complete full course of therapy.
- Take the drug on an empty stomach, 1 hr before or 2 hr after meals, with a full glass of water.
- Drink eight glasses of water per day.
- This drug is specific to this disease; do not self-treat any other infection.
- These side effects may occur: sensitivity to sunlight (use sunscreens; wear protective clothing); dizziness, drowsiness, difficulty walking, loss of sensation (avoid driving or performing tasks that require alertness); nausea, vomiting, diarrhea; loss of fertility.
- Report blood in the urine, rash, ringing in the ears, difficulty breathing, fever, sore throat, chills.

▽ **sulfasalazine**
(sul fa sal' a zeen)

Alti-Sulfasalazine (CAN), Azulfidine, Azulfidine EN-Tabs, Salazopyrin (CAN), S.A.S. (CAN)

PREGNANCY CATEGORY B

Drug classes

Antibiotic
Sulfonamide
Antirheumatic agent
Anti-inflammatory

Therapeutic actions

Bacteriostatic: competitively antagonizes PABA, an essential component of folic acid synthesis in susceptible gram-negative and gram-positive bacteria; one-third of the oral dose is absorbed from the small intestine; remaining two-thirds passes to the colon where it is split into 5-aminosalicylic acid and sulfapyridine; most of the sulfapyridine is absorbed; the 5-aminosalicylic acid acts locally as an anti-inflammatory agent.

Indications

- Treatment of ulcerative colitis
- Treatment of rheumatoid arthritis in patients intolerant or unresponsive to other anti-inflammatories (delayed-release)
- Treatment of children 6–16 yr with juvenile rheumatoid arthritis involving five joints who have not responded adequately to salicylates or other NSAIDS (*Azulfidine En-Tabs*)
- Unlabeled uses: Crohn's disease, ankylosing, spondylitis, psoriatic arthritis

Contraindications and cautions

- Contraindicated with allergy to sulfonamides, sulfonylureas, thiazides; pregnancy (teratogenic may cause kernicterus); lactation (risk of kernicterus, diarrhea, rash), intestinal or urinary obstruction, pediatric patients < 2 yr of age.
- Use cautiously with impaired renal or hepatic function, G-6-PD deficiency, porphyria.

Available forms

Tablets—500 mg; DR tablets—500 mg

Dosages

Administer around the clock; dosage intervals should not exceed 8 hr. Give after meals.
Adults
- *Ulcerative colitis:* Initial therapy, 3–4 g/day PO in evenly divided doses. Initial doses of 1–2 g/day PO may lessen adverse GI effects. Doses > 4 g/day increase risk of toxicity. Maintenance, 2 g/day PO in evenly spaced doses (500 mg qid).
- *Adult RA:* 2 g daily in 2 evenly divided doses.
Pediatric patients
- *Ulcerative colitis:* For ≥ 2 yr, initial therapy, 40–60 mg/kg/24 hr PO in 3 to 6 divided doses. Maintenance therapy, 30 mg/kg/24 hr PO in 4 equally divided doses. Maximum dosage, 2 g/day.
- *JRA—polyarticular course:* For ≥ 6 yr, 30–50 mg/kg daily in 2 evenly divided doses. Maximum, 2 g/day.

Pharmacokinetics

Route	Onset	Peak
Oral	Varies	1.5–6 hr, 6–24 hr metabolite

Metabolism: Hepatic; $T_{1/2}$: 5–10 hr
Distribution: Crosses placenta; enters breast milk
Excretion: Urine

Adverse effects

- **CNS:** Headache, peripheral neuropathy, mental depression, convulsions, ataxia, hal-

lucinations, tinnitus, vertigo, insomnia, hearing loss, drowsiness, transient lesions of posterior spinal column, transverse myelitis
- **Dermatologic:** Photosensitivity, cyanosis, petechiae, alopecia
- **GI:** *Nausea, emesis, abdominal pains,* diarrhea, bloody diarrhea, anorexia, pancreatitis, stomatitis, impaired folic acid absorption, hepatitis, **hepatocellular necrosis**
- **GU:** *Crystalluria, hematuria,* proteinuria, nephrotic syndrome, toxic nephrosis with oliguria and anuria, oligospermia, infertility
- **Hematologic:** Agranulocytosis, aplastic anemia, thrombocytopenia, leukopenia, hemolytic anemia, hypoprothrombinemia, methemoglobinemia, megaloblastic anemia
- **Hypersensitivity: Stevens-Johnson syndrome,** generalized skin eruptions, epidermal necrolysis, urticaria, serum sickness, pruritus, exfoliative dermatitis, anaphylactoid reactions, periorbital edema, conjunctival and scleral redness, photosensitization, arthralgia, allergic myocarditis, transient pulmonary changes with eosinophilia, decreased pulmonary function
- **Other:** Drug fever, chills, periarteritis nodosum

Interactions
✳ Drug-drug • Decreased absorption of digoxin with lessened therapeutic effect; monitor patient, space doses > 2 hr apart • Increased risk of folate deficiency, monitor for signs of folate deficiency

✳ Drug-lab test • Possible false-positive urinary glucose tests using Benedict's method

■ Nursing considerations
Assessment
- **History:** Allergy to sulfonamides, sulfonylureas, thiazides; pregnancy; lactation; impaired renal or hepatic function; G-6-PD deficiency; porphyria
- **Physical:** T; skin color, lesions; culture of infected site; orientation, reflexes, affect, peripheral sensation; R, adventitious sounds; mucous membranes, bowel sounds, liver

evaluation; liver and renal function tests, CBC and differential, urinalysis

Interventions
- Administer drug after meals or with food to prevent GI upset. Administer the drug around the clock.
- Ensure that patient swallows tablets whole; do not cut, crush, or chew.
- Ensure adequate fluid intake; sulfasalazine is very insoluble and may cause crystalluria if high concentrations occur in the urine; alkalinization of the urine may be necessary.
- Discontinue drug immediately if hypersensitivity reaction occurs.

Teaching points
- Complete full course of therapy. Swallow tablets whole; do not cut, crush, or chew.
- Take the drug with food or meals to decrease GI upset.
- Drink 8 glasses of water per day.
- These side effects may occur: sensitivity to sunlight (use sunscreen, wear protective clothing); dizziness, drowsiness, difficulty walking, loss of sensation (avoid driving or performing tasks that require alertness); nausea, vomiting, diarrhea; loss of fertility; yellow-orange urine.
- Report blood in the urine, rash, ringing in the ears, difficulty breathing, fever, sore throat, chills.

▽ **sulfinpyrazone**
(sul fin peer' a zone)

Anturan (CAN), Anturane, Apo-Sulfinpyrazone (CAN), Novopyrazone (CAN)

PREGNANCY CATEGORY C

Drug classes
Uricosuric agent
Antigout agent
Antiplatelet agent

Therapeutic actions

Inhibits the renal tubular reabsorption of uric acid, increasing the urinary excretion of uric acid, decreasing serum uric acid levels, retarding urate deposition, and promoting the resorption of urate deposits. Inhibits prostaglandin synthesis, which prevents platelet aggregation, but lacks analgesic and anti-inflammatory activity.

Indications

- Chronic gouty arthritis
- Intermittent gouty arthritis
- Unlabeled uses: post-MI therapy to decrease incidence of sudden death; in rheumatic mitral stenosis to decrease the frequency of systemic embolism

Contraindications and cautions

- Contraindicated with allergy to sulfinpyrazone, phenylbutazone, or other pyrazoles; blood dyscrasias; peptic ulcer or symptoms of GI inflammation.
- Use cautiously with renal failure, pregnancy, lactation.

Available forms

Tablets—100 mg; capsules—200 mg

Dosages

Adults

- *Gout:* 200–400 mg/day PO in 2 divided doses with meals or milk, gradually increase to maintenance dose over 1 wk. Maintenance, 400 mg/day PO in 2 divided doses. May increase to 800 mg/day or reduce to 200 mg/day. Regulate dose by monitoring serum uric acid levels.
- *Inhibition of platelet aggregation:* 200 mg PO tid or qid.

Pediatric patients

Safety and efficacy not established.

Pharmacokinetics

Route	Onset	Peak	Duration
Oral	Varies	1–2 hr	4–6 hr

Metabolism: $T_{1/2}$: 2.2–4 hr
Distribution: Crosses placenta; may enter breast milk
Excretion: Urine

Adverse effects

- **Dermatologic:** Rash
- **GI:** *Upper GI disturbances*
- **GU:** Exacerbation of gout and uric acid stones, renal failure
- **Hematologic:** Blood dyscrasias

Interactions

✳ **Drug-drug** • Decreased effectiveness with salicylates • Increased pharmacologic effects of tolbutamide, glyburide, warfarin • Increased risk of hepatotoxicity with acetaminophen

■ Nursing considerations

Assessment

- **History:** Allergy to sulfinpyrazone, phenylbutazone, or other pyrazoles; blood dyscrasias; peptic ulcer or symptoms of GI inflammation; renal failure; pregnancy; lactation
- **Physical:** Skin lesions, color; liver evaluation, normal output, gums; urinary output; CBC, renal and liver function tests, urinalysis

Interventions

- Administer drug with meals or antacids to prevent GI upset.
- Force fluids (2.5 to 3 L/day) to decrease the risk of renal stone development.
- Check urine alkalinity (urates crystallize in acid urine); use sodium bicarbonate or potassium citrate to alkalinize urine.
- Arrange for regular medical follow-ups and blood tests.
- Double-check any analgesics ordered for pain; avoid salicylates, acetaminophen.

Teaching points

- Take the drug with meals or antacids to prevent GI upset.
- These side effects may occur: exacerbation of gouty attack or renal stones (drink plenty of fluids, 2.5–3 L/day); nausea, vomiting, loss of appetite (take with meals, use antacids).
- Avoid the use of aspirin and aspirin-containing products; serious toxic effects could occur.
- Report flank pain, dark urine or blood in urine, acute gout attack, unusual fatigue or lethargy, unusual bleeding or bruising.

▽ sulfisoxazole

*(sul fi **sox'** a zole)*

Gantrisin, Novo-Soxazole (CAN)

PREGNANCY CATEGORY C

PREGNANCY CATEGORY D
(AT TERM)

Drug classes
Antibiotic
Sulfonamide

Therapeutic actions
Bacteriostatic: competitively antagonizes PABA, an essential component of folic acid synthesis in susceptible gram-negative and gram-positive bacteria, preventing cell replication.

Indications
- Treatment of acute infections caused by susceptible organisms: urinary tract infections, chancroid, inclusion conjunctivitis, trachoma, nocardiosis, toxoplasmosis (with pyrimethamine), malaria (as adjunctive therapy for chloroquine-resistant strains of *P. falciparum*), acute otitis media (due to *H. influenzae* when used with penicillin or erythromycin), *H. influenzae* meningitis (as adjunctive therapy with parenteral streptomycin), meningococcal meningitis
- Conjunctivitis, corneal ulcer, superficial ocular infections due to susceptible microorganisms
- CDC recommended for treatment of sexually transmitted diseases
- Unlabeled use: chemoprophylaxis for recurrent otitis media

Contraindications and cautions
- Contraindicated with allergy to sulfonamides, sulfonylureas, thiazides; pregnancy (teratogenic may cause kernicterus); lactation (risk of kernicterus, diarrhea, rash); patients < 2 mo of age except in congenital toxoplasmosis as an adjunct with pyrimethamine.
- Use cautiously with impaired renal or hepatic function, G-6-PD deficiency, porphyria.

Available forms
Tablets—500 mg; suspension—0.5 g/5 mL

Dosages
Adults
Oral
Loading dose: 2–4 g PO. Maintenance: 4–8 g/day PO in 4 to 6 divided doses.
- *CDC recommended treatment of sexually transmitted diseases—lymphogranuloma venereum:* As an alternative regimen to doxycycline, 500 mg PO qid for 21 days.
- *Treatment of uncomplicated urethral, endocervical, or rectal* Chlamydiatrachomatis *infections:* As an alternative regimen to doxycycline or tetracycline (if erythromycin is not tolerated), 500 mg PO qid for 10 days.

Pediatric patients > 2 mo
Oral
Initial dose, 75 mg/kg PO. Maintenance dose, 150 mg/kg/day PO in 4–6 divided doses with a maximum dose of 6 g/day.

Pharmacokinetics

Route	Onset	Peak
Oral	Varies	2–4 hr

Metabolism: Hepatic; $T_{1/2}$: 4.5–7.8 hr
Distribution: Crosses placenta; enters breast milk
Excretion: Urine

Adverse effects
Systemic
- **CNS:** *Headache,* peripheral neuropathy, mental depression, convulsions, ataxia, hallucinations, tinnitus, vertigo, insomnia, hearing loss, drowsiness, transient lesions of posterior spinal column, transverse myelitis
- **Dermatologic:** *Photosensitivity,* cyanosis, petechiae, alopecia
- **GI:** *Nausea, emesis, abdominal pains,* diarrhea, bloody diarrhea, anorexia, pancreatitis, stomatitis, impaired folic acid absorption, hepatitis, hepatocellular necrosis
- **GU:** *Crystalluria, hematuria,* proteinuria, nephrotic syndrome, toxic nephrosis with oliguria and anuria, oligospermia, infertility
- **Hematologic:** *Agranulocytosis,* aplastic anemia, thrombocytopenia, leukopenia, he-

---

Adverse effects in *Italics* are most common; those in **Bold** are life-threatening.

molytic anemia, hypoprothrombinemia, methemoglobinemia, megaloblastic anemia
- **Hypersensitivity: Stevens-Johnson syndrome,** generalized skin eruptions, epidermal necrolysis, urticaria, serum sickness, pruritus, exfoliative dermatitis, anaphylactoid reactions, periorbital edema, conjunctival and scleral redness, photosensitization, arthralgia, allergic myocarditis, transient pulmonary changes with eosinophilia, decreased pulmonary function
- **Other:** Drug fever, chills, periarteritis nodosum

Interactions
✴ **Drug-drug** • Increased risk of hypoglycemia with tolbutamide, tolazamide, glyburide, glipizide, acetohexamide, chlorpropamide • Increased risk of nephrotoxicity with cyclosporine • Possible increased bleeding with oral anticoagulants; monitor for bleeding
✴ **Drug-lab test** • False-positive urinary glucose tests using Benedict's method • False-positive results with *Urobilistix* test and sulfosalicylic acid tests for urinary protein

■ Nursing considerations
Assessment
- **History:** Allergy to sulfonamides, sulfonylureas, thiazides; impaired renal or hepatic function; G-6-PD deficiency; porphyria; pregnancy; lactation
- **Physical:** T; skin color, lesions; culture of infection; orientation, reflexes, affect, peripheral sensation; R, adventitious sounds; mucous membranes, bowel sounds, liver evaluation; liver and renal function tests, CBC and differential, urinalysis

Interventions
- Arrange for culture and sensitivity tests of infection before therapy; repeat cultures if response is not as expected.
- Administer oral drug on an empty stomach, 1 hr before or 2 hr after meals, with a full glass of water.
- Discontinue drug immediately if hypersensitivity reaction occurs.
- Monitor CBC, differential, urinalysis before and periodically during therapy.

Teaching points
- Complete full course of therapy.
- Take the drug on an empty stomach, 1 hr before or 2 hr after meals, with a full glass of water.
- This drug is specific to this disease. Do not self-treat any other infection.
- These side effects may occur: sensitivity to sunlight (use sunscreens, wear protective clothing); dizziness, drowsiness, difficulty walking, loss of sensation (avoid driving or performing tasks that require alertness); nausea, vomiting, diarrhea; loss of fertility.
- Report blood in the urine; rash; ringing in the ears; difficulty breathing; fever; sore throat; chills.

▽ **sulindac**
*(sul **in**' dak)*

Apo-Sulin (CAN), Clinoril, Novo-Sundac (CAN)

PREGNANCY CATEGORY B

Drug class
Nonsteroidal anti-inflammatory drug (NSAID)

Therapeutic actions
Anti-inflammatory, analgesic, and antipyretic activities largely related to inhibition of prostaglandin synthesis; exact mechanisms of action are not known.

Indications
- Acute or long-term use to relieve signs and symptoms of osteoarthritis, rheumatoid arthritis, acute gouty arthritis
- Acute or long-term use in relief of signs and symptoms of ankylosing spondylitis, acute painful shoulder

Contraindications and cautions
- Contraindicated with pregnancy, lactation.
- Use cautiously with allergies, renal, hepatic, CV, and GI conditions.

Available forms
Tablets—150, 200 mg

Dosages
Do not exceed 400 mg/day.

Adults

- *Rheumatoid arthritis or osteoarthritis, ankylosing spondylitis:* Initial dose of 150 mg bid PO. Individualize dosage.
- *Acute painful shoulder, acute gouty arthritis:* 200 mg bid PO. After adequate response, reduce dosage. Acute painful shoulder usually requires 7–14 days of therapy. Acute gouty arthritis, 7 days.

Pediatric patients

Safety and efficacy not established.

Pharmacokinetics

Route	Onset	Peak	Duration
Oral	Varies	2–4 hr	10–12 hr

Metabolism: Hepatic; $T_{1/2}$: 8–10 hr
Distribution: Crosses placenta; enters breast milk
Excretion: Urine and feces

Adverse effects

- **CNS:** *Headache, dizziness, somnolence, insomnia,* fatigue, tiredness, dizziness, tinnitus, ophthalmologic effects
- **Dermatologic:** *Rash,* pruritus, sweating, dry mucous membranes, stomatitis
- **GI:** *Nausea, dyspepsia, GI pain,* diarrhea, vomiting, *constipation,* flatulence
- **GU:** Dysuria, renal impairment
- **Hematologic:** Bleeding, platelet inhibition with higher doses, neutropenia, eosinophilia, leukopenia, pancytopenia, thrombocytopenia, agranulocytosis, granulocytopenia, aplastic anemia, decreased Hgb or Hct, bone marrow depression, menorrhagia
- **Respiratory:** Dyspnea, hemoptysis, pharyngitis, bronchospasm, rhinitis
- **Other:** Peripheral edema, **anaphylactoid reactions to fatal anaphylactic shock**

Interactions

✳ Drug-drug • Increased serum lithium levels and risk of toxicity • Decreased antihypertensive effects of beta-blockers • Decreased therapeutic effects of bumetanide, furosemide, ethacrynic acid

✳ Drug-food • Decreased rate but not extent of absorption when taken with food

■ Nursing considerations

Assessment

- **History:** Allergies, renal, hepatic, CV, and GI conditions; pregnancy; lactation
- **Physical:** Skin color and lesions; orientation, reflexes, ophthalmologic and audiometric evaluation, peripheral sensation; P, edema; R, adventitious sounds; liver evaluation; CBC, clotting times, renal and liver function tests; serum electrolytes, stool guaiac

Interventions

- Give with food or milk if GI upset occurs.
- Arrange for periodic ophthalmologic examination during long-term therapy.
- Institute emergency procedures if overdose occurs: gastric lavage, induction of emesis, supportive therapy.

Teaching points

- Take with food or meals if GI upset occurs.
- Take only the prescribed dosage.
- Dizziness, drowsiness can occur (avoid driving or the use of dangerous machinery).
- Report sore throat, fever, rash, itching, weight gain, swelling in ankles or fingers; changes in vision; black, tarry stools.

▷ sumatriptan succinate

*(sue mah **trip**' tan)*

Imitrex

PREGNANCY CATEGORY C

Drug classes

Antimigraine agent (triptan)
Serotonin-selective agonist

Therapeutic actions

Binds to serotonin receptors to cause vascular constrictive effects on cranial blood vessels, causing the relief of migraine in selective patients.

Indications

- Treatment of acute migraine attacks with or without aura
- Acute treatment of cluster headaches (SC)

Contraindications and cautions

- Contraindicated with allergy to sumatriptan, cerebrovascular or peripheral vascular syndromes, severe hepatic impairment, MAOIs, uncontrolled hypertension, hemiplegic migraine, pregnancy, coronary artery disease.
- Use cautiously with the elderly, lactation, renal function impairment.

Available forms

Tablets—25, 50, 100 mg; injection—12 mg/mL; nasal spray—5, 20 mg

Dosages
Adults
Oral
25, 50, or 100 mg; additional doses may be repeated in ≥ 2 hr; up to a maximum of 200 mg/day.
SC
6 mg, may be repeated in 1 hr. Maximum: 12 mg/24 hr.
Intranasal
5, 10, or 20 mg, may be repeated after 2 hr. Maximum: 40 mg/24 hr.
Pediatric patients
Safety and efficacy not established.
Patients with hepatic impairment
Maximum single dose: 50 mg.

Pharmacokinetics

Route	Onset	Peak
SC	Varies	5–20 min
Oral	1–1.5 hr	2–4 hr
Injection	Rapid	1.5 hr

Metabolism: Hepatic; $T_{1/2}$: 115 min
Distribution: Crosses placenta; enters breast milk
Excretion: Urine

Adverse effects

- **CNS:** *Dizziness, vertigo,* headache, anxiety, malaise or fatigue, *weakness, myalgia*
- **CV:** *Blood pressure alterations, tightness or pressure in chest*
- **GI:** Abdominal discomfort, dysphagia
- **Local:** *Injection site discomfort,* nose and throat discomfort (nasal spray)
- **Other:** *Tingling, warm/hot sensations, burning sensation, feeling of heaviness,*

pressure sensation, numbness, feeling of tightness, feeling strange, cold sensation
Nasal spray
- **GI:** Bad taste, nausea

Interactions

✲ Drug-drug • Prolonged vasoactive reactions with ergot-containing drugs • Increased serum levels and toxicity of sumatriptan with MAOIs; avoid this combination and for 2 wk after MAOI discontinuation

✲ Drug-alternative therapy • Increased risk of severe reaction if combined with St. John's wort therapy

■ Nursing considerations
Assessment

- **History:** Allergy to sumatriptan; active CAD; uncontrolled hypertension; hemiplegic migraine; pregnancy, lactation
- **Physical:** Skin color and lesions; orientation, reflexes, peripheral sensation; P, BP; renal and liver function tests

Interventions

- Administer to relieve acute migraine, not as a prophylactic measure.
- Administer as SC injection just below the skin as soon as possible after symptoms begin.
- Repeat injection only after 1 hr if relief is not obtained; only two injections may be given each 24 hr.
- Administer PO with fluids; may repeat in 2 hr if no relief.
- Repeat nasal spray after 2 hr if headache returns or does not respond.
- Monitor BP of patients with possible CAD; discontinue at any sign of angina, prolonged high BP.

Teaching points

- Learn to use the autoinjector; injection may be repeated only after 1 hr if relief is not obtained; do not administer more than two injections in 24 hr.
- Inject just below the skin as soon as possible after onset of migraine; this drug is for an acute attack only, not for use to prevent attacks.
- Administer nasal spray as a single dose; repeat if needed only after 2 hr.

- Take oral drug with fluids, may be repeated in 2 hr if no relief or return of headache.
- This drug should not be taken during pregnancy; if you suspect that you are pregnant, contact physician and refrain from using drug.
- These side effects may occur: dizziness, drowsiness (avoid driving or the use of dangerous machinery); numbness, tingling, feelings of tightness or pressure.
- Contact physician immediately if you experience severe or continuous chest pain or pressure.
- Report feelings of heat, flushing, tiredness, feelings of sickness, swelling of lips or eyelids.

▽tacrine hydrochloride (tetrahydroamino-acridine, THA)
(tay' krin)

Cognex

PREGNANCY CATEGORY C

Drug classes
Cholinesterase inhibitor
Alzheimer's drug

Therapeutic actions
Centrally acting reversible cholinesterase inhibitor, leading to elevated acetylcholine levels in the cortex, which slows the neuronal degradation that occurs in Alzheimer's disease.

Indications
- Treatment of mild to moderate dementia of the Alzheimer's type

Contraindications and cautions
- Contraindicated with allergy to tacrine or acridine derivatives, previous tacrine-associated jaundice, pregnancy.
- Use cautiously with renal or hepatic disease; bladder obstruction; seizure conditions; sick sinus syndrome; GI bleeding; anesthesia.

Available forms
Capsules—10, 20, 30, 40 mg

Dosages
Adults
10 mg PO qid; maintain this dose for 6 wk with regular monitoring of transaminase levels; after 6 wk, increase dose to 20 mg PO qid; if patient is tolerant to drug and transaminase levels are WNL, increase at 4-wk intervals at 10-mg increases to a total of 120–160 mg/day.
Pediatric patients
Safety and efficacy not established.
Patients with hepatic impairment
ALT levels > 3–≤ 5 times upper level of normal: Reduce dose to 40 mg/day, adjust up if levels improve.
ALT levels > 5 times upper level of normal: Stop treatment, rechallenge if levels become normal.

Pharmacokinetics

Route	Onset	Peak
Oral	Varies	1–2 hr

Metabolism: Hepatic; $T_{1/2}$: 2–4 hr
Distribution: Crosses placenta; may enter breast milk
Excretion: Urine

Adverse effects
- **CNS:** *Headache, fatigue, dizziness, confusion,* ataxia, insomnia, somnolence, tremor, agitation, depression, anxiety, abnormal thinking
- **CV:** Chest pain
- **Dermatologic:** *Rash,* flushing, purpura
- **GI:** *Nausea, vomiting, diarrhea, dyspepsia, anorexia, abdominal pain,* flatulence, constipation, **hepatotoxicity**
- **GU:** Urinary frequency, urinary tract infections
- **Respiratory:** *Rhinitis,* upper respiratory infections, coughing

Interactions
✳ Drug-drug • Increased effects and risk of toxicity of theophylline, cholinesterase inhibitors • Decreased effects of anticholinergics • Increased effects with cimetidine

✳ **Drug-food** • Decreased absorption and serum levels of tacrine if taken with food

■ Nursing considerations

CLINICAL ALERT!
Name confusion has occurred between tacrine and Tequin (gatifloxacin); use caution.

Assessment

- **History:** Allergy to tacrine or acridine derivatives; previous tacrine-associated jaundice; pregnancy; renal or hepatic disease; bladder obstruction; seizure conditions; sick sinus syndrome; GI bleed; anesthesia
- **Physical:** Orientation, affect, reflexes; BP, P; R, adventitious sounds; urinary output; abdominal exam; renal and liver function tests; serum transaminase levels

Interventions

- Arrange for regular transaminase level determination before and during therapy.
- Use with great care in patients with any history of hepatic dysfunction.
- Administer around the clock at regular intervals for best results.
- Administer on an empty stomach, 1 hr before or 2 hr after meals.
- Administer with meals only if severe GI upset occurs.
- Decrease dose and slowly discontinue drug if side effects become severe.
- Notify surgeons that patient is on tacrine; exaggerated muscle relaxation may occur if succinylcholine-type drugs are used.
- Do not suddenly discontinue high doses of drug.
- Monitor for any signs of neurologic change or deterioration; drug does not stop the disease but slows the degeneration.

Teaching points

- Take drug exactly as prescribed, around the clock. Work with your nurse to establish a schedule that is least disruptive. Do not take more than the prescribed dose.
- Take drug on an empty stomach, 1 hr before or 2 hr after meals. If severe GI upset occurs, drug may be taken with meals.

- This drug does not cure the disease but is thought to slow down the degeneration associated with the disease.
- Arrange for regular blood tests and follow-up visits while adjusting to this drug.
- These side effects may occur: nausea, vomiting (small, frequent meals may help); dizziness, confusion, light-headedness (use caution if driving or performing tasks that require alertness).
- Report nausea, vomiting, changes in stool or urine color, diarrhea, rash, changes in neurologic functioning, yellowing of eyes or skin.

▽ tacrolimus (FK 506)
*(tack **row'** lim us)*

Prograf, Protopic

PREGNANCY CATEGORY C

Drug classes
Immunosuppressant
Immunomodulator

Therapeutic actions
Immunosuppressant; inhibits T-lymphocyte activation; exact mechanism of action not known but binds to intracellular protein, which may prevent the generation of nuclear factor of activated T cells and suppress the immune activation and response of T cells.

Indications
- Prophylaxis for organ rejection in liver transplants in conjunction with adrenal corticosteroids
- Short-term treatment of moderate to severe atopic dermatitis when other therapies are not effective or contraindicated (topical)
- Unlabeled use: prophylaxis in kidney, bone marrow, cardiac, pancreas, pancreatic islet cell, and small bowel transplantation; treatment of autoimmune disease; recalcitrant psoriasis

Contraindications and cautions
- Contraindicated with allergy to tacrolimus, hypersensitivity to HCO-60 polyoxyl 60 hydrogenated castor oil, pregnancy, lactation.

T

- Use cautiously with impaired renal function, hyperkalemia, malabsorption, impaired hepatic function.

Available forms

Capsules—0.5, 1, 5 mg; injection—5 mg/mL; ointment—0.03%, 0.1%

Dosages
Adults
Oral

- *Kidney transplant:* 0.2 mg/kg/day divided q 12 hr.
- *Liver transplant:* 0.10–0.15 mg/kg/day divided q 12 hr; administer initial dose no sooner than 6 hr after transplant; If transferring from IV, give first dose 8–12 hr after discontinuing IV infusion. Adjust dose based on clinical assessment of rejection tolerance of drug.

Parenteral

Patients unable to take capsules: 0.03–0.05 mg/kg/day as continuous IV infusion begun no sooner than 6 hr after transplant. Switch to oral drug as soon as possible.

Topical

Apply thin layer of 0.03% or 0.1% ointment to affected area bid. Rub in gently and completely. Continue for 1 wk after resolution.

Pediatric patients

Children require the larger dose; begin treatment at higher end of recommended adult dose.

Oral

- *Liver transplant:* 0.15–0.20 mg/kg/day divided q 12 hr.

Parenteral

- *Liver transplant:* 0.03–0.05 mg/kg/day.

Topical

< 2 yr: Not recommended.

2–15 yr: Apply thin layer of 0.03% ointment bid. Rub in gently and completely. Continue treatment for 1 wk after resolution.

≥ 16 yr: Apply thin layer of 0.1% ointment bid.

Patients with hepatic or renal impairment

Start with lowest possible dose; delay therapy up to 48 hr in patients with postoperative oliguria.

Pharmacokinetics

Route	Onset	Peak
Oral	Varies	1.5–3.5 hr
IV	Rapid	1–2 hr

Metabolism: Hepatic; $T_{1/2}$: 5.7 hr then 11.7 hr
Distribution: Crosses placenta; enters breast milk
Excretion: Bile and urine

▼IV facts

Preparation: Dilute IV solution immediately before use; use 0.9% sodium chloride injection or 5% dextrose injection to a concentration between 0.004 and 0.02 mg/mL. Do not store in a PVC container; discard after 24 hr.
Infusion: Give by continuous IV infusion using an infusion pump.

Adverse effects

- **CNS:** *Tremor, headache, insomnia,* paresthesias
- **CV:** Hypertension
- **GI: Hepatotoxicity,** *constipation, diarrhea, nausea, vomiting,* anorexia
- **GU:** *Renal dysfunction,* nephrotoxicity, UTI, oliguria
- **Hematologic:** Leukopenia, anemia, hyperkalemia, hypokalemia, hyperglycemia
- **Other:** Abdominal pain, fever, asthenia, back pain, ascites, neoplasias, increased susceptibility to infection, lymphoma development, hyperkalemia, hyperglycemia

Interactions

✴ **Drug-drug** • Increased risk of nephrotoxicity with other nephrotoxic agents (erythromycin) • Risk of severe myopathy or rhabdomyolysis with any HMG-CoA inhibitor • Increased risk of toxicity with diltiazem, metoclopramide, nicardipine, cimetidine, clarithromycin, calcium channel-blockers • Decreased therapeutic effect with carbamazepine, phenobarbital, phenytoin, rifamycins

✴ **Drug-food** • Decreased metabolism and risk of toxic effects if combined with grapefruit juice; avoid this combination

---

■ Nursing considerations

Assessment

- **History:** Allergy to tacrolimus or polyoxyethylated castor oil; impaired renal function; malabsorption; lactation, pregnancy
- **Physical:** T; skin color, lesions; BP, peripheral perfusion; liver evaluation, bowel sounds, gum evaluation; renal and liver function tests, CBC

Interventions

- Use parenteral administration only if patient is unable to take the oral solution; transfer to oral solution as soon as possible.
- Apply thin layer of ointment to affected area; do not use occlusive dressings; do not apply to wet skin; encourage patient to avoid exposure to sunlight.
- Monitor renal and liver function tests before and periodically during therapy; marked decreases in function may require dosage changes or discontinuation.
- Monitor tacrolimus blood concentrations.
- Monitor liver function and hematologic tests to determine dosage.

Teaching points

- Avoid infections; avoid crowds or people with infections. Notify your health care provider at once if you injure yourself.
- Do not drink grapefruit juice while on this drug.
- These side effects may occur: nausea, vomiting (take drug with food); diarrhea; headache (request analgesics).
- This drug should not be taken during pregnancy. If you think that you are pregnant or you want to become pregnant, discuss this with your prescriber.
- Arrange to have periodic blood tests to monitor drug response and effects.
- Do not discontinue without your prescriber's advice. Continue use of topical ointment for one week after resolution of the infection.
- Report unusual bleeding or bruising, fever, sore throat, mouth sores, tiredness.

▽tamoxifen citrate
*(ta **mox'** i fen)*

Apo-Tamox (CAN), Nolvadex, Novo-Tamoxifen (CAN), Tamofen (CAN), Tamone (CAN)

PREGNANCY CATEGORY D

Drug class

Antiestrogen

Therapeutic actions

Potent antiestrogenic effects: competes with estrogen for binding sites in target tissues, such as the breast.

Indications

- Treatment of metastatic breast cancer in women and men; in premenopausal women with metastatic breast cancer, tamoxifen is an alternative to oophorectomy or ovarian irradiation
- Treatment of node-positive breast cancer in postmenopausal women following total mastectomy or segmental mastectomy, axillary dissection, and breast irradiation
- Treatment of axillary node-negative breast cancer in women following total mastectomy or segmental mastectomy, axillary dissection, and breast irradiation
- Reduction in risk of invasive breast cancer in women with ductal carcinoma in situ (DCIS) following breast surgery and radiation
- Reduction in occurrence of contralateral breast cancer in patients receiving adjuvant tamoxifen therapy for breast cancer
- Reduction in incidence of breast cancer in women at high risk for breast cancer
- Treatment of McCune–Albright syndrome and precocious puberty in female patients 2–10 yr
- Unlabeled uses: treatment of mastalgia; useful for decreasing size and pain of gynecomastia

Contraindications and cautions

- Contraindicated with allergy to tamoxifen, pregnancy, lactation, women who require concomitant coumarin-type anticoagulation therapy or in women with a history of DVT or PE.

T

- Use cautiously in women with a history of thromboembolic events.

Available forms
Tablets—10, 20 mg

Dosages
Adults
- *Breast cancer:* 20–40 mg/day PO for 5 yr. Dosages > 20 mg/day should be given in divided doses, morning and evening.
- *Reduction in breast cancer incidence:* 20 mg/day PO for 5 yr.
- *DCIS:* 20 mg/day PO for 5 yr.
- *McCune–Albright syndrome, precocious puberty:* 20 mg PO daily for ≤ 12 mo.

Pharmacokinetics

Route	Onset	Peak
Oral	Varies	4–7 hr

Metabolism: Hepatic; $T_{1/2}$: 7–14 days
Distribution: Crosses placenta; may enter breast milk
Excretion: Feces

Adverse effects
- **CNS:** Depression, light-headedness, dizziness, headache, corneal opacity, decreased visual acuity, retinopathy, **stroke**
- **Dermatologic:** *Hot flashes, rash,* **Stevens-Johnson syndrome**
- **GI:** *Nausea, vomiting,* food distaste
- **GU:** *Vaginal bleeding, vaginal discharge, menstrual irregularities,* pruritus vulvae, endometrial cancer, uterine sarcoma
- **Hematologic:** Hypercalcemia, especially with bone metastases, thrombocytopenia, leukopenia, anemia, **DVT**
- **Other:** Peripheral edema; increased bone and tumor pain and local disease (initially seen with a good tumor response, usually subsides); cancer in animal studies, changes in LFTs, **PE, CVA**

Interactions
✴ **Drug-drug** • Increased risk of bleeding with oral anticoagulants • Increased serum levels with bromocriptine • Increased risk of thromboembolic events if given with cytotoxic agents

✴ **Drug-food** • Decreased metabolism and risk of toxic effects if combined with grapefruit juice; avoid this combination
✴ **Drug-lab test** • Possible increase in calcium levels, T_4 levels without hyperthyroidism

■ Nursing considerations
Assessment
- **History:** Allergy to tamoxifen; pregnancy, lactation
- **Physical:** Skin lesions, color, turgor; pelvic exam; orientation, affect, reflexes; ophthalmologic exam; peripheral pulses, edema; liver function tests, CBC and differential, estrogen receptor evaluation of tumor cells

Interventions
- Administer bid, in the morning and the evening.
- Arrange for periodic blood counts.
- Arrange for initial ophthalmologic exam and periodic exams if visual changes occur.
- Counsel patient to use contraception while taking this drug; inform patient that serious fetal harm could occur.
- Decrease dosage if adverse effects become severe.

Teaching points
- In doses > 20 mg, take the drug twice a day, in the morning and evening. Do not drink grapefruit juice while on this drug.
- These side effects may occur: bone pain; hot flashes (staying in cool temperatures may help); nausea, vomiting (small, frequent meals may help); weight gain; menstrual irregularities; dizziness, headache, light-headedness (use caution if driving or performing tasks that require alertness).
- This drug can cause serious fetal harm and must not be taken during pregnancy. Contraceptive measures should be used. If you become pregnant or decide that you would like to become pregnant, consult with your health care provider immediately.
- Have regular gynecologic exams during therapy.
- Report marked weakness, sleepiness, mental confusion, pain or swelling of the legs, shortness of breath, blurred vision.

Adverse effects in *Italics* are most common; those in **Bold** are life-threatening.

▽tamsulosin hydrochloride
*(tam soo **low'** sin)*

Flomax

PREGNANCY CATEGORY B

Drug class
Alpha-adrenergic blocker (peripherally acting)

Therapeutic actions
Blocks the smooth muscle alpha$_1$-adrenergic receptors in the prostate, prostatic capsule, prostatic urethra, and bladder neck, leading to relaxation of the bladder and prostate and improving the flow of urine in cases of benign prostatic hypertrophy.

Indications
- Treatment of the signs and symptoms of benign prostatic hyperplasia (BPH)

Contraindications and cautions
- Contraindicated with hypersensitivity to tamsulosin, prostate cancer, pregnancy, lactation.

Available forms
Capsules—0.4 mg

Dosages
Adults
0.4 mg PO daily 30 min after the same meal each day; if response is not satisfactory in 2–4 wk, dosage may be increased to 0.8 mg PO daily 30 min after the same meal each day.
Pediatric patients
Safety and efficacy not established.

Pharmacokinetics

Route	Onset	Peak
Oral	Varies	4–6 hr

Metabolism: Hepatic; $T_{1/2}$: 9–13 hr
Distribution: May cross placenta; passes into breast milk
Excretion: Urine and feces

Adverse effects
- **CNS:** *Somnolence, insomnia,* amblyopia
- **CV:** *Orthostatic hypotension,* syncope
- **GI:** *Nausea,* dyspepsia
- **GU:** *Abnormal ejaculation, decreased libido,* increased urinary frequency
- **Other:** Cough, sinusitis, rhinitis

Interactions
❋ **Drug-drug** • Increased hypotensive effects with other alpha-adrenergic antagonists • Risk of increased toxic effects of cimetidine, warfarin

■ Nursing considerations

 CLINICAL ALERT!
Name confusion has occurred between Fosamax (alendronate) and Flomax (tamsulosin); use caution.

Assessment
- **History:** Allergy to tamsulosin; pregnancy, lactation; prostatic cancer
- **Physical:** Body weight; skin color, lesions; orientation, affect, reflexes; ophthalmologic exam; P, BP, orthostatic BP; R, adventitious sounds, status of nasal mucous membranes; voiding pattern, normal output, urinalysis

Interventions
- Ensure that patient does not have prostatic cancer before beginning treatment.
- Administer once a day, 30 min after the same meal each day.
- Resume therapy at 0.4 mg daily if therapy is interrupted for any reason.
- Ensure that patient does not crush, chew, or open capsule. Capsule should be swallowed whole.
- Monitor patient carefully for orthostatic hypotension; chance of orthostatic hypotension, dizziness, and syncope is high with the first dose. Establish safety precautions as appropriate.

Teaching points
- Take this drug exactly as prescribed, once a day. Do not chew, crush, or open capsules; capsules must be swallowed whole. Use care when beginning therapy; the chance of dizziness or syncope is greatest at that time. Change position slowly to avoid increased dizziness. Take the drug 30 min after the same meal each day.

T

• These side effects may occur: dizziness, weakness (more likely when you change position, in the early morning, after exercise, in hot weather, and when you have consumed alcohol; some tolerance may occur after you have taken the drug for a while; avoid driving or engaging in tasks that require alertness; change position slowly, use caution in climbing stairs, lie down if dizziness persists); GI upset (eat small, frequent meals); impotence (discuss this with your health care provider); stuffy nose. Most of these effects will disappear gradually with continued therapy.

• Report frequent dizziness or fainting, worsening of symptoms.

▽ tegaserod maleate

(teh gas' eh rod)

Zelnorm

PREGNANCY CATEGORY B

Drug class
5-HT4 Modulator

Therapeutic actions
Stimulates transmitter release at 5-HT4 (serotonin) receptors in the enteric nervous system of the gastrointestinal tract; interacting with these receptors results in normalization of intestinal peristalsis reflex and relief of abdominal pain and discomfort.

Indications
• Short-term treatment of women with irritable bowel syndrome (IBS) whose primary bowel symptom is constipation

Contraindications and cautions
• Contraindicated with hypersensitivity to the drug; lactation; bowel obstruction, gallbladder disease, hepatic impairment, severe renal impairment, abdominal adhesion, suspected sphincter of Oddi dysfunction, recent GI surgery.
• Use cautiously with diarrhea, pregnancy.

Available forms
Tablets—2, 6 mg

Dosages
Adults
6 mg PO bid before meals for 4–6 wk.
Pediatric patients < 18 yr
Safety and efficacy not established.

Pharmacokinetics

Route	Onset	Peak
Oral	1 hr	1–1.3 hr

Metabolism: Hepatic; $T_{1/2}$: 11 hr
Distribution: Crosses placenta; may pass into breast milk
Excretion: Feces and urine

Adverse effects
• **CNS:** *Headache,* dizziness, migraine
• **GI:** *Abdominal pain, nausea, vomiting, diarrhea, flatulence*
• **Other:** Back pain, arthropy, leg pain

■ Nursing considerations
Assessment
• **History:** Hypersensitivity to the drug; pregnancy, lactation; bowel obstruction, GI surgery, gallbladder disease, renal or hepatic impairment, abdominal adhesion, suspected sphincter of Oddi dysfunction, diarrhea
• **Physical:** Skin lesions; T; reflexes, affect; urinary output, abdominal exam; bowel patterns, renal and liver function test

Interventions
• Administer drug before a meal.
• Establish record of pain, frequency, and urgency of bowel movements.
• Arrange for further evaluation of patient after 4 wk of therapy to determine effectiveness of drug. Use of drug beyond one year has not been studied.
• Encourage the use of barrier contraceptives to prevent pregnancy while on this drug.
• Maintain supportive treatment as appropriate for underlying problem.
• Provide additional comfort measures to alleviate discomfort from GI effects, headache, and so on.

Adverse effects in *Italics* are most common; those in **Bold** are life-threatening.

Teaching points

- Take this drug before meals 2 times per day; if you miss a dose, do not make it up.
- Keep a record of your IBS symptoms to provide a monitor of drug effectiveness.
- Arrange to have regular medical follow-up while you are on this drug.
- Use barrier contraceptives while on this drug, serious adverse effects could occur during pregnancy; if you become or wish to become pregnant, consult with your physician.
- These side effects may occur: dizziness (avoid driving a car or performing hazardous tasks); headache (consult with your nurse if these become bothersome, medications may be available to help); nausea, vomiting, abdominal pain (proper nutrition is important, consult with your dietitian to maintain nutrition).
- Report severe headache, worsening of symptoms, severe diarrhea, constipation, fever, chills.
- Maintain all of the usual activities and restrictions that apply to your condition. If this becomes difficult, consult with your nurse or physician.

▷telmisartan
*(tell mah **sar'** tan)*

Micardis

PREGNANCY CATEGORY C
(FIRST TRIMESTER)

PREGNANCY CATEGORY D
(SECOND AND THIRD TRIMESTERS)

Drug classes
Angiotensin II receptor antagonist
Antihypertensive

Therapeutic actions
Selectively blocks the binding of angiotensin II to specific tissue receptors found in the vascular smooth muscle and adrenal gland; this action blocks the vasoconstriction effect of the renin–angiotensin system, as well as the release of aldosterone, leading to decreased blood pressure; appears to block the vascular remodeling that occurs with hypertension, decreasing the development of atherosclerosis.

Indications
- Treatment of hypertension, alone or in combination with other antihypertensive agents

Contraindications and cautions
- Contraindicated with hypersensitivity to telmisartan, pregnancy (use during the second or third trimester can cause injury or even death to the fetus), lactation.
- Use cautiously with hepatic or biliary dysfunction, hypovolemia.

Available forms
Tablets—20, 40, 80 mg

Dosages
Adults
Usual starting dose: 40 mg PO daily. Adjust dose based on patient response. Maximum dose: 80 mg/day. If response is still not as expected, a diuretic should be added.
Pediatric patients
Safety and efficacy not established.

Pharmacokinetics

Route	Onset	Peak	Duration
Oral	Rapid	0.5–1 hr	24 hr

Metabolism: Hepatic; $T_{1/2}$: 24 hr
Distribution: May cross placenta; may pass into breast milk
Excretion: Feces

Adverse effects
- **CNS:** *Headache, dizziness, light-headedness,* muscle weakness
- **CV:** Hypotension
- **Dermatologic:** Rash, inflammation, urticaria, pruritus, alopecia, dry skin
- **GI:** *Diarrhea, abdominal pain, nausea,* constipation, dry mouth, dental pain
- **Respiratory:** *URI symptoms,* cough, sinus disorders
- **Other:** Cancer in preclinical studies, back pain, fever, gout

Interactions
✱ Drug-drug • Increased serum levels and risk of toxicity of digoxin if combined

■ Nursing considerations
Assessment
- **History:** Hypersensitivity to telmisartan; pregnancy, lactation; hepatic or biliary dysfunction; hypovolemia
- **Physical:** Skin lesions, turgor;T; orientation, reflexes, affect; BP; R, respiratory auscultation; liver function tests

Interventions
- Administer without regard to meals.
- Ensure that patient is not pregnant before beginning therapy. Suggest the use of barrier birth control while using telmisartan; fetal injury and deaths have been reported.
- Find an alternate method of feeding the baby if given to a nursing mother. Depression of the renin–angiotensin system in infants is potentially very dangerous.
- Alert surgeon and mark patient's chart with notice that telmisartan is being taken. The blockage of the renin–angiotensin system following surgery can produce problems. Hypotension may be reversed with volume expansion.
- If blood pressure control does reach desired levels, diuretics or other antihypertensives may be added to telmisartan. Monitor patient's blood pressure carefully.
- Monitor patient closely in any situation that may lead to a decrease in blood pressure secondary to reduction in fluid volume—excessive perspiration, dehydration, vomiting, diarrhea—excessive hypotension can occur.

Teaching points
- Take drug without regard to meals. Do not stop taking this drug without consulting your health care provider.
- Use a barrier method of birth control while on this drug; if you become pregnant or desire to become pregnant, consult with your physician.
- These side effects may occur: dizziness (avoid driving a car or performing hazardous tasks); headache (medications may be available to help); nausea, vomiting, diarrhea (proper nutrition is important, consult with your dietitian to maintain nutrition); symptoms of upper respiratory tract infection; cough (do

not self-medicate, consult with your health care provider if this becomes uncomfortable).
- Report fever, chills, dizziness, pregnancy.

▽ temazepam
(te maz' e pam)

Apo-Temazepam (CAN), Novo-Temazepam (CAN), Restoril

PREGNANCY CATEGORY X

C-IV CONTROLLED SUBSTANCE

Drug classes
Benzodiazepine
Sedative/hypnotic

Therapeutic actions
Exact mechanisms of action not understood; acts mainly at subcortical levels of the CNS, leaving the cortex relatively unaffected; main sites of action may be the limbic system and mesencephalic reticular formation; benzodiazepines potentiate the effects of gamma-aminobutyrate (GABA), an inhibitory neurotransmitter.

Indications
- Insomnia characterized by difficulty falling asleep, frequent nocturnal awakenings, or early morning awakening
- Recurring insomnia or poor sleeping habits
- Acute or chronic medical situations requiring restful sleep

Contraindications and cautions
- Contraindicated with hypersensitivity to benzodiazepines, psychoses, acute narrow-angle glaucoma, shock, coma, acute alcoholic intoxication with depression of vital signs, pregnancy (risk of congenital malformations, neonatal withdrawal syndrome), labor and delivery ("floppy infant" syndrome), lactation (infants may become lethargic and lose weight).
- Use cautiously with impaired liver or kidney function, debilitation, depression, suicidal tendencies.

Available forms
Capsules—7.5, 15, 30 mg

Dosages
Adults
15–30 mg PO before retiring.
Pediatric patients
Not for use in patients < 18 yr.
Geriatric patients or patients with debilitating disease
Initially 15 mg PO; adjust dosage until individual response is determined.

Pharmacokinetics

Route	Onset	Peak
Oral	Varies	1.2–1.6 hr

Metabolism: Hepatic; $T_{1/2}$: 3.5–18.4 hr
Distribution: Crosses placenta; enters breast milk
Excretion: Urine

Adverse effects
- **CNS:** *Transient, mild drowsiness initially; sedation, depression, lethargy, apathy, fatigue, light-headedness, disorientation, restlessness, confusion,* crying, delirium, headache, slurred speech, dysarthria, stupor, rigidity, tremor, dystonia, vertigo, euphoria, nervousness, difficulty concentrating, vivid dreams, psychomotor retardation, extrapyramidal symptoms, *mild paradoxical excitatory reactions during first 2 wk of treatment* (especially in psychiatric patients, aggressive children, and with high dosage), visual and auditory disturbances, diplopia, nystagmus, depressed hearing, nasal congestion
- **CV:** *Bradycardia, tachycardia,* CV collapse, hypertension and hypotension, palpitations, edema
- **Dependence:** *Drug dependence with withdrawal syndrome* when drug is discontinued
- **Dermatologic:** Urticaria, pruritus, rash, dermatitis
- **GI:** *Constipation, diarrhea,* dry mouth, salivation, nausea, anorexia, vomiting, difficulty in swallowing, gastric disorders, elevations of blood enzymes; hepatic dysfunction, jaundice
- **GU:** *Incontinence, urinary retention, changes in libido,* menstrual irregularities
- **Hematologic:** Decreased Hct (primarily with long-term therapy), blood dyscrasias
- **Other:** Hiccups, fever, diaphoresis, paresthesias, muscular disturbances, gynecomastia

Interactions
✳ **Drug-drug** • Increased CNS depression with alcohol • Decreased sedative effects with theophylline, aminophylline, dyphylline, oxitriphylline

■ Nursing considerations
Assessment
- **History:** Hypersensitivity to benzodiazepines; psychoses; acute narrow-angle glaucoma; shock, coma; acute alcoholic intoxication; pregnancy, lactation, impaired liver or kidney function, debilitation, depression, suicidal tendencies
- **Physical:** Skin color, lesions; T; orientation, reflexes, affect, ophthalmologic exam; P, BP; R, adventitious sounds; liver evaluation, abdominal exam, bowel sounds, normal output; CBC, liver and renal function tests

Interventions
- Taper dosage gradually after long-term therapy, especially in epileptic patients.
- Caution patient to avoid pregnancy while on this drug; advise the use of barrier contraceptives.
- Prolonged therapy is generally not recommended.

Teaching points
- Take drug exactly as prescribed.
- Do not stop taking this drug (long-term therapy) without consulting your health care provider.
- Avoid pregnancy while taking this drug; use of contraceptive measures is advised; serious fetal harm could occur.
- These side effects may occur: drowsiness, dizziness (may lessen; avoid driving or engaging in other dangerous activities); GI upset (take drug with water); depression, dreams, emotional upset, crying.
- Nocturnal sleep may be disturbed for several nights after discontinuing the drug.
- Report severe dizziness, weakness, drowsiness that persists, rash or skin lesions, pal-

pitations, swelling of the extremities, visual changes, difficulty voiding.

▽temozolomide

See *Less Commonly Used Drugs,* p. 1352.

▽tenecteplase
(teh nek' ti plaze)

TNKase

PREGNANCY CATEGORY C

Drug class
Thrombolytic enzyme

Therapeutic actions
Enzyme that converts plasminogen to the enzyme plasmin (fibrinolysin), which degrades fibrin clots; lyses thrombi and emboli; is most active at the site of the clot and causes little systemic fibrinolysis.

Indications
• Reduction of mortality associated with acute MI

Contraindications and cautions
• Contraindicated with allergy to tenecteplase; active internal bleeding; history of CVA; intracranial or intraspinal surgery or trauma (within 2 mo); intracranial neoplasm, arteriovenous malformation, or aneurysm; known bleeding diathesis, severe uncontrolled HTN.
• Use cautiously with recent major surgery, previous puncture of noncompressible vessels, cerebrovascular disease, recent GI or GU bleeding, recent trauma, hypertension, high likelihood of left heart thrombus, acute pericarditis, subacute bacterial endocarditis, hemostatic defects, including those secondary to severe hepatic or renal disease, severe hepatic dysfunction, pregnancy, diabetic hemorrhagic retinopathy or other hemorrhagic ophthalmic conditions, septic thrombophlebitis or occluded AV cannula at seriously infected site, advanced age, patients currently receiving oral anticoagulants, recent administration of GP IIb/IIIa inhibitors, any other condition in which bleeding constitutes a significant hazard or would be particularly difficult to manage because of its location.

Available forms
Powder for injection—50 mg

Dosages
Adults
Do not exceed 50 mg/dose. Initiate treatment as soon as possible after onset of AMI.
< 60 kg: 30 mg IV by bolus over 5 sec.
60–< 70 kg: 35 mg IV.
70–< 80 kg: 40 mg IV.
80–< 90 kg: 45 mg IV.
≥ 90 kg: 50 mg IV.
Pediatric patients
Safety and efficacy not established.
Geriatric patients
Dosage adjustment is not recommended, but elderly patients have an increased risk of adverse effects. Monitor closely for early signs of bleeding.

Pharmacokinetics

Route	Onset	Peak
IV	Immediate	5–10 min

Metabolism: Hepatic; $T_{1/2}$: 90–130 min
Distribution: Crosses placenta; may enter breast milk
Excretion: Cleared by the liver

▼IV facts
Preparation: Reconstitute using the supplied 10 cc syringe with twinpack dual cannula device and 10 mL sterile water for injection. Do not shake. Slight foaming is normal and should dissipate if left standing for 10 min. Reconstituted solution is 5 mg/mL. Use immediately or may be refrigerated for up to 8 hr.
Infusion: Infuse as a bolus injection over 5 sec. Flush any dextrose-containing lines with saline before injecting and after administration. Discard any leftover solution.
Incompatibilities: Do not add other medications to infusion solution.

Adverse effects

- **CV:** Cardiac arrhythmias with coronary reperfusion, hypotension
- **Hematologic: Bleeding,** particularly at venous or arterial access sites; gastrointestinal bleeding; intracranial hemorrhage
- **Other:** Urticaria, nausea, vomiting, fever

Interactions

✳ Drug-drug • Increased risk of hemorrhage if used with heparin or oral anticoagulants, aspirin, dipyridamole, ticlopidine, clopidogrel; monitor patient very closely if these combinations are used • Decreased effectiveness if combined with aminocaproic acid

✳ Drug-lab test • During tenecteplase therapy, results of coagulation tests or measures of fibrinolytic activity may be unreliable unless specific precautions are taken to prevent in vitro artifacts

■ Nursing considerations
Assessment

- **History:** Allergy to tenecteplase; active internal bleeding; recent (within 2 mo) CVA; intracranial or intraspinal surgery or neoplasm; recent major surgery, obstetrical delivery, organ biopsy, or rupture of a noncompressible blood vessel; recent serious GI bleed; recent serious trauma, including CPR; SBE; hemostatic defects; cerebrovascular disease; early-onset, insulin-dependent diabetes; severe uncontrolled hypertension; liver disease; pregnancy, lactation.
- **Physical:** Skin color, temperature, lesions; orientation, reflexes; P, BP, peripheral perfusion, baseline ECG; R, adventitious sounds; liver evaluation, hematocrit, platelet count, thrombin time (TT), activated partial thromboplastin time (APTT), prothrombin time (PT).

Interventions

- Arrange to discontinue concurrent heparin and tenecteplase if serious bleeding occurs.
- Arrange for regular monitoring of coagulation studies.
- Apply pressure and/or pressure dressings to control superficial bleeding (at invaded or disturbed areas); avoid IM injections, invasive procedures, and excessive handling of the patient.

- Avoid any arterial invasive procedures during therapy.
- Arrange for typing and cross-matching of blood in case serious blood loss occurs and whole blood transfusions are required.
- Monitor patient for signs of bleeding, provide safety procedures to avoid injury.

Teaching points

- This drug can only be given IV and you will need to be closely monitored during drug treatment.
- These side effects may occur: tendency to bleed easily (use caution to avoid injury, use electric razor, a soft toothbrush, use caution with sharp objects), strict bed rest will help to decrease the risk of bleeding. If bleeding does occur, apply pressure to the site until bleeding stops.
- Report bruising or bleeding; blood in urine, stool, or with coughing; bleeding gums; changes in vision; difficulty breathing, chest pain.

▽**teniposide (VM-26)**
*(teh **nip'** oh side)*

Vumon

PREGNANCY CATEGORY D

Drug classes
Mitotic inhibitor
Antineoplastic

Therapeutic actions
Late S_2 and early G_2 specific cell toxic: lyses cells entering mitosis; inhibits cells from entering prophase; inhibits DNA synthesis, leading to cell death.

Indications

- In combination with other anticancer drugs for induction therapy with refractory childhood acute lymphoblastic leukemia

Contraindications and cautions

- Allergy to teniposide, *Cremophor EL*, bone marrow suppression, pregnancy, lactation.

T

Available forms
Injection—10 mg/mL

Dosages
Modify dosage based on myelosuppression.
Pediatric patients
165 mg/m^2 teniposide in combination with 300 mg/m^2 cytarabine IV twice weekly for eight to nine doses or 250 mg/m^2 teniposide in combination with 1.5 mg/m^2 vincristine IV weekly for 4–8 wk and prednisone 40 mg/m^2 orally for 28 days.
Pediatric patients with renal or hepatic impairment
Reduced dosage may be necessary.
Patients with Down syndrome
Reduce initial dosings; give the first course at half the usual dose.

Pharmacokinetics

Route	Onset	Peak
IV	30 min	60 min

Metabolism: Hepatic; T$_{1/2}$: 5 hr
Distribution: Crosses placenta; may enter breast milk
Excretion: Urine and bile

▽IV facts
Preparation: Dilute with 5% dextrose injection or 0.9% sodium chloride injection to give a concentration of 0.1, 0.2, 0.4, or 1 mg/mL. Use of glass or polyolefin plastic bags is recommended; PVC containers may crack or break; diluted solutions are stable for 24 hr at room temperature.
Infusion: Administer slowly over 30–60 min or longer. *Do not give by rapid IV infusion.*
Incompatibilities: Heparin may cause precipitation; do not mix with other drugs or in other solutions.

Adverse effects
- **CNS:** *Somnolence, fatigue,* peripheral neuropathy
- **CV:** Hypotension (after rapid IV administration)
- **Dermatologic:** *Alopecia*
- **GI:** *Nausea, vomiting, anorexia, diarrhea,* stomatitis, aftertaste, liver toxicity
- **Hematologic:** *Myelosuppression*

- **Hypersensitivity:** Chills, fever, tachycardia, bronchospasm, dyspnea, anaphylactic-like reaction
- **Other:** Potentially carcinogenic

■ Nursing considerations
Assessment
- **History:** Allergy to teniposide, *Cremophor EL*; bone marrow suppression; pregnancy; lactation
- **Physical:** T; weight; hair; orientation, reflexes; BP, P; mucous membranes, abdominal exam; CBC

Interventions
- Do not administer IM or SC because severe local reaction and tissue necrosis occur.
- Avoid skin contact with this drug. The use of rubber gloves is advised; if contact occurs, immediately wash with soap and water.
- Monitor patient for catheter occlusion, particularly during first 24 hr.
- Monitor blood pressure during administration; if hypotension occurs, discontinue dose and consult with physician. Fluids and other supportive therapy may be needed.
- Monitor patient before starting therapy and prior to each dose: platelet count, Hgb, WBC count, differential. If severe response occurs, discontinue therapy and consult with physician.

Teaching points
- Prepare a calendar showing return dates for specific treatments and additional courses of therapy.
- These side effects may occur: loss of appetite, nausea, vomiting, mouth sores (frequent mouth care, small, frequent meals may help; maintain good nutrition; request an antiemetic); loss of hair (obtain a wig or other suitable head covering before the hair loss occurs; keep the head covered in extremes of temperature).
- Have regular blood tests to monitor the drug's effects.
- Report severe GI upset, diarrhea, vomiting, unusual bleeding or bruising, fever, chills, sore throat, difficulty breathing.

Adverse effects in *Italics* are most common; those in **Bold** are life-threatening.

▽ tenofovir disoproxil fumarate
*(te **noe'** fo veer)*

Viread

PREGNANCY CATEGORY B

Drug class
Antiviral

Therapeutic action
- Antiviral activity; inhibits HIV reverse tran-scriptase activity, leading to a blocking of HIV reproduction.

Indications
- Treatment of HIV-1 infection in combina-tion with other antiretroviral drugs

Contraindications and cautions
- Contraindicated with allergy to tenofovir, re-nal insufficiency, lactation.
- Use cautiously in pregnancy, hepatic im-pairment, lactic acidosis.

Available forms
Tablets—300 mg

Dosages
Adults
300 mg/day PO with food. If administered with didanosine, give tenofovir 2 hr before or 1 hr after didanosine.
Pediatric patients
Safety and efficacy not established.

Pharmacokinetics

Route	Onset	Peak
Oral	Rapid	45–75 min

Metabolism: Unknown
Distribution: May cross placenta; may pass into breast milk
Excretion: Urine

Adverse effects
- **CNS:** Headache, asthenia
- **GI:** *Nausea, vomiting, diarrhea,* anorex-ia, abdominal pain, flatulence, **severe hepatomegaly with steatosis**
- **Metabolic: Lactic acidosis, some-times severe;** changes in body fat distri-bution (loss of fat from arms, legs, face and deposition of fat on trunk, neck, breasts)

Interactions
✳ **Drug-drug** • Potential increase in the serum level of tenofovir if combined with in-dinavir, lopinavir/ritonavir; monitor patient closely and consider decreasing dosage of teno-fovir • Potentially large increases in the serum level of didanosine if given with tenofovir; if these drugs are given together, give tenofovir 2 hr before or 1 hr after didanosine • Poten-tial decrease in serum levels and activity of lamivudine and ritonavir if combined with tenofovir

✳ **Drug-food** • Increased bioavailability and effectiveness if combined with food; tenofovir should be taken with food

■ Nursing considerations
Assessment
- **History:** Allergy to tenofovir, hepatic or he-patic dysfunction, pregnancy, lactation
- **Physical:** T, orientation, reflexes, abdom-inal exam, liver and renal function tests

Interventions
- Administer with other antiretroviral drugs; do not use as monotherapy.
- Administer with meals or food to increase absorption.
- Monitor patients with liver or renal prob-lems for possible adverse effects.
- Withdraw drug and monitor patient if signs or symptoms of lactic acidosis or hepato-toxicity develop, including hepatomegaly and steatosis. These are more common in women.
- Encourage women of child-bearing age to use barrier contraceptives while taking this drug because the effects of the drug on the fetus are not known.
- Advise women who are breast-feeding to find another method of feeding the baby.

Teaching points
- Take this drug once a day with meals or food.
- Take the full course of therapy as prescribed; if you miss a dose, take it as soon as you re-member and then take the next dose at the usual time. If it is almost time for the next dose when you remember, just take the next dose. Do not double any doses.

- If you are taking this drug with didanosine, take this drug 2 hr before or 1 hr after the didanosine. Do not take these drugs at the same time.
- This drug does not cure HIV infection; long-term effects are not yet known; continue to take precautions because the risk of transmission is not reduced by this drug.
- Avoid pregnancy while taking this drug; use of barrier contraceptives is advised.
- Do not take any other drug, prescription or OTC, without consulting your health care provider; this drug interacts with other drugs and serious problems can occur.
- These side effects may occur: nausea, vomiting, loss of appetite, diarrhea, abdominal pain, headache (try to maintain nutrition and fluid intake as much as possible; small, frequent meals may help); redistribution of fat on the body (arms and legs may become thin, a buffalo hump may develop on the back of the neck, and fat maybe distributed in the breasts and along the trunk; the meaning of these changes is not understood).
- Report severe diarrhea, changes in color of stool or urine, rapid respirations.

▽terazosin hydrochloride

(ter ay' zoe sin)

Hytrin

PREGNANCY CATEGORY C

Drug classes
Antihypertensive
Alpha-adrenergic blocker

Therapeutic actions
Selectively blocks postsynaptic alpha$_1$-adrenergic receptors, decreasing sympathetic tone on the vasculature, dilating arterioles and veins, and lowering supine and standing BP; unlike conventional alpha-adrenergic blocking agents (eg, phentolamine), it does not also block alpha$_2$ presynaptic receptors, does not cause reflex tachycardia.

Indications
- Treatment of hypertension alone or in combination with other drugs
- Treatment of symptomatic benign prostatic hyperplasia (BPH)

Contraindications and cautions
- Contraindicated with hypersensitivity to terazosin, lactation.
- Use cautiously with CHF, renal failure, pregnancy, other antihypertensive agents.

Available forms
Capsules—1, 2, 5, 10 mg; tablets (CAN)—1, 2, 5, 10 mg

Dosages
Adults
Adjust dose and dosing interval (12 or 24 hr) individually.
- *Hypertension:* Initial dose: 1 mg PO hs. Do not exceed 1 mg; strictly adhere to this regimen to avoid severe hypotensive reactions. Slowly increase dose to achieve desired BP response. Usual range: 1–5 mg PO daily. Up to 20 mg/day has been beneficial. Monitor BP 2–3 hr after dosing to determine maximum effect. If response is diminished after 24 hr, consider increasing dosage. If drug is not taken for several days, restart with initial 1-mg dose.
- *BPH:* Initial dose, 1 mg PO hs. Increase to 2, 5, or 10 mg PO daily. 10 mg/day for 4–6 wk may be required to assess benefit.
Pediatric patients
Safety and efficacy not established.

Pharmacokinetics

Route	Onset	Peak
Oral	Varies	1 hr

Metabolism: Hepatic; $T_{1/2}$: 12 hr
Distribution: Crosses placenta; may enter breast milk
Excretion: Feces and urine

Adverse effects
- **CNS:** *Dizziness, headache, drowsiness, lack of energy, weakness, somnolence,* nervousness, vertigo, depression, paresthesia

Adverse effects in *Italics* are most common; those in **Bold** are life-threatening.

- **CV:** *Palpitations,* sodium and water retention, increased plasma volume, *edema,* syncope, tachycardia, orthostatic hypotension, angina
- **Dermatologic:** Rash, pruritus, alopecia, lichen planus
- **EENT:** Blurred vision, reddened sclera, epistaxis, tinnitus, dry mouth, nasal congestion
- **GI:** *Nausea,* vomiting, diarrhea, constipation, abdominal discomfort or pain
- **GU:** Urinary frequency, incontinence, impotence, priapism
- **Respiratory:** *Dyspnea, nasal congestion, sinusitis*
- **Other:** Diaphoresis, lupus erythematosus

■ Nursing considerations
Assessment
- **History:** Hypersensitivity to terazosin; CHF; renal failure; pregnancy, lactation
- **Physical:** Weight; skin color, lesions; orientation, affect, reflexes; ophthalmologic exam; P, BP, orthostatic BP, supine BP, perfusion, edema, auscultation; R, adventitious sounds, status of nasal mucous membranes; bowel sounds, normal output; voiding pattern, urinary output; kidney function tests, urinalysis

Interventions
- Administer or have patient take first dose just before bedtime to lessen likelihood of first dose effect, syncope, believed due to excessive orthostatic hypotension.
- Have patient lie down, and treat supportively if syncope occurs; condition is self-limiting.
- Monitor patient for orthostatic hypotension, which is most marked in the morning, and is accentuated by hot weather, alcohol, exercise.
- Monitor edema, weight in patients with incipient cardiac decompensation, and add a thiazide diuretic to the drug regimen if sodium and fluid retention, signs of impending CHF, occur.

Teaching points
- Take this drug exactly as prescribed. Take the first dose just before bedtime. Do not drive or operate machinery for 4 hr after the first dose.
- These side effects may occur: dizziness, weakness (more likely when changing position,

in early morning, after exercise, in hot weather, and with alcohol use; some tolerance may occur after taking the drug for a while, but avoid driving or engaging in tasks that require alertness; change position slowly; use caution when climbing stairs; lie down for a while if dizziness persists); GI upset (frequent, small meals may help); impotence; dry mouth (sucking on sugarless lozenges, ice chips may help); stuffy nose. Most effects will gradually disappear.
- Report frequent dizziness or faintness.

▽ terbutaline sulfate
*(ter **byoo'** ta leen)*

Brethine

PREGNANCY CATEGORY B

Drug classes
Sympathomimetic
Beta$_2$-selective adrenergic agonist
Bronchodilator
Antiasthmatic agent
Tocolytic agent

Therapeutic actions
In low doses, acts relatively selectively at beta$_2$-adrenergic receptors to cause bronchodilation and relax the pregnant uterus; at higher doses, beta$_1$ selectivity is lost and the drug acts at beta$_2$ receptors to cause typical sympathomimetic cardiac effects.

Indications
- Prophylaxis and treatment of bronchial asthma and reversible bronchospasm that may occur with bronchitis and emphysema
- Unlabeled use: tocolytic to prevent preterm labor

Contraindications and cautions
- Contraindicated with hypersensitivity to terbutaline; tachyarrhythmias, tachycardia caused by digitalis intoxication; general anesthesia with halogenated hydrocarbons or cyclopropane, which sensitize the myocardium to catecholamines; unstable vasomotor system disorders; hypertension; labor and delivery (may inhibit labor; parenteral use of beta-adrenergic agonists can accel-

T

erate fetal heart beat, cause hypoglycemia, hypokalemia, and pulmonary edema in the mother and hypoglycemia in the neonate); lactation.

• Use cautiously with diabetes, coronary insufficiency, CAD, history of stroke, COPD patients who have developed degenerative heart disease, hyperthyroidism, history of seizure disorders, psychoneurotic individuals.

Pharmacokinetics

Route	Onset	Peak	Duration
SC	5–15 min	30–60 min	1.5–4 hr
Oral	30 min	2–3 hr	4–8 hr

Available forms

Tablets—2.5, 5 mg; injection—1 mg/mL

Dosages
Adults and patients > 15 yr
Oral
5 mg at 6-hr intervals tid during waking hours. If side effects are pronounced, reduce to 2.5 mg tid. Do not exceed 15 mg/day.
Parenteral
0.25 mg SC into lateral deltoid area. If no significant improvement in 15 min, give another 0.25-mg dose. Do not exceed 0.5 mg/4 hr. If patient fails to respond to second 0.25-mg dose within 15–30 min, other therapeutic measures should be considered.
Pediatric patients
Oral
12–15 yr: 2.5 mg tid. Do not exceed 7.5 mg/24 hr.
< 12 yr: Not recommended.
Geriatric patients
Patients > 60 yr are likely to experience adverse effects. Avoid use or use with extreme caution.

Adverse effects

• **CNS:** *Restlessness, apprehension, anxiety, fear,* CNS stimulation, hyperkinesia, insomnia, tremor, drowsiness, irritability, weakness, vertigo, headache
• **CV:** *Cardiac arrhythmias, palpitations,* anginal pain (less likely with bronchodilator doses of this drug than with broncho-

dilator doses of a nonselective beta-agonist (isoproterenol), changes in BP, ECG changes
• **GI:** *Nausea,* vomiting, heartburn, unusual or bad taste
• **Respiratory:** *Respiratory difficulties,* **pulmonary edema,** *coughing,* bronchospasm
• **Other:** Sweating, pallor, flushing, muscle cramps, elevated LFTs

Interactions

✳ **Drug-drug** • Increased likelihood of cardiac arrhythmias with halogenated hydrocarbon anesthetics (halothane), cyclopropane • Risk of bronchospasm if combined with diuretics • Increased risk of hypokalemia and ECG changes with MAOIs and TCAs

■ Nursing considerations
Assessment

• **History:** Hypersensitivity to terbutaline; tachyarrhythmias; general anesthesia with halogenated hydrocarbons or cyclopropane; unstable vasomotor system disorders; hypertension; CAD; history of stroke; COPD patients who have developed degenerative heart disease; hyperthyroidism; history of seizure disorders; psychoneurotic individuals; pregnancy; labor and delivery; lactation
• **Physical:** Weight; skin color, temperature, turgor; orientation, reflexes; P, BP; R, adventitious sounds; blood and urine glucose; serum electrolytes; thyroid function tests; ECG

Interventions

• Use minimal doses for minimal periods of time; drug tolerance can occur with prolonged use.
• Maintain a beta-adrenergic blocker (a cardioselective beta-blocker, such as atenolol, should be used in patients with respiratory distress) on standby in case cardiac arrhythmias occur.
• Do not exceed recommended dosage.

Teaching points

• Do not exceed recommended dosage; adverse effects or loss of effectiveness may result. Read product instructions, and ask your health care provider or pharmacist if you have any questions.

Adverse effects in *Italics* are most common; those in **Bold** are life-threatening.

- These side effects may occur: weakness, dizziness, inability to sleep (use caution when driving or performing activities that require alertness); nausea, vomiting (small, frequent meals may help); fast heart rate, anxiety.
- Report chest pain, dizziness, insomnia, weakness, tremor or irregular heartbeat, failure to respond to usual dosage.

▽terpin hydrate
(ter' pin)

PREGNANCY CATEGORY C

Drug classes
Antitussive
Expectorant

Therapeutic actions
Directly stimulates the respiratory tract secretory glands, increasing the production of respiratory fluids; used mainly as an ingredient in cough medications.

Indications
- Symptomatic relief of dry, nonproductive cough

Contraindications and cautions
- Contraindicated with diabetes, peptic ulcer, pregnancy (contains alcohol), lactation.
- Use cautiously with history of alcohol dependence.

Available forms
Elixir—85 mg/5 mL

Dosages
Adults
85–170 mg PO tid–qid.
Pediatric patients
1–4 yr: 20 mg PO tid–qid.
5–9 yr: 40 mg PO tid–qid.
10–12 yr: 85 mg PO tid–qid.

Pharmacokinetics
Not reported.

Adverse effects
- **CNS:** *Drowsiness, dizziness*
- **GI:** Nausea, vomiting, abdominal pain

■ Nursing considerations
Assessment
- **History:** Diabetes; peptic ulcer; alcohol abuse; pregnancy, lactation
- **Physical:** R, adventitious sounds; abdominal exam

Interventions
- Administer with food if severe GI upset occurs.
- Do not give water after administration to make the most of soothing effects.
- Do not give to pregnant or nursing women; contains alcohol which could adversely affect the fetus/baby.
- Ensure that patient is well hydrated during treatment; humidifier may be helpful in increasing bronchial secretions.

Teaching points
- Take this drug with food if severe GI upset occurs.
- Do not exceed recommended dose.
- These side effects may occur: drowsiness, dizziness (do not drive or operate dangerous machinery).
- Drink plently of fluids, and consider the use of a humidifier to help facilitate relief of bronchial irritation.
- Do not use if pregnant or nursing; consult with health care provider.
- Report vomiting, worsening of condition being treated, abdominal pain.

▽testolactone
*(tess toe **lak'** tone)*

Teslac

PREGNANCY CATEGORY C

C-III CONTROLLED SUBSTANCE

T

Drug classes
Androgen
Hormone
Antineoplastic

Therapeutic actions
Synthetic androgen; endogenous androgens are responsible for growth and development of male sex organs and the maintenance of secondary sex characteristics; administration

of androgen derivatives increases the retention of nitrogen, sodium, potassium, phosphorus, and decreases urinary excretion of calcium; increases protein anabolism and decreases protein catabolism; stimulates the production of red blood cells; exact mechanism by which antineoplastic effects are exerted is not known.

Indications

- Adjunctive therapy for palliation of advanced disseminated metastatic breast carcinoma in postmenopausal women when hormonal therapy is indicated
- Disseminated breast carcinoma in premenopausal women in whom ovarian function has been subsequently terminated

Contraindications and cautions

- Contraindicated with known sensitivity to androgens, pregnancy, lactation, carcinoma of the breast in males.
- Use cautiously with liver disease, cardiac disease, nephritis, nephrosis.

Available forms

Tablets—50 mg

Dosages
Adults

250 mg PO qid. Continue therapy for a minimum of 3 mo unless there is active disease progression.
Pediatric patients

Safety and efficacy not established.

Pharmacokinetics

Route	Onset
Oral	Rapid

Metabolism: Hepatic; $T_{1/2}$: unknown
Distribution: May cross placenta; may enter breast milk
Excretion: Urine

Adverse effects

- **CNS:** *Paresthesias*
- **CV:** Hypertension
- **Dermatologic:** Rash, dermatitis, aches of the extremities, edema

- **GI:** *Nausea, vomiting, anorexia, glossitis,* diarrhea, loss of appetite, swelling of the tongue
- **Hematologic:** Hypercalcemia
- **Virilization:** Hirsutism, hoarseness, deepening of the voice, clitoral enlargement, facial hair growth, affected libido

Interactions

✳ **Drug-drug** • Risk of increased bleeding with oral anticoagulants; monitor patient and adjust dosage as needed
✳ **Drug-lab test** • Physiologic effects of testolactone may result in decreased estradiol concentrations with radioimmunoassays for estradiol, increased plasma calcium concentrations, and increased 24 hr urinary excretion of creatine and 17-ketosteroids

■ Nursing considerations
Assessment

- **History:** Known sensitivity to androgens; liver or cardiac disease; nephritis; nephrosis; carcinoma of the breast; pregnancy, lactation
- **Physical:** Skin color, lesions, texture; hair distribution pattern; P, auscultation; abdominal exam, liver evaluation, mucous membranes; serum electrolytes, liver and renal function tests

Interventions

- Monitor tumor progression periodically.
- Monitor for occurrence of edema; arrange for diuretic therapy as needed.
- Arrange for periodic monitoring of urine and serum calcium during treatment of disseminated breast carcinoma, and arrange for treatment or discontinuation of the drug if hypercalcemia occurs.

Teaching points

- This drug will need to be taken for long term to evaluate effects.
- These side effects may occur: body hair growth, baldness, deepening of the voice, loss of appetite, edema or swelling, redness of the tongue.
- This drug is not intended to be taken during pregnancy; serious fetal effects can oc-

---

Adverse effects in *Italics* are most common; those in **Bold** are life-threatening.

cur. Use contraceptives during drug treatment.
- Report numbness or tingling of the fingers, toes, face; significant swelling; severe GI upset.

▽testosterone
*(tess **toss**'ter ohn)*

testosterone
Transdermal patch: Androderm, Testoderm, Testoderm TTS, Testoderm with Adhesive
Transdermal gel: AndroGel 1%, Testim
Testosterone pellets: Testopel

testosterone cypionate (long-acting)
Depo-Testosterone, Scheinpharm Testone-cyp (CAN)

testosterone enanthate (long-acting)
Delatestryl

PREGNANCY CATEGORY X

C-II! CONTROLLED SUBSTANCE

Drug classes
Androgen
Hormone

Therapeutic actions
Primary natural androgen; responsible for growth and development of male sex organs and the maintenance of secondary sex characteristics; administration of exogenous testosterone increases the retention of nitrogen, sodium, potassium, phosphorus; decreases urinary excretion of calcium; increases protein anabolism and decreases protein catabolism; stimulates the production of red blood cells.

Indications
- Replacement therapy in hypogonadism—primary hypogonadism, hypogonadotropic hypogonadism, delayed puberty (men) (testosterone pellets and testosterone enanthate only)

- Inoperable breast cancer (testosterone enanthate only)

Contraindications and cautions
- Contraindicated with known sensitivity to androgens, prostate or breast cancer in males, pregnancy, lactation, serious cardiac, hepatic, or renal disease.
- Use cautiously with MI.

Available forms
Transdermal system—2.5, 4, 5, 6 mg/24 hr; transdermal gel, 1%; pellets—75 mg; testosterone enanthate injection—200 mg/mL; testosterone cypionate injection—100, 200 mg/mL

Dosages
Adults
- *Carcinoma of the breast:* 200–400 mg IM q 2–4 wk.
- *Male hypogonadism (replacement therapy):* 50–400 mg IM every 2–4 wk or 150–450 mg pellets SC every 3–6 mo.
- *Males with delayed puberty:* 50–200 mg IM every 2–4 wk for a limited duration (4–6 mo) or 150 mg pellets SC every 3–6 mo (testosterone pellets).
- *Primary hypogonadism, hypogonadotropic hypogonadism in males:* Testosterone patch, initially 6 mg/day system applied to scrotal skin; then 4-mg/day system (*Testoderm* and *Testoderm with Adhesive*); 5-mg/day system applied to arm, back, or upper buttocks (*Testoderm TTS*); two 2.5-mg systems or one 5-mg system each night applied to nonscrotal skin (*Androderm*); testosterone gel—5 g/day (preferably in the morning) applied to clean, dry, intact skin of the shoulders, upper arms, or abdomen.

Pharmacokinetics

Route	Onset	Duration
IM	Slow	1–3 days
IM cypionate	Slow	2–4 wk
IM enanthate	Slow	2–4 wk
Dermal	Rapid	24 hr

Metabolism: Hepatic; $T_{1/2}$: 10–100 min; up to 8 days cypionate
Distribution: Crosses placenta; may enter breast milk
Excretion: Urine and feces

Adverse effects

- **CNS:** *Dizziness, headache, sleep disorders, fatigue,* tremor, sleeplessness, generalized paresthesia, sleep apnea syndrome, CNS hemorrhage
- **Dermatologic:** *Rash,* dermatitis, anaphylactoid reactions
- **Endocrine:** *Androgenic effects* (acne, edema, mild hirsutism, decrease in breast size, deepening of the voice, oily skin or hair, weight gain, clitoral hypertrophy or testicular atrophy), *hypoestrogenic effects* (flushing, sweating, vaginitis, nervousness, emotional lability)
- **GI:** *Nausea,* hepatic dysfunction; **hepatocellular carcinoma**
- **GU:** Fluid retention, decreased urinary output
- **Hematologic:** *Polycythemia, leukopenia,* hypercalcemia, altered serum cholesterol levels, retention of sodium, chloride, water, potassium, phosphates and calcium
- **Other:** Chills, premature closure of the epiphyses

Interactions

✳ **Drug-food** • Decreased metabolism and risk of toxic effects if combined with grapefruit juice; avoid this combination

✳ **Drug-lab test** • Altered glucose tolerance tests • Decrease in thyroid function tests, which may persist for 2–3 wk after therapy • Increased creatinine, creatinine clearance, which may last for 2 wk after therapy

■ Nursing considerations
Assessment

- **History:** Known sensitivity to androgens, prostate or breast cancer in males, MI, liver disease, pregnancy, lactation
- **Physical:** Skin color, lesions, texture; hair distribution pattern; injection site; affect, orientation, peripheral sensation; abdominal exam, liver evaluation; serum electrolytes, serum cholesterol levels, liver function tests, glucose tolerance tests, thyroid function tests, long-bone x-ray (in children)

Interventions

- Apply dermal patch to clean, dry skin as directed. *Testoderm* and *Testoderm with Adhesive* are to be applied to scrotal skin that has been dry shaved. Do not use chemical depilatories. *Testoderm TTS* and *Androderm* are to be applied to nonscrotal skin.
- Inject testosterone deeply into gluteal muscle.
- Shake vials well before use; crystals will redissolve.
- Do not administer frequently; these drugs are absorbed slowly; testosterone enanthate and cypionate are long acting and provide therapeutic effects for about 4 wk.
- Monitor effect on children with long-bone x-rays every 3–6 mo during therapy; discontinue drug well before the bone age reaches the norm for the patient's chronologic age.
- Monitor patient for occurrence of edema; arrange for diuretic therapy as needed.
- Monitor liver function, serum electrolytes periodically during therapy, and consult with physician for corrective measures as needed.
- Periodically measure cholesterol levels in patients who are at high risk for CAD.
- Monitor diabetic patients closely because glucose tolerance may change; adjustments may be needed in insulin, oral hypoglycemic dosage, and diet.
- Periodically monitor urine and serum calcium during treatment of disseminated breast carcinoma, and arrange for appropriate treatment or discontinuation of the drug.
- Monitor geriatric males for prostatic hypertrophy and carcinoma.
- Advise female patients, especially pregnant patients, that they should avoid contact with application site of testosterone gel as well as transdermal patches.
- Discontinue drug, and arrange for consultation if abnormal vaginal bleeding occurs.

Teaching points

- The injection forms of this drug can only be given IM. Mark calendar indicating days for injection. Patient receiving the dermal patch must apply the patch to dry, clean skin as directed. *Testoderm* and *Testoderm with Adhesive* are to be applied to scrotal skin that has been dry shaved. Do not use chemical depilatories. *Testoderm TTS* and *Androderm* are to be applied to nonscrotal skin. *Androgel* is to be applied to skin of the shoulders and upper arms. Do not shower or swim for at least 1 hr after application of gel.

- Avoid grapefruit juice while using this drug.
- These side effects may occur: body hair growth, baldness, deepening of the voice, loss of libido, impotence (reversible); excitation, confusion, insomnia (avoid driving or performing tasks that require alertness); swelling of the ankles, fingers (request medication).
- This drug cannot be taken during pregnancy; serious fetal effects could occur. Women should use contraceptive measures.
- Diabetic patients: Monitor urine sugar closely because glucose tolerance may change; report any abnormalities to prescriber, so corrective action can be taken.
- Report ankle swelling; nausea; vomiting; yellowing of skin or eyes; unusual bleeding or bruising; penile swelling or pain; hoarseness, body hair growth, deepening of the voice, acne, menstrual irregularities, pregnancy.

▷tetracycline hydrochloride
(tet ra sye' kleen)

Apo-Tetra (CAN), Novo-Tetra (CAN), Nu-Tetra (CAN), Panmycin, Sumycin, Tetracap, Tetracyn, Tetralan, Topicycline

PREGNANCY CATEGORY D

PREGNANCY CATEGORY B
(*TOPICYCLINE* ONLY)

Drug classes
Antibiotic
Tetracycline

Therapeutic actions
Bacteriostatic: inhibits protein synthesis of susceptible bacteria, preventing cell replication.

Indications
Systemic administration
- Infections caused by rickettsiae; *Mycoplasma pneumoniae;* agents of psittacosis, ornithosis, lymphogranuloma venereum and granuloma inguinale; *Borrelia recurrentis, Haemophilus ducreyi, Yersinia pestis, Yersinia tularensis, Bartonella bacilliformis, Bacteroides, Vibrio cholerae, Campylobacter fetus, Brucella, Escherichia coli, Enterobacter aerogenes, Shigella, Acinetobacter calcoaceticus, Haemophilus influenzae, Klebsiella, Streptococcus pneumoniae*
- When penicillin is contraindicated, infections caused by *Neisseria gonorrhoeae, Treponema pallidum, Treponema pertenue, Listeria monocytogenes, Clostridium, Bacillus anthracis, Fusobacterium fusiforme, Actinomyces, Neisseria meningitidis*
- Adjunct to amebicides in acute intestinal amebiasis
- Treatment of acne (oral)
- Uncomplicated urethral, endocervical or rectal infections in adults caused by *Chlamydia trachomatis*
- Instilled in a chest tube, unlabeled use: pleural sclerosing agent in malignant pleural effusions
- Treatment of trachoma
- Eradication of *H. pylori* in combination with other products (oral)

Ophthalmic administration
- Treatment of superficial ocular infections due to susceptible strains of microorganisms (ophthalmic preparations)
- Prophylaxis of ophthalmia neonatorum due to *N. gonorrhoeae* or *C. trachomatis* (ophthalmic preparations)

Topical administration
- Treatment of acne vulgaris (topical dermatologic solution)
- Treatment and prophylaxis of minor skin infections due to susceptible organisms (topical dermatologic ointment)

Contraindications and cautions
Systemic administration and dermatologic solution
- Contraindicated with allergy to any of the tetracyclines; allergy to tartrazine (in 250-mg capsules of *Panmycin*); pregnancy (toxic

to the fetus); lactation (causes damage to the teeth of infant).
• Use cautiously with hepatic or renal dysfunction.

Ophthalmic preparations
• Contraindicated with ocular viral, mycobacterial, or fungal infections.

Available forms
Capsules—100, 250, 500 mg; tablets—250, 500 mg; topical solution—2.2 mg/mL; oral suspension—125 mg/5 mL

Dosages
Systemic administration
Adults
1–2 g/day PO in two to four equal doses. Up to 500 mg PO qid.
• *Brucellosis:* 500 mg PO qid for 3 wk with 1 g streptomycin bid IM the first week and daily the second wk.
• *Syphilis:* 30–40 g PO in divided doses over 10–15 days.
• *Uncomplicated gonorrhea:* 1.5 g initially, then 500 mg q 6 hr PO to a total of 9 g.
• *Gonococcal urethritis:* 1.5 g PO initially, then 500 mg q 4–6 hr for 4–6 days.
• *Uncomplicated urethral, endocervical, or rectal infections with chlamydia trachomatis:* 500 mg qid PO for at least 7 days.
• *Severe acne:* 1 g/day PO in divided doses; then 125–500 mg/day.
• *Eradication of* H. pylori: 500 mg qid in combination with other products.
Pediatric patients > 8 yr
Oral
25–50 mg/kg/day PO in four equal doses.
Topical dermatologic solution
Apply generously to affected areas bid.

Pharmacokinetics

Route	Onset	Peak
Oral	Varies	2–4 hr
Topical: No general systemic absorption.		

Metabolism: $T_{1/2}$: 6–12 hr
Distribution: Crosses placenta; enters breast milk
Excretion: Urine

Adverse effects
Systemic administration
• **Dermatologic:** *Phototoxic reactions, rash,* exfoliative dermatitis
• **GI:** *Discoloring and inadequate calcification of primary teeth of fetus if used by pregnant women, discoloring and inadequate calcification of permanent teeth if used during period of dental development,* fatty liver, liver failure, *anorexia, nausea, vomiting, diarrhea, glossitis, dysphagia,* enterocolitis, esophageal ulcers
• **Hematologic:** Hemolytic anemia, thrombocytopenia, neutropenia, eosinophilia, leukocytosis, leukopenia
• **Hypersensitivity:** Reactions from urticaria to **anaphylaxis,** including intracranial hypertension
• **Other:** *Superinfections,* local irritation at parenteral injection sites
Ophthalmic preparations
• **Local:** *Transient irritation, stinging, itching,* angioneurotic edema, urticaria, dermatitis, superinfections
Topical dermatologic solutions
• **Local:** *Stinging, burning during application; skin irritation;* dermatitis; yellowing of areas of application

Interactions
✳ **Drug-drug** • Decreased absorption with calcium salts, magnesium salts, zinc salts, aluminum salts, bismuth salts, iron, urinary alkalinizers, food, dairy products, charcoal • Increased digoxin toxicity • Increased nephrotoxicity with methoxyflurane • Decreased effectiveness of hormonal contraceptives, though rare, has been reported with a risk of breakthrough bleeding or pregnancy • Decreased activity of penicillins

■ Nursing considerations
Assessment
• **History:** Systemic administration and dermatologic solution: allergy to any of the tetracyclines, tartrazine; hepatic or renal dysfunction, pregnancy, lactation. Ophthalmic preparations: ocular viral, mycobacterial, or fungal infections
• **Physical:** Systemic administration, topical dermatologic solution: site of infection,

---

Adverse effects in *Italics* are most common; those in **Bold** are life-threatening.

skin color, lesions; R, adventitious sounds; bowel sounds, output, liver evaluation; urinalysis, BUN, liver and renal function tests. Ophthalmic preparations, dermatologic ointment: site of infection

Interventions

- Administer oral medication on an empty stomach, 1 hr before or 2–3 hr after meals. Do not give with antacids. If antacids must be used, give them 3 hr after the dose of tetracycline.
- Culture infection before beginning drug therapy.
- Do not administer during pregnancy; drug is toxic to the fetus.
- Do not use outdated drugs; degraded drug is highly nephrotoxic and should not be used.
- Do not give oral drug with meals, antacids, or food.
- Arrange for regular renal function tests with long-term therapy.
- Use topical preparations of this drug only when clearly indicated. Sensitization from the topical use may preclude its later use in serious infections. Topical preparations containing antibiotics that are not ordinarily given systemically are preferable.

Teaching points
Oral preparations

- Take the drug throughout the day for best results. The drug should be taken on an empty stomach, 1 hr before or 2–3 hr after meals, with a full glass of water. Do not take the drug with food, dairy products, iron preparations, or antacids.
- Finish your complete prescription; if any is left, discard it immediately. Never take an outdated tetracycline product.
- There have been reports of pregnancy occurring when taking tetracycline with hormonal contraceptives. To be certain of avoiding pregnancy, use an additional type of contraceptive.
- This drug should not be used during pregnancy; use of barrier contraceptives is advised.
- These side effects may occur: stomach upset, nausea (reversible); superinfections in the mouth, vagina (frequent washing may help this problem; if severe, request medication); sensitivity of the skin to sunlight (use protective clothing and a sunscreen).
- Report severe cramps, watery diarrhea, rash or itching, difficulty breathing, dark urine or light-colored stools, yellowing of the skin or eyes.

Topical dermatologic solution

- Apply generously until skin is wet.
- Avoid the eyes, nose, and mouth.
- You may experience transient stinging or burning; this will subside quickly; skin in the treated area may become yellow; this will wash off.
- You may use cosmetics as you usually do.

▽ tetrahydrozoline hydrochloride
(tet rah hi draz' oh leen)

Tyzine, Tyzine Pediatric

OTC ophthalmic preparation: Collyrium Fresh Eye Drops, Eyesine, Geneye, Geneye Extra, Mallazine Eye Drops, Murine Plus, Optigene 3, Tetrasine, Tetrasine Extra, Visine Moisturizing

PREGNANCY CATEGORY C

Drug classes
Ophthalmic decongestant
Ophthalmic vasoconstrictor and mydriatic
Nasal decongestant

Therapeutic actions

Acts directly on alpha receptors to produce vasoconstriction of arterioles in nasal passages, which produces a decongestant response; no effect on beta receptors; dilates pupils; increases flow of aqueous humor, vasoconstricts in eyes.

Indications

- Symptomatic relief of nasal and nasopharyngeal mucosal congestion due to the common cold, hay fever, or other respiratory allergies (topical)
- Relief of redness of eyes due to minor irritations (ophthalmic)
- Temporary relief of burning and irritation due to dryness of the eye or discomfort due to minor irritations or to exposure to wind or sun (ophthalmic)

Contraindications and cautions

- Contraindicated with allergy to tetrahydro-zolozine, angle-closure glaucoma, anesthesia with cyclopropane or halothane, thyro-toxicosis, diabetes, hypertension, CV disorders, women in labor whose BP > 130/80.
- Use cautiously with angina, arrhythmias, prostatic hypertrophy, unstable vasomotor syndrome, lactation.

Available forms

Nasal solution—0.05%, 0.1%; ophthalmic solution—0.05%

Dosages

Adults

Nasal

2–4 drops of 0.1% solution in each nostril 3–4 times/day; or 3–4 sprays in each nostril q 4 hr as needed.

Ophthalmic

Instill 1–2 drops into eye(s) up to 4 times/day.

Pediatric patients

Nasal

≥ 6 yr: Adult dosage.

2–6 yr: 2–3 drops of 0.05% solution in each nostril q 4–6 hr as needed.

Ophthalmic

Safety and efficacy not established.

Pharmacokinetics

Route	Onset	Duration
Nasal	5–10 min	6–10 hr
Ophthalmic: No general systemic absorption.		

Metabolism: Hepatic; T$_{1/2}$: unknown
Distribution: Crosses placenta; may enter breast milk
Excretion: Urine

Adverse effects

- **CNS:** *Fear, anxiety, tenseness, restlessness, headache, light-headedness, dizziness,* drowsiness, tremor, insomnia, hallucinations, psychological disturbances, convulsions, CNS depression, weakness, blurred vision, ocular irritation, tearing, photophobia, symptoms of paranoid schizophrenia
- **CV:** Arrhythmias, hypertension resulting in intracranial hemorrhage, **CV collapse with hypotension,** palpitations, tachy-cardia, precordial pain in patients with ischemic heart disease
- **GI:** *Nausea,* vomiting, anorexia
- **GU:** Constriction of renal blood vessels, *dysuria, vesical sphincter spasm,* resulting in difficult and painful urination, urinary retention in males with prostatism
- **Local:** *Rebound congestion* with topical nasal application
- **Other:** *Pallor,* respiratory difficulty, orofacial dystonia, sweating

Interactions

✳ **Drug-drug** • Severe hypertension when taken with MAOIs, TCAs, furazolidone • Additive effects increase risk of toxicity with urinary alkalinizers • Decreased vasopressor response with reserpine, methyldopa, urinary acidifiers • Decreased hypotensive action of guanethidine

■ Nursing considerations

Assessment

- **History:** Allergy to tetrahydrozoline; angle-closure glaucoma; anesthesia with cyclopropane or halothane; thyrotoxicosis, diabetes, hypertension, CV disorders; prostatic hypertrophy, unstable vasomotor syndrome; lactation
- **Physical:** Skin color, temperature; orientation, reflexes, peripheral sensation, vision; P, BP, auscultation, peripheral perfusion; R, adventitious sounds; urinary output pattern, bladder percussion, prostate palpation; nasal mucous membrane evaluation

Interventions

- Do not administer ophthalmic solution if it is cloudy or changes color.
- Monitor CV effects carefully; patients with hypertension who take this drug may experience changes in BP because of the additional vasoconstriction. If a nasal decongestant is needed, pseudoephedrine is the drug of choice.

Teaching points

- Do not exceed recommended dose. Demonstrate proper administration technique for topical nasal application and administration of eye drops. Avoid prolonged use be-

---

Adverse effects in *Italics* are most common; those in **Bold** are life-threatening.

cause underlying medical problems can be disguised.

- These side effects may occur: dizziness, weakness, restlessness, light-headedness, tremor (avoid driving or operating dangerous equipment); urinary retention (empty bladder before taking drug).
- Rebound congestion may occur when this drug is stopped; drink plenty of fluids, use a humidifier, avoid smoke-filled areas.
- Report nervousness, palpitations, sleeplessness, sweating.

▽ thalidomide

See *Less Commonly Used Drugs,* p. 1352.

▽ theophylline
(thee off' i lin)

theophylline

Immediate-release capsules, tablets: Bronkodyl, Elixophyllin, Quibron-T Dividose, Slo-Phyllin, Theolair

Timed-release capsules: Slo-bid Gyrocaps, Slo-Phyllin Gyrocaps, Theo-24, Theobid, Theoclear L.A., Theospan-SR, Theovent

Timed-release tablets: Quibron-T/SR Dividose, Respbid, Sustaire, Theochron, Theo-Dur, Theolair-SR, Theo-X, T-Phyl, Uni-Dur, Uniphyl

Liquids: Accurbron, Aquaphyllin, Asmalix, Elixomin, Elixophyllin, Lanophyllin, Slo-Phyllin, Theoclear-80, Theolair, Theostat 80

theophylline sodium glycinate

Elixir: Acet-Amp (CAN)

PREGNANCY CATEGORY C

Drug classes

Bronchodilator
Xanthine

Therapeutic actions

Relaxes bronchial smooth muscle, causing bronchodilation and increasing vital capacity that has been impaired by bronchospasm and air trapping; actions may be mediated by inhibition of phosphodiesterase, which increases the concentration of cyclic adenosine monophosphate; in concentrations that may be higher than those reached clinically, it also inhibits the release of slow-reacting substance of anaphylaxis and histamine.

Indications

- Symptomatic relief or prevention of bronchial asthma and reversible bronchospasm associated with chronic bronchitis and emphysema
- Unlabeled use of 2 mg/kg/day to maintain serum concentrations between 3 and 5 mcg/mL: treatment of apnea and bradycardia of prematurity

Contraindications and cautions

- Contraindicated with hypersensitivity to any xanthines, peptic ulcer, active gastritis, pregnancy (neonatal tachycardia, jitteriness, and withdrawal apnea), underlying seizure disorders (unless receiving appropriate anticonvulsant medication).
- Use cautiously with cardiac arrhythmias, acute myocardial injury, CHF, cor pulmonale, severe hypertension, severe hypoxemia, renal or hepatic disease, hyperthyroidism, alcoholism, labor (may inhibit uterine contractions), lactation, status asthmaticus.

Available forms

Syrup—80, 150 mg/15 mL; elixir—80 mg/15 mL; oral solution—80 mg/15 mL; timed-release capsules—50, 75, 100, 125, 130, 200, 250, 260, 300 mg; timed-release tablets—100, 200, 250, 300, 400, 500 mg; injection in 5% dextrose—200, 400, 800 mg/container; extended-release tablets—100, 400, 450 mg; sustained-release tablets—100, 300 mg; controlled-release tablets—100, 200, 300 mg

Dosages

Maintain serum levels in the therapeutic range of 10–20 mcg/mL; base dosage on lean body mass.

Adults
Theophylline

• *Acute symptoms requiring rapid theo-phyllinization in patients not receiving theophylline:*

Young adult smokers: Oral loading dose of 6 mg/kg followed by 3 mg/kg q 4 hr for 3 doses. Maintenance: 3 mg/kg q 6 hr.

Otherwise healthy adult nonsmokers: Oral loading dose of 6 mg/kg, followed by 3 mg/kg q 6 hr for 2 doses. Maintenance: 3 mg/kg q 8 hr.

• *Acute symptoms requiring rapid theo-phyllinization in patients receiving the-ophylline:* A loading dose is required; each 0.5 mg/kg PO administered as a loading dose will result in about a 1 mcg/mL increase in serum theophylline. Ideally, defer loading dose until serum theophylline determination is made. Otherwise, base loading dose on clinical judgment and the knowledge that 2.5 mg/kg of a rapidly absorbed preparation will increase serum theophylline levels by about 5 mcg/mL and is unlikely to cause dangerous adverse effects if the patient is not experiencing theophylline toxicity before this dose; maintenance doses are as above.

• *Long-term therapy:* Initial dose of 16 mg/kg/24 hr PO or 400 mg/24 hr, whichever is less, in divided doses q 6–8 hr for immediate-release preparations or liquids, q 8–12 or 24 hr for timed-release preparations (consult manufacturer's recommendations for specific dosage interval). Increase dosage based on serum theophylline levels, or if these are unavailable, increase in 25% increments at 3-day intervals as long as drug is tolerated or until maximum dose of 13 mg/kg/day or 900 mg, whichever is less, is reached.

• *Dosage adjustment based on serum the-ophylline levels during long-term ther-apy:*

Serum theophylline levels < 10 mcg/mL are too low, levels of 10–20 mcg/mL are within normal limits, and levels > 20 mcg/mL are too high.

Serum theophylline level 5–7.5 mcg/mL: Increase dose by about 25%, recheck serum level; may need to increase dose.

Serum theophylline level 7.5–10 mcg/mL: Increase dose by 25%; may need to give total daily dose at more frequent intervals; recheck at 6- to 12-mo intervals.

Serum theophylline level 10–20 mcg/mL: Maintain dosage; recheck level at 6- to 12-mo intervals.

Serum theophylline level 20–25 mcg/mL: Decrease doses by about 10%; recheck level.

Serum theophylline level 25–30 mcg/mL: Skip next dose, and decrease subsequent doses by about 25%; recheck levels.

Serum theophylline level > 30 mcg/mL: Skip next two doses, and decrease subsequent doses by 50%; recheck level.

• *Measurement of serum theophylline lev-els during chronic therapy:* Measure serum theophylline in blood sample drawn 1–2 hr after administration of immediate-release preparations, 5–9 hr after administration of most sustained-release products.

Theophylline sodium glycinate (44.5%–47.3% theophylline)

330–660 mg PO q 6–8 hr after meals.

Pediatric patients

< 6 mo: Not recommended.

< 6 yr: Timed-release products not recommended.

Theophylline
Pediatric patients > 6 mo

• *Acute symptoms requiring rapid theo-phyllinization in patients not receiving theophylline:*

6 mo–9 yr: 6 mg/kg PO loading dose followed by 4 mg/kg q 4 hr for 3 doses. Maintenance: 2 mg/kg q 8 hr.

9–16 yr: 6 mg/kg PO loading dose followed by 2 mg/kg q 4 hr for 3 doses. Maintenance: 3 mg/kg q 6 hr.

Infants < 6 mo

Reduce initial and maintenance doses because elimination of theophylline appears to be delayed in these patients. Loading dose is 1 mg/kg for each 2 mcg/mL serum concentration desired.

Preterm infants: Maintenance: 1 mg/kg q 12 hr.

Term infants ≤ 4 wk: Maintenance: 1–2 mg/kg q 12 hr.

Infants 4–8 wk: Maintenance: 1–2 mg/kg q 8 hr.

Infants > 8 wk: Maintenance: 1–3 mg/kg q 6 hr.

- *Long-term therapy:* Initial dose of 16 mg/kg/24 hr PO or 400 mg/24 hr, whichever is less, in divided doses q 6–8 hr for immediate-release preparations or liquids, q 8–12 or 24 hr for timed-release preparations in children < 6 yr (consult manufacturer's recommendations for specific dosage interval). Increase dosage based on serum theophylline levels, or if these are unavailable, increase in 25% increments at 3-day intervals as long as drug is tolerated or until maximum dose given below is reached:

< 9 yr: Maximum daily dose: 24 mg/kg/day.
9–12 yr: Maximum daily dose: 20 mg/kg/day.
12–16 yr: Maximum daily dose: 18 mg/kg/day.
> 16 yr: Maximum daily dose: 13 mg/kg/day
Theophylline sodium glycinate
1–3 yr: 55–110 mg q 6–8 hr PO after meals.
3–6 yr: 110–165 mg q 6–8 hr PO after meals.
6–12 yr: 220–330 mg q 6–8 hr PO after meals.

Geriatric patients or impaired adults

Use caution, especially in elderly men, and in patients with cor pulmonale, CHF, or liver disease.

- *Acute symptoms requiring rapid theophyllinization in patients not receiving theophylline:*

Older patients and patients with cor pulmonale: Oral loading dose of 6 mg/kg, followed by 2 mg/kg q 6 hr for 2 doses. Maintenance: 2 mg/kg q 8 hr.
Patients with CHF: Oral loading dose of 6 mg/kg, followed by 2 mg/kg q 8 hr for 2 doses. Maintenance: 1–2 mg/kg q 12 hr.

Pharmacokinetics

Route	Onset	Peak
Oral	Varies	2 hr

Metabolism: Hepatic; $T_{1/2}$: 3–15 hr (nonsmoker) or 4–5 hr (smokers)
Distribution: Crosses placenta; enters breast milk
Excretion: Urine

Adverse effects

- **CNS:** *Irritability (especially children); restlessness,* dizziness, muscle twitching, convulsions, severe depression, stammering speech; abnormal behavior characterized by withdrawal, mutism and unresponsiveness alternating with hyperactive periods
- **CV:** Palpitations, sinus tachycardia, ventricular tachycardia, **life-threatening ventricular arrhythmias,** circulatory failure
- **GI:** *Loss of appetite,* hematemesis, epigastric pain, gastroesophageal reflux during sleep
- **GU:** Proteinuria, increased excretion of renal tubular cells and RBCs; diuresis (dehydration), urinary retention in men with prostate enlargement
- **Respiratory:** Tachypnea, **respiratory arrest**
- **Serum theophylline levels < 20 mcg/mL:** Adverse effects uncommon.
- **Serum theophylline levels > 20–25 mcg/mL:** *Nausea, vomiting, diarrhea, headache, insomnia, irritability* (75% of patients)
- **Serum theophylline levels > 35 mcg/mL:** Hyperglycemia, hypotension, cardiac arrhythmias, tachycardia (> 10 mcg/mL in premature newborns); seizures, brain damage, **death**
- **Other:** Fever, flushing, hyperglycemia, SIADH, rash, increased AST

Interactions

✳ Drug-drug • Increased effects and toxicity with cimetidine, erythromycin, troleandomycin, ciprofloxacin, norfloxacin, ofloxacin, hormonal contraceptives, ticlopidine, ranitidine • Possibly increased effects with rifampin • Increased serum levels and risk of toxicity in hypothyroid patients, decreased levels in patients who are hyperthyroid; monitor patients on thioamines, thyroid hormones for changes in serum levels as patients become euthyroid • Increased cardiac toxicity with halothane • Decreased effects in patients who are cigarette smokers (1–2 packs/day); theophylline dosage may need to be increased 50%–100% • Decreased effects with barbiturates, charcoal • Decreased effects of phenytoins, benzodiazepines, and theophylline preparations • Decreased effects of nondepolarizing neuromuscular blockers • Mutually antagonistic effects of beta-blockers and theophylline preparations
✳ Drug-food • Theophylline elimination is increased by a low-carbohydrate, high-protein

T

diet and by charcoal broiled beef • Theophylline elimination is decreased by a high-carbohydrate, low-protein diet • Food may alter bioavailability, absorption of timed-release theophylline preparations; these may rapidly release their contents with food and cause toxicity. Timed-release forms should be taken on an empty stomach

❋ **Drug-lab test** • Interference with spectrophotometric determinations of serum theophylline levels by furosemide, phenylbutazone, probenecid, theobromine; coffee, tea, cola beverages, chocolate, acetaminophen cause falsely high values • Alteration in assays of uric acid, urinary catecholamines, plasma free fatty acids

❋ **Drug-alternative therapy** • Decreased effectiveness if taken with St. John's wort

■ Nursing considerations
Assessment
- **History:** Hypersensitivity to any xanthines; peptic ulcer, active gastritis; status asthmaticus; cardiac arrhythmias, acute myocardial injury, CHF, cor pulmonale; severe hypertension; severe hypoxemia; renal or hepatic disease; hyperthyroidism; pregnancy, lactation
- **Physical:** Skin color, texture, lesions; reflexes, bilateral grip strength, affect; P, auscultation, BP, perfusion; R, adventitious sounds; bowel sounds, normal output; frequency, voiding pattern, normal urinary output; ECG; EEG; thyroid, liver, kidney function tests

Interventions
- Caution patient not to chew or crush enteric-coated timed-release preparations.
- Give immediate release, liquid dosage forms with food if GI effects occur.
- Do not give timed-release preparations with food; these should be given on an empty stomach, 1 hr before or 2 hr after meals.
- Advise patients that this drug should not be used during pregnancy; use of barrier contraceptives is recommended.
- Monitor results of serum theophylline level determinations carefully, and reduce dosage if serum levels exceed therapeutic range of 10–20 mcg/mL.

- Monitor carefully for clinical signs of adverse effects, particularly if serum theophylline levels are not available.
- Maintain diazepam on standby to treat seizures.

Teaching points
- Take this drug exactly as prescribed. If a timed-release product is prescribed, take it on an empty stomach, 1 hr before or 2 hr after meals. Do not chew or crush timed-release preparations; it may be necessary for you to take this drug around the clock for adequate control of asthma attacks.
- Avoid excessive intake of coffee, tea, cocoa, cola beverages, chocolate. These contain theophylline-related substances that may increase your side effects.
- Smoking cigarettes or other tobacco products may markedly influence the effects of theophylline. It is preferable not to smoke while you are taking this drug. Notify your health care provider if you change your smoking habits while you are taking this drug; it may be necessary to change your drug dosage.
- Have frequent blood tests to monitor drug effects and ensure safe and effective dosage.
- Do not use this drug during pregnancy; use of barrier contraceptives is advised.
- These side effects may occur: nausea, loss of appetite (take drug with food; applies only to immediate-release or liquid dosage forms); difficulty sleeping, depression, emotional lability.
- Report nausea, vomiting, severe GI pain, restlessness, convulsions, irregular heartbeat.

▽ **thiabendazole**
*(thye a **ben'** da zole)*

Mintezol

PREGNANCY CATEGORY C

Drug class
Anthelmintic

Therapeutic actions

Suppresses egg or larva production of helminths and may inhibit the subsequent development of eggs and larvae that are passed in the feces; inhibits a helminth-specific enzyme.

Indications

- Treatment of strongyloidiasis (threadworm infection), cutaneous larva migrans (creeping eruption), and visceral larva migrans. Not a primary therapy, but no other agent is usually needed with enterobiasis (pinworm) infection occurring with one of the above
- When more specific therapy cannot be used or a second agent is desirable, for the treatment of ascariasis (roundworm infection), uncinariasis (hookworm infection), trichuriasis (whipworm infection)
- Alleviation of symptoms of invasive trichinosis

Contraindications and cautions

- Contraindicated with allergy to thiabendazole, pregnancy.
- Use cautiously with renal or hepatic dysfunction, anemia, malnourishment or dehydration, lactation.

Available forms

Chewable tablets—500 mg; oral suspension—500 mg/5 mL

Dosages

Adults and pediatric patients

< 30 lb: Clinical experience with this group is limited.
> 30 lb–< 150 lb: 10 mg/lb per dose PO. See regimen below, based on indication.
≥ 150 lb: 1.5 g/dose PO. Maximum daily dose: 3 g. See regimen below, based on indication.

- *Enterobiasis:* 2 doses/day for 1 day; repeat in 7 days to reduce risk of reinfection (or 2 doses/day for 2 successive days).
- *Strongyloidiasis, ascariasis, uncinariasis, trichuriasis:* 2 doses/day for 2 successive days (or single dose of 20 mg/lb).
- *Cutaneous larva migrans:* 2 doses/day for 2 successive days (repeat treatment if lesions still present 2 days after therapy).
- *Trichinosis:* 2 doses/day for 2–4 successive days as needed.

- *Visceral larva migrans:* 2 doses/day for 7 successive days.

Pharmacokinetics

Route	Onset	Peak
Oral	Rapid	1–2 hr

Metabolism: Hepatic; $T_{1/2}$: unknown
Distribution: Crosses placenta; may enter breast milk
Excretion: Urine and feces

Adverse effects

- **CNS:** *Dizziness, drowsiness, giddiness, weariness, headache,* tinnitus, hyperirritability, numbness, abnormal sensation in eyes, blurred vision, xanthopsia
- **CV:** Hypotension, collapse
- **GI:** *Anorexia, nausea,* vomiting, epigastric distress, diarrhea, perianal rash, jaundice, cholestasis, parenchymal liver damage
- **GU:** Enuresis, *malodor of urine,* crystalluria, hematuria
- **Hematologic:** Rise in AST, hyperglycemia, leukopenia
- **Hypersensitivity:** Reactions ranging from rash, fever, chills, angioedema, lymphadenopathy, **anaphylaxis, Stevens-Johnson syndrome** (sometimes fatal)

Interactions

✴ **Drug-drug** ● Risk of increased serum levels and toxicity of xanthines if combined; monitor serum xanthine levels and adjust dosage appropriately

■ Nursing considerations
Assessment

- **History:** Allergy to thiabendazole; renal or hepatic dysfunction; anemia, malnourishment or dehydration; pregnancy, lactation
- **Physical:** Skin color, lesions, turgor; orientation, affect; bowel sounds, output; liver and renal function tests, urinalysis, CBC

Interventions

- Culture for ova and parasites.
- Administer drug with food; have patient chew tablets before swallowing them.
- Discontinue drug, and consult with physician if hypersensitivity reactions occur.
- Arrange for treatment of all family members (pinworm infestations).

- Arrange for disinfection of toilet facilities after patient use (pinworms).
- Arrange for daily laundry of bed linens, towels, nightclothes, and undergarments (pinworms).

Teaching points
- Take drug with food to decrease GI upset. Chew tablets before swallowing.
- Pinworms are easily transmitted; all family members should be treated for complete eradication.
- Strict handwashing and hygiene measures are important; launder undergarments, bedlinens, nightclothes daily; disinfect toilet facilities daily and bathroom floors periodically (pinworms).
- These side effects may occur: nausea, abdominal pain, diarrhea (small, frequent meals may help); drowsiness, dizziness, insomnia (avoid driving and using dangerous machinery); strange odor may develop in the urine (reversible).
- Report rash, joint pain, severe GI upset, fever, chills, swelling of feet or hands, yellow color to skin or eyes.

▽ thiethylperazine maleate
*(thye eth il **per'** a zeen)*

Norzine (CAN), Torecan

PREGNANCY CATEGORY X

Drug classes
Antiemetic
Antivertigo agent

Therapeutic actions
Mechanism of action not fully understood: acts directly on the CTZ and the vomiting center to suppress nausea and vomiting.

Indications
- Relief of nausea and vomiting
- Unlabeled use: treatment of vertigo

Contraindications and cautions
- Allergy to phenothiazines, comatose or severely depressed states, pregnancy, lactation, intracardiac or intracranial surgery, IV administration.

Available forms
Tablets—10 mg; injection—5 mg/mL

Dosages
Adults
Oral
10–30 mg/day in divided doses.
IM
2 mL, 1–3 times daily.
Pediatric patients
Safety and efficacy not determined for patients < 12 yr.

Pharmacokinetics

Route	Onset	Duration
Oral	60 min	4 hr
IM	30 min	4 hr

Metabolism: Hepatic; $T_{1/2}$: unknown
Distribution: Crosses placenta; enters breast milk
Excretion: Urine

Adverse effects
- **CNS:** *Drowsiness, insomnia, vertigo,* headache, weakness, tremors, ataxia, slurring, cerebral edema, seizures, exacerbation of psychotic symptoms, *extrapyramidal syndromes;* **neuroleptic malignant syndrome**
- **CV:** *Hypotension, orthostatic hypotension,* hypertension, tachycardia, bradycardia, cardiac arrest, CHF, cardiomegaly, refractory arrhythmias, **pulmonary edema**
- **EENT:** Nasal congestion, glaucoma, *photophobia, blurred vision,* miosis, mydriasis, deposits in the cornea and lens, pigmentary retinopathy
- **Endocrine:** Lactation, breast engorgement in females, galactorrhea, SIADH secretion, amenorrhea
- **GI:** *Dry mouth, salivation, nausea, vomiting, anorexia, constipation,* paralytic ileus, incontinence

---

Adverse effects in *Italics* are most common; those in **Bold** are life-threatening.

- **GU:** *Urinary retention,* polyuria, incontinence
- **Hematologic:** Eosinophilia, leukopenia, leukocytosis, *anemia,* aplastic anemia, hemolytic anemia, thrombocytopenic or nonthrombocytopenic purpura, pancytopenia, elevated serum cholesterol
- **Hypersensitivity:** Jaundice, *urticaria,* angioneurotic edema, laryngeal edema, photosensitivity, eczema, asthma, anaphylactoid reactions, exfoliative dermatitis
- **Respiratory:** Bronchospasm, laryngospasm, dyspnea, suppression of cough reflex and potential aspiration
- **Other:** Fever, heatstroke, pallor, flushed facies, sweating, *photosensitivity*

Interactions

✳ **Drug-drug** • Additive CNS depression, hypotension if given preoperatively with barbiturate anesthetics, alcohol, meperidine • Additive effects of both drugs with beta-blockers • Increased risk of tachycardia, hypotension with epinephrine, norepinephrine • Increased risk of seizure with metrizamide

✳ **Drug-lab test** • False-positive pregnancy tests (less likely if serum test is used) • Increase in PBI, not attributable to an increase in thyroxine

■ Nursing considerations
Assessment

- **History:** Allergy to phenothiazines; comatose or severely depressed states; lactation, pregnancy; intracranial or intracardiac surgery
- **Physical:** T, body weight, skin color, turgor; reflexes, orientation; P, BP, orthostatic BP, ECG; R, adventitious sounds; bowel sounds, normal output, liver evaluation; prostate palpation, normal urine output; CBC; urinalysis

Interventions

- For use after surgery; give slowly by deep IM injection into upper outer quadrant of buttock at or shortly before the termination of anesthesia.
- Do not administer to pregnant patients; serious fetal harm can occur.
- Keep the patient recumbent for 30 min after injection to avoid orthostatic hypotension.

- Be alert to potential for aspiration because of suppressed cough reflex.

Teaching points

- These side effects may occur: drowsiness (avoid driving or operating dangerous machinery; avoid alcohol, which will increase the drowsiness); faintness, dizziness (change position slowly, use caution climbing stairs).
- This drug can cause serious fetal harm; avoid use during pregnancy. Use of barrier contraceptives is advised.
- Report sore throat, fever, unusual bleeding or bruising, rash, weakness, tremors, impaired vision, dark urine, pale stools, yellowing of the skin and eyes.

▽**thioguanine (TG, 6-Thioguanine)**

(thye oh gwah' neen)

Lanvis (CAN)

PREGNANCY CATEGORY D

Drug classes

Antimetabolite
Antineoplastic

Therapeutic actions

Tumor-inhibiting properties, probably due to interference with a number of steps in the synthesis and use of purine nucleotides, which are normally incorporated into DNA and RNA.

Indications

- Remission induction, consolidation, and maintenance therapy of acute nonlymphocytic leukemias—usually used in combination therapy

Contraindications and cautions

- Contraindicated with allergy to thioguanine, prior resistance to thioguanine or mercaptopurine, hematopoietic depression, pregnancy (potential mutagen and teratogen), lactation.
- Use cautiously with impaired hepatic function.

Available forms

Tablets—40 mg

1132 ■ thioridazine hydrochloride

Dosages
Adults and pediatric patients
Initial dosage, 2 mg/kg/day PO daily for 4 wk.
If no clinical improvement is seen and there
are no toxic effects, increase dose to 3 mg/kg/
day. If complete hematologic remission is obtained, institute maintenance therapy. No adjustment of dosage is needed if used as part of
combination therapy.

Pharmacokinetics

Route	Onset	Peak
Oral	Slow	8 hr

Metabolism: Hepatic; T$_{1/2}$: 11 hr
Distribution: Crosses placenta; may enter
breast milk
Excretion: Urine

Adverse effects
- **GI:** Hepatotoxicity, *nausea, vomiting,
  anorexia,* diarrhea, stomatitis
- **Hematologic:** *Bone marrow suppression, immunosuppression, hyperuricemia*
  due to rapid lysis of malignant cells
- **Other:** Fever, weakness, cancer, chromosomal aberrations

■ Nursing considerations
Assessment
- **History:** Allergy to thioguanine, prior resistance to thioguanine; hematopoietic depression; impaired hepatic function; pregnancy, lactation
- **Physical:** Skin color; mucous membranes,
  liver evaluation, abdominal exam; CBC, differential, hemoglobin, platelet counts; liver
  function tests; serum uric acid

Interventions
- Evaluate hematopoietic status before and
  frequently during therapy.
- Discontinue drug therapy if platelet count
  < 50,000; polymorphonuclear granulocyte
  count < 1,000; consult physician for dosage
  adjustment.
- Arrange for discontinuation of this drug at
  any sign of hematologic or hepatic toxicity;
  consult physician.
- Ensure that patient is not pregnant before
  administration.

- Ensure that patient is well hydrated before
  and during therapy to minimize adverse effects of hyperuricemia; allopurinal and drugs
  to alkalinize the urine are sometimes prescribed.
- Administer as a single daily dose.

Teaching points
- Drink adequate fluids while you are on this
  drug; drink at least 8–10 glasses of fluid each
  day.
- These side effects may occur: mouth sores
  (use frequent mouth care); nausea, vomiting, loss of appetite (small, frequent meals
  may help); increased susceptibility to infection (avoid crowds and infections).
- This drug may cause miscarriages and birth
  defects. Use birth control; men also should
  use birth control measures while on this drug
  and for a time afterward.
- Have frequent, regular medical follow-up,
  including frequent blood tests to assess drug
  effects.
- Report fever, chills, sore throat, unusual
  bleeding or bruising, yellow discoloration of
  the skin or eyes, abdominal pain, flank pain,
  joint pain, swelling of the feet or legs.

▷thioridazine
hydrochloride
(thye oh rid' a zeen)

Apo-Thioridazine (CAN), Mellaril,
Mellaril-S

PREGNANCY CATEGORY C

Drug classes
Phenothiazine (piperidine)
Dopaminergic blocking agent
Antipsychotic
Antianxiety agent

Therapeutic actions
Mechanism of action not fully understood:
blocks postsynaptic dopamine receptors in the
brain, but this may not be necessary and sufficient for antipsychotic activity; depresses the
RAS, including the parts of the brain involved
with wakefulness and emesis; anticholinergic,

Adverse effects in Italics are most common; those in Bold are life-threatening.

antihistaminic (H₁), and alpha-adrenergic blocking activity also may contribute to some of its effects.

Indications

- Management of schizophrenic patients who fail to respond adequately to other antipsychotic drugs.

Contraindications and cautions

- Contraindicated with coma or severe CNS depression, hypersensitivity (cross-sensitivity between phenothiazines may occur), bone marrow depression, blood dyscrasia, subcortical brain damage, liver damage, cerebral arteriosclerosis, coronary disease, severe hypotension or hypertension; prolonged QTc interval; hypokalemia.
- Use cautiously with respiratory disorders ("silent pneumonia"); glaucoma, prostatic hypertrophy; epilepsy or history of epilepsy (drug lowers seizure threshold); breast cancer; thyrotoxicosis (severe neurotoxicity); peptic ulcer, decreased renal function; myelography within previous 24 hr or scheduled within 48 hr; exposure to heat or phosphorous insecticides; pregnancy; lactation; children < 12 yr, especially those with chickenpox, CNS infections (children are especially susceptible to dystonias that may confound the diagnosis of Reye's syndrome).

Available forms

Tablets—10, 15, 25, 50, 100, 150, 200 mg; concentrate—30, 100 mg/mL; suspension—25, 100 mg/5 mL

Dosages

Full clinical effects may require 6 wk–6 mo of therapy.

Adults

50–100 mg PO tid. Increase gradually to a maximum of 800 mg/day if necessary to control symptoms and then gradually reduce to minimum effective dose. Total daily dose ranges from 200–800 mg divided into two to four doses.

Pediatric patients 2–12 yr

0.5–3 mg/kg/day PO. Moderate disorders: 10 mg 2 or 3 times daily; hospitalized: 25 mg 2 or 3 times daily.

Pharmacokinetics

Route	Onset	Peak	Duration
Oral	Varies	2–4 hr	4–5 days

Metabolism: Hepatic; $T_{1/2}$: 21–25 hr
Distribution: Crosses placenta; may enter breast milk
Excretion: Urine

Adverse effects

- **Autonomic:** *Dry mouth, salivation, nasal congestion, nausea,* vomiting, anorexia, fever, pallor, flushed facies, sweating, constipation, paralytic ileus, urinary retention, incontinence, polyuria, enuresis, priapism, ejaculation inhibition, male impotence
- **CNS:** *Drowsiness,* insomnia, vertigo, headache, weakness, tremor, ataxia, slurring, cerebral edema, seizures, exacerbation of psychotic symptoms, extrapyramidal syndromes—*pseudoparkinsonism; dystonias; akathisia,* tardive dyskinesias, potentially irreversible **neuroleptic malignant syndrome** (NMS)
- **CV:** Hypotension, orthostatic hypotension, hypertension, tachycardia, bradycardia, cardiac arrest, CHF, cardiomegaly, **refractory arrhythmias,** pulmonary edema
- **EENT:** Glaucoma, *photophobia, blurred vision,* miosis, mydriasis, deposits in the cornea and lens (opacities), pigmentary retinopathy
- **Endocrine:** Lactation, breast engorgement, galactorrhea; SIADH secretion; amenorrhea, menstrual irregularities; gynecomastia; changes in libido; hyperglycemia or hypoglycemia; glycosuria; hyponatremia; pituitary tumor with hyperprolactinemia; inhibition of ovulation, infertility, pseudopregnancy; reduced urinary levels of gonadotropins, estrogens, progestins
- **Hematologic:** Eosinophilia, leukopenia, leukocytosis, anemia; aplastic anemia; hemolytic anemia; thrombocytopenic or nonthrombocytopenic purpura; pancytopenia
- **Hypersensitivity:** Jaundice, urticaria, angioneurotic edema, laryngeal edema, photosensitivity, eczema, asthma, anaphylactoid reactions, exfoliative dermatitis
- **Respiratory:** Bronchospasm, laryngospasm, dyspnea; suppression of cough reflex and potential for aspiration

T

- **Other:** *Urine discolored pink to red-brown*

Interactions

✳ **Drug-drug** • Additive CNS depression with alcohol • Additive anticholinergic effects and possibly decreased antipsychotic efficacy with anticholinergic drug • Increased likelihood of seizures with metrizamide • Increased effects from both drugs if given in combination with propranolol • Decreased antihypertensive effect of guanethidine • Increased risk of potentially fatal arrhythmias if combined with other drugs that prolong the QTc interval

✳ **Drug-lab test** • False-positive pregnancy tests (less likely if serum test is used) • Increase in PBI not attributable to an increase in thyroxine

■ Nursing considerations

Assessment

- **History:** Coma or severe CNS depression; blood dyscrasia; circulatory collapse; subcortical brain damage; Parkinson's disease; liver damage; cerebral arteriosclerosis; coronary disease; severe hypotension or hypertension; respiratory disorders; glaucoma, prostatic hypertrophy; epilepsy; breast cancer; thyrotoxicosis; peptic ulcer, decreased renal function; myelography within previous 24 hr or scheduled within 48 hr; exposure to heat or phosphorous insecticides; pregnancy; lactation; chickenpox; CNS infections; history of prolonged QTc interval
- **Physical:** Weight; T; reflexes, orientation, intraocular pressure; P, BP, orthostatic BP; R, adventitious sounds; bowel sounds and normal output, liver evaluation; urinary output, prostate size, CBC, urinalysis, thyroid, liver and kidney function tests, ECG, serum potassium levels

Interventions

- Ensure that patient has not responded to other antipsychotic drugs.
- Arrange for ophthalmologic (slit lamp) examination before and during drug therapy.
- Ensure that patient's baseline ECG shows a QTc interval < 450 msec; stabilize potassium levels before administering.

- Do not change brand names; bioavailability differences have been documented for different brands.
- Oral concentrate may be administered in distilled or acidified tap water or suitable juices, or use the flavored suspension.
- Do not change dosage in long-term therapy more often than weekly; drug requires 4–7 days to achieve steady-state plasma levels.
- Avoid skin contact with oral solution; contact dermatitis has occurred.
- Discontinue drug if serum creatinine, BUN become abnormal or if WBC count is depressed or if QTc interval is > 500 msec.
- Monitor elderly patients for dehydration, and institute remedial measures promptly; sedation and decreased sensation of thirst related to CNS effects can lead to severe dehydration.
- Consult physician regarding appropriate warning of patient or patient's guardian about tardive dyskinesias.
- Consult physician about dosage reduction, use of anticholinergic antiparkinsonian drugs (controversial) if extrapyramidal effects occur.

Teaching points

- Take drug exactly as prescribed.
- Avoid skin contact with drug solutions.
- Avoid driving or engaging in other dangerous activities if CNS, vision changes occur.
- Avoid prolonged exposure to sun, or use a sunscreen or covering garments.
- Maintain fluid intake and use precautions against heatstroke in hot weather.
- Arrange for ophthalmologic exams and ECGs periodically during therapy.
- Report sore throat, fever, unusual bleeding or bruising, rash, weakness, tremors, impaired vision, dark urine (pink or reddish brown urine is expected), pale stools, yellowing of the skin or eyes.

▷**thiotepa
(triethylenethiophos-
phoramide, TESPA,
TSPA)**

(thye oh tep' ah)

Thioplex

PREGNANCY CATEGORY D

Drug classes
Alkylating agent
Antineoplastic

Therapeutic actions
Cytotoxic: disrupts the bonds of DNA, causing cell death; cell cycle nonspecific.

Indications
- Treatment of adenocarcinoma of the breast, ovary
- Superficial papillary carcinoma of the urinary bladder
- Controlling intracavity effusions secondary to diffuse or localized neoplastic disease of various serosal cavities
- Treatment of lymphoma, including Hodgkin's disease; no longer a drug of choice

Contraindications and cautions
- Contraindicated with allergy to thiotepa, hematopoietic depression, pregnancy, lactation.
- Use cautiously with impaired hepatic or renal function, concomitant therapy with other alkylating agents or irradiation.

Available forms
Powder for injection—15 mg

Dosages
Adults
IV
0.3–0.4 mg/kg at 1- to 4-wk intervals.
Intratumor
Drug is diluted in sterile water to a concentration of 10 mg/mL, then 0.6–0.8 mg/kg is injected directly into the tumor after a local anesthetic is injected through the same needle. Maintainance doses of 0.07–0.8 mg/kg every 1–4 wk depending on patient's condition.

Intracavity
0.6–0.8 mg/kg through the same tube that is used to remove fluid from the cavity.
Intravesical
Dehydrate patient with papillary carcinoma of the bladder for 8–12 hr prior to treatment. Then instill 60 mg in 30–60 mL of sodium chloride injection into the bladder by catheter. Retain for 2 hr. If patient is unable to retain 60 mL, give the dose in 30 mL. Repeat once a week for 4 wk.

Pharmacokinetics

Route	Onset
IV	Gradual

Metabolism: Hepatic; $T_{1/2}$: 109 min
Distribution: Crosses placenta; may enter breast milk
Excretion: Urine

▼IV facts
Preparation: Reconstitute powder with sterile water for injection. 1.5 mL of diluent gives a drug concentration of 5 mg/0.5 mL of solution. May be further diluted with sodium chloride injection, dextrose injection, dextrose and sodium chloride injection, Ringer's injection, lactated Ringer's injection. Store powder in the refrigerator, reconstituted solution is stable for 8 hr if refrigerated. Sterile water for injection produces an isotonic solution, other diluents may produce a hypertonic solution that may cause mild to moderate discomfort on injection. Check solution before use; solution should be clear to slightly opaque; grossly opaque solutions or solutions with precipitates should not be used.
Infusion: Administer IV dose directly and rapidly, 60 mg over 1 min. There is no need for slow IV drip or the use of large volumes of fluid.

Adverse effects
- **CNS:** *Dizziness,* headache, blurred vision
- **Dermatologic:** Hives, rash, weeping from subcutaneous lesions, contact dermatitis at injection site
- **GI:** *Nausea, vomiting,* anorexia
- **GU:** *Amenorrhea, interference with spermatogenesis,* dysuria, urinary retention
- **Hematologic:** *Hematopoietic toxicity*
- **Other:** Febrile reactions, cancer

■ Nursing considerations
Assessment
- **History:** Allergy to thiotepa; hematopoietic depression; impaired renal or hepatic function; concomitant therapy with other alkylating agents or irradiation; pregnancy, lactation
- **Physical:** Weight; skin color, lesions; T; orientation, reflexes; CBC, differential; urinalysis; liver and renal function tests

Interventions
- Ensure that patient is not pregnant before administration; advise the use of barrier contraceptives.
- Arrange for blood tests to evaluate bone marrow function before therapy, weekly during therapy and for at least 3 wk after therapy.
- Mix solution with 2% procaine HCl, 1:1,000 epinephrine HCl, or both for local use into single or multiple sites.
- Reduce dosage with renal or hepatic impairment and for bone marrow depression.

Teaching points
- This drug can be given only parenterally. Prepare a calendar of treatment days.
- These side effects may occur: nausea, vomiting, loss of appetite (request an antiemetic; small frequent meals also may help); dizziness, headache (use special safety precautions to prevent falls or injury); amenorrhea in women, change in sperm production.
- This drug should not be taken during pregnancy; use birth control while you are on this drug. If you become pregnant, consult with your health care provider.
- Have regular medical follow-up, including blood tests, to assess drug effects.
- Report unusual bleeding or bruising, fever, chills, sore throat, stomach or flank pain, severe nausea and vomiting, skin rash or hives.

▷thiothixene (thiothixene hydrochloride)
(thye oh thix' een)

Navane

PREGNANCY CATEGORY C

Drug classes
Dopaminergic blocking agent
Antipsychotic
Thioxanthene

Therapeutic actions
Mechanism of action not fully understood: blocks postsynaptic dopamine receptors in the brain, but this may not be necessary and sufficient for antipsychotic activity.

Indications
- Management of manifestations of psychotic disorders

Contraindications and cautions
- Contraindicated with coma or severe CNS depression, blood dyscrasia, circulatory collapse, subcortical brain damage, Parkinson's disease, liver damage, cerebral arteriosclerosis, coronary disease, severe hypotension or hypertension, pregnancy, lactation.
- Use cautiously with respiratory disorders ("silent pneumonia"); glaucoma; prostatic hypertrophy; epilepsy or history of epilepsy (drug lowers seizure threshold); breast cancer; thyrotoxicosis (severe neurotoxicity); peptic ulcer, decreased renal function; myelography within previous 24 hr or scheduled within 48 hr; exposure to heat or phosphorous insecticides; children < 12 yr, especially those with chickenpox, CNS infections (children are especially susceptible to dystonias that may confound the diagnosis of Reye's syndrome).

Available forms
Capsules—1, 2, 5, 10, 20 mg; concentrate—5 mg/mL

Dosages

Full clinical effects may require 6 wk–6 mo of therapy.

Adults

Oral

Initially 2 mg tid (mild conditions) or 5 mg bid (more severe conditions). Increase dose as needed; the usual optimum dose is 20–30 mg/day. May increase to 60 mg/day, but further increases rarely increase beneficial response.

Pediatric patients

Not recommended for children < 12 yr.

Geriatric and debilitated patients

Use lower doses and increase more gradually.

Pharmacokinetics

Route	Onset	Duration
Oral	Slow	12 hr

Metabolism: Hepatic; $T_{1/2}$: 34 hr
Distribution: Crosses placenta; enters breast milk
Excretion: Bile and feces

Adverse effects

- **Autonomic:** *Dry mouth, salivation, nasal congestion, nausea,* vomiting, anorexia, fever, pallor, flushed facies, sweating, constipation, paralytic ileus, urinary retention, incontinence, polyuria, enuresis, priapism, ejaculation inhibition, male impotence
- **CNS:** *Drowsiness,* insomnia, vertigo, headache, weakness, tremor, ataxia, slurring, cerebral edema, seizures, exacerbation of psychotic symptoms, extrapyramidal syndromes—*pseudoparkinsonism; dystonias; akathisia,* tardive dyskinesias, potentially irreversible NMS; extrapyramidal symptoms, hyperthermia, **autonomic disturbances** (rare, but 20% fatal)
- **CV:** Hypotension, orthostatic hypotension, hypertension, tachycardia, bradycardia, cardiac arrest, CHF, cardiomegaly, **refractory arrhythmias** (some fatal), pulmonary edema
- **EENT:** Glaucoma, *photophobia, blurred vision,* miosis, mydriasis, deposits in the cornea and lens (opacities), pigmentary retinopathy
- **Endocrine:** Lactation, breast engorgement, galactorrhea; SIADH secretion; amenorrhea, menstrual irregularities; gynecomastia; changes in libido; hyperglycemia or hypoglycemia; glycosuria; hyponatremia; pituitary tumor with hyperprolactinemia; inhibition of ovulation, infertility, pseudopregnancy; reduced urinary levels of gonadotropins, estrogens, progestins
- **Hematologic:** Eosinophilia, leukopenia, leukocytosis, anemia; aplastic anemia; hemolytic anemia; thrombocytopenic or nonthrombocytopenic purpura; pancytopenia
- **Hypersensitivity:** Jaundice, urticaria, angioneurotic edema, laryngeal edema, photosensitivity, eczema, asthma, anaphylactoid reactions, exfoliative dermatitis
- **Respiratory:** Bronchospasm, laryngospasm, dyspnea, suppression of cough reflex and potential for aspiration
- **Other:** *Urine discolored pink to red-brown*

Interactions

✴ **Drug-lab test** • False-positive pregnancy tests (less likely if serum test is used) • Increase in PBI not attributable to an increase in thyroxine

■ Nursing considerations

Assessment

- **History:** Severe CNS depression; blood dyscrasia; circulatory collapse; subcortical brain damage; Parkinson's disease; liver damage; cerebral arteriosclerosis; coronary disease; severe hypotension or hypertension; respiratory disorders; glaucoma, prostatic hypertrophy; epilepsy; breast cancer; thyrotoxicosis; peptic ulcer, decreased renal function; myelography within previous 24 hr or scheduled within 48 hr; exposure to heat or phosphorous insecticides; pregnancy; lactation; chickenpox; CNS infections
- **Physical:** Weight, T; reflexes, orientation, intraocular pressure; P, BP, orthostatic BP; R, adventitious sounds; bowel sounds and normal output, liver evaluation; urinary output, prostate size. Arrange for CBC, urinalysis, thyroid, liver and kidney function tests

Interventions

- Avoid skin contact with oral solution; contact dermatitis has occurred.
- Discontinue drug if serum creatinine, BUN become abnormal or if WBC count is depressed.

T

- Monitor elderly patients for dehydration, and institute remedial measures promptly; sedation and decreased sensation of thirst related to CNS effects can lead to severe dehydration.
- Consult physician regarding appropriate warning of patient or patient's guardian about tardive dyskinesias.
- Consult physician about dosage reduction, use of anticholinergic antiparkinsonian drugs (controversial) if extrapyramidal effects occur.

Teaching points

- Take drug exactly as prescribed.
- Avoid skin contact with drug solutions.
- Avoid driving or engaging in other dangerous activities if CNS, vision changes occur.
- Avoid prolonged exposure to sun or use a sunscreen or covering garments.
- Maintain fluid intake, and use precautions against heatstroke in hot weather.
- Report sore throat, fever, unusual bleeding or bruising, rash, weakness, tremors, impaired vision, dark urine (pink or reddish brown urine is to be expected), pale stools, yellowing of the skin or eyes.

▽ thyroid desiccated
(thye' roid)

Armour Thyroid, Thyroid USP

PREGNANCY CATEGORY A

Drug class

Thyroid hormone preparation (contains T_3 and T_4 in their natural state and ratio)

Therapeutic actions

Increases the metabolic rate of body tissues, increasing oxygen consumption, respiratory and heart rate; rate of fat, protein, and carbohydrate metabolism; and growth and maturation; exact mechanism of action is not known.

Indications

- Replacement therapy in hypothyroidism
- Treatment of thyroid cancer
- Treatment or prevention of various types of euthyroid goiters
- Treatment of thyrotoxicosis with antithyroid drugs to prevent goitergenesis and hypothyroidism and thyrotoxicosis during pregnancy
- Diagnostic use in suppression tests

Contraindications and cautions

- Contraindicated with allergy to active or extraneous constituents of drug; thyrotoxicosis and acute MI uncomplicated by hypothyroidism.
- Use cautiously with Addison's disease (treatment of hypoadrenalism with corticosteroids should precede thyroid therapy), pregnancy, lactation, myxedema.

Available forms

Tablets—15, 30, 60, 90, 120, 180, 240, 300 mg

Dosages
Adults
- *Hypothyroidism:* Usual starting dose 30 mg; increase in 15-mg increments every 2–3 wk; usual maintenance dose 60–120 mg/day. Start with 15 mg/day in patients with long-standing myxedema.

Pediatric patients
0–6 mo: 15–30 mg/day PO.
6–12 mo: 30–45 mg/day PO.
1–5 yr: 45–60 mg/day PO.
6–12 yr: 60–90 mg/day PO.
> 12 yr: 90 mg/day PO.

Pharmacokinetics

Route	Onset	Peak
Oral	Varies	4 hr

Metabolism: Liver, kidney, and tissue; $T_{1/2}$: 1–2 days (T_3), 6–7 days (T_4)
Distribution: Does not readily cross placenta; minimally enters breast milk
Excretion: Urine and feces

Adverse effects

All adverse effects are rare at therapeutic doses.
- **Dermatologic:** Partial loss of hair in first few months of therapy in children
- **Endocrine:** Hyperthyroidism (palpitations, elevated pulse pressure, tachycardia, arrhythmias, angina pectoris, cardiac arrest;

tremors, headache, nervousness, insomnia; nausea, diarrhea, changes in appetite; weight loss, menstrual irregularities, sweating, heat intolerance, fever)
• **Hypersensitivity:** Allergic skin reactions

Interactions
* **Drug-drug** • Decreased absorption with cholestyramine • Increased risk of bleeding with warfarin • Decreased effectiveness of digitalis glycosides with thyroid replacement • Alterations in theophylline clearance occur in hypothyroid patients; if thyroid state changes during therapy, monitor patient carefully

■ Nursing considerations
Assessment
• **History:** Allergy to active or extraneous constituents of drug, bovine, or porcine products; thyrotoxicosis; acute MI uncomplicated by hypothyroidism; Addison's disease; lactation
• **Physical:** Skin lesions, color, temperature, texture; T; muscle tone, orientation, reflexes; P, auscultation, baseline ECG, BP; R, adventitious sounds; thyroid function tests

Interventions
• Monitor response carefully when beginning therapy, and adjust dosage accordingly.
• Administer as a single daily dose before breakfast.
• Arrange for regular, periodic blood tests of thyroid function.
• Monitor cardiac response throughout therapy. Reduce dose if angina occurs.

Teaching points
• Take as a single dose before breakfast.
• This drug replaces a very important hormone and will need to be taken for life. Do not discontinue this drug without consulting your nurse or physician; serious problems can occur.
• Wear or carry a medical alert tag to alert emergency medical personnel that you are on this drug.
• Nausea and diarrhea may occur (dividing the dose may help).
• Have periodic blood tests and medical evaluations while you are on this drug. Keep your scheduled appointments.

• Report headache, chest pain, palpitations, fever, weight loss, sleeplessness, nervousness, irritability, unusual sweating, intolerance to heat, diarrhea.

▽ tiagabine hydrochloride
(tye ag' ab bine)

Gabitril Filmtabs

PREGNANCY CATEGORY C

Drug class
Antiepileptic agent

Therapeutic actions
Increases GABA levels in the brain, which may result in antiseizure effects. GABA is the major inhibitory neurotransmitter in the CNS; tiagabine binds to GABA reuptake sites, preventing its reuptake, and increases levels in the presynaptic neurons and the glia.

Indications
• Adjunctive therapy in patients with partial seizures

Contraindications and cautions
• Contraindicated with hypersensitivity to tiagabine, hepatic disease or significant hepatic dysfunction.
• Use cautiously with pregnancy, lactation, and the elderly.

Available forms
Tablets—2, 4, 12, 16, 20 mg

Dosages
Adults
4 mg PO daily for 1 wk; may be increased by 4–8 mg/wk until desired response is seen; maximum dose 56 mg/day in 2–4 divided doses.
Pediatric patients 12–18 yr
4 mg PO daily for 1 wk; may be increased to 8 mg/day in 2 divided doses for 1 wk; then increased by 4–8 mg/wk up to a maximum of 32 mg/day in 2–4 divided doses.
Pediatric patients < 12 yr
Not recommended.

Pharmacokinetics

Route	Onset	Peak
Oral	Rapid	30–60 min

Metabolism: Hepatic; $T_{1/2}$: 7–9 hr
Distribution: Crosses placenta; may enter breast milk
Excretion: Feces and urine

Adverse effects

- **CNS:** *Dizziness, asthenia, somnolence,* nervousness, tremor, concentration difficulties
- **Dermatologic: Serious rash**
- **EENT:** Possible long-term ophthalmic effects
- **GI:** *GI upset, pain*
- **GU:** Irregular menses, secondary amenorrhea

Interactions

✳ **Drug-drug** • Decreased serum levels with carbamazepine, phenytoin, primidone; adjustment in tiagabine dosage may be necessary • Possible interaction with valproate; monitor patient closely

■ Nursing considerations
Assessment

- **History:** Hypersensitivity to tiagabine; hepatic disease or significant hepatic dysfunction; pregnancy, lactation
- **Physical:** Body weight; skin color, lesions; orientation, eye exam, affect, reflexes; hepatic function tests

Interventions

- Give drug with food.
- Reduce dosage and adjust more slowly if patient is not on comcomitant phenytoin, phenobarbital, carbamazepine.
- Provide frequent skin care if dermatologic effects occur.
- Avoid abrupt discontinuation; serious side effects could occur.
- Establish safety precautions (siderails, accompanying patient, etc.) if CNS changes occur.
- Arrange for appropriate counseling for women of childbearing age who wish to become pregnant.

Teaching points

- Take this drug exactly as prescribed.
- Do not discontinue this drug abruptly or change dosage, except on the advice of your health care provider.
- Avoid the use of alcohol and sleep-inducing or OTC drugs while you are on this drug; these could cause dangerous effects. If you feel that you need one of these preparations, consult your nurse or physician.
- Use contraceptive techniques at all times. If you wish to become pregnant while you are taking this drug, consult your health care provider.
- These side effects may occur: drowsiness (avoid driving or performing other tasks requiring alertness); GI upset (take the drug with food or milk; eat small, frequent meals).
- Wear a medical alert bracelet at all times so that any emergency medical personnel will know that you are an epileptic taking antiepileptic medication.
- Report bruising, yellowing of the skin or eyes, pale-colored feces, rash, pregnancy, vision changes.

▷ticarcillin disodium
*(tye kar **sill' in**)*

Ticar

PREGNANCY CATEGORY B

Drug classes
Antibiotic
Penicillin with extended spectrum

Therapeutic actions
Bactericidal: inhibits synthesis of cell wall of action-sensitive organisms, causing cell death.

Indications

- Severe infections caused by sensitive organisms, particularly *Pseudomonas aeruginosa, Proteus, E. coli*
- Infections caused by anaerobic bacteria
- GU infections caused by the above or *Enterobacter, Streptococcus faecalis*

Adverse effects in *Italics* are most common; those in **Bold** are life-threatening.

Contraindications and cautions

- Contraindicated with allergies to penicillins, cephalosporins, imipenem, or beta-lactamase inhibitors or other allergens.
- Use cautiously with renal disorders, pregnancy, lactation (may cause diarrhea or candidiasis in the infant).

Available forms

Powder for injection—1, 3, 6, 20, 30 g

Dosages

Maximum recommended dosage, 24 g/day. Maximum dose of single IM injection, 2 g.
Adults
- *UTIs:* 200–300 mg/kg/day IV in divided doses q 4–6 hr in severe cases.
- *Other infections:* 200–300 mg/kg/day IV in divided doses 3 g q 4 hr or 4 g q 6 hr.
Pediatric patients
- *UTIs (< 40 kg):* 50–100 mg/kg/day IM *or* direct IV in divided doses q 6–8 hr up to 150–200 mg/kg/day in divided doses q 4–6 hr IV.
- *Other infections (< 40 kg):* 200–300 mg/kg/day in divided doses q 4–6 hr IV.
Neonates
May be given IM or over 10–20 min IV.
< 2 kg, 0–7 days: 75 mg/kg q 12 hr initially; after 7 days old and < 2 kg, 75 mg/kg q 8 hr.
> 2 kg, 0–7 days: 75 mg/kg q 8 hr.
> 2 kg, > 7 days: 100 mg/kg q 8 hr.
Geriatric patients or patients with renal impairment
Patients on peritoneal dialysis should receive 3 g q 12 hr IV. Patients on hemodialysis should receive 2 g q 12 hr with 3 g after each dialysis. For patients with renal impairment, use an initial dose of 3 g IV followed by these doses:

Creatinine Clearance (mL/min)	Dosage
> 60	3 g q 4 hr IV
30–60	2 g q 4 hr IV
10–30	2 g q 8 hr IV
< 10	2 g q 12 hr IV or 1 g q 6 hr IM
< 10 with hepatic dysfunction	2 g daily or 1 g q 12 hr IM

Pharmacokinetics

Route	Onset	Peak
IM	Rapid	30–75 min
IV	Rapid	End of infusion

Metabolism: Hepatic; $T_{1/2}$: 0.8–1.4 hr
Distribution: Crosses placenta; enters breast milk
Excretion: Urine

▼IV facts
Preparation: Reconstitute each gram of ticarcillin for IV use with 4 mL of sodium chloride injection, 5% dextrose injection, or lactated Ringer's injection. Each 1 mL of solution will contain approximately 200 mg.
Date reconstituted solution. Reconstituted solution (10–50 mg/mL) is stable for 72 hr at room temperature if diluted with sodium chloride or 5% dextrose; 48 hr if diluted with lactated Ringer's; 14 days if refrigerated. Do not store for > 72 hr if for multidose purposes.
Infusion: Direct injection: administer as slowly as possible to avoid vein irritation—over 30 min preferred. Infusion should be run by continuous drip or intermittently from 30 min to 2 hr.
Incompatibilities: Do not mix with solution of gentamicin, tobramycin, amikacin.

Adverse effects
- **CNS:** Lethargy, hallucinations, seizures
- **GI:** *Glossitis, stomatitis, gastritis, sore mouth,* furry tongue, black "hairy" tongue, *nausea, vomiting, diarrhea,* abdominal pain, bloody diarrhea, enterocolitis, pseudomembranous colitis, nonspecific hepatitis
- **GU:** Nephritis—oliguria, proteinuria, hematuria, casts, azotemia, pyuria
- **Hematologic:** Anemia, thrombocytopenia, leukopenia, neutropenia, prolonged bleeding time, coagulation abnormalities
- **Hypersensitivity:** *Rash, fever, wheezing,* **anaphylaxis**
- **Local:** *Pain, phlebitis,* thrombosis at injection site
- **Other:** *Superinfections*—oral and rectal moniliasis, vaginitis, sodium overload

Interactions
✳ **Drug-drug** • Decreased effectiveness with tetracyclines • Inactivation of parenteral

aminoglycosides (amikacin, gentamicin, kanamycin, neomycin, metilmicin, streptomycin, tobramycin)

✳ **Drug-lab test** • False-positive Coombs' test with IV use

■ Nursing considerations
Assessment
- **History:** Allergies to penicillins, cephalosporins, other allergens; renal disorders; pregnancy; lactation
- **Physical:** Culture infection; skin color, lesion; R, adventitious sounds; bowel sounds; CBC, liver and renal function tests, serum electrolytes, Hct, urinalysis

Interventions
- Culture infection before beginning treatment; reculture if response is not as expected.
- Continue therapy for at least 2 days after signs of infection have disappeared, usually 7–10 days.
- Administer by IM or IV routes only.
- Reconstitute each gram for IM use with 2 mL sodium chloride injection, 5% dextrose injection, lactated Ringer's injection, or 1% lidocaine HCl without epinephrine. Each 2.6 mL will contain 1 g ticarcillin. Inject deep into a large muscle.
- Maintain epinephrine, IV fluids, vasopressors, bronchodilators, oxygen, and emergency equipment on standby in case of serious hypersensitivity reaction.

Teaching points
- This drug is given by injection.
- These side effects may occur: upset stomach, nausea, diarrhea (small, frequent meals may help); mouth sores (frequent mouth care may help); pain or discomfort at injection sites.
- Report difficulty breathing, rashes, severe diarrhea, severe pain at injection site, mouth sores.

▽ticlopidine hydrochloride
*(tye **klob'** pih deen)*

Ticlid

PREGNANCY CATEGORY B

Drug class
Antiplatelet agent

Therapeutic actions
Interferes with platelet membrane function by inhibiting fibrinogen binding and platelet-platelet interactions; inhibits platelet aggregation and prolongs bleeding time; effect is irreversible for life of the platelet.

Indications
- Reduces risk of thrombotic stroke in patients who have experienced stroke precursors and in patients who have had a completed thrombotic stroke; reserve use for patients who are intolerant to aspirin therapy because side effects may be life-threatening
- Unlabeled uses: intermittent claudication, chronic arterial occlusion, subarachnoid hemmorrhage, uremic patients with AV shunts or fistulas, open heart surgery, coronary artery bypass grafts, primary glomerulonephritis, sickle cell disease

Contraindications and cautions
- Contraindicated with allergy to ticlopidine, neutropenia, thrombocytopenia, hemostatic disorders, bleeding ulcer, intracranial bleeding, severe liver disease, lactation.
- Use cautiously with renal disorders, pregnancy, elevated cholesterol, recent trauma.

Available forms
Tablets—250 mg

Dosages
Adults
250 mg PO bid with food.
Pediatric patients
Safety and efficacy not established for patients < 18 yr.

Adverse effects in *Italics* are most common; those in **Bold** are life-threatening.

Pharmacokinetics

Route	Onset	Peak
Oral	Rapid	2 hr

Metabolism: Hepatic; $T_{1/2}$: 12.6 hr, then 4–5 days

Distribution: Crosses placenta; enters breast milk

Excretion: Urine and feces

Adverse effects

- **CNS:** Dizziness
- **GI:** *Diarrhea, nausea, vomiting, abdominal pain,* flatulence, dyspepsia, anorexia
- **Hematologic: Neutropenia, thrombotic thrombocytopenia,** bleeding
- **Local:** *Pain, phlebitis,* thrombosis at injection site
- **Other:** Rash, purpura

Interactions

✳ **Drug-drug** ● Decreased effectiveness of digoxin ● Increased serum levels and effects of theophylline, aspirin ● Increased effects with cimetidine ● Decreased absorption with antacids

✳ **Drug-food** ● Increased availability with food

■ Nursing considerations
Assessment

- **History:** Allergy to ticlopidine; neutropenia, thrombocytopenia; hemostatic disorders; bleeding ulcer, intracranial bleeding; severe liver disease; renal disorders; pregnancy, lactation, elevated cholesterol; recent trauma
- **Physical:** Skin color, lesions; orientation; bowel sounds, normal output; CBC, liver and renal function tests, serum cholesterol

Interventions

- Monitor WBC count before use and frequently while initiating therapy; if neutropenia is present or occurs, discontinue drug immediately.
- Administer with food or just after eating to minimize GI irritation and increase absorption.
- Maintain IV methylprednisolone (20 mg) on standby in case excessive bleeding occurs.

- Monitor patient for any sign of excessive bleeding (eg, bruises, dark stools), and monitor bleeding times.
- Provide increased precautions against bleeding during invasive procedures; bleeding will be prolonged.
- Mark patient's chart receiving drug to alert medical personnel of increased risk of bleeding in cases of surgery or dental surgery.

Teaching points

- Take drug with meals or just after eating.
- You will require regular blood tests to monitor your response to this drug.
- It may take longer than normal to stop bleeding; avoid contact sports, use electrical razors; apply pressure for extended periods to bleeding sites.
- These side effects may occur: upset stomach, nausea, diarrhea, loss of appetite (small, frequent meals may help).
- Notify dentist or surgeon that you are on this drug before invasive procedures.
- Report fever, chills, sore throat, rash, bruising, bleeding, dark stools or urine.

▽ **tiludronate disodium**

See *Less Commonly Used Drugs,* p. 1352.

▽ **timolol maleate**
(tye moe' lole)

Apo-Timol (CAN), Betimol, Blocadren, Novo-Timol, Timoptic, Timoptic-XE

PREGNANCY CATEGORY C

Drug classes
Beta-adrenergic blocker
Antihypertensive
Antiglaucoma agent

Therapeutic actions
Competitively blocks beta-adrenergic receptors in the heart and juxtaglomerular apparatus, decreasing the influence of the sympathetic nervous system on these tissues and decreasing the excitability of the heart, decreasing cardiac output and oxygen consumption, decreasing the release of renin, and

lowering BP; reduces intraocular pressure by decreasing the production of aqueous humor and possibly by increasing aqueous humor out-flow.

Indications
- Hypertension, used alone or in combination with other antihypertensives, especially thiazide-type diuretics
- Prevention of reinfarction in MI patients who are hemodynamically stable
- Prophylaxis of migraine
- Reduction of intraocular pressure in chronic open-angle glaucoma, some patients with secondary glaucoma, aphakic patients with glaucoma ocular HTN (ophthalmic solution)

Contraindications and cautions
- Contraindicated with sinus bradycardia (HR < 45 beats/min), second- or third-degree heart block (PR interval > 0.24 sec), cardiogenic shock, CHF, asthma, COPD, pregnancy, lactation.
- Use cautiously with diabetes or thyrotoxicosis (timolol can mask the usual cardiac signs of hypoglycemia and thyrotoxicosis).

Available forms
Tablets—5, 10, 20 mg; ophthalmic solution, gel—0.25%, 0.50%

Dosages
Adults
Oral
- *Hypertension:* Initially, 10 mg bid. Increase dosage at 1-wk intervals to a maximum of 60 mg/day divided into two doses, as necessary. Usual maintenance dose is 20–40 mg/day.
- *Prevention of reinfarction in MI (long-term prophylaxis in patients who survived the acute phase):* 10 mg bid PO.
- *Migraine:* 10 mg PO bid; during maintenance, the 20 mg/day may be given as a single dose. May be increased to a maximum of 30 mg/day in divided doses or decreased to 10 mg/day. Discontinue if satisfactory response is not obtained after 6–8 wk.

Ophthalmic
Initially 1 drop of 0.25% solution bid into the affected eye(s). Adjust dosage on basis of response to 1 drop of 0.5% solution bid or 1 drop of 0.25% solution daily. When replacing other agents, make change gradually and individualize dosage.
Pediatric patients
Safety and efficacy not established.

Pharmacokinetics

Route	Onset	Peak
Oral	Varies	1–2 hr
Ophthalmologic	Rapid	1–5 hr

Metabolism: Hepatic; $T_{1/2}$: 3–4 hr
Distribution: Crosses placenta; enters breast milk
Excretion: Urine

Adverse effects
Oral
- **Allergic reactions:** Pharyngitis, erythematous rash, fever, sore throat, laryngospasm, respiratory distress
- **CNS:** Dizziness, vertigo, tinnitus, fatigue, emotional depression, paresthesias, sleep disturbances, hallucinations, disorientation, memory loss, slurred speech
- **CV:** *CHF, cardiac arrhythmias, sinoatrial or AV nodal block,* peripheral vascular insufficiency, claudication, **CVA, pulmonary edema,** hypotension
- **Dermatologic:** Rash, pruritus, sweating, dry skin
- **EENT:** Eye irritation, dry eyes, conjunctivitis, blurred vision
- **GI:** *Gastric pain, flatulence, constipation, diarrhea, nausea, vomiting,* anorexia, ischemic colitis, renal and mesenteric arterial thrombosis, retroperitoneal fibrosis, hepatomegaly, acute pancreatitis
- **GU:** *Impotence, decreased libido,* Peyronie's disease, dysuria, nocturia, frequent urination
- **Musculoskeletal:** Joint pain, arthralgia, muscle cramp
- **Respiratory:** Bronchospasm, dyspnea, cough, bronchial obstruction, nasal stuffiness, rhinitis, pharyngitis (less likely than with propranolol)

Adverse effects in *Italics* are most common; those in **Bold** are life-threatening.

- **Other:** *Decreased exercise tolerance, development of antinuclear antibodies* (ANA), hyperglycemia or hypoglycemia, elevated serum transaminase

Ophthalmic
- **Local:** Ocular irritation, decreased corneal sensitivity, visual refractive changes, diplopia, ptosis

Interactions
✳ **Drug-drug** • Increased effects with verapamil • Increased risk of orthostatic hypotension with prazosin • Decreased antihypertensive effects with NSAIDs, clonidine • Decreased elimination of theophyllines with resultant decrease in expected actions of both drugs when taken concurrently • Peripheral ischemia and possible gangrene with ergotamine, methysergide, dihydroergotamine • Increased risk of hypoglycemia and masked signs of hypoglycemia with insulin • Hypertension followed by severe bradycardia with epinephrine • All of the above may occur with ophthalmic timolol; in addition, additive effects are possible with oral beta-blockers
✳ **Drug-lab test** • Possible false results with glucose or insulin tolerance tests (oral)

■ Nursing considerations
Assessment
- **History:** Sinus bradycardia, second- or third-degree heart block, cardiogenic shock, CHF, asthma, COPD, pregnancy, lactation, diabetes or thyrotoxicosis
- **Physical:** Weight, skin condition, neurologic status, P, BP, ECG, respiratory status, kidney and thyroid function, blood and urine glucose

Interventions
- Do not discontinue drug abruptly after long-term therapy (hypersensitivity to catecholamines may have developed, causing exacerbation of angina, MI, and ventricular arrhythmias). Taper drug gradually over 2 wk with monitoring.
- Consult with surgeon about withdrawal if patient is to undergo surgery (withdrawal is controversial).

Teaching points
- Do not stop taking this drug unless instructed to do so by a health care provider.

- Avoid driving or dangerous activities if CNS effects occur.
- Report difficulty breathing, night cough, swelling of extremities, slow pulse, confusion, depression, rash, fever, sore throat.
- Ophthalmic: Administer eye drops properly to minimize systemic absorption.

▽tinzaparin sodium
(ten zab' pear in)

Innohep

PREGNANCY CATEGORY B

Drug classes
Anticoagulant
Low-molecular-weight heparin

Therapeutic actions
Low-molecular-weight heparin that inhibits thrombus and clot formation by blocking factor Xa and factor IIa, preventing the formation of clots.

Indications
- Treatment of acute, symptomatic deep vein thrombosis with or without pulmonary emboli when given with warfarin sodium

Contraindications and cautions
- Contraindicated with hypersensitivity to any low-molecular-weight heparin, heparin, pork products; history of heparin-induced thrombocytopenia; uncontrolled bleeding.
- Use cautiously with pregnancy or lactation, history of GI bleed.

Available forms
Injection—20,000 IU/mL

Dosages
Adults
175 IU/kg/day SC given once daily for ≥ 6 days and until the patient has been successfully anticoagulated with warfarin (INR ≥ 2 for 2 consecutive days).
- *Treatment of overdose:* Protamine sulfate (1% solution). Each mg of protamine neutralizes 100 IU of tinzaparin. Give very slowly IV over 10 min.

Pediatric patients
Safety and efficacy not established.

Pharmacokinetics

Route	Onset	Peak	Duration
SC	2–3 hr	4–5 hr	12 hr

Metabolism: Cellular; $T_{1/2}$: 3–4 hr
Distribution: May cross placenta, may enter breast milk
Excretion: Urine

Adverse effects

- **Hematologic:** Hemorrhage; *bruising;* thrombocytopenia; elevated AST, ALT levels; hyperkalemia
- **Hypersensitivity:** Chills, fever, urticaria, asthma
- **Other:** Fever; pain; local irritation; hematoma; erythema at site of injection

Interactions

✳ Drug-drug • Increased bleeding tendencies with: oral anticoagulants, salicylates, penicillins, cephalosporins

✳ Drug-lab test • Increased AST, ALT levels

✳ Drug-alternative therapy • Increased risk of bleeding if combined with chamomile, garlic, ginger, ginkgo, and ginseng therapy

■ Nursing considerations
Assessment

- **History:** Recent surgery or injury; sensitivity to heparin, pork products, low-molecular-weight heparins; pregnancy, lactation; recent GI bleed
- **Physical:** Peripheral perfusion, R, stool guaiac test, partial thromboplastin time (PTT), INR or other tests of blood coagulation, platelet count, kidney function tests

Interventions

- Arrange to begin warfarin therapy within 1–3 days of starting tinzaparin.
- Give deep subcutaneous injections; do not give by IM or IV injection.
- Administer by deep SC injection; patient should be lying down; alternate administration between the left and right anterolateral and left and right posterolateral ab-

dominal wall. Introduce the whole length of the needle into a skin fold held between the thumb and forefinger; hold the skin fold throughout the injection.

- Apply pressure to all injection sites after needle is withdrawn; inspect injection sites for signs of hematoma.
- Do not massage injection sites.
- Do not mix with other injections or infusions.
- Store at room temperature; fluid should be clear, colorless to pale yellow.
- Provide for safety measures (electric razor, soft toothbrush) to prevent injury to patient who is at risk for bleeding.
- Check patient for signs of bleeding, monitor blood tests.
- Have protamine sulfate (tinzaparin antidote) on standby in case of overdose.

Teaching points

- Know that this drug must be given by a parenteral route (cannot be taken orally).
- Arrange for periodic blood tests that will be needed to monitor your response to this drug.
- Be careful to avoid injury while you are on this drug: use an electric razor, avoid activities that might lead to injury.
- Report nose bleed, bleeding of the gums, unusual bruising, black or tarry stools, cloudy or dark urine, abdominal or lower back pain, severe headache.

▷ tiopronin

See *Less Commonly Used Drugs,* p. 1352.

▷ tirofiban
*(tye row **feye' **ban)*

Aggrastat

PREGNANCY CATEGORY B

Drug class
Antiplatelet drug

Therapeutic actions
Inhibits platelet aggregation by binding to the platelet receptor glycoprotein, which prevents

the binding of fibrinogen and other adhesive ligands to the platelet.

Indications

- Treatment of acute coronary syndrome in combination with heparin
- Prevention of cardiac ischemic complications in patients undergoing elective, emergency, or urgent percutaneous coronary intervention

Contraindications and cautions

- Contraindicated with allergy to any component of this product, bleeding diasthesis, hemorrhagic stroke, active or abnormal bleeding or stroke within 30 days, uncontrolled or severe hypertension, major surgery within 6 wk, dialysis, low platelet count, aortic aneurysm, aortic dissection.
- Use cautiously with pregnancy, lactation, renal insufficiency, the elderly, platelet count < 150,000/mm^3.

Available forms

Injection concentrate—250 mcg/mL; injection—50 mcg/mL

Dosages

Adults

0.4 mcg/kg/min IV infusion over 30 min, then continue at rate of 0.1 mcg/kg/min.

Pediatric patients

Not recommended.

Patients with renal impairment

Use one-half the recommended adult dosage and monitor patient closely.

Pharmacokinetics

Route	Onset	Peak	Duration
IV	15 min	30 min	4–8 hr

Metabolism: Tissue; $T_{1/2}$: 2 hr
Distribution: Crosses placenta; may pass into breast milk
Excretion: Urine

▼IV facts

Preparation: Withdraw and discard 100 mL from a 500-mL bag of sterile 0.9% sodium chloride or 5% dextrose in water; replace this volume with 100 mL tirofiban injection (two- 50 mL vials) or remove 50 mL from 250-mL bag of sterile 0.9% sodium chloride or 5% dex-trose in water; replace this volume with 50 mL tirofiban injection, this will provide a concentration of 50 mcg/mL, mix well prior to administration. Protect from light; discard any remaining solution 24 hr after beginning of infusion. Premixed tirofiban is available in *IntraVia* containers at a concentration of 590 mcg/mL. To open, tear off dust cover; squeeze bag to ensure that no leaks occur— if fluid leaks out, discard solution as sterility has been compromised.
Infusion: Infuse loading dose over 30 min; continue infusion at rate of 0.1 mcg/kg/min.
Incompatibilities: Do not mix in solution with diazepam. May be given in same IV line as heparin, dopamine, lidocaine, potassium chloride, and famotidine.

Adverse effects

- **CNS:** *Dizziness*, weakness, syncope, flushing
- **CV:** Bradycardia
- **GI:** Nausea, GI distress, constipation, diarrhea
- **Other:** *Bleeding, hypotension,* edema, pain

Interactions

✳ Drug-drug • Increased risk of bleeding when combined with aspirin, heparin; monitor patient closely
✳ Drug-alternative therapy • Increased risk of bleeding if combined with chamomile, garlic, ginger, ginkgo and ginseng, turmeric, horse chestnut seed, green tea leaf, grape seed extract, feverfew, don qai; monitor patient closely

■ Nursing considerations

 CLINICAL ALERT!
Name confusion has been reported with Aggrastat (tirofiban) and argatroban. Use extreme caution.

Assessment

- **History:** Allergy to any component of this product, bleeding diasthesis, hemorrhagic stroke, active, abnormal bleeding or stroke within 30 days, uncontrolled or severe hypertension, major surgery within 6 wk, dialysis, low platelet count, aortic aneurysm, aortic dissection, pregnancy, lactation, renal dysfunction

• **Physical:** Skin color, temperature, lesions; orientation, reflexes, affect; P, BP, orthostatic BP, baseline ECG, peripheral perfusion; respiratory rate, adventitious sounds, aPTT, PT, active clotting time

Interventions

• Use tirofiban in conjunction with heparin.
• Minimize arterial and venous punctures, IM injections, catheterizations, intubations while using this drug to minimize blood loss.
• Avoid the use of noncompressible IV access sites to prevent excessive, uncontrollable bleeding.
• Do baseline and periodic CBC, PT, aPTT, and active clotting time. Maintain aPTT between 50–70 sec; and active bleeding time between 300–350 seconds.
• Properly care for femoral access site to minimize bleeding. Document aPTT of < 45 seconds and stop heparin for 3–4 hr before pulling sheath.

Teaching points

• This drug is given to minimize blood clotting and cardiac damage. It must be given IV.
• Know that you will be monitored closely and periodic blood tests will be done to monitor the effects of this drug on your body.
• These side effects may occur: dizziness, light-headedness, bleeding.
• Report light-headedness, palpitations, pain at IV site, bleeding.

▽ **tizanidine**

(tis an' i deen)

Zanaflex

PREGNANCY CATEGORY C

Drug classes

Antispasmodic
Sympatholytic, centrally acting

Therapeutic actions

Centrally acting alpha$_2$-agonist; antispasmodic effect thought to be a result of indirect depression of polysynaptic reflexes by blocking the excitatory actions of spinal interneurons.

Indications

• Acute and intermittent management of spasticity caused by MS, spinal cord injury, cerebral trauma

Contraindications and cautions

• Contraindicated with hypersensitivity to tizanidine, clonidine.
• Use cautiously with hepatic or renal impairment, hypotension, pregnancy, lactation.

Available forms

Tablets—2, 4 mg

Dosages

Adults
8 mg PO initial dose; repeat as needed q 6–8 hr; maximum dose 36 mg/day.
Pediatric patients
Safety and efficacy not established.
Patients with renal impairment
Use lower doses, monitor response.

Pharmacokinetics

Route	Onset	Peak	Duration
Oral	30–60 min	1–2 min	3–4 hr

Metabolism: Heptic; $T_{1/2}$: 2.7–4.2 hr
Distribution: Crosses placenta; may pass into breast milk
Excretion: Urine

Adverse effects

• **CNS:** *Drowsiness, sedation, dizziness, asthenia,* headache, hallucinations
• **CV:** *Hypotension, orthostatic hypotension,* bradycardia
• **GI:** *Dry mouth, constipation,* anorexia, malaise, nausea, vomiting, parotid pain, parotitis, mild transient abnormalities in liver function tests

Interactions

✳ **Drug-drug** • Potential risk of increased depression with alcohol, baclofen, other CNS depressants • Possible increased effects with

---

Adverse effects in *Italics* are most common; those in **Bold** are life-threatening.

hormonal contraceptives; monitor patient and decrease tizanidine dose

■ Nursing considerations
Assessment
- **History:** Hypersensitivity to tizanidine, clonidine; hepatic or renal impairment, hypotension; pregnancy, lactation
- **Physical:** Mucous membranes—color, lesions; orientation, affect; P, BP, orthostatic BP; perfusion; liver evaluation; liver and renal function tests

Interventions
- Administer drug q 6–8 hr around the clock for best effects.
- Adjust drug dosage slowly, which helps to decrease side effects.
- Continue all supportive measures used for spinal cord–injured or neurologically damaged patients.
- Provide sugarless lozenges or ice chips, as appropriate, if dry mouth or altered taste occurs.
- Establish safety precautions if CNS, hypotensive changes occur (side rails, accompany patient when ambulating, etc).
- Attempt to lower dose if side effects become severe or intolerable.

Teaching points
- Take this drug exactly as prescribed. It is important that you not miss doses. Consult your health care provider to determine a schedule that will not interfere with rest.
- Continue all other supportive measures used for your condition.
- These side effects may occur: drowsiness, dizziness, light-headedness, headache, weakness (use caution while driving or performing tasks that require alertness or physical dexterity); dry mouth (suck on sugarless lozenges or ice chips); GI upset (eat small, frequent meals); dizziness, light-headedness when changing position (rise slowly, use caution when transferring).
- Report changes in urine or stool, severe dizziness or passing out, changes in vision, difficulty swallowing.

▽tobramycin sulfate
(toe bra mye' sin)

Parenteral: Nebcin, Nebcin Pediatric
Nebulizer solution: TOBI
Ophthalmic: Tobrex Ophthalmic

PREGNANCY CATEGORY B

Drug class
Aminoglycoside antibiotic

Therapeutic actions
Bactericidal: inhibits protein synthesis in susceptible strains of gram-negative bacteria; mechanism of lethal action is not fully understood, but functional integrity of bacterial cell membrane appears to be disrupted.

Indications
- Serious infections caused by susceptible strains of *P. aeruginosa, E. coli, Proteus* species, *Providencia* species, *Klebsiella-Enterobacter-Serratia* group, *Citrobacter* species, and staphylococci (including *S. aureus*; parenteral)
- Staphylococcal infections when penicillin is contraindicated or when the bacteria are not susceptible
- Serious, life-threatening gram-negative infections when susceptibility studies have not been completed (sometimes concurrent penicillin or cephalosporin therapy)
- Management of cystic fibrosis patients with *P. aeruginosa* (nebulizer solution)
- Treatment of superficial ocular infections due to susceptible strains of organisms (ophthalmic)

Contraindications and cautions
- Contraindicated with allergy to aminoglycosides; pregnancy, lactation.
- Use cautiously with elderly or patients with diminished hearing, decreased renal function, dehydration, neuromuscular disorders (myasthenia gravis, parkinsonism, infant botulism); herpes, vaccinia, varicella, mycobacterial infections, fungal infections (ophthalmic solutions).

Available forms

Injection—10, 40 mg/mL; powder for injection—1.2 g, nebulizer solution—300 mg/5 mL; ophthalmic solution—0.3%; ophthalmic ointment—3 mg/g

Dosages
IM or IV
Adults

3 mg/kg/day in 3 equal doses q 8 hr. Up to 5 mg/kg/day in 3–4 equal doses can be used in life-threatening infections, but reduce to 3 mg/kg/day as soon as possible. Do not exceed 5 mg/kg/day unless serum levels are monitored.

Pediatric patients

6–7.5 mg/kg/day divided into 3–4 equal doses q 6–8 hr.

Premature infants or neonates ≤ 1 wk

Up to 4 mg/kg/day in 2 equal doses q 12 hr.

Geriatric patients or patients with renal failure

Reduce dosage, and carefully monitor serum drug levels and renal function tests throughout treatment. Reduced dosage nomogram is available; consult manufacturer's information.

Nebulizer solution

300 mg bid for adults and children ≥ 6 yr. Administer in 28-day cycles: 28 days on, 28 days of rest. Inhale over 10–15 min.

Ophthalmic solution

300 mg bid for adults and children ≥ 6 yr. Administer in 28-day cycles: 28 days on, 28 days of rest. Inhale over 10–15 min.

- *Mild to moderate disease:* 1–2 drops into conjunctival sac of affected eye(s) q 4 hr.
- *Severe disease:* 2 drops into conjunctival sac of affected eye(s) hourly until improvement occurs.

Ophthalmic ointment

One-half-inch ribbon bid–tid. Severe infection: one-half inch q 3–4 hr.

Pharmacokinetics

Route	Onset	Peak
IM, IV	Rapid	30–90 min
Ophthalmologic	Rapid	

Metabolism: Minimal hepatic; $T_{1/2}$: 2–3 hr
Distribution: Crosses placenta; enters breast milk
Excretion: Urine

▽▼ IV facts

Preparation: Dilute vials of solution for injection. Usual volume of diluent is 50–100 mL of 9% sodium chloride injection or 5% dextrose injection (less for children). Reconstitute powder for injection with sterile water for injection according to manufacturer's instructions.
Infusion: Infuse over 20–60 min.
Incompatibilities: Do not premix with other drugs; administer other drugs separately.

Adverse effects

- **CNS:** Ototoxicity, vestibular paralysis, confusion, disorientation, depression, lethargy, nystagmus, visual disturbances, headache, *numbness, tingling,* tremor, paresthesias, muscle twitching, convulsions, muscular weakness, neuromuscular blockade
- **CV:** Palpitations, hypotension, hypertension
- **EENT:** Localized ocular toxicity and hypersensitivity reactions; *lid itching, swelling;* conjunctival erythema; punctate keratitis
- **GI:** Hepatic toxicity, *nausea, vomiting, anorexia,* weight loss, stomatitis, increased salivation
- **GU:** *Nephrotoxicity*
- **Hematologic:** *Leukemoid reaction,* agranulocytosis, granulocytosis, leukopenia, leukocytosis, thrombocytopenia, eosinophilia, pancytopenia, anemia, hemolytic anemia, increased or decreased reticulocyte count, electrolyte disturbances
- **Hypersensitivity:** *Purpura, rash,* urticaria, exfoliative dermatitis, itching
- **Local:** *Pain, irritation, arachnoiditis at IM injection sites*
- **Other:** Fever, apnea, splenomegaly, joint pain, *superinfections*

Interactions

✳ **Drug-drug •** Increased ototoxic, nephrotoxic, neurotoxic effects with other aminoglycosides, cephalothin, potent diuretics • Increased neuromuscular blockade and muscular paralysis with anesthetics, nondepolarizing

---

*Adverse effects in Italics are most common; those in **Bold** are life-threatening.*

neuromuscular blocking drugs, succinylcholine • Potential inactivation of both drugs if mixed with beta-lactam-type antibiotics • Increased bactericidal effect with penicillins, cephalopsorins, carbenicillin, ticarcillin

■ Nursing considerations

Assessment

- **History:** Allergy to aminoglycosides; diminished hearing, decreased renal function, dehydration, neuromuscular disorders, lactation, pregnancy; infections (ophthalmic solutions)
- **Physical:** Weight; renal function, eighth cranial nerve function; state of hydration; hepatic function, CBC; skin color and lesions; orientation and affect; reflexes; bilateral grip strength; bowel sounds

Interventions

- Arrange culture and sensitivity tests of infection before beginning therapy.
- Limit duration of treatment to short term to reduce the risk of toxicity; usual duration of treatment is 7–14 days.
- Use ophthalmologic tobramycin only when indicated by sensitivity tests; use of opthalmologic tobramycin may cause sensitization that will contraindicate the systemic use of tobramycin or other aminoglycosides in serious infections.
- Monitor total serum concentration of tobramycin if ophthalmologic solution is used concurrently with parenteral aminoglycosides.
- Administer IM dose by deep IM injection.
- Administer nebulizer solution for 28 days—then 28 days of rest; have patient in upright position, inhale over 10–15 min.
- Ensure that patient is well hydrated before and during therapy.

Teaching points

Parenteral

- Report hearing changes, dizziness, pain at injection site.

Ophthalmic solution

- Tilt head back; place medication into conjunctival sac, and close eye; apply light finger pressure on lacrimal sac for 1 min.
- Solution may cause blurring of vision or stinging on administration.
- Report severe stinging, itching, or burning.

Nebulizer solution

- Inhale over 10–15 min while in an upright position.
- Mark calendar with 28 drug days followed by 28 nondrug days.
- Store drug in refrigerator; do not expose to intense light.

▷tocainide hydrochloride
(toe kay' nide)

Tonocard

PREGNANCY CATEGORY C

Drug class

Antiarrhythmic

Therapeutic actions

Type 1B antiarrhythmic: decreases the excitability of myocardial cells by a dose-dependent decrease in Na^+ and K^+ conductance.

Indications

- Treatment of life-threatening ventricular arrhythmias
- Unlabeled uses: treatment of myotonic dystrophy, trigeminal neuralgia

Contraindications and cautions

- Contraindicated with allergy to tocainide or amide-type local anesthetics, cardiac conduction abnormalities (heart block in the absence of an artificial ventricular pacemaker), pregnancy (abortions and stillbirths have occurred), lactation.
- Use cautiously with CHF, atrial fibrillation or atrial flutter, renal or hepatic disease, potassium imbalance, bone marrow failure, cytopenia.

Available forms

Tablets—400, 600 mg

Dosages

Careful patient assessment and evaluation with close monitoring of cardiac response are necessary for determining the correct dosage for each patient.

T

Adults
400 mg PO q 8 hr. 1,200–1,800 mg/day in 3 divided doses is the suggested therapeutic range.
Pediatric patients
Safety and efficacy not established.
Geriatric patients or patients with renal/hepatic impairment
Lower doses required; < 1,200 mg/day may suffice.

Pharmacokinetics

Route	Onset	Peak
Oral	Varies	30–120 min

Metabolism: Hepatic; $T_{1/2}$: 15 hr
Distribution: Crosses placenta; enters breast milk
Excretion: Urine

Adverse effects
- **CNS:** *Light-headedness, dizziness,* fatigue, drowsiness, disorientation, hallucinations, *numbness, paresthesias,* visual disturbances, *tremor*
- **CV:** CHF, cardiac arrhythmias
- **Dermatologic:** Sweating, hot flashes, night sweats
- **GI:** *Nausea,* vomiting, abdominal pain, diarrhea
- **Hematologic:** Leukopenia, agranulocytosis, hypoplastic anemia, thrombocytopenia
- **Respiratory:** Pulmonary fibrosis, **pneumonitis**

Interactions
✳ **Drug-drug** • Decreased pharmacologic effects with rifampin

■ Nursing considerations
Assessment
- **History:** Allergy to tocainide or amide-type local anesthetics, CHF, cardiac conduction abnormalities, atrial fibrillation or atrial flutter, hepatic or renal disease, potassium imbalance, pregnancy, lactation
- **Physical:** Weight; orientation, reflexes; P, BP, auscultation; ECG, edema; R, adventitious sounds; bowel sounds, liver evaluation; urinalysis, CBC, serum electrolytes, renal and liver function tests

Interventions
- Ensure that patient is not pregnant before administering tocainide; stillbirths and abortions have been reported.
- Carefully monitor patient response, especially when beginning therapy.
- Reduce dosage in patients with renal or hepatic disease.
- Check serum K^+ levels before administration.
- Carefully monitor cardiac rhythm.
- Arrange for regular follow-up of blood counts.
- Evaluate for safe and effective serum levels (4–10 mcg/mL).

Teaching points
- You will require frequent monitoring of cardiac rhythm.
- These side effects may occur: drowsiness, dizziness, numbness (avoid driving or working with dangerous machinery); nausea, vomiting, diarrhea (small, frequent meals may help); sweating, night sweats, hot flashes.
- Do not stop taking this drug for any reason without checking with your health care provider.
- This drug cannot be used during pregnancy; use of barrier contraceptives is advised.
- Have regular follow-up visits to check heart rhythm and blood cell counts.
- Report cough, wheezing, difficulty breathing, unusual bleeding or bruising, fever, chills, sore throat, tremors, visual changes, palpitations.

▽tolazamide
(tole az' a mide)

Tolinase

PREGNANCY CATEGORY C

Drug classes
Antidiabetic agent
Sulfonylurea, first generation

Adverse effects in *Italics* are most common; those in **Bold** are life-threatening.

Therapeutic actions
Stimulates insulin release from functioning beta cells in the pancreas; may improve binding between insulin and insulin receptors or increase the number of insulin receptors; has significant uricosuric activity.

Indications
- Adjunct to diet and exercise to lower blood glucose in patients with non–insulin-dependent diabetes mellitus (type 2)
- Adjunct to insulin therapy in the stabilization of certain cases of insulin-dependent maturity-onset diabetes, reducing the insulin requirement and decreasing the chance of hypoglycemic reactions

Contraindications and cautions
- Contraindicated with allergy to sulfonylureas; diabetes complicated by fever, severe infections, severe trauma, major surgery, ketosis, acidosis, coma (insulin is indicated in these conditions); type 1 or juvenile diabetes; serious hepatic or renal impairment; pregnancy.
- Use cautiously with uremia, thyroid or endocrine impairment, glycosuria, hyperglycemia associated with primary renal disease, lactation.

Available forms
Tablets—100, 250, 500 mg

Dosages
Adults
100 mg/day PO if fasting blood sugar (FBS) is < 200 mg/dL, or 250 mg/day if FBS is > 200 mg/dL. Adjust dose accordingly. If dose is larger than 500 mg/day, give in divided doses bid. Dosage greater than 1 g/day not recommended.
Pediatric patients
Safety and efficacy not established.
Geriatric patients
Geriatric patients tend to be more sensitive to the drug. Start with a lower initial dose, generally 100 mg/day; monitor for 24 hr, and gradually increase dose as needed.

Pharmacokinetics

Route	Onset	Peak	Duration
Oral	Varies	4–6 hr	12–24 hr

Metabolism: Hepatic; T₁/₂.
Distribution: Crosses placenta, milk
Excretion: Urine

Adverse effects
- **Dermatologic:** Allergic skin reaction, eczema, pruritus, erythema, urticaria, photosensitivity
- **GI:** *Anorexia, nausea, vomiting, epigastric discomfort, heartburn*
- **Hematologic:** *Hypoglycemia,* leukopenia, thrombocytopenia, anemia
- **Hypersensitivity:** Fever, eosinophilia, jaundice
- **Other: Increased risk of CV mortality** (potential)

Interactions
✷ **Drug-drug** • Increased risk of hypoglycemia with insulin, sulfonamides, chloramphenicol, oxyphenbutazone, phenylbutazone, salicylates, clofibrate, monoamine oxidase inhibitors • Decreased effectiveness of both tolazamide and diazoxide if taken concurrently • Increased risk of hyperglycemia with thiazides, other diuretics • Risk of hypoglycemia and hyperglycemia with ethanol; "disulfiram reaction" also has been reported
✷ **Drug-alternative therapy** • Increased risk of hypoglycemia if taken with juniper berries, ginseng, garlic, fenugreek, coriander, dandelion root, celery

■ Nursing considerations
Assessment
- **History:** Allergy to sulfonylureas; diabetes complicated by fever, severe infections, severe trauma, major surgery, ketosis, acidosis, coma; type 1 or juvenile diabetes; serious hepatic or renal impairment; uremia; thyroid or endocrine impairment; glycosuria; hyperglycemia associated with primary renal disease; pregnancy; lactation
- **Physical:** Skin color, lesions; T; orientation, reflexes, peripheral sensation; R, adventitious sounds; liver evaluation, bowel sounds; urinalysis, BUN, serum creatinine, liver function tests, blood glucose, CBC

Interventions
- Administer drug in the morning before breakfast. If severe GI upset occurs or if

dosage is > 500 g/day, dose may be divided with one dose before breakfast and one before the evening meal.
- Monitor urine or serum glucose levels frequently to determine effectiveness of drug and dosage.
- Transfer to insulin therapy during periods of high stress, infections, surgery, trauma, and so forth.
- Use IV glucose if severe hypoglycemia occurs due to overdose.

Teaching points
- Do not discontinue this medication without consulting health care provider.
- Monitor urine or blood for glucose and ketones as prescribed.
- This drug is not to be used during pregnancy.
- Avoid alcohol while on this drug.
- Report fever, sore throat, unusual bleeding or bruising, rash, dark urine, light-colored stools, hypoglycemic or hyperglycemic reactions.

▷tolazoline hydrochloride

See *Less Commonly Used Drugs,* p. 1352.

▷tolbutamide
(tole byoo' ta mide)

Apo-Tolbutamide (CAN), Novo-Butamide (CAN), Orinase, Orinase Diagnostic

PREGNANCY CATEGORY C

Drug classes
Antidiabetic agent
Sulfonylurea, first generation
Diagnostic agent

Therapeutic actions
Stimulates insulin release from functioning beta cells in the pancreas; may improve binding between insulin and insulin receptors or increase the number of insulin receptors.

Indications
- Adjunct to diet and exercise to lower blood glucose in patients with non–insulin-dependent diabetes mellitus (type 2)
- Adjunct to insulin therapy in the stabilization of certain cases of insulin-dependent type 1 diabetes, reducing the insulin requirement and decreasing the chance of hypoglycemic reactions
- Aid in the diagnosis of pancreatic islet cell adenoma (powder for injection)

Contraindications and cautions
- Contraindicated with allergy to sulfonylureas; diabetes complicated by fever, severe infections, severe trauma, major surgery, ketosis, acidosis, coma (insulin is indicated in these conditions); type 1 or juvenile diabetes; serious hepatic or renal impairment; uremia; thyroid or endocrine impairment; glycosuria; hyperglycemia associated with primary renal disease, pregnancy, lactation.

Available forms
Tablets—500 mg; powder for injection—1 g/vial

Dosages
Adults
Initial dose: 1–2 g/day. Maintenance dosage: 0.25–3 g/day PO in single morning or divided doses. Doses > 2 g/day are seldom required.
- *Diagnostic use:* 20 ml IV over 2–3 min.
Pediatric patients
Safety and efficacy not established.
Geriatric patients
Geriatric patients tend to be more sensitive to the drug. Start with a lower initial dose, monitor for 24 hr, and gradually increase dose as needed.

Pharmacokinetics

Route	Onset	Peak	Duration
Oral	1 hr	4–6 hr	6–12 hr

Metabolism: Hepatic; $T_{1/2}$: 7 hr
Distribution: Crosses placenta; enters breast milk
Excretion: Urine

Adverse effects

- **Dermatologic:** Allergic skin reactions, eczema, pruritus, erythema, urticaria, photosensitivity
- **GI:** *Anorexia, nausea, vomiting, epigastric discomfort, heartburn*
- **Hematologic:** *Hypoglycemia,* leukopenia, thrombocytopenia, anemia
- **Hypersensitivity:** Fever, eosinophilia, jaundice
- **Other: Increased risk of CV mortality**

Interactions

✳ Drug-drug • Increased risk of hypoglycemia with insulin, sulfonamides, chloramphenicol, fenfluramine, oxyphenbutazone, phenylbutazone, salicylates, clofibrate, MAOIs, dicumarol, rifampin • Decreased effectiveness of both tolbutamide and diazoxide if taken concurrently • Increased risk of hyperglycemia with thiazides, other diuretics • Risk of hypoglycemia and hyperglycemia with ethanol
✳ Drug-lab test • False-positive reaction for urine albumin if measured with acidification-after-boiling-test; no interference has been reported using sulfosalicylic acid test
✳ Drug-alternative therapy • Increased risk of hypoglycemia if taken with juniper berries, ginseng, garlic, fenugreek, coriander, dandelion root, celery

■ Nursing considerations
Assessment

- **History:** Allergy to sulfonylureas; diabetes complicated by fever, severe infections, severe trauma, major surgery, ketosis, acidosis, coma; type 1 or juvenile diabetes; serious hepatic or renal impairment, uremia; thyroid or endocrine impairment; glycosuria, hyperglycemia associated with primary renal disease; pregnancy; lactation
- **Physical:** Skin color, lesions; T; orientation, reflexes, peripheral sensation; R, adventitious sounds; liver evaluation, bowel sounds; urinalysis, BUN, serum creatinine, liver function tests, blood glucose, CBC

Interventions

- Administer drug in the morning before breakfast; if severe GI upset occurs, divide dose.

- Monitor urine or serum g[...] quently to determine effectiv[...] and dosage.
- Transfer patients from one oral hypo[...] agent to another with no transitiona[...] od or priming dose.
- Transfer to insulin therapy during perio[...] of high stress (eg, infections, surgery, trauma).
- Use IV glucose if severe hypoglycemia occurs due to overdose.

Teaching points

- Take this drug early in the morning before breakfast. If GI upset occurs, drug may be taken with food or in divided doses. Do not discontinue this medication without consulting your health care provider.
- These side effects may occur: nausea, GI upset, vomiting (take drug with food); diarrhea; rash, delays in healing (use good skin care; avoid injury).
- This drug is not to be used during pregnancy. If you become pregnant or want to become pregnant, consult your prescriber.
- Avoid alcohol while on this drug; serious reactions can occur.
- Report fever, sore throat, unusual bleeding or bruising, rash, dark urine, light-colored stools, hypoglycemic or hyperglycemic reactions.

▷**tolcapone**
*(toll **kap**' own)*

Tasmar

PREGNANCY CATEGORY C

T

Drug class
Antiparkinsonian agent

Therapeutic actions
Selectively and reversibly inhibits COMT, an enzyme that eliminates biologically active catecholamines including dopa, dopamine, norepinephrine, epinephrine; when given with levodopa, tolcapone's inhibition of COMT is believed to increase the plasma concentrations and duration of action of levodopa.

dications

Adjunct with levodopa and carbidopa in the treatment of the signs and symptoms of idiopathic Parkinson's disease

Contraindications and cautions

- Contraindicated with hypersensitivity to drug or its components, pregnancy, lactation, liver disease, patients with a history of nontraumatic rhabdomyolysis or hyperpyrexia and confusion.
- Use cautiously with hypertension, hypotension, or renal dysfunction.

Available forms

Tablets—100, 200 mg

Dosages
Adults
Initial dosage: 100 or 200 mg PO tid. Maximum daily dose: 600 mg.
Pediatric patients
Safety and efficacy not established.
Patients with hepatic impairment
Patients with moderate to severe hepatic dysfunction should not exceed 100 mg PO tid; patients with liver enzyme values > 4 times normal should not receive this drug.
Patients with renal impairment
Use caution.

Pharmacokinetics

Route	Onset	Peak
Oral	Varies	2 hr

Metabolism: Hepatic; T$_{1/2}$: 2–3 hr
Distribution: Crosses placenta; passes into breast milk
Excretion: Urine and feces

Adverse effects

- **CNS:** *Disorientation, confusion,* memory loss, *hallucinations,* psychoses, agitation, nervousness, delusions, delirium, paranoia, euphoria, excitement, *light-headedness, dizziness,* depression, drowsiness, weakness, giddiness, paresthesia, heaviness of the limbs, numbness of fingers
- **CV:** Hypotension, orthostatic hypotension
- **Dermatologic:** Rash, urticaria, other dermatoses
- **GI:** Acute suppurative parotitis, *nausea, vomiting,* epigastric distress, flatulence, **fulminant and possibly fatal liver failure**
- **Respiratory:** URIs, dyspnea, sinus congestion
- **Other:** Muscular weakness, muscular cramping

■ Nursing considerations
Assessment

- **History:** Hypersensitivity to drug or its components; hypertension, hypotension; hepatic or renal dysfunction; pregnancy, lactation
- **Physical:** Body weight; T; skin color, lesions; orientation, affect, reflexes, bilateral grip strength, visual exam; P, BP, orthostatic BP, auscultation; bowel sounds, normal output, liver evaluation; urinary output, voiding pattern, liver and kidney function tests

Interventions

- Administer in conjunction with levodopa and carbidopa. Monitor patient response; customary levodopa dosage may need to be decreased.
- Monitor liver enzymes prior to and every 2 wk during therapy; discontinue drug at any sign of liver failure.
- Provide sugarless lozenges, ice chips to suck if dry mouth is a problem.
- Give with meals if GI upset occurs; give before meals to patients bothered by dry mouth; give after meals if drooling is a problem or if drug causes nausea.
- Avoid abrupt withdrawal of drug, can lead to more serious complications. Taper drug slowly over 2 wk if possible.
- Advise patient to use barrier contraceptives, serious birth defects can occur while using this drug; advise nursing mothers to use another means of feeding the baby as drug can enter breast milk and adversely affect the infant.
- Establish safety precautions if CNS, vision changes, hallucinations, hypotension occur (use siderails, accompany patient when ambulating, etc).
- Provide additional comfort measures appropriate to patient with parkinsonism.

Adverse effects in *Italics* are most common; those in **Bold** are life-threatening.

Teaching points

- Take this drug exactly as prescribed. Take in conjuction with your levodopa and carbidopa.
- These side effects may occur: drowsiness, dizziness, confusion, blurred vision (avoid driving a car or engaging in activities that require alertness and visual acuity if these occur; rise slowly when changing positions to help decrease dizziness); nausea (frequent small meals may help); dry mouth (sucking sugarless lozenges or ice ice chips may help); hallucinations (it may help to know that this is a side effect of the drug; use care and have someone stay with you if this occurs); constipation (if maintaining adequate fluid intake and exercising regularly do not help, consult your nurse or physician).
- Use barrier contraceptives while on this drug, serious birth defects can occur. Do not nurse while on this drug, the drug passes into breast milk and can adversely affect the baby.
- Report constipation, rapid or pounding heartbeat, confusion, eye pain, hallucinations, rash; changes in color of urine or stools; fever, chills, fatigue; yellowing of skin or eyes.

▷tolmetin sodium
(tole' met in)

Novo-Tolmetin (CAN), Tolectin 200, Tolectin 600, Tolectin DS

PREGNANCY CATEGORY C

Drug class
Nonsteroidal anti-inflammatory drug (NSAID)

Therapeutic actions
Anti-inflammatory, analgesic, and antipyretic activities largely related to inhibition or prostaglandin synthesis; exact mechanisms of action are not known.

Indications
- Treatment of acute flares and long-term management of rheumatoid arthritis and osteoarthritis
- Treatment of juvenile rheumatoid arthritis

Contraindications and cautions
- Contraindicated with pregnancy, lactation.
- Use cautiously with allergies, renal, hepatic, CV and GI conditions, coagulation defects, patients taking anticoagulants.

Available forms
Tablets—200, 600 mg; capsules—400 mg

Dosages
Adults
Do not exceed 2,000 mg/day (rheumatoid arthritis) or 1,600 mg/day (osteoarthritis).
- *Rheumatoid arthritis or osteoarthritis:* Initial dose, 400 mg PO tid (1,200 mg/day) preferably including dose on arising and hs. Maintenance dose, 600–1,800 mg/day in 3–4 divided doses for rheumatoid arthritis, 600–1,600 mg/day in 3–4 divided doses for osteoarthritis.

Pediatric patients ≥ 2 yr
Initially, 20 mg/kg/day PO in 3–4 divided doses; when control has been achieved, the usual dose is 15–30 mg/kg/day. Do not exceed 30 mg/kg/day.

Pharmacokinetics

Route	Onset	Peak
Oral	Varies	30–60 min

Metabolism: Hepatic; $T_{1/2}$: 2–7 hr
Distribution: Crosses placenta; enters breast milk
Excretion: Urine

Adverse effects
- **CNS:** *Headache, dizziness, somnolence, insomnia,* fatigue, tiredness, dizziness, tinnitus, ophthalmologic effects
- **Dermatologic:** *Rash,* pruritus, sweating, dry mucous membranes, stomatitis
- **GI:** *Nausea, dyspepsia, GI pain, diarrhea,* vomiting, constipation, flatulence
- **GU:** Dysuria, renal impairment, including renal failure, interstitial nephritis, hematuria
- **Hematologic:** Bleeding, platelet inhibition with higher doses, neutropenia, eosinophilia, leukopenia, pancytopenia, thrombocytopenia, agranulocytosis, granulocytopenia, aplastic anemia, decreased Hgb or Hct, bone marrow depression, menorrhagia

T.

- **Respiratory:** Dyspnea, hemoptysis, pharyngitis, bronchospasm, rhinitis
- **Other:** Peripheral edema, **anaphylactoid reactions to fatal anaphylactic shock**

Interactions
✳ Drug-lab test • False-positive tests for proteinuria using acid precipitation tests; no interference has been reported with dye-impregnated reagent strips

■ Nursing considerations
Assessment
- **History:** Allergies, renal, hepatic, CV, and GI conditions; pregnancy, lactation
- **Physical:** Skin color, lesions; orientation, reflexes, ophthalmologic and audiometric evaluation, peripheral sensation; P, edema; R, adventitious sounds; liver evaluation; CBC, clotting times, renal and liver function tests; serum electrolytes, stool guaiac

Interventions
- Administer with milk if GI upset occurs; do not give with food—bioavailability is decreased by up to 16%.
- Use antacids other than sodium bicarbonate if GI upset occurs.
- Arrange for periodic ophthalmologic examination during long-term therapy.
- Institute emergency procedures if overdose occurs—gastric lavage, induction of emesis, supportive therapy.

Teaching points
- Take drug on an empty stomach; may be taken with milk or antacids other than sodium bicarbonate if GI upset occurs.
- Take only the prescribed dosage.
- These side effects may occur: dizziness, drowsiness (avoid driving or using dangerous machinery).
- Report sore throat, fever, rash, itching, weight gain, swelling in ankles or fingers; changes in vision; black, tarry stools.

▽tolterodine tartrate
*(toll **tear'** oh dyne)*

Detrol, Detrol LA

PREGNANCY CATEGORY C

Drug class
Antimuscarinic

Therapeutic actions
Competitively blocks muscarinic receptor sites; bladder contraction is mediated by muscarinic receptors—blocking these receptors decreases bladder contraction.

Indications
- Treatment of overactive bladder in patients with symptoms of urinary frequency, urgency or incontinence

Contraindications and cautions
- Contraindicated with urinary retention, uncontrolled narrow angle glaucoma, allergy to the drug or any of its components.
- Use cautiously with renal or hepatic impairment, pregnancy, lactation.

Available forms
Tablets—1, 2 mg; ER capsules—2, 4 mg

Dosages
Adults
2 mg PO bid, may be lowered to 1 mg PO bid based on individual response; ER capsules—4 mg PO taken once a day.
Pediatric patients
Safety and efficacy not established.
Patients with hepatic impairment
Reduce dosage to 1 mg PO bid (2 mg daily ER capsules) and monitor patient.

Pharmacokinetics

Route	Onset	Duration
Oral	1–2 hr	6–8 hr

Metabolism: Hepatic; $T_{1/2}$: 1.9–3.7 hr
Distribution: Crosses placenta; passes into breast milk
Excretion: Urine

Adverse effects in *Italics* are most common; those in **Bold** are life-threatening.

Adverse effects

- **CNS:** *Blurred vision,* headache, dizziness, somnolence
- **Dermatologic:** Pruritus, rash, erythema, dry skin
- **GI:** *Nausea, vomiting, constipation, dyspepsia,* flatulence, *dry mouth,* abdominal pain
- **GU:** *Dysuria,* urinary retention; impotence, UTIs
- **Other:** Weight gain, pain, fatigue, acute myopia and secondary angle closure glaucoma (pain, visual changes, redness, increased IOP)

Interactions

✳ **Drug-drug** • Risk of increased serum levels and toxicity if given with drugs that inhibit cytochrome P450; reduce dose to 1 mg PO bid (2 mg daily ER capsules)

■ Nursing considerations
Assessment

- **History:** Presence of urinary retention; uncontrolled narrow angle glaucoma; allergy to the drug or any of its components; renal or hepatic impairment; pregnancy, lactation
- **Physical:** Bowel sounds, normal output; normal urinary output, prostate palpation; intraocular pressure, vision; liver function tests; renal function tests; skin color, lesions, texture; weight

Interventions

- Provide small, frequent meals if GI upset is severe.
- Provide frequent mouth hygiene, skin care if dry mouth, skin occur.
- Arrange for safety precautions if blurred vision occurs.
- Monitor bowel function and arrange for bowel program if constipation occurs.

Teaching points

- Take drug exactly as prescribed.
- These side effects may occur: constipation (ensure adequate fluid intake, proper diet, consult your nurse or physician if this becomes a problem); dry mouth (sugarless lozenges, frequent mouth care may help, this effect sometimes lessens over time); blurred vision (it may help to know that these are drug effects that will go away when you

discontinue the drug, avoid ... quire acute vision); difficulty ... (it may help to empty the bladde... ately before taking each dose of dru...
- Report rash, flushing, eye pain, diffi... breathing, tremors, loss of coordination,... regular heartbeat, palpitations, headache, abdominal distention.

▽ topiramate
*(toe **pie'** rah mate)*

Topamax

PREGNANCY CATEGORY C

Drug class
Antiepileptic agent

Therapeutic actions
Mechanism of action not understood; antiepileptic effects may be due to the actions of blocking sodium channels in neurons with sustained depolarization; increasing GABA activity at receptors, thus potentiating the effects of this inhibitory neurotransmitter; and blocking excitatory neurotransmitters at neuron receptor sites.

Indications
- Adjunctive therapy for partial-onset seizure treatment in adults and children 2–16 yr
- Adjunctive therapy for seizures associated with Lennox-Gastaut syndrome in adults and children
- Adjunctive therapy for primary generalized tonic-clonic seizures in adults and children 2–16 yr
- Unlabeled uses: cluster headaches, infantile spasms

Contraindications and cautions
- Contraindicated with hypersensitivity to any component of the drug.
- Use cautiously with pregnancy (use only if benefits outweigh potential risks to fetus), lactation, renal or hepatic impairment, renal stones.

Available forms
Tablets—25, 100, 200 mg; sprinkle capsules—15, 25 mg

Dosages

Adults

400 mg PO daily in 2 divided doses; begin adjustment of dose at 25–50 mg/day in the evening for wk 1; 50 mg AM and PM for wk 2; 50 mg AM and 100 mg PM for wk 3; 100 mg AM and PM for wk 4; 100 mg AM and 150 mg PM for wk 5; 150 mg AM and PM for wk 6; 150 mg AM and 200 mg PM for wk 7; and 200 mg AM and PM for wk 8 and beyond.

Pediatric patients 2–16 yr

5–9 mg/kg/day PO in 2 divided doses, as adjunctive therapy for Lennox-Gastaut syndrome; begin therapy at ≤ 25 mg and increase in increments of 1–3 mg/kg/day every 1–2 wk.

Patients with renal impairment

Creatinine clearance < 70 mL/min: use one-half the usual dose; allow increased time to reach desired level.

Patients with hepatic impairment

Adjust slowly, monitor patient carefully.

Pharmacokinetics

Route	Onset	Peak
Oral	Rapid	2 hr

Metabolism: Hepatic; $T_{1/2}$: 21 hr
Distribution: Crosses placenta; enters breast milk
Excretion: Urine

Adverse effects

- **CNS:** *Ataxia, somnolence, dizziness, nystagmus,* nervousness, anxiety, tremor, speech impairment, paresthesias, confusion, depression
- **GI:** *Nausea, dyspepsia,* anorexia, vomiting
- **GU:** Dysmenorrhea
- **Hematologic:** Leukopenia
- **Respiratory:** *Upper respiratory infection,* pharyngitis, sinusitis
- **Other:** *Fatigue,* rash, acute myopia and secondary angle closure glaucoma (pain, visual disturbances, pupil dilation, redness, increased intraocular pressure), weight loss

Interactions

✳ **Drug-drug** • Increased CNS depression if taken with alcohol or CNS depressants; use extreme caution • Increased risk of renal stone development with carbonic anhydrase inhibitors • Decreased effects of hormonal contraceptives with topiramate; suggest use of barrier contraceptives instead

■ Nursing considerations

CLINICAL ALERT!
Name confusion has occurred between Topamax and Toprol-XL (metoprolol); use caution.

Assessment

- **History:** Hypersensitivity to any component of the drug; pregnancy, lactation; renal or hepatic impairment; renal stones
- **Physical:** Skin color, lesions; orientation, affect, reflexes, vision exam; R, adventitious sounds; liver and renal function tests

Interventions

- Reduce dosage, discontinue or substitute other antiepileptic medication gradually; abrupt discontinuation may precipitate status epilepticus.
- Stop the drug immediately and arrange for appropriate consults at first sign of blurred vision, periorbital edema, redness.
- Administer with food if GI upset occurs.
- Caution patient not to chew or break tablets because of bitter taste.
- Have patient swallow sprinkle capsules whole or by carefully opening capsule and sprinkling onto a soft food. Swallow this immediately; do not allow it to be chewed.
- Encourage patients with a history of renal stone development to maintain adequate fluid intake while on this drug.
- Suggest the use of barrier contraceptives to patients using this drug.
- Arrange for consultation with appropriate epilepsy support groups as needed.

Teaching points

- Take this drug exactly as prescribed. Do not break or chew tablets; they have a very bitter taste. If using sprinkle capsules, open carefully and sprinkle onto soft food and swallow immediately; do not chew.

Adverse effects in *Italics* are most common; those in **Bold** are life-threatening.

- Do not discontinue this drug abruptly or change dosage except on the advice of your health care provider.
- Arrange for frequent check-ups to monitor your response to this drug. It is very important that you keep all appointments for check-ups.
- These side effects may occur: drowsiness, dizziness, sleepiness (avoid driving or performing other tasks that require alertness; symptoms may occur initially but usually disappear with continued therapy); vision changes (avoid performing tasks that require visual acuity); GI upset (take drug with food; eat small, frequent meals).
- Wear a medical alert bracelet at all times so that any emergency medical personnel will know that you are an epileptic taking antiepileptic medication.
- Avoid using alcohol while you are on this drug; serious sedation could occur.
- Report fatigue, vision changes, speech problems, personality changes.

▽ topotecan hydrochloride

See *Less Commonly Used Drugs,* p. 1352.

▽ toremifene
(tore em' ah feen)

Fareston

PREGNANCY CATEGORY D

Drug classes
Estrogen receptor modulator
Antineoplastic

Therapeutic actions
Binds to estrogen receptors, has anti-estrogen effects, and inhibits growth of estrogen receptor–positive and estrogen receptor–negative breast cancer cell lines.

Indications
- Treatment of advanced breast cancer in post-menopausal women with estrogen receptor–positive disease or estrogen-receptor unknown tumors

Contraindications and cautions
- Contraindicated with allergy to toremifene, pregnancy, lactation.
- Use cautiously with history of hypercalcemia, liver dysfunction.

Available forms
Tablets—60 mg

Dosages
Adults
60 mg PO daily.

Pharmacokinetics

Route	Onset	Peak
Oral	Rapid	1–6 hr

Metabolism: Hepatic; $T_{1/2}$: 5–6 days
Distribution: Crosses placenta; enters breast milk
Excretion: Feces

Adverse effects
- **CNS:** Depression, light-headedness, *dizziness,* headache, hallucinations, vertigo
- **Dermatologic:** *Hot flashes, skin rash*
- **GI:** *Nausea, vomiting,* food distaste
- **GU:** Vaginal bleeding, vaginal discharge
- **Other:** Peripheral edema, hypercalcemia, cataracts, sweating

Interactions
✳ **Drug-drug** • Increased risk of bleeding if taken with oral anticoagulants

■ Nursing considerations
Assessment
- **History:** Allergy to toremifene, pregnancy, lactation, hypercalcemia, liver dysfunction
- **Physical:** Skin lesions, color, turgor; pelvic exam; orientation, affect, reflexes; BP, peripheral pulses, edema; liver function tests, serum electrolytes

Interventions
- Administer daily without regard to food.
- Counsel patient about the need to use contraceptive measures while taking this drug; inform patient that serious fetal harm could occur.
- Provide comfort measures to help patient deal with drug effects: hot flashes (environmental temperature control); headache, de-

pression (monitoring of light and noise); vaginal bleeding (hygiene measures).

Teaching points

* Take this drug as prescribed.
* These side effects may occur: hot flashes (stay in cool temperatures); nausea, vomiting (eat small, frequent meals); weight gain; dizziness, headache, light-headedness (use caution if driving or performing tasks that require alertness).
* This drug can cause serious fetal harm and must not be taken during pregnancy. Contraceptive measures should be used while you are taking this drug. If you become pregnant or decide that you would like to become pregnant, consult with your physician immediately.
* Report marked weakness, sleepiness, mental confusion, changes in color of urine or stool, rash.

▽torsemide
(tor' seh myde)

Demadex

PREGNANCY CATEGORY B

Drug class
Loop (high-ceiling) diuretic

Therapeutic actions
Inhibits the reabsorption of sodium and chloride from the proximal and distal renal tubules and the loop of Henle, leading to a natriuretic diuresis.

Indications
* Treatment of hypertension and edema associated with CHF, hepatic cirrhosis, renal failure

Contraindications and cautions
* Allergy to torsemide; known hypersensitivity to sulfonylureas; electrolyte depletion; anuria, severe renal failure; hepatic coma; SLE; gout; diabetes mellitus; lactation.

Available forms
Tablets—5, 10, 20, 100 mg; injection—10 mg/mL

Dosages
Adults
Do not exceed 200 mg/day.
* *CHF:* 10–20 mg PO or IV daily. Dose may be titrated upward until desired results are seen. Do not exceed 200 mg/day.
* *Chronic renal failure:* 20 mg PO or IV daily. Dose may be titrated upward until desired results are seen. Do not exceed 200 mg/day.
* *Hepatic failure:* 5–10 mg PO or IV daily. Do not exceed 40 mg/day.
* *Hypertension:* 5 mg PO daily. May be increased to 10 mg if response is not sufficient.

Pediatric patients
Safety and efficacy not established.

Pharmacokinetics

Route	Onset	Peak	Duration
Oral	60 min	60–120 min	6–8 hr
IV	10 min	60 min	6–8 hr

Metabolism: Hepatic; $T_{1/2}$: 210 min
Distribution: Crosses placenta; may enter breast milk
Excretion: Unchanged in the urine

▽IV facts
Preparation: May be given direct IV or diluted in solution with 5% dextrose in water, 0.9% sodium chloride, lactated Ringer's solution. Discard unused solution after 24 hr.
Infusion: Give by direct injection slowly, over 1–2 min. Further diluted in solution, give slowly, each 200 mg over 2 min.

Adverse effects
* **CNS:** *Asterixis, dizziness,* vertigo, paresthesias, confusion, fatigue, nystagmus, *weakness, headache, drowsiness,* fatigue, blurred vision, tinnitus, irreversible hearing loss
* **CV:** *Orthostatic hypotension,* volume depletion, cardiac arrhythmias, thrombophlebitis
* **GI:** *Nausea, anorexia, vomiting, diarrhea,* gastric irritation and pain, dry mouth, acute pancreatitis, jaundice

---

Adverse effects in *Italics* are most common; those in **Bold** are life-threatening.

- **GU:** *Polyuria, nocturia,* glycosuria, renal failure
- **Hematologic:** *Hypokalemia,* leukopenia, anemia, thrombocytopenia
- **Local:** *Pain, phlebitis at injection site*
- **Other:** Muscle cramps and muscle spasms, weakness, arthritic pain, fatigue, hives, photosensitivity, rash, pruritus, sweating, nipple tenderness

Interactions

✳ **Drug-drug** • Decreased diuresis and natriuresis with NSAIDs • Increased risk of cardiac glycoside toxicity (secondary to hypokalemia) • Increased risk of ototoxicity with aminoglycoside antibiotics, cisplatin

■ Nursing considerations
Assessment

- **History:** Allergy to torsemide; electrolyte depletion; anuria; severe renal failure; hepatic coma; SLE; gout; diabetes mellitus; lactation
- **Physical:** Skin color, lesions; edema; orientation, reflexes, hearing; pulses, baseline ECG, BP, orthostatic BP, perfusion; R, pattern, adventitious sounds; liver evaluation, bowel sounds; urinary output patterns; CBC, serum electrolytes, blood sugar, liver and renal function tests, uric acid, urinalysis

Interventions

- Administer with food or milk to prevent GI upset.
- Mark calendars or other reminders of drug days if intermittent therapy is optimal for treating edema.
- Administer single daily doses early in the day so increased urination will not disturb sleep.
- Avoid IV use if oral use is at all possible.
- Measure and record regular weights to monitor fluid changes.
- Monitor serum electrolytes, hydration, liver function during long-term therapy.
- Provide diet rich in potassium or supplemental potassium.

Teaching points

- Record alternate-day or intermittent therapy on a calendar or dated envelopes.
- Take the drug early in the day so increased urination will not disturb sleep.

- Take the drug with food or meals to prevent GI upset.
- Weigh yourself on a regular basis, at the same time and in the same clothing, and record the weight on your calendar.
- These side effects may occur: increased volume and frequency of urination; dizziness, feeling faint on arising, drowsiness (avoid rapid position changes, hazardous activities [eg, driving a car] and alcohol consumption); sensitivity to sunlight (use sunglasses and sunscreen, wear protective clothing when outdoors); increased thirst (sucking on sugarless lozenges, frequent mouth care may help); loss of body potassium (a potassium-rich diet, or even a potassium supplement, will be necessary).
- Report weight change of more than 3 lb in one day; swelling in ankles or fingers; unusual bleeding or bruising; nausea, dizziness, trembling, numbness, fatigue; muscle weakness or cramps.

▷ **tramadol hydrochloride**
(tram' ah doll)

Ultram

PREGNANCY CATEGORY C

Drug class
Centrally acting analgesic

Therapeutic actions
Binds to mu-opioid receptors and inhibits the reuptake of norepinephrine and serotonin; causes many effects similar to the opioids—dizziness, somnolence, nausea, constipation—but does not have the respiratory depressant effects.

Indications
- Relief of moderate to moderately severe pain

Contraindications and cautions
- Contraindicated with pregnancy; allergy to tramadol; acute intoxication with alcohol, opioids, psychotropic drugs or other centrally acting analgesics; lactation.

- Use cautiously with seizures, concomitant use of CNS depressants or MAOIs, renal or hepatic impairment.

Available forms
Tablets—50 mg

Dosages
Adults
50–100 mg PO q 4–6 hr; do not exceed 400 mg/day.
Pediatric patients
Safety and efficacy not established.
Geriatric patients and patients with renal or hepatic impairment
50 mg PO q 12 hr. Do not exceed 200 mg/day.
> 75 yr: Do not exceed 300 mg/day.

Pharmacokinetics

Route	Onset	Peak
Oral	1 hr	2 hr

Metabolism: Hepatic; $T_{1/2}$: 6–7 hr
Distribution: Crosses placenta; enters breast milk
Excretion: Urine

Adverse effects
- **CNS:** *Sedation, dizziness/vertigo, headache,* confusion, dreaming, sweating, anxiety, **seizures**
- **CV:** *Hypotension*, tachycardia, bradycardia
- **Dermatologic:** *Sweating,* pruritus, rash, pallor, urticaria
- **GI:** *Nausea, vomiting,* dry mouth, constipation, flatulence
- **Other:** Potential for abuse, **anaphylactoid reactions**

Interactions
✳ Drug-drug • Decreased effectiveness with carbamazepine • Increased risk of tramadol toxicity with MAOIs

■ Nursing considerations
Assessment
- **History:** Hypersensitivity to tramadol; pregnancy; acute intoxication with alcohol, opioids, psychotropic drugs or other centrally acting analgesics; lactation; seizures; concomitant use of CNS depressants or MAOIs;

renal or hepatic impairment; past or present history of opioid addiction
- **Physical:** Skin color, texture, lesions; orientation, reflexes, bilateral grip strength, affect; P, auscultation, BP; bowel sounds, normal output; liver and kidney function tests

Interventions
- Provide environmental control (temperature, lighting) if sweating, CNS effects occur.

Teaching points
- Limit use in patients with past or present history of addiction to or dependence on opioids.
- These side effects may occur: dizziness, sedation, drowsiness, impaired visual acuity (avoid driving or performing tasks that require alertness); nausea, loss of appetite (lie quietly, eat small frequent meals).
- Report severe nausea, dizziness, severe constipation.

▽ trandolapril
*(tran **dole'** ah pril)*

Mavik

PREGNANCY CATEGORY C
(FIRST TRIMESTER)

PREGNANCY CATEGORY D
(SECOND AND THIRD TRIMESTERS)

Drug classes
Antihypertensive
Angiotensin converting enzyme inhibitor (ACE inhibitor)

Therapeutic actions
Blocks ACE from converting angiotensin I to angiotensin II, a powerful vasoconstrictor, leading to decreased blood pressure, decreased aldosterone secretion, a small increase in serum potassium levels, and sodium and fluid loss; increased prostaglandin synthesis may also be involved in the antihypertensive action.

Adverse effects in *Italics* are most common; those in **Bold** are life-threatening.

Indications

- Treatment of hypertension, alone or in combination with other antihypertensives
- Treatment of post-MI patients with evidence of left-ventricular dysfunction and symptoms of CHF

Contraindications and cautions

- Contraindicated with allergy to ACE inhibitors, history of ACE-associated angioedema.
- Use cautiously with impaired renal function, CHF, CAD, salt/volume depletion, surgery, pregnancy, lactation.

Available forms

Tablets—1, 2, 4 mg

Dosages

Adults

- *Hypertension:* African-American patients: 2 mg PO daily. Non–African-American patients: 1 mg PO daily. Maintenance: 2–4 mg/day.
- *Patients on diuretics:* Stop diuretic 2–3 days before beginning trandolapril. Resume diuretic only if BP is not controlled; start at 0.5 mg PO daily and adjust upward as needed.
- *Heart failure post-MI:* 1 mg/day PO, adjust to a target of 4 mg/day.

Pediatric patients

Safety and efficacy not established.

Patients with renal or hepatic impairment

0.5 mg PO daily, adjust at 1-wk intervals to control BP; usual range is 2–4 mg PO daily.

Pharmacokinetics

Route	Onset
Oral	4 hr

Metabolism: $T_{1/2}$: 6–10 hr
Distribution: Crosses placenta; passes into breast milk
Excretion: Urine and feces

Adverse effects

- **CNS:** Headache, fatigue
- **CV:** *Tachycardia,* angina pectoris, **MI,** Raynaud's syndrome, CHF, hypotension in salt- or volume-depleted patients
- **Dermatologic:** *Rash*
- **GI:** *Diarrhea,* GI upset
- **GU:** Renal insufficiency, renal failure, polyuria, oliguria, urinary frequency, UTI
- **Other:** *Cough, dizziness,* malaise, dry mouth

Interactions

✳ **Drug-drug** • Excessive hypotension may occur with diuretics; monitor closely • Hyperkalemia may occur with potassium supplements, potassium-sparing diuretics, salt substitutes; monitor serum potassium levels • Potential increase in lithium levels if taken concurrently; decreased lithium dose may be needed

■ Nursing considerations

Assessment

- **History:** Allergy to ACE inhibitors; impaired renal or hepatic function; CAD; CHF; salt or volume depletion; surgery; pregnancy, lactation
- **Physical:** Skin color, lesions, turgor; T; P, BP, peripheral perfusion; mucous membranes, bowel sounds, liver evaluation; urinalysis, renal and liver function tests, CBC and differential

Interventions

- Ensure that patient is not pregnant before administering; advise the use of barrier contraceptives.
- Administer once a day at same time each day.
- Alert surgeon and mark patient's chart with notice that trandolapril is being taken; angiotensin II formation subsequent to compensatory renin release during surgery will need to be blocked; hypotension may be reversed with volume expansion.
- Monitor patient closely in any situation that may lead to fall in BP secondary to reduction in fluid volume—excessive perspiration and dehydration, vomiting, diarrhea—as excessive hypotension may occur.
- Reduce dosage in patients with impaired renal or hepatic function.
- Discontinue immediately if laryngeal edema, angioedema, or jaundice occurs.

Teaching points

- Take drug once a day at the same general time each day. Do not stop taking this medication without consulting your health care provider.

- These side effects may occur: GI upset, diarrhea (limited effects that will pass); dizziness, light-headedness (usually passes after first few days; change position slowly and limit your activities to those that do not require alertness and precision); cough (can be very irritating and does not respond to cough suppressants; notify health care provider if very uncomfortable).
- This drug cannot be used during pregnancy; use of barrier contraceptives is recommended.
- Be careful in any situation that may lead to a drop in BP (diarrhea, sweating, vomiting, dehydration); if light-headedness or dizziness occurs, consult your health care provider.
- Avoid use of OTC medications while on this drug, especially cough, cold, allergy medications; they may contain ingredients that will interact with this drug. If you feel that you need one of these preparations, consult your nurse or physician.
- Report sore throat, fever, chills; swelling of the hands or feet; irregular heartbeat, chest pains; swelling of the face, eyes, lips, tongue; difficulty breathing; yellowing of skin.

▷tranylcypromine sulfate

*(tran ill **sip'** roe meen)*

Parnate

PREGNANCY CATEGORY C

Drug classes
Antidepressant
MAOI, hydrazine derivative

Therapeutic actions
Irreversibly inhibits MAO, an enzyme that breaks down biogenic amines, such as epinephrine, norepinephrine, and serotonin, allowing these biogenic amines to accumulate in neuronal storage sites; according to the biogenic amine hypothesis, this accumulation of amines is responsible for the clinical efficacy of MAOIs as antidepressants.

Indications
- Treatment of adult outpatients with reactive depression; efficacy in endogenous depression has not been established

Contraindications and cautions
- Contraindicated with hypersensitivity to any MAOI; pheochromocytoma, CHF; history of liver disease or abnormal liver function tests; severe renal impairment; confirmed or suspected cerebrovascular defect; CV disease, hypertension; history of headache (headache is an indicator of hypertensive reaction to drug); myelography within previous 24 hr or scheduled within 48 hr; lactation.
- Use cautiously with seizure disorders; hyperthyroidism; impaired hepatic, renal function; psychiatric patients (agitated or schizophrenic patients may show excessive stimulation; manic-depressive patients may shift to hypomanic or manic phase); patients scheduled for elective surgery (MAOIs should be discontinued 10 days before surgery); pregnancy or in women of childbearing age.

Available forms
Tablets—10 mg

Dosages
Adults
Usual effective dose is 30 mg/day PO in divided doses. Improvement should be seen within 48 hr to 3 wk. If no improvement is seen within 2 wk, increase dosage in 10 mg/day increments every 1 to 3 wk. May be increased to a maximum of 60 mg/day.
Pediatric patients
Not recommended for patients < 16 yr.
Geriatric patients
Patients > 60 yr are more prone to develop adverse effects; use with caution.

Pharmacokinetics

Route	Onset	Duration
Oral	Rapid	10 days

Metabolism: Hepatic; $T_{1/2}$: unknown

Adverse effects in *Italics* are most common; those in **Bold** are life-threatening.

Distribution: Crosses placenta; enters breast milk
Excretion: Urine

Adverse effects

- **CNS:** *Dizziness, vertigo, headache, overactivity, hyperreflexia, tremors, muscle twitching, mania, hypomania, jitteriness, confusion, memory impairment, insomnia, weakness, fatigue, drowsiness, restlessness, overstimulation, increased anxiety, agitation, blurred vision, sweating,* akathisia, ataxia, coma, euphoria, neuritis, repetitious babbling, chills, glaucoma, nystagmus
- **CV: Hypertensive crises, sometimes fatal,** sometimes with intracranial bleeding, usually attributable to tyramine ingestion (see Drug–food interactions below); symptoms include occipital headache, which may radiate frontally; palpitations; neck stiffness or soreness; vomiting; sweating (sometimes with fever, cold and clammy skin); dilated pupils; photophobia; tachycardia or bradycardia; chest pain; *orthostatic hypotension, sometimes associated with falling; disturbed cardiac rate and rhythm,* palpitations, tachycardia
- **Dermatologic:** Minor skin reactions, spider telangiectases, photosensitivity
- **GI:** *Constipation, diarrhea, nausea, abdominal pain, edema, dry mouth, anorexia, weight changes*
- **GU:** Dysuria, incontinence, urinary retention, sexual disturbances
- **Other:** Hematologic changes, black tongue, hypernatremia

Interactions

✴ **Drug-drug** ● Increased sympathomimetic effects (hypertensive crisis) with sympathomimetic drugs (norepinephrine, epinephrine, dopamine, dobutamine, levodopa, ephedrine), amphetamines, other anorexiants, local anesthetic solutions containing sympathomimetics ● Hypertensive crisis, coma, severe convulsions with TCAs (eg, imipramine, desipramine) ● Additive hypoglycemic effect with insulin, oral sulfonylureas (eg, tolbutamide) ● Increased risk of adverse interactive actions with meperidine ● Potentially dangerous hypotension with general anesthetics; avoid this combination ● Reduce dose of barbiturates if given with MAOIs ● Toxic levels of buspirone and bupropion if combined with MAOIs; separate use by 10 or 14 days, respectively ● Increased hypertension effects with carbamazepine, levodopa ● Risk of hypotension with thiazide diuretics

✴ **Drug-food** ● Tyramine (and other pressor amines) contained in foods are normally broken down by MAO enzymes in the GI tract; in the presence of MAOIs, these vasopressors may be absorbed in high concentrations; in addition, tyramine releases accumulated norepinephrine from nerve terminals; thus, hypertensive crisis may occur when the following foods that contain tyramine or other vasopressors are ingested by a patient on an MAOI: dairy products (blue, camembert, cheddar, mozzarella, parmesan, romano, roquefort, Stilton chesses; sour cream; yogurt); meats, fish (liver, pickled herring, fermented sausages [bologna, pepperoni, salami], caviar, dried fish, other fermented or spoiled meat or fish); undistilled beverages (imported beer, ale; red wine, especially Chianti; sherry; coffee, tea, colas containing caffeine; chocolate drinks); fruit/vegetables (avocado, fava beans, figs, raisins, bananas, yeast extracts, soy sauce, chocolate)

■ Nursing considerations
Assessment

- **History:** Hypersensitivity to any MAOI; pheochromocytoma, CHF; abnormal liver function tests; severe renal impairment; confirmed or suspected cerebrovascular defect; CV disease, hypertension; history of headache, myelography within previous 24 hr or scheduled within 48 hr; lactation; seizure disorders; hyperthyroidism; impaired hepatic, renal function; psychiatric patients; patients scheduled for elective surgery; pregnancy
- **Physical:** Weight; T; skin color, lesions; orientation, affect, reflexes, vision; P, BP, orthostatic BP, perfusion; bowel sounds, normal output, liver evaluation; urine flow, normal output; liver, kidney function tests, urinalysis, CBC, ECG, EEG

Interventions
- Limit amount of drug that is available to suicidal patients.

- Monitor BP and orthostatic BP carefully; arrange for more gradual increase in dosage initially in patients who show tendency for hypotension.
- Arrange for periodic liver function tests during therapy; discontinue drug at first sign of hepatic dysfunction or jaundice.
- Monitor BP carefully (and if appropriate, discontinue drug) if patient reports unusual or severe headache.
- Provide phentolamine or another alpha-adrenergic blocking drug on standby in case of hypertensive crisis.

Teaching points

- Take drug exactly as prescribed.
- Do not stop taking drug abruptly or without consulting health care provider.
- Avoid ingesting tyramine-containing foods or beverages while on this drug and for 10 days afterward (patient and significant other should receive a list of such foods and beverages; see Appendix N, *Important Dieary Guidelines for Patient Teaching*).
- These side effects may occur: dizziness, weakness or fainting when arising from a horizontal or sitting position (transient; change position slowly); drowsiness, blurred vision (reversible; safety measures may need to be taken if severe; avoid driving or performing tasks that require alertness); nausea, vomiting, loss of appetite (small, frequent meals, frequent mouth care may help); nightmares, confusion, inability to concentrate, emotional changes; changes in sexual function.
- Report headache, rash, darkening of the urine, pale stools, yellowing of the eyes or skin, fever, chills, sore throat, or any other unusual symptoms.

▽trastuzumab
*(trass too **zoo'** mab)*

Herceptin

PREGNANCY CATEGORY B

Drug classes
Monoclonal antibody
Antineoplastic agent

Therapeutic actions
Humanoid anticlonal antibody to the HER2 (human epidermal growth factor receptor 2) protein. This protein is often overexpressed in patients with aggressive, metastatic breast cancer.

Indications
- Treatment of metastatic breast cancer with tumors that overexpress HER2 protein (a genetic defect) as a first-line therapy in combination with paclitaxel and as a single agent in second- and third-line therapy

Contraindications and cautions
- Contraindicated with allergy to trastuzumab or any component of the drug; breast cancers without HER2 overexpression.
- Use cautiously with known cardiac disease, bone marrow depression, lactation and pregnancy.

Available forms
Powder for injection—440 mg

Dosages
Adults
4 mg/kg IV once by IV infusion over 90 min; maintenance: 2 mg/kg IV once weekly over at least 30 min as tolerated. Do not exceed 500 mg/dose.

Pharmacokinetics

Route	Onset	Duration
IV	Slow	Days

Metabolism: Tissue; T$_{1/2}$: 2–9 days
Distribution: Crosses placenta, may enter breast milk

▼IV facts
Preparation: Reconstitute powder with diluent provided; dilute in 0.9% sodium chloride injection. Solution should be colorless to pale yellow. Use within 24 hr.
Infusion: Infuse initial dose over 90 min; maintenance doses may be infused over 30 minutes.
Incompatibilities: Do not mix with any other drug solution or add any other drugs to the IV line.

Adverse effects in *Italics* are most common; those in **Bold** are life-threatening.

Adverse effects
- **CNS:** Malaise, headache, tremor, insomnia
- **CV: Serious cardiac toxicity**
- **GI:** Vomiting, nausea, *diarrhea, abdominal pain*
- **Other:** Anemia, pain, edema, *increased susceptibility to infection, leukopenia, local reaction at infusion site, infusion reaction* (flushing, sweating, chills, fever), *fever, chills,* hypersensitivity reactions

■ Nursing considerations
Assessment
- **History:** Allergy to trastuzumab or any component of the product; known cardiac disease, bone marrow depression; pregnancy, lactation
- **Physical:** T; P, BP; R, adventitious sounds; baseline ECG; orientation, affect, CBC with differential, tumor testing for HER2 status

Interventions
- Monitor patient at time of infusion and provide comfort measures and analgesics as appropriate if infusion reaction occurs.
- Monitor cardiac status, especially if patient is receiving chemotherapy; have emergency equipment on standby if cardiac toxicity occurs.
- Protect patient from exposure to infections and maintain sterile technique for invasive procedures.

Teaching points
- This drug is given IV to help fight your breast cancer. It will be given once a week. Mark calendar with return dates for repeat infusion.
- Avoid infection while you are on this drug; stay away from crowded areas or people with known infections.
- These side effects may occur: discomfort, sweating, fever during infusion (comfort measures and analgesics may help); diarrhea, nausea, abdominal pain.
- Report chest pain, difficulty breathing, chills, fever.

▽trazodone hydrochloride
(traz' oh done)

Alti-Trazodone (CAN), Apo-Trazodone (CAN), Desyrel, Desyrel Dividose, Nu-Trazodone (CAN)

PREGNANCY CATEGORY C

Drug classes
Antidepressant
Selective serotonin reuptake inhibitor (SSRI)

Therapeutic actions
Mechanism of action unknown; differs from other antidepressants in that it is a triazo compound, not a TCA, an amphetamine-like CNS stimulant, or an MAOI; inhibits the presynaptic reuptake of the neurotransmitter serotonin and potentiates the behavioral effects of the serotonin precursor; the relation of these effects to clinical efficacy is unknown.

Indications
- Treatment of depression in inpatient and outpatient settings and for depressed patients with and without anxiety
- Unlabeled uses: treatment of aggressive behavior, cocaine withdrawal

Contraindications and cautions
- Contraindicated with hypersensitivity to trazodone, EST, recent MI, pregnancy (congenital abnormalities reported).
- Use cautiously with preexisting cardiac disease (arrhythmias, including ventricular tachycardia, may be more likely), lactation.

Available forms
Tablets—50, 100, 150, 300 mg

Dosages
Adults
Initially 150 mg/day PO. May be increased by 50 mg/day every 3–4 days. Maximum dose for outpatients should not exceed 400 mg/day in divided doses. Maximum dose for inpatients or those severely depressed should not exceed 600 mg/day in divided doses. Use lowest effective dosage for maintenance.

Pediatric patients 6–18 yr
Initially 1.5–2 mg/kg/day PO in divided doses. May be increased every 3–4 days. Do not exceed 6 mg/kg/day.

Geriatric patients
Initially 75 mg/day PO in divided doses. Monitor patient closely.

Pharmacokinetics

Route	Onset	Peak
Oral	Varies	1–2 hr

Metabolism: Hepatic; $T_{1/2}$: 3–6 hr and then 5–9 hr
Distribution: Crosses placenta; may enter breast milk
Excretion: Urine and feces

Adverse effects

- **CNS:** *Anger, hostility, agitation, nightmares/vivid dreams, hallucinations, delusions, hypomania, confusion, disorientation, decreased concentration, impaired memory, impaired speech, dizziness, incoordination, drowsiness, fatigue,* excitement, insomnia, nervousness, paresthesia, tremors, akathisia, headache, grand mal seizures, tinnitus, blurred vision, red eyes, nasal/sinus congestion, *malaise*
- **CV:** *Hypertension, hypotension, shortness of breath, syncope, tachycardia, palpitations,* chest pain, **MI,** ventricular ectopic activity, occasional sinus bradycardia with long-term use
- **GI:** *Abdominal/gastric disorder, decreased/increased appetite, bad taste in mouth, dry mouth, hypersalivation, nausea, vomiting, diarrhea, flatulence, constipation*
- **GU:** *Decreased libido,* impotence, priapism, retrograde ejaculation, early menses, missed periods, hematuria, delayed urine flow, increased urinary frequency
- **Hematologic:** Anemia, neutropenia, leukopenia, liver enzyme alterations
- **Hypersensitivity:** *Allergic skin conditions, edema,* rash
- **Musculoskeletal:** Musculoskeletal aches and pains, muscle twitches
- **Other:** Sweating, clamminess

Interactions

✳ **Drug-drug** ● Increased serum levels and toxicity of alcohol, CNS depressants, digoxin, phenytoin ● Risk of serotonin syndrome if combined with other SSRIs ● Increased risk of toxicity with phenothiazines ● Decreased effectiveness with carbamazepine

✳ **Drug-alternative therapy** ● Increased risk of severe reaction if combined with St. John's wort therapy

■ Nursing considerations
Assessment

- **History:** Hypersensitivity to trazodone; EST; recent MI, preexisting cardiac disease; pregnancy, lactation
- **Physical:** Skin color, lesions; orientation, affect, reflexes, vision and hearing; P, BP, orthostatic BP, perfusion; bowel sounds, normal output, liver evaluation; urine flow, normal output; usual sexual function, frequency of menses; liver function tests, urinalysis, CBC, ECG

Interventions

- Ensure that depressed and potentially suicidal patients have access to only limited quantities of drug.
- Administer shortly after a meal or light snack to enhance absorption.
- Administer major portion of dose hs if drowsiness occurs.
- Anticipate symptomatic relief during the first week of therapy with optimal effects within 2 wk (some patients require 2–4 wk to respond).
- Monitor patient for orthostatic hypotension during therapy.
- Discontinue therapy immediately if priapism occurs.
- Arrange for CBC if patient develops fever, sore throat, or other signs of infection.

Teaching points

- Take drug with food or a snack to enhance absorption and decrease likelihood of dizziness.
- Avoid alcohol, sleep-inducing drugs, and OTC drugs.
- These side effects may occur: ringing in the ears, headache, dizziness, drowsiness, weak-

---

Adverse effects in *Italics* are most common; those in **Bold** are life-threatening.

ness (reversible; safety measures may need to be taken if severe; avoid driving or performing tasks that require alertness); nausea, vomiting, loss of appetite (small, frequent meals, frequent mouth care may help); dry mouth (sucking sugarless candies may help); changes in sexual function and abilities; nightmares, dreams, confusion, inability to concentrate (may lessen).
- Report dizziness, light-headedness, faintness, blood in urine, fever, chills, sore throat, rash, prolonged or inappropriate penile erection (discontinue immediately).

▽ treprostinil sodium
*(tra **pros'** tin ill)*

Remodulin

PREGNANCY CATEGORY B

Drug classes
Endothelin receptor antagonist
Antihypertensive

Therapeutic actions
Specifically blocks receptor sites for endothelin (ET_A and ET_B) in the endothelium and vascular smooth muscles; these endothelins are elevated in plasma and lung tissue of patients with pulmonary arterial hypertension; also inhibits platelet aggregation.

Indications
- Treatment of pulmonary arterial hypertension in patients with class II–class IV symptoms, to improve exercise ability and to decrease the rate of clinical worsening

Contraindications and cautions
- Contraindicated with allergy to treprostinil or any component of the drug.
- Use cautiously with liver or renal dysfunction, lactation, pregnancy, elderly patients.

Available forms
Multi-use vials—1, 2.5, 5, 10 mg/mL

Dosages
Adults
Administered by continuous SC infusion. Initially the rate is 1.25 ng/kg/min. Rate is in-creased in increments of no more than 1.25 ng/kg/min/wk for the first 4 wk, then by 2.5 ng/kg/min per wk. Do not exceed 40 ng/kg/min. Dosage is based on clinical response and patient tolerance. See manufacturer's instructions for infusion weight charts.
Pediatric patients
Safety and efficacy not established.
Patients with hepatic impairment
Decrease initial dose to 0.625 ng/kg/min and increase slowly.

Pharmacokinetics

Route	Onset	Peak
SC infusion	Gradual	10 hr

Metabolism: Hepatic; $T_{1/2}$: 2–4 hr
Distribution: Crosses placenta; may enter breast milk
Excretion: Urine

Adverse effects
- **CNS:** *Headache, diarrhea, jaw pain*
- **CV:** Vasodilation, edema, hypotension, dyspnea, chest pain
- **GI:** *Nausea, diarrhea*
- **Skin:** Pruritis, *rash*
- **Other:** *Pain at injection site, local reaction at infusion site,* increased bleeding, *jaw pain*

Interactions
✳ Drug-drug • Potential for increased hypotensive effects if combined with other drugs that decrease blood pressure; monitor patient carefully • Potential for increased bleeding tendencies if combined with drugs that alter blood clotting

■ Nursing considerations
Assessment
- **History:** Allergy to treprostinil or any component of the drug, hepatic or renal dysfunction, pregnancy, lactation, advanced age
- **Physical:** Skin color, lesions; injection site; orientation, BP; liver and renal function tests, CBC

Interventions
- Evaluate the patient for the ability to accept, place, and care for a subcutaneous catheter and to use a continuous infusion pump.

- Ensure that patient is reevaluated weekly for possible adjustments in dosage.
- Inspect solution to make sure no particulate matter is present before use. Use vial within 14 days of initial introduction into the vial.
- Monitor injection site for any sign of reaction of infection.
- Monitor patients who are discontinuing treprostinil; tapering of dose may be needed to avoid sudden worsening of disease.
- Provide analgesics as appropriate for patients who develop headache or injection site pain.
- Monitor patient's functional level to note improvement in exercise tolerance.
- Maintain other measures used to treat pulmonary arterial hypertension.

Teaching points

- This drug must be given by a continuous subcutaneous infusion pump. It may be needed for prolonged periods, possibly years. The pump is lightweight and attached to a catheter that goes into your skin. You will need to care for the insertion site and set and monitor the pump. It would be wise to have a significant other who is also able to care for and maintain the site and the pump as a backup for you.
- Be aware that this drug should not be taken during pregnancy; use of a barrier contraceptive is advised.
- Keep a chart of your exercise tolerance to help monitor improvement in your condition.
- These side effects may occur: headache (analgesics may be available that will help); stomach upset (taking the drug with food may help); pain at the injection site (analgesics may also help, monitor the site for any sign of redness, heat, or swelling).
- This drug should not be discontinued abruptly. It must be tapered. Notify your health care provider if anything happens that you are unable to get your continuous infusion of the drug.
- Maintain any procedures you usually use for treating your pulmonary arterial hypertension.
- Know that you will need to be followed closely to determine the correct dose of the drug that is best for your situation.

- Report swelling of the extremities, dizziness, chest pain, fever, changes in the appearance of the catheter insertion site.

▷tretinoin (retinoic acid)
(tret' i noyn)

Avita, Renova, Retin-A, Retin-A Micro, Stieva-A (CAN), Vesanoid

PREGNANCY CATEGORY D

Drug classes
Antineoplastic
Retinoid (topical form, see Appendix J, *Topical Drugs*)

Therapeutic actions
Induces cell differentiation and decreases proliferation of acute promyelocytic leukemia (APL) cells, leading to an initial maturation of the primitive promyelocytes, followed by a repopulation of the bone marrow and peripheral blood by normal hematopoietic cells in patients achieving complete remission; exact mechanism of action is not understood.

Indications
- Induction of remission in acute promyelocytic leukemia (APL)
- Topical treatment of acne vulgaris
- Adjunctive agent for use in mitigation of fine wrinkles, mottled hyperpigmentation in select patients

Contraindications and cautions
- Contraindicated with allergy to retinoids or parabens, suicidal tendencies; pregnancy, lactation.
- Use cautiously with liver disease, hypercholesterolemia, hypertriglyceridemia.

Available forms
Capsule—10 mg; cream—0.02%, 0.025%, 0.05%, 0.1%; gel—0.025%, 0.01%, 0.1%; liquid—0.05%

Dosages
Adults
Oral
45 mg/m²/day PO administered in 2 evenly divided doses until complete remission is documented; discontinue therapy 30 days after complete remission is obtained or after 90 days, whichever comes first.

Topical
Apply once a day before bedtime. Cover entire affected area lightly.

Pediatric patients
Not recommended.

Pharmacokinetics

Route	Onset	Peak
Oral	Slow	1–2 hr

Metabolism: Hepatic; $T_{1/2}$: 0.5–2 hr
Distribution: Crosses placenta; may enter breast milk
Excretion: Urine and feces

Adverse effects
- **CNS:** *Fever, headache,* **pseudotumor cerebri** (papilledema, headache, nausea, vomiting, visual disturbances), *earache, visual disturbances, malaise, sweating,* suicidal ideation
- **CV:** Arrhythmias, flushing, hypotension, CHF, **MI, cardiac arrest**
- **Dermatologic:** *Skin fragility, dry skin, pruritus, rash,* thinning hair, peeling of palms and soles, skin infections, photosensitivity, nail brittleness, petechiae
- **GI:** *Hemorrhage, nausea, vomiting, abdominal pain,* anorexia, inflammatory bowel disease
- **GU:** Renal insufficiency, dysuria, frequency, enlarged prostate
- **Hematologic: Rapid and evolving leukocytosis,** *liver function, elevated lipids, elevated liver enzymes*
- **Musculoskeletal:** Skeletal hyperostosis, arthralgia, *bone and joint pain* and stiffness
- **Respiratory: RA-APL syndrome** (fever, dyspnea, weight gain, pulmonary infiltrates, pleural and/or pericardial effusion, hypotension may progress to death)

Interactions
✳ **Drug-drug** • Increased risk of high serum levels and toxicity with ketoconazole

■ Nursing considerations
Assessment
- **History:** Allergy to retinoids or parabens; pregnancy, lactation; liver disease; hypercholesterolemia, hypertriglyceridemia, suicidal tendencies
- **Physical:** Skin color, lesions, turgor, texture; joints—range of motion; orientation, reflexes, affect, ophthalmologic exam; mucous membranes, bowel sounds; R, adventitious sounds, auscultation; serum triglycerides, HDL, sedimentation rate, CBC and differential, urinalysis, pregnancy test, chest x-ray

Interventions
- Ensure that patient is not pregnant before administering; arrange for a pregnancy test within 2 wk of beginning therapy. Advise patient to use two forms of contraception during treatment and for 1 mo after treatment is discontinued.
- Monitor patient for any suicidal ideation or tendencies. The risk of suicide should be explained and the *Medguide* brochure given as the patient signs the release affirming that he or she understands the potential risk.
- Oral tretinoin is for induction of remission only; arrange for consolidation or maintenance chemotherapy for APL after induction therapy.
- Arrange for baseline recording of serum lipids and triglyceride levels, liver function tests, chest x-ray, CBC with differential and coagulation profile; monitor for changes frequently.
- Discontinue drug and notify physician if liver function tests are > 5 times upper range of normal, pulmonary infiltrates appear, or patient has difficulty breathing.
- Discontinue drug if signs of papilledema occur; consult with a neurologist for further care.
- Discontinue drug if visual disturbances occur, and arrange for an ophthalmologic exam.
- Discontinue drug if abdominal pain, rectal bleeding, or severe diarrhea occurs, and consult with physician.

T

- Monitor triglycerides during therapy; if elevations occur, institute other measures to lower serum triglycerides: weight reduction, reduction in dietary fat, exercise, increased intake of insoluble fiber, decreased alcohol consumption.
- Maintain high-dose steroids on standby in case of severe leukocytosis or liver damage.
- Administer drug with meals; do not crush capsules.
- Do not administer vitamin supplements that contain vitamin A.
- Maintain supportive care appropriate for APL patients: monitor for and treat infections, prophylaxis for bleeding, etc.
- Topical form should be applied lightly to entire area before bed. Cleanse area thoroughly before use.

Teaching points

- Take the oral drug with meals; do not crush capsules.
- Frequent blood tests will be necessary to evaluate the drug's effects on your body.
- This drug has been associated with severe birth defects and miscarriages; it is contraindicated for pregnant women. Use contraceptives during treatment and for 1 mo after treatment is discontinued. If you think that you are pregnant, consult with your physician immediately.
- You will not be permitted to donate blood while on this drug because of its possible effects on the fetus of a blood recipient.
- These side effects may occur: dizziness, lethargy, headache, visual changes (avoid driving or performing tasks that require alertness); sensitivity to the sun (avoid sunlamps, exposure to the sun; use sunscreens and protective clothing); diarrhea, abdominal pain, loss of appetite (take drug with meals); dry mouth (sucking sugarless lozenges may help); eye irritation and redness, inability to wear contact lenses; dry skin, itching, redness.
- Avoid the use of vitamin supplements containing vitamin A; serious toxic effects may occur. Limit alcohol consumption. You may also need to limit your intake of fats and increase exercise to limit the drug's effects on blood triglyceride levels.

- Report headache with nausea and vomiting, difficulty breathing, severe diarrhea or rectal bleeding, visual difficulties, suicidal ideas or feelings.
- Apply topical form lightly to entire affected area before bed. Cleanse area thoroughly before use.

▷triamcinolone
*(trye am **sin'** oh lone)*

triamcinolone
Oral: Aristocort, Atolone

triamcinolone acetonide
IM, intra-articular, or soft-tissue injection; respiratory inhalant; dermatologic ointment, cream, lotion, aerosol: Azmacort, Flutex, Kenaject 40, Kenalog, Nasacort, Nasacort AQ, Oracort (CAN), Tac-3, Tac-40, Triacet, Triamonide, Triam-A, Triderm, Tri-Kort, Trilog, Tri-Nasal

triamcinolone diacetate
IM, intra-articular, intrasynovial, intralesional injection: Amcort, Aristocorte Forte, Aristocort Intralesional, Clinacort, Triam-Forte, Trilone, Tristoject

triamcinolone hexacetonide
Intra-articular, intralesional injection: Aristospan Intra-articular, Aristospan Intralesional

PREGNANCY CATEGORY C

Drug classes
Corticosteroid (intermediate acting)
Glucocorticoid
Hormone

Therapeutic actions

Enters target cells and binds to cytoplasmic receptors, thereby initiating many complex reactions that are responsible for its anti-inflammatory and immunosuppressive effects.

Indications

- Hypercalcemia associated with cancer (systemic)
- Short-term management of various inflammatory and allergic disorders, such as rheumatoid arthritis, collagen diseases (eg, SLE), dermatologic diseases (eg, pemphigus), status asthmaticus, and autoimmune disorders
- Hematologic disorders: thrombocytopenia purpura, erythroblastopenia
- Ulcerative colitis, acute exacerbations of multiple sclerosis, and palliation in some leukemias and lymphomas
- Trichinosis with neurologic or myocardial involvement
- Pulmonary emphysema with bronchial spasm or edema; diffuse interstitial pulmonary fibrosis; with diuretics in CHF with refractory edema and in cirrhosis with refractory ascites
- Postoperative dental inflammatory reactions
- Arthritis, psoriatic plaques, and so forth (intra-articular, soft-tissue administration)
- Control of bronchial asthma requiring corticosteroids in conjunction with other therapy (respiratory inhalant)
- Prophylactic therapy in the maintenance treatment of asthma (bid use)
- To relieve inflammatory and pruritic manifestations of dermatoses that are steroid responsive (dermatologic preparations)
- Treatment of seasonal and perennial allergic-rhinitis symptoms (nasal spray)

Contraindications and cautions

- Contraindicated with infections, especially tuberculosis, fungal infectons, amebiasis, vaccinia and varicella, and antibiotic-resistant infections; lactation.
- Use cautiously with pregnancy (teratogenic in preclinical studies); kidney or liver disease, hypothyroidism, ulcerative colitis with impending perforation, diverticulitis, active or latent peptic ulcer, inflammatory bowel disease, CHF, hypertension, thromboembol-

ic disorders, osteoporosis, convulsive disorders, diabetes mellitus.

Available forms

Tablets—1, 2, 4, 8 mg; syrup—4 mg/5 mL; injection—5, 20, 25, 40 mg/mL; aerosol—100 mcg/actuation; topical ointment—0.25, 0.1, 0.5%; cream—0.25, 0.1, 0.5%; lotion—0.025, 0.1%; nasal spray—50, 55 mcg/actuation

Dosages

Systemic

Adults: Individualize dosage, depending on the severity of the condition and the patient's response. Administer daily dose before 9 AM to minimize adrenal suppression. If long-term therapy is needed, consider alternate-day therapy. After long-term therapy, withdraw drug slowly to avoid adrenal insufficiency. For maintenance therapy, reduce initial dose in small increments at intervals until the lowest effective dose is reached.

Pediatric patients: Individualize dosage, depending on the severity of the condition and the patient's response rather than by formulae that correct adult doses for age or body weight. Carefully observe growth and development in infants and children on prolonged therapy.

Oral (triamcinolone)

- *Adrenal insufficiency:* 4–12 mg/day, plus a mineralocorticoid.
- *Rheumatic, dermatologic, allergic, ophthalmologic, hematologic disorders and asthma:* 8–60 mg/day.
- *TB meningitis:* 32–48 mg/day.
- *Acute leukemia:*

Adults: 16–40 mg up to 100 mg/day.
Pediatric patients: 1–2 mg/kg/day.

IM

Triamcinolone acetonide: 2.5–60 mg/day.
Triamcinolone diacetate: 40 mg/wk. A single parenteral dose 4–7 times oral daily dose provides control for 4 days–4 wk.

Intra-articular, intralesional

Dose will vary with joint or soft-tissue site to be injected.
Triamcinolone acetonide: 2.5–15 mg.
Triamcinolone diacetate: 5–40 mg intra-articular; 5–48 mg intralesional; do not use

T

> 12.5 mg per injection site or 25 mg per lesion.
Triamcinolone hexacetatonide: 2–20 mg intraarticular; up to 0.5 mg/square inch of affected area intralesional.

Respiratory inhalant (triamcinolone acetonide)
200 mcg released with each actuation delivers about 100 mcg to the patient.
Adults: 2 inhalations tid–qid, not to exceed 16 inhalations/day.
Pediatric patients 6–12 yr: 1–2 inhalations tid–qid, not to exceed 12 inhalations/day.

Nasal spray
2 sprays in each nostril daily—maximum of 4 sprays/day.

Topical dermatologic preparations
Apply sparingly to affected area bid–qid.

Pharmacokinetics

Route	Onset	Peak	Duration
Oral	24–48 hr	1–2 hr	2.25 days
IM	24–48 hr	8–10 hr	1–6 wk

Metabolism: Hepatic; $T_{1/2}$: 2–5 hr
Distribution: Crosses placenta; enters breast milk
Excretion: Urine

Adverse effects
Effects depend on dose, route, and duration of therapy.

- **CNS:** *Vertigo, headache,* paresthesias, insomnia, convulsions, psychosis, cataracts, increased intraocular pressure, glaucoma (long-term therapy)
- **CV:** Hypotension, shock, hypertension and CHF secondary to fluid retention, thromboembolism, thrombophlebitis, fat embolism, cardiac arrhythmias
- **Electrolyte imbalance:** *Na+ and fluid retention,* hypokalemia, hypocalcemia
- **Endocrine:** Amenorrhea, irregular menses, growth retardation, decreased carbohydrate tolerance, diabetes mellitus, cushingoid state (long-term effect), increased blood sugar, increased serum cholesterol, decreased T_3 and T_4 levels, hypothalamic-pituitary-adrenal (HPA) suppression with systemic therapy longer than 5 days

- **GI:** Peptic or esophageal ulcer, pancreatitis, abdominal distention, nausea, vomiting, *increased appetite, weight gain* (long-term therapy)
- **Hypersensitivity:** Hypersensitivity or anaphylactoid reactions
- **Musculoskeletal:** Muscle weakness, steroid myopathy, loss of muscle mass, osteoporosis, spontaneous fractures (long-term therapy)
- **Other:** *Immunosuppression, aggravation, or masking of infections; impaired wound healing;* thin, fragile skin; petechiae, ecchymoses, purpura, striae; subcutaneous fat atrophy

Intra-articular
- **Local:** Osteonecrosis, tendon rupture, infection

Intralesional (face and head)
- **Local:** Blindness (rare)

Respiratory inhalants
- **Local:** Oral, laryngeal, and pharyngeal irritation; fungal infections

Topical dermatologic ointments, creams, sprays
- **Local:** Local burning, irritation, acneiform lesions, striae, skin atrophy

Interactions
✷ Drug-drug • Increased therapeutic and toxic effects with troleandomycin • Risk of severe deterioration of muscle strength when given to myasthenia gravis patients who are also receiving ambenonium, edrophonium, neostigmine, pyridostigmine • Decreased steroid blood levels with barbiturates, phenytoin, rifampin • Decreased effectiveness of salicylates
✷ Drug-lab test • False-negative nitrobluetetrazolium test for bacterial infection • Suppression of skin test reactions

■ Nursing considerations
Assessment
- **History:** Infections; kidney or liver disease; hypothyroidism; ulcerative colitis with impending perforation; diverticulitis; active or latent peptic ulcer; inflammatory bowel disease; CHF; hypertension; thromboembolic disorders; osteoporosis; convulsive disorders; diabetes mellitus; pregnancy; lactation

- **Physical:** Weight, T, reflexes and grip strength, affect and orientation, P, BP, peripheral perfusion, prominence of superficial veins, R, adventitious sounds, serum electrolytes, blood glucose

Interventions

- Administer once-a-day doses before 9 AM to mimic normal peak corticosteroid blood levels.
- Increase dosage when patient is subject to stress.
- Taper doses when discontinuing high-dose or long-term therapy.
- Do not give live virus vaccines with immunosuppressive doses of corticosteroids.
- Taper systemic steroids carefully during transfer to inhalational steroids; deaths caused by adrenal insufficiency have occurred.
- Use caution when occlusive dressings, tight diapers, and so forth cover affected area; these can increase systemic absorption when using topical preparations.
- Avoid prolonged use of topical preparations near the eyes, in genital and rectal areas, and in skin creases.

Teaching points

- Do not stop taking the drug without consulting your health care provider.
- Avoid exposure to infections.
- Report unusual weight gain, swelling of the extremities, muscle weakness, black or tarry stools, fever, prolonged sore throat, colds or other infections, worsening of your disorder.

Intra-articular administration
- Do not overuse joint after therapy, even if pain is gone.

Respiratory inhalant
- Do not use during an acute asthmatic attack or to manage status asthmaticus.
- Do not use with systemic fungal infections.
- Do not use more often than prescribed.
- Do not stop using this drug without consulting your health care provider.
- Administer inhalational bronchodilator drug first, if receiving concomitant bronchodilator therapy; rinse mouth after use.

Nasal spray
- Do not spray in eyes.

- Prime pump before first use and again if not used for > 2 wk.

Topical dermatologic preparations
- Apply drug sparingly, avoid contact with eyes.
- Report irritation or infection at the site of application.

▽ triamterene
*(trye **am**' ter een)*

Dyrenium

PREGNANCY CATEGORY B

Drug class
Potassium-sparing diuretic

Therapeutic actions
Inhibits sodium reabsorption in the renal distal tubule, causing loss of sodium and water and retention of potassium.

Indications
- Edema associated with CHF, nephrotic syndrome, hepatic cirrhosis; steroid-induced edema, edema from secondary hyperaldosteronism (alone or with other diuretics for added diuretic or antikaliuretic effects)

Contraindications and cautions
- Contraindicated with allergy to triamterene, hyperkalemia, renal disease (except nephrosis), liver disease, lactation.
- Use cautiously with diabetes mellitus, pregnancy.

Available forms
Capsules—50, 100 mg

Dosages
Adults
100 mg bid PO if used alone. Reduce dosage if added to other diuretic or antihypertensive therapy. Maintenance dosage should be individualized, may be as low as 100 mg every other day. Do not exceed 300 mg/day.

Pediatric patients
Safety and efficacy not established.

Pharmacokinetics

Route	Onset	Peak	Duration
Oral	2–4 hr	6–8 hr	12–16 hr

Metabolism: Hepatic; T$_{1/2}$: 3 hr
Distribution: Crosses placenta; enters breast milk
Excretion: Urine

Adverse effects

- **CNS:** *Headache,* drowsiness, fatigue, *weakness*
- **Dermatologic:** Rash, photosensitivity
- **GI:** *Nausea, anorexia, vomiting, dry mouth,* diarrhea
- **GU:** Renal stones, interstitial nephritis
- **Hematologic: Hyperkalemia,** blood dyscrasias

Interactions

✳ Drug-drug • Increased hyperkalemia with potassium supplements, diets rich in potassium, ACE inhibitors • Increased serum levels and possible toxicity with cimetidine, indomethacin • Increased risk of amantadine toxicity

✳ Drug-lab test • Interference with fluorescent measurement of serum quinidine levels

■ Nursing considerations
Assessment

- **History:** Allergy to triamterene, hyperkalemia, renal or liver disease, diabetes mellitus, pregnancy, lactation
- **Physical:** Skin color, lesions, edema; orientation, reflexes, muscle strength; pulses, baseline ECG, BP; R, pattern, adventitious sounds; liver evaluation, bowel sounds; urinary output patterns; CBC, serum electrolytes, blood sugar, liver and renal function tests, urinalysis

Interventions

- Administer with food or milk if GI upset occurs.
- Mark calendars or provide other reminders of drug days for outpatients if alternate-day or 3- to 5-day/wk therapy is optimal for treating edema.
- Administer early in the day so that increased urination does not disturb sleep.
- Measure and record regular weights to monitor mobilization of edema fluid.
- Arrange for regular evaluation of serum electrolytes, BUN.

Teaching points

- Record alternate-day therapy on a calendar, or make dated envelopes. Take the drug early in the day as increased urination will occur. The drug may be taken with food or meals if GI upset occurs.
- Weigh yourself on a regular basis, at the same time and in the same clothing, and record the weight on your calendar.
- These side effects may occur: increased volume and frequency of urination; drowsiness (avoid rapid position changes; do not engage in hazardous activities [eg, driving a car]; this problem is often made worse by the use of alcohol); avoid foods that are rich in potassium (eg, fruits, *Sanka*); sensitivity to sunlight and bright lights (wear sunglasses, use sunscreens and protective clothing).
- Report weight change of more than 3 lb in one day, swelling in ankles or fingers, fever, sore throat, mouth sores, unusual bleeding or bruising, dizziness, trembling, numbness, fatigue.

▽**triazolam**
(trye ay' zoe lam)

Alti-Triazolam (CAN), Apo-Triazo (CAN), Halcion, Novo-Triolam (CAN)

PREGNANCY CATEGORY X

C-IV CONTROLLED SUBSTANCE

Drug classes
Benzodiazepine
Sedative and hypnotic

Therapeutic actions
Exact mechanisms of action not understood; acts mainly at subcortical levels of the CNS, leaving the cortex relatively unaffected; main sites of action may be the limbic system and

mesencephalic reticular formation; benzodiazepines potentiate the effects of GABA, an inhibitory neurotransmitter.

Indications

- Insomnia characterized by difficulty falling asleep, frequent nocturnal awakenings, or early morning awakening (short-term use: 7–10 days)
- Recurring insomnia or poor sleeping habits
- Acute or chronic medical situations requiring restful sleep

Contraindications and cautions

- Contraindicated with hypersensitivity to benzodiazepines; pregnancy (risk of congenital malformations, neonatal withdrawal syndrome); labor and delivery ("floppy infant" syndrome); lactation (infants may become lethargic and lose weight).
- Use cautiously with impaired liver or kidney function, debilitation, depression, suicidal tendencies.

Available forms

Tablets—0.125, 0.25 mg

Dosages
Adults
0.125–0.5 mg PO before retiring.
Pediatric patients
Not for use in patients < 18 yr.
Geriatric patients or patients with debilitating disease
Initially, 0.125–0.25 mg PO. Adjust as needed and tolerated.

Pharmacokinetics

Route	Onset	Peak
Oral	Varies	30 min–2 hr

Metabolism: Hepatic; $T_{1/2}$: 1.5–5.5 hr
Distribution: Crosses placenta; enters breast milk
Excretion: Urine

Adverse effects

- **CNS:** *Transient, mild drowsiness initially; sedation, depression, lethargy,* apathy, fatigue, *light-headedness, disorientation, restlessness, confusion,* crying, delirium, headache, slurred speech, dysarthria, stupor, rigidity, tremor, dystonia, vertigo, euphoria, nervousness, difficulty in concentration, vivid dreams, psychomotor retardation, extrapyramidal symptoms; *mild paradoxical excitatory reactions during first 2 wk of treatment* (especially in psychiatric patients, aggressive children, and with high dosage), visual and auditory disturbances, diplopia, nystagmus, depressed hearing, nasal congestion, retrograde amnesia, "traveler's amnesia"
- **CV:** *Bradycardia, tachycardia,* CV collapse, hypertension and hypotension, palpitations, edema
- **Dependence:** *Drug dependence with withdrawal syndrome* when drug is discontinued (more common with abrupt discontinuation of higher dosage used for longer than 4 mo)
- **Dermatologic:** Urticaria, pruritus, rash, dermatitis
- **GI:** *Constipation, diarrhea,* dry mouth, salivation, nausea, anorexia, vomiting, difficulty in swallowing, gastric disorders, elevations of blood enzymes: hepatic dysfunction, jaundice
- **GU:** *Incontinence, urinary retention, changes in libido,* menstrual irregularities
- **Hematologic:** Decreased Hct, blood dyscrasias
- **Other:** Hiccups, fever, diaphoresis, paresthesias, muscular disturbances, gynecomastia

Interactions

✷ Drug-drug • Increased CNS depression and sedation with alcohol, cimetidine, omeprazole, disulfiram, hormonal contraceptives • Decreased sedative effects with theophylline, aminophylline, dyphylline, oxitriphylline • Potentially serious to fatal reactions with ketoconazole, itraconazole; avoid this combination

✷ Drug-food • Decreased metabolism and risk of toxic effects if combined with grapefruit juice; avoid this combination

■ Nursing considerations
Assessment

- **History:** Hypersensitivity to benzodiazepines; pregnancy, lactation; impaired liver or kidney function; debilitation, depression, suicidal tendencies

- **Physical:** Skin color, lesions; T; orientation, reflexes, affect, ophthalmologic exam; P, BP; R, adventitious sounds; liver evaluation, abdominal exam, bowel sounds, normal output; CBC, liver and renal function tests

Interventions
- Arrange for periodic blood counts, urinalyses, and blood chemistry analyses with protracted treatment.
- Taper dosage gradually after long-term therapy, especially in epileptic patients.

Teaching points
- Take drug exactly as prescribed. Do not drink grapefruit juice while on this drug.
- Do not stop taking this drug (long-term therapy) without consulting your health care provider.
- Avoid alcohol, sleep-inducing, and OTC drugs.
- Avoid pregnancy while taking this drug; use of contraceptives is advised; serious fetal harm could occur.
- These side effects may occur: drowsiness, dizziness (may lessen; avoid driving or engaging in hazardous activities); GI upset (take drug with food); depression, dreams, emotional upset, crying; disturbance of nocturnal sleep for several nights after discontinuing the drug.
- Report severe dizziness, weakness, drowsiness that persists, rash or skin lesions, palpitations, swelling of the extremities, visual changes, difficulty voiding.

▽ trichlormethiazide
(trye klor meth eye' a zide)

Diurese, Metahydrin, Naqua, Trichlorex (CAN)

PREGNANCY CATEGORY C

Drug class
Thiazide diuretic

Therapeutic actions
Inhibits reabsorption of sodium and chloride in distal renal tubule, thereby increasing excretion of sodium, chloride, and water by the kidney.

Indications
- Adjunctive therapy in edema associated with CHF, cirrhosis, corticosteroid and estrogen therapy, renal dysfunction
- Hypertension, as sole therapy or in combination with other antihypertensives
- Unlabeled uses: calcium nephrolithiasis alone or with amiloride or allopurinol to prevent recurrences in hypercalciuric or normal calciuric patients, diabetes insipidus, especially nephrogenic diabetes insipidus

Contraindications and cautions
- Contraindicated with hypersensitivity to thiazides or related diuretics or sulfonamide-derived drugs, fluid or electrolyte imbalances, pregnancy, lactation, allergy to tartrazine or aspirin (tartrazine contained in tablets marketed under the name *Metahydrin*).
- Use cautiously with renal or liver disease, gout, SLE, glucose tolerance abnormalities, hyperparathyroidism, manic-depressive disorders.

Available forms
Tablets—2, 4 mg

Dosages
Adults
- *Edema, hypertension:* 2–4 mg PO daily.
- *Calcium nephrolithiasis:* 4 mg/day PO.

Pediatric patients
0.07 mg/kg/day PO or 2 mg/m^2/day PO in divided doses.

Pharmacokinetics

Route	Onset	Peak	Duration
Oral	2 hr	6 hr	24 hr

Metabolism: Hepatic; $T_{1/2}$: 2.3–7.3 hr
Distribution: Crosses placenta; enters breast milk
Excretion: Urine

Adverse effects

- **CNS:** *Dizziness, vertigo,* paresthesias, weakness, headache, drowsiness, fatigue, leukopenia, thrombocytopenia, agranulocytosis, aplastic anemia, neutropenia
- **CV:** Orthostatic hypotension, venous thrombosis, volume depletion, cardiac arrhythmias, chest pain
- **Dermatologic:** Photosensitivity, rash, purpura, exfoliative dermatitis, hives
- **GI:** *Nausea, anorexia, vomiting, dry mouth,* diarrhea, constipation, jaundice, hepatitis, pancreatitis
- **GU:** *Polyuria, nocturia,* impotence, decreased libido
- **Other:** Muscle cramps and muscle spasms, fever, gouty attacks, flushing, weight loss, rhinorrhea

Interactions

✳ Drug-drug • Risk of hyperglycemia with diazoxide • Decreased absorption with cholestyramine, colestipol • Increased risk of digitalis glycoside toxicity if hypokalemia occurs • Increased risk of lithium toxicity with thiazides • Increased fasting blood glucose leading to need to adjust dosage of antidiabetic agents

✳ Drug-lab test • Decreased PBI levels without clinical signs of thyroid disturbances

■ Nursing considerations
Assessment

- **History:** Fluid or electrolyte imbalances; renal or liver disease; gout; SLE; glucose tolerance abnormalities; hyperparathyroidism; manic-depressive disorders; pregnancy, lactation; allergy to tartrazine or aspirin
- **Physical:** Skin color and lesions; orientation, reflexes, muscle strength; P, BP, orthostatic BP, perfusion, edema, baseline ECG; R, adventitious sounds; liver evaluation, bowel sounds; CBC, serum electrolytes, blood glucose, liver and renal function tests, serum uric acid, urinalysis

Interventions

- Do not use this drug during pregnancy.
- Administer with food or milk if GI upset occurs.
- Mark calendars or provide other reminders of drug days for outpatients on alternate-day or 3- to 5-day/wk therapy.
- Administer early in the day so increased urination will not disturb sleep.

Teaching points

- Take drug early in the day so sleep will not be disturbed by increased urination.
- Weigh yourself daily, and record weights on your calendar.
- Protect skin from exposure to sun or bright lights.
- Increased urination will occur.
- This drug cannot be taken during pregnancy; use of contraceptive measures is advised.
- Use caution if dizziness, drowsiness, feeling faint occur.
- Report rapid weight change, swelling in ankles or fingers, unusual bleeding or bruising, muscle cramps.

▽ trientine hydrochloride

See *Less Commonly Used Drugs,* p. 1354.

▽ trifluoperazine hydrochloride

*(trye floo oh **per**' a zeen)*

Apo-Trifluoperazine (CAN), Stelazine

PREGNANCY CATEGORY C

Drug classes

Phenothiazine (piperazine)
Dopaminergic blocking agent
Antipsychotic
Antianxiety agent

Therapeutic actions

Mechanism of action not fully understood: antipsychotic drugs block postsynaptic dopamine receptors in the brain, but this may not be necessary and sufficient for antipsychotic activity; depresses the RAS, including the parts of the brain involved with wakefulness and emesis; anticholinergic, antihistaminic (H_1), and alpha-adrenergic blocking activity also may contribute to some of its therapeutic (and adverse) actions.

Indications

- Management of schizophrenia

- Short-term treatment of nonpsychotic anxiety (not drug of choice)

Contraindications and cautions
- Contraindicated with coma or severe CNS depression, bone marrow depression, blood dyscrasia, circulatory collapse, subcortical brain damage, Parkinson's disease, liver damage, cerebral arteriosclerosis, coronary disease, severe hypotension or hypertension, sensitivity to phenothiazines.
- Use cautiously with respiratory disorders ("silent pneumonia"); glaucoma, prostatic hypertrophy; epilepsy or history of epilepsy (lowers seizure threshold); breast cancer; thyrotoxicosis (severe neurotoxicity); peptic ulcer, decreased renal function; myelography within previous 24 hr or scheduled within 48 hr; exposure to heat or phosphorous insecticides; pregnancy; lactation; children < 12 yr, especially those with chickenpox, CNS infections (children are especially susceptible to dystonias that may confound the diagnosis of Reye's syndrome).

Available forms
Tablets—1, 2, 5, 10 mg; concentrate—10 mg/mL; injection—2 mg/mL

Dosages
Adults
- *Schizophrenia:*
Oral
2–5 mg bid. Start small or emaciated patients on the lower dosage. Most patients will show optimum response with 15 or 20 mg/day. Optimum dosage should be reached within 2–3 wk. Do not exceed 40 mg/day.
IM
For prompt control of severe symptoms, 1–2 mg by deep IM injection q 4–6 hr, as needed. Do not give more often than q 4 hr. More than 6 mg/day is rarely needed. More than 10 mg/day should be given only in exceptional cases.
Pediatric patients
Adjust dosage to weight of child and severity of symptoms. The following dosages are for hospitalized or closely supervised children 6–12 yr:

Oral
Initially, 1 mg daily–bid. It is usually not necessary to exceed 15 mg/day. Older children with severe symptoms may require higher dosage.
IM
For prompt control of severe symptoms, 1 mg daily–bid.
Geriatric patients
Use lower doses, and increase dosage more gradually than in younger patients.
- *Nonpsychotic anxiety:* Usual dose 1–2 mg bid. Do not administer > 6 mg/day or for > 12 wk.

Pharmacokinetics

Route	Onset	Peak	Duration
Oral	Varies	2–4 hr	< 12 hr
IM	Rapid	1–2 hr	< 12 hr

Metabolism: Hepatic; $T_{1/2}$: 47–100 hr
Distribution: Crosses placenta; enters breast milk
Excretion: Bile and feces

Adverse effects
- **Autonomic:** *Dry mouth, salivation, nasal congestion, nausea,* vomiting, anorexia, fever, pallor, flushed facies, sweating, constipation, paralytic ileus, urinary retention, incontinence, polyuria, enuresis, priapism, ejaculation inhibition, male impotence
- **CNS:** *Drowsiness,* insomnia, vertigo, headache, weakness, tremor, ataxia, slurring, cerebral edema, seizures, exacerbation of psychotic symptoms, extrapyramidal syndromes—*pseudoparkinsonism; dystonias; akathisia;* tardive dyskinesias, potentially irreversible (no known treatment), **neuroleptic malignant syndrome**
- **CV:** Hypotension, orthostatic hypotension, hypertension, tachycardia, bradycardia, cardiac arrest, CHF, cardiomegaly, **refractory arrhythmias, pulmonary edema**
- **EENT:** Glaucoma, *photophobia, blurred vision,* miosis, mydriasis, deposits in the cornea and lens (opacities), pigmentary retinopathy
- **Endocrine:** Lactation, breast engorgement, galactorrhea; SIADH; amenorrhea, menstrual irregularities; gynecomastia; changes in libido; hyperglycemia or hypoglycemia;

Adverse effects in *Italics* are most common; those in **Bold** are life-threatening.

glycosuria; hyponatremia; pituitary tumor with hyperprolactinemia; inhibition of ovulation, infertility, pseudopregnancy; reduced urinary levels of gonadotropins, estrogens, progestins

- **Hematologic:** Eosinophilia, leukopenia, leukocytosis, anemia; aplastic anemia; hemolytic anemia; thrombocytopenic or nonthrombocytopenic purpura; pancytopenia
- **Hypersensitivity:** Jaundice, urticaria, angioneurotic edema, laryngeal edema, photosensitivity, eczema, asthma, anaphylactoid reactions, exfoliative dermatitis
- **Respiratory:** Bronchospasm, laryngospasm, dyspnea, suppression of cough reflex and potential for aspiration
- **Other:** *Urine discolored pink to red-brown*

Interactions

✳ Drug-drug • Additive CNS depression with alcohol • Additive anticholinergic effects and possibly decreased antipsychotic efficacy with anticholinergic drugs • Increased likelihood of seizures with metrizamide • Increased frequency and severity of neuromuscular excitation and hypotension in patients who are premedicated with trifluoperazine and are given barbiturate anesthetics (methohexital, thiamylal, phenobarbital, thiopental) • Decreased antihypertensive effect of guanethidine

✳ Drug-lab test • False-positive pregnancy tests (less likely if serum test is used) • Increase in PBI, not attributable to an increase in thyroxine

■ Nursing considerations
Assessment

- **History:** Coma or severe CNS depression; bone marrow depression; blood dyscrasia; circulatory collapse; subcortical brain damage; Parkinson's disease; liver damage; cerebral arteriosclerosis; coronary disease; severe hypotension or hypertension; respiratory disorders; glaucoma, prostatic hypertrophy; epilepsy; breast cancer; thyrotoxicosis; peptic ulcer, decreased renal function; myelography within previous 24 hr or scheduled within 48 hr; exposure to heat or phosphorous insecticides; pregnancy; lactation; chickenpox; CNS infections
- **Physical:** Weight; T; reflexes, orientation, intraocular pressure; P, BP, orthostatic BP; R, adventitious sounds; bowel sounds and normal output, liver evaluation; urinary output, prostate size; CBC; urinalysis; thyroid, liver, and kidney function tests

Interventions

- Do not change brand names; bioavailability differences have been documented.
- Dilute oral concentrate (for institutional use only) immediately before use by adding the dose to 60 mL of one of the following: tomato or fruit juice, milk, simple syrup, orange syrup, carbonated beverages, coffee, tea, or water; semisolid foods (soup, pudding) also may be used.
- Avoid skin contact with drug solution; contact dermatitis has occurred.
- Discontinue drug if serum creatinine, BUN become abnormal or WBC count is depressed.
- Monitor elderly patients for dehydration, and institute remedial measures promptly; sedation and decreased sensation of thirst related to CNS effects can lead to severe dehydration.
- Consult physician regarding appropriate warning of patient or patient's guardian about tardive dyskinesias.
- Consult physician about dosage reduction, use of anticholinergic antiparkinsonian drugs (controversial) if extrapyramidal effects occur.

Teaching points

- Take drug exactly as prescribed.
- Avoid skin contact with drug solutions.
- Avoid driving or engaging in other hazardous activities if CNS, vision changes occur.
- Avoid prolonged exposure to sun, or use a sunscreen or covering garments.
- Maintain fluid intake, and use precautions against heatstroke in hot weather.
- Report sore throat, fever, unusual bleeding or bruising, rash, weakness, tremors, impaired vision, dark urine (pink or reddish brown urine is expected), pale stools, yellowing of the skin or eyes.

▷ triflupromazine hydrochloride

*(trye flu **proe'** ma zeen)*

Vesprin

PREGNANCY CATEGORY C

Drug classes
Phenothiazine
Dopaminergic blocking agent
Antipsychotic
Antiemetic
Antianxiety agent

Therapeutic actions
Mechanism of action not fully understood: blocks postsynaptic dopamine receptors in the brain; depresses the parts of the brain involved with wakefulness and emesis; anticholinergic, antihistaminic (H_1), and alpha-adrenergic blocking.

Indications
- Control of severe nausea and vomiting
- Management of manifestations of psychotic disorders

Contraindications and cautions
- Contraindicated with allergy to triflupromazine, comatose or severely depressed states, bone marrow depression, circulatory collapse, subcortical brain damage.
- Use cautiously with Parkinson's disease; liver damage; cerebral or coronary arteriosclerosis; severe hypotension or hypertension; respiratory disorders; glaucoma; epilepsy or history of epilepsy; peptic ulcer or history of peptic ulcer; decreased renal function; prostate hypertrophy; breast cancer; thyrotoxicosis; myelography within 24 hr or scheduled within 48 hr; lactation; exposure to heat, phosphorous insecticides; children with chickenpox, CNS infections (such children are more susceptible to dystonias, which may confound the diagnosis of Reye's syndrome or other encephalopathy; may mask symptoms of Reye's syndrome, encephalopathies).

Available forms
Injection—10, 20 mg/mL

Dosages
Adults
- *Nausea and vomiting:* 5–15 mg IM q 4 hr, up to a maximum of 60 mg/day. 1 mg IV up to a maximum of 3 mg/day.
- *Psychotic disorders:* 60 mg IM, up to 150 mg/day.

Pediatric patients > 2 yr
- *Nausea and vomiting:* 0.2–0.25 mg/kg IM up to a maximum of 10 mg/day. Do not give IV.
- *Psychotic disorders:* 0.2–0.25 mg/kg IM to a maximum of 10 mg/day. Do not give IV.

Pharmacokinetics

Route	Onset	Peak	Duration
IM	10–15 min	15–20 min	4–6 hr

Metabolism: Hepatic; $T_{1/2}$: 10–20 hr
Distribution: Crosses placenta; enters breast milk
Excretion: Urine

▼ IV facts
Preparation: No further preparation required.
Infusion: Inject slowly into tubing of actively running IV over 5–10 min.

Adverse effects
- **CNS:** *Drowsiness, insomnia, vertigo,* headache, weakness, tremors, ataxia, slurring, cerebral edema, seizures, exacerbation of psychotic symptoms, *extrapyramidal syndromes;* **neuroleptic malignant syndrome**
- **CV:** *Hypotension, orthostatic hypotension,* hypertension, tachycardia, bradycardia, **cardiac arrest,** CHF, cardiomegaly, **refractory arrhythmias,** pulmonary edema
- **EENT:** Nasal congestion, glaucoma, *photophobia, blurred vision,* miosis, mydriasis, deposits in the cornea and lens, pigmentary retinopathy
- **Endocrine:** Lactation, breast engorgement, galactorrhea, SIADH secretion, amenorrhea, menstrual irregularities; gynecomastia; changes in libido, hyperglycemia, inhibi-

---

Adverse effects in *Italics* are most common; those in **Bold** are life-threatening.

tion of ovulation, infertility, pseudopregnancy, reduced urinary levels of gonadotropins, estrogens, and progestins
- **GI:** *Dry mouth, salivation, nausea, vomiting, anorexia, constipation,* paralytic ileus, incontinence
- **GU:** *Urinary retention,* polyuria, incontinence, priapism, ejaculation inhibition, male impotence, urine discolored pink to redbrown
- **Hematologic:** Eosinophilia, leukopenia, leukocytosis, *anemia,* aplastic anemia, hemolytic anemia, thrombocytopenic or nonthrombocytopenic purpura, pancytopenia, elevated serum cholesterol
- **Hypersensitivity:** Jaundice, *urticaria,* angioneurotic edema, laryngeal edema, photosensitivity, eczema, asthma, anaphylactoid reactions, exfoliative dermatitis, contact dermatitis with drug solutions
- **Respiratory:** Bronchospasm, laryngospasm, dyspnea, suppression of cough reflex and potential aspiration
- **Other:** Fever, heatstroke, pallor, flushed facies, sweating, *photosensitivity*

Interactions
✱ **Drug-drug** • Additive anticholinergic effects and possibly decreased antipsychotic efficacy with anticholinergic drugs • Additive CNS depression, hypotension if given preoperatively with barbiturate anesthetics, alcohol, meperidine • Additive effects of both drugs with beta-blockers •; Increased risk of tachycardia, hypotension with epinephrine, norepinephrine • Increased risk of seizure with metrizamide • Decreased hypotension effect with guanethidine

✱ **Drug-lab test** • False-positive pregnancy tests (less likely if serum test is used) • Increase in protein-bound iodine, not attributable to an increase in thyroxine

■ Nursing considerations
Assessment
- **History:** Allergy to trifluromazine; comatose or severely depressed states; bone marrow depression; circulatory collapse; subcortical brain damage, Parkinson's disease; liver damage; cerebral or coronary arteriosclerosis; severe hypotension or hypertension; respiratory disorders; glaucoma; epilepsy; peptic ulcer; decreased renal function; prostate hypertrophy; breast cancer; thyrotoxicosis; myelography within 24 hr or scheduled within 48 hr; lactation; exposure to heat, phosphorous insecticides; chickenpox, CNS infections
- **Physical:** T; weight, skin color, turgor; reflexes, orientation, intraocular pressure, ophthalmologic exam; P, BP, orthostatic BP, ECG; R, adventitious sounds; bowel sounds, normal output, liver evaluation; prostate palpation, normal urine output; CBC; urinalysis; thyroid, liver, and kidney function tests; EEG (as appropriate)

Interventions
- Do not give by SC injection; give slowly by deep IM injection into upper outer quadrant of buttock.
- Reserve IV use for situations when IM use is not possible. Do not use IV in children.
- Keep the patient recumbent for 30 min after injection to avoid orthostatic hypotension.
- Avoid skin contact with drug solutions; may cause contact dermatitis.
- Be alert to potential for aspiration because of suppressed cough reflex.
- Monitor renal function tests and discontinue if serum creatinine, BUN become abnormal.
- Monitor CBC and discontinue if WBC count is depressed.
- Withdraw drug gradually after high-dose therapy; gastritis, nausea, dizziness, headache, tachycardia, insomnia have occurred after abrupt withdrawal.
- Monitor elderly patients for dehydration: sedation and decreased sensation of thirst due to CNS effects can lead to dehydration, hemoconcentration, and reduced pulmonary ventilation; promptly institute remedial measures.
- Avoid use of epinephrine as vasopressor if drug-induced hypotension occurs.

Teaching points
- This drug can be given only by injection.
- These side effects may occur: drowsiness (avoid driving or operating dangerous machinery; avoid alcohol, which will increase the drowsiness); sensitivity to the sun (avoid prolonged sun exposure, and wear protective garments or use a sunscreen); pink or

T

reddish-brown urine (expected effect); faintness, dizziness (transient; change position slowly, use caution climbing stairs).
- Use caution in hot weather; you may be prone to heatstroke; keep up fluid intake, and do not exercise unduly in a hot climate.
- Report sore throat, fever, unusual bleeding or bruising, rash, weakness, tremors, impaired vision, dark urine, pale stools, yellowing of the skin and eyes.

▷trihexyphenidyl hydrochloride
*(trye hex ee **fen'** i dill)*

Apo-Trihex (CAN), Trihexy-2, Trihexy-5

PREGNANCY CATEGORY C

Drug class
Antiparkinsonian agent (anticholinergic type)

Therapeutic actions
Has anticholinergic activity in the CNS that is believed to help normalize the hypothesized imbalance of cholinergic and dopaminergic neurotransmission created by the loss of dopaminergic neurons in the basal ganglia of the brain of parkinsonism patients; reduces severity of rigidity and reduces to a lesser extent the akinesia and tremor that characterize parkinsonism; less effective overall than levodopa; peripheral anticholinergic effects suppress secondary symptoms of parkinsonism, such as drooling.

Indications
- Adjunct in the treatment of parkinsonism (postencephalitic, arteriosclerotic, and idiopathic)
- Adjuvant therapy with levodopa
- Control of drug-induced extrapyramidal disorders

Contraindications and cautions
- Contraindicated with hypersensitivity to trihexyphenidyl; glaucoma, especially angle-closure glaucoma; pyloric or duodenal obstruction, stenosing peptic ulcers, achalasia (megaesophagus); prostatic hypertrophy or bladder neck obstructions; myasthenia gravis; lactation.
- Use cautiously with cardiac arrhythmias, hypertension, hypotension, hepatic or renal dysfunction, alcoholism, chronic illness, people who work in hot environment, pregnancy.

Available forms
Tablets—2, 5 mg; SR capsules—5 mg

Dosages
Adults
Tablets
- *Parkinsonism:* 1–2 mg PO the first day. Increase by 2-mg increments at 3- to 5-day intervals until a total of 6–10 mg is given daily. Postencephalitic patients may require 12–15 mg/day. Tolerated best if daily dose is divided into three (or four) doses administered at mealtimes (and bedtime).
- *Concomitant use with levodopa:* Usual dose of each may need to be reduced; however, trihexyphenidyl has been shown to decrease bioavailability of levodopa. Adjust dosage on basis of response. 3–6 mg/day PO of trihexyphenidyl is usually adequate.
- *Concomitant use with other anticholinergics:* Gradually substitute trihexyphenidyl for all or part of the other anticholinergic and reduce dosage of the other anticholinergic gradually.
- *Drug-induced extrapyramidal symptoms:* Initially 1 mg PO. If reactions are not controlled in a few hours, progressively increase subsequent doses until control is achieved. Dose of tranquilizer may need to be reduced temporarily to expedite control of extrapyramidal symptoms. Adjust dosage of both drugs subsequently to maintain ataractic effect without extrapyramidal reactions.
Sustained-release capsules
- Do not use for initial therapy. Substitute on a milligram for milligram of total daily dose basis after patient is stabilized on conventional dosage forms. A single PO dose after breakfast or two divided doses 12 hr apart may be given.
Pediatric patients
Safety and efficacy not established.

Adverse effects in *Italics* are most common; those in **Bold** are life-threatening.

Geriatric patients
Patients > 60 yr often develop increased sensitivity to the CNS effects of anticholinergic drugs.

Pharmacokinetics

Route	Onset	Peak	Duration
Oral tablet	1 hr	2–3 hr	6–12 hr

Metabolism: Hepatic; $T_{1/2}$: 5.6–10.2 hr
Distribution: Crosses placenta; enters breast milk
Excretion: Urine

Adverse effects

- **CNS (some CNS effects are characteristic of centrally acting anticholinergic drugs):** *Disorientation, confusion,* memory loss, hallucinations, psychoses, agitation, nervousness, delusions, delirium, paranoia, euphoria, excitement, *lightheadedness, dizziness,* depression, drowsiness, weakness, giddiness, paresthesia, heaviness of the limbs, numbness of fingers, *blurred vision, mydriasis,* diplopia, increased intraocular tension, angle-closure glaucoma
- **CV:** Tachycardia, palpitations, hypotension, orthostatic hypotension
- **Dermatologic:** Rash, urticaria, other dermatoses
- **GI:** *Dry mouth, constipation,* dilation of the colon, paralytic ileus, acute suppurative parotitis, nausea, vomiting, epigastric distress
- **GU:** *Urinary retention,* urinary hesitancy, dysuria, difficulty achieving or maintaining an erection
- **Other:** Muscular weakness, muscular cramping, *flushing, decreased sweating,* elevated T

Interactions

✳ **Drug-drug** • Additive adverse CNS effects; toxic psychosis with phenothiazines • Possible masking of the development of persistent extrapyramidal symptoms, tardive dyskinesia, in patients on long-term therapy with antipsychotic drugs, such as phenothiazines, haloperidol • Decreased therapeutic efficacy of antipsychotic drugs (phenothiazines, haloperidol)

■ Nursing considerations
Assessment

- **History:** Hypersensitivity to trihexyphenidyl; glaucoma; pyloric or duodenal obstruction, stenosing peptic ulcers; achalasia; prostatic hypertrophy or bladder neck obstructions; myasthenia gravis, tachycardia, cardiac arrhythmias; hypertension, hypotension; hepatic or renal dysfunction; alcoholism; chronic illness; people who work in hot environments; pregnancy, lactation
- **Physical:** Weight; T; skin color, lesions; orientation, affect, reflexes, bilateral grip strength, visual exam, including tonometry; P, BP, orthostatic BP, auscultation; bowel sounds, normal output, liver evaluation; urinary output, voiding pattern, prostate palpation; liver and kidney function tests

Interventions

- Decrease dosage or discontinue drug temporarily if dry mouth is so severe that swallowing or speaking becomes difficult.
- Reserve use of sustained-release preparations for patients who have been stabilized on the drug.
- Give with caution and arrange dosage reduction in hot weather; drug interferes with sweating and ability of body to maintain body heat equilibrium; anhidrosis and fatal hyperthermia have occurred.
- Ensure that patient voids before receiving each dose if urinary retention is a problem.

Teaching points

- Take this drug exactly as prescribed.
- These side effects may occur: drowsiness, dizziness, confusion, blurred vision (avoid driving or engaging in activities that require alertness and visual acuity); nausea (frequent, small meals may help); dry mouth (sucking sugarless lozenges or ice chips may help); painful or difficult urination (emptying the bladder immediately before each dose may help); constipation (if maintaining adequate fluid intake and exercising regularly do not help, consult your health care provider).
- Use caution in hot weather (this drug makes you more susceptible to heat prostration).
- Report difficult or painful urination, constipation, rapid or pounding heartbeat, confusion, eye pain, or rash.

▷ trimethobenzamide hydrochloride

*(trye meth oh **ben'** za mide)*

Oral preparations: Tigan, Trimazide

Suppositories: Tebamide, T-Gen, Tigan, Triban, Trimazide

Parenteral preparations: Tigan

PREGNANCY CATEGORY C

Drug class
Antiemetic drug (anticholinergic)

Therapeutic actions
Mechanism of action not understood; antiemetic action may be mediated through the chemoreceptor trigger zone (CTZ); impulses to the vomiting center do not appear to be affected.

Indications
• Control of nausea and vomiting

Contraindications and cautions
• Contraindicated with allergy to trimethobenzamide, benzocaine, or similar local anesthetics; uncomplicated vomiting in children (drug may contribute to development of Reye's syndrome or unfavorably influence its outcome; extrapyramidal effects of drugs may obscure diagnosis of Reye's syndrome); pregnancy.
• Use cautiously with lactation; acute febrile illness, encephalitis, gastroenteritis, dehydration, electrolyte imbalance, especially when these occur in children, the elderly, or debilitated; narrow-angle glaucoma; stenosing peptic ulcer; symptomatic prostatic hypertrophy; bronchial asthma; bladder neck obstruction; pyloroduodenal obstruction; cardiac arrhythmias; recent use of CNS-acting drugs (phenothiazine, barbiturates, belladonna alkaloids).

Available forms
Capsules—100, 250 mg; suppositories—100, 200 mg; injection—100 mg/mL

Dosages
Adults
Oral
250 mg tid–qid.
Rectal suppositories
200 mg tid–qid.
Parenteral
200 mg IM tid–qid.
Pediatric patients
Do not administer parenterally to children.
Oral
30–90 lb: (13.6–40.9 kg): 100–200 mg tid–qid.
Rectal suppositories
30–90 lb: 100–200 mg tid–qid.
< 30 lb: 100 mg tid–qid.
Premature infants and neonates
Not recommended.
Geriatric patients
More likely to cause serious adverse reactions in elderly patients; use with caution.

Pharmacokinetics

Route	Onset	Duration
Oral	10–40 min	3–4 hr
IM	15 min	2–3 hr

Metabolism: Hepatic; $T_{1/2}$: unknown
Distribution: Crosses placenta; enters breast milk
Excretion: Urine

Adverse effects
• **CNS:** Parkinsonlike symptoms, coma, convulsions, opisthotonus, depression, disorientation, *dizziness, drowsiness, headache, blurred vision*
• **CV:** Hypotension
• **GI:** Diarrhea
• **Hematologic:** Blood dyscrasias, jaundice
• **Hypersensitivity:** Allergic-type skin reactions
• *Local: Pain following IM injections*

■ Nursing considerations
Assessment
• **History:** Allergy to trimethobenzamide, benzocaine, or similar local anesthetics; uncomplicated vomiting in children; pregnancy; lactation; acute febrile illness, encephalitis, gastroenteritis, dehydration,

---

Adverse effects in *Italics* are most common; those in **Bold** are life-threatening.

electrolyte imbalance; narrow-angle glaucoma; stenosing peptic ulcer; symptomatic prostatic hypertrophy; bronchial asthma; bladder neck obstruction; pyloroduodenal obstruction; cardiac arrhythmias

- **Physical:** Skin color, lesions, texture; T; orientation, reflexes, affect; vision exam; P, BP; R, adventitious sounds; bowel sounds; prostate palpation; CBC, serum electrolytes

Interventions
- Administer IM injections deep into upper outer quadrant of the gluteal region.
- Teach patient technique of administering rectal suppositories, as appropriate.
- Ensure adequate hydration.

Teaching points
- Take as prescribed. Use proper technique for administering rectal suppositories. Avoid excessive dosage.
- These side effects may occur: dizziness, sedation, drowsiness (use caution if driving or performing tasks that require alertness); diarrhea; blurred vision (reversible).
- Avoid alcohol while taking this drug; serious sedation could occur.
- Report difficulty breathing, tremors, loss of coordination, sore muscles or muscle spasms, unusual bleeding or bruising, sore throat, visual disturbances, irregular heartbeat, yellowing of the skin or eyes.

▽trimethoprim (TMP)
(trye **meth'** oh prim)

Primsol, Proloprim, Trimpex

PREGNANCY CATEGORY C

Drug class
Antibacterial

Therapeutic actions
Inhibits the synthesis of nucleic acids and proteins in susceptible bacteria; the bacterial enzyme involved in this reaction is more readily inhibited than the mammalian enzyme.

Indications
- Uncomplicated urinary tract infections caused by susceptible strains of E. coli, Pro-

teus mirabilis, Klebsiella pneumoniae, Enterobacter species, and coagulase-negative Staphylococcus species, including Staphylococcus saprophyticus
- Treatment of acute otitis media due to susceptible strains of S. pneumoniae and H. influenza in children

Contraindications and cautions
- Contraindicated with allergy to trimethoprim, pregnancy (teratogenic in preclinical studies), megaloblastic anemia due to folate deficiency.
- Use cautiously with hepatic or renal dysfunction, lactation.

Available forms
Tablets—100, 200 mg; solution—50 mg/5 mL

Dosages
Adults
100 mg PO q 12 hr or 200 mg q 24 hr for 10 days.
Pediatric patients
- Otitis media: 10 mg/kg/day in divided doses q 12 hr for 10 days.
Geriatric patients or patients with renal impairment
Creatinine clearance of 15–30 mL/min, 50 mg PO q 12 hr; creatinine clearance of < 15 mL/min, not recommended.

Pharmacokinetics

Route	Onset	Peak
Oral	Varies	1–4 hr

Metabolism: Hepatic; $T_{1/2}$: 8–10 hr
Distribution: Crosses placenta; enters breast milk
Excretion: Urine

Adverse effects
- **Dermatologic:** Rash, pruritus, exfoliative dermatitis
- **GI:** Epigastric distress, nausea, vomiting, glossitis
- **Hematologic:** Thrombocytopenia, leukopenia, neutropenia, megaloblastic anemia, methemoglobinemia, elevated serum transaminase and bilirubin, increased BUN and serum creatinine levels
- **Other:** Fever

■ Nursing considerations
Assessment
- **History:** Allergy to trimethoprim, megaloblastic anemia due to folate deficiency, renal or hepatic dysfunction, pregnancy, lactation
- **Physical:** Skin color, lesions; T; status of mucous membranes; CBC; liver and renal function tests

Interventions
- Perform culture and sensitivity tests before beginning drug therapy.
- Protect the 200-mg tablets from exposure to light.
- Arrange for regular, periodic blood counts during therapy.
- Discontinue drug, consult with physician if any significant reduction in any formed blood element occurs.

Teaching points
- Take the full course of the drug; take all the tablets prescribed.
- These side effects may occur: epigastric distress, nausea, vomiting (small, frequent meals may help); rash (consult with your health care provider for appropriate skin care).
- Have periodic medical checkups, including blood tests.
- Report fever, sore throat, unusual bleeding or bruising, dizziness, headaches, rash.

▽ trimetrexate glucuronate
(tri meh trex' ate)

Neutrexin

PREGNANCY CATEGORY D

Drug classes
Antineoplastic
Folic acid antagonist

Therapeutic actions
Inhibits the enzyme responsible for folate activity and DNA, RNA, and protein production, leading to cell death.

Indications
- Alternate therapy with leucovorin for the treatment of moderate-to-severe *Pneumocystis carinii* pneumonia in immunocompromised patients, including patients with AIDS, who are intolerant to or refractory to trimethoprim-sulfamethoxazole therapy
- Unlabeled use: treatment of non–small-cell lung, prostate, and colorectal cancer

Contraindications and cautions
- Contraindicated with allergy to trimetrexate, leucovorin, or methotrexate; pregnancy (teratogenic in preclinical studies); lactation.
- Use cautiously with hepatic or renal dysfunction, myelosuppression.

Available forms
Powder for injection—25 mg/5 mL

Dosages
Adults
45 mg/m^2 IV once a day over 60–90 min with leucovorin IV at a dose of 20 mg/m^2 over 5–10 min q 6 hr or orally as four doses of 20 mg/m^2. Treatment course is 21 days of trimetrexate and 24 days of leucovorin.
Pediatric patients
Effectiveness for patients < 18 yr has not been established.
Geriatric patients or patients with renal, hepatic, or hematologic impairment
Reduce dosage, and monitor blood tests before proceeding to next dose.

Pharmacokinetics

Route	Onset
IV	Rapid

Metabolism: Hepatic; T$_{1/2}$: 7–15 hr
Distribution: Crosses placenta; enters breast milk
Excretion: Urine

▽ IV facts
Preparation: Reconstitute with 2 mL of 5% dextrose injection or sterile water for injection for a concentration of 12.5 mg/mL; solution should be pale greenish-yellow with no par-

---

Adverse effects in *Italics* are most common; those in **Bold** are life-threatening.

ticulates; may be further diluted with 5% dextrose to a concentration of 0.25–2 mg/mL; store at room temperature, protect from light; stable for up to 24 hr; discard after that time.
Infusion: Flush IV line with 10 mL of 5% dextrose injection before and after infusing trimetrexate; infuse diluted solution over 60 min; give leucovorin separately.

Adverse effects
- **CNS:** Confusion
- **GI:** Nausea, vomiting
- **Hematologic:** Hyponatremia, hypocalcemia; increased AST, ALT, alkaline phosphatase, bilirubin, serum creatinine, *neutropenia, thrombocytopenia,* anemia
- **Other:** *Fever,* rash, fatigue

■ Nursing considerations
Assessment
- **History:** Allergy to trimetrexate, leucovorin, or methotrexate; pregnancy, lactation; use cautiously with hepatic or renal dysfunction, myelosuppression
- **Physical:** Skin color, lesions; T; CBC; liver and renal function tests; serum electrolytes

Interventions
- Ensure that patient is not pregnant before administering; advise the use of contraceptive measures.
- Avoid contact with solution; if drug contacts skin, flush with soap and water.
- Arrange for proper disposal of drug, using disposal techniques for cytotoxic drugs.
- Ensure that leucovorin is administered as scheduled while on this drug; it is essential for safe use of trimetrexate.
- Arrange for regular, periodic blood counts and liver function tests.
- Protect patient from exposure to infection.
- Consult with physician for changes in drug dose or timing if significant reduction in formed blood elements occurs.
- Monitor for signs of electrolyte disturbances, and arrange for replacement therapy.

Teaching points
- This drug must be given IV in conjunction with another drug, leucovorin. The treatment will last for 21 and 24 days.
- These side effects may occur: nausea, vomiting (small, frequent meals may help); rash.

- This drug cannot be taken during pregnancy; contraceptive measures should be used.
- You will need regular blood tests during the drug treatment.
- Avoid exposure to infections; you may be more susceptible to infections.
- Report fever, sore throat, unusual bleeding or bruising, extreme fatigue.

▽ **trimipramine maleate**
*(trye **mi'** pra meen)*

Apo-Trimip (CAN), Novo-Tripramine (CAN), Rhotrimine (CAN), Surmontil

PREGNANCY CATEGORY C

Drug class
Tricyclic antidepressant (TCA) (tertiary amine)

Therapeutic actions
Mechanism of action unknown; the TCAs are structurally related to the phenothiazine antipsychotic drugs (eg, chlorpromazine); TCAs inhibit the presynaptic reuptake of the neurotransmitters norepinephrine and serotonin; anticholinergic at CNS and peripheral receptors; the relation of these effects to clinical efficacy is unknown.

Indications
- Relief of symptoms of depression (endogenous depression most responsive); sedative effects of tertiary amine TCAs may be helpful in patients whose depression is associated with anxiety and sleep disturbance
- Unlabeled uses: treatment of peptic ulcer disease, dermatologic disorders

Contraindications and cautions
- Contraindicated with hypersensitivity to any tricyclic drug, concomitant therapy with an MAOI, recent MI, myelography within previous 24 hr or scheduled within 48 hr, pregnancy (limb reduction abnormalities may occur), lactation.
- Use cautiously with EST; preexisting CV disorders (eg, severe CAD, progressive CHF, angina pectoris, paroxysmal tachycardia); angle-closure glaucoma, increased intraocular pressure; urinary retention, ureteral or urethral spasm (anticholinergic effects of TCAs

may exacerbate these conditions); seizure disorders (TCAs lower the seizure threshold); hyperthyroidism (predisposes to CVS toxicity, including cardiac arrhythmias); impaired hepatic, renal function; psychiatric patients (schizophrenic or paranoid patients may exhibit a worsening of psychosis); manic-depressive patients (may shift to hypomanic or manic phase); elective surgery (TCAs should be discontinued as long as possible before surgery).

Available forms
Capsules—25, 50, 100 mg

Dosages
Adults
Hospitalized patients: Initially, 100 mg/day PO in divided doses. Gradually increase to 200 mg/day as required. If no improvement in 2–3 wk, increase to a maximum dose of 250–300 mg/day.
Outpatients: Initially 75 mg/day PO in divided doses. May increase to 150 mg/day. Do not exceed 200 mg/day. Total daily dosage may be administered hs. Maintenance dose is 50–150 mg/day given as a single hs dose. After satisfactory response, reduce to lowest effective dosage. Continue therapy for 3 mo or longer to lessen possibility of relapse.
Pediatric patients
< 12 yr: Not recommended.
≥12 yr: 50 mg/day PO with gradual increases up to 100 mg/day.
Geriatric patients
50 mg/day PO with gradual increases up to 100 mg/day PO.

Pharmacokinetics

Route	Onset	Peak
Oral	Varies	2 hr

Metabolism: Hepatic; $T_{1/2}$: 7–30 hr
Distribution: Crosses placenta; enters breast milk
Excretion: Urine and feces

Adverse effects
- **CNS:** *Sedation and anticholinergic (atropine-like) effects; confusion* (especially in elderly), *disturbed concentration,*

hallucinations, disorientation, decreased memory, feelings of unreality, delusions, anxiety, nervousness, restlessness, agitation, panic, insomnia, nightmares, hypomania, mania, exacerbation of psychosis, drowsiness, weakness, fatigue, headache, numbness, tingling, paresthesias of extremities, incoordination, motor hyperactivity, akathisia, ataxia, tremors, peripheral neuropathy, extrapyramidal symptoms, *seizures,* speech blockage, dysarthria, tinnitus, altered EEG
- **CV:** *Orthostatic hypotension,* hypertension, syncope, tachycardia, palpitations, **MI**, arrhythmias, heart block, **precipitation of CHF, stroke**
- **Endocrine:** Elevated or depressed blood sugar, elevated prolactin levels, SIADH secretion
- **GI:** *Dry mouth, constipation,* paralytic ileus, *nausea,* vomiting, anorexia, epigastric distress, diarrhea, flatulence, dysphagia, peculiar taste, increased salivation, stomatitis, glossitis, parotid swelling, abdominal cramps, black tongue, hepatitis, jaundice (rare), elevated transaminase, altered alkaline phosphatase
- **GU:** Urinary retention, delayed micturition, dilation of the urinary tract, gynecomastia, testicular swelling; breast enlargement, menstrual irregularity and galactorrhea; increased or decreased libido; impotence
- **Hematologic:** Bone marrow depression including agranulocytosis; eosinophila, purpura, thrombocytopenia, leukopenia
- **Hypersensitivity:** Rash, pruritus, vasculitis, petechiae, photosensitization, edema (generalized, facial, tongue), drug fever
- **Withdrawal:** Symptoms with abrupt discontinuation of prolonged therapy: nausea, headache, vertigo, nightmares, malaise
- **Other:** Nasal congestion, excessive appetite, weight gain or loss, sweating, alopecia, lacrimation, hyperthermia, flushing, chills

Interactions
✳ Drug-drug • Increased TCA levels and pharmacologic (especially anticholinergic) effects with cimetidine, fluoxetine, ranitidine • Risk of arrhythmias and hypertension with sympathomimetics • Risk of severe hypertension with clonidine • Decreased hypoten-

sive activity of guanethidine ● Risk of life-threatening cardiac arrhythmias if combined with fluoroquinolone antibiotics; avoid this combination ● Hyperpyretic crises, severe convulsions, hypertensive episodes and deaths with MAOIs. *Note:* MAOIs and TCAs have been used successfully in some patients resistant to therapy with single agents; however, case reports indicate that the combination can cause serious and potentially fatal adverse effects

■ Nursing considerations
Assessment
- **History:** Hypersensitivity to any tricyclic drug; concomitant therapy with an MAOI; recent MI; myelography within previous 24 hr or scheduled within 48 hr; pregnancy; lactation; EST; preexisting CV disorders; angle-closure glaucoma, increased intraocular pressure; urinary retention, ureteral or urethral spasm; seizure disorders; hyperthyroidism; impaired hepatic, renal function; psychiatric patients; manic-depressive patients; elective surgery
- **Physical:** Weight; T; skin color, lesions; orientation, affect, reflexes, vision and hearing; P, BP, orthostatic BP, perfusion; bowel sounds, normal output, liver evaluation; urine flow, normal output; usual sexual function, frequency of menses, breast and scrotal examination; liver function tests, urinalysis; CBC, ECG

Interventions
- Ensure that depressed and potentially suicidal patients have access to limited quantities of the drug.
- Administer major portion of dose at bedtime if drowsiness, severe anticholinergic effects occur.
- Reduce dosage if minor side effects develop; discontinue if serious side effects occur.
- Arrange for CBC if patient develops fever, sore throat, or other sign of infection.

Teaching points
- Take drug exactly as prescribed.
- Do not stop taking this drug abruptly or without consulting your health care provider.
- Avoid alcohol, other sleep-inducing drugs, and OTC drugs.
- Avoid prolonged exposure to sunlight or sunlamps; use a sunscreen or protective garments.

- These side effects may occur: headache, dizziness, drowsiness, weakness, blurred vision (reversible; safety measures may need to be taken if severe; avoid driving or performing tasks that require alertness); nausea, vomiting, loss of appetite, dry mouth (small, frequent meals, frequent mouth care, sucking sugarless candies may help); nightmares, inability to concentrate, confusion; changes in sexual function.
- Report dry mouth, difficulty in urination, excessive sedation.

▷ tripelennamine hydrochloride
(tri pel enn' a meen)

PBZ, PBZ-SR, Pyribenzamine (CAN)

PREGNANCY CATEGORY C

Drug class
Antihistamine (ethylenediamine type)

Therapeutic actions
Competitively blocks the effects of histamine at H_1 receptor sites; has anticholinergic (atropine-like), antipruritic, and sedative effects.

Indications
- Symptomatic relief of perennial and seasonal allergic rhinitis, vasomotor rhinitis, allergic conjunctivitis, mild, uncomplicated urticaria and angioedema, pruritus
- Amelioraton of allergic reactions to blood or plasma
- Dermatographism
- Adjunctive therapy in anaphylactic reactions

Contraindications and cautions
- Contraindicated with allergy to any antihistamines, pregnancy, lactation.
- Use cautiously with narrow-angle glaucoma, stenosing peptic ulcer, symptomatic prostatic hypertrophy, asthmatic attack, bladder neck obstruction, pyloroduodenal obstruction.

Available forms
Tablets—25, 50 mg; ER tablets—100 mg

Dosages

Adults
25–50 mg PO q 4–6 hr. Up to 600 mg/day has been used. Sustained-release preparation: 100 mg PO in the morning and the evening; 100 mg q 8–12 hr may be needed.

Pediatric patients
5 mg/kg/day PO or 150 mg/m^2/day PO divided into 4–6 doses. Maximum total dose of 300 mg/day. Do not use sustained-release preparations with children.

Geriatric patients
More likely to cause dizziness, sedation, syncope, toxic confusional states and hypotension in elderly patients; use with caution.

Pharmacokinetics

Route	Onset	Peak	Duration
Oral	15–30 min	1–2 hr	4–6 hr

Metabolism: Hepatic; $T_{1/2}$: unknown
Distribution: Crosses placenta; enters breast milk
Excretion: Urine

Adverse effects

- **CNS:** *Drowsiness, sedation, dizziness, disturbed coordination,* fatigue, confusion, restlessness, excitation, nervousness, tremor, headache, blurred vision, diplopia, vertigo, tinnitus, acute labyrinthitis, hysteria, tingling, heaviness and weakness of the hands
- **CV:** Hypotension, palpitations, bradycardia, tachycardia, extrasystoles
- **Dermatologic:** Urticaria, rash, **anaphylactic shock,** photosensitivity, excessive perspiration, chills
- **GI:** *Epigastric distress,* anorexia, increased appetite and weight gain, nausea, vomiting, diarrhea or constipation
- **GU:** Urinary frequency, dysuria, urinary retention, early menses, decreased libido, impotence
- **Hematologic:** Hemolytic anemia, hypoplastic anemia, thrombocytopenia, leukopenia, agranulocytosis, pancytopenia
- **Respiratory:** *Thickening of bronchial secretions,* chest tightness, wheezing, nasal stuffiness, dry mouth, dry nose, dry throat, sore throat

- **Other:** Drug abuse when used with pentazocine ("Ts and Blues") as a heroin substitute

■ Nursing considerations

Assessment
- **History:** Allergy to any antihistamines, narrow-angle glaucoma, stenosing peptic ulcer, symptomatic prostatic hypertrophy, asthmatic attack, bladder neck obstruction, pyloroduodenal obstruction, pregnancy, lactation
- **Physical:** Skin color, lesions, texture; orientation, reflexes, affect; vision exam; P, BP; R, adventitious sounds; bowel sounds; prostate palpation; CBC with differential

Interventions
- Administer with food if GI upset occurs.
- Caution patient not to crush or chew sustained-release tablets.

Teaching points
- Avoid excessive dosage.
- Take with food if GI upset occurs.
- Do not crush or chew sustained-release tablets.
- These side effects may occur: dizziness, sedation, drowsiness (use caution if driving or performing tasks that require alertness); epigastric distress, diarrhea, or constipation (take drug with meals); dry mouth (frequent mouth care, sucking sugarless lozenges may help); thickening of bronchial secretions, dryness of nasal mucosa (use a humidifier).
- Avoid alcohol; serious sedation could occur.
- Report difficulty breathing, hallucinations, tremors, loss of coordination, unusual bleeding or bruising, visual disturbances, irregular heartbeat.

▷triptorelin pamoate
*(trip toe **rell***' *in)*

Trelstar Depot, Trelstar LA

PREGNANCY CATEGORY X

Drug classes
Antineoplastic agent
Hormonal agent

Adverse effects in Italics *are most common; those in* **Bold** *are life-threatening.*

Therapeutic actions

An analog of luteinizing hormone–releasing hormone (LHRH); causes a decrease in FSH and LH levels, leading to a suppression of ovarian and testicular hormone production, which causes decreased levels of estrogens (females) and testosterone (males); after continuous use, a sustained decrease in FSH and LH levels occurs.

Indications

- Palliative treatment of advanced prostatic cancer when orchiectomy or estrogen administration are not indicated or are unacceptable to the patient
- Treatment of advanced-stage prostatic cancer

Contraindications and cautions

- Pregnancy, lactation, hypersensitivity to LHRH or any component.

Available forms

Powder for depot injection—3.75 mg, 11.25 mg

Dosages
Adults

- *Palliative treatment:* 3.75 mg IM once monthly.
- *Treatment:* 11.25 mg depot injection IM every 3 mo.

Pediatric patients

Safety and efficacy not established.

Pharmacokinetics

Route	Onset	Peak
IM	Slow	1–3 hr

Metabolism: Hepatic; $T_{1/2}$: 2.8–4 hr
Distribution: Crosses placenta; may pass into breast milk
Excretion: Urine and bile

Adverse effects

- **CNS:** Insomnia, dizziness, lethargy, anxiety, depression, headache
- **CV:** CHF, edema, hypertension, arrhythmia, chest pain
- **GI:** Nausea, anorexia
- **GU:** *Hot flashes, sexual dysfunction, decreased erections, lower urinary tract symptoms*

- **Other:** *Bone pain,* rash, sweating, cancer, angioedema, **anaphylaxis**

Interactions

✳ **Drug-drug** • Do not administer with drugs that increase prolactin production—antipsychotics, metoclopropamide; risk of severe hyperprolactinemia

■ Nursing considerations
Assessment

- **History:** Pregnancy, lactation, hypersensitivity to LHRH or other LHRH drugs
- **Physical:** Skin temperature, lesions; reflexes, affect; BP, P; urinary output; serum testosterone levels, PSA levels

Interventions

- Reconstitute with 2 mL sterile water for injection. Shake well. Withdraw the entire contents of the vial into the syringe and inject immediately.
- Monitor testosterone and PSA levels prior to and periodically during therapy.
- Ensure repeat injection each month or every 3 mo—it is important to keep as close to this schedule as possible.
- Offer appropriate comfort measures (temperature control, analgesics, etc.) to help patient cope with hot flashes, urinary retention, and bone pain. Most likely to occur at initiation of therapy.

Teaching points

- Be aware that this drug will need to be injected each month or every 3 mo.
- These side effects may occur: hot flashes (a cool temperature may help you to cope with this); sexual dysfunction—regression of sex organs, impaired fertility, decreased erections (it may help to know that these are drug effects; if these become worrisome, consult with your nurse or physician); bone pain, urinary retention, blood in the urine (these usually resolve within the first week of treatment; analgesics may be ordered to help you cope with the pain).
- Do not take this drug if pregnant—if you are pregnant or wish to become pregnant, consult with your physician.
- Report chest pain, rapid heartbeat, numbness or tingling, breast pain, difficulty breath-

T

ing, unresolved nausea and vomiting, signs of infection at the injection site.

▷ tromethamine
(troe meth' a meen)

Tham

PREGNANCY CATEGORY C

Drug class
Systemic alkalinizer

Therapeutic actions
Sodium-free organic amine that acts as a buffer, preventing the occurrence of acidosis; acts as a weak osmotic diuretic; may be preferable to sodium bicarbonate in the treatment of metabolic acidosis when sodium restriction is important.

Indications
- Prevention or correction of systemic acidosis; metabolic acidosis associated with coronary artery bypass surgery; correction of acidity of acid dextrose blood in cardiac bypass surgery; cardiac arrest

Contraindications and cautions
- Contraindicated with anuria, uremia, pregnancy.
- Use cautiously with respiratory depression, impaired renal function.

Available forms
Injection—18 g/500 mL

Dosages
Adults and patients > 12 yr
- *Acidosis during cardiac bypass surgery:* Single dose of 500 mL IV is usually sufficient; 9 mL/kg IV; do not exceed 500 mg/kg/hr.
- *Acidity of ACD blood:* 0.5–2.5 g (15–77 mL) IV added to each 500 mL of ACD blood.
- *Acidosis of cardiac arrest:* Inject 2–6 g directly into ventricular cavity if chest is open; Inject 3.6–10.8 g IV into a large peripheral vein if chest is not open.

Pharmacokinetics

Route	Onset	Duration
IV	Rapid	8 hr

Metabolism: $T_{1/2}$: unknown
Distribution: Crosses placenta; enters breast milk
Excretion: Urine

▽ IV facts
Preparation: Use as provided by manufacturer.
Infusion: Infuse slowly, 5 mL over 1 min, into pump oxygenator, ACD blood, priming fluid or ventricular cavity; infuse slowly into peripheral vein.

Adverse effects
- **GI:** Hemorrhagic hepatic necrosis
- **Hematologic:** Decreased blood glucose
- **Local:** Phlebitis, infection of injection site
- **Respiratory:** Respiratory depression

■ Nursing considerations
Assessment
- **History:** Anuria, uremia, pregnancy, respiratory depression, impaired renal function
- **Physical:** P, BP; R, adventitious sounds; CBC, blood gases, electrolytes, glucose

Interventions
- Monitor blood pH, pCO_2, bicarbonate, glucose, electrolytes before and during administration.
- Provide supportive or replacement therapy as needed for hematologic changes.
- Use a large needle in the biggest vein available for peripheral use; alkalinity is very irritating to tissues.

Teaching points
- Patients receiving this drug will be unconscious and unaware of its use. If local irritation occurs after use, incorporate some information about the drug into the wound care of the injection site.

Adverse effects in *Italics* are most common; those in **Bold** are life-threatening.

▽trovafloxacin
*(troh va **flox'** a sin)*

trovafloxacin
Trovan

alatrofloxacin mesylate
Trovan IV

PREGNANCY CATEGORY C

Drug class
Fluoroquinolone-like antibiotic

Therapeutic actions
Bactericidal; interferes with DNA replication in susceptible gram-negative and gram-positive aerobic and anaerobic bacteria, preventing cell reproduction.

Indications
- Nosocomial pneumonia caused by *E. coli, Pseudomonas aeruginosa, Haemophilus influenzae, Staphylococcus aureus*
- Treatment of adults with community-acquired pneumonia caused by *Streptococcus pneumoniae, H. influenzae, Klebsiella pneumonia, S. aureus, Mycoplasma pneumoniae, Moraxella catarrhalis, Legionella pneumophila, Chlamydia pneumoniae*
- Treatment of complicated intra-abdominal infections, including postoperative infections caused by susceptible bacteria
- Treatment of gynecologic and pelvic infections including endomyometritis, parametritis, cervicitis, septic abortion, and postpartum infections caused by susceptible bacteria
- Complicated skin and skin structure infections, including diabetic foot infections caused by *S. aureus, Streptococcus agalactiae, P. aeruginosa, E. faecalis, E. coli, Proteus mirabilis*
- Treatment of chronic bacterial prostatitis caused by *E. coli, E. faecalis, Staphylococcus epidermidis*
- Treatment of urethral gonorrhea in males, endocervical and rectal gonorrhea in females

Contraindications and cautions
- Contraindicated with allergy to any fluoroquinolones, pregnancy, lactation.

- Use cautiously with renal or hepatic dysfunction, seizures.

Available forms
Tablets—100, 200 mg; solution for injection: 5 mg/mL

Dosages
Adults
- *Nosocomial pneumonia:* 300 mg IV followed by 200 mg PO daily for 10–14 days.
- *Community-acquired pneumonia:* 200 mg PO or IV followed by 200 mg PO daily for 7–14 days.
- *Complicated intra-abdominal infections:* 300 mg IV followed by 200 mg PO daily for 7–14 days.
- *Gynecologic and pelvic infections:* 300 mg IV followed by 200 mg PO daily for 7–14 days.
- *Skin infection, complicated:* 200 mg PO or IV followed by 200 mg PO daily for 10–14 days.

Pediatric patients
Not recommended in patients < 18 yr.

Patients with hepatic impairment
For normal recommended dose of 300 mg IV, use 200 mg IV; for 200 mg IV or PO, use 100 mg IV or PO.

Pharmacokinetics

Route	Onset	Peak
Oral	Varies	0.5–1 hr
IV	Rapid	1 hr

Metabolism: Hepatic; $T_{1/2}$: 9–11 hr
Distribution: Crosses placenta; passes into breast milk
Excretion: Bile

▼IV facts
Preparation: Inspect vial for any discoloration or particulate matter; aseptic technique must be used in preparation of the final solution. Dilute with appropriate amount of 5% dextrose injection, 0.45% sodium chloride injection, 5% dextrose and 0.45% sodium chloride injection, 5% dextrose and 0.2% sodium chloride injection, or lactated Ringer's and 5% dextrose injection to reach a final concentration of 1–2 mg/mL. Discard any unused portion of the vial. Diluted solution is stable for up to 7 days if refrigerated, for 3 days at room temperature.

T

Infusion: Administer slowly over at least 60 min; avoid rapid or bolus injections.

Incompatibilities: Do not administer in solution with or in the same line with any other drug. If other drugs are given through the same line, the line should be flushed between drugs.

Adverse effects
- **CNS:** *Light-headedness, dizziness, insomnia,* fatigue, somnolence, depression, headache
- **CV:** Chest pain, peripheral edema
- **GI:** *Nausea,* vomiting, dry mouth, *diarrhea,* abdominal pain, **liver toxicity, possibly leading to death**
- **Other:** Fever, rash, *pruritus,* photosensitivity (low potential for this effect compared with other fluoroquinolones), pain and sensitivity at injection site

Interactions
✳ **Drug-drug** • Decreased therapeutic effect with iron salts, sucralfate, antacids, zinc, magnesium; separate by at least 2 hr • Decreased absorption of oral trovafloxacin with IV morphine; give IV morphine at least 2 hr after oral trovafloxacin given on an empty stomach or 4 hr after trovafloxacin given with food

■ Nursing considerations
Assessment
- **History:** Allergy to fluoroquinolones; hepatic dysfunction; seizures; lactation, pregnancy
- **Physical:** Skin color, lesions; T; orientation, reflexes, affect; mucous membranes, bowel sounds; liver function tests

Interventions
- Arrange for culture and sensitivity tests before beginning therapy.
- Monitor liver function before and during therapy; discontinue drug at first sign of liver toxicity.
- Continue therapy as indicated for condition being treated; do not exceed 2 wk duration.
- Separate oral drug from other cation administration, including antacids, by at least 2 hr.

- Ensure that patient is well hydrated during course of drug therapy.
- Discontinue drug at any sign of hypersensitivity (rash, photophobia) or at complaint of tendon pain, inflammation, or rupture.
- Monitor clinical response; if no improvement is seen or a relapse occurs, repeat culture and sensitivity.

Teaching points
- Take oral drug without regard to meals. If an antacid is needed, do not take it within 2 hours of trovafloxacin dose.
- Drink plenty of fluids while you are on this drug.
- These side effects may occur: nausea, vomiting, abdominal pain (eat small, frequent meals); diarrhea or constipation (consult nurse or physician); drowsiness, blurring of vision, dizziness (use caution if driving or operating dangerous equipment); sensitivity to the sun (avoid exposure; use a sunscreen if necessary).
- Report rash, visual changes, severe GI problems, weakness, tremors, sensitivity to light, tendon pain, fatigue, changes in color of stool or urine.

▷**urea**
(yoor ee' a)

Ureaphil

PREGNANCY CATEGORY C

Drug class
Osmotic diuretic

Therapeutic actions
Elevates the osmolarity of the glomerular filtrate, hindering the reabsorption of water and leading to a loss of water, sodium, and chloride; creates an osmotic gradient in the eye between plasma and ocular fluids, reducing intraocular pressure.

Indications
- Reduction of intracranial pressure and treatment of cerebral edema
- Reduction of elevated intraocular pressure

Adverse effects in *Italics* are most common; those in **Bold** are life-threatening.

• Unlabeled use: induction of abortion when used by intra-amniotic injection

Contraindications and cautions
• Active intracranial bleeding (except during craniotomy), marked dehydration, severe renal or hepatic disease, pregnancy, lactation.

Available forms
Injection—40 g/150 mL

Dosages
Adults
Slow IV infusion of 30% solution only: 1–1.5 g/kg. Do not exceed 120 g/day.
Pediatric patients
0.5–1.5 g/kg IV. As little as 0.1 g/kg may be adequate in children < 2 yr.

Pharmacokinetics

Route	Onset	Peak	Duration
IV	30–45 min	60 min	5–6 hr

Metabolism: $T_{1/2}$: unknown
Distribution: Crosses placenta; enters breast milk
Excretion: Urine

▼IV facts
Preparation: For 135 mL of a 30% solution of sterile urea, mix one 40-g vial with 105 mL of 5% or 10% dextrose injection or 10% invert sugar in water; each mL of a 30% solution provides 300 mg of urea; use only fresh solution; discard any solution within 24 hr after reconstitution.
Infusion: Administer 30% solution by slow IV infusion; do not exceed 4 mL/min.
Incompatibilities: Do not administer urea through the same IV set as blood or blood products.

Adverse effects
• **CNS:** *Dizziness, headache,* syncope, disorientation
• **GI:** *Nausea, vomiting*
• **Hematologic:** Hyponatremia, hypokalemia
• **Local:** Tissue necrosis if extravasation occurs at IV site
• **Other:** Thrombophlebitis, febrile response, hypervolemia if improperly administered

■ Nursing considerations
Assessment
• **History:** Active intracranial bleeding, marked dehydration, hepatic or renal disease, pregnancy, lactation
• **Physical:** Skin color, edema; orientation, reflexes, muscle strength, pupillary reflexes; pulses, BP, perfusion; R, pattern, adventitious sounds; urinary output patterns; serum electrolytes, urinalysis, renal and liver function tests

Interventions
• Do not infuse in veins of lower extremities of elderly patients.
• Monitor urinary output carefully.
• Monitor BP regularly and carefully.
• Monitor serum electrolytes periodically.
• Use an indwelling catheter in comatose patients.

Teaching points
• This drug can only be given IV.
• These side effects may occur: increased urination, GI upset (eat small, frequent meals), dry mouth (sugarless lozenges to suck may help), headache, blurred vision (use caution when moving around; ask for assistance).
• Report pain at the IV site, severe headache, chest pain.

▷urofollitropin
See *Less Commonly Used Drugs,* p. 1354.

▷urofollitropin, purified
See *Less Commonly Used Drugs,* p. 1354.

▷urokinase
(yoor oh kin' ase)

Abbokinase, Abbokinase Open-Cath

PREGNANCY CATEGORY B

U

Drug class
Thrombolytic agent

Therapeutic actions
Enzyme isolated from human urine; converts plasminogen to the enzyme plasmin (fibri-

nolysin), which degrades fibrin clots, fibrinogen, and other plasma proteins; lyses thrombi and emboli.

Indications
- Lysis of pulmonary emboli
- Coronary artery thrombosis within 6 hr of onset of symptoms of coronary occlusion
- IV catheter clearance

Contraindications and cautions
- Contraindicated with hypersensitivity to urokinase, active internal bleeding, recent (within 2 mo) CVA, intracranial or intraspinal surgery, intracranial neoplasm; recent trauma, including pulmonary resuscitation, arteriovenous malformation or aneurysm, known bleeding diathesis, severe uncontrolled hypertension.
- Use cautiously with recent major surgery, obstetric delivery, organ biopsy, or rupture of a noncompressible blood vessel; recent serious GI bleed; SBE; hemostatic defects; cerebrovascular disease; diabetic hemorrhagic retinopathy; septic thrombosis; pregnancy; lactation.

Available forms
Powder for injection—250,000 IU/vial; powder for catheter clearance—5,000, 9,000 IU

Dosages
Adults
- *Pulmonary embolism:* Give through constant infusion pump: Priming dose of 4,400 IU/kg as an admixture with 5% dextrose injection or 0.9% sodium chloride at a rate of 90 mL/hr over 10 min. Then give 4,400 IU/kg/hr at a rate of 15 mL/hr for 12 hr. At end of infusion, flush the tubing with 0.9% sodium chloride or 5% dextrose injection equal to the volume of the tubing. At the end of the infusion, treat with continuous heparin IV infusion, beginning heparin when the thrombin time has decreased to less than twice the normal control.
- *Lysis of coronary artery thrombi:* Before therapy, administer heparin bolus of 2,500–10,000 IU IV; infuse urokinase into occluded artery at rate of 6,000 IU/min for up to 2 hr. Continue infusion until the artery is maximally opened, usually 15–30 min after initial opening.
- *IV catheter clearance:* For clearing a central venous catheter; have patient exhale and hold his or her breath any time catheter is not connected to IV tubing. Disconnect catheter and after determining amount of occlusion, attach tuberculin syringe with urokinase solution and inject amount equal to volume of catheter. Wait 5 min and aspirate; repeat aspirations every 5 min for up to 1 hr. A repeat infusion of urokinase may be necessary in severe cases. When patency is restored, aspirate 4–5 mL of blood to ensure removal of drug and residual clot. Irrigate gently with 0.9% sodium chloride in fresh 10 mL syringe and reconnect IV tubing.

Pediatric patients
Safety and efficacy not established.

Pharmacokinetics

Route	Onset	Peak
IV	Immediate	End of infusion

Metabolism: Plasma, $T_{1/2}$: unknown
Distribution: Crosses placenta; enters breast milk
Excretion: Unknown

▼IV facts
Preparation: Reconstitute vial with 5.2 mL of sterile water for injection without preservatives. Avoid shaking during reconstitution; gently roll or tilt vial to reconstitute; consult manufacturer's directions for further dilution. Solution may be filtered through 0.45 or smaller cellulose membrane filter in administration set. Use immediately and discard any unused portion of drug; do not store. Refrigerate vials.
Infusion: Maintain infusion via an infusion pump to ensure accurate delivery over 12 hr.
Incompatibilities: Do not add other medications to reconstituted solutions.

Adverse effects
- **CNS:** Headache
- **CV:** Angioneurotic edema, arrhythmias (with intracoronary artery infusion)
- **Dermatologic:** Skin rash, urticaria, itching, flushing

- **Hematologic:** *Bleeding (minor or surface* to major internal bleeding)
- **Respiratory:** Breathing difficulty, bronchospasm
- **Other:** Musculoskeletal pain, *fever*

Interactions

✳ Drug-drug • Increased risk of hemorrhage if used with heparin or oral anticoagulants, aspirin, indomethacin, phenylbutazone

✳ Drug-lab test • Marked decrease in plasminogen, fibrinogen; increases in thrombin time, activated partial thromboplastin time (APTT), prothrombin time (PT)

■ Nursing considerations
Assessment

- **History:** Hypersensitivity to urokinase; active internal bleeding; recent CVA, intracranial or intraspinal surgery; intracranial neoplasm; recent major surgery, obstetric delivery, organ biopsy, or rupture of a noncompressible blood vessel; GI bleed; recent serious trauma; severe hypertension; SBE; hemostatic defects; cerebrovascular disease; diabetic hemorrhagic retinopathy; septic thrombosis; pregnancy; lactation
- **Physical:** Skin color, temperature, lesions; T; orientation, reflexes; P, BP, peripheral perfusion, baseline ECG; R, adventitous sounds; liver evaluation; Hct, platelet count, thrombin time, APTT, PT

Interventions

- Discontinue heparin unless ordered specifically for coronary artery infusion.
- Regularly monitor coagulation studies.
- Apply pressure or pressure dressings to control superficial bleeding (at invaded or disturbed areas).
- Avoid any arterial invasive procedures.
- Arrange for typing and cross-matching of blood if serious blood loss occurs and whole blood transfusions are required.
- Institute treatment within 6 hr of onset of symptoms for evolving MI and within 7 days of other thrombotic event.
- Monitor cardiac rhythm continually during coronary artery infusion.

Teaching points

- You will require frequent blood tests; this drug can only be given IV.

- Report rash, difficulty breathing, dizziness, disorientation, numbness, tingling.

▽ursodiol
(ursodeoxycholic acid)
*(ur soe **dye'** ole)*

Actigall, URSO, Ursofalk (CAN)

PREGNANCY CATEGORY B

Drug class
Gallstone solubilizing agent

Therapeutic actions
A naturally occurring bile acid that suppresses hepatic synthesis of cholesterol and inhibits intestinal absorption of cholesterol, leading to a decreased cholesterol concentration in the bile and a bile that is cholesterol solubilizing and not cholesterol precipitating.

Indications

- Treatment of selected patients with radiolucent, noncalcified gallstones in gallbladders in whom elective surgery is contraindicated
- Prevention of gallstone formation in obese patients experiencing rapid weight loss
- Orphan drug use: treatment of primary biliary cirrhosis (*URSO*)

Contraindications and cautions

- Contraindicated with allergy to bile salts, hepatic dysfunction, calcified stones, radiopaque stones or radiolucent bile pigment stones, unremitting acute cholecystitis, cholangitis, biliary obstruction, gallstone pancreatitis, biliary gastrointestinal fistula (cholecystectomy required), pregnancy.
- Use cautiously with lactation.

Available forms
Capsules—300 mg, tablets—250 mg (*URSO*)

Dosages
Adults

- *Solubilization of gallstones:* 8–10 mg/kg/day PO given in 2 to 3 divided doses. Resolution of the gallstones requires months of therapy; condition needs to be monitored with ultrasound at 6-mo and 1-yr intervals.

U

- *Treatment of biliary cirrhosis:* 250 mg PO daily (*URSO*).
- *Prevention of gallstones:* 300 mg PO bid or 8–10 mg/kg/day PO in 2–3 divided doses.

Pediatric patients
Safety and efficacy not established.

Pharmacokinetics

Route	Onset	Peak
Oral	Varies	Days

Metabolism: Hepatic; $T_{1/2}$: unknown
Distribution: Crosses placenta; may enter breast milk
Excretion: Feces

Adverse effects

- **CNS:** Headache, fatigue, anxiety, depression, sleep disorder
- **Dermatologic:** Pruritus, rash, urticaria, dry skin, sweating, hair thinning
- **GI:** *Diarrhea,* cramps, heartburn, constipation, nausea, vomiting, anorexia, epigastric distress, dyspepsia, flatulence, abdominal pain
- **Respiratory:** Rhinitis, cough
- **Other:** Back pain, arthralgia, myalgia

Interactions

✱ Drug-drug • Absorption decreased if taken with bile acid sequestering agents (cholestyramine, colestipol), aluminum-based antacids

■ Nursing considerations
Assessment

- **History:** Allergy to bile salts, hepatic dysfunction, calcified stones, radiopaque stones or radiolucent bile pigment stones, unremitting acute cholecystitis, cholangitis, biliary obstruction, gallstone pancreatitis, biliary-gastrointestinal fistula, pregnancy, lactation
- **Physical:** Liver evaluation, abdominal exam; affect, orientation; skin color, lesions; liver function tests, hepatic and biliary radiological studies, biliary ultrasound

Interventions

- Assess patient carefully for suitability of ursodiol therapy. Alternative therapy should be reviewed before using ursodiol.

- Give drug in 2 to 3 divided doses.
- Do not administer drug with aluminum-based antacids. If such drugs are needed, administer 2–3 hr after ursodiol.
- Schedule patients for periodic oral cholecystograms or ultrasonograms to evaluate drug effectiveness at 6-mo intervals until resolution, then every 3 mo to monitor stone formation. Stones recur within 5 yr in more than 50% of patients. If gallstones appear to have dissolved, continue treatment for 3 mo and perform follow-up ultrasound.
- Monitor liver function tests periodically. Carefully assess patient if any change in liver function occurs.

Teaching points

- Take drug 2 to 3 times a day. Take the drug as long as prescribed. It may be needed for a prolonged period.
- This drug may dissolve your gallstones; it does not "cure" the problem that caused the stones, and in many cases, the stones can recur; medical follow-up is important.
- Arrange to receive periodic x-rays or ultrasound tests of your gallbladder; you also will need periodic blood tests to evaluate your response to this drug. Keep follow-up appointments.
- These side effects may occur: diarrhea; rash (skin care may help); headache, fatigue (request analgesics).
- Do not take with any aluminum-based antacids.
- Report gallstone attacks (abdominal pain, nausea, vomiting), yellowing of the skin or eyes.

▷ valacyclovir hydrochloride
(val ah sye' kloe ver)

Valtrex

PREGNANCY CATEGORY B

Drug class
Antiviral

Therapeutic actions

Antiviral activity; inhibits viral DNA replication and deactivates viral DNA polymerase.

Indications

- Treatment of herpes zoster (shingles) in immunocompromised adults
- Episodic treatment of first-episode or recurrent genital herpes
- Suppression of recurrent episodes of genital herpes
- Treatment of cold sores (herpes labialis) in healthy adults

Contraindications and cautions

- Contraindicated with allergy to valacyclovir or acyclovir, lactation.
- Use cautiously with pregnancy, renal impairment, thrombotic thrombocytopenic purpura.

Available forms

Tablets—500 mg, 1 g.

Dosages

Systemic
Adults
- *Herpes zoster:* 1 g tid PO for 7 days; most effective if started within 48 hr of onset of symptoms.
- *Genital herpes:* 500 mg PO bid for 5 days.
- *Episodic treatment of recurrent genital herpes:* 500 mg PO bid for 3 days.
- *Suppression of recurrent episodes of genital herpes:* 1 g PO daily; patients with history of < 9 episodes in 1 yr may respond to 500 mg PO daily.
- *Cold sores:* 2 g PO bid for one day.
Pediatric patients
Safety and efficacy not established.
Geriatric patients or patients with renal impairment

Creatinine Clearance (mL/min)	Dose
≥ 50	1 g q 8 hr
30–49	1 g q 12 hr
10–29	1 g q 24 hr
< 10	500 mg q 24 hr

Pharmacokinetics

Route	Onset	Peak
Oral	Rapid	3 hr

Metabolism: $T_{1/2}$: 2.5–3.3 hr
Distribution: Crosses placenta: passes into breast milk
Excretion: Unchanged in the urine and feces

Adverse effects

- **CNS:** Headache, dizziness
- **GI:** *Nausea, vomiting,* diarrhea, anorexia

Interactions

✴ **Drug-drug** • Decreased rate of effectiveness with probenecid, cimetidine

■ Nursing considerations

 CLINICAL ALERT!
Name confusion has been reported with Valtrex (valacyclovir) and Valcyte (valganciclovir); use caution.

Assessment

- **History:** Allergy to valacyclovir, acyclovir; renal disease; lactation; thrombotic thrombocytopenic purpura
- **Physical:** Orientation; urinary output; abdominal exam, normal output; BUN, creatinine clearance

Interventions

- Begin treatment within 72 hr of onset of symptoms of shingles.
- Administer without regard to meals; administer with meals to decrease GI upset if necessary.
- Provide appropriate analgesics for headache, discomfort of shingles.

Teaching points

- Take this drug without regard to meals; if GI upset is a problem, take with meals.
- Take the full course of therapy as prescribed.
- Avoid contact with lesions and avoid intercourse when lesions or symptoms are present to avoid infecting others.
- Start therapy at first sign of an episode when treating recurrent herpes.

V

- These side effects may occur: nausea, vomiting, loss of appetite, diarrhea; headache; dizziness.
- Report severe diarrhea, nausea; headache; worsening of the shingles.

▽valdecoxib
(val dah cox' hib)

Bextra

PREGNANCY CATEGORY C

Drug classes
NSAID (nonsteroidal anti-inflammatory drug)
Analgesic
Specific COX-2 enzyme blocker

Therapeutic actions
Analgesic and anti-inflammatory activities related to inhibition of COX-2 enzyme, which is activated in inflammation to cause the signs and symptoms associated with inflammation; not thought to affect the COX-1 enzyme, which protects the lining of the GI tract and has blood clotting and renal functions.

Indications
- Relief of signs and symptoms of osteoarthritis and adult rheumatoid arthritis
- Treatment of primary dysmenorrhea

Contraindications and cautions
- Contraindicated with allergy to valdecoxib, salicylates, other NSAIDs (more common in patients with rhinitis, asthma, chronic urticaria, nasal polyps), sulfonamides, or any component of the drug; lactation.
- Use cautiously with impaired renal or hepatic function, fluid retention, hypertension or CHF, history of ulcer or GI bleeding, pregnancy (teratogenic effects and lack of closure of the ductus arteriosus have been reported with use in late pregnancy).

Available forms
Tablets—10, 20 mg

Dosages
Adults
- *Osteoarthritis and rheumatoid arthritis:* 10 mg/day PO.
- *Primary dysmenorrhea:* 20 mg PO bid as needed.
Pediatric patients
Safety and efficacy not established in patients < 18 yr.

Pharmacokinetics

Route	Onset	Peak
Oral	Varies	2–3 hr

Metabolism: Hepatic; $T_{1/2}$: 8–11 hr
Distribution: Crosses placenta; passes into breast milk
Excretion: Urine

Adverse effects
- **CNS:** *Headache,* dizziness, neuralgia, neuropathy, tremors, anxiety
- **CV:** Arrhythmia, hypertension, **CHF,** hypotension, edema
- **Dermatologic:** Rash, pruritus, sweating, **Stevens–Johnson syndrome, toxic epidermal necrolysis,** dry mucous membranes, urticaria, exfoliative dermatitis, erythema multiforme
- **GI:** *Abdominal pain, diarrhea, dyspepsia,* nausea, flatulence, hemorrhoids, abdominal fullness
- **Hematologic:** Bleeding, platelet inhibition with higher doses, neutropenia, eosinophilia, leukopenia, pancytopenia, thrombocytopenia, agranulocytosis, altered hepatic function
- **Respiratory:** *URI,* sinusitis, coughing, dyspnea, rhinitis
- **Other:** Back pain, flulike illness, myalgia, **anaphylaxis, angioedema**

Interactions
✳ **Drug-drug** • Increased risk of GI bleeding if combined with aspirin • Risk of decreased antihypertensive effect if given with ACE inhibitors; monitor patient closely and adjust dosage as needed • Increased lithium levels and risk of toxicity if taken concomitantly; monitor patient closely • Risk of increased anticoagulant effects if taken with warfarin; mon-

itor INR closely and adjust dosage accordingly • Increased serum levels of valdecoxib with fluconazole and ketoconazole; monitor patient closely

■ Nursing considerations
Assessment
- **History:** Allergy to valdecoxib, salicylates, other NSAIDs, sulfonamides, any component of the drug; pregnancy; lactation; impaired renal or hepatic function; fluid retention; hypertension; CHF; ulcer; GI bleeding
- **Physical:** Skin (color, lesions), T, orientation, reflexes, peripheral sensation, P, BP, edema, R, adventitious sounds, liver evaluation, CBC, clotting times, liver and renal function tests

Interventions
- Administer drug with food or after meals if GI upset occurs.
- Discontinue drug at first sign of skin rash or hypersensitivity.
- Establish safety measures if CNS, visual disturbances occur.
- Institute emergency procedures (gastric lavage, induction of emesis, supportive therapy) if overdose occurs.
- Provide further comfort measures to reduce pain (positioning, environmental control, etc.), and to reduce inflammation (warmth, positioning, rest, etc.).

Teaching points
- Take the drug with food or after meals if GI upset occurs.
- Do not exceed the prescribed dosage.
- These side effects may occur: drowsiness, dizziness (use caution when driving or operating dangerous machinery if these occur); GI upset, diarrhea (small frequent meals may help; consult with health care provider if severe).
- Report sore throat, fever, rash, itching, weight gain, swelling in ankles or fingers, severe abdominal pain, changes in color of urine or stool.

▽valganciclovir hydrochloride
(val gan sigh' kloe veer)

Valcyte

PREGNANCY CATEGORY C

Drug class
Antiviral

Therapeutic action
Antiviral activity; inhibits viral DNA replication in cytomegalovirus (CMV).

Indications
- Treatment of CMV retinitis in patients with AIDS

Contraindications and cautions
- Contraindicated with hypersensitivity to valganciclovir, ganciclovir, or acyclovir; lactation.
- Use cautiously with cytopenia, history of cytopenic reactions, impaired renal function, pregnancy, the elderly.

Available forms
Tablets—450 mg

Dosages
Adults
900 mg PO bid for 21 days; maintenance, 900 mg PO daily.
Pediatric patients
Safety and efficacy not established.
Patients with renal impairment
Do not administer to patients on hemodialysis. For patients with renal impairment, see the following table:

Creatinine Clearance (mL/min)	Initial Dose	Maintenance Dose
≥ 60	900 mg PO bid	900 mg PO daily
40–59	450 mg PO bid	450 mg PO daily
25–39	450 mg PO daily	450 mg PO every other day
10–24	450 mg PO q 2 days	450 mg PO twice weekly

Pharmacokinetics

Route	Onset	Peak
Oral	Slow	1–3 hr

Metabolism: Hepatic transformation to ganciclovir; $T_{1/2}$: 4 hr
Distribution: Crosses placenta; may pass into breast milk
Excretion: Urine

Adverse effects

- **CNS:** *Headache, insomnia,* neuropathy, paresthesias, confusion, hallucinations
- **GI:** *Nausea, vomiting,* anorexia, *diarrhea,* abdominal pain
- **Hematologic:** *Neutropenia, anemia,* thrombocytopenia
- **Other:** *Fever,* retinal detachment

Interactions

✷ **Drug-drug** • Increased ganciclovir effects if taken with probenecid • Use with extreme caution with cytotoxic drugs because the accumulation effect could cause severe bone marrow depression and other GI and dermatologic problems • Increased risk of seizures if taken concurrently with imipenem-cilastatin • Extreme drowsiness and risk of bone marrow depression if taken with zidovudine; avoid this combination

■ Nursing considerations

 CLINICAL ALERT!
Name confusion has been reported with Valcyte (valganciclovir) and Valtrex (valacyclovir); use caution.

Assessment

- **History:** Hypersensitivity to valganciclovir, ganciclovir, or acyclovir; cytopenia; history of cytopenic reactions; impaired renal function; pregnancy; lactation
- **Physical:** T, orientation, reflexes, urinary output, CBC, BUN, creatinine clearance

Interventions

- Administer drug with food to maximize absorption and to decrease GI upset.
- Do not exceed the recommended dosage, frequency; note that valganciclovir cannot be

substituted for ganciclovir capsules on a one-to-one basis.
- Arrange for decreased dosage in patients with impaired renal function.
- Arrange for CBC before beginning therapy and at least weekly thereafter. Consult with physician and arrange for reduced dosage if WBCs or platelets fall.
- Consult with pharmacy for proper disposal of unused tablets. Precautions are required for disposal of nucleoside analogues. Do not cut, crush, or chew tablets. Avoid handling broken tablets.
- Arrange for periodic ophthalmic examinations during therapy. Drug is not a cure of the disease and deterioration may occur.
- Provide comfort measures for patients who develop fever, rash, headache.
- Advise patients that valganciclovir can decrease sperm production in men and birth defects in pregnant women. Advise the patient to use some form of contraception during ganciclovir therapy. Men receiving valganciclovir therapy should use some form of barrier contraception during and for at least 90 days after therapy.
- Advise patient that valganciclovir has caused cancer in animals and that risk is possible in humans.
- Maintain support therapy and program for AIDS patients who are receiving this drug as part of their overall treatment plan.

Teaching points

- Take this drug with food. This will help the absorption of the drug and may decrease GI upset.
- Make appointments for frequent blood tests that will need to be done to determine the effects of the drug on your blood count and to determine the appropriate dosage needed. It is important that you keep appointments for these tests.
- Arrange for periodic eye examinations (every 4–6 wk) during therapy to evaluate progress of the disease. This drug is not a cure for your retinitis.
- Be aware that if you are also receiving zidovudine, the two drugs cannot be given concomitantly; severe adverse effects may occur.

Adverse effects in *Italics* are most common; those in **Bold** are life-threatening.

- These side effects may occur: decreased blood count leading to susceptibility to infection (frequent blood tests will be needed; avoid crowds and exposure to disease as much as possible); birth defects and decreased sperm production (drug cannot be taken during pregnancy); sedation, dizziness, confusion (avoid driving or operating dangerous machinery if these effects occur). If you think you are pregnant or wish to become pregnant, consult with your physician. Use contraception during drug therapy. Male patients should use barrier contraceptives during drug therapy and for at least 90 days after therapy.
- Report bruising, bleeding, infection, extreme fatigue, edema.

▽valproic acid
(val proe' ik)

valproic acid
Capsules: Alti-Valproic (CAN), Depakene, Deproic (CAN)

sodium valproate
Syrup: Depakene

valproate acid
Injection: Depacon

divalproex sodium
Tablets, enteric coated: Depakote, Depakote ER, Depakote Sprinkle, Epival (CAN)

PREGNANCY CATEGORY D

Drug class
Antiepileptic agent

Therapeutic actions
Mechanism of action not understood: antiepileptic activity may be related to the metabolism of the inhibitory neurotransmitter, gamma-aminobutyric acid (GABA); divalproex sodium is a compound containing equal proportions of valproic acid and sodium valproate.

Indications
- Sole and adjunctive therapy in simple (petit mal) and complex absence seizures

- Adjunctive therapy with multiple seizure types, including absence seizures
- Treatment of mania (divalproex)
- Prophylaxis of migraine headaches (divalproex-DR tablets)
- Treatment of complex partial seizures as monotherapy or with other antiepilepsy drugs (divalproex, sodium valproate injection)
- Unlabeled uses: sole and adjunctive therapy in atypical absence, myoclonic and grand mal seizures; possibly effective therapy in atonic, elementary partial, and infantile spasm seizures; prophylaxis for recurrent febrile seizures in children

Contraindications and cautions
- Contraindicated with hypersensitivity to valproic acid, hepatic disease or significant hepatic dysfunction.
- Use cautiously with children < 18 mo; children < 2 yr, especially with multiple antiepileptic drugs, congenital metabolic disorders, severe seizures accompanied by severe mental retardation, organic brain disorders (higher risk of developing fatal hepatotoxicity); pregnancy (fetal neural tube defects; do not discontinue to prevent major seizures; discontinuing such medication is likely to precipitate status epilepticus, hypoxia and risk to both mother and fetus); lactation.

Available forms
Capsules—250 mg; syrup—250 mg/5 mL; DR tablets—125, 250, 500 mg; sprinkle capsules—125 mg; injection—100 mg/mL; ER tablets—500 mg

Dosages
Adults
Dosage is expressed as valproic acid equivalents. Initial dose is 10–15 mg/kg/day PO, increasing at 1-wk intervals by 5–10 mg/kg/day until seizures are controlled or side effects preclude further increases. Maximum recommended dosage is 60 mg/kg/day PO. If total dose > 250 mg/day, give in divided doses.
- *Mania:* 750 mg PO daily in divided doses; do not exceed 60 mg/kg/day (DR tablets only).
- *Migraine:* 250 mg PO bid; up to 1,000 mg/day has been used (divalproex DR tablets); 500 mg ER tablet once a day.

V

Pediatric patients

Use extreme caution. Fatal hepatotoxicity has occurred. Children < 2 yr are especially susceptible. Monitor all children carefully.

Pharmacokinetics

Route	Onset	Peak
Oral	Varies	1–4 hr
IV	Rapid	1 hr

Metabolism: Hepatic; $T_{1/2}$: 6–16 hr
Distribution: Crosses placenta; enters breast milk
Excretion: Urine

▽ IV facts

Preparation: Dilute vial in 5% dextrose injection, 0.9% sodium chloride injection or lactated Ringer's injection. Stable for 24 hr at room temperature. Discard unused portions.
Infusion: Administer over 60 min, not more than 20 mg/min. Do not use > 14 days; switch to oral products as soon as possible.

Adverse effects

- **CNS:** *Sedation,* tremor (may be dose-related), emotional upset, depression, psychosis, aggression, hyperactivity, behavioral deterioration, weakness
- **Dermatologic:** Transient increases in hair loss, rash, petechiae
- **GI:** *Nausea, vomiting, indigestion,* diarrhea, abdominal cramps, constipation, anorexia with weight loss, increased appetite with weight gain, **life-threatening pancreatitis, hepatic failure**
- **GU:** Irregular menses, secondary amenorrhea
- **Hematologic:** Slight elevations in AST, ALT, LDH; increases in serum bilirubin, abnormal changes in other liver function tests, altered bleeding time; thrombocytopenia; bruising; hematoma formation; frank hemorrhage; relative lymphocytosis; hypofibrinogenemia; leukopenia, eosinophilia, anemia, bone marrow suppression

Interactions

✳ **Drug-drug** ● Increased serum phenobarbital, primidone, ethosuximide, diazepam, zidovudine levels ● Complex interactions with phenytoin; breakthrough seizures have occurred with the combination of valproic acid and phenytoin ● Increased serum levels and toxicity with salicylates, cimetidine, chlorpromazine, erythromycin, felbamate ● Decreased effects with carbamazepine, rifampin, lamotrigine ● Decreased serum levels with charcoal ● Increased sedation with alcohol, other CNS depressants
✳ **Drug-lab test** ● False interpretation of urine ketone test

■ Nursing considerations

 CLINICAL ALERT!
Confusion has occurred between delayed release *Depakote* and *Depakote ER.* Dosage is very different and serious adverse effects can occur; use extreme caution.

Assessment

- **History:** Hypersensitivity to valproic acid; hepatic dysfunction; pregnancy, lactation
- **Physical:** Weight; skin color, lesions; orientation, affect, reflexes; bowel sounds, normal output; CBC and differential, bleeding time tests, hepatic function tests, serum ammonia level, exocrine pancreatic function tests, EEG

Interventions

- Give drug with food if GI upset occurs; substitution of the enteric-coated formulation also may be of benefit; have patient swallow SR tablet whole; do not cut, crush, or chew.
- Reduce dosage, discontinue, or substitute other antiepileptic medication gradually; abrupt discontinuation of all antiepileptic medication may precipitate absence status.
- Arrange for frequent liver function tests; discontinue drug immediately with significant hepatic dysfunction, suspected or apparent; hepatic dysfunction has progressed in spite of drug discontinuation.
- Arrange for patient to have platelet counts, bleeding time determination before therapy, periodically during therapy, and prior to surgery. Monitor patient carefully for clotting defects (bruising, blood tinged toothbrush). Discontinue if there is evidence of hemorrhage, bruising, or disorder of hemostasis.

Adverse effects in *Italics* are most common; those in **Bold** are life-threatening.

- Monitor ammonia levels, and discontinue if there is clinically significant elevation in level.
- Monitor serum levels of valproic acid and other antiepileptic drugs given concomitantly, especially during the first few weeks of therapy. Adjust dosage on the basis of these data and clinical response.
- Arrange for counseling for women of childbearing age who wish to become pregnant.
- Discontinue drug at any sign of pancreatitis.
- Evaluate for therapeutic serum levels—usually 50–100 mcg/mL.

Teaching points
- Take this drug exactly as prescribed. Do not chew tablets or capsules before swallowing them. Swallow them whole to prevent local irritation of mouth and throat.
- Do not discontinue this drug abruptly or change dosage, except on the advice of your physician.
- Avoid alcohol and sleep-inducing and OTC drugs. These could cause dangerous effects.
- Have frequent checkups, including blood tests, to monitor your drug response. Keep all appointments for checkups.
- Use contraceptive techniques at all times. If you wish to become pregnant, you should consult your physician.
- These side effects may occur: drowsiness (avoid driving or performing other tasks requiring alertness; take at bedtime); GI upset (take with food or milk, eat frequent, small meals; if problem persists, substitute enteric-coated drug); transient increase in hair loss.
- Wear a medical ID tag to alert emergency medical personnel that you are an epileptic taking antiepileptic medication.
- This drug may interfere with urine tests for ketones (diabetic patients).
- Report bruising, pink stain on the toothbrush, yellowing of the skin or eyes, pale feces, rash, pregnancy; abdominal pain with nausea, vomiting, anorexia.

▽ valrubicin

See *Less Commonly Used Drugs,* p. 1354.

▽ valsartan
*(val **sar'** tan)*

Diovan

PREGNANCY CATEGORY C
(FIRST TRIMESTER)

PREGNANCY CATEGORY D
(SECOND AND THIRD TRIMESTERS)

Drug classes
Angiotensin II receptor blocker (ARB)
Antihypertensive

Therapeutic actions
Selectively blocks the binding of angiotensin II to specific tissue receptors found in the vascular smooth muscle and adrenal gland; this action blocks the vasoconstricting effect of the renin–angiotensin system as well as the release of aldosterone, leading to decreased BP; may prevent the vessel remodeling associated with the development of atherosclerosis.

Indications
- Treatment of hypertension, alone or in combination with other antihypertensive agents
- Treatment of heart failure in patients who are intolerant of ACE inhibitors

Contraindications and cautions
- Contraindicated with hypersensitivity to valsartan, pregnancy (use during second or third trimester can cause injury or even death to fetus), lactation.
- Use cautiously with hepatic or renal dysfunction, hypovolemia.

Available forms
Tablets—40, 80, 160, 320 mg

Dosages
Adults
80 mg PO daily; range 80–320 mg/day.
- *Heart failure:* Starting dose is 40 mg bid, titration to 80 mg and 160 mg bid should be done to the highest dose, as tolerated by the patient. Maximum daily dose is 320 mg daily. Concomitant use with an ACE inhibitor and a beta blocker is not recommended.
Pediatric patients
Safety and efficacy not established.

V

Patients with hepatic or renal impairment
Exercise caution and monitor patient frequently.

Pharmacokinetics

Route	Onset	Peak
Oral	Varies	2–4 hr

Metabolism: Hepatic; $T_{1/2}$: 6 hr
Distribution: Crosses placenta; passes into breast milk
Excretion: Feces and urine

Adverse effects
- **CNS:** *Headache, dizziness,* syncope, muscle weakness
- **CV:** Hypotension
- **Dermatologic:** Rash, inflammation, urticaria, pruritus, alopecia, dry skin
- **GI:** *Diarrhea, abdominal pain, nausea,* constipation, dry mouth, dental pain
- **Respiratory:** *URI symptoms, cough,* sinus disorders
- **Other:** Cancer in preclinical studies, back pain, fever, gout

■ Nursing considerations
Assessment
- **History:** Hypersensitivity to valsartan; pregnancy, lactation; hepatic or renal dysfunction; hypovolemia
- **Physical:** Skin lesions, turgor; T; reflexes, affect; BP; R, respiratory auscultation; liver and renal function tests

Interventions
- Administer without regard to meals.
- Ensure that patient is not pregnant before beginning therapy; suggest use of barrier birth control while on drug; fetal injury and deaths have been reported.
- Find alternative method of feeding infant if drug is being given to nursing mother. Depression of renin–angiotensin system in infants is potentially very dangerous.
- Alert surgeon and mark patient's chart that valsartan is being given. Blockage of renin–angiotensin system following surgery can produce problems. Hypotension may be reversed with volume expansion.

- Monitor patient closely in any situation that may lead to decrease in BP secondary to reduction in fluid volume—excessive perspiration, dehydration, vomiting, diarrhea—as excessive hypotension can occur.

Teaching points
- Take this drug without regard to meals. Do not stop taking drug without consulting your nurse or physican.
- Use a barrier method of birth control while on this drug; if you become pregnant or desire to become pregnant, consult your physician.
- These side effects may occur: dizziness (avoid driving or performing hazardous tasks); headache (medications may be available to help); nausea, vomiting, diarrhea (proper nutrition is important; consult your dietitian); symptoms of upper respiratory tract infection, cough (do not self-medicate; consult your nurse or physician if this becomes uncomfortable).
- Report fever, chills, dizziness, pregnancy.

▷ vancomycin hydrochloride
(van koe mye' sin)

Vancocin, Vancoled

PREGNANCY CATEGORY C

CATEGORY B (PULVULES)

Drug class
Antibiotic

Therapeutic actions
Bactericidal: inhibits cell wall synthesis of susceptible organisms, causing cell death.

Indications
- Potentially life-threatening infections not treatable with other less toxic antibiotics (parenteral)
- Severe staphylococci infections in patients who cannot receive or have failed to respond to penicillins and cephalosporins
- Prevention of bacterial endocarditis in penicillin-allergic patients undergoing den-

tal, upper respiratory, GI, or GU surgery or invasive procedures
• Staphylococcal enterocolitis and antibiotic-associated pseudomembranous colitis caused by *Clostridium difficile* (oral)

Contraindications and cautions
• Contraindicated with allergy to vancomycin.
• Use cautiously with hearing loss, renal dysfunction, pregnancy, lactation.

Available forms
Pulvules—125, 250 mg; powder for oral solution—1, 10 g; powder for injection—500 mg, 1, 5, 10 g

Dosages
Adults
500 mg–2 g/day PO in 3–4 divided doses for 7–10 days; 500 mg IV q 6 hr or 1 g IV q 12 hr.
Pediatric patients
40 mg/kg/day PO in 3–4 divided doses for 7–10 days. 10 mg/kg/dose IV q 6 hr. Do not exceed 2 g/day.
Premature and full-term neonates: Use with caution because of incompletely developed renal function. Initial dose of 15 mg/kg, followed by 10 mg/kg q 12 hr in first week of life and q 8 hr thereafter up to age of 1 mo.
• *Pseudomembranous colitis caused by C. difficile:*
Adults
500 mg to 2 g/day PO in 3 to 4 divided doses for 7–10 days or 125 mg PO tid–qid.
Pediatric patients
40 mg/kg/day in 4 divided doses PO for 7–10 days. Do not exceed 2 g/day.
• *Prevention of bacterial endocarditis in penicillin-allergic patients undergoing dental or upper respiratory procedures:*
Adults and pediatric patients
> 27 kg: 1 g IV slowly over 1 hr, beginning 1 hr before the procedure. May repeat in 8–12 hr.
< 27 kg: 20 mg/kg IV slowly over 1 hr beginning 1 hr before the procedure. May repeat in 8–12 hr.
• *Prevention of bacterial endocarditis in patients undergoing GI or GU procedures:*
Adults and pediatric patients
> 27 kg: 1 g IV slowly over 1 hr plus 1.5 mg/kg gentamicin IM or IV concurrently 1 hr before the procedure. May repeat in 8–12 hr.

< 27 kg: 20 mg/kg IV slowly over 1 hr and 2 mg/kg gentamicin IM or IV concurrently 1 hr before the procedure. May repeat in 8–12 hr.
Geriatric patients or patients with renal failure
Monitor dosage and serum levels very carefully. Dosage nomogram is available for determining the dose according to creatinine clearance (see manufacturer's insert).

Pharmacokinetics
Route	Onset	Peak
Oral	Varies	Varies
IV	Rapid	End of infusion

Metabolism: Hepatic; $T_{1/2}$: 4–6 hr
Distribution: Crosses placenta; may enter breast milk
Excretion: Urine

▼ IV facts
Preparation: Not for IM administration. Reconstitute with 10 mL sterile water for injection; 500 mg/mL concentration results. Dilute reconstituted solution with 100–200 mL of 0.9% sodium chloride injection or 5% dextrose in water for intermittent infusion. For continuous infusion (use only if intermittent therapy is not possible), add 2–4 (1–2 g) vials reconstituted solution to sufficiently large volume of 0.9% sodium chloride injection or 5% dextrose in water to permit slow IV drip of the total daily dose over 24 hr. Refrigerate reconstituted solution; stable over 14 days. Further diluted solution is stable for 24 hr.
Infusion: For intermittent infusion, infuse q 6 hr, over at least 60 min to avoid irritation, hypotension, throbbing back and neck pain. Give continuously slowly over 24 hr.
Incompatibilities: Do not mix with amobarbital, chloramphenicol, dexamethasone, heparin, barbiturates, warfarin.
Y-site incompatibility: Do not give with foscarnet.

Adverse effects
• **CNS:** *Ototoxicity*
• **CV:** Hypotension (IV administration)
• **Dermatologic:** *Urticaria,* macular rashes
• **GI:** *Nausea*
• **GU:** *Nephrotoxicity*

- **Hematologic:** Eosinophilia
- **Other:** Superinfections; "**red neck or red man syndrome**" (sudden and profound fall in BP, fever, chills, paresthesias, erythema of the neck and back)

Interactions
* Drug-drug • Increased neuromuscular blockade with atracurium, pancuronium, tubocurarine, vecuronium

■ Nursing considerations
Assessment
- **History:** Allergy to vancomycin, hearing loss, renal dysfunction, pregnancy, lactation
- **Physical:** Site of infection, skin color, lesions; orientation, reflexes, auditory function; BP, perfusion; R, adventitious sounds; CBC, renal and liver function tests, auditory tests

Interventions
- Oral solution: Add 115 mL distilled water to contents of 10-g container. Each 6 mL of solution will contain 500 mg vancomycin. Alternatively, dilute the contents of 500-mg vial for injection in 30 mL of water for oral or nasogastric tube administration.
- Observe the patient very closely when giving parenteral solution, particularly the first doses; "red neck" syndrome can occur (see adverse effects); slow administration decreases the risk of adverse effects.
- Culture site of infection before beginning therapy.
- Monitor renal function tests with prolonged therapy.
- Evaluate for safe serum levels; concentrations of 60–80 mcg/mL are toxic.

Teaching points
- This drug is available only in the IV and oral forms.
- Do not stop taking this drug without notifying your health care provider.
- Take the full prescribed course of this drug.
- These side effects may occur: nausea (small, frequent meals may help); changes in hearing; superinfections in the mouth, vagina (frequent hygiene measures will help).

- Report ringing in the ears, loss of hearing, difficulty voiding, rash, flushing.

▽**vasopressin (8-arginine-vasopressin)**
(vay soe press' in)

Pitressin, Pressyn (CAN)

PREGNANCY CATEGORY C

Drug class
Hormone

Therapeutic actions
Purified form of posterior pituitary having pressor and antidiuretic hormone activities; promotes resorption of water in the renal tubular epithelium, causes contraction of vascular smooth muscle, increases GI motility and tone.

Indications
- Neurogenic diabetes insipidus
- Prevention and treatment of postoperative abdominal distention
- To dispel gas interfering with abdominal roentgenography
- Unlabeled uses: control acute variceal hemorrhage; treatment of refractory septic shock; to treat ventricular fibrillating cardiac arrest

Contraindications and cautions
- Contraindicated with allergy to vasopressin or any components, chronic nephritis.
- Use cautiously with vascular disease (may precipitate angina or MI), epilepsy, migraine, asthma, CHF, pregnancy, lactation.

Available forms
Injection—20 units/mL

Dosages
Adults
5–10 units IM or SC. Repeat at 3- to 4-hr intervals as needed.
- *Diabetes insipidus:*
Intranasal
Administer on cotton pledgets by nasal spray or dropper *or* 5–10 units bid or tid, IM or SC.

- *Abdominal distention:* 5 units IM initially. Increase to 10 units at subsequent injections given IM at 3- to 4-hr intervals.
- *Abdominal roentgenography:* Administer 2 injections of 10 units IM or SC each. Give 2 hr and 30 min before films are exposed. An enema may be given prior to first dose.

Pediatric patients
Decrease dose proportionately for children.

Pharmacokinetics

Route	Onset	Duration
IM, SC	Varies	2–8 hr

Metabolism: Hepatic; $T_{1/2}$: 10–20 min
Distribution: Crosses placenta; enters breast milk
Excretion: Urine

Adverse effects

- **CNS:** *Tremor, sweating, vertigo,* circumoral pallor, "pounding" in the head
- **GI:** Abdominal cramps, passage of gas, nausea, vomiting
- **Hypersensitivity:** Reactions ranging from urticaria, bronchial constriction to **anaphylaxis**
- **Other:** *Water intoxication* (drowsiness, light-headedness, headache, coma, convulsions), local tissue necrosis

■ Nursing considerations
Assessment

- **History:** Allergy to vasopressin or any components; vascular disease; chronic nephritis; epilepsy; migraine; asthma, CHF; pregnancy
- **Physical:** Skin color, lesions; nasal mucous membranes (if used intranasally); injection site; orientation, reflexes, affect; P, BP, rhythm, edema, baseline ECG; R, adventitous sounds; bowel sounds, abdominal exam; urinalysis, renal function tests, serum electrolytes

Interventions

- Administer injection by IM route; SC may be used if necessary.
- Monitor condition of nasal passages during long-term intranasal therapy; inappropriate administration can lead to nasal ulceration.

- Monitor patients with CV diseases very carefully for cardiac reactions.
- Monitor fluid volume for signs of water intoxication and excess fluid load; arrange to decrease dosage if this occurs.

Teaching points

- Give nasally on cotton pledgets, by nasal spray, or dropper. (Watch and review drug administration periodically with patient.) Other routes must be IM or SC.
- These side effects may occur: GI cramping, passing of gas; anxiety, tinnitus, vision changes (avoid driving or performing tasks that require alertness); nasal irritation (proper administration may decrease problem).
- Report swelling, difficulty breathing, chest tightness or pain, palpitations, running nose, painful nasal passages (intranasal).

▽**venlafaxine hydrochloride**
(vin lah facks' in)

Effexor, Effexor XR

PREGNANCY CATEGORY C

Drug class
Antidepressant

Therapeutic actions
Potentiates the neurotransmitter activity in the CNS; inhibits serontonin, norepinephrine, and dopamine reuptake leading to prolonged stimulation at neuroreceptors.

Indications

- Treatment of depression
- Treatment of generalized anxiety disorder (ER form)
- Prevention of major depressive disorder relapse

Contraindications and cautions

- Allergy to venlafaxine, use of MAOIs, pregnancy, lactation.

Available forms
Tablets—25, 37.5, 50, 75, 100 mg; ER capsules—37.5, 75, 150 mg

V

Dosages
Adults
- *Depression:* Starting dose, 75 mg/day PO in 2 to 3 divided doses (or once a day, ER capsule) taken with food. May be increased slowly up to 225 mg/day to achieve desired effect.
- *Transfer to or from MAOI:* At least 14 days should elapse from the discontinuation of the MAOI and the starting of venlafaxine; allow at least 7 days to elapse from the stopping of venlafaxine to the starting of an MAOI.
- *Generalized anxiety disorder:* 75–225 mg/day PO should be taken on a daily basis, not as needed.
- *Prevention of major depressive disorder relapse:* 75–225 mg/day PO or 75–150 mg/day PO extended-release capsule.

Pediatric patients
Safety and efficacy not established.
Geriatric patients
No dosage adjustment required.
Patients with hepatic or renal impairment
Reduce total daily dose by 50%, and increase very slowly to achieve desired effect.

Pharmacokinetics

Route	Onset	Duration
Oral	Slow	48 hr

Metabolism: Hepatic; $T_{1/2}$: 1.3–2 hr
Distribution: Crosses placenta; may enter breast milk
Excretion: Urine

Adverse effects
- **CNS:** *Somnolence, dizziness, insomnia, nervousness,* anxiety, tremor, dreams
- **CV:** Vasodilation, hypertension, tachycardia
- **Dermatologic:** *Sweating,* rash, pruritus
- **GI:** *Nausea, constipation, anorexia,* diarrhea, vomiting, dyspepsia, *dry mouth,* flatulence
- **GU:** *Abnormal ejaculation,* impotence, urinary frequency
- **Other:** *Headache, asthenia,* infection, chills, chest pain

Interactions
✳ **Drug-drug** • Increased serum levels and risk of toxicity with MAOIs, cimetidine • Serotonin syndrome may occur if combined with trazodone • Increased sedation with alcohol
✳ **Drug-alternative therapy** • Increased sedation and hypnotic effects with St. John's wort

■ Nursing considerations
Assessment
- **History:** Allergy to venlafaxine; use of MAOIs; pregnancy, lactation
- **Physical:** Skin color, temperature, lesions; reflexes, gait, sensation, cranial nerve evaluation; mucous membranes, abdominal exam, normal output; P, BP, peripheral perfusion

Interventions
- Give with food to decrease GI effects.
- Advise patient to use contraceptives.

Teaching points
- Take with food to decrease GI upset.
- These side effects may occur: loss of appetite, nausea, vomiting, dry mouth (frequent mouth care, small, frequent meals, sucking sugarless lozenges may help); constipation (request bowel program); dizziness, drowsiness, tremor (avoid driving or operating dangerous machinery).
- Avoid alcohol while on this drug.
- This drug cannot be taken during pregnancy; use birth control. If you become pregnant, consult with your health care provider.
- Report rash, hives, increased depression, pregnancy.

▽ verapamil hydrochloride
*(ver **ap'** a mill)*

Calan, Calan SR, Covera-HS, Isoptin, Isoptin SR, Verelan, Verelan PM

PREGNANCY CATEGORY C

Drug classes
Calcium channel-blocker

Adverse effects in *Italics* are most common; those in **Bold** are life-threatening.

Antianginal agent
Antiarrhythmic
Antihypertensive

Therapeutic actions

Inhibits the movement of calcium ions across the membranes of cardiac and arterial muscle cells; calcium is involved in the generation of the action potential in specialized automatic and conducting cells in the heart, in arterial smooth muscle, and in excitation-contraction coupling in cardiac muscle cells; inhibition of transmembrane calcium flow results in the depression of impulse formation in specialized cardiac pacemaker cells, slowing of the velocity of conduction of the cardiac impulse, the depression of myocardial contractility, and the dilation of coronary arteries and arterioles and peripheral arterioles; these effects lead to decreased cardiac work, decreased cardiac energy consumption, and in patients with vasospastic (Prinzmetal's) angina, increased delivery of oxygen to myocardial cells.

Indications

- Angina pectoris due to coronary artery spasm (Prinzmetal's variant angina)
- Effort-associated angina
- Chronic stable angina in patients who cannot tolerate or do not respond to beta-adrenergic blockers or nitrates
- Unstable, crescendo, preinfarction angina
- Essential hypertension (sustained-release oral only)
- Treatment of supraventricular tachyarrhythmias (parenteral)
- Temporary control of rapid ventricular rate in atrial flutter or atrial fibrillation (parenteral)
- Unlabeled oral uses: paroxysmal supraventricular tachycardia, migraine headache, nocturnal leg cramps, hypertrophic cardiomyopathy

Contraindications and cautions

- Contraindicated with allergy to verapamil; sick sinus syndrome, except with ventricular pacemaker; heart block (second- or third-degree); hypotension; pregnancy; lactation.
- Use cautiously with idiopathic hypertrophic subaortic stenosis, cardiogenic shock, severe CHF, impaired renal or hepatic function, and in patients with atrial flutter or atrial fibrillation and an accessory to bypass tract.

Available forms

Tablets—40, 80, 120 mg; SR tablets—120, 180, 240 mg; ER tablets—120, 180, 240 mg; SR capsules—120, 180, 240, 360 mg; injection—2.5 mg/mL; ER capsules—100, 120, 180, 200, 240, 300, 360 mg

Dosages
Adults
Oral

Initial dose: 80–120 mg tid; increase dose every 1–2 days to achieve optimum therapeutic effects. Usual maintenance dose: 320–480 mg/day.

- *Hypertension:* 120–240 mg PO daily, sustained-release form in morning. 80 mg PO tid; ER capsules—100–300 mg PO hs.

Parenteral

IV use only. Initial dose: 5–10 mg over 2 min; may repeat dose of 10 mg 30 min after first dose if initial response is inadequate.

Pediatric patients
IV

≤ *1 yr:* Initial dose: 0.1–0.2 mg/kg over 2 min. *1–15 yr:* Initial dose: 0.1–0.3 mg/kg over 2 min. Do not exceed 5 mg. Repeat above dose 30 min after initial dose if response is not adequate. Repeat dose should not exceed 10 mg.

Geriatric patients or patients with renal impairment

Reduce dosage, and monitor patient response carefully. Give IV doses over 3 min to reduce risk of serious side effects. Administer IV doses very slowly, over 2 min.

Pharmacokinetics

Route	Onset	Peak	Duration
Oral	30 min	1–2.2 hr	3–7 hr
IV	1–5 min	3–5 min	2 hr

Metabolism: Hepatic; $T_{1/2}$: 3–7 hr
Distribution: Crosses placenta; enters breast milk
Excretion: Urine

▼ IV facts

Preparation: No further preparation required.
Infusion: Infuse very slowly over 2–3 min.

Y-site incompatibilities: Do not give with albumin, ampicillin, mezlocillin, nafcillin, oxacillin, sodium bicarbonate, amphotericin B, hydralazine, aminophylline, trimethoprim and sulfamethoxazole.

Adverse effects
- **CNS:** *Dizziness,* vertigo, emotional depression, sleepiness, *headache*
- **CV:** *Peripheral edema, hypotension,* arrhythmias, bradycardia; AV heart block
- **GI:** *Nausea,* constipation
- **Other:** Muscle fatigue, diaphoresis, rash

Interactions
✳ **Drug-drug** • Increased cardiac depression with beta-adrenergic blocking agents • Additive effects of verapamil and digoxin to slow AV conduction • Increased serum levels of digoxin, carbamazepine, prazosin, quinidine • Increased respiratory depression with atracurium, gallamine, pancuronium, rucuronium, tubocurarine, vecuronium • Risk of serious cardiac effects with IV beta-adrenergic blocking agents; do not give these drugs within 48 hr before or 24 hr after IV verapamil • Decreased effects with calcium, rifampin
✳ **Drug-food** • Decreased metabolism and risk of toxic effects if combined with grapefruit juice; avoid this combination

■ Nursing considerations
Assessment
- **History:** Allergy to verapamil; sick sinus syndrome; heart block; IHSS; cardiogenic shock, severe CHF; hypotension; impaired hepatic or renal function; pregnancy, lactation
- **Physical:** Skin color, edema; orientation, reflexes; P, BP, baseline ECG, peripheral perfusion, auscultation; R, adventitious sounds; liver evaluation, normal output; liver function tests, renal function tests, urinalysis

Interventions
- Monitor patient carefully (BP, cardiac rhythm, and output) while drug is being titrated to therapeutic dose. Dosage may be increased more rapidly in hospitalized patients under close supervision.

- Ensure that patient swallows SR tablets whole: do not cut, crush, or chew.
- Monitor BP very carefully with concurrent doses of antihypertensives.
- Monitor cardiac rhythm regularly during stabilization of dosage and periodically during long-term therapy.
- Administer sustained-release form in the morning with food to decrease GI upset.
- Protect IV solution from light.
- Monitor patients with renal or hepatic impairment carefully for possible drug accumulation and adverse reactions.

Teaching points
- Take sustained-release form in the morning with food; swallow whole, do not cut, crush, or chew. Do not drink grapefruit juice while on this drug.
- These side effects may occur: nausea, vomiting (eat small, frequent meals); headache (monitor the lighting, noise, and temperature; request medication); dizziness, sleepiness (avoid driving or operating dangerous equipment); emotional depression (reversible); constipation (request aid).
- Report irregular heart beat, shortness of breath, swelling of the hands or feet, pronounced dizziness, nausea, constipation.

▷ verteporfin
See *Less Commonly Used Drugs,* p. 1354.

▷ vinblastine sulfate (VLB)
(vin blas' teen)

Velban, Velbe (CAN)

PREGNANCY CATEGORY D

Drug classes
Mitotic inhibitor
Antineoplastic

Therapeutic actions
Affects cell energy production required for mitosis and interferes with nucleic acid synthe-

sis; has antimitotic effect and causes abnormal mitotic figures.

Indications

- Palliative treatment for generalized Hodgkin's disease (stages III and IV), lymphocytic lymphoma, histiocytic lymphoma, mycosis fungoides, advance testicular carcinoma, Kaposi's sarcoma, Letterer-Siwe disease
- Palliation of choriocarcinoma, breast cancer unresponsive to other therapies
- Hodgkin's disease (advanced) alone or in combination therapies
- Advanced testicular germinal-cell cancers alone or in combination therapy

Contraindications and cautions

- Contraindicated with allergy to vinblastine, leukopenia, acute infection, pregnancy, lactation.
- Use cautiously with liver disease.

Available forms

Powder for injection—10 mg; injection—1 mg/mL

Dosages

Do not administer more than once a week because of leukopenic response.

Adults

Initial dose, 3.7 mg/m² as a single IV dose, followed at weekly intervals by increasing doses; a conservative regimen follows:

Dose	Adult Dose (mg/m²)	Pediatric Dose (mg/m²)
First	3.7	2.5
Second	5.5	3.75
Third	7.4	5
Fourth	9.25	6.25
Fifth	11.1	7.5

Use these increments until a maximum dose of 18.5 mg/m² for adults or 12.5 mg/m² for children is reached; do not increase dose after WBC is reduced to 3,000/mm³.

- *Maintenance therapy:* When dose produces WBC of 3,000/mm³, use a dose one increment smaller for weekly maintenance. Do not give another dose until WBC is 4,000/mm³ even if 7 days have passed. Du-

ration of therapy depends on disease and response; up to 2 yr may be necessary.

Pediatric patients

Initial dose, 2.5 mg/m² as a single IV dose, followed at weekly intervals by increasing doses (see adult regimen).

Pharmacokinetics

Route	Onset
IV	Slow

Metabolism: Hepatic; $T_{1/2}$: 3.7 min, then 1.6 hr, then 24.8 hr.
Distribution: Crosses placenta; enters breast milk
Excretion: Bile

▼ IV facts

Preparation: Add 10 mL of sodium chloride injection preserved with phenol or benzyl alcohol to the vial for a concentration of 1 mg/mL. Refrigerate drug; opened vials are stable for 30 days when refrigerated.
Infusion: Inject into tubing of a running IV or directly into the vein over 20–30 min or as a prolonged infusion over up to 96 hr. Rinse syringe and needle with venous blood prior to withdrawing needle from vein (to minimize extravasation). Do not inject into an extremity with poor circulation or repeatedly into the same vein.
Y-site incompatibilities: Do not give with furosemide.

Adverse effects

- **CNS:** Numbness, paresthesias, peripheral neuritis, mental depression, loss of deep tendon reflexes, headache, seizures, malaise, weakness, dizziness
- **Dermatologic:** Topical epilation (loss of hair), vesiculation of the skin
- **GI:** Nausea, vomiting, pharyngitis, vesiculation of the mouth, ileus, diarrhea, constipation, anorexia, abdominal pain, rectal bleeding, hemorrhagic enterocolitis
- **GU:** Aspermia
- **Hematologic:** Leukopenia
- **Local:** Local cellulitis, phlebitis, sloughing if extravasation occurs
- **Other:** Pain in tumor site

V

Interactions

❋ **Drug-drug** • Decreased serum concentrations of phenytoins • Risk of toxicity if combined with erythromycin

❋ **Drug-food** • Decreased metabolism and risk of toxic effects if combined with grapefruit juice; avoid this combination

■ Nursing considerations

 CLINICAL ALERT!
Confusion has occurred between vinblastine and vincristine; use extreme caution if giving either drug.

Assessment

- **History:** Allergy to vinblastine; leukopenia; acute infection; liver disease; pregnancy, lactation
- **Physical:** Weight; hair; T; reflexes, gait, sensation, orientation, affect; mucous membranes, abdominal exam, rectal exam; CBC, liver function tests, serum albumin

Interventions

- Ensure that patient is not pregnant before administering; advise patients to use contraceptive measures.
- Do not administer IM or SC due to severe local reaction and tissue necrosis.
- Avoid extravasation; if it occurs, discontinue injection immediately, and give remainder of dose in another vein. Consult physician to arrange for hyaluronidase injection into local area, after which apply moderate heat to disperse drug and minimize pain.
- Avoid contact with the eyes; if contact occurs, immediately wash thoroughly with water.
- Consult with physician if antiemetic is needed for severe nausea and vomiting.
- Check CBC before each dose.

Teaching points

- Prepare a calendar for dates to return for treatment and drug therapy. Avoid grapefruit juice while you are on this drug.
- These side effects may occur: loss of appetite, nausea, vomiting, mouth sores (frequent mouth care, small, frequent meals may help; maintain nutrition; request an antiemetic);

constipation (a bowel program may be ordered); malaise, weakness, dizziness, numbness and tingling (avoid injury); loss of hair, rash (obtain a wig; keep the head covered in extremes of temperature).
- This drug should not be used during pregnancy. Use birth control. If you become pregnant, consult your physician.
- Have regular blood tests to monitor the drug's effects.
- Report severe nausea, vomiting, pain or burning at injection site, abdominal pain, rectal bleeding, fever, chills, acute infection.

▷vincristine sulfate (LCR, VCR)
*(vin **kris'** teen)*

Oncovin, Vincasar PFS

PREGNANCY CATEGORY D

Drug classes
Mitotic inhibitor
Antineoplastic

Therapeutic actions
Mitotic inhibitor: arrests mitotic division at the stage of metaphase; exact mechanism of action unknown.

Indications
- Acute leukemia
- Hodgkin's disease, non-Hodgkin's lymphoma, rhabdomyosarcoma, neuroblastoma, Wilms' tumor as part of combination therapy

Contraindications and cautions
- Contraindicated with allergy to vincristine, leukopenia, acute infection, pregnancy, lactation, demyelinating form of Charcot-Marie-Tooth syndrome.
- Use cautiously with neuromuscular disease, diabetes insipidus, hepatic dysfunction.

Available forms
Injection—1 mg/mL

Dosages
Adults
1.4 mg/m^2 IV at weekly intervals.
Pediatric patients
2 mg/m^2 IV weekly.
< 10 kg: 0.05 mg/kg once a week.
Geriatric patients or patients with hepatic insufficiency
Serum bilirubin 1.5–3.0, reduce dosage by 50%.

Pharmacokinetics

Route	Onset	Peak
IV	Varies	15–30 min

Metabolism: Hepatic; T$_{1/2}$: 5 min, then 2.3 hr, then 85 hr
Distribution: Crosses placenta; enters breast milk
Excretion: Feces and urine

▽ IV facts
Preparation: No further preparation required; drug should be refrigerated.
Infusion: Inject solution directly into vein or into the tubing of a running IV infusion. Infusion may be completed within 1 min.
Y-site incompatibility: Do not give with furosemide.

Adverse effects
- **CNS:** *Ataxia, cranial nerve manifestations;* foot drop, headache, convulsions, bladder neuropathy, paresthesias, sensory impairment, *neuritic pain, muscle wasting,* SIADH, optic atrophy, transient cortical blindness, ptosis, diplopia, photophobia
- **GI:** *Constipation,* oral ulcerations, abdominal cramps, vomiting, diarrhea, intestinal necrosis
- **GU:** Acute uric acid nephropathy, polyuria, dysuria
- **Hematologic:** *Leukopenia*
- **Local:** Local irritation, cellulitis if extravasation occurs
- **Other:** *Weight loss, loss of hair,* fever, **death** with serious overdose

Interactions
✱ **Drug-drug** • Decreased serum levels and therapeutic effects of digoxin • If L-asparaginase is administered first, the hepatic clearance of vincristine may be reduced. Give vincristine 12–24 hr before L-asparaginase to minimize toxicity
✱ **Drug-food** • Decreased metabolism and risk of toxic effects if combined with grapefruit juice; avoid this combination

■ Nursing considerations

CLINICAL ALERT!
Confusion has occurred between vincristine and vinblastine; use extreme caution if giving either drug.

Assessment
- **History:** Allergy to vincristine; leukopenia; acute infection; neuromuscular disease; diabetes insipidus; hepatic dysfunction; pregnancy, lactation
- **Physical:** Weight; hair; T; reflexes, gait, sensation, cranial nerve evaluation, ophthalmic exam; mucous membranes, abdominal exam; CBC, serum sodium, liver function tests, urinalysis

Interventions
- Ensure that patient is not pregnant before administering; use of barrier contraceptives is advised.
- Avoid grapefruit juice while you are on this drug.
- Do not administer IM or SC due to severe local reaction and tissue necrosis.
- Take care to avoid extravasation; if it occurs, discontinue injection immediately and give remainder of dose in another vein. Consult with physician to arrange for hyaluronidase injection into local area, and apply heat to disperse the drug and to minimize pain.
- Arrange for wig or suitable head covering if hair loss occurs; ensure that patient's head is covered in extremes of temperature.
- Monitor urine output and serum sodium; if SIADH occurs, consult with physician, and arrange for fluid restriction and perhaps a potent diuretic.

Teaching points
- Prepare a calendar of dates to return for treatment and additional therapy.
- Avoid grapefruit juice while you are on this drug.

V

- These side effects may occur: loss of appetite, nausea, vomiting, mouth sores (frequent mouth care, small frequent meals may help; maintain nutrition; request an antiemetic); constipation (bowel program may be ordered); sensitivity to light (wear sunglasses; avoid bright lights); numbness, tingling, change in style of walking (reversible; may persist for up to 6 wk); hair loss (transient; obtain a wig or other suitable head covering; keep the head covered at extremes of temperature).
- This drug cannot be taken during pregnancy; use birth control. If you become pregnant, consult with your physician.
- Have regular blood tests to monitor the drug's effects.
- Report change in frequency of voiding; swelling of ankles, fingers, and so forth; changes in vision; severe constipation, abdominal pain.

▷vinorelbine tartrate
(vin oh rel' been)

Navelbine

PREGNANCY CATEGORY D

Drug classes
Mitotic inhibitor
Antineoplastic

Therapeutic actions
Affects cell energy production required for mitosis and interferes with nucleic acid synthesis; has antimitotic effect, prevents the formation of microtubules and leads to cell death; cell cycle specific.

Indications
- First line treatment of ambulatory patients with unresectable advanced non–small-cell lung cancer
- Treatment of stage IV non–small-cell lung cancer alone or with cisplatin
- Treatment of stage III non–small-cell lung cancer with cisplatin

- Unlabeled uses: breast cancer, ovarian cancer, Hodgkin's disease, desmoid tumors and fibromatosis, advanced Kaposi's sarcoma

Contraindications and cautions
- Contraindicated with allergy to vinca alkaloids, pretreatment granulocyte counts ≤ 1,000 cells/mm³, pregnancy, lactation.
- Use cautiously with liver disease.

Available forms
Injection—10 mg/mL

Dosages
Adults
Do not administer more than once a week because of leukopenic response.
- *Initial dose:* 30 mg/m² as single IV dose; repeat once a week until progression of disease or toxicity limits use.
- *With cisplatin:* 120 mg/m² cisplatin on days 1 and 29 and then every 6 wk.

Patients with hepatic impairment
Reduce dose.

Pharmacokinetics

Route	Onset
IV	Slow

Metabolism: Hepatic; $T_{1/2}$: 22–66 hr
Distribution: Crosses placenta; passes into breast milk
Excretion: Bile and feces

▽IV facts
Preparation: Dilute for 50 or 10 mg solution. Supplied as single use vials only. Discard after withdrawing solution.
Infusion: Inject into tubing of a running IV or directly into the vein over 6–10 min. Rinse syringe and needle with venous blood prior to withdrawing needle from vein (to minimize extravasation). Do not inject into an extremity with poor circulation or repeatedly into the same vein.

Adverse effects
- **CNS:** Numbness, paresthesias (less common than with other vinca alkaloids); headache, weakness, dizziness

---

Adverse effects in *Italics* are most common; those in **Bold** are life-threatening.

- **Dermatologic:** Topical epilation (loss of hair), vesiculation of the skin
- **GI:** Nausea, vomiting, pharyngitis, vesiculation of the mouth, ileus, diarrhea, constipation, anorexia, abdominal pain, *increased liver enzymes*
- **Hematologic:** Granulocytopenia, leukopenia
- **Local:** Local cellulitis, phlebitis, sloughing with extravasation
- **Other:** Myalgia, arthralgia

Interactions
* **Drug-drug** • Acute pulmonary reactions with mitomycin • Increased risk of granulocytopenia with cisplatin • Risk of neuropathies if combined or given sequentially with paclitaxel; monitor patient closely

■ Nursing considerations
Assessment
- **History:** Allergy to vinca alkaloids; leukopenia; acute infection; liver disease; pregnancy, lactation
- **Physical:** Weight; hair; T; reflexes, gait, sensation, orientation, affect; mucous membranes, abdominal exam; CBC, liver function tests, serum albumin

Interventions
- Ensure that patient is not pregnant before use; advise patient to use barrier contraceptives.
- Do not administer IM or SC—severe local reaction and tissue necrosis occur.
- Avoid extravasation; if it should occur, discontinue injection immediately and give remainder of dose in another vein. Consult physician to arrange for hyaluronidase injection into local area, after which apply moderate heat to disperse drug and minimize pain.
- Avoid contact with the eyes; if contact occurs, immediately wash thoroughly with water.
- Consult with physician if antiemetic is needed for severe nausea and vomiting.
- Check CBC before each dose.

Teaching points
- Prepare a calendar for dates to return for treatment and additional therapy.

- These side effects may occur: loss of appetite, nausea, vomiting, mouth sores (frequent mouth care, small frequent meals may help; maintain nutrition; request an antiemetic); constipation (bowel program may be ordered); malaise, weakness, dizziness, numbness and tingling (avoid injury); loss of hair, rash (obtain a wig; keep the head covered in extremes of temperature).
- This drug should not be used during pregnancy. Use birth control. If you become pregnant, consult your health care provider.
- Have regular blood tests to monitor the drug's effects.
- Report severe nausea, vomiting, pain or burning at injection site, abdominal pain, rectal bleeding, fever, chills, acute infection.

▽ voriconazole
*(vor ah **kon'** ah zole)*

Vfend

PREGNANCY CATEGORY D

Drug class
Triazole antifungal

Therapeutic actions
Inhibits fungal ergosterol biosynthesis leading to cell membrane rupture and cell death in susceptible fungi.

Indications
- Treatment of invasive aspergillosis
- Treatment of serious fungal infections caused by *Scedosproim apiospermum* and *Fusarium* species in patients intolerant of or refractory to other therapy

Contraindications and cautions
- Contraindicated with hypersensitivity to voriconazole, treatment with other drugs that could prolong the QTc interval, severe hepatic dysfunction, galactose intolerance; patients taking the following drugs: ergot alkaloids, sirolimus, rifabutin, rifampin, carbamazepine, and long-acting barbiturates.
- Use cautiously with known allergies to other azoles, pregnancy, lactation.

Available forms
Tablets—50, 200 mg; powder for injection—200 mg to be reconstituted to 10 mg/mL

Dosages
Adults
Loading dose of 6 mg/kg IV q 12 hr for 2 doses, then 4 mg/kg IV q 12 hr. Switch to oral dose as soon as patient is able:
> *40 kg:* 200 mg PO q 12 hr; may increase to 300 mg PO q 12 hr if necessary.
< *40 kg:* 100 mg PO q 12 hr; may increase to 150 mg PO q 12 hr if necessary.
Pediatric patients < 12 yr
Safety and efficacy not established.

Pharmacokinetics

Route	Peak	Duration
Oral	1–2 hr	96 hr
IV	Onset of infusion	96 hr

Metabolism: Hepatic; $T_{1/2}$: 24 hr
Distribution: Crosses placenta; may enter breast milk
Excretion: Urine

▼IV facts
Preparation: Reconstitute powder with 19 mL of water for injection, resulting solution contains 10 mg/mL. Shake the vial until powder is dissolved. Further dilute VFEND to obtain a concentration of 5 mg/mL using 0.9% sodium chloride, lactated Ringer's, 5% dextrose and lactated Ringer's, 5% dextrose and 0.45% sodium chloride, 5% dextrose, 5% dextrose and 20 mEq potassium chloride, 0.45% sodium chloride, 5% dextrose and 0.9% sodium chloride. Do not use if solution is not clear or if it contains particulate matter. Use immediately after reconstitution. Discard any unused solution.
Infusion: Infuse over 1–2 hr at no more than 3 mg/kg/hr.
Incompatibilities: Do not infuse with parenteral nutrition, blood products, electrolyte supplements, any alkaline solution, other drug infusions.

Adverse effects
- **CNS:** Headache, *visual disturbance,* hallucinations, dizziness
- **CV:** Tachycardia, blood pressure changes, vasodilation, chest pain, peripheral edema
- **GI:** Nausea, vomiting, diarrhea, dry mouth, abnormal liver function tests, abdominal pain
- **Hematologic:** Anemia, thrombocytopenia, leukopenia
- **Other:** *Fever,* chills, rash pruritis, **Stevens-Johnson syndrome, anaphylactic reactions**

Interactions
✳ **Drug-drug** • Decreased serum levels and effectiveness of voriconazole if combined with rifampin, rifabutin, carbamazepine, phenobarbital, mephobarbital; avoid these combinations • Increased serum levels of sirolimus, terfenidine, pimozide, quinidine, ergot alkaloids if taken with voriconazole; avoid these combinations • Possible alterations in serum levels and effectiveness of warfarin, tacrolimus, statins, oral anticoagulants, benzodiazepine, calcium channel blockers, sulfonylureas, vincristine, vinblastine, when taken with voriconazole; patients should be monitored closely and appropriate dosage adjustments made • Altered serum levels and risk of adverse effects from both drugs when voriconazole is taken concomitantly with phenytoin, omeprazole, protease inhibitors; patients should be monitored frequently and appropriate dosage adjustments made • Increased plasma levels of cyclosporine; reduce cyclosporine dose to one-half of the starting dose and monitor cyclosporine blood levels frequently; after voriconazole therapy ends, increase cyclosporine dose as needed • Increased plasma concentration of ergot alkaloids, which may lead to ergotism; avoid this combination

■ Nursing considerations
Assessment
- **History:** Hypersensitivity to *E. coli* products, filgrastim, sickle cell disease, pregnancy, lactation
- **Physical:** Skin color, lesions, hair; T; orientation, affect; abdominal exam, status of mucous membranes; liver and kidney function tests, CBC, platelets

---

Adverse effects in *Italics* are most common; those in **Bold** are life-threatening.

Interventions

- Obtain baseline liver function before beginning therapy and repeat during the course of therapy. Stop drug at first sign of significant liver toxicity.
- Check patient's medications carefully before beginning drug therapy, voriconazole is associated with many drug-drug interactions.
- Administer oral drug on an empty stomach, at least 1 hour before or 2 hours after meals.
- Monitor vision changes. Advise patient not to drive at night or perform potentially hazardous tasks because of possible visual disturbances.
- Protect patient from exposure to strong sunlight while on this drug.
- Women of childbearing age should be advised to use barrier contraceptives while on this drug because of the risk of fetal death or abnormalities.
- Provide appropriate comfort and supportive measures for headache, GI discomfort.
- Arrange for small, frequent meals if nausea and vomiting are a problem.

Teaching points

- This drug will be started by IV infusion and then you will switch to an oral form.
- Take the drug on an empty stomach one hour before or two hours after a meal.
- Avoid exposure to strong sunlight while you are on this drug.
- Women of childbearing age should use barrier contraceptives while on this drug, it has been associated with fetal abnormalities.
- These side effects may occur: nausea and vomiting (small, frequent meals may help); headache, fever (analgesics may be available that will help); visual changes (do not drive at night, avoid performing potentially hazardous tasks while on this drug).
- Tell any other health care provider that you see that you are taking this drug; it has been associated with many drug interactions when taken with other drugs. Adjustments may need to be made.
- Report fever, chills, changes in color of stool or urine, visual disturbances.

▽ warfarin sodium
(war' far in)

Coumadin, Warfilone (CAN)

PREGNANCY CATEGORY X

Drug classes
Oral anticoagulant
Coumarin derivative

Therapeutic actions
Interferes with the hepatic synthesis of vitamin K-dependent clotting factors (factors II-prothrombin, VII, IX, and X), resulting in their eventual depletion and prolongation of clotting times.

Indications
- Venous thrombosis and its extension, treatment, and prophylaxis
- Treatment of thromboembolic complications of atrial fibrillation with embolization, and cardiac valve replacement
- Pulmonary embolism, treatment, and prophylaxis
- Prophylaxis of systemic embolization after acute MI
- Unlabeled uses: prevention of recurrent TIAs, prevention of recurrent MI, adjunct to therapy in small-cell carcinoma of the lung

Contraindications and cautions
- Contraindicated with allergy to warfarin; SBE; hemorrhagic disorders; TB; hepatic diseases; GI ulcers; renal disease; indwelling catheters, spinal puncture; aneurysm; diabetes; visceral carcinoma; uncontrolled hypertension; severe trauma (including recent or contemplated CNS, eye surgery; recent placement of IUD); threatened abortion, menometrorrhagia; pregnancy (fetal damage and death); lactation (suggest using heparin if anticoagulation is required).
- Use cautiously with CHF, diarrhea, fever; thyrotoxicosis; senile, psychotic, or depressed patients.

Available forms
Tablets—1, 2, 2.5, 3, 4, 5, 6, 7.5, 10 mg; powder for injection—2 mg

W

Dosages

Adjust dosage according to the one-stage PT to achieve and maintain 1.5–2.5 times the control value or prothrombin activity 20%–30% of normal; PT ratio of 1.3–1.5 or INR of 2–3. IV use is reserved for situations in which oral warfarin is not feasible. Dosages are the same for oral and IV forms.

Adults

Initial: 2–5 mg/day PO. Adjust dose according to PT response. Maintenance: 2–10 mg/day PO based on PT ratio or INR.

Geriatric patients

Lower doses are usually needed; begin with smaller doses than those recommended for adults, and closely monitor PT ratio or INR.

Pharmacokinetics

Route	Peak	Duration
Oral	1.5–3 days	2–5 days

Metabolism: Hepatic; $T_{1/2}$: 1–2.5 days
Distribution: Crosses placenta; enters breast milk
Excretion: Feces and urine

▽IV facts

Preparation: Reconstitute vial with 2.7 mL of sterile water. Protect from light. Use within 4 hr of reconstitution.
Infusion: Inject slowly over 1–2 min; switch to oral preparation as soon as possible.

Adverse effects

- **Bleeding: Hemorrhage:** GI or urinary tract bleeding (hematuria, dark stools; paralytic ileus, intestinal obstruction from hemorrhage into GI tract); petechiae and purpura, bleeding from mucous membranes; hemorrhagic infarction, vasculitis, skin necrosis of female breast; adrenal hemorrhage and resultant adrenal insufficiency; compressive neuropathy secondary to hemorrhage near a nerve
- **Dermatologic:** *Alopecia, urticaria, dermatitis*
- **GI:** *Nausea,* vomiting, anorexia, abdominal cramping, diarrhea, retroperitoneal hematoma, hepatitis, jaundice, mouth ulcers
- **GU:** Priapism, nephropathy, red-orange urine
- **Hematologic:** Granulocytosis, leukopenia, eosinophilia
- **Other:** Fever, "purple toes" syndrome

Interactions

✳ Drug-drug • Increased bleeding tendencies with salicylates, chloral hydrate, phenylbutazone, clofibrate, disulfiram, chloramphenicol, metronidazole, cimetidine, ranitidine, co-trimoxazole, sulfinpyrazone, quinidine, quinine, oxyphenbutazone, thyroid drugs, glucagon, danazol, erythromycin, androgens, amiodarone, cefamandole, cefoperazone, cefotetan, moxalactam, cefazolin, cefoxitin, ceftriaxone, meclofenamate, mefenamic acid, famotidine, nizatidine, nalidixic acid • Decreased anticoagulation effect may occur with barbiturates, griseofulvin, rifampin, phenytoin, glutethimide, carbamazepine, vitamin K, vitamin E, cholestyramine, aminoglutethimide, ethchlorvynol • Altered effects with methimazole, propylthiouracil • Increased activity and toxicity of phenytoin when taken with oral anticoagulants
✳ Drug-lab test • Red-orange discoloration of alkaline urine may interfere with some lab tests
✳ Drug-alternative therapy • Increased risk of bleeding if combined with chamomile, garlic, ginger, ginkgo, and ginseng therapy • Increased bleeding with turmeric, horse chestnut seed, green tea leaf, grape seed extract, feverfew, don quai

■ Nursing considerations
Assessment

- **History:** Allergy to warfarin; SBE; hemorrhagic disorders; TB; hepatic diseases; GI ulcers; renal disease; indwelling catheters; spinal puncture; aneurysm; diabetes; visceral carcinoma; uncontrolled hypertension; severe trauma; threatened abortion, menometrorrhagia; pregnancy; lactation; CHF, diarrhea, fever; thyrotoxicosis; senile, psychotic or depressed patients
- **Physical:** Skin lesions, color, temperature; orientation, reflexes, affect; P, BP, peripheral perfusion, baseline ECG; R, adventitious sounds; liver evaluation, bowel sounds, nor-

mal output; CBC, urinalysis, guaiac stools, PT, renal and hepatic function tests

Interventions

- Do not use drug if patient is pregnant (heparin is anticoagulant of choice); advise patient to use contraceptives.
- Monitor PT ratio or INR regularly to adjust dosage.
- Administer IV form to patients stabilized on *Coumadin* who are not able to take oral drug. Dosages are the same. Return to oral form as soon as feasible.
- Do not change brand names once stabilized; bioavailability problems exist.
- Evaluate patient regularly for signs of blood loss (petechiae, bleeding gums, bruises, dark stools, dark urine). Maintain PT ratio of 1.3–1.5, 1.5–2 with mechanical prosthetic valves or recurrent systemic embolism; INR ratio of 2–3, 3–4.5 with mechanical prosthetic valves or recurrent systemic emboli.
- Do not give patient any IM injections.
- Double check all drugs ordered for potential drug–drug interaction; dosage of both drugs may need to be adjusted.
- Use caution when discontinuing other medications; warfarin dosage may need to be adjusted; carefully monitor PT values.
- Maintain vitamin K on standby in case of overdose.
- Arrange for frequent follow-up, including blood tests to evaluate drug effects.
- Evaluate for therapeutic effects: PT 1.5–2.5 times the control value; PT ratio, INR within therapeutic range.

Teaching points

- Many factors may change your body's response to this drug—fever, change of diet, change of environment, other medications. Your dosage may have to be changed repeatedly. Write down changes that are prescribed.
- Do not change any medication that you are taking (adding or stopping another drug) without consulting your health care provider. Other drugs can affect your anticoagulant; starting or stopping another drug can cause excessive bleeding or interfere with the desired drug effects.
- Carry or wear a medical ID tag to alert emergency medical personnel that you are taking this drug.
- Avoid situations in which you could be easily injured (contact sports, shaving with a straight razor).
- These side effects may occur: stomach bloating, cramps (transient); loss of hair, rash; orange-red discoloration to the urine (if upsetting, add vinegar to your urine and the color should disappear).
- Have periodic blood tests to check on the drug action. These tests are important.
- Use contraception; do not become pregnant while taking this drug.
- Report unusual bleeding (from brushing your teeth, excessive bleeding from injuries, excessive bruising), black or bloody stools, cloudy or dark urine, sore throat, fever, chills, severe headaches, dizziness, suspected pregnancy.

▷ xylometazoline hydrochloride
(zye low met az' oh leen)

Natru-Vent, Otrivin Nasal Drops or Spray, Otrivin Pediatric Nasal Drops

PREGNANCY CATEGORY C

Drug class
Nasal decongestant

Therapeutic actions
Acts directly on alpha receptors to produce vasoconstriction of arterioles in nasal passages, which produces a decongestant response; no effect on beta receptors.

Indications
- Symptomatic relief of nasal and nasopharyngeal mucosal congestion due to the common cold, hay fever, or other respiratory allergies (topical)

Contraindications and cautions

- Contraindicated with allergy to xylometazoline, angle-closure glaucoma, anesthesia with cyclopropane or halothane, thyrotoxicosis, diabetes, hypertension, CV disorders, women in labor whose BP > 130/80.

- Use cautiously with angina, arrhythmias, prostatic hypertrophy, unstable vasomotor syndrome, lactation.

Available forms
Nasal solution—0.05%, 0.1%

Dosages
Adults and children ≥ 12 yr
2–3 sprays or 2–3 drops in each nostril q 8–10 hr (0.1% solution).
Pediatric patients 2–12 yr
2–3 drops of 0.05% solution in each nostril q 8–10 hr (0.05% solution).

Pharmacokinetics

Route	Onset	Duration
Nasal	5–10 min	5–6 hr

Metabolism: Hepatic; $T_{1/2}$: unknown
Distribution: Crosses placenta; may enter breast milk
Excretion: Urine

Adverse effects
Systemic effects are less likely with topical administration than with systemic administration, but because systemic absorption can take place, the systemic effects should be considered.
- **CNS:** *Fear, anxiety, tenseness, restlessness, headache, light-headedness, dizziness,* drowsiness, tremor, insomnia, hallucinations, psychological disturbances, convulsions, CNS depression, weakness, blurred vision, ocular irritation, tearing, photophobia, symptoms of paranoid schizophrenia
- **CV:** Arrhythmias, hypertension resulting in intracranial hemorrhage, CV collapse with hypotension, palpitations, tachycardia, precordial pain in patients with ischemic heart disease
- **GI:** *Nausea,* vomiting, anorexia
- **GU:** Constriction of renal blood vessels, *dysuria, vesical sphincter spasm,* resulting in difficult and painful urination, urinary retention in males with prostatism
- **Local:** *Rebound congestion* with topical nasal application
- **Other:** *Pallor,* respiratory difficulty, orofacial dystonia, sweating

Interactions
* **Drug-drug** • Severe hypertension with MAOIs, TCAs, furazolidone • Additive effects and increased risk of toxicity with urinary alkalinizers • Decreased vasopressor response with reserpine, methyldopa, urinary acidifiers • Decreased hypotensive action of guanethidine

■ Nursing considerations
Assessment
- **History:** Allergy to xylometazoline; angle-closure glaucoma; anesthesia with cyclopropane or halothane; thyrotoxicosis, diabetes, hypertension, CV disorders; prostatic hypertrophy, unstable vasomotor syndrome; lactation
- **Physical:** Skin color, temperature; orientation, reflexes, peripheral sensation, vision; P, BP, auscultation, peripheral perfusion; R, adventitious sounds; urinary output pattern, bladder percussion; prostate palpation; nasal mucous membrane evaluation

Interventions
- Monitor CV effects carefully in hypertensive patients; change in BP may be from additional vasoconstriction. If a nasal decongestant is needed, pseudoephedrine is the drug of choice.

Teaching points
- Do not exceed recommended dose. Demonstrate proper administration technique for topical nasal application. Avoid prolonged use because underlying medical problems can be disguised.
- These side effects may occur: dizziness, weakness, restlessness, light-headedness, tremor (avoid driving or operating dangerous equipment); urinary retention (empty bladder before taking drug).
- Rebound congestion may occur when this drug is stopped; drink plenty of fluids, use a humidifier, avoid smoke-filled areas.
- Report nervousness, palpitations, sleeplessness, sweating.

Adverse effects in *Italics* are most common; those in **Bold** are life-threatening.

sounds, liver evaluation; renal and hepatic function tests; CBC and differential

Interventions

- Monitor hematologic indices every 2 wk.
- Monitor for signs of peripheral neuropathy (numbness, tingling), and reduce drug dose by 50% until sensation returns; gradually reintroduce drug. Permanently discontinue if patient experiences severe discomfort and loss of sensation.
- Monitor liver function before and periodically during therapy; stop drug if signs of liver failure develop.
- Administer the drug every 8 hr in combination with other antiretroviral agents.

Teaching points

- Take drug every 8 hr, around the clock. Use an alarm clock to wake you up at night; rest periods during the day may be necessary. Do not share this drug; take exactly as prescribed.
- Zalcitabine does not cure AIDS or ARC; opportunistic infections may occur, obtain continuous medical care.
- Arrange for frequent blood tests; results of blood counts may indicate a need for decreased dosage or discontinuation of the drug for a period of time.
- These side effects may occur: nausea, loss of appetite, change in taste (eat small, frequent meals); dizziness, loss of feeling (use precautions); headache, fever, muscle aches.
- These drugs do not reduce the risk of transmission of HIV to others by sexual contact or blood contamination; use precautions.
- Report extreme fatigue, lethargy, severe headache, severe nausea, vomiting, difficulty breathing, rash, numbness, tingling, pain in extremities.

▽ zaleplon
(*zal' ah plon*)

Sonata

PREGNANCY CATEGORY C

C-IV CONTROLLED SUBSTANCE

Drug class
Sedative and hypnotic (nonbarbiturate)

Therapeutic actions
Interacts with GABA-B2 receptor complex to cause suppression of neurons leading to sedation and hypnosis.

Indications
- Short-term treatment of insomnia

Contraindications and cautions
- Contraindicated with hypersensitivity to zaleplon, lactation.
- Use cautiously with impaired hepatic or respiratory function, depressed patients, pregnancy, labor and delivery.

Available forms
Capsules—5, 10 mg

Dosages
Adults
10 mg PO hs. Patient must remain in bed for 4 hr after taking the drug. Do not exceed 20 mg/day.
Pediatric patients
Safety and efficacy not established.
Geriatric patients or patients with hepatic impairment
5 mg PO hs. Do not exceed 10 mg/day.

Pharmacokinetics

Route	Onset	Peak
Oral	Rapid	1 hr

Metabolism: Hepatic; $T_{1/2}$: 1 hr
Distribution: Crosses placenta; may pass into breast milk
Excretion: Urine

Adverse effects
- **CNS:** Headache, depression, drowsiness, somnolence, abnormal vision, lack of coordination, *short-term memory impairment*
- **GI:** Diarrhea
- **Hypersensitivity:** Generalized allergic reactions; pruritus, rash

Interactions
✳ **Drug-drug** • Increased sedation with alcohol or other CNS depressants; avoid this combination • Risk of increased serum levels and toxicity with cimetidine

Z

■ Nursing considerations
Assessment

- **History:** Hypersensitivity to zaleplon; impaired hepatic or respiratory function, pregnancy, labor or delivery, lactation; depression
- **Physical:** T, orientation, affect, reflexes, vision exam; P, BP; bowel sounds, normal output, liver evaluation; hepatic function tests

Interventions

- Do not prescribe or dispense more than 1 month's supply at a time.
- Limit amount of drug dispensed to depressed patients.
- Administer to patient at bedtime, onset of action is rapid and sleep usually occurs within 20 min; encourage patient to remain in bed for 4 hr after taking drug to ensure patient safety.
- Help patients with prolonged insomnia to seek the cause of their problem and not to rely on drugs for sleep (eg, ingestion of stimulants such as caffeine shortly before bedtime, fear, etc.).
- Institute appropriate additional measures for rest and sleep (back rub, quiet environment, warm milk, reading, etc.).

Teaching points

- Take this drug exactly as prescribed. Do not exceed prescribed dosage. Long-term use is not recommended. Time your drug dose to allow you to go to bed immediately after taking the drug. Drug effects will be felt for 4 hours; after that time you may safely become active again.
- These side effects may occur: drowsiness, dizziness, blurred vision (avoid driving a car or performing other tasks requiring alertness or visual acuity if these occur); diarrhea (ensure ready access to bathroom facilities).
- Report rash, sore throat, fever, bruising.

▽ zanamivir
(zan am' ah ver)

Relenza

PREGNANCY CATEGORY C

Drug classes
Antiviral drug
Neuroaminidase inhibitor

Therapeutic action
Selectively inhibits influenza virus neuroaminidase; by blocking the actions of this enzyme, there is decreased viral release from infected cells, increased formation of viral aggregates, and decreased spread of the virus.

Indications
- Treatment of uncomplicated acute illness due to influenza virus in adults and children ≥ 7 yr who have been symptomatic for ≤ 2 days

Contraindications and cautions
- Contraindicated with allergy to any component of the drug.
- Use cautiously with pregnancy, lactation, asthma, COPD, or other severe medical conditions.

Available forms
Powder blister for inhalation—5 mg

Dosages
Adults and patients ≥ 7 yr
2 inhalations (one 5-mg blister per inhalation administered with a *Diskhaler* device, for a total of 10 mg) bid at 12 hr intervals for 5 days. Should be started within 2 days of onset of flu symptoms, 2 doses should be given the first treatment day, at least 2 hr apart; subsequent doses should be separated by 12 hr.

Pharmacokinetics

Route	Onset	Peak
Inhalation	Rapid	1–2 hr

Metabolism: Hepatic; $T_{1/2}$: 2.5–5 hr

Distribution: Crosses placenta; may pass into breast milk
Excretion: Urine and feces

Adverse effects
- **CNS:** *Headache,* dizziness
- **GI:** *Nausea,* vomiting, *diarrhea, anorexia*
- **Respiratory:** Cough, *rhinitis,* bronchitis, ENT infections, **bronchospasm, serious respiratory effects**
- **Other:** Flulike symptoms, bacterial infections

■ Nursing considerations
Assessment
- **History:** Allergy to any components of the drug; COPD, asthma; pregnancy, lactation
- **Physical:** T; orientation, reflexes; R, adventitious sounds; bowel sounds

Interventions
- Administer using a *Diskhaler* delivery system. Demonstrate the use of the system to the patient.
- Encourage patient to complete full 5-day course of therapy; advise patient that treatment does not decrease the risk of transmission of the flu to others.
- Administer bronchodilators before using zanamivir if they are due at the same time as zanamivir dose.
- Caution patients with asthma or COPD of the risk of bronchospasm; a fast-acting inhaled bronchodilator should be on hand in case bronchospasm occurs; zanamivir should be discontinued and physician consulted promptly if respiratory symptoms worsen.

Teaching points
- Take this drug every 12 hr, at the same time each day, for 5 days. Use the *Diskhaler* delivery system provided.
- Take the full course of therapy as prescribed; be advised that this drug does not decrease the risk of transmitting the virus to others.
- If a bronchodilator is being used to treat a respiratory problem, the bronchodilator should be used before this drug.
- These side effects may occur: nausea, vomiting, loss of appetite, diarrhea; headache, dizziness (use caution if driving an automobile or operating dangerous machinery).

- Report severe diarrhea, severe nausea, worsening of respiratory symptoms.

▷ zidovudine (azidothymidine, AZT, Compound S)
(zid o vew' den)

Apo-Zidovudine (CAN), Aztec, Novo-AZT (CAN), Retrovir

PREGNANCY CATEGORY C

Drug class
Antiviral

Therapeutic actions
Thymidine analogue isolated from the sperm of herring; drug is activated to a triphosphate form that inhibits replication of some retroviruses, including HIV, HTLV III, LAV, ARV.

Indications
- Management of certain adult patients with symptomatic HIV infection in combination with other antiretrovirals
- Prevention of maternal–fetal HIV transmission

Contraindications and cautions
- Contraindicated with life-threatening allergy to any component, pregnancy, lactation.
- Use cautiously with compromised bone marrow, impaired renal or hepatic function.

Available forms
Capsules—100 mg; tablets—300 mg; CR tablets—30 mg; syrup—50 mg/5 mL; injection—10 mg/mL

Dosages
Adults
- *Symptomatic HIV infection:* Initially: 100 mg q 4 hr (2.9 mg/kg q 4 hr) PO, around the clock. Monitor hematologic indices every 2 wk. If significant anemia (Hgb < 7.5 g/dL, reduction of > 25%) or reduction of granulocytes > 50% below baseline occurs, dose interruption is necessary until evidence of bone marrow recovery is seen. If less severe bone marrow depression occurs, a dosage

Z

reduction may be adequate; *or* 1–2 mg/kg q 4 hr IV.

- *Asymptomatic HIV infection:* 100 mg q 4 hr PO while awake (500 mg/day).
- *Maternal–fetal transmission:* 100 mg PO 5 times/day from ≤ 14 wk gestation to the start of labor.

IV
1–2 mg/kg q 4 hr infused over 1 hr.

Pediatric patients

3 mo–12 yr: Initial dose, 180 mg/m² q 6 hr PO or IV (720 mg/m²/day, not to exceed 200 mg q 6 hr).

Infants born to HIV mothers: 2 mg/kg q 6 hr starting within 12 hr of birth to 6 wk of age or 1.5 mg/kg IV over 30 min q 6 hr.

Pharmacokinetics

Route	Onset	Peak
Oral	Varies	30–90 min
IV	Rapid	End of infusion

Metabolism: Hepatic; $T_{1/2}$: 30–60 min
Distribution: Crosses placenta; may enter breast milk
Excretion: Urine

▼IV facts

Preparation: Remove desired dose from vial, and dilute in 5% dextrose in water to a concentration no greater than 4 mg/mL. Discard after 24 hr. Protect from light.
Infusion: Administer over 60 min; avoid rapid infusion.
Incompatibilities: Do not mix with blood or blood products.

Adverse effects

- **CNS:** *Headache,* insomnia, myalgia, *asthenia,* malaise, dizziness, paresthesias, somnolence
- **GI:** *Nausea, GI pain, diarrhea,* anorexia, vomiting, dyspepsia
- **Hematologic:** *Agranulocytopenia,* severe anemia requiring transfusions
- **Other:** *Fever,* diaphoresis, dyspnea, *rash,* taste perversion

Interactions

✻ **Drug-drug** • Increased risk of hematologic toxicity if combined with nephrotoxic,

cytotoxic, or bone marrow suppressing drugs, ganciclovir, interferon alfa • Severe drowsiness and lethargy with cyclosporine
✻ **Drug-alternative therapy** • Decreased effectiveness if taken with St. John's wort

■ Nursing considerations

CLINICAL ALERT!
Name confusion has been reported between ritonavir and Retrovir (zidovudine); use caution.

Assessment

- **History:** Life-threatening allergy to any component; compromised bone marrow; impaired renal or hepatic function; pregnancy, lactation
- **Physical:** Skin rashes, lesions, texture; T; affect, reflexes, peripheral sensation; bowel sounds, liver evaluation; renal and hepatic function tests, CBC and differential

Interventions

- Monitor hematologic indices every 2 wk.
- Give the drug around the clock; rest periods may be needed during the day due to interrupted sleep.

Teaching points

- Take drug every 4 hr, around the clock. Use an alarm clock to wake you up at night; rest periods during the day may be necessary. Do not share this drug; take exactly as prescribed.
- Zidovudine is not a cure for AIDS or ARC; opportunistic infections may occur; obtain continuous medical care.
- Arrange for frequent blood tests; results of blood counts may indicate a need for decreased dosage or discontinuation of the drug for a period of time.
- These side effects may occur: nausea, loss of appetite, change in taste (eat small, frequent meals); dizziness, loss of feeling (use precautions); headache, fever, muscle aches.
- Zidovudine does not reduce the risk of transmission of HIV to others by sexual contact or blood contamination; use precautions.
- Report extreme fatigue, lethargy, severe headache, severe nausea, vomiting, difficulty breathing, rash.

Adverse effects in *Italics* are most common; those in **Bold** are life-threatening.

▽**zileuton**
(zye loot' on)

Zyflo

PREGNANCY CATEGORY C

Drug classes
Antiasthmatic agent
Leukotriene formation inhibitor

Therapeutic actions
Selectively and competitively blocks the receptor that inhibits leukotriene formation, thus blocking many of the signs and symptoms of asthma (neutrophil and eosinophil migration, neutrophil and monocyte aggregation, leukocyte adhesion, increased capillary permeability, and smooth muscle contraction). These actions contribute to inflammation, edema, mucus secretion and bronchoconstriction caused by cold air challenge in patients with asthma.

Indications
• Prophylaxis and long-term treatment of bronchial asthma in adults and children ≥ 12 yr

Contraindications and cautions
• Contraindicated with hypersensitivity to zileuton or any of its components; acute asthma attacks; status asthmaticus; pregnancy and lactation; severe hepatic impairment.
• Use cautiously with hepatic impairment.

Available forms
Tablets—600 mg

Dosages
Adults and patients > 12 yr
600 mg PO qid for a total of 2,400 mg/day.
Patients with hepatic impairment
Use caution; contraindicated if liver enzymes ≥ 3 times normal.

Pharmacokinetics

Route	Onset	Peak
Oral	Rapid	1.7 hr

Metabolism: Hepatic; $T_{1/2}$: 2.5 hr
Distribution: Crosses placenta; enters breast milk
Excretion: Metabolism

Adverse effects
• **CNS:** *Headache,* dizziness, myalgia
• **GI:** Nausea, diarrhea, abdominal pain, vomiting, **elevation of liver enzymes**
• **Other:** Generalized pain, fever, myalgia

Interactions
✳ **Drug-drug** • Increased effects of propranolol, theophylline, warfarin; monitor patient and decrease dose as appropriate
✳ **Drug-food** • Bioavailability decreased markedly by the presence of food; administer at least 1 hr before or 2 hr after meals

■ Nursing considerations
Assessment
• **History:** Hypersensitivity to zileuton; impaired hepatic function; lactation; pregnancy; acute asthma or bronchospasm
• **Physical:** T; orientation, reflexes; R, adventitious sounds; GI evaluation; liver function tests

Interventions
• Obtain baseline hepatic function tests before beginning therapy; monitor liver enzymes on a regular basis during therapy; discontinue drug and consult prescriber if enzymes rise more than three times normal.
• Administer without regard to food.
• Ensure that drug is taken continually for optimal effect.
• Do not administer for acute asthma attack or acute bronchospasm.

Teaching points
• Take this drug regularly as prescribed; do not stop taking this drug during symptom-free periods; do not stop taking this drug without consulting your health care provider. Continue taking any other antiasthma drugs that have been prescribed for you.
• Do not take this drug for an acute asthma attack or acute bronchospasm; this drug is not a bronchodilator; routine emergency procedures should be followed during acute attacks.
• These side effects may occur: dizziness (use caution when driving or performing activities that require alertness); nausea, vomiting (eat small, frequent meals; take drug with food); headache (analgesics may be helpful).

Z

- Avoid the use of OTC drugs while you are on this medication; many of them contain products that can interfere with or cause serious side effects when used with this drug. If you feel that you need one of these products, consult your nurse or physician.
- Report fever, acute asthma attacks, flulike symptoms, lethargy, pruritus, changes in color of urine or stool.

▽**zinc**
(zink')

zinc

zinc acetate
Halls Zinc Defense

zinc gluconate

zinc sulfate
OTC and prescription drug:
Orazinc, PMS-Egozinc (CAN), Verazinc, Zincate

PREGNANCY CATEGORY C

Drug class
Mineral

Therapeutic actions
Natural element that is essential for growth and tissue repair; acts as an integral part of essential enzymes in protein and carbohydrate metabolism.

Indications
- Dietary supplement to treat or prevent zinc deficiencies
- Treatment of Wilson's disease
- Unlabeled uses: acrodermatitis enteropathica and delayed wound healing associated with zinc deficiency; treatment of acne, rheumatoid arthritis; treatment of the common cold

Contraindications and cautions
- Contraindicated with pregnancy and lactation (recommended dietary allowance is needed, but not supplemental replacement).

Available forms
Tablets—zinc sulfate, 15, 25, 45, 50 mg zinc; zinc gluconate, 1.4, 2, 7, 11 mg zinc

Dosages
Adults
- *Recommended dietary allowance (RDA):* 12–15 mg/day PO; pregnancy RDA, 15 mg/day PO; lactation RDA, 6 mg/day PO for the first 6 mo; then 4 mg/day for the next 6 mo.
- *Dietary supplement:* 25–50 mg zinc/day PO.
Pediatric patients
- *RDA:* 5–10 mg/day PO.

Pharmacokinetics

Route	Onset	Peak
Oral	Slow	Delayed

Metabolism: Hepatic; $T_{1/2}$: unknown
Distribution: Crosses placenta; may enter breast milk
Excretion: Feces

Adverse effects
- **GI:** Vomiting, *nausea*

■ Nursing considerations
Assessment
- **History:** Lactation, pregnancy
- **Physical:** Bowel sounds, normal output; serum zinc levels

Interventions
- Give with food if GI upset occurs; avoid bran and other high-fiber foods, calcium and phosphates that may interfere with absorption.
- Ensure that patient receives only the prescribed dosage. Avoid overdose.

Teaching points
- Take this drug exactly as prescribed. Do not exceed prescribed dosage.
- Take with food, but avoid taking it with bran and other high-fiber foods, dairy products that may interfere with absorption.
- These side effects may occur: nausea, vomiting (take drug with food).
- Report severe nausea and vomiting, restlessness, fatigue, lethargy.

▽ziprasidone
(zih praz' i done)

Geodon

PREGNANCY CATEGORY C

Drug classes
Antipsychotic drug
Benzisoxazole

Therapeutic actions
Mechanism of action not fully understood;
blocks dopamine and serotonin receptors in
the brain, depresses the reticular activating
system; effective in suppressing many of the
negative aspects of schizophrenia (blunted affect, social withdrawal, lack of motivation,
anger).

Indications
- Treatment of schizophrenia and to delay the
time and rate of relapse
- Rapid control of agitated behavior and psychotic symptoms in patients with acute schizophrenia exacerbations (IM)

Contraindications and cautions
- Contraindicated with allergy to ziprasidone,
pregnancy, lactation, prolonged QTc interval, history of severe cardiac disease.
- Use cautiously with renal or hepatic impairment, cardiovascular disease.

Available forms
Capsules—20, 40, 60, 80 mg; injection—
20 mg/mL

Dosages
Adults
Initially 20 mg PO bid with food. Adjust as
needed. Effective range: 20–80 mg PO bid.
- *Rapid control of agitated behavior:*
10–20 mg IM; doses of 10 mg may be re-
peated q 2 hr; doses of 20 mg may be re-
peated in 4 hr. Maximum dose: 40 mg/day.
Pediatric patients
Safety and efficacy not established.

Pharmacokinetics

Route	Onset	Peak	Duration
Oral	Varies	1 hr	6–8 hr

Metabolism: Hepatic; $T_{1/2}$: 3 hr
Distribution: Crosses placenta; passes into
breast milk
Excretion: Urine

Adverse effects
- **CNS:** *Somnolence, drowsiness, sedation,
headache,* extrapyramidal reactions
- **CV: Arrhythmias,** hypotension, ECG
changes, hypertension
- **GI:** *Nausea, dyspepsia, constipation,* ab-
dominal discomfort, dry mouth
- **GU:** Polyuria
- **Other:** *Fever,* weight gain (not as likely as
with other antipsychotics), rash

Interactions
✳ **Drug-drug** • Increased risk of severe cardiac arrhythmias if taken with other drugs that
prolong the QTc interval
✳ **Drug-alternative therapy** • Possibility
of increased toxicity if taken with St. John's
wort

■ Nursing considerations
Assessment
- **History:** Allergy to ziprasidone, pregnancy, lactation, cardiac disease, hepatic or renal dysfunction, prolonged QTc interval
- **Physical:** T, weight; reflexes, orientation;
P, ECG; bowel sounds, normal output, liver
evaluation; normal urine output; urinalysis, liver, and kidney function tests

Interventions
- Ensure that patient is not pregnant before
beginning therapy; advise the use of contraceptive measures while on this drug.
- Obtain baseline ECG to rule out prolonged
QTc interval; monitor periodically throughout therapy.
- Monitor weight before beginning therapy
and periodically during therapy. Weight gain
is not usually a concern with this drug.
- Follow patients with renal or hepatic impairment carefully throughout therapy.
- Continue other measures used to deal with
schizophrenia.

Teaching points
- This drug cannot be taken during pregnancy. If you think you are pregnant, or wish to

Z

become pregnant, contact your health care provider.
- These side effects may occur: somnolence, drowsiness, dizziness, sedation (avoid driving a car, operating machinery, or performing tasks that require concentration); nausea, dyspepsia (small, frequent meals may help); headache (analgesics may be available to help, consult with your health care provider).
- Report lethargy, weakness, fever, sore throat, palpitations, return of symptoms.

▽zoledronic acid

*(zoh-leh-**droh**'-nik)*

Zometa

PREGNANCY CATEGORY D

Drug classes
Bisphosphonate
Calcium regulator

Therapeutic actions
A bisphonic acid that inhibits bone resorption, possibly by inhibiting osteoclast activity and promoting osteoclast cell apoptosis; this action leads to a decrease in the release of calcium from bone and a decrease in serum calcium.

Indications
- Intravenous treatment of the hypercalcemia of malignancy
- Treatment of patients with multiple myelomas and patients with documented bone metastases from solid tumors in conjuction with standard antineoplastic therapy

Contraindications and cautions
- Contraindicated with allergy to any components of the drug or to bisphosphonates.
- Use cautiously with renal dysfunction (do not exceed single doses of 4 mg, and duration of infusion must not be less than 15 min), hepatic dysfunction, aspirin-sensitive asthmatic patients, pregnancy, or lactation.

Available forms
Injection—4 mg/vial

Dosages
Adults
4 mg IV as a single-dose infusion of not less than 15 min for hypercalcemia of malignancy with albumin-corrected serum calcium levels of ≥ 12 mg/dL. Retreatment may be done with 4 mg IV if needed; a minimum of 7 days should elapse between doses with careful monitoring of serum creatinine levels. Patients with prostate cancer should have progressed after treatment with at least 1 hormonal therapy. Patients with solid tumors should receive 4 mg IV q 3–4 wk.
Pediatric patients
Safety and efficacy not established.
Patients with renal impairment
Contraindicated in severe renal impairment; no data are available. Patients with normal creatinine before therapy who increase level by 0.5 mg/dL within 2 wk should have drug withheld until creatinine returns to within 10% of baseline. Patients with abnormal serum creatinine before therapy with an increase of 1 mg/dL within 2 wk of next dose should have dose held until creatinine returns to within 10% of baseline value.

Pharmacokinetics

Route	Onset	Peak
IV	Slow	8 hr

Metabolism: Hepatic; $T_{1/2}$: 0.23 hr then 1.75 hr
Distribution: May cross placenta; may enter breast milk
Excretion: Urine

▼IV facts
Preparation: Reconstitute by adding 5 mL sterile water for injection to vial; swirl to dissolve. Withdraw solution, equivalent to 4 mg *Zometa*, further dilute in 100 mL 0.9% sodium chloride, 5% dextrose injection. May be refrigerated and stored for up to 24 hr before the time of the end of the infusion.
Infusion: Infuse over not less than 15 min.
Incompatibilities: Do not mix with any other drug solution; always administer via a

separate line. Physically incompatible with calcium-containing infusions.

Adverse effects
- **CNS:** Agitation, confusion, *insomnia,* anxiety
- **CV:** *Hypotension*
- **GI:** *Nausea, constipation,* vomiting, diarrhea, abdominal pain, anorexia
- **Hematologic:** Hypophosphatemia, hypokalemia, hypomagnesemia, hypocalcemia
- **Respiratory:** *Dyspnea,* coughing, pleural effusion
- **Other:** *Infections* (UTI, candidiasis), *fever,* progression of cancer

Interactions
✻ Drug-drug • Possible increased risk of hypocalcemia if taken with aminoglycosides, loop diuretics. If this combination is used, monitor serum calcium levels closely

■ Nursing considerations
Assessment
- **History:** Allergy to components of the drug or any bisphosphonate, hepatic or renal dysfunction, aspirin-sensitive asthma, pregnancy, lactation
- **Physical:** T, BP, R, orientation and affect, adventitious sounds, CBC and electrolytes

Interventions
- Make sure that patient is well hydrated before use; vigorous saline hydration to establish a urine output of about 2 L/day is suggested.
- Monitor urinary output and assess patient for hydration status continually.
- Monitor serum creatinine levels prior to each dose of zoledronic acid; follow dosage guidelines for any indication of renal toxicity.
- Ensure that reconstituted solution is infused within 24 hr of reconstitution.
- Ensure that drug infuses over not less than 15 min.
- Provide small, frequent meals if GI upset occurs.
- Arrange for nutritional consult if nausea and vomiting are persistent.
- Monitor patient for any sign of infection, and arrange for appropriate interventions.

Teaching points
- This drug must be given by IV infusion; you will be closely monitored prior to and following the infusion.
- If you are returning for every 3–4 wk infusions, mark a calendar with your return dates.
- It is important to maintain your fluid levels before using this drug; fluids may be pushed to ensure that you are hydrated.
- These side effects may occur: nausea, vomiting (small, frequent meals may help); agitation, confusion, anxiety (consult with your health care provider if this becomes a problem).
- Report difficulty breathing, muscle pain, tremors, pain at injection site.

▽ zolmitriptan
*(zohl mah **trip'** tan)*

Zomig, Zomig ZMT

PREGNANCY CATEGORY C

Drug classes
Antimigraine agent
Serotonin selective agonist

Therapeutic actions
Binds to serotonin receptors to cause vascular constrictive effects on cranial blood vessels, causing the relief of migraine in selected patients.

Indications
- Treatment of acute migraine attacks with or without aura

Contraindications and cautions
- Contraindicated with allergy to zolmitriptan, active coronary artery disease, Printzmetal's angina, pregnancy.
- Use cautiously with the elderly and with lactation.

Available forms
Tablets—2.5, 5 mg; orally disintegrating tablet—2.5 mg

Dosages

Adults

2.5 mg PO at onset of headache or with beginning of aura; may repeat dose if headache persists after 2 hr, do not exceed 10 mg in 24 hr. Orally disintegrating tablets: 2.5 mg PO, may repeat after 2 hr; do not exceed 10 mg/24 hr.

Pediatric patients

Safety and efficacy not established.

Patients with hepatic impairment

Use caution, keep doses ≤ 2.5 mg. Significant increases in BP can occur.

Pharmacokinetics

Route	Onset	Peak
PO	Varies	2–4 hr

Metabolism: Hepatic; $T_{1/2}$: 2.5–3.7 hr
Distribution: Crosses placenta; may pass into breast milk
Excretion: Urine and feces

Adverse effects

- **CNS:** *Dizziness, vertigo,* headache, anxiety, malaise/fatigue, *weakness, myalgia*
- **CV:** *Blood pressure alterations, tightness or pressure in chest*
- **GI:** Abdominal discomfort, dysphagia
- **Other:** *Tingling, warm/hot sensations, burning sensation, feeling of heaviness, pressure sensation, numbness, feeling of tightness,* feeling strange, cold sensation

Interactions

✳ Drug-drug • Prolonged vasoactive reactions with ergot-containing drugs • Risk of severe effects with or within < 2 wk of discontinuation of an MAO inhibitor • Increased risk of toxic effects with cimetidine, hormonal contraceptives • A serotonin syndrome may occur when sibutramine is coadministered

■ Nursing considerations

Assessment

- **History:** Allergy to zolmitriptan; active CAD; Printzmetal's angina; pregnancy, lactation
- **Physical:** Skin color and lesions; orientation, reflexes, peripheral sensation; P, BP; renal and liver function tests

Interventions

- Administer to relieve acute migraine, not as prophylactic measure.
- Establish safety measures if CNS, visual disturbances occur.
- Provide environmental control as appropriate to help relieve migraine (lighting, temperature, etc.).
- Monitor BP of patients with possible CAD; discontinue at any sign of angina, prolonged high blood pressure, etc.

Teaching points

- Take this drug exactly as prescribed, at the onset of headache or aura.
- This drug should not be taken during pregnancy; if you suspect that you are pregnant, contact physician and refrain from using drug.
- These side effects may occur: dizziness, drowsiness (avoid driving or using dangerous machinery); numbness, tingling, feelings of tightness or pressure.
- Maintain any procedures you usually use during a migraine (controlled lighting, noise, etc.).
- Contact your physician immediately if you experience chest pain or pressure that is severe or does not go away.
- Report feelings of heat, flushing, tiredness, feelings of sickness, swelling of lips or eyelids.

▷ zolpidem tartrate
(zol' pih dem)

Ambien

PREGNANCY CATEGORY B

C-IV CONTROLLED SUBSTANCE

Drug class

Sedative or hypnotic (nonbarbiturate)

Therapeutic actions

Modulates GABA receptors to cause suppression of neurons, leading to sedation, anticonvulsant, anxiolytic, and relaxant properties.

Indications

- Short-term treatment of insomnia

Contraindications and cautions

- Contraindicated with hypersensitivity to zolpidem.
- Use cautiously with acute intermittent porphyria, impaired hepatic or renal function, addiction-prone patients, pregnancy, lactation.

Available forms

Tablets—5, 10 mg

Dosages

Adults
10 mg PO hs. Do not exceed 10 mg/day.
Pediatric patients
Safety and efficacy not established.
Geriatric patients
Increased chance of confusion, acute brain syndrome; initiate treatment with 5 mg PO.

Pharmacokinetics

Route	Onset	Peak
Oral	45 min	1.6 hr

Metabolism: Hepatic; $T_{1/2}$: 2.6 hr
Distribution: Crosses placenta; may enter breast milk
Excretion: Urine

Adverse effects

- **CNS:** Convulsions, hallucinations, ataxia, EEG changes, pyrexia, *morning drowsiness, hangover, headache, dizziness*, vertigo, acute brain syndrome and confusion; paradoxical excitation, anxiety, depression, nightmares, dreaming, diplopia, blurred vision, *suppression of REM sleep;* REM rebound when drug is discontinued
- **GI:** Esophagitis, vomiting, *nausea,* diarrhea, constipation
- **Hypersensitivity:** Generalized allergic reactions; pruritus, rash
- **Other:** Influenza-like symptoms, dry mouth, infection

■ Nursing considerations
Assessment

- **History:** Hypersensitivity to zolpidem, acute intermittent porphyria, impaired hepatic or renal function, addiction-prone patients, lactation, pregnancy
- **Physical:** T; skin color, lesions; orientation, affect, reflexes, vision exam; P, BP; bowel sounds, normal output, liver evaluation; CBC with differential; hepatic and renal function tests

Interventions

- Limit amount of drug dispensed to patients who are depressed or suicidal.
- Withdraw drug gradually if patient has used drug long-term or if patient has developed tolerance. Supportive therapy similar to that for withdrawal from barbiturates may be necessary to prevent dangerous withdrawal symptoms.

Teaching points

- Take this drug exactly as prescribed. Do not exceed prescribed dosage. Long-term use is not recommended.
- These side effects may occur: drowsiness, dizziness, blurred vision (avoid driving or performing tasks requiring alertness or visual acuity); GI upset (eat frequent, small meals).
- Report rash, sore throat, fever, bruising.

▽**zonisamide**
*(zoh **niss'** ah mide)*

Zonegran

PREGNANCY CATEGORY C

Drug class

Antiepileptic

Therapeutic actions

Mechanism of action not fully understood; inhibits voltage-sensitive sodium and calcium channels, stabilizing the neuronal membrane and modulating calcium-dependent presynaptic release of excitatory amino acids; may also have dopaminergic effects.

Indications

- Adjuvant therapy in the treatment of partial seizures in adults with epilepsy

Z

Contraindications and cautions

- Contraindicated with lactation, history of sulfonamide hypersensitivity.
- Use cautiously with impaired hepatic; renal, or cardiac function; pregnancy.

Available forms

Capsules—100 mg

Dosages

Adults

Initial dose: 100–200 mg PO daily as a single dose or divided into 2–3 doses; may increase by 100 mg/day every 1–2 weeks to achieve control. Maximum dose: 600 mg/day.

Pediatric patients

Not recommended in patients < 16 yr.

Pharmacokinetics

Route	Onset	Peak
Oral	Rapid	2–6 hr

Metabolism: Hepatic; $T_{1/2}$: 49.7–130 hr
Distribution: Crosses placenta; may pass into breast milk
Excretion: Urine

Adverse effects

- **CNS:** *Dizziness,* insomnia, headache, somnolence, *ataxia*, diplopia, blurred vision, nystagmus, *decrease in mental functioning*
- **Dermatologic:** *Rash*
- **GI:** *Nausea,* vomiting, *dry mouth, unusual taste*
- **Other:** Bone marrow depression, *renal calculi*

Interactions

✳ **Drug-drug** ● Rapid elimination of zonisamide if taken with enzyme-inducing antiepileptic agents: carbamazepine, phenytoin, phenobarbital, primidone ● Increased levels and potential for toxicity with carbamazepine if taken with zonisimide; adjust dosage and monitor patient carefully

∎ Nursing considerations

Assessment

- **History:** Lactation; impaired hepatic, renal, or cardiac function; pregnancy
- **Physical:** Body weight; T; skin color, lesions; orientation, affect, reflexes; P, BP, perfusion; bowel sounds, normal output; liver and renal function test, CBC

Interventions

- Monitor drug doses carefully when starting therapy and with each increase in dose; special care will need to be taken when changing the dose or frequency of any other antiepileptic.
- Taper drug slowly, over a 2-wk period, when discontinuing.
- Ensure that patient is well hydrated to prevent formation of renal calculi.
- Provide safety measures if CNS effects occur.

Teaching points

- Take this drug exactly as prescribed. Dosage may be increased slowly.
- Do not discontinue this drug abruptly or change dosage, except on the advice of your physician.
- These side effects may occur: dizziness, drowsiness, decreased mental functioning (avoid driving a car or performing other tasks requiring alertness or visual acuity if this occurs); GI upset (taking the drug with food or milk and eating frequent small meals may help); headache (medication can be ordered); rash (skin care and lotions may be helpful).
- You should wear a medical alert tag at all times so that any emergency medical personnel taking care of you will know that you are an epileptic taking antiepileptic medication.
- Report yellowing of skin, abdominal pain, changes in color of urine or stools, flank pain, painful urination.

Adverse effects in *Italics* are most common; those in **Bold** are life-threatening.

Appendices

APPENDIX A:

Alternative and Complementary Therapies

Many natural substances are used by the public for self-treatment of many complaints. These substances, derived from folklore of various cultures, often have ingredients that have been identified and have known therapeutic activities. Some of these substances have unknown mechanisms of action but over the years have been reliably used to relieve specific symptoms. There is an element of the placebo effect in using some of these substances. The power of believing that something will work and that there is some control over the problem is often very beneficial in achieving relief from pain or suffering. Some of these substances may contain yet unidentified ingredients, which, when discovered, may prove very useful in the modern field of pharmacology. Because these products are not regulated or monitored, there is always a possibility of toxic effects. Some of these products may contain ingredients that interact with prescription drugs. A history of the use of these alternative therapies may explain unexpected reactions to some drugs.

Substance	Reported use
alfalfa	Topical: healing ointment, relief of arthritis pain Oral: arthritis treatment, strength giving
allspice	Topical: anesthetic for teeth and gums; soothes sore joints and muscles Oral: treatment of indigestion, flatulence, diarrhea, fatigue Seizures have been reported with excessive dosage.
aloe leaves	Topical: treatment of burns, healing of wounds Oral: treatment of chronic constipation
angelica	Oral: "cure all" for gynecological problems, headaches and backaches; increases circulation in the periphery Risk of bleeding if combined with anticoagulants.
anise	Oral: relief of dry cough, treatment of flatulence
apple	Oral: control of blood glucose, constipation
arnica gel	Topical: relief of pain from muscle or soft tissue injury
ashwagandha	Oral: enhancement of mental and physical functioning; general tonic; used to protect cells during cancer chemotherapy and radiation therapy Avoid use during pregnancy and lactation.
astragalus	Oral: increases stamina and energy; improves immune function and resistance to disease Do not use with fever or acute infection.
barberry	Oral: antidiarrheal, antipyretic, cough suppressant Risk of spontaneous abortion if taken during pregnancy.
bayberry	Topical: to promote wound healing Oral: stimulant, emetic, antidiarrheal

Substance	Reported use
bee pollen	Oral: treatment of allergies, asthma, impotence, prostatitis; suggested use to decrease cholesterol levels Risk of hyperglycemia; do not use in diabetic patients or with anti-diabetic drugs.
bilberry	Oral: treatment of diabetes; cardiovascular problems; lowers cholesterol and triglycerides; treatment of diabetic retinopathy; treatment of cataracts, night blindness
birch bark	Topical: treatment of infected wounds, cuts Oral: as tea for relief of stomachache
blackberry	Oral: as tea for generalized healing; treatment of diabetes
black cohosh root	Oral: treatment of PMS, menopausal disorders, rheumatoid arthritis Contains estrogen-like components. Do not use with hormone replacement therapy or hormonal contraceptives; avoid use in pregnancy and lactation.
bromelain	Oral: treatment of inflammation, sports injuries, URIs, PMS, and adjunctive therapy in cancer treatments Associated with nausea, vomiting, diarrhea, menstrual disorders.
burdock	Oral: treatment of diabetes; atropine-like side effects, uterine stimulant
capsicum	Topical: external analgesic Oral: treatment of bowel disorders, chronic laryngitis, peripheral vascular disease
catnip leaves	Oral: treatment of bronchitis, diarrhea
cat's claw	Oral: treatment of allergies, arthritis; adjunct in the treatment of cancers and AIDS Do not use with pregnancy, lactation, transplant recipients; increased risk of bleeding episodes if taken with oral anticoagulants.
cayenne pepper	Topical: treatment of burns, wounds, relief of toothache
celery	Oral: lowers blood glucose, acts as a diuretic; may cause potassium depletion
chamomile	Topical: treatment of wounds, ulcer, conjunctivitis Oral: treatment of migraines, gastric cramps, relief of anxiety Contains coumarin–closely monitor patients taking anticoagulants. May cause depression; monitor patients on antidepressants. Cross-reaction with ragweed allergies may occur. Do not use during pregnancy or lactation.
chaste-tree berry	Oral: progesterone-like effects; used to treat PMS and menopausal problems, and to stimulate lactation Use caution with hormone replacement therapy and hormonal contraceptives.
chicken soup	Oral: breaks up respiratory secretions, bronchodilator, relieves anxiety

(continued)

Substance	Reported use
chicory	Oral: treatment of digestive tract problems, gout; stimulates bile secretions
Chinese angelica (dong quai)	Oral: general tonic; treatment of anemias, PMS, menopause, antihypertensive, laxative Use caution with the flu, hemorrhagic diseases. Monitor patients on antihypertensives or vasodilators for toxic effects. Use caution with hormone replacement therapy.
chondroitin	Oral: treatment of osteoarthritis and related disorders Risk of increased bleeding if combined with anticoagulants.
chong cao fungi	Oral: antioxidant, promotes stamina, sexual function Avoid use in children.
coleus forskohlii	Oral: treatment of asthma, hypertension, eczema Use caution with antihypertensives or antihistamines, severe additive effects can occur. Avoid use with hypotension or peptic ulcers.
comfrey	Topical: treatment of wounds, cuts, ulcers Oral: gargle for tonsillitis
coriander	Oral: weight loss, lowers blood glucose
creatine monohydrate	Oral: enhancement of athletic performance
dandelion root	Oral: treatment of liver and kidney problems; decreases lactation (after delivery or with weaning); lowers blood glucose
DHEA	Oral: slows aging, improves vigor ("Fountain of Youth"); androgenic side effects
di huang	Oral: treatment of diabetes mellitus
dried root bark of lycium Chinese mill	Oral: lowers cholesterol, lowers blood glucose
echinacea (cone flower)	Oral: treatment of colds, flu; stimulates the immune system, attacks viruses; causes immunosuppression May be liver toxic. Do not use longer than 8 wk. Do not give with liver-toxic drugs or immunosuppressants. Avoid use with antifungals; serious liver injury could occur. Avoid use in patients with SLE, tuberculosis, AIDS.
elder bark and flowers	Topical: gargle for tonsillitis, pharyngitis Oral: treatment of fever, chills
ephedra	Oral: increases energy, relieves fatigue Associated with serious complications, withdrawn in some states; do not use with any known CV disease.
ergot	Oral: treatment of migraine headaches, treatment of menstrual problems, hemorrhage

Substance	Reported use
eucalyptus	Topical: treatment of wounds Oral: decreases respiratory secretions, suppresses cough
evening primrose	Oral: treatment of PMS, menopause, rheumatoid arthritis, diabetic neuropathy Do not use with phenothiazines, antidepressants—increases risk of seizures; avoid use in patients with epilepsy, schizophrenia.
false unicorn root	Oral: treatment of menstrual and uterine problems Do not use during pregnancy or lactation.
fennel	Oral: treatment of colic, gout, flatulence; enhances lactation
fenugreek	Oral: lowers cholesterol levels; reduces blood glucose; aids in healing
feverfew	Oral: treatment of arthritis, fever, migraine Use caution with anticoagulants; may increase bleeding. Avoid use before or immediately after surgery because of bleeding risk.
fish oil	Oral: treatment of coronary diseases, arthritis, colitis, depression, aggression, attention deficit disorder
gamboge	Oral: appetite suppressant, lowers cholesterol, promotes weight loss
garlic	Oral: treatment of colds, diuretic; prevention of coronary artery disease, intestinal antiseptic; lowers blood glucose, anticoagulant Use caution with diabetic patients, oral anticoagulants Known to affect blood clotting. Do not use with warfarin.
ginger	Oral: treatment of nausea, motion sickness, postoperative nausea (may increase risk of miscarriage) Affects blood clotting. Do not give with anticoagulants.
ginkgo	Oral: vascular dilation; increases blood flow to the brain, improving cognitive function; used in treating Alzheimer's disease; antioxidant Can inhibit blood clotting. Do not give with aspirin or NSAIDs. Can interact with phenytoin, carbamazepine, phenobarbital, TCAs, and MAOIs; use caution.
ginkobe	Oral: increases cerebral blood flow, improves concentration and memory
ginseng	Oral: aphrodisiac, mood elevator, tonic; antihypertensive; decreases cholesterol levels; lowers blood glucose; adjunct in cancer chemotherapy and radiation therapy May cause irritability if combined with caffeine. Inhibits clotting. Do not use with anticoagulants, aspirin, NSAIDs. Do not use for longer than 3 months. May cause headaches, manic episodes if used with phenelzine, MAOIs. Additive effects of estrogens and corticosteroids. May also interfere with cardiac effects of digoxin. Monitor patients closely.
glucosamine	Oral: treatment of osteoarthritis and joint diseases, usually combined with chondroitin

(continued)

Substance	Reported use
goldenrod leaves	Oral: treatment of renal disease, rheumatism, sore throat, eczema
goldenseal	Oral: lowers blood glucose, aids healing; treatment of bronchitis, colds, flulike symptoms, cystitis. High doses may cause paralysis. Affects blood clotting; do not give with anticoagulants.
gotu kola	Topical: treatment of cellulitis, scleroderma, open wounds, pressure sores
grape seed extract	Oral: treatment of allergies, asthma; improves circulation; decreases platelet aggregation Use caution with oral anticoagulants; may increase bleeding.
green tea leaf	Oral: antioxidant, used as a preventative for cancer and cardiovascular disease Use caution with oral anticoagulants; may increase bleeding.
guayusa	Oral: lowers blood glucose; promotes weight loss
hawthorn	Oral: treatment of angina, arrhythmias, blood pressure problems; decreases cholesterol Use with caution with digoxin, ACE inhibitors; may potentiate effects.
hop	Oral: sedative; aids healing; alters blood glucose
horehound	Oral: expectorant; treatment of respiratory problems, GI disorders
horse chestnut seed	Oral: treatment of varicose veins, hemorrhoids Use caution with oral anticoagulants; may increase bleeding.
hyssop	Topical: treatment of cold sores, genital herpes, burns, wounds Oral: treatment of coughs, colds, indigestion, and flatulence
Java plum	Oral: treatment of diabetes mellitus
jojoba	Topical: promotion of hair growth, relief of skin problems Toxic if ingested.
juniper berries	Oral: increases appetite, aids digestion; diuretic; urinary tract disinfectant; lowers blood glucose
kava	Oral: treatment of nervous anxiety, stress, restlessness; tranquilizer Do not use with alprazolam—may cause coma. Do not use with Parkinson's disease or history of stroke. Do not combine with St. John's wort, antianxiety drugs, or alcohol.
kudzu	Oral: reduces cravings for alcohol; being researched for use with alcoholics
lavender	Topical: astringent for minor cuts, burns Oral: treatment of insomnia, restlessness
ledum tincture	Topical: treatment of insect bites, puncture wounds; dissolves some blood clots and bruises

Substance	Reported use
licorice	Oral: prevents thirst, soothes coughs; treats "incurable" chronic fatigue syndrome; treatment of duodenal ulcer. Acts like aldosterone. Blocks spironolactone effects. Can lead to digoxin toxicity because of effects of lowering aldosterone. Use extreme caution. Contraindicated with renal or liver disease, hypertension, CAD, pregnancy, lactation. Do not combine with thyroid drugs, antihypertensives, hormonal contraceptives.
ma huang	Oral: treatment of colds, nasal congestion, asthma. Contains ephedrine. Do not use with antihypertensives, diabetes, MAOIs, or digoxin. Serious side effects could occur.
mandrake root	Oral: treatment of fertility problems
marigold leaves and flowers	Oral: relief of muscle tension, increases wound healing
melatonin	Oral: relief of jet lag, treatment of insomnia
milk thistle	Oral: treatment of hepatitis, cirrhosis, fatty liver due to alcohol or drugs
milk vetch	Oral: improves resistance to disease; adjunct therapy in cancer chemotherapy and radiation therapy
mistletoe leaves	Oral: promotes weight loss; relief of signs and symptoms of diabetes
momordica charantia (Karela)	Oral: blocks intestinal absorption of glucose; lowers blood glucose; weight loss
nettle	Topical: stimulation of hair growth, treatment for bleeding Oral: treatment of rheumatism, allergic rhinitis; antispasmodic; expectorant Do not use during pregnancy or lactation.
nightshade leaves and roots	Oral: stimulates circulatory system; treatment of eye disorders
octacosanol	Oral: treatment of parkinsonism, enhancement of athletic performance Do not use during pregnancy or lactation.
parsley seeds and leaves	Oral: treatment of jaundice, asthma, menstrual difficulties, conjunctivitis
passionflower vine	Oral: sedative and hypnotic May increase sedation with other CNS depressants, MAOIs. Avoid alcohol while using this drug.
peppermint leaves	Oral: treatment of nervousness, insomnia, dizziness, cramps, coughs Topical: rubbed on forehead to relieve tension headaches
psyllium	Oral: treatment of constipation; lowers cholesterol Can cause severe gas and stomach pain; may interfere with nutrient absorption. Avoid use with warfarin, digoxin, lithium—absorption of drug may be blocked. Do not combine with laxatives.

(continued)

Substance	Reported use
raspberry	Oral: healing of minor wounds; control and treatment of diabetes
rose hips	Oral: laxative, to boost the immune system and prevent illness
rosemary	Topical: relief of rheumatism, sprains, wounds, bruises, eczema Oral: gastric stimulation, relief of flatulence, stimulation of bile release, relief of colic
rue extract	Topical: relief of pain associated with sprains, groin pulls, whiplash
saffron	Oral: treatment of menstrual problems, abortifacient
sage	Oral: lowers blood pressure; lowers blood glucose
SAM-e (adomet)	Oral: promotion of general well being and health Associated with frequent GI complaints and headache.
sarsaparilla	Oral: treatment of skin disorders, rheumatism
sassafras	Topical: treatment of local pain, skin eruptions Oral: enhancement of athletic performance, "cure" for syphilis Oil has been toxic to fetus, children, and adults when ingested.
saw palmetto	Oral: treatment of benign prostatic hyperplasia Do not use with estrogen-replacement or hormonal contraceptives—may greatly increase side effects. May decrease iron absorption. Do not combine with finasteride; toxicity could occur.
schisandra	Oral: health tonic, liver protectant; adjunct in cancer chemotherapy and radiation therapy Do not use in pregnancy; causes uterine stimulation.
squaw vine	Oral: diuretic, tonic, aid in labor and childbirth, treatment of menstrual problems Associated with hepatic toxicity.
St. John's wort	Oral: treatment of depression, PMS symptoms; antiviral Topical: treatment of puncture wounds, insect bites, crushed fingers or toes Avoid tyramine-containing foods; hypertensive crisis is possible. Can increase sensitivity to light; do not combine with drugs that cause photosensitivity. Severe photosensitivity can occur in light-skinned people. Serious drug interactions have been reported with SSRIs, MAOIs, kava, digoxin, theophylline, AIDS antiviral agents, antineoplastics, hormonal contraceptives. Avoid these combinations.
sweet violet flowers	Oral: treatment of respiratory disorders, emetic
tarragon	Oral: weight loss; prevents cancer; lowers blood glucose
tea tree oil	Topical: antifungal, antibacterial; used in the treatment of burns, insect bites; used as a mouth wash

Substance	Reported use
thyme	Topical: liniment, treatment of wounds, gargle Oral: antidiarrheal, relief of bronchitis and laryngitis Can increase sensitivity to light; do not combine with drugs that cause photosensitivity. Do not use with MAOIs or with SSRIs—can cause serious side effects.
turmeric	Oral: antioxidant, anti-inflammatory; used to treat arthritis May cause GI distress. Do not use with known biliary obstruction. May cause increased bleeding with oral anticoagulants.
Valerian	Oral: sedative and hypnotic; reduces anxiety, relaxes muscles Can cause severe liver damage. Do not use with barbiturates, alcohol, CNS depressants, or antihistamines; can cause serious sedation.
went rice	Oral: cholesterol- and triglyceride-lowering effects Do not use in pregnancy, liver disease, alcoholism, or acute infections.
white willow bark	Oral: treatment of fevers
xuan shen	Oral: lowers blood glucose; slows heart rate; treatment of congestive heart failure
yohimbe	Oral: treatment of erectile dysfunction Can affect blood pressure; CNS stimulant; has cardiac effects; use caution, manic episodes have been reported in psychiatric patients.

Commonly Used Biologicals

▷ diphtheria and tetanus toxoids, combined, adsorbed (DT, Td) (available in adult and pediatric preparations)

Therapeutic actions

Contains reduced dose of inactivated diphtheria toxin and full dose of inactivated tetanus toxin to provide adequate immunization in adults without the severe sensitivity reactions caused when full pediatric doses of diphtheria toxoid are given to adults.

Indications

- Active immunization of adults and children ≥ 7 yr against diphtheria and tetanus. Trivalent DTP is preferred for use in most children; DT can be used for children ≥ 6 wk when pertussis vaccine is contraindicated.

Adverse effects

Fretfulness; drowsiness; anorexia; vomiting; transient fever; malaise; generalized aches and pains; edema of injection area with redness, swelling, induration, pain (may persist for a few days); hypersensitivity reactions.

Dosage

Two primary IM doses of 0.5 mL each given at 4- to 8-wk intervals, followed by a third 0.5-mL IM dose given in 6–12 mo. Routine booster of 0.5 mL IM every 10 yr for maintenance of immunity.

Nursing considerations

- Use caution in pregnant women. **Pregnancy Category C**—safety not established.
- Defer administration of routine immunizing or booster doses in case of acute infection.
- Arrange to interrupt immunosuppressive therapy if emergency booster doses of Td are required after injury.
- Not for treatment of acute tetanus or diphtheria infections.
- Administer by IM injection only; avoid SC or IV injection. Deltoid muscle is the preferred site. Do not administer into the same site more than once.
- Arrange for epinephrine 1:1,000 to be immediately available at time of injection in case of hypersensitivity reactions.
- Provide comfort measures to help patient cope with discomforts of injection: analgesics, warm soaks for injection site, small meals, environmental control—temperature, stimuli.
- Provide patient with written record of immunization and reminder of when booster injection is needed.

▷ diphtheria and tetanus toxoids and acellular pertussis vaccine, adsorbed (DTaP)

Certiva, Daptacel, Infanrix, Tripedia

Therapeutic actions

Provides detoxified diphtheria and tetanus toxins and acellular pertussis vaccine to stimulate an immunologic response in children leading to an active immunity against these diseases. For active immunization of children 6 wk to 7 yr (*Infanrix*).

Indications
- Primary immunization of children ≥ 6 wk–7 yr. Induction of immunity against diphtheria, tetanus, and pertussis. Being considered for immunization of adults against pertussis.

Adverse effects
Hypersensitivity reactions; erythema, induration, redness, pain, swelling of the injection area; nodule at the injection site, which may persist for several weeks; temperature elevations, malaise, chills, irritability, fretfulness, drowsiness, anorexia, vomiting, persistent crying; rarely—fatal reactions.

Dosage
- As primary immunization: 3 IM doses of 0.5 mL at 4- to 8-wk intervals. Start doses by 6–8 wk of age; finish by 7th birthday. Use the same vaccine for all 3 doses.
- Fourth dose: 0.5 mL IM at 15–20 mo, at least 6 mo after previous dose (*Certiva, Infanrix, Tripedia*).
- Fifth dose: 0.5 mL IM at 4–6 years of age or preferably before entry into school. If fourth dose was given after the 4-yr birthday, however, the preschool dose may be omitted. Booster injections every 10 yr should be given after this, using the adult diphtheria and tetanus toxoids combination. Do not give pertussis vaccine to person ≥ 7 yr.

Nursing considerations
- Do not use for treatment of acute tetanus, diphtheria, or whooping cough infections.
- Do not administer to any person ≥ 7 yr.
- Do not attempt routine immunization with DTaP if the child has a personal history of CNS disease or convulsions.
- Do not administer DTaP after recent blood transfusions or receipt of immune globulin, in immunodeficiency disorders or with immunosuppressive therapy, or to patients with malignancy.
- Question the parent concerning occurrence of any symptoms or signs of adverse reactions after the previous dose before administering a repeat dose of the vaccine. If temperature > 39°C (103°F), convulsions with or without fever, alterations of consciousness, focal neurologic signs, screaming episodes, shock, collapse, somnolence, or encephalopathy has occurred, DTP is contraindicated and diphtheria and tetanus toxoids without pertussis should be used for immunization.
- Administer by IM injection only. Avoid SC or IV injection. Midlateral muscle of the thigh is preferred site for infants; deltoid muscle is the preferred site for older children. Do not administer at same site more than once.
- Arrange for epinephrine 1:1,000 to be immediately available at time of injection in case of hypersensitivity reactions.
- DTaP products are not generically equivalent and are not interchangeable. Use vaccines from the same manufacturer for at least the first 3 doses.
- Provide comfort measures and teach parents to provide comfort measures to help the patient cope with the discomforts of the injection: analgesics, warm soaks for injection site, small meals, environmental control—temperature, stimuli.
- Provide parent with written record of immunization and reminder of when booster injection is needed.

▷ diphtheria and tetanus toxoids and acellular pertussis adsorbed, hepatitis B (recombinant), and inactivated poliovirus vaccine combined

Pediarix

Therapeutic actions

Contains diphtheria and tetanus toxoids, acellular pertussis vaccine, recombinant antigenic hepatitis B vaccine and inactivated poliovirus vaccine in one injection to stimulate active immunity against these diseases in children who have received all doses of the vaccine.

Indications

- Active immunization against diphtheria, tetanus, pertussis, hepatitis B virus and poliomyelitis caused by poliovirus Types 1, 2 and 3 as a three-dose primary series in infants born to HBsAg-negative mothers.

Adverse effects

Hypersensitivity reactions: erythema, induration, redness, pain, swelling of the injection area; nodule at the injection site, which may persist for several weeks; temperature elevations, malaise, chills, irritability, fretfulness, drowsiness, anorexia, vomiting, persistent crying; rarely—fatal reactions.

Dosage

- Infants with HBsAG-negative mothers, three 0.5-mL doses IM given at 6- to 8- (preferably 8-) wk intervals beginning at 2 mo.
- Children previously vaccinated with one dose of hepatitis B vaccine should receive the three-dose series.
- Children previously vaccinated with one or more doses of *Infanrix* or *IPV*. *Pediarix* may be used to complete the series.

Nursing considerations

- Administer only to children of HbsAg-negative mothers.
- Do not administer to children with immunodeficiency, immunosuppression, or malignancy.
- Do not administer to any person > 7 yr or < 6 wk.
- Do not administer if patient is febrile.
- Administer by IM injection only; avoid SC or IV injection. Midlateral muscle of the thigh is the preferred site for infants; deltoid muscle is preferred site for older children.
- Shake the vial vigorously to suspend the drug; do not use if particles are apparent; do not re-enter the vial; discard any unused portion.
- Do not administer into the same site more than once.
- Arrange for epinephrine 1:1,000 to be immediately available at time of injection because of risk of hypersensitivity reactions.
- Provide comfort measures and teach parents to provide comfort measures to help the patient cope with the discomforts of the injection: analgesics, warm soaks for the injection site, small meals, environmental control—temperature, stimuli.
- Provide parents with written record of immunization and reminder of when booster injections are needed.
- Do not use this drug as a booster injection after the completion of the three-shot series; use appropriate single vaccines for boosters.

▽haemophilus b conjugate vaccine

HibTITER, Liquid PedvaxHIB, ActHIB

Therapeutic actions

Provides antigenic combination of *Haemophilus* b conjugate vaccine to stimulate an immunologic response in children, leading to an active immunity against these diseases.

Indications

- Active immunization of infants and children against *H. influenzae* b for primary immunization and routine recall; 2–71 mo (*HibTITER, Pedvax HIB*), 2–18 mo (*ActHIB* with DPT), or 15–18 mo (*ActHIB* with *Tripedia*)

Adverse effects

Hypersensitivity reactions; erythema, induration, redness, pain, swelling of the injection area; nodule at the injection site, which may persist for several weeks; temperature elevations, malaise, chills, irritability, fretfulness, drowsiness, anorexia, vomiting, persistent crying; rarely—fatal reactions.

Dosage

ActHIB: Reconstitute with DTP, *Tripedia*, or saline.
- *2–6 mo:* 3 IM injections of 0.5 mL at 2, 4, and 6 mo; 0.5 mL at 15–18 mo and DPT alone at 4–6 yr.
- *7–11 mo:* 2 IM injections of 0.5 mL at 8-wk intervals; booster dose at 15–18 mo.
- *12–14 mo:* 0.5 mL IM with a booster 2 mo later.
- *15–18 mo:* 0.5 mL IM, booster of *Tripedia* at 4–6 yr.

HibTITER
- *2–6 mo:* 3 separate IM injections of 0.5 mL at 2-mo intervals.
- *7–11 mo:* 2 IM injections of 0.5 mL; give 2 mo apart.
- *12–14 mo:* 0.5 mL IM.

Booster dose at ≥ 15 mo but not < 2 mo from last dose. Unvaccinated children 15–71 mo: 0.5 mL IM.

Pedvax HIB
- *2–14 mo:* 2 IM injections of 0.5 mL at 2 mo of age and 2 mo later; 0.5-mL booster at 12 mo (if 2 doses complete before 12 mo, not < 2 mo after last dose).
- *≥ 15 mo:* 0.5 mL IM, single injection.

Nursing considerations

- Do not administer to children with immunodeficiency, immunosuppression, or malignancy.
- Do not administer to adults.
- Do not administer in the presence of febrile illness.
- Administer by IM injection only. Avoid SC or IV injection. Midlateral muscle of the thigh is preferred site for infants; deltoid muscle is preferred site for older children. Do not administer at same site more than once.
- Arrange for epinephrine 1:1,000 to be immediately available at time of injection in case of hypersensitivity reaction.
- Provide comfort measures and teach parents to provide comfort measures to help patient cope with the discomforts of the injection: analgesics, warm soaks for injection site, small meals, environmental control—temperature, stimuli.
- Provide parents with written record of immunization and reminder of when booster injection is needed.

- Conjugate vaccines can be given simultaneously with other routine vaccines using separate sites and syringes.

▷ haemophilus b conjugate vaccine with hepatitis B surface antigen (recombinant)

Comvax

Therapeutic actions

Provides antigenic hepatitis B vaccine to stimulate an immunologic response in children, leading to an active immunity against the disease.

Indications

- Active immunization of infants and children against hepatitis B, for primary immunization and routine recall for ages 2–15 mo.

Adverse effects

Hypersensitivity reactions: erythema, induration, redness, pain, swelling of the injection area; nodule at the injection site, which may persist for several weeks; temperature elevations, malaise, chills, irritability, fretfulness, drowsiness, anorexia, vomiting, persistent crying; rarely—fatal reactions.

Dosage

- Infants with HBsAg-negative mothers: Three 0.5-mL doses at 2, 4, and 12–15 mo.
- Children previously vaccinated with one or more doses of hepatitis B vaccine or haemophilus b vaccine: 0.5-mL doses at 2, 4, and 12–15 mo.

Nursing considerations

- Administer only to children of HBsAg-negative mothers.
- Do not administer to children with immunodeficiency, immunosuppression, or malignancy.
- Do not administer to adults.
- Do not administer if patient has febrile illness.
- Administer by IM injection only. Avoid SC or IV injection. Midlateral muscle of the thigh is preferred site for infants; deltoid muscle is preferred site for older children.
- Do not administer into same site more than once.
- Arrange for epinephrine 1:1,000 to be immediately available at time of injection because of risk of hypersensitivity reactions.
- Provide comfort measures and teach parents to provide comfort measures to help patient cope with the discomforts of the injection: analgesics, warm soaks for injection site, small meals, environmental control—temperature, stimuli.
- Provide parents with written record of immunization and reminder of when booster injection is needed.
- Conjugate vaccines can be given simultaneously with other routine vaccines, using separate sites and syringes.

▷ hepatitis A vaccine, inactivated

Havrix, Vaqta

Therapeutic effects

Contains hepatitis A antigen that stimulates production of specific antibodies against HAV, which protects against HAV infection. The immunity does not protect against hepatitis caused by other agents.

Indications
- Active immunization of adults and children ≥ 2 yr against disease caused by HAV in situations that warrant immunization (eg, travel, institutionalization); used with IG for immediate and long-term protection against hepatitis A.

Adverse effects
Transient fever; edema of injection area with redness, swelling, induration, pain (may persist for a few days); upper respiratory illness, headache, rash.

Dosage
- Adults: *Havrix*—1440 EL.U (1 mL) IM; same dose booster in 6–12 mo. *Vaqta*—50 units (1 mL) IM; same dose booster in 6–12 mo.
- Pediatric patients 2–18 yr: 25 units/0.5 mL IM with a repeat dose in 6–12 mo. (*Vaqta*); 720 EL.U (0.5 mL) IM; repeat dose in 6–12 mo (*Havrix*) or 360 EL.U (0.5 mL) at 0 and 1 mo; repeat dose in 6–12 mo.

Nursing considerations
- Use caution in pregnancy. **Pregnancy Category C**—safety not established.
- Defer administration in case of acute infection.
- Administer by IM injection only. Deltoid muscle is the preferred site; do not give in the gluteal site.
- Arrange for epinephrine 1:1,000 to be immediately available at time of injection in case of hypersensitivity reaction.
- Provide comfort measures to help patient cope with the discomforts of the injection: analgesics, warm soaks for injection site, small meals, environmental control—temperature, stimuli.
- Provide patient with written record of immunization and timing for booster immunization.

▷ hepatitis A inactivated and hepatitis B recombinant vaccine

Twinrix

Therapeutic actions
Provides inactivated hepatitis A antigens that stimulate production of specific antibodies against HAV, which protect against hepatitis A, and inactivated human hepatitis B surface antigen particles, which stimulate active immunity and production of antibodies against hepatitis B surface antigens.

Indications
- Active immunization against disease caused by hepatitis A virus and hepatitis B virus in persons ≥ 18 yr who desire protection against or are at high risk of exposure to the viruses.

Adverse effects
Soreness, swelling, erythema, warmth, induration at injection site; malaise, fatigue, headache, nausea, vomiting, dizziness; myalgia, arthralgia, rash, low-grade fever; pharyngitis, rhinitis, cough; lymphadenopathy; hypotension; dysuria.

Dosage
- 3 doses (1 mL by IM injection) given on a 0-, 1-, and 6-month schedule.

- Safety for use in patients < 18 yr not established.

Nursing considerations
- Do not administer to any patient with a known hypersensitivity to hepatitis A vaccine or hepatitis B vaccine or any components used in the solution.
- Use cautiously in patients with bleeding disorders, immunosuppressed patients, pregnancy, and lactation. **Pregnancy Category C**.
- Postpone injection in the presence of moderate to severe illness.
- Administer IM, preferably in the deltoid region. Do not administer in the gluteal region.
- Shake vial or syringe well before withdrawal; observe for any particulate matter or discoloration. Should appear as a white, homogenous, turbid suspension; discard if it appears otherwise.
- Administer drug as provided; do not dilute.
- Provide comfort measures—analgesics, antipyretics, care of injection site—to help patient cope with the effects of the injection.
- Provide patient with a written record of the immunization and the dates that repeat vaccinations and antibody tests are needed.

▷hepatitis B immune globulin (HBIG)
BayHep B, Nabi-HB

Therapeutic actions
Globulin contains a high titer of antibody to hepatitis B surface antigen (HBsAg), providing a passive immunity to HBsAg.

Indications
- Postexposure prophylaxis following parental exposure (accidental "needle-stick"), direct mucous membrane contact (accidental splash), or oral ingestion (pipetting accident) involving HBsAg-positive materials such as blood, plasma, serum, or sexual exposure to an HbsAg-positive person.
- Prophylaxis of infants born to HBsAg-positive mothers.
- Adjunct to hepatitis B vaccine when rapid achievement of protective levels of antibodies is desirable.

Adverse effects
Hypersensitivity reactions; tenderness, muscle stiffness at the injection site; urticaria, angioedema; fever, chills, nausea, vomiting, chest tightness.

Dosage
- Perinatal exposure: 0.5 mL IM within 12 hr of birth; repeat dose at 1 mo and 6 mo after initial dose.
- Percutaneous exposure: 0.06 mL/kg IM immediately (within 7 days) and repeat 28–30 days after exposure. Usual adult dose is 3–5 mL.
- Individuals at high risk of infection: 0.06 mL/kg IM at same time (but at a different site) as hepatitis B vaccine is given.
- IV use approved only for prophylaxis against hepatitis B virus reinfection in liver transplant patients.
- Sexual exposure: a single dose of 0.06 mL/kg IM within 14 days of last sexual contact.

Nursing considerations
- Do not administer to patients with history of allergic response to gamma globulin or with anti–immunoglobulin A antibodies.

- Use caution in pregnant women. **Pregnancy Category C**—safety not established, if benefits outweigh potential unknown risks to the fetus.
- HBIG may be administered at the same time or up to 1 mo preceding hepatitis B vaccination without impairing the active immune response from the vaccination.
- Administer IM in the deltoid region or anterolateral aspect of upper thigh. Do not administer IV.
- Administer the appropriate dose as soon after exposure as possible (within 7 days is preferable); repeat 28–30 days after exposure.
- Have epinephrine 1:1,000 immediately available at time of injection in case of anaphylactic reaction.
- Provide comfort measures to help patient deal with discomfort of drug therapy—analgesics, antipyretics, environmental control.

▽ hepatitis B vaccine

Engerix-B, Recombivax HB

Therapeutic actions

Provides inactivated human hepatitis B surface antigen particles to stimulate active immunity and production of antibodies against hepatitis B surface antigens using surface antigen produced by yeast.

Indications

- Immunization against infection caused by all known subtypes of hepatitis B virus, especially those at high risk for infection—health care personnel, military personnel identified to be at risk, prisoners, users of illicit drugs, populations with high incidence (Eskimos, Indochinese refugees, Haitian refugees), morticians and embalmers, persons at increased risk because of their sexual practices (repeated sexually transmitted diseases, homosexually active males, prostitutes), patients in hemodialysis units, patients requiring frequent blood transfusions, residents of mental institutions, household contacts of people with persistent hepatitis B antigenemia.
- All infants, adolescents 11–12 yr, and older unvaccinated adolescents at high risk.

Adverse effects

Soreness, swelling, erythema, warmth, induration at injection site; malaise, fatigue, headache, nausea, vomiting, dizziness; myalgia, arthralgia, rash; low-grade fever, pharyngitis, rhinitis, cough; lymphadenopathy; hypotension; dysuria.

Dosage

- *Birth–10 yr:* Initial dose—0.5 mL IM, followed by 0.5 mL IM at 1 mo and 6 mo after initial dose.
- *11–19 yr:* 0.5 mL IM, followed by 0.5 mL IM at 1 mo and 6 mo after initial dose.
- *Adults:* Initial dose—1 mL IM, followed by 1 mL IM at 1 mo and 6 mo after initial dose, all types.
- *Dialysis or predialysis patients:* Initial dose—40 mcg IM; repeat dose at 1 mo, 2 mo, and 6 mo after initial dose (*Engerix-B*). Or, 40 mcg IM; repeat dose at 1 mo and 6 mo (*Recombivax HB*).
- Revaccination (a booster dose should be considered if anti-HBs levels < 10 mIU/mL 1 to 2 mo after third dose). *Children < 10 yr:* 10 mcg. *Adults and patients > 10 yr:* 20 mcg. *Hemodialysis patients (when antibody testing indicates need):* two 20-mcg doses.

Nursing considerations

- Do not administer to any patient with known hypersensitivity to any component of the vaccine or allergy to yeast.
- Use caution in pregnant or nursing women. **Pregnancy Category C**—safety not established. Use only if clearly needed and benefits outweigh potential unknown effects.
- Use caution in any patient with active infection. Delay use of vaccine if possible. Use with caution in any patient with compromised cardiopulmonary status or patients in whom a febrile or systemic reaction could present a significant risk.
- Administer IM, preferably in the deltoid muscle in adults or the anterolateral thigh muscle in infants and small children. Do not administer IV or intradermally; SC route may be used in patients who are at high risk for hemorrhage following IM injection, but increased incidence of local effects has been noted.
- Shake vaccine container well before withdrawing solution; no dilution is needed. Use vaccine as supplied. Vaccine appears as a slightly opaque, white suspension. Refrigerate vials; do not freeze.
- Have epinephrine 1:1,000 immediately available at time of injection in case of severe anaphylactic reaction.
- Provide comfort measures—analgesics, antipyretics, care of injection site—to help patient cope with effects of the drug.
- Provide patient or parent with a written record of the immunization and dates that repeat injections and antibody tests are needed.

▷immune globulin intramuscular (IG; gamma globulin; IGIM)

BayGam

immune globulin intravenous (IGIV)

Gamimune N, Gammagard S/D, Gammar-P IV, Iveegam, Panglobulin, Polygam S/D, Sandoglobulin, Venoglobulin-S

Therapeutic actions

Contains human globulin (16.5% IM, 5% IV), which provides passive immunity through the presence of injected antibodies. IM gamma globulin involves a 2- to 5-day delay before adequate serum levels are obtained. IV gamma globulin provides immediate antibody levels. Mechanism of action in idiopathic thrombocytopenic purpura not determined.

Indications

- Prophylaxis after exposure to hepatitis A, measles (rubeola), varicella, rubella; IM route is preferred.
- Prophylaxis for patients with immunoglobulin deficiency—IM; IV if immediate increase in antibodies is necessary.
- Idiopathic thrombocytopenic purpura. IV route has produced temporary increase in platelets in emergency situations (*Gamimune N, Gammagard S/D, Polygam S/D, Sandoglobulin, Venoglobulin-S, Panglobulin*).
- B-cell chronic lymphocytic leukemia (CLL) (*Gammagard S/D, Polygam S/D*).
- Kawasaki syndrome (*Iveegam, Venoglobulin-S, Gammagard S/D, Polygam S/D*).
- Bone marrow transplant (*Gamimune N* only).
- Pediatric HIV infection (*Gamimune N* only).

Adverse effects
Tenderness, muscle stiffness at injection site; urticaria, angioedema, nausea, vomiting, chills, fever, chest tightness; anaphylactic reactions, precipitous fall in blood pressure—more likely with IV administration. Risk of acute renal failure with IV products.

Dosage
- Hepatitis A: 0.02 mL/kg IM for household and institutional contacts. Persons traveling to areas where hepatitis A is common: 0.02 mL/kg IM if staying < 2 mo; 0.06 mL/kg IM repeated every 5 mo for prolonged stay.
- Measles (rubeola): 0.25 mL/kg IM if exposed < 6 days previously; immunocompromised child exposed to measles: 0.5 mL/kg to a maximum of 15 mL IM given immediately.
- Varicella: 0.6–1.2 mL/kg IM given promptly if zoster immune globulin is unavailable.
- Rubella: 0.55 mL/kg IM given to those pregnant women who have been exposed to rubella and will not consider a therapeutic abortion may decrease likelihood of infection and fetal damage.
- Immunoglobulin deficiency: Initial dosage of 1.3 mL/kg IM, followed in 3–4 wk by 0.66 mL/kg IM every 3–4 wk; some patients may require more frequent injections.
- *Sandoglobulin:* 200 mg/kg IV once a month by IV infusion; if insufficient response, increase dose to 300 mg/kg by IV infusion or repeat more frequently. Idiopathic thrombocytopenic purpura: 400 mg/kg IV for 5 consecutive days.
- *Gamimune N:* 100 mg/kg IV once a month by IV infusion. May be increased to 200 mg/kg IV or infusion may be repeated more frequently.
- *Gammagard S/D:* 200–400 mg/kg IV; monthly doses of at least 100 mg/kg are recommended. B-cell CLL: 400 mg/kg IV every 3–4 wk. Idiopathic thrombocytopenic purpura: 1,000 mg/kg IV; base dose on clinical response. Give up to 3 doses on alternate days if required.
- *Gammar-P IV:* 100–200 mg/kg IV every 3–4 wk.
- *Venoglobulin-S:* 200 mg/kg IV administered monthly. If response is inadequate, dose may be increased to 300–400 mg/kg/mo. Idiopathic thrombocytopenic purpura: 500 mg/kg/day for 2–7 consecutive days.
- *Iveegam:* 200 mg/kg IV per month.

Nursing considerations
- Do not administer to patients with history of allergy to gamma globulin or anti-immunoglobulin A antibodies.
- Use IM gamma globulin with caution in patients with thrombocytopenia or any coagulation disorder that would contraindicate IM injections. Use only if benefits outweigh risks.
- Use with caution in pregnant women. **Pregnancy Category C**—safety not established.
- Administer 2 wk before or 3 mo after immune globulin administration because antibodies in the globulin preparation may interfere with the immune response to the vaccination.
- Have epinephrine 1:1,000 immediately available at time of injection in case of anaphylactic reaction, which is more likely with IV immune globulin, large IM doses, and repeated injections.
- Refrigerate drug; do not freeze. Discard partially used vials.
- Administer IM preparation by IM injection only; do not administer SC or intradermally.
- Administer IV preparation with extreme caution as follows:
Sandoglobulin: Give the first infusion as a 3% solution (reconstitute by inverting the two bottles so that solvent flows into the IV bottle). Start with a flow rate of 0.5–1 mL/min; after 15–30 min, increase infusion rate to 1.5–2.5 mL/min. Administer subsequent infusions at a rate of 2–2.5 mL/min; if high doses must be administered repeatedly after the first infusion of 3% solution, use a 6% solution (reconstitute 1-g vial with 16.5 mL diluent, 3-g vial with 50 mL diluent, 6-g vial with 100 mL diluent) with an initial infusion rate of 1–1.5 mL/min, increased after 15–30 min to a maximum of 2.5 mL/min.

Gamimune N: May be diluted with 5% dextrose, infusion rate of 0.01–0.02 mL/kg/min for 30 min. If patient does not experience any discomfort, the rate may be increased to 0.02–0.04 mL/kg/min. If side effects occur, reduce the rate or interrupt the infusion until the symptoms subside and resume at a rate tolerable to the patient.

Gammagard S/D: Initially administer at a rate of 0.5 mL/kg/hr. If rate causes no distress, may be gradually increased, not to exceed 4 mL/kg/hr.

Gammar-P IV: Administer at 0.01 mL/kg/min, increasing to 0.02 mL/kg/min after 15–30 min. If adverse reactions occur, slow the infusion rate.

Venoglobulin-S: Infuse at a rate of 0.01–0.02 mL/kg/min for the first 30 min. If patient experiences no distress, 5% solution may be increased to 0.08 mL/kg/min; 10% solution may be increased to 0.05 mL/kg/min.

Iveegam: Infuse at rate of 1 mL/min up to a maximum of 2 mL/min of the 5% solution. Drug may be further diluted with 5% dextrose or saline.

- Do not mix immune globulin with any other medications.
- Monitor patient's vital signs continuously and observe for any symptoms during IV administration. Adverse effects appear to be related to the rate of infusion.
- Provide comfort measures or teach patient to provide comfort measures—analgesics, antipyretics, warm soaks to injection site—to help patient to cope with the discomforts of drug therapy.
- Provide patient with written record of injection and dates for follow-up injections as needed.

▽ influenza virus vaccine

Fluzone, Fluvirin

Therapeutic effects

Inactivated influenza virus antigens stimulate an active immunity through the production of antibodies specific to the antigens used; the antigens used vary from year to year depending on which influenza virus strains are anticipated to be prevalent.

Indications

- Prophylaxis for people at high risk of developing complications from infection with influenza virus—adults and children with chronic cardiovascular or pulmonary disorders, chronic metabolic disorders, renal dysfunction, anemia, immunosuppression, asthma; residents of chronic care facilities; medical personnel with extensive contact with high-risk patients, to prevent their transmitting the virus to these patients; children on chronic aspirin therapy who are at high risk of developing Reye's syndrome; people who provide essential community services (to decrease the risk of disruption of services).

Adverse effects

Tenderness, redness, and induration at the injection site; fever, malaise, myalgia; allergic responses—flare, wheal, respiratory symptoms; Guillain-Barré syndrome.

Dosage

- *6–35 mo:* Split virus or purified surface antigen only—0.25 mL IM repeated in 4 wk.
- *3–8 yr:* Split virus or purified surface antigen only—0.5 mL IM repeated in 4 wk.
- *≥ 9 yr:* Split virus or purified surface antigen—0.5 mL IM.

Nursing considerations

- Do not administer to patients with sensitivities to eggs, chicken, chicken feathers, or chicken dander. If an allergic condition is suspected, administer a scratch test or an intradermal injec-

tion (0.05–0.1 mL) of vaccine diluted 1:100 in sterile saline. A wheal greater than 5 mm justifies withholding immunization.
- Do not administer to patient with a hypersensitivity to any component of the vaccine or history of Guillain-Barré syndrome.
- Do not administer to infants and children at the same time as diphtheria, tetanus toxoid, and pertussis vaccine (DTP) or within 14 days after measles virus vaccine.
- Delay administration in the presence of acute respiratory disease or other active infection or acute febrile illness.
- Use caution in pregnant women. **Pregnancy Category C**—safety not established. Delay use until the second or third trimester to minimize concern over possible teratogenicity.
- Monitor patient for enhanced drug effects and possible toxicity of theophylline, warfarin sodium for as long as 3 wk after vaccine injection.
- Administer IM only. The deltoid muscle is preferred for adults and older children, the anterolateral aspect of the thigh for infants and younger children.
- Consider the possible need for amantadine for therapeutic use for patients in high-risk groups who develop illness compatible with influenza during a period of known influenza A activity in the community.
- Have epinephrine 1:1,000 immediately available at time of injection in case of anaphylactic reaction.
- Provide comfort measures or teach patient to provide comfort measures—analgesics, antipyretics, warm soaks to injection site—to help patient cope with effects of the drug.
- Provide patient with written record of vaccination and dates of second injection as appropriate.
- Do not use vaccine supplies remaining from previous years for current year vaccination.

▽ measles (rubeola) virus vaccine, live, attenuated
Attenuvax

Therapeutic actions
Attenuated measles virus produces a modified measles infection and stimulates an active immune reaction with antibodies to the measles virus.

Indications
- Immunization against measles (rubeola) immediately after exposure to natural measles; more effective if given before exposure—children ≥ 15 mo (immunization with trivalent MMR vaccine is the preferred product for routine vaccinations).
- Revaccination for children immunized before the age of 12 mo or vaccinated with inactivated vaccine alone.
- Prophylaxis for high school or college age persons in epidemic situations or for adults in isolated communities where measles is not endemic.

Adverse effects
Moderate fever, rash; high temperature (less common); febrile convulsions, Guillain-Barré syndrome, ocular palsies (less common); burning or stinging wheal or flare at injection site.

Dosage
Inject the total volume of the reconstituted vaccine or 0.5 mL of multi-dose vial SC into the outer aspect of the upper arm; dose is the same for all patients.

Nursing considerations
- Do not administer to patients with a history of anaphylactic hypersensitivity to neomycin (contained in injection), to patients with immune deficiency conditions (immunosuppressive ther-

apy with corticosteroids, antineoplastics; neoplasms; immunodeficiency states), to patients receiving immune serum globulin.
- Do not administer to pregnant women. **Pregnancy Category C**—advise patients to avoid pregnancy for 3 mo following vaccination. If measles exposure occurs during pregnancy, provide passive immunity with immune serum globulin.
- Use caution if administering to children with history of febrile convulsions, cerebral injury, or other conditions in which stress due to fever should be avoided.
- Use caution if administering to patient with a history of sensitivity to eggs, chicken, chicken feathers.
- Do not administer within 1 mo of immunization with other live virus vaccines; may be administered concurrently with monovalent or trivalent polio vaccine, rubella vaccine, mumps vaccine.
- Do not administer for at least 3 mo following blood or plasma transfusions or administration of serum immune globulin.
- Monitor for possible depression of *tuberculin skin sensitivity;* administer test before or simultaneously with vaccine.
- Administer with a sterile syringe free of preservatives, antiseptics, and detergents for each injection (these may inactivate the live virus vaccine). Use a 23-gauge, 5/8-inch needle.
- Refrigerate unreconstituted vial; protect from exposure to light. Use only the diluent supplied with the vaccine and reconstitute just before using. Discard reconstituted vaccine if not used within 8 hr.
- Have epinephrine 1:1,000 immediately available at time of injection in case of anaphylactic reaction.
- Provide comfort measures or teach patient or parent to provide comfort measures to help patient to cope with the discomforts of drug therapy: analgesics, antipyretics, warm soaks to injection site.
- Provide patient or parent with a written record of immunization.

▽measles (rubeola) and rubella virus vaccine, live

M-R-Vax II

Therapeutic actions

Viral antigens stimulate active immunity against measles (rubeola) and rubella through production of antibodies to both the rubeola and rubella viruses.

Indications

- Simultaneous immunization against measles and rubella in children ≥ 15 mo.

Adverse effects

Fretfulness; drowsiness; anorexia; vomiting; transient fever; malaise; generalized aches and pains; edema of injection area with redness, swelling, induration, pain (may persist for a few days); hypersensitivity reactions.

Dosage

0.5 mg SC preferably injected in the outer aspect of the upper arm. Booster doses during outbreaks of measles or rubella are best done with the appropriate monovalent vaccine. Boosters recommended for entry into kindergarten or middle school are best done with the MMR trivalent vaccine.

Nursing considerations

- Defer administration of routine immunizing or booster doses in case of acute infection.

- Use only the diluent supplied to reconstitute. Protect from light. Discard after 8 hr.
- Not for treatment of acute infections.
- Administer by SC injection only; not for IM or IV injection.
- Arrange for epinephrine 1:1,000 to be immediately available at time of injection in case of hypersensitivity reaction.
- Provide comfort measures to help the patient cope with the discomforts of the injection: analgesics, warm soaks for injection site, small meals, environmental control—temperature, stimuli.
- Provide parent with written record of immunization and reminder of when additional injections are needed.

▽ measles, mumps, rubella vaccine, live
M-M-R II

Therapeutic actions

Attenuated measles, mumps, and rubella viruses produce a modified infection and stimulate an active immune reaction with antibodies to these virus.

Indications

- Immunization against measles, mumps, rubella in children > 15 mo and adults.

Adverse effects

Moderate fever, rash, burning or stinging wheal or flare at injection site, high temperature; less common: febrile convulsions, Guillain-Barré syndrome, ocular palsies.

Dosage

0.5 mL reconstituted vaccine SC into the outer aspect of the upper arm. Dose is the same for all patients. Booster dose is recommended on entry into school and again at entry into junior high school.

Nursing considerations

- Do not administer to patients with a history of anaphylactic hypersensitivity to neomycin (contained in injection), to patients with immune deficiency conditions (immunosuppressive therapy with corticosteroids, antineoplastics; neoplasms; immunodeficiency states), to patients receiving immune serum globulin.
- Do not administer to pregnant women. **Pregnancy Category C**—advise patients to avoid pregnancy for 3 mo following vaccination. If measles exposure occurs during pregnancy, provide passive immunity with immune serum globulin.
- Use caution if administering to children with history of febrile convulsions, cerebral injury, or other conditions in which stress due to fever should be avoided.
- Use caution if administering to patient with a history of sensitivity to eggs, chicken, chicken feathers.
- Do not administer within 1 mo of immunization with other *live virus vaccines;* may be administered concurrently with monovalent or trivalent polio vaccine, rubella vaccine, mumps vaccine.
- Do not administer for at least 3 mo following blood or plasma transfusions or administration of serum immune globulin.
- Monitor for possible depression of tuberculin skin sensitivity. Administer the test before or simultaneously with the vaccine.
- Administer with a sterile syringe free of preservatives, antiseptics, and detergents for each injection (these may inactivate the live virus vaccine). Use a 25-gauge, 5/8-inch needle.

- Refrigerate unreconstituted vial. Protect from exposure to light. Use only the diluent supplied with the vaccine and reconstitute just before using. Discard reconstituted vaccine if not used within 8 hr.
- Have epinephrine 1:1,000 immediately available at time of injection in case of anaphylactic reaction.
- Provide comfort measures or teach patient or parent to provide comfort measures to help patient cope with the discomforts of drug therapy: analgesics, antipyretics, warm soaks to injection site.
- Provide patient or parent with a written record of immunization.
- MMR is the vaccination of choice for routine vaccinations. Other combinations that are available—rubella and mumps vaccine (*Biavax II*) and measles and rubella (*MR Vax-II*)—are used for specific situations.

▷ mumps virus vaccine, live
Mumpsvax

Therapeutic actions
Viral antigen stimulates active immunity through production of antibodies to the mumps virus.

Indications
- Immunization against mumps in children > 12 mo and adults. (Trivalent MMR vaccine is the drug of choice for routine vaccinations.)

Adverse effects
Fever, parotitis, orchitis; purpura and allergic reactions such as wheal and flare at injection site; febrile seizures, unilateral nerve deafness, encephalitis—rare; anaphylactic reactions.

Dosage
Inject total volume (0.5 mL) of reconstituted vaccine SC into the outer aspect of the upper arm; each dose contains not less than 20,000 TCID$_{50}$ (Tissue Culture Infectious Doses) of mumps virus vaccine. (Vaccine is available only in single-dose vials of diluent.)

Nursing considerations
- Do not administer to patients with history of hypersensitivity to neomycin (each single-dose vial of vaccine contains 25 mcg neomycin); immune deficiency conditions. **Pregnancy Category C**—advise patient to avoid pregnancy for 3 mo after vaccination.
- Use caution if administering to patient with history of allergy to eggs, chicken, chicken feathers.
- Delay administration in the presence of active infection.
- Do not administer within 1 month of immunization with other live virus vaccines, but it may be administered concurrently with live monovalent or trivalent polio vaccine, live rubella vaccine, live measles vaccine.
- Do not administer for at least 3 mo following blood or plasma transfusions or administration of serum immune globulin.
- Monitor for possible depression of tuberculin skin sensitivity; administer test before or simultaneously with the vaccine.
- Administer with a sterile syringe free of preservatives, antiseptics, and detergents for each injection (these may inactivate the live virus vaccine). Use a 25-gauge, five-eighths inch needle.
- Refrigerate unreconstituted vial. Protect from exposure to light.
- Use only the diluent supplied with the vaccine and reconstitute just before using. Discard reconstituted vaccine if not used within 8 hr.

- Have epinephrine 1:1,000 immediately available at time of injection in case of anaphylactic reaction.
- Provide comfort measures or teach patient or parent to provide comfort measures to help patient cope with the discomforts of drug therapy—analgesics, antipyretics, warm soaks to injection site.
- Provide patient or parent with a written record of vaccination.

▽ pneumococcal vaccine, polyvalent
Pneumovax 23

Therapeutic actions
Polysaccharide capsules of the 23 most prevalent or invasive pneumococcal types stimulate active immunity through antipneumococcal antibody production against the capsule types contained in the vaccine.

Indications
- Immunization against pneumococcal pneumonia and bacteremia caused by the types of pneumococci included in the vaccine, specifically in children > 2 yr and adults with chronic illnesses or who are immunocompromised and at increased risk for pneumococcal infections.
- Prophylaxis in children ≥ 2 yr with asymptomatic or symptomatic HIV infections.
- Prophylaxis in community groups at high risk for pneumococcal infections—institutionalized persons, groups in an area of outbreak, patients at high risk of influenza complications, including pneumococcal infection.

Adverse effects
Erythema, induration, soreness at injection site; fever, myalgia; acute febrile reactions, rash, arthralgia (less common); paresthesias, acute radiculoneuropathy (rare); anaphylactic reaction.

Dosage
One 0.5-mL dose SC or IM. Not recommended for children < 2 yr.

Nursing considerations
- Do not administer to patients with hypersensitivity to any component of the vaccine or with previous immunization with any polyvalent pneumococcal vaccine.
- Do not administer < 10 days prior to or during treatment for Hodgkin's disease.
- Use caution if administering to patients who nursing or pregnant. **Pregnancy Category C**—safety not established.
- Use caution if administering to patients with cardiac, pulmonary disorders; systemic reaction could pose a significant risk.
- May be administered concomitantly with influenza virus vaccine by separate injection in the other arm.
- Administer SC or IM only, preferably in the deltoid muscle or lateral mid-thigh; do not give IV.
- Refrigerate vials. Use directly as supplied; do not dilute (reconstitution is not necessary).
- Have epinephrine 1:1,000 immediately available at time of injection in case of anaphylactic reaction.
- Provide or teach patient to provide appropriate comfort measures—analgesics, antipyretics, warm soaks to injection site—to help patient to cope with effects of the drug therapy.
- Provide patient with written record of immunization and caution patient not to have another polyvalent pneumococcal vaccine injection.

▷ pneumococcal 7-valent conjugate vaccine

(diphtheria CRM$_{197}$ protein) Prevnar

Therapeutic actions

Stimulates active immunity against disease caused by *Streptococcus pneumoniae* by introduction of 7 capsular serotypes.

Indications

- Prevention of invasive pneumococcal disease in infants and toddlers; for use in all children < 23 mo of age. For high-risk populations age 24–59 mo, including children with sickle cell anemia, HIV, functional or anatomic asplenia, other immunocompromised conditions, and Native Americans and Alaskan natives.
- Active immunization of infants and toddlers against otitis media caused by vaccine serotypes.
- Prevention of otitis media caused by resistant strains.

Adverse effects

Fretfulness; drowsiness; anorexia; vomiting; transient fever; malaise; generalized aches and pains; edema of injection area with redness, swelling, induration, pain (may persist for a few days); hypersensitivity reactions.

Dosage

0.5 mg IM, preferably injected in the anterolateral aspect of the thigh in infants and the deltoid muscle of the upper arm in older children.

- *7–11 mo:* 3 doses with 2 doses at least 4 wk apart and last dose at > 1 yr of age.
- *12–23 mo:* 2 doses spaced at least 2 mo apart.
- *24 mo–9 yr:* 1 dose.

Nursing considerations

- Defer administration of routine immunizing or booster doses in case of acute infection or febrile illness.
- Not for treatment of acute pneumococcal infections.
- Shake vigorously prior to use. Do not use if a uniform suspension is not attained.
- Administer by IM injection only; avoid SC or IV injection. Do not inject vaccine in gluteal area.
- Arrange for epinephrine 1:1,000 to be immediately available at time of injection because of risk of hypersensitivity reactions.
- Provide comfort measures to help patient cope with the discomforts of the injection: analgesics, warm soaks for injection site, small meals, environmental control—temperature, stimuli.
- Provide parent with written record of immunization and reminder of when additional injections are needed.

▷ poliovirus vaccine, inactivated (IPV, Salk)

IPOL

Therapeutic actions

Inactivated, attenuated sterile suspension of three types of polio virus used to produce antibody response against poliomyelitis infection.

Indications

- Prevention of poliomyelitis caused by poliovirus types 1, 2, and 3 as routine immunization of infants and children; for adults at risk in whom OPV is contraindicated.

Adverse effects

Local reaction at site of injection within 48 hr.

Dosage

- *Children:* 0.5 mL SC at 2 mo, 4 mo, and 12–15 mo. A booster dose is needed at time of entry into elementary school.
- *Adults:* Not usually needed in adults in the United States; if unimmunized adult is exposed, is traveling to a high-risk area, or is a household contact of children receiving IPV (inactivated polio virus vaccine; Salk vaccine) immunization is recommended. 0.5 mL SC: two doses given at 1- to 2-mo intervals and a third dose given 6 to 12 mo later. Previously vaccinated adults at risk for exposure should receive a 0.5-mL dose of this drug.

Nursing considerations

- Do not administer to patients with known hypersensitivity to streptomycin or neomycin (each dose contains < 25 mcg of each).
- Defer administration in the presence of persistent vomiting or diarrhea and in patients with acute illness or any advanced debilitating condition.
- Do not administer to any patient with immune deficiency conditions; do not administer shortly after immune serum globulin unless necessary because of travel or exposure; if given with or shortly after ISG dose should be repeated after 3 mo.
- Use caution if administering to pregnant patients. **Pregnancy Category C**—safety not established; use only if clearly needed and benefits outweigh potential unknown effects on the fetus; if immediate protection is needed, TOPV is the recommended therapy.
- Refrigerate vaccine. Do not freeze.
- Provide patient or parent with a written record of the vaccination and information on when additional doses are needed.

▽**RH₀ (D) immune globulin**

BayRho-D Full Dose, RhoGAM

RH₀ (D) immune globulin micro-dose

BayRho-D Mini-Dose, MICRhoGAM

RH₀ (D) immune globulin IV (human) (RH₀ D IGIV)

WinRho SDF

Therapeutic actions

Suppresses the immune response of nonsensitized Rh_0-negative individuals who receive Rh_0-positive blood as the result of a fetomaternal hemorrhage or a transfusion accident; each vial of Rh_0-immune globulin completely suppresses immunity to 15 mL of Rh-positive packed RBCs (about 30 mL whole blood); each vial Rh_0 immune globulin micro-dose suppresses immunity to 2.5 mL Rh-positive packed RBCs.

Indications

- Prevention of sensitization to the Rh_0 factor.
- To prevent hemolytic disease of the newborn (erythroblastosis fetalis) in a subsequent pregnancy—mother must be Rh_0 negative; mother must not be previously sensitized to Rh_0 factor; infant must be Rh_0 positive and direct antiglobulin negative—used at full-term delivery, for incomplete pregnancy, for antepartum prophylaxis in case of abortion or ectopic pregnancy.
- To prevent Rh_0 sensitization in Rh_0-negative patients accidentally transfused with Rh_0-positive blood.

• Orphan drug use—immune thrombocytopenic purpura (ITP) (IV).

Adverse effects
Pain and soreness at injection site.

Dosage
• *Postpartum prophylaxis:* 1 vial IM or IV (*WinRho*) within 72 hr of delivery.
• *Antepartum prophylaxis:* 1 vial IM or IV (*WinRho*) at 28 wk gestation and one vial within 72 hr after an Rh-incompatible delivery to prevent Rh isoimmunization during pregnancy.
• *Following amniocentesis, miscarriage, abortion, ectopic pregnancy at or beyond 13 wk gestation:* 1 vial IM or IV.
• *Transfusion accidents:* Multiply the volume in mL of Rh-positive whole blood administered by the hematocrit of the donor unit and divide this volume (in mL) by 15 to obtain the number of vials to be administered. If results of calculation are a fraction, administer the next whole number of vials.
• *ITP:* 250 IU/kg IV; base therapy on response.
• *Spontaneous abortion or induced abortion or termination of ectopic pregnancy up to and including 12 wk gestation (unless the father is Rh negative):* 1 vial micro-dose IM given as soon as possible after termination of pregnancy.

Nursing considerations
• Rh_0 globulin is not needed in Rh_0-negative mothers if the father can be determined to be Rh_0 negative.
• Do not administer to the Rh_0-positive postpartum infant, to an Rh_0-positive individual, to an Rh_0-negative individual previously sensitized to the Rh_0 antigen (if it is not known whether a woman is Rh_0 sensitized, administer the Rh_0 globulin).
• Before administration, determine the infant's blood type and arrange for a direct antiglobulin test using umbilical cord, venous, or capillary blood; confirm that the mother is Rh_0 negative.
• Do not administer *BayRho* IV; administer IM within 72 hr after Rh_0-incompatible delivery, miscarriage, abortion, or transfusion.
• For *BayRho*, prepare one vial dose by withdrawing entire contents of vial; inject entire contents IM.
• For *BayRho*, prepare two or more vial doses using 5- to-10 mL syringes. Withdraw contents from the vials to be administered at one time and inject IM. Contents of the total number of vials may be injected as a divided dose at different injection sites at the same time, or the total dosage may be divided and injected at intervals, as long as the total dose is administered within 72 hr postpartum or after a transfusion accident.
• Refrigerate vials; do not freeze.
• Provide appropriate comfort measures if injection sites are painful.
• Reassure patient and explain what has been given and why; the patient needs to know what was given in the event of future pregnancies.

▽rubella virus vaccine, live
Meruvax II

Therapeutic actions
Live virus stimulates active immunity through development of antibodies against the rubella virus.

Indications
• Immunization against rubella—children 12 mo of age to puberty, adolescent and adult males, nonpregnant adolescent and adult females, rubella-susceptible women in the postpartum pe-

riod, leukemia patients in remission whose chemotherapy has been terminated for at least 3 mo, susceptible persons traveling abroad.
- Revaccination of children vaccinated when < 12 mo.

Adverse effects

Burning, stinging at injection site; regional lymphadenopathy, urticaria, rash, malaise, sore throat, fever, headache, polyneuritis—symptoms similar to natural rubella; arthritis, arthralgia—often 2 to 4 wk after receiving the vaccine.

Dosage

Inject total volume of reconstituted vaccine SC into the outer aspect of the upper arm; each dose contains not less than 1,000 $TCID_{50}$ of rubella.

Nursing considerations

- Do not administer to patients with a history of anaphylactic hypersensitivity to neomycin (each dose contains 25 mcg neomycin), to patients with immune deficiency conditions, to patients receiving immune serum globulin or blood transfusions.
- Do not administer to pregnant women. **Pregnancy Category C**—advise patients to avoid pregnancy for 3 mo following vaccination.
- Defer administration in the presence of acute respiratory or other active infections; susceptible children with mild illnesses may be vaccinated.
- Do not administer within 1 mo of immunization with other live virus vaccines, except that rubella vaccine may be administered concurrently with live monovalent or trivalent polio vaccine live measles virus vaccine, live mumps vaccine.
- Do not administer for at least 3 mo following blood or plasma transfusions or administration of serum immune globulin.
- Monitor for possible depression of *tuberculin skin sensitivity;* administer the test before or simultaneously with the vaccine.
- Refrigerate vials and protect from light. Reconstitute using only the diluent supplied with the vial; use as soon as possible after reconstitution; discard reconstituted vaccine if not used within 8 hr.
- Provide or instruct patient to provide appropriate comfort measures to help patient cope with the adverse effects of the drug—analgesics, antipyretics, fluids, rest.
- Provide patient or parent with a written record of immunization; advise that revaccination is not necessary.

▽ rubella and mumps virus vaccine, live

Biavax II

Therapeutic actions

Viral antigens stimulate active immunity against rubella and mumps through production of antibodies to both the rubella and mumps viruses.

Indications

- Simultaneous immunization against rubella and mumps in children > 12 mo, preferably at 15 mo.

Adverse effects

Fretfulness; drowsiness; anorexia; vomiting; transient fever; malaise; generalized aches and pains; edema of injection area with redness, swelling, induration, pain (may persist for a few days); hypersensitivity reactions

Dosage
0.5 mg SC preferably injected in the outer aspect of the upper arm. Booster doses at the age of entry into kindergarten and again in junior high school are preferably done using a trivalent MMR vaccine.

Nursing considerations
- Defer administration of routine immunizing or booster doses in case of acute infection.
- Use only the diluent supplied to reconstitute. Protect from light. Discard after 8 hr.
- Not for treatment of acute infections.
- Administer by SC injection only; not for IM or IV injection.
- Arrange for epinephrine 1:1,000 to be immediately available at time of injection in case of hypersensitivity reaction.
- Provide comfort measures to help patient cope with the discomforts of the injection: analgesics, warm soaks for injection site, small meals, environmental control—temperature, stimuli.
- Provide parent with written record of immunization and reminder of when additional injections are needed.

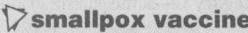

▽ smallpox vaccine
Dryvax

Therapeutic actions
A live-virus preparation of vaccinia virus prepared from calf lymph, which stimulates immunity and cellular hypersensitivity to the smallpox virus.

Indications
- Active immunization against smallpox disease.

Adverse effects
Fever, regional lymphadenopathy, malaise; generalized rashes (erythematous, urticarial nonspecific) spread of inoculation to sites other than site administered; rarely: Stevens-Johnson syndrome or other severe reactions including encephalitis, encephalopathy, progressive vaccinia, eczema vaccinatum with severe disability or death.

Dosage
- Primary vaccination: Using the vaccinating needle, two or three punctures into a prepared, dried area on the upper deltoid muscle or the posterior aspect of the arm over the triceps muscle onto which a drop of the live vaccine has been placed. Inspect the site for reaction after 6–8 days; if a major reaction has occurred, the site will scab over and heal, leaving a scar. If a mild or equivocal reaction has occurred, review the vaccination technique and repeat the process using 15 punctures into the area where a drop of vaccine has been placed.

Nursing considerations
- Follow the procedure for reconstitution of the vaccine precisely. Date vial and store only up to 15 days.
- Using strict aseptic technique and wearing protective gloves, follow guidelines for use of the vaccine: clean and dry area, place one drop of vaccine on the area, and use the supplied bifurcated needle to puncture the skin enough to see blood appear.
- Dispose of the needles and vaccine appropriately.
- Do not administer if the patient has a febrile illness.
- Do not administer by IM, SC, or IV routes.

- Do not administer to anyone with allergies to any component of the vaccine, including polymyxin B sulfate, dihydrostreptomycin, chlortetracycline, or neomycin.
- Do not administer to anyone with eczema or with a past history of eczema or those with household contact with people who have eczema or exfoliative skin conditions.
- Do not administer to anyone taking systemic corticosteroids or immunosuppressive drugs or who is immunocompromised.
- Do not administer to anyone who is pregnant or to household contacts of anyone who is pregnant.
- Provide comfort measures and teach parents to provide comfort measures to help the patient cope with the discomforts of the injection: analgesics, small meals, environmental control—temperature, stimuli.
- Leave the vaccination area uncovered, or cover the area with a loose bandage until the scab has fallen off and the area is healing. Do not use salves or lotions on the site. Caution the patient not to touch or scratch the area. Strict handwashing technique is advised after changing the dressing or touching the area. Bandages should be disposed of properly to avoid contact with other areas or other people.
- Arrange for the patient to have the site inspected 6–8 days after the inoculation. If a major reaction does not occur, the patient should be revaccinated.
- Provide parents with written record of immunization and reminder of when booster injection is needed.

▷typhoid vaccine

Typhim Vi, Typhoid Vaccine (H-P), Vivotif Berna

Therapeutic actions

Contains live attenuated strains of typhoid bacteria; produces a humoral antibody response against the causative agent of typhoid fever. Precise mechanism of action is not understood.

Indications

- Active immunization against typhoid fever (parenteral) (*Typhim Vi*); oral (*Vivotif Berna*).
- Immunization of adults and children against disease caused by *Salmonella typhi* (routine immunization is not recommended in the United States but is recommended for travelers, workers in microbiology fields, or those who may come into household contact with typhoid fever).

Adverse effects

Transient fever; edema of injection area with redness, swelling, induration, pain (may persist for a few days); headache, malaise.

Dosage

- Parenteral (*H-P*). *> 10 yr:* 2 doses of 0.5 mL SC at intervals of ≥ 4 wk. *≤ 10 yr:* 2 doses of 0.25 mL SC at ≥ 4-wk intervals.
- Booster dose (given every 3 yr in cases of continued exposure). *> 10 yr:* 0.5 mL SC or 0.1 mL intradermally. *6 mo–10 yr:* 0.25 mL SC or 0.1 mL intradermally.
- Parenteral (*Typhim Vi*). *Children ≥ 2 yr:* 0.5 mL IM; booster dose every 2 yr: 0.5 mL IM.
- Oral (*Vivotif Berna*). *Patients > 6 yr:* One capsule on days 1, 3, 5, and 7 taken 1 hr before a meal with a cold or lukewarm drink. There are no data on the need for a booster dose at this time; 4 capsules on alternating days—once every 5 yr is suggested.
- Complete vaccine regimen 1–2 wk before potential exposure.

Nursing considerations

- Use caution with pregnancy. **Pregnancy Category C**—safety not established.
- Defer administration in case of acute infection, GI illness, nausea, vomiting.
- Have patient swallow capsules whole; do not chew. All 4 doses must be taken to ensure antibody response.
- Administer *Typhim Vi* parenteral doses by IM injection; deltoid muscle is the preferred site. *Typhoid vaccine H-P* is administered SC. Booster doses may be given intradermally.
- Arrange for epinephrine 1:1,000 to be immediately available at time of injection because of risk of hypersensitivity reactions.
- Provide comfort measures to help patient cope with the discomforts of the injection: analgesics, warm soaks for injection site, small meals, environmental control—temperature, stimuli.
- Provide patient with written record of immunization and information on booster immunization if appropriate.
- Vaccines must be kept refrigerated. Do not freeze injectable products.

▽ varicella virus vaccine, live
Varivax

Therapeutic actions
Contains live attenuated varicella virus obtained from human or guinea pig cell cultures. Varicella virus causes chickenpox in children and adults. Vaccine produces an active immunity to the virus; longevity of immunity is not known.

Indications
- Active immunization of adults and children ≥ 12 mo against chickenpox (varicella).

Adverse effects
Transient fever; edema of injection area with redness, swelling, induration, pain (may persist for a few days); upper respiratory illness, cough, rash.

Dosage
- *Adult and patients ≥ 13 yr:* 0.5 mL SC in the deltoid area followed by 0.5 mL 4 to 8 wk later.
- *Children 1–12 yr:* Single 0.5-mL dose SC.

Nursing considerations
- Use caution with allergy to neomycin or gelatin; use caution in pregnancy. **Pregnancy Category C**—safety not established.
- Defer administration in case of acute infection and for at least 5 mo after plasma transfusion or receipt of immune globulin, other immunizations.
- Do not administer salicylates for up to 6 wk after immunization; cases of Reye's syndrome have been reported.
- Use reconstituted vaccine within 30 minutes. Only use diluent supplied.
- Administer by SC injection. Outer aspect of upper arm is preferred site.
- Arrange for epinephrine 1:1,000 to be immediately available at time of injection because of risk of hypersensitivity reactions.
- Provide comfort measures to help patient cope with the discomforts of the injection: analgesics, warm soaks for injection site, small meals, environmental control—temperature, stimuli.
- Provide patient with written record of immunization. It is not known whether booster immunization will be needed.

Other biologicals

Name	Indications	Instructions
Immunoglobulins		
anti-thymocyte globulin (*Thymoglobulin*)	Treatment of renal transplant acute rejection in conjunction with immunosuppression.	1.5 mg/kg/day for 7–14 days as 6-hr IV infusion for first dose and ≥ 4 hr each subsequent dose. Store in refrigerator and use within 4 hr of reconstitution.
cytomegalovirus immune globulin IV (CMV-IGIV) (*CytoGam*)	Attenuation of primary CMV disease following renal, lung, liver, pancreas, and heart transplant.	15 mg/kg IV over 30 min, increase to 30 mg/kg IV for 30 min, then 60 mg/kg IV to a max of 150 mg/kg. Infuse at 72 hr, 2 wk, and then 4, 6, 8, 12, and 16 wk. Monitor for allergic reactions. Use within 6 hr of entering vial. Administer through an IV line with an in-line filter.
lymphocyte, immune globulin (*Atgam*)	Management of allograft rejection in renal transplants; treatment of aplastic anemia.	10–30 mg/kg/day IV adult transplant; 5–25 mg/kg/day IV pediatric transplant, 10–20 mg/kg/day IV for 8–14 days for aplastic anemia. Stable for up to 12 hr after reconstitution. Administer a skin test prior to administration of first dose.
rabies immune globulin (*BayRab, Imogam Rabies-HT*)	Passive protection against rabies in nonimmunized patients with exposure to rabies.	20 IU/kg IM. Refrigerate vial. Infuse wound area if possible. Give in conjunction with rabies vaccine. Never give in same site as vaccine.
respiratory syncytial virus immune globulin (human) (RSV-IGIV) (*RespiGam*)	Prevention of serious lower respiratory tract infection caused by RSV in children < 24 mo with bronchopulmonary dysplasia or history of premature birth.	1.5 mL/kg/hr for 15 min; may increase to 3 mL/kg/hr if needed for 15 min; may then increase to 6 mL/kg/hr to a total monthly infusion of 750 mg/kg. Administer using infusion pump; use at start of RSV season. Increase rate of infusion only if clinical condition is stable; critically ill children may require a slower rate. Begin infusion within 6 hr of entering vial.
tetanus immune globulin (*BayTet*)	Passive immunization against tetanus, useful at time of injury.	250 units IM. Do not give IV. Arrange proper medical care of wound.
varicella-zoster immune globulin (*Varicella-Zoster Immune Globulin*)	Passive immunity for immunosuppressed patients with significant exposure to varicella.	125 units/10 kg IM to a maximum of 625 units. Administer within 96 hr of exposure to chicken pox. Not for use in nonimmunosuppressed individuals. Give no more than 2.5 mL at a single site.
Antitoxins and antivenins		
antivenin (crotalidae) polyvalent	Neutralize the venom of pit vipers, including rattlesnakes, copperheads.	20 to 40 mL IV; up to 100–150 mL IV in severe cases. Removal of venom should be done at once; antivenin to rare breeds of snake may be available from the CDC.

(continued)

Name	Indications	Instructions
Antitoxins and antivenins (continued)		
antivenin (micrurus fulvius)	Neutralize the venom of coral snakes in the United States	30-50 mL by slow IV injection. Give first 1 to 2 mL over 3 to 5 min and observe for allergic reaction. Flush with IV fluids after antivenin has been infused. May require up to 100 mL.
Black Widow spider species antivenin (*Antivenin*) (*Latrodectus mactans*)	Treatment of symptoms of Black Widow spider bites.	2.5 mL IM; may be given IV in 10–50 mL saline over 15 min. Ensure supportive therapy and use of muscle relaxants.
crotalidae polyvalent immune fab (ovine) (*CroFab*)	Treatment of rattlesnake bites.	4–6 vials IV; may be repeated based on patient response. Dilute each vial with 10 mL sterile water, then with 250 mL 0.9% sodium chloride. Give each 250 mL over 60 min. Contains specific antibody fragments that bind to four different rattlesnake toxins. Removal of venom should be done at once. Monitor patient carefully for hypersensitivity reaction. Most effective if given within first 6 hr after snake bite.
Bacterial vaccines		
BCG (*Tice BCG*)	Exposure to TB of skin test—negative infants and children; treatment of groups with high rates or TB; travel to areas with high rates of endemic TB.	0.2–0.3 mL percutaneous using a sterile multipuncture disc. Refrigerate, protect from light; keep the vaccination site clean until reaction disappears.
Meningococcal polysaccharide vaccine (*Menomune-A/C/Y/W-135*)	Prevention of meningitis in patients at risk in epidemic or highly endemic areas. Prophylaxis for college freshmen living in dormitories.	0.5 mL SC. May revaccinate with 0.5 mL in high-risk patients. Consider revaccination within 3–5 yr. Reconstitute with diluent provided.
Viral vaccines		
Japanese encephalitis vaccine (*JE-VAX*)	Active immunization in persons > 1 yr who will reside or travel in areas where it is endemic or epidemic.	3 SC doses of 1 mL given at days 0, 7, and 30; Children 1–3 yr: 3 SC doses of 0.5 mL. Refrigerate vial. Do not remove rubber stopper. Do not travel within 10 days of vaccination.
rabies vaccine (*Imovax Rabies, RabAvert*)	Preexposure rabies immunization for patients in high-risk area; postexposure antirabies regimen in conjunction with rabies immunoglobulin.	Preexposure: 1 mL IM on days 0, 7, 21, and 28. Postexposure: 1 mL IM on days 0, 3, 7, 21, and 28. Refrigerate. If titers are low, booster may be needed.
yellow fever vaccine (*YF-Vax*)	Immunization of travelers to endemic areas.	0.5 mL SC. Booster dose suggested q 10 yr. Caution with allergy to chicken or egg products.

Recommendations for Pediatric Immunizations

Vaccine	Birth	1 mo	2 mo	4 mo	6 mo	12 mo	15 mo	18 mo	24 mo	4-6 yr	11-12 yr	14-18 yr
Hepatitis B*	X		X			X				0		
Hepatitis B†	X	X			X							
DTaP			X	X	X		X			X		
Tetanus Booster												X
H. influenzae type b 2‡			X	X	X	X						
Poliovirus (IPV)			X	X		X				X		
Measles, mumps, rubella						X				X	0	
Varicella						X				0		
Hepatitis A‡										X		

0 = suggested timing of immunization if recommended immunizations have been missed or given early.
*Infants born to HBsAg-negative mothers.
†Infants born to HBsAg-positive mothers or HBsAg-unknown mothers.
‡Recommended in selected areas only; check with your local health department.
Suggested by the American Academy of Pediatrics, 2003.

Recommendations for Adult Immunizations

Adults often need immunizations because of being exposed or being immunocompromised. These vaccines should not be given to patients who have had any previous anaphylactic reaction to any vaccine or who have moderate or severe infections. These vaccines can be given with other vaccines, but separate injection sites should be used.

Vaccine and route	Recommendation
Influenza, IM	All people ≥ 65 yr; people with chronic medical conditions; all health care workers; pregnant women who will be in second or third trimester during the flu season; anyone wishing to avoid the flu
Pneumococcal, IM or SC	All people ≥ 65 yr; people with chronic medical conditions; people in immune-suppressed or debilitated states
Hepatitis B, IM	High-risk adults; all adolescents
Hepatitis A, IM	Adults who travel outside the United States; people with chronic liver disease, hepatitis C; IV drug users; food handlers
	In many areas of the country, prevaccination titers may remove the need for this vaccine.
Td, IM	After a primary series, a booster dose every 10 years; may give a booster after 5 yr. For wound management.
MMR, SC	Adults born in 1957 or later and > 18 yr should receive one dose of MMR. High-risk adults, including health care workers, college students, and international travelers should receive a second dose. Adults born before 1957 or with a positive titer are considered immune and do not need the vaccine. Should be spaced 4 wk apart from varicella vaccine.
Varicella, SC	All susceptible adults should be vaccinated, including people living in institutional settings and nonpregnant women of child-bearing age.
	Reliable proof of having had chickenpox, or positive titers can be an assumption of immunity.
Polio (IPV), IM or SC	Not recommended for adults ≥ 18 yr. Adults traveling to endemic areas with reported outbreaks may receive one booster dose.

Adapted from Advisory Committee on Immunization Practices (ACIP), October 2001

Schedule	Schedule for those fallen behind
October–November; any time during the flu season.	May be given any time during the flu season.
Usually a one-time dose. May be repeated in 5 yr for people in the highest risk group, or for people who received first dose at < 65 yr of age.	
Three-dose series. Must be 4 wk between first and second doses, and 5 mo between second and third doses.	If series is delayed, do not start over. Continue series from last dose.
Two-dose series. At least 6 mo between first and second doses.	If second dose is delayed, do not repeat first dose; give second dose when possible.
Booster every 10 yr; make sure the patient has received the three-dose primary series.	If no primary series has been given, give second dose 4 wk after first dose; give third dose 6–12 mo after second dose.
Second dose, if recommended, is given no sooner than 4 wk after first dose.	Second dose may be given as early as 4 wk after first dose if needed.
Two-dose series. Second dose should be given 4–8 wk after first dose.	Give second dose no sooner than 4 wk after first dose.
Should be given 4 wk apart from MMR. Should not be given to immunocompromised people.	

Therapeutic Class Combination Products

Commonly Prescribed Fixed-Combination Drugs: Dosages

AMPHETAMINES

▷ dextroamphetamine and amphetamine

C-II CONTROLLED SUBSTANCE

Adderall, Adderall XL

1.25 mg (5-mg tablet), 2.5 mg (10-mg tablet), 5 mg (20-mg tablet), or 7.5 mg (30-mg tablet) mg each of dextroamphetamine sulfate and saccharate, amphetamine aspartate, and sulfate; ER capsules with 2.5, 5, or 7.5 mg of each.
Usual adult dosage: 5 to 60 mg per day to control symptoms; ER capsules: 10 to 30 mg per day.

ANALGESICS

▷ acetaminophen and codeine

C-III CONTROLLED SUBSTANCE

Tylenol with Codeine

Elixir: 12 mg codeine; 120 mg acetaminophen
Tablets No. 2: 15 mg codeine, 300 mg acetaminophen
Tablets No. 3: 30 mg codeine, 300 mg acetaminophen
Tablets No. 4: 60 mg codeine, 300 mg acetaminophen
Usual adult dosage: 1 to 2 tablets q 4 to 6 hr as needed or 15 mL q 4 to 6 hr.

▷ aspirin and codeine

C-III CONTROLLED SUBSTANCE

Empirin with Codeine

Tablets No. 3: 30 mg codeine, 325 mg aspirin
Tablets No. 4: 60 mg codeine, 325 mg aspirin
Usual adult dosage: 1 to 2 tablets q 4 to 6 hr as needed.

C-III CONTROLLED SUBSTANCE

Fiorinal with Codeine

Capsules: 30 mg codeine, 325 mg aspirin, 40 mg caffeine, 50 mg butabarbital
Usual adult dosage: 1 to 2 capsules as needed for pain, up to 6 per day.

▷ diclofenac sodium and misoprostol

PREGNANCY CATEGORY X

Arthrotec

Tablets:
'50': 50 mg diclofenac, 200 mcg misoprostol
'75': 75 mg diclofenac, 200 mcg misoprostol
Usual adult dosage:
- *Osteoarthritis:* Arthrotec '50': PO tid; *Arthrotec* '50' or '75': PO bid.
- *Rheumatoid arthritis:* Arthrotec '50' PO tid or qid; *Arthrotec* '50' or '75' PO bid.

▷ hydrocodone bitartrate and acetaminophen

C-III CONTROLLED SUBSTANCE

Anexsia, Ceta-Plus, Co-Gesic, Duocet, Hydrocet, Hydrogesic, Lorcet Plus Tablets, Lortab Tablets, Margesic H, Norco, Panacet 5/500, Stagesic, Vicodin, Vicodin ES, Zydone

Capsules or tablets:
5 mg hydrocodone, 500 mg acetaminophen
7.5 mg hydrocodone, 650 mg acetaminophen
10 mg hydrocodone, 650 mg acetaminophen
Norco tablets:
5 mg hydrocodone, 325 mg acetaminophen
7.5 mg hydrocodone, 325 mg acetaminophen
10 mg hydrocodone, 325 mg acetaminophen
10 mg hydrocodone, 660 mg acetaminophen
Usual adult dosage: 1 to 2 tablets or capsules q 4 to 6 hr, up to 8 per day.

▷ hydrocodone and aspirin

C-III CONTROLLED SUBSTANCE

Alor 5/500, Azdone, Damason-P, Lortab ASA, Panasal 5/500

Tablets: 5 mg hydrocodone, 500 mg ASA
Usual adult dosage: 1 tablet q 4 to 6 hr as needed.

▷ hydrocodone and ibuprofen

C-III CONTROLLED SUBSTANCE

Vicoprofen

Tablets: 7.5 mg hydrocodone, 200 mg ibuprofen
Usual adult dosage: 1 tablet q 4 to 6 hr as needed.

▽ oxycodone and acetaminophen

C-II CONTROLLED SUBSTANCE

Percocet, Roxicet, Roxilox, Tylox

Tylox capsules: 5 mg oxycodone, 500 mg acetaminophen
Tablets: 5 mg oxycodone, 325 mg acetaminophen
Usual adult dosage: 1 to 2 tablets q 4 to 6 hr as needed.

▽ oxycodone and aspirin

C-II CONTROLLED SUBSTANCE

Percodan, Roxiprin

Tablets: 4.5 mg oxycodone, 325 mg aspirin
Usual adult dosage: 1 to 2 tablets q 6 hr as needed.

▽ tramadol hydrochloride and acetaminophen

Ultracet

Tablets: 37.5 mg tramadol, 325 mg acetaminophen
Usual adult dosage: 2 tablets PO q 4 to 6 hr as needed. Do not exceed 8 tablets per day. Reduce dosage with geriatric or renally impaired patients.

ANTIACNE DRUGS

▽ ethinyl estradiol and norethindrone

Estrostep

Tablets:
   1 mg norethindrone, 20 mcg ethinyl estradiol
   1 mg norethindrone, 30 mcg ethinyl estradiol
   1 mg norethindrone, 35 mcg ethinyl estradiol
Usual adult dosage: 1 tablet PO each day (21 tablets contain active ingredients and 7 are inert).
See also **norethindrone, estradiol.**

▽ norethindrone and ethinyl estradiol

Estrostep-21

Tablets:
   1 mg norethindrone, 20 mcg estradiol (5 tablets)
   1 mg norethindrone, 30 mcg estradiol (7 tablets)
   1 mg norethindrone, 35 mcg estradiol (9 tablets)
Usual adult dosage: 1 tablet PO per day in sequence.
See also **estradiol.**

▽norgestimate and estradiol

Ortho Tri-Cyclen tablets

Tablets:
    0.18 mg norgestimate, 35 mcg ethinyl estradiol (7 tablets)
    0.215 mg norgestimate, 35 mcg estradiol (7 tablets)
    0.25 mg norgestimate, 35 mcg estradiol (7 tablets)
Usual adult dosage: For women >15 yr: 1 tablet PO per day.
Birth control agent used cyclically.
See also **estradiol.**

ANTIBACTERIALS

▽amoxicillin and clavulanic acid

Augmentin, Augment ES-600

Tablets:
    '250': 250 mg amoxicillin, 125 mg clavulanic acid
    '500': 500 mg amoxicillin, 125 mg clavulanic acid
    '875': 875 mg amoxicillin, 125 mg clavulanic acid
Powder for oral suspension:
    '125' powder: 125 mg amoxicillin, 31.25 mg clavulanic acid
    '200' powder: 200 mg amoxicillin, 28.5 mg clavulanic acid
    '250' powder: 250 mg amoxicillin, 62.5 mg clavulanic acid
    '400' powder: 400 mg amoxicillin, 57 mg clavulanic acid
Solution (*Augmentin ES-600*):
    ES-600: 600 mg amoxicillin, 125 mg clavulanic acid
Chewable tablets:
    '125': 125 mg amoxicillin, 31.25 mg clavulanic acid
    '200': 200 mg amoxicillin, 28.5 mg clavulanic acid
    '250': 250 mg amoxicillin, 62.5 mg clavulanic acid
    '400': 400 mg amoxicillin, 57 mg clavulanic acid
Usual adult dosage: One 250-mg tablet or one 500-mg tablet q 8 hr. For severe infections: 875-mg tablet q 12 hr.
Usual pediatric dosage: In children weighing 40 kg: 20 to 40 mg amoxicillin/kg per day in divided doses q 8 hr (pediatric dosage is based on amoxicillin content) or q 12 hr; 90 mg/kg per day PO oral solution (*Augmentin ES-600*).
See also **amoxicillin.** Clavulanic acid protects amoxicillin from breakdown by bacterial beta-lactamase enzymes and is given only in combination with certain antibodies that are broken down by beta-lactamase.

▽carbapenem

Primaxin

Powder for injection (IV):
    250 mg imipenem and 250 mg cilastatin
    500 mg imipenem and 500 mg cilastatin

Powder for injection (IM):
   500 mg imipenem and 500 mg cilastatin
   750 mg imipenem and 750 mg cilastatin
- Follow manufacturer's instructions for reconstituting and diluting the drug.
- Administer each 250- to 500-mg dose by IV infusion over 20 to 30 min; infuse each 1-g dose over 40 to 60 min. Give 500 to 750 mg IM q 12 hr. Do not exceed 1,500 mg/day.
- Dosage recommendations represent the amount of imipenem to be given. Initial dose should be individualized on the basis of the type and severity of infection. Subsequent dosage is individualized on the basis of the severity of the patient's illness, the degree of susceptibility of the pathogens, and the patient's age, weight, and creatinine clearance. Dosage for adults with normal renal function ranges from 250 mg to 1 g q 6 to 8 hr. Dosage should not exceed 50 mg/kg per day or 4 g/day, whichever is less.
- Dosage for patients with renal impairment is based on creatinine clearance and weight. Consult manufacturer's guidelines.
- Imipenem is an antibiotic that inhibits cell wall synthesis in susceptible bacteria; cilastatin inhibits the renal enzyme that metabolizes imipenem; these drugs are commercially available only in the combined formulation.

▷ co-trimoxazole (TMP-SMZ)

Bactrim, Bactrim DS, Cotrim, Septra, Sulfatrim

Tablets:
   80 mg trimethoprim (TMP), 400 mg sulfamethoxazole (SMZ)
   160 mg trimethoprim, 800 mg sulfamethoxazole
Oral suspension:
   40 mg trimethoprim, 200 mg sulfamethoxazole per 5 mL
IV infusion:
   80 mg trimethoprim, 400 mg sulfamethoxazole per 5 mL
   80 mg/mL sulfamethoxazole, 16 mg/mL trimethoprim per 5 mL

Usual adult dosage:
- *Urinary tract infections, shigellosis, and acute otitis media:* 160 mg TMP and 800 mg sulfamethoxazole PO q 12 hr; 8 to 10 mg/kg per day (based on TMP component) in 2 to 4 divided doses of q 6, 8, or 12 hr IV. Treat for up to 14 days (urinary tract infection) or for 5 days (shigellosis).
- *Acute exacerbations of chronic bronchitis:* 160 mg TMP and 800 mg SMZ PO q 12 hr for 14 days.
- Pneumocystis carinii *pneumonitis*: 20 mg/kg TMP and 100 mg/kg SMZ q 24 hr PO in divided doses q 6 hr; 15 to 20 mg/kg per day (based on TMP component) in 3 to 4 divided doses q 6 to 8 hr IV. Treat for 14 days.
- *Traveler's diarrhea:* 160 mg TMP/800 mg SMZ q 12 hr for 5 days

Usual pediatric dosage:
- *Urinary tract infections, shigellosis, acute otitis media:* 8 mg/kg per day TMP and 40 mg/kg per day SMZ PO in 2 divided doses q 12 hr; 8 to 10 mg/kg per day (based on TMP component) in 2 to 4 divided doses q 6, 8, or 12 hr IV. Treat for 10 to 14 days (urinary tract infections and acute otitis media) or for 5 days (shigellosis).
- Pneumocystis carinii *pneumonitis:* 20 mg/kg TMP and 100 mg/kg SMZ q 24 hr PO in divided doses q 6 hr; 15 to 20 mg/kg per day (based on TMP component) in 3 to 4 divided doses q 6 to 8 hr IV. Treat for 14 days.

Impaired renal function:

Creatinine Clearance (mL/min)	Dosage
> 30	Use standard dosage.
15–30	Use 1/2 standard dosage.
< 15	Not recommended.

- Administer IV over 60 to 90 min. Thoroughly flush IV line after each use; do not refrigerate. IV solution must be diluted before use. See manufacturer's instructions. Do not give IM.

See also **trimethoprim**, **sulfamethoxazole.**

▽ erythromycin and sulfisoxazole

Eryzole, Pediazole

Granules for oral suspension: erythromycin ethylsuccinate (equivalent of 200 mg erythromycin activity) and 600 mg sulfisoxazole per 5 mL when reconstituted according to manufacturer's directions.

- Usual dosage for acute otitis media: 50 mg/kg per day erythromycin and 150 mg/kg per day sulfisoxazole in divided doses qid for 10 days.
- Administer without regard to meals.
- Refrigerate after reconstitution; use within 14 days.

See also **erythromycin, sulfisoxazole.**

▽ piperacillin sodium and tazobactam sodium

Zosyn

Tazobactam is a beta-lactamase inhibitor used in combination with the broad-spectrum penicillin.
Powder for injection:

    2 g piperacillin, 0.25 g tazobactam
    3 g piperacillin, 0.375 g tazobactam
    4 g piperacillin, 0.5 g tazobactam

Usual adult dosage: 12 g/1.5 g IV given as 3.375 g q 6 hr.

- Recommended for appendicitis, peritonitis, postpartum endometritis and PID, community-acquired pneumonia, nosocomial pneumonia if agent is responsive in sensitivity testing.
- Reduced dosage required for renal impairment or dialysis.
- Administer by IV infusion over 30 min. Reconstitute with 5 mL of suitable diluent per 1 g piperacillin. Discard after 24 hr.

See also **piperacillin.**

▽ quinupristin and dalfopristin

Synercid

New class of drugs available only as this combination product.
Streptogramin antibiotics: 500-mg/10-mL vial contains 150 mg quinupristin, 350 mg dalfopristin

- Treatment of life-threatening, susceptible infections associated with vancomycin-resistant *E. faecium* bacteremia (VREF), complicated skin infections due to *S. aureus, S. pyogenes.*
- Skin infections in patients >16 yr: 7.5 mg/kg IV q 12 hr for 7 days.
- VREF in patients >16 yr: 7.5 mg/kg IV q 8 hr.
- Dangerous when used with drugs that prolong the QTc interval.
- May cause pseudomembranous colitis.

▽ sulbactam and ampicillin

Unasyn

Powder for injection:
    1.5-g vial: 1 g ampicillin, 0.5 g sulbactam
    3-g vial: 2 g ampicillin, 1 g sulbactam
Usual adult dosage: 0.5 to 1 g sulbactam with 1 to 2 g ampicillin IM or IV q 6 to 8 hr.
Pediatric dosage:
    < 40 kg: 300 mg/kg per day IV in divided doses q 6 hr.
    ≥ 40 kg: adult dosage, do not exceed 4 g per day.
See also **ampicillin.** Sulbactam inhibits many bacterial penicillinase enzymes, thus broadening the spectrum of ampicillin; sulbactam is also weakly antibacterial alone.

▽ ticarcillin and clavulanic acid

Timentin

Powder for injection, solution for injection: 3.1-g vial (3 g ticarcillin, 0.1 g clavulanic acid)
• Administer by IV infusion over 30 min.
• Dosage for 60-kg adults: 3.1 g (3 g ticarcillin, 0.1 g clavulanic acid) q 4 to 6 hr. Dosage for adults < 60 kg: 200 to 300 mg ticarcillin/kg per day in divided doses q 4 to 6 hr.
• Urinary tract infections: 3.1 g (3 g ticarcillin, 0.1 g clavulanic acid) q 8 hr.
• Pediatric dosage in children ≥ 3 mo: 3.1 g (3 g ticarcillin, 0.1 g clavulanic acid) q 4 to 6 hr or 200 to 300 mg/kg per day in divided doses q 4 to 6 hr.
• Geriatric or renal failure patients: For patients on hemodialysis, give 2 g q 12 hr, supplemented with 3.1 g after each dialysis. For patients with renal impairment, give initial loading dose of 3.1 g, then as follows:

Creatinine Clearance (mL/min)	Dosage
> 60	3.1 g q 4 hr
30–60	2 g q 4 hr
10–30	2 g q 8 hr
< 10	2 g q 12 hr
< 10 with hepatic disease	2 g q 24 hr

• Continue treatment for 2 days after signs and symptoms of infection have disappeared. Usual duration of therapy is 10 to 14 days.
See also **ticarcillin.** Clavulanic acid protects ticarcillin from breakdown by bacterial beta-lactamase enzymes and is given only in combination with certain antibiotics that are broken down by beta-lactamase.

ANTIDEPRESSANTS

▽ chlordiazepoxide and amitriptyline

Limbitrol DS 10–25

Tablets:
    5 mg chlordiazepoxide, 12.5 mg amitriptyline
    10 mg chlordiazepoxide, 25 mg amitriptyline

Usual adult dosage: 10 mg chlordiazepoxide with 25 mg amitriptyline 3 to 4 times per day up to 6 times daily. For patients who do not tolerate the higher doses, 5 mg chlordiazepoxide with 12.5 mg amitriptyline 3 to 4 times per day. Reduce dosage after initial response.
See also **amitriptyline, chlordiazepoxide.**

▽ perphenazine and amitriptyline
Etrafon, Triavil

Tablets:
    2 mg perphenazine, 10 mg amitriptyline
    2 mg perphenazine, 25 mg amitriptyline
    4 mg perphenazine; 10 mg amitriptyline
    4 mg perphenazine, 25 mg amitriptyline
    4 mg perphenazine, 50 mg amitriptyline (*Triavil* only)
Usual adult dosage: 2 to 4 mg perphenazine with 10 to 50 mg amitriptyline 3 to 4 times daily. Reduce dosage after initial response.
See also **amitriptyline, perphenazine.**

ANTIDIABETIC DRUGS

▽ glyburide and metformin
Glucovance

Tablets:
    1.25 mg glyburide, 250 mg metformin
    2.5 mg glyburide, 500 mg metformin
    5 mg glyburide, 500 mg metformin
Usual adult dosage: 1 tablet daily PO, usually in the morning.
Not for initial therapy; drug should be adjusted using the individual products, switching to appropriate dosage of this combination product.

▽ glypizide and metformin
Metaglip

Tablets:
    2.5 mg glipizide, 250 mg metformin
    2.5 mg glipizide, 500 mg metformin
    5 mg glipizide, 500 mg metformin
Usual adult dosage: 1 tablet per day with a meal; adjust dose based on patient response. Do not exceed maximum dose of 20 mg glipizide with 2,000 mg metformin per day.
See also **glipizide, metformin.**

▽ rosiglitazone and metformin
Avandamet

Tablets:
    1 mg rosiglitazone, 500 mg metformin
    2 mg rosiglitazone, 500 mg metformin

4 mg rosiglitazone, 500 mg metformin

Usual adult dosage: 4 mg rosiglitazone with 500 mg metformin, once a day or in divided doses. Not for initial therapy; dosage should be adjusted using individual drugs alone and then switching to the appropriate dosage of the combination product. See package insert for details on adjusting dosage based on use of other agents and previous dosage levels.

See also **rosiglitazone, metformin.**

ANTIDIARRHEAL DRUG

▷diphenoxylate hydrochloride and atropine sulfate

C-V CONTROLLED SUBSTANCE

Logen, Lomanate, Lomotil, Lonox

Tablets: 2.5 mg diphenoxylate hydrochloride, 0.025 mg atropine sulfate
Liquid: 2.5 mg diphenoxylate hydrochloride, 0.025 mg atropine sulfate/5 mL
• Individualized dosage.
Usual adult dosage: 5 mg qid.
• Pediatric initial dosage (use only liquid in children 2–12 yr): 0.3 mg/kg daily in 4 divided doses.

Age	Weight	Dose	Frequency
2–5	13–20 kg	2 mg, 4 mL	3 times daily
5–8	20–27 kg	2 mg, 4 mL	4 times daily
8–12	27–36 kg	2 mg, 4 mL	5 times daily

• Reduce dosage as soon as initial control of symptoms is achieved. Maintenance dosage may be as low as one-fourth of the initial dosage.

See also **atropine sulfate.**

ANTIHYPERTENSIVES

▷atenolol and chlorthalidone

Tenoretic

Tablets: 50 or 100 mg atenolol with 25 mg chlorthalidone
Usual adult dosage: 1 tablet PO daily in the morning.
Drug should be adjusted using the individual products, then switched to appropriate dosage.
See also **atenolol, chlorthalidone.**

▷amlodipine and benazepril

Lotrel

Capsule:
    2.5 mg amlodipine, 10 mg benazepril
    5 mg amlodipine, 10 mg benazepril
    5 mg amlodipine, 20 mg benazepril
    10 mg amlodipine, 20 mg benazepril
Usual adult dosage: 1 tablet PO daily in the morning.

Monitor patient for hypertension and adverse effects closely over first 2 wk and regularly thereafter.
See also **amlodipine, benazepril.**

▷ bisoprolol and hydrochlorothiazide

Ziac

Tablets: 2.5, 5, or 10 mg bisoprolol and 6.25 mg hydrochlorothiazide
Usual adult dosage: 1 tablet per day PO in the morning. Initial dose is 2.5/6.25 mg tablet PO per day.
Dosage should be adjusted within 1 wk; optimal antihypertensive effect may require 2 to 3 wk.
See also **bisoprolol, hydrochlorothiazide.**

▷ candesartan and hydrochlorothiazide

Atacand HCT

Tablets:
   16 mg candesartan, 12.5 mg hydrochlorothiazide
   32 mg candesartan, 12.5 mg hydrochlorothiazide
Usual adult dosage: 1 tablet PO daily in the morning.
Drug should be adjusted using the individual products, then switched to appropriate dosage.
See also **candesartan, hydrochlorothiazide.**

▷ chlorthalidone and clonidine

Combipres

Tablets: 15 mg chlorthalidone with 0.1, 0.2, or 0.3 mg clonidine HCl
Usual adult dosage: 1 to 2 tablets per day PO in the morning.
Dosage should be adjusted with the individual products, switching to this combination product when patient's condition is stabilized on the dosage of each drug available in this combination.
See also **clonidine.**

▷ enalapril and diltiazem

Teczem Extended-Release Tablets

ER Tablets: 5 mg enalapril maleate, 180 mg diltiazem maleate
Usual adult dosage: 1 to 2 tablets per day PO taken in the morning.
Dosage should be adjusted with the individual products, switching to this combination product when the patient is stabilized on the dosage of each drug available in this combination. Ensure that patient swallows tablet whole. Do not cut, crush, or chew.
See also **enalapril, diltiazem.**

▷ enalapril and felodipine

Lexxel Extended-Release Tablets

ER Tablets: 5 mg enalapril, 2.5 or 5 mg felodipine

Usual adult dosage: 1 tablet per day PO.
Dosage should be adjusted with the individual products, switching to the combination product when the patient's condition is stabilized on the dosage of each drug that is available in this combination. Ensure that patient swallows tablet whole. Do not cut, crush, or chew.
See also **enalapril, felodipine.**

▷ enalapril and hydrochlorothiazide

Vaseretic

Tablets:
>10 mg enalapril maleate, 25 mg hydrochlorothiazide
5 mg enalapril maleate, 12.5 mg hydrochlorothiazide
Usual adult dosage: 1 to 2 tablets per day PO in the morning.
Dosage should be adjusted with individual products, switching to combination product after patient's condition is stabilized on the dosage of each drug that is available in this combination.
See also **enalapril maleate, hydrochlorothiazide.**

▷ eprosartan and hydrochlorothiazide

Teveten HCT

Tablets:
600 mg eprosartan, 12.5 mg hydrochlorothiazide
600 mg eprosartan, 25 mg hydrochlorothiazide
Usual adult dosage: 1 tablet PO each day. Dosage should be established with each component alone before using the combination product; if blood pressure is still not controlled, 300 mg eprosartan may be added each evening.
See also **eprosartan mesylate, hydrochlorothiazide.**

▷ fosinopril and hydrochlorothiazide

Monopril-HCT

Tablets:
10 mg fosinopril, 12.5 mg hydrochlorothiazide
20 mg fosinopril, 12.5 mg hydrochlorothiazide
Usual adult dosage: 1 tablet PO per day in the morning.
Drug should be adjusted using the individual products, switching to appropriate dosage of this combination product.
See also **fosinopril, hydrochlorothiazide.**

▷ hydrochlorothiazide and benazepril

Lotensin HCT

Tablets:
25 mg hydrochlorothiazide, 20 mg benazepril
12.5 mg hydrochlorothiazide, 20 mg benazepril
12.5 mg hydrochlorothiazide, 10 mg benazepril
6.25 mg hydrochlorothiazide, 5 mg benazepril

Usual adult dosage: 1 tablet per day PO in the morning.
Dosage should be adjusted with the individual products, switching to this combination product once the patient's condition is stabilized.
See also **hydrochlorothiazide, benazepril.**

▷ hydrochlorothiazide and captopril

Capozide

Tablets:
25 mg hydrochlorothiazide and 25 or 50 mg captopril
15 mg hydrochlorothiazide and 25 or 50 mg captopril
Usual adult dosage: 1 to 2 tablets PO daily, in the morning.
Dosage should be adjusted with individual products, switching to this combination product when patient's condition is stabilized on the dosage of each drug available in this combination
See also **hydrochlorothiazide, captopril.**

▷ hydrochlorothiazide and propranolol

Inderide

Tablets: 25 mg hydrochlorothiazide with 40 or 80 mg propranolol HCl
Usual adult dosage: 1 to 2 tablets bid.
Dosage should be adjusted with individual products, switching to combination product when patient's condition is stabilized on the dosage of each drug available in this combination.
See also **hydrochlorothiazide, propranolol.**

▷ irbesartan and hydrochlorothiazide

Avalide

Tablets:
150 mg irbesartan, 12.5 mg hydrochlorothiazide
300 mg irbesartan, 12.5 mg hydrochlorothiazide
Usual adult dosage: 1 to 2 tablets per day PO.
Dosage should be adjusted with individual products, switching to combination product when patient's condition is stabilized.
See also **irbesartan, hydrochlorothiazide.**

▷ lisinopril and hydrochlorothiazide

Prinzide, Zestoretic

Tablets:
10 mg lisinopril, 12.5 mg hydrochlorothiazide
20 mg lisinopril, 12.5 mg hydrochlorothiazide
20 mg lisinopril, 25 mg hydrochlorothiazide
Usual adult dosage: 1 tablet per day PO taken in the morning.
Dosage should be adjusted with individual products, switching to combination product when patient's condition is stabilized.
See also **lisinopril, hydrochlorothiazide.**

▷ losartan and hydrochlorothiazide
Hyzaar

Tablets:
   50 mg losartan, 12.5 mg hydrochlorothiazide
   100 mg losartan, 25 mg hydrochlorothiazide
Usual adult dosage: 1 tablet per day PO in the morning.
Not for initial therapy; start using each component and if desired effects are obtained, *Hyzaar* may be used.
See also **losartan, hydrochlorothiazide.**

▷ methyldopa and chlorothiazide
Aldoclor

Tablets: 250 mg methyldopa with 150 or 250 mg chlorothiazide
Usual adult dosage: 1 tablet PO per day taken in the morning.
Drug should be adjusted using the individual products, switching to appropriate dosage of this combination product.
See also **methyldopa, chlorothiazide.**

▷ methyldopa and hydrochlorothiazide
Aldoril D

Tablets: 500 mg methyldopa with 30 or 50 mg hydrochlorothiazide; 250 mg methyldopa with 25 mg hydrochlorothiazide; 250 mg methyldopa with 15 mg hydrochlorothiazide
Usual adult dosage: 1 tablet PO daily, in the morning.
Drug should be adjusted using the individual products, switching to appropriate dosage of this combination product.
See also **methyldopa, hydrochlorothiazide**.

▷ metoprolol and hydrochlorothiazide
Lopressor HCT

Tablets: 50 mg metoprolol with 25 mg hydrochlorothiazide; 100 mg metoprolol with 25 or 50 mg hydrochlorothiazide
Usual adult dosage: 1 tablet PO per day.
Drug should be adjusted using the individual products, switching to appropriate dosage of this combination product.
See also **metoprolol, hydrochlorothiazide.**

▷ moexipril and hydrochlorothiazide
Uniretic

Tablets:
   7.5 mg moexipril, 12.5 mg hydrochlorothiazide
   15 mg moexipril, 25 mg hydrochlorothiazide

Usual adult dosage: 1 to 2 tablets per day 1 hr before or 2 hr after a meal.
Not for initial therapy. Adjust dose to maintain appropriate BP.
See also **moexipril, hydrochlorothiazide.**

nadolol and bendroflumethiazide
Corzide

Tablets: 40 or 80 mg nadolol with 5 mg bendroflumethiazide
Usual adult dosage: 1 tablet PO per day in the morning.
Drug should be adjusted using the individual products, switching to appropriate dosage of this combination product.
See also **nadolol, bendroflumethiazide.**

prazosin and polythiazide
Minizide

Tablets: 0.5 mg polythiazide with 1, 2, or 5 mg prazosin
Usual adult dosage: 1 capsule PO bid to tid.
Drug should be adjusted using the individual products, switching to appropriate dosage of this combination product.
See also **prazosin, polythiazide.**

quinapril and hydrochlorothiazide
Accuretic

Tablets: 10 or 20 mg quinapril, 12.5 mg hydrochlorothiazide
Usual adult dosage: 1 tablet PO per day in the morning.
Drug should be adjusted using the individual products, switching to appropriate dosage of this combination product.
See also **quinapril, hydrochlorothiazide.**

telmisartan and hydrochlorothiazide
Micardis HCT

Tablets:
    40 mg telmisartan, 12.5 mg hydrochlorothiazide
    80 mg telmisartan, 12.5 mg hydrochlorothiazide
Usual adult dosage: 1 tablet PO per day; may be adjusted up to 160 mg telmisartan and 25 mg hydrochlorothiazide, based on patient's response.
See also **telmisartan, hydrochlorothiazide.**

trandolapril and verapamil
Tarka

Tablets:
    1 mg trandolapril, 240 mg verapamil
    2 mg trandolapril, 180 mg verapamil

4 mg trandolapril, 240 mg verapamil
Usual adult dosage: 1 tablet PO per day.
Take with food.
Dosage should be adjusted with the individual products, switching to this combination product when the patient's condition is stabilized on the dosage of each drug available in combination. Ensure that patient swallows tablet whole. Do not cut, crush, or chew.
See also **trandolapril, verapamil.**

▽ valsartan and hydrochlorothiazide

Diovan HCT

Tablets:
80 mg valsartan, 12.5 mg hydrochlorothiazide
160 mg valsartan, 12.5 mg hydrochlorothiazide
Usual adult dosage: 1 tablet per day PO.
Not for initial therapy; start using each component first.
See also **valsartan, hydrochlorothiazide.**

ANTIMIGRAINE DRUGS

▽ ergotamine and caffeine

Cafergot, Cafatine-PB, Ercaf, Wigraine

Tablets: 1 mg ergotamine tartrate, 100 mg caffeine
Usual adult dosage: 2 tablets at first sign of attack. Follow with 1 tablet every 30 minutes, if needed. Maximum dose is 6 tablets per attack. Do not exceed 10 tablets per week.
Suppositories: 2 mg ergotamine tartrate, 100 mg caffeine
Usual adult dosage: 1 at first sign of attack; follow with second dose after 1 hr, if needed. Maximum dose is 2 per attack. Do not exceed 5 per week.
Do not combine this drug with ritonavir, nelfinavir, indinavir, erythromycin, clarithromycin, or troleandomycin—serious vasospasm events could occur.
See also **ergotamine.**

ANTIPARKINSONISM DRUGS

▽ levodopa and carbidopa

Sinemet, Sinemet CR

Tablets:
10 mg carbidopa, 100 mg levodopa
25 mg carbidopa, 100 mg levodopa
25 mg carbidopa, 250 mg levodopa
Controlled release:
25 mg carbidopa, 100 mg levodopa
50 mg carbidopa, 200 mg levodopa
Usual adult dosage: Starting dose for patients not presently receiving levodopa: 1 tablet of 10 mg carbidopa/100 mg levodopa or 25 mg carbidopa/100 mg levodopa tid. For patients receiving levodopa: start combination therapy with the morning dose at least 8 hr after the last dose of levodopa and choose a daily dosage of carbidopa and levodopa that will provide 25% of the pre-

vious levodopa daily dose. Dosage must be adjusted based on the patient's clinical response. See manufacturer's directions for adjusting the combination and single-agent drugs.

Carbidopa is available alone only by a specific request to the manufacturer from physicians who have a patient who needs a different dosage of carbidopa than is provided by the fixed combination drug; carbidopa is a peripheral inhibitor of dopa decarboxylase, an enzyme that converts dopa to dopamine, which cannot penetrate the CNS. The addition of carbidopa to the levodopa regimen reduces the dose of levodopa needed and decreases the incidence of certain adverse reactions to levodopa.

See also **levodopa.**

ANTIPLATELET DRUGS

▷ **aspirin and dipyridamole**

Aggrenox

Capsules: 25 mg aspirin, 200 mg dipyridamole
Usual adult dosage: 1 capsule PO daily to decrease risk of stroke in patients with known cerebrovascular disease.

ANTIULCER DRUGS

▷ **bismuth subsalicylate, metronidazole, and tetracycline**

Helidac

Tablets: 262.4 mg bismuth subsalicylate, 250 mg metronidazole, 500 mg tetracycline HCl
Usual adult dosage: 1 tablet PO qid for 14 days along with a prescribed H_2 antagonist. Indicated for the treatment of active duodenal ulcers associated with *Helicobacter pylori* infection.

See also **bismuth subsalicylate, metronidazole, tetracycline.**

▷ **lansoprazole, amoxicillin, and clarithromycin**

Prevpac

Daily administration pack: two 30-mg lansoprazole capsules, four 500-mg amoxicillin capsules, and two 500-mg clarithromycin tablets.
Usual adult dosage: Divide pack equally to take twice daily, morning and evening.

▷ **ranitidine, trivalent bismuth, and citrate**

Tritec (ranitidine bismuth citrate)

Tablets: 162 mg ranitidine, 128 mg trivalent bismuth, 110 mg citrate
Usual adult dosage: 400 mg PO bid for 4 wk in combination with clarithromycin, 500 mg PO bid or tid for the first 2 wk.
Indicated for the treatment of active duodenal ulcers associated with *Helicobacter pylori* infection.

See also **ranitidine.**

ANTIVIRAL DRUGS

▷ abacavir, zidovudine, and lamivudine
Trizivir

Tablets: 300 mg abacavir, 300 mg zidovudine, 150 mg lamivudine
Usual adult dosage: 1 tablet PO bid.
Carefully monitor patient for hypersensitivity reactions.
See also **lamivudine.**

▷ lamivudine and zidovudine
Combivir

Tablets: 150 mg lamivudine, 300 mg zidovudine
Usual adult dose: 1 tablet PO twice daily.
Not recommended for children or adults weighing < 50 kg.
May be taken with food.
Does not decrease risk of spreading infections; use caution.
See also **lamivudine, zidovudine.**

▷ ribavirin and interferon alfa-2b
Rebetron

Capsules: 200 mg ribavirin
Injection: 3 million IU interferon alfa-2b
Usual adult dosage: 400 mg ribavirin per day PO in the morning and 600 mg per day PO in the evening with 3 million IU interferon alfa-2b SC 3 times per week for patients weighing < 75 kg; 600 mg ribavirin per day PO in the morning, 600 mg per day PO in evening with 3 million IU interferon alfa-2b SC 3 times per week for patients weighing > 75 kg.
For treatment of chronic hepatitis C in patients who relapse after interferon alfa therapy.
See also **ribavirin, interferon alfa-2b.**

DIURETICS

▷ amiloride and hydrochlorothiazide
Moduretic

Tablets: 5 mg amiloride, 50 mg hydrochlorothiazide
Usual adult dosage: 1 to 2 tablets per day with meals.
See also **amiloride, hydrochlorothiazide.**

▷ hydrochlorothiazide and triamterene
Dyazide

Capsules: 37.5 mg triamterene, 25 mg hydrochlorothiazide
Usual adult dosage: 1 tablet per day or bid after meals.

See also **hydrochlorothiazide**, **triamterene**.

Maxzide

Tablets: 75 mg triamterene, 50 mg hydrochlorothiazide
Usual adult dosage: 1 tablet per day.
Also see **hydrochlorothiazide**, **triamterene**

▷ spironolactone and hydrochlorothiazide
Aldactazide

Tablets: 25 mg spironolactone, 25 mg hydrochlorothiazide
Usual adult dosage: 1 to 8 tablets daily.
Tablets: 50 mg spironolactone, 50 mg hydrochlorothiazide
Usual adult dosage: 1 to 4 tablets daily.
Also see **hydrochlorothiazide, spironolactone.**

HORMONAL CONTRACEPTIVES

For a list of hormonal contraceptives by trade name, see Appendix F, pp. 1299–1302.

Usual dosage for oral contraceptives: Take 1 tablet PO daily for 21 days, beginning on day 5 of the cycle (day 1 of the cycle is the first day of menstrual bleeding). Inert tablets or no tablets are taken for the next 7 days. Then start a new course of 21 days.
Suggested measures for missed doses of oral contraceptives:
One tablet missed: take tablet as soon as possible, or take 2 tablets the next day.
Two consecutive tablets missed: take 2 tablets daily for the next 2 days, then resume the regular schedule.
Three consecutive tablets missed: begin a new cycle of tablets 7 days after the last tablet was taken; use an additional method of birth control until the start of the next menstrual period.
Postcoital contraception ("morning after" pills): Safe and effective for emergency contraception. Dosing regimen starts within 72 hr of unprotected intercourse with a follow-up dose of the same number of pills 12 hr after the first dose.
Ovral: 2 white tablets
Nordette: 4 light orange tablets
Lo/Ovral: 4 white tablets
Triphasil: 4 yellow tablets
Levlen: 4 light orange tablets
Tri-Levlin: 4 yellow tablets
Preven: postcoital contraceptive kit—includes pregnancy kit, used first to assure no pregnancy; four tablets containing 0.25 mg levonorgestrel and 0.05 mg ethinyl estradiol: two pills taken within 72 hr of intercourse, 2 taken 12 hr later.
Plan B: 0.75 mg levonorgestrel; take 1 tablet within 72 hr of sexual intercourse, take the second tablet 12 hr later.

LIPID-LOWERING DRUGS

▷ niacin and lovastatin
Advicor

Tablets: 500, 750, or 1,000 mg niacin, 20 mg lovastatin
Usual adult dosage: 1 tablet daily at night.
Also see **niacin**, **lovastatin.**

MENOPAUSE DRUGS

▷ estradiol and norgestimate
Ortho-Prefest

Tablets: 1 mg estradiol, 0.09 mg norgestimate
Usual adult dosage: 1 tablet per day PO (3 days of pink tablets: estradiol alone; followed by 3 days of white tablets: estradiol and norgestimate combination; continue cycle uninterrupted).
Treatment of moderate to severe symptoms of menopause and prevention of osteoporosis in women with intact uterus.

▷ ethinyl estradiol and norethindrone acetate
femhrt 1/5

Tablets: 5 mcg ethinyl estradiol, 1 mg norethindrone acetate
Usual adult dosage: 1 tablet per day PO.
Treatment of signs and symptoms of menopause and prevention of osteoporosis in women with intact uterus.

▷ estrogens and medroxyprogesterone
Premphase

Tablets: 0.625 mg conjugated estrogens, 5 mg medroxyprogesterone
Usual adult dosage: 1 tablet per day PO.
Treatment of moderate to severe symptoms of menopause and prevention of osteoporosis in women with intact uterus.
See also **estrogen, medroxyprogesterone.**

▷ estrogen, medroxyprogesterone, and conjugated estrogens
Prempro

Tablets: 0.625 mg estrogen, 2.5 mg medroxyprogesterone; 0.625 mg conjugated estrogen; 5 mg medroxyprogesterone
Usual adult dosage: 1 tablet per day PO.
For relief of symptoms of menopause and prevention of osteoporosis in women with intact uterus.
See also **estrogen.**

▽estrogen and norethindrone
CombiPatch

Patch: 0.05 mg per day estradiol, 0.14 mg per day norethindrone or 0.25 mg per day norethindrone
Usual adult dosage: Change patch twice a week.
For relief of symptoms of menopause.
See also **estrogens.**

NARCOTIC AGONIST

▽buprenorphine and naloxone

C-III CONTROLLED SUBSTANCE

Suboxone

Sublingual tablets: 2 mg buprenorphine with 0.5 mg naloxone, or 8 mg buprenorphine with 2 mg naloxone
Usual adult dosage: 12–16 mg sublingually once each day following induction with sublingual buprenorphine for treatment of opioid dependence.
See also **buprenorphine, naloxone.**

RESPIRATORY DRUGS

▽azatadine and pseudoephedrine
Trinalin Repetabs

Tablets: 1 mg azatadine maleate and 120 mg pseudoephedrine sulfate
Usual adult dosage: 1 tablet q 12 hr for relief of upper respiratory symptoms of colds, allergies.
See also **pseudoephedrine. Azatadine** is an antihistamine.

▽fluticasone and salmeterol
Advair Diskus

Inhalation: 100, 250, or 500 mcg fluticasone with 50 mcg salmeterol
Usual dosage in patients ≥ 12 yr: one inhalation bid to manage asthma.
See also **fluticasone, salmeterol.**

▽ipratropium and albuterol
Combivent

Metered dose inhaler: 18 mcg ipratropium bromide, 90 mcg albuterol
Usual adult dosage: 2 inhalations 4 times per day
Not for use during acute attack.
Use caution with known sensitivity to atropine, soy beans, joya lecithin, peanuts.

Treatment of bronchospasm with COPD in patients who require more than a single bronchodilator. See also **ipratropium, albuterol.**

▽loratadine and pseudoephedrine
Claritin-D

ER Tablets: 5 mg loratadine, 120 mg pseudoephedrine
Usual adult dosage: 1 tablet every 12 hr.
See also **loratadine, pseudoephedrine.**

Claritin-D 24 Hour

ER Tablets: 10 mg loratadine, 240 mg pseudoephedrine
Usual adult dosage: 1 tablet every day.
See also **loratadine, pseudoephedrine**

TENSION HEADACHE DRUGS

▽butalbital, acetaminophen and caffeine
Esgic-Plus

Capsules: 50 mg butalbital, 500 mg acetaminophen, 40 mg caffeine
Usual adult dosage: 1 capsule q 4 hr as needed, up to 6 per day. May be habit-forming; avoid driving and dangerous tasks.
See also **acetaminophen, caffeine.**

APPENDIX F

Hormonal Contraceptives

Oral contraceptives

Trade name	Combination
Monophasic	
Alesse, Aviane	20 mcg estradiol and 0.10 mg levonorgestrel
Brevicon, Modicon	35 mcg ethinyl estradiol (estrogen) and 0.5 mg norethindrone (progestin)
Demulen 1/50, Zovia 1/50E	50 mcg ethinyl estradiol (estrogen) and 1 mg ethynodiol diacetate (progestin)
Demulen 1/35, Zovia 1/35E	35 mcg ethinyl estradiol (estrogen) and 1 mg ethynodiol diacetate (progestin)
Apri, Desogen, Ortho-Cept	30 mcg ethinyl estradiol and 0.15 mg desogestrel
Levlen, Levora 0.15/30, Nordette	30 mcg ethinyl estradiol (estrogen) and 0.15 mg levonorgestrel (progestin)
Levlite	0.10 mg levonorgestrel and 0.02 mg ethinyl estradiol
Loestrin 21 1.5/30, Microgestin Fe 1.5/30	30 mcg ethinyl estradiol (estrogen) and 1.5 mg norethindrone acetate (progestin)
Loestrin 21 1/20, Microgestin Fe 1/20	20 mcg ethinyl estradiol (estrogen) and 1 mg norethindrone (progestin)
Lo/Ovral, Low-Ogestrel	30 mcg ethinyl estradiol (estrogen) and 0.3 mg norgestrel
Necon 1/50, Norinyl 1 + 50	50 mcg mestranol (estrogen) and 1 mg norethindrone (progestin)
Necon 1/35, Norinyl 1 + 35, Ortho-Novum 1/35	35 mcg ethinyl estradiol (estrogen) and 1 mg norethindrone (progestin)
Ortho-Cyclen, Sprintec	35 mcg ethinyl estradiol (estrogen) and 0.25 mg norgestimate (progestin)
Ortho-Novum 1/50, Ovcon-50	50 mcg ethinyl estradiol (estrogen) and 1 mg norethindrone acetate (progestin)
Ovcon-35	35 mcg ethinyl estradiol (estrogen) and 0.4 mg norethindrone (progestin)
Ovral-28, Ogestrel	50 mcg ethinyl estradiol (estrogen) and 0.5 mg norgestrel (progestin)
Yasmin	3 mg drospirenone (progestin) and 30 mcg ethinyl estradiol (estrogen)

(continued)

Trade name	Combination
Biphasic	
Jenest-28	phase 1—10 tablets: 0.5 mg norethindrone (progestin) and 35 mcg ethinyl estradiol (estrogen);
	phase 2—11 tablets: 1 mg norethindrone (progestin) and 35 mcg ethinyl estradiol (estrogen)
Necon 10/11, Ortho-Novum 10/11	phase 1—10 tablets: 0.5 mg norethindrone and 35 mcg ethinyl estradiol;
	phase 2—11 tablets: 1 mg norethindrone and 35 mcg ethinyl estradiol
Mircette	phase 1—21 tablets: 0.15 mg desogesinel and 20 mcg ethinyl estradiol;
	phase 2—5 tablets: 0.01 mg ethinyl estradiol
Tri-phasic	
Cyclessa	phase 1—7 tablets, 0.1 mg desogestrel, 25 mcg ethinyl estradiol;
	phase 2—7 tablets, 0.125 mg desogestrel, 25 mcg ethinyl estradiol;
	phase 3—7 tablets, 0.15 mg desogestrel, 25 mcg ethinyl estradiol
Estrostep 21, Estrostep Fe	phase 1—5 tablets, 1 mg norethindrone and 20 mcg ethinyl estradiol;
	phase 2—7 tablets, 1 mg norethindrone and 30 mcg ethinyl estradiol;
	phase 3—9 tablets, 1 mg norethindrone and 35 mcg ethinyl estradiol
Ortho-Novum 7/7/7, Nortel 7/7/7	phase 1—7 tablets, 0.5 mg norethindrone (progestin) and 35 mcg ethinyl estradiol (estrogen);
	phase 2—7 tablets, 0.75 mg norethindrone (progestin) and 35 mcg ethinyl estradiol (estrogen);
	phase 3—7 tablets, 1 mg norethindrone (progestin) and 35 mcg ethinyl estradiol (estrogen)
Ortho Tri-Cyclen	phase 1—7 tablets, 0.18 mg norgestimate and 35 mcg ethinyl estradiol;
	phase 2—7 tablets, 0.215 mg norgestimate and 35 mcg ethinyl estradiol;
	phase 3—7 tablets, 0.25 mg norgestimate and 35 mcg ethinyl estradiol

Trade name	Combination
Tri-phasic (continued)	
Ortho Tri-Cyclen Lo	phase 1—7 tablets, 0.18 mg norgestimate and 25 mcg ethinyl estradiol;
	phase 2—7 tablets, 0.215 mg norgestimate and 25 mcg ethinyl estradiol;
	phase 3—7 tablets, 0.25 mg norgestimate and 25 mcg ethinyl estradiol
Enpresse, Tri-Levlen, Triphasil, Portia	phase 1—6 tablets, 0.05 mg levonorgestrel (progestin) and 30 mcg ethinyl estradiol (estrogen);
	phase 2—5 tablets, 0.075 mg levonorgestrel (progestin) and 40 mcg ethinyl estradiol (estrogen);
	phase 3—10 tablets, 0.125 mg levonorgestrel (progestin) and 30 mcg ethinyl estradiol (estrogen)
Tri-Norinyl	phase 1—7 tablets, 0.5 mg norethindrone (progestin) and 35 mcg ethinyl estradiol (estrogen);
	phase 2—9 tablets, 1 mg norethindrone (progestin) and 35 mcg ethinyl estradiol (estrogen);
	phase 3—5 tablets, 0.5 mg norethindrone (progestin) and 35 mcg ethinyl estradiol (estrogen)
Trivora-28	phase 1—6 tablets, 0.5 mg levonorgestrel (progestin) and 30 mcg ethinyl estradiol (estrogen);
	phase 2—5 tablets, 0.075 mg levonorgestrel (progestin) and 40 mcg ethinyl estradiol (estrogen);
	phase 3—10 tablets, 0.125 mg levonorgestrel (progestin) and 30 mcg ethinyl estradiol (estrogen)

Injectable Contraceptives

Trade name	Combination
Lunelle	5 mg estradiol (estrogen), 25 mg medroxyprogesterone (progestin)/0.5 mL; give 0.5 mL IM within first 5 days of menstrual period, then 0.5 mL IM q 28 to 30 days
Depo-Provera	150 mg medroxyprogesterone Give 1-mL injection deep IM, repeated every 3 mo.

(continued)

Vaginal Ring

Trade name	Combination
NuvaRing	0.12 mg etonogestrel (progestin), 0.015 mg ethinyl estradiol (estrogen) per day; insert ring into vagina on or before the 5th day of menstrual period; remove after 3 wk. Insert new ring after 1-wk rest.

Transdermal System

Trade name	Combination
Ortho Evra	6 mg norelgestromin, 0.75 ethinyl estradiol in a patch form, which releases 150 mcg norelgestromin and 20 mcg ethinyl estradiol each 24 hr for 1 wk. Patch is applied on the same day of the wk for 3 consecutive wk, followed by a patch-free week.

Levonorgestrel Implants

Trade name	Combination
Norplant System	6 capsules containing 36 mg levonorgestrel implanted within first 7 days of start of menses. Provides contraception for 5 yr, at which time capsules need to be removed.

Intrauterine Systems

Trade name	Combination
Progestasert	38 mg progesterone inserted into the uterus, replaced each year.
Mirena	52 mg levonorgestrel inserted into the uterus for up to 5 yr.

Frequently Used Combination Products by Trade Name

Many products are available on the market in combination form. Many of these are OTC preparations used frequently by consumers. It is helpful to have a guide to the ingredients of these products when instructing patients or assessing for drug interactions. The following is a list of brand names, active ingredients, and common usage. Nursing process information can be checked by looking up the active ingredient.

Trade name	Active ingredients	Common usage
Accuretic	quinapril, hydrochlorothiazide	Antihypertensive
Actifed Cold & Allergy	pseudoephedrine, triprolidine	Decongestant
Actifed Cold & Sinus Maximum Strength	pseudoephedrine, chlorpheniramine, acetaminophen	Decongestant
Adderall	dextroamphetamine sulfate and saccharate, amphetamine aspartate and sulfate	Amphetamine
Adderall XL	dextroamphetamine sulfate and saccharate, amphetamine aspartate, and sulfate	Treatment of ADHA
Advair Diskus	fluticasone, salmeterol	Antiasthmatic
Advicor	niacin, lovastatin	Antihyperlipidemic
Advil Cold and Sinus	ibuprofen, pseudoephedrine	Decongestant
Advil Flu & Body Ache	ibuprofen, pseudoephedrine	Decongestant, analgesic
Aggrenox	aspirin, dipyridamole	Stroke prevention
Aldactazide	spironolactone, hydrochlorothiazide	Diuretic
Aldoclor	methyldopa, chlorothiazide	Antihypertensive
Aldoril D	methyldopa, hydrochlorothiazide	Antihypertensive
Alka-Seltzer Plus Cold & Flu Medicine	pseudoephedrine, dextromethorphan, acetaminophen	Decongestant, analgesic
Alka-Seltzer Plus Cold and Cough	chlorpheniramine, dextromethorphan, phenylephrine	Decongestant, antihistamine, antitussive, analgesic
Alka-Seltzer Plus Flu Medicine	dextromethorphan, chlorpheniramine, aspirin	Antitussive, analgesic, decongestant
Allegra-D	pseudophedrine, fexofenadine	Decongestant, antihistamine

(continued)

Trade name	Active ingredients	Common usage
Allerest Maximum Strength	pseudoephedrine, chlorpheniramine	Decongestant, antihistamine
Alor 5/500	hydrocodone, aspirin	Analgesic
Anacin	aspirin, caffeine	Analgesic
Anacin Aspirin Free	diphenhydramine, acetaminophen	Analgesic
Anexsia	hydrocodone, acetaminophen	Analgesic
Antrocol	atropine, phenobarbital	Sedative, GI anticholinergic
Apresazide	hydralazine, hydrochlorothiazide	Antihypertensive
Apri	ethinyl estradiol, desogestrel	Oral contraceptive
Atacand HCT	candesartan, hydrochlorothiazide	Antihypertensive
Augmentin	amoxicillin, clavulanic acid	Antibiotic
Augmentin ES-600	amoxicillin, clavulanic acid	Antibiotic
Avalide	irbesartan, hydrochlorothiazide	Antihypertensive
Avandamet	rosiglitazone, metformin	Antidiabetic
Aviane	estradiol, levonorgestrel	Oral contraceptive
Azdone	hydrocodone, aspirin	Analgesic
Bactrim	trimethoprim, sulfamethoxazole	Antibiotic
Bayer Plus Extra Strength	aspirin, calcium carbonate	Analgesic
Bayer Select Maximum Strength Backache	magnesium tetrahydrate, aspirin	Analgesic
Bayer Select Maximum Strength Night Time Pain Relief	acetaminophen, diphenhydramine	Analgesic
Bellergal-S	belladonna, phenobarbital, ergotamine	GI anticholinergic, sedative
Benadryl Allergy & Sinus	diphenhydramine, pseudoephedrine, acetaminophen	Decongestant
Benylin Decongestant	diphenhydramine, pseudoephedrine	Decongestant
Bromfed	brompheniramine, pseudoephedrine	Decongestant, antihistamine
Bromo Seltzer	acetaminophen, sodium bicarbonate, citric acid	Analgesic, antacid

Trade name	Active ingredients	Common usage
Bronkaid Dual Action	theophylline, ephedrine, guaifenesin	Antiasthmatic
Bufferin	aspirin, magnesium carbonate, calcium carbonate, magnesium oxide	Analgesic, antacid
Bufferin AF Nite Time	diphenhydramine, acetaminophen	Decongestant, analgesic
Cafatine-PB	ergotamine, caffeine	Antimigraine
Cafergot	ergotamine, caffeine	Antimigraine
Capozide	captopril, hydrochlorothiazide	Antihypertensive
Ceta-Plus	hydrocodone, acetaminophen	Analgesic
Cheracol Plus	codeine, guaifenesin, alcohol	Antitussive, expectorant
Chlor-Trimeton Allergy-D 4-Hr	pseudoephedrine, chlorpheniramine	Antihistamine, decongestant
Chlor-Trimeton Allergy-D 12-H	pseudoephedrine, chlorpheniramine	Antihistamine, decongestant
Claritin-D 12 Hour	loratadine, pseudoephedrine	Decongestant, antihistamine
Claritin-D 24 Hour	loratadine, pseudoephedrine	Decongestant, antihistamine
Codimal DH	phenylephrine, pyrilamine, hydrocodone	Antitussive
Codimal PH	codeine, pyrilamine, phenylephrine	Antitussive, antihistamine, decongestant
Co-Gesic	hydrocodone, acetaminophen	Analgesic
CombiPatch	estrogen, norethindrone	Menopause drug
Combipres	chlorthalidone, clonidine	Antihypertensive
Combivent	ipratropium, albuterol	Asthma drug
Combivir	lamivudine, zidovudine	Antiviral
Comtrex Acute Head Cold & Sinus Pressure Relief	pseudoephedrine, brompheniramine, acetaminophen	Antihistamine, decongestant, analgesic
Comtrex Cough & Cold Relief	pseudoephedrine, dextromethorphan, chlorpheniramine, acetaminophen	Decongestant, antitussive, analgesic
Contac 12 Hour Day & Night	pseudoephedrine, diphenhydramine, acetaminophen	Decongestant, antihistamine

(continued)

Trade name	Active ingredients	Common usage
Contac Severe Cold Plus Flu Maximum	pseudoephedrine, chlorpheniramine, dextromethorphan, acetaminophen	Antihistamine, decongestant
COPE	aspirin, caffeine, magnesium hydroxide, aluminum hydroxide	Analgesic, antacid
Coricidin "D" Cold, Flu & Sinus	chlorpheniramine, acetaminophen, pseudoephedrine	Antihistamine, decongestant, analgesic
Coricidin HBP Cold & Flu Tablets	chlorpheniramine, acetaminophen	Antihistamine, analgesic
Corzide	nadolol, bendroflumethiazide	Antihypertensive
Cosamin DS	glucosamine, chondroitin sulfate, manganese ascorbate	Antiarthritis
Cotrim	trimethoprim, sulfamethoxazole	Antibiotic
Cyclessa	desogestrel, ethinyl estradiols	Oral contraceptive
Cyclomydril	cyclopentolate, phenylephrine	Ophthalmic
Cylex	methenamine, sodium salicylate, benzoic acid	Urinary anti-infective
Damason-P	hydrocodone, aspirin	Analgesic
Deconamine	pseudoephedrine, chlorpheniramine	Antihistamine, decongestant
Dermoplast	benzocaine, menthol, methyl-paraben	Local anesthetic
Di Gel	magnesium hydroxide, aluminum hydroxide, magnesium carbonate, simethicone	Local anesthetic, antacid
Dilaudid Cough Syrup	hydromorphone, guaifenesin	Antitussive
Dimetapp	brompheniramine, pseudoephedrine	Antihistamine, decongestant
Dimetapp Cold & Allergy	pseudoephedrine, brompheniramine	Antihistamine, decongestant
Diovan HCT	valsartan, hydrochlorothiazide	Antihypertensive
Doxidan	docusate, phenolphthalein	Laxative
Dristan Cold Multi-Symptom	phenylephrine, chlorpheniramine, acetaminophen	Antihistamine, decongestant
Dristan Sinus Tablets	pseudoephedrine, ibuprofen	Decongestant, analgesic
Drixoral Allergy Sinus	pseudoephedrine, dexbrompheniramine, acetaminophen	Antihistamine, decongestant

Trade name	Active ingredients	Common usage
Duocet	hydrocodone, acetaminophen	Analgesic
Dyazide	triamterene, hydrochlorothiazide	Diuretic
Elixophyllin GG	guaifenesin, theophylline	Antiasthmatic
Empirin with Codeine	aspirin, codeine	Analgesic
Enduronyl	methyclothiazide, deserpidine	Antihypertensive
E-Pilo	pilocarpine, epinephrine	Antiglaucoma
Ercaf	ergotamine, caffeine	Antimigraine
Eryzole	erythromycin, sulfisoxazole	Antibiotic
Esgic Plus	butalbital, acetaminophen, caffeine	Tension headache
Esimil	guanethidine, hydrochlorothiazide	Antihypertensive
Estrostep FE	ethinyl estradiol, norethindrone	Oral contraceptive
Etrafon	perphenazine, amitriptyline	Antidepressant
Excedrin Extra Strength	aspirin, acetaminophen, caffeine	Analgesic
Excedrin P.M.	acetaminophen, dimenhydramine	Analgesic
Fansidar	sulfadoxine, pyrimethamine	Antimalarial
fembrt	ethinyl estradiol, norethindrone	Menopause drug
Fioricet	acetaminophen, butalbital, caffeine	Analgesic
Fiorinal	aspirin, butalbital, caffeine	Analgesic
Fiorinal with Codeine	aspirin, butalbital, caffeine, codeine	Analgesic
Gaviscon	aluminum hydroxide, magnesium carbonate	Antacid
Gelusil	aluminum hydroxide, magnesium hydroxide, simethicone	Antacid
Glucovance	glyburide, metformin	Antidiabetic
Granulex	trypsin, Balsam Peru, castor oil	Topical enzyme
Haley's MO	mineral oil, magnesium hydroxide	Laxative
Halotussin-AC	guaifenesin, codeine	Antitussive, expectorant
Helidac	bismuth subsalicylate, metronidazole, tetracycline	Antiulcer

(continued)

Trade name	Active ingredients	Common usage
Hydrocet	hydrocodone, acetaminophen	Analgesic
Hydrogesic	hydrocodone, acetaminophen	Analgesic
Hyzaar	losartan, hydrochlorothiazide	Antihypertensive
Inderide	hydrochlorothiazide, propranolol	Antihypertensive
Kapectolin	kaolin, pectin	Antidiarrheal
Kondremul Plain	mineral oil, Irish moss, glycerin, acacia	Laxative
Lexxel ER Tablets	enalapril, felodipine	Antihypertensive
Librax	chlordiazepoxide, clidinium	Anticholinergic
Limbitrol DS 10-25	chlordiazepoxide, amitriptyline	Antidepressant
Logen	diphenoxylate, atropine	Antidiarrheal
Lomanate	diphenoxylate, atropine	Antidiarrheal
Lomotil	diphenoxylate, atropine	Antidiarrheal
Lonox	diphenoxylate, atropine	Antidiarrheal
Lopressor HCT	metoprolol, hydrochlorothiazide	Antihypertensive
Lorcet Plus Tablets	hydrocodone, acetaminophen	Analgesic
Lorcet Tablets	hydrocodone, acetaminophen	Analgesic
Lortab ASA	hydrocodone, aspirin	Analgesic
Lotensin HCT	hydrochlorothiazide, benazepril	Antihypertensive
Lotrel	amlodipine, benazepril	Antihypertensive
Low-Ogestrel	ethinyl estradiol, norgestrel	Oral contraceptive
Lufyllin EPG	dyphylline, ephedrine, guaifenesin, phenobarbital	Bronchodilator
Lufyllin GG	dyphylline, guaifenesin	Bronchodilator, expectorant
Lunelle	estradiol, medroxyprogesterone	Contraceptive
Maalox Suspension	aluminum hydroxide, magnesium hydroxide	Antacid
Maalox Therapeutic	aluminum hydroxide, magnesium hydroxide	Antacid
Malarone	atovaquone, proguanil	Antimalarial

Trade name	Active ingredients	Common usage
Marax	theophylline, ephedrine, hydroxyzine	Antiasthmatic
Margesic H	hydrocodone, acetaminophen	Analgesic
Maxitrol	dexamethasone, neomycin, polymyxin B	Ophthalmic
Maxzide	triamterene, hydrochlorothiazide	Diuretic
Metaglip	glipizide, metformin	Antidiabetic
Micardis HCT	telmisartan, hydrochlorothiazide	Antihypertensive
Micrainin	meprobamate, aspirin	Analgesic
Microgestin Fe 1.5/30	ethinyl estradiol, norethindrone	Oral contraceptive
Microgestin Fe 1/20	ethinyl estradiol, norethindrone	Oral contraceptive
Midol Maximum Strength	acetaminophen, caffeine	Analgesic
Midol Teen	acetaminophen, pamabrom	Analgesic
Minizide	prazosin, polythiazide	Antihypertensive
Moduretic	amiloride, hydrochlorothiazide	Diuretic
Monopril-HCT	fosinopril, hydrochlorothiazide	Antihypertensive
Mycolog-II	triamcinolone, nystatin	Antifungal
Mylagen Gelcaps	magnesium carbonate	Antacid
Mylagen Liquid	aluminum hydroxide, simethicone	Antacid
Mylagen II Liquid	aluminum hydroxide, magnesium hydroxide, simethicone	Antacid
Mylanta	aluminum hydroxide, magnesium hydroxide simethicone, sorbitol	Antacid
Mylanta Gelcaps	calcium carbonate, magnesium hydroxide	Antacid
Mylanta II	aluminum hydroxide, magnesium hydroxide simethicone	Antacid
Necon 1/50	mestranol, norethindrone	Oral contraceptive
Necon 1/35E	norethindrone, ethinyl estradiol	Oral contraceptive
Necon 10/11	ethinyl estradiol, norethindrone	Oral contraceptive

(continued)

Trade name	Active ingredients	Common usage
Neo Dexameth	neomycin, dexamethasone	Antibiotic, steroid
Neosporin	polymyxin B, neomycin, bacitracin	Antibiotic
Norgesic	orphenadrine, aspirin, caffeine	Skeletal muscle relaxant
Nortrel 7/7/7	norethindrone, ethinyl estradiol	Oral contraceptive
NuvaRing	etonogestrel, ethinyl estradiol	Contraceptive ring
Nyquil Cold/Cough Relief	pseudoephedrine, chlorpheniramine, dextromethorphan	Antihistamine, decongestant
Ogestrel	ethinyl estradiol, norgestrel	Oral contraceptive
Ortho-Cyclen	ethinyl estradiol, norgestimate	Oral contraceptive
Ortho-Evra	norgestimate, ethinyl estradiol	Contraceptive patch
Ortho-Novum 1/35	ethinyl estradiol, norethindrone	Oral contraceptive
Ortho-Novum 1/50	ethinyl estradiol, norethindrone	Oral contraceptive
Ortho-Novum 10/11	ethinyl estradiol, norethindrone	Oral contraceptive
Ortho-Prefest	estradiol, norgestimate	Menopause drug
Ortho Tri-Cyclen	norgestimate, ethinyl estradiol	Antiacne
Ortho Tri-Cyclen Lo	ethinyl estradiol, norgestimate	Oral contraceptive
Otocort	hydrocortisone, neomycin, polymyxin B	Antibiotic, steroid
Ovcon-50	ethinyl estradiol, ethynodiol diacetate	Oral contraceptive
Pamprin	acetaminophen, pamabrom, pyrilamine	Analgesic
Panacet 5/500	hydrocodone, acetaminophen	Analgesic
Panasal 5/500	hydrocodone, aspirin	Analgesic
Pediazole	erythromycin, sulfisoxazole	Antibiotic
Pepcid Complete	famotidine, calcium carbonate, magnesium hydroxide	Antacid
Percocet	oxycodone, acetaminophen	Analgesic
Percodan	oxycodone, aspirin	Analgesic
Peri-Colace	docusate, casanthranol	Laxative

Trade name	Active ingredients	Common usage
Phrenilin	acetaminophen, butalbital	Analgesic
Polaramine	guaifenesin, dexchlorpheniramine, pseudoephedrine	Antihistamine, decongestant, expectorant
Polysporin	polymyxin B, bacitracin	Antibiotic
Portia	levonorgestrel, ethinyl estradiol	Oral contraceptive
Premphase	estrogen, medroxyprogesterone	Menopause drug
Prempro	estrogen, medroxyprogesterone	Menopause drug
Premsyn PMS	acetaminophen, pamabrom, pyrilamine	Analgesic
Prevpac	lansoprazole, amoxicillin, clarithromycin	Ulcer treatment
Primatene	theophylline, ephedrine	Antiasthma
Primaxin	imipenem, cilastin	Antibiotic
Prinzide	lisinopril, hydrochlorothiazide	Antihypertensive
Quadrinal	ephedrine, theophylline, potassium iodide, phenobarbital	Bronchodilator
Quibron	theophylline, guaifenesin	Antiasthma, expectorant
R & C Shampoo	pyrethrins, piperonyl butoxide	Pediculicide
Rebetron	ribavirin, interferon alfa-2b	Antiviral
Repan	acetaminophen, caffeine, butalbital	Analgesic
RID	pyrethrins, piperonyl butoxide	Pediculicide
Rifamate	isoniazid, rifampin	Antituberculosis
Riopan Plus	magaldrate, simethicone	Antacid
Robitussin Allergy & Cold	dextromethorphan, brompheniramine, pseudoephedrine	Antitussive, antihistamine, decongestant
Robitussin CF	pseudoephedrine, guaifenesin, alcohol, dextromethorphan	Antitussive, expectorant
Robitussin Cold, Sinus & Congestion	acetaminophen, guaifenesin, alcohol, pseudoephedrine	Antitussive, expectorant
Robitussin DM	guaifenesin, dextromethorphan, alcohol	Antitussive, expectorant

(continued)

Trade name	Active ingredients	Common usage
Robitussin PE	pseudoephedrine, guaifenesin, alcohol	Antitussive, expectorant
Rondec	pseudophedrine, carbinoxamine	Antihistamine, decongestant
Roxilox	oxycodone, acetaminophen	Analgesic
Roxiprin	oxycodone, aspirin	Analgesic
Rulox	aluminum hydroxide, magnesium hydroxide	Antacid
Ryna	pseudoephedrine, chlorpheniramine	Antihistamine, decongestant
Ryna-C	codeine, pseudoephedrine, chlorpheniramine	Antihistamine, decongestant
Sedapap	acetaminophen, butalbital	Analgesic
Senokot-S	senna, docusate	Laxative
Septra	trimethoprim, sulfamethoxazole	Antibiotic
Sinemet	carbidopa, levodopa	Antiparkinsonism drug
Sinemet-CR	carbidopa, levodopa	Antiparkinsonism drug
Sine-Off No Drowsiness	pseudoephedrine, acetaminophen	Decongestant
Sinutab	pseudoephedrine, chlorpheniramine, acetaminophen	Decongestant
Soma Compound	aspirin, carisoprodol	Skeletal muscle relaxant
Sprintec	norgestimate, ethinyl estradiol	Oral contraceptive
Stagesic	hydrocodone, acetaminophen	Analgesic
Suboxone	buprenorphine, naloxone	Narcotic agonist
Sudafed Sinus Headache	pseudoephedrine, acetaminophen	Antihistamine, analgesic
Sulfatrim	trimethoprim, sulfamethoxazole	Antibiotic
Synalgos DC	aspirin, caffeine, dihydrocodeine	Analgesic
Synercid	quinupristin/dalfopristin	Antibiotic
Talacen	pentazocine, acetaminophen	Analgesic
Talwin Compound	aspirin, pentazocine	Analgesic
Talwin NX	pentazocine, naloxone	Analgesic

Trade name	Active ingredients	Common usage
Tarka	trandolapril, verapamil	Antihypertensive
Tavist Sinus	pseudoephedrine, acetaminophen	Antihistamine, analgesic
Teczem ER Tablets	enalapril, diltiazem	Antihypertensive
Tenoretic	atenolol, chlorthalidone	Antihypertensive
Teveten HCT	eprosartan, hydrochlorothiazide	Antihypertensive
Theodrine	ephedrine, theophylline, phenobarbital	Antiasthma
TheraFlu Flu and Cold	pseudoephedrine, chlorpheniramine, acetaminophen	Antihistamine, decongestant
TheraFlu Flu, Cold & Cough	pseudoephedrine, chlorpheniramine, dextromethorphan, acetaminophen	Antihistamine, decongestant, antitussive
Timolide	hydrochlorothiazide, timolol	Antihypertensive
TMP-SMZ	trimethoprim, sulfamethoxazole	Antibiotic
Triacin C	pseudoephedrine, triprolidine, codeine	Antitussive
Triad	acetaminophen, caffeine, butalbital	Analgesic
Triaminic Cold & Allergy	chlorpheniramine, pseudoephedrine	Antihistamine, decongestant
Triaminic Cold & Cough	chlorpheniramine, pseudoephedrine, dextromethorphan	Antihistamine, decongestant
Triaminic Cough & Congestion	dextromethorphan, pseudoephedrine	Antihistamine, decongestant
Triaminic Throat Pain & Cough	dextromethorphan, pseudoephedrine, acetaminophen	Antihistamine, decongestant, analgesic
Triavil	perphenazine, amitriptyline	Antidepressant
Trinalin Repetabs	azatadine, pseudoephedrine	Antihistamine
Tritec	ranitidine, trivalent bismuth, citrate	Antiulcer
Trivora-28	ethinyl estradiol, levonorgestrel	Oral contraceptive
Trizivir	abacavir, zidovudine, lamivudine	Antiviral, AIDS drug
Tylenol Multi-Symptom	acetaminophen, pseudoephedrine, dextromethorphan, guaifenesin	Antihistamine, decongestant, expectorant, analgesic

(continued)

Trade name	Active ingredients	Common usage
Tylenol Flu	acetaminophen, pseudoephedrine, dextromethorphan	Antihistamine, decongestant
Tylenol with Codeine	acetaminophen, codeine	Analgesic
Tylox	oxycodone, acetaminophen	Analgesic
Ultracet	tramadol, acetaminophen	Analgesic
Unasyn	ampicillin, sulbactam	Antibiotic
Uniretic	moexipril, hydrochlorothiazide	Antihypertensive
Vanex-HD	chlorpheniramine, hydrocodone, phenylephrine	Antihistamine, decongestant
Vaseretic	enalapril, hydrochlorothiazide	Antihypertensive
Vicks Cough Silencer	dextromethorphan, benzocaine	Antitussive, local anesthetic
Vicks DayQuil	dextromethorphan, pseudoephedrine, acetaminophen	Antihistamine, decongestant
Vicks Formula 44	dextromethorphan, benzocaine	Antihistamine, decongestant
Vicks Nyquil Multi-Symptom	dextromethorphan, doxylamine, pseudoephedrine, acetaminophen	Antihistamine, antitussive, decongestant
Vicodin	hydrocodone, acetaminophen	Analgesic
Vicoprofen	hydrocodone, ibuprofen	Analgesic
Wigraine	caffeine, ergotamine	Antimigraine
Yasmin	drospirenone, ethinyl estradiol	Oral contraceptive
Zestoretic	lisinopril, hydrochlorothiazide	Antihypertensive
Ziac	bisoprolol, hydrochlorothiazide	Antihypertensive
Zosyn	piperacillin, tazobactam	Antibiotic
Zovia 1/35E	ethinyl estradiol, ethynodiol diacetate	Oral contraceptive
Zovia 1/50E	ethinyl estradiol, ethynodiol diacetate	Oral contraceptive
Zydone	hydrocodone, acetaminophen	Analgesic
Zyrtec-D	cetirizine, pseudoephedrine	Antihistamine, decongestant

APPENDIX H

Topical Agents

Topical agents are drugs that are intended for surface use, not ingestion or injection. They may be very toxic if absorbed into the system, but they serve several purposes when used topically.

Pregnancy Category C
Contraindicated with allergy to these drugs, open wounds, or abrasions.

Adverse effects
Local irritation (common), stinging, burning, dermatitis, toxic effects if absorbed systemically.

Teaching points
Apply sparingly to affected area as directed. Do not use with open wounds or broken skin. Avoid contact with eyes. Report any local irritation, allergic reaction, worsening of condition being treated.

Drug	Selected trade names	Instructions
Emollients		
boric acid ointment	*Borofax*	Relieves burns, itching, irritation. Apply as needed.
dexpanthenol	*Panthoderm*	Relieves itching and aids in healing for mild skin irritations. Apply once or twice daily.
urea	*Aquacare* *Carmol 10* *Carmol 20* *Gordon's Urea 40%* *Nutraplus* *Ureacin*	Apply two to four times per day to area affected; rub in completely. Also used to restore nails (*Gordon's Urea 40%*)—cover with plastic wrap; keep dry and remove in 3, 7, 10, or 14 days.
vitamins A and D		Relieves minor burns, chafing skin irritations. Apply locally with gentle massage 2 to 4 times daily. Consult physician if not improved within 7 days.
zinc oxide	*Borofax Skin Protectant*	Relieves burns, abrasions, diaper rash. Apply as needed.
Growth factor		
becaplermin	*Regranex*	Increases incidence of healing of diabetic foot ulcers as adjunctive therapy. Apply to diabetic foot ulcers daily; patient must have an adequate blood supply.

(continued)

Drug	Selected trade names	Instructions
Lotions and solutions		
Burow's solution aluminum acetate	*Bluboro Powder* *Boropak Powder* *Buro-Sol* *Domeboro Powder* *Pedi-Boro Soak Paks*	Astringent wet dressing for relief of inflammatory conditions, insect bites, athlete's foot, bruises. Dissolve one packet or tablet in a pint of water, apply every 15 to 30 min for 4 to 8 hr; do not use occlusive dressing. Do not use in plastic containers.
calamine lotion	*Calamatum* *Calamox*	Relieves itching, pain of poison ivy, poison sumac, and poison oak, insect bites, and minor skin irritations. Apply to affected area 3 to 4 times daily.
hamamelis water	*A-E-R* *Witch Hazel*	Relieves itching and irritation of vaginal infection, hemorrhoids, postepisiotomy discomfort, posthemorrhoidectomy care. Apply locally up to 6 times per day.
Antiseptics		
benzalkonium chloride	*Benza* *Mycocide NS* *Zephiran*	Mix in solution as needed. Spray for preoperative use; store instruments in solution. Thoroughly rinse detergents and soaps from skin before use. Add antirust tablets for instruments stored in solution; dilute solution as indicated for use.
chlorhexidine gluconate	*BactoShield* *Dyna-Hex* *Exidine* *Hibiclens* *Hibistat*	Use for surgical scrub, preoperative skin prep, wound cleansing, preoperative bathing and showering. Scrub or rinse. Leave on for 15 seconds; for surgical scrub, leave on for 3 min.
hexachlorophene	*pHisoHex* *Septisol*	Use for surgical wash, scrub. Apply as wash; do not use with burns or on mucous membranes. Rinse thoroughly. Do not use routinely for bathing infants.
iodine		Wash affected area with solution. Solution is highly toxic; avoid occlusive dressings; stains skin and clothing.
povidone iodine	*ACU-dyne* *Aerodine* *Betadine* *Betagen* *Biodine* *Etodine* *Iodex* *Mallisol* *Minidyne* *Operand* *Polydine*	HIV may be inactivated in this solution. Apply as needed; treated areas may be bandaged. Causes less irritation than iodine and is less toxic.

Drug	Selected trade names	Instructions

Antiseptics (continued)

sodium hypochlorite	Dakin's	Apply as antiseptic. Caution: Chemical burns can occur.
thimerosal	Aeroaid Mersol	Used preoperatively and as first aid for abrasions, wounds. Apply every day up to 3 times per day. Contains mercury compound.

Antibiotics

mupirocin	Bactroban	Used to treat impetigo caused by *Staphylococcus aureus, Streptococcus,* and *Staphylococcus pyogenes.* Apply small amount to affected area 3 times per day; may be covered with a gauze dressing. Monitor for signs of superinfection; reevaluate if no clinical response in 3 to 5 days.
	Bactroban Nasal	Used to eradicate the nasal colonization of MRSA. Apply one-half of the ointment from single-use tube between nostrils and apply bid for 5 days.

Antivirals

acyclovir	Zovirex	Apply 0.5-inch ribbon to affected area and rub in gently 6 times daily for 7 days.
docosanol	Abreva	Used to treat oral and facial herpes simplex cold sores, fever blisters. Apply 5 times per day for 10 days. Caution patient not to overuse.
imiquimod	Aldara	Used to treat external genital warts and perianal warts. Apply a thin layer to warts and rub in 3 times per week at bedtime for 16 wk; remove with soap and water after 6 to 10 hr.
penciclovir	Denavir	Used to treat cold sores in healthy patients. Reserve use for herpes labialis on lips and face; avoid mucous membranes. Use at first sign of cold sore. Apply thin layer to affected area q 2 hr while awake for 4 days.

Antipsoriatics

anthralin	Anthra-Derm Drithocreme Dritho-Scalp Micanol	Apply every day only to psoriatic lesions. Use protective dressing. Avoid contact with eyes. May stain fabrics, skin, hair, fingernails.
calcipotriene	Dovonex	Used as a synthetic vitamin D_2. Use only for disorder prescribed. Apply thin layer once or twice a day. Monitor serum calcium levels with extended use. May cause local irritation.

(continued)

Drug	Selected trade names	Instructions
Antiseborrheics		
selenium sulfide	*Exsel* *Selsun Blue*	Massage 5 to 10 mL into scalp; rest 2 to 3 minutes, rinse, repeat. May damage jewelry; remove jewelry before use. Discontinue use if local irritation occurs.
chloroxine	*Capitrol*	Do not use on active lesions. Massage into wet scalp; leave lather on for 3 minutes. May discolor blond, gray, bleached hair.
Antifungals		
amphotericin B	*Fungizone*	Used to treat cutaneous mycotic infections. Apply liberally 2 to 4 times per day. May cause drying and discoloration of skin.
butenafine hydrochloride	*Mentax*	Used to treat intradigital pedia (athlete's foot), tinea corporis, ringworm, tinea cruris. Apply to affected area only once a day for 4 wk.
butoconazole nitrate	*Gynazole-1*	Apply intravaginally as one dose. Culture fungus; if no response, reculture. Ensure use of full course of therapy. May cause irritation, burning.
ciclopirox	*Loprox* *Penlac Nail Lacquer*	Used to treat onychomycosis of fingernails and toenails in immunocompromised patients. Apply directly to affected fingernails or toenails.
clotrimazole	*Cruex* *Desenex* *Lotrimin* *Mycelex*	Cleanse area before applying. Gently massage into affected area up to twice daily. Use for up to 4 wk. Discontinue if irritation, worsening of condition occurs.
econazole nitrate	*Spectazole*	Apply locally once or twice daily. Cleanse area before applying. Treat for 2 to 4 wk. Discontinue if irritation, burning, or worsening of condition occurs. For athlete's foot, change socks and shoes at least once a day.
gentian violet		Do not apply to active lesions. Apply locally up to twice daily. May stain skin and clothing.
ketoconazole	*Nizoral*	Apply topically up to twice a day or shampoo daily. Itching or stinging of the scalp may occur.
naftifine HCl	*Naftin*	Gently massage into affected area twice daily. Avoid occlusive dressings. Wash hands thoroughly after application. Do not use longer than 4 wk.
oxiconazole	*Oxistat*	Apply every day up to twice daily. May be needed for up to 1 month.

Drug	Selected trade names	Instructions
Antifungals *(continued)*		
terbinafine	*Lamisil*	Apply to area twice daily until clinical signs are improved, 1 to 4 wk. Do not use occlusive dressings. Report local irritation. Discontinue if local irritation occurs.
tolnaftate	*Absorbine* *Aftate* *Genaspor* *Quinsana Plus* *Tinactin* *Ting*	Apply small amount twice daily for 2 to 3 wk; 4 to 6 wk may be needed if skin is very thick. Cleanse skin with soap and water before applying drug, dry thoroughly, wear loose, well-fitting shoes, change socks at least 4 times a day.
Pediculicides and scabicides		
crotamiton	*Eurax*	For external use only. Shake well before using. Thoroughly massage into skin of entire body; repeat in 24 hr. Take a cleansing bath or shower 48 hr after last application. Change bed linens and clothing the next day. Contaminated clothing can be dry cleaned or washed on hot cycle.
lindane	*G-Well*	For external use only. Do not use in premature neonates. Apply thin layer to entire body; leave on 8 to 12 hr, then wash thoroughly. Shampoo 1 to 2 oz into dry hair and leave in place 4 minutes. Single application is usually sufficient, reapply after 7 days at signs of live lice. Teach hygiene and prevention; treat all contacts. Assure parents that this is a readily communicable disease.
malathion	*Ovide Lotion*	Avoid use with open lesions. Apply to dry hair; leave on 8 to 12 hr. Repeat in 7 to 9 days. Change bed linens and clothing. Treat all contacts. Contains flammable alcohol.
permethrin	*Acticin* *Elimite* *Nix*	For external use only. Approved for prophylactic use during head lice epidemics. Thoroughly massage into all skin areas (30 g/adult); wash off after 8 to 14 hr. Shampoo into freshly washed, rinsed, and towel-dried hair. Leave on for 10 minutes; rinse. Single application is usually curative. Notify health care provider if rash, itching become worse.
Keratolytics		
podophyllum resin	*Podocon-25* *Podofin*	Applied only by physician. Do not use if wart is inflamed or irritated. Very toxic; use minimum amount possible to avoid absorption.
podofilox	*Condylox*	Apply q 12 hr for 3 consecutive days. Allow to dry before using area. Dispose of used applicator. May cause burning and discomfort.

(continued)

Drug	Selected trade names	Instructions
Topical hemostatics		
absorbable gelatin (also comes in powder form)	*Gelfoam*	Prepare paste by adding 3 to 4 mL sterile saline to contents of jar. Apply sponge dry or saturated with saline. Smear or press paste to cut surface; when bleeding stops, remove excess. Apply sponge and allow to remain in place; it will be absorbed. Assess continually for any sign of infection; agent may act as site of infection or abscess formation. Do not use with infection.
microfibrillar collagen	*Avitene Hemostat* *Hemopad* *Hemotene*	Use dry. Apply directly to the source of bleeding; apply pressure. Time will vary from 3 to 5 minutes depending on the site. Discard any unused product; monitor for infection; do not use with infection. Remove any excess material once bleeding has been controlled.
thrombin	*Thrombinar* *Thrombin JMI* *Thrombogen* *Thrombostat*	Prepare in sterile distilled water or isotonic saline; 100 to 1,000 units/mL. Mix freely with blood on the surface of injury; contraindicated with any bovine allergies. Watch for any sign of severe allergic reaction in sensitive individuals.
Pain relief		
capsaicin	*Capsin* *Dolorac* *Pain-X* *Pain Doctor* *R-Gel* *Zostrix*	Apply not more than 3 or 4 times per day. Applied locally, provides temporary relief from the pain of osteoarthritis, rheumatoid arthritis, neuralgias. Do not bandage tightly. Stop use and seek health care if condition worsens or persists after 14 to 28 days.
Burn preparations		
mafenide	*Sulfamylon*	Apply to a clean, debrided wound, 1 or 2 times per day with a gloved hand. Cover burn at all times with drug, reapply as needed. Bathe patient in a whirlpool daily to aid debridement. Continue mafenide until healing occurs; monitor for infection and toxicity—acidosis. May cause marked discomfort on application.
nitrofurazone	*Furacin*	Apply directly to burn or place on gauze; reapply daily. Flushing the dressing with sterile saline facilitates removal. Monitor for signs of superinfections; treat supportively. Rash frequently occurs.
silver sulfadiazine	*Silvadene* *SSD cream* *Thermazene*	Apply once or twice a day to a clean, debrided wound. Use a 1/16th-inch thickness. Bathe patient in a whirlpool to aid debridement. Dressings are not necessary but may be used; reapply whenever necessary. Monitor for fungal superinfections.

Drug	Selected trade names	Instructions
Estrogen		
dienestrol	*Ortho Dienestrol*	Treats postmenopausal atrophic vaginitis and kraurosis vulvae. Use 1 to 2 applicators intravaginally daily for 1 to 2 wk; reduce to one-half initial dose every other day for 1 to 2 wk. Maintenance: 1 applicator 1 to 3 times per week. Lie down for 15 minutes after dose; wear a pad to protect clothing.
estradiol hemihydrate	*Vagifem*	For treatment of atrophic vaginitis. Use 1 tablet inserted vaginally every day for 2 wk; then 1 tablet inserted vaginally 2 times per week. Attempt to taper every 3 to 6 months.
Acne, rosacea, and melasma products		
adapalene	*Differin*	Do not use on cuts or any open area. Avoid use on sunburned skin, in combination with other products, or exposure to sun. Apply a thin film to affected area after washing every night at bedtime. Less drying than other products.
alitretinoin	*Panretin*	Used for treatment of lesions of Kaposi's sarcoma. 1% gel; apply as needed to cover lesions twice daily. Inflammation, peeling, redness may occur.
azelaic acid	*Azelex* *Finevin (20%)*	Wash and dry skin. Massage a thin layer into affected area twice daily. Wash hands thoroughly after application. Improvement usually occurs within 4 wk. Initial irritation usually occurs but passes with time.
clindamycin and benzoyl peroxide	*BenzaClin*	Apply gel to affected areas twice daily. Wash area and pat dry before application.
flucinolone acetonide, hydroquinone, and tretinoin	*Tri-Luma*	Do not use during pregnancy. Apply to depigmented area of melasma once each evening, at least 30 min before bedtime after cleansing and patting dry; avoid occlusive dressings. Use a sunscreen and protective clothing if outside; skin dryness and peeling may occur.
metronidazole	*MetroGel* *MetroLotion* *Noritate*	For treatment of rosacea. Apply cream to affected area twice daily.
sodium sulfacetamide	*Klaron*	Apply a thin film twice daily to affected areas. Wash affected area with mild soap and water; pat dry. Avoid use in denuded or abraded areas.

(continued)

Drug	Selected trade names	Instructions
Acne, rosacea, and melasma products (continued)		
tazarotene	_Tazorac_	Avoid use in pregnancy. Apply thin film once daily in the evening. Do not use with irritants or products with high alcohol content. Drying causes photosensitivity.
tretinoin, 0.025% cream	_Avita_	Apply thin layer once daily. Discomfort, peeling, redness may occur for the first 2 to 4 wk. Worsened acne may occur in first few weeks.
tretinoin, 0.05% cream	_Renova_	Used for removal of fine wrinkles. Apply thin coat in the evening.
tretinoin, gel	_Retin-A* Micro_	Apply to cover once daily after cleansing. Exacerbation of inflammation may occur at first. Therapeutic effects usually seen in first 2 wk.
Oral preparations		
amlexanox	_Aphthasol_	Apply to aphthous ulcers 4 times a day—after meals, at bedtime, following oral hygiene—for 10 days; consult with dentist if ulcers are not healed within 10 days. May cause local pain.
Antihistamine		
azelastine hydrochloride	_Astelin_	Use 2 sprays per nostril twice daily. Avoid use of alcohol and OTC antihistamines; dizziness and sedation can occur.
Nasal corticosteroid		
fluticasone propionate	_Flonase_	Used as preventive treatment of asthma, not as primary treatment. May take several weeks to work. Clean nasal spray adapter weekly. _Adult:_ 2 sprays each nostril daily. Approved for children 4 to 11 years old.
	Flovent Rotadisk	Used as treatment of allergic rhinitis. ≥ _4 yr:_ 2 sprays in each nostril daily.
	Flovent Diskus	Used as prophylactic treatment of asthma for patients who require a corticosteroid. ≥ _4 yr:_ 88–220 mcg twice daily using provided inhalation device.
Hair removal		
Eflornithine	_Vaniqa_	Approved for use in women only. Apply to unwanted facial hair twice daily for up to 24 wk. Do not wash treated areas until at least 4 hr after treatment.

APPENDIX I

Topical Corticosteroids

Drug classes
Hormonal agents
Corticosteroids
Glucocorticoids and mineralocorticoids

Therapeutic actions
Enter cells and bind cytoplasmic receptors, thereby initiating complex reactions that are responsible for the anti-inflammatory, antipruritic, and antiproliferative effects.

Indications
- Relief of inflammatory and pruritic manifestations of corticosteroid-sensitive dermatoses.
- Temporary relief of minor skin irritations, itching, and rashes—nonprescription products.

Adverse effects
- **Local:** Burning, irritation, acneiform lesions, striae, skin atrophy, secondary infection.
- **CNS:** Glaucoma, cataracts after prolonged periorbital use that allows the drug to enter the eyes.
- **Systemic:** Systemic absorption can occur, leading to the adverse effects experienced with systemic use; growth retardation and suppression of the HPA (more likely to occur with occlusive dressings, in patients with liver failure, and with children who have a larger skin surface-to-body weight ratio).

Dosage
Apply sparingly to affected area 2 to 3 times daily.

Teaching points
- Apply sparingly in a light film; rub in gently. Washing the area before application may increase drug penetration.
- Do not use occlusive dressings, tight-fitting diapers, or plastic pants unless otherwise indicated. This may increase systemic absorption (except with alclometasone used to treat psoriasis).
- Avoid prolonged use, especially near the eyes, in genital or rectal areas, on the face, and in skin creases. Avoid any direct contact with eyes.
- Use this drug only for the purpose indicated. Do not apply to open lesions.
- Notify nurse or physician if condition becomes worse or persists, if burning or irritation occurs, or if infection occurs in the area.

Drug	Trade name	Preparations
alclometasone dipropionate	*Aclovate*	Ointment, cream: 0.05% concentration
amcinonide	*Cyclocort*	Ointment, cream, lotion: 0.1% concentration
betamethasone dipropionate	*Alphatrex, Diprosone, Maxivate, Rhoprosone (CAN), Taro-Sone (CAN), Teladar*	Ointment, cream, gel, lotion, aerosol: 0.05% concentration

(continued)

Drug	Trade name	Preparations
betamethasone dipropionate augmented	*Diprolene*	Ointment, cream, lotion: 0.05% concentration
betamethasone valerate	*Betacort (CAN), Betaderm (CAN), Betatrex, Beta-Val, Betnovate (CAN), Celestroderm (CAN), Luxiq, Prevex, B(CAN), Rholosone (CAN), Valisone*	Ointment, cream, lotion: 0.1% concentration Foam: 0.12%
clobetasol propionate	*Cormax, Dermovate (CAN), Embeline E, Olux, Temovate*	Ointment, cream, foam, gel: 0.05% concentration
clocortolone pivalate	*Cloderm*	Cream: 0.1% concentration
desonide	*DesOwen, Tridesilon*	Ointment, lotion, cream: 0.05% concentration
desoximetasone	*Topicort*	Ointment, cream: 0.25% concentration Cream, gel: 0.05% concentration
dexamethasone	*Aeroseb-Dex, DecaSpray*	Aerosol: 0.01%, 0.04% concentration
dexamethasone sodium phosphate		Cream: 0.1% concentration
diflorasone diacetate	*Florone, Maxiflor, Psorcon E, Florone E*	Ointment, cream: 0.05% concentration Cream: 0.05% concentration
fluocinolone acetonide	*Flurosyn, Synalar*	Ointment: 0.025% concentration Cream: 0.01% concentration
	Flurosyn, Synalar	Cream: 0.025% concentration
	Fluonid, Flurosyn, Synalar	Solution: 0.01% concentration
fluocinonide	*Lidex*	Ointment: 0.05% concentration
	Fluonex, Lidex, Lyderm Cream (CAN)	Cream: 0.05% concentration
	Lidex, Topsyn Gel (CAN)	Solution, gel: 0.05% concentration
flurandrenolide	*Cordran*	Ointment, cream: 0.025% concentration Ointment, cream, lotion: 0.05% concentration Tape: 4 mcg/cm^2
fluticasone propionate	*Cutivate*	Cream: 0.05% concentration Ointment: 0.005% concentration

Drug	Trade name	Preparations
halcinonide	*Halog*	Ointment, cream, solution: 0.1% concentration Cream: 0.025% concentration
halobetasol propionate	*Ultravate*	Ointment, cream: 0.05% concentration
hydrocortisone	*Cortizone-5, Bactine Hydrocortisone, Cort-Dome, Dermolate, Dermtex HC, HydroTex*	Lotion: 0.25%, 0.5%, 1%, 2%, 2.5%
	Cortizone-10, Hycort, Tegrin-HC	Cream, lotion, ointment, aerosol: 0.5%
	Hytone	Cream, lotion, ointment, solution: 1%
hydrocortisone acetate	*Cortaid, Lanacort-5*	Ointment: 0.5% concentration
	Corticaine (R_x), Gynecort, Lanacort-5	Cream: 0.5% concentration
	Anusol-HC, *Cortaid with Aloe*	Cream: 1% concentration Cream: 0.5% concentration
hydrocortisone buteprate	*Pandel*	Cream: 0.1%
hydrocortisone butyrate	*Locoid*	Ointment, cream: 0.1% concentration
hydrocortisone valerate	*Westcort*	Ointment, cream: 0.2% concentration
mometasone furoate	*Elocon*	Ointment, cream, lotion: 0.1% concentration
	Nasonex	Nasal spray: 0.2%
prednicarbate	*Dermatop*	Cream: 0.1% concentration: preservative free
triamcinolone acetonide	*Flutex, Kenalog*	Ointment: 0.025% concentration
	Aristocort	Ointment: 0.1% concentration and 0.5% concentration Cream: 0.025% concentration and 0.5% concentration
	Triacet, Triderm	Cream: 0.1% concentration Lotion: 0.025% and 0.1% concentration

Ophthalmic Agents

Ophthalmic agents are drugs that are intended for direct administration into the conjunctiva of the eye. These drugs are used to treat glaucoma (miotics constrict the pupil and decrease the resistance to aqueous flow), to aid in diagnosis of eye problems (mydriatics—dilate the pupil for examination of the retina; cyclopegics paralyze the muscles that control the lens to aid refraction), or to treat local ophthalmic infections or inflammation; and to provide relief from the signs and symptoms of allergic reactions.

Pregnancy category C
Contraindicated in cases of allergy to these drugs. These drugs are seldom absorbed systemically, but caution should be taken with any patient who would have problems with the systemic effects of the drug if it were absorbed systemically.

Adverse effects
Local irritation, stinging, burning, blurring of vision (prolonged when using ointment), tearing; headache.

Dosage
1–2 drops to each eye bid to qid or 0.25–0.5 inch of ointment to each eye is the usual dosage.

Solution or drops
Wash hands thoroughly before administering; do not touch dropper to eye or to any other surface; have patient tilt head backward or lie down and stare upward; gently grasp lower eyelid and pull the eyelid away from the eyeball; instill drop(s) into pouch formed by eyelid; release lid slowly; have patient close eye and look downward; apply gentle pressure to the inside corner of the eye for 3–5 min to retard drainage; do not rub eyes; do not rinse eyedropper. Do not use eyedrops that have changed color; if more than one type of eyedrop is used, wait 5 min before administration.

Ointment
Wash hands thoroughly before administering; hold tube between hands for several minutes to warm the ointment; discard the first cm of ointment when opening the tube for the first time; tilt head backward or lie down and stare upward; gently pull out lower lid to form pouch; place 0.25–0.5 inch of ointment inside the lower lid; have patient close eyes for 1–2 min and roll eyeball in all directions; remove any excess ointment from around eye. If using more than one kind of ointment, wait 10 min between administration.

Teaching points
Teach patient the proper administration technique for the ophthalmic agent ordered; caution patients that transient stinging or burning may occur and that blurring vision may also occur—appropriate safety measures should be taken; sensitivity to sun will occur with mydriatic agents which cause pupils to dilate; sunglasses may be needed. Report severe eye discomfort, palpitations, nausea, headache.

Drug	Trade names	Usage	Special considerations
apraclonidine	*Iopidine*	To control or prevent postsurgical elevations of IOP in patients after argon-laser eye surgery; short-term adjunct in patients on maximum tolerated therapy who need additional IOP reduction	Monitor for the possibility of vasovagal attack; do not give to patients with allergy to clonidine.
azelastine HCl	*Optivar*	Treatment of ocular itching associated with allergic conjunctivitis	Antihistamine, mast cell stabilizer. ≥ 3 yr: 1 drop bid. Rapid onset, 8 hr duration.
bimatoprost	*Lumigan*	Treatment of open-angle glaucoma and ocular hypertension; prostamide	Use when patient unresponsive to other agents; darkening of iris may occur; 1 drop daily.
brimonidine tartrate	*Alphagan*	Treatment of open-angle glaucoma and ocular hypertension; selective alpha$_2$-antagonist	Selective alpha$_2$-antagonist; minimal effects on CV and pulmonary systems; may stain soft contact lenses. Do not use with MAOIs. 1 drop tid.
brinzolamide	*Azopt*	Decrease IOP in open-angle glaucoma	May be given with other agents; 1 drop tid. Give 10 min apart from other agents.
carbachol	*Carbastat Carboptic Isopto Carbachol Miostat*	Direct-acting miotic; for treatment of glaucoma; for miosis during surgery	Surgical dose a one-use only portion; 1 or 2 drops up to tid as needed for glaucoma.
cyclopentolate	*AK-Pentolate Cyclogyl Pentolair*	Mydriasis or cycloplegia in diagnostic procedures	Individuals with dark pigmented irides may require higher doses; compress lacrimal sac for 1–2 min after administration to decrease any systemic absorption.
cyclosporine emulsion 0.05%	*Restasis*	Increase tear production in patients whose tear production is presumed to be suppressed due to ocular inflammation associated with keratoconjunctivitis sicca	1 drop in each eye twice a day, approximately 12 hr apart; remove contact lenses before using.

(continued)

Drug	Trade names	Usage	Special considerations
dapiprazole	*Rev-Eyes*	Miotic: iatrogenically induced mydriasis produced by adrenergic or parasympathetic agents	Not for use to reduce IOP; do not use if constriction is undesirable. Do not use more than once a week.
demecarium	*Humorsol*	Treatment of glaucoma and strabismus; cholinesterase inhibitor	If response is not adequate in first 24 hr, consider another drug. Do not use more often than necessary—1 or 2 drops/wk up to 1 or 2 drops/day have been used.
diclofenac sodium	*Voltaren*	Photophobia; for use in patients undergoing incisional refractive surgery	Apply 1 drop qid beginning 24 hr after cataract surgery; continue through the first 2 wk postoperatively.
dipivefrin	*Propine* *AKPro*	Control of IOP in chronic open-angle glaucoma	1 drop q 12 hr. Monitor closely with tonometry.
dorzolamide	*Trusopt*	Treatment of elevated IOP in patients with ocular hypertension or open-angle glaucoma	A sulfonamide; monitor patients on parenteral sulfonamides for possible additive effects.
dorzolamide 2% and timolol 0.5%	*Cosopt*	Decrease IOP in open-angle glaucoma or ocular hypertension in patients who do not respond to beta-blockers alone	Administer 1 drop in affected eye bid. Monitor for cardiac failure; if absorbed, may mask symptoms of hypoglycemia or thyrotoxicosis.
echothiophate	*Phospholine Iodide*	Treatment of open-angle glaucoma; irreversible cholinesterase inhibitor; long-acting. Accommodative esotropia	Given only once or twice a day because of long action; tolerance may develop with prolonged use, usually responds to a rest period.
emedastine	*Emadine*	Temporary relief of signs and symptoms of allergic conjunctivitis	1 drop in affected eye or eyes up to qid. Do not wear contact lenses if eyes are red; may cause headache, blurred vision.
fluorometholone	*Flarex* *Fluor-Op* *FML*	Topical corticosteroid used for treatment of inflammatory conditions of the eye	Improvement should occur within several days, discontinue if no improvement is seen. Monitor IOP if used > 10 days. Discontinue if swelling of the eye occurs.
fomivirsen sodium	*Vitravene*	Treatment of CMV in AIDS patients who cannot tolerate other treatments for CMV retinitis	Injected into affected eye every other wk for two doses, then every 4 wk. Do not use if treated with cidofovir within the past 2–4 wk.

Drug	Trade names	Usage	Special considerations
homatropine	*Isopto-Homatropine* *Homatropine HBr*	Long-acting mydriatic and cycloplegic used for refraction and treatment of inflammatory conditions of the uveal tract; preoperative and postoperative states when mydriasis is required	Individuals with dark pigmented irides may require larger doses; 5–10 min is usually required for refraction.
ketotifen	*Zaditor*	Temporary relief of itching due to allergic conjunctivitis	Remove contact lenses before use—may be replaced within 10 min. An antihistamine and mast cell stabilizer.
latanoprost	*Xalatan*	Treatment of open-angle glaucoma or ocular hypertension in patients intolerant or nonresponsive to other agents	Remove contact lenses before use and for 15 min after use; allow at least 5 min between this and the use of any other agents; expect burning, blurred vision.
levobetaxolol	*Betaxon*	Reduction of IOP with chronic open-angle glaucoma, ocular hypertension	1 drop bid; may take up to 2 wk to see results, do not combine with beta adrenergics.
levocabastine	*Livostin*	Relief of allergic conjunctivitis	Treatment may be needed for up to 2 wk. Do not wear soft contact lenses during use of this drug. Shake well before use and do not use any discolored solution.
levobunolol	*AKBeta* *Betagan Liquifilm*	Lowering of IOP with chronic, open-angle glaucoma, ocular hypertension	1 or 2 drops bid. Do not combine with other beta-blockers.
levofloxacin	*Quixin*	Treatment of bacterial conjunctivitis caused by susceptible bacteria	1 or 2 drops in affected eye q 2 hr while awake, days 1 and 2; then q 4 hr while awake, up to 4 times per day for days 3 to 7.
lodoxamide tromethamine	*Alomide*	Treatment of vernal conjunctivitis and keratitis for patients > 2 yr	Patients should not wear contact lenses while using this drug; discontinue if stinging and burning persist after instillation.

(continued)

Drug	Trade names	Usage	Special considerations
loteprednol etabonate	*Lotemax (0.5%)*	Treatment of steroid-resistant ocular disease	1 or 2 drops qid.
	Alrex (0.2%)	Treatment of postoperative inflammation after ocular surgery	1 or 2 drops qid beginning 24 hr after surgery and continuing for 2 wk. Shake vigorously before use. Discard after 14 days; prolonged use may cause nerve or eye damage.
metipranolol	*OptiPranolol*	Beta-blocker; used in treating chronic open-angle glaucoma and ocular hypertension	Concomitant therapy may be needed; caution patient about possible vision changes.
natamycin	*Natacyn*	Antibiotic used to treat fungal blepharitis, conjunctivitis, and keratitis; drug of choice for *Fusarium sotani* keratitis	Shake well before each use; store at room temperature; failure to improve in 7–10 days suggests a nonsusceptible organism, reevaluate.
nedocromil sodium	*Alocril*	Treatment of itching of allergic conjunctivitis	Use at regular intervals through the entire allergic season: 1 or 2 drops in each eye bid.
olopatadine hydrochloride	*Patanol*	Mast cell stabilizer and antihistamine; provides fast onset of relief of itching due to conjunctivitis with prolonged action	Not for use with contact lenses; headache is common side effect.
pemirolast potassium	*Alamast*	Prevention of itchy eyes due to allergic conjunctivitis	1 or 2 drops qid.
pilocarpine	*Adsorbocarpine* *Akarpine* *Isopto Carpine* *Pilocar* *Piloptic* *Pilostat*	Chronic and acute glaucoma; treatment of mydriasis caused by drugs; direct-acting miotic agent	Can be stored at room temperature for up to 8 wk, then discard. 1 or 2 drops up to 6 times per day may be needed, based on patient response.
polydimethyl-siloxane	*AdatoSil 5000*	Treatment of retinal detachments where other therapy is not effective or is inappropriate; primary choice for retinal detachment due to AIDS-related CMV retinitis or viral infection	Monitor for cataracts; must be injected into aqueous humor.

Drug	Trade names	Usage	Special considerations
primexolone	*Vexol*	Corticosteroid; postoperative ocular surgery and for treatment of anterior uveitis	Monitor for signs of steroid absorption.
suprofen	*Profenal*	NSAID; used to inhibit intraoperative miosis	Local burning may occur; monitor patient for any cross sensitivities to other NSAIDs.
travoprost	*Travatan*	Treatment of open-angle glaucoma and ocular hypertension	1 drop in affected eye or eyes each evening; eye discomfort, pain, darkening of iris, growth of eyelashes common.
trifluridine	*Viroptic*	Antiviral; used to treat primary keratoconjunctivitis and recurrent epithelial keratitis due to herpes simplex virus types 1 and 2	Transient burning and stinging may occur; reconsider drug if improvement is not seen within 7 days. Do not administer for longer than 21 days at a time.
tropicamide	*Mydriacy Opticyl Tropicacyl*	Mydriatic and cycloplegic used for refraction	1 or 2 drops of 1% solution; repeat in 5 min. May repeat in 30 min for prolonged effects.
unoprostone isopropyl	*Rescula*	Treatment of open-angle glaucoma, ocular hypertension in patients who have not responded to other agents	1 drop bid; not for use in children, pregnancy, lactation. Remove contact lenses.
vidarabine	*Vira-A*	Acute keratoconjunctivitis and recurrent epithelial keratitis due to herpes simplex types 1 and 2; superficial keratitis caused by herpes simplex virus and not responding to idoxuridine	Treat an additional 7 days after epithelialization has occurred; if no improvement in 21 days, consider other therapy.

Laxatives

Laxative use has been replaced by the use of proper diet and exercise in many clinical situations. Most laxatives are available as OTC preparations and are often abused by people who become dependent on them for GI movement.

Indications

Short-term relief of constipation; to prevent straining; to evacuate the bowel for diagnostic procedures; to remove ingested poisons from the lower GI tract; as adjunct in anthelmintic therapy.

Drug	Selected trade names	Type
bisacodyl	*Bisco-Lax* *Dulcolax*	Stimulant
cascara		Stimulant
castor oil	*Emulsoil* *Neoloid* *Purge*	Stimulant
docusate	*Colace* *Diocto-C* *Ex-Lax Stool Softener* *Genasoft* *Modane Soft* *Phillips' Liqui-Gels*	Detergent, softener
glycerin	*Fleet Babylax* *Sani-Supp*	Hyperosmolar
lactulose	*Cephulac* *Chronulac* *Constilac* *Constulose*	Hyperosmolar
magnesium citrate	*Citrate of Magnesia*	Saline
magnesium hydroxide	*Milk of Magnesia* *MOM* *Philip's MOM*	Saline
magnesium sulfate	*Epsom Salts*	Saline
mineral oil	*Kondremul Plain*	Emollient

Pregnancy Category C
Contraindicated in cases of allergy to these drugs, third trimester of pregnancy, acute abdominal pain.

Adverse effects
Excessive bowel activity, perianal irritation, abdominal cramps, *weakness, dizziness,* cathartic dependence.

Teaching points
Use as a temporary measure. Swallow tablets whole. Do not take this drug within 1 hr of any other drugs. Report sweating, flushing, muscle cramps, excessive thirst.

Dosage	Onset	Special considerations
10–15 mg PO 2.5 g in water via enema	6–10 hr Rapid	Allergy to tartrazine in *Dulcolax* tablets; may discolor urine.
325–650 mg PO	6–10 hr	
15–30 mL	2–6 hr	May be very vigorous; abdominal cramping.
50–240 mg	24–72 hr	Gentle; beneficial with anorectal conditions that are painful and with dry or hard feces.
Suppository; 4 mL liquid	15–30 min	Insert suppository high into rectum, retain 15 min; insert liquid dispenser and apply gentle, steady pressure until all liquid is gone, then remove.
15–30 mL PO	24–48 hr	Also used for treatment of portal system encephalopathy. May be more palatable mixed with fruit juice, water, or milk.
1 glassful	0.5–3 hr	Reduce pediatric dosage by one-half.
15–30 mL	0.5–3 hr	Take with liquids; flavored varieties vary.
10–25 g	0.5–3 hr	Take mixed with glass of water; reduce pediatric dose to 5–10 g in glass of water.
5–45 mL PO	6–8 hr	Reduce pediatric dose to 5–20 mL. May decrease absorption of fat-soluble vitamins. Use caution to avoid lipid pneumonia with aspiration.

(continued)

Drug	Selected trade names	Type
polycarbophil	*Equalactin* *FiberCon* *Konsyl Fiber*	Bulk
polyethylene glycol	*MiraLax*	Bulk
polyethylene glycol- electrolyte solution	*CoLyte* *GoLYTELY* *NuLytely*	Bulk
psyllium	*Fiberall Fruit* *Hydrocil Instant* *Metamucil*	Bulk
senna	*Agoral* *Black-Draught* *Fletcher's Castoria* *Senna-Gen* *Senokot*	Stimulant

Dosage	Onset	Special considerations
1 g PO 1–4 times per day as needed; do not exceed 6 g per day in adults or 3 g per day in children	12–24 hr	Good with irritable bowel syndrome, diverticulitis. Abdominal fullness may occur. Smaller doses more frequently may alleviate discomfort.
Dissolve 17 g in 8 oz water and drink every day for up to 2 wk	48–72 hr	Do not use with bowel obstruction; diarrhea common.
4 L oral solution before GI examination	1 hr	Used as bowel evacuant before GI examinations. Do not use with GI obstruction, mega colon. GI discomfort common.
1 tsp or packet in cool water or juice, 1–3 times per day in children	12–24 hr	Safest and most physiologic. Ensure that patient has sufficient water to completely swallow dose.
1–8 tablets per day at bedtime; suppository; syrup—10–25 mL	6–10 hr	May be very aggressive; abdominal cramps and discomfort may occur.

Less Commonly Used Drugs

Generic and trade names	Drug class and indications
acitretin *Soriatane*	Antipsoratic agent, retinoic acid Treatment of severe psoriasis
albendazole *Albenza*	Anthelmintic Treatment of parenchymal neurocysticercosis due to active lesions caused by larval forms of Taenia solium (pork tapeworm) Treatment of cystic hydatid disease from Echinococcus granulosus (dog tapeworm)
alefacept *Amevive*	Immune suppressant Treatment of adults with moderate to severe chronic plaque psoriasis who are candidates for systemic therapy or phototherapy
alemtuzumab *Campath*	Monoclonal antibody; antineoplastic Treatment of B cell chronic lymphocytic leukemia in patients treated with alkylating agents who have failed fludarabine therapy
alglucerase *Ceredase*	Enzyme Long-term replacement in Gaucher's disease in patients with anemia, hepatic, or spleen disease
alpha₁-proteinase inhibitor *Prolastin*	Blood product Treatment of congenital alpha1-antitrypsin deficiency, chronic treatment of adults with early evidence of panacinar emphysema
amifostine *Ethyol*	Cytoprotective agent Reduction of renal toxicity associated with repeated administration of cisplatin in patients with advanced ovarian cancer; reduction of incidence of xerostomia in patients receiving radiation for head and neck cancer Unlabeled use: protection of lung fibroblasts from effects of paclitaxel
aminolevulinic acid hydrochloride *Levulan Kerastick*	Photosensitizer Treatment of nonkeratotic actinic keratoses of the face and scalp
antithrombin III *Thrombate III*	Coagulation inhibitor Treatment of patients with hereditary antithrombin III deficiency in connection with surgical or obstetric procedures or when they have thromboembolism Replacement therapy in congenital antithrombin III deficiency

Dosages and special alerts

25–50 mg/day PO with the main meal. Pregnancy category X. Numerous adverse effects. Stop drug when lesions resolve. Do not crush capsules. Do not allow patient to donate blood. Monitor vision periodically; protect patient from sun exposure.

> 60 kg: 400 mg PO bid with meals for 8–30 days.< 60 kg: 15 mg/kg/day divided bid PO for 8–30 days.

> 60 kg: 400 mg PO bid with meals for 28 days, then 14 drug-free days, repeat for 3 cycles.< 60 kg: 15 mg/kg/day divided bid PO following the same cycle. Avoid using during pregnancy; GI upset, nausea and vomiting common; use analgesics to relieve headache.

7.5 mg as an IV bolus once a week or 15 mg IM given once a week; recommended course is 12 weekly injections. An additional 12-wk course may be initiated if CD4+ T lymphocytes are within normal range and 12 wk have passed since first course. Patient has increased risk of infection; monitor closely.

3 mg/day as a 2-hr IV infusion, increase up to 30 mg/day as a 2-hr infusion 3 times weekly, every other day for 12 wk. Premedicate with diphenhydramine and acetaminophen; ensure that patient is well hydrated; use of prophylactic antibiotic and antiviral therapy may be used to prevent serious infections.

60 U/kg IV over 1–2 hr. Repeat every 2–4 wk; may attempt to decrease dosage every 3–6 mo.

60 mg/kg IV once a week to achieve functional levels of alpha1-proteinase inhibitor in lower respiratory tract. Monitor for possible hepatitis related to use of human blood products.

910 mg/m^2 IV daily as a 15-min infusion. Start within 30 min of starting chemotherapy. Monitor BP carefully; severe hypotension has been reported.

Must be applied in timing with blue light photodynamic illuminator; clean and dry area to be treated, break ampule and apply solution with applicator provided. Light treatment must be done within the next 14–18 hr. One application of solution and one dose illumination per treatment site per 8-wk treatment session.

Dosage units = desired antithrombin level (%)—baseline ATIII level (%) × body weight divided by 1.4 q 2–8 day. Dosage varies greatly; frequent blood tests are needed.

(continued)

Generic and trade names	Drug class and indications
argatroban *Argatroban*	Anticoagulant Prophylaxis or treatment of thrombosis in heparin-induced thrombocytopenia; as an anticoagulant in patients at risk of heparin-induced thrombocytopenia undergoing percutaneous coronary intervention (PCI)
arsenic trioxide *Trisenox*	Antineoplastic Induction and remission of PML in patients refractory to retinoid or anthracycline chemotherapy and whose leukemia is characterized by t(15;17) translocation or PML/RAR-alpha gene expression
basiliximab *Simulect*	Immunosuppressive; monoclonal antibody Prophylaxis of acute rejection in renal transplant patients in combination with cyclosporine and corticosteroids
BCG intravesical *Pacis* *TheraCys* *Tice BCG*	Antineoplastic Treatment and prophylaxis for carcinoma in situ of the urinary bladder; prophylaxis of primary or recurrent Ta and T1 papillary tumors following TUR; administered intravesically only
betaine anhydrous *Cystadane*	Homocysteine reducer Treatment of homocystinuria to decrease homocysteine levels, mostly seen in children with genetic deficiencies
bexarotene *Targretin*	Antineoplastic Treatment of the cutaneous manifestations of cutaneous T-cell lymphoma in patients refractory to at least one other systemic therapy
bicalutamide *Casodex*	Antiandrogen Treatment of advanced prostatic carcinoma in combination with LHRH analogue
bivalirudin *Angiomax*	Anticoagulant, thrombin inhibitor Anticoagulation of patients undergoing percutaneous transluminal angioplasty who have unstable angina
botulinum toxin type B *Myobloc*	Skeletal muscle relaxant, direct acting Reduction of the severity of abnormal head position and neck pain associated with cervical dystonia
bretylium *Bretylate* (CAN)	Antiarrhythmic Adrenergic neuron blocker Prevention and treatment of ventricular fibrillation Treatment of serious ventricular arrhythmias resistant to other treatment

Dosages and special alerts

Dilute to concentration of 1 mg/mL; administer 2 mcg/kg/min as a continuous infusion. Monitor aPTT, usually achieves desired level within 1–3 hr; adjust dose of infusion to maintain a steady state aPPT that is 1.5–3 times the initial baseline value; do not exceed 10 mcg/kg/hr. Reduce initial dose to 0.05 mg/kg/min with hepatic impairment. With PCI—25 mcg/kg/min with a bolus of 350 mcg/kg over 3–5 min. Excessive bleeding and hemorrhage may occur; monitor patient carefully for any sign of excess bleeding, decrease infusion rate or stop drug if excessive bleeding occurs.

Induction: 0.15 mg/kg/day IV until bone marrow remission (maximum, 60 doses).Consolidation: 0.15 mg/kg/day IV starting 3–6 wk after completion of induction (maximum, 25 doses over 5 wk).Cardiac and CNS toxicity common; baseline and weekly ECG; biweekly electrolytes, CBC with differential and clotting profiles advised.
Avoid seafood and many alternative therapies (arsenic in many of these). Advise patient to avoid pregnancy, driving, or dangerous activities. Drug can be very toxic and carcinogenic.

2 doses of 20 mg IV with the first dose 2 hr before transplant, then 4 days after transplant. Must be given in combination with other immunosuppressant drugs. GI effects common.

Do not drink fluids for 4 hr before treatment; empty bladder before treatment. Instill 1 ampule, diluted as indicated in saline solution by catheter, allow to flow slowly; have patient lie down for first hour, turning side to side, then stay upright for 1 hr; try to retain solution for 2 hr; void retained solution trying not to splash liquid. Increase fluid intake for next few days. Monitor patient for local discomfort and reactions. Monitor for bone marrow depression and infection.

6 g/day PO in divided doses of 3 g bid. Up to 20 g/day may be required. In patients < 3 yr, may start at 100 mg/kg/day and increase weekly in 100-mg/kg/day increments. Regular blood tests are needed to monitor homocysteine levels. May cause GI upset.

300 mg/m^2 PO daily, may be increased to 400 mg/m^2 PO daily; pregnancy category X; risk of serious pancreatitis, photosensitivity.

50 mg/day PO at the same time each day. Monitor liver function regularly. Administer only with LHRH analogue.

1 mg/kg IV bolus then 2.5 mg/kg/hr IV infusion over 4 hr; begin just before PCTA procedure; may then give 0.2 mg/kg/hr IV infusion for up to 20 hr. Reduce dosage with renal dysfunction. Give with aspirin. Monitor for excessive bleeding, which would indicate need to discontinue drug.

2,500–5,000 units IM, injected locally into affected muscles. Blocks cholinergic transmission between the nerve and muscle. Monitor for lack of muscle function, infection at injection site.

Immediate life-threatening ventricular arrythmias—Adults: 5 mg/kg (undiluted) IV. Increase to 10 mg/kg and repeat as needed. Maintenance, 1-2 mg/min diluted solution via IV infusion, or 5–10 mg/kg diluted solution over > 8 min q 6 hr. Children: 5 mg/kg IV then 10 mg/kg q 15–30 min, maximum, 30 mg/kg. Other ventricular arrhythmias—Adults: 5–10 mg/kg IV infusion over > 8 min. Repeat q 1–2 hr. May repeat q 6 hr for maintenance or continuous infusion of 1–2 mg/min. Or, 5–10 mg/kg undiluted solution IM, repeat q 1–2 hr, as needed. Children: 5–10 mg/kg/dose q 6 hr. Monitor cardiac rhythm and blood pressure continually keep patient supine during infusion; monitor for safe and effective serum levels—0.5–1.5 mcg/mL.

(continued)

Generic and trade names	Drug class and indications
cabergoline *Dostinex*	Dopamine receptor agonist Treatment of hyperprolactinemia disorders
caspofungin acetate *Cancidas*	Echinocandin antifungal Treatment of invasive aspergillosis in patients unresponsive to or who cannot tolerate standard therapy
cetrorelix acetate *Cetrotide*	Fertility drug Inhibition of premature LH surges in women undergoing controlled ovarian stimulation
cevimeline HCL *Evoxac*	Parasympathomimetic Treatment of symptoms of dry mouth in patients with Sjorgen's syndrome
chenodiol *Chenix*	Gallstone solubilizer Treatment of selected patients with radiolucent gallstones in well-opacifying gallbladders when elective surgery is contraindicated
chorionic gonadotropin alfa (recombinant) *Ovidrel*	Fertility drug Induction of ovulation in infertile females who have been pretreated with FSH Induction of final follicular maturation and early luteinization in infertile women who have undergone pituitary desensitization and who have been appropriately pretreated with follicle-stimulating hormones.
chymopapain *Chymodiactin*	Enzyme Treatment of hernitated lumbar intervertebral disks unresponsive to conservative therapy
clofazimine *Lamprene*	Leprostatic Treatment of leprematous leprosy including dapsone-resistant Part of combination therapy in initial treatment of multibacillary leprosy to prevent development of drug-resistant strains
coagulation factor VIIa (recombinant) *NovoSeven*	Antihemophilic Treatment of bleeding episodes in hemophilia A or B patients with inhibitors to Factor VIII or Factor IX
cosyntropin *Cortrosyn* *Synacthen Depot* (CAN)	Diagnostic agent Diagnostic tests of adrenal function
cysteamine bitartrate *Cystagon*	Urinary tract agent Treatment of adults and children with nephropathic cystinosis, an inherited defect of lysosomal transport
daclizumab *Zenapax*	Immunosuppressive monoclonal antibody Prophylaxis of acute rejection in renal transplant patients in combination with cyclosporine and corticosteroids

Dosages and special alerts

0.25 mg PO 2 times per week with a maximum dose of 1 mg 2 times per week. Base dose on target prolactin levels of <20 mcg/L for women and <15 mcg/L for men. Patients should use contraceptives. Orthostatic hypotension is a common adverse effect; monitor patient closely.

Daily IV infusion of 50 mg/day preceded by 75 mg loading dose IV for up to 7 days. Monitor for IV complications. Use with cyclosporin is not recommended.

3 mg SC given when serum estradiol levels show appropriate stimulation, given with gonadotropins; if HCG is not given within 4 days, continue giving 0.25 mg/day SC until HCG is given or 0.25 mg SC morning or evening of stimulation day 5, or morning of stimulation day 6, continue daily until HCG is given. Patient or significant other should learn to give SC injections using the proper technique. Given only as part of overall fertility program.

30 mg PO tid; administer with food if GI upset is severe; monitoring swallowing; monitor patient for dehydration and provide supportive therapy.

13–16 mg/kg/day in 2 doses, AM and PM. Start with 250 mg PO bid for 2 wk, then increase by 250 mg/day each week. Monitor liver function carefully. Discontinue if hepatitis occurs; caution patient to use barrier contraceptives and avoid pregnancy.

250 mcg SC given 1 day following the last dose of a follicle-stimulating agent. Administer only when adequate follicular development has occurred. Do not administer if there is an excessive ovarian response. Inject into stomach area. Alert patient to risk of multiple births; patient should report shortness of breath, sudden abdominal pain, nausea, vomiting.

2–4 nKat units/disk injected by physician skilled in this technique. To be used only in hospital setting with emergency equipment available. CNS adverse effects are common.

100 mg/day PO with other drugs for 2–3 yr, then use same dose for monotherapy. If dapsone-resistant, give with other antileprosy drug. Protect drug from moisture and heat; always give with meals. Alert patient that tears, sputum, sweat, and urine may be discolored. Skin will darken, may be reversible in months to years after drug discontinued.

90 mcg/kg as an IV bolus q2hr until hemostasis is achieved; continue dosing at 3- to 6-hr intervals after hemostasis in severe bleeds. Monitor for early signs of hypersensitivity reactions (hives, wheezing, hypotension, anaphylaxis).

0.25–0.75 mg IV or IM or as an IV infusion of 0.04 mg/hr. Monitor for seizures, anaphylactoid reactions, excessive adrenal effects. Monitor plasma and urinary corticosteroid levels to determine adrenal function.

Initial dose 1/4 to 1/6 of maintenance dose increased slowly over 4–6 wk. Maintenance dose for patients > 12 yr and weighing > 50 kg is 2 g/day PO in 4 divided doses. For children < 12 yr, 1.3 g/m2/day PO in 4 divided doses. Obtain leukocyte cysteine measurements 3–6 hr after first dose and then at 2-wk intervals; progress to q 3 mo. Monitor for seizures, GI intolerance; monitor liver function.

1 mg/kg IV—5 doses, with the first dose within 24 hr of transplant, last doses within 14 days. Protect patient from infections and invasive procedures; GI effects common.

(continued)

Generic and trade names	Drug class and indications
dapsone *Avlosulfon* (CAN)	Leprostatic Treatment of Hansen's disease Treatment of dermatitis herpetiformis
deferoxamine mesylate *Desferal*	Chelating agent Treatment of acute iron toxicity and chronic iron overload
denileukin diftitox *Ontak*	Biological protein Treatment of cutaneous T-cell lymphoma in patients whose cells express the CD25 component of the IG-2-receptor
dexmedetomidine hydrochloride *Precedex*	Sedative and hypnotic Sedation of initially intubated and mechanically ventilated patients during treatment in an ICU setting
dimercaprol *BAL in Oil*	Antidote; chelating agent Treatment of arsenic, gold, mercury poisoning Treatment of acute lead poisoning when used with calcium edetate disodium Treatment of acute mercury poisoning if used within the first 1–2 hr
doxercalciferol *Hectorol*	Vitamin D analogue Reduction of elevated intact parathyroid hormone (iPTH) levels in the management of secondary hyperparathyroidism in patients undergoing chronic renal dialysis
epoprostenol sodium prostacyclin, PGX, PGI_2 *Flolan*	Prostaglandin Treatment of primary pulmonary hypertension in patients unresponsive to standard therapy
exemestane *Aromasin*	Antineoplastic Treatment of advanced breast cancer in postmenopausal women whose disease has progressed following tamoxifen therapy
follitropin alfa *Gonal-F*	Fertility drug Induction of ovulation, stimulation, and development of multiple follicles for in vitro fertilization Also used to increase spermatogenesis in men with hypogonadism
follitropin beta *Follistim* *Puregon* (CAN)	Fertility drug Induction of ovulation, stimulation, and development of multiple follicles for in vitro fertilization

Dosages and special alerts

50–100 mg/day PO (leprosy). 50 mg/day PO (dermatitis herpetiformis), 50–300 mg/day has been used. Children should not receive >100 mg/day. Monitor patients for bone marrow suppression and for the development of resistance if relapse occurs; give with food to decrease GI upset. Will need to be used for prolonged time.

Acute toxicity: 1 g IM or IV, followed by 0.5 g q 4 hr for 2 doses, then q 4–12 hr based on patient response. Chronic overload: 0.5–1 g IM qid; 2 g IV with each unit of blood or 20-40 mg/kg/day as a continuous SC infusion over 8 to 24 hr. IM preferred for acute intoxication; slow IV infusion. Monitor serum iron levels. Note that injection can be very painful.

Adults: 9 or 18 mcg/kg/day IV over ≥ 15 min for 5 consecutive days every 21 days. Severe hypersensitivity reactions may occur. Monitor for capillary leak syndrome.

1 mcg/kg infused over 10 min, then 0.2–0.7 mcg/kg/hr using a controlled infusion device for ≤ 24 hr; drug is not indicated for use > 24 hr.

2.5–5 mg/kg IM qid for 2 days, taper to bid for 10 days. Can cause severe renal damage; alkalinize urine to increase chelated complex excretion; use extreme caution with children.

Adults: 10 mcg 3 times per week at dialysis. Maximum, 20 mcg 3 times per week. Regulate dose by iPTH levels. Monitor carefully for hypercalcemia (arrhythmias, seizures, calcifications).

2 ng/kg/min with increases in increments of 2 ng/kg as tolerated using a portable infusion pump through a central venous catheter; 20–40 ng/kg/min common dosage after 6 mo of continuous therapy. Teach patient and significant other the proper maintenance and use of infusion pump, ensure that therapy is continuous. Headache, muscle aches, and pains are common.

25 mg PO every day with meals. May be antagonized by estrogens. Avoid use premenopause or with renal or hepatic dysfunction. Hot flashes, GI upset, anxiety, depression, headache are common.

Ovulation induction: 75 IU/day SC, increase by 37.5 IU/day after 14 days; may increase again after 7 days; do not exceed 35 days of treatment. Follicle development: 150 IU/day SC of days 2 or 3 and continue for 10 days. In patients whose endogenous gonadotropin levels are suppressed, initiate at 225 IU/day SC. Adjust dose after 5 days based on patient response; dosage should be adjusted no more than q 3–5 days and by no more than 75–150 IU at each adjustment. Maximum, 450 IU/day; then give 5,000–10,000 units HCG. Spermatogenesis: 150 IU SC 3 times per week in conjunction with HCG. May increase to 300 IU 3 times per week, as needed. May administer up to 18 mo for adequate effect. Pregnancy category X; explain risk of multiple births; risk of arterial thromboembolism.

Ovulation induction: 75 IU/day SC, increase by 37.5 IU/day after 14 days; do not exceed 35 days of treatment. Follicle development: 150–225 IU/day SC or IM for at least 4 days of treatment. Adjust dose based on ovarian response; then give 5,000–10,000 IU. HCG: maintenance dosage of 375–600 IU/day SC or IM may be necessary. Pregnancy category X. Give SC in navel or abdomen. Warn patients of risk of multiple births.

(continued)

Generic and trade names	Drug class and indications
fomepizole *Antizol*	Antidote Antidote for antifreeze (ethylene glycol) poisoning or for use in suspected poisoning Antidote for methanol poisoning
ganirelix acetate *Antagon*	Fertility drug Inhibition of premature LH surges in women undergoing controlled ovarian overstimulation as part of a fertility program
gemtuzumab ozogamicin *Mylotarg*	Monoclonal antibody Treatment of CD33-positive AML in the first relapse in patients ≥ 60 yr who are not candidates for cytotoxic chemotherapy
gonadorelin hydrochloride *Factrel*	Diagnostic agent Evaluation of functional capacity and response of the gonadotropes of the anterior pituitary Testing for suspected gonadotropin deficiency Evaluating residual activity following pituitary removal or irradiation
griseofulvin *Fulvicin* *Grifulvin* *Gris-PEG*	Antifungal drug Treatment of ringworm infections
hylan G-F 20 *Synvisc*	Hyaluronic acid derivative Treatment of pain in osteoarthritis of the knee in patients who have failed to respond to conservative therapy
ibritumomab *Zevalin*	Monoclonal antibody Treatment of patients with relapsed or refractory low-grade follicular transformed B-cell non-Hodgkin's lymphoma
infliximab *Remicade*	Monoclonal antibody To reduce the signs and symptoms of moderate to severe Crohn's disease in patients who do not adequately respond to conventional therapy, monoclonal antibody to tumor necrosis factor-alpha Treatment of rheumatoid arthritis together with methotrexate in patients who failed on methotrexate alone Treatment of patients with fistulizing Crohn's disease
interferon alfa-n3 *Alferon N*	Interferon Treatment of phase I/II ARC, AIDS, asymptomatic AIDS
Alferon LDO	Antineoplastic Treatment of condylomata acummata (vaginal and genital warts)
iron sucrose *Venofer*	Iron salt Treatment of iron deficiency anemia in patients undergoing chronic hemodialysis who are receiving supplemental erythropoetin therapy

Dosages and special alerts

15 mg/kg loading dose followed by doses of 10 mg/kg q 12 hr for 12 doses given as a slow IV infusion over 30 min. Start immediately after diagnosis is made. Headache, nausea, and dizziness are common. Consider hemodialysis as added therapy.

250 mcg SC once daily starting on day 2 or 3 of the cycle. Pregnancy category X. Teach patient to administer SC injections. Abdominal pain is a common adverse effect.

9 mg/m2 IV over 2 hr for a total of 2 doses given 14 days apart. Administer diphenhydramine, acetaminophen before each dose. Ensure patient is hydrated; GI problems, fever common. Protect patient from infection. Monitor vital signs for 4 hr following infusion.

100 mg SC or IV; in females, perform test days 1–7 of the menstrual cycle; have patient report any difficulty breathing.

Adults: Single or divided dose of 500 mg (330–375 mg ultramicrosize) for tinea corporis cruris (treat for 2–4 wk), capitis (treat for 4–6 wk), 0.75–1 g/day PO (660–750 ultramicrosize) in divided doses for tinea pedis, unguium. Pediatric patients ≥ 2 yr: 11 mg/kg/day PO or 7.3 mg/kg/day ultramicrosize. Verify cause of infection before use. Not effective in bacterial infections. Photosensitivity, lupuslike syndrome may occur. Monitor for allergic reactions, cross-sensitivity to penicillin. Women should avoid pregnancy; men should wait ≥ 6 mo after therapy before fathering a child.

2 mL by intra-articular injection once per week for 3 wk. Do not use in patients with known hypersensitivity to chicken products. Do not use in any other joint or in severely inflamed joint.

Single infusion of 250 mg/m^2 rituximab preceding a fixed dose of 0.4 mCi/kg Zevalin as a 10-min IV push. Premedicate with acetaminophen and diphenhydramine before each rituximab infusion. Monitor for severe cytopenia.

5 mg/kg IV over 2 hr given once (Crohn's disease). May repeat dose with fistulating disease at 2 wk and 6 wk after first dose. 3 mg/kg IV followed by 3 mg/kg at 2 and 6 wk, then every 8 wk (RA). Do not use in patients with allergy to mouse protein; discontinue if lupus-like reaction occurs.

Investigational drug with this indication, orphan drug status.
100 mg (5 mL) IV, 1–3 times per week, during dialysis. Administer slowly, 1 mL over 1 min. Serious to fatal hypersensitivity reactions have occurred. Administer test dose and monitor patient carefully during administration.

0.05 mL per wart 2 times per week for 8 wk.

100 mg (5mL) IV, 1–3 times per week, during dialysis. Administer slowly, 1 mL over 1 min. Serious to fatal hypersensitivity reaction have occurred. Administer test dose and monitor patient carefully during administration.

(continued)

Generic and trade names	Drug class and indications
isocarboxazid *Marplan*	Monoamine oxidase inhibitor (MAOI) Treatment of depression (not a first choice for initial treatment)
ivermectin *Stromectol*	Anthelmintic Treatment of intestinal strongyloidiasis Treatment of onchocerciasis
lepirudin *Refludan*	Anticoagulant Treatment of heparin-induced thrombocytopenia associated with thromboembolic disease; a rare allergic reaction to heparin; directly inhibits thrombin.
levamisole HCl *Ergamisol*	Antineoplastic Adjunctive treatment in combination with fluorouracil after surgical resection in patients with Dukes' Stage C colon cancer
L-hyoscyamine sulfate *Anaspaz* *Levsin* *Cystospaz* *Gastrosed*	Anticholinergic and antispasmodic Treatment of functional GI disorders, irritable bowel syndrome, infant colic, pancreatitis
mesna *Mesnex*	Cytoprotective agent Prophylaxis to reduce the incidence of ifosfamide-induced hemorrhagic cystitis Unlabeled use: Reduction of the incidence of cyclophosphamide-induced hemorrhagic cystitis
methoxsalen *Oxsoralen-Ultra* *Uvadex*	Psorlen Symptomatic treatment of severe disabling psoriasis refractory to other forms of therapy; repigmentation of vitiliginous skin Treatment of cutaneous cell lymphoma Unlabeled use: with UVAR, treatment of mycosisfungoides Orphan drug use: with UVAR photophoresis to treat diffuse systemic sclerosis; prevention of acute rejection of cardiac allografts
metyrosine *Demser*	Enzyme inhibitor Preoperative preparation for surgery for pheochromocytoma Management of pheochromocytoma when surgery is contraindicated Chronic treatment of malignant pheochromocytoma
monoctanoin *Moctanin*	Gallstone solubilizer Dissolution of cholesterol gallstones retained in the biliary tract after cholecystectomy when other means of stone removal are unsuccessful or contraindicated Orphan drug use: dissolution of cholesterol gallstones in the common duct

Dosages and special alerts

Up to 40 mg PO daily. Dosage can usually be reduced after 3–4 wk because drug effects are cumulative. Not a first-line treatment for depression because of potential for serious side effects and food interactions. Might be useful in patients unable to tolerate newer and safer antidepressants. Patient must be given list of tyramine-containing foods.

Strongyloidiasis: 200 mcg/kg PO as a single dose. Oonchocerciasis: 150 mcg/kg PO as a single dose may be repeated in 3–12 mo if needed. Give with a full glass of water. Nausea and vomiting very common. Instruct patient to use barrier contraceptives while on this drug.

0.4 mg/kg initial IV bolus followed by a continuous infusion of 0.15 mg/kg for 2–10 days. Monitor for bleeding from any sites; watch for hepatic injury. Reduce dosage with renal failure. Increased risk of bleeding if combined with chamomile, garlic, ginger, ginkgo, and ginseng therapy.

Initial therapy is 50 mg PO q 8 hr for 3 days starting 7–30 days after surgery with fluorouracil 450 mg/m^2/day IV for 5 days. Maintenance is 50 mg PO q 8 hr for 3 days q 2 wk with fluorouracil 450 mg/m^2/day IV once a week beginning 28 days after first course. GI upset common. Monitor patient for bone marrow depression. Avoid exposure to infection.

Adults: 0.125–0.25 mg PO or SL tid or qid; determine pediatric dosage based on weight. May cause dry mouth, dizziness, blurred vision.

20% ifosfamide dose IV at the time of ifosfamide injection and at 4 and 8 hr after that. Timing needs to be exact. Monitor for any signs of bladder hemorrhage.

Oral: Dosage varies with weight; dosing must be timed to coincide with ultraviolet (UV) light exposure. Do not expose patient to additional UV light. GI effects are very common.

250–500 mg PO qid. Preoperative: 2–3 g/day PO for 5–7 days. Maximum, 4 g/day. Ensure a liberal intake of fluids. Severe diarrhea may occur; use antidiarrheals if needed.

3–5 mL/hr continually via a perfusion pump at a pressure of 10 cm water in the common bile duct for 7–21 days. Monitor liver function carefully; monitor for allergic reaction. Must be given under strict medical supervision.

(continued)

Generic and trade names	Drug class and indications
nitisinone *Orfadin*	Tyrosine catabolism inhibitor Adjunct to dietary restriction of tyrosine and phenylalanine in the treatment of children with hereditary tyrosinemia type 1
nitazoxanide *Alinia*	Antiprotozoal Treatment of diarrhea caused by *Cryptosporidium parvum* or *Giardia lamblia* in pediatric patients 1–11 yr
oprelvekin *Neumega*	Interleukin Prevention of severe thrombocytopenia and reduction of platelet transfusions following myelosuppressive chemotherapy in patients with non-myeloid malignancies at high risk to develop severe thrombocytopenia
oxaliplatin *Eloxatin*	Antineoplastic Treatment of patients with metastatic carcinoma of the colon or rectum whose disease has progressed during or within 6 mo of completion of first-line therapy with 5-FU/LV and irinotecan
paricalcitol *Zemplar*	Vitamin Prevention and treatment of secondary hyperparathyroidism associated with chronic renal failure
pegaspargase *Oncaspar*	Antineoplastic Treatment of ALL in patients hypersensitive to native forms of L-asparaginase
peginterferon alfa-2b *Peg-Intron*	Interferon Treatment of patients > 18 yr with chronic hepatitis C, who have not received alpha interferon and who have compensated liver function Unlabeled use: renal carcinoma
pentosan polysulfate sodium *Elmiron*	Bladder protectant Relief of bladder pain associated with interstitial cystitis
pentostatin *Nipent* 2′ deoxycoformycin (DCF)	Antineoplastic Antibiotic Treatment of adults with alpha interferon refractory hairy cell leukemia, CLL, cutaneous T-cell lymphoma, peripheral T-cell lymphoma
pilocarpine hydrochloride *Salagen*	Parasympathomimetic Mouth and throat product Treatment of symptoms of xerostomia from salivary gland dysfunction caused by radiation therapy for cancer of the head and neck
pimozide *Orap*	Antipsychotic diphenylbutylpiperidine Suppression of severely compromising motor or phonic tics in patients with Tourette's syndrome who have not responded to other therapy

Dosages and special alerts

1 mg/kg/day PO divided into morning and evening doses. Monitor plasma tyrosine levels carefully. Slit lamp eye exams should be done prior to and periodically during therapy. Monitor CBC for bone marrow suppression, provide appropriate supportive therapy.

12–47 mo: 5 mL (100 mg nitazoxanide) PO q 12 hr for 3 days. 4–11 yr: 10 mL (200 mg nitazoxanide) PO q 12 hr for 3 days. Obtain stool for O & P testing before beginning therapy. To reconstitute, tap bottle until all powder flows freely; add approximately 24 mL of water to bottle and shake vigorously to suspend powder; add remaining 24 mL of water and shake vigorously again. Use cautiously with diabetic patients; suspension contains sucrose. Give drug with food. Advise parents to use good hand-washing technique and to dispose of diapers properly, when appropriate.

50 mcg/kg/day SC starting 1 day after chemotherapy and continuing for 14–21 days or until platelet count is ≥ 50,000 cells/mg. Protect patient from exposure to infection; urge the use of contraceptives.

85 mg/m^2 IV infusion in 250–500 mL D$_5$W with leucovorin 200 mg/m^2 in D$_5$W both given over 2 hr followed by 5-FU 400 mg/m^2 IV bolus over 2–4 min, followed by 5-FU 600 mg/m^2 IV infusion in 500 mL D$_5$W as a 22-hr continuous infusion on day one, then leucovorin 200 mg/m^2 IV infusion over 2 hr followed by 5-FU 400 mg/m^2 bolus given over 2–4 min, followed by 5-FU 600 mg/m^2 IV infusion in 500 mL D$_5$W as a 22-hr continuous infusion on day 2; repeat cycle every 2 wk. Premedicate with antiemetics and dexamethasone. Monitor for potentially dangerous anaphylactic reactions.

0.04–0.1 mcg/kg injected during dialysis, not more often than every other day. Monitor for hypercalcemia, treat appropriately. Ensure adherence to dietary regimen and use of calcium supplements.

2,500 IU/m^2 IM or IV q 14 days. < 0.6 m^2: 825 IU/kg IM or IV q 14 days. Associated with pancreatitis, bone marrow depression, and renal toxicity. Monitor patient closely. Save IV use for extreme situations; IM use preferred.

1 mcg/kg SC once per week for 1 yr; flulike symptoms common. Monitor bone marrow and liver function.

100 mg PO tid on an empty stomach. May cause loss of hair (suggest wig); increased bleeding (is a low-molecular-weight heparin).

4 mg/m^2 IV every other week, decrease to 2 mg/m^2 with renal impairment. Associated with fatal pulmonary toxicity and bone marrow depression. Hydrate patient before each dose and monitor closely.

5–10 mg PO tid. Can cause blurred vision, parasympathomimetic effects. Monitor susceptible patients carefully.

1–2 mg/day PO; up to a maximum of 10 mg/day. Monitor for prolonged QTc interval. Has been associated with severe cardiac complications; may cause dizziness, sedation, Parkinson-like symptoms.

(continued)

Generic and trade names	Drug class and indications
porfimer sodium *Photofrin*	Antineoplastic Photodynamic therapy for palliation of patients with complete or partially obstructing esophageal cancer or transitional cancer who cannot be treated with laser alone, transitional cell carcinoma in situ of urinary bladder, endobronchial non–small-cell lung cancer
praziquantel *Biltricide*	Anthelmintic Treatment of Schistosoma infections, liver flukes Orphan drug use: treatment of neurocysticercosis
procarbazine *Matulane* *Natulan* (CAN)	Antineoplastic Used in combination with other antineoplastics for treatment of stage II and IV Hodgkin's disease (part of MOPP).
rasburicase *Elitek*	Enzyme Initial management of plasma uric acid levels in pediatric patients with leukemia, lymphoma, and solid tumor malignancies who are receiving anti-cancer therapy expected to result in tumor lysis and subsequent elevation of plasma uric acid
rifabutin *Mycobutin*	Antibiotic Prevention and treatment of disseminated Mycobacterium avium complex (MAC) disease in patients with advanced HIV infection
riluzole *Rilutek*	ALS agent Treatment of ALS; extends survival time or time to tracheostomy Orphan drug use: Treatment of Huntington's disease
ritodrine hydrochloride *Yutopar*	Sympathomimetic, tocolytic drug Management of preterm labor in select patients ≥ 20 wk gestation
rituximab *Rituxan*	Antineoplastic Monoclonal antibody Treatment of relapsed or refractory, low-grade or follicular CD20-positive non-Hodgkin's B cell lymphoma
sacrosidase *Sucraid*	Enzyme Oral replacement of genetically determined sucrase deficiency
secretin *SecreFlo*	Diagnostic agent Stimulation of pancreatic secretions to aid in the diagnosis of pancreatic exocrine dysfunction Stimulation of gastrin secretion to aid in the diagnosis of gastrinoma
sermorelin acetate *Geref* *GHRH*	Hormone Treatment of idiopathic growth hormone deficiency in children with growth failure who are prepubescent with a bone age of 7.5 yr (F) or 8 yr (M), AIDS-associated catabolism or weight loss, adjunct to gonadotropin for ovulation induction

Dosages and special alerts

2 mg/kg IV given as a slow injection over 3–5 min; must be followed in 40–50 hr and again in 96–120 hr by laser therapy. Monitor for pleural effusion and respiratory complications. Avoid any contact with the drug. Protect patient from exposure to light for 30 days after treatment.

3 doses of 20 mg/kg PO as a one-day treatment; allow 4–6 hr between doses. Administer with food. Do not cut, crush, or chew tablets; swallow whole. GI upset is common.

2–4 mg/kg/day PO for first week, then 4–6 mg/kg/day PO. Maintenance dosage is 1–2 mg/kg/day. Monitor bone marrow and adjust dosage accordingly, stress need for barrier contraceptives; advise patient to avoid alcohol and foods high in tyramine.

0.15 or 0.2 mg/kg IV as a single daily infusion over 30 min for 5 days. Chemotherapy should be started 4–24 hr after the first dose. Blood drawn to monitor uric acid levels must be collected in prechilled, heparinized vials and kept in an ice-water bath. Analysis must be done within 4 hr.

Adults: 300 mg PO daily. Children: 5 mg/kg/day. GI effects, bone marrow depression common. Body fluids turn a reddish-orange; contact lenses may be stained. Do not use with active TB.

50 mg PO q 12 hr. Slows disease, does not cure it. Take on an empty stomach at the same time each day. Protect drug from light. Often causes nausea and vomiting.

0.05 mg/min IV, gradually increase by 0.05 mg/min every 10 min until desired result is attained; usual effective dose between 0.15 and 0.35 mg/min continued for at least 12 hr after uterine contractions cease; monitor maternal pulse and R closely. P > 140/min or R >20 /min may be signs of impending pulmonary edema. Maintain patient in left lateral position during infusion; avoid fluid overload; avoid use of corticosteroids, potentially fatal pulmonary edema has occurred with this combination

Adults: 375 mg/m^2 IV, once weekly for 4 doses. Premedicate patient with acetaminophen and diphenhydramine to decrease fever, chills associated with infusion. Protect patient from exposure to infection.

≤ 15 kg: 1 mL or 22 drops per meal or snack. >15 kg: 2 ml or 44 drops per meal or snack. Do not use in patients with known allergy to yeast. Refrigerate bottle; discard 4 wk after opening.

0.2–0.4 mcg/kg IV over 1 min.

30 mcg/kg/day SC hs. Discontinue when epiphyses close. Monitor for hypothyroidism. Evaluate bone growth regularly.

(continued)

Generic and trade names	Drug class and indications
sevelamer hydrochloride *Renagel*	Calcium-phosphate binder Reduction of serum phosphorus levels in hemodialysis patients in end-stage renal disease
sodium ferric gluconate complex *Ferrlecit*	Iron product Treatment of iron deficiency in patients undergoing chronic hemodialysis who are also receiving erythropoietin therapy
sodium hyaluronate *Hyalgan*	Hyaluronic acid derivative Treatment of pain in osteoarthritis of the knee in patients who have failed to respond to conservative therapy and analgesics
stanozolol *Winstrol*	Anabolic steroid, hormone Prophylactic use to decrease the frequency and severity of hereditary angioedema attacks
streptomycin sulfate (generic only)	Antibiotic Fourth drug in the treatment of TB Treatment of tularemia, plague SBE (if less toxic agents are not appropriate)
temozolomide *Temodar*	Antineoplastic Treatment of refractory astrocytoma in patients at first relapse with disease progression on a drug regimen including a nitrosourea and procarbazine; treatment of advanced metastatic melanoma
thalidomide *Thalomid*	Immune modulator Treatment of erythema nodosum leprosum—painful inflammatory condition related to an immune reaction to dead bacteria following treatment of leprosy; multiple myeloma; brain tumors; Crohn's disease; HIV-wasting syndrome; graft-host reaction in bone marrow transplant
tiludronate disodium *Skelid*	Bisphosphonate Treatment of Paget's disease in patients with alkaline phosphatase at least 2 times the upper limit, who are asymptomatic and at risk for future complications
tiopronin *Thiola*	Thiol compound Prevention of cystine kidney stone formation in patients with severe homozygous cystinuria with urine cystine levels > 500 mg/day who are resistant to other therapy
tolazoline hydrochloride *Priscoline*	Vasodilator Antihypertensive Treatment of persistent pulmonary hypertension of the newborn when systemic arterial oxygenation cannot be maintained by the usual methods
topotecan hydrochloride *Hycamtin*	Antineoplastic Treatment of metastatic ovarian cancer after failure of traditional chemotherapy Treatment of small-cell lung cancer after failure of first-line treatment

Dosages and special alerts

4–5 capsules with each meal; may be increased by 1 capsule per meal to achieve desired serum phosphorus level. Does not cause increase in calcium levels.

Test dose: 2 mL diluted in 50 mL 0.9% sodium chloride for injection, given IV over 60 min. Adults: 10 mL diluted in 100 mL 0.9% sodium chloride for injection given IV over 60 min. Most patients will initially require 8 doses given at sequential dialysis sessions, then periodic use based on hematocrit. Flushing and hypertension are common effects.

2 mL by intra-articular injection once a week for 5 wk. Do not use in any other joint; remove effusions. Before injection, use strict aseptic technique. Avoid any weight bearing after injection.

2 mg PO tid, with favorable response, decrease dose to 2 mg/day over 1–3 mo. Pregnancy category X. Monitor liver function, cholesterol level and blood glucose levels regularly during therapy. Monitor long-bone x-rays of children every 3–6 mo; discontinue well before the bone age reaches the norm for patient's age.

Adults: 15 mg/kg/day IM, or 25–30 mg/kg IM 2 or 3 times a week. Pediatric patients: 20–40 mg/kg/day IM or 25–30 mg/kg/IM 2 or 3 times a week. Tularemia: 1–2 g/day IM for 7–14 days. Plague: 2 g/day IM in two divided doses for at least 10 days. Tinnitus, dizziness, ringing in the ears, hearing loss common. Monitor patient for renal toxicity; injection site infections.

PO: Dose is based on body surface area. Taken for 5 consecutive days for a 28-day treatment cycle. Adjusted dose is based on neutrophil and platelet counts. Monitor bone marrow function closely. Especially toxic in women and the elderly.

100–300 mg/day PO. Taken once daily with water hs for at least 2 wk. Taper off in increments of 50 mg q 2–4 wk. Associated with severe birth defects; women must have a pregnancy test and sign consent agreeing to use birth control to avoid pregnancy while on this drug (STEPS program).

400 mg/day PO for 3 mo taken with 6–8 oz of plain water at least 2 hr before any other food or beverage. Monitor serum calcium closely; patient should increase intake of vitamin D and calcium; allow a 3-mo rest period if retreatment is needed.

800 mg/day PO; increase to 100 mg/day in divided doses; take on an empty stomach. Monitor cystine levels at 1 mo and then q 3 mo. Patient should drink fluids liberally to 3 L/day.

1–2 mg/kg IV through scalp needle over 10 min followed with infusion of 1–2 mg/kg/hr for no longer than 36–48 hr. Monitor for severe pulmonary or GI hemorrhage.

1.5 mg/m^2 IV over 30 min daily for 5 days, starting on day 1 of a 21-day course; minimum of 4 courses recommended; monitor bone marrow carefully; provide analgesics; suggest use of wig or head covering; protect patient from exposure to infection; barrier contraceptives should be urged.

(continued)

Generic and trade names	Drug class and indications
trientine hydrochloride *Syprine*	Chelating agent Treatment of patients with Wilson's disease who are intolerant of penicillamine
urofollitropin *Fertinex* *Metrodin* *Fertinorm HP* (CAN)	Fertility drug Sequentially with HCG for the stimulation of follicular recruitment and induction of ovulation in patients with polycystic ovary syndrome and infertility Follicle stimulation in ovulatory patients undergoing ART
urofollitropin, purified *Bravelle*	Fertility drug Sequentially with HCG to induce ovulation in patients who have previously received pituitary suppression Stimulation of multiple follicle development in ovulatory patients
valrubicin *Valstar*	Antineoplastic agent Treatment of bacillus Calmette-Guerin (BCG) refractory carcinoma in situ of the bladder in patients who are not candidates for cystectomy
verteporfin *Visudyne*	Ophthalmic agent Treatment of age-related macular degeneration, pathologic myopia, ocular histoplasmosis

Dosages and special alerts

Adults: 750–1,250 mg/day PO in divided doses; maximum dose, 2 g/day. Pediatric: 500–750 mg/day PO; maximum dose, 1,500 mg/day. Interruption of therapy can lead to severe hypersensitivity reactions when drug is restarted. If iron supplements are taken, separate by $\geq$ 2 hr.

Polycystic ovary syndrome and infertility: 75 IU/day SC for first cycle. Adjust dose q 5–7 days based on response. In absence of LH surge, give 5,000–10,000 units HGC one day after the last dose of urofollitropin. Follicle stimulation: 150 IU/day cycle day 2 or 3 until follicles are ready; therapy should not exceed 10 days. Monitor patient for ovarian overstimulation; warn patient of risk of multiple births.

Patients who have received GnRH agonist or antagonist suppression is 150 IU daily SC or IM for the first 5 days of treatment. Subsequent dosing should be adjusted according to individual patient response, should not be made more frequently than once every 2 days, and should not exceed more than 75 to 150 IU per adjustment. The maximum daily dose is 450 IU; treatment beyond 12 days is not recommended. If patient response is appropriate, give HGC 5,000 to 10,000 units 1 day following the last dose of Bravelle. Monitor patient for ovarian overstimulation; warn patient of risk of multiple births.

800 mg per week intravesically for 6 wk. If no response or recurrence in 3 mo, consider need for cystectomy.

6 mg/m^2 diluted in D$_5$W to total 30 mL IV into a free-flowing IV over 10 min at a rate of 3 mL/min using an inline filter and syringe pump. Laser light therapy should begin within 15 min of the start of the IV; may be repeated in 3 mo if needed. Protect patient from exposure to bright light for at least 5 days following the treatment. Avoid use with hepatic impairment or sensitivity to eggs.

APPENDIX M

Federal Drug Classifications

FDA pregnancy categories

The Food and Drug Administration has established five categories to indicate the potential for a systemically absorbed drug to cause birth defects. The key differentiation among the categories rests upon the degree (reliability) of documentation and the risk-benefit ratio.

Category A: Adequate studies in pregnant women have not demonstrated a risk to the fetus in the first trimester of pregnancy, and there is no evidence of risk in later trimesters.

Category B: Animal studies have not demonstrated a risk to the fetus but there are no adequate studies in pregnant women. *Or,* animal studies have shown an adverse effect, but adequate studies in pregnant women have not demonstrated a risk to the fetus during the first trimester of pregnancy, and there is no evidence of risk in later trimesters.

Category C: Animal studies have shown an adverse effect on the fetus but there are no adequate studies in humans; the benefits from the use of the drug in pregnant women may be acceptable despite its potential risks. *Or,* there are no animal reproduction studies and no adequate studies in humans.

Category D: There is evidence of human fetal risk, but the potential benefits from the use of the drug in pregnant women may be acceptable despite its potential risks.

Category X: Studies in animals or humans demonstrate fetal abnormalities or adverse reaction; reports indicate evidence of fetal risk. The risk of use in a pregnant woman clearly outweighs any possible benefit.

Regardless of the designated Pregnancy Category or presumed safety, *no* drug should be administered during pregnancy unless it is clearly needed.

DEA schedules of controlled substances

The Controlled Substances Act of 1970 regulates the manufacturing, distribution, and dispensing of drugs that are known to have abuse potential. The Drug Enforcement Agency (DEA) is responsible for the enforcement of these regulations. The controlled drugs are divided into five DEA schedules based on their potential for abuse and physical and psychological dependence.

Schedule I *(C-I):* High abuse potential and no accepted medical use (heroin, marijuana, LSD)

Schedule II *(C-II):* High abuse potential with severe dependence liability (narcotics, amphetamines, and barbiturates)

Schedule III *(C-III):* Less abuse potential than Schedule II drugs and moderate dependence liability (nonbarbiturate sedatives, nonamphetamine stimulants, limited amounts of certain narcotics)

Schedule IV *(C-IV):* Less abuse potential than Schedule III and limited dependence liability (some sedatives, antianxiety agents, and nonnarcotic analgesics)

Schedule V *(C-V):* Limited abuse potential. Primarily small amounts of narcotics (codeine) used as antitussives or antidiarrheals. Under federal law, limited quantities of certain Schedule V drugs may be purchased without a prescription directly from a pharmacist. The purchaser must be at least 18 years of age and must furnish suitable identification. All such transactions must be recorded by the dispensing pharmacist.

Prescribing physicians and dispensing pharmacists must be registered with the DEA, which also provides forms for the transfer of Schedule I and II substances and establishes criteria for the inventory and prescribing of controlled substances. State and local laws are often more stringent than federal law. In any given situation, the more stringent law applies.

Important Dietary Guidelines for Patient Teaching

Tyramine-rich foods (important to avoid with MAO inhibitors, some antihypertensives)

Aged cheese	Bologna	Liver	Red wine	Smoked fish
Avocados	Caffeinated	Pepperoni	(Chianti)	Yeast
Bananas	beverages	Pickled fish	Ripe fruit	Yogurt
Beer	Chocolate		Salami	

Potassium-rich foods (important to eat with potassium-wasting diuretics)

Avocados	Dried fruit	Navy beans	Prunes	Spinach
Bananas	Grapefruit	Oranges	Rhubarb	Tomatoes
Broccoli	Lima beans	Peaches	Sanka coffee	
Cantaloupe	Nuts	Potatoes	Sunflower seeds	

Calcium-rich foods (important after menopause, in children, in hypocalcemic states)

Bok choy	Canned sar-	Cream soup	Spinach	Molasses
Broccoli	dines	(made with	Dairy products	Oysters
Canned salmon	Clams	milk)	Milk	Tofu

Urine acidifiers (important in maintaining excretion of some drugs)

Cheese	Eggs	Grains	Poultry	Red meat
Cranberries	Fish	Plums	Prunes	

Urine alkalinizers (important in maintaining excretion of some drugs)

Apples	Berries	Citrus fruit	Milk	Vegetables

Iron-rich foods (important in maintaining RBC)

Beets	Dried beans	Dried fruit	Leafy green	Organ meats
Cereals	and peas	Enriched grains	vegetables	(liver, heart, kidney)

Low-sodium foods (important in CHF, hypertension, fluid overload)

Egg yolks	Honey	Macaroons	Puffed rice	Sherbet
Fresh vegetables	Jam and jelly	Potatoes	Puffed wheat	Unsalted nuts
Fresh fruit	Lean meat	Poultry	Red kidney	
Grits	Lima beans	Pumpkin	beans	

High-sodium foods (important to avoid in CHF, hypertension, fluid overload)

BBQ	Canned seafood	Cured meat	Sauces	Snack foods
Beer	Canned	Fast food	Pickles	Tomato
Buttermilk	spaghetti	Microwave	Sauerkraut	ketchup
Butter	Prepackaged	dinners	Cookies	TV dinners
Canned soup	dinners	Pretzels	Mixes	

NANDA-Approved Nursing Diagnoses

The North American Nursing Diagnosis Association (NANDA) endorsed its first nursing diagnosis taxonomic structure, NANDA Taxonomy I, in 1986. This taxonomy has been revised several times, most recently in 2002. The new Taxonomy II has a code structure that is compliant with recommendations from the National Library of Medicine concerning health care terminology codes. The taxonomy that appears here represents the currently accepted classification system for nursing diagnosis.

Imbalanced nutrition: More than body requirements

Imbalanced nutrition: Less than body requirements

Risk for imbalanced nutrition: More than body requirements

Risk for infection

Risk for imbalanced body temperature

Hypothermia

Hyperthermia

Ineffective thermoregulation

Autonomic dysreflexia

Risk for autonomic dysreflexia

Constipation

Perceived constipation

Diarrhea

Bowel incontinence

Risk for constipation

Impaired urinary elimination

Stress urinary incontinence

Reflex urinary incontinence

Urge urinary incontinence

Functional urinary incontinence

Total urinary incontinence

Risk for urge urinary incontinence

Urinary retention

Ineffective tissue perfusion (specify type: renal, cerebral, cardiopulmonary, gastrointestinal, peripheral)

Risk for imbalanced fluid volume

Excess fluid volume

Deficient fluid volume

Risk for deficient fluid volume

Decreased cardiac output

Impaired gas exchange

Ineffective airway clearance

Ineffective breathing pattern

Impaired spontaneous ventilation

Dysfunctional ventilatory weaning response

Risk for injury

Risk for suffocation

Risk for poisoning

Risk for trauma

Risk for aspiration

Risk for disuse syndrome

Latex allergy response

Risk for latex allergy response

Ineffective protection

Impaired tissue integrity

Impaired oral mucous membrane

Impaired skin integrity

Risk for impaired skin integrity

Impaired dentition

Decreased intracranial adaptive capacity

Disturbed energy field

Impaired verbal communication

Impaired social interaction

Social isolation

Risk for loneliness

Ineffective role performance

Impaired parenting

Risk for impaired parenting

Risk for impaired parent/infant/child attachment

Sexual dysfunction

Interrupted family processes

Caregiver role strain

Risk for caregiver role strain

Dysfunctional family processes: Alcoholism

Parental role conflict

Ineffective sexuality patterns

Spiritual distress

Risk for spiritual distress

Readiness for enhanced spiritual well-being

Ineffective coping

Impaired adjustment

Defensive coping

Ineffective denial

Disabled family coping

Compromised family coping

Readiness for enhanced family coping

Readiness for enhanced community coping

Ineffective community coping

Ineffective therapeutic regimen management

Noncompliance (specify)

Ineffective family therapeutic regimen management

Ineffective community therapeutic regimen management

Effective therapeutic regimen management

Decisional conflict (specify)

Health-seeking behaviors (specify)

Impaired physical mobility

Risk for peripheral neurovascular dysfunction

Risk for perioperative-positioning injury

Impaired walking

Impaired wheelchair mobility

Impaired transfer ability

Impaired bed mobility

Activity intolerance

Fatigue

Risk for activity intolerance

Disturbed sleep pattern

Sleep deprivation

Deficient diversional activity

Impaired home maintenance

Ineffective health maintenance

Delayed surgical recovery

Adult failure to thrive

Feeding self-care deficit

Impaired swallowing

Ineffective breast-feeding

Interrupted breast-feeding

Effective breast-feeding

Ineffective infant feeding pattern

Bathing or hygiene self-care deficit

Dressing or grooming self-care deficit

Toileting self-care deficit

Delayed growth and development

Risk for delayed development

Risk for disproportionate growth

Relocation stress syndrome

Risk for disorganized infant behavior

Disorganized infant behavior

Readiness for enhanced organized infant behavior

Disturbed body image

Chronic low self-esteem

Situational low self-esteem

Disturbed personal identity

Disturbed sensory perception (specify: visual, auditory, kinesthetic, gustatory, tactile, olfactory)

Unilateral neglect

Hopelessness

Powerlessness

Deficient knowledge (specify)

Impaired environmental interpretation syndrome

Acute confusion

Chronic confusion

Disturbed thought processes

Impaired memory

Acute pain

Chronic pain

Nausea

Dysfunctional grieving

Anticipatory grieving

Chronic sorrow

Risk for other-directed violence

Risk for self-mutilation

Risk for self-directed violence

Posttrauma syndrome

Rape-trauma syndrome

Rape-trauma syndrome: Compound reaction

Rape-trauma syndrome: Silent reaction

Risk for posttrauma syndrome

Anxiety

Death anxiety

Fear

Risk for relocation stress syndrome

Risk for suicide

Self-mutilation

Risk for powerlessness

Risk for situational low self-esteem

Wandering

Risk for falls

Risk for sudden infant death syndrome

APPENDIX P

Tablets and Capsules That Cannot Be Cut, Crushed, or Chewed

acitretin (*Soriatane*)

alendronate (*Fosamax*)

aminophylline-SR

aspirin-SR (*ZORprin, Bayer Extended Release*)

benzonatate (*Tessalon Perles, Benzonatate Softgels*)

bisacodyl (numerous preparations)

budesonide (*Entocort E C*)

bupropion SR (*Wellbutrin SR, Zyban*)

carbamazepine (T*egretol-XR*)

cefaclor (*Ceclor CD*)

cefuroxime (*Ceftin*)

chloral hydrate (*Aquachloral Supprettes*)

chlorpheniramine-SR (*Chlor-Trimeton Allergy*)

chlorpromazine-SR (*Thorazine Spansules*)

clarithromycin (*Biaxin XL*)

colestipol (*Colestid*)

dexchlorpheniramine TR (*Polaramine Repetabs*)

dextroamphetamine (*Dexedrine Spansules*)

diethylpropion (*Tenuate*)

diflunisal (*Dolobid*)

diltiazem (*Dilacor XR* and others)

dirithromycin (*Dynabac*)

disopyramide (*Norpace CR*)

divalproex (*Depakote*)

enalapril with felodipine (*Lexxel ER*)

esomeprazole (*Nexium*)

felodipine (*Plendil*)

fluphenazine (*Prolixin*)

gatifloxacin (*Tequin*)

hyoscyamine CR (*Cystospaz-M, Levsin*)

isosorbide (SR and ER preparation)

isotretinoin (*Accutane*)

lansoprazole (*Prevacid*)

lovastatin ER (*Altocor*)

meprobamate-SR (*Equanil*)

mesalamine (*Asacol, Pentasa*)

methylphenidate-SR (*Ritalin-SR, Concerta, and others*)

metoprolol-XL (*Toprol XL*)

morphine-SR (*MS Contin, Oramorph SR*)

nifedipine-SR (*Adalat CC, Procardia XL*)

nisoldipine (*Sular*)

nitroglycerin (*Nitroglyn, Nitrong, Nitro-Time*)

norfloxacin (*Noroxin*)

omeprazole (*Prilosec*)

ondansetron (*Zofran*)

orphenadrine (*Norflex*)

oxtriphylline-SA (*Choledyl SA*)

oxybutynin SR (*Ditropan XL*)

oxycodone-SR (*OxyContin*)

pancrelipase (*Cotazym, Creon, Ku-Zyme*)

pancreatin (*Creon Capsules, Donnazyme*)

pantoprazole (*Protonix*)

paroxetine CR (*Paxil CR*)

pentoxifylline (*Trental*)

potassium chloride tablets (*Kaon-Cl, Slow-K, Ten-K, K-Dur*) procainamide SR (*Procanbid, Pronestyl-SR*)

prochlorperazine-SR (*Compazine*)

quinidine SR (*Quinidex Extentabs, Quinaglute Dura-Tabs*)

rabeprazole (*AcipHex*)

sulfasalazine (*Azulfidine EN-Tabs*)

tamsulosin (*Flomax*)

temozolomide (*Temodar*)

theophylline-SR (numerous brand names)

topiramate (*Topamax*)

tripelennamine SR (*PBZ-SR*)

typhoid vaccine, oral (*Vivotif Berna*)

valproic acid (*Depakote* and others)

verapamil (*Calan SR, Isoptin SR, Covera-HS*)

Canadian regulations

Narcotic, controlled drugs, benzodiazepines, and other targeted substances

Table 1 summarizes the requirements for prescribing, dispensing, and record keeping for narcotic, controlled drugs, benzodiazepines, and other targeted substances. This information is not intended to present a comprehensive review; the reader is therefore encouraged to seek additional and confirmatory information (eg, Controlled Drugs and Substances Act, Narcotic Control Regulations, Controlled Drugs Regulations, Benzodiazepines, and Other Targeted Substances Regulations).

Classification and description	Legal requirements
Narcotic drugs*	
• 1 narcotic (eg, cocaine, codeine, hydromorphone, morphine) • 1 narcotic + 1 active non-narcotic ingredient (eg, *Cophylac, Empracel-30, Penntuss, Tylenol No. 4*) • All narcotics for parenteral use (eg, fentanyl, pethidine) • All products containing diamorphine (hospitals only), hydrocodone, oxycodone, methalone, or pentazocine • Dextropropoxyphene, propoxyphene (straight) (eg, *Darvon-N, 642*)	• Written prescription required. • Verbal prescriptions not permitted. • Refills not permitted. • Written prescription may be prescribed to be dispensed in divided portions (part-fills). • For part-fills, copies of prescriptions should be made in reference to the original prescription. Indicate on the original prescription: the new prescription number, the date of the part-fill, the quantity dispensed, and the pharmacist's initials. • Transfers not permitted. • Exempted codeine compounds when dispensed pursuant to a prescription follow the same regulations as for verbal prescription narcotics. • Record and retain all documents pertaining to all transactions in a manner that permits an audit. • Sales reports required except for dextropropoxyphene, propoxyphene. • Report the loss or theft of narcotic drugs as well as forged prescriptions within 10 days to the Office of Controlled Substances at the address indicated at the back of the form.
Narcotic Preparations*	
• Verbal prescription narcotics: 1 narcotic + 2 or more active non-narcotic ingredients (eg, *Cophylac Expectorant, Darvon-N Compound, Fiorinal with Codeine, 692, 282, 292, Tylenol No. 2* and *No. 3.*) • Exempted codeine compounds contain codeine up to 8 mg/solid dosage form or 20 mg/30 mL liquid + 2 or more	• Written or verbal prescriptions permitted. • Refills not permitted. • Written or verbal prescriptions may be prescribed to be dispensed in divided portions (part-fills). • For part-fills, copies of prescriptions should be made in reference to the original prescription. Indicate on the original prescription: the new prescription number, the date of the part-fill, the quantity dispensed, and the pharmacist's initials. • Transfers not permitted. • Record and retain all documents pertaining to all transactions in a manner that permits an audit. • Sales reports not required.

(continued)

Classification and description	Legal requirements

Narcotic drugs* *(continued)*

active non-narcotic ingredients (eg, *Atasol-8, Robutussin with Codeine*)
- Report the loss or theft of narcotic drugs as well as forged prescriptions in 10 days to the Office of Controlled Substances at the address indicated at the back of the form.

Controlled Drugs*

• Part I
eg, amphetamines *(Dexedrine)*
methylphenidate *(Ritalin)*
pentobarbital *(Nembutal)*
secobarbital *(Seconal, Tuinal)*
preparations: 1 controlled drug + 1 or more active noncontrolled drug(s) *(Cafergot-PB)*

- Written or verbal prescriptions permitted.
- Refills not permitted for verbal prescriptions.
- Refills permitted for written prescriptions if the prescriber has indicated in writing the number of refills and dates for, or intervals between, refills.
- Written or verbal prescriptions may be prescribed to be dispensed in divided portions (part-fills).
- For refills and part-fills, copies of prescriptions should be made in reference to the original prescription. Indicate on the original prescription: the new prescription number, the date of the repeat or part-fill, the quantity dispensed, and the pharmacist's initials.
- Transfers not permitted.
- Record and retain all documents pertaining to all transactions in a manner that permits an audit.
- Sales reports required except for controlled drug preparations.
- Report any loss or theft of controlled drugs as well as forged prescriptions within 10 days to the Office of Controlled Substances at the address indicated on the forms.

• Part II
eg, barbiturates (amobarbital, phenobarbital)
butorphanol *(Stadol NS)*
diethylpropion *(Tenuate)*
nalbuphine *(Nubain)*
phenteramine *(Lonamin)*
preparations (1 controlled drug + 1 or more active noncontrolled ingredients *(Fiorinal, Neo-Pause, Tecnal)*

- Written or verbal prescriptions permitted.
- Refills permitted for written or verbal prescriptions if the prescriber has authorized in writing or verbally (at the time of issuance) the number of refills and dates for, or intervals between, refills.
- Written or verbal prescriptions may be prescribed to be dispensed in divided portions (part-fills).
- For refills and part-fills, copies of prescriptions should be made in reference to the original prescription. Indicate on the original prescription: the new prescription number, the date of the refill or part-fill, the quantity dispensed, and the pharmacist's initials.
- Transfers not permitted.
- Record and retain all documents pertaining to all transactions in a manner that permits an audit.

• Part III
eg, anabolic steroids (methyltestosterone, nandrolone decanoate)

- Sales reports not required.
- Report the loss or theft of controlled drugs as well as forged prescriptions within 10 days to the Office of Controlled Substances at the address indicated at the back of the forms.

Benzodiazepines and Other Targeted Substances*

eg, alprazolam *(Xanax)*
bromazepam *(Lectopam)*
chlordiazepoxide *(Librium)*
clobazam *(Frisium)*
ethchlorvynol
lorazepam *(Ativan)*
mazindol

- Written and verbal prescriptions permitted.
- Refills for written or verbal prescriptions permitted if indicated by prescriber.
- Part-fills permitted as per prescriber's instructions.
- For refills or part-fills of prescriptions, the following information should be recorded: date of the repeat or part-fill, prescription number, quantity dispensed, and the pharmacist's initials.

*The products noted are examples only.

Classification and description	Legal requirements
Benzodiazepines and Other Targeted Substances* *(continued)*	
meprobamate oxazepam (*Serax*)	• Transfer of prescriptions permitted except a prescription that has been already transferred. • Sales reports not required. • Report loss or theft of benzodiazepines and other targeted substances within 10 days to the Office of Controlled Substances at the address indicated on the forms.

Reprinted by permission from the *Compendium of Pharmaceuticals and Specialties.* Ottawa, Canada: Canadian Pharmacists Association, 2002: A5–A6.
Reviewed 2002 by the Office of Controlled Substances, Health Canada.

Adverse Drug Reactions: Surveillance and Reporting

The following is a description of the Canadian Adverse Drug Reaction Monitoring Program (CADRMP). This information is not intended to present a comprehensive review.
Reviewed 2002 by the Bureau of License Product Assessment, Health Canada.

Canadian Adverse Drug Reaction Monitoring Program: Although drugs are carefully tested before licensing to ensure safety and efficacy, there is insufficient information to detect rare adverse events that may occur. Only once a drug is on the market is it exposed to sufficient numbers of patients to uncover these events. Through assessment and surveillance of suspected adverse drug reaction reports, the Canadian Adverse Drug Reaction Monitoring program can detect early trends in suspected adverse drug reactions (ADR). For more information on the program contact one of the centers listed below.

What to Report? An ADR is a noxious and unintended response to a drug which occurs with use or testing for the diagnosis, treatment, or prevention of a disease or the modification of an organic function. This includes any undesirable patient effect suspected to be associated with drug use. ADRs as a result of prescription, nonprescription, biological (including blood products), complementary medicines (including herbals) and radiopharmaceutical drug products are monitored. Drug abuse, drug overdoses, drug interactions, and unusual lack of therapeutic efficacy are also considered to be reportable as ADRs. ADR reports are, for the most part, only suspected associations. A temporal or possible association is sufficient for a report to be made. Reporting of an ADR does not imply a causal link.

ADRs that should be reported include all suspected adverse drug reactions which are:

- **unexpected,** regardless of their severity, i.e., not consistent with the product information or labeling; or
- **serious,** whether expected or not. The Canadian Regulations pertaining to reporting ADRs for marketed drug products define a serious adverse drug reaction as "a noxious and unintended response to a drug, which occurs at any dose and requires inpatient hospitalization or prolongation of existing hospitalization, causes congenital malformation, results in persistent or significant disability or incapacity, is life-threatening or results in death"; or
- **reactions to recently marketed drugs** (on the market for less than 5 years) regardless of their nature or severity.

How to Report? To report a suspected ADR for drug products marketed in Canada, health professionals should complete a copy of the ADR Reporting Form provided in this section. This form

*The products noted are examples only.

may also be obtained from your Regional ADR Centre or from the National ADR Unit (see addresses below) or from Health Canada's web site (www.hc-sc.gc.ca/hpb-dgps/therapeut) under Forms. The Canadian Adverse Drug Reaction Newsletter is also available on-line through the same web site, under Publications.

Health professionals may also report ADRs to the manufacturer and should indicate on the ADR report sent to Health Canada if a case was also reported to the manufacturer.

The success of the program depends on the quality and accuracy of the information sent in by the reporter.

Electronic subscription to the Canadian Adverse Drug Reaction Newsletter and drug advisories is now available: You may now join the Health_Prod_Info mailing list to subscribe electronically to this Newsletter and to receive notices of health professional advisories. Go to www.hc-sc.gc.ca/hpb-dgps/therapeut/htmleng/adr.html, click "subscribe" and follow the instructions.

Regional ADR Centres

To facilitate the receipt of drug safety information, health professionals and consumers may use the following toll-free numbers to report ADRs. Calls will be automatically routed to the appropriate regional or national ADR centre.
Telephone: 1-866-234-2345
Fax: 1-866-678-6789

British Columbia
BC Regional ADR Centre
c/o BC Drug and Poison
 Information Centre
1081 Burrard St.
Vancouver BC V6Z 1Y6
(604) 806-8625
Fax: (604) 806-8262
E-mail: adr@dpic.bc.ca

New Brunswick, New-foundland, Nova Scotia and Prince Edward Island
Atlantic Regional ADR Centre
c/o Queen Elizabeth II Health
 Sciences Centre
Drug Information Centre
1796 Summer St., Rm. 2421
Halifax NS B3H 3A7
(902) 473-7171
Fax: (902) 473-8612
E-mail: adr@qe2-hsc.ns.ca

Ontario
Ontario Regional ADR Centre
LonDIS Drug Information
 Centre
London Health Sciences Centre
339 Windermere Rd.
London ON N6A 5A5
(519) 663-8801
Fax: (519) 663-2968
E-mail: adr@lhsc.on.ca

Quebec
Quebec Regional ADR Centre
Drug Information Centre
Hôpital du Sacré-Coeur de
 Montréal
5400 boul. Gouin ouest
Montréal QC H4J 1C5
(514) 338-2961 or 1-888-265-
 7692
Fax: (514) 338-3670
E-mail: cip.hscm@sympatico.ca

Saskatchewan
Sask ADR Regional Centre
Dial Access Drug Information
 Service
College of Pharmacy and
 Nutrition
University of Saskatchewan
110 Science Pl.
Saskatoon SK S7N 5C9
(306) 966-6340 or 1-800-667-
 3425
Fax: (306) 966-6377
E-mail: vogt@duke.usask.ca

Other provinces and territories
National ADR Unit
Adverse Reaction Information
 Unit
Bureau of Licensed Product
 Assessment
Finance Building
Tunney's Pasture
AL 0201C2
Ottawa ON K1A 1B9
(613) 957-0337
Fax: (613) 957-0335
E-mail: cadrmp@hc-sc.gc.ca

Calculating Pediatric Dosages

Children often require different doses of drugs than adults because children's bodies often handle drugs very differently from adults' bodies. The standard drug dosages listed in package inserts and references such as the PDR refer to the adult dosage. In some cases, a pediatric dosage is suggested, but in many cases it will need to be calculated based on the child's age, weight, or body surface. The following are some standard formulae for calculating the pediatric dose.

Fried's rule

$$\text{Infant's dose } (< 1 \text{ yr}) = \frac{\text{infant's age (in mo)}}{150 \text{ mo}} \times \text{ average adult dose}$$

Young's rule

$$\text{Child's dose } (1-12 \text{ yr}) = \frac{\text{child's age (in yr)}}{\text{child's age (in yr)} + 12} \times \text{ average adult dose}$$

Clark's rule

$$\text{Child's dose} = \frac{\text{weight of child (lb)}}{150 \text{ lb}} \times \text{ average adult dose}$$

Surface area rule

$$\text{Child's dose} = \frac{\text{surface area of child (in square meters)}}{1.73} \times \text{ average adult dose}$$

The surface area of a child is determined using a nomogram that determines surface area based on height and weight measurements.

Pediatric dosage calculations should be checked by two persons. Many institutions have procedures for double checking the dosage calculation of those drugs (eg, digoxin) used most frequently in the pediatric area.

Adverse Drug Effects

All drugs are potentially dangerous. Even though chemicals are carefully screened and tested on animals and in people before they are released as drugs, drug products often cause unexpected or unacceptable reactions when they are given to people in the clinical situation. The nurse, being the caregiver who most frequently administers medications, must be constantly alert for signs of drug reactions of different types. Patients and their families need to be taught what to look for when patients are taking drugs at home. Some adverse effects can be countered with specific comfort measures or precautions. Knowing how to recognize these effects and what action can be taken to prevent or cope with these drug effects may be the critical factor in helping the patient be compliant with drug therapy and adjust to it successfully.

ALLERGIC REACTIONS

Anaphylactic type
Hives, rash, difficulty breathing, increased BP, dilated pupils, diaphoresis, "panic" feeling, increased heart rate, respiratory arrest

Interventions
Epinephrine, 0.3 mL of a 1:1,000 solution, SC, repeated every 15 to 20 minutes.

Cytotoxic type
Damage to blood forming cells (decreased Hct, decreased WBC, decreased platelets); elevated liver enzymes; decreased renal function

Interventions
Discontinue drug.

Serum-sickness type
Itchy rash, high temperature, swollen lymph nodes, swollen and painful joints, edema of the face and limbs

Interventions
Discontinue drug; provide comfort measures, such as cool environment, skin care, positioning, ice to joints, antipyretic, or anti-inflammatory.

Delayed reactions
Rash, hives, swollen joints (similar to the reaction to poison ivy)

Interventions
Discontinue drug; provide skin care and comfort measures, such as antihistamines or topical corticosteroids.

OTHER REACTIONS

Dermatologic reactions
Moderate: Hives, rash, lesions
Exfoliative dermatitis: Rash and scaling, fever, enlarged lymph nodes, enlarged liver
Erythema multiforme exudativum (Stevens-Johnson syndrome): Dark red papules on the extremities with no pain or itching, often appearing in rings or disk-shaped patches

Interventions

Mild case: Frequent skin care; avoid rubbing skin; avoid tight or rough clothing; avoid harsh soaps or perfumed lotions; antihistamines. Severe case: Discontinue drug; topical corticosteroids, antihistamines, emollients.

Stomatitis

Inflammation of the mucous membranes, swollen gums, inflamed gums (gingivitis), swollen and red tongue (glossitis), difficulty swallowing, bad breath, pain in mouth and throat

Interventions

Frequent mouth care with a nonirritating solution, nutrition evaluation, dental consult, antifungal agents, or local anesthetics

Superinfections

Fever, diarrhea, black "hairy" tongue, inflamed swollen tongue (glossitis), mucous membrane lesions, vaginal discharge or itching

Interventions

Frequent mouth care, skin care, access to bathroom facilities, small and frequent meals, antifungal therapy.

Blood dyscrasias (bone marrow depression)

Fever, chills, sore throat, weakness, back pain, dark urine, decreased Hct (anemia), thrombocytopenia (low platelet count), leukopenia (low WBC count), pancytopenia (a reduction of all cellular elements of the CBC)

Interventions

Monitor blood counts, rest, protection from exposure to infections, protection from injury, avoidance of activities that might result in injury or bleeding. Severe case: Discontinue drug or stop drug until bone marrow recovers to a safe level.

Liver injury

Fever, malaise, nausea, vomiting, jaundice, change in color of urine or stools, abdominal pain or colic, elevated liver enzymes (AST, ALT), alterations in bilirubin levels, PTT changes

Interventions

Discontinue drug, small and frequent meals, skin care, cool environment, rest.

Hypoglycemia

Fatigue, drowsiness, hunger, anxiety, headache, cold or clammy skin, tremulousness (shaking and lack of coordination), increased heart rate, increased BP, numbness and tingling of the mouth, tongue, or lips, confusion, rapid and shallow respirations. Severe case: Seizure or coma.

Interventions

Restore glucose; skin care, environmental control of light and temperature, rest; prevention of injury or falls.

Hyperglycemia

Fatigue, increased urination (polyuria), increased thirst (polydipsia), deep respirations (Kussmaul's respirations), restlessness, increased hunger (polyphagia), nausea, hot or flushed skin, fruity odor to breath.

Interventions
Insulin therapy to decrease blood glucose, carefully monitor blood glucose levels; access to bathroom facilities, controlled environment, reassurance, mouth care.

Renal injury
Elevated BUN, elevated creatinine levels, decreased Hct, electrolyte imbalances, fatigue, malaise, edema, irritability, skin rash

Interventions
Discontinue drug, positioning, diet and fluid restrictions, skin care, electrolyte therapy, rest periods, controlled environment. Severe case: Dialysis.

Hypokalemia
Serum potassium less than 3.5 mEq/L, weakness, numbness and tingling in the extremities, muscle cramps, nausea, vomiting, diarrhea, decreased bowel sounds, irregular pulse, weak pulses, orthostatic hypotension, disorientation. Severe case: Paralytic ileus (absent bowel sounds, abdominal distention, acute abdomen).

Interventions
Replacement of serum potassium with careful monitoring of serum levels and patient response; prevention of injury or falls; orientation of patient; comfort measures for pain and discomfort.

Hyperkalemia
Serum potassium level greater than 5.0 mEq/L, weakness, muscle cramps, diarrhea, numbness and tingling, slow heart rate, low blood pressure, decreased urine output, difficulty breathing.

Interventions
Measures to decrease serum potassium including use of sodium polystyrene sulfonate; prevention of injury or falls; monitor cardiac effects and be prepared for cardiac emergency. Severe case: Dialysis.

Ocular toxicity
Blurred vision, color vision changes, corneal damage, blindness

Interventions
Discontinue drug; supportive measures; monitor lighting and exposure to sunlight.

Auditory damage
Dizziness, "ringing in the ears," loss of balance, loss of hearing

Interventions
Protective measures to prevent falling or injury, supportive measures to cope with drug effects.

CNS effects
Confusion, delirium, insomnia, drowsiness, hyperreflexia or hyporeflexia, bizarre dreams, hallucinations

Interventions
Safety measures to prevent injury; caution patient to avoid dangerous situations such as driving a car or operating dangerous machinery.

Atropine-like or cholinergic effects
Dry mouth, altered taste perception, dysphagia, heartburn, constipation, bloating, paralytic ileus, urinary hesitancy and retention, impotence, blurred vision, cycloplegia, photophobia, headache, mental confusion, nasal congestion, palpitations, decreased sweating, dry skin

Interventions
Sugarless lozenges, mouth care to help mouth dryness; bowel program as appropriate; void before taking drug to aid voiding; safety measures if vision changes occur; medication for headache, nasal congestion; avoidance of hot environments and protective measures if exposed to heat due to decreased sweating.

Parkinson-like syndrome
Lack of activity, akinesia, muscular tremors, drooling, changes in gait, rigidity, akathisia (extreme restlessness, "jitters"), dyskinesia (spasms)

Interventions
Anticholinergics or antiparkinsonians; small, frequent meals if swallowing becomes difficult; safety measures if ambulation or motor coordination becomes a problem.

Neuroleptic malignant syndrome (NMS)
Extrapyramidal symptoms, hyperthermia, autonomic disturbances

Interventions
Anticholinergics or antiparkinsonians, supportive care to lower body temperature, safety precautions.

Drugs That Interact with Grapefruit Juice

Grapefruit juice inhibits the cytochrome CYP-3A4 system in the liver which can cause a decrease in the metabolism of several drugs. Decreasing the metabolism of the drug can lead to increased serum drug levels and toxicity. If any of these drugs are being given, the patient should avoid the use of grapefruit juice. If the combination cannot be avoided, space the drug as far away from the grapefruit juice as possible during the day and monitor the patient closely for signs of drug toxicity. If a patient has been stabilized on one of these drugs and suddenly begins to develop signs of drug toxicity, ask the patient specifically if he has been drinking grapefruit juice. If a patient is receiving one of these drugs, a key point of patient education should be to avoid the use of grapefruit juice.

17 beta-estradiol	progesterone
alfentanil	quinidine
alprazolam	ritonavir
amprenavir	saquinavir
atorvastatin	sildenafil
budesonide	sufentanil
clarithromycin	tacrolimus
cortisol	tamoxifen
cyclophosphamide	testosterone
cyclosporine A	triazolam
diltiazem	troleandomycin
erythromycin	verapamil
felodipine	vinblastine
fentanyl	vincristine
fluvastatin	warfarin
ifosfamide	
indinavir	
lovastatin	
midazolam	
nelfinavir	
nifedipine	
nimodipine	
nisoldipine	

Bibliography

Carpenito, L.J. *Nursing Diagnosis* (8th ed.). Philadelphia: Lippincott-Raven, 1999.

Drug Evaluations Subscription. Chicago: American Medical Association, 2003.

Drug Facts and Comparisons. St. Louis, MO: Facts and Comparisons, 2003.

Drug Facts Update: Physicians On-Line. Multimedia, 2003.

Eisenhauer, L.A., Nichols, L.W., Spencer, R.T., & Bergan, F.W. *Clinical Pharmacology and Nursing Management* (6th ed.). Philadelphia: Lippincott-Raven, 2002.

Fetrow, C.W. & Avila, J. *Professional's Handbook of Complementary and Alternative Medicines* (2nd ed.). Springhouse, PA: Lippincott Williams & Wilkins, 2004.

Gilman, A.G., Hardman, J.G., & Limbird, L.E. (Eds). *Goodman and Gilman's The Pharmacological Basis of Therapeutics* (10th ed.). New York: McGraw-Hill, 2002.

Griffiths, M.C. (Ed). *USAN 1999 and the USP Dictionary of Drug Names*. Rockville, MD: United States Pharmacopeial Convention, 1999.

Handbook of Adverse Drug Interactions. New Rochelle, NY: The Medical Letter, 2002.

ISMP Medication Safety Alert! Huntington Valley, PA: Institute for Safe Medication Practices, 2003.

Karch, A.M. *Focus on Pharmacology* (2nd ed.). Philadelphia: Lippincott Williams & Wilkins, 2002.

Levine, R.R. *Pharmacology: Drug Actions and Reactions* (3rd ed.). Boston: Little, Brown, 1993.

Lindberg, J.B., Hunter, M.L., & Kruszewski, A.Z. *Introduction to Nursing: Concepts, Issues, and Opportunities* (3rd ed.). Philadelphia: Lippincott-Raven, 1998.

PDR for Nonprescription Drugs. Oradell, NJ: Medical Economics Company, 2003.

PDR for Ophthalmology. Oradell, NJ: Medical Economics Company, 2003.

Physicians' Desk Reference (48th ed.). Oradell, NJ: Medical Economics Company, 2003.

Smeltzer, S.C., & Bare, B.G. *Brunner and Suddarth's Textbook of Medical-Surgical Nursing* (10th ed.). Philadelphia: Lippincott Williams & Wilkins, 2002.

Tatro, D.S. (Ed). *Drug Interaction Facts*. St. Louis, MO: Facts and Comparisons, 2003.

The Medical Letter on Drugs and Therapeutics. New Rochelle, NY: Medical Letter, 2003.

Acknowledgments

Abbott Laboratories
Biaxin®, Biaxin® XL, Depakote®,
Depakote® Sprinkle, E-Mycin®,
Ery-Tab®, Hytrin®, Isoptin® SR,
Kaletra™, Synthroid®, Vicodin®,
Vicodin ES®

AstraZeneca LP
Elavil®, Nolvadex®, Prilosec®,
Tenormin®, Toprol-XL®, Zestril®

Aventis Pharmaceuticals
Allegra®, Carafate®, DiaBeta®, Lasix®,
Trental®

Bayer Corporation
Cipro®

Biovail Corporation
Cardizem®, Cardizem® CD, Cardizem®
SR, Vasotec®

Bristol-Myers Squibb Company
Abilify™, BuSpar®, Capoten®, Cefzil®,
Coumadin®, Desyrel®, Glucophage®,
Glucophage® XR, Monopril®,
Pravachol®, Serzone®

Elan Pharmaceuticals, Inc.
Frova®

Forest Pharmaceuticals, Inc.
Celexa™, Lexapro™

Geneva Pharmaceuticals
Pen-Vee-K

Gilead Sciences
Viread®

GlaxoSmithKline
Amoxil®, Augmentin®, Augmentin®
Chewable, Avandia®, Ceftin®, Combivir®,
Compazine®, Coreg®, Imitrex®,
Lanoxicaps®, Lanoxin®, Lotronex®,
Paxil®, Relafen®, Retrovir®, Tagamet®,
Wellbutrin®, Wellbutrin SR®, Zovirax®,
Zyban®

Janssen Pharmaceutica, Inc.
Risperdal®

King Pharmaceuticals, Inc.
Levoxyl®

Eli Lilly and Company
Evista®, Prozac®, Sarafem®, Strattera™

Mallinckrodt, Inc.
Pamelor®, Restoril®

McNeil-PPC, Inc.
Concerta®

Merck & Co., Inc.
Cozaar®, Crixivan®, Fosamax®,
HydroDIURIL®, Mevacor®, Pepcid®,
Prinivil®, Sinemet®, Sinemet CR®,
Singulair®, Vioxx®, Zocor®

**Merck/Schering-Plough
Pharmaceuticals**
Zetia™

**Novartis Pharmaceuticals
Corporation**
Gleevec®, Lescol®, Lotensin®, Ritalin®,
Ritalin SR®

Ortho-McNeil Pharmaceutical
Floxin®, Levaquin®, Tylenol® with
Codeine No. 3, Ultracet®

Parke-Davis
Accupril®, Dilantin® Infatabs®,
Dilantin® Kapseals®, Lipitor®, Lopid®,
Neurontin®, Nitrostat®

Pfizer, Inc.
Cardura®, Celebrex®, Diflucan®,
Glucotrol®, Glucotrol XL®, Norvasc®,
Procardia®, Procardia XL®, Viagra®,
Zantac®, Zithromax®, Zoloft®, Zyrtec®

Pharmacia Corporation
Bextra®, Calan®, Deltasone®,
Demulen®, Detrol®, Medrol®,
Micronase®, Motrin, Pletal®, Provera®,
Xanax®

**Procter and Gamble
Pharmaceuticals, Inc.**
Actonel®, Macrobid®

Purdue Pharma L.P.
OxyContin®

Roche Laboratories, Inc.
Bumex®, Klonopin®, Naprosyn®,
Ticlid®, Valium®

Sanofi-Synthelabo, Inc.
Ambien®, Demerol®

Sankyo Pharma
Benicar™

**Schering Corporation and Key
Pharmaceuticals, Inc.**
Clarinex™, Claritin®, Claritin®
Reditabs®, K-Dur®

Schwarz Pharma
Verelan®

Tap Pharmaceuticals, Inc.
Prevacid®

UCB Pharmaceuticals, Inc.
Lortab®

Wallace Pharmaceuticals
Soma®

Warner Chilcott Laboratories, Inc.
Duricef, Eryc®, Estrace®, Ovcon® 35

Women First HealthCare, Inc.
Bactrim DS®

Wyeth Pharmaceuticals
Cordarone®, Effexor®, Effexor® XR,
Inderal®, Inderal® LA, Phenergan®,
Premarin®, Sonata®

Index

Generic names and alternative therapies are boldface in main entries. *Brand names* of drugs are italics, followed by the generic name in parentheses. Brand names of drugs that are Canadian are followed by (CAN). Chemical or nonofficial names appear in regular typeface. **DRUG CLASSES** appear in bold capital letters with the drugs that fall in that class listed as official names under the class heading.

Advil Migraine (ibuprofen): 614
A-E-R (hamamelis water): 1316
Aerobid (flunisolide): 527
Aerobid-M (flunisolide): 527
Aerodine (povidone iodine): 1316
Aeroid (thimersol): 1317
Aeroseb-Dex (dexamethasone): 372, 1324
Aerosporin (CAN) (polymyxin B): 973
Afrin (oxymetazoline): 905
Afrin (pseudoephedrine): 1013
Afrin Children's Pump Mist (oxymetazoline): 905
Afrin Children's Pump Mist (phenylephrine): 958
Afrin Sinus (oxymetazoline): 905
Aftate (tolnaftate): 1319
Agenerase (amprenavir): 30
Agoral (senna): 1334
Aggrastat (tirofiban): 1146
Aggrenox (aspirin and dipyridamole): 1293, 1303
Agrylin (anagrelide): 132
AHA (acetohydroxamic acid): 74
AH-Chew D (phenylephrine): 958
AHF (antihemophilic factor): 137
A-hydroCort (hydrocortisone): 599
a-2-interferon (interferon alfa-2b): 634
AK-Beta (levobunolol): 1329
Ak-Chlor (chloramphenicol): 276
AK-Dilate (phenylephrine): 958
AK-Nefrin (phenylephrine): 958
Aknemycin (erythromycin): 464
Ak-Pentolate (cyclopentolate): 1327
AK-Pred (prednisolone): 985
AK Pro (dipivefrin): 1328
AK-Tracin (bacitracin): 163
Akarpine (pilocarpine): 1330
Akineton (biperiden): 183
Alamast (pemirolast): 1330
alatrofloxacin mesylate: 1197
Alavert (loratadine): 712
albendazole: 1336
Albenza (albendazole): 1336
Albert Glyburide (CAN) (glyburide): 574
Albert Oxybutynin (CAN) (oxybutynin): 902
albumin, human: 80
Albuminar-5 (albumin): 80
Albuminar-25 (albumin): 80
Albunex (albumin 5%): 80
Albutein 5% (albumin): 80
Albutein 25% (albumin): 80

albuterol sulfate: 82
alclometasone dipropionate: 1323
Alcomicin (CAN) (gentamicin): 565
Aldactazide (spironolactone and hydrochlorothiazide): 1295, 1303
Aldactone (spironolactone): 1082
Aldara (imiquimod): 1317
aldesleukin: 84
Aldoclor (methyldopa, chlorothaizide): 1290, 1303
Aldomet (methyldopa): 776
Aldoril D (methyldopa, hydrochlorothiazide): 1290, 1303
ALDOSTERONE ANTAGONIST
  spironolactone: 1082
**ALDOSTERONE RECEPTOR
  BLOCKER**
  eplerenone: 455
alefacept: 1336
alemtuzumab: 1336
alendronate sodium: 86, C2
Alesse (levonorgestrel and estradiol): 1299
Aleve (naproxen): 837
alfalfa: 1242
Alferon LDO (interferon alfa-n3): 1344
Alferon N (interferon alfa-n3): 1344
alglucerase: 1336
Alinia (nitazoxanide): 1348
alitretinoin: 1321
Alka-Seltzer (aspirin): 143
Alka-Seltzer Plus Cold & Flu Medicine
  (combo): 1303
*Alka-SeltzerPlus Cold and Cough
  Medicine* (combo): 1303
Alka-Seltzer Plus Flu Medicine (combo):
  1303
Alkeran (melphalan): 739
**ALKYLATING AGENTS (see page
  10)**
  busulfan: 205
  carboplatin: 226
  carmustine: 230
  chlorambucil: 275
  cisplatin: 303
  cyclophosphamide: 344
  ifosfamide: 619
  lomustine: 707
  mechlorethamine: 730
  melphalan: 739
  streptozocin: 1086
  thiotepa: 1135
Allegra (fexofenadine): 513, C12

ANTIDEPRESSANTS
citalopram: 305
escitalopram: 468
fluoxetine: 530
fluvoxamine: 541
maprotiline: 725
mirtazapine: 802
nefazodone: 843
paroxetine: 922
phenelzine: 951
sertraline: 1060
tranylcypromine: 1166
trazodone: 1169
venlafaxine: 1213
ANTIDIABETIC AGENTS (see page 19)
acarbose: 63
acetohexamide: 69
chlorpropamide: 288
glimepiride: 569
glipizide: 570
glyburide: 574
insulin: 630
metformin: 760
miglitol: 796
nateglinide: 840
pioglitazone: 967
repaglinide: 1031
rosiglitazone: 1048
tolazamide: 1152
tolbutamide: 1154
ANTIDIARRHEAL AGENTS
bismuth subsalicylate: 185
loperamide: 708
octreotide: 880
opium: 889
ANTIDOTES
acetylcysteine: 72
atropine: 152
charcoal: 272
deferoxamine: 1342
digoxin immune fab: 398
dimercaprol: 1342
edetate disodium: 437
edrophonium: 439
flumazenil: 526
fomepizole: 1344
mesna: 1346
methylene blue: 778
neostigmine: 847
pralidoxime: 979

ANTIDOTES (continued)
pyridostigmine: 1017
succimer: 1088
ANTIEMETICS
buclizine: 196
chlorpromazine: 285
cyclizine: 342
dolasetron: 417
dronabinol: 431
granisetron: 581
hydroxyzine: 611
meclizine: 732
metoclopramide: 784
ondansetron: 888
perphenazine: 947
prochlorperazine: 994
promethazine: 1001
thiethylperazine: 1130
triflupromazine: 1184
trimethobenzamide: 1188
ANTIEPILEPTIC DRUGS
acetazolamide: 67
carbamazepine: 222
clonazepam: 317
clorazepate: 322
diazepam: 385
ethosuximide: 493
ethotoin: 494
fosphenytoin: 550
gabapentin: 556
lamotrigine: 673
levetiracetam: 683
mephenytoin: 746
mephobarbital: 748
methsuximide: 773
oxcarbazepine: 900
phenobarbital: 953
phensuximide: 955
phenytoin: 961
primidone: 989
tiagabine: 1139
topiramate: 1159
valproic acid: 1207
zonisamide: 1239
ANTIESTROGEN DRUGS
anastrozole: 135
letrozole: 678
tamoxifen: 1103
ANTIFLATULENT
simethicone: 1064

ANTIFUNGALS (see page 20)
amphotericin B: 125
fluconazole: 521
flucytosine: 522
griseofulvin: 1344
itraconazole: 661
ketoconazole: 664
miconazole: 792
nystatin: 878
voriconazole: 1221

ANTIFUNGALS, TOPICAL
amphotericin B: 1318
butenafine: 1318
butoconazole: 1318
ciclopirox: 1318
clotrimazole: 324, 1318
econazole: 1318
gentian violet: 1318
ketoconazole: 1318
naftitine: 1318
oxiconazole: 1318
terbinafine: 1319
tolnaftate: 1319

ANTIGLAUCOMA AGENTS
acetazolamide: 67
betaxolol: 180
brimonidine: 1327
brinzolamide: 1327
epinephrine: 449
latanoprost: 1329
methazolamide: 763
timolol: 1143

ANTIGONADOTROPIC DRUGS
cetrorelix: 1340

ANTIGOUT DRUGS
allopurinol: 87
colchicine: 329
probenecid: 991
sulfinpyrazone: 1094

ANTIHEMOPHILIC AGENTS
antihemophilic factor: 137
coagulation factor VIIa: 1340
factor IX concentrates: 502
antihemophilic factor: 137
Antihist-1 (clemastine): 309

ANTIHISTAMINES (see page 22)
azatadine: 157
azelastine: 1322, 1327
brompheniramine: 195
buclizine: 196
cetirizine: 271

ANTIHISTAMINES *(continued)*
chlorpheniramine: 284
clemastine: 309
cyclizine: 342
cyproheptadine: 349
desloratadine: 369
dexchlorpheniramine: 376
dimenhydrinate: 403
diphenhydramine: 406
fexofenadine: 513
hydroxyzine: 611
loratadine: 712
meclizine: 732
promethazine: 1001
tripelennamine: 1193

ANTIHYPERLIPIDEMIC AGENTS
atorvastatin: 149
cholestyramine: 292
clofibrate: 313
colesevelam: 331
colestipol: 332
fenofibrate: 508
fluvastatin: 540
gemfibrozil: 564
lovastatin: 717
niacin: 853
pravastatin: 982
simvastatin: 1065

ANTIHYPERTENSIVE DRUGS
acebutolol: 64
amlodipine: 117
atenolol: 146
benazepril: 168
betaxolol: 180
bisoprolol: 186
bosentan: 190
candesartan: 217
captopril: 221
carteolol: 232
carvedilol: 233
clonidine: 319
diazoxide: 388
diltiazem: 401
doxazosin: 424
enalapril: 442
eplerenone: 455
eprosartan: 458
felodipine: 507
fosinopril: 549
guanabenz: 583
guanadrel: 584
guanethidine: 585

ANTIPROTOZOALS
atovaquone: 151
metronidazole: 789
nitazoxanide: 1348
pentamidine: 938
ANTIPSORIATIC AGENT
acitretin: 1336
ANTIPSORIATICS, TOPICAL
anthralin: 1317
calcipotriene: 1317
ANTIPSYCHOTIC DRUGS
chlorpromazine: 285
clozapine: 326
fluphenazine: 534
haloperidol: 588
loxapine: 718
mesoridazine: 755
molindone: 812
olanzapine: 883
perphenazine: 947
pimozide: 1348
prochlorperazine: 994
quetiapine: 1020
risperidone: 1040
thioridazine: 1132
thiothixene: 1136
trifluoperazine: 1181
triflupromazine: 1184
ziprasidone: 1235
ANTIPYRETIC DRUGS
acetaminophen: 66
aspirin: 143
choline magnesium trisalicylate: 293
choline salicylate: 294
diclofenac: 390
diflunisal: 395
etodolac: 498
oxaprozin: 898
salsalate: 1051
sodium thiosalicylate: 1075
ANTIRHEUMATIC AGENTS
aspirin: 143
auranofin: 154
aurothioglucose: 156
hydroxychloroquine: 607
methotrexate: 768
penicillamine: 929
salsalate: 1051
sodium thiosalicylate: 1075
ANTISEBORRHEICS
chloroxine: 1318
selenium: 1318

ANTISECRETORY AGENTS
esomeprazole: 470
lansoprazole: 675
omeprazole: 887
pantoprazole: 918
rabeprazole: 1025
ANTISEPTICS
benzalkonium: 1316
chlorhexidine: 1316
hexachlorophene: 1316
iodine: 1316
povidone iodine: 1316
sodium hypochlorite: 1317
thimersol: 1317
Antispas (dicyclomine): 392
ANTISPASMODICS
dicyclomine: 392
glycopyrrolate: 576
hyoscyamine: 613, 1346
methscopolamine: 772
propantheline: 1004
tizanidine: 1148
antithrombin III: 1336
ANTITHROMBOTICS
dalteparin: 355
danaparoid: 357
enoxaparin: 444
fondaparinux: 543
anti-thymocyte globulin: 1273
ANTITHYROID DRUGS
methimazole: 766
propylthiouracil: 1010
ANTITUBERCULOUS DRUGS
capreomycin: 219
cycloserine: 346
ethambutol: 489
ethionamide: 492
isoniazid: 651
pyrazinamide: 1016
rifampin: 1035
rifapentine: 1036
streptomycin: 1352
Anti-Tuss (guaifenesin): 582
ANTITUSSIVES
benzonatate: 171
codeine: 328
dextromethorphan: 384
terpin hydrate: 1117
Antivert (meclizine): 732
antivenin (crotalidae) polyvalent:
1273

BIOLOGICAL RESPONSE MODIFIER
  etanercept: 486
Biologicals, Commonly Used (see pages 1250-1274)
biperiden: 183
biperiden hydrochloride: 183
biperiden lactate: 183
birch bark: 1243
bisacodyl: 1332
Bisco-Lax (bisacodyl): 1332
Bismatrol (bismuth subsalicylate): 185
Bismatrol Extra Strength (bismuth subsalicylate): 185
bismuth subsalicylate: 185
bisoprolol fumarate: 186
BISPHOSPHONATES (see page 32)
  alendronate: 86
  etidronate: 496
  pamidronate: 916
  risedronate: 1039
  tiludronate: 1352
  zoledronic acid: 1236
bitolterol mesylate: 187
bivalirudin: 1338
blackberry: 1243
black cohosh root: 1243
Black Draught (senna): 1334
Black Widow spider species antivenin: 1274
BLADDER PROTECTANT
  pentosan: 1348
Blenoxane (bleomycin): 189
bleomycin sulfate: 189
BLM (bleomycin): 189
Blocadren (timolol): 1143
BLOOD PRODUCTS
  albumin: 80
  alpha$_1$-proteinase inhibitor: 1336
  factor IX concentrates: 502
  plasma protein fraction: 972
Bluboro Powder (Burow's solution): 1316
Bonamine (CAN) (meclizine): 732
Bonine (meclizine): 732
boric acid ointment: 1315
Borofax (boric acid): 1315
Borofax Skin Protectant: 1315
Boropak Powder (Burow's solution): 1316
bosentan: 190

Botox Cosmetic (botulinum toxin type A): 191
botulinum toxin type A: 191
botulinum toxin type B: 1338
BPH AGENT
  dutasteride: 434
4% BranchAmin (amino acids): 105
Bravelle (urofollitropin): 1354
Breeze Mist Antifungal (miconazole): 792
Breonesin (guaifenesin): 582
Brethine (terbutaline): 1115
Bretylate (CAN) (bretylium): 1338
bretylium tosylate: 1338
Brevibloc (esmolol): 469
Brevicon (combo OC): 1299
brimonidine tartrate: 1327
brinzolamide: 1327
bromelain: 1243
Bromfed (combo): 1304
bromocriptine mesylate: 193
Bromo Seltzer (combo): 1304
brompheniramine maleate: 195
Bronalide (CAN) (flunisolide): 527
BRONCHODILATORS
  albuterol: 82
  aminophylline: 109
  bitolterol: 187
  dyphylline: 435
  ephedrine: 447
  epinephrine: 449
  isoetharine: 650
  isoproterenol: 653
  levalbuterol: 682
  metaproterenol: 757
  pirbuterol: 970
  terbutaline: 1115
  theophylline: 1125
Bronkaid Dual Action (combo): 1305
Bronkaid Mist (epinephrine): 449
Bronkodyl (theophylline): 1125
Bucladin-S Softabs (buclizine): 196
buclizine hydrochloride: 196
budesonide: 197
Bufferin (aspirin): 143
Bufferin (combo): 1305
Bufferin AF Nite Time (combo): 1305
Buffex (aspirin): 143
bumetanide: 199, C5
Bumex (bumetanide):199, C5
Buminate 5% (albumin): 80
Buminate 25% (albumin): 80

Eurax (crotamiton): 1319
evening primrose: 1245
Evista (raloxifene): 1026, C26
Evoxac (cevimeline): 1340
Exelon (rivastigmine): 1043
Exelon Oral Solution (rivastigmine): 1043
exemestane: 1342
Excedrin Extra Strength (combo): 1307
Excedrin PM (combo): 1307
Exidine (chlorhexidine): 1316
ex-lax Stool Softener (docusate): 1332
Exna (benzthiazide): 172
Exosurf Neonatal (colfosceril): 333
EXPECTORANTS
  guaifenesin: 582
  terpin hydrate: 1117
Exsel (selenium): 1318
Eyesine (tetrahydrozoline): 1123
ezetimibe: 500, C12
Ezide (hydrochlorothiazide): 597

F

factor IX concentrates: 502
Factor VIII (antihemophilic factor): 137
FACTOR Xa INHIBITOR
  fondaparinux: 543
Factrel (gonadorelin): 1344
Falapen (CAN) (penicillin G potassium): 933
false unicorn root: 1245
famciclovir sodium: 503
famotidine: 504, C12
Famvir (famciclovir): 503
Fansidar (combo): 1307
Fareston (toremifene): 1161
Faslodex (fulvestrant): 553
fat emulsion, intravenous: 505
5-FC (flucytosine): 522
FDA Pregnancy Categories: 1356
FE 50 (ferrous sulfate, exsiccated): 512
Feldene (piroxicam): 971
felodipine: 507
Femara (letrozole): 678
femhrt 1/5 (estradiol/norethindrone): 1296, 1307
Femiron (ferrous fumarate): 512
FemPatch (estradiol): 473
Fenesin (guaifenesin): 582
fennel: 1245

fenofibrate: 508
fenoprofen: 509
fentanyl: 510
Fentanyl Oralet (fentanyl): 510
fenugreek: 1245
Feosol (ferrous sulfate): 512
Feostat (ferrous fumarate): 512
Feratab (ferrous sulfate excissated): 512
Fer-gen-Sol (ferrous sulfate): 512
Fergon (ferrous gluconate): 512
Fer-In-Sol (ferrous sulfate): 512
Fer-Iron (ferrous sulfate): 512
Ferodan (CAN) (ferrous salts): 512
Fero-Grad (CAN) (ferrous salts): 512
Ferrlecit (sodium ferric gluconate complex): 1352
ferrous fumarate: 512
ferrous gluconate: 512
ferrous sulfate: 512
ferrous sulfate exsiccated: 512
FERTILITY DRUGS
  cetrorelix: 1340
  chorionic gonadotropin, recombinant: 1340
  clomiphene: 314
  follitropin alfa: 1342
  follitropin beta: 1342
  ganirelix acetate: 1344
  menotropins: 741
  urofollitropin: 1354
  urofollitropin purified: 1354
Fertinex (urofollitropin): 1354
Fertinorm HP (CAN) (urofollitropin): 1354
feverfew: 1245
fexofenadine: 513, C12
Fiberall Fruit (psyllium): 1334
Fiber Con (polycarbophil): 1334
filgrastim: 514
finasteride: 516
Finevin 20% (azelaic acid): 1321
Fioricet (combo): 1307
Fiorinal (combo): 1307
Fiorinal with Codeine (combo): 1278, 1307
fish oil: 1245
FK 506 (tacrolimus): 1101
Flagyl (metronidazole): 789
Flagyl 375 (metronidazole): 789
Flagyl ER (metronidazole): 789
Flagyl IV (metronidazole): 789

Grifulvin (griseofulvin): 1344
Gris-PEG (griseofulvin): 1344
griseofulvin: 1344
GROWTH FACTOR
  becaplermin: 1315
guaifenesin: 582
Guaifenex LA (guaifenesin): 582
guanabenz acetate: 583
guanadrel sulfate: 584
guanethidine monosulfate: 585
guanfacine hydrochloride: 587
guayusa: 1246
G-Well (lindane): 1319
Gynazole-1 (butoconazole): 1318
Gynecort (hydrocortisone): 1325
Gynecort Female Creme (hydrocortisone): 599
Gyne-Lotrimin-3(clotrimazole): 324
Gyne-Lotrimin-7 (clotrimazole): 324
Gynodiol (estradiol): 473
Gynogen L.A. 20 (estradiol): 473

H

5-HT4 MODULATOR
  tegaserod: 1106
Habitrol (nicotine): 856
haemophilus b conjugated with hepatitis
  B surface antigen vaccine: 1254
HAIR GROWTH RETARDANT
  eflornithine: 1322
halcinonide: 1325
Halcion (triazolam): 1178
Haldol (haloperidol): 588
Haldol Decanoate (haloperidol): 588
Haldol LA (CAN) (haloperidol): 1307
Halls Zinc Defense (zinc): 1234
halobetasol propionate: 1325
Halfprin 81 (aspirin): 143
1/2 Halfprin (aspirin): 143
Halog (halcinonide): 1325
haloperidol: 588
haloperidol decanoate: 588
Halotestin (fluoxymesterone): 532
Halotussin-AC (combo): 1307
Haltran (ibuprofen): 614
hamamelis water: 1316
Havrix (hepatitis A vaccine): 1254
hawthorn: 1246
HBIG (hepatitis B immune globulin):
  1256

hBNP (nesiritide): 849
HCG (human chorionic gonadotropin):
  295
Heartline (aspirin): 143
Hectoral (doxercalciferol): 1342
Helidac (combo): 1293, 1307
Helixate FS (antihemophilic factor): 137
Hemabate (carboprost): 228
Hemocyte (ferrous fumarate): 512
Hemofil-M (antihemophilic factor): 137
Hemopad (microfibrillar collagen): 1320
HEMORHEOLOGIC DRUG
  pentoxifylline: 944
HEMOSTATIC AGENTS
  absorbable gelatin: 1320
  microfibrillar collagen: 1320
  thrombin: 1320
Hemotene (microfibrillar collagen): 1320
Hepalean (CAN) (heparin): 591
Hepalean-Lok (CAN) (heparin): 591
HEPARIN ANTAGONIST
  protamine sulfate: 1011
Heparin Leo (CAN) (heparin): 591
heparin sodium injection: 591
**heparin sodium and 0.9% sodium
    chloride:** 591
**heparin sodium lock flush solu-
    tion:** 591
HepatAmine (amino acids): 105
hepatitis A vaccine, inactivated:
  1254
**hepatitis A vaccine, inactivated
    with hepatitis B, recombinant
    vaccine:** 1255
hepatitis B immune globulin: 1256
hepatitis B vaccine: 1257
Hep-Lock (heparin): 591
Hep-Lock U/P (heparin): 591
Hepsera (adefovir): 78
Herceptin (trastuzumab): 1168
HES (hetastarch): 593
Hespan (hetastarch): 593
hetastarch: 593
hexachlorophene: 1316
Hexadrol (dexamethasone): 372
Hexadrol Phosphate (dexamethasone):
  372
Hexalen (altretamine): 97
hexamethylenamine (altretamine): 97
Hibiclens (chlorhexidine): 1316
Hibistat (chlorhexidine): 1316

Modecate Deconate (CAN)
(fluphenazine): 534
Modicon (combo OC): 1299
Moditen Enanthate (CAN)
(fluphenazine): 534
Moditen Hydrochloride (fluphenazine):
534
Moduretic (amiloride and hydrochloroth-
iazide): 1294, 1309
moexipril: 810
Moi-stir (saliva): 1049
Moi-stir Swabsticks (saliva): 1049
molindone hydrochloride: 812
MOM (magnesium hydroxide): 1332
mometasone furoate: 1325
momordica charantia: 1247
Monafed (guaifenesin): 582
Monazole 7 (CAN) (miconazole): 792
Mononine (factor IX): 502
Monistat 3 (miconazole): 792
Monistat 7 (miconazole): 792
Monistat-Derm (miconazole): 792
Monistat Dual Pak (miconazole): 792
Monitan (CAN) (acebutolol): 64
MONOAMINE OXIDASE INHIBITORS
(MAO Inhibitors)
isocarboxazid: 1346
phenelzine: 951
tranylcypromine: 1166
MONOBACTAM ANTIBIOTICS
aztreonam: 161
Monocid (cefonicid): 245
Monoclate-P (antihemophilic factor):
137
MONOCLONAL ANTIBODIES
adalimumab: 76
alemtuzumab: 1336
basiliximab: 1338
daclizumab: 1340
gemtuzumab: 1344
ibritumomab: 1344
infliximab: 1344
muromonab-CD 3: 821
palivizumab: 915
rituximab: 1350
trastuzumab: 1168
monoctanoin: 1346
Mono-Gesic (salsalate): 1051
Monoket (isosorbide mononitrate): 656
Monopril (fosinopril): 549, C13
Monopril HCT (fosinopril and hydrochlorothiazide): 1288, 1309

montelukast sodium: 814, C21
Monurol (fosfomycin): 548
moricizine hydrochloride: 815
Morning-After Pill Schedule: 1295
morphine sulfate: 817
Motrin (ibuprofen): 615, C15
Motrin IB (ibuprofen): 615
Motrin Migraine Pain (ibuprofen): 615
MOUTH AND THROAT PRODUCTS
pilocarpine hydrochloride: 1348
MouthKote (saliva): 1049
MouthKote F/R (sodium flouride): 1071
moxifloxacin: 819
M-Oxy (oxycodone): 903
6-MP (mercaptopurine): 751
M-R-Vax II (measles and rubella vac-
cine): 1262
MS Contin (morphine): 817
MSIR (morphine): 817
MTC (mitomycin): 805
MTX (methotrexate): 768
Muco-Fen-LA (guaifenesin): 582
MUCOLYTICS
acetylcysteine: 72
dornase alfa : 421
Mucomyst (acetylcysteine): 72
Mucomyst 10 IV (acetylcysteine): 72
Mucosil-10 (acetylcysteine): 72
Mucosil-20 (acetylcysteine): 72
Multipax (CAN) (hydroxyzine): 611
MULTIPLE SCLEROSIS DRUG
glatiramer: 568
Mumpsvax (mumps virus vaccine): 1264
mumps virus vaccine, live: 1264
mupirocin: 1317
Murine Plus (tetrahydrozoline): 1123
muromonab-CD3: 821
MUSE (alprostadil): 93
Mustargen (mechlorethamine): 730
Mutamycin (mitomycin): 805
Myambutol (ethambutol): 489
Mycelex (clotrimazole): 324, 1318
Mycelex-7 (clotrimazole): 324
Mycelex-7 Combination Pack (clotrima-
zole): 324
Mycelex OTC (clotrimazole): 324
Mycifradin (CAN) (neomycin): 845
Myciguent (neomycin): 845
Mycil (CAN) (chlorphenesin): 283
Myclo (CAN) (clotrimazole): 324
Mycobutin (rifabutin): 1350
Mycocide NS (benzalkonium): 1316

O

Ting (tolnaftate): 1319
tinzaparin sodium: 1145
tiopronin: 1352
tirofiban: 1146
tissue-type plasminogen activator (alteplase): 95
tizanidine: 1148
TMP (trimethoprim): 1189
TMP-SMZ (co-trimoxazole): 1282, 1313
TNKase (tenecteplase): 1110
TOBI (tobramycin): 1149
tobramycin sulfate: 1149
Tobrex Ophthalmic (tobramycin): 1149
tocainide hydrochloride: 1151
TOCOLYTIC AGENTS
  ritodrine: 1350
  terbutaline: 1115
Tofranil (imipramine): 622
Tofranil-PM (imipramine): 622
tolazamide: 1152
tolazoline hydrochloride: 1352
tolbutamide: 1154
tolcapone: 1155
Tolectin 200 (tolmetin): 1157
Tolectin 600 (tolmetin): 1157
Tolectin DS (tolmetin): 1157
Tolinase (tolazamide): 1152
tolmetin sodium: 1157
tolnaftate: 1319
tolterodine tartrate: 1158, C30
Tonocard (tocainide): 1151
Topamax (topiramate): 1159
Topical Corticosteroids (see page 1323)
  alclometasone: 1323
  amcinonide: 1323
  betamethasone dipropionate: 177, 1323
  betamethasone dipropionate, augmented: 1324
  betamethasone valerate: 178, 1324
  clobetasol: 1324
  clocortolone: 1324
  desonide: 1324
  desoximetasone: 1324
  dexamethasone: 372, 1324
  dexamethasone sodium phosphate: 372, 1324
  diflorasone: 1324
  fluocinolone: 1324
  fluocinonide: 1324

Topical Corticosteroids
  (continued)
  flurandrenolide: 1324
  fluticasone: 1322, 1324
  halcinonide: 1325
  halobetasol: 1325
  hydrocortisone: 599, 1325
  hydrocortisone acetate: 599, 1325
  hydrocortisone buteprate: 1325
  hydrocortisone butyrate: 599, 1325
  hydrocortisone valerate: 599, 1325
  mometasone: 1325
  prednicarbate: 1325
  triamcinolone: 1174, 1325
Topical Lotions and Solutions (see pages 1315-1322)
  aluminum acetate: 1316
  Burow's solution: 1316
  calamine lotion: 1316
  hamamelis water: 1316
  malathion: 1319
TOPICAL GROWTH AGENT
  becaplermin: 1315
Topicort (desoximetasone): 1324
Topicycline (tetracycline): 1121
topiramate: 1159
Toposar (etoposide): 499
topotecan hydrochloride: 1352
Toprol XL (metoprolol): 787, C21
Topsyn Gel (CAN) (fluocinonide): 1324
Toradol (ketorolac): 667
Torecan (thiethylperazine): 1130
toremifene: 1161
Tornalate (bitolterol): 187
torsemide: 1162
Totacillin (ampicillin): 127
Touro-EX (guaifenesin): 582
TPA (alteplase): 95
T-phyl (theophylline): 1125
Tracleer (bosentan): 190
tramadol: 1163
Trandate (labetalol): 669
trandolapril: 1164
Transderm-Nitro (nitroglycerin): 865
Transderm-Scop (scopolamine): 1056
tranylcypromine sulfate: 1166
Tranxene SD (clorazepate): 322
Tranxene SD Half Strength (clorazepate): 322
Tranxene-T (clorazepate): 322
trastuzumab: 1168

Trasylol (aprotinin): 139
Travasol (amino acids): 105
Travatan (travoprost): 1331
Traveltabs (CAN) (dimenhydrinate): 403
travoprost: 1331
trazodone hydrochloride: 1169, C30
Trecator S.C. (ethionamide): 492
Trelstar Depot (triptorelin): 1194
Trelstar LA (triptorelin): 1194
Trental (pentoxifylline): 944, C24
treprostinil sodium: 1171
tretinoin: 1172, 1322
Trexan (CAN) (naltrexone): 834
Triacet (triamcinolone): 1174, 1325
Triacin C (combo): 1313
Triad (combo): 1313
Triadapin (CAN) (doxepin): 425
Triam-A (triamcinolone): 1174
triamcinolone: 1174
triamcinolone acetonide: 1174, 1325
triamcinolone diacetate: 1174
triamcinolone hexacetonide: 1174
Triam-Forte (triamcinolone): 1174
Triaminic Allergy Congestion (pseudo-
    ephedrine): 1013
Triaminic Cold & Allergy (combo): 1313
Triaminic Cold & Congestion (combo):
    1313
Triaminic Cold & Cough (combo): 1313
Triaminic-Throat Pain & Cough (com-
    bo): 1313
Triamonide (triamcinolone): 1174
triamterene: 1177
Triavil (perphenazine and amitriptyline):
    1285, 1313
triazolam: 1178
Triban (trimethobenzamide): 1188
Trichlorex (CAN) (trichlormethiazide):
    1180
trichlormethiazide: 1180
Tricor (fenofibrate): 508
Tricosal (choline magnesium trisalicy-
    late): 293
**TRICYCLIC ANTIDEPRESSANTS
    (TCAs) (see page 59)**
    amitriptyline: 115
    amoxapine: 121
    clomipramine: 315
    desipramine: 368
    doxepin: 425
    imipramine: 622

TRICYCLIC ANTIDEPRESSANTS
    (continued)
    nortriptyline: 876
    protriptyline: 1012
    trimipramine maleate: 1191
Triderm (triamcinolone): 1174, 1325
Tridesilon (desonide): 1324
Tridil (nitroglycerin): 865
trientine hydrochloride: 1352
triethylenethiophosphoramide (thiotepa):
    1135
trifluoperazine hydrochloride:
    1181
triflupromazine hydrochloride:
    1184
trifluridine: 1331
trihexyphenidyl hydrochloride:
    1186
Trihexy-2 (trihexyphenidyl): 1186
Trihexy-5 (trihexyphenidyl): 1186
triiodothyronine (liothyronine): 698
Tri-K (potassium): 978
Trikacide (CAN) (metronidazole): 789
Tri-Kort (triamcinolone): 1174
Trilafon (perphenazine): 947
Trileptal (oxcarbazepine): 900
Tri-Levlen (combo OC): 1301
Trilisate (choline magnesium trisalicy-
    late): 293
Trilog (triamcinolone): 1174
Trilone (triamcinolone): 1174
Tri-Luma (combo): 1321
Trimazide (trimethobenzamide): 1188
**trimethobenzamide hydrochlo-
    ride:** 1188
trimethoprim: 1189
trimetrexate glucuronate: 1190
trimipramine maleate: 1191
Trimox (amoxicillin): 123
Trimox Pediatric Drops (amoxicillin):
    123
Trimpex (trimethoprim): 1189
Trinalin Repetabs (azatadine and
    pseudoephedrine): 1297, 1313
Tri-Nasal (triamcinolone): 1174
Tri-Norinyl (combo, OC): 1301
Twinrix (hepatitis A and hepatitis B vac-
    cine): 1255
Triptone (dimenhydrinate): 403
triptorelin pamoate: 1194
Triostat (liothyronine): 698